SELF ASSESSMENT AND REVIEW OF
Short Subjects

Skin & STDs, Anaesthesia, Radiodiagnosis & Radiotherapy, Psychiatry *plus* Orthopaedics

SELF ASSESSMENT AND REVIEW OF
Short Subjects

Skin & STDs, Anaesthesia, Radiodiagnosis & Radiotherapy, Psychiatry *plus* Orthopaedics

Sixth Edition

Dr. Vivek Jain
MBBS, Maulana Azad Medical College, New Delhi
MD (Community Medicine), Lady Hardinge Medical College, New Delhi

Formerly
Senior Resident VMMC & SJH & UCMS & GTB Hospital
Faculty GFIMSR, Faridabad, Haryana
Consultant UN Office on Drugs & Crime – South Asia

Editors
Dr. Rashmi Naudiyal MBBS DCH
Paediatrician & Director, Kidz Care Clinic & Immunisation Centre

Dr. Pritam Roy MBBS MD (PSM)
Public Health Specialist, NCDC

Dr. Shanthan V MBBS
Author & Teacher

Dr. Snigdha Reddy MBBS MD (Psychiatry)
Bhaskar Medical College, Hyderabad

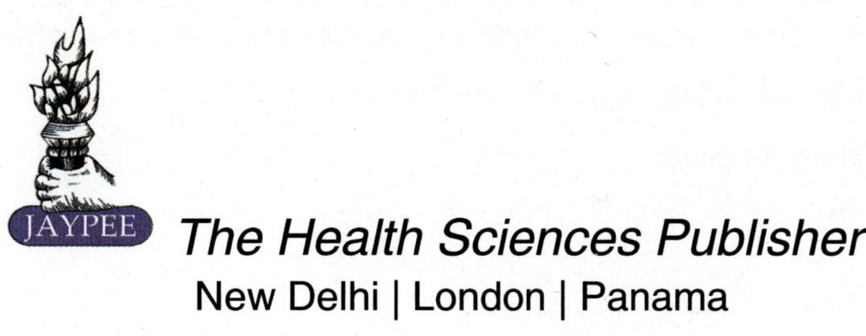

The Health Sciences Publisher
New Delhi | London | Panama

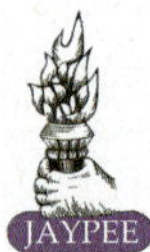

Jaypee Brothers Medical Publishers (P) Ltd

Headquarters
Jaypee Brothers Medical Publishers (P) Ltd.
4838/24, Ansari Road, Daryaganj
New Delhi 110 002, India
Phone: +91-11-43574357
Fax: +91-11-43574314
E-mail: jaypee@jaypeebrothers.com

Overseas Offices
JP Medical Ltd.
83, Victoria Street, London
SW1H 0HW (UK)
Phone: +44-20 3170 8910
Fax: +44(0)20 3008 6180
E-mail: info@jpmedpub.com

Jaypee-Highlights Medical Publishers Inc.
City of Knowledge, Bld. 235, 2nd Floor, Clayton
Panama City, Panama
Phone: +1 507-301-0496
Fax: +1 507-301-0499
E-mail: cservice@jphmedical.com

Jaypee Brothers Medical Publishers (P) Ltd.
17/1-B, Babar Road, Block-B, Shyamoli
Mohammadpur, Dhaka-1207
Bangladesh
Mobile: +08801912003485
E-mail: jaypeedhaka@gmail.com

Jaypee Brothers Medical Publishers (P) Ltd.
Bhotahity, Kathmandu, Nepal
Phone: +977-9741283608
E-mail: kathmandu@jaypeebrothers.com

Website: www.jaypeebrothers.com
Website: www.jaypeedigital.com

Inquiries for bulk sales may be solicited at: jaypee@jaypeebrothers.com

Self Assessment and Review of Short Subjects

Sixth Edition: 2018

ISBN: 978-93-5270-523-8

Printed at: Samrat Offset Pvt. Ltd.

Disclaimer

This book contains questions based on topics asked in previous years' State and National Level PG Entrance and Medical Officer Examinations in India. Often repeated topics and sub-topics have been included for students' benefit. We do not claim that these questions are exact or similar to questions asked in recent examinations in India. If any such similarity is found, it is purely coincidental and by chance.

Preface to the Sixth Edition

'Success in Entrance Exams is not difficult, provided you are guided throughout your preparation by Experienced teachers and Exam-pattern specific books'
A PGMEE student

Dear Students,

First-of-all let me thank you for accepting Previous editions of **Self Assessment & Review of Short Subjects (erstwhile PROAFS®)** and making it a grand success among PG-aspirants (both National & State level) and FMGE-aspirants in India. It gives me immense pleasure to share with you an updated and highly-improvised NEW Sixth Edition of **Self Assessment & Review of Short Subjects**.

In any PG Entrance examination in India, **Five Clinical Short Subjects (Skin & STDs, Anaesthesia, Radiodiagnosis & Radiotherapy, Psychiatry, Orthopaedics)** contribute around 35-45 MCQs (12-18% of total paper) which easily play a big role in qualification of a candidate. Also without scoring higher in this part, it becomes impossible to achieve success in most important step of your life.

- **Importance of Short Subjects:** These five subjects are considered BACKBONE of your preparation for any medical entrance examination in India. Besides being of scoring nature, their application in Medicine, Surgery, PSM, Pathology and other subjects make them vital-base to score good marks in para-clinical and clinical parts too. I may sound too harsh, but attempting PG Entrance examination without **Short Subjects** is invitation for a disastrous result.
- **Paucity of time:** Each of the 5 subjects is comprehensive and major in itself (good enough for keeping specialised and super-specialised courses post-MBBS). Due to limited time during PG Entrance examination preparation, students are not able to devote a lot of time to theory of **Short Subjects** as they can do for major subjects of Medicine, Surgery, Gyn-Obs and PSM.
- **Unavailability of NBE-specific books:** All books available in the market for **Short Subjects** are based on older examination pattern MCQs with high-difficulty-level questions and extremely detailed explanations. In contrast, Recent examinations have started focusing on concept-based basic questions only MOSTLY in form of short MCQs. So these books end up wasting crucial time of students.
  Keeping this in mind, I have written this book considering a student's invaluable time, requirements, and a result-oriented approach.
  Each of the Short Subjects' has been subdivided into sub-sections,
- **Theoretical concepts:** Brief, concise yet comprehensive theory specifically arranged topic and sub-topic wise. Important points (previous NBE MCQs and potential MCQs) have been marked bold and as^{Q} for easy filtering. Images have been integrated for comprehensive understanding.
- **Image based questions:** Based on Recent Examinations
- **NEET/ NBE Pattern MCQs:** All authentic MCQs till date (1991-2018) have been given TOPIC-WISE and SUB-TOPIC WISE.
- **High Yield MCQs:** Last 27 years (1991-2018) PGMEE MCQs have been given to give students a cutting edge over others and make a thorough-comprehensive preparation. Includes AIPGMEE, AIIMS, Karnataka PG, Kerala PG, PGI (Multiple response), DPG, Rajasthan PG, Andhra Pradesh PG, Bihar PG, JIPMER PG and other State PGMEE/ UPSC/ MO Examination MCQs.
- **NEET/NBE Pattern MCQs & High Yield MCQs - Answers:** All standard textbooks have been used to provide referenced explanatory answers. Deliberate use of multiple books for reference so as to provide you with best concepts at a single station.
- **Annexures:** For quick review, high yield topics based on Recent Questions given in tabular form.
- **Golden points:** FOR LAST MINUTE QUICK REVISION based on prior most frequently asked MCQs.

In a NUTSHELL, I am making an attempt to provide **Short Subjects** book as a COMPLETE PACKAGE; you won't need to look beyond it! With changing pattern of PG examinations in India, this book is surely a **One-Stop Junction** for all Examinations in India & abroad. Hopefully you will find all relevant theory and MCQs in this user-friendly book.

Features of Sixth Edition of Self Assessment & Review of Short Subjects

- **Topic and Sub-topic wise** arrangement of Simplified Theory and all MCQs
- **Important points in Bold** and marked^{Q}
- **User-friendly layout** with Integrated Image Based Questions
- **Wider coverage of MCQs** as per Recent Examination pattern
- **ALL MCQs in Market** Over 6700 MCQs with Explained, Referenced Answers
- **'Recent Pattern' Questions (2012-2018)** with Explained, Referenced Answers
- **AIIMS, PGI, UPSC, State PG, MO Exams (1991-2018)** with Explained, Referenced Answers
- **Image-based MCQs** Over 430 given Subject- & Chapter-wise
- **New Images added** Over 700 Images in theoretical concepts
- **Topper's Edge** High yield theoretical concepts for scoring over competitors in Examinations
- **Latest, changing, evolving pattern** of PG Examinations in India
- **Annexures** subject-wise for High yield topics

- **Golden Points** based on Recent MCQs
- **Tables and Mnemonics** High yield text for easy memorization
- **Differential Diagnosis** for tackling challenging clinical MCQs
- **MULTI-COLOUR** Whole book design and print

Although every possible effort has been undertaken to ensure no technical or typographical errors in the book, such are bound to be present in any book. If you come across any such error or if you have any comment, suggestions, queries or views, you are most welcome to e-mail to us for a prompt response. Do share your experiences while reading this book and the subject.

Hope you have a successful career ahead.
Wish you Success, *not just in Examination, but in Life!*

Dr. Vivek Jain MBBS MD (Community Medicine)
e-mail: docvivekjain@gmail.com, docvivekjain2@gmail.com
New Delhi, India

Author support Get regular updates on Short Subjects

- *E-mail:* docvivekjain@gmail.com; docvivekjain2@gmail.com
- **Facebook** Type <**Dr Vivek Jain Short Subjects**> in Search box: Like Like the page, Follow the posts
- **WhatsApp** Join Dr Vivek Jain's Updates group: Send your Name, College & Current city to **+91-9871960266**
- **Website** Visit the webpage **www.drvivekjainpsm.com**

Acknowledgements

I am sincerely thankful to my wife Dr. Rashmi Naudiyal and Baby Mischka for being a constant source of inspiration for completion of this book. Dr. Rashmi played an important role in completion of this product and her technical, academic and personal support has been instrumental in helping me reach this milestone. Without blessings of my parents, parents-in-laws and GOD this endeavour would not have been possible.

A heart-felt thanks to my grandfather Late Mr RD Jain who has made me what I am today.

I am grateful to Dr Saudan Singh, Director Professor & Head, Department of Community Medicine, North DMC Medical College & Hindu Rao Hospital, New Delhi, Former DG (Medical Education), Government of Uttar Pradesh, and Director NOTTO for being a source of support, guidance and motivation for myself.

I am thankful to Dr SK Pradhan, former Director Professor, Department of Community Medicine, VMMC, New Delhi for providing me with academic opportunities to help me understand the finer nuances of the subject throughout my PGship and SRship. I also appreciate the support and encouragement by Dr DK Raut, former Director Professor, VMMC SJH, Dr AT Kannan, former Director Professor and Head, Department of Community Medicine, UCMS, Dr GK Ingle, Director Professor and Head, Department of Community Medicine, MAMC, Dr Vibha, Former Professor and Head, Department of Community Medicine, LHMC, Dr SK Rasania, Director Professor & Head, LHMC and respected Faculty of Department of Community Medicine of these colleges respectively. Dr Rajesh Kumar, Faculty, MAMC has always inspired me to excel academically.

Words of thanks for Mr Rajesh Sharma (PG-DIAMS), Dr Sumer Sethi (DAMS) and Dr Bhatia (DBMCI) for helping me gain entry into the competitive world of academics. I am thankful to Mr Rajesh Sharma for his germ-idea for the book.

Sincere thanks to Dr Rashmi Naudiyal (Paediatrician & Director, Kidz Care Clinic & Immunisation Centre), Dr. Pritam Roy (Public Health Specialist, NCDC), Dr Shanthan V (Author & Teacher) and Dr Snigdha Reddy (Psychiatrist, Bhaskara Medical College, Hyderabad) for helping me with editing work. A vote of thanks to Mr. Sameer Kohli (M/s 120 Kohli Printers, Delhi), Mr. Deepak Bhardwaj (Shivam Graphics) and Mr Arora for support towards the genesis and development of initial phase of this book.

I am highly grateful to Shri Jitendar P Vij (Group Chairman), Jaypee Brothers Medical Publishers (P) Ltd, New Delhi, India for his wholehearted support in publication of this book. I thank Ms Chetna Malhotra Vohra (Associate Director–Content Strategy), Ms Payal Bharti (Senior Manager Professional Publishing) and Mr Ravinder (Typesetter) and their team at Jaypee Brothers Medical Publishers (P) Ltd, New Delhi, India for working on the current edition.

I also take this opportunity to express my gratitude to Dr Gobind Rai Garg (Author & Teacher, Pharmacology) and Dr Sparsh Gupta (Author & Teacher, Pathology), my close friends and True Legends in the Field of Academics in India & Abroad.

Words will fall short of my true gratitude feelings for:

Dr Abhay Mitkane, SSMA, Russia
Dr Ajay Arora, Jaipur
Dr Amrit Chattopadhyay, RG Kar Medical College, Kolkata
Dr Ankur Rana, Shimla
Dr Animesh Hore, NRS Medical College, Kolkata
Mr. Anurag, M/s Medical Book Store, MAMC and LHMC, Delhi
Dr Asharaf Abdul Rahuman, Kollam District Hospital
Dr Ashwani Kanoria
Dr Avinash Dubey
Dr Awadhesh Kumar, Bilaspur, Chattisgarh
Dr Bhavana Surya
Dr Bichitra Kr Mondal, KPC Medical College, Kolkata
Dr Feroz Ahamed, Taishan Medical University
Dr Gagan Dabas, BM Patil Medical College
Dr Geeta Singh, GSVM, Kanpur
Dr Hardik D Patel, BJ Medical College, Ahmedabad
Dr Harshika Singh, ELMCH, Lucknow
Dr Hemant R Kanase, TNMC & BYL Nair Ch. Hospital, Mumbai
Dr Humera Fatima, Hyderabad
Dr Jaspreet Kaur
Dr Jeffery Abraham Douglous
Dr Jitender Jakhar, MLB Medical College, Jhansi
Dr Jyoti Prakash Panda, SCB Medical College, Cuttack

Dr Kalyan Penta
Dr Kaushik Biswas, RG Kar Medical College, Kolkata
Dr Kushal Patel, MP Shah Medical College, Jamnagar
Dr Kushal MR, TNMC, Mumbai
Dr Manisha Agrawal, NRSMCH
Dr Mohinder Kumar Goutam
Dr Naushad Alam, HIMS Hospital, Kaithal
Dr Neelima, GSVM, Kanpur
Dr Nikhil Kr Gupta, KGMC, Lucknow
Dr P. Sai Kumar, Global Fund, Geneva
Dr Pace Chaitu
Dr Pijush Kanti Roy, NBMC, Siliguri
Dr Pankaj Sharma, Shimla
Dr Prashant Agrawal, JNMC, Raipur
Dr Pritam Bhattacharya
Dr Raj Kumar, Aysha Hospitals Pvt Ltd
Dr Rakesh Kumar Naik
Dr (Late) Ravi Shankar Bishnoi, Rajasthan
Dr Revanth Kumar, Dalian Medical University, China
Dr Richa Agrawal, JNMC, Raipur
Dr Ronak Patel, SSG Hospital, Vadodara
Dr Sagar Kotkar
Dr Sahu
Dr Sam Rohan
Dr Samata Mylavarapu, AIMU, St. Lucia
Dr Sarvoday Sinha, Gant Medical College, Mumbai
Dr Sapna Jain, JNM College, Raipur
Dr Shiffali Chabbra, GMC & Rajindra Hospital, Patiala
Dr Shrikant Patil
Dr SK Wasim Raza, CNMC & Hospital
Dr Spandana Katakam, Louzhou Medical College, China
Dr Subodh Kumar, Nalanda Medical College, Patna
Dr Sultan Gunga, Zhengzhou University, China
Dr Sumedh Joshi, ESIC, New Delhi
Dr Sumit De, IPGMER, Kolkata
Dr Sumit Gajjar, CCMU, China
Dr Swati Soni, University of Northern Philippines
Dr Vaibhav Goriya
Dr Upendra Uppi, Osmania General Hospital
Dr Vidhata Vidhu, Patna Medical College, Patna
Dr Vinay Kumar, VMMC SJH, New Delhi
Dr Vinod Jaiswal, JNMC, Raipur
Dr Vishal Sawale, TNMC, Mumbai
Dr Vivek Sinha

Last but definitely not the least, no words can describe the role of all Medical Graduate Students in India and abroad, with whom I ever have had interacted, in helping me give this book, its final shape.

Dr. Vivek Jain
New Delhi, India

Contents

Skin and STDs

ANNEXURES

CHAPTERS

EACH CHAPTER DIVIDED INTO FOLLOWING SECTIONS

Theoretical Concepts (Including Images)
Image-Based Questions
Answers with Explanations of IBQs
NEET/NBE Pattern MCQs
High Yield MCQs
NEET/NBE Pattern MCQs Answers with Explanations
High Yield MCQs Answers with Explanations
AIIMS PG 2018 MCQs with Explanatory Answers

Anesthesiology

ANNEXURES

CHAPTERS

EACH CHAPTER DIVIDED INTO FOLLOWING SECTIONS

Theoretical Concepts (Including Images)
Image-Based Questions
Answers with Explanations of IBQs
NEET/NBE Pattern MCQs
High Yield MCQs
NEET/NBE Pattern MCQs Answers with Explanations
High Yield MCQs Answers with Explanations
AIIMS PG 2018 MCQs with Explanatory Answers

Radiodiagnosis and Radiotherapy

ANNEXURES

CHAPTERS

EACH CHAPTER DIVIDED INTO FOLLOWING SECTIONS

Theoretical Concepts (Including Images)
Image-Based Questions
Answers with Explanations of IBQs
NEET/NBE Pattern MCQs
High Yield MCQs
NEET/NBE Pattern MCQs Answers with Explanations
High Yield MCQs Answers with Explanations
AIIMS PG 2018 MCQs with Explanatory Answers

Psychiatry

ANNEXURES

CHAPTERS

EACH CHAPTER DIVIDED INTO FOLLOWING SECTIONS

Theoretical Concepts (Including Images)
Image-Based Questions
Answers with Explanations of IBQs
NEET/NBE Pattern MCQs
High Yield MCQs
NEET/NBE Pattern MCQs Answers with Explanations
High Yield MCQs Answers with Explanations
AIIMS PG 2018 MCQs with Explanatory Answers

Orthopedics

ANNEXURES

CHAPTERS

EACH CHAPTER DIVIDED INTO FOLLOWING SECTIONS

Theoretical Concepts (Including Images)
Image-based Questions
Answers with Explanations of IBQs
NEET/NBE Pattern MCQs
High Yield MCQs
NEET/NBE Pattern MCQs Answers with Explanations
High Yield MCQs Answers with Explanations
AIIMS PG 2018 MCQs with Explanatory Answers

Skin and STDs

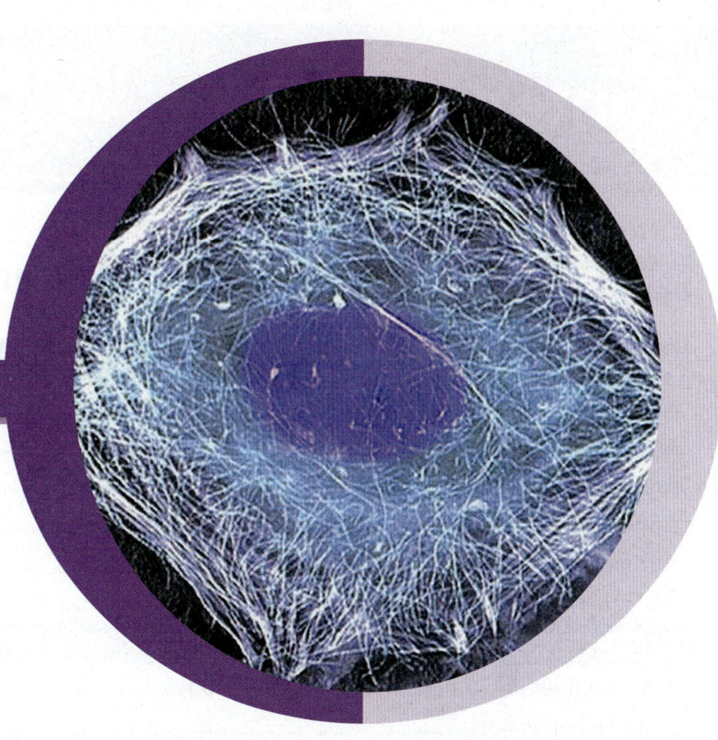

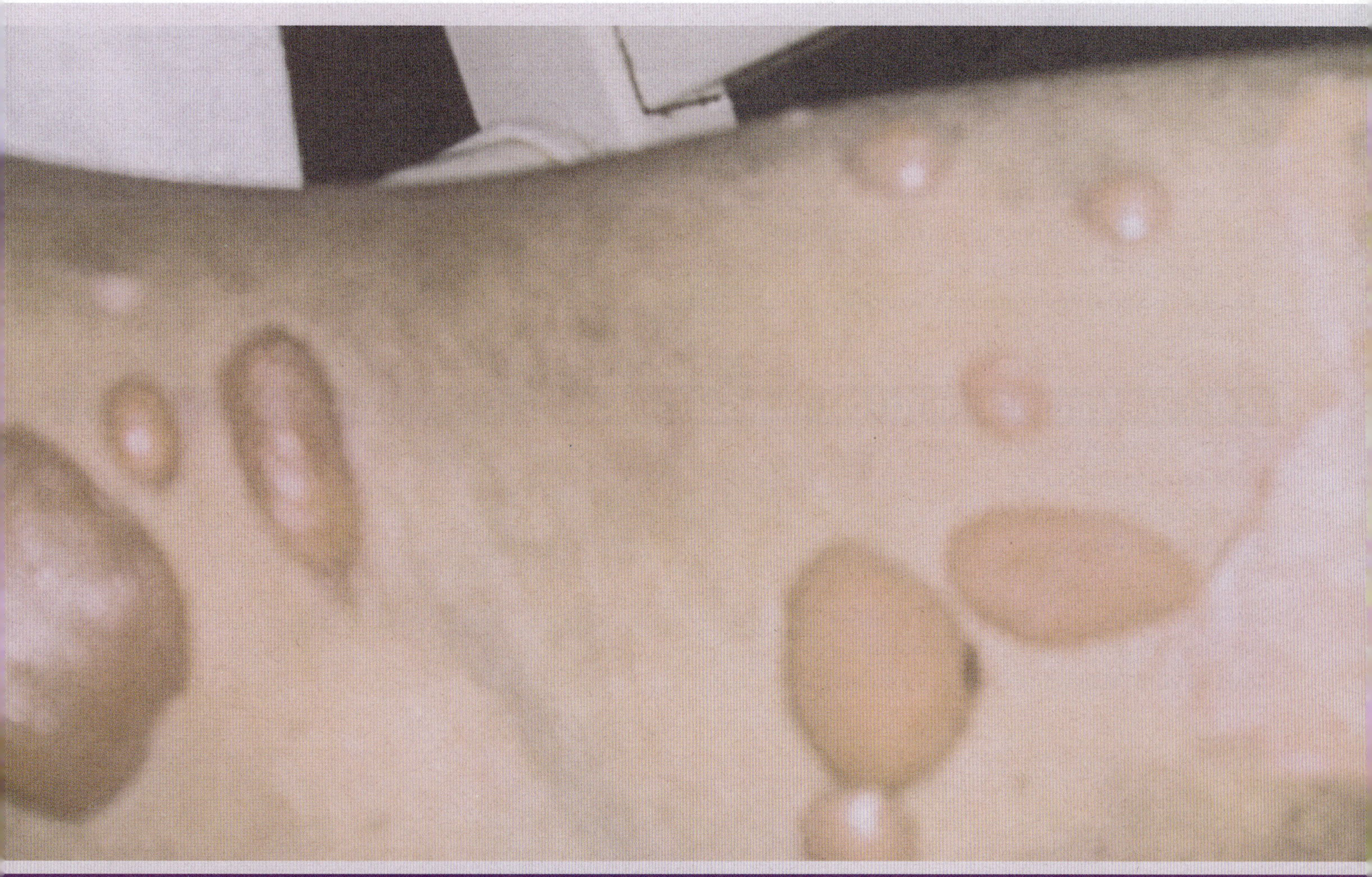

Contents

Skin and STDs

EACH CHAPTER DIVIDED INTO FOLLOWING SECTIONS

Theoretical Concepts (Including Images)
Image-Based Questions
Answers with Explanations of IBQs
NEET/NBE Pattern MCQs
High Yield MCQs
NEET/NBE Pattern MCQs Answers with Explanations
High Yield MCQs Answers with Explanations
AIIMS PG 2018 MCQs with Explanatory Answers

Annexures

ANNEXURE 1. CLINICAL SIGNS IN DERMATOLOGY

Asboe-Hansen sign	Pemphigus, Bullous pemphigoid, Bullous drug eruptions
Auspitz sign	Psoriasis vulgaris
Battle sign	Basal skull fracture (posterior fossa)
Blue dot sign	Testicular sign
Bulla spread sign	Pemphigus vulgaris
Butterfly sign	Systemic lupus erythematosus (SLE)
Button-hole sign	Cutaneous neurofibroma
Carpet tack (Tic tack) sign	Discoid lupus erythematosus
Casal's necklace sign	Pellagra
Crowe's sign (Axillary freckling)	Type 2 Neurofibromatosis
Cullens' sign	Intraperitoneal hemorrhage
Darier's sign	Urticaria pigmentosa, Systemic mastocytosis, Insect bite
Dennie-Morgan fold	Atopic dermatitis
Doughnut sign	Scleromyxedema
Dimple (Fitzpatrick) sign	Dermatofibroma
Drip sign	Corrosive liquids
Dubois sign	Congenital syphilis
Enamle paint sign	Kwashiorkar
Exclamation mark hair sign	Alopecia areata
Flag sign	Protein energy malnutrition
Forchheimer's sign	Rubella
Gottron's sign	Dermatomyositis
Grey turner sign	Retroperitoneal hemorrhage
Hanging curtain sign	Pityriasis rosea
Heliotrope sign	Dermatomyositis
Hertoghe sign	Atopic dermatitis
Hoaglande's sign	Infectious mononucleosis
Holster sign	Dermatomyositis
Hutchinson's (Nose) sign	Herpes zoster
Jeelinek's sign	Hyperthyroidism
Koebner (True) phenomenon*	Lichen planus, Vitiligo, Psoriasis
Koebner (Pseudo) phenomenon*	Warts, Molluscum contagiosum, Behcet's syndrome, Pyoderma gangrenosum
Koebner (Occasional) phenomenon*	Hailey-Hailey disease, Erythema multiforme, Lichen sclerosus et atrophicus, Pellagra, Darier's disease, Cancers, Kaposi's sarcoma
Leser-Trélat sign	Internal malignancy
Nikolsky sign	Pemphigus vulgaris, Pemphigus foliaceus, SSSS*

Contd...

Contd...

Oil-drop sign	Psoriasis
Pastia (Thomson) sign	Scarlet fever
Pseudo-Darier sign	Smooth muscle hamartoma, Becker's nevus
Racoon' sign	Basilar skull fracture
Romana sign	Chagas disease
Round finger pad sign	Scleroderma
Russels' sign	Bulimia nervosa
Shawl sign	Dermatomyositis
Sign of Groove	Lymphogranuloma venerum (LGV)
Slapped cheek sign	Fifth disease (Erythema infectiosum)
Sternberg's thumb sign	Marfans' syndrome
Thumbprint sign	Strongyloidosis
Triple palm sign	Internal malignancy (Lungs/ Stomach)
Trousseau's sign	Internal malignancy/ Hypocalcemic tetany
V sign	Dermatomyositis
Walzel sign	Acute and Chronic Pancreatitis

*(*SSSS Staphylococcal scalded skin syndrome; Koebner = Isomorphic phenomenon)*

ANNEXURE 2. TESTS USED IN DERMATOLOGY

Test	Use in Dermatology
Diascopy (Apple jelly nodules)	Lupus vulgaris
Grattage test	Psoriasis vulgaris
Kahn Flocculation test	Syphilis
Lepromin test	Cell mediated immunity in Leprosy
Porphobilinogen urine test	Acute intermittent porphyria
Patch (provocative) test	Sensitivity of penicillin, neomycin, benzocaine
Patch (vapor) test	Sensitivity of volatile substances (perfumes)
Patch (mucus membrane) test	Sensitivity of local sensitizing agents of mouth
Patch (photo) test	Sensitivity to photosensitizing substances
Prick test	Routine allergy test
Rapid plasma reagin (RPR) test	Syphilis
Tzanck test	Bullous eruptions, Pemphigus, Herpes zoster
VDRL flocculation test	Syphilis
Wasserman Complement Fixation test	Syphilis
Wood's lamp (Brilliant green)	Tinea capitis
Wood's lamp (Dull yellow)	Pityriasis versicolor
Wood's lamp (Coral pink/ red)	Erythrasma
Wood's lamp (White)	Vitiligo
Wood's lamp (Blue-white)	Tuberous sclerosis
Wood's lamp (Pale blue-green)	Pseudomonas infection
Wood's lamp (Pinkish-red Urine)	Porphyrea cutanea tarda
Wood's lamp (Orange)	Acne (Propionibacterium acne)

ANNEXURE 3. TYPES OF EPITHELIUM IN BODY

Simple squamous epithelium • Blood vessels • Lymph vessels • Mesothelium of body cavities • Kidney ascending thin limb	**Stratified squamous (non-keratinised) epithelium** • Oesophagus • Oropharynx • Vocal cords • Cornea • Cervix (ectocervix) • Vagina • External urethral orifice Anus (above Hilton's line)
Stratified squamous (keratinised) epithelium • Skin • Gingiva • Tongue • Hard palate • Labia majora • Anus (below Hilton's line)	**Transitional epithelium** • Renal pelvis • Ureter • Urinary bladder • Prostatic urethra
Simple columnar epithelium • Stomach (non-ciliated) • Small intestine (non-ciliated) • Large intestine (non-ciliated) • Rectum (non-ciliated) • Bulbourethral glands • Ejaculatory duct • Cervix (endocervix) (non-ciliated) • Endometrium • Fallopian tubes • Gallbladder (non-ciliated)	**Pseudostratified columnar epithelium** • Nose • Larynx • Trachea • Seminal vesicles • Vas deferens • Epididymis • Ductuli efferentis • Penile urethra (non-ciliated) • Membranous urethra (non-ciliated)
Stratified columnar epithelium • Ducts of submandibular glands **Stratified cuboidal epithelium** • Sweat glands ducts	**Simple cuboidal epithelium** • Respiratory bronchioles • Thyroid follicles • Kidney PCT (with microvilli) • Kidney DCT • Kidney Collecting ducts • Ependyma • Ovaries • Tubuli recti • Rete testes

ANNEXURE 4. COMMON DERMATOLOGICAL DRUG REACTIONS

Reaction	Drug(s) Responsible
Allergic vasculitis	Sulphonamides, Phenytoin, Propylthiouracil
Drug related lupus erythematosus	Diltiazem, Etanercept, Hydrochlorothiazide, Lisinopril, Terbinafine
Exfoliative dermatitis/ Erythroderma	Allopurinol, Anticonvulsants, Carbamazepine, Isoniazid, Sulphonamides
Erythema nodosum	Oral contraceptive pills
Fixed drug eruptions	Various drugs
Lichenoid/ Lichen planus like eruptions	Beta blockers, Carbamazepine, Furosemide, Phenothiazines, Quinine, Tetracycline, Thiazides
Photosensitivity	Amiodarone, NSAIDs, Phenothiazines, Sulphonamides, Sulindac, Thiazides, Tetracyclines
Pigmentary changes (Flat hypopigmented)	Oral contraceptive pills
Pigmentary changes (Blue gray)	Chlorpromazine

Contd...

Contd...

Reaction	Drug(s) Responsible
Pigmentary changes (Brown)	Silver, Gold, Bismuth, Arsenic heavy metals
Pigmentary changes (Yellow)	Quinacrine
Pigmentary changes (Blue-black shins)	Chloroquine, Minocycline
Pigmentary changes (Blue-black nails/ palate)	Chloroquine
Pigmentary changes (Slate gray)	Amiodarone
Pigmentary changes (Brown nails)	Hydroxyurea
Psoriasiform eruptions	Chloroquine, Beta-blockers, Lithium
Stevens Johnson Syndrome/ TEN	Allopurinol, Anticonvulsants, NSAIDs, Sulphonamides
Toxic erythema	Ampicillin, Cotrimoxazole, Barbiturates, Sulphonamides
Urticaria	Penicillin, NSIADs, Opioids, Salicylates, Sulphonamides

ANNEXURE 5. DISEASES AND DISORDERS OF NAILS

Disorders of nails	Disease condition(s) responsible
Onycholysis	Hyperthyroidism, Psoriasis, Fungal infections
Koilonychia	Iron deficiency anaemia, Syphilis, Ischaemic heart disease
Splinter haemorrhages	Trauma, Nail psoriasis, Subacute bacterial endocarditis
Pterygium of nails	Lichen planus, Idiopathic
Half-and-half nails	Chronic renal failure
Pitting of nails	Psoriasis, Alopecia areata, Hand eczema
Beau's lines	Acute systemic illnesses
Terry's nails	Cirrhosis
Hippocratic nails	Clubbing of nails
Mee's lines on nails	Chronic arsenic poisoning, Hypoalbuminemia
Hyperpigmentation of nails	Zidovudine, Mephalan, Daunorubicin, Bleomycin, Hydroxyurea
Blue nails	Chloroquine, Wilson's disease, Subungal hematoma
Yellow nail syndrome	Pleural effusion, Sinusitis, Ankle oedema
Nail fold telengiactasia	Dermatomyositis

Golden Points

Most consistent immunological finding in Atopic dermatitis	Raised IgE levels
Dennie-morgan folds under eyes are seen in	Atopic dermatitis
Hanifin and Rajka's Criteria are used for diagnosis of	Atopic dermatitis
MC type of Pemphigus is	Pemphigus vulgaris
In Pemphigus, antibodies are found against	Desmoglobins
Hailey Hailey disease is	Familial benign Pemphigus
MC drug causing Pemphigus	Penicillamine
In Bullous pemphigoid there are antibodies against	IgG and c3
MC Pemphigus type seen in Indian population	Pemphigus vulgaris
Underlying causative organism in Dandruff	Malassezia furfur
Dermatitis herpetiformis is always associated with	Gluten-sensitive enteropathy
HLA associated with Psoriasis	HLA-DW6
MC type of Psoriasis is	Chronic/ Stable plaque psoriasis
Skin lesions on site of lines of trauma	Koebner (Isomorphic) phenomenon
Oil-drop nails are seen in	Psoriasis
Grattage sign is positive in	Psoriasis
Auspitz sign is positive in	Psoriasis
Rain-drop skin lesions are seen in	Guttate psoriasis
Herald/ mother patch is first lesion in	Pityriasis rosea
Fir-tree/ Christmas-tree appearance of scales is seen in	Pityriasis rosea
Pityriasis simplex capillitii is	Dandruff
Underlying causative organism in Dandruff	Malassezia furfur
Target/ Iris/ Bull's-eye lesion is charateristic of	Erythema multiforme
Causative organism of Erythrasma	Corynebacterium minutissimum
Honey-coloured crusts are seen in	Impetigo contagiosa
Sycosis barbae is	Deep folliculitis of beard area
Impetigo contagiosa is caused by	Staphylococcus/ Streptococcus
Bullous impetigo is caused by	Staphylococcus aureus
Ecthyma is caused by	Staphylococcus aureus
Furuncles (Boils) is caused by	Staphylococcus aureus
Apple-jelly nodules are seen in	Lupus vulgaris (TB skin)
Lichen scrofulosorum (Tuberculides) is	Hypersensitivity to TB bacterium
Verruca vulgaris is caused by	Human Papilloma Virus
Pleomorphism (All stages of rash at same time) is seen in	Varicella Zoster/ Chicken pox
Dew-drop on rose-petal appearance of rash is seen in	Varicella Zoster/ Chicken pox
MC type of infective genital ulcer disease in adults	Herpes genitalis
Tzanck smear is generally used to diagnose	Herpes simplex, Chicken pox
Hand-foot-mouth disease is caused in animals by	Picorna virus
Bacterial superinfection of interdigital Tinea pedis	Athlete's foot
MC form of Oral candidiasis	Thrush
MC site of Mycetoma in human body	Foot
MC cause of Acquired Icthyosis in India	Leprosy
Malignant pustule is	Anthrax of skin

Contd...

Contd...

Inflammatory tinea capitis of scalp is known as	Kerion
Pathogonomic lesion of Scabies	Burrows
Norwegian/ Crusted scabies is seen in	Immunocompromised patients
Rodent ulcer is a type of	Basal cell carcinoma
Treatment of choice for Basal cell carcinoma	Surgical excision
Treatment of choice for Squamous cell carcinoma	Surgical excision
MC type of Malignant melanoma	Superficial spreading MM
Most aggressive type of Malignant melanoma	Nodular MM
Breslow's method, Clark's method is used for	Malignant melanoma
MC vascular malformation present at birth	Salmon patch
MC site of Port-wine strain	Face
Cutaneous venous malformations with enchondromas seen in	Maffucci's syndrome
MC site for Arterio-venous malformation is	Head
Mycosis fungoides is a lymphoma of	Helper T-lymphocytes of skin
Pautrier's microabscesses are seen in	Mycosis fungoides (CTCL)
Letterer-Siwe disease is	Langerhan's cell histiocytosis
MC mode of Syphilis transmission	Sexual transmission
Hunterian chancre is a characteristic lesion of	Primary syphilis
Syphilitic rhinitis seen in Congenital syphilis is known as	Snuffles
Soft sore is characteristic of	Chancroid
Causative organism of Soft sore/ Soft chancre (Chancroid)	Hemophilus ducreyi
Pseudo-buboes (Donovanosis/ Granuloma inguinale) is due to	Klebsiella granulomatis
Sign of groove is seen in	Lymphogranuloma venerum (LGV)
Lymphogranuloma venerum (LGV) is caused by	Chlamydia trachomatis (L1/L2/L3)
MC symptom of Gonococcal infection in males	Anterior urethritis
MC cause of Non-gonococcal urethritis	Chlamydia trachomatis (D-K)
MC cause of ano-genital warts	Human papilloma virus (HPV 6, 11)
MC type of anogenital warts	Condylomata acuminata
MC type of HIV seen in India	HIV type 1 (Subtype C)
MC cutaneous infection in HIV	Candidiasis
MC dermatosis in AIDS patients	Seborrhoeic dermatitis
MC type of Vitiligo seen	Vitiligo vulgaris
MC dermatomal involvement in Vitiligo segmental	Trigeminal nerve
Melasma/ chloasma is a disorder of	Hyper-pigmentation
Normal melanocytes producing more melanosomes lead to	Freckles
MC dermatological cause of Pruritis	Xerosis of skin
Cock's peculiar tumor is a type of	Sebaceous cyst epithelioma
Ashleaf spots are characteristic of	Tuberous sclerosis
MC manifestation of Tuberous sclerosis	Angiofibroma
Earliest manifestation of Tuberous sclerosis	Ash-leaf macules
Shagreen patch may be seen in	Tuberous sclerosis
MC systemic manifestation of Tuberous sclerosis	Seizures
MC cause of erythroderma	Idiopathic
MC skin manifestation of Scleroderma	Raynaud's phenomenon
Earliest manifestation of Scleroderma	Raynaud's phenomenon
Drug of choice for Dermatitis herpetiformis	Dapsone
Pathogonomic lesions of acne vulgaris	Comedones

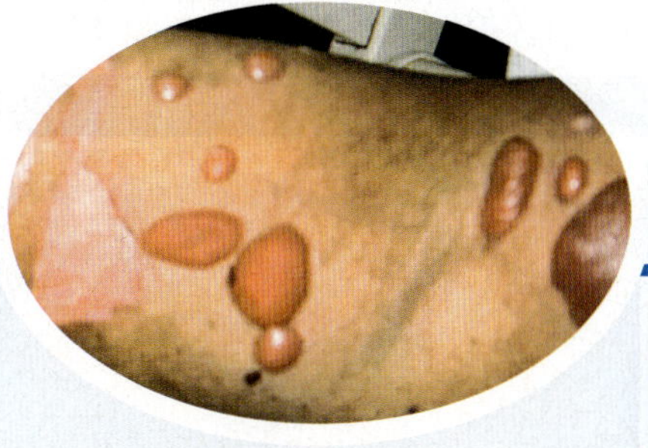

Chapter 1

Epithelium, Tumors, General Dermatology

THEORETICAL CONCEPTS

I A. EPITHELIUM

- *Definition*: A vascular type of body tissue which lines cavities and surface of body structures and forms many glands
- *Components*:
  - Basement membrane: All epithelial membrane rest on basement membrane on which it can grow and regenerate after injuries
  - Call junctions: Contact points between plasma membrane and tissue cells e.g. **tight junctions and desmosomes**[Q]
- *Types of epithelium*:
  - ***Simple epithelium***: Epithelium that is one cell thick and every cell is in contact with basement membrane
    - Simple squamous epithelium: Lining areas where passive diffusion of gases occur; e.g. walls of capillaries, linings of the pericardial, pleural, peritoneal cavities, alveoli of the lungs
    - Simple cuboidal epithelium: Cells with secretory, absorptive, or excretory functions; e.g. collecting ducts of kidney, pancreas, salivary gland
    - Simple columnar epithelium: Seen in high secretive (as in wall of the stomach), or absorptive (as in small intestine) areas
    - Pseudostratified epithelium: Exclusive confinement to the larger respiratory airways i.e. the nasal cavity, trachea, bronchi
  - ***Stratified epithelium***: Epithelium that is multi-layered
    - Keratinized epithelium: Most apical/ exterior layer cells are dead, making it water-proof; e.g. oesophageal; lining
    - Transitional epithelium: Found in tissues that can stretch; e.g. urinary bladder, ureters, urethra

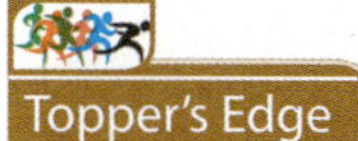

Topper's Edge

Epithelium
- One of the four basic types of animal tissue, along with connective tissue, muscle tissue and nervous tissue
  - Epithelial tissues line the cavities and surfaces of blood vessels and organs throughout the body
  - All glands are made up of epithelial cells
- **Epithelial layers contain no blood vessels**[Q], so they must receive nourishment via diffusion of substances from the underlying connective tissue, through the basement membrane
  - Cell junctions are well-employed in epithelial tissues

Principal shapes associated
- Squamous epithelium: Cells are wider than their height (flat and scale-like)
- Cuboidal epithelium: Cells height and width are approximately the same (cube shaped)
- Columnar epithelium: Cells taller than they are wide (column-shaped)

Types of epithelium
- Simple epithelium: Arranged in a single layer of cells
- Stratified (layered) epithelium: Arranged in layers of two or more cells deep

Embryological Development

- **Epithelial tissues are derived from all of the embryological germ layers[Q]:**
  - Ectoderm (e.g., the epidermis)
  - Endoderm (e.g., the lining of the gastrointestinal tract)
  - Mesoderm (e.g., the inner linings of body cavities)

Primary functions of Epithelial tissues[Q]

- Protect the tissues that lie beneath it from radiation, desiccation, toxins, invasion by pathogens, and physical trauma
- Regulation and exchange of chemicals between the underlying tissues and a body cavity
- Secretion of hormones into the blood vascular system, and/ or the secretion of sweat, mucus, enzymes, and other products that are delivered by ducts
- Provide sensation

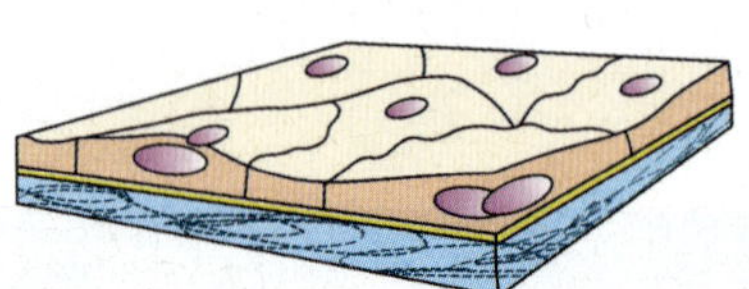
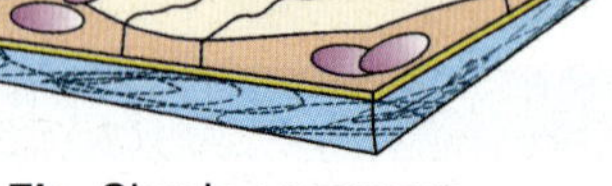

Fig. Simple squamous

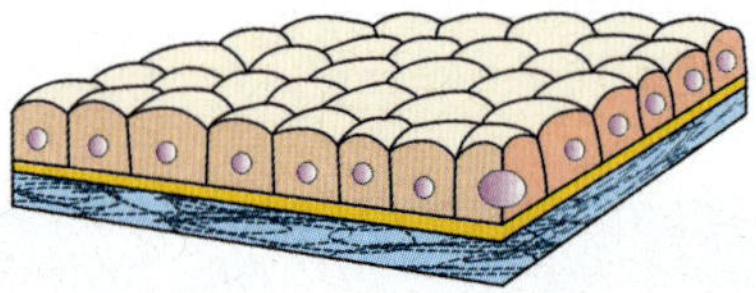

Fig. Simple cuboidal

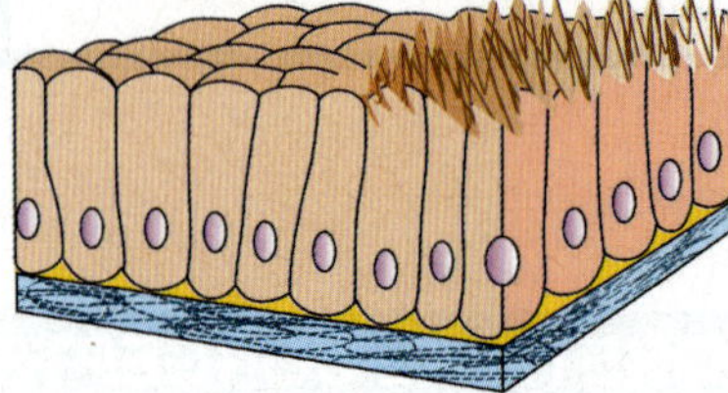

Fig. Simple columnar

I B. LAYERS OF SKIN

I B1. Epidermis: Outermost Layer of Skin

- Epidermis consist of:
  - Melanocytes
  - Langerhans cells
  - Merkel cells
  - Sensory nerves
- Layers of epidermis: [Bottom to top]
  - ***Stratum germinativum/Basal cell layer***:
    - Contains **Melanocytes** which produce melanin[Q]
    - Contains **Merkel cells**: Cells of neuro-ectodermal origin[Q]
    - Sun exposure increase melanocyte production to prevent damage from UV rays (sun tanning)[Q]
  - ***Stratum spinosum/Squamous cell layer***:
    - **Thickest layer of epidermis[Q]**
    - Contains **Keratinocytes** which produce keratin, the major structure in skin, hair, nails[Q]
    - Contains **Langerhans cells** which alert immune system from antigens that invade skin[Q]
  - ***Stratum lucidum and Stratum granulosum***:
    - Formed by pushing up of keratinocytes through these two layers to form durable material
    - Cells become bigger, flatter and adhere together
  - ***Stratum corneum/ Horny layer***:
    - Outermost layer of epidermis[Q]
    - Contains 10-30 thin layers of continuously shedding dead keratinocytes
    - Complete cell turnover in 28-30 days

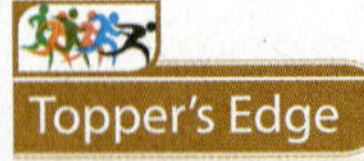

Topper's Edge

EPIDERMIS

Key Features of Epidermis

- **Epidermis has no blood supply** and is nourished almost exclusively by diffused oxygen from the surrounding air[Q]
- **95% keratinocytes[Q]**, also contain Melanocytes, Langerhans cells, Merkel cells, Inflammatory cells
- Rete ridges (or Rete pegs) are epidermal thickenings that extend downward between dermal papillae[Q]
- Blood capillaries are found beneath epidermis, and are linked to an arteriole and a venule

Layers of Epidermis

- Stratum corneum: 10-30 layers of polyhedral, anucleated corneocytes, with palms and soles having the most layers, attached together through Corneodesmosomes[Q]
- Most of the barrier functions of the epidermis localize to S. corneum
- Skin found in the palms and soles is "thick skin" as it has 5 epidermal layers instead of 4 (Stratum lucidum is only found in palms and soles[Q])
- **Langerhans cells are located in middle of Stratum spinosum[Q]**
- Malpighian layer (Stratum malpighi[Q]): Usually defined as both Stratum basale and Stratum spinosum

Functions of Epidermis

- Barrier against pathogens, oxidant stress (UV light) and chemical compounds and provides mechanical resistance
- Mechanical strength, Chemical barrier, Immunologically active barrier
- Skin hydration: Ability of skin to hold water is primarily due to Stratum corneum & Lipids form a barrier to transepidermal water loss
- Skin color: Amount and distribution of melanin pigment in epidermis is the main reason for variation in skin color

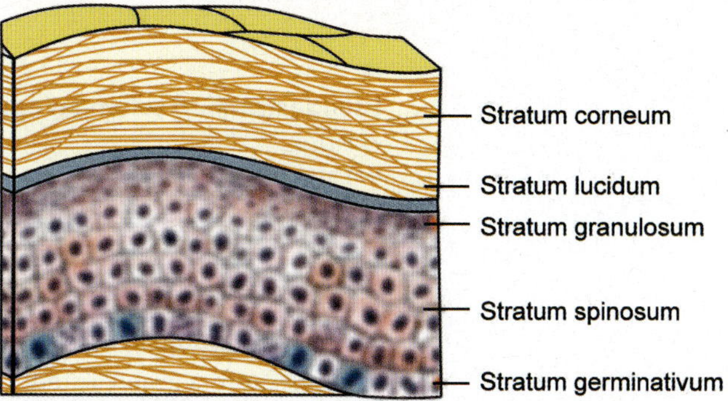

Fig. Layers of epidermis

I B2. Dermis

- **Dermis consist of:**
  - Blood vessels
  - Lymph vessels
  - Hair follicles
  - Sweat glands
    - Apocrine glands
    - Eccrine glands
  - Sebaceous glands
  - Nerve endings
  - Collagen and elastin
- **Layers of epidermis**: [Bottom to top]
  - *Papillary layer*:
    - Contains thin collagen fibres
    - Supplies nutrients to select layers of epidermis and regulates temperature
  - *Reticular layer*:
    - Contains thick collagen fibres
    - Provides strength, structure, elasticity and supports other components

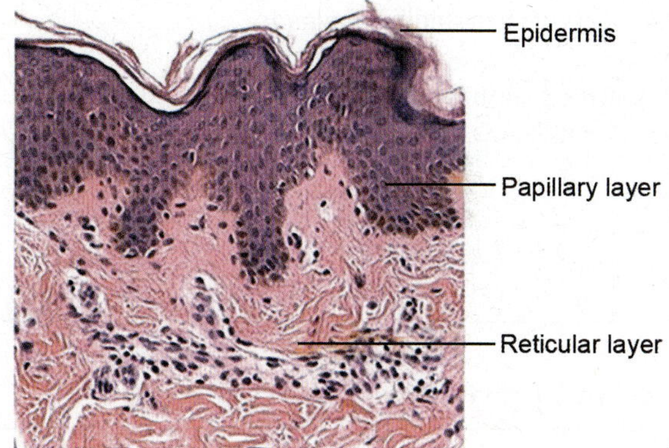

Fig. Layers of dermis

I B3. Cutis

- *Cutis/ Hypodermis/ Subcutaneous layer consist of*:
  - Fat
  - Collagen cells
- *Functions of cutis*:
  - Insulator: Conserves body heat
  - Shock absorber: Protects inner organs
  - Stores fat as an energy reserve

I C. TYPES OF EPITHELIUM IN BODY

Simple squamous epithelium[Q]	**Stratified squamous (non-keratinised[Q]) epithelium**
• Blood vessels • Lymph vessels • Mesothelium of body cavities • Kidney Ascending thin limb	• Oesophagus • Oropharynx • Vocal cords • Cornea • Cervix (ectocervix) • Vagina • External urethral orifice Anus (above Hilton's line)
Stratified squamous (keratinised[Q]) epithelium • Skin • Gingiva • Tongue • Hard palate • Labia majora • Anus (below Hilton's line)	**Transitional epithelium[Q]** • Renal pelvis • Ureter • Urinary bladder • Prostatic urethra
Simple columnar epithelium[Q] • Stomach (non-ciliated) • Small intestine (non-ciliated) • Large intestine (non-ciliated) • Rectum (non-ciliated) • Bulbourethral glands • Ejaculatory duct • Cervix (endocervix) (non-ciliated) • Endometrium • Fallopian tubes • Gallbladder (non-ciliated)	**Pseudostratified columnar epithelium[Q]** • Nose • Larynx • Trachea • Seminal vesicles • Vas deferens • Epididymis • Ductuli efferentis • Penile urethra (non-ciliated) • Membranous urethra (non-ciliated)
Stratified columnar epithelium[Q] • Ducts of submandibular glands **Stratified cuboidal epithelium[Q]** • Sweat glands ducts	**Simple cuboidal epithelium[Q]** • Respiratory bronchioles • Thyroid follicles • Kidney PCT (with microvilli) • Kidney DCT • Kidney Collecting ducts • Ependyma • Ovaries • Tubuli recti • Rete testes

I D. TYPES OF CELLS IN THE SKIN

I D1. Cells in the Epidermis

- **Keratinocytes:**
  - Hallmark feature[Q]: Keratin filament
  - Proliferate in Basal layer, Differentiation in Stratum spinosum/ Stratum granulosum, Maturation and death in Stratum corneum
- **Melanocytes:**
  - Function: Synthesis of melanin[Q]
  - Location: Basal layer, Hair follicles
  - Highest number: Genitals
- **Langerhans cells:**
  - Location: Stratum spinosum[Q]
  - Function: Macrophages/Antigen presenting cells[Q]
  - **Histologic hallmark[Q]: Birbeck granules (Tennis racket shaped)**
- **Merkel/Touch cells:**
  - Location: Basal layer
  - Function[Q]: Touch sensation

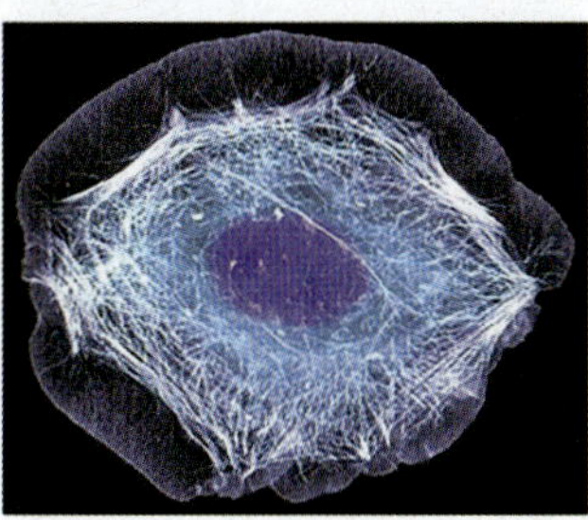
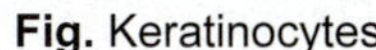

Fig. Keratinocytes

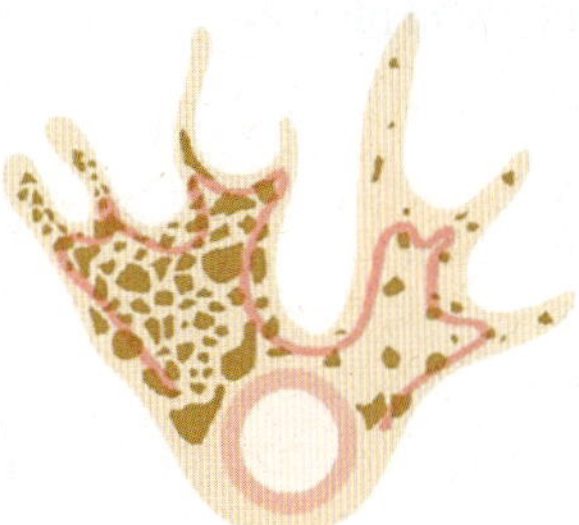

Fig. Melanocytes

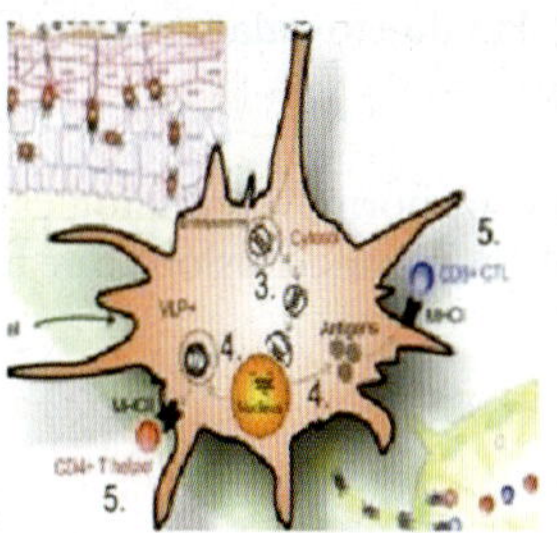

Fig. Langerhans cells

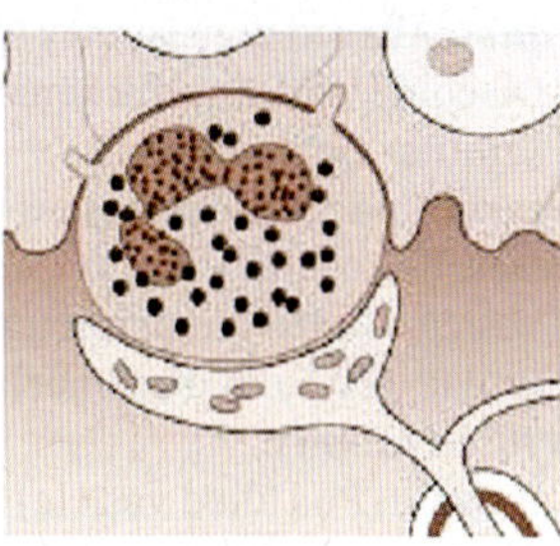

Fig. Merkel/Touch cells

I D2. Cells in the Dermis

- Dermal dendritic cells
- Tissue macrophages/ Histiocytes
- Fibroblasts

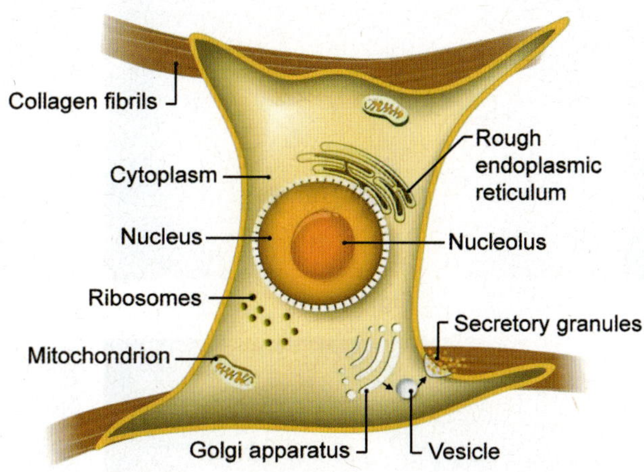

Fig. Fibroblast

Topper's Edge

Normal Resident Flora of Skin[Q]

- Staphylococcus epidermidis: On surface of skin, moist sites
- Corynebacterium spp.: Aerobic, moist sites
- Propionibacterium spp.: Anaerobic, depth of hair follicle
- Brevibacterium spp.: Aerobic, moist sites
- Malassezia spp.: Superficial part of hair follicle

I E. MORPHOLOGY OF SKIN LESIONS

- ***Macules***: Circumscribed flat lesion of skin seen due to change in colour
  - Hyperpigmented (Café au lait spots)
  - Hypopigmented (Piebaldism)
  - Erythematous (Purpura)
- ***Papules***: Small solid elevated lesion < 0.5 cm diameter
  - May be due to hyperplasia, cellular deposits or cellular infiltrate in dermis
- ***Nodules***: Solid lesions > 0.5 cm diameter having a deeper component

- ***Plaques***: Altered consistency of skin due to enlargement/ confluence of plaques
  - Discoid (Uniform thickening)
  - Annular (Ring shaped)
- ***Tumors***: Enlarged tissue mass due by normal/ pathological cells
- ***Blisters***: Fluid-filled, circumscribed, elevated lesions due to split in skin
  - Vesicles (< 0.5 cm diameter)
  - Bullae (> 0.5 cm diameter)
- ***Pus filled lesions***:
  - Pustule (Pus filled vesicle)
  - Abscess (Pus filled nodule)
- ***Dermal/subcutaneous edema***:
  - Wheal (Elevated lesion due to dermal edema)
  - Angioedema (Wheal extending into subcutaneous tissue and lasts > 48 hours)

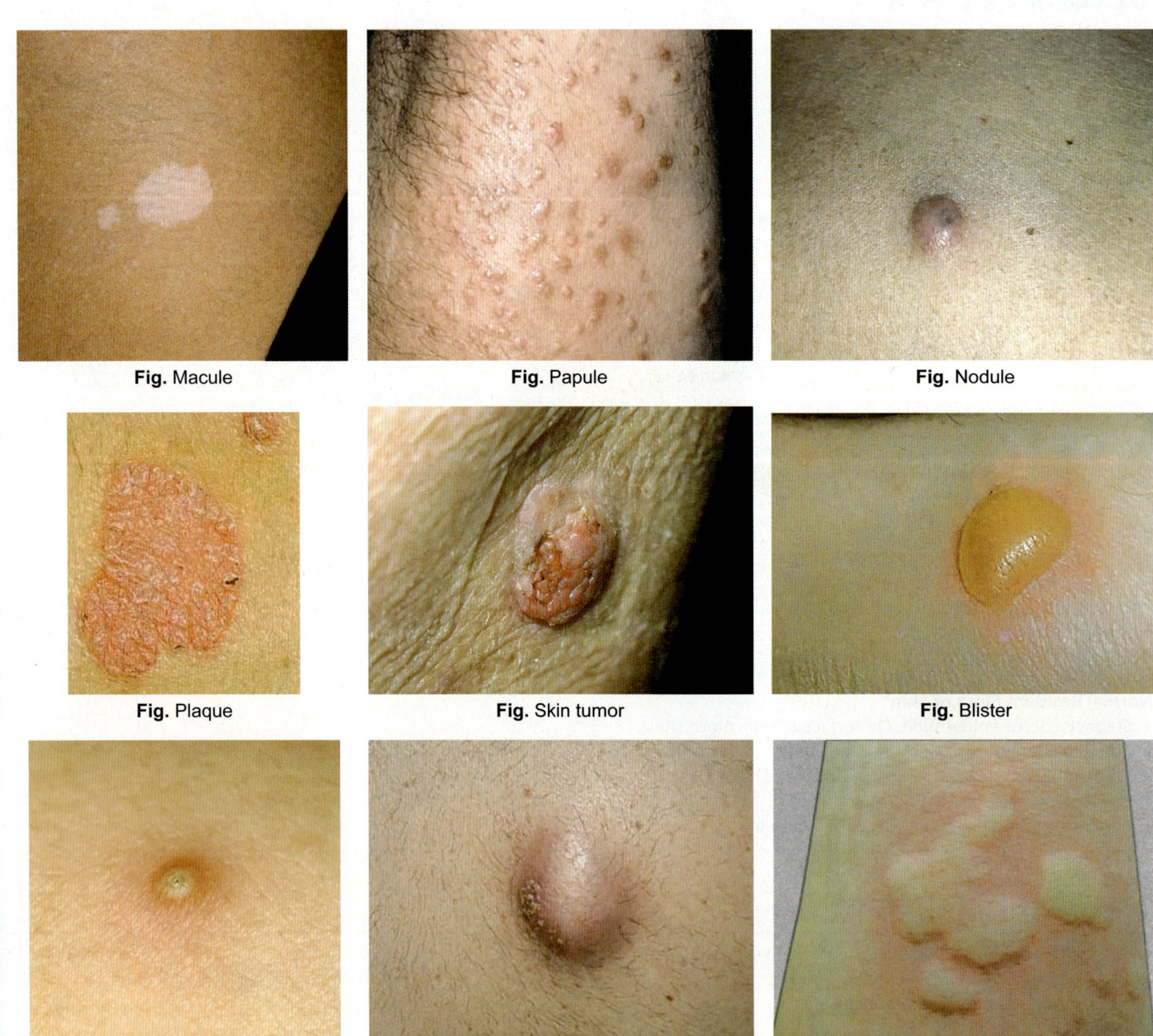

Fig. Macule

Fig. Papule

Fig. Nodule

Fig. Plaque

Fig. Skin tumor

Fig. Blister

Fig. Pustule

Fig. Abscess

Fig. Wheal

- ***Lesions due to extravasated blood***:
  - Purpura (Erythematous macule due to extravasated RBCs in dermis)
  - Hematoma (Swelling due to extravasated blood)
- ***Lesions due to dilatation of vessels***:
  - Telangiectasia (Visible dilation of small blood vessels of skin)
  - Poikiloderma (Atrophy of skin, reticulate hyperpigmentation, telangiectasia)
- ***Specific lesions***:
  - Burrow (Serpentine thread-like curvilinear lesion in scabies)
  - Comedones (Inspissated plugs of keratin and sebum in pilosebaceous orifices)
- ***Secondary changes due to collection of cells/ exudate***:
  - Scales (Flakes due to collection of cells in horny layer of skin)
  - Crust (Collection of dead epidermal cells with dried serum/ blood)
- ***Secondary changes due to loss of continuity of skin***:
  - Erosion (Complete/ partial loss of viable epidermis)
  - Ulcer (Loss of epidermis and upper dermis)
  - Fissure (Epidermis slit)
  - Excoriation (Linear erosion/ulcer when skin is scratched)
  - Sinus (Blind track in skin)

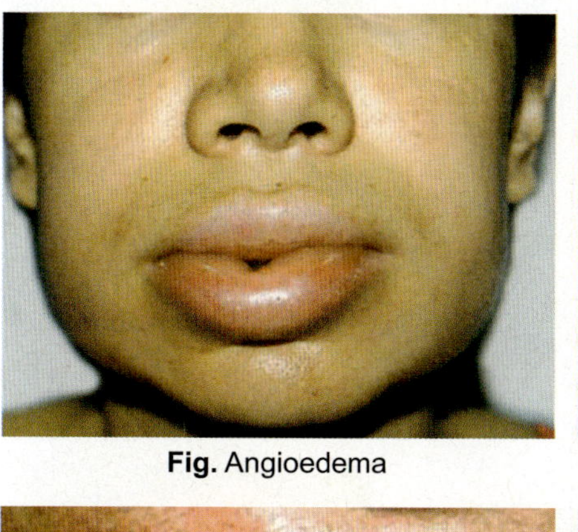

Fig. Angioedema

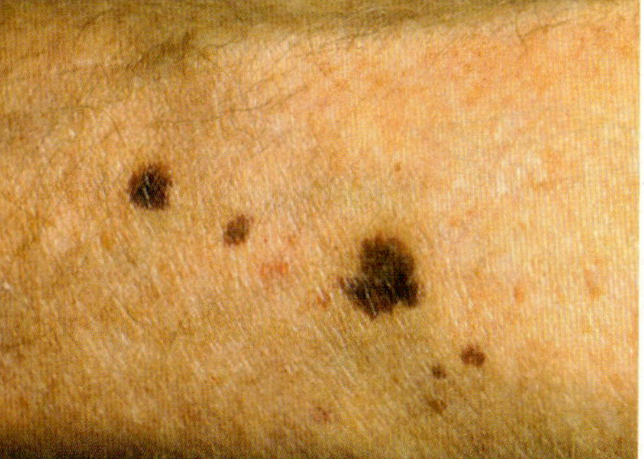

Fig. Purpura

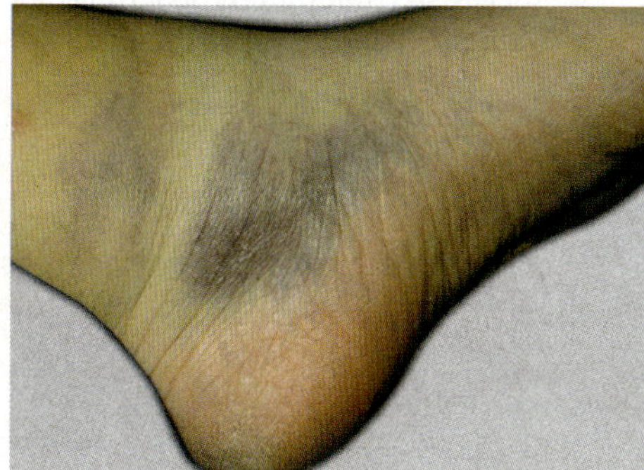

Fig. Hematoma

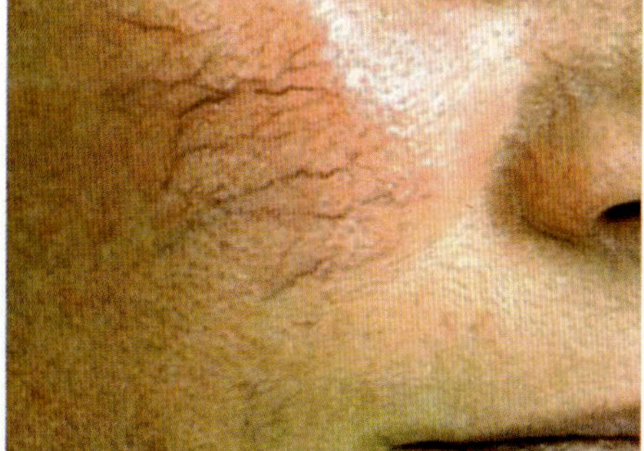

Fig. Telengiectasia

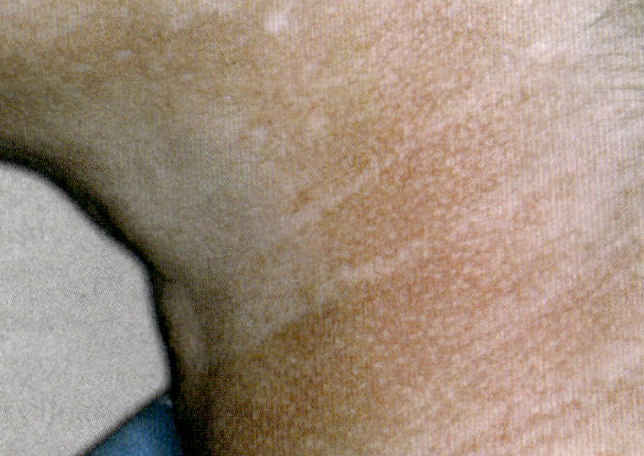

Fig. Poikiloderma

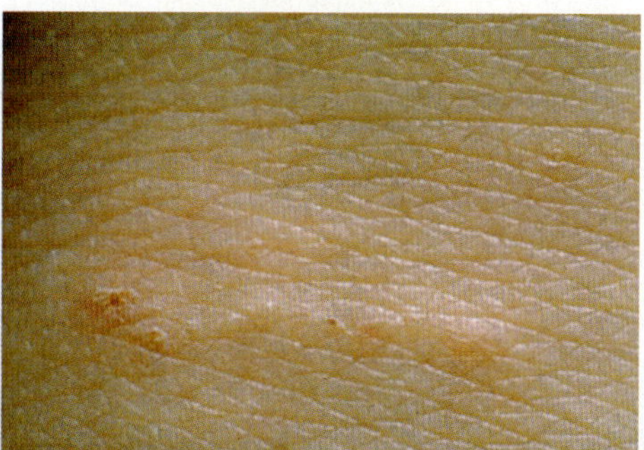

Fig. Skin burrow

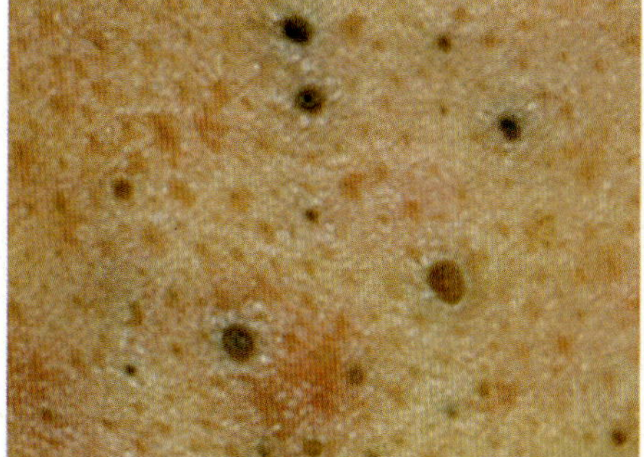

Fig. Comedone

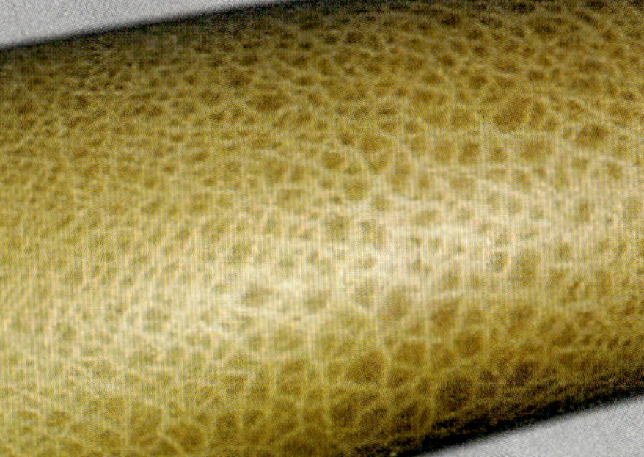

Fig. Scaling

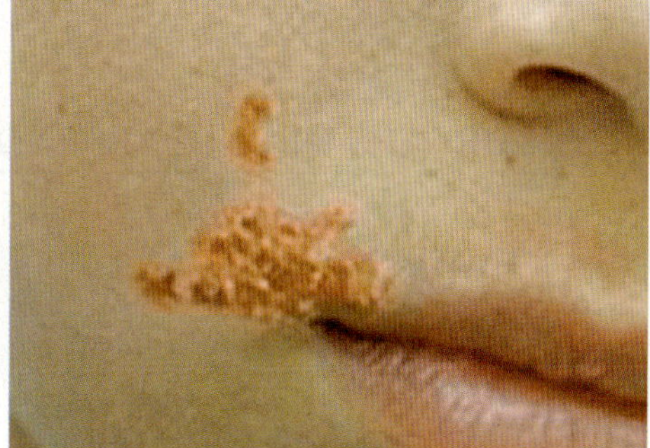

Fig. Crusting

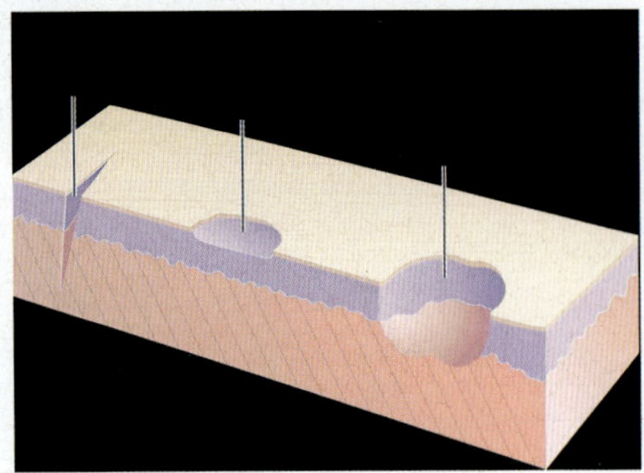

Fig. Fissure, Ulcer, Erosion

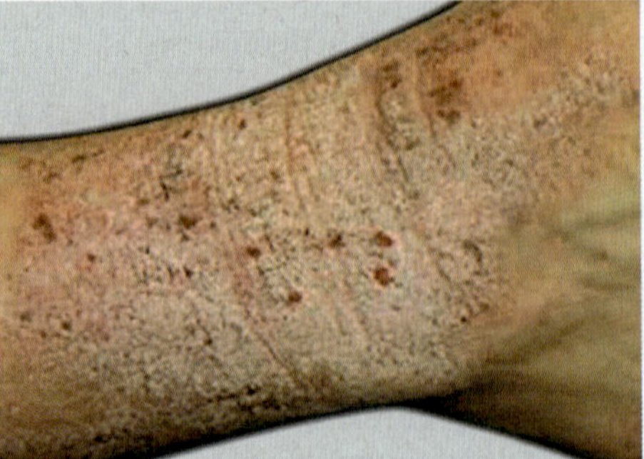

Fig. Lichenification

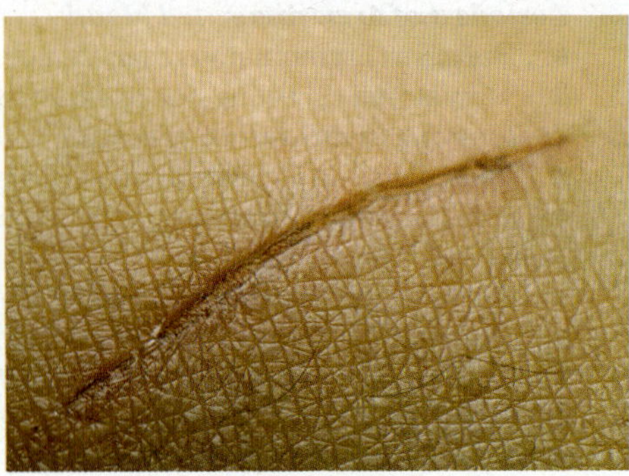

Fig. Skin scar

- ***Miscellaneous changes***:
  - Atrophy (Epidermal or dermal)
  - Lichenification (Thickening and hyperpigmentation of skin on repeated scratching)
  - Scar (Normal structures of skin replaced by fibrous tissue)
  - Sclerosis (Indurations of dermis/ subcutaneous tissue)
  - Colour changes (hyperpigmentation or hypopigmentation)

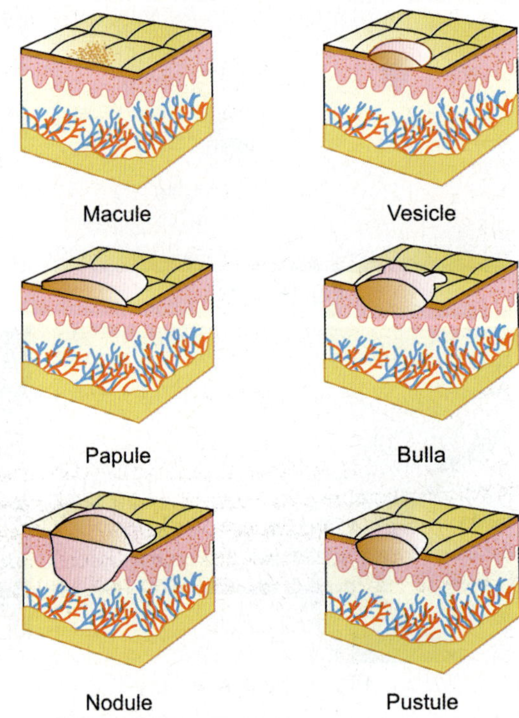

Fig.

I F. DISORDERS OF SKIN APPENDAGES

- ***Disorders of Sebaceous glands***[Q]:
  - Acne vulgaris
  - Rosacea
- ***Disorders of Eccrine sweat glands***[Q]:
  - Hyperhidrosis
  - Hypohidrosis
  - Anhidrosis
  - Miliaria

- ***Disorders of Apocrine glands*** [Q]:
  - Hidradentis suppurativa
- ***Disorders of Hair***:
  - Alopecia areata
  - Androgenetic areata
  - Miscellaneous alopecia
    - Telogen effluvium
    - Traction alopecia
    - Cicatricial alopecia
    - Trichotillomania
  - Hirsutism
  - Hypertrichosis
- ***Disorders of Nails***:
  - Congenital disorders: Paronychia congenital
  - Infective disorders
    - Onchomycosis
    - Paronychia
  - Traumatic disorders
    - Splinter hemorrhages
    - Subungal hematomas
    - Chronic injury
    - Nervous tics
    - Chemical injury
  - Skin disorders
    - Psoriasis
    - Lichen planus
    - Dermatitis
    - Trachyonychia
  - Neoplastic disorders
  - Systemic disorders

I G. SKIN TUMORS

I G1. Seborrheic Keratosis

- *Clinical presentation*:
  - Usually on face, upper trunk, upper extremities
  - Multiple brown-black papules with ***'Stuck-on' appearance*** [Q]
  - *Currant bun appearance*: Scattered keratin plugs on greasy skin [Q]
  - Hyperkeratosis, Papillomatosis, Horn cysts
- Treatment: None should be done

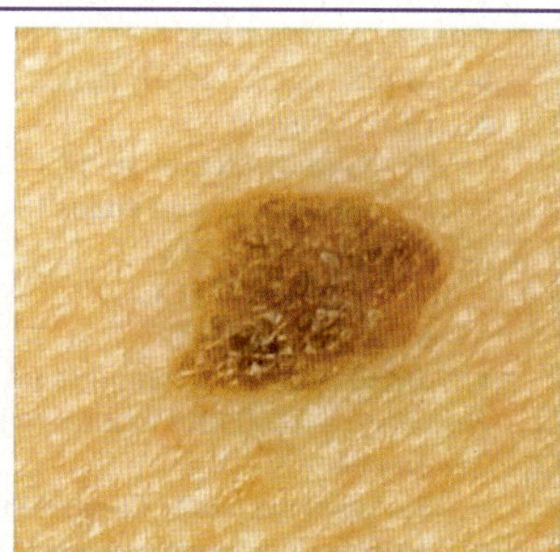

Fig. Seborrheic keratitis

I G2. Milia

- *Definition*: Sub-epidermal keratin cysts [Q]
- ***Most common site*: Face** [Q]

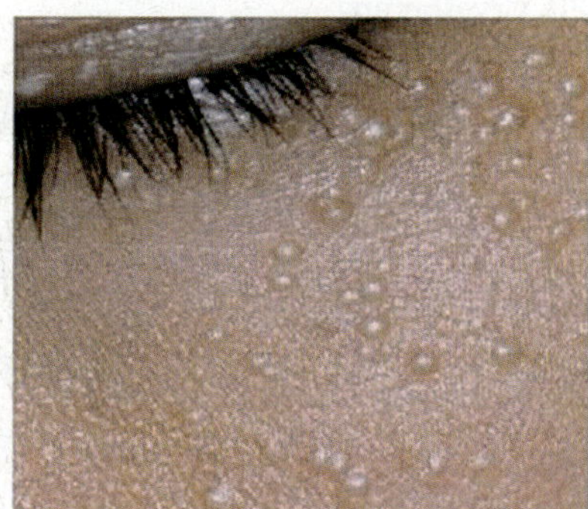

Fig. Milia

Skin and STDs

I G3. Keratoacanthoma

- *Underlying cause*:
  - Photosensitizing chemicals
  - Radiation
  - Immunosuppression
- *Clinical presentation*: Rapidly growing skin-coloured nodule with a ***'central horny plug'***[Q]
- *Most common site*: Photo-exposed parts

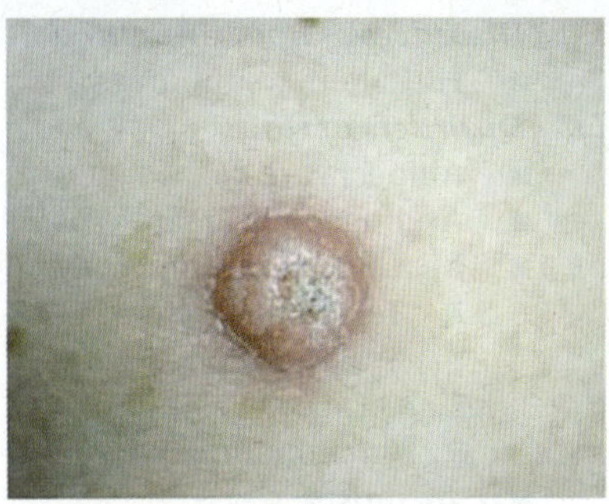

Fig. Keratoacanthoma

I G4. Bowen's Disease

- *Underlying cause*:
  - UV rays
  - Chronic arsenic poisoning
- *Clinical presentation*: Single enlarging psoriasiform plaque with ***'reniform margins'***[Q]
- *Most common site*: Face or trunk

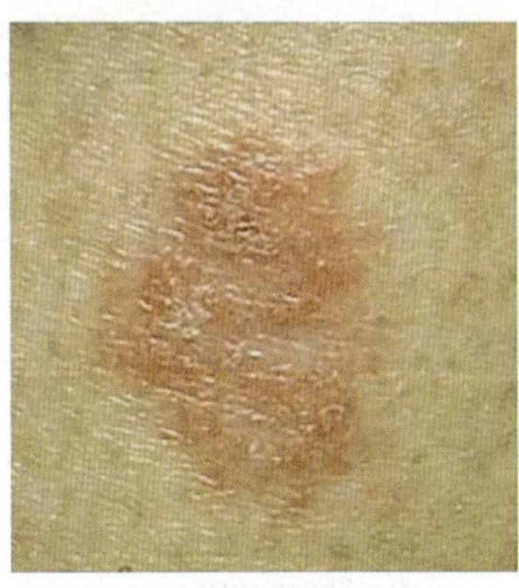

Fig. Bowen's disease

I G5. Actinic Keratoses

- *Underlying cause*:
  - UV rays
  - Vitiligo
- *Clinical presentation*: Multiple irregular pink macules/ papules
- *Most common site*: Face, scalp, dorsum of hand

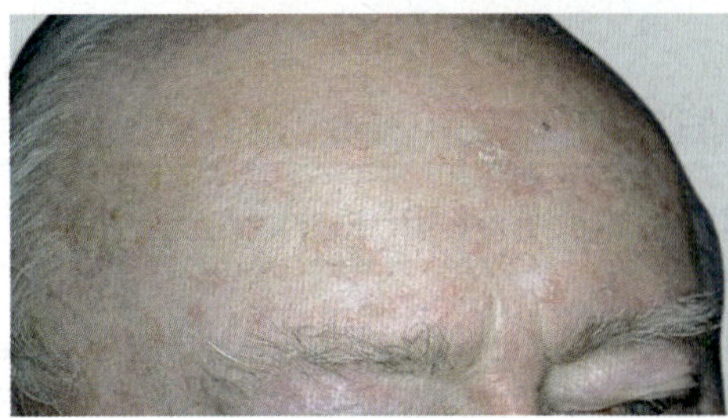

Fig. Actinic keratoses

I G6. Basal Cell Carcinoma

- *Underlying cause*: [Q]
  - Albinism
  - Arsenic
  - Psoralens + UVA
  - UV rays
  - Tar
  - Xeroderma pigmentosum
- *Clinical presentation*:
  - Middle aged/ elderly males
  - *Clinical types*:
    - Nodulo-ulcerative BCC **(*Rodent ulcer*): Ulcerated nodule with rolled, pearly, beaded edges**[Q]
    - Superficial BCC
    - Morphoeic BCC
    - Pigmented BCC
  - ***Site*: Face** (except Superficial BCC)[Q]
- *Histology*: Islands and lobules of basaloid cells in *'Palisading arrangement'*[Q]
- *Treatment*:
  - ***Surgical excision*: Treatment of choice**[Q]
  - *Moh's microscopic surgery*: If BCC at high risk site, > 2 cm size, recurrent or morpheic variant
  - *Other treatments*: Cryosurgery, Topical 5-FU, Cryotherapy

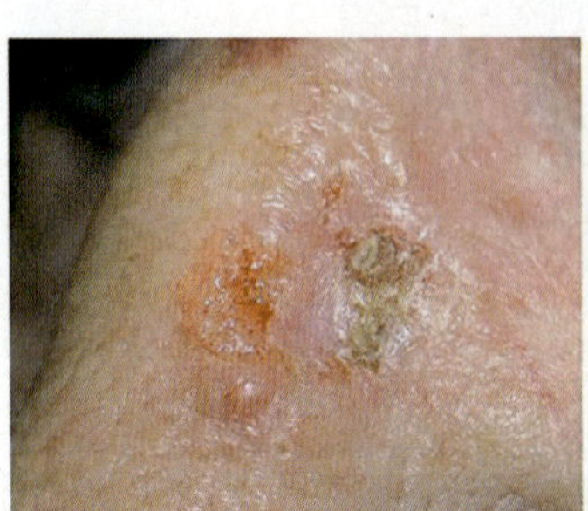

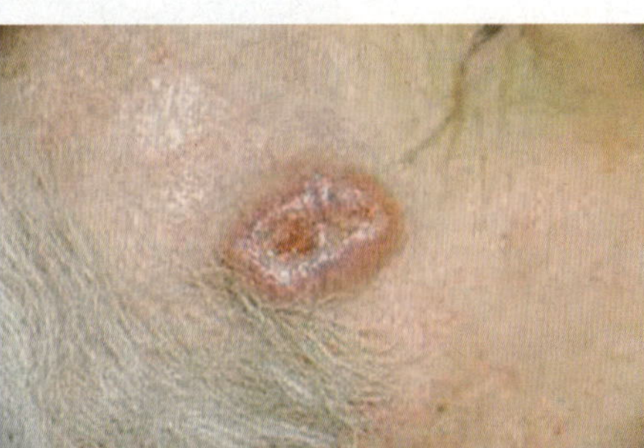

Fig. Basal cell carcinoma

I G7. Squamous cell carcinoma

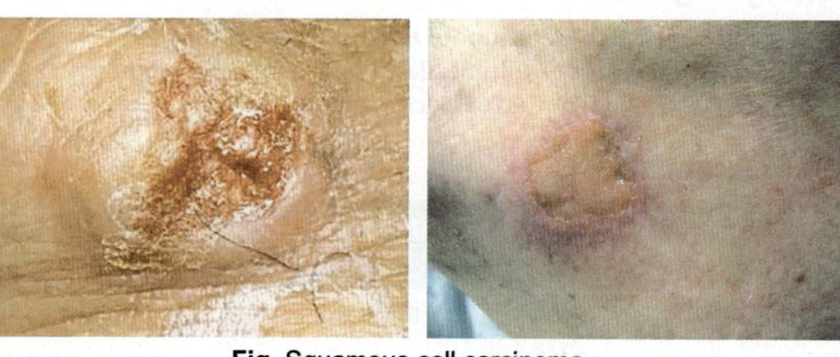
Fig. Squamous cell carcinoma

- *Underlying cause*:
  - Damaged skin **[Mnemonic: BLENDS]** [Q]
    - **B**urn scars
    - **L**eucoplakia
    - **E**rythroplakia
    - **N**on-healing ulcers
    - **D**ermatitis
    - **S**unlight induced Actinic keratoses
  - *Carcinogens*: Tar, Arsenic, Mineral oil
  - Xeroderma pigmentosum
  - HPV
  - Immunosuppression
- *Clinical presentation*:
  - Verrucous plaque with shallow ulcer having red granular floor
  - Regional lymphadenopathy
- *Histology*: Invading malignant keratinocytes with horn cysts, hyperkeratosis[Q]
- *Treatment*:
  - ***Surgical excision*: Treatment of choice**[Q]
  - *Radiotherapy*: Older patients

I G8. Malignant Melanoma

- *Underlying cause*:
  - UV radiation[Q]
  - Xeroderma pigmentosum
  - Melanocytic nevi
- *Clinical presentation*: **[Mnemonic: ABCDE]** [Q]
  - **A**symmetrical pigmented nodule
  - **B**order irregularity
  - **C**olour variability
  - **D**iameter size > 5 mm
  - **E**levation irregularity
  - Clinical types:
    - ***Superficial spreading melanoma*: Most common type**[Q]
    - *Lentigo maligna melanoma*
    - *Acral lentiginous melanoma*
    - *Nodular malignant melanoma*: Most aggressive type
- *Histology*: Invading malignant keratinocytes with horn cysts, hyperkeratosis
- *Treatment*:
  - ***Surgical excision*: Treatment of choice**[Q]

Thickness of tumor	Excision with margins[Q]
< 0.5 mm	5 mm
0.5 – 1 mm	1 cm
1 – 2 mm	2 cm
> 2 mm	3 cm

  - *Chemotherapy*: Dacarbazine
  - Radiotherapy

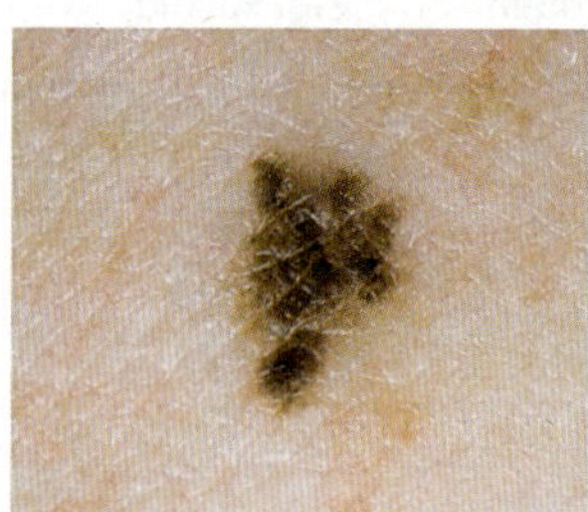
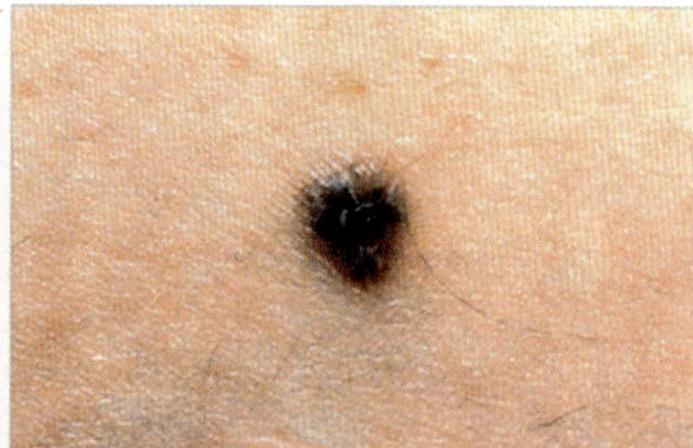
Fig. Malignant melanoma

Skin and STDs

I G9. Syringoma

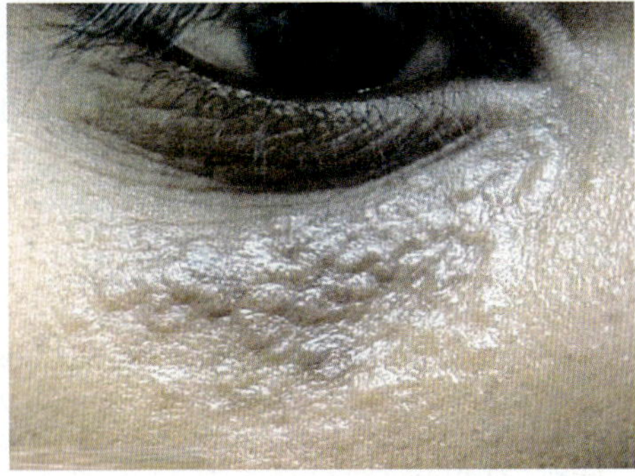
Fig. Syringoma

- *Type of tumor*: **Benign tumor of eccrine sweat glands**[Q]
- *Clinical presentation*: Multiple, flat-topped angulated papules
- *Treatment*: None required or electrocautery

I G10. Paget's Disease

Paget's disease		
	Breast	**Extramammary**
Age-sex distribution	Females – fourth decade	Females – fifth decade
Origin	Ductal carcinoma breasts[Q]	Apocrine gland duct[Q]
Site	Around areola of breast[Q]	Vulva, peri-anal area[Q]
Lesion	Sharp margin plaque with raised edge, irregular outline	
Treatment	For breast carcinoma	Surgical excision

I G11. Benign Tumors of Dermis

- ***Salmon patch***:
  - **Is most common type of vascular malformation**[Q]
  - Is a type of Capillary malformation presenting as telengiactic macules
  - Seen on neck, forehead, eyelids[Q]
- ***Port-wine stain/Telengiactic nevus/ Nevus flammeus***:
  - Is a type of Capillary malformation presenting as deep-red telengiactic macules which turn darker and nodular
  - Seen on face[Q]
  - *Sturge Weber syndrome*: Trigeminal port-wine strain associated with vacular hamartomas of CNS (seizures) and eyes (glaucoma)[Q]
  - *Treatment*: Pulse tunable dye laser
- ***Keloid***:
  - Is abnormal response of skin to trauma/ surgical wounds/ insect bites/ acne lesions
  - Itchy, irregular, firm nodules/ plaques with ***'claw like projections'***[Q]
  - Presternal-area[Q], neck, upper back, deltoid
- ***Leiomyoma***:
  - Is tumor of smooth muscles[Q]
  - Painful, red, tender nodules
- ***Lipoma***:
  - Is tumor of adipose tissue[Q]
  - Asymptomatic, soft, slippery, lobulated sub-cutaneous nodules
- ***Dermatofibroma***:
  - Is benign tumor of fibrous tissue[Q]
  - Single, firm, ***'button-like'***[Q], dermal nodules

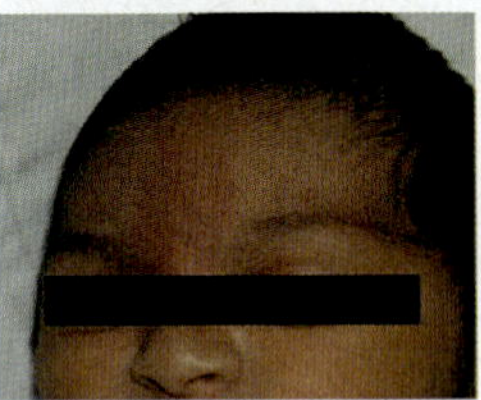
Fig. Salmon patch

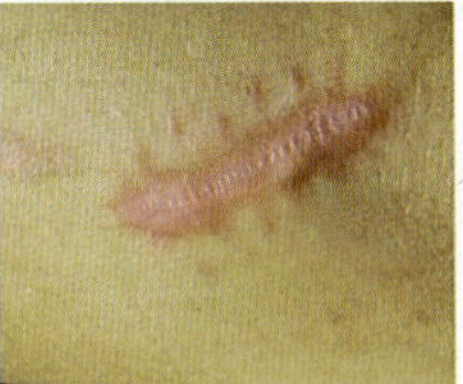
Fig. Port-wine stain

Fig. Keloid

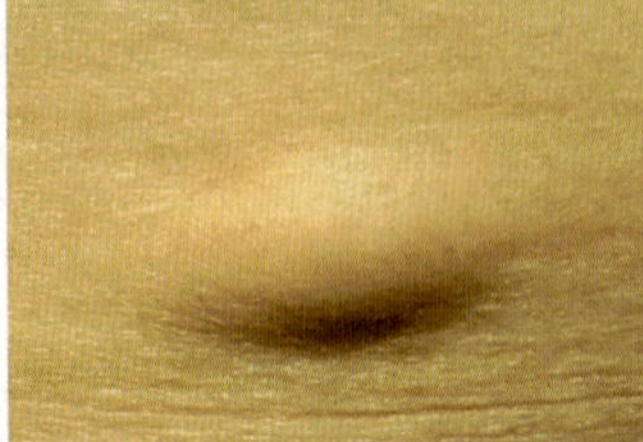
Fig. Lipoma

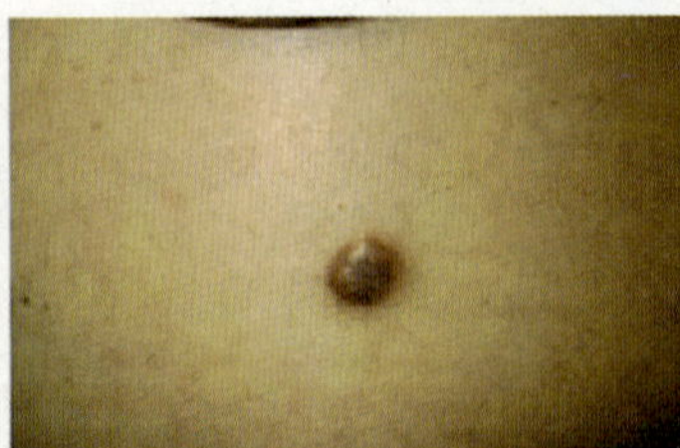
Fig. Dermatofibroma

I G12. Cutaneous T-cell Lymphoma/ Mycosis Fungoides

- Type of tumor: **Lymphoma of Helper T-cells of skin**[Q]
- Underlying cause: Infection with HTLV-I[Q]
- Clinical presentation:
  - *Patch stage*: Minimally erythematous, pigmented plagues with *'Cigarette paper atrophy'* and *'Piokiloderma'*[Q]
  - *Plaque stage*
  - *Tumor stage*: Tumor d' emblee
- ***Histology*: Pautrier's microabscesses**[Q]
- *Treatment*:
  - Patch stage: Corticosteroids, UV-B, PUVA
  - Plaque stage: Electron beam, PUVA, Acitretin
  - Tumor stage: Radiotherapy, Chemotherapy

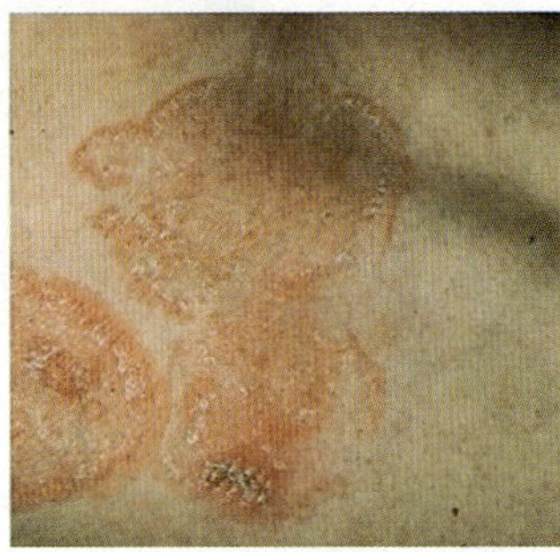
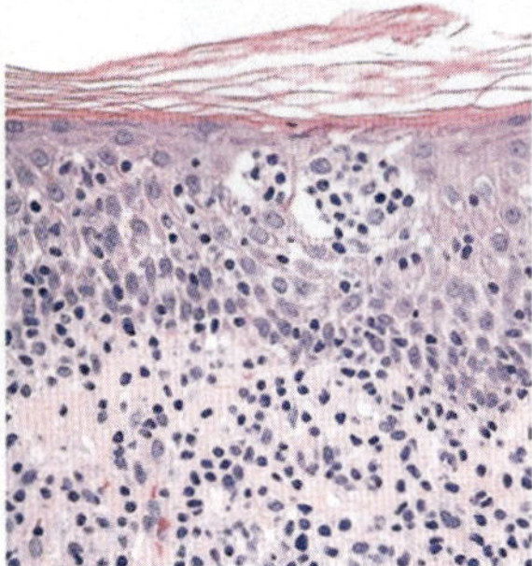

Fig. Mycosis fungoides

I G13. Acanthosis Nigricans

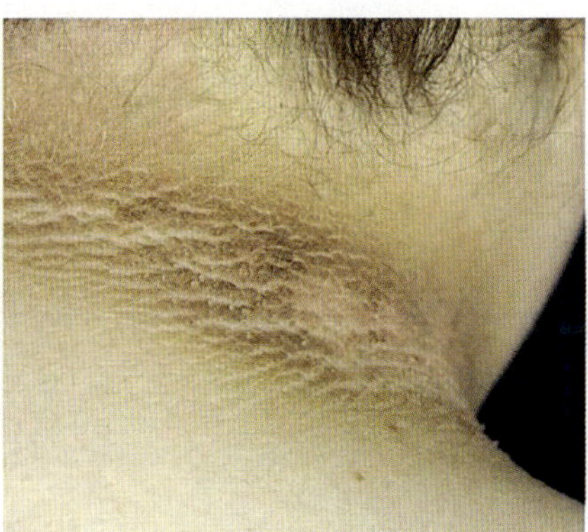

Fig. Acanthosis nigricans

- *Etiological classification*:
  - *Hereditary AN*: Autosomal dominant disorder
  - *HAIR-AN syndrome*:
    - **H**yper-**A**ndrogenism
    - **I**nsulin **R**esistance
    - **A**canthosis **N**igricans
  - *Benign acquired AN*: Obesity
  - *Drug induced AN*:
    - Nicotinic acid
    - Stilbesterol
    - Corticosteroids
    - Oral contraceptives
  - *Malignant AN*:
    - Adenocarcinoma stomach
    - Carcinoma genitor-urinary tract
- *Clinical presentation*: Thick, velvety, hyper-pigmented skin with feathered edges of lesions in flexures
- *Treatment*: Retinoic acid

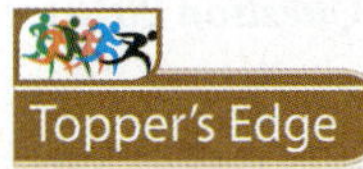

Topper's Edge

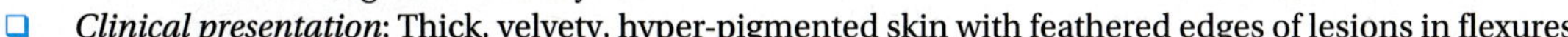

Dermatological Stains

Tissue/ organism/ Deposit	Stain
Collagen[Q]	Masson's trichome, Verhoeff-van Gieson
Elastic fibres	Verhoeff-van Gieson
Mast cell granules	Toluidine blue
Mycobacteria[Q]	Fite
Fungi	Periodic acid Schiff
Glycogen[Q]	Periodic acid Schiff
Acid mucopolysaccharides	Toluidine blue, Alcian blue
Amyloid[Q]	Congo red

IMAGE-BASED QUESTIONS

1. Dermatological test shown in the Photograph is ***[Recent Question 2012]***

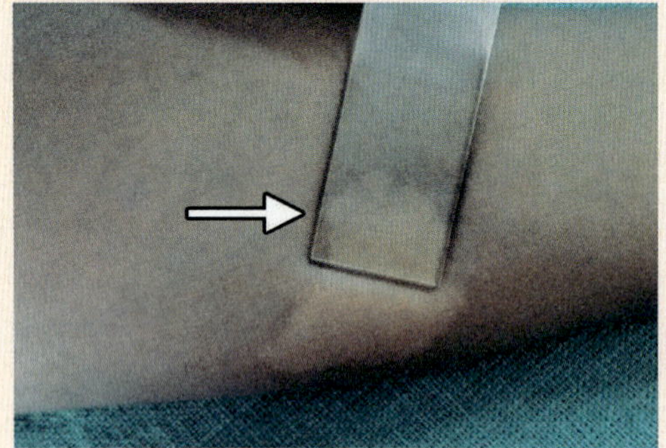

a. Wood lamp examination
b. Patch testing
c. Diascopy
d. Blanch test

2. Identify Skin lesion shown in Photograph ***[Recent Question 2014]***

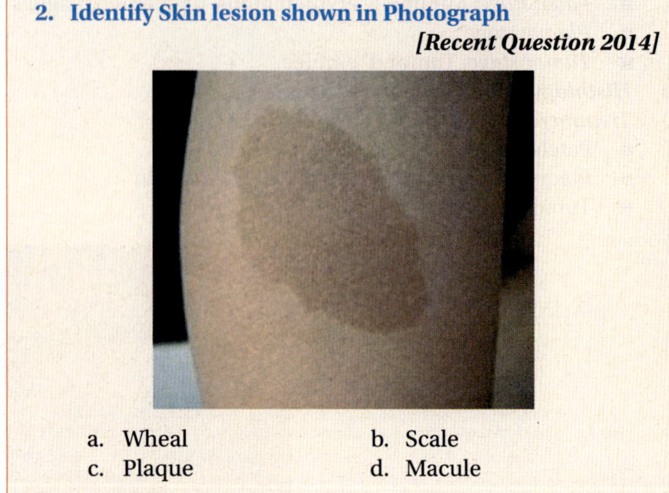

a. Wheal
b. Scale
c. Plaque
d. Macule

3. Identify the Morphology of Skin lesion shown in Photograph

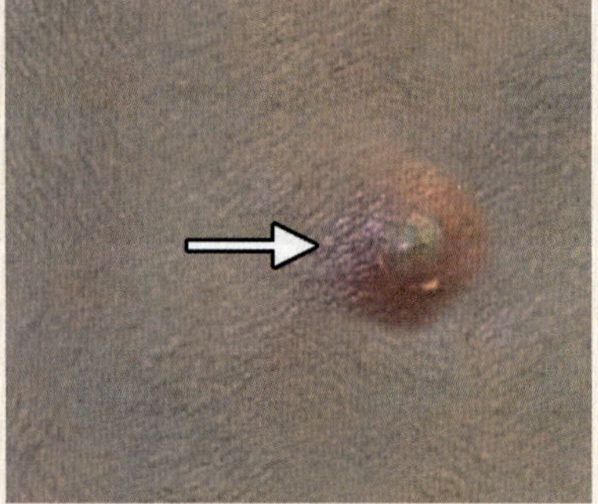

a. Pustule
b. Wheal
c. Blister
d. Purpura

4. Microscopic Test shown in Photograph is used for ***[Recent Question 2014]***

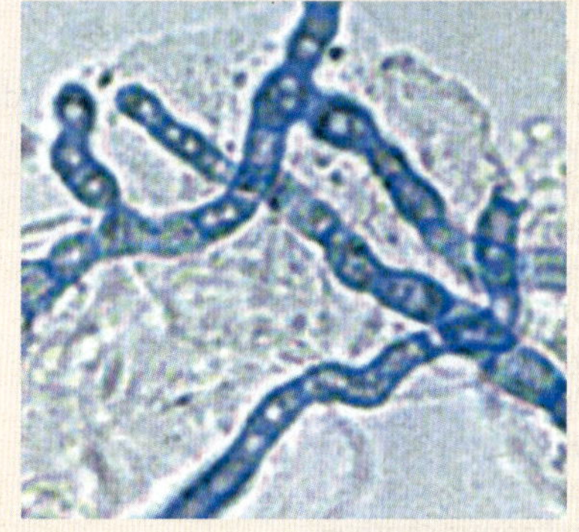

a. Bacteria
b. Virus
c. Fungi
d. Rickettsiae

5. Identify the Morphology of Skin lesion shown in Photograph

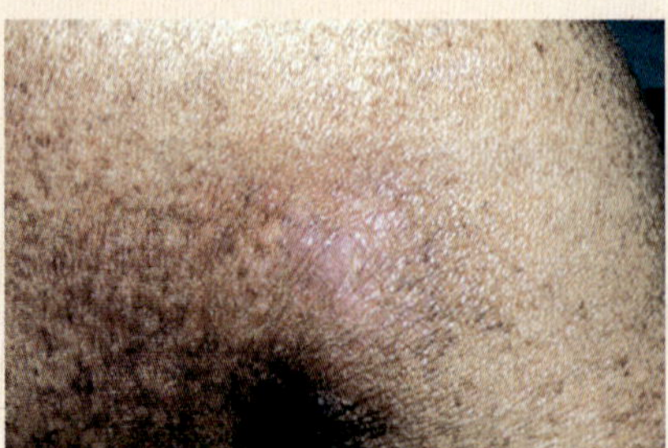

a. Poikiloderma
b. Purpura
c. Comedones
d. Burrows

6. Identify the Morphology of Skin lesion shown in Photograph ***[Recent Question 2012]***

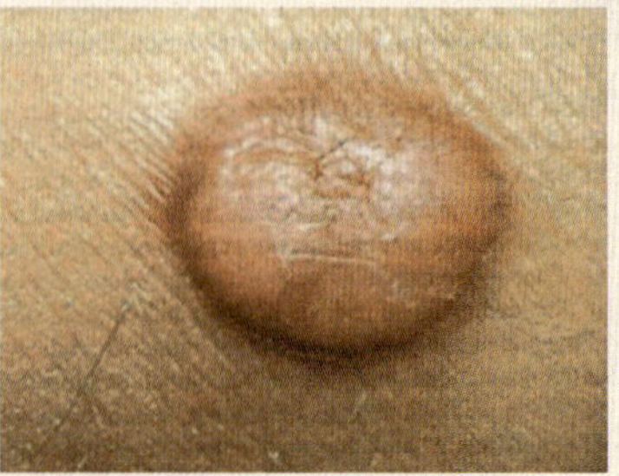

a. Macule
b. Papule
c. Nodule
d. Plaque

7. Identify Dermatological test shown in Photograph ***[Recent Question 2013]***

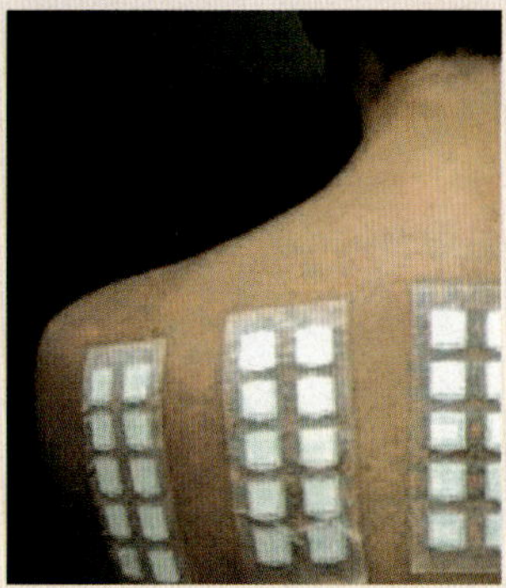

a. Dermascopy
b. Diascopy
c. Skin biopsy
d. Patch test

8. Identify the Morphology of Skin lesion shown in Photograph

a. Wheal
b. Papule
c. Plaque
d. Blister

9. Identify the Morphology of Skin lesion shown in Photograph ***[Recent Question 2014]***

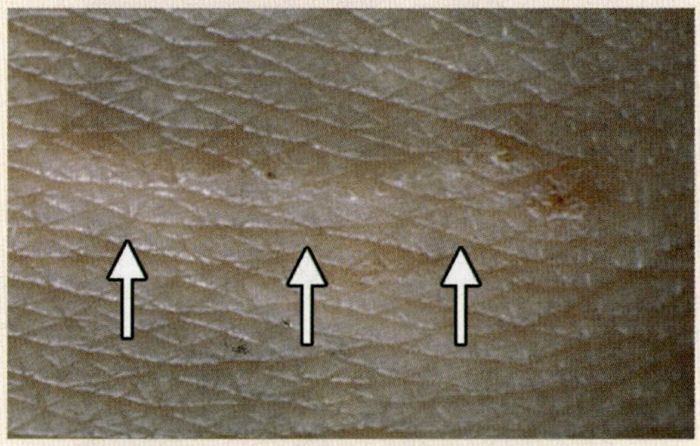

a. Erosion
b. Crust
c. Burrow
d. Fissure

10. Identify the Dermatological test shown in Photograph

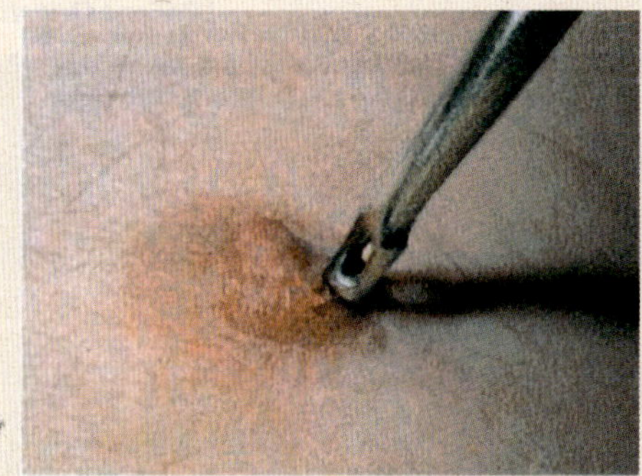

a. Dermascopy
b. Photo-patch test
c. Skin biopsy
d. Patch test

11. Identify Feature of Tuberous sclerosis shown ***[Recent Question 2012]***

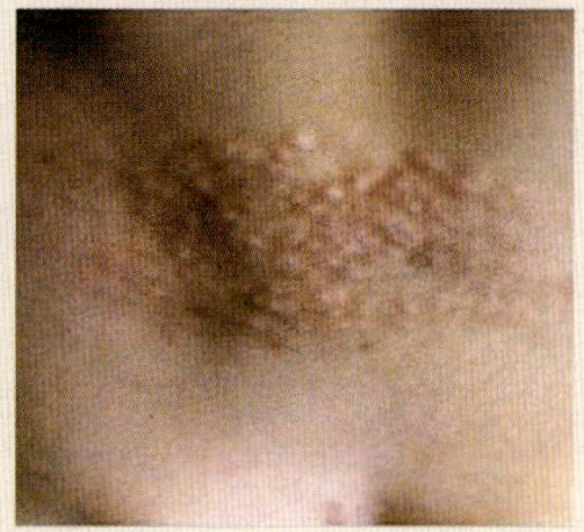

a. Angiofibroma
b. Shagreen patch
c. Ash leaf macule
d. Koenen's tumor

12. Diagnose the Skin disorder shown in Photograph

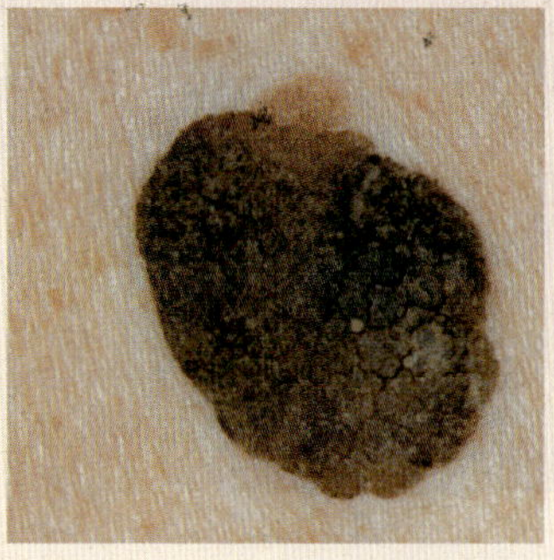

a. Seborrheic keratosis
b. Melanocytic nevus
c. Skin tags
d. Nevus of Ota

13. Skin tumor shown in Photograph is

[Recent Question 2012, 2013]

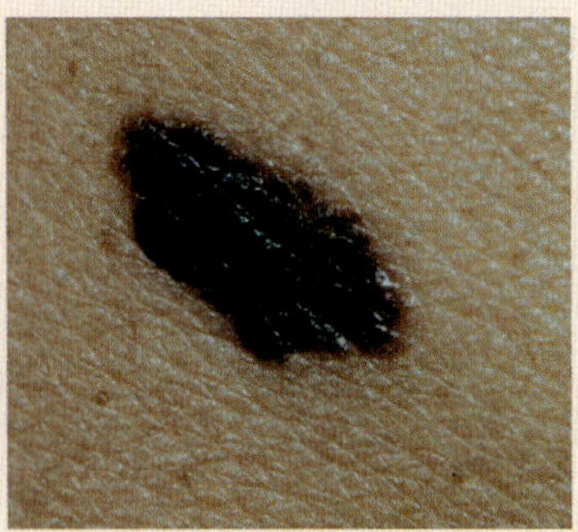

a. Syringoma
b. Malignant melanoma
c. Basal cell carcinoma
d. Squamous cell carcinoma

14. Diagnose the Skin disorder shown in Photograph

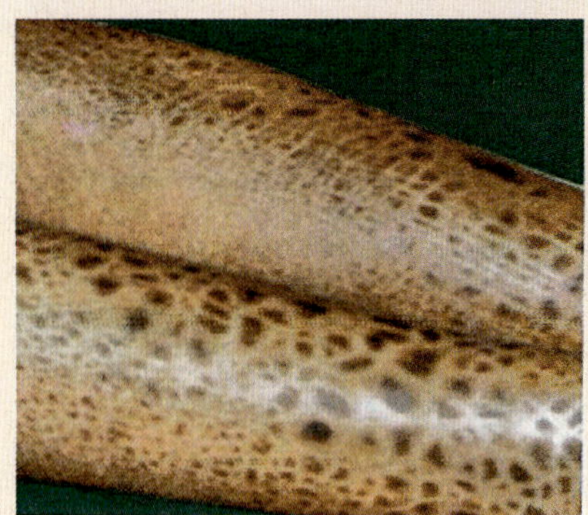

a. Scabies
b. Vitiligo
c. Ichthyosis
d. Hemangioma

15. Diagnose the Vascular birthmark shown in Photograph

[Recent Question 2013]

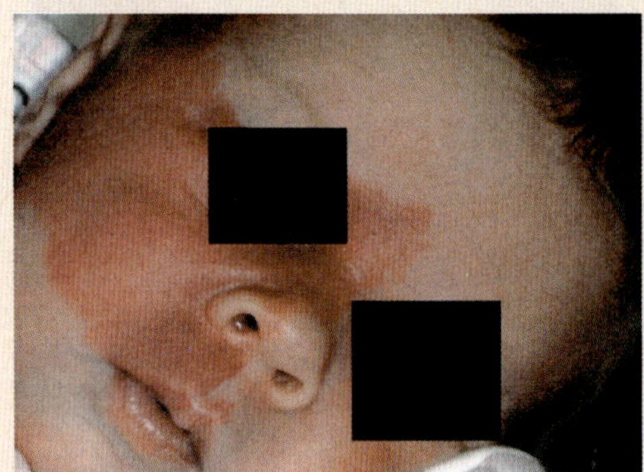

a. Infantile hemangioma
b. Salmon patch
c. Port wine stain
d. Lymphangioma

16. Diagnose the Skin disorder shown in Photograph

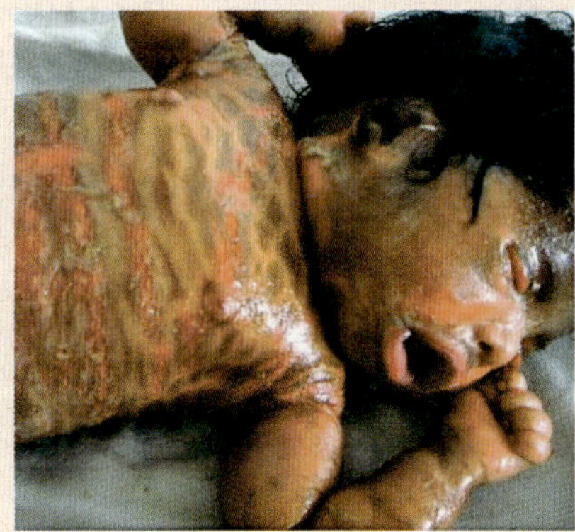

a. Ichthyosis vulgaris
b. X-linked Ichthyosis
c. Acquired Ichthyosis
d. Lamellar Ichthyosis

17. Diagnose the Skin disorder shown in Photograph

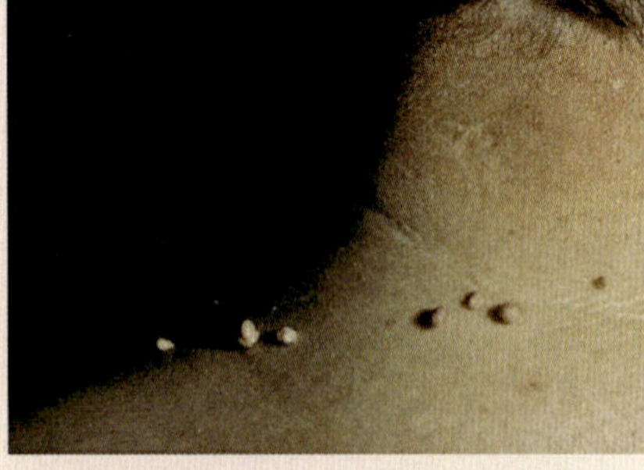

a. Melanocytic nevus
b. Seborrheic keratosis
c. Skin tags
d. Nevus of Ota

18. Identify the Skin tumor as shown in Photograph

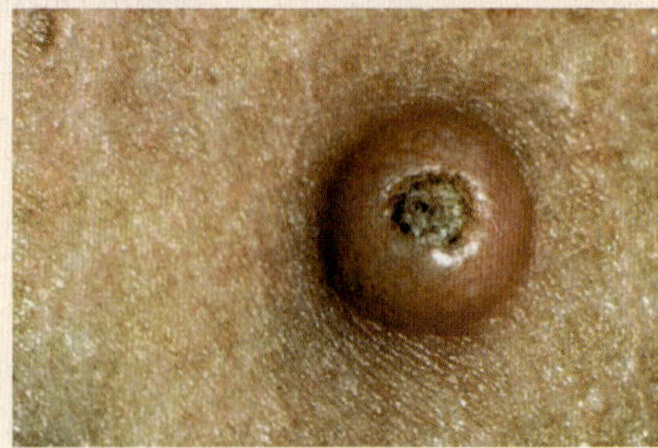

a. Corn
b. Horn
c. Nevus
d. Keratoacanthoma

19. Identify the Feature of Tuberous sclerosis shown in Photograph ***[Recent Question 2014]***

a. Angiofibroma
b. Shagreen patch
c. Ash leaf macule
d. Koenen's tumor

20. Identify the Skin tumor as shown in Photograph ***[Recent Question 2013, 2012]***

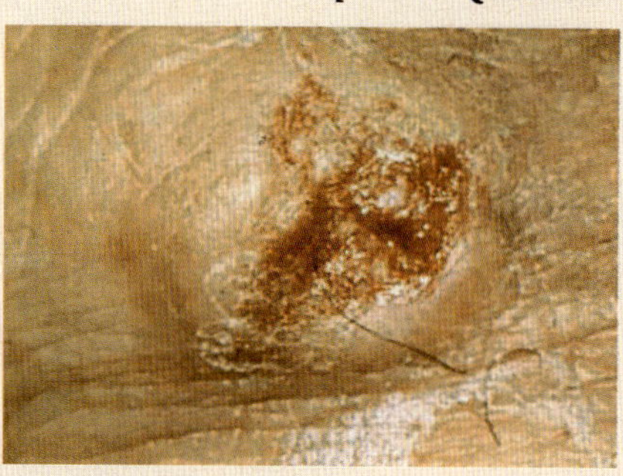

a. Syringoma
b. Malignant melanoma
c. Basal cell carcinoma
d. Squamous cell carcinoma

21. Identify the Skin tumor as shown in Photograph ***[Recent Question 2014, 2012]***

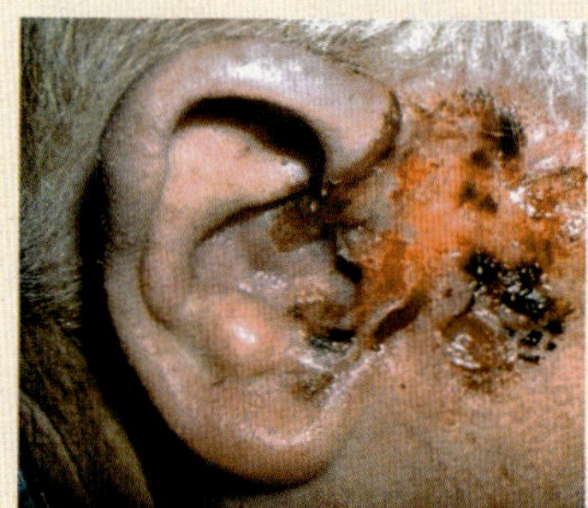

a. Syringoma
b. Malignant melanoma
c. Basal cell carcinoma
d. Squamous cell carcinoma

22. Identify the Skin disorder as shown in Photograph ***[Recent Question 2013, 2012]***

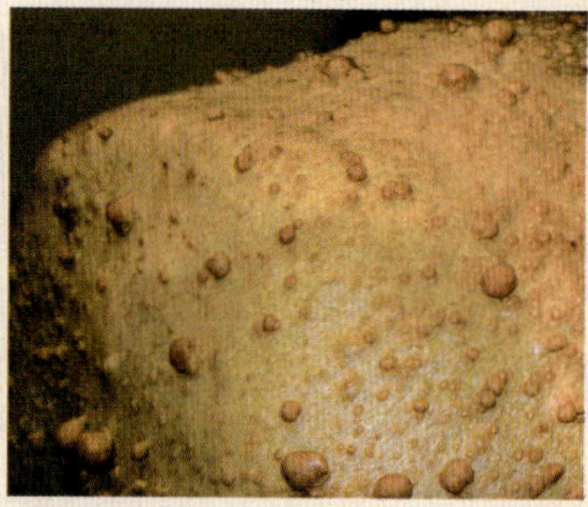

a. Angiofibroma
b. Neurofibromatosis
c. Xeroderma pigmentosum
d. Acanthosis nigricans

23. Identify the unit of skin shown in the Photograph

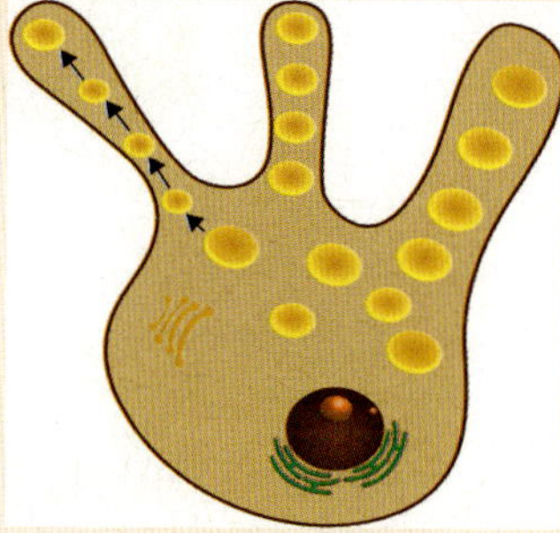

a. Melanocyte
b. Keratinocyte
c. Melanosome
d. Promelanosome

24. A child presents to OPD (Photograph) with Glaucoma. On CT scan there is Tram-track subcortical calcification. Diagnosis is ***[Recent Question 2015]***

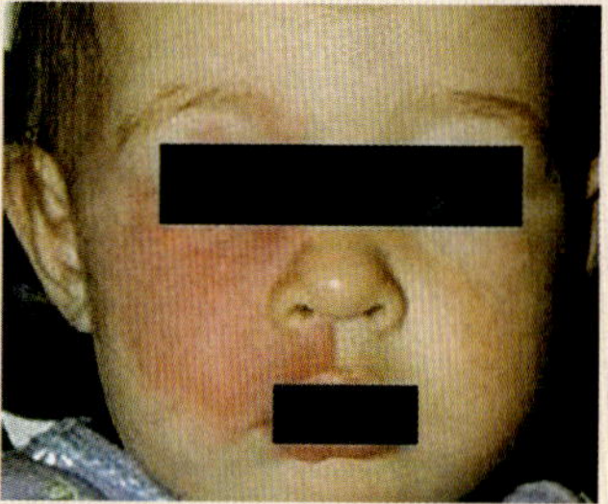

a. Von Hippel-Landau disease
b. Tuberous sclerosis
c. Sturge-Weber syndrome
d. Peutz-Jeghers syndrome

25. Identify the condition shown in the photograph given below which is present from birth ***[AIIMS May 2017]***

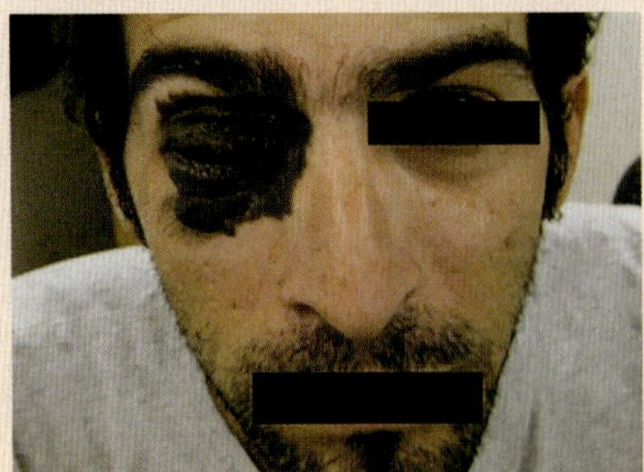

Congenital Melanocytic Nevus

a. Epidermal verrucous nevus
b. Melanoacanthoma
c. Congenital nevus
d. Malignant melanoma

26. Which of the following layer of Epidermis has maximum Desmosomes? ***[AIIMS November 2017]***

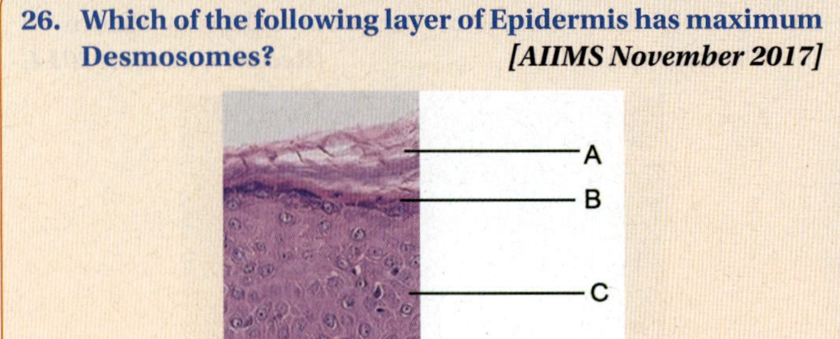

a. A
b. B
c. C
d. D

27. Identify the malformation shown in Photograph ***[Recent Question 2017]***

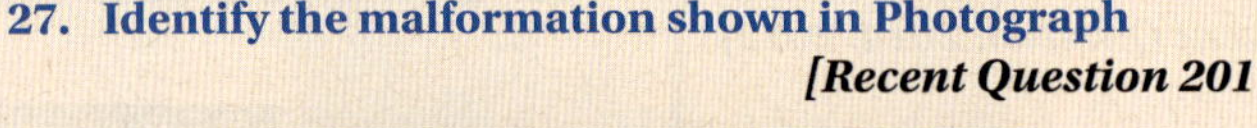

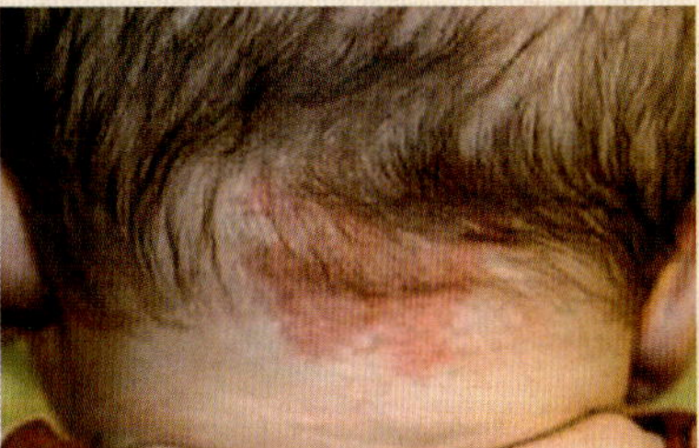

a. Port-wine stain
b. Hemangioma
c. Salmon patch
d. Lymphangioma

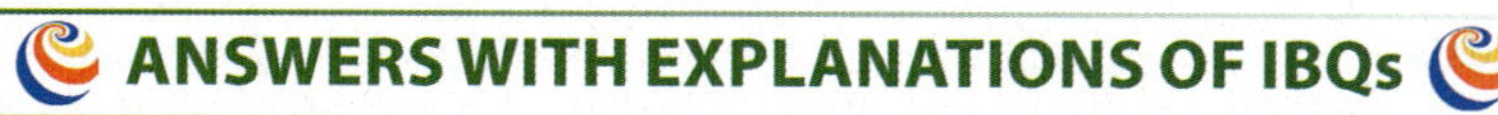

1. Ans. (c) Diascopy *[Ref. Neena Khanna, 4/e p13-14]*

Diascopy

- Description: Firm pressure applied with a hard, transparent instrument, such as a plastic or glass spatula or two microscope slides, may be used to blanch the skin temporarily
- Use in Dermatology:
  - Differentiate Purpuric lesions (Does not blanch) from Erythema (Blanches)
  - Granulomatous lesions

2. Ans. (d) Macule *[Ref. Neena Khanna, 4/e p5]*

- Macules: Circumscribed flat lesion of skin seen due to change in colour
  - Hyperpigmented (Café au lait spots)
  - Hypopigmented (Piebaldism)
  - Erythematous (Purpura)

3. Ans. (a) Pustule *[Ref. Neena Khanna, 4/e p7]*

- Pustule: Pus filled vesicle which can be Follicular or Extrafollicular

4. Ans. (c) Fungi *[Ref. Dermatology by Dykes, 1/e p162]*

- Potassium hydroxide (KOH) preparation: Rapidly diagnose fungal infections of the hair, skin, or nails
- Method: A sample of the infected area is analyzed under a microscope following the addition of a few drops of KOH

5. Ans. (a) Poikiloderma *[Ref. Neena Khanna, 4/e p9]*

- Poikiloderma: Skin lesion with hypopigmentation/ hyperpigmentation with a Classical Triad of Telengiectasia, Atrophy, Reticulate pigmentation

6. Ans. (c) Nodule *[Ref. Neena Khanna, 4/e p6]*

- Nodule is a Solid lesion of skin > 0.5 cm diameter having a deeper component

7. Ans. (d) Patch test *[Ref. Neena Khanna, 4/e p16]*

Patch Test

- Description: Detection of antigens responsible for Type IV hypersensitivity
- Method:
  - Antigens in standardized dilutions are applied on back if body as occlusions
  - Patches removed after 48 hours and sites marked
  - Inspection is done after ½ -1 hour and then at 96 hours
- Reading: Reaction (erythema/ Edema/ Papulation/ Vesiculation) noted with grading

8. Ans. (d) Blister *[Ref. Neena Khanna, 4/e p7]*

- *Blisters*: Fluid-filled, circumscribed, elevated lesions due to split in skin
  - Vesicles (< 0.5 cm diameter)
  - Bullae (> 0.5 cm diameter)

9. Ans. (c) Burrow *[Ref. Neena Khanna, 4/e p9]*

Burrow

- Serpentine thread-like curvilinear lesion seen in scabies
- Varies in length few mm to a cm
- Open end marked by a papule

10. Ans. (c) Skin biopsy *[Ref. Neena Khanna, 4/e p17]*

Skin Biopsy

- Description: Useful diagnostic technique in dermatology
- Techniques:
- Punch biopsy: For Superficial skin lesions
- Scalpel biopsy: For Deep skin lesions
- Processing of skin biopsy:
  - Specific staining
  - Specific procedures (immunofluorescence/ Electron microscopy)
  - Culture

11. Ans. (b) Shagreen patch *[Ref. Neena Khanna, 4/e p33]*

Shagreen Patch

- Leathery cobble-stoned yellow-black pig-skin like plaques
- Sites: Lumbosacral area, Face
- Occurrence: 40% patients of Tuberous sclerosis

12. Ans. (a) Seborrheic keratosis *[Ref. Neena Khanna, 4/e p351]*

Seborrheic Keratosis

- Skin colored, sharply demarcated brown macules
- Progress to dark brown-black papules with 'Stuck-on' appearance
- Greasy surface with scattered keratin plugs (Currant bun appearance)

13. Ans. (b) Malignant melanoma *[Ref. Neena Khanna, 4/e p367]*

Malignant Melanoma: [Mnemonic: ABCDE]

- **A**symmetrical pigmented nodule
- **B**order irregularity
- **C**olour variability
- **D**iameter size > 5 mm
- **E**levation irregularity

14. Ans. (c) Ichthyosis *[Ref. Neena Khanna, 4/e p21]*

Ichthyosis

- Fish-like scales worse in winters
- Fish scale disease: Dead skin accumulates in a similar pattern to a fish's scales
- Distribution: Majority of cases are mild and confined to specific areas of the body; Few cases are severe and can cover large areas of the body, including the abdomen, back, arms, and legs

15. Ans. (c) Port wine stain *[Ref. Neena Khanna, 4/e p372]*

Port-wine Stain

- Synonyms: Telengiectatic nevus, Nevus flammeus
- Description: Pink-red telengiectatic papules which may be become darker, nodulated
- MC site: Face

16. Ans. (d) Lamellar Ichthyosis *[Ref. Clinical Dermatology by Mann, 5/e p47]*

Lamellar Ichthyosis

- Description: All non-bullous (non-epidermolytic) and isolated types of congenital ichthyoses, except for harlequin fetus
- Collodion baby: An infant who is born with membrane like covering resembling collodion generally associated
- Autosomal recessive

17. Ans. (c) Skin tags *[Ref. Neena Khanna, 4/e p352]*

Skin Tags

- Soft papules in flexures of Obese individual
- Skin coloured/ pigmented pedunculated papules
- Associated features: Obesity, Diabetes, Acanthosis nigricans

18. Ans. (d) Keratoacanthoma *[Ref. Neena Khanna, 4/e p360]*

Keratoacanthoma

- Underlying cause: Photosensitizing chemicals, Radiation, Immunosuppression
- Clinical presentation: Rapidly growing skin-colored nodule with a 'central horny plug'
- MC site: Photo-exposed parts

19. Ans. (c) Ash leaf macule *[Ref. Neena Khanna, 4/e p33]*

Ash-leaf Macules

- Earliest manifestation of Tuberous sclerosis, often present at birth
- Hypopigmented macules on trunk
- Seen in 80% patients

20. Ans. (d) Squamous cell carcinoma *[Ref. Neena Khanna, 4/e p365]*

Squamous Cell Carcinoma

- Clinical presentation:
  - Verrucous plaque with shallow ulcer having red granular floor
  - Regional lymphadenopathy
- Histology: Invading malignant keratinocytes with horn cysts, hyperkeratosis

21. Ans. (c) Basal cell carcinoma *[Ref. Neena Khanna, 4/e p362]*

Basal Cell Carcinoma

- Middle aged/ elderly males
- Clinical types:
  - Nodulo-ulcerative BCC (Rodent ulcer): Ulcerated nodule with rolled, pearly, beaded edges
  - Superficial BCC
  - Morphoeic BCC

- Pigmented BCC
- Site: Face (except Superficial BCC)
- Histology: Islands and lobules of basaloid cells in 'Pallisading arrangement'

22. Ans. (b) Neurofibromatosis *[Ref. Clinical Dermatology by Mann, 5/e p345]*

Neurofibromatosis Type-1 (> 1 criteria required)

- Café au lait spots >5 mm in children, >15 mm in adults (Six or more)
- Cutaneous/ Subcutaneous neurofibroma (Six or more) OR Plexiform neurofibroma (One)
- Axillary/ groin freckling
- Optic pathway glioma
- Lisch nodules (Two or more)
- Bony dysplasia
- Relative (First degree) with NF-1

23. Ans. (a) Melanocyte *[Ref. Dermatology by Rapini, 1/e]*

Melanocytes

- Melanin-producing cells located in Stratum basale of skin's epidermis, middle layer of the eye (the uvea), inner ear, meninges, bones, heart
- Melanin is the pigment primarily responsible for skin color
- Once synthesised, melanin is contained in a special organelle called a melanosome and moved along arm-like structures called dendrites, so as to reach the keratinocytes

24. Ans. (c) Sturge-Weber syndrome *[Ref. Syndromes of Head and Neck by Regents, 4/e p456]*

Sturge-Weber Syndrome (Encephalotrigeminal Angiomatosis)

- Description: Phakomatosis characterised by facial port wine stains and pial angiomas
- Clinical presentation:
  - Congenital facial cutaneous haemangioma (Port wine stain)
  - Childhood seizures
  - Hemiplegia/hemiparesis and/or hemianopsia
  - Retinal detachment, buphthalmos, glaucoma
- CT scan: 'Tram track' subcortical calcifications

25. Ans. (c) Congenital nevus *[Ref. Rook's dermatology, 9/e p72]*

Congenital Melanocytic Nevus

- Garment nevus, Nevus pigmentosus et pilosus, Giant nevus, verrucous nevus, Giant pigmented nevus
- Present at birth or shortly thereafter
- Lesions may be small or cover a substantial portion of the body surface
- Nevi are generally darker than the surrounding skin, have a rugose or smooth elevated surface and may demonstrate long, darker, thicker hairs
- Large lesions have a significant risk of melanoma development
- Cranial or midline lesions and large congenital nevomelanocytic nevus lesions with satellite lesions have an increased risk of leptomeningeal involvement
- Often exhibit extensive nevomelanocytic infiltration of the dermis with potential involvement of the underlying adipose and muscular tissue

26. Ans. (c) C *[Ref. DiFiore's Atlas of Histology, 12/e p262]*

- Stratum spinosum layer of the epidermis is formed from 8 to 10 layers of irregularly shaped cells with very prominent intercellular bridges, or Desmosomes
- **In the given Photograph,** A: Stratum corneum, B: Stratum granulosum, C: Startum spinosum, D: Stratum basale, E: Dermis

27. Ans. (c) Salmon patch *[Ref Pediatric Dermatology by Weston, 3/e p308]*

Capillary Vascular Malformations

- Salmon patch (Naevus simplex):
  - Commonly seen malformations
  - Small flat patches of pink or red skin with poorly defined borders
  - Commonly found at the nape of the neck (stork bite, erythema nuchae), on the forehead between the eyebrows (angel's kiss) or on the eyelids
  - Most lesions will spontaneously disappear within the first year of life
- Port wine stain (Naevus flammeus):
  - Large flat patch of purple or dark red skin with well-defined borders
  - Face is most commonly affected although they can occur anywhere on the body
  - Most remain unchanged or may even deepen in colour

NEET/NBE PATTERN MCQs

1. **Sunscreen lotion contains** *[Recent Question 2016]*
   a. Mercury b. Selenium
   c. Sulfide d. Zinc oxide
2. **Thickening of the epidermis and/or dermis is:** *[Recent Question 2016]*
   a. Callus
   b. Lichenification
   c. Scaling
   d. Lacking in sensitive people
3. **All of the following are premalignant except** *[Recent Question 2016]*
   a. Actinic solar keratosis b. Bowens disease
   c. Bowenoid papulosis d. Rhinophyma
4. **Acanthosis involves** *[Recent Question 2016]*
   a. Stratum corneum b. Stratum spinosum
   c. Stratum granulosum d. Stratum basale
5. **Gorlin's syndrome is** *[Recent Question 2016]*
   a. Squamous cell carcinoma
   b. Basal cell carcinoma
   c. Sarcoma
   d. Guttate psoriasis
6. **Desmosomes are helpful in connecting** *[Recent Question 2016]*
   a. Keratinocytes b. Lichen planus
   c. Pemphigus d. Langerhans cells
7. **Epulis is** *[Recent Question 2016]*
   a. Benign b. Malignant
   c. Pre-cancerous d. Reactive process
8. **Haascheiben cells in epidermis are responsible for** *[Recent Question 2016]*
   a. Touch b. Temperature
   c. Pressure d. Proprioception
9. **Carpet tack sign seen in** *[Recent Question 2016]*
   a. Syphilis b. Psoriasis
   c. Lupus vulgaris d. DLE
10. **FDA approved drug for the treatment of Superficial basal cell carcinoma is** *[Recent Question 2016]*
    a. Imiquimod b. Acyclovir
    c. Clobesterol d. Terbinafine
11. **Lichenification occurs in which layer of skin** *[Recent Question 2016]*
    a. Stratum malpighi b. Stratum corneum
    c. Stratum lucidum d. Stratum granulosum
12. **Desmoglein is an autoantigen in** *[Recent Question 2016]*
    a. Pemphigus b. Eczema
    c. Sarcoidosis d. Vitiligo
13. **Patient with pruritic lesion over left shoulder showing cigarette paper atrophy and poikiloderma with generalized lymphadenopathy. Histopathology examination of lesion shows CD4 positive Sezary lutzner cells. What is the dermoepidermal manifestation of the disease?** *[Recent Question 2016]*
    a. Pautrier's microabscess
    b. Pin point ulcers
    c. Discharging sinus
    d. Miliaria
14. **Telogen phase of hair growth lasts for** *[Recent Question 2016]*
    a. 1 day b. 10 day
    c. 100 days d. 1000 days
15. **Premalignant skin lesions are all except** *[Recent Question 2016]*
    a. Bowen's disease b. Actinic keratoses
    c. DLE d. Miliaria
16. **Stratified squamous epithelium is found in all except** *[NBE FMGE March 2009]*
    a. Skin b. Vagina
    c. Oesophagus d. Gallbladder
17. **Which one of the following is a capillary malformation?** *[NBE DNB 2011]*
    a. Arterial plexiform angiomas
    b. Cirsoid aneurysm
    c. Port wine stain
    d. Visceral haemangioma
18. **Icthyosis vulgaris is transmitted as** *[NBE FMGE September 2008]*
    a. Autosomal dominant b. Autosomal recessive
    c. Sex linked dominant d. Sex linked recessive
19. **Pre-malignant condition of the skin include all of the following EXCEPT** *[NBE DNB 2011]*
    a. Leukoplakia b. Solar keratosis
    c. Acanthosis nigricans d. Bowen's disease
20. **Not a primary skin disease** *[Recent Question 2012, 2013]*
    a. Lichen planus b. Psoriasis
    c. Reiter's disease d. Vitiligo
21. **Drug which may cause Acanthosis nigricans** *[NBE FMGE September 2005]*
    a. Amphotericin B b. Ketoconazole
    c. Nicotinic acid d. Nalidixic acid
22. **Koebner's phenomenon is seen in** *[NBE DNB 2006, 2007]*
    a. Psoriasis b. Icthyosis
    c. Psoriasis d. Pemphigus
23. **Desmosomes are helpful in connecting** *[Recent Question 2012, 2013]*
    a. Keratinocytes b. Melanocytes
    c. Dermis and epidermis d. Langerhans cells
24. **Degeneration of basal cells occurs in** *[NBE DNB 1996]*
    a. Pemphigoid
    b. Lichen planus
    c. Pemphigus
    d. Psoriasis
25. **Stage 1 Cutaneous T cell lymphoma treatment is** *[Recent Question 2012, 2013]*
    a. PUVA
    b. Biological response modifiers
    c. Systemic chemotherapy
    d. Extracorporial photopheresis
26. **All of the following are lined by Stratified squamous epithelium except** *[NBE FMGE September 2012]*
    a. Cornea b. Vagina
    c. Cervix d. Uterus
27. **Which of the following is/are associated with Acanthosis nigricans?** *[Recent Questions 2016, UPSC 2012]*
    1. Carcinoma stomach
    2. Obesity
    3. Insulin resistance
    4. Hemochromatosis
    a. 1 only b. 4 only
    c. 1, 2, 3 d. 2, 3, 4

28. Pruritis is seen in all except *[NBE FMGE September 2005]*
a. Atopic dermatitis b. Lichen planus
c. Urticaria d. Pityriasis versicolor

29. Koebner phenomenon present in which of the following *[Recent Question 2012]*
a. Plane warts b. Pemphigus vulgaris
c. Lupus vulgaris d. Lichen simplex chronicus

30. Mycosis fungoides is a *[NBE DNB 1992, 2003, 2007]*
a. T-cell lymphoma
b. T-cell and B-cell lymphoma
c. Same as Hodgkin's lymphoma but seen only in skin
d. Derived from stem cell

31. Dyskeratosis of dermo-epidermal junction and saw-tooth appearance of rete-ridges is seen in *[NBE FMGE September 2012]*
a. Vitiligo b. Lichen planus
c. Dermatomyositis d. Pityriasis rosea

32. Tzank cell is *[Recent Question 2012, 2013]*
a. Keratinocyte b. Neutrophil
c. Fibroblast d. Lymphocyte

33. Cock's peculiar tumor is *[NBE FMGE March 2005]*
a. Carcinoma b. Epithelioma
c. Lipoma d. Corn

34. Auspitz sign is seen in *[Recent Question 2013, 2014]*
a. Psoriasis b. Lichen Planus
c. Alopecia aerata d. Lichen sclerosus

35. Alopecia areata *[NBE DNB 1992]*
a. Requires chronic use of steroids
b. Requires chronic use of antifungal
c. Spontaneous recovery will occur within 3-6 months in the majority of patients
d. Chronic unremitting disease

36. Lucio reaction is seen in *[Recent Question 2012, 2013]*
a. TB b. Leprosy
c. Syphilis d. LGV

37. Sun burns are *[NBE FMGE March 2004]*
a. First degree burns b. Second degree burns
c. Third degree burns d. Any of the above

38. Darier sign is seen in *[Recent Question 2017, 2016, 2014]*
a. Becker's melanosis b. Urticaria pigmentosa
c. Alopecia areata d. Papular urticaria

39. Loss of Intercellular cohesion between keratinocytes is called as *[Recent Question 2012]*
a. Acanthosis b. Acantholysis
c. Keratinolysis d. Spongiosis

40. Common cutaneous lesions of Hodgkin's disease are *[NBE DNB 1994]*
a. Ulcers b. Tumors
c. Secondary to pruritus d. Ichthyosis vulgaris

41. Epulis is *[Recent Question 2014]*
a. Precancerous
b. Benign
c. Malignant
d. Reactive process

42. Not true about Skin tag *[Recent Question 2012]*
a. Associated with Seborrhoeic keratosis
b. Pedunculated
c. Most common site is neck and axilla
d. Premalignant

43. Icthyosis is associated with *[NBE FMGE September 2003]*
a. AIDS b. Hypothyroidism
c. Hodgkin's disease d. All of the above

44. Which of the following histological type is most sensitive in cold? *[NBE DNB 1996]*
a. Meissner's corpuscle b. Merkel's disc
c. Langerhans cell d. Melanocyte

45. Spider telengectacia false is
a. More common in males *[Recent Question 2012, 2013]*
b. Can be caused by trauma
c. Light therapy for treatment
d. May be associated with liver disease

46. Tzanck smear is used for diagnosis of
a. Molluscum contagiosum *[Recent Question 2014]*
b. Herpes simplex
c. Pemphigus vulgaris
d. All of the above

47. Loss of Intercellular cohesion between keratinocytes is called as *[Recent Question 2012]*
a. Acanthosis b. Acantholysis
c. Keratinolysis d. Spongiosis

48. Which of the following structure in the skin give protection from UV radiation? *[NBE FMGE September 2011]*
a. Horny layer b. Langerhan's layer
c. Keratinocyte d. Melanocyte

49. Pomphylox affects *[Recent Question 2012]*
a. Palms & soles b. Groin
c. Scalp d. Trunk

50. Acanthosis nigricans is most common due to carcinoma of *[NBE DNB 1996, 2003, 2007]*
a. Bronchus b. Breast
c. Colon d. Testis

51. Immediate hypersensitivity reaction is mediated by which of the following immunoglobulin *[NBE FMGE September 2011]*
a. IgG b. IgA
c. IgM d. IgE

52. Acanthosis involves *[Recent Question 2012]*
a. Stratum spinosum b. Stratum granulosum
c. Stratum Basale d. Stratum corneum

53. Implantation dermoid is most commonly seen in *[NBE FMGE September 2011]*
a. Finger b. Skull
c. Scalp d. Hip

54. Tzanck smear is for *[Recent Question 2012, 2013]*
a. HZV b. Psittacosis
c. Cryptococcus d. Rickettsia

55. Which is not a primary cutaneous disorder? *[NBE DNB 2009]*
a. Lichen planus b. Psoriasis
c. Reiter syndrome d. Bowen disease

56. Angioedema is characterized by swelling of the *[NBE FMGE March 2012]*
a. Subcutaneous tissue b. Epidermis
c. Dermis d. Blood vessels

57. Epidermoid cysts are lined by *[NBE FMGE March 2012]*
a. Cuboidal epithelium
b. Squamous epithelium

c. Columnar epithelium
d. Pseudo epithelium

58. Most common malignant degeneration in Marjolin's ulcer is
a. Squamous cell carcinoma *[NBE FMGE March 2012]*
b. Basal cell carcinoma
c. Sarcoma
d. Melanoma

59. Stratified squamous epithelium is found in all the following structures EXCEPT *[NBE FMGE March 2012]*
a. Oesophagus b. Gallbladder
c. Vagina d. Skin

60. Gorlin' syndrome is *[Recent Question 2015]*
a. Squamous cell carcinoma
b. Basal cell carcinoma
c. Lichen planus
d. Guttate psoriasis

61. Ear papilloma is a type of *[Recent Question 2015]*
a. Wart b. Exostosis
c. Cutaneous horn d. Dermoid cyst

62. Cystic swelling at Outer Canthus eroding underlying bone is *[Recent Question 2015]*
a. Squamous cell carinoma
b. Basal cell carcinoma
c. Dermoid cyst
d. Mycetoma

63. Match List-I with List-II and select the correct answer using the code given below the lists *[UPSC CMS 2015]*

List-I (disease state)	List-II (clinical feature)
A. Pemphigus vulgaris	1. Acro-osteolysis
B. Psoriasis	2. Brachydactyly
C. Turner syndrome	3. Koebner phenomenon
D. Primary hyperparathyroidism	4. Nikolsky sign

Codes
a. A B C D 1 2 3 4 b. A B C D 1 3 2 4
c. A B C D 4 2 3 1 d. A B C D 4 3 2 1

64. All of the following are Premalignant lesions except *[UPSC CMS 2015]*
a. Actinic Solar Keratosis b. Bowen's Disease
c. Giant Hairy Naevus d. Rhinophyoma

65. A 70-year-old man with history of smoking has a 1 cm ulcerative lesion over the vermilion of his upper lip. What is he likely to be suffering from? *[UPSC CMS 2015]*
a. Squamous cell carcinoma
b. Basal cell carcinoma
c. Spindle cell carcinoma
d. Adenoid squamous carcinoma

66. Which of the following Epidermal layer is dead layer? *[Recent Question 2017]*
a. Stratum Basale b. Stratum spinosum
c. Stratum corneum d. Stratum granulosum

67. Substance common is skin and hair is? *[Recent Question 2017]*
a. Keratin b. Laminin
c. Nectin d. Vimentin

68. Increase in the thickness of the prickle cell layer of the epidermis is called? *[Recent Question 2017]*
a. Spongiosis b. Acanthosis
c. Hypergranulosis d. Hyperkeratosis

69. Langerhans cell are seen in which layer of skin? *[Recent Question 2017]*
a. Stratum basal b. Stratum carneum
c. Stratum granulosum d. Stratum spinosum

70. Treatment of choice for Mycosis fungoides in tumor stage is? *[Recent Question 2017]*
a. PUVA therapy b. Chemotherapy
c. Electron beam therapy d. Topical corticosteroids

71. False about Langer's lines is? *[Recent Question 2017]*
a. Remain constant throughout life of a person
b. Correspond to the collagen fibers in dermis
c. Incision along these lines produces better scar
d. Skin along these lines is least flexible

72. Which of the following is true about Xeroderma pigmentosa? *[Recent Question 2017]*
a. Autosomal dominant
b. Good long term prognosis
c. Purine dimmers
d. DNA repair defect

73. True about Erythema toxicum is? *[Recent Question 2017]*
a. Common in pre-term baby
b. Lesions contain many lymphocytes
c. Can be life threatening condition
d. Occurs mainly in neonatal period

74. Nevus simplex commonly presents at *[Recent Question 2017]*
a. Face b. Trunk
c. Legs d. Hand

75. Which antibody is least commonly seen in Keloid? *[Recent Question 2017]*
a. IgG b. IgM
c. IgE d. None

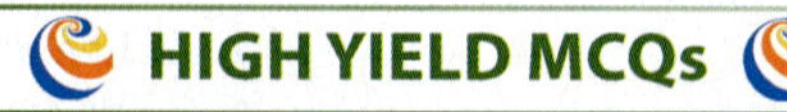

1. True about Skin is/ are *[PGI June 2016]*
a. Epidermis is highly vascular
b. Melanocyte is derived from neural crest
c. Sebaceous gland are holocrine and absent in palm
d. Apocrine gland presents in axilla and groin
e. Hidradenitis suppurativa is infection of apocrine gland

2. True about Corneum lucidum *[PGI 2009]*
a. Sandwitched between c.spinosum and c. granulosum
b. Sandwitched between c.corneum and c. granulosum
c. Contain hair follicle
d. Also known as prickle cell layer
e. Contain degenerated cells

3. Acantholytic cells are *[SGPGI 2001]*
a. Epidermal cells b. Plasma cells
c. Keratinocytes d. Giant cells

4. A girl child with verrucous lesions at an age of 2 weeks later on developed linear bands of hyperkeratotic papules and nodules followed by whorled pigmentation. Her mother had history of in-utero child death and hypopigmented atrophic linear lesions. The diagnosis is *[AIIMS PGMEE 2008]*
a. Neurofibromatosis
b. Xeroderma pigmentosa
c. Tuberous sclerosis
d. Incontinentia pigmenti

5. True about Acanthosis nigricans *[PGI 2003]*
a. Most commonly seen in obesity
b. Seen in axilla
c. It signifies internal malignancy
d. It is associated with insulin resistance
e. Seen in old age

6. Hypopigmented patches present in *[SGPGI 2002]*
a. Nevus Ota
b. Nevus Ito
c. Nevus anemicus
d. Becker nevus

7. All are true about Langerhans' histocytosis except?
a. Common before 3 years of age *[AIIMS PGMEE 2009]*
b. Letterer-Siwe disease is systemic manifestation
c. Radio sensitive
d. Testis is commonly involved

8. Which layer of epidermis is underdeveloped in the VLBW infants in the initial 7 days *[AIIMS PGMEE 2002]*
a. Stratum germinativum b. Stratum granulosum
c. Stratum lucidum d. Stratum corneum

9. Growth phase of hair is *[Recent Question 2017]* *[PGI 1997, 1999, All India PGMEE 1998]*
a. Anagen b. Metagen
c. Telogen d. None

10. 2-month-old girl present with verrucous plague on the trunk. What is your most probable diagnosis?
a. Incontinentia pigmentosa *[AIIMS PGMEE 2008]*
b. Darier disease
c. Congenital naevus
d. Icthyosis

11. Acantholysis involves
a. Epidermis *[All India PGMEE 1995, PGI 2008]*
b. Dermis
c. Epidermis-Dermis junction
d. Subcutaneous tissue
e. Adipose tissue

12. Hypo-depigmented lesion seen in *[PGI 2004]*
a. Naevus Ito b. Naevus depigmentosa
c. Naevus Ota d. Naevus anaemicus
e. Freckles

13. Scabies, an infection of the skin caused by Sarcoptes scabie, is an example of *[AIIMS PGMEE 2002]*
a. Water borne disease b. Water washed disease
c. Water based disease d. Water related disease

14. Bleeding spots seen on removal of scales in psoriasis is called as *[Recent Question 2017, PGI 2008]*
a. Auspitz sign b. Punctuate hemorrhage
c. Nikolyski's sign d. Darier sign

15. Which of the following stains is used to study fungal morphology in tissue sections? *[All India PGMEE 2010]*
a. PAS b. Von-Kossa
c. Alizarin Red d. Masson's Trichrome

16. All of the following may lead to plaque formation except *[PGI 1999, SGPGI 2003]*
a. Psoriasis b. Lichen planus
c. Pityriasis rosea d. Pemphigus

17. Acantholysis is due to destruction of *[AIIMS PGMEE 1997]*
a. Epidermis b. Subepidermis
c. Basement membrane d. Intercellular substance

18. Mycosis cells are altered *[All India PGMEE 1989]*
a. T Lymphocytes b. Monocytes
c. B lymphocytes d. Eosinophils

19. All are seen in Tuberous sclerosis except
a. Iris nodule *[All India PGMEE 2000]*
b. Renal Cortical Cyst
c. Rhabdomyoma of heart and lung
d. Adenoma Sebaceum

20. Ash leaf maculae is found in *[Jharkand PGMEE 2005]*
a. Tuberous sclerosis b. Neurofibromatosis
c. Lymphangioma d. None

21. Mouth Lesion are seen in *[All India PGMEE 1994, 1999]*
a. Psoriasis b. Lichen planus
c. Rasal cell CA d. Icthyosis vulgaris

22. Oral examination is done in case of *[PGI 1997]*
a. Peutz-Jeghers syndrome
b. Psoriasis
c. Beri-beri
d. Plummer-Vinson syndrome

23. An auto immune disease is *[All India PGMEE 2000]*
a. Pemphigus Vulgaris b. Psoriasis
c. Lichen planus d. Acne vulgaris

24. Which of the following are pruritic lesions? *[PGI 2000]*
a. Lichen planus b. Sun burns
c. Pemphigoid d. Psoriasis
e. SLE

25. Basal cell degeneration characteristically seen in *[JIPMER PGMEE 1998, 2002, PGI 2002]*
a. Lichen planus b. Psoriasis
c. Pemphigus d. DLE

26. Genetic predisposition is seen in which disease? *[PGI 1997]*
a. Lichen planus b. Bullous pemphigoid
c. Pemphigus vulgaris d. Epidermolysis bullosa

27. Which layer of skin causes vesicular change in case of burn? *[AIIMS PGMEE 1997]*
a. Basal layer b. Papillary layer
c. Epidermis d. Dermis

28. Genodermal disease that can cause skin malignancy are: *[PGI 2003]*
a. Xeroderma pigmentosa b. Neurofibromatosis
c. Actinic keratosis d. Porphyria cutanea tarda

29. Cells cultured from patients with this disorder exhibit low activity for the nucleotide excision repair proxess. This autosomal recessive genetic disease includes marked sensitivity to sunlight (Ultra violet light) with subsequent formation of multiple skin cancers and premature death, the disorder is

[Karnataka PGMEE 1998, TN PGMEE 2003]

a. Acute intermittent Porphyria *[UP PGMEE 2002]*
b. Alkaptonuria
c. Xeroderma Pigmentosa
d. Ataxia - Telangiectasia

30. The mode of inheritance of incontinentia pigment is *[Kerala PGMEE 2004, J&K PGMEE 2007]* *[UP PGMEE 2006]*

a. Autosomal dominant b. Autosomal recessive
c. X-linked dominant d. X-linked recessive

31. All statements are true regarding skin except *[PGI 1999]*

a. Skin is stratified squamous epithelium
b. Melanocyte & merkel cells are immigrant cells
c. Keratin filaments are a hall mark of epidermal cells
d. Keratinization process cause hydration of cells
e. Spines of spinous cells are formed from house keeping organelle

32. Which among is not a primary skin lesion? *[Bihar PGMEE 2006]*

a. Plaque b. Macule
c. Abscess d. None

33. Mycosis fungoides which is not true

a. It is the most common form of cutaneous lymphoma
b. Pautriers microabscess *[AIIMS PGMEE 2006]*
c. Indolent course and good prognosis, easily amenable to treatment
d. Erythroderma seen and spreads to peripheral circulation

34. Pautrier's microabscess is a histological feature of

a. Sarcoidosis *[AIIMS PGMEE 2005]*
b. TB
c. Mycosis fungoides
d. Ptyriasis lichenoides chronica

35. Actinic keratosis is seen in *[AIIMS PGMEE 2002]*

a. Basal cell carcinoma
b. Squamous cell carcinoma
c. Malignant melanoma
d. Epithelial cell carcinoma

36. Normal turnover time of epidermis (skin doubling time) is *[Recent Question 2017, AIIMS PGMEE 1991]*

a. 2 weeks b. 4 weeks
c. 6 weeks d. 8 weeks

37. Neither raised nor depressed is *[PGI 1997]*

a. Macule b. Plaque
c. Nodule d. Papule

38. A flat discolouration on skin as 1 cm is called *[Rohtak PGMEE 1997]*

a. Macule b. Plague
c. Boil d. Papule
e. Wheel

39. TOC in mycosis fungoides *[AIIMS PGMEE 1991]*

a. 5 - FU
b. Radiotherapy
c. Full skin electron therapy
d. Intravenous adriamycin

40. Which of the following statements about mycosis fungoides is not true? *[All India PGMEE 2007]*

a. It is the most common skin lymphoma
b. Pautriers micro abscesses are common
c. It has a indolent course and good prognosis
d. It presents with diffuse erythroderma

41. Underlying internal malignancy is not shown by *[All India PGMEE 1996]*

a. Acanthosis nigricans & Annular erythema
b. Bullous pyoderma & migratory necrotizing erythema
c. Granuloma annulare
d. Erythema gyratum repens

42. Acanthosis Nigricans in old patient usually indicate

a. Skin disorder *[JHARKHAND PGMEE 2004)*
b. Malignancy c. Senile brain
d. Usually found in negro

43. False regarding Acanthosis nigricans is *[PGI 2007]*

a. Prognostic indicator
b. Velvety plaques on dirty hyperpigmentation
c. Confirmatory sign of malignancy
d. Gastric adenocarcinoma is commonest malignant association
e. Indicate hyper androgenic state

44. Tzank cell is a *[All India PGMEE 1998]*

a. Lymphocyte b. Monocyte
c. Neutrophil d. Keratinocyte
e. Eosinophil

45. All are true regarding LCH except *[PGI 2007]*

a. Papular trunk lesions with scaling & crusting
b. Ulcerative nodules on mucosa
c. Calvarial defect with map lesions & floating teeth
d. CD-68 positive
e. Polyostotis bone lesions treatment by polychemotherapy

46. Treatment of Refractory histiocytosis?

a. Cladarabine *[AIIMS PGMEE 2008]*
b. High dose MTX
c. High dose cytosine arabinoside
d. Fludarabine

47. Pathogonomic sign of neurofibromatosis is *[All India PGMEE 1989]*

a. Cafe-au-lait macules b. Axillary freckling
c. Shagreen patch d. None of the above

48. Child presents with linear verrucous plaques on the trunk with vacuolization of keratinocytes in S. spinosum and S. granulosum. Diagnosis is *[AIIMS PGMEE 2008]*

a. In continentia pigmenti
b. Delayed hypersensitivity reaction
c. Linear epidermal naevus
d. Linear Darier's disease

49. Gottron's papules or sign seen in *[Recent Questions 2016, 2017, AIIMS PGMEE 1993]*

a. Dermatomyositis b. Multiple myeloma
c. Acute myeloid leukemia d. Psoriasis

50. Common sites of Mongolian spot are *[PGI 2008]*

a. Face b. Neck
c. Lumbosacral area d. Leg
e. Thigh

51. Which of the following condition resolves spontaneously in an infant? *[PGI 2008]*
a. Erythema toxicum
b. Mongolian spot
c. Lymphoma
d. Milia
e. Port wine stain

52. Mongolian spots is usually seen at region *[All India PGMEE 1998]*
a. Cervicofacial
b. Lumbosacral
c. Deltoid
d. Thoracolumbar

53. Normal commensal of skin is/ are *[PGI 2009]*
a. Staphylococcus aureus
b. Candida
c. Propionibacterium acnes
d. Diphtheria
e. Streptococcus pyogenes

54. Following are signs of internal malignancy except *[PGI 1997]*
a. Tuberous sclerosis
b. Acanthosis nigricans
c. Clubbing
d. Dermatomyositis

55. Predisposing factors for skin carcinoma are *[PGI 2002]*
a. Lichen planus
b. Bowen's disease
c. Psoriasis
d. Behcet's disease
e. UV rays

56. Changes of squamous cell carcinoma are seen in *[PGI 1997]*
a. Seborrheic keratosis
b. Bowen's disease
c. Lichen planus
d. DLE

57. Acanthosis nigricans is indicative of *[PGI 1998]* *[Kerala PGMEE 1997]*
a. Internal malignancy
b. Endocrine disorder
c. Blooms syndrome
d. Pigmentation of face, neck etc.
e. All are correct

58. Langerhans' cells in skin are *[All India PGMEE 1996]*
a. Antigen presenting cells
b. Pigment producing cells
c. Keratin synthesising cells
d. Sensory neurons

59. Maculopapular rash is seen in *[PGI May 2014]*
a. Measles
b. Rubella
c. HIV
d. Chicken pox
e. Parvovirus B19

60. Which of the following is NOT a Primary skin disease? *[ESI IMO 2014]*
a. Reiter's syndrome
b. Bowen's disease
c. Psoriasis
d. Lichen planus

61. Which of the following is associated with Skin cancer? *[CGPG 2015]*
a. Erythropoietic porphyria
b. Epidermolysis bullosa
c. Leprosy
d. Dermatomyositis

62. Dense irregular connective tissue is present in *[AIIMS November 2017]*
a. Tendon
b. Ligament
c. Lamina propria
d. Dermis

63. All of the following statements are true for Keloids EXCEPT *[UPSC CMS 2017]*
a. It is rarely seen in white skinned persons and is more common over the sternum
b. True keloid continues to become worse even after one year
c. True keloid does not spread into surrounding tissue
d. The maturation and stabilization of the collagen fibrils is inhibited

NEET/NBE PATTERN MCQs ANSWERS WITH EXPLANATIONS

1. Ans. (d) Zinc Oxide
[Ref. DVL by Thappa, 4/e p261,262]

Sunscreens

- Medications used topically or systemically to block ultraviolet rays
- Physical sunscreens:
  - Reflect and scatter UV rays, IR rays and visible light
  - Examples: Zinc oxide, titanium dioxide, iron oxide, magnesium silicate, red veterinary petrolatum
- Chemical sunscreens:
  - Absorb various length of UV rays
  - Examples: PABA, PABA esters, cinnamates, salicylates and those protect against UVA are benzphenones and avobenzene

2. Ans. (b) Lichenification
[Ref. Clinical Dermatology by Habif, 6/e p18]

Lichenification

- An area of thickened epidermis induced by scratching; skin lines are accentuated so the surface looks like a washboard
- Involve both dermis and epidermis and is characterized by both hardening and thickening

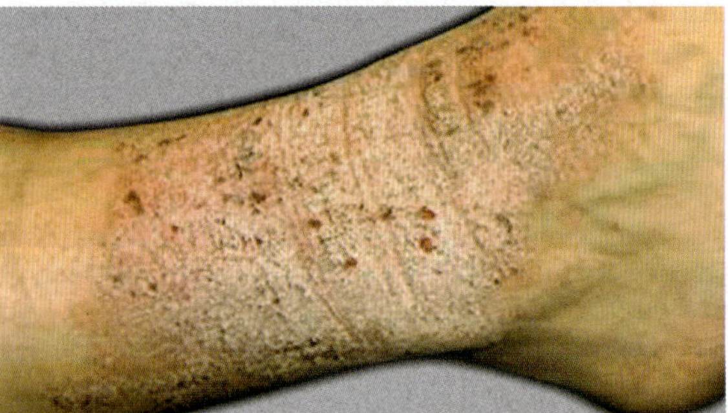

Fig. Lichenification

3. Ans. (d) Rhinophyma
[Ref. Clinical Dermatology by Habif, 6/e p257, 809]

Rhinophyma

- Rosacea of nose: Painless benign swelling due to hypertrophy of the sebaceous gland of the face and nose in particular
- Non-neoplastic hypertrophic tumor of nose

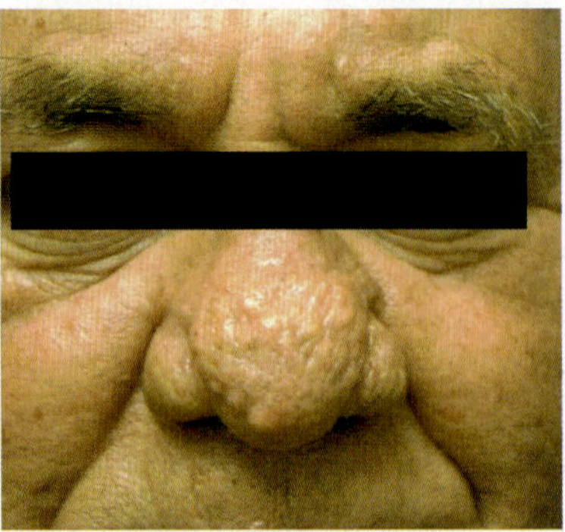

Fig. Rhinophyma

Also Remember

Premalignant Conditions

- Basal cell carcinoma
- Actinic keratosis
- Squamous cell carcinoma in situ
- Bowen's disease
- Erythroplasia of queyrat
- Arsenical keratoses and other arsenic related skin diseases
- Squamous cell carcinoma
- Leukoplakia
- Verrucous carcinoma, Primary cutaneous lymphomas, Cutaneous t-cell lymphoma Paget's disease of the breast, Extramammary Paget's disease

4. Ans. (b) S. Spinosum
[Ref. Clinical Dermatology by Habif, 6/e p990]

Acanthosis Nigricans (AN)

- Nonspecific reaction pattern that may accompany obesity; diabetes; excess corticosteroids; pineal tumors; other endocrine disorders; multiple genetic variants; drugs such as nicotinic acid, estrogens, and corticosteroids; and adenocarcinoma
- Pathology: Papillary hypertrophy, hyperkeratosis, and an increased number of melanocytes in the S. Spinosum

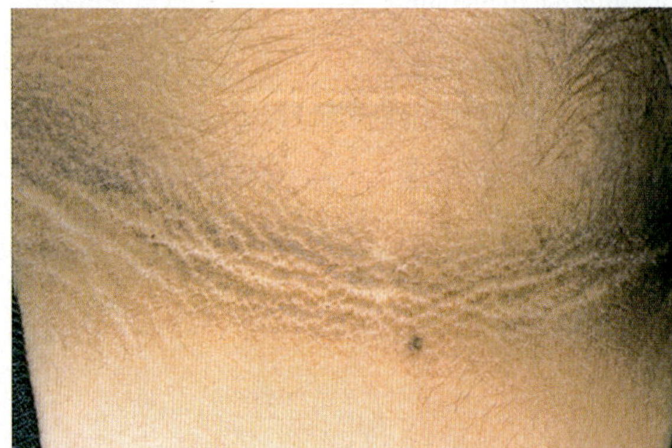

Fig. Acanthosis nigricans

5. Ans. (b) Basal cell carcinoma
[Ref. Clinical Dermatology by Habif, 6/e p835]

Gorlin- Goltz Syndrome

- Nevoid Basal Cell Carcinoma Syndrome
- Rare disease inherited as an autosomal dominant trait with high penetrance and variable expressivity
- Gene is located on chromosome 9q22.3-q31
- Major features: Multiple BCCs appear at birth or in early childhood; numerous small pits on the palms and soles, epithelium-lined jaw cysts, ectopic calcification with lamellar calcification of falx cerebri; and a variety of skeletal abnormalities, especially of the ribs, skull, and spine
- Characteristic facies: "Coarse face", relative macrocephaly, hypertelorism, and frontal bossing

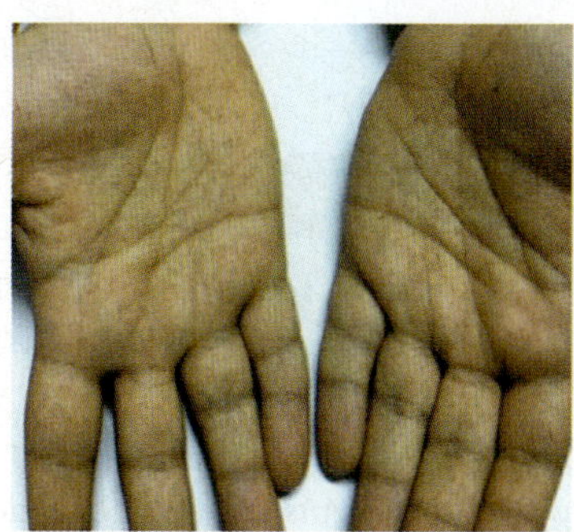

Fig. Gorlin-Goltz syndrome

6. Ans. (a) Keratinocytes

[Ref. Clinical Dermatology by Habif, 6/e p658]

- Desmosomes contribute to epidermal cell-cell adhesion (keratinocytes)

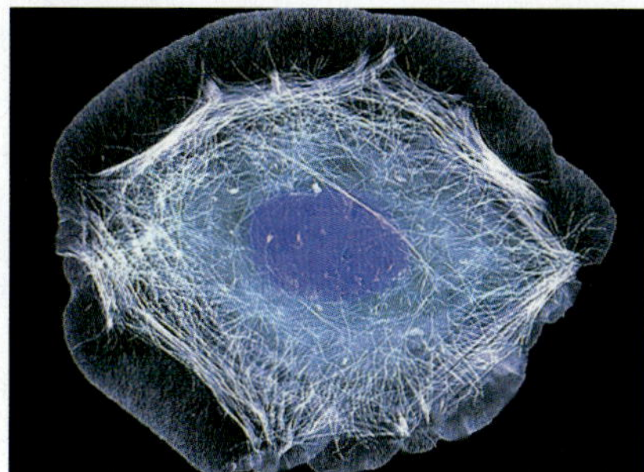

Fig. Keratinocyte

Also Remember

- Desmosomal proteins (desmoglein 1, desmoglein 3) are the autoantigens of pemphigus foliaceus and pemphigus vulgaris respectively
- Paraneoplastic pemphigus (PNP) is associated with auto-antibodies to the desmosomal plaque protein desmoplakin
- These diseases have intra-epidermal blistering

7. Ans. (a) Benign

[Ref. Clinical Dermatology by Habif, 6/e p936]

Epulis

- A localized growth on the gingiva
- Benign tumor-like growth of the gingival tissues
- May be present at birth or develop secondary to inflammatory conditions of the periodontal tissues

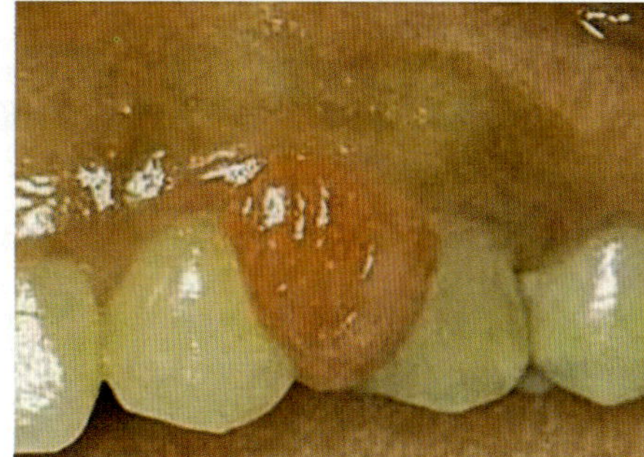

Fig. Epulis

8. Ans. (a) Touch

[Ref. Merkel Cell by Baumann, 1/e]

- In addition to keratinocytes, melanocytes, Langerhan cell and indeterminate cell in the epidermis, Merkel cell/ Haascheiben/Touch cells are found at the base of the epidermal rete ridges and they are in contact with nerve fibrils
- They are mostly present in palms, soles, nail beds, oral and genital epithelium and act as slow touch receptors

9. Ans. (d) DLE

[Ref. Clinical Dermatology by Habif, 6/e p684,951]

Discoid Lupus Erythematosus (DLE)

- MC chronic form of cutaneous lupus
- Persistent scaly, disk-like plaques on scalp, face and ears that may cause pigmentary changes, scarring and hair loss.
- Initial lesions are dry red patches evolve to indurated red or hyperpigmented plaques with adherent scale
- Follicular keratosis, i.e. plugs of keratin within hair follicles, is noted when surface scale is removed, e.g. with tape **(Carpet-tack sign)**
- Scarring results in central loss of pigment (white patches) and skin atrophy (tissue loss)
- Hypertrophic (warty) lupus erythematous describes red, very thickened plaque

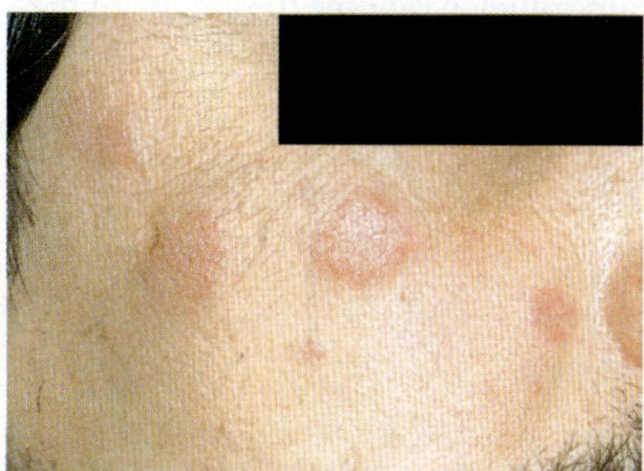

Fig. DLE

10. Ans. (a) Imiquimod

[Ref. Clinical Dermatology by Habif, 6/e p814]

- In 2004, imiquimod 5% cream was approved by the Food and Drug Administration for the treatment of superficial basal cell carcinoma

11. Ans. (a) Stratum malpighi

[Ref, DVL by Thappa, 4/e p. 43]

- Lichenfication is characterized by thickening of skin with increased skin markings and pigmentation in Stratum Malpighi
- Seen in Chronic dermatitis

12. Ans. (a) Pemphigus

[Ref. Clinical Dermatology by Habif, 6/e p648]

- Desmosomes contribute to Epidermal cell-cell adhesion (keratinocytes)
- Desmosomal proteins (desmoglein 1, desmoglein 3) are the autoantigens of pemphigus foliaceus and pemphigus vulgaris respectively
- Paraneoplastic pemphigus (PNP) is associated with autoantibodies to the desmosomal plaque protein desmoplakin
- These diseases have intra-epidermal blistering

13. Ans. (a) Pautrier microabscess

[Ref. Clinical Dermatology by Habif, 6/e p845]

- Sézary syndrome is an erythrodermic form of cutaneous T-Cell lymphoma (CTCL), a term that collectively includes all cutaneous lymphomas arising from T lymphocytes
- In mycosis fungoides, T cells characteristically form band like aggregates within the superficial dermis and invade the epidermis as single cells and small clusters called as Pautrier micro abscess

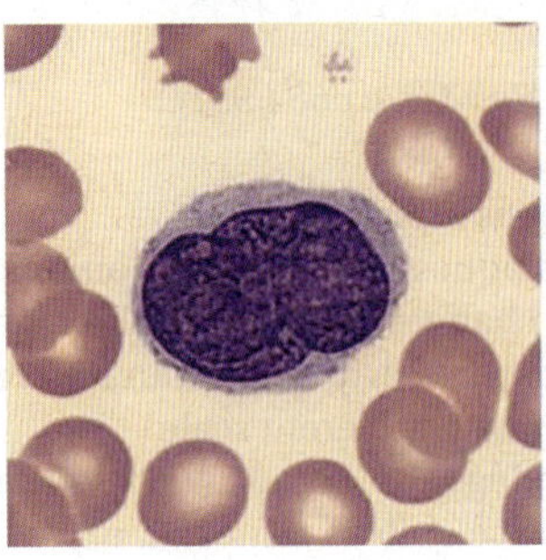

Fig. Lutzner cell

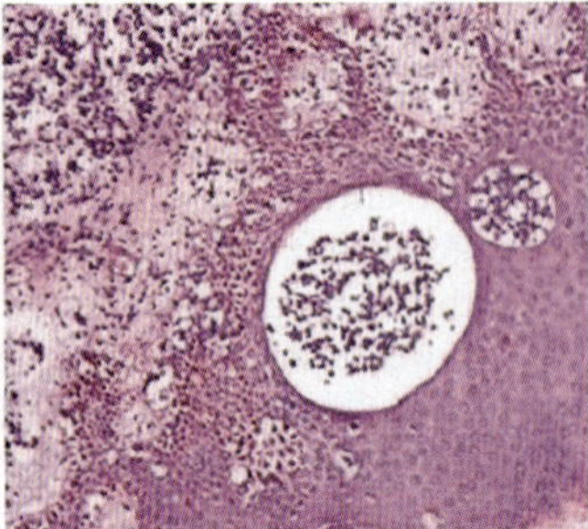

Fig. Pautrier microabscesses

14. Ans. (c) 100 days

[Ref. Clinical Dermatology by Habif, 6/e p571]

- Telogen phase in the scalp lasts for 2 to 3 months before the scalp follicles reenter the anagen stage and the cycle is repeated

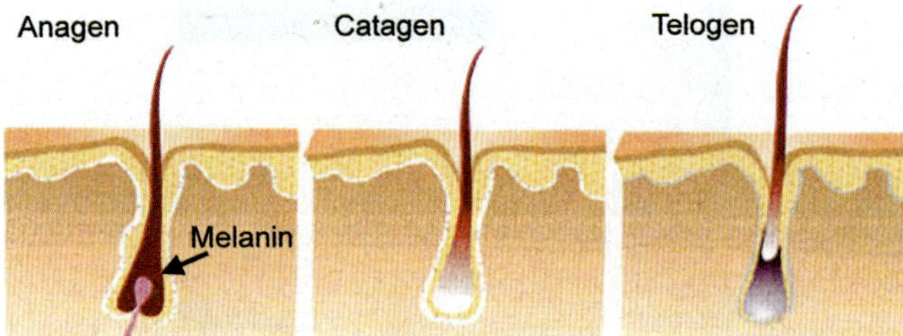

Fig. Hair growth cycle

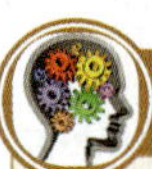

Also Remember

- Anagen or growth phase begins with resumption of mitotic activity in the hair bulb and dermal papilla; hair grows at an average rate of 0.35 mm/day, or 1 cm in 28 days; this rate diminishes with age
- Scalp hair remains in an active growing phase for an average of 2 to 6 years
- Catagen is a process of involution that occurs with cell death in follicular keratinocytes
- It is the phase of acute follicular regression that signals the end of anagen
- Less than 1% of scalp hairs are in this 2-3 week transitional phase at any one time

15. Ans. (d) Miliaria

[Ref. DVL by Thappa, 4/e p285,286]

Premalignant Tumors

- Actinic keratosis
- Cutaneous horn
- Bowen's disease
- DLE
- Leukoplakia

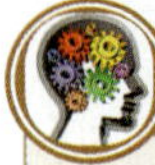

Also Remember

- Benign tumors include seborrheic keratosis, nevi, melanocytic nevi, keloids, milia, granuloma pyogenicum, skin tags

16. Ans. (d) Gallbladder

[Ref. Handy Anatomical Answers Book by Balban and Bobick, 2008]

Epithelium Types in Human Body

Epithelium	Tissue
Simple squamous epithelium	Blood vessels, Lymph vessels Mesothelium of body cavities Kidney ascending thin limb
Simple cuboidal epithelium	Thyroid follicles Respiratory bronchioles Ovaries, Rete testes Ependyma Kidneys – PCT, DCT, Collecting ducts
Simple columnar epithelium	Fallopian tubes, Cervix, Endometrium (Uterus) Ejaculatory duct, Bulbourethral glands Stomach, Small intestine, Large intestine, Rectum Gallbladder
Pseudostratified epithelium	Epididymis, Vas deferens, Seminal vesicles Larynx, Trachea, Nose Membranous urethra, Penile urethra
Keratinized stratified epithelium	Tongue, Hard palate, Oesophagus Oropharynx, Larynx Ectocervix, Vagina Cornea, Skin Anus
Transitional stratified epithelium	Renal pelvis, Ureter, Bladder, Prostatic urethra

17. Ans. (c) Port wine stain

[Ref. Neena Khanna, 5/e p450]

- Vascular naevi lesions are seen in Port wine stain

18. Ans. (a) Autosomal dominant

[Ref. Neena Khanna, 4/e p21]

Ichthyosis

- *Definition*: Presence of fish-like scales, worse in winters
- *Causes of Ichthyosis*:
  - *Congenital Icthyosis*:
    1. Ichthyosis vulgaris
    2. X-linked ichthyosis

3. Lamellar Ichthyosis
4. Epidermolytic hyperkeratosis

- *Acquired Ichthyosis*:
  1. Infections: Leprosy, HIV, TB, Typhoid
  2. Drugs: Clofazimine
  3. Malignancies: Lymphomas (Hodgkin's), Kaposi sarcoma
  4. Endocrine disorders: Hypothyroidism
  5. Systemic diseases: Sarcoidosis
  6. Nutritional deficiencies:

- *Inheritance in Ichthyosis*:
  - Ichthyosis vulgaris: Autosomal dominant
  - X-linked Ichthyosis: X-linked recessive
  - Lamellar Ichthyosis: Autosomal recessive
  - Non-bullous ichthyosiform erythroderma: Autosomal recessive
  - Epidermolytic hyperkeratosis: Autosomal dominant
  - Colloidan baby: X-linked

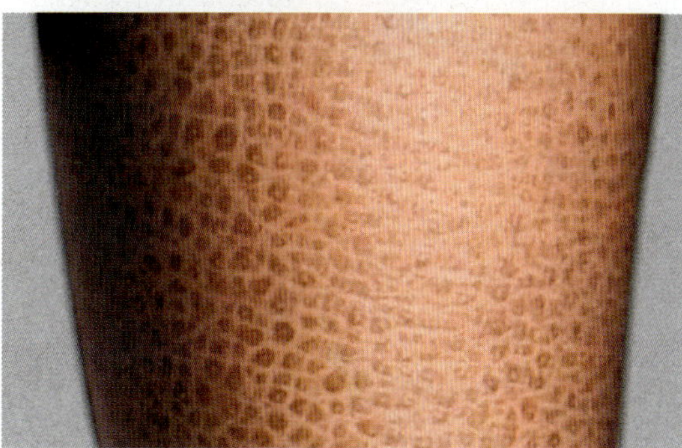

Fig. Ichthyosis

19. Ans. (c) Acanthosis nigricans

[Ref. Neena Khanna, 5/e p38, 385]

- **Acanthosis nigricans is not pre malignant**: It is either benign or malignant
- Pre-malignant skin lesions: Cutaneous horns, Keratoacanthoma, Bowen's disease, Actinic keratoses, Arsenical keratoses, Leukoplakia

20. Ans. (c) Reiter's disease

[Ref. Neena Khanna, 5/e p48]

- Reiter's disease is mainly HLA B27 linked arthritis

21. Ans. (c) Nicotinic acid

[Ref. Neena Khanna, 4/e p37]

Drug Induced Acanthosis Nigricans [Mnemonic: Cons]

- **C**orticosteroids
- **O**ral contraceptives
- **N**icotinic acid
- **S**tilbesterol

22. Ans. (a) Psoriasis

[Ref. Neena Khanna, 5/e p45; Differential Diagnosis in Dermatology by Ashton, 3/e p179]

- Koebner's phenomenon or Isomorphic phenomenon: New lesions of the original disease develop at sites of trauma (scratches, surgical incisions, & injury) and indicates active disease
- Types of Koebner phenomena: **[Mnemonic: L**eft **V**entricular **P**ulsations **W**ill **M**ake **B**lood **P**ressure]

True isomorphic phenomena	Pseudo-isomorphic phenomena
Lichen planus **V**itiligo **P**soriasis	**W**arts **M**olluscum contagiosum **B**ehcet's syndrome **P**yoderma gangrenosum

23. Ans. (a) Keratinocytes

[Ref. Neena Khanna, 5/e p79]

Desmogleins (Dsg)

- Description: Present in desmosomes which are involved in keratinocyte - keratinocyte adhesion in the epidermis
- Dsg 1 & 3 are important in Pemphigus:
  - **Antibodies to Dsg 3 & 1** are pathognomonic in Pemphigus vulgaris
  - **Antibodies to Dsg 1** are pathognomonic in pemphigus foliaceus

24. Ans. (b) Lichen planus

[Ref. Neena Khanna, 5/e p67]

Lichen Planus Histopathology

- Thickened granular layer
- Saw toothing of rete pegs
- Basal cell degeneration (leading to Max Joseph's spaces and colloid/ Civatte body formation)
- Band like upper dermal infiltrate of lymphocytes

25. Ans. (a) PUVA

[Ref. Evidence-Based Dermatology edited by Hywel Williams, 2/e p283]

26. Ans. (d) Uterus

[Ref. Histology by Jo Ann Eurell, 1/e p57]

27. Ans. (c) 1, 2, 3

[Ref. Neena Khanna, 5/e p38]

Associated Features of Acanthosis Nigricans

- Obesity
- HAIR -AN syndrome
- Diabetes mellitus, Hyperandrogenism, Cushings syndrome
- Nicotinic acid, Stilbestrol, Corticosteroids, Oral contraceptives
- Gastric adenocarcinoma and Genitourinary tract malignancy

28. Ans. (d) Pityriasis versicolor

[Ref. Pruritis by James S Taylor, Cleveland Clinic]

Dermatological Causes of Pruritis

- Autoimmune causes:
  - Dermatitis herpetiformis
  - Dermatomyositis
  - Pemphigoid
  - Sjogren's syndrome
- *Infectious causes*:
  - Dermatophytosis
  - Folliculitis
  - Impetigo
  - Insect bites
  - Pediculosis
  - Scabies

- *Neoplastic causes*:
  - Cutaneous T-cell lymphoma (Mycosis fungoides)
  - Cutaneous B-cell lymphoma
  - Leukemia cutis
- *Genetic causes*:
  - Darier's disease
  - Hailey-Hailey disease
  - Icthyosis
  - Sjogren-Larsson syndrome
- *Inflammatory causes*:
  - Atopic dermatitis
  - Contact dermatitis
  - Drug reactions
  - Lichen planus
  - Mastocytosis
  - Miliaria
  - Psoriasis
  - Scars
  - Urticaria
- *Pregnancy causes*:
  - Pemphigoid gestationis
  - Polymorphic eruption of pregnancy

29. Ans. (a) Plane warts
[Ref. Neena Khanna, 5/e p45; Differential Diagnosis in Dermatology by Richard Ashton,3/e p179]

30. Ans. (a) T-cell lymphoma
[Ref. Evidence-Based Dermatology edited by Hywel Williams, 2/e p283]

31. Ans. (b) Lichen planus
[Ref. Neena Khanna, 5/e p67]

32. Ans. (a) Keratinocyte
[Ref. European Handbook of Dermatological Treatments by Katsambas, 3/e p708]

33. Ans. (b) Epithelioma
[Ref. SRB's Clinical Methods in Surgery by Sriram Bhat M, 2/e p125]

Cock's Peculiar Tumor

- Type of growth: Trichilemmal (Sebaceous) cyst linked growth arising from hair-follicle epithelium
  - Is not a type of tumor
- Most common sites: Hairs of scalp, scrotum
- Clinical importance: Resembles Squamous cell carcinoma

34. Ans. (a) Psoriasis
[Ref. Neena Khanna, 5/e p46]

3 Steps of Auspitz Sign

- Gently scrape lesion with a glass slide: This accentuates the silvery scale **(Grattage test)**
- On scraping the lesion: A listening white adherent membrane appears **(Berkley's membrane)**
- On removing the membrane, punctuate bleeding points become visible: **Positive Auspitz sign**

35. Ans. (c) Spontaneous recovery will occur within 3-6 months in majority of patient
[Ref. Neena Khanna, 5/e p145]

36. Ans. (b) Leprosy
[Ref. Textbook of Pediatric Dermatology by Arun C Inamadar, 2/e p175]

- IL-1 and TNF-α, and antibodies against M. leprae are implicated in Type 2 and Type 3 (Lucio phenomenon) Lepra reactions that are seen in LL

37. Ans. (d) Any of the above
[Ref. Neena Khanna, 4/e p192]

Sunburns

- Underlying cause: UVB rays produce cytokines in skin
- Clinical presentation:
  - First (Most common), second or third degree burns
  - Seen in skin types I and II
  - Seen in light skin
  - Redness followed by scaling and hyperpigmentation
- Treatment:
  - Calamine lotion
  - Topical steroids
  - NSAIDs

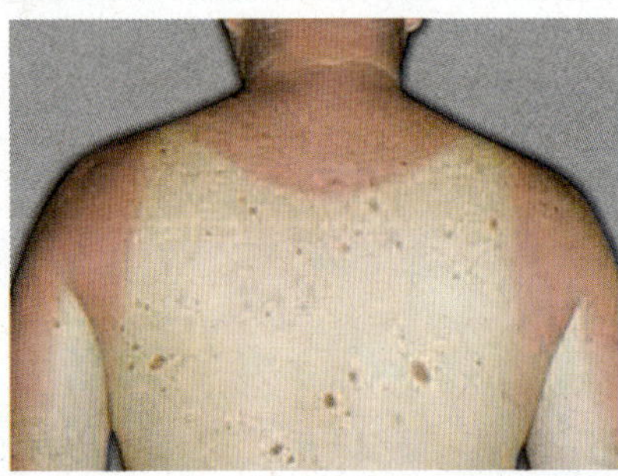

Fig. Sunburn

38. Ans. (b) Urticaria pigmentosa
[Ref. Textbook of Dermatology, Leprology & Venereology by Thappa, 4/e p19]

- Darier's sign: When Dermographism is limited to skin overlying a lesion (macule or papule): Diagnostic of Urticaria pigmentosa (mast cell disease)
- Pseudo Darier's sign: It is seen in congenital smooth muscle hamartoma

39. Ans. (b) Acantholysis
[Ref. Neena Khanna, 5/e p78]

40. Ans. (c) Secondary to pruritus
[Ref. Diagnosis: A Symptom-based Approach in Internal Medicine by Madgaonkar, 1/e p246]

- Of all the malignancies known to induce pruritus, Hodgkin's disease is the most common

41. Ans. (b) Benign
[Ref. SRB's Clinical Methods in Surgery by Bhat, 2/e p309]

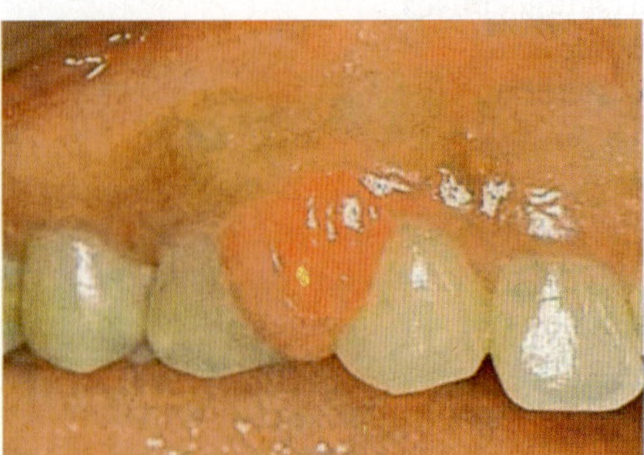

Fig. Epulis

Epulis

- Swelling arising from the gums is called as Epulis (gumboil, upon the gum—Greek)
- **Congenital epulis**: It is a benign condition seen in a newborn arising from gum pads
  - It is a variant of granular cell myoblastoma originating from gums.

42. Ans. (d) Premalignant
[Ref. Neena Khanna, 5/e p378]

43. Ans. (d) All of the above

44. Ans. (d) Melanocyte
[Ref. Manual of Dermatologic Therapeutics by Kenneth A. Arndt, 7/e p113]

- Melanocytes are more sensitive to cold injury than keratinocytes and may be selectively damaged by this technique

45. Ans. (a) More common in males
[Ref. Current Dermatologic Diagnosis & Treatment by Irwin, 1/e p206]

46. Ans. (d) All of the above
[Ref. Neena Khanna, 5/e p77]

47. Ans. (b) Acantholysis
[Ref. Neena Khanna, 5/e p78]

48. Ans. (d) Melanocyte
[Ref. Dermatology in Clinical Practice by Zaidi, 1/e p4]

Stratum Germinativum/ Basal Cell Layer

- Contains Melanocytes which produce melanin
- Contains Merkel cells: Cells of neuro-ectodermal origin
- Sun exposure increase melanocyte production to prevent damage from UV rays (sun tanning)

49. Ans. (a) Palm & soles
[Ref. Neena Khanna, 5/e p116]

- Pompholyx aggravates in summer and involves fingers and palms and sometime soles

50. Ans. (c) Colon
[Ref. Neena Khanna, 5/e p38]

51. Ans. (d) IgE
[Ref. Neena Khanna, 4/e p179]

- Hypersensitivity Urticaria is due to IgE mediation

52. Ans. (a) Stratum spinosum
[Ref. Rook's Textbook of Dermatology by Burns,7/e 7.36]

- Acanthosis: Describe an increase in number of cells in the spinous cell layer or prickle cell layer of the epidermis

53. Ans. (a) Finger
[Ref. Textbook of Surgery by Roshan Lall Gupta, 2/e, p337]

Implantation Dermoid

- Underlying cause: Acquired cyst formed by indriving of surface epithelium usually due to a needle prick
- Underlying pathology:
  - Lined by squamous epithelium
  - Absence of hair follicles, sweat/ sebaceous glands
  - Cyst contains amorphous material (desquamated epithelial cells)
- Commonly seen in: Gardeners, tailors
- Common site: Pulp of fingers
- Complications:
  - Infection
  - Rupture
  - Pressure effect on digital nerves
- Treatment: Excision of cyst under digital local anesthetic block

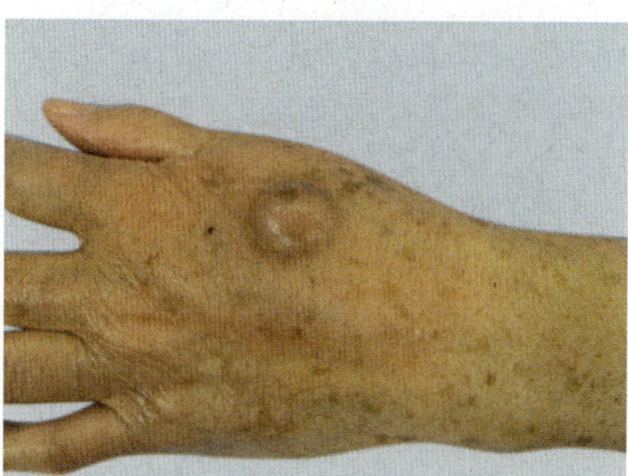

Fig. Implantation dermoid

54. Ans. (a) HZV
[Ref. Neena Khanna, 5/e p77]

- Multinucleated giant cells are Tzanck smear findings in HZV

55. Ans. (c) Reiter syndrome
[Ref. Neena Khanna, 5/e p48]

56. Ans. (a) Subcutaneous tissue
[Ref. Neena Khanna, 4/e p8]

- Angioedema occurs when wheal extends into subcutaneous tissue and lasts > 48 hours

Also Remember

- *Difference between Angioedema and Urticaria:*

Angioedema	Urticaria	
Tissue involved	Subcutaneous, submucosal	Epidermis, dermis
Organs affected	Skin, mucosa (eyelids, lips)	Skin
Duration	24-48 hours	< 24 hours
Signs	Red swellings below skin	Red patches/ wheals on skin
Symptoms	Pain, tender	Itchy

57. Ans. (b) Squamous epithelium
[Ref. Neena Khanna, 4/e p358]

Cysts In Skin

- *Keratinous cyst*: Lining of cyst is keratinous
  - *Epidermoid cyst*: Lining of cyst resembles normal epidermis
  - *Trichilemmal cyst*: Lining of cyst resembles external root sheath
- *Sebaceous cyst/ Steatocystoma multiplex*

58. Ans. (a) Squamous cell carcinoma
[Ref. Cancer Symptom Management by Goodman, 3/e p295]

- *Majorlin's Ulcer*: Malignant transformation of a scar
  - MC carcinoma type: Squamous cell carcinoma
  - Overall chances of metastasis: 33%
  - Overall chances of death: 33%

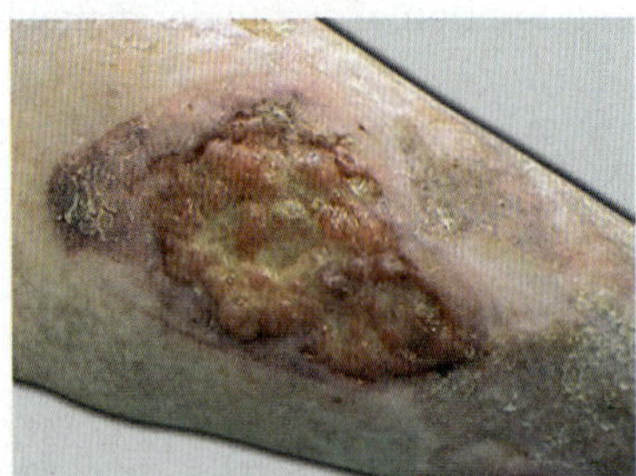

Fig. Marjolin's ulcer

59. Ans. (b) Gallbladder
[Ref. Barron's Anatomy and Physiology, 2/e p74]

- *Simple squamous epithelium*: Blood vessels, Lymph vessels, Mesothelium of body cavities, Kidney Ascending thin limb
- *Stratified squamous (keratinised) epithelium*: Skin, Gingiva, Tongue, Hard palate, Labia majora, Anus (below Hilton's line)
- *Stratified squamous (non-keratinised) epithelium*: Oesophagus, Oropharynx, Vocal cords, Cornea, Cervix (ectocervix), Vagina, External urethral orifice Anus (above Hilton's line)

60. Ans. (b) Basal cell carcinoma
[Ref. Skin Tumors by Baykal, 1/e p311]

Gorlin Syndrome
- Synonym: Naevoid Basal Cell Carcinoma
- Inheritance: Autosomal dominant
- Underlying cause: Germline mutation of PTCH1, a tumor suppressing gene
- Features: Genodermatoses with Basal cell carcinomas and Multiorgan abnormalities

61. Ans. (a) Wart
[Ref. ENT by Dhingra, 6/e p106]

Tumors of External Ear

Benign tumors of Pinna	Benign tumors of External ear canal
• Dermoid cyst • Hemangioma • Keloid • Papilloma • Neurofibroma • Cutaneous horn • Keratoacanthoma • Sebaceous cyst • Preauricular cyst/ sinus	• Osteoma • Exostosis • Papilloma • Ceruminoma • Sebaceous adenoma
Malignant tumors of Pinna	**Malignant tumors of External ear canal**
• Squamous cell carcinoma • Basal cell carcinoma • Melanoma	• Squamous cell carcinoma • Basal cell carcinoma • Melanoma • Adenocarcinoma • Malignant ceruminoma

62. Ans. (c) Dermoid cyst
[Ref. Modern Ophthalmology by Sorsby, 1/e p863]

Dermoid Cyst
- Presents clinically as a cystic swelling at the outer and less commonly the inner canthus
- Attached to the underlying bone in which a defect can be demonstrated
- Extension of tumors outside the sac area may cause intranasal symptoms, and radiographic changes are noted with erosion in the bone

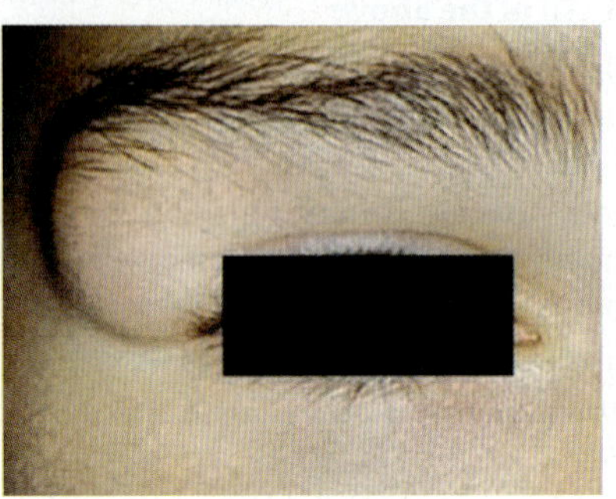

Fig. Dermoid cyst

63. Ans. (d) A B C D 4 3 2 1
[Ref. Neena Khanna, 4/e]

64. Ans. (d) Rhinophyoma
[Ref. Plastic and Reconstructive Surgery, 1/e p118]

- Rhinophyma has no malignant potential but may be associated with BCC

65. Ans. (a) Squamous cell carcinoma
[Ref. Dermatology in General Medicine: 2, p1200]

66. Ans. (c) Stratum corneum
[Ref. DiFiore's Atlas of Histology, 11/2 p214]

- Epidermis is made up of two layers; a basal layer known as the Stratum germinativum, which is living, and an outer dead layer called the Stratum corneum
- Composed mainly of dead keratinocytes, the Stratum corneum is the final stop for skin cells before they are shed

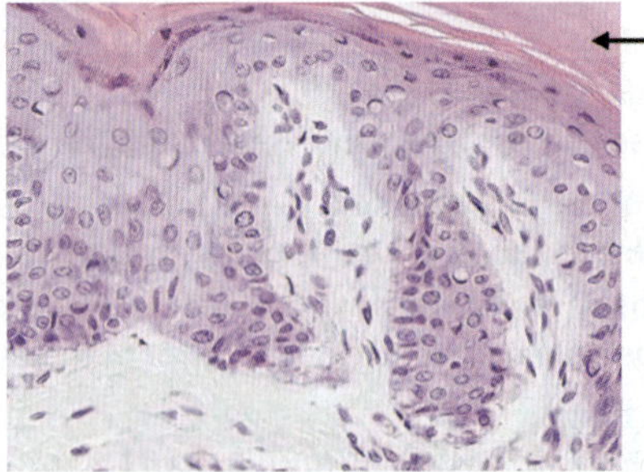

Fig. Stratum corneum

67. Ans. (a) Keratin
[Ref. Maternity & Pediatric Nursing E-Book by Leifer, 6/e p294]

- Keratin is a protein produced by skin cells
- Outermost layer of skin cells contains keratin
- Hair and claws/nails are also made of keratin
- Dermatophytosis is a contagious fungal infection that can affect the skin, hair, and claws

68. Ans. (b) Acanthosis
[Ref. Rook's Textbook of Dermatology, 9/e p3.34]

Acanthosis

- An increase in number of cells in the Malpighian or Prickle cell layer of the epidermis (from the Greek for prickle or thorn)
- Acanthosis is diffuse epidermal hyperplasia
- It is a disease of the prickle cell layer of the skin, where warts appear on the skin or inside the mouth
  - True acanthosis: Increased number of acanthocytes
  - Pseudo-acanthosis: Enlarged acanthocytes

69. Ans. (d) Stratum spinosum
[Ref. Textbook of Histology by Gartner, 4/e p378]

Stratum spinosum/ Squamous cell layer

- Thickest layer of epidermis
- Contains Keratinocytes which produce keratin, the major structure in skin, hair, nails
- Contains Langerhans cells which alert immune system from antigens that invade skin (Langerhans cells sometimes called Dendritic cells because of their numerous long processes)

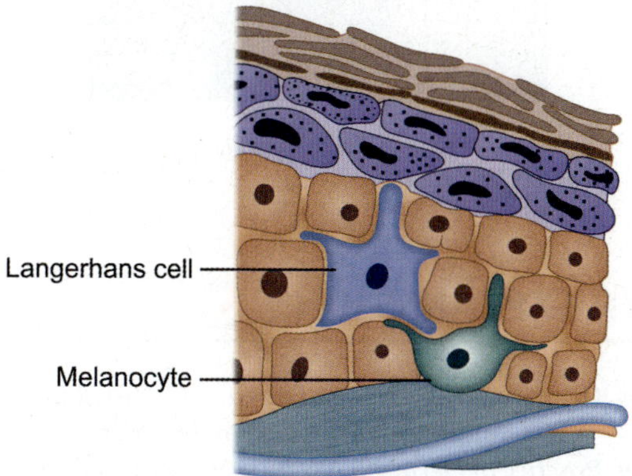

Fig. Langerhans cell

70. Ans. (b) Chemotherapy
[Ref. Rook's Textbook of Dermatology, 9/e p140.53]

Treatment of Mycosis Fungoides

- Patch stage: Corticosteroids, UV-B, PUVA
- Plaque stage: Electron beam, PUVA, Acitretin
- Tumor stage: Radiotherapy, Chemotherapy

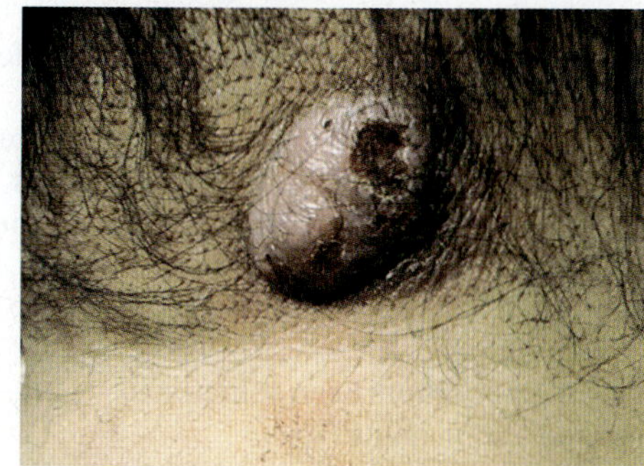

Fig. Mycosis fungoides (Tumor stage)

71. Ans. (a) Remain constant throughout life of a person
[Ref. Anatomy and Human Movement by Palastanga, 2/e p47]

Langer's lines/Cleavage lines

- Skin is subjected to internal stresses varying from region to region leading to stress lines known as Langer's lines
- Formed by the collagen bundles that lie parallel in the dermis
- Incisions along these lines heal with a minimum of scar, whereas in wounds across them the scar may become thicker, with the possible risk of scar contraction, because the wound edges are being pulled apart by the internal stresses of the skin
- Langer's lines do not always correspond with the stress lines of life; they merely reflect the stresses within the skin at rest

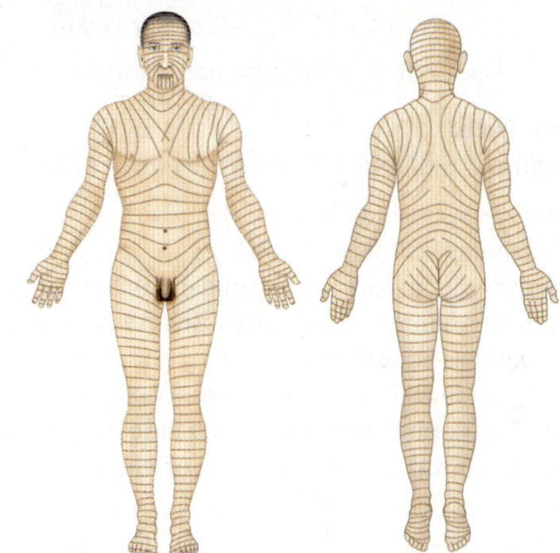

Fig. Langer lines

72. Ans. (d) DNA repair defect
[Ref. DNA Repair and Human Disease by Balajee, 1/e p138]

Xeroderma Pigmentosum

- A human disease in which an initial stage of DNA repair is defective
- Autosomal recessive genetic disorder of DNA repair in which the ability to repair damage caused by ultraviolet (UV) light is deficient

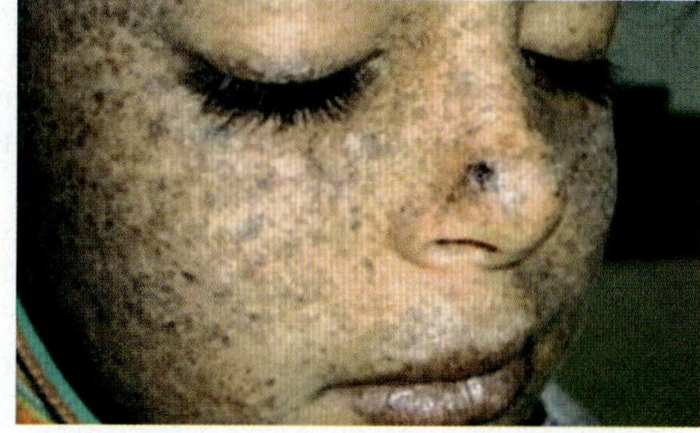

Fig. Xeroderma Pigmentosum

73. Ans. (d) Occurs mainly in neonatal period
[Ref. Dermatology by Falco, 2/e p702]

Erythema Toxicum Neonatorum

- Common short-lived erythematous eruption of newborn in first 2 days of life
- Flea bitten rash of newborn: Widespread erythematous macules, coalesce to become urticarial pustules
- Occurrence: 30-50% of newborns develop ETN

- Underlying cause: Transition from watery womb to dry external environment
- Treatment Generally not required, Zinc oxide lotion may be used

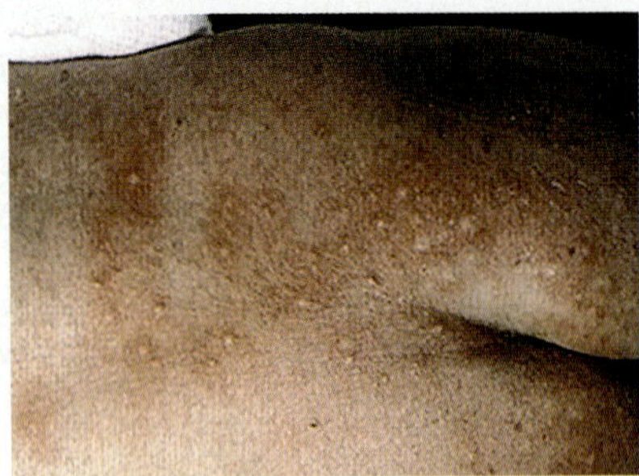

Fig. Erythema toxicum neonatorum

74. Ans. (a) Face
[Ref. Pediatric Systemic Disease by Levin, 1/e p214]

Salmon Patch (Nevus Simplex)

- MC vascular lesion of infancy
- Presents as a flat salmon to pinkish faint colored patch that occurs frequently on the posterior neck, around the face and eyelids and glabellar region
- Can be present in up to 40% of newborn infants
- These "stork bite" lesions usually fade on the face, but can persists around the orbit or back of the neck

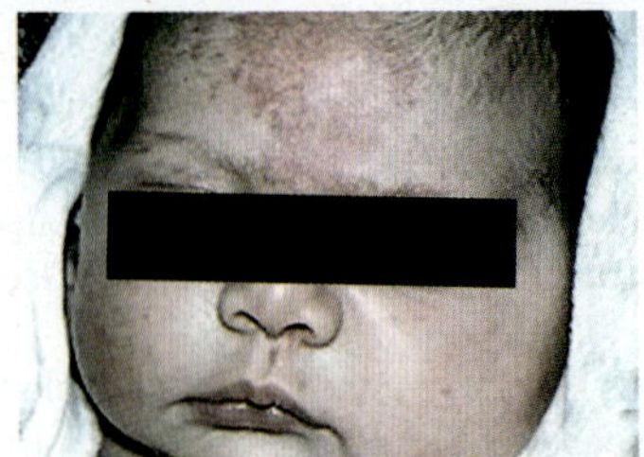

Fig. Nevus simplex

75. Ans. (c) IgE
[Ref. Intercollegiate MRCS by Ramachandran, 1/e p13]

Immunology in Keloid

- Increased IgG, IgM and C3 levels
- Antinuclear antibodies to keloid fibroblasts

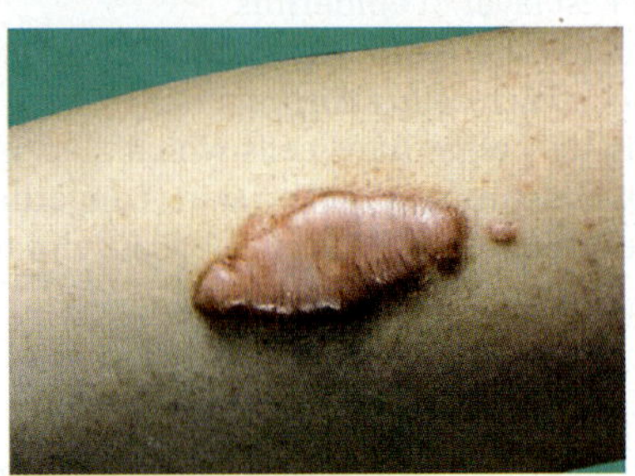

Fig. Keloid

HIGH YIELD MCQs ANSWERS WITH EXPLANATIONS 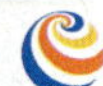

1. Ans. (b) Melanocyte is derived...; (c) Sebaceous gland are holocrine and...; (d) Apocrine gland presents...; (e) Hidradenitis suppurativa...
[Ref. DVL by Thappa, 4/e p125,126]

Epidermis and Appendages

- Non-vascularized Epidermis and Epidermal appendages are separated from the highly vascularized Dermis by a complex basement membrane
  - Highly vascular Dermis nourishes the Epidermis
- Melanocytes are derived from neural crest cells that follow a dorsal migration route under the ectoderm
- Sebaceous glands:
  - Holocrine glands that drain into the pilosebaceous unit in hair-bearing skin
  - Most prevalent on forehead, nose and cheek; absent from palms and soles
- **Apocrine glands:**
  - Part of the odoriferous or accessory sex gland system
  - Normally present in the skin, particularly in the groin, axilla, and anogenital region
  - Modified apocrine glands occur in the ears **(Ceruminous glands)** and eyelids **(Moll's glands)**
  - Hidradenitis suppurativa: Chronic acneiform infection of the cutaneous apocrine glands that also can involve adjacent subcutaneous tissue and fascia of the axillae, groin, or wherever apocrine glands are concentrated

2. Ans. (b) Sandwitched between c. corneum and c. granulosum; (e) Contain degenerated cells
[Ref. Practice of Dermatology by P N Behal, 10/e p7]

- Between stratum granulosum and corneum in palms and soles, there is an additional layer called stratum lucidum

3. Ans. (c) Keratinocytes
[Ref. Neena Khanna, 5/e p79 & Figure 5.5]

- Acantholytic cells (Tzank cell) are separated keratinocytes

4. Ans. (d) Incontinentia pigmenti
[Ref. Neena Khanna, 5/e p37]

Incontinentia Pigmenti

- Rare X-linked dominant disorder seen only in female
- Stages of skin lesion
  - Vesicular: Initial stage, Usually occur in uterus
  - Verrucous papules: Broad linear bands of hyper keratotic papules, seen after healing of the vesicular stage
  - Pigmentation: Typical whorls of brown to slate grey pigmentation
  - Hypopigmentation: Seen sometimes
- Associated abnormality:
  - Mental retardation, seizures, microcephaly
  - Skeletal abnormality
  - Delayed and abnormal dentition
  - Ocular defects in 33% of cases.

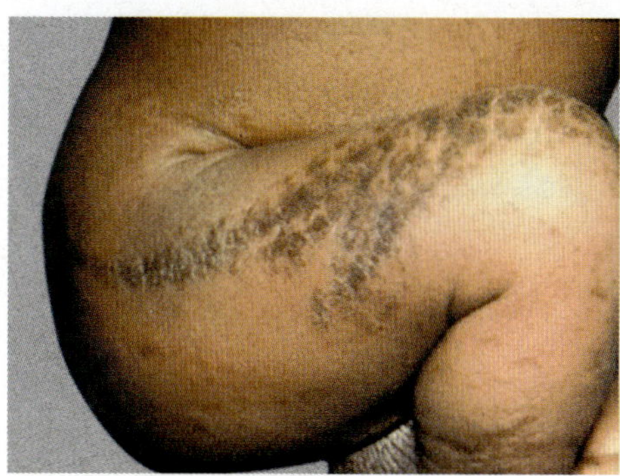

Fig. Incontinentia pigmenti

5. Ans. (a) Most commonly seen in obesity; (b) Seen in axilla; (c) It signifies internal malignancy; (d) It is associated with insulin resistance

[Ref. Neena Khanna, 5/e p38-39]

6. Ans. (c) Nevus anemicus

[Ref. Dermatology by Otto Braun-Falco, 2/e p997]

- Nevus anemicus is a congenital vascular anomaly that presents clinically as a hypopigmented macule or patch
- Lesional pallor is due to a localized hypersensitivity to catecholamines with resultant vasoconstriction
- Nevus anemicus is an uncommon disorder, first described by Vorner (1906)

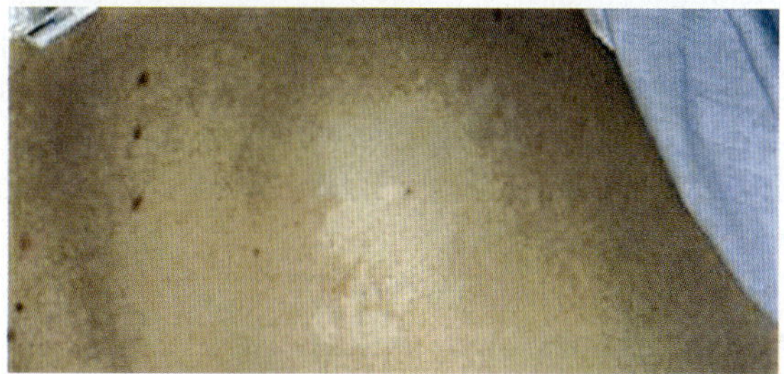

Fig. Nevus anemicus

7. Ans. (d) Testis is commonly involved

[Ref. Neena Khanna, 5/e p406]

Langerhans' Histocytosis

- Seen mostly in infants
- It includes LettererSiwe disorder, Hand Schuller Christian disease, Eosinophilic granuloma

8. Ans. (d) Stratum corneum

[Ref. Practice of Dermatology by P N Behal, 10/e p18-19]

- First layer to develop is Stratum basale and the last one is the Stratum corneum
- In preterm infants, Stratum corneum is underdeveloped and permeable

9. Ans. (a) Anagen

[Ref. Neena Khanna, 5/e p140]

Stages of Hair Cycle

- Anagen: Phase of activity & growth, Hair shows pigmented angulated bulb
- Catagen : Phase of involution
- Telogen: Phase of resting, Hair shows depigmented club-shaped bulb

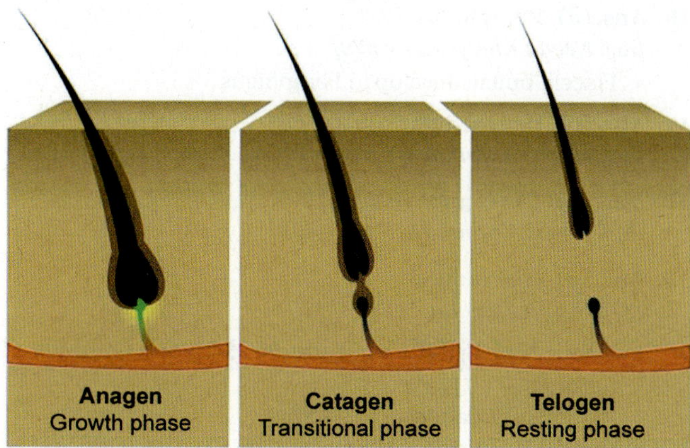

Fig. Hair growth cycle

10. Ans. (a) Incontinentia pigmentosa

[Ref. Neena Khanna, 5/e p37]

11. Ans. (a) Epidermis

[Ref. Neena Khanna, 5/e p78]

12. Ans. (b) Nevus depigmentosa; (d) Naevas anaemicus

[Ref. Dermatology by Otto, 2/e p997]

- Nevus depigmentosus or Nevus achromicus is a depigmentation problem in skin

13. Ans. (b) Water washed disease

[Ref. Text Book of Public Health and Community Medicine by RajVirBhalwar, 1/e p654]

Public Health Classification of Water Borne Diseases

- Water borne diseases: Caused by the ingestion of water contaminated by human or animal faeces or urine containing pathogenic bacteria or viruses.
  - Cholera, Typhoid, Amoebic and bacillary dysentery, Viral hepatitis, Leptospirosis, Giardiasis
- Water washed diseases: Diseases due to lack of water, Poor personal hygiene favours spread
  - Scabies, Skin sepsis & ulcers, Yaws, Trachoma, Conjunctivitis, Flea/ Lice/ Tick- borne diseases
- Water based diseases: Caused by parasites found in intermediate organisms living in water, Infecting agents spread by contact or ingestion of water
  - An essential part of life cycle of agent takes place in aquatic animal
  - Schistosomiasis, Dracunculiasis
- Water related diseases: Transmitted by insect vectors which breed in water
  - Yellow fever, Dengue, Encephalitides, Filariasis, Malaria, Onchocerciasis, Trypanosomiasis, Sleeping sickness

14. Ans. (a) Auspitz sign

[Ref. Neena Khanna, 5/e p46]

15. Ans. (a) PAS

[Ref. Neena Khanna, 5/e p18]

- Stains used in dermatology:

Organism	Stain	Colour
Mycobacteria	Fite stain	Pink
Fungi	PAS	Red

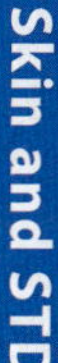

16. Ans. (d) Pemphigus
[Ref. Neena Khanna, 5/e p79]
- Flaccid bullae develop in Pemphigus

17. Ans. (d) Intercellular substance
[Ref. Neena Khanna, 5/e p79]

18. Ans. (a) T Lymphocytes
[Ref. Neena Khanna, 5/e p404-405]

19. Ans. (a) Iris Nodule
[Ref. Neena Khanna, 5/e p34-35]

Systemic Manifestation of Tuberous Sclerosis Complex
- Seizures
- Mental retardation
- Retinal & optic nerve hamartomas
- Achromic retinal patches
- Involvement of skull, spine and pelvis
- Dental pits
- Tumors of heart (rhabdomyomas)
- Tumors (angiomyolipomas) and cysts in kidneys
- Rectal polyps
- Bone cysts

20. Ans. (a) Tuberous sclerosis
[Ref. Neena Khanna, 5/e p34]

Ash Leaf Macule
- Seen in 80% of patients
- Are the earliest manifestation, being present at birth
- ≥ 3 dull, hypopigmented macules, rounded at one end and pointed at the other
- Frequently on trunk

Fig. Ash leaf macule

21. Ans. (b) Lichen planus
[Ref. Neena Khanna, 5/e p67]

Oral Lesion of Lichen Planus
- Asymptomatic or complain of intolerance to spicy food
- White, reticulate lacey patter on the buccal mucosa, tongue and gingival
- White plaques in buccal mucosa and tongue
- Erosive gingivitis

22. Ans. (a) Peutz-Jeghers syndrome
[Ref. Neena Khanna, 5/e p170]

Peutz-Jeghers syndrome
- Autosomal dominant
- Scattered oral and acral lentigines
- Small intestinal polyps and ovarian tumors

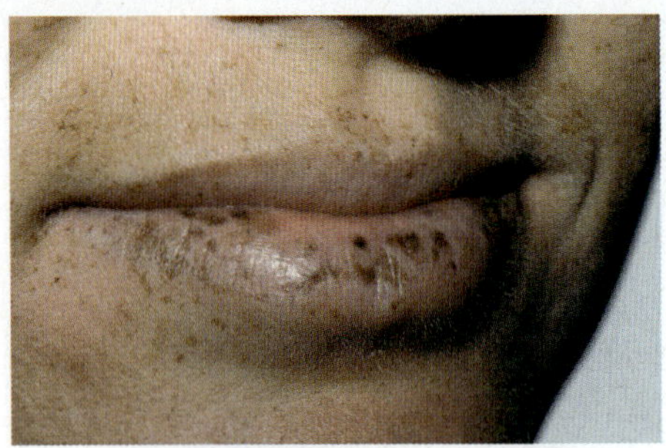

Fig. Peutz-Jeghers syndrome

23. Ans. (a) Pemphigus vulgaris
[Ref. Neena Khanna, 5/e p81]
- Pemphigus vulgaris is characterized by deposit of Ig A antibodies in epidermis.

24. Ans. (a) Lichen planus; (b) Sun burns; (c) Pemphigoid
[Ref. Fundamentals of Pathology of Skin by Venkataram, 1/e p29]

Itching

None/ Mild itching	Psoriasis, Pityriasisrosea, SLE, Parapsoriasis, Secondary syphilis, Pemphigus
Moderate itching	Contact dermatitis, Dry skin, Bullous pemphigoid, Photosensitivity/ Sunburn
Severe itching	Lichen planus, Mastocytosis, Scabies, Lichen simplex chronicus, Dermatitis herpetiformis, Herpes gestations, Prurigonodularis

25. Ans. (a) Lichen planus
[Ref. Neena Khanna, 5/e p67]

26. Ans. (d) Epidermolysis Bullosa
[Ref. Neena Khanna, 5/e p32]

27. Ans. (d) Dermis
[Ref. NCLEX-RN Review Made Incredibly Easyby Springhouse, 2/e p337]

28. Ans. (a) Xeroderma Pigmentosa
[Ref. Neena Khanna, 5/e p38]

29. Ans. (c) Xeroderma Pigmentosa
[Ref. Neena Khanna, 5/e p38]
- Normally, exposure to ultraviolet rays damages DNA (due to production of covalent linkages between adjacent pyrimidines), which is normally rectified by excision and repair, but in XP the repair of UV-damaged DNA is defective

30. Ans. (c) X-linked dominant
[Ref. Neena Khanna, 5/e p37]

31. Ans. (d) Keratinization process cause hydration of cell; (e) Spines of spinous cells are formed from housekeeping organelle
[Ref. Textbook of Dermatology, Leprology & Venereology by Thappa, 3/e p4]

32. Ans. (c) Abscess
[Ref. Neena Khanna, 5/e p4-6]

33. Ans. (c) Indolent course and good prognosis, easily...
[Ref. Neena Khanna, 5/e p406]
- Only patch stage has good response whereas plaque stage has moderate response and tumor stage has poor response.

34. Ans. (c) Mycosis fungoides
[Ref. Neena Khanna, 5/e p405]
- Histopathology shows collection of atypical lymphocytes (Pautrier'smicroabscesses) in epidermis and band of lymphoid cells in upper dermis

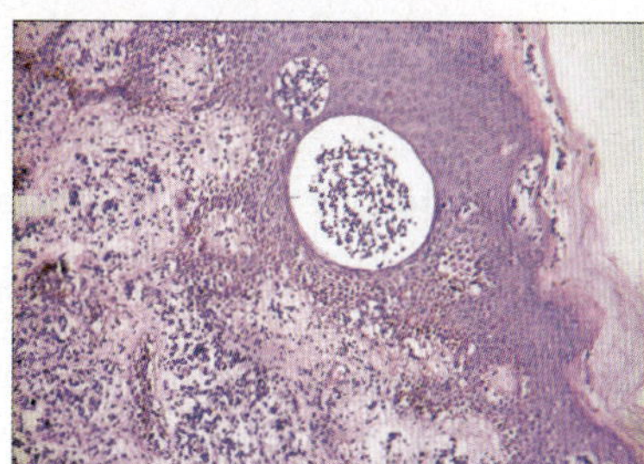

Fig. Pautrier microabscess

35. Ans. (b) Squamous cell carcinoma
[Ref. Neena Khanna, 5/e p387]
- Suspect transformation into squamous cell carcinoma, if the lesions of Acitinic Keratosis enlarges rapidly, ulcerates and bleed

36. Ans. (b) 4 weeks
[Ref. Introduction to Cosmetic Formulation and Technology byBaki, 1/e p131]
- Normal turn-over of epidermis / Skin doubling time is 4 weeks or roughly 1 month

37. Ans. (a) Macule
[Ref. Neena Khanna, 5/e p4]

38. Ans. (a) Macule
[Ref. Neena Khanna, 5/e p4]

39. Ans. (c) Full skin electron therapy
[Ref. Neena Khanna, 5/e p406]

40. Ans. (c) It has a indolent course and good prognosis
[Ref. Neena Khanna, 5/e p406]
- Only patch stage has good response, whereas plaque stage has moderate response and tumor stage has poor response

41. Ans. (c) Granuloma annulare
[Ref. Neena Khanna, 5/e p411]

42. Ans. (b) Malignancy
[Ref. Neena Khanna, 5/e p39]

43. Ans. (c) Confirmatory sign of malignancy
[Ref. Neena Khanna, 5/e p38-39]

44. Ans. (d) Keratinocyte
[Ref. Neena Khanna, 5/e p79 & Figure 5.5]

45. Ans. (d) CD-68 positive; (e) Polyostosis bone lesions treatment by polychemotherapy
[Ref. Neena Khanna, 5/e p406]

46. Ans. (a) Caladarbine
[Ref. Histiocytic Disorders of Children and Adults by Weitzman, 1/e p179]
- Caladarbine or 2-chlorodeoxyadenosine [Ref. 2-CdA] is active as salvage therapy for LCH, but that it is more effective in low-risk patients or patients with multifocal bone disease
- Those patients with risk-organ involvement who responded to 2-CdA therapy had a good prognosis, while those who were refractory typically had grim outcomes
- Notably, patients older than 2 years and those with a longer time between diagnosis and 2-CdA therapy had better responses, presumably because their disease was less aggressive

47. Ans. (b) Axillary freckling
[Ref. Neena Khanna, 5/e p36]
- Intertriginous freckling (Crowe's sign)/ Axillary and inguinal freckling: Pathognomonic of NF1
- Presence of ≥ 6 Café au lait macules (CALMs) is diagnostic of NF1

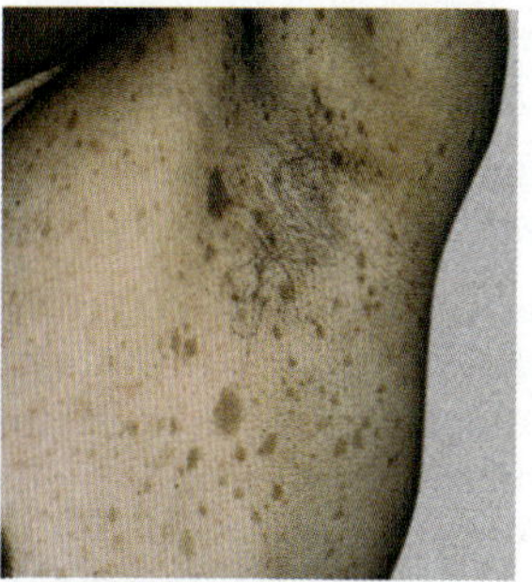

Fig. Axillary freckling

48. Ans. (c) Linear Epidermal naevus
[Ref. Male Genital Lesions by Belda, 1/e p259]

Verrucous Epidermal Nevi
- Benign lesions due to Mutations in fetal life
- Hyperplasia of Epidermal components
- Circumscribed hamartomatous lesion composed of Keratinocytes
- Linear distribution affecting any region of the body

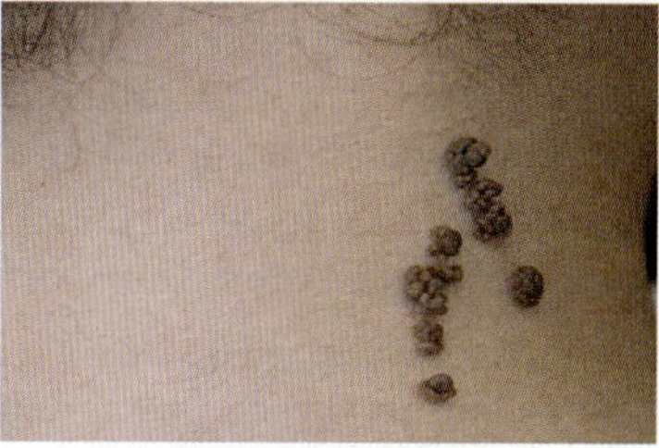

Fig. Epidermal nevus

49. Ans. (a) Dermatomyositis
[Ref. Neena Khanna, 5/e p243]
- Gottron's sign: Symmetrical, somewhat linear, papulo-squamous plaques over interphalangeal or metacarpo-phalangeal joints, elbow and knees

50. Ans. (c) Lumbosacral area; (d) Leg; (e) Thigh
[Ref. Neena Khanna, 5/e p381]

51. Ans. (a) Erythema toxicum; (b) Mongolian spot; (d) Milia
[Ref. Neena Khanna, 5/e p32, 381]

52. Ans. (b) Lumbosacral
[Ref. Neena Khanna, 5/e p381]

53. Ans. (b) Candida; (c) Propionibacterium acnes
[Ref. Neena Khanna, 5/e p120, 312]

- Candida albicans is present as commensal in oral mucosa (50% of normal humans) and vagina (25% of normal woman)

54. Ans. (a) Tuberous sclerosis
[Ref. Neena Khanna, 5/e p34]

55. Ans. (a) Lichen planus; (b) Bowen's disease; (e) UV
[Ref. ABC of Skin Cancer by SajjadRajpar, 1/e p6, 7; Neena Khanna, 5/e p387]

56. Ans. (b) Bowens disease; (c) Lichen planus; (d) DLE
[Ref. Neena Khanna, 5/e p63-65, 381; Rook's Textbook of Dermatology by Burns,7/e 36.26]

- DLE is a premalignant lesion for SCC of skin

57. Ans. (e) All correct
[Ref. Neena Khanna, 5/e p38-39]

58. Ans. (a) Antigen presenting cells
[Ref. Epidermal Langerhans Cells by Schuler, 1/e p276]

59. Ans. (a) Measles; (b) Rubella; (c) HIV; (e) Parvovirus B19
[Ref. API Textbook of Medicine by Munjal, 10/e p120]

- Acute maculopapular rashes in children are usually caused by viral infections whereas in adults they are usually caused by drug reactions
- Viral infections: Measles, Rubella, Chickenpox, Herpes simplex and zoster, Dengue and Chikungunya, HIV, EBV, Parvovirus B19, Coxsackie A16, Arenavirus

60. Ans. (a) Reiter's syndrome
[Ref. Sauer's Manual of Skin Diseases, 1/e]

- Primary skin lesions are present at the onset of a disease
  - Primary lesions: Bulla, Cyst, Macule, Nodule, Papule, Plaque, Pustule, Vesicle, Wheal, Patch, Tumor, Petechiae, Purpura,
- Secondary skin lesions result from changes over time caused by disease progression, manipulation (scratching, picking, rubbing), or treatment
  - Secondary lesions: Crust, Excoriation, Lichenification, Scale, Fissure, Induration, Ulcer, Scar, Keloid

61. Ans. (b) Epidermolysis bullosa
[Ref. Perez and Brady's Radiation, 5/e p690]

Skin Conditions Associated with Skin Cancer

- Chronic skin damage: Ulcers, Osteomyelitis, Sinus tracts, Burns (Majorlin's ulcer), Vaccination scars
- Chronic skin inflammation: DLE, Lichen sclerosus, Lichen planus, Dystrophic epidermolysis bullosa, Lupus vulgaris.

62. Ans. (d) Dermis
[Ref. Histology by Ash, 1/e p30]

- Dense irregular connective tissue is found in the dermis of the skin, the submucosa of the gut, below the loose connective tissue of the lamina propria, and in the capsule surrounding organs
- Extensive collagen fibers allow this type of tissue to withstand tension exerted in many directions, which provides structural strength and flexibility to organs

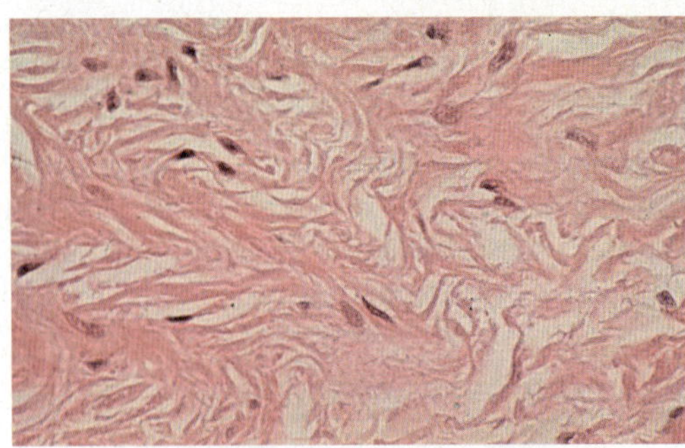

Fig. Dense irregular connective tissue

63. Ans. (c) True keloid does not spread into surrounding tissue
[Ref. Surgery by Prasad, 1/e p12]

Keloids

- Common in people of African and Asian descent as compared to white-skinned populations
- Prevalence among men and women is approximately equal, with occurrence predominantly in younger individuals, ages 10-30 years age
- MC site is Sternal region, but keloids also occur frequently on the neck, ears, extremities, or trunk and rarely on the face, palms, or soles
- More common in burns, vaccination scars, or healing of an ulcer
- Maturation and stabilization of collagen fibers is inhibited
- Continues to grow and may become worse even after one year
- True keloid spread into surrounding tissue (In contrast Hypertrophic scar does not)

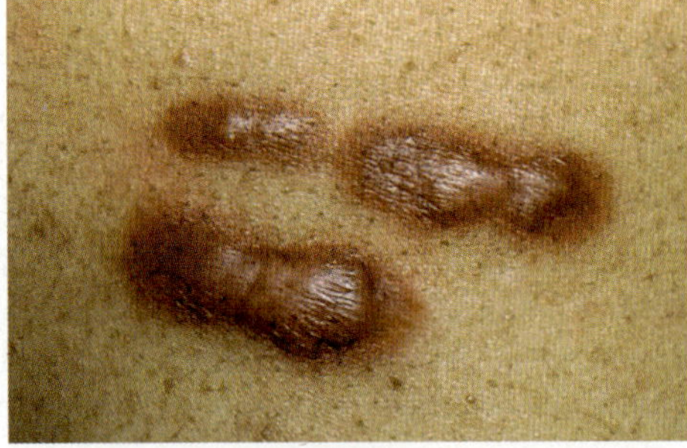

Fig. Keloid

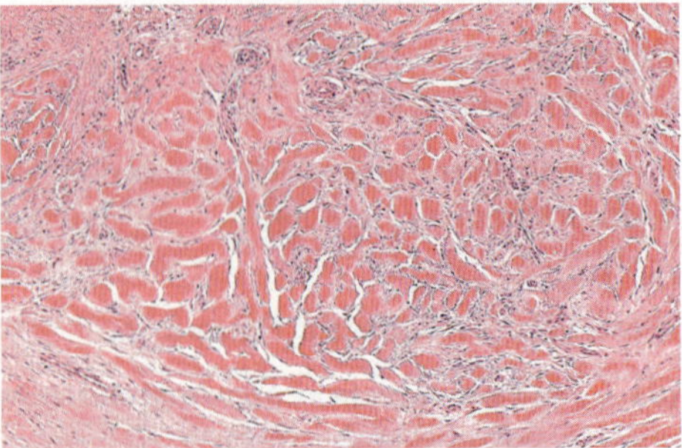

Fig. Thick collagen bundles of keloid

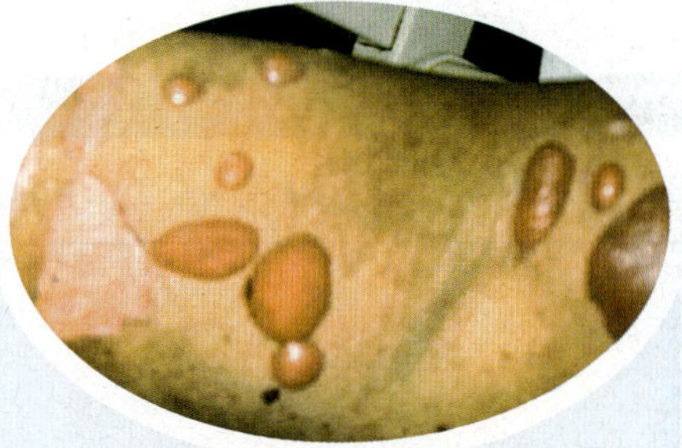

Chapter 2

Lichen Planus

THEORETICAL CONCEPTS

II A. TYPE OF DISORDER

- Papulosquamous, cell-mediated, unknown origin

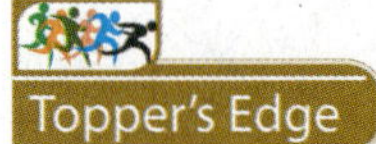

Topper's Edge

Types of Lichen Planus

Variant	Morphology
Annular[Q]	**'Ring-shaped' lesions**, Hyperpigmented skin in center, Elevated periphery, Face/ Glans penis
Linear	Papules arranged in line **(Blaschko line**[Q]**)**, Face/ Dorsal aspect of upper extremities
Hypertrophic	Verrucous hyperkeratotic papules/ nodules, Most pruritic variant, Extremities, Shins, IP joints ***"Lichen planus verrucosus"***[Q]
Atrophic	Demarcated, white-bluish papules/ plaques, Central superficial atrophy, Rare variant
Bullous	Vesicles/bullae with skin lesions, Rare variant ***"Vesiculobullous lichen planus"***[Q]
Ulcerative	Chronic, painful bullae, Ulceration of the feet, Cicatricial sequelae, Rare variant
Pigmented	Hyperpigmented, dark-brown macules in sun-exposed areas/ flexural folds, Rare variant

II B. CHARACTERISTICS OF LESIONS: [MNEMONIC: P5][Q]

- **P**lain top (Flat)
- **P**urple (Violaceous)
- **P**olygonal
- **P**ruritic (Itchy)
- **P**apular

II C. SITES

- Wrists and ankles (medial aspect)
- Flexor aspects of limbs
- Lumbar region
- Oral mucosa
- Genitalia

II D. ASSOCIATIONS

- Hepatitis C
- Autoimmune diseases
- Drugs: Gold, Penicillamine, Phenothiazines, Diuretics, Anti-malarials

II E. PRESENTATION

- ***Wickham's striae***: Grey-white lines on lesions[Q]
- ***Koebner's phenomenon***: New lesions appear on sites of trauma[Q]
- *Lichen piloplanaris*
- *Scarring alopecia*
  - White lace-like or net-like eruption in oral mucosa
  - Residual pigmentation and scarring
- *Nail changes*:[Q] Hyperpigmentation, Hyperkeratosis, ***Pterygium***[Q], Onchylolysis, Longitudinal grooves, Oil spots, Trachyonychia, Pup-tent sign
- *Histology*:
  - ***Civatte (Colloid) bodies***[Q]
  - 'Sawtooth' dermoepidermal junction
  - 'Bunch-of grapes' pattern on immunofluorescence

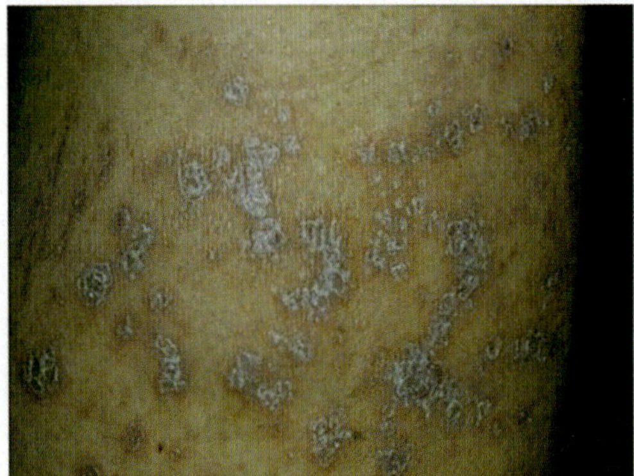

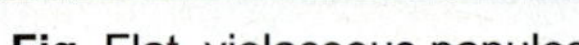

Fig. Flat, violaceous papules

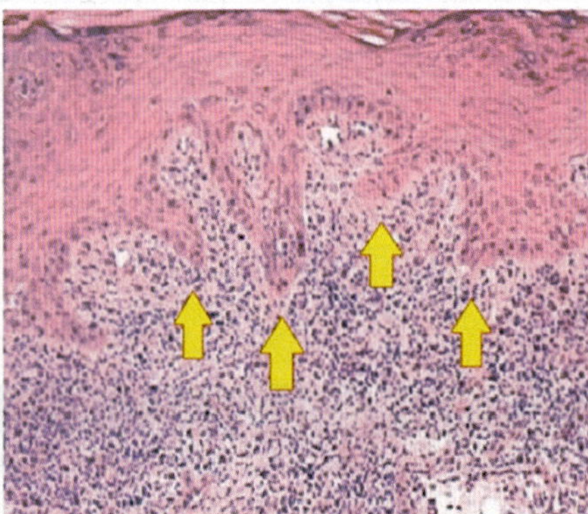

Fig. Saw-tooth Rete-ridges

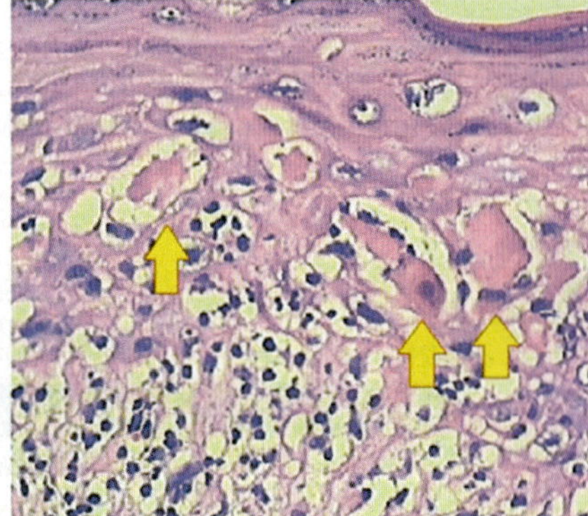

Fig. Civatte (Colloid) bodies

IMAGE-BASED QUESTIONS

1. Polygonal, violaceous lesion on arms (Image). What is the likely diagnosis? ***[Recent Question 2016]***

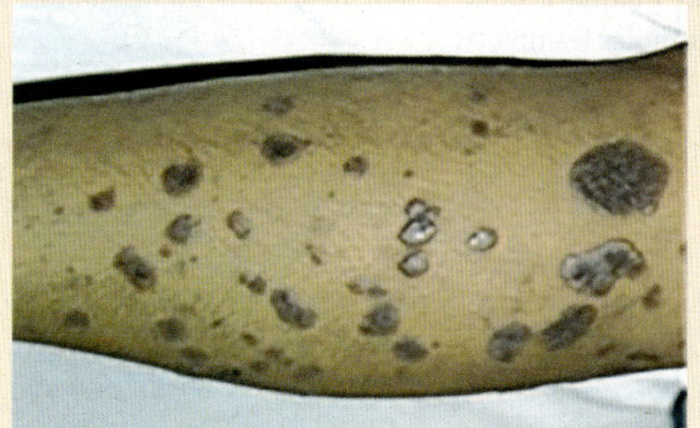

a. Psoriasis
b. Pityriasis rosea
c. Lichen planus
d. Dermatophytosis

2. Diagnose the skin disorder as shown in photograph ***[Recent Questions 2012, 2014]***

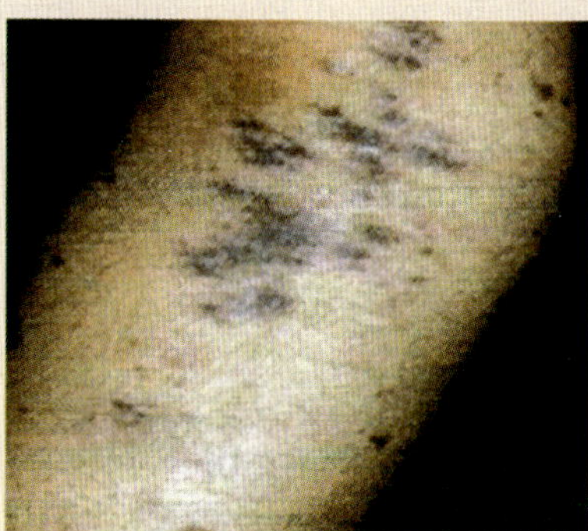

a. Miliaria profunda
b. Seborrhoeic dermatitis
c. Lichen planus
d. Vitiligo

3. Identify the phenomenon shown by a Lichen planus case (photograph)

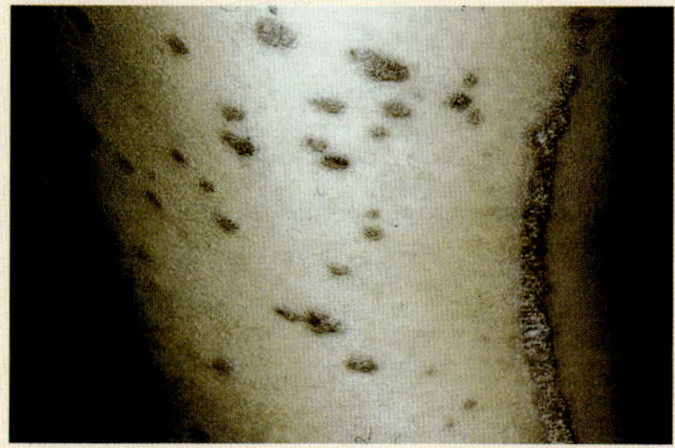

a. Auspitz sign
b. Koebner phenomenon
c. Gottron's sign
d. Darier's sign

4. Lines (Arrow) seen in a case of Lichen planus (photograph) ***[Recent Question 2012]***

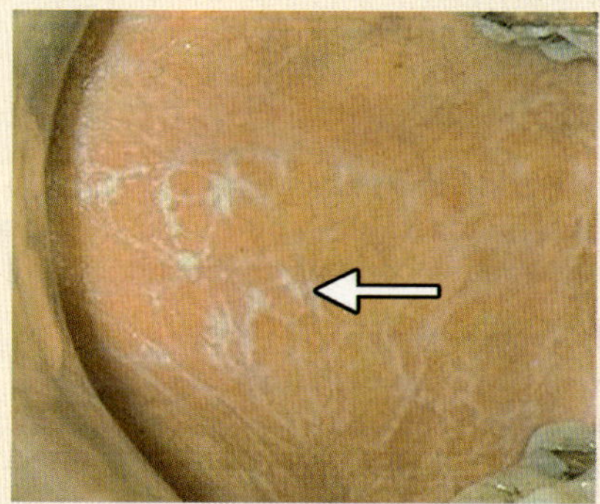

a. Mees lines
b. Nikolsky's sign
c. Wickham's striae
d. Beau lines

5. A Woman presents with bilateral buccal reticulate white streaks. Pain increases on spicy food intake. No history of tobacco exposure. Amalgam on 3rd molar. Diagnosis is ***[AIIMS November 2015]***

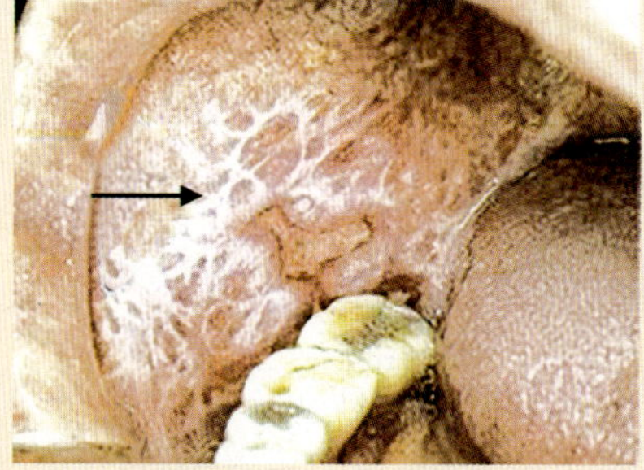

a. Candidiasis
b. Leukoplakia
c. Aphthous stomatitis
d. Lichen planus

ANSWERS WITH EXPLANATIONS OF IBQs

1. Ans. (c) Lichen planus *[Ref. DVL by Thappa, 4/e p130]*

Lichen planus (photograph)

- Unique papulosquamous disorder classically remembered as **9Ps**
- **P**ruritic, **P**lane topped, **P**olyangular, **P**urple coloured, **P**apules and **P**laque lesions which heal with **P**igmentation and has characteristic nail changes known as **P**terygium ungium and **P**enile annular lesions.

2. Ans. (c) Lichen planus *[Ref. Neena Khanna, 4/e p56]*

Lichen Planus Lesions: [Mnemonic: P5]

- Plain top (Flat)
- Purple (Violaceous)
- Polygonal
- Pruritic (Itchy)
- Papular

3. Ans. (b) Koebner phenomenon *[Ref. Neena Khanna, 4/e p41]*

Isomorphic/Koebner Phenomenon

- Definition: Are skin lesions appearing on lines of trauma
- Underlying causes:
  - Thermal trauma
  - Dermatoses
  - Allergic reactions
  - Therapy
- True isomorphic phenomena:
  - Lichen planus
  - Vitiligo
  - Psoriasis

4. Ans. (c) Wickham's striae *[Ref. Neena Khanna, 4/e p57]*

- Wickham's striae: Grey-white lines/ streaks on lesions of Lichen planus when viewed under magnifying glass
- Enhancement on putting drop of mineral oil on lesions

5. Ans. (d) Lichen planus *[Ref. Neena Khanna, 4/e p57]*

Patches of Oral Lichen Planus

- Usually appear as white lines and puncta in a reticulated (lace-like) pattern
- Occasionally, these patches become confluent, producing a solid plaque
- Blisters and erosions occur less often

NEET/NBE PATTERN MCQs

1. **Lichen planus all true except** *[Recent Question 2016]*
   a. Pruritic lesion
   b. Involves nails
   c. Involves mucus membranes
   d. Steroid is not used in treatment
2. **Complication of Chronic Lichen planus** *[Recent Question 2016]*
   a. Dermatofibroma b. Malignant melanoma
   c. Basal cell carcinoma d. Squamous cell carcinoma
3. **Histological finding of Lichen planus** *[Recent Question 2016]*
   a. Acanthosis b. Hyperkeratosis
   c. Basal cell degeneration d. All of the above
4. **Itchy polygonal violaceous papular lesions are seen in** *[NBE FMGE September 2008]*
   a. Lichen planus b. Psoriasis
   c. Pityriasis rosea d. Pityriasis rubra pilaris
5. **Diagnostic histology of lichen planus is** *[NBE DNB 1997]*
   a. Dyskeratosis b. Basal cell proliferation
   c. Hyperkeratosis d. Lymphocytic infiltration
6. **Characteristic nail involvement in lichen planus is** *[NBE DNB 2011]*
   a. Pterygium formation
   b. Subungual hyperkeratosis
   c. Coarse pining
   d. Salmon patch formation
7. **Not a histological feature of lichen planus is** *[Recent Question 2012]*
   a. Acanthosis b. Interface dermatitis
   c. Neutrophils in stratum d. Pigment incontinence
8. **In Lichen planus, nails deformities include all except** *[NBE FMGE March 2009]*
   a. Beau's lines
   b. Pterygium
   c. Longitudinal grooves
   d. Oncholysis
9. **All of the following regarding classical lichen planus are true EXCEPT that** *[NBE DNB 2011]*
   a. Lesions commonly occur on the flexor aspect or wrists
   b. Plaques occur on the palm and soles
   c. Koebnerisation of skin lesions occur
   d. Pruritis occurs rarely
10. **Wickham's striae are seen in** *[NBE FMGE September 2009, September 2010]* *[Recent Question 2016]*
    a. Vitiligo
    b. Lichen planus
    c. Psoriasis
    d. Pityriasis rosea
11. **Max-Joseph cleft are seen in** *[Recent Question 2015]*
    a. Vitiligo
    b. Lichen planus
    c. Psoriasis
    d. Pityriasis rosea
12. **Which of the following is not a feature of Lichen planus?** *[Recent Question 2017]*
    a. Pterygium b. Spontaneous healing
    c. Scarring alopecia d. Not premalignant
13. **Wickham's striae are usually seen in?** *[Recent Question 2017]*
    a. Nails b. Mucosa
    c. Hair d. Skin

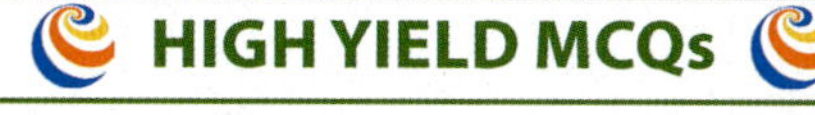

HIGH YIELD MCQs

1. **Mucosa is involved in** *[PGI 2007]*
   a. Psoriasis b. Lichen planus
   c. Alopecia d. Scabies
   e. Porphyria
2. **Max. Joseph's space is a histopathological feature of** *[Recent Question 2016, AIIMS PGMEE 2006]*
   a. Psoriasis vulgaris b. Lichen planus
   c. Pityriasis rosea d. Parapsoriasis
3. **A young lady presents with lacy lesions in oral cavity and her proximal nail fold has extended onto the nail bed. What is the likely diagnosis** *[All India PGMEE 2010]*
   a. Psoriasis b. Geographic tongue
   c. Lichen planus d. Candidiasis
4. **Regarding Lichen planus all are true, except** *[All India PGMEE 2000]*
   a. Hypopigmentation in residual disease
   b. Lymphatic infiltration on supradermal layer
   c. Itchy polygonal, purple papule
   d. Skin, hair and oral mucosa commonly involved
5. **Most characteristic finding in lichen planus is** *[PGI 1999]*
   a. Civatte bodies b. Basal cell degeneration
   c. Thinning of nail plate d. Violaceous lesions
6. **All of the following regarding Lichen planus are true** *[MP PGMEE 2005]*
   a. Does not involve mucous membrane
   b. Associated with Hepatitis 'C'
   c. Topical steroid are the mainstay of therapy
   d. Spontaneous remissions 6 months to 2 years
7. **A patient presented with scarring alopecia, thinned nails, hypopigmented macular lesions over the trunk and oral mucosa. The diagnosis is** *[AIIMS PGMEE 2001]*
   a. Psoriasis b. Leprosy
   c. Lichen planus d. Pemphigus
8. **Characteristic nail finding in Lichen planus** *[AIIMS PGMEE 2001]*
   a. Pitting b. Pterygium
   c. Beau's lines d. Hyperpigmentation of nails
9. **Wickehm's striae seen in** *[SGPGI 2002]* *[Bihar PGMEE 2003, All India PGMEE 2002]*
   a. Lichen niditus b. Lichenoid eruption
   c. Lichen striates d. Lichen planus
10. **In Lichen planus TOC is** *[AIIMS PGMEE 1993]*
    a. Topical salicyclic acid b. UV ray
    c. Systemic steroids d. Erythromycin

11. A 10-year-old child has violaceous papule and pterygium of nails. The diagnosis is *[AIIMS PGMEE 1999]*
a. Psoriasis b. Pemphigus
c. Pemphigoid d. Lichen planus

12. Itchy polygonal violaceous papules seen in *[All India PGMEE 1998]*
a. Psoriasis b. Pemphigus
c. Lichen planus d. Pityriasis rosea

13. True about lichen planus *[PGI 2004]*
a. Basal cell degeneration
b. Colloid bodies seen
c. Epidermal hyperplasia in chronic cases
d. Wickham's striae seen
e. Autoimmune disease

14. Civatte bodies are found in *[Recent Question 2017, Kerala PGMEE 1998]*
a. Lichen planus b. Psoriasis
c. Dermatophytosis d. Vitiligo

15. A 30-year-old male present with pruritic flat-topped polygonal, shiny violaceous papules with flexural distribution the most likely diagnosis is *[Bihar PGMEE 2005, J&K PGMEE 2006]*
a. Psoriasis b. Pityriasis
c. Lichen planus d. Lichenoid dermatitis

16. Regarding Lichen planus all are true except *[All India PGMEE 2000]*
a. Hypopigmentation in residual disease
b. Lymphatic infiltration in supradermal layer
c. Itchy, polygonal, purple, papule
d. Skin Hair & Oral mucosa commonly involved

17. Which of the following is pruritic? *[PGI 1993, Kerala PGMEE 1998]*
a. Lichen planus
b. Psoriasis
c. Ichthyosis
d. Secondary syphilis

18. Lacy while lesion in mouth with pterygium is seen in *[SGPGI 2001]*
a. Psoriasis b. Pityriasis alba
c. Lichen planus d. Leprosy

19. Most characteristic feature of lichen planus is *[PGI 1998]*
a. Thinning of nail plate is most common
b. Non-scarring alopecia
c. Violaceous lesions on skin and mucous membrane
d. Wickham striae

20. Nails in Lichen planus *[PGI November 2014]*
a. Pup-tent b. Beau lines
c. Trachyonychia d. Telangiectasia
e. Pterygium

21. Not a variant of lichen is *[AIIMS November 2014]*
a. Lichen planus actinus
b. Lichen scrofulosorum
c. Lichen planopilaris
d. Oral lichen planus

22. Wickham's striae are seen in *[PGMCET 2015]*
a. Lichen planus
b. Lichen aureus
c. Lichen nitidus
d. Lichen sclerosus et atrophicus

NEET/NBE PATTERN MCQs ANSWERS WITH EXPLANATIONS

1. Ans. (d) Steroid is not used in treatment
[Ref. DVL by Thappa, 4/e p135]
- Specific treatment protocol of Lichen planus includes Steroids (topical, intralesional, systemic), PUVA therapy, Cyclosporine, Dapsone, Tacrolimus

2. Ans. (d) Squamous cell carcinoma
[Ref. Lookingbill and Marks' Principles of Dermatology, 5/e p149]
- Complications of mucous membrane Lichen planus include Candidiasis and Squamous cell carcinoma

3. Ans. (d) All of the above
[Ref. DVL by Thappa, 4/e p129]

Lichen Planus Histopathology
- Hyperkeratosis
- Hypertrophic basal cell degeneration
- Saw-tooth rete pegs
- Band-like infiltrates in lamina propria
- Colloid bodies
- Acanthosis
- Papillomatosis

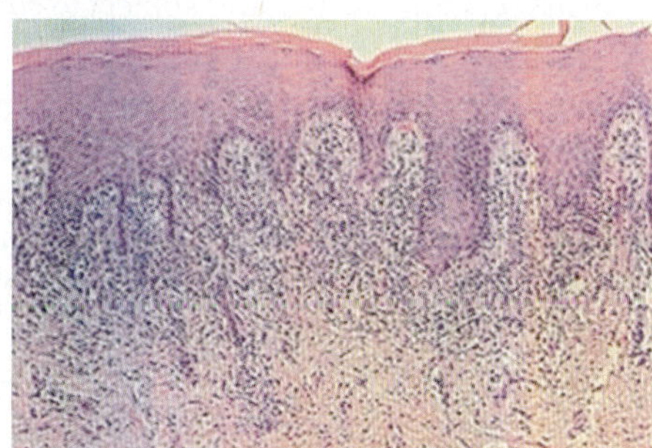

Fig. Lichen planus

4. Ans. (a) Lichen planus
[Ref. Neena Khanna, 4/e p56]
- Characteristics of lesions of Lichen planus: **[Mnemonic: P5]**
  - **P**lain top (Flat)
  - **P**urple (Violaceous)
  - **P**olygonal
  - **P**ruritic (Itchy)
  - **P**apular

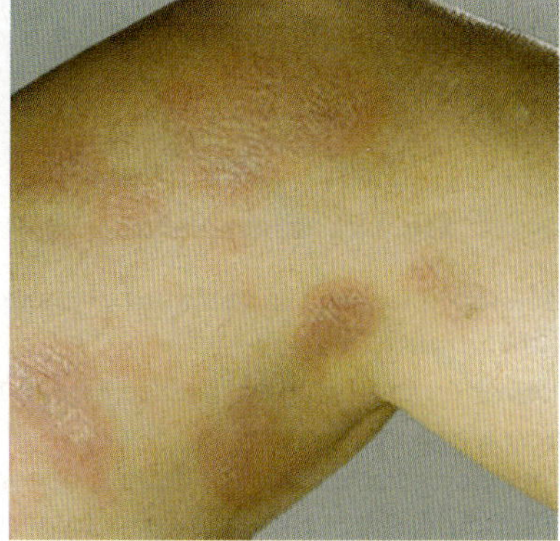

Fig. Lichen planus

Also Remember
- ***Clinical presentation of Psoriasis***: Extensor, pressure points
  - Well-demarcated, indurated, scaly, silvery, discoid lesions
  - Erythrematous (*Ring of Woronoff*)
  - *Koebner's/Isomorphic phenomenon* (lesions at site of trauma)
  - Nail changes: Thickened nail-plates, Oil-spots/ Oil-drop sign, Dystrophy, Discolouration, Onycholysis, Thimble-pitting, Subungal hyperkeratosis
  - *Bed-side tests*:
    1. *Grattage test*: Accentuation of scales with glass-slide
    2. *Auspitz sign*: Bleeding points on removing membrane
- ***Clinical presentation of Pityriasis rosea***: Flexures in trunks
  - *Herald/ Mother patch*:
    1. Cigarette papery scales
    2. *Trailing/ Collarette of scales*
  - Secondary lesions: (Lesions resemble secondary syphilis)
    1. *Fir-tree/ Christmas-tree appearance of scales*
- ***Clinical presentation of Pityriasis rubra pilaris***: Trunks, Dorsal aspects of digits
  - Erythroderma with islands of normal skin
  - Orange-pink follicular papules
  - Keratodermic sandals (Orangish thickening of palms/ soles)
  - Yellow-brown nails with thick nail-plates

5. Ans. (c) Hyperkeratosis; (d) Lymphocytic infiltration
[Ref. Rook's Textbook of Dermatology edited by Tony Burns, 7/e 42.3, 42.4; Neena Khanna, 5/e p67]
- Thickening of stratum corneum leads to Hyperkeratosis in Lichen planus
- Band like upper dermal infiltrate of lymphocytes is characteristic of Lichen planus

6. Ans. (a) Pterygium formation
[Ref. Neena Khanna, 5/e p64]

Nail Changes in Lichen planus
- Thinning and distal splitting of nail plates
- Trachyonychia: Sand paper nails (Irregular longitudinal grooves and ridges in nail plate resulting in roughness of nail)
- Tenting of nail plate: Puptent sign
- Pterygium: Diagnostic and manifestation of severe LP of nails

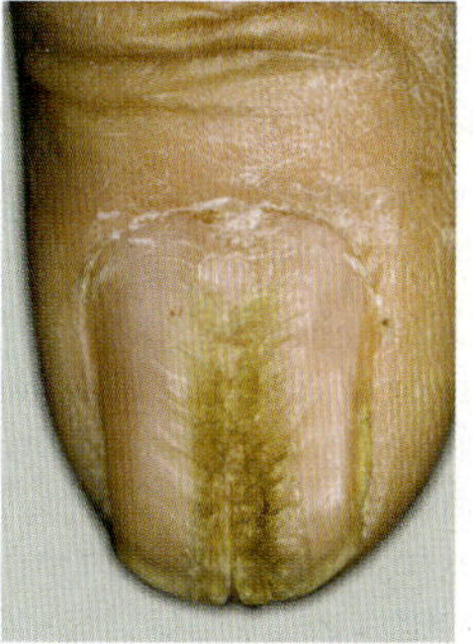

Fig. Pterygium nails

7. **Ans. (c) Neutrophils in stratum**
[Ref. Neena Khanna, 5/e p67]
   - Band like upper dermal infiltrate of lymphocytes is characteristic of Lichen planus.

8. **Ans. (a) Beau's lines**
[Ref. Neena Khanna, 4/e p58]

Nail Changes in Lichen Planus
- Hyperpigmentation
- Hyperkeratosis
- Pterygium
- Onchylolysis
- Longitudinal grooves
- Oil spots
- Trachyonychia
- Pup-tent sign

9. **Ans. (d) Pruritis occurs rarely**
[Ref. Neena Khanna, 5/e p65]

Characteristic 5Ps of Lichen planus
- **P**ruritic
- **P**urple
- **P**olygonal
- **P**lane topped
- **P**apules

10. **Ans. (b) Lichen planus**
[Ref. Neena Khanna, 4/e p57]

Clinical Presentation of Lichen planus
- ***Wickham's striae***: Grey-white lines on lesions
- *Koebner's phenomenon*: New lesions appear on sites of trauma
- *Lichen piloplanaris*
- *Scarring alopecia*
  - White lace-like or net-like eruption in oral mucosa
  - Residual pigmentation and scarring
- *Nail changes*: Hyperpigmentation, Hyperkeratosis, *Pterygium*, Onchylolysis, Longitudinal grooves, Oil spots, Trachyonychia, Pup-tent sign
- *Histology*:
  - *Civatte (Colloid) bodies*
  - 'Sawtooth' dermo-epidermal junction
  - 'Bunch-of grapes' pattern on immunofluorescence

11. **Ans. (b) Lichen planus**
[Ref. Inflammatory Skin Disorders by Plaza, 1/e p20]
   - **Max-Joesph clefts**: Liquefactive degeneration of the stratum basale, with separation from the underlying lamina propria, as a result of desmosome loss, creating small spaces in Lichen planus

12. **Ans. (d) Not premalignant**
[Ref. Oral Cancer by Werning, 1/e p32]
   - Premalignant lesions of the oral cavity include Leukoplakia, Erythroplakia, Lichen planus, Keratosis of the palate, Oral submucous fibrosis
   - Most important complication of oral lichen planus (OLP) is the development of squamous cell carcinoma (SCC); his being an association that remains subject to controversy

13. **Ans. (b) Mucosa**
[Ref. A Manual of Dermatology by Zaidi, 2/e p275]
   - MC form of Wickham's striae is a reticular pattern with a network of white striae, principally on the buccal mucosa
   - Lesions sometimes appear as white plaques on the buccal mucosa or tongue, but these are often associated with radiating peripheral white striae.

HIGH YIELD MCQs ANSWERS WITH EXPLANATIONS 

1. **Ans. (b) Lichen planus**
[Ref. Neena Khanna, 5/e p63]
   - Both oral and genital mucosa are involved in LP

2. **Ans. (b) Lichen planus**
[Ref. Neena Khanna, 5/e p67]

Lichen Planus Histopathology
- Thickened granular layer
- Saw toothing of rete pegs
- Basal cell degeneration (leading to Max Joseph's spaces and colloid/Civatte body formation)
- Band like upper dermal infiltrate of lymphocytes

3. **Ans. (c) Lichen planus**
[Ref. Neena Khanna, 5/e p63,64, 67]

Oral Lesion of Lichen Planus
- Asymptomatic or complain of intolerance to spicy food
- White, reticulate lacey pattern on the buccal mucosa, tongue and gingival
- White plaques in buccal mucosa and tongue
- Erosive gingivitis

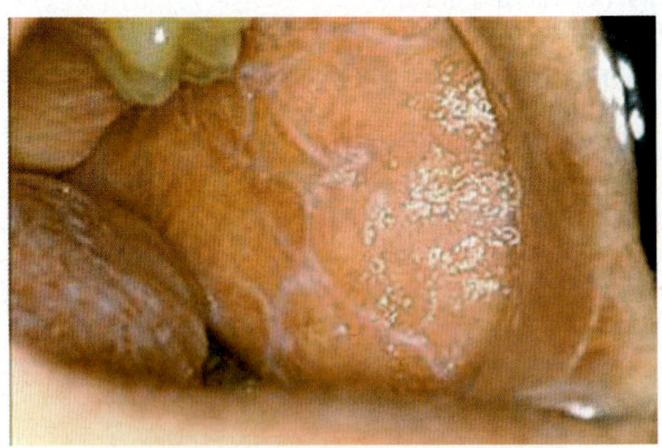

Fig. Oral lichen planus

4. **Ans. (a) Hypopigmented in residual disease**
[Ref. Neena Khanna, 5/e p65]
   - LP is a chronic, self-limiting disease, which may last many months to a couple of years
   - Over a period of time, papules flatten, become darker and leave behind discrete grayish areas of hyperpigmentation

5. Ans. (b) Basal cell degeneration
[Ref. Neena Khanna, 5/e p67]

6. Ans. (a) Does not involve mucous membrane
[Ref. Neena Khanna, 5/e p63]

7. Ans. (c) Lichen planus
[Ref. Neena Khanna, 5/e p62-65]

8. Ans. (b) Pterygium
[Ref. Neena Khanna, 5/e p64, 65]

9. Ans. (d) Lichen planus
[Ref. Neena Khanna, 5/e p62]

- When viewed under magnifying lens, surface of the lesion has white streaks (Wickham's striae)

10. Ans. (c) Systemic steroids
[Ref. Neena Khanna, 5/e p68]

- Steroid as Oral Mini Pulse **(OMP)** - Weekly steroids, given as 3-5 mg of betamethasone, once or twice (then on 2 consecutive days) a week

11. Ans. (d) Lichen planus
[Ref. Neena Khanna, 5/e p62-65]

12. Ans. (c) Lichen planus
[Ref. Neena Khanna, 5/e p62-65]

13. Ans. ALL CHOICES
[Ref. Neena Khanna, 5/e p62-65]

14. Ans. (a) Lichen planus
[Ref. Neena Khanna, 5/e p67]

15. Ans. (c) Lichen planus
[Ref. Neena Khanna, 5/e p62-65]

16. Ans. (a) Hypopigmented in residual disease
[Ref. Neena Khanna, 5/e p65]

17. Ans. (a) Lichen planus
[Ref. Neena Khanna, 5/e p65]

18. Ans. (c) Lichen planus
[Ref. Neena Khanna, 5/e p62-65]

19. Ans. (d) Wickham's striae
[Ref. Neena Khanna, 5/e p62]

- When viewed under magnifying lens, surface of the lesion has white streaks (Wickham's striae) which can be enhanced by putting a drop of mineral oil on the surface of lesion.

20. Ans. (a) Pup-tent; (c) Trachyonychia; (e) Pterygium
[Ref. DVL by Bansal, 1/e p293]

Lichen Planus of the Nails

- Nail involvement occurs in 10 to 15 percent of patients
- Thinning, Longitudinal ridging, Distal splitting of nail plate (Onychoschizia)
- Onycholysis, Longitudinal striation (Onychorrhexis), Subungual hyperkeratosis, or Absence (Anonychia) of nail plate
- Trachyonychia
- Pterygium
- "Tenting" or **"pup-tent" sign**: Nail bed involvement that elevates the nail plate and may cause longitudinal splitting

21. Ans. (b) Lichen scrofulosorum
[Ref. Dermatology by Zaidi, 2/e p276]

Variants of Oral Lichen Planus

- Hypertrophic LP
- Follicular LP (Lichen planoplanaris)
- LP Actinus
- Annular LP
- Atrophic LP
- Ulcerative/ Erosive LP
- Bullous LP
- LP Pigmentosus
- Invisible LP

22. (a) Lichen planus
[Ref. Dermatology by Wolff, 1/e p448]

- **Wickham's striae**: Presence of fine, white or gray lines or dots (Striae) seen on the top of the pruritic papular rash on the skin in lichen planus.

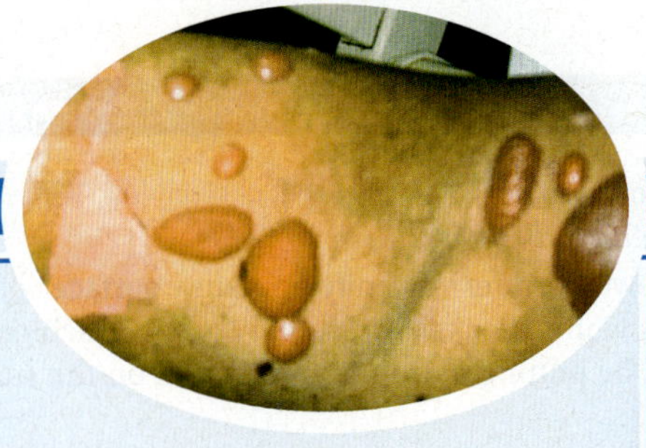

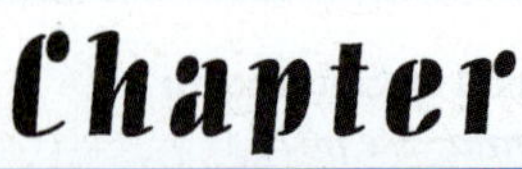

Chapter 3

Nutritional and Environmental Factors in Dermatology

THEORETICAL CONCEPTS

III A. SKIN MANIFESTATIONS OF PROTEIN ENERGY MALNUTRITION (PEM)

- *'Crazy pavement'* like skin (parchment)
- ***'Flag sign'*** in hair (alternate bands of light and dark colours)[Q]

Topper's Edge

Flag Sign

- Peculiar change in hair color
- Hair becomes discolored in a band perpendicular to its long axis
- **Seen in: Kwashiorkor**[Q]
- Indicates: Period of Severe malnutrition[Q]

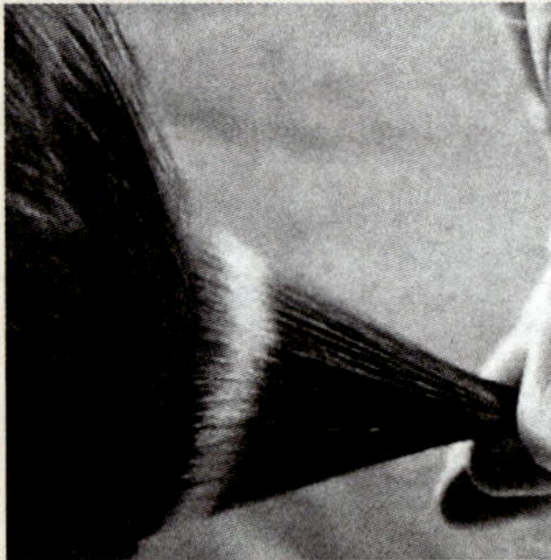

Fig. Flag sign

III B. SKIN MANIFESTATIONS OF VITAMIN A DEFICIENCY

- *'Xerosis of skin'*[Q]
- ***'Phrynoderma'*** (Toad like skin)[Q]

III C. SKIN MANIFESTATIONS OF VITAMIN B_1 (RIBOFLAVIN) DEFICIENCY

- **Angular stomatitis**[Q]
- Cheilitis[Q]
- Seborrheic dermatitis like rash

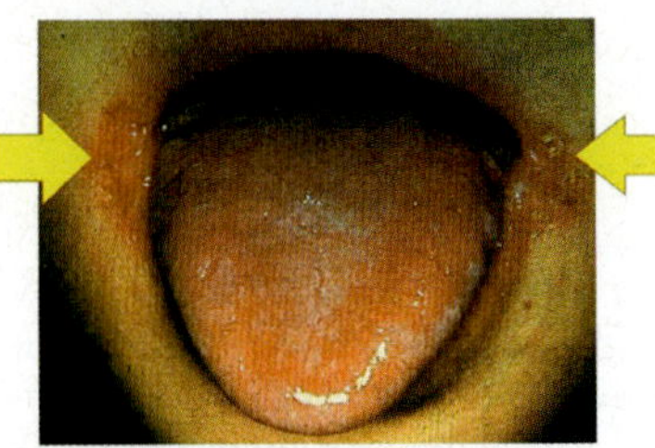

Fig. Cheilitis

III D. SKIN MANIFESTATIONS OF VITAMIN B_3 (NICOTINIC ACID) DEFICIENCY [PELLAGRA]

- *Dermatitis*[Q]
- **Casal's necklace**[Q]
- Erythema
- Dyssebacia

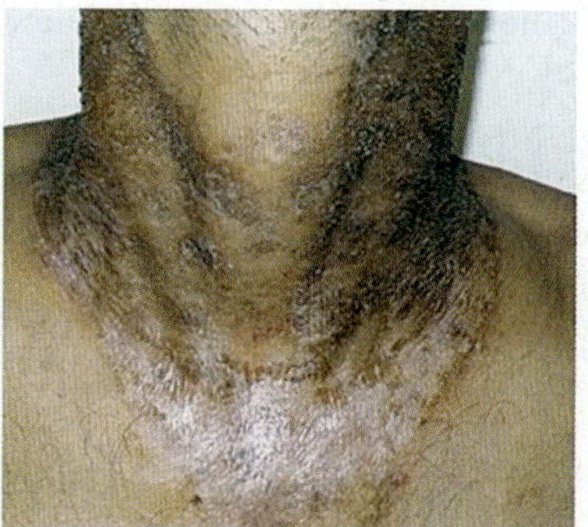

Fig. Casal's necklace

III E. SKIN MANIFESTATIONS OF VITAMIN C (ASCORBIC ACID) DEFICIENCY [SCURVY]

- Follicular hyperkeratosis
- ***Corkscrew hair***[Q]
- Perifollicular hemorrhages
- Ecchymosis on feet, ankles

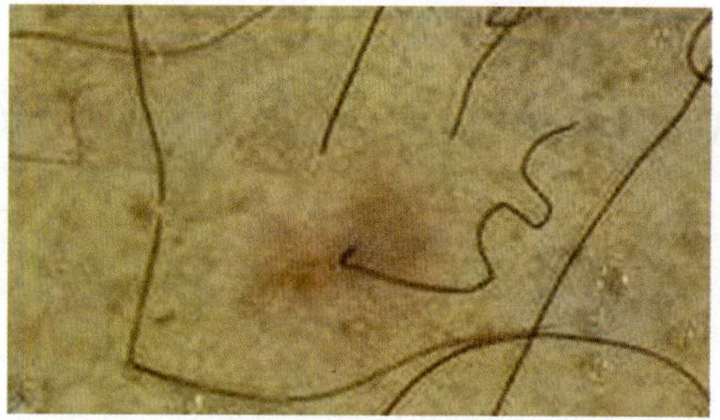

Fig. Corkscrew hair

III F. SKIN MANIFESTATIONS OF ZINC DEFICIENCY [ACRODERMATITIS ENTEROPATHICA][Q]

- Scaly eczematous plaques in **periorificial regions**[Q], acral areas and bony prominences
- Pustular and hemorrhagic paronychia
- Non-scarring alopecia of scalp

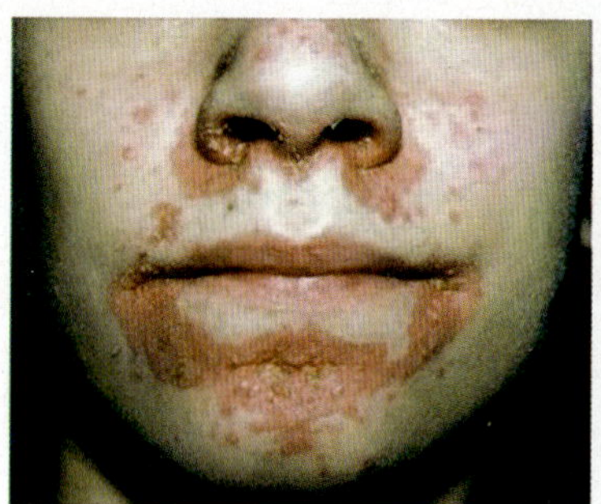

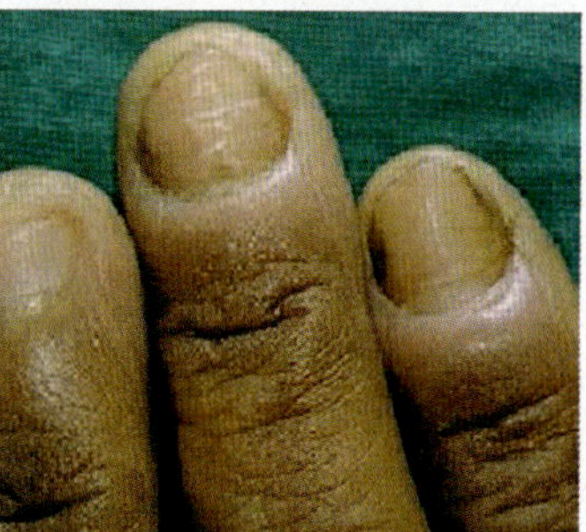

Fig. Acrodermatitis enteropathica

III G. SKIN MANIFESTATIONS OF ESSENTIAL FATTY ACID DEFICIENCY

- Dry skin, eczematous dermatitis
- ***Phrynoderma***[Q]

IMAGE-BASED QUESTION

1. **Condition shown in photograph occurs due to deficiency of**

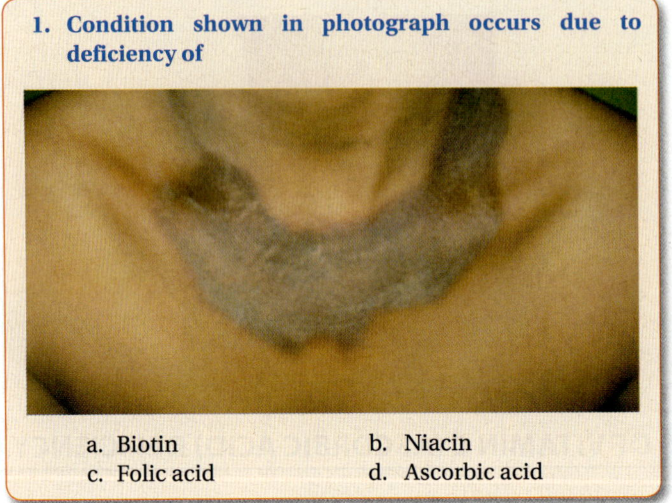

a. Biotin
b. Niacin
c. Folic acid
d. Ascorbic acid

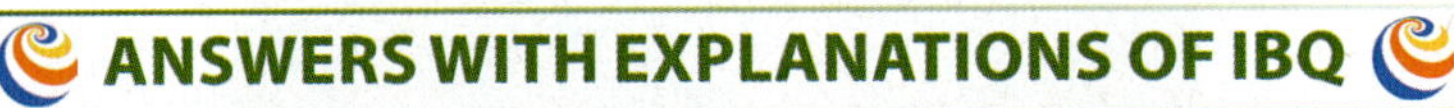

ANSWERS WITH EXPLANATIONS OF IBQ

1. **Ans. (b) Niacin** *[Ref. Neena Khanna, 4/e p392]*
   - Casal collar/ Casal necklace: A clinical sign in which there is an erythematous pigmented skin rash in the distribution of a broad collar (dermatomes C3 and C4), Seen in patients with pellagra.

NEET/NBE PATTERN MCQs

1. **Flag sign in hair is characteristic of** *[NBE FMGE September 2007]*
   a. Zinc deficiency b. Vitamin C deficiency
   c. Xerophthalmia d. PEM
2. **Acrodermatitis enteropathica is due to deficiency of** *[NBE FMGE September 2012, Recent Questions 2012, 2017]*
   a. Molybdenum b. Copper
   c. Zinc d. Calcium
3. **Phrynoderma is NOT due to deficiency of** *[Recent Questions 2012, 2013]*
   a. EFA b. Vitamin A
   c. Vitamin C d. Vitamin D
4. **Vitamin playing a role in preventing miliaria rubra** *[NBE DNB 1992]*
   a. A
   b. B
   c. C
   d. E
5. **Raynaud's phenomenon has typical progression of Colour change as follows** *[NBE FMGE March 2012]*
   a. Red, Blue, White
   b. Red, White, Blue
   c. Blue, Red, White
   d. White, Blue, Red

HIGH YIELD MCQs

1. **Gluten free diet is beneficial in** *[Kerala PGMEE 1996]*
   a. Psoriasis
   b. Exfoliative dermatitis
   c. Dermatitis herpetiformis
   d. Pemphigoid
2. **What can patient with gluten sensitive hypersensitivity consume as food?** *[PGI 2006]*
   a. Rice b. Barley
   c. Oat d. Corn
   e. Rye
3. **Dermatitis and alopecia are due to deficiency of** *[SGPGI 2001]*
   a. Zinc b. Molybodenum
   c. Magnesium d. Calcium
4. **Casal's paint necklace is caused by** *[Recent Question 2017, PGI 1997]*
   a. Lichen planus b. Pellagra
   c. Pernicious anemia d. SLE
5. **All are true about Acrodermatitisenteropathica except** *[AIIMS PGMEE 2008]*
   a. Decreased Zinc level
   b. Reverse with Zn supplement
   c. Triad of acral dermatitis, dementia & diarrhea
   d. Autosomal recessive
6. **Phrynoderma is a cutaneous manifestation of severe deficiency of vitamin** *[DPG 1999, AMU PGMEE 1998]*
   a. A b. B
   c. C d. D
7. **Acrodermatitis enteropathica is due to deficiency of** *[AIIMS PGMEE 1993, TN PGMEE 1997]*
   a. Zn b. Se
   c. Cu d. Cr
8. **Flaky pain appearance of skin is seen in** *[All India PGMEE 1995]*
   a. Dermatitis b. Pellagra
   c. Marasmus d. Kwashiorkor

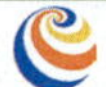 NEET/NBE PATTERN MCQs ANSWERS WITH EXPLANATIONS 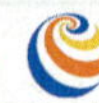

1. **Ans. (d) PEM**
   [Ref. Neena Khanna, 4/e p389]

   Skin Manifestations of Protein Energy Malnutrition (PEM)
   - *'Crazy pavement'* like skin (parchment)
   - *'Flag sign'* in hair (alternate bands of light and dark colours)

2. **Ans. (c) Zinc**
   [Ref. Neena Khanna, 5/e p 422]
   - **Acrodermatitis enteropathica**: Autosomal recessive trait with to deficient zinc transporter protein

3. **Ans. (d) Vitamin D**
   [Ref. Neena Khanna, 5/e p 422; Ragunatha S, Kumar VJ, Murugesh SB. A Clinical Study of 125 Patients with Phrynoderma. IJD, 2011;56(4): 389-392]

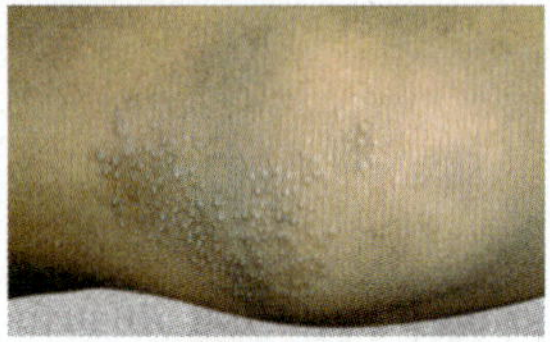

Fig. Phrynoderma

   Phrynoderma
   - Phrynoderma (toad skin) characterized by spiny hyperkeratotic follicular papules
   - Distribution of lesions is bilateral and symmetrical in 70% of patients
   - Disease is localized elbows, knees, extensor extremities, and/or buttocks
   - Deficiencies of vitamins A and E, B complex vitamins, and essential fatty acids have all been implicated in the etiology of follicular hyperkeratosis
   - Phrynoderma is associated with nutritional deficiencies
   - It is endemic to poor populations but is rare in developed countries
   - In developed countries, phrynoderma most often occurs as a result of malabsorption due to surgical or medical causes, such as small-bowel bypass surgery, colectomy and pancreatic insufficiency.

4. **Ans. (c) C**
   [Ref. Illustrated Textbook of Dermatology by JS Pasricha, 4/e p142]
   - Vitamin C in a dose of 500 mg twice daily helps to prevent miliaria rubra

5. **Ans. (d) White, Blue, Red**
   [Ref. Neena Khanna, 4/e p162]

   Triphasic/ Colour Changes in Raynaud's Phenomenon
   [Mnemonic: PCR]
   - **P**allor/White: Skin turns pale upon exposure to cold due to markedly reduced blood supply
   - **C**yanosis/Blue: Depletion of oxygen supply
   - **R**ubor/Red: If episode subsides or skin is warmed, skin becomes red then returns to normal due to return of blood flow

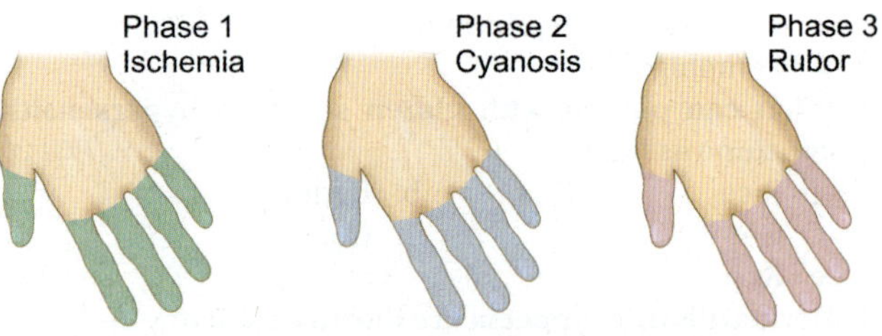

Fig. Raynaud's phenomenon

 HIGH YIELD MCQs ANSWERS WITH EXPLANATIONS

1. **Ans. (c) Dermatitis herpetiformis**
   [Ref. Neena Khanna, 5/e p 91]
   - Gluten-free diet is slow to act on the skin lesion (several months) of Dermatitis herpetiformis though the bowel changes revert to normal quickly

2. **Ans. (a) Rice; (d) Corn**
   [Ref. Neena Khanna, 5/e p 91]
   - **Gluten** is found in grains such as wheat, barley, rye, and a cross between wheat and rye called triticale
   - A gluten-free diet is a diet that excludes the protein gluten
   - Intake of oat is controversial

3. **Ans. (a) Zinc**
   [Ref. Nutrition for Healthy Skin by Krutmann, 1/e p8]
   - Zinc deficiency is known for the Classic Triad of,
     - Dermatitis
     - Alopecia
     - Diarrhoea

4. **Ans. (b) Pellagra**
   [Ref. API Textbook of Medicine by Y P Munjal, 9/e p533]
   - Deficiency of Niacin leads to Pellagra
   - Sharply outlined brownish plaques around the neck leads to the typical **"Casal's necklace"**

5. **Ans. (c) Triad of Acral dermatitis, dementia & diarrhea**
   [Ref. Neena Khanna, 5/e p 422]

6. **Ans. (a) A**
   [Ref. Neena Khanna, 5/e p 422; Ragunatha S, Kumar VJ, Murugesh SB. A Clinical Study of 125 Patients with Phrynoderma. IJD, 2011;56(4):389-392]
   - Deficiencies of vitamins A and E, B complex vitamins, and essential fatty acids have all been implicated in the etiology of **follicular hyperkeratosis**
   - Most characteristic is EFA deficiency and Vitamin A deficiency

7. **Ans. (a) Zinc**
   [Ref. Neena Khanna, 5/e p 422]

8. **Ans. (d) Kwashiorkor**
   [Ref. Therapeutic Pediatric Nutrition by Sharma Madhu, 1/e p5]
   - Children with Kwashiorkor have characteristic skin lesions, with alternating zones of hyperpigmentation, areas of desquamation, and hypopigmentation, giving a ***"flaky paint" appearance***.

Chapter 4

Infective Disorders

THEORETICAL CONCEPTS

IV A. CLASSIFICATION OF INFECTIVE DISORDERS[Q]

Diseases caused by resident flora
Pitted keratolysis Erythrasma Trichomycosis axillaris
Bacterial infections
Pyodermas (Impetigo, SSSS, Ecthyma, Folliculitis, Furuncle, Carbuncle, Erysipelas) Cutaneous TB (Lupus vulgaris, Scrofuloderma, TB verrucosa cutis) Leprosy
Viral infections
Warts Molluscum contagiosum Varicella-Zoster infections (Varicella, Herpes zoster) Herpes simplex infections (Type I, Type II) Viral exanthems (Measles, Rubella, Kawasaki syndrome)
Fungal infections
Dermatophytic infections (Tinea capitis, T. corporis, T. cruris, T. unguium) Pityriasis versicolor Candidiasis Deep fungal infections (Mycetoma, Sporotrichosis)

IV B. DISEASES CAUSED BY RESIDENT FLORA

IV B1. Pitted Keratolysis

Causative agent: **Corynebacterium spp (Micrococcus sedentarius)**
Characteristic feature: **Cribriform pattern of punched-out pits due to digestion of keratin by bacteria**

IV B2. Erythrasma

Causative agent: **Corynebacterium minutissimum[Q]**
Characteristic feature: **Creasing/ crinkling of lesions in inter-digital, groin, axillary areas**
Wood's lamp examination: **Coral-red fluorescence[Q]**

Fig. Coral-red fluorescence

IV C. BACTERIAL INFECTIONS

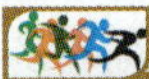

Topper's Edge

Bacterial Pyodermas

Staphylococcus aureus[Q]	
Follicular	Superficial folliculitis, Deep folliculitis, Carbuncle, Furuncle
Non-follicular	Bullous impetigo, Impetigo contagiosa, Ecthyma
Streptococcus pyogenes[Q]	
Localised	Impetigo contagiosa, Ecthyma
Spreading	Erysipelas, Cellulitis

IV C1. Impetigo Contagiosa

- *Causative agent*:
  - Staphylococcus aureus[Q]
  - Streptococcus pyogenes[Q]
- *Characteristic feature*: **Honey-coloured crusts**[Q]

IV C2. Bullous Impetigo

- *Causative agent*: Staphylococcus aureus[Q]
- *Characteristic feature*: Bullae with turbid fluid leading to **'varnish-like crusts'** in infants

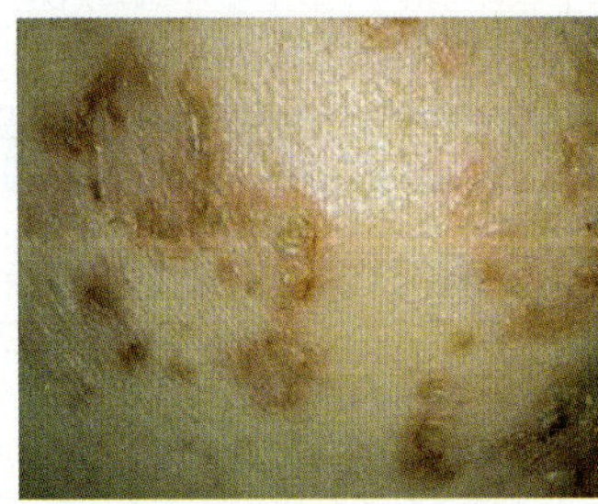

Fig. Impetigo contagiosa

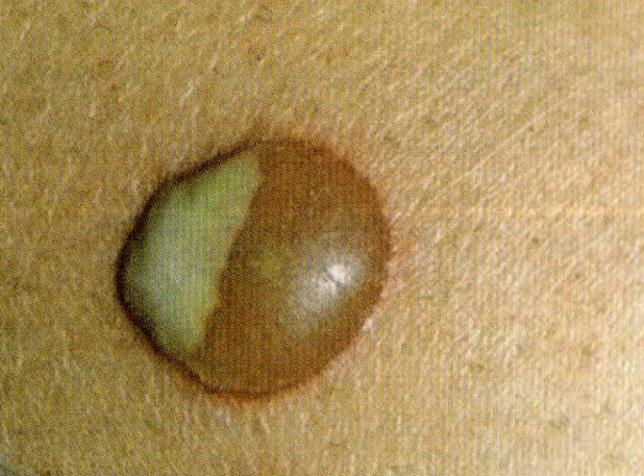

Fig. Bullous impetigo

Topper's Edge

Impetigo Contagiosa Vs Bullous Impetigo

	Impetigo Contagiosa	Bullous Impetigo
Cause[Q]	Staph aureus/ Staph pyogenes	Staph aureus
Age	Children	Infants
Bullae	Thin-walled, transient	Thick-walled, persistent
Erythematous halo	Common	Absent
Crusts	**Thick, Honey-coloured**[Q]	**Thin, Varnish-like**[Q]
Central clearing	Absent	Present
Site	Face	Face, Other parts

IV C3. Staphylococcus Scalded Skin Syndrome (SSSS)

- *Causative agent*: Staphylococcus aureus[Q]
- *Characteristic feature*: **Superficial peeling of skin in infants**

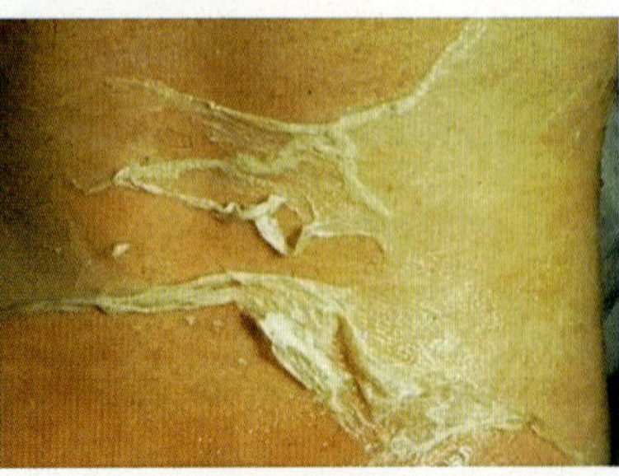

Fig. SSSS

Topper's Edge

Staphylococcal Scalded Skin Syndrome Vs Epidermal Necrolysis

	SSSS	EN
Etiology	**Staph aureus**	**Drugs**
Age	Infancy[Q]	All age groups
Skin lesions	Superficial[Q]	Deep seated
Mucosal involvement	Absent	Present
Constitutional symptoms	Absent	Present
Treatment	Antibiotics	Avoid drug, Steroids

IV C4. Ecthyma

- *Causative agent*:
  - Staphylococcus aureus[Q]
  - Streptococcus pyogenes
- *Characteristic feature*: Consequence of neglected Impetigo contagiosa[Q]

IV C5. Superficial Folliculitis

- *Causative agent*:
  - Staphylococcus aureus
  - Mineral oils, Vegetable oils
- *Characteristic feature*: Dome-shaped follicular pustules

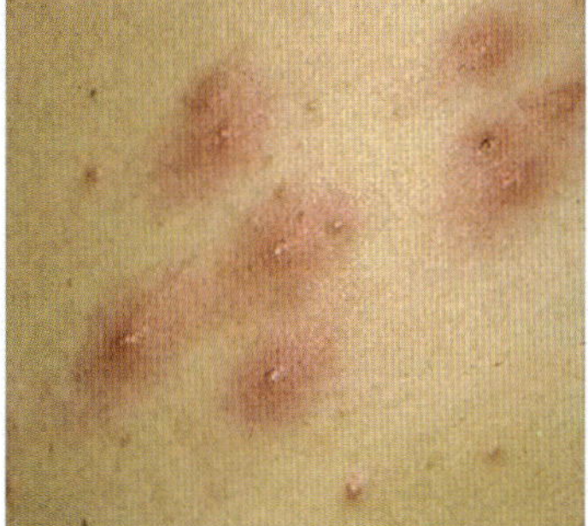

Fig. Folliculitis

IV C6. Deep Folliculitis

- *Causative agent*: Staphylococcus aureus
- *Characteristic feature*:
  - Deep-seated erythematous follicular pustules
  - Common in beard area (Sycosis barbae) and scalp

IV C7. Furuncles/ Boils

- ***Causative agent*: Staphylococcus aureus**[Q]
- *Predisposing factors*:[Q]
  - Nasal carriage
  - HIV, Diabetes mellitus
  - Scabies, Atopic dermatitis
- *Characteristic feature*:
  - Tender, firm, red, follicular nodules
  - Common in hair-bearing friction-prone sites in adolescent boys
- *Treatment*:
  - *Acute form*: Topical Mupirocin/ Sodium-flusidate, Systemic Flucloxacillin
  - *Chronic (recurrent) form*: Antibiotics, Rifampicin[Q]

IV C8. Carbuncle

- *Causative agent*: **Staphylococcus aureus**[Q]
- *Predisposing factors*:
  - Diabetes mellitus
  - Systemic steroids
- *Characteristic feature*:
- Multiple erythrematous pus-discharging plaques

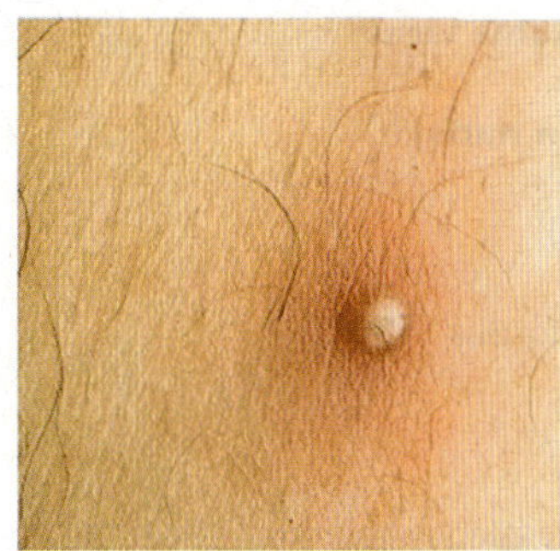

Fig. Furuncle

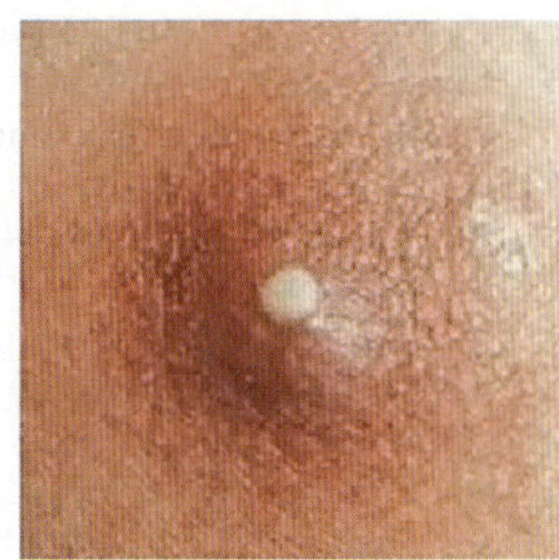

Fig. Carbuncle

Skin and STDs

IV C9. Erysipelas and Cellulitis

- *Causative agent*:
  - **Streptococcus pyogenes**[Q]
  - Staphylococcus aureus (less frequent)
- *Predisposing factors*:
  - Lymphoedema
  - Venous stasis
  - Intertrigo
  - Obesity
- *Characteristic feature*:
  - Warm indurated plaques
  - Commonly in lower limbs

IV C10. Cutaneous Tuberculosis

- *Causative agent*: Mycobacterium tuberculosis
- *Clinical types*:[Q]

Lupus vulgaris[Q]	Annular plaques with peripheral nodules **Apple-jelly nodules**[Q]
Scrofuloderma[Q]	Skin connected from underlying TB focus Chronic sinus with hyperpigmented edges
Tuberculosis verrucosa cutis	Single, indurated plaque on acral parts Inoculation tuberculosis
Tuberculides *Lichen scrofulosorum*[Q] *Papulonecrotic tuberculide*	Hypersensitivity reactions to Mycobacterium TB[Q]

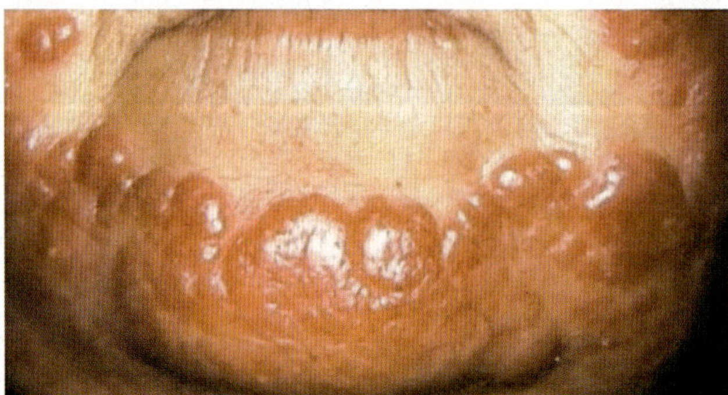

Fig. Apple-jelly nodules

IV D. VIRAL INFECTIONS

IV D1. Warts

- *Causative agent*: **Human Papilloma Virus**[Q]
- *Clinical types*:
  - **Verruca vulgaris (Common warts)**[Q]
  - Palmoplantar warts
  - Verruca plana (Plane warts)
  - Filiform warts
  - Epidermodysplasia verruciformis
  - Anogenital warts (STD)
- *Treatment*:
  - Cryotherapy
  - Electric cautery and radiofrequency ablation (RFA)
  - Topical agents: Salicylic acid, Wart paint, Retinoic acid, Formalin soaks

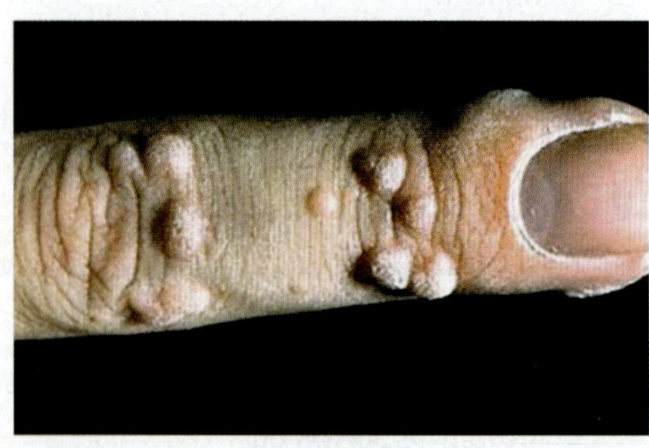

Fig. Warts

IV D2. Molluscum Contagiosum

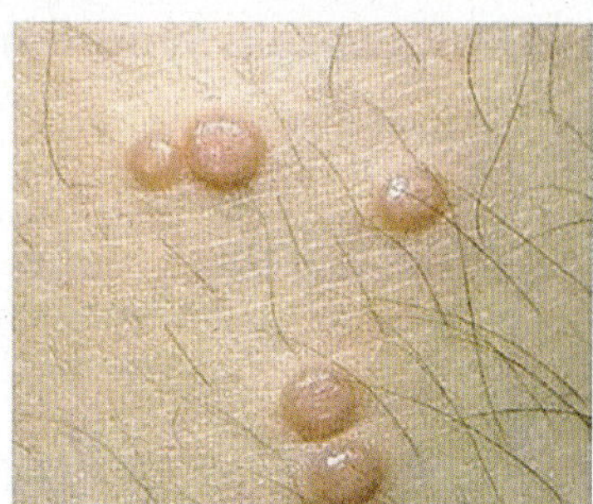
Fig. Molluscum contagiosum

- *Causative agent*: Pox Virus[Q]
- *Clinical presentation*:
  - Pearly white, ***'umblicated'* dome-shaped papules**[Q]
  - Pseudo-isomorphic phenomenon
  - White cheesy material on incision
- *Treatment*:
  - Cryotherapy
  - Chemical cautery
  - Wart paint

IV D3. Varicella Zoster/ Chicken Pox

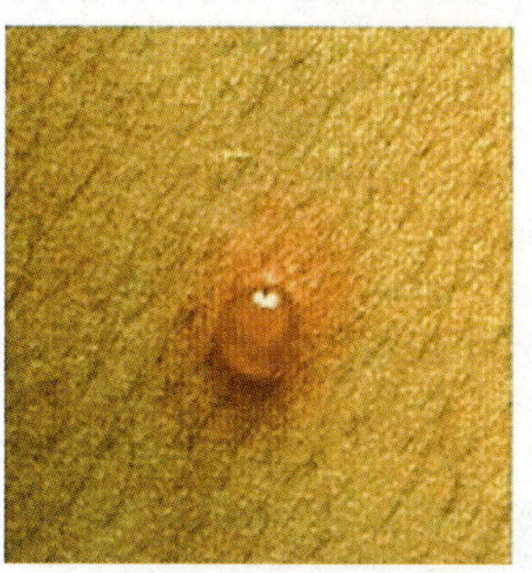
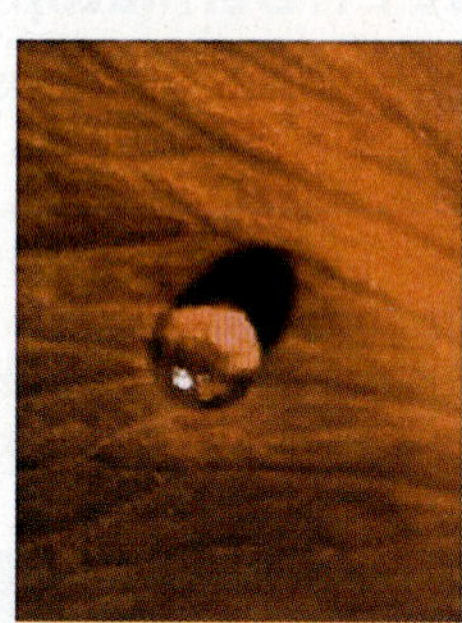
Fig. Dew-drop on Rose-petal appearance

- *Causative agent*: Varicella-Zoster Virus
- *Clinical presentation*:
  - Pleomorphism (All stages of rash at same time on body)[Q]
  - ***Dew-drop on rose-petal'* appearance**[Q]
  - Centripetal distribution[Q]
  - Superficial, unilocular, axilla/ flexor surfaces rash
- *Treatment*:
  - Calamine, Antihistamine
  - Severe cases: Acyclovir, Famciclovir

IV D4. Herpes Zoster/ Shingles

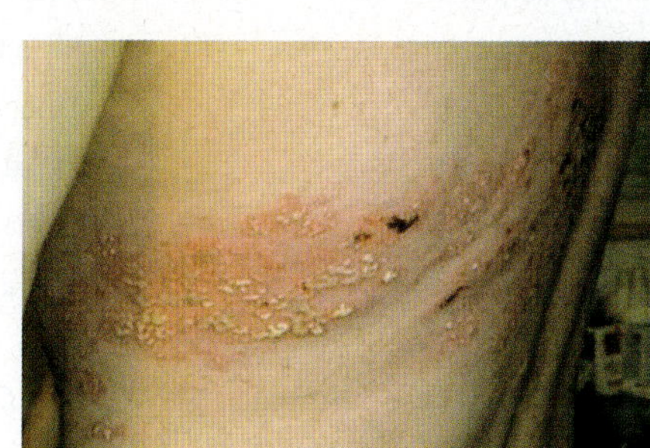
Fig. Dermatomal distribution

- *Causative agent*: Varicella-Zoster Virus (reactivation after dormancy in sensory root ganglion)[Q]
- *Clinical presentation*:
  - Severe pain
  - Grouped vesicles in segmental/ dermatomal distribution[Q]
- *Complications*: Post-herpetic neuralgia, Hutchison's sign
- *Treatment*:
  - NSAIDs
  - Acyclovir, Famciclovir, Valcyclovir

IV D5. Herpes Simplex Virus Infections

- *Causative agent*: HSV hominis
  - **Type I**: Cause Herpes labialis and infections above waist[Q]
  - **Type II**: Causes peri-genital infection[Q]
- *Clinical presentation*:
  - Primary infection: Acute gingivostomatitis (Type I), Grouped painful vesicles (Type II)
  - Recurrent infection: Grouped vesicles with polycyclic margins on lips/ genitals
- *Complications*: [Q]
  - Erythema multiforme
  - Eczema herpeticum[Q]
  - Herpetic encephalitis
  - Herpes simplex keratitis/ Dendritic ulcers
  - Disseminated cutaneous HSV infection
- *Treatment*:
  - Symptomatic treatment
  - Acyclovir, Famciclovir, Valcyclovir

IV D6. Measles

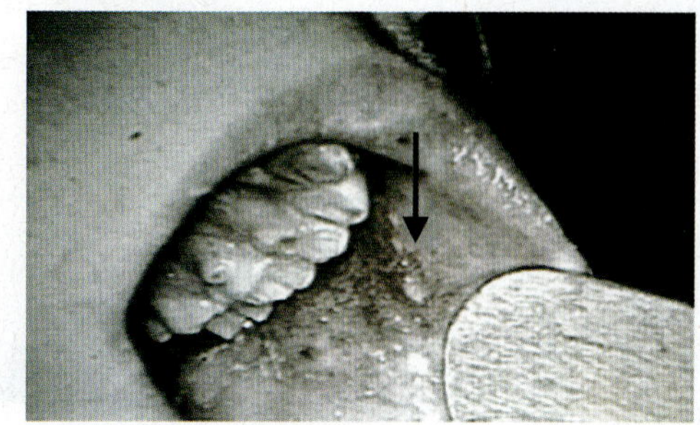
Fig. Koplik spot

- *Causative agent*: Rubeolla virus (Paramyxovirus)
- *Clinical presentation*:
  - Maculo-papular confluent rash
  - **Koplik spots** (on buccal mucosa opposite Lower 2nd molar)[Q]
- *Treatment*: Symptomatic treatment

IV D7. Kawasaki Syndrome (Mucocutaneous Lymph Node Syndrome)

- *Causative agent*: Antecedent Corona virus infection (possibly)[Q]
- *Clinical presentation*:
  - Non-exudative conjunctivitis
  - Oropharyngeal lesions, fissured lips, **strawberry tongue**
  - Cervical lymphadenopathy
- *Treatment*: Aspirin, Gamma-globulin

IV E. FUNGAL INFECTIONS

IV E1. Dermatophytic/ Ring-worm Infections

- *Causative agent*: Keratinophilic fungi[Q]
  - Trichophyton
  - Microsporum
  - Epidermophyton
- *Clinical presentation*:
  - Annular lesion with lichenification in centre
  - Centrifugal spread
- *Types of Tinea*: [Q]

Type of Tinea	Body part affected	Feature
Tinea capitis[Q]	Tinea of scalp	Discoid alopecia
Tinea corporis	Tinea of trunk and limbs	In hairless skin
Tinea incognito[Q]	Modified by steroid therapy	-
Tinea cruris[Q]	Tinea of groin	Inner region of thighs
Tinea pedis	Tinea of feet	Athlete's foot[Q]
Tinea mannum	Tinea of hands	Plaques or Erythema
Tinea unguium[Q]	Tinea of nails (Onchomycosis)	Tunneling, Subungal hyperkeratosis, Oncholysis

- *Treatment*:
  - Topical antifungals: Miconazole, Clotrimazole, Ketoconazole, Terbinafine, Ciclopirox
  - Systemic antifungals: Terbinafine, Griseofulvin, Itraconazole

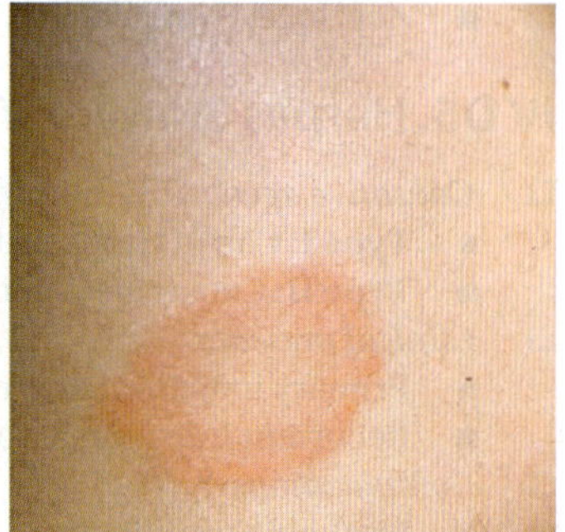

Fig. Ringworm

IV E2. Pityriasis Versicolor

- *Causative agent*: **Malassezia furfur**[Q]
- *Clinical presentation*:
  - Asymptomatic[Q]
  - Scaly, perifollicular macules
  - *KOH mount*: **Spaghetti and meat balls appearance**[Q]
- *Treatment*:
  - Topical antifungals: Ketoconazole, Selenium sulphide
  - Systemic antifungals: Ketoconazole, Fluconazole, Itraconazole

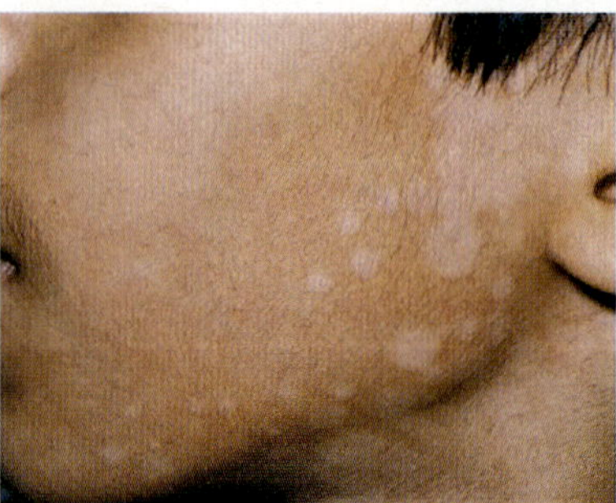

Fig. Scaly perifollicular macules

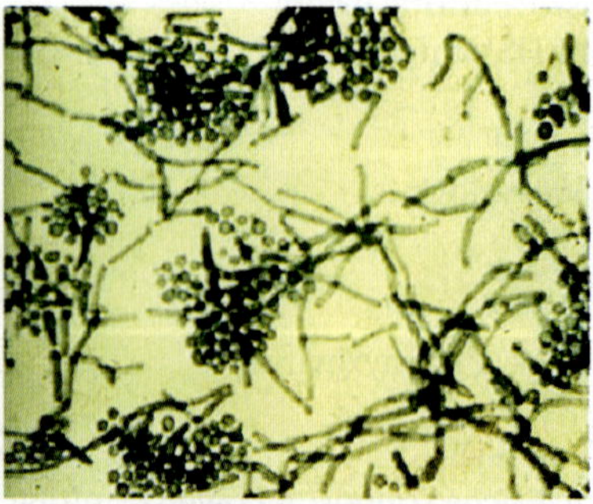

Fig. KOH: Spaghetti and meatballs

IV E3. Candidiasis

- *Causative agent*: Candida albicans
- *Predisposing factors*: **[Mnemonic: M**an **I**n **P**leasant **MOOD]**[Q]
  - **M**oisture
  - **I**mmuno-compromised states (HIV)
  - **P**regnancy
  - **M**etronidazole
  - **O**besity
  - **O**ral contraceptive pills (OCPs)
  - **D**iabetes
- *Clinical presentation*:

Type of candidiasis	Body part	Feature
Acute mucocutaneous candidiasis		
Intertrigo candidiasis	**Flexures**[Q]	Frayed scaling, pustules
Candidial paronychia	Nails	Red, swollen nail-fold
Genital candidiasis	Genitalia	Vulvovaginitis Balanoposthitis[Q]
Oral candidiasis	Oral mucosa	Thrush (Most common)[Q] Angular stomatitis Leucoplakia
Chronic mucocutaneous candidiasis		In endocrinopathies
Systemic candidiasis		In leucopenia, HIV patients[Q]

- *Treatment*:
  - Topical antifungals: Imidazoles, Amphotericin, Nystatin
  - Systemic antifungals: Fluconazole

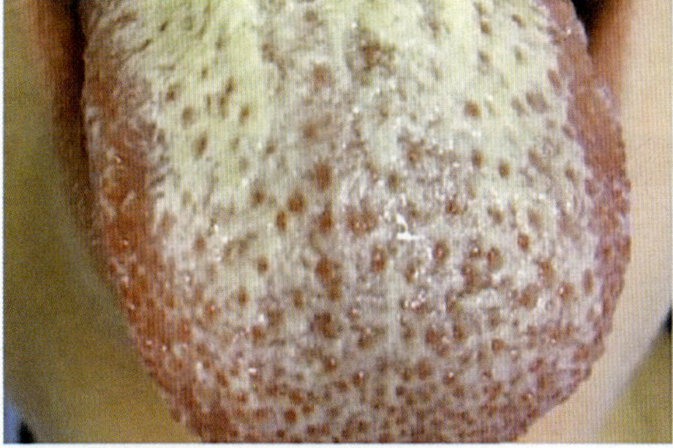
Fig. Oral thrush

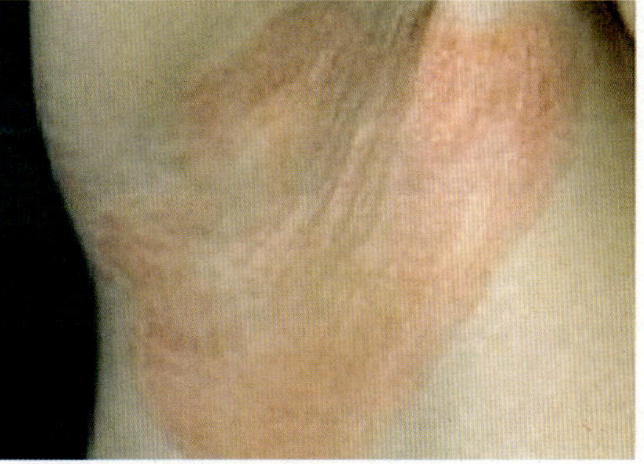
Fig. Intertrigo candidiasis

IV E4. Mycetoma

- *Causative agent*:[Q]

Actinomycetoma	Eumycetoma
Nocardia braziliensis	Madurelle mycetomatis
Streptomyces	Madurelle grisea
Actinomadura madurae	Petriellidium boydii

- *Clinical presentation*:
- Subcutaneous nodules, abscesses, sinuses
- *Most common site*: **Foot**[Q]
- *Treatment*:

Skin and STDs

Actinomycetoma	Eumycetoma
Streptomycin Dapsone Cotrimoxazole Penicillin Tetracyclines	Ketoconazole Itraconzole Amphotericin B

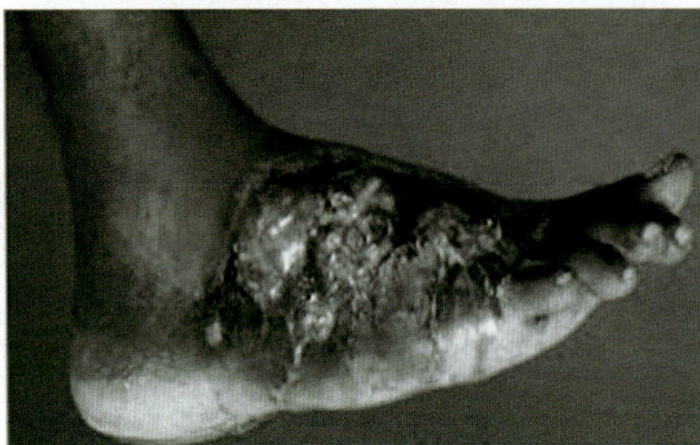
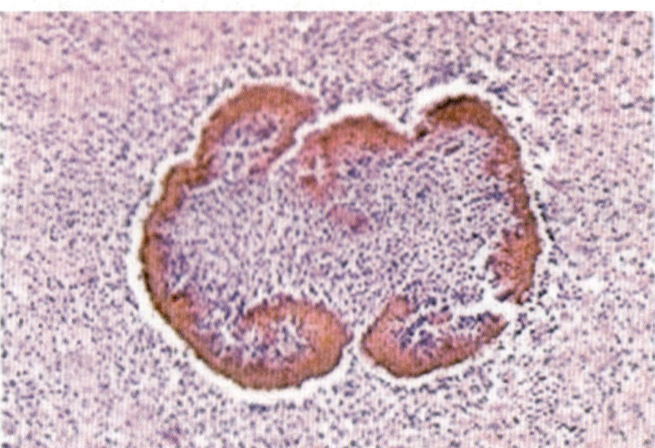

Fig. Mycetoma

IV F. SCABIES

- *Underlying cause*: Sarcoptes scabei var. hominis **(Itch mite)**[Q]
- *Route of transmission*:
  - Skin contact
  - Sexual transmission
  - Fomite transmission
  - Mite burrows through stratum corneum and lays eggs
  - *Clinical presentation*:
  - Asymptomatic
  - Sever itching more severe at night[Q]

Primary lesions	Secondary lesions
Burrows (Pathogonomic lesion)	Pustules
Papules	Eczema
Papulo-vesicles	Nodular lesions

- *Sites involved*: Webs of fingers, Flexures
- *Complications*:
  - Eczematization
  - Acute post-streptococcal glomerulonephritis[Q]
  - Secondary infection with Staph. aureus and Strep. pyogenes
- *Treatment of Scabies*:

Topical applications	
5% Permethrin	**Drug of choice for Scabies**[Q]
25% Benzyl benzoate	Older drug of choice
1% Gammaxene/ BHC	Can cause seizures, avoided in infants[Q]
10% Crotamiton	Useful in children
10% Sulphur	Useful in children
Oral medications Ivermectin	Useful in epidemic, Norwegian form[Q]

Skin and STDs

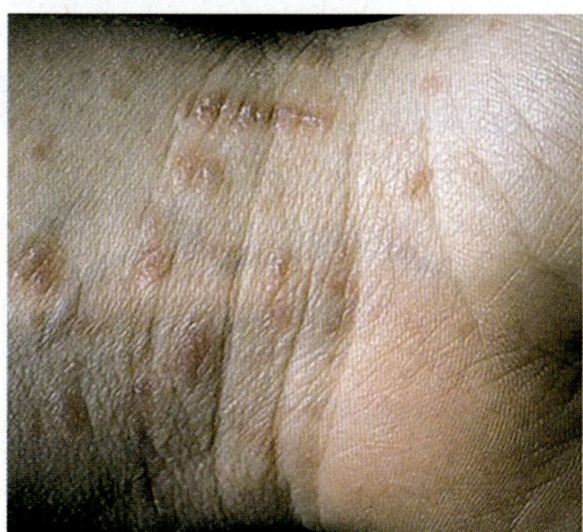

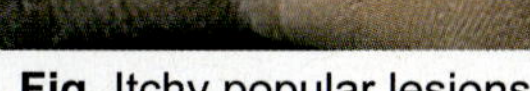

Fig. Itchy popular lesions

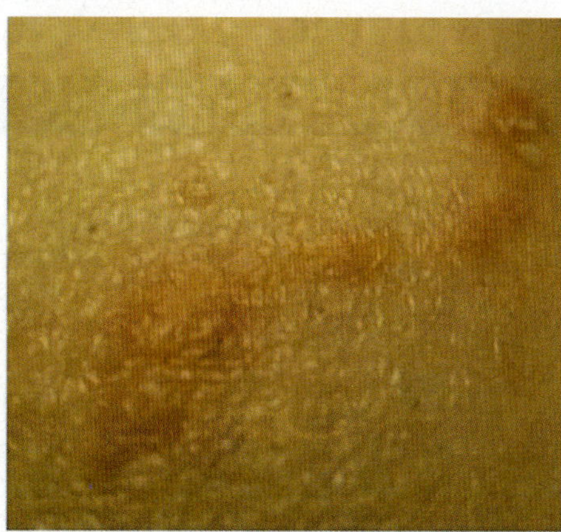

Fig. Burrow

IV G. EXANTHEMATA

CAUSES OF EXANTHEMATA				
Morbilliform				**Scantiliform**
Bacterial	**Viral**	**Drugs**	**Others**	
Typhoid Syphilis Meningococcus Rickettsia	Measles Rubella Cytomegalovirus Ebstein barr virus HIV Parvovirus B19	Penicillin Ampicillin Phenylbutazone Sulphonamides Phenytoin Gold	Kawasaki disease	Toxic shock syndrome SSSS Scarlet fever Kawasaki disease

(SSSS Staphylococcal scalded skin syndrome)

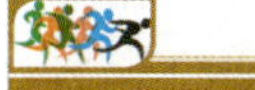

Topper's Edge

INFECTIVE DISORDERS OF SKIN

HPV types associated with Warts

- Verruca vulgaris: HPV 2, 4, 27
- Palmoplantar warts: HPV 1, 2, 4, 57
- Verruca plana[Q]: HPV 3, 10
- Epidermodysplasia verruciformis[Q]: HPV 3, 5, 8, 9
- Anogenital warts[Q]: HPV 6, 11, 16, 18, 31, 33 (6, 11 have low oncogenic potential)

Cause of Tinea capitis

- Inflammatory capitis: Zoophilic dermatophytes (M. canis)
- Non-inflammatory capitis: Anthrophilic organisms (T. verrucosum)
- Favus: T. schoenleinii[Q]
- Tinea incognito: Dermatophytic infection of skin modified by Steroid therapy[Q]

Sites of Dermatophytic infections

- Trichophyton: Skin, Hair, Nails
- Microsporum: Skin, Hair
- Epidermophyton: Skin, Nails

Must know facts

- Vertical transmission of Anogenital warts in infants (Vagina delivery) manifest as: Laryngeal papilloma[Q]
- Myrmecia: Deep palmoplantar warts[Q]
- Plane warts: Verruca plana

IMAGE-BASED QUESTIONS

1. **Organism causing Condition shown in Photograph is**

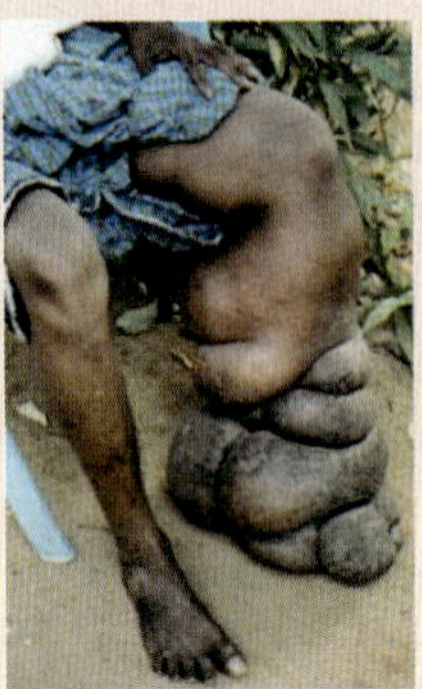

a. Mycobacterium tuberculosis
b. Mycobacterium leprae
c. Wuchereria bancrofti
d. HIV

2. **Identify the Infective disorder of skin as shown in Photograph**

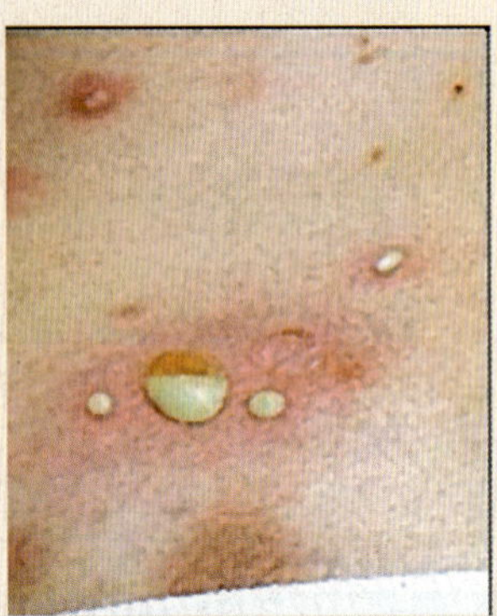

a. Pyoderma
b. SSSS
c. Bullous impetigo
d. Impetigo contagiosa

3. **Identify the Infective disorder of skin as shown in Photograph**

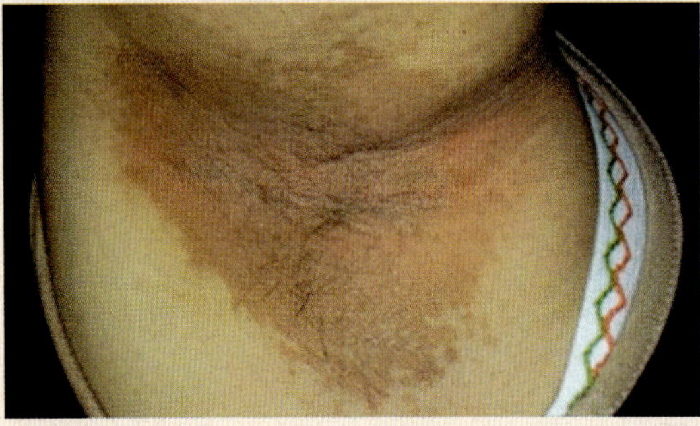

a. Leprosy
b. Pyoderma
c. Erythrasma
d. Impetigo

4. **Identify Infective disorder of skin as shown** ***[Recent Question 2013]***

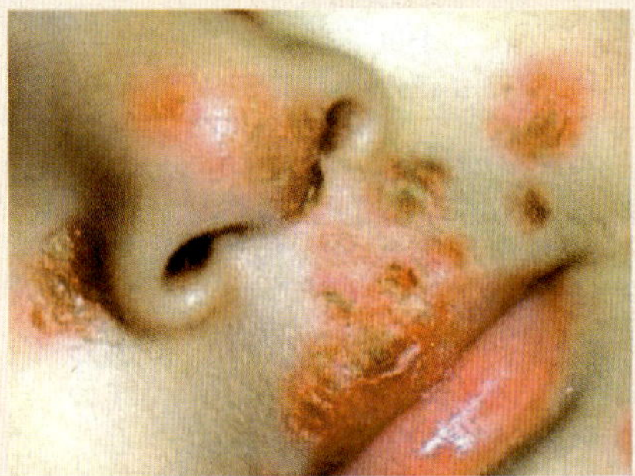

a. Pyoderma
b. SSSS
c. Bullous impetigo
d. Impetigo contagiosa

5. **Identify the Infective disorder of skin as shown in Photograph** ***[Recent Question 2013]***

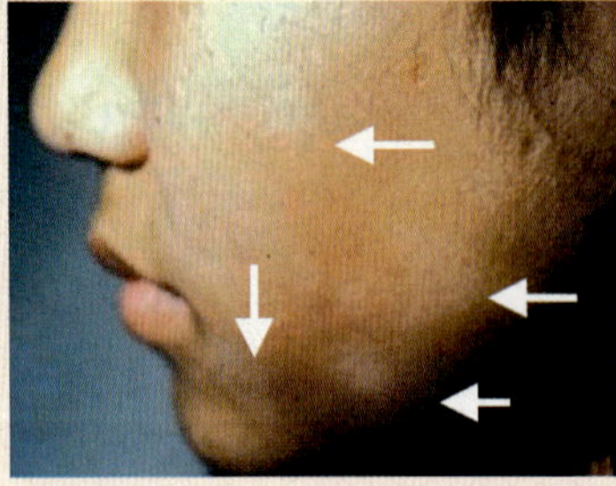

a. Verruca plana
b. Tuberculoid leprosy
c. P. alba
d. TB scrofuloderma

6. **Identify the Infective disorder of skin as shown in Photograph** ***[Recent Question 2014]***

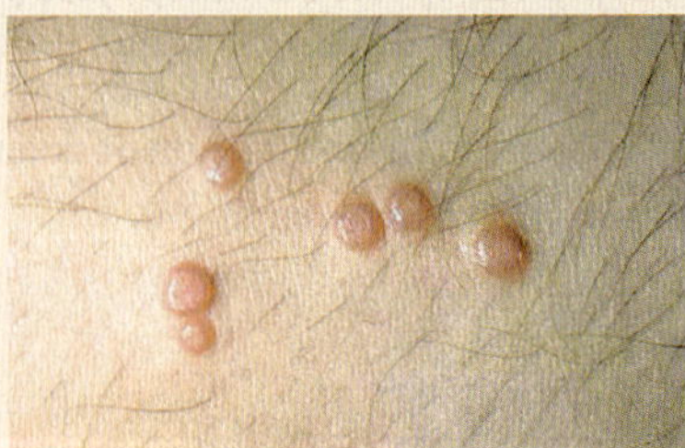

a. Verruca plana
b. Varicella
c. Warts
d. Molluscum contagiosum

7. Identify the Infective disorder of skin as shown in Photograph

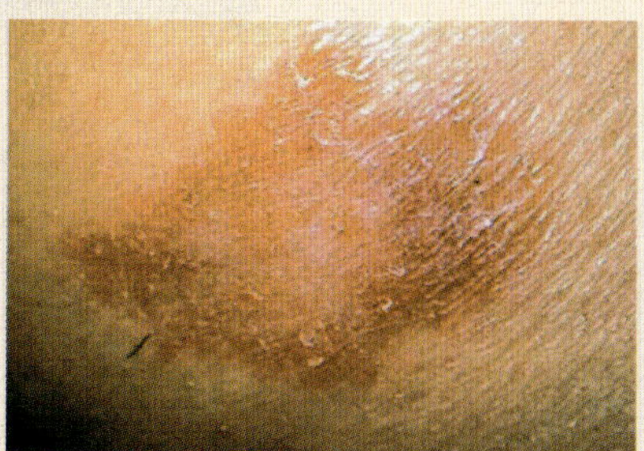

a. Scrofuloderma
b. Lupus vulgaris
c. Tuberculous verrucosa cutis
d. Lichen scrofulosum

8. Identify the Infective disorder of skin as shown in Photograph ***[Recent Question 2013]***

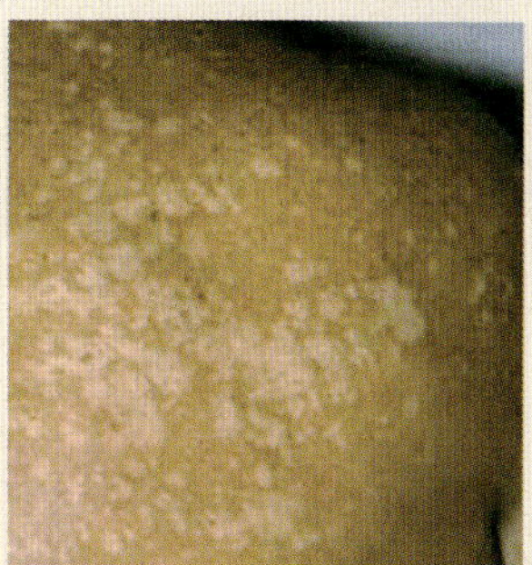

a. P. alba
b. P. versicolor
c. Tuberculosis scrofuloderma
d. Leprosy tuberculoid

9. Identify the Infective disorder of skin as shown in Photograph

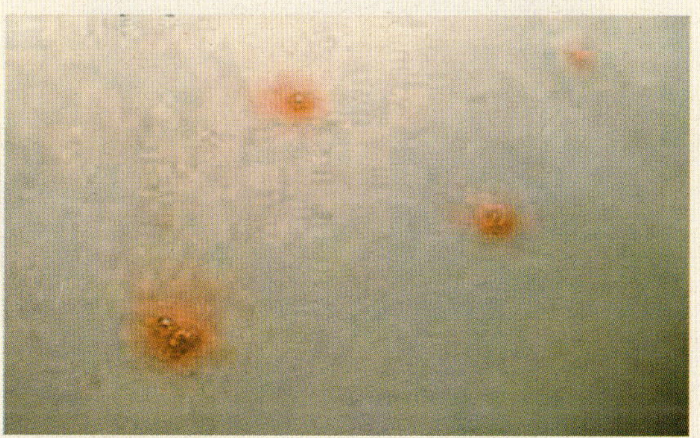

a. Verruca plana
b. Varicella
c. Warts
d. Molluscum contagiosum

10. Identify the Infective disorder of skin as shown in Photograph

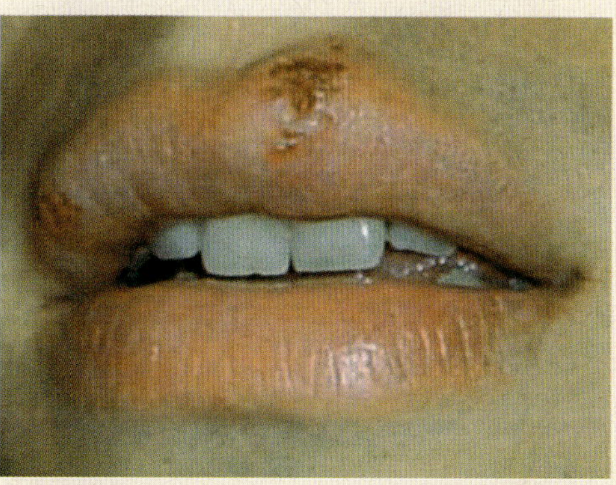

a. Varicella
b. Herpes zoster
c. Herpes simplex
d. Eczema herpeticum

11. Identify the Infective disorder of skin as shown in Photograph

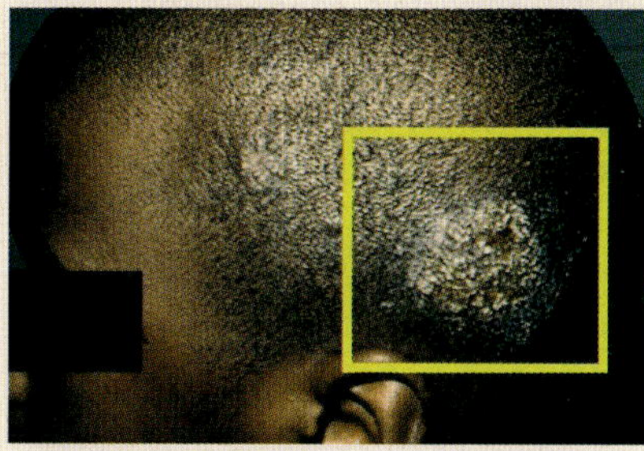

a. Non-inflammatory Tinea capitis
b. Kerion
c. Verruca plana
d. TB Scrofuloderma

12. Identify the Infective disorder of skin as shown in Photograph

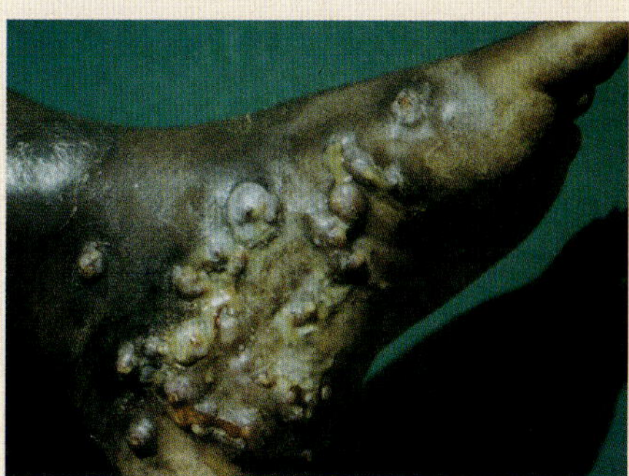

a. Candida
b. Sporotrichosis
c. Mycetoma
d. T. pedis

13. Identify the Infective disorder of skin as shown in Photograph ***[Recent Question 2012]***

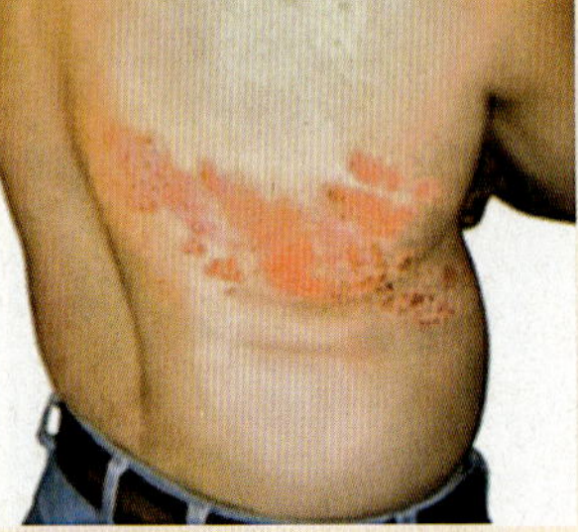

a. Herpes zoster
b. Lepromatous leprosy
c. Tinea corporis
d. Eczema herpticum

14. Itchy papular lesions on Wrist as shown in Photograph is ***[Recent Question 2012]***

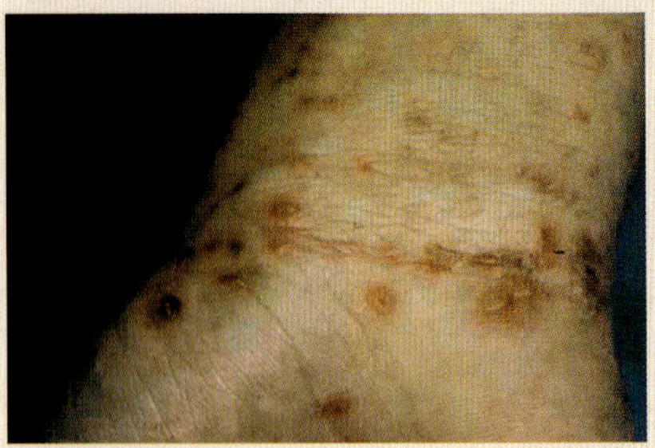

a. Myiasis
b. Pediculus corporis
c. Scabies
d. Larva migrans

15. Identify the condition shown for Penis ***[Recent Question 2014]***

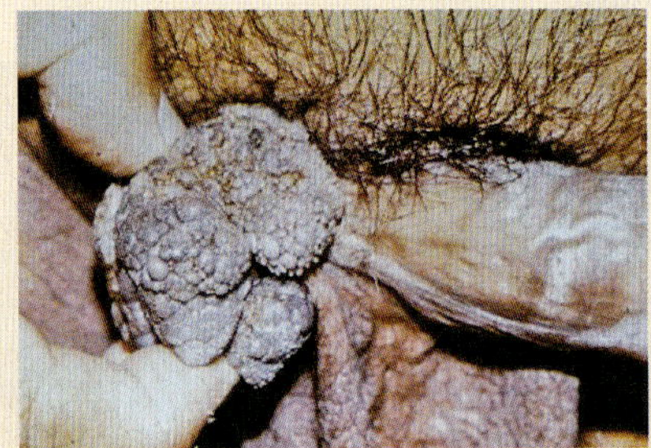

a. Herpes genitalis
b. Genital wart
c. Buschke-Lowenstein tumour
d. HIV

16. Identify condition of a 1 day old newborn child in Photograph ***[Recent Question 2014]***

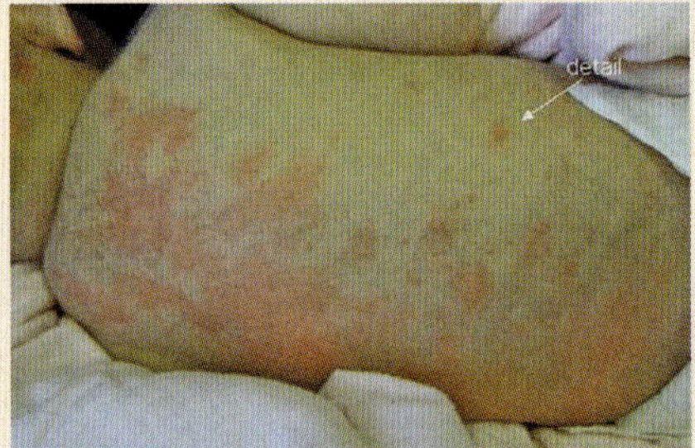

a. Measles
b. Erythema neonatorum
c. Drug eruption
d. Scabies

17. A 28 years old Lady has small dome shaped asymptomatic papules on her forehead since last 2 months. Her 2 year old daughter also has similar lesions. Probable diagnosis ***[AIIMS November 2015]***

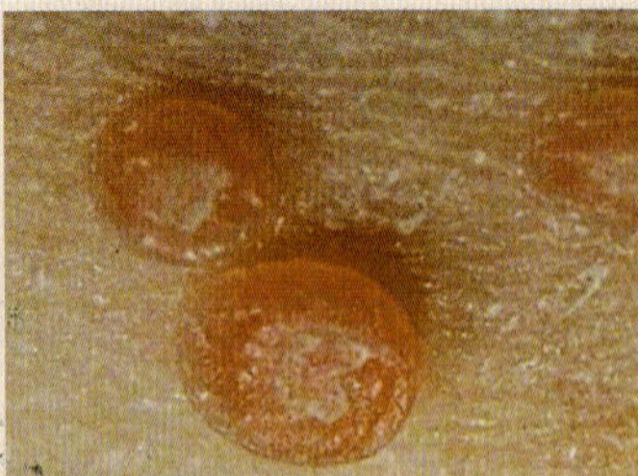

a. HHV 6
b. Papilloma virus
c. Pox virus
d. Coxsackie virus

18. A 26 years old man from Bihar presented with juicy looking papules over face (See Photograph) and back of neck. Papules were hypopigmented and normoaesthetic with no nerve thickening. History of prolonged fever in childhood was reported. Diagnosis is ***[AIIMS PG May 2015]***

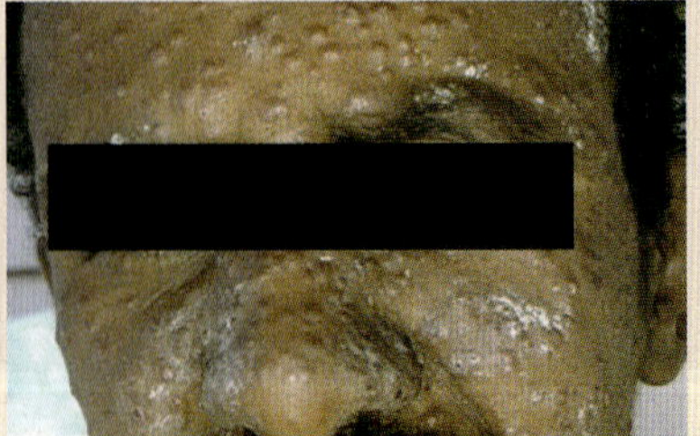

a. Tuberculoid leprosy
b. Histoid leprosyt
c. PKDL
d. Lepromatous leprosy

19. A 30 years old woman has history of fever and joint pains. She was started on NSAIDS. After 8-10 days, she presented with the following skin lesions as shown in the Photograph. Diagnosis of underlying disorder is ***[AIIMS November 2017]***

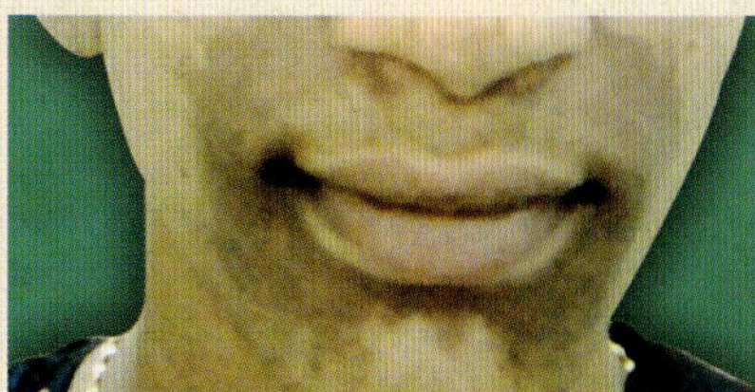

a. Dengue
b. Melasma
c. Chikungunya fever
d. Fixed drug eruption

20. Middle aged main presents with Itchy rash. Clinical presentation and Causative organism are shown in Photograph below. Diagnose the condition. ***[AIIMS November 2017]***

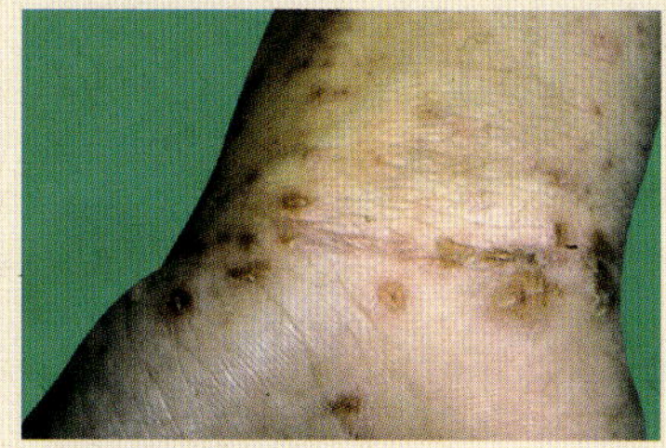

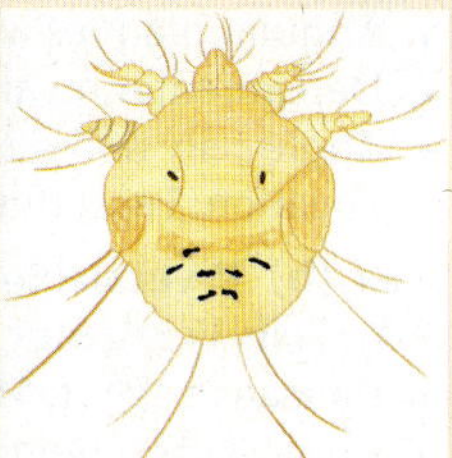

a. Tinea
b. Pediculoses
c. Scabies
d. Insect bite hypersensitivity

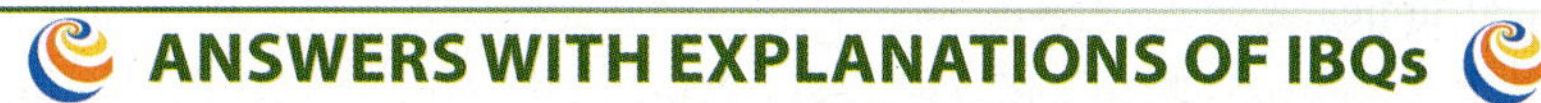

ANSWERS WITH EXPLANATIONS OF IBQs

1. Ans. (c) Wuchereria bancrofti *[Ref. Neena Khanna, 4/e p345]*

Elephantiasis
- Description: A parasitic infection that causes extreme swelling in the arms and legs
- Causative agent: Wuchereria bancrofti (Filaria worm)
- Route of transmission: Culex quinquefasciatus (fatigans) mosquito

2. Ans. (c) Bullous impetigo *[Ref. Neena Khanna, 4/e p246]*

Bullous Impetigo
- Causative agent: Staphylococcus aureus
- Characteristic feature: Bullae with turbid fluid leading to 'varnish-like crusts' in infants

3. Ans. (c) Erythrasma *[Ref. Neena Khanna, 4/e p242]*

Erythrasma
- Causative agent: Corynebacterium minutissimum
- Characteristic feature: Creasing/ crinkling of lesions in inter-digital, groin, axillary areas
- Wood's lamp examination: Coral-red fluorescence

4. Ans. (d) Impetigo contagiosa *[Ref. Neena Khanna, 4/e p245]*

Impetigo Contagiosa
- Causative agent:
  - Staphylococcus aureus
  - Streptococcus pyogenes
- Characteristic feature: Honey-coloured crusts

5. Ans. (c) P. alba *[Ref. Neena Khanna, 4/e p267]*

Pityriasis Alba
- Affects: Children and young adults
- Associated with: Atopic dermatitis
- Appearance:
  - Hypopigmented spots on face (lateral cheeks) and other areas of skin (upper forearms)
  - Dark skinned children
  - More in summer

6. Ans. (d) Molluscum contagiosum *[Ref. Neena Khanna, 4/e p274]*

Molluscum Contagiosum
- Underlying cause: Molluscum contagiosum virus
- Clinical presentation: Pearly-white 'umblicated' papules

- Treatment:
  - Cryotherapy
  - Mechanical removal with curette

7. Ans. (b) Lupus vulgaris *[Ref. Neena Khanna, 4/e p252]*

Lupus Vulgaris
- Annular plaques with peripheral nodules
- Depigmentation and scarring
- Apple-jelly nodules
- Location: Face, Buttocks

8. Ans. (b) P. versicolor *[Ref. Neena Khanna, 4/e p290]*

Pityriasis Versicolor
- Causative agent: Malassezia furfur
- Clinical presentation:
- Asymptomatic
- Scaly, perifollicular macules
- KOH mount: Spaghetti and meat balls appearance

9. Ans. (b) Varicella *[Ref. Neena Khanna, 4/e p275]*

Varicella Zoster/ Chicken Pox
- Causative agent: Varicella-Zoster Virus
- Clinical presentation:
  - Pleomorphism (All stages of rash at same time on body)
  - 'Dew-drop on rose-petal' appearance
  - Centripetal distribution
  - Superficial, unilocular, axilla/ flexor surfaces rash

10. Ans. (c) Herpes simplex *[Ref. Neena Khanna, 4/e p279]*
- Acute gingivostomatitis: Closely grouped vesicles which rapidly form polycyclic ulcers covered with a yellow pseudomembrane caused by Herpes simplex virus

11. Ans. (b) Kerion *[Ref. Neena Khanna, 4/e p284]*

Kerion
- Cause: Zoophilic dermatophytes (M. canis)
- Features:
  - Boggy swelling with postulation, pus discharge from multiple orifices
  - Pluckable hair
  - Lymphadenopathy (Occipital)

12. Ans. (c) Mycetoma *[Ref. Neena Khanna, 4/e p296]*

Mycetoma
- Subcutaneous nodules evolve as abscesses and draining sinuses
- Serosanguinous/ Seropurulent discharge
- Sites: Foot, Hands

13. Ans. (a) Herpes zoster *[Ref. Neena Khanna, 4/e p277]*

Herpes Zoster
- Dermatomal distribution of vesicles on erythematous base
- Vesicles become pustular and crusty
- Minimal scarring

14. Ans. (c) Scabies *[Ref. Neena Khanna, 4/e p341]*
- Scabies: Multiple itchy papular lesions on flexural areas especially wrists
- Primary lesions: Burrows Pathognomonic), Papules, Papulo-vesicles
- Secondary lesions: Pustules, Eczema, Nodular lesions

15. Ans. (c) Buschke-Lowenstein tumour *[Ref. Bedside Clinics in Surgery by Saha, 1/e p498]*

Buschke Lowenstein Tumour
- Giant condyloma
- A form of verrucous carcinoma of Penis
- Locally destructive invasive lesion
- Displaces, invades and destroys adjacent structure by compression
- Does not spread to Lymph nodes
- No potential for metastasis

16. Ans. (b) **Erythema neonatorum** *[Ref. Dermatology by Falco, 2/e p702]*

Erythema Toxicum Neonatorum

- Description:
- Common short-lived erythematous eruption of newborn in first 2 days of life
- *Flea bitten rash of newborn*: Widespread erythematous macules, coalesce to become urticarial pustules
- Occurrence: 30-50% of newborns develop ETN
- Underlying cause: Transition from watery womb to dry external environment
- Treatment Generally not required, Zinc oxide lotion may be used

17. Ans. (c) **Pox virus** *[Ref. Neena Khanna, 4/e p274]*

Molluscum Contagiosum

- Underlying cause: Molluscum contagiosum (Pox) virus
- Clinical presentation: Smooth dome shaped, Pearly-white 'Umblicated' papules

18. Ans. (c) **PKDL** *[Ref. Dermatology by Winkelmann, 1/e p206]*

Post Kala Azar Dermal Leishmaniasis

- Generally presents after 2-3 years of treatment of Kala azar
- Macular/ Maculo-papular/ Nodular rash start around mouth, spread to other parts of body
- Triad: Hypopigmented macules, Erythematous macules, Nodules
- High infectivity

19. Ans. (c) **Chikungunya fever** *[Ref. Pediatric Dermatology by Inamadar, 1/e p188]*

Cutaneous Lesions in Chikungunya

- Hyperpigmentation: Centrofacial/ Generalized, Freckle/ Melasma-like, Flagellate/ Streaky, Addisonian type
- Maculopapular eruption, Transient/ generalized erythema
- Pruritis, Palmoplantar desquamation
- Vesicobullous lesions, Aphthous like ulcers, Vasculitic lesions
- Lymphadenopathy, Ecchymosis, Hemorrhages

20. Ans. (c) **Scabies** *[Ref. Neena Khanna, 4/e p341]*

Scabies

- Cause: Sarcoptes scabei var. hominis (Itch mite)
- Route of transmission: Skin contact, Sexual transmission, Fomite transmission
- Clinical presentation: Asymptomatic, Severe itching more severe at night, Burrows (Pathogonomic lesion), Papules, Papulo-vesicles, Pustules, Eczema, Nodular lesions
- Sites involved: Webs of fingers, Flexures
- Treatment of Scabies: 5% Permethrin Drug of choice for Scabies

NEET/NBE PATTERN MCQs

1. **Ear papilloma is a type of** *[Recent Question 2016]*
   a. Wart b. Exostosis
   c. Cutaneous horn d. Dermoid cyst
2. **True about Chicken pox rash** *[Recent Question 2016]*
   a. Polymorphic b. Pleomorphic
   c. Centripetal d. Cytoplasmic inclusion
3. **Exanthema subitum is caused by** *[Recent Question 2016]*
   a. HSV b. HCV
   c. HIV d. HPV
4. **Characteristic lesion in Scabies is** *[Recent Question 2016, 2017]*
   a. Vesicle b. Papule
   c. Pustule d. Burrows
5. **Burrow in Scabies is in** *[Recent Question 2016]*
   a. S. germinatum b. S. granulosum
   c. Malpighian layer d. None of the above
6. **Which of the following is not a Tuberculid?** *[Recent Question 2016]*
   a. Lichen scrofuloderma
   b. Lichen nitidus
   c. Papulonecrotic tuberculide
   d. Erythema nodosum
7. **Tinea mannum affects** *[Recent Question 2016]*
   a. Face b. Hands
   c. Nails d. Foot
8. **Myrmecia warts are** *[Recent Question 2016]*
   a. Plantar warts b. Palmar warts
   c. Verrucous warts d. Plane warts
9. **Esthiomine is seen in** *[Recent Question 2016]*
   a. Chancroid b. Granuloma inguinale
   c. LGV d. Syphilis
10. **Drug of choice for Genital warts is** *[Recent Question 2016]*
    a. Acyclovir b. Podophyllin
    c. Minocycline d. Interferon alpha
11. **Not a feature of Scabies is** *[Recent Question 2016]*
    a. Serpentine burrow b. Severe itching
    c. Web space affection d. Genitalia are not affected
12. **Bullous impetigo is caused by** *[Recent Question 2016]*
    a. Streptococcus b. Staphylococcus
    c. Pseudomonas d. Yersinia pestis
13. **Most common infectious cause of Erythema multiforme** *[Recent Question 2016]*
    a. Staphylococcus b. TB
    c. HSV d. EBV
14. **Dermatophytes affect** *[Recent Question 2016]*
    a. Keratin b. Dermis of skin
    c. Stratum basal d. Stratum spongiosum
15. **Sabin Feldman dye test is used for** *[Recent Question 2016]*
    a. Toxoplasmosis
    b. Syphilis
    c. Herpes genitalis
    d. Gardnerella vaginalis
16. **Multinucleate giant cells are seen in Tzanck smear in** *[Recent Question 2016]*
    a. Herpes genitalis
    b. Bullous pemphigoid
    c. Toxic epidermal necolysis
    d. Pemphigus
17. **Drug not given in treatment of Tinea versicolor is** *[Recent Question 2016]*
    a. Miconazole b. Selenium sulfide
    c. Sodium thiosulfate d. Griseofulvin
18. **Hair infection with scutula formation is seen in case of** *[Recent Question 2016]*
    a. Tinea capitis b. Jock itch
    c. Tinea glabrosa d. Tinea barbae
19. **Tinea corporis is commonly caused by all the following except** *[Recent Question 2016]*
    a. T. rubrum b. T. verrucosum
    c. E. floccosum d. M. canis
20. **Koplik spots are pathognomonic of** *[Recent Question 2016]*
    a. Measles b. Diphtheria
    c. Donovanosis d. Gonorrhoea
21. **All of the following are caused by Staphylococcus aureus except** *[NBE FMGE September 2008]*
    a. Impetigo b. Erysipelas
    c. Ecthyma d. Furuncle
22. **A 26 years old unmarried, female patient presented with asymptomatic, whitish, homogenous vaginal discharge of 1 month duration. She denied history of sexual contact. On laboratory examination, the amine test was found to be positive. The diagnosis is** *[NBE DNB 2011]*
    a. Trichomonas vaginalis vaginitis
    b. Bacterial vaginosis
    c. Candidial vulvovaginitis
    d. Chlamydial infection
23. **Norwegian scabies is caused by** *[NBE DNB 1995]*
    a. Female acarus scabiei b. Male acarus scabiei
    c. Demodex mite d. Harvest mite
24. **Tinea capitis is not caused by** *[NBE FMGE September 2008]*
    a. Trichophytin rubrum
    b. Micropolyspora rubrum
    c. Epidermophyton flociosum
    d. Trichophyton scoliosis
25. **Cutaneous manifestations of tuberculosis may include all EXCEPT** *[NBE DNB 2011]*
    a. Lupus pernio
    b. Erythema induratum
    c. Lupus vulgaris
    d. Erythema nodosum
26. **Malignant pustule is** *[NBE FMGE September 2007]*
    a. An infected malignant melanoma
    b. Anthrax of skin
    c. A rapidly spreading rodent ulcer
    d. A carbuncle
27. **Exanthema subitum is caused by** *[Recent Question 2012, 2013]*
    a. HSV b. HPV
    c. HIV d. HCV

28. Oral drug used in treatment of scabies is *[Recent Question 2017, NBE DNB 2011]*
a. Cotrimoxazole b. Penicillin
c. Ivermectin d. Levamisole

29. Most common cause of Cellulitis is *[NBE FMGE September 2007]*
a. Streptococcus pyogenes
b. Streptococcus viridans
c. Streptococcus faecalis
d. Microaerophilic Streptococci

30. A 4-month old infant presents with itchy papules and burrows on wrist, web spaces, genitals and trunk. The most appropriate treatment for this is *[UPSC 2012]* *[Recent Question 2017]*
a. Permethrin 1% cream
b. Permethrin 5% cream
c. Gamma benzene hexachloride 1% lotion
d. Benzyl benzoate 25% lotion

31. Characteristic lesion in scabies *[Recent Question 2013]*
a. Burrows b. Vesicle
c. Papule d. Pustule

32. Kerion is a form of *[Recent Question 2016]* *[NBE FMGE September 2006, NBE DNB 2011]*
a. Bacterial infection b. Viral infection
c. Fungal infection d. Parasitic infection

33. Oral drug used in treatment of Scabies is *[NBE FMGE September 2006]*
a. Cotrimoxazole b. Penicillin
c. Ivermectin d. Levamisole

34. Felon is commonly seen in *[NBE DNB 2011]*
a. Index finger b. Ring finger
c. Little finger d. Middle finger

35. Common conditions due to Herpes simplex include all except *[NBE FMGE September 2005]*
a. Eczema herpeticum b. Genital lesion
c. Oral lesion d. Tender lesion

36. All are true about Bacterial vaginosis except *[NBE FMGE September 2012]*
a. Fishy smell white discharge
b. Clue cells on mount
c. Abundant lactobacillus d. Alkaline pH in vagina

37. Molluscum contagiosum skin infection is caused by a *[NBE FMGE September 2012]*
a. Bacterium b. Virus
c. Fungus d. Rickettsia

38. H. ducreyi causes *[NBE DNB 2002]*
a. Soft chancre b. Hard chancre
c. Pustule d. Painless chancre

39. 'Apple-jelly nodules' are seen in *[Recent Question 2016, 2017]* *[NBE DNB 1992, NBE FMGE September 2005]*
a. Lupus vulgaris
b. Erythroplakia
c. Actinic keratosis
d. Paget's disease

40. Candida is most often implicated in causation of *[NBE FMGE March 2005]*
a. Tinea capitis b. Conjunctivitis
c. Thrush d. Desert rheumatism

41. Herpes infection of Ulcer is known as *[Recent Question 2014]*
a. Epithelial keratitis b. Stromal keratitis
c. Keratouveitis d. None

42. What is the causative organism for common warts? *[UPSC 2010]*
a. Human papilloma virus
b. Cytomegalovirus
c. Human immunodeficiency virus
d. Herpes virus

43. Most commonly seen fungal infection in Neutropenic patients is *[NBE FMGE September 2005]*
a. Candidiasis b. Aspergillosis
c. Histoplasmosis d. None of the above

44. Shingles is caused by *[Recent Question 2016, 2014]*
a. Hepatitis B virus
b. Ureaplasma urealyticum
c. Molluscum contagiosum
d. Varicella zoster

45. Fungus affecting hair is *[NBE FMGE March 2009]*
a. Microsporum b. Trichophyton
c. Both d. None

46. A young female complains of genital wart, the agent implicated is *[NBE DNB 2002, 2007]*
a. Treponema pallidum b. Adenovirus
c. Human papilloma virus d. Pox virus

47. Characteristic lesion in scabies *[Recent Question 2012]*
a. Burrows b. Vesicle
c. Papule d. Pustule

48. Molluscum contagiosum is caused by *[NBE FMGE September 2009]*
a. Bacterium b. Virus
c. Fungus d. Prion

49. Tuberculides are seen in *[NBE DNB 2009]*
a. Lupus vulgaris b. Serofuloderma
c. Lichen scrofulososum d. Erythema nodosum

50. Dermatophytosis is not *[Recent Question 2012]*
a. Scaly b. Itchy
c. Superficial d. Subdermal

51. A child presented with severe itching over webs of fingers, especially more so at night. Local examination revealed presence of burrows. It indicate a diagnosis of *[NBE FMGE September 2009]*
a. Infantile eczema b. Tinea cruris
c. Papular urticaria d. Scabies

52. Tinea versicolor is caused by *[NBE DNB 1995, 2000]*
a. Malassezia furfur
b. Candida
c. Trichophyton rubra
d. Trichophyton mentagrophyte

53. Not a feature of scabies *[Recent Question 2012]*
a. Burrows are seen in Stratum Corneum
b. Itching is more severe at night
c. Family history is found
d. Fever is a common finding

54. Which of the following structure is affected by dermatophytes? *[NBE FMGE March 2012]*
a. Skin b. Hair
c. Nail d. All of the above

55. The burrow is scabies is in the *[NBE DNB 1997]*
a. Stratum germinatum b. Stratum corneum
c. Malphigian layer d. Rheumatic fever

56. Best diagnostic test for fungal skin infection *[Recent Question 2012]*
a. KOH test b. Diascopy
c. Wood's lamp d. Patch test

57. Human herpes virus 8 infection is associated with *[NBE FMGE March 2012]*
a. Hairy cell leukemia
b. Kaposi sarcoma
c. Oral hairy leucoplakia
d. Molluscum contagiosum

58. Definitive diagnosis of sporotrichosis generally depends on *[NBE DNB 2007]*
a. Serology
b. Culture
c. Biopsy
d. KOH preparation from the lesion

59. Treatment for Stage 1 Mycosis fungoides *[Recent Question 2012, 2013]*
a. PUVA
b. Biological response modifiers
c. Systemic chemotherapy
d. Extracorporial photopheresis

60. Molluscum contagiosum is caused by *[Recent Question 2014]*
a. Rhabdovirus
b. Bunya virus
c. Pox virus
d. Flavivirus

61. MC Oral fungal infection *[Recent Question 2014]*
a. Histoplasma
b. Candida
c. Aspergillus
d. None

62. Ritter's disease is caused by *[Recent Question 2015]*
a. Staphylococcus aureus
b. Staphylococcus epidermidis
c. Staphylococcus albus
d. Staphylococcus saprophyticus

63. Tinea mannum affects *[Recent Question 2015]*
a. Face b. Nails
c. Hands d. Foot

64. Cutaneous viral infection which is commonly seen in children and characterized by single or multiple pearly-white skin colored smooth dome shaped papules with central pitting is *[UPSC CMS 2015]*
a. Chicken pox
b. Herpes zoster
c. Molluscum contagiosum
d. Verruca vulgaris

65. Not a feature of Candidal intertrigo is *[Recent Question 2017]*
a. Obesity is a risk factor
b. C. albicans is the most common causative species
c. Central scaling
d. Satellite lesions

66. A 32 years old lady from Chhattisgarh tribal area came with an erythematous indurated plaque with scarring on right side of face and extension to ear lobe. Most likely diagnosis is? *[Recent Question 2017]*
a. Lepromatous leprosy
b. Molluscum contagiousum
c. Lupus vulgaris
d. Pityriasis rubra pilaris

67. Which of the following is not true for Scabies? *[Recent Question 2017]*
a. Wrist is common site in children
b. Burrows are intradermal lesions
c. Papules and pustules are due to hypersensitivity to mite
d. Itching generalized

68. Treatment for Impetigo includes all except? *[Recent Question 2017]*
a. Topical Mupirocin
b. Systemic Erythromycin
c. Topical Gentamycin
d. Systemic Cephalosporins

69. Jock itch is caused by? *[Recent Question 2017]*
a. Epidermophyton floccosum
b. Candida albicans
c. Trichophyton tonsurans
d. Malassezia furfur

70. Volcano sign is seen in? *[Recent Question 2017]*
a. Leprosy b. Leishmaniasis
c. Lupus vulgaris d. DLE

71. Treatment of choice for Oral candidiasis is? *[Recent Question 2017]*
a. Terbinafin b. Nystatin
c. Griesofulvin d. Selenium sulphide

72. Treatment for Pityriasis versicolor includes? *[Recent Question 2017]*
a. Griesofulvin b. Terbinafine
c. Itraconazole d. All of the above

73. Plane skin warts are caused by HPV type? *[Recent Question 2017]*
a. HPV 6 & 11 b. HPV2 & 4
c. HPV 3 & 10 d. HPV 5 & 8

74. Incubation period of Sarcoptes scabiei is? *[Recent Question 2017]*
a. 1-2 weeks b. 2-3 weeks
c. 3-4 weeks d. 4-5 weeks

75. Scabies is caused by? *[Recent Question 2017]*
a. Mite b. Tic
c. Virus d. Fungus

76. Which of the following color is characteristic of Tinea versicolor on Wood's lamp examination? *[Recent Question 2017]*
a. Bright green b. Milky white
c. Golden yellow d. Blue white

77. A 15-year-old boy presented with a tender erythematous plaque on his left buttock. It has been there for 4 years and slowly progressing. Annular shaped plaque with irregular borders with peripheral crusting. It was progressing towards the medial side of the buttock and with scarring on healed lateral border. There was no regional lymphadenopathy, and systemic examination revealed no abnormalities. No other family members had similar lesions. Most likely diagnosis is? *[Recent Question 2017]*
a. Lupus vulgaris b. Granuloma annulare
c. Psoriasis d. SCC

78. A diabetic male with red, tender & painful swelling on right buttock with multiple discharging points. Swelling is hard and indurated. There is high grade fever with malaise. Most likely diagnosis is? *[Recent Question 2017]*
a. Folliculitis b. Furuncle
c. Carbuncle d. Impetigo

79. Most common infecting organism responsible for boils on face is *[Recent Question 2017]*
a. Streptococcus b. Staphylococcus
c. Pseudomonas d. None of the above

80. Maculae ceruleae are seen in? *[Recent Question 2017]*
a. Pediculosis b. Leishmaniasis
c. Scabies d. Tinea

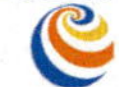 HIGH YIELD MCQs 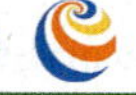

1. A 35-year-old factory worker developed itchy, annular scaly plaques in both groins. The lesion healed temporarily to topical steroids but continue to extend at the periphery. The most likely diagnosis is *[AIIMS May 2016]*
a. Annular lichen planus
b. Granuloma annulare
c. Tinea cruris
d. Erythema annular centrifugum

2. To diagnose a case of post-herpetic neuralgia, pain must persist for *[AIIMS November 2016]*
a. 1 week
b. 2 weeks
c. 3 weeks
d. 4 weeks

3. A young boy presents with circular granulomatous lesion with central scarring on buttock. Most likely cause is *[AIIMS November 2016]*
a. Tinea corporis b. Lupus vulgaris
c. Granuloma annulare d. Annular psoriasis

4. Which one of the following is tuberculid? *[AIIMS PGMEE 2006]*
a. Lichen scrofulosorum b. Erythema nodosum
c. Lupus vulgaris d. Scrofuloderma

5. A 8-year-old child has localized non cicatrial alopecia over scalp with itching and scales. The diagnosis is *[AIIMS PGMEE 1993]*
a. Tinea Barbae b. Alopecia areata
c. Tinea capitis d. Lichen planus

6. Involvement of sweat gland, dermal appendages, and hair follicles with epithelioid granuloma are typical features of which of the following? *[All India PGMEE 2009]*
a. Lichen scrofulosorum b. Miliary TB
c. Papulonecrotic type d. Lupus vulgaris

7. A 12-year-old boy had a gradually progressive plaque on a buttock for the last 3 years. The plaque was 15 cm in diameter, annular in shape, with crusting and induration at the periphery and scarring at the center. The most likely diagnosis *[AIIMS PGMEE 2003]*
a. Tinea corporis b. Granuloma annulare
c. Lupus vulgaris d. Borderline leprosy

8. A young boy presented with a lesion over his right buttock which had peripheral scaling and central clearing with scarring. The investigation of choice would be *[AIIMS PGMEE 2001]*
a. Tzank smear b. KOH preparation
c. Biopsy d. Sabourad's agar

9. An 8-year-old boy present with well-defined annular lesion over the buttock with central scarring that is gradually progressive over the last 8 months. The diagnosis is *[AIIMS PGMEE 2001]*
a. Annular psoriasis
b. Lupus vulgaris
c. Tinea corporis
d. Chronic granulomatous disease

10. Which of the following is/are tuberculides? *[PGI 2000]*
a. Lichen scrofuloderma b. Lichen nitidus
c. Lichen aureus d. Erythema nodosum

11. Erysipeloid is transmitted by *[PGI 1999]*
a. Droplet b. Feco-oral
c. Mosquito bite d. Contact with animal

12. Staphylococcus causes all except *[PGI 1999]*
a. Scarlet fever b. TSS
c. Carbuncle d. Sycosis barbae

13. After 3 days of fever patient developed maculo erythematous rash lasting for 48 hrs diagnosis is *[All India PGMEE 2002]*
a. Fifth disease b. Rubella
c. Measles d. Roseola infantum

14. Dermatophytes are *[PGI 2003]*
a. Trichophyton rubrum b. Tinea versicularis
c. Sporothrix d. Micosporidium

15. Dermatophytes infection to *[BIHAR PGMEE 2006]*
a. Superficial b. Subdermal
c. Subfascial d. Muscular

16. All cause Tinea capitis except *[AIIMS PGMEE 1992]*
a. Trichophyton b. Epidermophyton
c. Microsporum d. All

17. An 8-year-old boy presents with boggy swelling and easily pluckable hair, Diagnosis is *[AIIMS PGMEE 1998]*
a. Tinea capitis b. Alopecia areata
c. Tuberculoid leprosy d. Pityriasis alba

18. A boggy swelling over scalp with easily pluckable hairs in a child, the investigation done is *[AIIMS PGMEE 1994, 1996]*
a. Giemsa staining
b. Bacterial culture
c. KOH preparation
d. Gram staining/Tzank smear

19. A 10-year-old boy presented with painful boggy swelling of scalp, multiple sinuses with purulent discharge, easily pluckable hair, and lymph nodes enlarged in occipital

region. Which one of the following would be most helpful for diagnostic evaluation? *[All India PGMEE 2001, AIIMS PGMEE 2009]*

a. Biopsy b. Bacterial culture
c. KOH mount d. Patch test

20. Tinea Capitis is caused by all except *[JIPMER PGMEE 1997]*

a. Epidermophyton
b. Microsporum
c. T. Violaceum
d. T. Schoenleinii

21. An 11-year-old boy is having tinea capitis on his scalp. The most appropriate line of treatment is *[All India PGMEE 2003]*

a. Oral griseofulvin therapy
b. Topical griseofulvin therapy
c. Shaving of the scalp
d. Selenium sulphide shampoo

22. A 22-year-old male patient presents with a complaints of severe itching and white scaly lesions in the groin for past month. Which of the following is most likely to be the causative agent? *[AIIMS PGMEE 2003]*

a. Trichophyton rubrum
b. Candida albicans
c. Candida glabrata
d. Malassezia furfur

23. Which of the following is/ are bacterial infection of skin? *[PGI 2005]*

a. Pyoderma gangrenosum
b. Piedra
c. Impetigo contagiosa
d. Impetigo herpetiformis
e. Ecthyma

24. A 6-month-old infant had itchy erythematous papules and exudative lesions on the scalp, face, groins and axillae for one month. She also had vesicular lesions on the palms. The most likely diagnosis is *[All India PGMEE 2006]*

a. Congenital syphilis b. Seborrhoeic dermatitis
c. Scabies d. Psoriasis

25. Ring worm fungi live in *[AIIMS PGMEE 1992), UP PGMEE 1997]*

a. Stratum corneum b. Dermis
c. Prickle Cell layer d. Basal Cell layer

26. Tinea versicolour is caused by *[All India PGMEE 1992]*

a. E. Floccosum b. Malassezia furfur
c. T. rubrum d. T. Schonleini

27. A 36-year-old factory worker developed itchy annular scaly plaques in both groins. Application of a corticosteroid ointment led to temporary relief but the plaques continued to extend at the periphery. The most likely diagnosis is *[All India PGMEE 2005]*

a. Erythema annulare centrifugam
b. Granuloma annulare
c. Annular lichen planus
d. Tinea cruris

28. A 3-year-old female child develops umblicated nodule over face, following a trivial infection, probable diagnosis *[AIIMS PGMEE 1999]*

a. Molluscum contagiosum
b. Scabies
c. Chicken pox
d. L. planus

29. A 30-year-old female presents with history of itching under right breast. On examination annular ring lesion was present under the breast. The diagnosis is *[AIIMS PGMEE 2002]*

a. Trichophyton rubrum b. Candida albicans
c. Epidermophyton d. Microsporum

30. A 6-month-old infant presented with multiple papules & exudative lesions on the face, scalp, trunk and few vesicles on palms and soles for 2 weeks. His mother has history of itchy lesions. The most likely diagnosis is *[AIIMS PGMEE 2005]*

a. Scabies
b. Infantile exzema
c. Infantile seborrhoeic dermatitis
d. Impetigo contagiosa

31. Causative organism of Molluscum contagiosum is *[AIIMS PGMEE 1999]*

a. Papova virus b. Pox virus
c. Orthomyxo virus d. Parvo virus

32. Which of the following is true of Molluscum contagiosum? *[Kerala PGMEE 1997]*

a. Treatment is extirpation
b. Is an STD
c. Viral infection
d. Central umbilication
e. All are correct

33. Herpes zoster is commonly seen in a *[All India PGMEE 1999]*

a. Cervical region b. Thoracic region
c. Lumbar region d. Geniculate ganglion

34. Test likely to help in diagnosis of a patient who presents with an itchy annular plaque on the face is *[All India PGMEE 2003]*

a. Gram's stain
b. Potassium hydroxide mount
c. Tissue smear
d. Wood's lamp examination

35. A 24-year-old man had multiple, small hypopigmented macules on the upper chest and back for the last three months. The macules were circular, arranged around follicles and many had coalesced to form large sheets. The surface of the macules showed fine scaling. He had similar lesions one year ago which subsided with treatment. The most appropriate investigation to confirm the diagnosis is *[AIIMS PGMEE 2003]*

a. Potassium hydroxide preparation of scales
b. Slit skin smear from discrete macules
c. Tzanck test
d. Skin biopsy of coalesced macules

36. Most common site of affection of Herpes simplex *[UP PGMEE PGMEE 1996]*

a. Thorax b. Abdomen
c. Face d. Extremities

37. Following drug is indicated in the treatment of pityriasis versicolar *[AIIMS PGMEE 2003]*

a. Ketoconazole b. Metronidazole
c. Griseofulvin d. Chloroquine

38. Most common age group to suffer from T. Cruris *[AIIMS PGMEE 1991]*

a. Infant b. Male child
c. Adult male d. Adult female

39. Which of the following is/ are fungal infection of skin? *[PGI 2005]*
a. Sporotrichosis
b. Molluscum contagiousm
c. Madura foot
d. Tinea

40. Drug of choice in Herpes zoster *[AIIMS PGMEE 1999]*
a. Acyclovir b. Vidarabine
c. Idoxuridine d. Actinomycin

41. Skin manifestations of T.B. *[PGI 2004]*
a. Lupus vulgaris
b. Lupus pernio
c. Scrofuloderma
d. Butcher warts

42. Rash in measles occurs first in occurs first in ...... region *[Kerala PGMEE 1990]*
a. Forehead b. Postauricular
c. Chest d. Neck

43. Papulovesicular lesion on face, trunk, palm and sole in a 9 month old child is seen in *[AIIMS PGMEE 1995]*
a. Scabies b. Drug reaction
c. Atopic dermatitis d. Seborrheic dermatitis

44. An otherwise healthy male presents with a creamy curd like white patch on the tongue. The probable diagnosis is *[All India PGMEE 2010]*
a. Candidiasis b. Histoplasmosis
c. Lichen planus d. Aspergillosis

45. Erythema marginatum is seen in *[Bihar PGMEE 2005, Kerala PGMEE 1997]*
a. Drug reactions b. Typhoid fever
c. Enteric fever d. Rheumatic fever

46. An infant presented with itchy eczematous crusted lesions with exudation on palm, sole, glans penis and face. All are true except *[PGI 2002]*
a. Family should be examined
b. Only patient needs drug treatment
c. All clothing & linen should be discarded or burnt
d. Distribution of lesion help in diagnosis making
e. Drug should be applied to affected areas for whole day

47. Tuberculosis verrucosa cutis is a form of *[SGPGI 2005]*
a. Tuberculid
b. Primary tuberculosis
c. Postprimary tuberculosis with good resistance
d. Post primary tuberculosis with poor resistance

48. Which of the following is/are tuberculides? *[PGI 2007]*
a. Lichen scrofulosorum b. Lichen nitidus
c. Lichen aureus d. Erythema nodosum

49. Tuberculosis of skin is called as *[AIIMS PGMEE 1998, SGPGI 2004]*
a. Lupus vulgaris b. Lupus Pernio
c. Lupus profundus d. Scrofuloderma

50. True about Lupus vulgaris *[PGI 2004]*
a. Apple jelly nodule at root of nose
b. TB of skin & mucosa
c. Also known as scrofuloderma
d. ATT is helpful
e. Is most common type of cutaneous tuberculosis

51. Scabies in children differs from that in adults in that it affects *[JIPMER PGMEE 2000]*
a. Webspace b. Face
c. Genitalia d. Axilla

52. Nodular scabies is found in *[AIIMS PGMEE 1997]*
a. Web space of finger b. Axilla
c. Abdomen d. Scrotum

53. Cutaneous Tuberculosis secondary in underlying tissue is called as *[All India PGMEE 1999]*
a. Lupus vulgaris
b. Scrofuloderma
c. Spina ventosa
d. Tuberculous verrucosa cutis

54. Mycobacterium causing skin ulcer *[PGI 2002]*
a. M. smegmatis b. M. scrofulaceum
c. M. ulcerans d. M. fortuitum
e. M. marinum

55. Skin hazards of swimming are *[PGI 2001]*
a. Verrucae
b. Pyoderma gangrenosum
c. M. marinum infection
d. M. ulcerans infection

56. Staphylococcal infection causes all disease except *[All India PGMEE 1997]*
a. Impetigo b. Erysipelas
c. Ecthyma d. Scaldy skin syndrome

57. Toxic shock syndrome is caused by *[All India PGMEE 1993]*
a. Staphylococcal infection
b. Streptococcus
c. Pseudomonas
d. E. Coli

58. An infant presenting with itchy lesions over groin and prepuce all is indicated except *[All India PGMEE 2001]*
a. Bathe & apply scabicidal solution
b. Treatment of all family members
c. Dispose all clothes by boiling
d. IV antibiotics

59. Rose spot are seen in *[Kerala PGMEE 1998, UP PGMEE 2006]*
a. Typhus fever b. Typhoid fever
c. Enteric fever d. Rheumatic fever

60. False statement about Impetigo *[PGI 2001]*
a. Mostly caused by staphylococcus or streptococcus or both
b. B. predisposes to glumerulonephritis
c. Produces scar on healing
d. Erythromycin is drug of choice
e. It is infectious lesion

61. Commonest skin infection is children is *[All India PGMEE 1989]*
a. Scabies b. Impetigo contagiosa
c. Molluscum contagiosa d. Warts

62. Characteristic lesion of scabies is *[Kerala PGMEE 1987, Bihar PGMEE 2003]*
a. Burrow b. Fissure
c. Vesicle d. Papule

63. *'Honey colour'* crusts are characteristic of *[JIPMER PGMEE 1979, PGI 1981]*
a. Nummular eczema b. Impetigo
c. Herpes zoster d. Cutaneous diphtheria

64. 'Slapped cheeks' appearance is seen in *[PGI 1998, AIIMS PGMEE 1997]*
a. Roseloa infantum b. Erythema subitum
c. Erythema infectiosum d. Erythema multiforme

65. An 8-month old child presented with itchy, exudative lesions on the face, palms and soles. The siblings also have similar complaints. The treatment of choice is such a patient is *[All India PGMEE 2003]*
a. Systemic ampicillin b. Topical betamethasone
c. Systemic prednisolone d. Topical permethrin

66. Dermatophytes are *[PGI 2006]*
a. Sporothrix b. Timex versicularis
c. Microsporidium d. Trichophyton rubrum
e. All of the above

67. Which does not cause Tinea capitis? *[AIIMS PGMEE 1994]*
a. Epidermophyton b. Microsporum
c. Trichophyton rubrum d. Trichophyton violaceum

68. Most common organism causing T. capitis is *[All India PGMEE 2003]*
a. Trichophyton tonsurans b. Microsporum
c. Epidermophyton d. Candida albicans

69. Kerion is seen in *[AIIMS PGMEE 1998]*
a. Candida infection b. Trichomoniasis
c. Pityriasis d. Dermatophytosis

70. DOC for Tinea unguium *[All India PGMEE 1993, UP PGMEE 2005]*
a. Amphotericin B b. Miconazole
c. Griseofulvin d. Nystatin

71. A child has multiple itchy popular lesions on the genitalia and fingers. Similar lesions are also seen in the younger brother. Which of the following is most possible diagnosis? *[AIIMS PGMEE 2002]*
a. Papular urticaria b. Scabies
c. Atopic dermatitis d. Allergic contact dermatitis

72. Regarding Athlete's foot which is correct? *[PGI 1996, Kerala PGMEE 1997]*
a. 4th tow web is commonly involved
b. Severe itching
c. Caused by Trichophyton mentagrophyte
d. Hyperthyroidism is present
e. All of the above

73. Tinea incognito is seen with *[PGI 1999, WB PGMEE 2002]*
a. Steroid treatment b. 1% BHC
c. 5% Permethrin d. Antibiotics

74. A child has itchy vesicles on face, palm and sole the diagnosis is *[AIIMS PGMEE 1996]*
a. Scabies b. Seborrheic dermatitis
c. Chicken pox d. Atopic dermatitis

75. About dermatophytes all are true except *[AIIMS PGMEE 1993]*
a. Candida albicans usually cause systemic infection
b. Dermatophytes involve superficial layers of skin
c. Microsporum doesn't involve nail
d. Epidermophyte doesn't involve hair

76. Black dot ring worm is caused by *[PGI 1999, AIIMS PGMEE 1995]*
a. Microsporon b. Trichophyton
c. Epidermophyton d. Candida

77. HPV vaccine is *[AIIMS PGMEE 2009]*
a. Monovalent b. Bivalent
c. Quadrivalent d. Bivalent and quadrivalent

78. True about Impetigo is *[PGI 2008]*
a. Contagious b. Bacterial infection
c. Non contagious d. Honey coloured crusts
e. Viral infection

79. A washerman presents with thickness erosion & discolouration of web space of toes diagnosis is *[Rajasthan PGMEE 2003]*
a. Psoriasis b. Tinea unguium
c. Both d. Candidiasis

80. Permethrin is used in treatment of *[Recent Question 2017, All India PGMEE 1999]*
a. Scabies b. Leprosy
c. Body Louse d. Leishmaniaris

81. Skin TB which involves skin after involving lymph nodes *[AIIMS PGMEE 1996]*
a. Scrofuloderma b. Lupus vulgaris
c. Lupus erythematous d. Lupus pernio

82. A 20-year-old male from Jaipur with erythematous lesion on cheek with central crusting likely diagnosis is *[All India PGMEE 2001]*
a. SLE b. Lupus vulgaris
c. Chill blain d. Cutaneous leishmaniasis

83. Linear lesion is seen in *[PGI 1997]*
a. Sporotrichosis b. Lichen planus
c. Psoriasis d. Pemphigus

84. Burrows in scabies is in *[Karnataka PGMEE 1998, Kerala PGMEE 1990]*
a. Straum germination b. Stratum corneum
c. Malphigian layer d. Dermis

85. Dhobi's itch is *[JIPMER PGMEE 1992]*
a. Tinea corfioris b. Tinea cruris
c. Tinea barbae d. Tinea capitis

86. Drug used for scabies is/ are *[All India PGMEE 1988]*
a. Sulphur ointment
b. Benzyl benzoate
c. Gamma benzene hexachloride
d. Crotamiton
e. All of the above

87. Tinea unguium effects *[All India PGMEE 1995]*
a. Nail fold b. Nail plate
c. Joints d. Inter digital space

88. Most severe form of scabies *[AP PGMEE 1998]*
a. Norwegian scabies b. Nodular scabies
c. Animal scabies d. Genital
e. Generalised scabies

89. Incubation period of Scabies is *[WB PGMEE 2000]*
a. 7 days b. 2 weeks
c. 4 weeks d. 2–3 days

90. Circle of hebra is associated with *[PGI 2008]*
a. Syphilis b. Scabies
c. Leprosy d. Lichen planus

91. Adult scabies is characterized by *[PGI 2004]*
a. Involve palm & soles b. Involve face
c. Involve anterior abdomen
d. Involve web space e. Involve genitalia

92. Which of these statements is false for Erytherma marginatum? *[MP PGMEE 2004]*
a. Lesions are serpiginous
b. Characteristically it is an evanescent
c. Rash worsens on application of heart
d. Rash is itchy

93. M.C. type of cutaneous T.B. is *[PGI 2006]*
a. Lupus vulgaris
b. Scrofuloderma
c. T.B. verruca cutis
d. Erythema induratum

94. Vagabond's disease is *[WB PGMEE 2000]*
a. Pediculosis corporis b. Scabies
c. Eczema d. Ringworm

95. Impetigo contagiosa most commonly due to
a. Group B Streptococcous *[Jharkhand PGMEE 2004]*
b. Staphylococcus
c. Moniliasis
d. Streptococcus viridans

96. TOC in Pediculosis corporis is *[AIIMS PGMEE 1993]*
a. 3 applications of Gamma BHC
b. One application of Benzyl Benzoate
c. 4 application of Benzyl Benzoate
d. Disinfection of Clothes only

97. Condylomata acuminata is caused by
[WB PGMEE 2004, J&K PGMEE 2004]
a. HPV b. HSV
c. HIV d. All

98. True about Impetigo is *[PGI May 2014]*
a. Caused by Staphylococcus aureus
b. Always bullous
c. Most common around genitelia
d. Caused by Staphylococcus pyogenes
e. Honey coloured crusts

99. Tinea capitis in India is mainly caused by
a. Microsporum canis *[JIPMER PGMEE 2014]*
b. T. tonsurans
c. T. soudanense
d. T. violaceum

100. Verruga peruana is caused by *[PGI November 2014]*
a. Molluscum contagiosum
b. Bartonella bacilliformis
c. Klebsiella pneumoniae
d. Human papilloma virus
e. Bartonella qunitana

101. Correct regarding Tinea capitis is/ are
a. Caused by Trichophyton *[PGI November 2014]*
b. Caused by Microsporum
c. Absent alopecia
d. Black dot hair
e. Oral antifungals useful

102. Rash is seen in which of the following Viral exanthems?
[PGI November 2014]
a. Rubella b. Erythema infectiosum
c. Measles d. Varicella
e. Exanthem subitum

103. Fungal keratomycosis treatment is
[AIIMS November 2014]
a. Silver sulphadiazine b. Doxycycline
c. Vancomycin d. Linezolid

104. An Athletic male presents with Itchy lesion at Groin. Causative organism can include all except
[AIIMS November 2015]
a. Trichophyton b. Aspergillus
c. Epidermophyton d. Microsporum

105. Oral candidiasis presents with white patch in all of the following except *[AIIMS November 2015]*
a. Acute pseudomembranous candidiasis
b. Chronic hyperplastic candidiasis
c. Chronic mucocutaneous candidiasis
d. Chronic atrophic candidiasis

106. An otherwise healthy male presents with a Creamy curd like white patch on the tongue. The probable diagnosis is
[ESI IMO 2014]
a. Candidiasis b. Histoplasmosis
c. Lichen planus d. Aspergillosis

107. Organism playing pathogenic role in Seborrheic dermatitis is *[PGMCET 2015]*
a. Pityrosporum
b. Sarcoptes
c. Corynebacterium
d. Trichophyton

108. Causative organism of Erythrasma is
[Recent Question 2016, PGMCET 2015]
a. Corynebacterium b. Staphylococcus
c. Streptococcus d. Pseudomonas

109. Tuberculids are seen in *[CGPG 2015]*
a. Miliary tuberculosis
b. Lichen scrofulosorum
c. PKDL
d. Leprosy

110. Mycetoma false is *[CGPG 2015]*
a. Starts as small nodule
b. Involves bone in early stages
c. Caused by fungus
d. Tendons and nerves are resistant to invasion

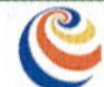

NEET/NBE PATTERN MCQs ANSWERS WITH EXPLANATIONS

1. Ans. (a) Wart

[Ref. Rubin's Pathology, 5/e p301]

- Warts are common and are known to be caused by the DNA human papilloma virus (HPV), of which there are seven recognized types
- Warts can occur anywhere on the face, neck, or elsewhere on the body, and clinically are hyperkeratotic

2. Ans. (b) Pleomorphic

[Ref. DVL by Thappa, 4/e p67,68]

Chicken pox (Varicella) Rash

- Starts on trunk (Centripetal distribution)
- Spreads to face and extremities (Centrifugal spread)
- Characteristic appearance: Pleomorphic; **'Dew drop on a rose petal'** appearance

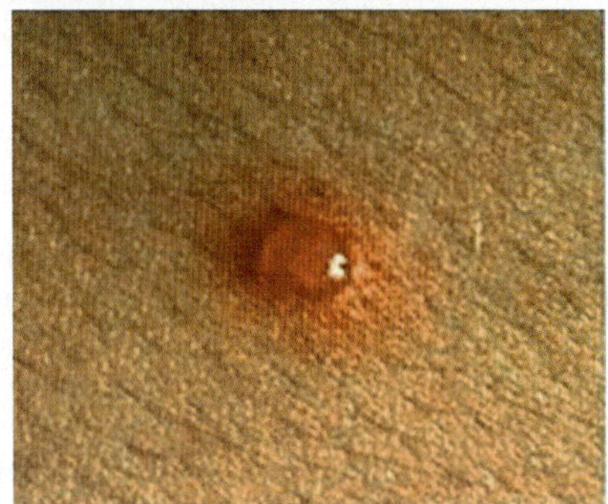

Fig. Dew drop appearance

3. Ans. (a) HSV

[Ref. Clinical Dermatology by Habif, 6/e p567]

Roseola Infantum

- Exanthema subitum, Sudden rash, Sixth disease, Rose rash of infants, **3-day fever**
- Caused primarily by Human herpesvirus 6 **(HHV-6)**, which is epidemiologically and biologically like cytomegalovirus

4. Ans. (d) Burrows

[Ref. DVL by Thappa, 4/e p21, 362]

Burrows in Scabies

- Serpentine caves of scabies mite at the level of Stratum granulosum
- Visible as S- shaped brownish-black lesion that have a papule housing the mite at their distal end
- Commonly in finger web spaces, wrist, shaft of penis

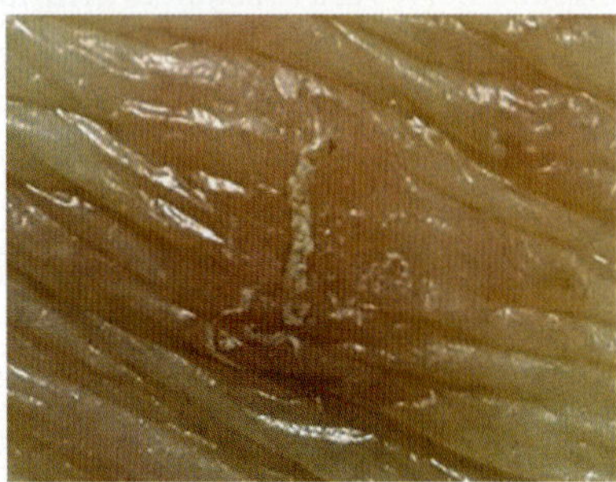

Fig. Burrow

5. Ans. (b) S. granulosum

[Ref. DVL by Thappa, 4/e p21, 362]

- **Typical burrow of the S. scabei** is a short, linear, curved, or S-shaped line
- After impregnation of skin surface, gravid female burrows Stratum corneum within 30 min and gradually extends the tract along the boundary with Stratum granulosum depositing 10-25 eggs over 4-5 weeks period

6. Ans. (b) Lichen nitidus

[Ref. DVL by Thappa, 4/e p84]

- Multiple, tiny, discrete, flat-topped papules that are uniform in size and usually skin- colored; may occasionally be pink to brown in color or hypopigmented (darkly pigmented individuals)
- Histologically, characteristic finding of a 'ball' consisting of a superficial circumscribed infiltrate of lymphocytes and epithelioid cells (2–3 dermal papillae in width) surrounded by a 'claw' of epidermis is typical feature of Lichen nitidus

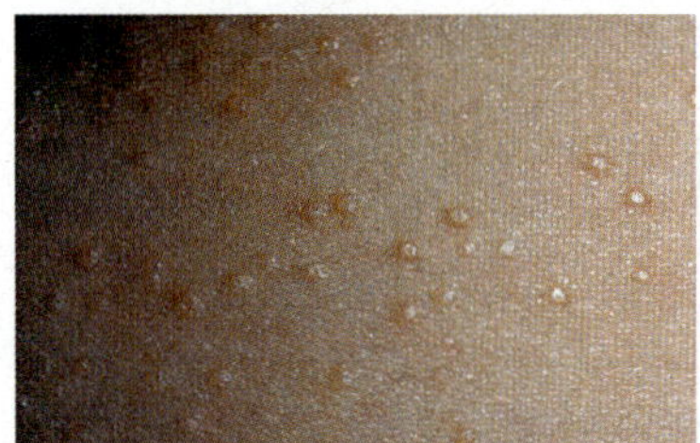

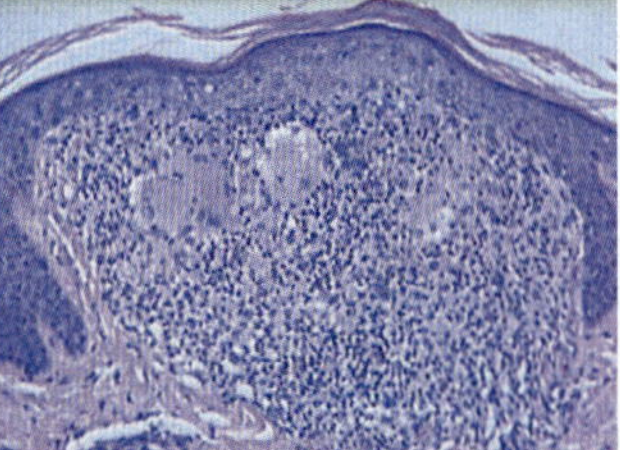

Fig. Lichen nitidus

7. Ans. (d) Foot

[Ref. DVL by Thappa, 4/e p84]

Tinea Pedis / Tinea Mannum

- Commonly affects shoe-bearing population and is rare in those who are bare footed
- Typical manifestations:
  - **Intertriginous type:** Commonly occurs in fourth or third toe web space in form of itchy maceration, scales, fissuring
  - **Hyperkeratotic type:** Scaly erythematous plaque lesion occur on soles or palms
  - **Vesicular type:** Painful multiple vesico-bullous lesions occur on soles

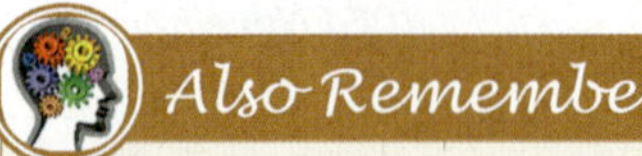

Also Remember

- Trichophyton rubrum causes majority of Tinea of hands and feet

8. Ans. (a) Plantar warts

[Ref. DVL by Thappa, 4/e p72]

Plantar Warts (Myrmecia warts)

- Hyperkeratotic lesion found particularly over pressure areas of feet
- Also known as plantar warts or verrucae plantaris.
- Differ from other warts by being painful

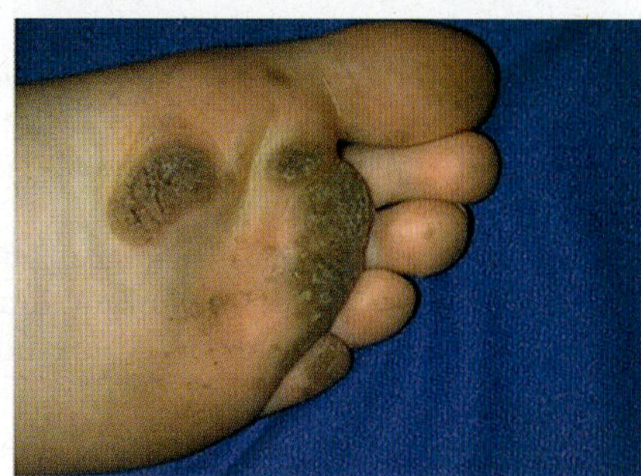

Fig. Plantar warts

9. Ans. (c) LGV
[Ref. DVL by Thappa, 4/e p307,309]

Lymphogranuloma Venereum (LGV)

- Mainly a disease of lymphatic tissue that spreads to tissue surrounding lymphatics
- Genitoanorectal Syndrome is late stage occurs more often in women who were previously asymptomatic
- The enlargement, thickening, and fibrosis of the labia are termed Esthiomene
- Penile and/or scrotal edema and gross distortion of the penis are called "saxophone penis"

10. Ans. (b) Podophyllin
[Ref. Netter's Obstetrics and Gynecology, 3/e p134]

Drug of Choice for Genital Warts

- Podophyllin (20-25% tincture benzoin, 25% ointment)
- Podophyllotoxin (0.5% solution)
- Bichloro- or Trichloroacetic acid (80-100% solution)

11. Ans. (d) Genitalia are not affected
[Ref. Netter Collection of Medical Illustrations, 2/e p184]

- Scabies is a common infestation of the skin caused by the mite Sarcoptes scabiei
- Majority of cases of scabies are not sexually transmitted
- However, the genitals are the third most common body site affected by scabies
- Red papules on Glans penis, Shaft of penis or Scrotum are virtually pathognomonic of Scabies

12. Ans. (b) Staphylococcus
[Ref. Clinical Dermatology by Habif, 6/e 330]

Bullous Impetigo

- Bullous impetigo / Staphylococcal impetigo is caused by an epidermolytic toxin produced at the site of infection and usually is not secondarily contaminated by streptococci
- Toxin causes intraepidermal cleavage below or within the stratum granulosum.
- MC in infants and children but may occur in adults
- It typically occurs on the face, but it may infect anybody surface
- There may be a few lesions localized in one area, or the lesions may be so numerous and widely scattered that they resemble poison ivy
- One or more vesicles enlarge rapidly to form bullae in which the contents turn from clear to cloudy
- The center of the thin-roofed bulla collapses, but the peripheral area may retain fluid for many days in an inner tube shaped rim
- A thin, flat, honey-colored, "varnish-like" crust may appear in the center and, if removed, discloses a bright red, inflamed, moist base that oozes serum

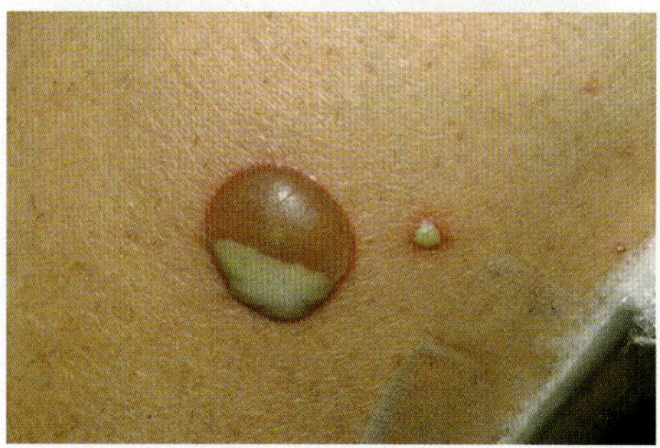

Fig. Bullous impetigo

13. Ans. (c) HSV
[Ref. Clinical Dermatology by Habif, 6/e p713]

- MCC of Erthema multiforme are infectious (viral, bacterial, and fungal)
- Herpes simplex virus (HSV) is MC infectious etiology followed by Mycoplasma pneumoniae

14. Ans. (a) Keratin
[Ref. DVL by Thappa, 4/e p78]

Dermatophytes (Ring worm or Tinea)

- Skin lesions are annular, resulting from progressive central clearing
- Dermatophytes are keratinophilic, so they grow in keratin of stratum corneum

15. Ans. (a) Toxoplasmosis
[Ref. Neurology by Navneet, 1/e p220]

- A Sabin–Feldman dye test is a serologic test to diagnose for toxoplasmosis
- The test is based on the presence of certain antibodies that prevent methylene blue dye from entering the cytoplasm of Toxoplasma organisms

16. Ans. (a) Herpes genitalis
[Ref> DVL by Thappa, 4/e p64,66]

Herpes Genitalis

- It is a sexually transmitted disease and involves genitals
- Tzanck smear from lesion show multinucleated giant cells formed due to fusion of ballooned keratinocytes

17. Ans. (d) Griseofulvin
[Ref. DVL by Thappa, 4/e p96]

- Systemic therapy is only indicated in resistant cases and extensive cases of Tinea versicolor
- Griseofulvin is not effective in treatment.
- Other treatment options: Ketoconazole, fluconazole, itraconazole

18. Ans. (a) Tinea Capitis
[Ref. DVL by Thappa, 4/e p83]

- Inflammatory type of Tinea capitis, Favus is caused by Trichophyton schoenleinii
- On scalp active lesion demonstrates concave sulphur yellow crust called as "scutula" formed around loose wiry hairs
- Later they heal with thin smooth atrophic scarring

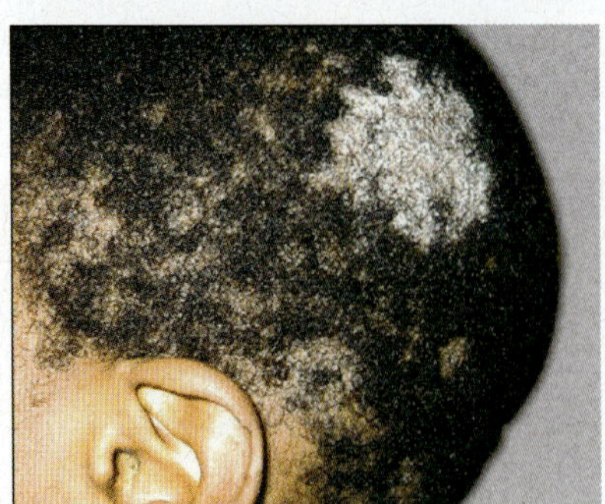

Fig. Tinea capitis

19. Ans. (d) M. canis

[Ref. DVL by Thappa, 4/e p130]

- Tinea corporis is a dermatophyton infection of the non-hair bearing skin on body.
- Species of dermatophyton involved are T. verrucosum, Trichophyton mentagrophytes, Microsporium, Epidermophyton.
- An epidemic of Tinea corporis caused by Trichophyton tonsurans was reported in student wrestlers

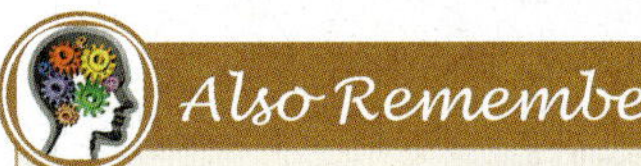

- Microsporum canis and Trichophyton mentagrophytes are zoophilic dermatophytes which can cause skin infections in animals and humans

20. Ans. (a) Measles

[Ref. Clinical Dermatology by Habif, 6/e 779]

Koplik Spots (Koplik's Sign)

- Prodromic viral small spots of measles manifesting two to three days before the measles rash itself
- Clustered, white lesions on the buccal mucosa opposite to lower 1st and 2nd molars and are **pathognomonic for measles**

21. Ans. (b) Erysipelas

[Ref. Neena Khanna, 4/e p245]

- *Bacteria causing pyodermas*:

Staphylococcus aureus Scientist	
Non-follicular	Bullous impetigo Impetigo contagiosa Ecthyma
Follicular	Superficial folliculitis Deep folliculitis Furuncle Carbuncle
Streptococcus pyogenes	
Localised	Impetigo contagiosa Ecthyma
Spreading	Erysipelas Cellulitis

22. Ans. (b) Bacterial vaginosis

[Ref. Infectious Diseases of the Female Genital Tract by Richard L. Sweet, 5/e p204]

Bacterial Vaginosis

- Disorder of Vaginal ecosystem characterized by a shift in the vaginal flora from the normally predominant *Lactobacillus* to one dominated by sialidase enzyme-producing mixed flora
- MC cause of abnormal vaginal discharge in adult women
- Demonstrating three of the following four **AMSEL'S CRITERIA** is considered necessary to diagnose BV most accurately
  - Demonstration of clue cells on a saline smear: Most specific criterion
    1. **Clue cells**: Vaginal epithelial cells with bacteria adherent to their surfaces
    2. Edges of the squamous epithelial cells, which normally have a sharply defined cell border, become studded with bacteria
    3. Epithelial cells appear to be peppered with coccobacilli
  - A pH greater than 4.5 indicates infection, and pH may be elevated in upto 90% of patients with BV
  - Characteristic discharge appearance is thin, gray, and homogeneous
  - Whiff test may be positive in upto 70% of BV patients
    1. This test is performed by placing a drop of 10% KOH on the speculum after the vaginal examination or mixing vaginal fluid with a drop of KOH on a microscope slide
    2. KOH, by virtue of its alkaline properties, causes the release of volatile amines from the vaginal fluid
    3. The amines are products of anaerobic bacterial metabolism

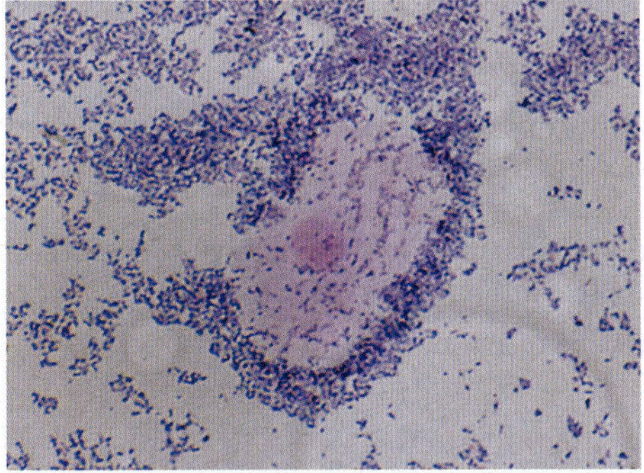

Fig. Clue cells

23. Ans. (a) Female acarus scabiei

[Ref. Neena Khanna, 5/e p366, 367]

24. Ans. (c) Epidermophyton flociosum

[Ref. Sure Success in PGMEE by Ramgopal, 1/e p223]

- *Causative agent of Dermatophytic infections*: Keratinophilic fungi
  - Trichophyton
  - Microsporum
  - Epidermophyton
  - Tinea capitis is caused by dermatophytes of Trichophyton and Microsporum species only

25. Ans. (a) Lupus pernio

[Ref. Neena Khanna, 5/e p268]

Common Presentations of Cutaneous Tuberculosis

- Lupus vulgaris
- Scrofuloderma
- Tuberous verrucosa cutis
- Tuberculides
- Miliary TB

26. Ans. (b) Anthrax of skin

[Ref. Competitive science vision, 2001, 4(11), p1211]

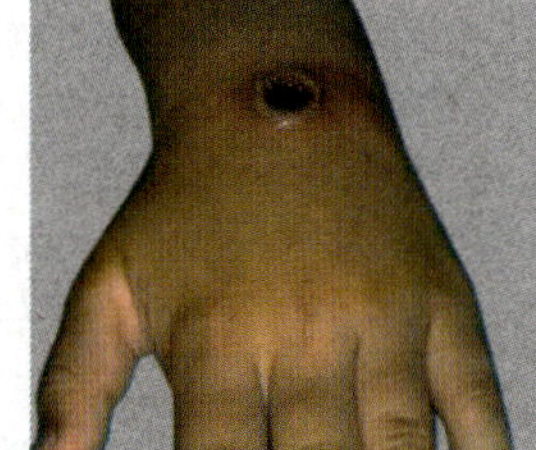

Fig. Malignant pustule

Malignant Pustule/ Cutaneous Anthrax

- *Malignant pustule*: A septic and gangrenous affection of skin, caused by Bacillus anthracis, confined in beginning to cutaneous tissues and on uncovered parts of body
- *Malignant pustule is the* ***most common type of anthrax***
- *Course of malignant pustule*: Begins as a papule and soon becomes a vesicle and breaks, discharging a bloody serum; the seat of this vesicle, in about 36 hours, becomes a bluish black necrotic mass; constitutional symptoms of septicaemia are severe: high fever, vomiting, profuse sweating, and extreme prostration; the infection is often fatal

27. Ans. (a) HSV

[Ref. Biosafety in Microbiological and Biomedical Laboratories by Casey Chosewood, 2/e p217]

- HHV-6 is the causative agent of exanthema subitum (Roseola), a common childhood exanthem

28. Ans. (c) Ivermectin

[Ref. Neena Khanna, 5/e p370]

- Ivermectin 200 μg/ kg, SOD. Repeat after 2 wks

29. Ans. (a) Streptococcus pyogenes

[Ref. Neena Khanna, 4/e p251]

30. Ans. (b) Permethrin 5% cream

[Ref. Neena Khanna, 5/e p370]

Permethrin 5%

- Apply X 8 hrs on day 1 & 8
- Second application is to reduce potential for reinfestation from fomites and to kill any nymphs which may have hatched after treatment, as some eggs may have survived

31. Ans. (a) Burrows

[Ref. Neena Khanna, 5/e p367]

- Mites burrow through the stratum corneum
- Copulation occurs in burrow.

32. Ans. (c) Fungal infection

[Ref. Neena Khanna, 4/e p284]

Types of Tinea Capitis (Tinea of Scalp)

- Non-inflammatory tinea capitis:
  - Caused by T. verrucosum (anthrophilic)
  - Occurs in epidemics (human-to-human spread)
  - Partially bald with scaling at periphery, broken hairs appear as gray/ black dots
- *Inflammatory tinea capitis*: (Kerion)
  - Caused by M. canis (zoophilic)
  - Boggy swelling with pustules
- *Favus*:
  - Caused by T. schoenleinii
  - Yellow cup-shaped, foul-smelling crusts
  - Results in cicatricial alopecia

33. Ans. (c) Ivermectin

[Ref. Neena Khanna, 4/e p344]

- *Treatment of Scabies*:

Topical applications	
5% Permethrin	Drug of choice for Scabies
25% Benzyl benzoate	Older drug of choice
1% Gammaxene/ BHC	Can cause seizures, avoided in infants
10% Crotamiton	Useful in children
10% Sulphur	Useful in children
Oral medications	
Ivermectin	Useful in epidemic, Norwegian form

34. Ans. (a) Index finger

[Ref. Textbook of Pediatric Emergency Procedures by King, 2/e p1090]

- Felon: An abscess of the distal pulp or pad of the fingertip
- MC affected digits: Thumb and index finger

35. Ans. (a) Eczema herpeticum

[Ref. Neena Khanna, 4/e p279-280]

Herpes Simplex Virus Infections

- *Causative agent*: HSV hominis
  - Type I: Cause Herpes labialis and infections above waist
  - Type II: Causes peri-genital infection
- *Clinical presentation*:
  - *Primary infection*: Acute gingivostomatitis (Type I), Grouped painful vesicles (Type II)
  - *Recurrent infection*: Grouped vesicles with polycyclic margins on lips/ genitals
- *Complications*:
  - Erythema multiforme
  - Eczema herpeticum
  - Herpetic encephalitis
  - Herpes simplex keratitis/ Dendritic ulcers
  - Disseminated cutaneous HSV infection

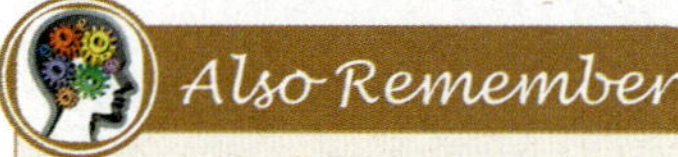

Eczema Herpeticum

- Predisposing factors: Generalised HSV infection in patients with
  - Extensive atopic eczema
  - Pemphigus
  - Pre-existing dermatosis
- *Underlying causes*:
  - Herpes simplex virus I or II
  - Coxsackie virus A16
  - Vaccinia virus

36. Ans. (c) Abundant lactobacillus

[Ref. Infectious Diseases of the Female Genital Tract by Sweet, 5/e p204]

Bacterial Vaginosis (BV)

- Description: A disorder of the vaginal ecosystem characterized by a shift in the vaginal flora from the normally predominant *Lactobacillus* to one dominated by sialidase enzyme-producing mixed flora
- It is the most common cause of abnormal vaginal discharge in adult women

37. Ans. (b) Virus

[Ref. Neena Khanna, 5/e p292]

- Agent: Pox virus

38. Ans. (a) Soft chancre

[Ref. Koneman's Color Atlas and Textbook of Diagnostic Microbiology, 6/e p444]

Haemophius Ducreyi

- H. ducreyi is the causative agent of chancroid, a highly contagious sexually transmitted infection
- Genital lesions caused by this organism are also called "soft chancres" because, the borders of the lesion are ragged and pliable

39. Ans. (a) Lupus vulgaris

[Ref. Neena Khanna, 4/e p253]

Manifestations of Cutaneous Tuberculosis

Types	Remarks
Lupus vulgaris	Annular plaques with peripheral nodules Apple-jelly nodules
Scrofuloderma	Skin connected from underlying TB focus Chronic sinus with hyperpigmented edges
Tuberculosis verrucosa cutis	Single, indurated plaque on acral parts Inoculation tuberculosis
Tuberculides *Lichen scrofulosorum* *Papulonecrotic tuberculide*	Hypersensitivity reactions to Mycobacterium TB

40. Ans. (c) Thrush

[Ref. Neena Khanna, 4/e p294]

Clinical Presentation of Candidiasis

Type of Candidiasis	Body Part	Feature
Acute mucocutaneous candidiasis		
Intertrigo candidiasis	Flexures	Frayed scaling, pustules
Candidial paronychia	Nails	Red, swollen nail-fold
Genital candidiasis	Genitalia	Vulvovaginitis Balanoposthitis
Oral candidiasis	Oral mucosa	Thrush (Most common) Angular stomatitis Leucoplakia
Chronic mucocutaneous candidiasis		In endocrinopathies
Systemic candidiasis		In leucopenia, HIV patients

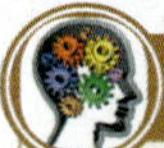

Also Remember

- Cause of Tinea capitis:
  - Non-inflammatory tinea capitis: Trichophyton verrucosum
  - Inflammatory tinea capitis/ Kerion: Microphyton canis
  - Favus: Trichosporum schoenleinii
- *Cause of Conjunctivitis*: Allergic, Bacterial, Viral, Chemical, Neonatal
- *Cause of Desert rheumatism*: Coccidiomycosis

41. Ans. (a) Epithelial keratitis

[Ref. Principles and Practice of Infectious Diseases by Bennett, 8/e p1409]

42. Ans. (a) Human papilloma virus

[Ref. Neena Khanna, 5/e p287]

- Human Papiloma virus (HPV) is a DNA virus of more than 120 genotypes having clinical association with common wart

43. Ans. (a) Candidiasis

[Ref. Medscape]

- Candidiasis is the **most frequent fungal infection in setting of Neutropenia**
- Staphylococcus aureus skin infection is the most frequent bacterial infection in setting of Neutropenia

44. Ans. (d) Varicella zoster

[Ref. Pelvic Pain: Diagnosis and Management by Howard, 1/e p466]

- Varicella-zoster virus: Virus that causes chickenpox and shingles

45. Ans. (c) Both

[Ref. Sure Success in PGMEE by B. Ramgopal, 1st Ed., Pg 223]

46. Ans. (c) Human papiloma virus

[Ref. Neena Khanna, 5/e p287]

- Human Papilloma virus (HPV) is a DNA virus of more than 120 genotypes having clinical association with common wart

47. Ans. (a) Burrows

[Ref. Neena Khanna, 5/e p367]

- Mites burrow through the Stratum corneum
- Copulation occurs in burrow

48. Ans. (b) Virus

[Ref. Neena Khanna, 4/e p274]

Molluscum Contagiosum

- *Causative agent*: Pox Virus
- *Clinical presentation*:
  - Pearly white, ***'umblicated'* dome-shaped papules**
  - Pseudo-isomorphic phenomenon
  - White cheesy material on incision
- *Treatment*:
  - Cryotherapy
  - Chemical cautery
  - Wart paint

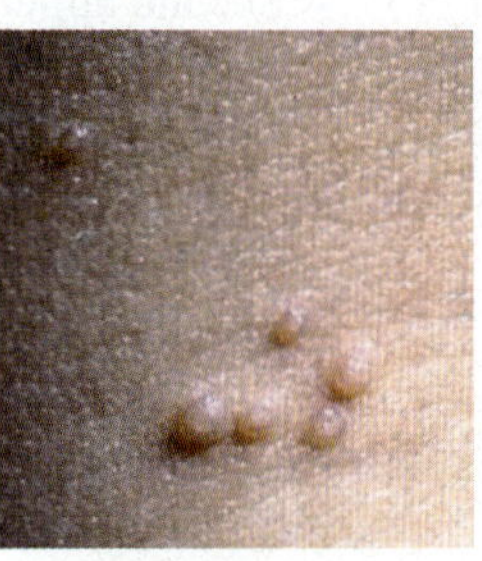

Fig. Molluscum contagiosum

49. Ans. (c) Lichen scrofulososum
[Ref. Neena Khanna, 5/e p270]

Well Established Tuberculides

- Lichen scrofulosorum: characterized by grouped popular lesion on trunk
- Papulonecrotic tuberculide: characterized by papules surmounted with pustules/crusts and healing with scarring

50. Ans. (d) Subdermal
[Ref. Principles and Practice of Infectious Diseases by Bennett, 8/e p2985]

- Dermatophyte infections are superficial infections of the stratum corneum of the skin

51. Ans. (d) Scabies
[Ref. Neena Khanna, 4/e p341]

Scabies

- *Underlying cause*: Sarcoptes scabei var. hominis (Itch mite)
- *Route of transmission*:
  - Skin contact
  - Sexual transmission
  - Fomite transmission
  - Mite burrows through stratum corneum and lays eggs
- *Clinical presentation*:
  - Asymptomatic
  - Severe itching more severe at night

Primary lesions	Secondary lesions
Burrows (Pathogonomic lesion) Papules Papulo-vesicles	Pustules Eczema Nodular lesions

- *Sites involved*: Webs of fingers, Flexures
- *Complications*:
  - Eczematization
  - Acute post-streptococcal glomerulonephritis
  - Secondary infection with Staph. aureus and Strep. pyogenes
- *Treatment of Scabies*:

Topical applications	
Topical applications	
5% Permethrin	Drug of choice for Scabies
25% Benzyl benzoate	Older drug of choice
1% Gammaxene/ BHC	Can cause seizures, avoided in infants
10% Crotamiton	Useful in children
10% Sulphur	Useful in children
Oral medications	
Ivermectin	Useful in epidemic, Norwegian form

52. Ans. (a) Malassezia furfur
[Ref. Neena Khanna, 5/e p310]

- Malassezia furfur (earlier classified as *Pityrosporum ovale*), a commensal yeast is causative agent of Tinea versicolor

53. Ans. (d) Fever is a common finding

54. Ans. (d) All of the above
[Ref. Neena Khanna, 4/e p283]

Dermatophytic Infections

- *Definition*: Fungal infection that affects skin, hair and nails DUE TO their ability to obtain nutrients from keratinized material
- *Causative agents*:
  - Microsporum
  - Trichophyton
  - Epidermophyton
- *Types of Tinea*:

Type of Tinea	Body Part Affected	Feature
Tinea capitis	Tinea of scalp	Discoid alopecia
Tinea corporis	Tinea of trunk and limbs	In hairless skin
Tinea incognito	Modified by steroid therapy	-
Tinea cruris	Tinea of groin	Inner region of thighs
Tinea pedis	Tinea of feet	Athlete's foot
Tinea mannum	Tinea of hands	Plaques or Erythema
Tinea unguium	Tinea of nails (Onchomycosis)	Tunneling, Subungal hyperkeratosis, oncholysis

Also Remember

Synonymous Names

Type of Tinea	Synonymous name
Tinea capitis	**Blackdot ringworm**, Scalp ring worm
Tinea corporis	Ringworm of body
Tinea cruris	**Jock itch**
Tinea pedis	**Athlete's foot**
Tinea mannum	Ringworm of hands
Tinea unguium	Ringworm of nails/ Onchomycosis
Tinea faciei	Ringworm of face

55. Ans. (b) Stratum corneum
[Ref. Neena Khanna, 5/e p367]

56. Ans. (a) KOH test
[Ref. Neena Khanna, 5/e p4]

- This simple bedside test should always be done if a fungal infection is suspecte(d)

57. Ans. (b) Kaposi sarcoma
[Ref. Neena Khanna, 4/e p380]

Causative Organisms

- *Hairy cell leukemia*: Tobacco/ radiation/ chemical/ HTLV-2
- *Kaposi sarcoma*: Human herpes virus 8
- *Oral hairy leukoplakia*: Ebstein barr virus
- *Molluscum contagiosum*: Pox virus

58. Ans. (b) Culture
[Ref. Fungal Infection by Richardson, 4/e p357]

- Definitive diagnosis of Sporotrichosis depends on the isolation of the aetiological agent from material aspirated from a lesion or a tissue biopsy specimen

- Clinical material should be inoculated onto several media, including glucose peptone (Sabouraud's dextrose) agar and brain -heart infusion agar, and incubation at 25-30° C

59. Ans. (a) PUVA
[Ref. Neena Khanna, 5/e p406]

Treatment of Stage I Mycosis Fungoides

- Potent topical corticosteroid
- Narrow band UVB
- Psoralens + UVA (PUVA)

60. Ans. (c) Pox virus
[Ref. Neena Khanna, 4/e p274]

61. Ans. (b) Candida
[Ref. Head and Neck Pathology by Wenig, 3/e p244]

62. Ans. (a) Staphylococcus aureus
[Ref. Neena Khanna, 4/e p247]

- **Ritter's disease** (Staphylococcus scalded skin syndrome **SSSS**):
  - *Causative agent*: Staphylococcus aureus
  - *Characteristic feature*: Superficial peeling of skin in infants

63. Ans. (c) Hands
[Ref. Neena Khanna, 4/e p286]

64. Ans. (c) Molluscum contagiosum
[Ref. Podiatric Dermatology, 1/e p156]

Molluscum Contagiosum

- Causative agent: Pox Virus
- Clinical presentation:
  - Pearly white, 'umblicated' dome-shaped papules
  - Pseudo-isomorphic phenomenon
  - White cheesy material on incision

65. Ans. (c) Central scaling
[Ref. Dermatology by Fry L, 1/e p6]

Candida Intertrigo

- Candida albicans is the most common causative species
- Usually affects the groins, and submammary, perianal and perivulval skin
- Erythematous macerated skin
- Occurs almost exclusively in obese individuals
- Can be distinguished from simple Seborrheic eczema because there are **Satellite lesions**
- Skin involvement may spread to the buttocks or down the thighs
- Candidal.intertrigo.is more uniformly red with no central clearing

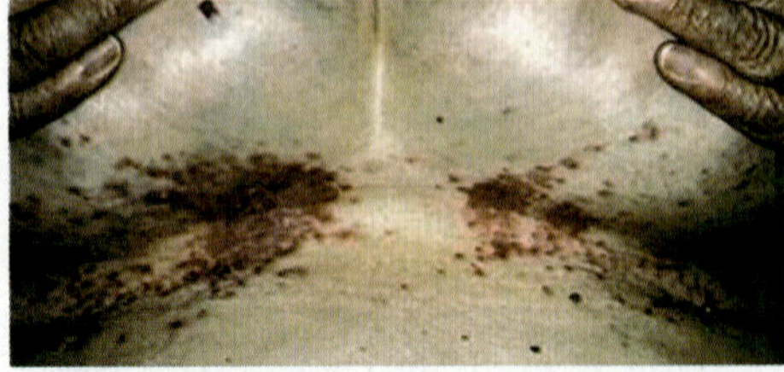

Fig. Candida intertrigo with satellite lesions

66. Ans. (c) Lupus vulgaris
[Ref. Dermatology by Braun-Falco, 2/e p211]

Lupus Vulgaris

- MC morphological variant of Cutaneous tuberculosis
- Classical lupus lesions are often seen in the head and neck region
- **Turkey ear**: A clinically descriptive term, previously being used for the earlobe with reddish indurated plaque lesions

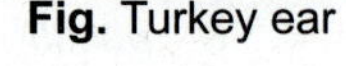

Fig. Turkey ear

67. Ans. (b) Burrows are intradermal lesions
[Ref. Diagnostic Pathology by Milner, 1/e pVI1/4]

- Classical scabies Burrows: Wavy gray-brown lines on epidermal surface Predilection for palms, soles, wrists, nipples, inframammary folds, waist, and male genitalia
- Norwegian scabies: Crusted lesions and scaly plaques infected with hundreds to millions of female mites
- Nodular scabies: Subcutaneous nodules on trunk, thighs, abdomen

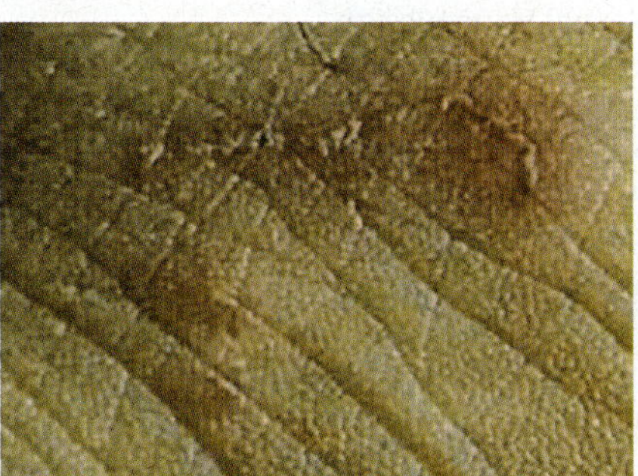

Fig. Scabies burrow

68. Ans. (c) Topical gentamycin
[Ref. Neena Khanna, 5/e p367]

Treatment of Impetigo

- Topical antibiotics like Sodium fusidate or Mupirocin
- Systemic antibiotics like Azithromycin for 5-7 days
- In poor response, Cloxacillin or Amoxicillin-Clavulanic acid or Cephalexin

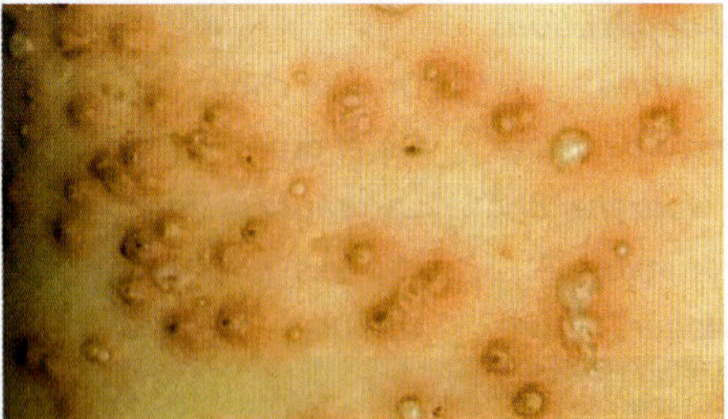

Fig. Impetigo

69. Ans. (a) Epidermophyton floccosum
[Ref. Pediatric Nurse Practitioner by Silbert-Flagg, 5/e]

Tinea Cruris (Jock Itch)

- Superficial dermatophyte fungal skin infection of the groin, upper thighs, and/or inguinal folds
- Caused by Epidermophyton floccosum, Trichophyton rubrum, Trichophyton mentagrophytes

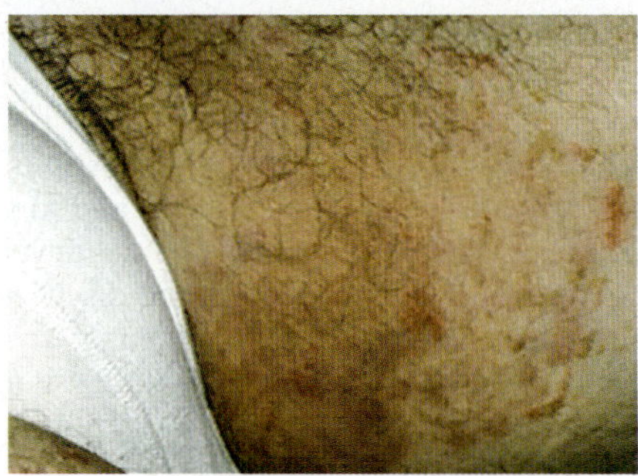

Fig. Jock's itch

70. Ans. (b) Leishmaniasis
[Ref. Conn's Current Therapy 2016, p282]

Volcano sign

- Cutaneous leishmaniasis is characterized by an ulcerated nodule with a raised and indurated border
- It begins as a small erythematous papule at the site of the bite of the Sandfly
- Look like Volcano from above

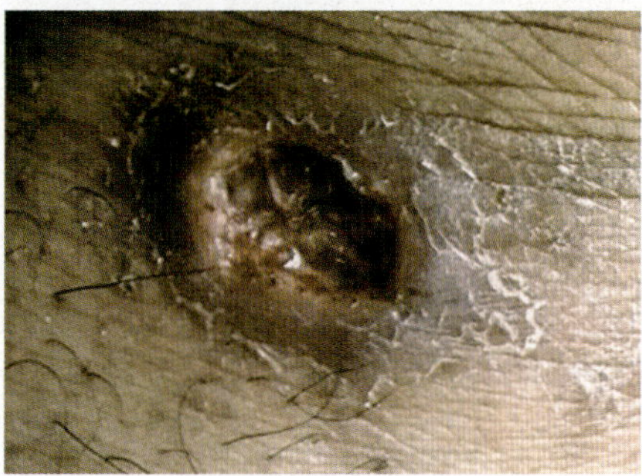

Fig. Volcano sign

71. Ans. (b) Nystatin
[Ref. AHFS Drug Information, 2000, p120]

- Topical therapy with Oral clotrimazole or Oral nystatin the treatment of choice for uncomplicated Oropharyngeal candidiasis in HIV-infected patients
- Systemic antifungal agents (Oral fluconazole/itraconazole/ketoconazole) be reserved for the treatment of Oropharyngeal candidiasis unresponsive to topical agents or for the treatment of severe Oropharyngeal candidiasis with esophageal involvement

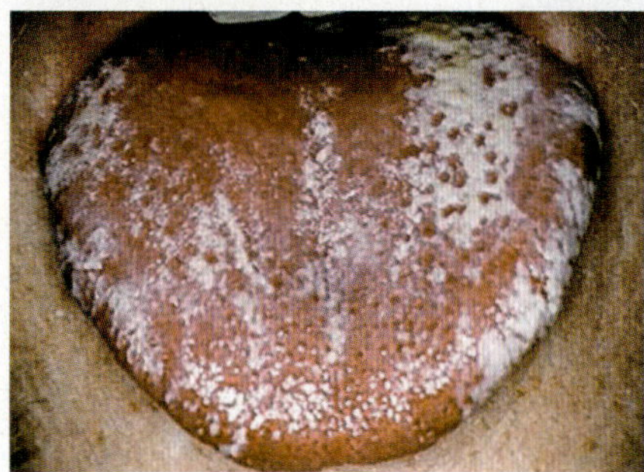

Fig. Oral candidiasis

72. Ans. (c) Itraconazole
[Ref. Neena Khanna, 5/e p311-312]

Treatment of Pityriasis Versicolor

- Topical agents: 2% Ketokonazole, 2.5% selenium sulphide
- Systemic agents: Fluconazole – 300 mg once weekly × 2 week, Itraconazole – 200 mg OD × 5 days, Ketokonazole - 400 mg OD

Fig. Pityriasis versicolor

73. Ans. (c) HPV 3 & 10
[Ref. Taylor and Kelly's Dermatology for Skin of Color, 2/e p652]

- Plane/Flat warts are mainly caused by HPV-3 and HPV-10, while Common warts are mainly caused by HPV-2 and HPV-4

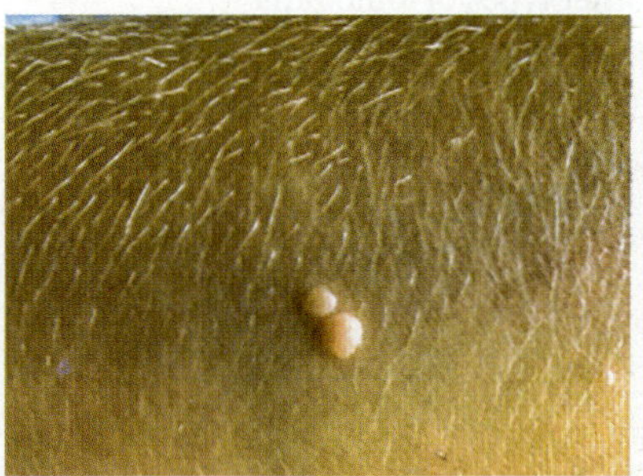

Fig. Flat warts

74. Ans. (d) 4-5 weeks
[Ref. Manson's Tropical Diseases, 22/e p1591]

- Incubation period of Scabies is 4 to 6 weeks with initial exposure; 1 to 5 days with re-exposure

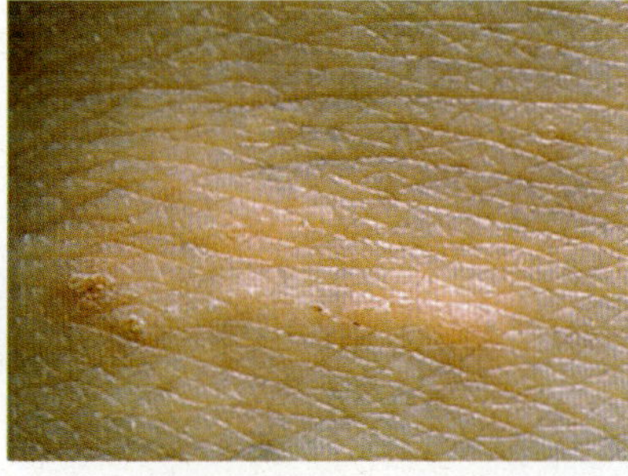

Fig. Scabies burrows

75. Ans. (a) Mite
[Ref. Lippincott's Guide to Infectious Diseases, 1/e p288]

- Scabies is a contagious disease caused by the mite Sarcoptes scabiei (Itch mite)
- Scabies is a highly transmissible skin infection that is characterized by burrows, pruritus, and excoriations with secondary bacterial infection

- Mites that cause this disorder can live their entire life cycle in human skin, causing chronic infection
- Female mite burrows into the skin to lay eggs, from which larvae emerge to copulate and then re-burrow under the skin

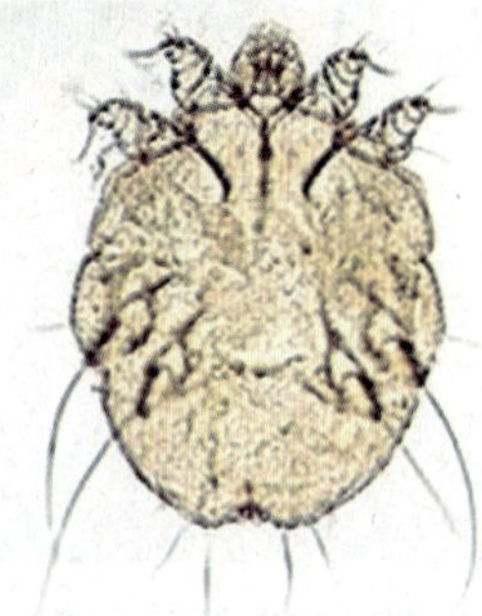

Fig. Sarcoptes scabiei

76. Ans. (c) Golden yellow

[Ref. Textbook of Medical Mycology by Chander, 4/e p179]

- Wood's Lamp shows golden yellow fluorescence in Pityriasis versicolor and Malassezia folliculitis to differentiate from other types of folliculitis

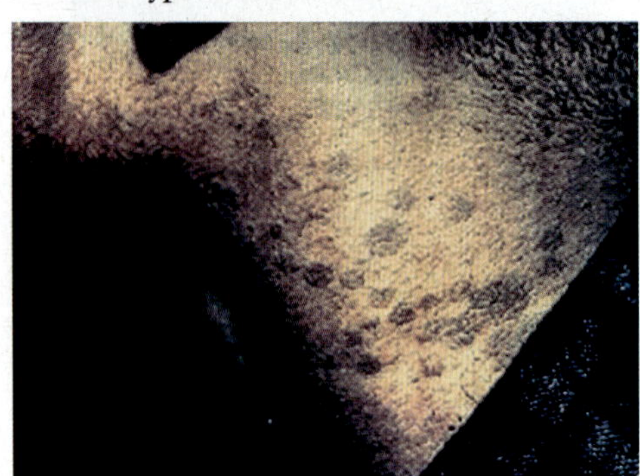

Fig. Golden yellow fluorescence

77. Ans. (a) Lupus vulgaris

[Ref. Neena Khanna, 4/e p252]

Lupus Vulgaris

- Annular plaques with peripheral nodules
- Depigmentation and scarring
- Apple-jelly nodules
- Location: Face, Buttocks

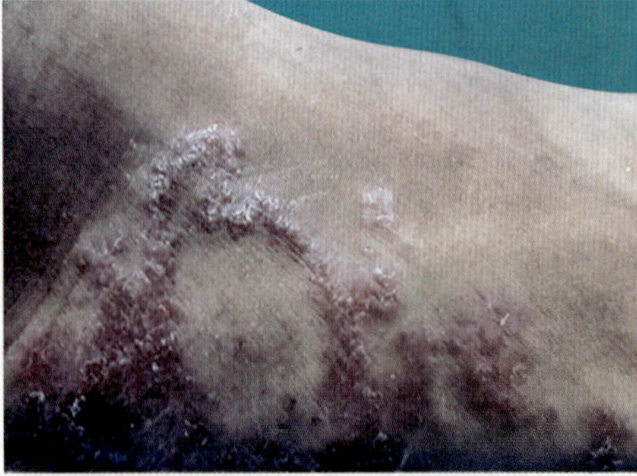

Fig. Lupus vulgaris (Annular plaques)

78. Ans. (c) Carbuncle

[Ref. Dermatology by Rycroft, 2/e p208]

- Carbuncle
- Carbuncles are more extensive lesions with infection and necrosis spreading to several follicles and to surrounding soft tissues; an inflammatory nodule develops into a follicular pustule which will point and discharge
- Causative agent: Staphylococcus aureus
- Predisposing factors: Diabetes mellitus, Systemic steroids
- Characteristic feature: Multiple erythrematous pus-discharging plaques

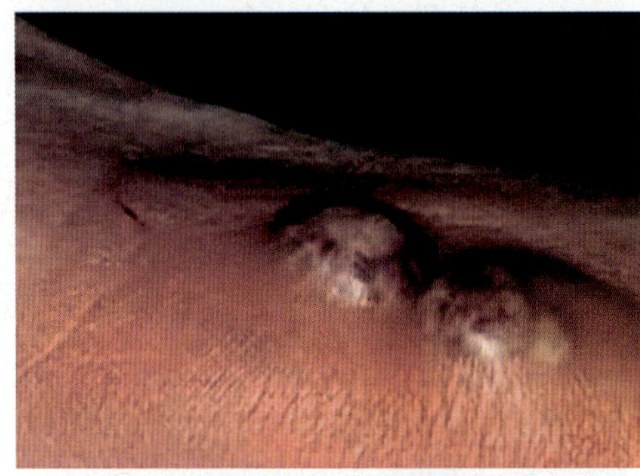

Fig. Carbuncle

79. Ans. (b) Staphylococcus

[Ref. Rook's Textbook of Dermatology, 9/e p26.6]

- A boil is a bacterial infection that begins deep in a hair follicle or a sebaceous gland, one of the skin's oil-producing glands, and gradually works its way up to the surface of the skin
  - Boils are a common and more severe form of folliculitis, often affecting sebaceous and sweat glands
  - A boil is a painful, tender, elevated red-rimmed pustule that grows until it discharges or is opened with a sterile needle or blade
- Staphylococcus aureus is the bacteria most frequently responsible for boils

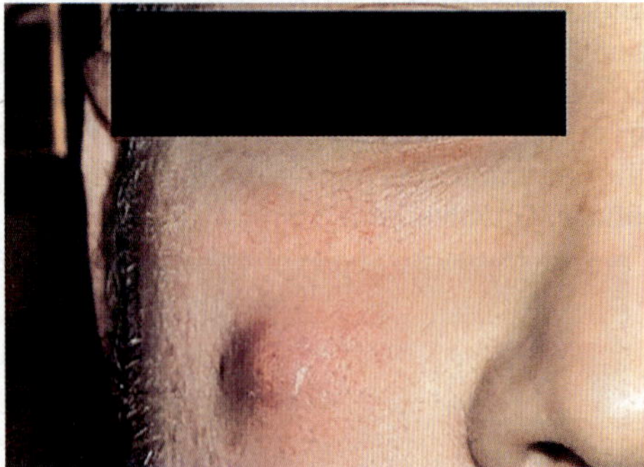

Fig. Boil on face

80. Ans. (a) Pediculosis

[Ref. Lippincott's Guide to Infectious Diseases, 1/e p236]

- Patient with Pediculosis corporis may have excoriated red papules on the axilla, groin, and trunk and small, gray-blue spots (Maculae ceruleae) on the thighs or upper body
- Present in areas where clothing most commonly contacts a person, such as the waistband and on buttocks and thighs

 HIGH YIELD MCQs ANSWERS WITH EXPLANATIONS 

1. Ans. (c) Tinea cruris
[Ref. DVT by Thappa, 4/e p80]

Aggravation of Lesions in Tinea Cruris

- Presence of annular plaques over the groins suggests tinea cruris
- Application of steroid creams gives symptomatic relief but aggravate the underlying dermatophytosis

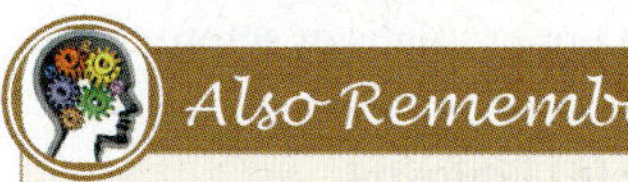

- Annular lichen planus is usually present on glans penis and topical steroids help in resolution of lesions
- Granuloma annulare is usually asymptomatic
- Erythema annulare centrifugum, which is a hypersensitivity reaction to dermatophytes, can present with annular urticarial plaques, which heal with pigmentation, itching is variable

2. Ans. (d) 4 weeks
[Ref. Oral and Maxillofacial Pathology by Neville, 4/e p228]

- In defining Post-herpetic neuralgia, there is a lack of consensus regarding the duration of pain persistence following the rash, although many investigators consider 1-3 months
- Risk factors: Old age, females, Prodromal pain, Moderate-severe rash, Pain during acute phase, Ophthalmic involvement

3. Ans. (b) Lupus vulgaris
[Ref. Neena Khanna, 4/e p221]

Lupus vulgaris

- Annular plaques with peripheral nodules
- Well demarcated annular lesions extending centrifugally
- Apple-jelly nodules on periphery
- Atrophic, depigmented and scarred centre
- Sites: Buttocks (Most common), Upper extremities, Face

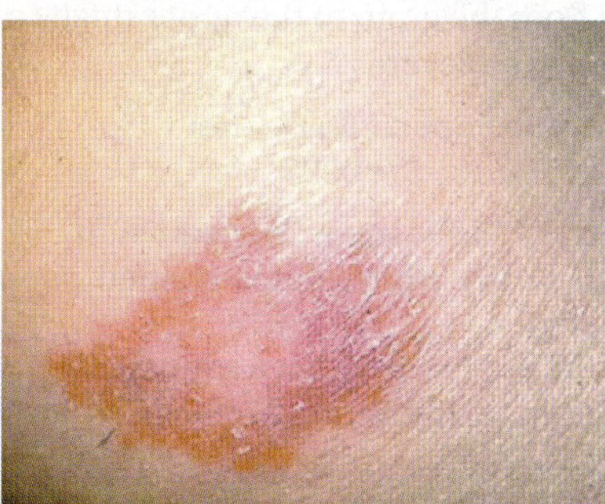

Fig. Lupus vulgaris

4. Ans. (a) Lichen scrofulosorum
[Ref. Neena Khanna, 5/e p270]

5. Ans. (c) Tinea capitis
[Ref. Neena Khanna, 5/e p301]

Tinea Capitis

- Invariably children
- Discoid patch of partial alopecia with scaling

6. Ans. (a) Lichen scrofulosorum
[Ref. Rook's Textbook of Dermatology, 7/e 28.20; Weedon's Skin Pathology, 2/e p627]

Lichen Scrofulosorum

- Presence of non caseating epithelioid granulomas and localization around hair follicles and sweat ducts suggests a diagnosis of Lichen Scrofulosorum
- It is a tuberculid that has a tendency to cause inflammation around hair follicles and sweat ducts
- Granulomas with epithelioid and giant cells are seen but there is no caseous necrosis
- Characteristic features are
  - Discrete cutaneous lesions occurring in the superficial dermis in patients with tuberculosis elsewhere in the body
  - Perifollicular and eccrine localization of hair follicles and sweat ducts in the dermis
  - Epithelioid Granulomas without Caseous necrosis-Non caseating granulomas
  - Acid fast organisms are usually not seen
  - Cell mediate immunity to tubercular antigen is usually strongly positive
  - Papulonecrotic tuberculides often present with central necrosis and are not typically localized to hair follicles and sweat ducts

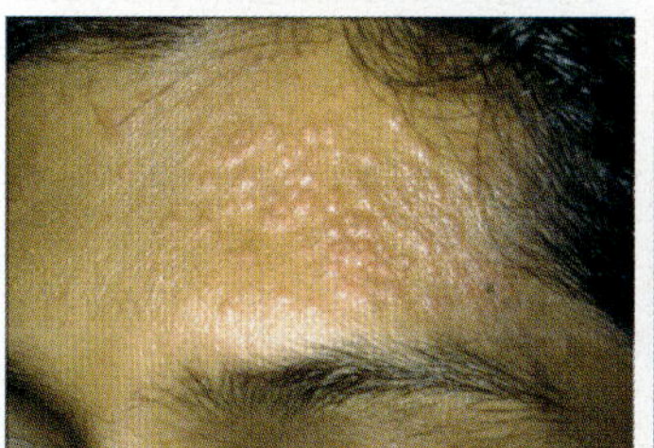
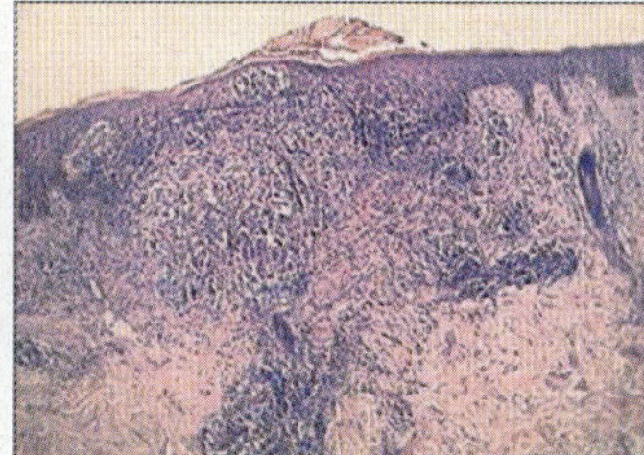

Fig. L. scrofulosorum

7. Ans. (c) Lupus vulgaris
[Ref. Neena Khanna, 5/e p234]

Characteristic Features of Lupus Vulgaris

- Distribution: face & buttocks
- Absent follicular plug
- Atrophic and scarred
- Nodules characteristically present in scarred area
- Annular or arcuate plaque with an indurated border

8. Ans. (c) Biopsy
[Ref. Roxburgh's Common Skin Diseases, 16/e p41]

- The subject is having lupus vulgaris because the lesions have central scarring (characteristic of lupus vulgaris)
- Diagnosis of lupus vulgaris is biopsy

9. Ans. (b) Lupus vulgaris
[Ref. Neena Khanna, 5/e p234]

10. Ans. (a) Lichen scrofulosorum; (d) Erythema nodosum
[Ref. Neena Khanna, 5/e p270; Fitzpatrick's Dermatology in General Medicine, 7/e p1774; Rook's Textbook of Dermatology by Burns, 7/e 28.20]

Tuberculids

- True tuberculides: Mycobacterium tuberculosis plays a major etiologic role
- Facultative tuberculides: Mycobacterium tuberculosis is one of several possibly etiologic agents
    - All were once believed to be a consequence of hypersensitivity to the presence of mycobacterial antigens within a host of previously acquired immunity to TB
- Well established tuberculides:
    - Lichen scrofulosorum: Grouped popular lesion on trunk
    - Papulonecrotic tuberculide: Papules surmounted with pustules/ crusts and healing with scarring
    - Erythema nodosum, Erythema induratum (Bazin's disease): Facultative tuberculides

11. Ans. (d) Contact with animal
[Ref. Dermatology by Braun-Falco, 1/e p211]

12. Ans. (a) Scarlet fever
[Ref. The Encyclopedia of Skin and Skin Disorders by Turkington, 3/e p321]

- Scarlet fever is caused by infection with Group A streptococcus.

13. Ans. (d) Roseola infantum
[Ref. Infectious Diseases by Ramsay, 1/e p167]

14. Ans. (a) Trichophyton rubrum
[Ref. Principles and Practice of Infectious Diseases by Bennett, 8/e p2985]

15. Ans. (a) Superficial
[Ref. Principles and Practice of Infectious Diseases by Bennett, 8/e p2985]

- Dermatophyte infections are superficial infections of the stratum corneum of the skin

16. Ans. (b) Epidermophyton
[Ref. Neena Khanna, 5/e p302-303]

Tinea Capitis Causes

- Microsporum: M. audouinii, M. canis
- Trichophyton: T. tonsurans, T. violaceum, T. verrucosum

17. Ans. (a) Tinea capitis
[Ref. Neena Khanna, 5/e p301,302]

Characteristics of Tinea Capitis

- Invariably a child
- Discoid patch of partial alopecia from which the hair can be easily and painlessly be plucked
- Varied degree of inflammation depending on the strain of fungus

18. Ans. (c) KOH preparation
[Ref. Neena Khanna, 5/e p301,302]

- The diagnosis is suggestive of Tinea capitis
- Potassium Hydroxide (KOH) scrapping is simple, inexpensive quick and sensitive investigation

19. Ans. (c) KOH mount
[Ref. Neena Khanna, 5/e p301,302]

20. Ans. (a) Epidermophyton
[Ref. Neena Khanna, 5/e p302-303]

21. Ans. (a) Oral griseofulvin therapy
[Ref. Neena Khanna, 5/e p309]

Treatment Protocol for Tinea Capitis

- Oral griseofulvin (8 wks)
- Oral terbinafine (4-8 wks)

22. Ans. (a) Trichophyton rubrum
[Ref. Oxford Textbook of Medicine by Warrell, 5/e p621]

- Tinea cruris / Tinea of groin is often caused by Trichophyton rubrum
- An erythematous and scaly rash with a distinct margin extends from the groin to the upper thighs or scrotum
- Itching may be severe

23. Ans. (c) Impetigo contagiosa; (e) Ecthyma
[Ref. Neena Khanna, 5/e p260, 263]

- **Impetigo Contagiosa**: Staphylococcus aureus &/or Streptococcus pyogenes
- **Ecthyma**: Staphylococcus aureus &/or Streptococcus pyogenes

24. Ans. (c) Scabies
[Ref. Neena Khanna, 5/e p367]

25. Ans. (a) Stratum corneum
[Ref. Neena Khanna, 5/e p301]

- Ring worm fungi/ Dermatophytes are keratinophilic fungi, living on dead keratin (o in stratum corneum)

26. Ans. (b) Malassezia furfur
[Ref. Neena Khanna, 5/e p310]

27. Ans. (d) Tinea cruris
[Ref. Oxford Textbook of Medicine by Warrell, 5/e p621]

- Tinea cruris/Tinea of groin is often caused by **Trichophyton rubrum**

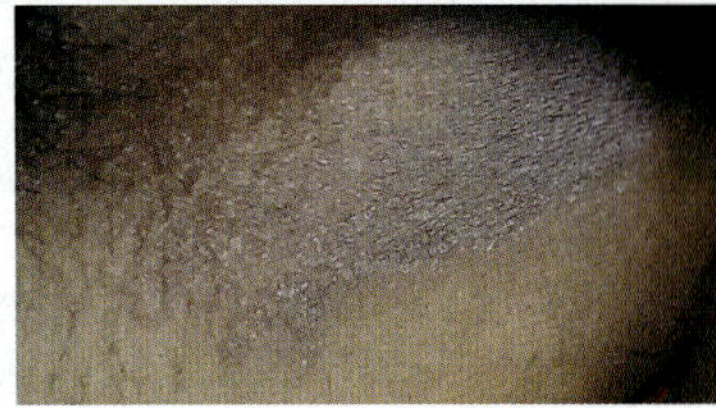

Fig. Tinea cruris

- An erythematous and scaly rash with a distinct margin extends from the groin to the upper thighs or scrotum
- Itching may be severe.

28. Ans. (a) Molluscum contagiosum
[Ref. Neena Khanna, 5/e p292]

Morphology of Molluscum Contagiosum

- Multiple, pearly white, dome-shaped papules which are umbilicated
- Under a hand lens, may have a mosaic appearance
- On piercing the umbilicated center, a white cheesy material can be extruded

29. Ans. (a) Trichophyton rubrum

30. Ans. (a) Scabies
[Ref. Neena Khanna, 5/e p367]

31. Ans. (b) Pox virus
[Ref. Neena Khanna, 5/e p292]

32. Ans. (e) All are correct
[Ref. Neena Khanna, 5/e p292]

33. Ans. (b) Thoracic region
[Ref. Neena Khanna, 5/e p295]

- Sites of predilection: Uni/ multidermatomal. Thoracic intercostals nerves and ophthalmic division of trigeminal nerve

34. Ans. (b) Potassium hydroxide mount
[Ref. Neena Khanna, 5/e p4]

35. Ans. (a) Potassium hydroxide preparation of scales
[Ref. Neena Khanna, 5/e p311]

Pityriasis Versicolor to be Suspected
- Adolescent or young adult
- Hypopigmented (sometimes hyperpigmented), perifollicular macules that become confluent
- Lesions appear to be sitting on neck
- Branny scales, accentuated by scratching with glass slide
- Upper trunk and neck

Fig. Pityriasis versicolor

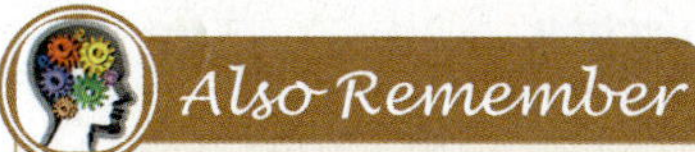

Also Remember
- KOH mount confirmatory shows a mixture of short, branched hyphae and spores (Spaghetti and meat ball appearance)

36. Ans. (c) Face
[Ref. Neena Khanna, 5/e p296, 297]
- HSV1: Orofacial
- HSV2: Anogenital

37. Ans. (a) Ketoconazole
[Ref. Neena Khanna, 5/e p311]
- Ketoconazole, 2% applied daily for 1-4 weeks

38. Ans. (c) Adult male
[Ref. Oxford Textbook of Medicine by Warrell, 5/e p621]
- Adult Males more affected than females

39. Ans. (a) Sporotrichosis; (c) Madras foot; (d) Tinea
[Ref. Neena Khanna, 5/e p292]
- Molluscum contagiousum is due to Pox virus

40. Ans. (a) Acyclovir
[Ref. Neena Khanna, 5/e p300]

Principles of Treatment of HSV Infection
- Acyclovir, 400 mg TDS × 7-10 days
- Famciclovir, 250 mg TDS × 7-10 days
- Valacyclovir, 1gm BD × 7-10 days

41. Ans. (a) Lupus vulgaris; (c) Scrofuloderma
[Ref. Neena Khanna, 5/e p268]

Common Presentations of Cutaneous Tuberculosis
- Lupus vulgaris
- Scrofuloderma
- Tuberous verrucosa cutis
- Tuberculides
- Miliary TB

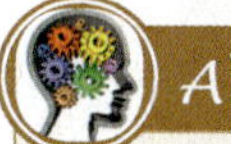

Also Remember
- MC type of cutaneous TB in adult population: Lupus Vulgaris.

42. Ans. (b) Post auricular
[Ref. Neena Khanna, 5/e p300]

43. Ans. (a) Scabies
[Ref. Neena Khanna, 5/e p367]

44. Ans. (a) Candidiasis
[Ref. Neena Khanna, 5/e p313]

45. Ans. (d) Rheumatic fever
[Ref. Dermatology, Volume 1 by Jean Bolognia, 1/e p306]
- Erythema marginatum is seen in less than 10% of patients acute rheumatic fever
- The target-like lesions of erythema multiforme evolve over a period of 1 week

46. Ans. (a) Family should be examined; (c) All clothing & linen...; (e) Drug should be applied to...
[Ref. Neena Khanna, 5/e p367]
- It is suspected of scabies and preventive management should be followed

47. Ans. (c) Postprimary tuberculosis with good resistance
[Ref. Neena Khanna, 5/e p269]
- TVC is cutaneous tuberculosis in a patient with good immunity (resistance towards disease) , with bacillus reaching the skin by inoculation (i.e. from exogenous source)

48. Ans. (a) Lichen scrofulosorum; (d) Erythema nodosum
[Ref. Neena Khanna, 5/e p270; Fitzpatrick's Dermatology in General Medicine, 7/e p1774]

49. Ans. (a) Lupus vulgaris
[Ref. Neena Khanna, 5/e p268]

50. Ans. (a) Apple jelly nodule at root of nose; (b) TB of skin & mucosa; (d) ATT helpful; (e) Is most common type of cutaneous tuberculosis
[Ref. Neena Khanna, 5/e p268]

51. Ans. (b) Face
[Ref. Neena Khanna, 5/e p367]
- In adults , scalp, face, palms and soles are characteristically spared but typically involved in infants/ children

52. Ans. (d) Scrotum
[Ref. Neena Khanna, 5/e p367]
- Persistent nodular lesions, sometime by a burrow, may be seen on scrotum and penis, anterior axillary folds and in groins

53. Ans. (b) Scrofuloderma
[Ref. Neena Khanna, 5/e p269]

- Scrofuloderma is cutaneous tuberculosis due to direct extension of infection from an underlying tuberculosis focus present either in lymph nodes, bone or a joint
- It generally occurs in a patient with poor moderate immunity

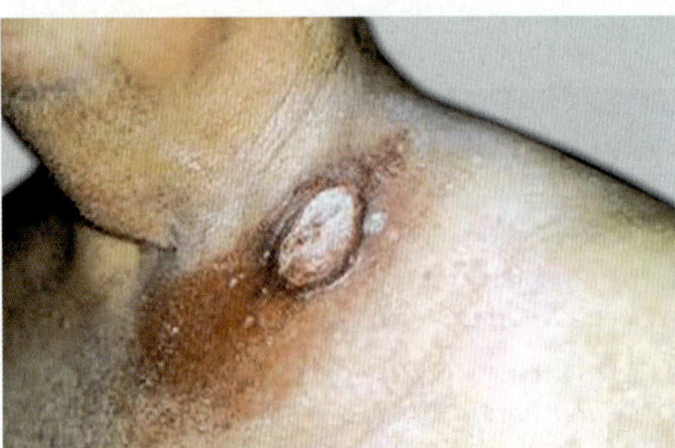

Fig. Scrofuloderma

54. Ans. (c) M. ulcerans; (e) M. marinum
[Ref. Granulomatous Disorders of Adult Skin, an Issue of Dermatologic Clinics by Joseph C. English, Vol/33 p565]

- Clinical settings for skin and soft tissue infections caused by nontuberculous mycobacteria include 2 distinctive species specific clinical disorder:
  - **"Fish-tank" granuloma caused by M marinum**
  - **Buruli ulcer (BU) caused by M ulcerans**

55. Ans. (a) Verrucae; (c) M. marinum infection
[Ref. Granulomatous Disorders of Adult Skin by English, Vol/33 p565; Foot Problems in Older People by Menz, 1/e p86]

Verrucae

- Cause: Human papillomavirus **(HPV) types 1, 2, 4, 27 and 5**
- Affect epithelial cells causing small rough papules
- Replication of the virus within the epithelial cells causes a proliferative reaction and formation of plaque or papule
- Incubation is very variable, ranging from one month to over a year
- HPV infection is acquired from direct contact with an affected individual or from the environment (e.g., from contaminated floors in communal showers/changing areas or swimming pools
- It appears the virus can survive outside the body for a significant length of time, probably months or even years
- Damaged or wet skin predisposes to infection

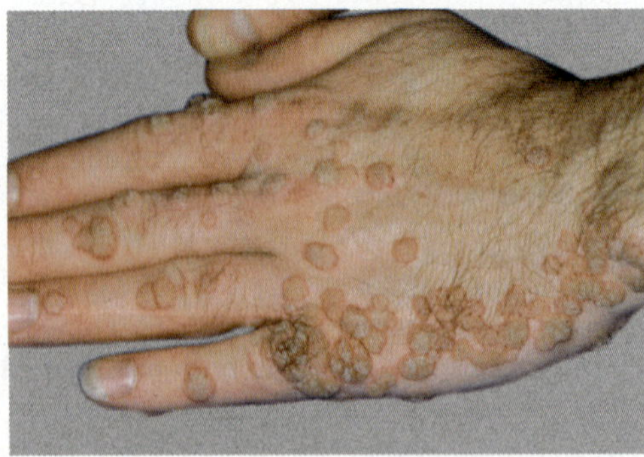

Fig. Verruca vulgaris

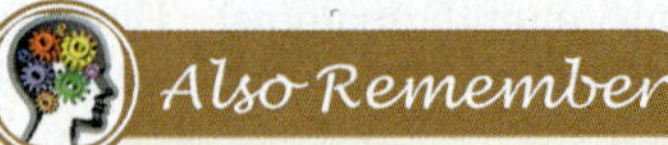

Also Remember

- Fish tank (or swimming pool) granuloma: Caused by M. marinum infection, which infects fish and is also found in swimming pools.
  - Typically, it causes a reddish, slightly scaly plaque on the hand or arm of someone who keeps tropical fish
  - M. marinum is sensitive to minocycline, clarithromycin, amikacin, rifampicin, ethambutol and doxycycline.

56. Ans. (b) Erysipelas
[Ref. Neena Khanna, 5/e p269]

- **Erysipelas** is seen only occasionally with Staphylococcus aureus as a sequelae of manipulated furuncle or in surgical wound
- In rest of the options, staph is an important etiological agent

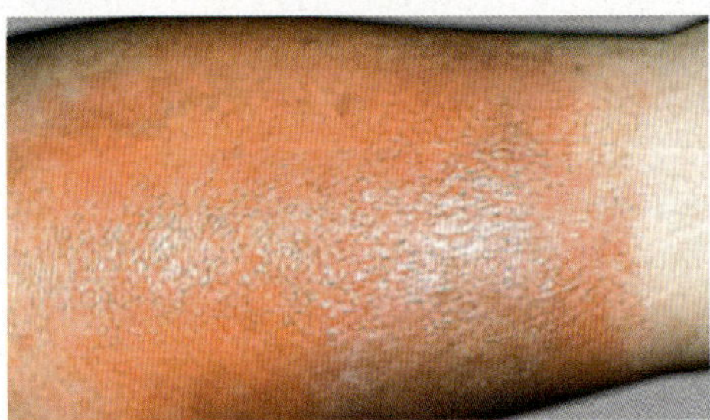

Fig. Erysipelas

57. Ans. (a) Staphylococcal infection
[Ref. Toxic Shock Syndrome by Shmaefsky, 1/e p32]

58. Ans. (d) IV antibodies
[Ref. Neena Khanna, 5/e p367]

- Diagnosis is clear cut Scabies
- IV antibiotic has no role in management of scabies.

59. Ans. (b) Typhoid fever
[Ref. Nelson Textbook of Pediatrics by Robert M. Kliegman, 20/e p1390]

Rose Spots in Typhoid

- In approximately 25% of cases, a macular or maculopapular rash (rose spots) may be visible around the 7th-10th day of the illness, and lesions may appear in crops of 10-15 on the lower chest and abdomen and last 2-3 days
- These lesions may be difficult to see in darker skinned children.

60. Ans. (c) Produces scar on healing; (d) Erythromycin is drug of choice
[Ref. Neena Khanna, 5/e p367]

Impetigo

- On drying, the crust falls leaving erythema which fades without scarring
- Management: Topical antibiotics like Sodium fusidate or Mupirocin
- Systemic antibiotics like Azithromycin for 5-7 days
- In poor response, Cloxacillin or Amoxicillin-Clavulanic acid or Cephalexin

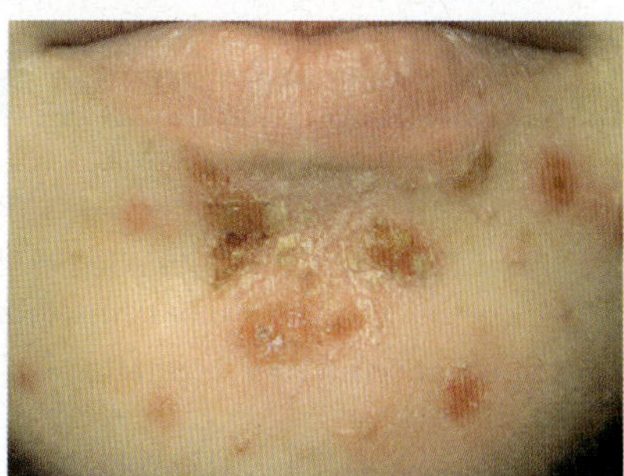

Fig. Impetigo

61. Ans. (b) Impetigo contagiosa
[Ref. Rapid Paediatrics and Child Health by Helen, 1/e p90]

62. Ans. (a) Burrow
[Ref. Neena Khanna, 5/e p367]

- Mites burrow through the Stratum corneum
- Copulation occurs in burrow

63. Ans. (b) Impetigo
[Ref. Neena Khanna, 5/e p260]

- Thin walled bulla with an erythematous halo, ruptures rapidly to form an exudative plaque covered with thick, honey coloured crusts

64. Ans. (c) Erythema infectiosum
[Ref. Nursing Care of Children by James, 4/e p362]

- Erythema infectiosum (also known as fifth disease) is usually a benign childhood condition characterized by a classic slapped-cheek appearance and lacy exanthema
- It results from infection with human parvovirus (PV) B19, an erythrovirus

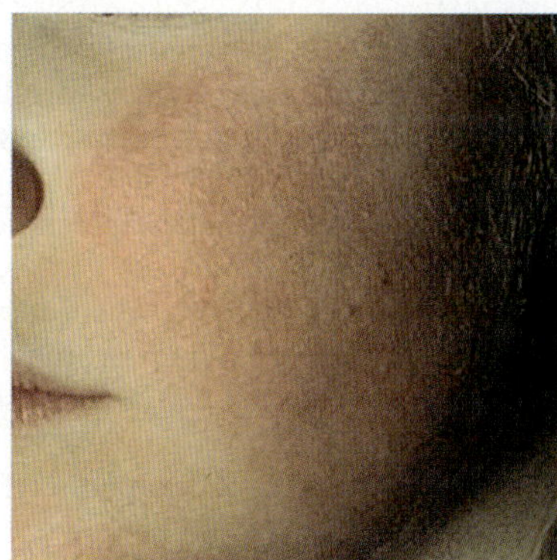

Fig. Erythema infectiosum

65. Ans. (d) Topical permethrin
[Ref. Neena Khanna, 5/e p370]

- The diagnosis is Scabies
- Management is Topical Permethrin 5% : Apply × 8 hours on day 1 & 8
  - Second application is to reduce potential for re-infestation from fomites and to kill any nymphs which may have hatched after treatment, as some eggs may have survived

66. Ans. (c) Microsporidium; (d) Trichophyton rubrum
[Ref. Principles and Practice of Infectious Diseases by Bennett, 8/e p2985]

67. Ans. (a) Epidermophyton
[Ref. Neena Khanna, 5/e p302-303]

68. Ans. (b) Microsporum
[Ref. Neena Khanna, 5/e p302-303]

69. Ans. (d) Dermatophytosis
[Ref. Dermatology by Rapini, 2/e. Mosby Elsevier]

Kerion

- A kerion is an abscess caused by fungal infection
  - It is often misdiagnosed as bacterial infection
- Occurrence: **MC on scalp** (Tinea capitis), but it may also arise on any site exposed to the fungus such as face (Tinea faciei) and upper limbs (Tinea corporis)
- Causation: Dramatic immune response to a dermatophyte fungal infection (Tinea); MC fungi found in Kerion,
  - Microsporum canis
  - Trichophyton tonsurans
  - Trichophyton verrucosum
  - Trichophyton mentagrophytes

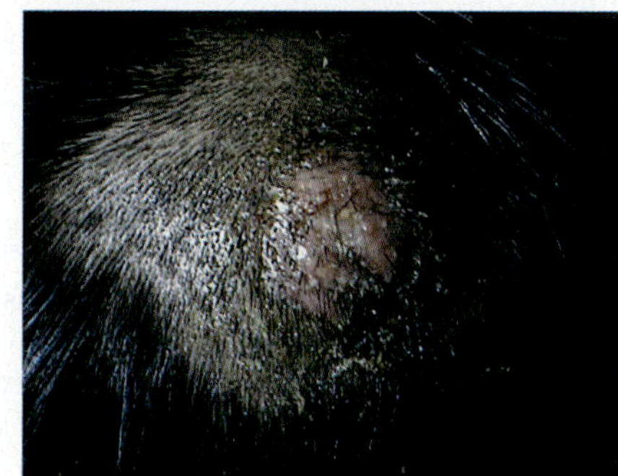

Fig. Kerion

70. Ans. (c) Griseofulvin
[Ref. Neena Khanna, 5/e p302-303]

- Treatment protocol of Tinea unguium:
  - Oral Terbinafine (6wks for finger nails & 12 weeks for toe nails)
  - Oral Griseofulvin (6wks for finger nails & 12 weeks for toe nails)

71. Ans. (b) Scabies
[Ref. Neena Khanna, 5/e p367]

72. Ans. (e) All of the above
[Ref. Introduction to Sports Medicine and Athletic Training by France, 2/e p624]

73. Ans. (a) Steroid treatment
[Ref. Neena Khanna, 5/e p304]

74. Ans. (a) Scabies
[Ref. Neena Khanna, 5/e p367]

75. Ans. (a) Candida albicans usually cause systemic infection
[Ref. Neena Khanna, 5/e p312]

76. Ans. (b) Trichophyton
[Ref. Oxford Textbook of Medicine, Volume 1 by Warrell, 4/e p690]

77. Ans. (d) Bivalent and quadrivalent
[Ref. Cervical Cancer: Contemporary Management by Rajaram, 1/e p69]

- GARDASIL (tradename) Human Papillomavirus Quadrivalent (Types 6, 11, 16, and 18) Vaccine
- CERVARIX (tradename) is designed to prevent infection from HPV types 16 and 18

78. Ans. (a) Contagious; (b) Bacterial infection; (d) Honey coloured crust
[Ref. Neena Khanna, 5/e p260]

79. Ans. (d) Candidiasis
[Ref. Neena Khanna, 5/e p312-314]

80. Ans. (a) Scabies
[Ref. Neena Khanna, 5/e p370]

81. Ans. (a) Scrofuloderma
[Ref. Neena Khanna, 5/e p269]

- **Scrofuloderma** is cutaneous tuberculosis due to direct extension of infection from an underlying tuberculosis focus present either in lymph nodes, bone or a joint
- It generally occurs in a patient with poor moderate immunity
- Sites of predilection: Cervical (most frequently), Axillary and Inguinal

82. Ans. (d) Cutaneous Leishmaniasis
[Ref. Neena Khanna, 5/e p373]

Cutaneous Leishmaniasis (Oriental Sore)

- Incubation period varies from weeks to months
- Frequently occurs on face and hands
- Asymptomatic, solitary (usually) edematous, erythematous nodule which ulcerates to form a crateriform ulcer and ultimately heals with a depressed scar (within 2 years)

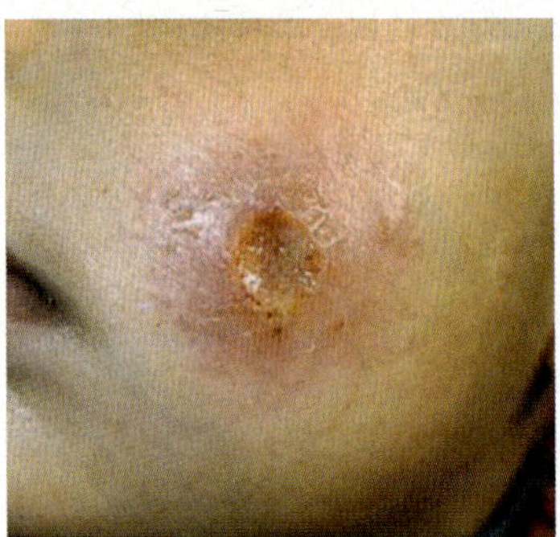

Fig. Oriental sore

83. Ans. (a) Sporotrichosis
[Ref. Neena Khanna, 5/e p373]

- Think of Sporotrichiosis when granulomatous plaques/nodules are aligned in a linear arrangement

84. Ans. (b) Stratum corneum
[Ref. Neena Khanna, 5/e p367]

85. Ans. (b) Tinea cruris
[Ref. Scientific Basis for Ayurvedic Therapies edited by Lakshmi C. Mishra, 1/e p482]

- Tinea cruris: This infection is also known as Dhobi's itch, Ringworm of the groin, Jock itch, or Eczema marginatum

86. Ans. (e) All of the above
[Ref. Neena Khanna, 5/e p370]

Use of Scabicides

Scabicide	Method of use	Comments
Permethrin 5%	8hrs × Day 1 & day 8	Scabicide of choice Resistance reported
GBHC 1%	8hrs × Day 1 & day 8	Avoided in seizure patients, infants
Benzyl benzoate 25%	3 applications, 12 hourly interval	Irritation is a common side effect
Crotamiton 10%	8 hourly on days 1, 2, 3 &8	Marginal efficacy, useful in children
Precipitated Sulphur 10%	BD × 14 days	Marginal efficacy, useful in children
Ivermectin	200 mcg/ kg, SOD Repeat after 2 weeks	Use in Epidemics in Orphanages & Norwegian

87. Ans. (b) Nail plate
[Ref. Neena Khanna, 5/e p305]

- Tinea ungum is known as Tinea of nails

88. Ans. (a) Norwegian scabies
[Ref. Neena Khanna, 5/e p367]

Crusted (Norwegian) Scabies

- Description:
  - Rare, severe form of scabies
  - Extremely contagious: Large number of mites found in and on the skin
- Seen in: Nutritional disorders, Infectious diseases, Leukemia, or Weakened immune systems (such as people who have AIDS)
- Characteristics:
  - Scaly, crusted sores on the hands, feet, scalp, face, torso, and pressure-bearing areas such as the elbows
  - Facial skin may flake off, and significant hair loss can result
  - Mild itching despite the heavy infestation of mites is characteristic
  - Mental or nervous system disorders may mask the itching sensation: When scabies itching goes undetected, the infestation can become severe
- Treatment:
  - Slow response to treatment compared with other forms of scabies
  - When multiple treatments are ineffective: Oral Ivermectin

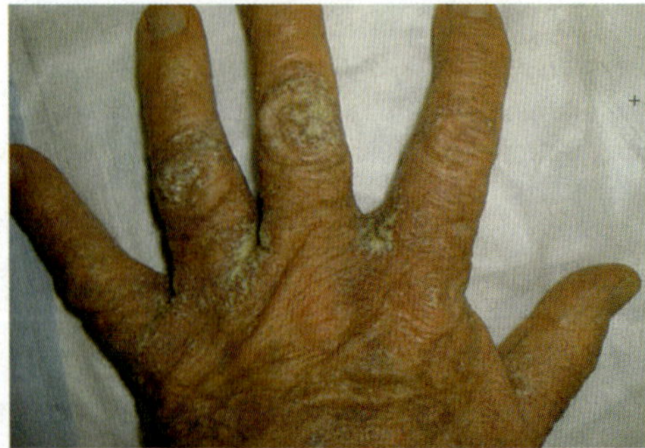

Fig. Norwegian scabies

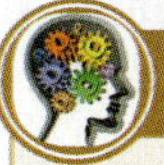

Also Remember

- Crusted scabies has been called Norwegian scabies because the condition was first described in Norway in the mid-19th century

89. Ans. (c) 4 weeks
[Ref. Neena Khanna, 5/e p367]
- Incubation period is 4-6 weeks

90. Ans. (b) Scabies
[Ref. Textbook of Dermatology, Leprology & Venereology by Thappa, 3/e p97]
- Main sites of predilection in scabies like axillae, elbows, wrists, hands, and crotch form a circle called the 'Circle of Hebra'

91. Ans. (c) Involve anterior abdomen; (d) Involve web space; (e) Involve genitalia
[Ref. Textbook of Dermatology, Leprology & Venereology by Thappa, 3/e p97]

92. Ans. (d) Rash is itchy
[Ref. Neena Khanna, 5/e p185]

93. Ans. (a) Lupus vulgaris
[Ref. Issues in Dermatology and Cosmetic Medicine, 2013 e p167]
- MC type of cutaneous TB in adult population: Lupus Vulgaris

94. Ans. (a) Pediculosis corporis
[Ref. API Textbook of Medicine by Munjal, 10/e p672]
- Pediculosis Corporis **(Vagabond's Disease)**: It is a disease of people with poor hygiene who are not regular in bathing and changing clothes and living in overcrowded condition

95. Ans. (b) Staphylococcus
[Ref. Neena Khanna, 5/e p260]

96. Ans. (a) 3 application of Gamma BHC
[Ref. API Textbook of Medicine by Munjal, 10/e p672]
- Previously TOC was GBHC, but now it is Permethrin 5% or 1% cream applied 8-10 hourly
- GHBC used is 1%

97. Ans. (a) HPV
[Ref. Anorectal and Colon Diseases: Textbook and Color Atlas of Proctology by E. Stein, 1/e p158]
- Condylomata Acuminata: Lesions caused by HPV and arising on or near mucosal surfaces, be it genital, perianal, or oral

98. Ans. (a) Caused by Staphylococcal aureus; (d) Caused by Staphylococcal pyogenes; (e) Honey coloured crusts
[Ref. Neena Khanna, 5/e p260-262]

99. Ans. (d) T. violaceum
[Ref. Neena Khanna, 5/e p302-303]

100. Ans. (b) Bartonella bacilliformis
[Ref. Andrew's Diseases of Skin, 12/e p274]

Bartonella Bacilliformis
- Diseases caused:
  - Oroya fever **(Carrion's disease)**: Acute febrile stage
  - Verruga peruana: Chronic delayed stage
- Vector: Lutzomyia verrucarum (Sandfly)

101. Ans. (a) Caused by Trichophyton; (b) Caused by Microsporum; (d) Black dot hair; (e) Oral antifungals useful
[Ref. Neena Khanna, 4/e p283]

102. Ans. ALL CHOICES
[Ref. Textbook of Family Medicine by Rakel, 8/e p32]

103. Ans. (a) Silver sulphadiazine
[Ref. Clinical Pharmacology by Maddison, 1/e p567]

104. Ans. (b) Aspergillus
[Ref. Neena Khanna, 4/e p285]
- Causative agents of Tinea Cruris:
  - Trichophyton
  - Microsporum
  - Epidermophyton

105. Ans. (d) Chronic atrophic candidiasis
Ref. Neena Khanna, 4/e p294]

Types of Oral Candidiasis
- Angular stomatitis: White plaques at angle of mouth (Seen in Dentures use)
- Acute pseudomembranous candidiasis **(Thrush)**:
  - White erythematous plaques revealing erythematous base on removal
  - Seen on tongue, palate, gingiva, mucosa
  - MC type of Candidiasis
- Acute atrophic candidiasis: Patch depapillated areas on dorsal tongue
- Chronic atrophic candidiasis: Sharply defined erythematous, edematous areas on plate (Denture mouth)
- Candidal leukoplakia:
  - Rough white-grey plaque with erythematous halo on buccal mucosa and tongue
  - Cannot be removed
  - Premalignant potential

106. Ans. (a) Candidiasis
[Ref. ENT Secrets by Murrow, 3/e p32]

107. Ans. (a) Pityrosporum
[Ref. Weeedon's Skin Pathology, 4/e p122]
- Pityrosporum/ Malassezia play a pathogenic role in Seborrheic dermatitis

108. Ans. (a) Corynebacterium
[Ref. Lippincott's Infectious Diseases, 1/e p120]
- Erythrasma, a skin disease that causes brown, scaly skin patches, is caused by the Gram-positive bacterium Corynebacterium minutissimum

109. Ans. (b) Lichen scrofulosorum
[Ref. Textbook of DVL by Thappa, 3/e p160]

Tuberculids
- Heterogeneous group of cutaneous disorders associated with TB infections elsewhere in body

- Composition:
  - Erythema induratum
  - Lichen scrofulosorum
  - Papulonecrotic tuberculids

110. Ans. (b) **Involves bone in early stages**
[Ref. Manson's Tropical Disease, 23/e p447]

Mycetoma

- Typically begins as a small subcutaneous nodule, the size of a groundnut, or an induration of the skin of exposed areas
- Madura foot) is a chronic subcutaneous infection caused by Actinomycetes/ Fungi in which the organisms form into aggregates (Grains)
- Lesion involves the subcutaneous tissues primarily but it may extend into the bones in the later stages
- Tendons and nerves are resistant to invasion

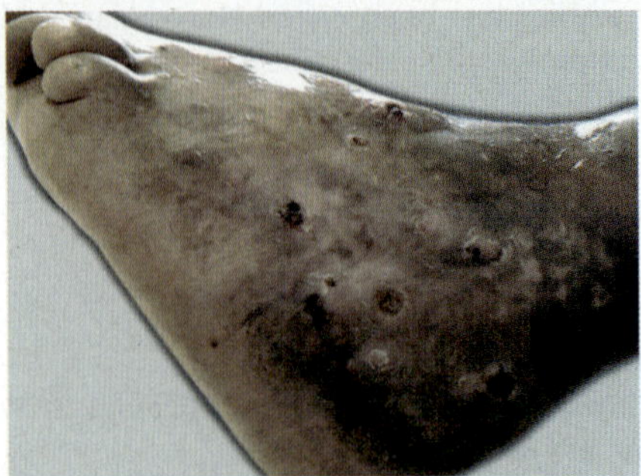

Fig. Mycetoma

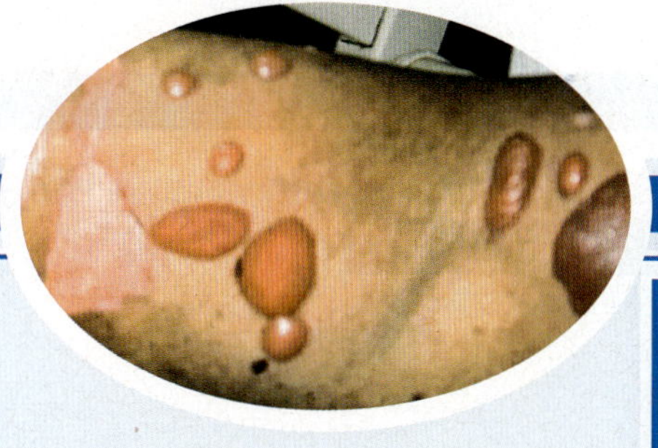

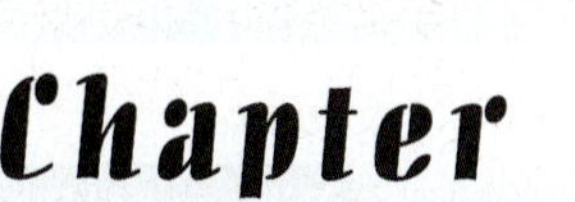

Chapter 5

Melanocytes, Pigment Metabolism and Disorders of Pigmentation

THEORETICAL CONCEPTS

V A. CLASSIFICATION OF PIGMENT DISORDERS

V A1. Hypopigmentation Disorders

Absent/damaged melanocytes[Q]	Defective tyrosinase metabolism[Q]
Vitiligo	Pityriasis versicolor
Piebaldism	Endocrine disorders
Chemicals (rubber)	Albinism
Post-inflammatory	

Primary skin disorders[Q]	Systemic diseases[Q]
Pityriasis alba	Tuberous sclerosis
Pityriasis versicolor	Scleroderma
Nevus anemicus	Tuberculoid Leprosy
Nevus achromicus/depigmentosus	Indeterminate leprosy
Piebaldism	CTC lymphoma
Vitiligo	Onchocerciasis
Chemical leukoderma	Sarcoidosis

Differential Diagnosis of Hypopigmentation Disorders

Albinism
- Location: Diffuse hypopigmented hair/ skin throughout the body
- Associated eye defects[Q]

Vitiligo
- Location: Anywhere on body
- Non-pigmented patch
- **Sharp scalloped hyperpigmented margins[Q]**
- Koebner phenomenon
- Leucotrichia (Loss of pigment in affected hair[Q])

Pityriasis alba
- **Location: Face** of children 6-12 years age
- Hypopigmented macule with fine scales[Q]

Contd...

Contd...

Differential Diagnosis of Hypopigmentation Disorders
Pityriasis versicolor • Location: Trunk and shoulders of young adults • Multiple, small, hypopigmented macules with fine scales • Start around hair follicles
Leprosy • Seen in geographical areas with presence of disease • Sharply demarcated, hypopigmented patch with no scales • Hypoesthesia/ Anesthesia in patch with Epidermal atrophy[Q]
Tuberous sclerosis • **Ash-leaf spots**[Q] (Hypopigmented macules) • **Shagreen patch**[Q] (Leathery skin on back) • **Café-au-lait macules** • Angiofibroma (Facial)
Nevus achromicus • Location: Trunk, Extremities (Proximal parts) • Unilateral hypopigmented macule with Feathery margins • Erythema on massage
Nevus anemicus • Location: Upper chest • Vascular anomaly as Hypopigmented patch • Disappears on massage/ pressure
Piebaldism • Location: Forehead, trunk extremities with sacral sparing[Q] • Localized depigmented/ hypopigmented macule with Hyperpigmented islands • **White forelock**[Q] • Present since birth

V A2. Hyperpigmentation Disorders

Epidermal pigmentation	Dermal pigmentation
Increased no. of melanocyte[Q]	
Lentigines Café au lait macules Malignant melanoma	Mongolian spots Nevus of Ota Post-inflammatory hyperpigmentation
Increased activity of melanocytes[Q]	
Freckles Exposure to UV light PUVA treatment Endocrine disorders	

Primary skin disorders[Q]	Systemic diseases[Q]
Freckles	Addison's disease
Nevus of Ito	Cushing's syndrome
Nevus of Ota	Hyperthyroidism
Becker's nevus	Vitamin B3, B9, B12 deficiency
Acanthosis nigricans	Hemochromatosis
Seborrhoeic keratosis	Whipple's disease
Melanoma	Argyria (Silver deposition)

V B. OCULOCUTANEOUS ALBINISM

- *Type of disorder*: Autosomal recessive, hypopigmentation disorder
- *Underlying cause*: **Complete/ partial absence of Tyrosinase**[Q] at birth leading to no melanin production[Q]
- *Clinical presentation*: [Q]
  - Little/ none melanin produced in skin, hair, eyes (iris, retina)
  - Photophobia, poor eye sight, nystagmus
  - Small stature, mental retardation
  - Tyrosinase positive have less severity
- *Complication*: **Squamous cell carcinoma of skin**[Q]
- *Treatment*: No effective treatment

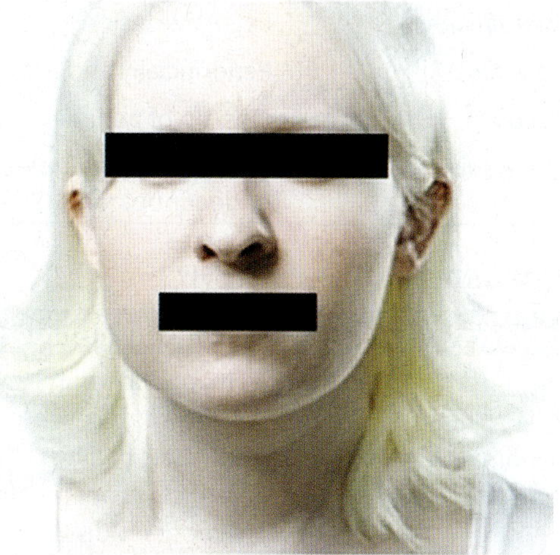

Fig. Oculocutaneous albinism

V C. PIEBALDISM

- *Type of disorder*: Autosomal dominant, hypopigmentation disorder
- *Underlying cause*: **Melanocytes absent in affected areas**[Q]
- *Clinical presentation*:
  - Depigmented macules with normo/hyper-pigmented island areas
  - **White forelock**[Q]
- *Treatment*:
  - Photoprotection
  - PUVA
  - Grafting

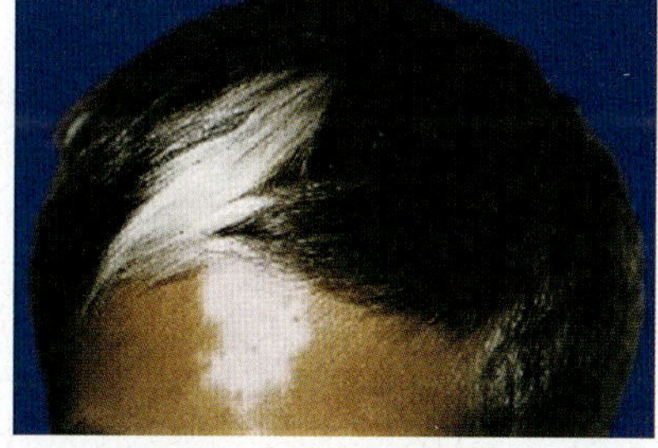

Fig. White forelock

Topper's Edge

Oculocutaneous Albinism Vs Piebaldism

	Oculocutaneous Albinism	Piebaldism
Onset	At birth	At birth
Morphology	Generalized depigmentation, Some pigmentation in sun-exposed areas	Localised depigmentation symmetrically with hyperpigmented areas[Q]
Hair	Pigment dilution	White forelock[Q]
Eye	Universal	Depigmented eye-brows and lashes

V D. VITILIGO

- *Type of disorder*: Polygenic inheritance, hypo-pigmentation disorder usually in children and young adults
- *Underlying cause*: Genetic, autoimmune, neurogenic origin
- *Clinical presentation*:

- **Depigmented chalky-white macules with 'scalloped outline'**[Q]
- Leucotrichia (loss of hair pigment) ONLY in older lesions
- Koebner/ Isomorphic phenomenon[Q]

❑ *Site*: Dorsal aspect of hands, feet, elbows, knees

Type of Vitiligo	Features
Vitiligo vulgaris	**Most common type**[Q]
Segmental vitiligo	Seen in children[Q] Most frequent in Trigeminal nerve distribution[Q]
Generalised vitiligo	Extensive lesions
Acrofacial vitiligo	Periorificially and acral parts
Lip-tip vitiligo	Lips, tip of penis, vulva, nipples
Vitiligo universalis	Widespread, multiple endocrinopathies

❑ *Vitiligo associations*: **[Mnemonic: HAMAM HAD P**ure **H**erbal **H**oney**]**[Q]

Cutaneous Disorders	Endocrine disorders
Halo nevus **A**lopecia areata **M**alignant melanoma **A**topic dermatitis **M**orphea	**H**ypoparathyroidism **A**ddison's disease **D**iabetes mellitus **P**ernicious anemia **H**ypothyroidism **H**yperthyroidism

❑ *Treatment*:[Q]
- Steroids
- Psoralens
- Narrow band UVB
- PUVA
- Monobenzyl ether of Hydroquinone
- Other drugs:
  - Tacrolimus
  - Levamisole
  - Khellin
  - Placental extract
  - Depigmentation agents

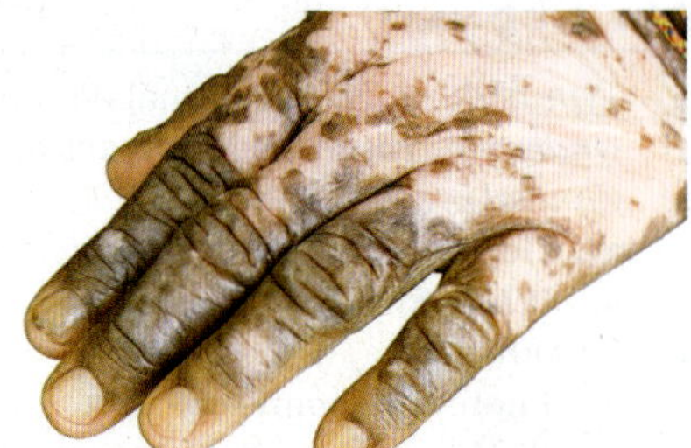

Fig. Vitiligo

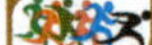

Topper's Edge

Oculocutaneous Albinism Vs Vitiligo

	Oculocutaneous Albinism	Vitiligo
Onset	At birth	Later life
Morphology	Freckling on photo-exposed parts[Q]	Depigmentation progress/ regress
Eye changes	Present[Q]	Absent
Response to treatment	Absent	Present

V E. MELASMA/CHLOASMA

❑ *Type of disorder*: Hyper-pigmentation disorder mainly in females 30–50 years[Q]

❑ *Underlying cause*:

- Estrogens (Pregnancy/ OCPs) [Q]
- Sunlight[Q]

- *Clinical presentation*:
  - Brown macular pigmentation with scalloped margins
  - Symmetric distribution on cheeks, nose, chin, forehead
- *Treatment*:
  - Photoprotection
  - Hydroquinone
  - Azelaic acid
  - Glycolic acid
  - Kojic acid
  - Chemical peeling with Glycolic acid/ Trichloroacetic acid

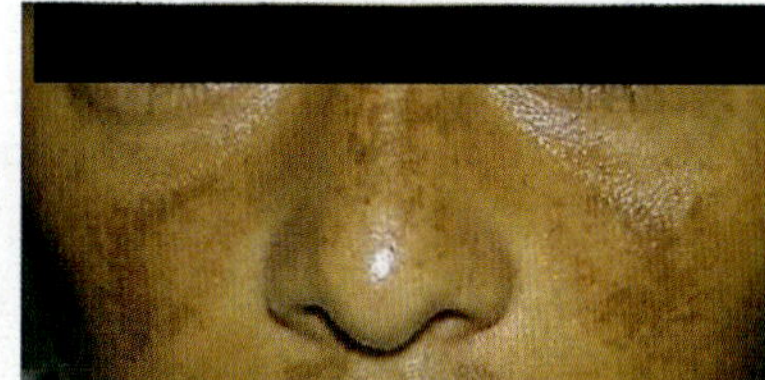

Fig. Melasma/Chloasma

V F. FRECKLES

- *Type of disorder*: Autosomal dominant geno-dermatoses of hyperpigmentation
- *Underlying cause*: **Normal melanocytes producing more melanosomes**[Q]
- *Clinical presentation*:
  - Multiple brown macules turning darker on sun exposure
  - Seen in photo-exposed areas
- *Treatment*:
  - Photoprotection
  - Hydroquinone
  - Azelaic acid
  - Chemical peeling

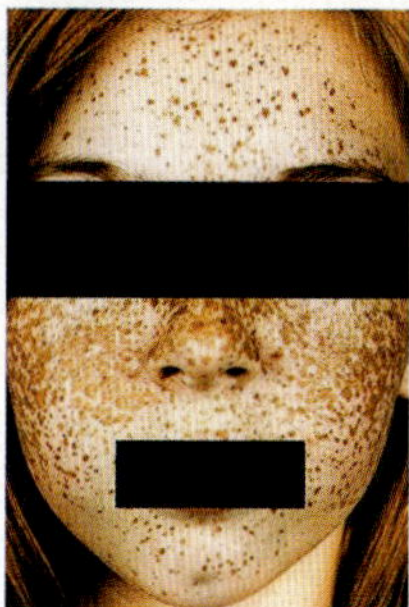

Fig. Freckles

V G. LENTIGINES

- *Type of disorder*: Hyper-pigmentation disorder
- *Underlying cause*: **Increased number of melanocytes**[Q]
  - Brown uniformly coloured macules with irregular sharp margin
  - Seen in any part of body
- *Lentigines associations*:[Q]
  - Peutz-Jeghers syndrome
  - Cronkhite-Canada syndrome
  - LAMB syndrome
  - LEOPARD syndrome
- *Treatment*: None required

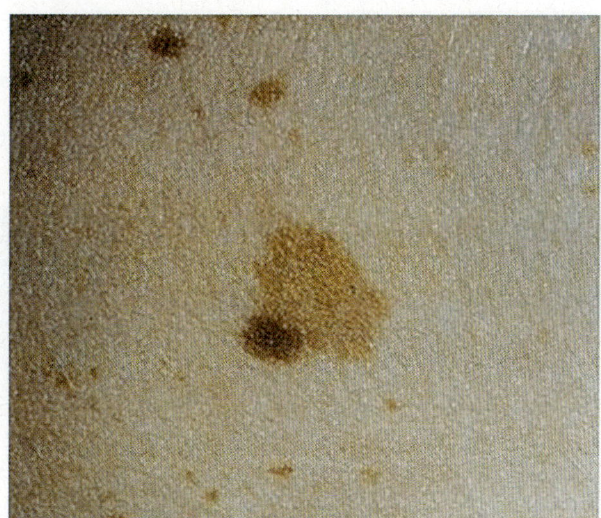

Fig. Lentigines

IMAGE-BASED QUESTIONS

1. Diagnose the Underlying Pigment disorder as shown in Photograph

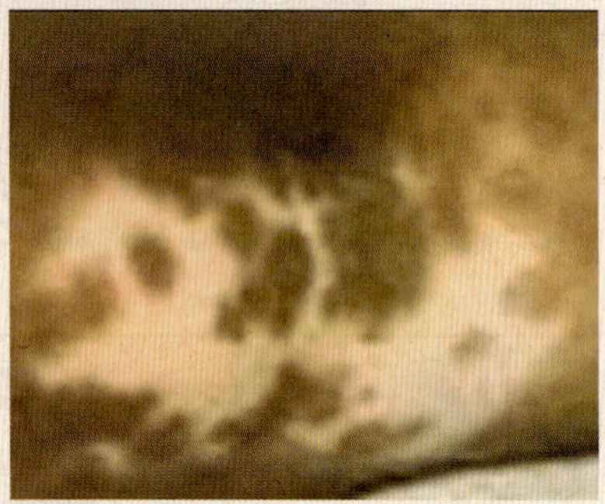

a. Piebaldism
b. Vitiligo
c. Trichrome vitiligo
d. Segmental vitiligo

2. Diagnose the Underlying Pigment disorder as shown in Photograph

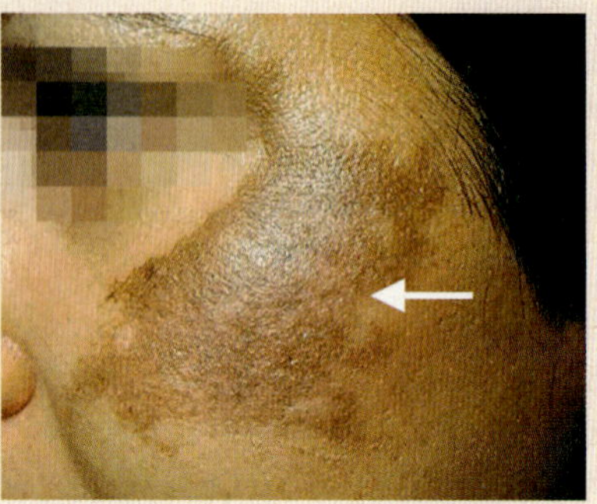

a. Lentigines
b. Freckles
c. Phototoxic reaction
d. Melasma

3. Diagnose the Underlying Pigment disorder as shown in Photograph

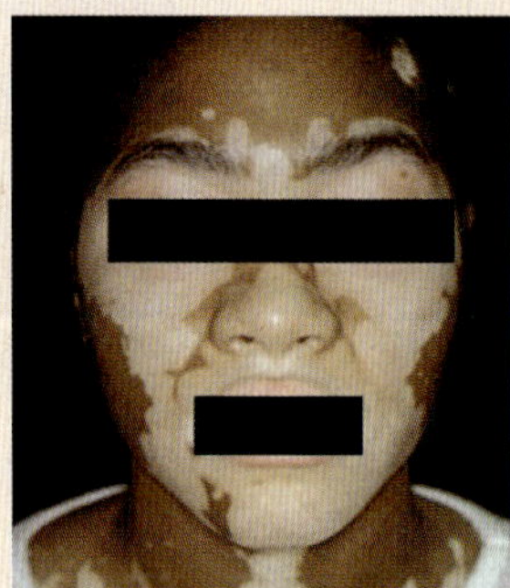

a. Piebaldism
b. Vitiligo
c. Trichrome vitiligo
d. Segmental vitiligo

4. Diagnose the Underlying Pigment disorder as shown in Photograph

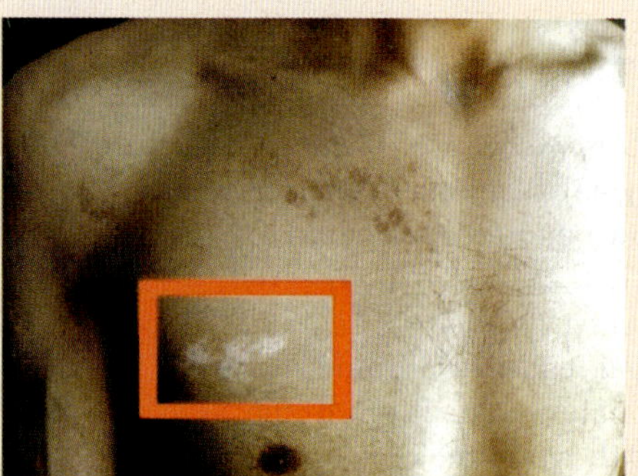

a. Lentigines
b. Phototoxic reaction
c. Trichrome vitiligo
d. Segmental vitiligo

5. Diagnose the Underlying Pigment disorder as shown in Photograph

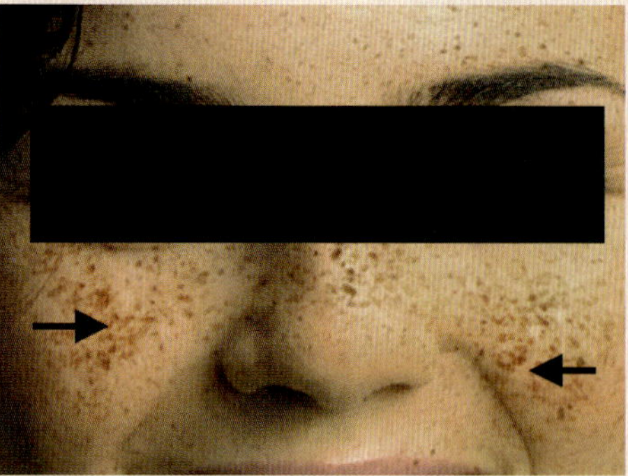

a. Lentigines
b. Freckles
c. Phototoxic reaction
d. Melasma

6. An 18 years old woman presented with Hypopigmented patches on bilateral ankles (See Photograph) Which of the following would NOT be used for treatment?
[AIIMS November 2015]

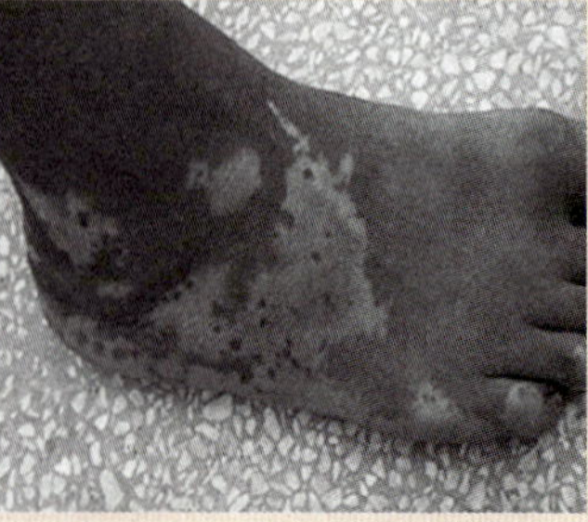

a. Topical Clobetasol
b. Topical Tretinoin
c. Topical Tacrolimus
d. Topical Methoxsalen

7. A 24 years old woman presents with Unilateral white skin lesions with Leucotrichia, as shown in the photograph. Diagnosis is ***[AIIMS PG May 2015]***

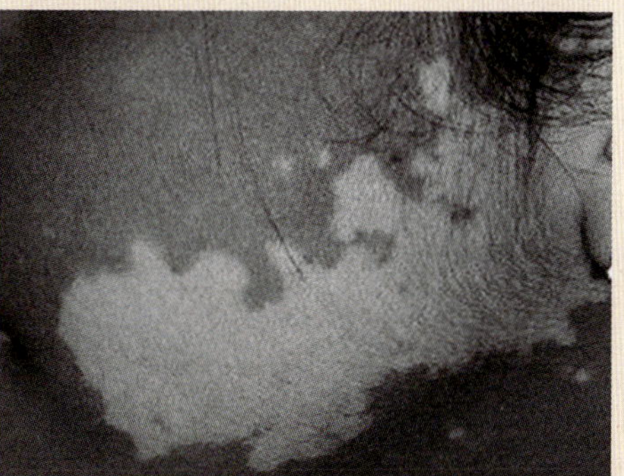

a. Focal vitiligo
b. Segmental vitiligo
c. Piebaldism
d. Waardenburg syndrome

8. A woman presented in Dermatology OPD with a bluish lesion over left side of forehead and left eye (See Photograph). Diagnosis is ***[AIIMS PG May 2015]***

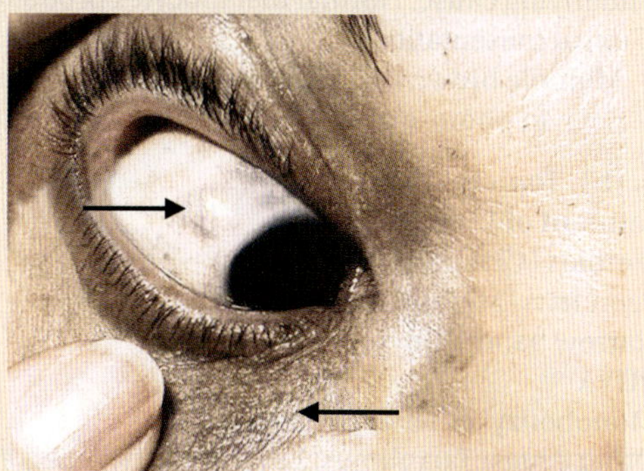

a. Nevus of Ota
b. Nevus of Ito
c. Becker's nevus
d. Mongolian spots

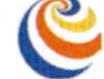 ANSWERS WITH EXPLANATIONS OF IBQs 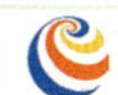

1. Ans. (a) Piebaldism *[Ref. Neena Khanna, 4/e p149]*

Piebaldism

- Type of disorder: Autosomal dominant, hypo-pigmentation disorder
- Underlying cause: Melanocytes absent in affected areas
- Clinical presentation:
  - Depigmented macules with normo/hyper-pigmented island areas
  - White forelock

2. Ans. (d) Melasma *[Ref. Dermatology by Bigby, 2/e p497]*

Melasma/Chloasma

- Type of disorder: Hyper-pigmentation disorder mainly in females 30–50 years
- Underlying cause: Estrogens (Pregnancy/ OCPs), Sunlight
- Clinical presentation:
  - Brown macular pigmentation with scalloped margins
  - Symmetric distribution on cheeks, nose, chin, forehead

3. Ans. (b) Vitiligo *[Ref. Neena Khanna, 4/e p149]*

Vitiligo

- Type of disorder: Polygenic inheritance, hypo-pigmentation disorder usually in children and young adults
- Underlying cause: Genetic, autoimmune, neurogenic origin
- Clinical presentation:
  - Depigmented chalky-white macules with 'scalloped outline'
  - Leucotrichia (loss of hair pigment) ONLY in older lesions
  - Koebner/Isomorphic phenomenon
  - Site: Dorsal aspect of hands, feet, elbows, knees

4. Ans. (d) Segmental vitiligo *[Ref. Neena Khanna, 4/e p151]*

Segmental Vitiligo

- Usually occur in children
- Dermatomal/ Quasi-dermatomal depigmentation
- Leucotrichia on depigmented areas
- Feathery margins

5. Ans. (b) Freckles *[Ref. Neena Khanna, 4/e p157]*

Freckles

- Type of disorder: Autosomal dominant geno-dermatoses of hyper-pigmentation
- Underlying cause: Normal melanocytes producing more melanosomes
- Clinical presentation:
  - Multiple brown macules turning darker on sun exposure
  - Seen in photo-exposed areas

6. Ans. (b) Topical Tretinoin *[Ref. Neena Khanna, 4/e p154]*

Treatment of Vitiligo

- Steroids (Clobetasol)
- Psoralens (Methoxsalen)
- Narrow band UVB
- PUVA
- Monobenzyl ether of Hydroquinone
- Other drugs: Tacrolimus, Levamisole, Khellin, Placental extract, Depigmentation agents

7. Ans. (b) Segmental vitiligo *[Ref. Vitiligo by Ortonne, 1/e p24]*

Segmental Vitiligo (Photograph)

- Early onset in life
- Non-progressive course
- Spreads rapidly within affected area
- Area limited to one segment of integument, i.e. part of face, part of trunk and extremity or one extremity
- Lesion stop abruptly at midline of affected segment

8. Ans. (a) Nevus of Ota *[Ref. Oski's Pediatrics, p829]*

Nevus of Ota

- An uncommon, bluish or gray-brown patch of pigmentation that occurs on the skin of the face, usually in the distribution of the first and second branches of the trigeminal nerve
- Ipsilateral bluish discoloration of sclera (Photograph)
- Can develop Glaucoma, Rarely malignant transformation

NEET/NBE PATTERN MCQs

1. **Hypopigmented patches are seen in** *[Recent Question 2016]*
   a. Nevus ota b. Nevus Ito
   c. Nevus anemicus d. Becker nevus
2. **Melanocytes are reduced in number in all of the following except** *[Recent Question 2016]*
   a. Albinism
   b. Piebaldism
   c. Vitiligo
   d. Chemical induced hypopigmentation
3. **Vitiligo vulgaris best treatment is** *[Recent Question 2016]*
   a. PUVA b. Steroids
   c. Coal tar d. All
4. **Depigmenting agent of choice in treatment of Dermatological disorders is** *[Recent Question 2016]*
   a. Hydroquinone b. Zinc
   c. Kojic acid d. Azelaic acid
5. **Vitiligo is associated with the following except** *[Recent Question 2016]*
   a. Addison's disease b. MEN syndrome
   c. Pernicious anemia d. Crohn's disease
6. **Mainstay of treatment of Vitiligo is** *[Recent Question 2016]*
   a. PUVA b. Imiquimod
   c. Acyclovir d. Coal tar
7. **Following are the differential diagnosis of Congenital disorders of pigmentation** *[Recent Question 2016]*
   a. Tietze syndrome b. Piebaldism
   c. Tuberous sclerosis d. All the above
8. **Causes of Localized hypopigmented macule or patch are all except** *[Recent Question 2016]*
   a. Vitiligo b. Piebaldism
   c. Pityriasis alba d. Freckle
9. **Increased incidence of vitiligo is found in** *[Recent Question 2017, NBE FMGE September 2005]*
   a. Old age b. Coronary heart disease
   c. Diabetes mellitus d. Hypertension
10. **Number of melanocytes is decreased in** *[NBE DNB 2011]*
    a. Albinism
    b. Nevus anemicus
    c. Piebaldism
    d. Waardenburg's Syndrome
11. **Which of the following is not a NEVUS of melanocyte?** *[Recent Question 2012, 2013]*
    a. Mongolian spot
    b. Nevus of Ito
    c. Nevus of ota
    d. Becker nevus
12. **Albinism is an** *[NBE DNB 2011]*
    a. Autosomal dominant disorder
    b. Autosomal recessive disorder
    c. X-linked dominant disorder
    d. X-linked recessive disorder
13. **Melanocytes number is reduced in all except** *[NBE FMGE March 2005]*
    a. Albinism
    b. Vitiligo
    c. Piebaldism
    d. Chemical induced hypopigmentation
14. **Which of the following is untrue regarding piebaldism?** *[Recent Question 2012]*
    a. Autosomal dominant condition
    b. Amelanotic skin associated with a white forelock
    c. Islands of normal or hypermelanotic skin
    d. Usually improves with age
15. **All statements are true regarding Albinism except** *[NBE FMGE March 2009]*
    a. Autosomal recessive inheritance
    b. Can develop squamous cell carcinoma
    c. Tyrosinase positive have less severity
    d. Melanin production is normal
16. **PUVA therapy is used for all except** *[NBE FMGE March 2010]*
    a. Psoriasis
    b. Vitiligo
    c. Albinism
    d. Atopic dermatitis
17. **All are true about Oculocutaneous albinism type I except** *[Recent Question 2017]*
    a. Tyrosinase deficiency
    b. Increased risk of skin cancer
    c. White hair and skin
    d. Iris may retain color in OCAI
18. **Oculocutaneous albinism is associated with?** *[Recent Question 2017]*
    a. Squamous cell carcinoma
    b. Basal cell carcinoma
    c. Melanoma
    d. All of the above
19. **Hypomelanosis of Ito is associated with?** *[Recent Question 2017]*
    a. Mental retardation
    b. Seizures
    c. Visual abnormalities
    d. All of the above
20. **Acanthosis nigricans is associated with?** *[Recent Question 2017]*
    a. Insulin resistance
    b. Gastric carcinoma
    c. Hyperpigmentation
    d. All of the above

HIGH YIELD MCQs

1. **Melanocytes are present in** *[PGI 1999]*
   a. Stratum corneum b. Stratum basale
   c. Stratum granulosum d. Dermis
2. **A 19-year-old girl presents with light brown pigmentation over Malar eminence, likely diagnosis is** *[All India PGMEE 2001]*
   a. Chloasma b. SLE
   c. Melasma d. Melanoma
3. **An increased incidence of vitiligo is found in** *[Karnataka PGMEE 98, AIIMS PGMEE 1994]*
   a. Psoriasis b. Nutritional deficiency
   c. Old age d. Diabetes mellitus
4. **Female presents with history of color change from pallor to cyanosis on exposure to cold in fingers. This condition is mostly associated with?** *[AIIMS PGMEE 2008]*
   a. Scleroderma b. Leukemia
   c. Lung infections d. Hepatosplenomegaly
5. **A 23-year-old lady develops brown macular lesions over bridge of nose and cheek following exposure to light. The probable diagnosis is** *[AIIMS PGMEE 1999]*
   a. SLE b. Acne Rosacea
   c. Chloasma d. Photodermatitis
6. **The concentration of hydroquinone for treating chloasma should be** *[AIIMS PGMEE 1996, NBE DNB 1998]*
   a. 1% b. 1 to 2%
   c. 2 to 5% d. 10%
7. **In a patch of vitiligo** *[AIIMS PGMEE 2004, PGI 1994]*
   a. Melanin synthesis is inhibited
   b. Melanosomes are absent
   c. Melanocytes are absent
   d. Melanocytes are reduced
8. **Exposure to sunlight can precipitate** *[UPSC 2000]*
   a. Chloasma
   b. Discoid lupus erythematosus
   c. Dermatitis herpetiformis
   d. Lupus vulgaris
9. **Melanocytes are present in** *[PGI 1999]*
   a. Stratum corneum
   b. Stratum basale
   c. Stratum granulosum
   d. Dermis
10. **True about Vitiligo are all except** *[JIPMER PGMEE 2004, WB PGMEE 2005]*
    a. Genetic predisposition is known
    b. Leucotrichia is associated with good prognosis
    c. PUVA-B is used for treatment
    d. Topical steroids give good results
11. **Vitiligo vulgaris, treatment is** *[Jharkhand PGMEE 2006]*
    a. PUVA b. Steroids
    c. Coal tar d. All
12. **Vitiligo vulgaris, best treatment is** *[Bihar PGMEE 2003]*
    a. PUVA b. Steroids
    c. Coal tar d. All

 NEET/NBE PATTERN MCQs ANSWERS WITH EXPLANATIONS 

1. **Ans. (c) Nevus anemicus**
   [Ref. Clinical Dermatology by Habif, 6/e p776]

Nevus Anemicus

- Congenital localized pharmacologic cutaneous anomaly most often seen on the trunk
- Hypopigmented patches are seen
- Lesion usually consists of a well-defined white macule with an irregular border, often surrounded by smaller white macules beyond the border of the major lesion

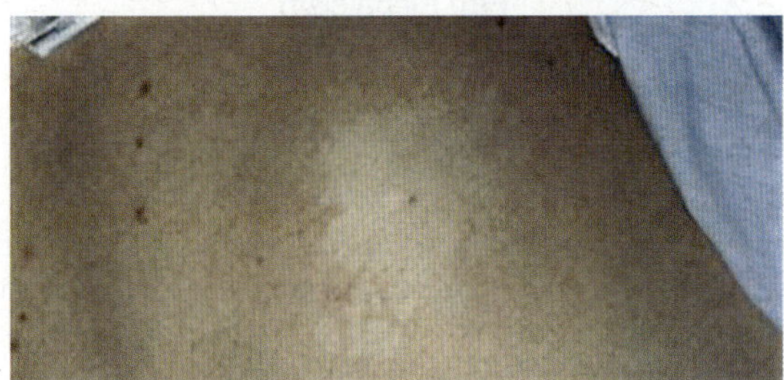

Fig. Nevus anemicus

2. **Ans. (a) Albinism**
   [Ref. DVL by Thappa, 4/e p220]

Albinism

- AR disorder resulting from absence of activity of the enzyme Tyrosinase
- Partial or complete failure of melanin production in skin and eyes in oculocutaneous albinism
- Melanocytes are present in normal distribution but they fail to synthesize melanin adequately

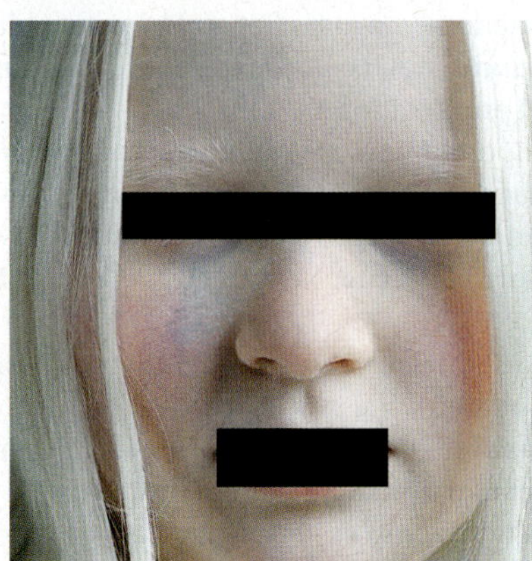

Fig. Albinism

3. **Ans. (b) Steroids**
   [Ref. DVL by Thappa, 4/e p225]

Vitiligo Vulgaris

- Most common form of vitiligo in which widespread macules are often symmetrically placed over limbs and trunk
- Topical treatments used in the treatment of Vitiligo: Steroids, Calcineurin inhibitors, Vitamin D analogues, Pseudocatalase, Depigmenting agents
- Treatment of choice: Steroids

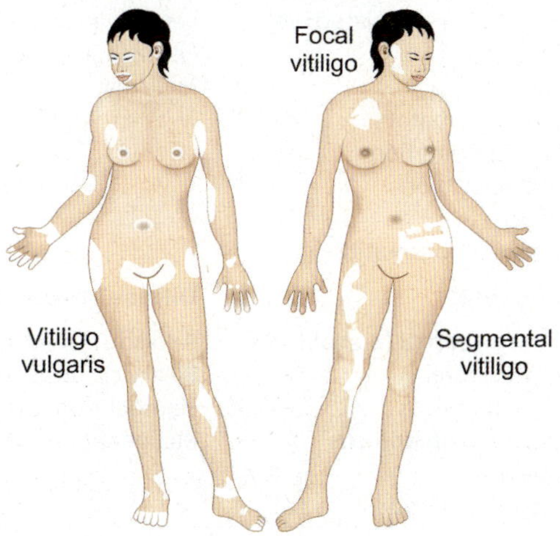

Fig. Vitiligo

4. **Ans. (a) Hydroquinone**
   [Ref. Clinical Dermatology by Habif, 6/e p782]

Hypopigmenting Agents

- **Hydroquinone** is the most effective topically applied bleaching agent
  - Hydroquinone is thought to inhibit tyrosinase, which leads to altered melanosome formation and increased melanosome destruction.
- **Kojic acid (KA)** is an antibiotic produced by many species of *Aspergillus* and *Penicillium* that inhibits tyrosinase
  - Azelaic acid (Finacea is 15% azelaic acid) is used to treat acne and melisma
  - It has selective effects on hyperactive and abnormal melanocytes and minimal effects on normally pigmented human skin, freckles, and senile lentigines

5. **Ans. (d) Crohn's disease**
   [Ref. DVL by Thappa 4/e p223]
   - Vitiligo is associated with auto immune diseases such as Hashimoto's thyroiditis, Graves's disease, DM, Pernicious anaemia, Addison's disease, Alopecia areata etc

6. **Ans. (a) PUVA**
   [Ref. Clinical Dermatology by Habif, 6/e p770]
   - Photochemotherapy with psoralens with UVA exposure (PUVA) forms the mainstay of therapy in vitiligo
   - Recently Narrow band Ultraviolet B (NUVB) rays have become mainstay of treatment for Generalized and Nonsegmental vitiligo

7. **Ans. (d) All of the above**
   [Ref. Clinical Dermatology by Habif, 6/e p790]

Hypopigmentation	Hyperpigmentation
Acquired	**Circumscribed brown**
Chemical induced Halo nevus Idiopathic guttate hypomelanosis Leprosy	Cafe-au-lait spots, freckles Diabetic dermopathy, erythema ab igne Fixed drug eruption

Contd...

Contd...

Hypopigmentation	Hyperpigmentation
Leukoderma associated with melanoma Pityriasis alba Post-inflammatory hypopigmentation Tinea versicolor Vitiligo Phytophotodermatitis	Lentigo in children Peutz-jeghers syndrome Melisma
Congenital	**Diffuse brown**
Albinism, partial (piebaldism) Albinism total Nevus anemicus Nevus depigmentosus Piebaldism Tuberous sclerosis	Addison's disease Biliary cirrhosis Hemochromatosis Malignant melanoma

8. Ans. (d) Freckle

[Ref. DVL by Thappa, 4/e p219]

Hyperpigmentation	Hypopigmentation
Addison's disease Nelson syndrome Hyperthyroidism Cushing syndrome Ectopic ACTH syndrome Freckles	Vitiligo, Piebaldism Nevus anemicus Nevus depigmentosus Pityriasis Scleroderma Sarcoidosis

9. Ans. (c) Diabetes mellitus

[Ref. Neena Khanna, 4/e p152]

- *Vitiligo associations*: **[Mnemonic: HAMAM HAD** Pure **H**erbal **H**oney]

Cutaneous Disorders	Endocrine Disorders
Halo nevus	**H**ypoparathyroidism
Alopecia areata	**A**ddison's disease
Malignant melanoma	**D**iabetes mellitus
Atopic dermatitis	**P**ernicious anemia
Morphea	**H**ypothyroidism
	Hyperthyroidism

10. Ans. (c) Piebaldism; (d) Waardenburg's syndrome

[Ref. Practical Dermatopathology by Rapini, 1/e p165]

Piebaldism

- Description: Rare autosomal dominant disorder characterized by the congenital absence of melanocytes in affected areas of the skin and hair
- Cause: Mutations of the c-kit gene, located on Chromosome 4q12, which affects the differentiation and migration of melanoblasts from the neural crest during the embryonic life
- Presentation: Affected individuals present at birth with a white forelock and relatively stable, persistent depigmentation of skin with a characteristic distribution

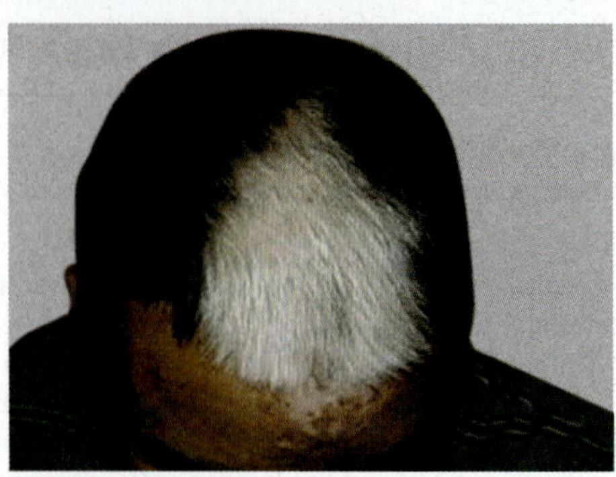

Fig. Piebaldism

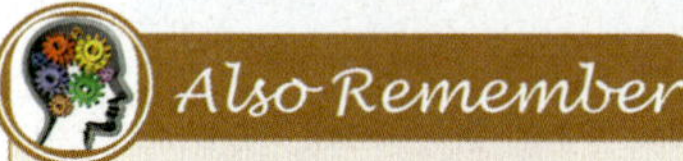

Waardenburg's Syndrome

- Description: An autosomal dominant disorder is characterized by a congenital white forelock, lateral displacement of the medial canthi, a hypertrophic nasal root, partial or total heterochromia of the iris and sensorineural deafness
- All anomalies of **Waardenburg's syndrome** involve the neural crest from which are derived not only melanocytes, but also gut enteric plexus ganglion cells and other neural tissue as well as connective tissue of the head and neck

11. Ans. (d) Becker nevus

[Ref. Pathology of Melanocytic Nevi and Melanoma by Barnhill, 3/e p275]

Nevus of Melanocytes

- **Junctional nevus**: Nevus cells are located along the junction of the epidermis and the underlying dermis
  - A junctional nevus is flat and brown to black.
- **Compound nevus**: A mixture of junctional and intradermal proliferation
  - Compound nevi are slightly raised and brown to black
  - Beauty marks are usually compound nevi of either the acquired variety or congenital variety.
- **Intradermal nevus**: Nevus cells are located in the dermis only
  - Intradermal nevi are raised, most are flesh-colored (not pigmented)
- **Dysplastic nevus (Nevus of Clark)**: A compound nevus with cellular and architectural dysplasia
  - Like typical moles, dysplastic nevi can be flat or raised
  - Dysplastic nevi are markers of risk when they are numerous (Atypical mole syndrome)
- **Blue nevus**: It is blue in color as its melanocytes are very deep in the skin
  - Nevus cells are spindle shaped and scattered in deep layers of the dermis
  - Covering epidermis is normal.
- **Spitz nevus**: A distinct variant of intradermal nevus, usually in a child
  - Raised and reddish (non-pigmented)
  - A pigmented variant, called the 'Nevus of Reed': Typically appears on the leg of young women

- **Acquired nevus**: Any melanocytic nevus that is not a congenital nevus or not present at birth or near birth
  - Includes junctional, Compound and Intradermal nevus.
- **Congenital nevus**: Small to large nevus present at or near time of birth
  - Small ones have low potential for forming melanomas, however the risk increases with size, as in the giant pigmented nevus
- **Giant pigmented nevus**: Large, pigmented, often hairy congenital nevi
  - Melanoma may occasionally (10 to 15%) appear in them
- **Intramucosal nevus**: Junctional nevus of the mucosa of the mouth or genital areas
  - In the mouth, they are found most frequently on the hard palate
- **Nevus of Ito and Nevus of Ota**: Congenital, flat brownish lesions on the face or shoulder
- **Mongolian spot**: Congenital large, deep, bluish discoloration which generally disappears by puberty
  - Named for its association with East Asian ethnic groups but is not limited to them
- **Recurrent nevus**: Any incompletely removed nevus with residual melanocytes left in the surgical wound
  - It creates a dilemma for the patient and physician, as these scars cannot be distinguished from a melanoma

12. Ans. (b) Autosomal recessive disorder
[Ref. Neena Khanna, 5/e p40]

13. Ans. (a) Albinism
[Ref. Neena Khanna, 4/e p147]

Hypopigmentation Disorders

Absent/ Damaged Melanocytes	Defective Tyrosinase Metabolism
Vitiligo Piebaldism Chemicals (rubber) Post-inflammatory	Pityriasis versicolor Endocrine disorders Albinism

14. Ans. (d) Usually improves with age
[Ref. Practical Dermatopathology by Rapini, 1/e p165]

15. Ans. (d) Melanin production is normal
[Ref. Neena Khanna, 4/e p148]

Oculocutaneous Albinism

- *Type of disorder*: Autosomal recessive, hypo-pigmentation disorder
- *Underlying cause*: Complete/ partial absence of Tyrosinase at birth leading to no melanin production
- *Clinical presentation*:
  - Little/ none melanin produced in skin, hair, eyes (iris, retina)
  - Photophobia, poor eye sight, nystagmus
  - Small stature, mental retardation
  - Tyrosinase positive have less severity
- *Complication*: Squamous cell carcinoma of skin
- *Treatment*: None is effective

16. Ans. (c) Albinism
[Ref. Various sources]

PUVA Therapy

- *Definition*: PUVA is a combination of Psoralen and UVA treatment
- *Uses of PUVA therapy*:
  - Psoriasis
  - Mycosis fungoides (Cutaneous T-cell lymphoma)
  - Vitiligo
  - Graft-versus-host disease
  - Piebaldiam
  - Atopic dermatitis

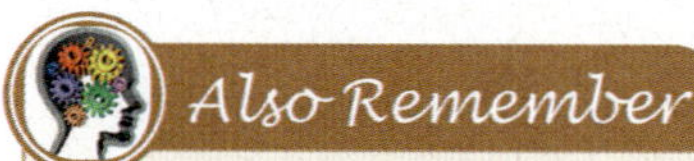

Management of Albinism is protection from UV rays by UV protective sunglass broad spectrum sunscreen lotion with clothing

17. Ans. (d) Iris may retain color in OCAI
[Ref. Neena Khanna, 4/e p148]

Oculocutaneous Albinism

- Autosomal recessive, hypopigmentation disorder
- Occur due to complete/ partial absence of Tyrosinase at birth leading to no melanin production
- *Clinical presentation*: Little/none melanin produced in skin, hair, eyes (iris, retina), Photophobia, poor eye sight, nystagmus, Small stature, mental retardation, Tyrosinase positive have less severity
- *Complication*: Squamous cell carcinoma of skin
- *Treatment*: No effective treatment

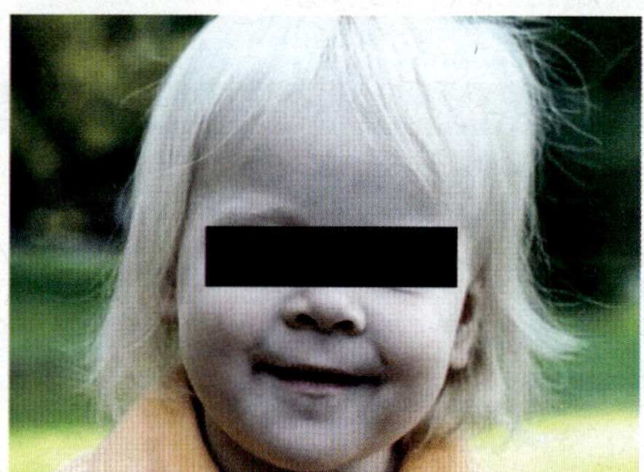

Fig. Oculocutaneous albinism

18. Ans. (d) All of the above
[Ref. Dermatopathology in Systemic Disease by Smoller, 1/e p357]

- Incidences of Squamous cell carcinoma, Basal cell carcinoma, and Actinic keratosis are markedly increased in patients with Oculocutaneous albinism
- Interestingly, although rare cases of malignant melanoma are reported in these patients, the incidence does not appear to be markedly elevated

19. Ans. (d) All of the above
[Ref. Encyclopedia of the Neurological Sciences, 2/e p691]

Associated manifestations in Hypomelanosis of Ito

- Mental retardation, epilepsy, language disabilities, motor system dysfunction, psychiatric symptoms including autism, cortical visual impairment
- Visual problems including cataracts, a cleft along the edge of the iris of the eye, near-sightedness, and crossed eyes

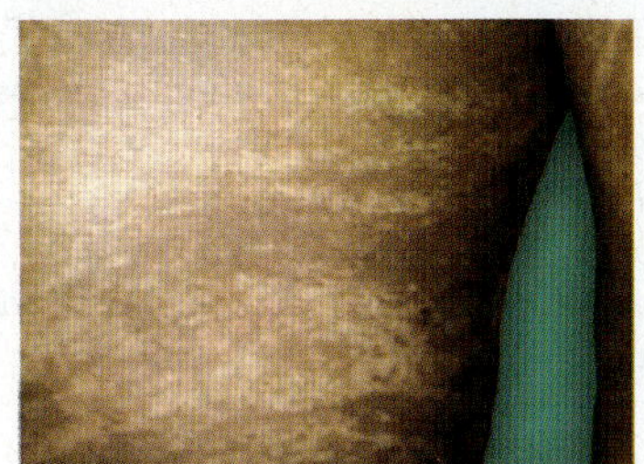

Fig. Hypomelanosis of Ito

20. Ans. (d) All of the above

[Ref. Palliative Care and Supportive Oncology, 1/e p234]

Acanthosis Nigricans

- Characterized by velvety, hyperpigmented plaques involving intertriginous areas
- Associated with internal cancers, particularly Gastric adenocarcinoma, as well as Endocrinopathies resulting in Hyperinsulinemia and Insulin resistance

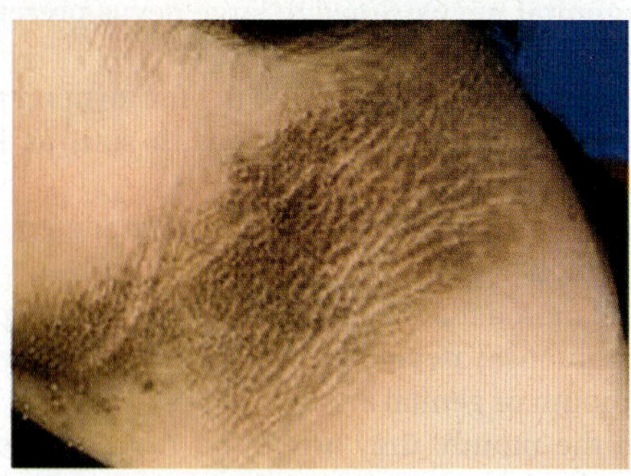

Fig. Acanthosis nigricans

HIGH YIELD MCQs ANSWERS WITH EXPLANATIONS

1. Ans. (b) Stratum basale

[Ref. Neena Khanna, 5/e p157]

- Melanocytes are present in basal layer of epidermis, interspread between keratinocytes

2. Ans. (a) Chloasma

[Ref. Neena Khanna, 5/e p168]

3. Ans. (d) Diabetes mellitus

[Ref. Neena Khanna, 5/e p163]

Vitiligo Associations

Endocrine disorders	Cutaneous disorders
Diabetes mellitus	Alopecia areata
Addison's disease	Halo nevus
Hypoparathyroidism	Atopic dermatitis
Hypo and hyper thyroidism	Malignant melanoma
Pernicious anemia	Morphea

4. Ans. (a) Scleroderma

[Ref. Neena Khanna, 5/e p246]

- In scleroderma, the most frequent and earliest symptom is Raynaud's phenomenon
- Characterized by pallor → cyanosis → redness (PCR) of finger tips and toes on exposure to cold
- It is worse in winter and eventually leads to stellate ulcers, loss of finger pulp, gangrene

5. Ans. (c) Chloasma

[Ref. Neena Khanna, 5/e p168]

6. Ans. (c) 2 to 5%

[Ref. Neena Khanna, 5/e p169]

Medical Treatment of Chloasma

- Hydroquinone 2–4% topically: Used alone or as combination with Retinoic acid (0.025-0.05%) and a topical steroid
- Azelaic acid topically as 10–20% cream: As efficacious as hydroquinone.
- Other agents:
  - Glycolic acid (6-12%)
  - Kojic acid (1-4%)

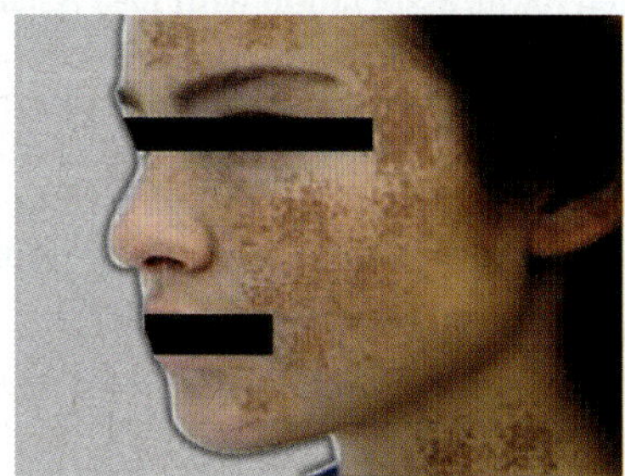

Fig. Chloasma

7. Ans. (c) Melanocytes are absent

[Ref. Encyclopedia of Health, Volume 15, p879]

8. Ans. (b) Discoid lupus erythematosus

[Ref. Neena Khanna, 5/e p168]

UVR Exacerbate DLE (70% of Patients)

- Inducing neoantigen expression which triggers a dysregulated immune response.
- Inducing a heat shock protein in keratinocytes which acts as a target for T cell-mediated cytotoxicity
- Releasing immune mediators which induce inflammation

9. Ans. (b) Stratum basale

10. Ans. (b) Leucotrichia is associated with good prognosis

[Ref. Neena Khanna, 5/e p163]

Poor Prognostic Factors of Vitiligo

- Long standing disease
- Acrofacial lesion
- Lesions on resistant areas
  - Bony prominences (ankles and elbow)
  - Non fleshy areas (periungual areas)
  - Non hairy areas (nipple and areola)
  - Mucosae (lips and genitalia)
- Presence of leucotrichia

11. Ans. (d) All

[Ref. Neena Khanna, 5/e p164-166]

12. Ans. (a) PUVA

[Ref. Neena Khanna, 5/e p165]

Photo therapy and PUVA are mainstay of therapy in Vitiligo

Chapter 6

Allergic and Reactive Disorders, Dermatitis, Hypersensitivity

THEORETICAL CONCEPTS

VI A. ATOPIC DERMATITIS

- *Definition*: Eczema with pruritus and recurrent eczematous lesions
- *Underlying cause*:
  - Increased IgE levels
  - Decreased T-lymphocytes
- *Clinical presentation*:
  - Papulo-vesicular lesions in infants
  - Itchy plaques on elbow and knee flexors in children
  - Lichenified plaques in adults in cubital/Popliteal fossae[Q]
  - Ichthyosis
  - ***Dennie-Morgan fold***: Atopic skin folds under eye[Q]
  - ***Hertoghe's sign***[Q]: Thinning of lateral part of eyebrows
  - White dermatographism
  - Hyper-pigmented eyelids
- *Complications*: Increased susceptibility to infections[Q]
  - Impetigo
  - Herpes simplex (Eczema herpeticum/Kaposi varicelliform eruption)
  - Molluscum contagiosum
  - Human papilloma virus
- *Treatment*: **[Mnemonic: TIE A HIP]**[Q]
  - **T**opical steroids
  - **I**mmuno-modulators (Calcineurin inhibitors) topical
  - Pimecrolimus
  - Tacrolimus
  - **E**mollients
  - **A**void triggers/irritants
  - **H**ydration of skin
  - **I**mmunosuppressives
  - Cyclosporine
  - Azathioprine
  - Mycophenolate mofetil
  - **P**hototherapy: Narrow-band UVB or PUVA

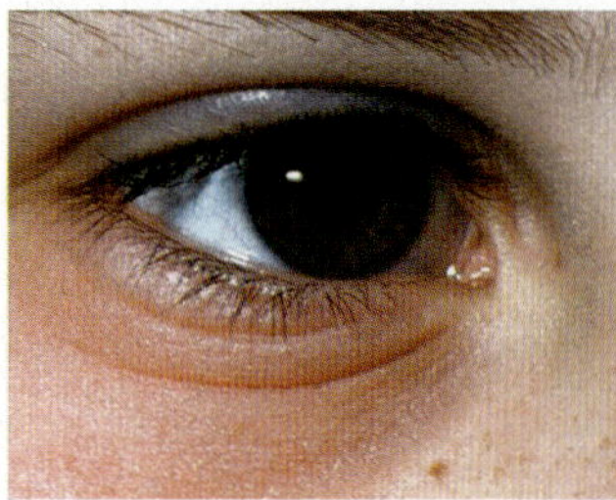

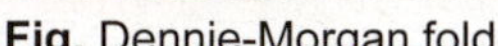

Fig. Dennie-Morgan fold

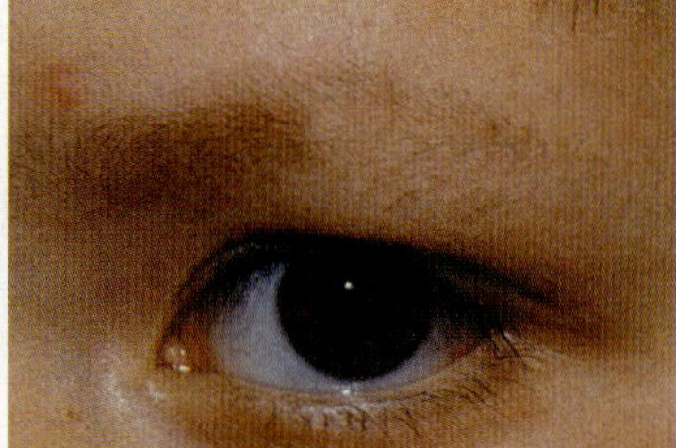

Fig. Hertoghe's sign

Differential Diagnosis of Atopic Dermatitis[q]

Atopic dermatitis (Infants)
- Pruritic, itchy papules/vesicles
- Location: **Face** (Initiation [q]), Neck, Extensor surfaces with sparing of diaper area
- Family/personal history of atopy [q]

Atopic dermatitis (Children/Adolescents)
- Pruritic lesions
- Location: Flexural areas [q]
- **Dennie-Morgan fold** [q]
- Family/personal history of atopy [q]

Seborrheic dermatitis (Infants)
- **Stuck-on appearance** [q] of Greasy-yellow scales [q] on erythematous papules
- Location: Scalp, Face
- Cradle cap, Dandruff present

Seborrheic dermatitis (Adults)
- **Cradle cap** [q] (Most common) with Scaly erythematous lesions
- Location: Scalp (Most common [q]), Flexural areas
- Dandruff present

Irritant Contact Dermatitis (Adults)
- Location: Hands, Forearms of Housewives [q]
- History of contact with irritants (soap, water, detergents) [q]

Allergic Contact Dermatitis (Adults)
- Location: Wrist, hand, forehead, foot [q]
- History of contact with allergen at site of lesions[q]

Airborne Contact Dermatitis (Adults)
- Location: Face, neck, forearm, eyelids, cubital fossa [q]
- History of contact with Parthenium/Congress grass[q]
- Seasonal nature, Common in Farmers, Labourers

Erosive napkin dermatitis (Infants)
- Fissured erythematous, eroded lesions
- Location: Diaper area
- Ammoniac smell present [q]

Xerotic dermatitis (Infants)
- Dry erythema with Fine scales
- Location: Cheeks, Extensor aspect of extremities
- Associated with Winter season [q]

Topper's Edge

Eczema
- To boil out
- Group of diseases that results in inflammation of skin, characterized by itchiness, red skin, and a rash
- In cases of short duration, there may be small blisters while in long-term cases the skin may become thickened
- Area of skin involved can vary from small to the entire body

Clinical presentation
- Pruritus, erythema, edema
- Papules, vesicles, scaling, lichenification

Histology[q]
- Spongiosis (**Hallmark feature[q]**)
- Hyperkeratosis, Acanthosis

Types of Eczema
- Endogenous eczema: Constitutional symptoms predispose acute discoid presentation
- Exogenous eczema: Exogenous stimuli predispose chronic hyperkeratotic presentation
- Combined eczema: Both Constitutional and Exogenous stimuli predispose lichenified/seborrheic presentation

Complications of Eczema
- Skin complications: Infection, Ide eruption, Contact dermatitis, Erythroderma
- Psychosocial complications: Anxiety, Depression, Wage loss, Debility

Tests of Eczema[Q]
- **Patch tests: Detect antigens for Type IV hypersensitivity**[Q]
- Photopatch tests: Establish cause of Photoallergic contact dermatitis[Q]
- Prick tests: Detect Type I hypersensitivity[Q]
- Serological tests: Serum IgE levels, RAST[Q]

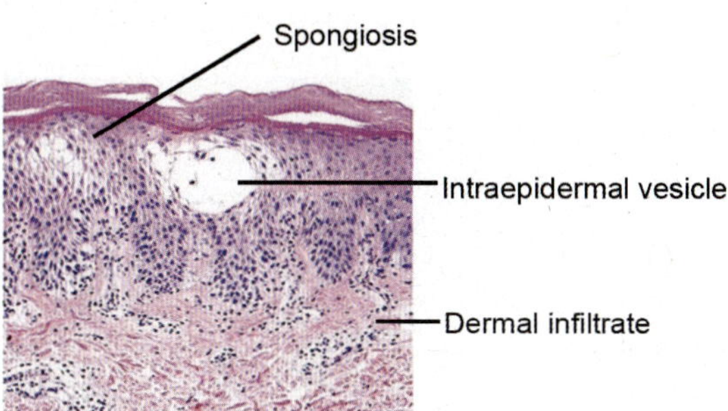

Fig. Eczema

VI B. ETIOLOGICAL CLASSIFICATION OF ECZEMA

Endogenous eczema	Exogenous eczema	Combined eczema
Seborrheic dermatitis Nummular/Discoid dermatitis Lichen simplex chronicus Pityriasis alba Stasis dermatitis	Contact/Irritant dermatitis Allergic dermatitis Photodermatitis Radiation dermatitis Infective dermatitis	Atopic dermatitis Pompholyx

VI C. PHASES OF ECZEMA

Acute phase	Sub-acute phase	Chronic phase
Vesicles Erythema[Q] Edema[Q] Crusts	Plaques Scales Crusts	Lichenification[Q] Hyperpigmentation Skin thickening Skin marking increase
Spongiosis edema[Q]	Parakeratosis	S. malpighi thickening

VI D. HANIFIN AND RAJKA DIAGNOSTIC CRITERIA FOR ATOPIC DERMATITIS[Q]

(At least 3 Major and 3 Minor must be present)

Major Criteria[Q]

- Pruritus
- Chronic or chronically-relapsing dermatitis
- Personal or family history of atopy
- Typical morphology, distribution
  - Flexural lichenification/linearity (Adult)
  - Facial and extensor involvement (Infant/Child)

Minor Criteria

- Xerosis/Dry skin
- Ichthyosis, Palmar hyperlinearity, Keratosis pilaris
- Immediate (Type 1) skin-test reactivity
- Raised serum IgE

- Early age of onset
- Tendency toward cutaneous infections (especially *S. aureus* and herpes simplex)
- Impaired CMI
- Non-specific hand or foot dermatitis
- Nipple eczema
- Cheilitis
- Recurrent conjunctivitis
- Dennie-Morgan infraorbital fold
- Keratoconus
- Anterior subcapsular cataracts
- Orbital darkening
- Facial pallor or facial erythema
- Pityriasis alba
- Anterior neck folds
- Itch when sweating
- Intolerance to wool and lipid solvents
- Perifollicular accentuation
- Food intolerance
- Influenced by environmental or emotional factors
- White dermographism or delayed blanch

VI E. URTICARIA/HIVES

- Description: Type I hypersensitivity reaction due to histamine release[Q]
- Causes of Urticaria[Q]:
  - Food borne: Milk, Egg, Meat, Fish
  - Drugs: Penicillin, Aspirin, ACE inhibitors, NSAIDs, Opiates
  - Systemic disorders: Serum sickness[Q], SLE, Thyrotoxicosis
  - Contact disease: Pollen, Animals
  - Infectious organisms: Hepatitis B, Hepatitis C, Tuberculosis, Worm infestations, *H. pylori*
  - Physical/Environmental causes: Cold, Heat, Colar, Cholinergic, Dermographism
  - Pregnancy, Exercise
  - Insect bite

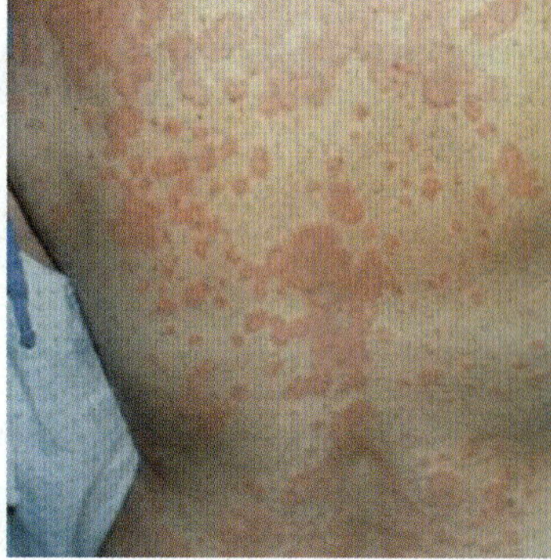

Fig. Urticaria

VI F. ANGIONEUROTIC EDEMA VS ANAPHYLAXIS

Characteristic	Angioneurotic edema	Anaphylaxis
Family history	Present	Absent
Upper respiratory obstruction	Present	Absent
Pruritus	Not present	Present
Hypotension	Absent	Present
Progression	Slow	Rapid

(Both may have Upper respiratory tract obstruction, Angioedema and Association with food allergy)

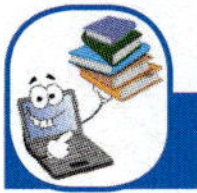

IMAGE-BASED QUESTIONS

1. Identify the Skin disorder shown in Photograph

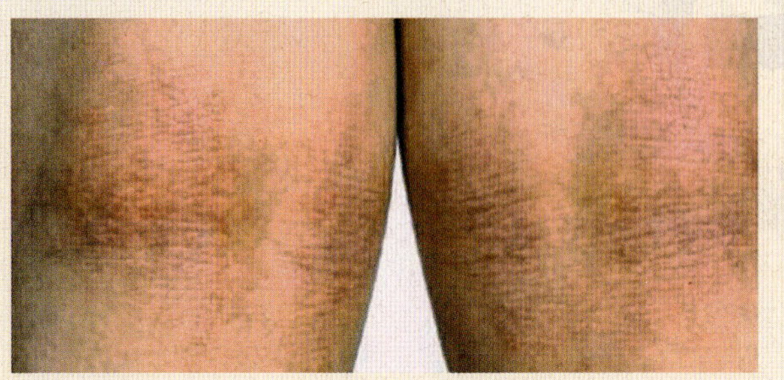

a. SSSS
b. Seborrheic dermatitis
c. Atopic dermatitis
d. Pompholyx

2. Diagnose the Skin disorder shown in the Photograph

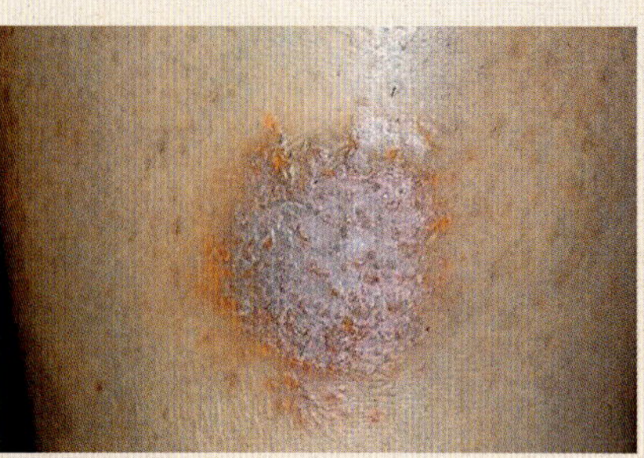

a. Pompholyx
b. Nummular eczema
c. Lichen simplex chronicus
d. Allergic contact dermatitis

3. Identify the Skin disorder shown in Photograph

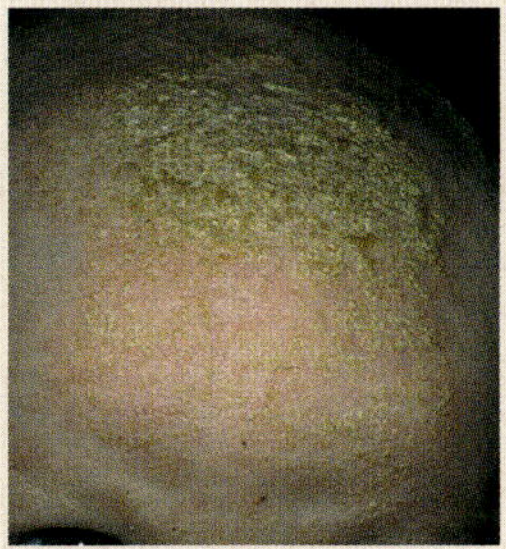

a. Irritant contact dermatitis
b. Seborrheic dermatitis
c. Atopic dermatitis
d. Pompholyx

4. Diagnose the Skin disorder shown in the Photograph

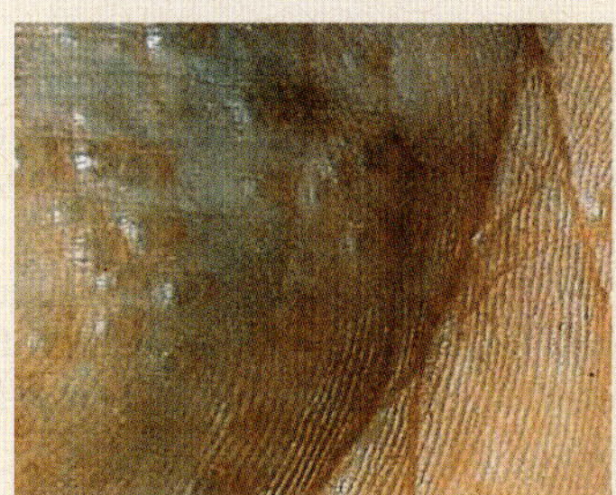

a. Pompholyx
b. Nummular eczema
c. Lichen simplex chronicus
d. Allergic contact dermatitis

5. Plant shown in Photograph is a common cause of

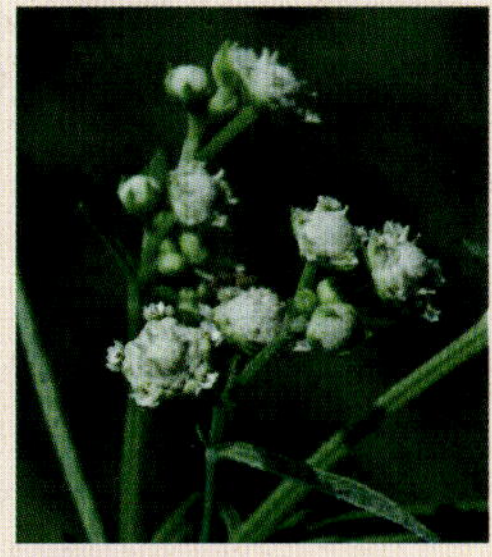

a. Atopic dermatitis
b. Seborrheic dermatitis
c. Allergic contact dermatitis
d. Stasis eczema

6. Identify the Skin disorder shown in the Photograph
[Recent Question 2014]

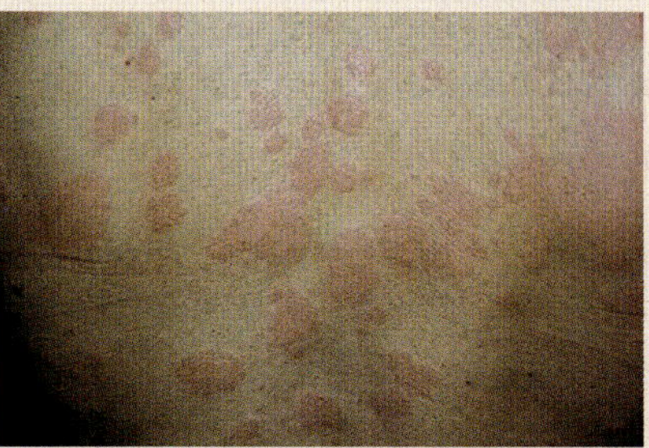

a. Scabies
b. Urticaria
c. Angioedema
d. Erythema multiforme

7. Identify Skin disorder shown in the Photograph
[Recent Question 2014]

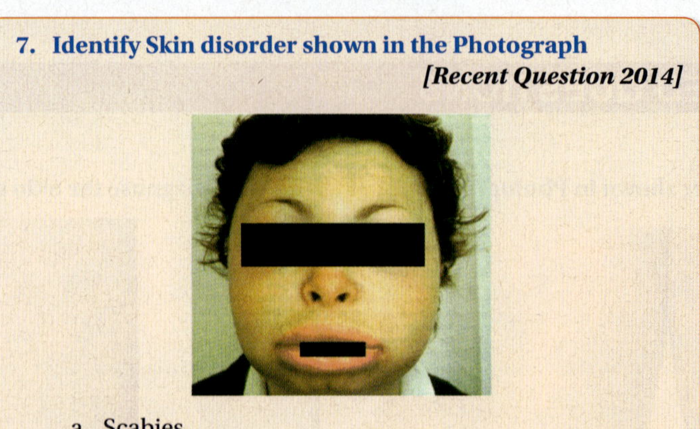

a. Scabies
b. Urticaria
c. Angioedema
d. Erythema multiforme

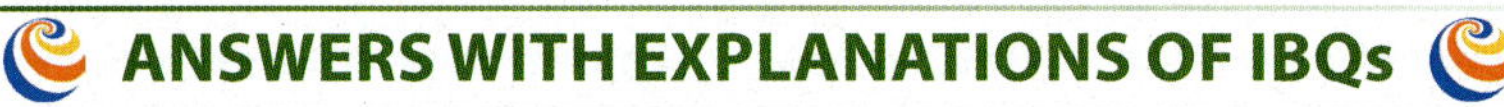

ANSWERS WITH EXPLANATIONS OF IBQs

1. Ans. (c) Atopic dermatitis *[Ref. Neena Khanna, 4/e p92-93]*

Atopic Dermatitis
- Papulo-vesicular lesions in infants
- Itchy plaques on elbow and knee flexors in children
- Lichenified plaques in adults in cubital/Popliteal fossae
- Ichthyosis
- *Dennie-Morgan fold*: Atopic skin folds under eye
- *Hertoghe's sign*: Thinning of lateral part of eyebrows
- White dermatographism
- Hyper-pigmented eyelids

2. Ans. (b) Nummular eczema *[Ref. Neena Khanna, 4/e p104]*
- Nummular eczema: Extremely itchy, multiple, sharply demarcated, coin-shaped vesicular/crusted plaques

3. Ans. (b) Seborrheic dermatitis *[Ref. Neena Khanna, 4/e p98]*
- Seborrheic dermatitis: Scalp erythema and greasy scale chronic dermatitis
- Characterized by erythematous skin with overlying greasy scale concentrated in the seborrheic areas of the face and scalp

4. Ans. (a) Pompholyx *[Ref. Neena Khanna, 4/e p104]*
- Pompholyx: Recurrent episodes of Deep seated, bland looking vesicles without inflammation
- Sites: Fingers, Palms, Soles

5. Ans. (c) Allergic contact dermatitis *[Ref. Neena Khanna, 4/e p101]*
- Common allergens for Allergic contact dermatitis: Parthenium pant (Photograph), Metals (Nickel, Silver), Cosmetics (Hair dyes, Fragrances), Medicines, Rubber

6. Ans. (b) Urticaria *[Ref. Neena Khanna, 4/e p179]*

Urticaria
- Erythematous macules rapidly evolve into pale pink edematous wheals with surrounding flare
- Shapes can be circular, annular, serpiginous, bizarre, linear

7. Ans. (c) Angioedema *[Ref. Neena Khanna, 4/e p179]*

Angioedema
- Pale pink swellings on face affecting lips and eyelids
- Swelling of tongue, pharynx, larynx

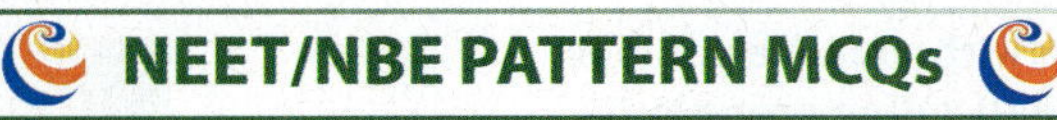

NEET/NBE PATTERN MCQs

1. **Exposure to sunlight can precipitate** *[Recent Question 2016]*
   a. Chloasma b. Discoid LE
   c. Dermatitis herpetiformis d. Lupus vulgaris
2. **In Atopic dermatitis all are seen except** *[Recent Question 2016]*
   a. Pruritus b. Eczema
   c. Mica-like scales d. Lichenification
3. **Sago grain like lesions between fingers is** *[Recent Question 2016]*
   a. Pompholyx b. Erythema multiforme
   c. Scabies d. Papular urticaria
4. **Kaposi varicelliform lesions is seen in** *[Recent Question 2016]*
   a. Varicella zoster b. Darier's disease
   c. Lichen planus d. Lichen nitidus
5. **Patch test is read after** *[Recent Question 2016]*
   a. 2 hours b. 2 days
   c. 2 months d. 2 weeks
6. **Quincke's disease is** *[Recent Question 2016]*
   a. Norwegian scabies b. Angioneurotic edema
   c. Seborrhea olesa d. Saddle nose
7. **MC plant implicated in the causation of dermatitis is** *[Recent Question 2016]*
   a. Cotton fibres b. Poison ivy
   c. Parthenium grass d. Ragweed
8. **Pompholyx affects** *[Recent Question 2016, 2017]*
   a. Palms and soles b. Groin
   c. Scalp d. Trunk
9. **RAST test is used in diagnosis of** *[Recent Question 2016]*
   a. Allergic dermatitis b. Seborrhoeic dermatitis
   c. Mycosis fungoides d. Squamous cell carcinoma
10. **Lesions of Childhood Atopic Dermatitis are located in** *[NBE FMGE September 2010]*
    a. Scalp
    b. Axilla and groin
    c. Cubital and Popliteal fossae
    d. Nasolabial folds
11. **'Itch is disease' is true for** *[UPSC 2000]*
    a. Atopic dermatitis b. Insect bites
    c. Seborrheic dermatitis d. Tinea cruris
12. **Perioral pallor and Dennie's line are seen in** *[NBE DNB 2009]*
    a. Atopic dermatitis
    b. Chronic actinic dermatitis
    c. Blood dyscrasia
    d. Perioral contact dermatitis
13. **Commonest site of atopic dermatitis is** *[Recent Question 2016, NBE DNB 2007]*
    a. Scalp b. Elbow
    c. Ante-cubital fossa d. Trunk
14. **True about atopic dermatitis are all except** *[Recent Question 2012]*
    a. Pruritus b. Scratching
    c. Mica-like scales d. Eczema
15. **Hereditary angioneurotic edema false is** *[Recent Question 2012]*
    a. C4 for screening
    b. Deficiency of C1 inhibitor
    c. Excessive production of C2 kinin
    d. C3 level are reduced
16. **Atopic dermatitis all are seen except** *[Recent Question 2012, Recent Question 2013]*
    a. Pruritis b. Eczema
    c. Mica like scales d. Lichenification
17. **Cradle cap in babies is** *[NBE DNB 1992]*
    a. Burns of scalp b. Seborrheic dermatitis
    c. Fracture skull d. Newborn
18. **Two year old with rash on extensor surface, diagnosis** *[Recent Question 2012]*
    a. Infantile eczema b. Atopic dermatitis
    c. Contact dermatitis d. Viral exanthema
19. **Most common cause of plant induced dermatitis in India** *[NBE DNB 2009]*
    a. Poison ivy b. Parthenium
    c. Ragweed d. Cotton fibres
20. **Term 'Atopy' was introduced by** *[NBE FMGE September 2007]*
    a. Ehrlich b. Ovary
    c. Coca d. Dale
21. **Which of the following is an example of endogenous eczema?** *[NBE FMGE September 2011]*
    a. Photodermatitis
    b. Contact dermatitis
    c. Atopic dermatitis
    d. Infective eczema
22. **Pityriasis alba is a type of** *[NBE FMGE March 2012]*
    a. Vitiligo b. Atopic eczema
    c. Photodermatosis d. Malassezia furfur infection
23. **Sago grain like lesions in between Fingers of hands is** *[Recent Question 2016. 2015]*
    a. Pompholyx b. Erythema multiforme
    c. Scabies d. Papular urticarial
24. **Hertoghe's sign is seen in?** *[Recent Question 2017]*
    a. Atopic dermatitis b. Cutaneous TB
    c. Lichen planus d. Psoriasis
25. **Most common type of Cutaneous mastocytosis is?** *[Recent Question 2017]*
    a. Soiitary mastocltoma
    b. Urticaria pigmentosa
    c. Telangiectasia rnacularis eruptive perstans
    d. Diffuse ervthrodermic

26. **40 years old diabetic patient presents with round lesions for 2 weeks on abdomen. HPE shows palisading granuloma. What is the diagnosis?** *[Recent Question 2017]*
   a. Granuloma annulare b. Pemphigus erythematosus
   c. Leprosy d. Tinea
27. **Which of the following is characteristically associated with Dermatitis?** *[Recent Question 2017]*
   a. Spongiosis b. Orthokeratosis
   c. Hypergranulosis d. Acanthosis
28. **A 12-year-old presented with history of red lesions with itching and discharges on flexure aspect of elbow as shown below. Your diagnosis is** *[AIIMS May 2017]*

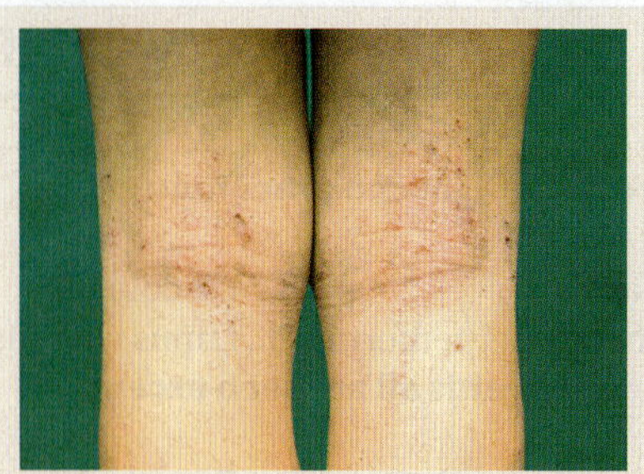

   a. Psoriasis b. Atopic dermatitis
   c. Pemphigus vulgaris

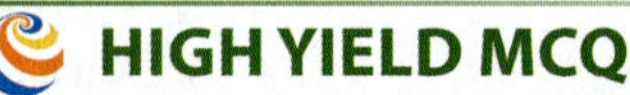

HIGH YIELD MCQs

1. **Which of the following statement(s) is/are true about Urticaria?** *[PGI November 2016]*
   a. Cholinergic urticaria is precipitated by cold mostly
   b. Solar urticaria is skin sign of Erythropoietic protoporphyria
   c. Dermatographism is an example
   d. Cholinergic urticaria is precipitated by emotion
   e. None of the above
2. **A 40-year-old farmer has itchy erythematous popular lesions on face, neck, V area of chest. The lesions were aggravated during summer and 75% reduced during winter. The most appropriate investigation to arrive at a diagnosis is** *[AIIMS May 2016]*
   a. IgE levels in blood b. Skin biopsy
   c. Intradermal patch test d. Serology
3. **A 22-year-old woman developed small itchy wheals after physical exertion, sun exposure, spicy food and anger. Diagnosis is** *[AIIMS May 2016]*
   a. Chronic idiopathic urticaria
   b. Heat-induced urticaria
   c. Solar urticaria
   d. Cholinergic urticaria
4. **A female presents with rash increasing in severity on taking spicy food, becoming angry, sun exposure and sweating. Most likely diagnosis is**
   a. Cholinergic urticaria *[AIIMS November 2016]*
   b. Heat urticaria
   c. Solar urticaria
   d. Hypersensitivity urticaria
5. **Dennie-Morgan fold is seen in** *[Karnataka PGMEE 1996, Bihar PGMEE 2006]*
   a. Mastocytosis b. Seborrhoeic dermatitis
   c. Sarcoidosis d. Atopic dermatitis
6. **A 3-year-old child has eczematous dermatitis on extensor surfaces. His mother has a history of bronchial asthma. Diagnosis could be** *[AIIMS PGMEE 2006]*
   a. Atopic dermatitis b. Contact dermatitis
   c. Seborrhoeic dermatitis
   d. Infantile eczematous dermatitis
7. **Rakesh, a 7-year-old boy had itchy, excoriated papules on the forehead and the exposed parts of the arms and legs for 3 years. The disease was most severe in the rainy season and improved completely in winter. Most likely diagnosis is** *[AIIMS PGMEE 2004]*
   a. Insect bite hypersensitivity
   b. Scabies
   c. Urticaria d. Atopic dermatitis
8. **A 25-year-old man presents with recurrent episodes of flexural eczema contact urticaria, recurrent skin infections and severe abdominal cramps and diarrhoea upon taking sea foods. He is suffering from**
   a. Seborrheic dermatitis *[All India PGMEE 2004]*
   b. Atopic dermatitis
   c. Airborne contact dermatitis
   d. Nummular dermatitis
9. **An infant presented with erythematous lesions on cheek, extensor aspect of limbs, mother has history of bronchial asthma, the probable diagnosis is** *[All India PGMEE 2007)*
   a. Airborne contact dermatitis
   b. Atopic dermatitis
   c. Seborrhoeic dermatitis
   d. Infectious eczematoid dermatitis
10. **Kaposi varicelliform lesion seen in** *[PGI 2005]*
   a. Atopic dermatitis b. Darier's disease
   c. Lichen planus d. Varicella zoster
11. **A 22-year-old woman developed small itchy wheals after physical exertion, walking in the sun, eating hot spicy food and when she was angry. The most likely diagnosis is** *[AIIMS PGMEE 2003]*
   a. Chronic idiopathic urticaria
   b. Heat urticaria
   c. Solar urticaria
   d. Cholinergic urticaria
12. **A 5-year-old male child has multiple hyperpigmented macules over the trunk. On rubbing the lesion with the rounded end of a pen, he developed urticarial wheal, confined to the border of the lesion. The most likely diagnosis is** *[All India PGMEE 2004]*
   a. Fixed drug eruption b. Lichen planus
   c. Urticaria pigmentosa d. Urticarial vasculitis
13. **A 9-year-old has multiple itchy erythematous wheals all over the body for 2 days. There is no respiratory difficulty. Which is the best treatment?** *[AIIMS PGMEE 2004]*

a. Antihelminthics b. Systemic corticosteroids
c. Antihistamines d. Adrenaline

14. Recurrent orogenital ulceration with arthritis is seen in *[PGI 1996]*
a. Behçet's syndrome b. Gonorrhoea
c. Reiter's syndrome d. Syphilis

15. A patient presents with history of episodic painful edema of face and larynx and abdominal pain associated with stress. Which of the following is likely to be deficient? *[All India PGMEE 2009, 2010]*
a. Complement C3 b. Complement C5
c. C1 Esterase Inhibitor d. Properidin

16. Immediately after eating, a man develops swelling of face and lips, respiratory distress, intense pruritus, hypotension and feeling of impending doom. The most likely diagnosis is *[All India PGMEE 2009]*
a. Angioneurotic Edema b. Anaphylaxis
c. Myocardial Infarction d. Food stuck in throat

17. Alopecia areata is presumed to be *[AIIMS PGMEE 1992]*
a. Androgenic in nature
b. Autoimmune in etiology
c. Infective in etiology
d. Part of lichenoid in spectrum

18. Laboratory evaluation of a patient with recurrent lip edema shows decreased C4 and C1INH (quantity & function) with normal C1q. Diagnosis is *[All India PGMEE 2009]*
a. Hereditary angioedema type II
b. Hereditary angioedema type I
c. Acquired AE type II
d. Acquired AE type I

19. Characteristic feature of Atopic dermatitis is *[MP PGMEE 2005]*
a. Pruritus
b. Dennie's Lines
c. Scaling of skin (Lichenification)
d. Rash

20. Not true about angioneurotic edema? *[All India PGMEE 2009]*
a. Pitting edema of face, lips and mucous membrane
b. C1 Esterase inhibitor deficiency can cause it
c. Extreme temperature exposure can provoke it
d. Known with ACE inhibitors

21. A man takes peanut and develops, tongue swelling, neck swelling, stridor, hoarseness of voice. What is the probable diagnosis? *[AIIMS PGMEE 2006]*
a. Angioneurotic edema b. FB bronchus
c. Parapharyngeal abscess d. FB in larynx

22. Air-borne contact dermatitis can be diagnosed by *[AIIMS PGMEE 2006]*
a. Skin biopsy
b. Patch test
c. Prick test
d. Estimation of serum IgE levels

23. Exfoliative dermatitis can be due to all of the following disease except *[All India PGMEE 2002]*
a. Drug hypersensitivity b. Pityriasis rubra pilaris
c. Pityriasis rosea d. Psoriasis

24. Patch testing is done for *[PGI 2008]*
a. Atopic dermatitis
b. Irritant contact dermatitis
c. Allergic contact dermatitis
d. Discoid eczema
e. Seborrhoeic dermatitis

25. True regarding Reactive arthritis is all except *[PGI 2008]*
a. HLA B27 & HIV affects severity
b. Dactylitis & enthesitis
c. Keratoderma mostly on glans
d. Asymmetrical sacroiliitis
e. Onycholysis & hyperkeratosis of nails

26. All are neutrophilic dermatosis, except *[PGI 2008]*
a. Subcorneal pustular dermatosis
b. Kimura disease c. Granuloma facial
d. Sweet's syndrome e. Pyoderma gangrenosum

27. Erythema nodosum is not seen in *[AIIMS PGMEE 1991]*
a. Primary TB b. Sulfonamides
c. Giant cell arteritis d. Streptococcal Infection

28. False about Sweet syndrome *[PGI 2009]*
a. Be a/w high fever
b. Neutrophilia not present
c. Be a/w hematological malignancy
d. Pseudovesication
e. Tender erythematous nodule/plaque

29. A child with fever had multiple skin lesions, an on microscopic examination, the skin lesions are seen to have neutrophilic and histiocytic infiltration in the dermis. What is the diagnosis? *[All India PGMEE 2009]*
a. Sweet syndrome b. Behcet's syndrome
c. Pyoderma gangrenosum d. Juvenile dermatosis

30. Commonest site of Atopic dermatitis is *[JIPMER PGMEE 2003]*
a. Scalp b. Elbow
c. Trunk d. Anterior cubital fossa

31. A 25 years old male having fever & malaise since 2 weeks, arthritis of ankle joint and tender erythematous nodules over the shin. Diagnosis is *[AIIMS PGMEE 2010]*
a. Erythema nodosum b. Hansen's disease
c. Weber-Christian disease d. Nodular Vasculitis

32. Erythema nodosum is due to *[Jharkhand PGMEE 2004]*
a. Contraceptive pills b. Barbiturates
c. Penicillin d. Sulphonamides

33. Atopic Dermatitis is diagnosed by *[Recent Question 2016, 2017, All India PGMEE 1999]*
a. Patch test b. Wood Lamp
c. Clinical Examination d. IgE

34. Commonest metal causing Skin hypersensitivity *[Recent Question 2016, 2017]* *[AIIMS PGMEE 1998, All India PGMEE 1993]*
a. Nickel b. Cu
c. Iron d. Brass

35. Most common cause of Allergic contact dermatitis in Indian female is *[AIIMS PGMEE 2007]*
a. Vegetables b. Nail polish
c. Detergents d. Dyes

36. Commonest cause of Air-borne contact dermatitis in India is *[AIIMS PGMEE 1994]*
a. Parthenium b. Garden grass
c. Oleander d. Yellow oleander

37. In India, the plant which causes Dermatitis most commonly is *[AIIMS PGMEE 1998]*
a. Parthenium grass b. Cotton fibers
c. Poison Ivy d. Ragweed

38. All may lead to hives and wheels, except *[PGI 1997]*
a. Cold b. Hepatitis C
c. Serum Sickness d. Typhoid fever

39. A patient gets Recurrent urticaria while doing exercise and on exposure to sunlight. Which of the following is most likely cause? *[AIIMS PGMEE 2000]*
a. Chronic Idiopathic Urticaria
b. Universal dermographism
c. Cholinergic Urticaria d. Photodermatitis

40. Which of these statements is false for lesions of Erythema nodosum? *[MP PGMEE 2004]*
a. They are considered as hypersensitivity reaction
b. The skin overlying the lesions is red, smooth and shiny
c. They are usually non tender
d. They can be associated with tuberculosis

41. Darier's sign is seen in *[Recent Question 2016, JIPMER PGMEE 1998, PGI 1999]*
a. Xeroderma pigmentosa b. Urticaria pigmentosa
c. Herpes zoster d. Glucagonoma

42. Epithelioid granuloma is characteristic of *[AIIMS PGMEE 1994]*
a. Sarcoidosis b. Eosinophilia
c. T.B. d. Mycosis Fungoides

43. All are true regarding hereditary angioedema, except *[PGI 1998]*
a. Dysfunction of enzyme is most common cause
b. Enzyme involved in C1 INH
c. C1 inhibitor targets Hageman factor
d. Complement C4 & C2 decrease
e. Bradykinin level decrease during attack

44. A person presents with recurrent swelling on face and lips due to emotional stress, cause is
a. C1 esterase inhibitor deficiency *[AIIMS PGMEE 2009]*
b. Allergy
c. Anaphylaxis
d. None of the above

45. Quincke's disease is popularly known as *[PGI 1995, AIIMS PGMEE 1998]*
a. Norwegian scabies b. Angioneurotic oedema
c. Seborrhoea oleosa d. Saddle nose

46. What is not seen in Reiter's syndrome?
a. Subcutaneous nodules *[AIIMS PGMEE 2008]*
b. Keratoderma blennorrhagicum
c. Circinate balanitis
d. Oral ulcers

47. Exfoliative dermatitis is seen in all the following, except *[PGI 2006]*
a. Pityriasis rosea b. Pityriasis rubra pilaris
c. Psoriasis d. Drug hypersensitivity
e. Eczema

48. Causes of Erythroderma *[PGI 2005]*
a. Pityriasis alba b. Pityriasis versicolor
c. Psoriasis d. Lichen planus
e. Eczema

49. Erythema nodosum is seen in all, except *[AIIMS PGMEE 1992]*
a. Rheumatoid arthritis b. Tuberculosis
c. Enteric fever d. Aspirin therapy

50. Patch test is a type of *[AIIMS PGMEE 2009]*
a. Immediate hypersensitivity
b. Antibody-mediated hypersensitivity
c. Immune complex-mediate hypersensitivity
d. Delayed type hypersensitivity

51. Berloque dermatitis is due to contact with *[JIPMER PGMEE 1999, AMU PGMEE 1999] [All India PGMEE 1998]*
a. Metals b. Cosmetics
c. Food d. Plants

52. Patch test is read after *[All India PGMEE 1999]*
a. 2 hours b. 2 days
c. 2 weeks d. 2 months

53. Minor clinical feature in diagnosis of Atopic dermatitis all, except *[PGI 1994]*
a. Dry skin b. Pruritus
c. Morgagnian fold d. Pityriasis alba
e. Dermographism

54. IgA deposits on skin biopsy *[AIIMS PGMEE 1999]*
a. Henoch-Schonlein purpura
b. Giant cell arteritis
c. Microscopic polyangiitis
d. Wegener's granulomatosis

55. Which of the following is not included in the Triad of Reiter's syndrome? *[Karnataka PGMEE 1996]*
a. Conjunctivitis
b. Urethritis
c. Arthritis
d. Keratoderma blennorrhagica

56. Chloroquine is indicated in treatment of *[All India PGMEE 1991]*
a. Pemphigus b. Pemphigoid
c. Psoriasis d. DLE

57. A girl of 19 years with arthritis and photosensitive rash on cheeks, likely diagnosis is *[All India PGMEE 2001, Bihar PGMEE 2003]*
a. SLE
b. Chloasma
c. Stevens-Johnson syndrome
d. Lyme's disease

58. Which of the organisms most commonly causes reactive arthritis? *[AIIMS PGMEE 2008]*
a. Ureaplasma urealyticum
b. Group A beta hemolytic streptococci
c. *Borrelia burgdorferi*
d. *Chlamydia*

59. Erythema nodosum is seen in all, except *[AIIMS PGMEE 1994]*
a. Salicylate poisoning b. Typhoid
c. Tuberculosis d. Leprosy

60. M.C. site of Atopic dermatitis *[AIIMS PGMEE 1998]*
a. Scalp b. Elbow
c. Antecubital fossa d. Trunk

61. After hepatitis B vaccination child with allergic family history and pruritus involving face & convexities developed

numerous umbilicated vesicles; which became pustular, haemorrhagic & crusted. After 2 days, child developed high fever and lymphadenopathy. The diagnosis is *[AIIMS PGMEE 2007]*

a. Secondary infected atopic dermatitis
b. Molluscum contagiosum
c. Eczema herpeticum
d. Eczema vaccinatum

62. Eczema herpeticum seen with *[PGI 2007]*

a. HSV
b. EBV
c. CMV
d. VZV

63. Eczema herpeticum is caused by *[PGI 2000]*

a. Herpes simplex virus 1
b. Coxsackie
c. HSV-2
d. Vaccinia
e. HSV-6

64. A 3-year-old child has eczematous dermatitis on extensor surfaces. His mother has a history of Bronchial asthma. Diagnosis should be *[AIIMS PGMEE 2007]*

a. Atopic dermatitis
b. Contact dermatitis
c. Seborrheic dermatitis
d. Infantile eczematous dermatitis

65. Spongiosis is seen in *[Karnataka PGMEE 2003, All India PGMEE 2001]*

a. Acute eczema
b. Lichen planus
c. Psoriasis
d. Pemphigus

66. Coin-shaped eczema is *[Jharkhand PGMEE 2005]*

a. Nummular eczema
b. Atopic eczema
c. Infantile eczema
d. Endogenous eczema

Skin and STDs

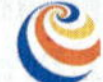 NEET/NBE PATTERN MCQs ANSWERS WITH EXPLANATIONS 

1. **Ans. (a) Chloasma; (b) Discoid LE**
   [Ref. Dermatopathology by Fuchs, 1/e]
   - Diseases can be exacerbated by sunlight (Rosacea, Cutaneous discoid lupus erythematosus) or improved with sunlight (Psoriasis)
   - Photosensitivity is one of the major clinical symptoms of the disease
   - Skin lesions are frequently associated with solar exposure and are also aggravated by UV. UVB and sunlight can precipitate or exacerbate the disease
   - Exposure to sunlight intensifies chloasma, especially among fair-skinned individuals

2. **Ans. (c) Mica-like scales**
   [Ref. DVL by Thappa, 4/e p143]

   Atopic Dermatitis
   - An eczematous eruption that is itchy, recurrent & symmetric
   - Scales: dry & excoriations are frequent

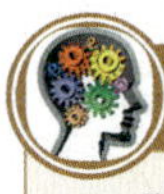

Also Remember

- Yellow and greasy scales are diagnostic of seborrheic dermatitis

3. **Ans. (a) Pompholyx**
   [Ref. DVL by Thappa, 4/e p149,150]

   Pompholyx (Dyshidrosis)
   - Characterized by itchy deep-seated vesiculation (sago grain) on palms & sides of fingers
   - Topical steroids are first line
   - Second-line agents are tacrolimus, pimecrolimus, calcipotriene

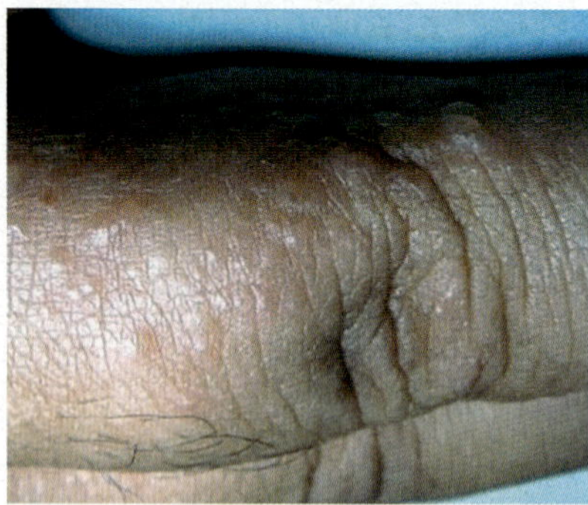

Fig. Pompholyx

4. **Ans. (b) Darier's disease**
   [Ref. DVL by Thappa, 4/e p.234,235)

   Darier's Disease
   - Genodermatosis of AD inheritance
   - Characterized by dirty, warty, popular lesions in the seborrheic areas of the body, mainly involving the trunk, face, flexures of extremities in a symmetrical fashion
   - Hard palate may demonstrate **"Pebble stone appearance"** and palms show pits

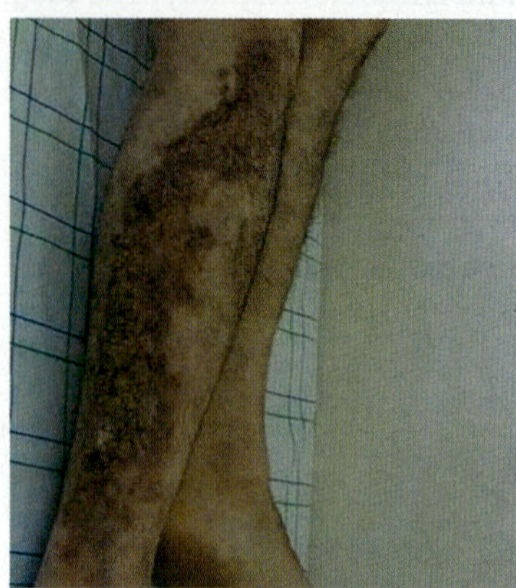

Fig. Darier's disease

5. **Ans. (b) 2 days**
   [Ref. DVL by Thappa, 4/e p. 43]

   Patch Testing
   - A diagnostic procedure in which the patient's skin is exposed to various substances and reaction is then observed
   - It is helpful in confirming a clinical diagnosis of allergic contact dermatitis and in identifying the specific chemical allergens
   - Results of patch test are read after 48 hours

6. **Ans. (b) Angioneurotic edema**
   [Ref. DVL by Thappa, 4/e p208)

   Angioedema
   - Giant Edema, Giant Urticaria, Hives, Nettle Rash, **Quincke's disease**
   - A vascular reaction, which involves subcutaneous or submucosal tissues so the skin overlying the swelling is normal in color & margins of swelling are indistinct
   - It commonly results in swelling of the lips, eyelids but may also affect pharynx, larynx

7. **Ans. (c) Parthenium grass**
   [Ref. DVL by Thappa, 4/e p154]
   - In allergic contact, dermatitis patch test helps to identify the allergens, commonly encountered allergens include nickel, chromate, rubber chemicals, paraphenylene-diamine, plants (Parthenium)

8. **Ans. (a) Palms and soles**
   [Ref. Clinical Dermatology by Habif, 6/e p109]

   Pompholyx
   - Type of eczema that causes tiny blisters to develop across the fingers, palms of the hands and sometimes the soles of the feet
   - It's also known as dyshidrotic eczema
   - Moderate to severe itching precedes the appearance of vesicles on the palms and sides of the fingers
   - Vesicles slowly resolve in 3–4 weeks and are replaced by 1–3 mm rings of scale

- Treatment:
  - Topical steroids cold, wet compresses and oral antibiotics are used as the initial treatment
  - Resistant cases PUVA therapy

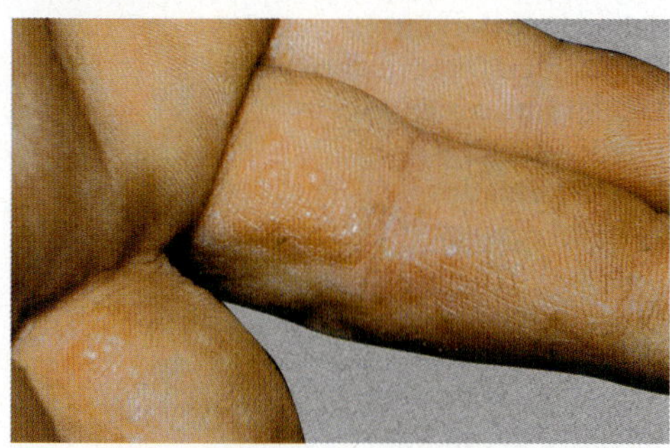

Fig. Pompholyx

9. Ans. (a) Allergic dermatitis

[Ref. Clinical Dermatology by Habif, 6/e p155]

- Allergic contact dermatitis is a type of delayed hypersensitivity reaction
- Latex allergy occurs in up to 10% of operating room nurses
- Patients with a history of symptoms from rubber exposure can be screened with a radio allegro sorbent test **(RAST)** to detect latex-specific IgE
- If the RAST is positive, no further testing should be done

10. Ans. (c) Cubital and Popliteal fossae

[Ref. Neena Khanna, 4/e p93]

Clinical Presentation of Atopic Dermatitis

- Papulo-vesicular lesions in infants
- Itchy plaques on elbow and knee flexors in children
- Lichenified plaques in adults in cubital/Popliteal fossae
- Ichthyosis
- White dermatographism
- Hyper-pigmented eyelids
- ***Dennie-Morgan fold***: Atopic skin folds under eye
- ***Hertoghe's sign***: Thinning of lateral part of eyebrows

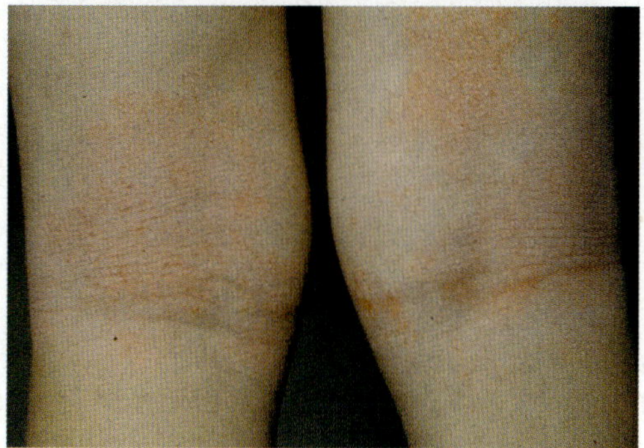

Fig. Pompholyx

11. Ans. (a) Atopic dermatitis

[Ref. Neena Khanna, 5/e p100-101]

- It is one of the itchiest disorders

12. Ans. (a) Atopic dermatitis

[Ref. Lookingbill and Marks' Principles of Dermatology, 5/e p91]

- Atopic dermatitis have a characteristic expression: Face has mild to moderate erythema, perioral pallor, and infraorbital folds (Dennie-Morgan lines) associated with dermatitis and hyperpigmentation

13. Ans. (c) Ante-cubital fossa

[Ref. Neena Khanna, 5/e p102]

- Cubital or antecubital fossa and popliteal fossa along with neck is the common site for Atopic dermatitis in adults

14. Ans. (c) Mica-like scales

[Ref. Neena Khanna, 5/e p100-101]

15. Ans. (d) C3 level are reduced

[Ref. Immunological and Clinical Aspects of Allergy by Lessof, 1/e p187; Hereditary Angioedema by Frank, Medscape Article135604]

Hereditary Angioneurotic Edema (HAE)

- Concept:
  - C1 esterase is the activated form of C1: Patients who lack the C1 esterase inhibitor therefore have excess circulating C1 esterase activity
  - Substrates for C1 esterase are C4 and C2 which are split into C4a, C4b and C2a respectively: Levels of both C4 and C2 are therefore low during attacks and C4 levels are also reduced during asymptomatic periods, thus a useful screening test for the disease
  - Combination of C4b and C2a produces the enzyme C3 convertase which is responsible for activation of C3 and the continuing complement activation cascade
  - In the process of formation of C2a, a kinin-like substance, C2-kinin is also produced and it is this C2-kinin which is thought to be the mediator of the disease process
  - Production of C2-kinin appears also to be dependent on Hageman factor, a protein which is itself involved both in coagulation and in the plasma bradykinin-forming system
- Diagnosis of Hereditary Angioedema depends on the demonstration of the C1 esterase inhibitor in serum
  - A low absolute level, which is the usual abnormality, can be detected by a quantitative immunochemical method
  - However, in a minority of affected families this quantitative method gives normal results but the protein is functionally inactive: Defect can only be confirmed using a chemical esterolytic assay
  - Low levels of C4 in the presence of normal quantities of the inhibitor detected immunochemically: Functional defect and lead to further investigation
  - Measurement of C4 is also a useful screening test: Levels are low even between attacks and C4 levels are usually normal in other forms of angioedema
- Imaging studies can be used in the diagnosis of HAE:
  - Abdominal radiography: Features of ileus
  - Chest radiography: Pleural effusions
  - Abdominal ultrasonography or CT: Edematous thickening of the intestinal wall, a fluid layer around the bowel, and large amounts of free peritoneal fluid

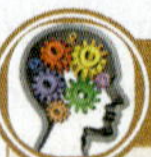

Also Remember

3 Types of HAE

- Type I HAE is characterized by the following:
  - Low C1 esterase inhibitor (C1-INH) protein level
  - Low C4 level
  - Normal C1q level
- Type II HAE is characterized by the following:
  - Normal or elevated, but dysfunctional, C1-INH level
  - Low C4 level
  - Normal C1q level
- Type III HAE with normal C1 inhibitor levels is characterized by the following:
  - Normal C1-INH level
  - Normal C1-INH functional assay
  - Normal C4 and C1q level
  - Factor XII mutation may be present

16. Ans. (c) Mica-like scales
[Ref. Neena Khanna, 5/e p100-101]

17. Ans. (b) Seborrheic dermatitis
[Ref. Caring for Your Baby & Young Child by Shelov, 1/e p630]

Cradle Cap

- Infantile seborrhoeic dermatitis that is confined to the scalp
- Patchy, greasy, scaly and crusty skin rash that occurs on the scalp of recently born babies
- May also affect other areas of the body such as behind the ears, in the creases of the neck, armpits and diaper area

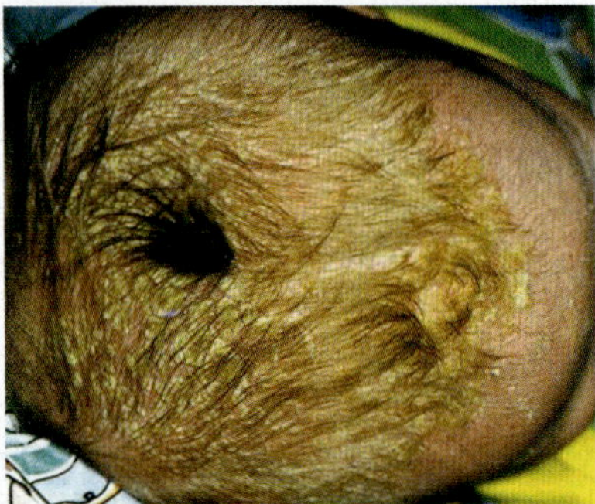

Fig. Cradle cap

18. Ans. (b) Atopic dermatitis
[Ref. Neena Khanna, 5/e p102]

AD in Children

- Extremely itchy, dry, leathery plaques
- Mainly on elbow and knee flexors: Reversed (extensor) pattern

19. Ans. (b) Parthenium
[Ref. Neena Khanna, 5/e p114]

- Parthenium hysterophorus is common cause of air-borne contact dermatitis in India

20. Ans. (c) Coca
[Ref. Neena Khanna, 4/e p 91]

- *Atopy*: Predisposition towards certain allergic hypersensitivity
- *Term was coined by*: Coca and Crooke

21. Ans. (c) Atopic dermatitis
[Ref. Neena Khanna, 4/e p86]

Etiological Classification of Eczema

- *Endogenous eczema*:
  - Seborrheic dermatitis
  - Nummular/Discoid dermatitis
  - Lichen simplex chronicus
  - Pityriasis alba
  - Stasis dermatitis
- *Exogenous eczema*:
  - Contact/ Irritant dermatitis
  - Allergic dermatitis
  - Photodermatitis
  - Radiation dermatitis
  - Infective dermatitis
- *Combined eczema*:
  - Atopic dermatitis
  - Pompholyx

22. Ans. (b) Atopic eczema
[Ref. Differential Diagnosis by Goodheart, 1/e p83]

Pityriasis Alba

- *Affects*: Children and young adults
- *Associated with*: Atopic dermatitis
- *Appearance*:
  - Hypopigmented spots on face (lateral cheeks) and other areas of skin (upper forearms)
  - Dark skinned children
  - More in summer season
  - Absence of scaling
- *Treatment*:
  - No treatment
  - Moisturising cream
  - 1% Hydrocortisone cream

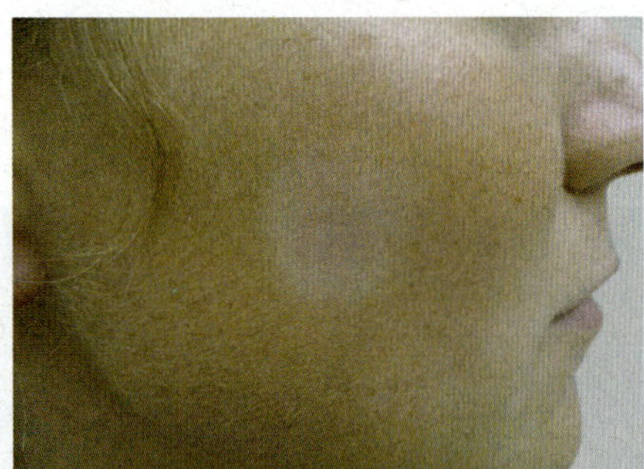

Fig. Pityriasis alba

23. Ans. (a) Pompholyx
[Ref. French's Index of Differential Diagnosis by Douthwaite, 7/e p56]

- Pompholyx: Numerous minute vesicles are deeply imbedded in the skin and show through the epidermis like 'boiled sago grains' on both hands, mostly in the palms and volar surfaces

24. Ans. (a) Atopic dermatitis
[Ref. Neena Khanna, 4/e p93]

- Hertoghe's sign occurs in Atopic dermatitis
- Characterised by thinning of lateral part of eyebrows

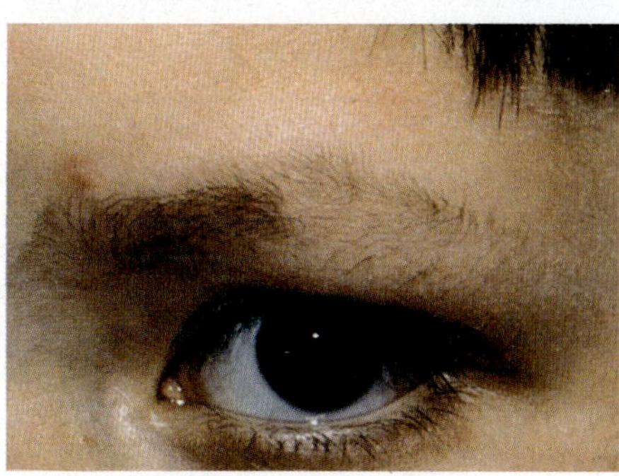

Fig. Hertoghe's sign

25. Ans. (b) Urticaria pigmentosa
[Ref. Clinical Dermatology by Habif, 6/e p209]

Cutaneous Mastocytosis (CM)

- Most cases of Pediatric mastocytosis are sporadic and appear during the first 2 years of life, especially on the trunk
- Urticaria pigmentosa is the most frequent variant
- Three main forms of CM (defined by the WHO)
  - Urticaria pigmentosa (UP - Maculopapular cutaneous mastocytosis MPCM)
  - Diffuse cutaneous mastocytosis (DCM)
  - Mastocytoma of skin

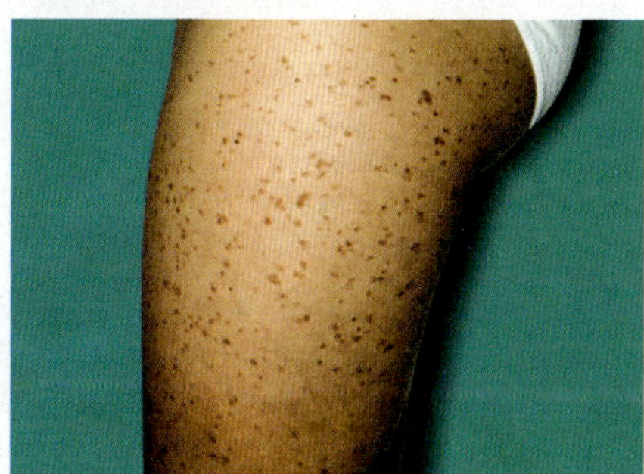

Fig. Urticaria pigmentosa

26. Ans. (a) Granuloma annulare
[Ref. Shimizu's Dermatology, 2/e p374]

Granuloma Annulare

- Doughnut-shaped eruption with elevated rim
- Palisading granuloma on histopathology
- When involves whole body, it may be associated with Diabetes
- Types: Localised, Generalized, Perforating, Subcutanoeus

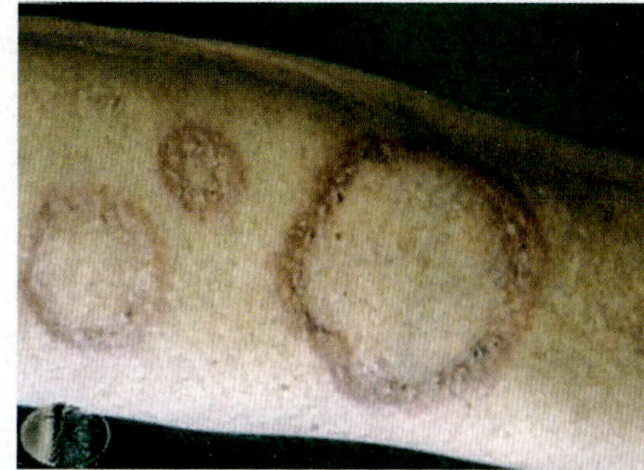

Fig. Granuloma annulare

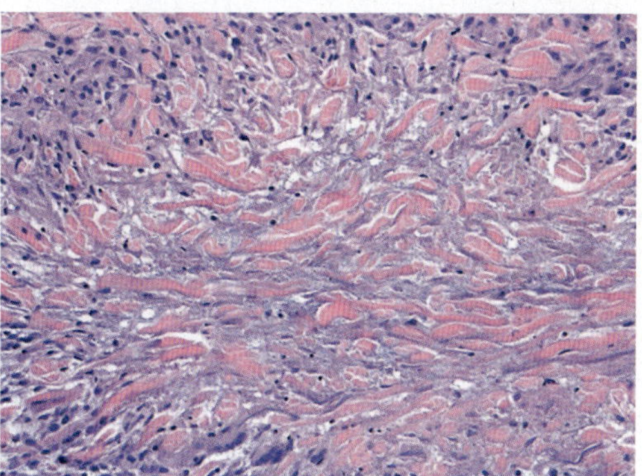

Fig. Palisading granuloma

27. Ans. (a) Spongiosis
[Ref. Irritant Dermatitis by Chew, 1/e p13]

Allergic Contact Dermatitis is a Spongiotic Dermatitis

- Early allergic reactions: Dermal inflammatory infiltrates around the dilated venules of the superficial plexus, edema, and spongiosis
- Inflammatory cells in epidermis characteristically adopt a focal distribution
- Fully developed spongiosis becomes organized in focal microvesicles and the infiltrate becomes denser
- If the process evolves more slowly, the spongiosis propels the epidermis to become more hyperplastic

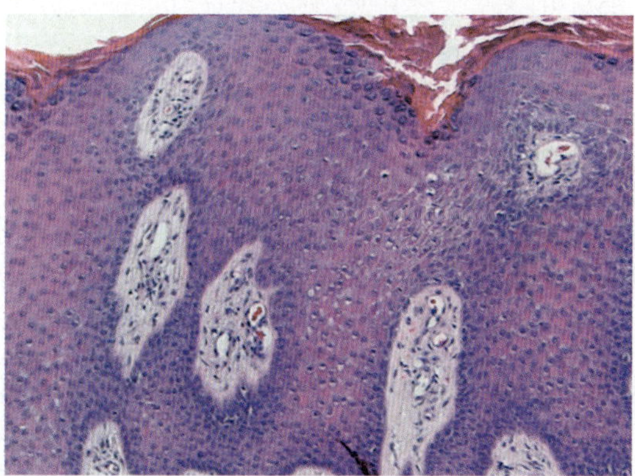

Fig. Spongiotic dermatitis

28. Ans. (b) Atopic dermatitis
[Ref. Fitzpatrick's Dermatology, 8/e p165]

Atopic Dermatitis

- Chronic or chronically relapsing disorder with major features of:
  - Pruritus
  - Eczematous dermatitis: Facial and extensor involvement in infancy; and flexural eczema/lichenification in children and adults
- Commonly associated with the following:
  - Personal or family history of atopy (allergic rhinitis, asthma, atopic dermatitis)
  - Xerosis/skin barrier dysfunction
  - Immunoglobulin E reactivity

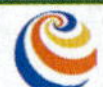 HIGH YIELD MCQs ANSWERS WITH EXPLANATIONS 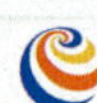

1. **Ans. (b) Solar urticaria is skin sign of Erythropoietic protoporphyria; (c) Dermatographism is an example; (d) Cholinergic urticaria is precipitated by emotion**
[Ref. Clinical Dermatology by Habif, 6/e p14]

Urticarias

- Cholinergic urticaria, from elevation in core body temperature, is precipitated by exercise or use of hot tubs or emotional stress
- Solar urticaria:
  - Virtually always idiopathic
  - Rarely, medications such as tetracycline (but not minocycline), chlorpromazine, progestational agents, and repirinast have been reported to induce solar urticaria
  - Erythropoietic protoporphyria and Porphyria cutanea tarda simulate lesions like Solar urticaria
- Dermatographism, the most common form of physical urticaria (seen in 2–5% of the population), results in a linear wheal at site of friction

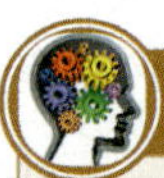

Also Remember

Physical (Inducible) Urticaria

- Due to mechanical stimuli: Dermographism, delayed pressure urticarial
- Due to temperature changes
- Due to sweating/physical exertion: Cholinergic > adrenergic urticaria, exercise-induced anaphylaxis, solar urticarial is skin sign of Erythropoietic protoporphyria

2. **Ans. (c) Intradermal patch test**
[Ref. DVT by Thappa, 4/e p43]

- Occupation of farming, history of aggravation in summer probably indicates Photodermatitis due to Parthenium
- Ideal investigation would be a Patch test/Photopatch test
- Extracts of the plant allergens can be used either alone or with the Indian Standard Series used for Patch testing (ISS)

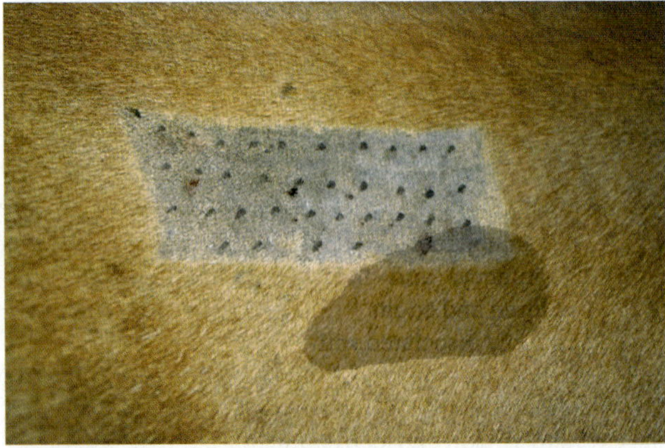

Fig. Intradermal skin test

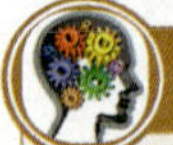

Also Remember

- Patch testing is a diagnostic procedure in which the patient's skin is exposed to various substances and reaction is then observed
- It is helpful in confirming a clinical diagnosis of allergic contact dermatitis and in identifying the specific chemical allergens

3. **Ans. (d) Cholinergic urticaria**
[Ref. Clinical Dermatology by Habif, 6/e p213]

Cholinergic Urticaria

- MC of the physical urticarias
- Typically presents with numerous small wheals, aggravated by mental stress, exercise (e.g. cycling, gymming, hot climates, hot and spicy foods, steam baths)

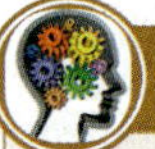

Also Remember

- Solar urticaria develops only on exposure to sunlight and not by other causes
- Chronic idiopathic urticaria usually does not have any specific triggering agents
- Heat urticaria develops only on contact with heat

4. **Ans. (a) Cholinergic urticaria**
[Ref. Neena Khanna, 4/e p178]

Cholinergic Urticaria

- Typical lesions: Small, short-lasting hives but may also involve cutaneous inflammation (wheals) and pain which develops usually in response to exercise, bathing, staying in a heated environment, or emotional stress
- Small (2–4 mm), punctate, very pruritic wheals on a large surrounding bright macular erythematous base
- Classically start on the neck, upper trunk, and arms, but can spread distally to include the whole body
- Although the symptoms subside rapidly, commonly within 1 hour, CU may significantly impair quality of life
- Causes:
  - Sweat hypersensitivity
  - Acquired anhidrosis and/or hypohidrosis
  - Idiopathic

5. **Ans. (d) Atopic dermatitis**
[Ref. Lookingbill and Marks' Principles of Dermatology, 5/e p91]

6. **Ans. (a) Atopic dermatitis**
[Ref. Neena Khanna, 5/e p102]

7. **Ans. (d) Atopic dermatitis**
[Ref. Neena Khanna, 5/e p102]

8. **Ans. (b) Atopic dermatitis**
[Ref. Neena Khanna, 5/e p102]

9. **Ans. (b) Atopic dermatitis**
[Ref. Neena Khanna, 5/e p102]

10. Ans. (a) Atopic dermatitis; (b) Darier's disease

[Ref. Cutaneous Medicine by Provost, 1/e p599; Neena Khanna, 5/e p103]

- Kaposi's varicelliform eruption: A serious infection occurring in atopic eczema and Darier's disease patients
  - Also seen in pemphigus vulgaris patients receiving high-dose oral steroids (> 100 mg prednisolone)
- Atopics have a greater susceptibility to viral infections like Herpes simplex, Molluscum contagiosum and Human papilloma virus infection
  - In the presence of active dermatitis, herpes simplex infection may become generalized (Kaposi's vericelliform), manifesting as generalized grouped vesicles which rapidly evolve into polycyclic erosions

11. Ans. (d) Cholinergic urticaria

[Ref. Anaphylaxis and Hypersensitivity Reactions by Castells, 1/e p278]

Cholinergic Urticaria

- Presentation:
  - Typical lesions: Small, short-lasting hives but may also involve cutaneous inflammation (wheals) and pain which develops usually in response to exercise, bathing, staying in a heated environment, or emotional stress
  - Lesions: Small (2–4 mm), punctate, very pruritic wheals on a large surrounding bright macular erythematous base
  - Lesions: Classically start on the neck, upper trunk, and arms, but can spread distally to include the whole body
  - Although the symptoms subside rapidly, commonly within 1 hour, CU may significantly impair quality of life (Sporting and sexual activities)
- Causes:
  - Sweat hypersensitivity
  - Acquired anhidrosis and/or hypohidrosis
  - Idiopathic
- Treatment
  - Proposed first-line treatment: Rapid desensitization protocol using autologous sweat
  - Non-pharmacological treatment: Forced perspiration by excessive body warming (hot bath or exercise) used daily may reduce the symptoms through exhaustion of inflammatory mediators (Contraindicated in those with hypohidrosis)
  - Antihistamines are first-line treatment for Conventional urticaria, but limited effectiveness: First-generation antihistamines with anticholinergic properties such as Diphenhydramine are most successful
  - Treatment(s) with mixed success: Omalizumab (Anti-IgE therapy), Danazol (Synthetic androgen), Propranolol (Beta blocker), Zileuton (Anti-leukotriene)

12. Ans. (c) Urticaria pigmentosa

[Ref. Anaphylaxis and Hypersensitivity Reactions by Castells, 1/e p253]

13. Ans. (c) Antihistamines

[Ref. Rook's Textbook of Dermatology by Burns, 7/e 47.1 -47.29]

- Acute araucaria is a self-limiting disease
- As the pathophysiology is histamine release, antihistaminics is given
- Had there been respiratory distress due to laryngeal oedema, 0.5 mL epinephrine is the initial drug of choice

14. Ans. (a) Behcet's syndrome; (c) Reiter's syndrome

[Ref. CMDT, 51/e p831,871,876] & [Ref. Textbook of Ophthalmology by HV Nema, 6/e p210]

15. Ans. (c) C1esterase inhibitor

[Ref. Immunological and Clinical Aspects of Allergy by Lessof, 1/e p187; Hereditary Angioedema by Frank, Medscape Article135604]

16. Ans. (b) Anaphylaxis

[Ref. Harrison's Principles of Internal Medicine by by Dennis L. Kasper, 18/e p2710]

- Intense pruritus and hypotension is characteristic of anaphylaxis
- Besides immediate onset, welling of face and respiratory distress is conclusive of Anaphylaxis

17. Ans. (b) Autoimmune in etiology

[Ref. Neena Khanna, 5/e p142]

- Alopecia aerate is a skin specific autoimmune disease, due to inappropriate response to hair follicle associated antigens
- Cytokines produced by dermal papillae in lesions, attract lymphocytes to perifollicular region and stimulate them to multiply

18. Ans. (b) Hereditary angioedema type I

[Ref. Immunological and Clinical Aspects of Allergy by Lessof, 1/e p187; Hereditary Angioedema by Frank, Medscape Article135604]

19. Ans. (a) Pruritus

[Ref. Neena Khanna, 5/e p100-101]

20. Ans. (a) Pitting edema of face, lips and mucosa membrane

[Ref. Neena Khanna, 5/e p190]

21. Ans. (a) Angioneurotic edema

[Ref. Neena Khanna, 5/e p190-191]

22. Ans. (b) Patch test

[Ref. Neena Khanna, 5/e p15]

- Patch test detects antigens (allergens) responsible for allergic contact dermatitis (type IV hypersensitivity)

23. Ans. (c) Pityriasis rosea

[Ref. Neena Khanna, 5/e p60]

- Herald patch followed by secondary eruptions are seen in P. rosea

24. Ans. (c) Allergic contact dermatitis

[Ref. Neena Khanna, 5/e p15]

25. Ans. (c) Keratoderma mostly on glans

[Ref. Psoriatic and Reactive Arthritis by Ritchlin, 1/e p133]

26. Ans. (b) Kimura disease; (c) Granuloma facial

[Ref. Neena Khanna, 5/e p202-203; Cohen PR. Neutrophilic dermatoses: a review of current treatment options. Am J Clin Dermatol. 2009;10(5):301-12]

Neutrophilic Dermatoses

- Description: A group of disorders characterized by skin lesions for which histologic examination reveals

intense epidermal, dermal, or hypodermal inflammatory infiltrates composed primarily of neutrophils (mature polymorphonuclear leukocytes) with no evidence of infection or true vasculitis
- Examples:
  - Sweet syndrome (Acute febrile neutrophilic dermatosis): Neutrophils in dermis
  - Pyoderma gangrenosum: Neutrophils in dermis
  - Behcet's syndrome
  - Subcorneal pustular dermatosis: Neutrophils in upper layers of epidermis

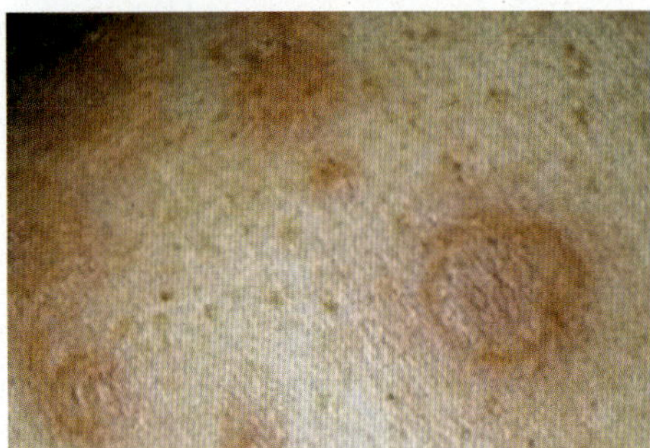

Fig. Neutrophilic dermatosis

27. Ans. (c) Giant cell arteritis
[Ref. Neena Khanna, 5/e p201]

Causes of Erythema Nodosum

Idiopathic (55%)	Tissue
Bacteria	*Streptococcus*, TB & *Yersinia* Rarely: Campylobacter, Rickettsia, *Salmonella*, Psittacosis, *Bartonella*, Syphilis
Fungi	Coccidioidomycosis
Viruses	Infectious mononucleosis, Hepatitis B & C Rarely: HSV, Epstein Barr virus & HIV
Other infections	Amoebiasis, Giardiasis & *Chlamydia*
Enteropathies	Regional enteritis, Ulcerative colitis
Drugs	Sulfonamides, Amoxycillin, Bromides & OCP
Miscellaneous	Sarcoidosis, Behcet's syndrome, Rheumatoid arthritis, Congenital tissue diseases, Leprosy Malignancy, Pregnancy

28. Ans. (b) Neutrophilia not present
[Ref. Neena Khanna, 5/e p202-203; Cohen PR. Neutrophilic dermatoses: a review of current treatment options. Am J Clin Dermatol. 2009;10(5):301-12]

Sweet Syndrome/Acute Febrile Neutrophilic Dermatosis
- Pyrexia, elevated neutrophil count, painful erythematous cutaneous lesions that have an infiltrate of mature neutrophils typically located in the upper dermis
- Prompt clinical improvement following the initiation of Systemic corticosteroid therapy
- Classical, malignancy-associated, and drug-induced variants of Sweet syndrome exist

29. Ans. (a) Sweet syndrome
[Ref. Neena Khanna, 5/e p202-203; Cohen PR. Neutrophilic dermatoses: a review of current treatment options. Am J Clin Dermatol. 2009;10(5):301-12]

30. Ans. (d) Anterior cubital fossa
[Ref. Neena Khanna, 5/e p102]
- Cubital or antecubital fossa and popliteal fossa along with neck is the common site for Atopic dermatitis in adults

31. Ans. (a) Erythema nodosum
[Ref. Neena Khanna, 5/e p201]

32. Ans. (a) Contraceptive pills; (d) Sulphonamides
[Ref. Neena Khanna, 5/e p201; Schwartz RA. Erythema Nodosum: A Sign of Systemic Disease. Am Fam Physician. 2007;75(5):695-700.]

33. Ans. (c) Clinical examination
[Ref. Neena Khanna, 5/e p104]

34. Ans. (a) Nickel
[Ref. Neena Khanna, 5/e p131]

Agents Causing Allergic Dermatitis

Plants	Parthenium
Metals	Nickel, Chromates, Cobalt
Cosmetics	Paraphenylenediamine, Fragrances, Formaldehyde, Parabens
Medicine	Neomycin, Benzocaine
Rubber	Mercapto mix (Additives in shoe soles), Thiuram mix (Additives in rubber gloves)

35. Ans. (c) Detergent

36. Ans. (a) Parthenium
[Ref. Neena Khanna, 5/e p114]

37. Ans. (a) Parthenium grass
[Ref. Neena Khanna, 5/e p114]

38. Ans. (d) Typhoid fever
[Ref. Cutis, Volume 10 p300]

Hives and Wheel Triggers
- Some food (especially peanuts, eggs, nuts and shellfish)
- Medications, such as antibiotics (especially penicillin and sulfa), aspirin and ibuprofen
- Insect stings or bites
- Physical stimuli, such as pressure, cold, heat, exercise or sun exposure
- Latex
- Blood transfusions
- Type III hypersensitivity reaction—Serum sickness
- Bacterial infections, including urinary tract infections and strep throat
- Viral infections, including the common cold, infectious mononucleosis and hepatitis
- Pet dander
- Pollen
- Some plants, such as poison oak and poison ivy

39. Ans. (c) Cholinergic Urticaria
[Ref. Anaphylaxis and Hypersensitivity Reactions by Castells, 1/e p278]

40. Ans. (c) They are usually non tender
[Ref. Neena Khanna, 5/e p201]

41. Ans. (b) Urticaria pigmentosa
[Ref. Textbook of Pediatric Emergency Medicine by Fleisher, 6/e p523]

- Darier's sign: A change observed after stroking the skin of a person with systemic mastocytosis or urticaria pigmentosa
  - In general, the skin becomes swollen, itchy and red: A result of compression of mast cells, which are hyperactive in these diseases
  - These mast cells release inflammatory granules which contain histamine, responsible for the response seen after rubbing the skin

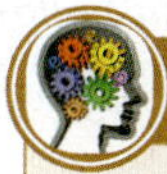

Also Remember

- Darier's sign is named after the French dermatologist Ferdinand-Jean Darier
- In classical Darier's sign, gentle rubbing or stroking of the lesions, is followed by local itching, erythema and weal formation within 2–5 minutes: This may persist from 30 minutes to several hours

42. Ans. (a) Sarcoidosis
[Ref. Dail and Hammar's Pulmonary Pathology by Dail, 1/e p422]

- Characteristic microscopic finding in sarcoidosis:
  - Discrete, compact, non-caseating epithelioid cell granuloma
  - CD4+, CD8+ T lymphocytes and, to a lesser extent, B lymphocytes form a concentric rim around the epithelioid granuloma

43. Ans. (a) Dysfunction of enzyme is most common cause; (e) Bradykinin level decrease during attack
[Ref. Immunological and Clinical Aspects of Allergy by Lessof, 1/e p187; Hereditary Angioedema by Frank, Medscape Article135604]

44. Ans. (a) C1 esterase inhibitor deficiency
[Ref. Immunological and Clinical Aspects of Allergy by Lessof, 1/e p187; Hereditary Angioedema by Frank, Medscape Article135604]

45. Ans. (b) Angioneurotic oedema
[Ref. Oral and Maxillofacial Pathology by Brad W. Neville, 4/e p326]

- Angioedema is a diffuse edematous swelling of the soft tissues that most commonly involves the subcutaneous and submucosal connective tissue
- Referred as **Quincke disease**, after the clinician who initially related the changes to an alteration in vascular permeability

46. Ans. (a) Subcutaneous nodules
[Ref. Encyclopedia of STDs by Moore, 1/e p209]

47. Ans. (b) Pityriasis rubra pilaris; (c) Psoriasis; (d) Drug hypersensitivity; (e) Eczema
[Ref. Harrison's Principles of Internal Medicine, 18/e p400; Fitzpatrick's Dermatology in General Medicine, 7/e p164]

Causes of Erythroderma (Generalized Exfoliative Dermatitis)

- Skin disorders: Psoriasis, Pityriasis rubra pilaris, Lichen planus, Eczema
- Systemic disease: Cutaneous T-cell lymphoma
- Drugs: Gold, Allopurinol, Phenytoin, Sulfonamide
- Idiopathic: Secondary to solid tumors of Lung, Liver, Prostrate, Thyroid & Colon

48. Ans. (c) Psoriasis; (d) Lichen planus; (e) Eczema
[Ref. Dermatology by Braun-Falco,1/e p621; Gupta LK, Garg A, Khare AK, Mittal A. Lichen planus presenting as erythroderm(a). Indian J Dermatol Venereol Leprol 2012;78:409]

Erythroderma

- Description: Intense and usually widespread reddening of the skin due to inflammatory skin disease
  - It often precedes or is associated with exfoliation (skin peeling off in scales or layers) when it may also be known as exfoliative dermatitis (ED)
  - It is sometimes called 'Red man syndrome' when no primary cause can be found (Idiopathic erythroderma)
- Common pre-existing dermatoses to result in erythroderma:
  - Dermatitis especially atopic dermatitis, contact dermatitis (allergic or irritant) and stasis dermatitis (gravitational eczema) and in babies, seborrhoeic dermatitis
  - Psoriasis
  - Pityriasis rubra pilaris
  - Blistering diseases including pemphigus and bullous pemphigoid
  - Sezary syndrome (Erythrodermic form of cutaneous T-cell lymphoma)
  - Internal malignancies (Carcinoma of rectum, lung, fallopian tubes, colon)
  - Haematological malignancies (Lymphoma, leukaemia)
  - Graft vs Host disease
  - HIV infection
  - Drugs
  - Lichen planus (Rare)

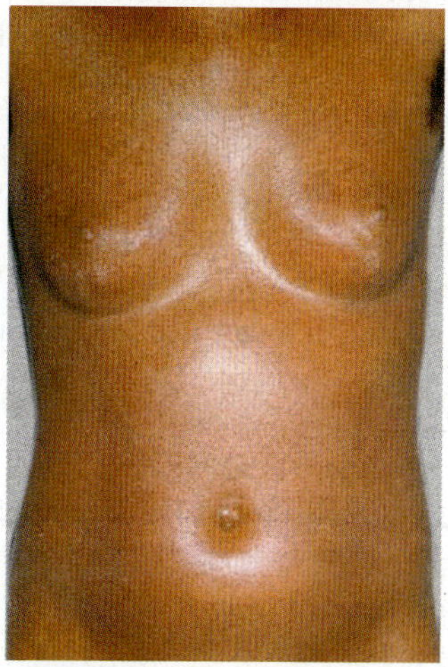

Fig. Psoriatic erythroderma

Skin and STDs

49. Ans. (d) Aspirin therapy
[Ref. Neena Khanna, 5/e p201; Schwartz RA. Erythema Nodosum: A Sign of Systemic Disease. Am Fam Physician. 2007;75(5):695-700]

50. Ans. (d) Delayed type hypersensitivity
[Ref. Neena Khanna, 5/e p15]

- Patch test detects antigens (allergens) responsible for allergic contact dermatitis (type IV hypersensitivity/ delayed type hypersensitivity)

51. Ans. (b) Cosmetics
[Ref. Colour Atlas of Tropical Dermatology and Venereology by Schaller, p13-19]

Berloque Dermatitis

- German word berlock or the French berloque, meaning trinket or charm
    - Rosenthal coined the term (1925): Pendant like streaks of pigmentation on the neck, face, arms, or trunk
- Phototoxic ingredient: Bergapten (A component of oil of bergamot, derived from the rind of Citrus bergamia, the bergamot lime)
    - Since the introduction of artificial oil of bergamot and the reduced use of the natural product in perfumes, berloque dermatitis has become rare

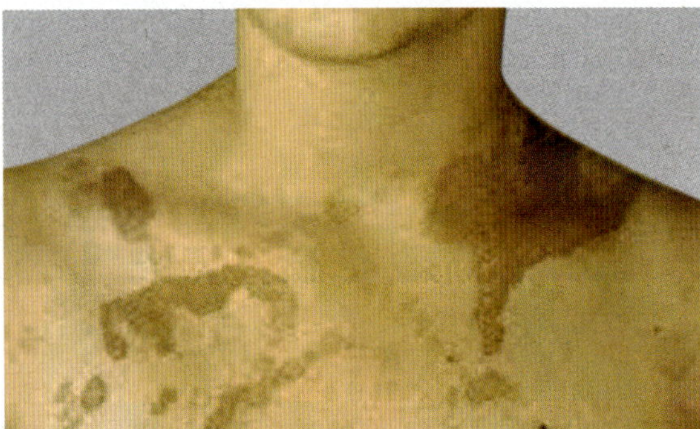

Fig. Berloque dermatitis

52. Ans. (b) 2 days
[Ref. Neena Khanna, 5/e p15]

Techniques of Patch Test

- Antigens in standardized dilutions are applied to the back and occluded
- Patches are removed after 48 hours and read after half an hour
- Another reading done at 96 hours detects delayed reaction

53. Ans. (b) Pruritus
[Ref. Neena Khanna, 5/e p104]

- Pruritus is a major factor and not minor feature of Atopic dermatitis

54. Ans. (a) Henoch-Schonlein purpura
[Ref. Neena Khanna, 5/e p195]

- Henoch-Schonlein purpura is characterized by deposition of IgA in vessel walls

55. Ans. (d) Keratoderma blennorrhagica

56. Ans. (d) DLE
[Ref. Neena Khanna, 5/e p215, 449]

- Chloroquine & hydroxychloroquine uses
    - Systemic & discoid lupus erythematosus
    - Dermatomyositis
    - Polymorphous light eruption
    - Porphyria cutanea tarda (PCT)

57. Ans. (a) SLE
[Ref. Neena Khanna, 5/e p237]

- Adult female having typical description of butterfly rash is suggestive of SLE

58. Ans. (d) *Chlamydia*
[Ref. Chlamydia: Genomics and Pathogenesis by Bavoil, 1/e p402]

59. Ans. (a) Salicylate poisoning
[Ref. Neena Khanna, 5/e p201; Schwartz RA. Erythema Nodosum: A Sign of Systemic Disease. Am Fam Physician. 2007; 75(5):695-700.]

60. Ans. (c) Antecubital fossa
[Ref. Neena Khanna, 5/e p102]

61. Ans. (c) Eczema herpeticum
[Ref. Medscape]

Eczema Herpeticum

- Eczema herpeticum starts with clusters of itchy and/or painful blisters
    - It may affect any site but is most often seen on face and neck
    - Blisters can occur in normal skin or in sites actively or previously affected by atopic dermatitis or other skin disease
    - New patches form and spread over a period of 7–10 days and may rarely be widely disseminated throughout the body
- Blisters:
    - The blisters are monomorphic, i.e. they all appear similar to each other
    - They may be filled with clear yellow fluid or thick purulent material
    - They are often blood-stained, i.e. red, purple or black in colour
    - New blisters have central dimples (umbilication)
    - They may weep or bleed
    - Older blisters crust over and form sores (erosions)
    - Lesions heal over a period of 2–6 weeks
- In severe cases where the skin has been destroyed by infection, small white scars may persist long term

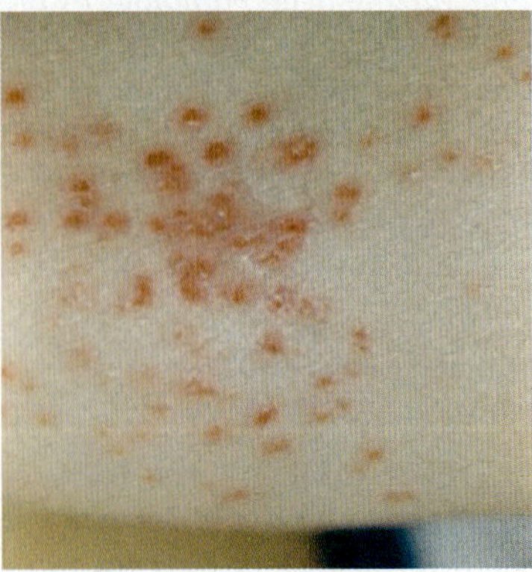

Fig. Eczema herpeticum

62. Ans. (a) HSV

[Ref. Neena Khanna, 5/e p 298]

- Generalized HSV infection in patients with extensive atopic eczema and pemphigus.

63. Ans. (a) Herpex simplex virus 1; (b) Coxsackie; (c) HSV2; (d) Vaccinia

- Eczema herpeticum: A rare but severe disseminated infection that generally occurs at sites of skin damage produced by, for example, atopic dermatitis, burns, long-term usage of topical steroids or eczema
- It is also known as Kaposi varicelliform eruption, Pustulosis varioliformis acuta and Kaposi-Juliusberg dermatitis
- MC cause: Herpes simplex virus type 1 or 2 (but may also be caused by Coxsackievirus A16, or Vaccinia virus)
- It appears as numerous umbilicated vesicles superimposed on healing atopic dermatitis. It is often accompanied by fever and lymphadenopathy
- Eczema herpeticum can be life-threatening in babies

64. Ans. (a) Atopic dermatitis

[Ref. Neena Khanna, 5/e p 107]

65. Ans. (a) Acute eczema

[Ref. Neena Khanna, 5/e p 95]

- Histologically, the hallmark of acute dermatitis is spongiosis (due to intercellular edema resulting in loss of cohesion between epidermal cells).

66. Ans. (a) Nummular eczema

[Ref. Goodheart's Photoguide to Common Skin Disorders by Goodheart, 3/e p71]

- The round lesions of nummular eczema often have the shape of coins
- Word "nummular" comes from the same root as "numismatic," meaning **"coin-shaped"**

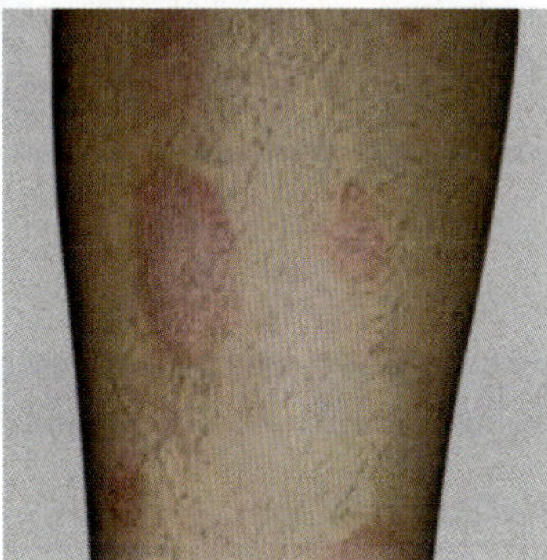

Fig. Nummular eczema

Skin and STDs

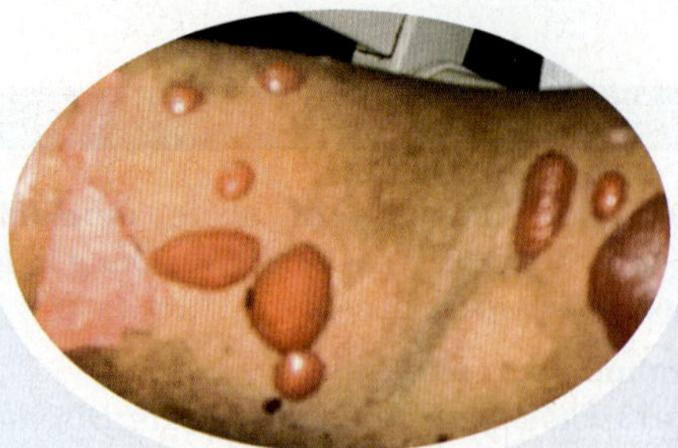

Chapter 7

Dermatological Therapy, Side Effects

THEORETICAL CONCEPTS

VII A. RETINOIDS

- *Definition*: Chemical compounds related chemically to Vitamin A
- *Types of Retinoids*:

Retinoids	Use(s)
First generation retinoids	
Retinol	Vision, bone/tooth/reproductive system development
Retinal	
Tretinoin (Retinoic acid)	Acnevulgaris
Isotretinoin	Nodulocystic acne, Acne rosacea
Alitretinoin	Kaposi sarcoma, Chronic hand eczema/ dermatitis
Second generation retinoids	
Etretinate	Psoriasis[Q]
Acitretin	Psoriasis[Q]
Third generation retinoids	
Tazarotene	Psoriasis[Q], Breast/Lung carcinoma
Bexarotene	Cutaneous T cell lymphoma, Breast/Lung carcinoma
Adapelene	Acne vulgaris

VII B. ERYTHRODERMA

- *Definition*: Generalised Exfoliative dermatitis covering more than 90% of skin
- *Causes*: **[Mnemonic: ID SCALP]**[Q]
  - **I**diopathic (Most common)[Q]
  - **S**eborrheic dermatitis
  - **A**topic dermatitis
  - **P**soriasis
  - **D**rug reactions
  - **C**ontact dermatitis
  - **L**ymphoma and leukemia
- *Drugs causing Erythroderma*:[Q]
  - Sulphonamides[Q]
  - Barbiturates
  - Phenylbutazone
  - Gold
  - Penicillins
  - Carbamazepine
  - Isoniazid

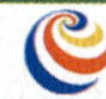 NEET/NBE PATTERN MCQs 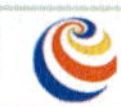

1. Prolonged use of Topical steroids causes *[Recent Question 2016]*
a. Open angle glaucoma b. Uveitis
c. Macular oedema d. Conjunctival papillae

2. Photochemotherapy is useful in *[Recent Question 2016]*
a. P rosea b. Psoriasis
c. Lichen planus d. Ichthyosis vulgaris

3. Maximum dose of Isoretinion should not exceed *[Recent Question 2016]*
a. 30-60 mg/kg b. 60-90 mg/kg
c. 90-120 mg/kg d. 120-150 mg/kg

4. At which wavelength Phototherapy is most effective *[Recent Question 2016]*
a. 150 nm b. 250 nm
c. 350 nm d. 450 nm

5. Lupus like picture is caused by all except *[Recent Question 2016]*
a. Chloroquine b. Procainamide
c. Hydralazine d. Isoniazid

6. Exfoliative dermatitis due to gold poisoning is treated by *[Recent Question 2016]*
a. Chloroquine b. Steroid
c. Antibiotics d. Anti-histaminic

7. Exanthema is caused by which drug *[Recent Question 2016]*
a. Phenytoin b. Valproate
c. Digoxin d. NTG

8. Whitfield's ointment consists of *[Recent Question 2016]*
a. 3% Salicylic acid + 6% benzoic acid
b. 3% Benzoic acid + 6% Salicylic acid
c. 2% Salicylic acid + 4% Benzoic acid
d. 2% Benzoic acid + 4% salicylic acid

9. Vitamin D analogue Calcitriol is useful in the treatment of *[Recent Question 2016]*
a. Lichen planus b. Psoriasis
c. Pemphigus d. Leprosy

10. Erythroderma is NOT related with *[NBE FMGE September 2008]*
a. Sulphonamides b. Air-borne dermatitis
c. Psoriasis d. Lepromatous leprosy

11. Prolonged use of topical steroids can result in *[NBE DNB 2011]*
a. Open angle glaucoma b. Uveitis
c. Macular edema d. Conjunctival papillae

12. Treatment of primary syphilis is *[NBE FMGE September 2012]*
a. Benzathine penicillin b. Procaine penicillin
c. Procaine penicillin d. Tetracycline

13. Dapsone is used in the treatment of all except *[NBE DNB 1998]*
a. Dermatitis herpetiformis
b. Leprosy
c. Pityriasis rosea
d. Pemphigus vulgaris

14. Commonest complication of synthetic retinoid is *[NBE DNB 1992]*
a. Dryness of skin and mucosa
b. Increased intracranial tension
c. Diffuse alopecia
d. Bone pain

15. Drugs producing erythoma nodosum are *[NBE DNB 1997]*
a. Barbiturates b. Sulfonamides
c. Penicillin d. Tetracycline

16. Ivermectin is indicated in the treatment of *[NBE DNB 2009]*
a. Syphilis b. Scabies
c. Tuberculosis d. Dermatophytosis

17. Which of the following skin conditions is treated with PUVA therapy? *[NBE DNB 2003, NBE DNB 2006]*
a. Psoriasis b. Tinea versicolor
c. Lichen planus d. Porphyria cutaneatarda

18. A topical retinoid recently introduced for the treatment of psoriasis is *[NBE DNB 2011]*
a. Adapalene b. Tazarotene
c. Alitretinoin d. Bexarotine

19. The oral drug used in treatment of scabies is *[NBE DNB 2011]*
a. Cotrimaxazole b. Penicillin
c. Ivermectin d. Levamisole

20. Drug causing exanthematous skin eruption *[Recent Question 2012]*
a. Phenytoin b. Hydrocortisone
c. Ampicillin d. Phenylbutazone

21. Photochemotherapy is useful in *[NBE DNB 1994, 1995, 1999, 2001, 2005, 2007]*
a. Pityriasis rosea b. Psoriasis
c. Lichen planus d. Ichthyosis vulgaris

22. Following drugs produce fixed drug eruptions EXCEPT *[NBE DNB 1997, 1999, 2001]*
a. Phenolphthalein b. Aspirin
c. Dapsone d. Furosemide
e. Mepacrine

23. Maximum cumulative dose of Isotretinoin shouldn't exceed for acne treatment *[Recent Question 2012]*
a. 30-60 mg/kg b. 60-90 mg/kg
c. 90-120 mg/kg d. 120-150 mg/kg

24. Following drugs produce fixed drug eruption *[NBE DNB 2004]*
a. Phenolphthalein b. Aspirin
c. Dapsone d. All of the above

25. Photosensitivity may be caused by the following, except *[NBE DNB 1997, 1999]*
a. Sulphonamides b. Promethazine
c. Chloropromazine d. Chloroquine

26. Selenium sulfide is indicated for treating *[Recent Question 2017, NBE DNB 2008]*
a. Tines versicolor
b. Tinea corporis
c. Mixed myocotic infections
d. Condidiasis only

27. Oral retinoid is indicated in the treatment of *[NBE DNB 1994, 2000, 2001, 2007]*
a. Acne vulgaris b. Pemphigus vulgaris
c. Lupus vulgaris d. Erythema multiforme

28. **All are used in the treatment of visceral leishmaniasis except** *[NBE DNB 2010]*
    a. Hydroxychloroquine b. Miltefosine
    c. Paromomycin d. Sitamaquine
29. **At which wavelength is Phototherapy most effective?** *[UPSC 2012]*
    a. 150 nm b. 250 nm
    c. 350 nm d. 450 nm
30. **All are true for Transdermal drug delivery except** *[Recent Question 2015]*
    a. Useful for drugs with poor bioavailability
    b. Useful for drugs with high molecular weights
    c. Steady drug serum concentration
    d. Minimal gastric discomfort
31. **Consider the following** *[UPSC CMS 2015]*
    1. Psoriasis 2. Atopic dermatitis
    3. Leprosy 4. Vitiligo

    PUVA therapy can be used to treat which of the above?
    a. 1 and 2 only b. 2 and 3
    c. 1, 2 and 4 d. 3 and 4
32. **Which of the following is a Melanising agent?** *[Recent Question 2017]*
    a. Methoxsalen b. Dapsone
    c. Minocycline d. Kojic acid
33. **Residual Hypopigmentation following a drug reaction, is best known as?** *[Recent Question 2017]*
    a. Vitiligo
    b. Chemical leukoderma
    c. Post inflammatory hypomelanosis
    d. Piebaldism
34. **First generation Topical retinoid is?** *[Recent Question 2017]*
    a. Retinoic acid b. Adapalene
    c. Tazarotene d. Acitretin
35. **Resorcinol is used in the treatment of** *[Recent Question 2017]*
    a. Lichen planus b. Acne
    c. Vitiligo d. Scabies
36. **Which of the following antifungal agent is used topically?** *[Recent Question 2017]*
    a. Griesofulvin b. Itraconazole
    c. Voriconazoie d. Nystatin
37. **Methoxsalen is** *[Recent Question 2017]*
    a. Melanising agent b. Depigmenting agent
    c. Photo Protective agent d. None of the above
38. **Which of the following steroid cream has maximum efficacy?** *[Recent Question 2017]*
    a. Hydrocortisone butyrate cream 0.1%
    b. Betamethasone propionate cream 0.1%
    c. Betamethasone valerate cream 0.17%
    d. Fluticasone propionate cream 0.05%

HIGH YIELD MCQs

1. **Acneiform eruption is/ are side effect of** *[PGI June 2016]*
   a. Tetracycline b. Phenytoin
   c. Isoniazid d. Steroid
   e. Potassium iodide
2. **Wavelength of UVB is** *[PGI November 2016]*
   a. 250-280 nm b. 280-320 nm
   c. 320-400 nm d. 400-700 nm
   e. 100-200 nm
3. **A patient presented with multiple nodulocystic lesions on the face. The drug of choice is** *[Recent Question 2016, AIIMS PGMEE 2002]*
   a. Retinoids b. Antibiotics
   c. Steroids d. UV light
4. **Psoralen A is used in treatment of** *[JIPMER PGMEE 1991]*
   a. Pemphigus b. Vitiligo
   c. Pityriasis alba d. Ichthyosis
5. **A female has hypopigmented lesion on centre of forehead drug, responsible is** *[AIIMS PGMEE 2008]*
   a. Hydroquinone
   b. Mono benzene metabolite of hydroquinone
   c. Para tetra butyl catechol
   d. Para tetra butyl phenol
6. **A 55-year-old male, with uncontrolled diabetes mellitus and hypertension, developed severe air-borne contact dermatitis. The most appropriate drug for his treatment would be** *[AIIMS PGMEE 2004]*
   a. Systemic corticosteroids
   b. Thalidomide
   c. Azathioprine
   d. Cyclosporine
7. **A patient of hypertension on ACE inhibitors developed rosea skin eruptions. True statement regarding this situation is** *[SGPGI 2003]*
   a. Drug may be the cause and discontinuation may improve the skin condition
   b. High dose steroids are needed initially
   c. ACE inhibitors are safe and cannot lead to skin eruptions
   d. Drug may be the cause discontinuation is not required
8. **Gold poisoning leading to exfoliative dermatitis is treated by** *[AIIMS PGMEE 1995]*
   a. Chloroquine b. Steroid
   c. Antibiotics d. Antihistaminics
9. **Podophyllum is useful for the treatment of the following types of warts** *[AIIMS PGMEE 2002, NBE DNB 2004]*
   a. Genital warts b. Plantar warts
   c. Verruca vulgaris d. Filiform warts
10. **Uses of PUVA** *[PGI 2004]*
    a. Pigmented purpuric lesion
    b. Herpes zoster
    c. Mycosis fungoides
    d. Lupus panniculitis
    e. Lichenoid dermatitis of Gougerot & Blum
11. **Photochemotherapy is used in** *[All India PGMEE 1992]*
    a. Pityriasis rosea b. Erythroderma
    c. Scabies d. Psoriasis
12. **Circulating lymphocytes are most sensitive to** *[AIIMS PGMEE 1994] [UP PGMEE 2002]*
    a. UV-A b. UV-B
    c. UV-C d. 760-800 mm

13. Most effective treatment of pruritus in uremia is *[AIIMS PGMEE 1995, PGI 2002]*
a. Ultraviolet light b. Cholestyramine
c. Eskazine d. Topical benzocaine

14. Regarding podophyllin resin which of following statement is true? *[PGI 2008]*
a. Derived from plant source
b. Safe in pregnancy
c. Teratogenic
d. High recurrence rate of wart after podophyllin resin treatment
e. Individual variation in response rate

15. DOC for lepra II reaction is *[All India PGMEE 2008]*
a. Steroids b. Thalidomide
c. Clofazimine d. Dapsone

16. Toxic epidermo-necrolysis is caused by *[PGI 2004]*
a. Phenytoin b. Penicillin
c. Erythromycin d. Gold

17. All are considered to be high risk agents for TEN except *[PGI 2007]*
a. Sulfonamide b. Sulfonyl urea
c. Aspirin d. Oxicam
e. Phenytoin

18. A 3 months old male infant developed otitis media for which he was given a course of Co-trimoxazole. A few days later, he developed extensive peeling of the skin; there were no mucosal lesions and the baby was not toxic. The most likely diagnosis is *[AIIMS PGMEE 2004]*
a. Toxic epidermal necrolysis
b. Staphylococcal scalded skin syndrome
c. Steven Johnson syndrome
d. Infantile pemphigus

19. First line antileprosy drugs include all except *[PGI 1997] [Delhi PGMEE 2003]*
a. Dapsone b. Thiacetazone
c. Clofazimine d. Rifampicin

20. Thalidomide is drug of choice for *[All India PGMEE 1999]*
a. Lepra I reaction b. Lepra II reaction
c. Both d. Nerve Abscess

21. A 27-year-old sexually active male develops a vesiculo-bullous lesion on the glass soon after taking tab paracetamol for fever. The lesion healed with hyperpigmentation. The most likely diagnosis is *[All India PGMEE 2005]*
a. Behcet's syndrome b. Herpes genitalis
c. Fixed drug eruption d. Pemphigus vulgaris

22. Ciclipirox olamine is used in *[AP PGMEE 1996]*
a. Dermatophytosis b. Acne
c. Psoriasis d. Lichen Planus

23. Treatment of tinea unguium *[PGI 2005]*
a. Fluticasone b. Itraconazole
c. Oleamine oil d. Terbinafine
e. Neomycin

24. Griseofulvin given for the treatment of fungal infection in the finger nail dermatophytosis for how much duration *[All India PGMEE 2002]*
a. 4 weeks b. 6 weeks
c. 2 months d. 3 months

25. Herpes resistant to acyclovir is treated by *[JIPMER PGMEE 2002]*
a. Foscarnet b. Lamivudine
c. Ganciclovir d. Valocyclovir

26. Dose of Dapsone is *[All India PGMEE 1988]*
a. 1-2 mg/kg b. 5 mg/kg
c. 10 mg/kg d. 20 mg/kg

27. Which of the following not a feature of dermatomyositis? *[AIIMS PGMEE 2009]*
a. Gottron's papules b. Periungua telangiectasia
c. Salmon rash d. Mechanic's hand

28. Daily dose of thalidomide for controlling E.N.L. is *[PGI 1979] [NBE DNB 1991]*
a. 100 mg b. 200-300 mg
c. 500 mg d. 1000 mg only

29. A 40-year-old woman presented with a 8 month history of erythema and swelling of the periorbital region & papules & plaques and the dorsolateral aspect of forearms & knuckles with ragged cuticles. There was no muscle weakness. The most likely diagnosis is *[AIIMS PGMEE 2004]*
a. SLE
b. Dermatomyositis
c. Systemic sclerosis
d. Mixed connective tissue disorder

30. Antibody that is strongly associated with polymyositis? *[AIIMS PGMEE 2008]*
a. Anti-jo1 b. Anti-ku
c. Anti-Scl-70 d. Anti-sm

31. Lupus like picture is causes by all except *[All India PGMEE 1991]*
a. Chloroquine b. Procanamide
c. Hydralazine d. Isoniazid

32. Which of the following not photosensitive? *[AP PGMEE 2004]*
a. Porphyria b. DLE
c. SLE d. Lichen Planus

33. Recurrent erythematous plaques on glans penis in a 19 yrs old sexually active male which heals with residual hyperpigmentation, is suggestive of? *[AIIMS PGMEE 2009]*
a. Apthous Balanitica b. Fixed Drug Eruption
c. Herpes Gestations d. Chlamydial infective

34. TOC for Pediculosis corporis (non-sensitized) is *[AIIMS PGMEE 1998]*
a. 3 application of BHC
b. 4 application of BHC
c. Disinfection of all clothes and beddings
d. DDT application

35. Podophylline is used in treatment of *[AIIMS PGMEE 1992, 2003, AIIMS PGMEE 1994]* *[Recent Question 2017]*
a. Plantar warts
b. Palmar warts
c. Comdylomata accuminata
d. Condylomata lata

36. Thalidomide is not used in *[AIIMS PGMEE 2008]*
a. ENL
b. Behcet's syndrome
c. HIV associated Oral ulcers
d. HIV associated neuropathy

37. Most common side effects of Retinoids is *[AIIMS PGMEE 1994]*
a. Headache b. Skin rashes
c. Photosensitivity d. Diarrhoea

38. A 17-year-old girl with Acne has been taking a drug for the last two years. Show now presents with blue black pigmentation of nails. The likely medication causing the above pigmentation is *[All India PGMEE 2010]*
a. Tetracycline b. Minocycline
c. Doxycycline d. Azithromycin

39. Skin pigmentation is caused by *[AIIMS PGMEE 1993]*
a. Methotrexate b. Dactinomycin
c. Cyclophosphamide d. Busulphan

40. Slate like discolouration of the skin is caused by all these drugs except *[PGI 1979, AIIMS PGMEE 1980]*
a. Chlorpromazine b. Minocycline
c. Amiodarone d. Thiacetazone

41. Photosensitive lichenoid drug eruption is seen in .... therapy *[Kerala PGMEE 1990]*
a. Rifampicin b. Tetracycline (old)
c. Gold d. Streptomycin

42. Vitamin D analogue calcitriol is useful in the treatment of *[All India PGMEE 1994, UP PGMEE 2004]* *[Jharkhand PGMEE 2005]*
a. Lichen Planus b. Psoriasis
c. Phemphigus d. Leprosy

43. Chloroquine cause exacerbation of *[All India PGMEE 1991]*
a. Malaria b. Psoriasis
c. DLE d. Photosensitivity

44. DOC of pustular psoriasis *[AIIMS PGMEE 1991]*
a. PUVA b. Methotrexate
c. Steroid d. Cyclophosphamide

45. Which is not a complication of PUVA therapy? *[AIIMS PGMEE 1997] [PGI 2000]*
a. Premature aging of skin b. Cataracts
c. Skin cancers d. Exfoliative

46. PUVA therapy is used in *[PGI 2002]*
a. Psoriasis b. Lichen planus
c. Freckles d. Melasma
e. Vitiligo

47. Toxic Epidermal Necrolysis is also called *[PGI 1992, AIIMS PGMEE 1993]*
a. Sweet's syndrome
b. Lyell's syndrome
c. Hailey and Hailey's disease
d. Duhring's disease

48. Photochemotherapy is useful in *[AIIMS PGMEE 1995]*
a. Psoriasis b. Lichen planus
c. Tinea d. Ichthyosis

49. True about drug induced SLE is *[PGI 2000]*
a. CNS manifestation are common
b. Renal involvement is common
c. Antihistone antibodies are found
d. All with antibodies progress to lupus
e. Sex ratio is nearly equal

50. The following drug is not used for the treatment of type II lepra reaction *[AIIMS PGMEE 2006]*
a. Chloroquine b. Thalidomide
c. Cyclosporine d. Corticosteroids

51. Reversal lepra reaction shown no response to *[JIPMER PGMEE 1995]*
a. Clofazimine b. Chloroquine
c. Glucocorticoids d. Thalidomide

52. Which of the following drugs is not antifungal? *[All India PGMEE 2008]*
a. Caspofungin b. Undecylenic acid
c. Ciclopirox d. Clofazimine

53. Not used topically *[DPG 2004]*
a. Nystatin b. Ketoconazole
c. Griseofulvin d. Micronazole

54. Griseofulvin is not useful in one of the following *[Kerala PGMEE 1990]*
a. Tinea capitis b. Tinea cruris
c. Tinea versicolor d. Tinea pedis

55. Drug of choice in Systemic candidiasis is *[JIPMER PGMEE 1993]*
a. Amphotericin b. Griseofulvin
c. Nystatin d. Ketoconazole

56. Medically most important form of UV radiation is *[All India PGMEE 1999]*
a. UV-A b. UV-B
c. UV-C d. None of the above

57. Range of light which causes maximum skin damage is *[JIPMER PGMEE 1998, AIIMS 1999]*
a. 360-400 nm b. 290-360 nm
c. 240-290 nm d. 760-800 nm

58. Griseofulvin is used in all except *[AIIMS PGMEE 1990]*
a. Tinea capitis
b. Tinea versicolor & Candida
c. Tinea corporis
d. Tinea unguium

59. Ivermectin in indicated in the treatment of *[AIIMS PGMEE 2006]*
a. Syphilis b. Scabies
c. Tuberculosis d. Dermatophytosis

60. Treatment of both partners is recommended in all except *[PGI 1999]*
a. Candida infection b. Gardnerella
c. Herpes d. Trichomonas vaginalis

61. Recurrent fever followed by ulcers on genitalia and hyperpigmentation is suggestive of *[AIIMS November 2014]*
a. Eczema b. Allergic contact dermatitis
c. Fixed drug eruption d. Lichen planus

62. A 20-year-old patient with Nerurocysticercosis develops generalized peeling of skin (except palms and soles) Starting one month after taking medications for seizures. What is the most probable diagnosis? *[AIIMS PG November 2015]*
a. SJS b. TEN
c. Fixed drug eruption d. Pemphigus vulgaris

NEET/NBE PATTERN MCQs ANSWERS WITH EXPLANATIONS

1. Ans. (a) Open angle glaucoma
[Ref. DVL by Thappa, 4/e p381]

Ocular side effects of Topical steroids
- Open angle glaucoma
- Posterior subcapsular cataract
- Aggravation of existing infection

2. Ans. (b) Psoriasis
[Ref. DVL by Thappa, 4/e p417]

Indications of Photochemotherapy
- Psoriasis
- Vitiligo
- Photodermatoses
- Cutaneous T-cell lymphoma

3. Ans. (d) 120-150 mg/kg
[Ref. DVL by Thappa, 4/e p419]

Dosage of Retinoid
- Isotretinoin: 0.5-2 mg/kg body weight/ day
- Acitretin: 0.5-1mg/kg body weight/ day

4. Ans. (c) 350 nm
[Ref. DVL by Thappa, 4/e p429]
- Phototherapy is most effective at 350 nm

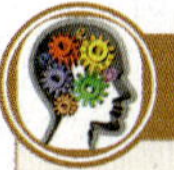

Also Remember

Types of Phototherapy
- Psoralen and UVA therapy
- Broadband UVB (290-320 nm)
- Narrowband UVB (311 nm) most effective for psoriasis & vitiligo
- UVA1 (340-400 nm)

5. Ans. (a) Chloroquine
[Ref. Clinical dermatology by Habif, 6/e p595]

Drug-induced Lupus (DIL)
- Rare adverse reaction to a large variety of drugs
- Minocycline induced lupus occurs in young patients (median age, 21 years) and 80% of patients with minocycline-induced lupus are women
- More than 80 drugs have been implicated; MC being hydralazine, procainamide, isoniazid, methyldopa, quinidine, minocycline, and chlorpromazine
- Drug-induced lupus caused by anti–tumor necrosis factor-α agents (TNF-α) (infliximab, etanercept, adalimumab)

6. Ans. (b) Steroid
[Ref. Clinical Pharmacology and Therapeutics by Maronde, 1/e p308]
- In the event of exfoliative dermatitis, gold nephropathy, thrombocytopenia, pneumonitis, hepatotoxicity, enterocolitis, and anaphylaxis, gold therapy should never be resumed
- In addition, severe toxicity constitutes indication for steroid therapy and/or gold chelation

7. Ans. (a) Phenytoin
[Ref. Litt's Drug Eruption and Reaction Manual, 2/e p404]

Drugs causing Exanthem

Commonly associated drugs	Other drugs associated
Penicillin Ampicillin Phenylbutazone Sulphonamides Phenytoin Gold	Amoxycillin Bleomycin Captopril Carbamazepine Chlorpromazine Cotrimoxazole Nalidixic acid Naproxen Piroxicam

8. Ans. (a) 3% Salicylic acid + 6% benzoic acid
[Ref. Dermatological Drug Therapy by Khopkar, 1/e p258]

Whitfield's ointment
- 3% Salicylic acid + 6% benzoic acid
- Salicyclic acid is keratolytic
- Useful in treating superficial fungal infections

9. Ans. (b) Psoriasis
[Ref. DVL by Thappa, 4/e p126]
- Calcipotriol is a vitamin D3 analogue which is effective for short & long term treatment of Psoriasis
- It is used in combination with corticosteroids

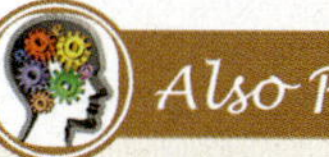

Also Remember

- Other topical therapy includes Tars, Tazarotene, Topical steroids, Emollients, Tacrolimus, Pimerolimus, Dithranol, Salicylic acid

10. Ans. (d) Lepromatous leprosy
[Ref. Neena Khanna, 4/e p207]

Erthroderma
- *Definition*: Generalised Exfoliative dermatitis covering more than 90% of skin

Causes

[Mnemonic: ID SCALP]
- **I**diopathic
- **D**rug reactions
- **S**eborrheic dermatitis
- **C**ontact dermatitis
- **A**topic dermatitis
- **L**ymphoma and leukemia
- **P**soriasis

- *Drugs causing Erythroderma*:
  - Sulphonamides
  - Penicillins
  - Barbiturates
- Carbamazepine
  - Phenylbutazone
  - Isoniazid
  - Gold

11. Ans. (a) Open angle glaucoma
[Ref. Textbook of Ophthalmology by Sunita Agarwal, 1/e p1351]

Skin and STDs

Complications of Topical Steroids

- Elevated IOP (steroid induced open glaucoma)
- Cataract
- Delayed wound healing
- Infection and ulceration
- Periocular dermatitis

12. Ans. (a) Benzathine penicillin

[Ref. Textbook of Family Medicine by David Rakel, 9/e p217]

- Primary syphilis typically presents 2-6 weeks after exposure as a painless, indurated ulcer (Chancre)
- Benzathine penicillin G is used for non-penicillin-allergic patients with early syphilis and their recent partners
- High-dose penicillin G given intravenously remains the treatment of choice for non-penicillin-allergic patients with late syphilis

13. Ans. (c) Pityriasisrosea

[Ref. Neena Khanna, 5/e p449]

Dapsone is Drug of Choice

- Dermatitis herpetiformis
- Erythema elevatum diutinum

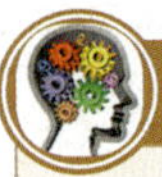

Also Remember

- Dapsone is also used for:
  - Leprosy
  - Chronic bullous dermatosis of childhood & pemphigus group
  - Pyoderma gangrenosum
  - Oral Lichen planus

14. Ans. (a) Dryness of skin and mucosa

[Ref. Neena Khanna, 5/e p440]

- Side effects of newer retinoids (Avoid in pregnancy):
  - Irritation
  - Photosensitivity
  - Dryness

15. Ans. (b) Sulfonamides

[Ref. Neena Khanna, 5/e p201]

Causes of Erythema Nodosum

Bacteria	Streptococcus, TB, Yersinia
Fungi	Coccidioidomycosis
Viruses	Infectious mononucleosis,Hepatitis B
Other infections	Amoebiasis, Giardiasis, Chlamydia
Drugs	Sulfonamides, Bromides, OCP
Miscellaneous	Sarcoidosis, Behcet's syndrome, Ulcerative colitis, Congenital tissue diseases, Malignancy, Pregnancy

16. Ans. (b) Scabies

[Ref. Neena Khanna, 5/e p370]

Use of Scabicides

Scabicides	Method of use	Comments
Permethrin 5%	8 hours X Day 1 & Day 8	**Scabicide of choice,** Resistance reported
GBHC 1%	8 hours X Day 1 & Day 8	Avoided in seizure patients, infants

Contd...

Contd...

Scabicides	Method of use	Comments
Benzyl benzoate 25%	3 applications X 12 hourly interval	Irritation is a common side effect
Crotamiton 10%	8 hourly on days 1,2,3 & 8	Marginal efficacy, Useful in children
Precipitated sulphar 10%	BD X 14 days	Marginal efficacy, Useful in children
Ivermectin	200 mcg/ kg, Repeat after 2 weeks	Use in Orphanages & Norwegian scabies

17. Ans. (a) Psoriasis

[Ref. Neena Khanna, 5/e p58]

18. Ans. (b) Tazarotene

[Ref. Neena Khanna, 5/e p56]

- Newer topical retinoid used in psoriasis is Tazarotene, 0.05-0.1% formulation
- It is Keratolytic & Keratoplastic agent.

19. Ans. (c) Ivermectin

[Ref. Neena Khanna, 5/e p370]

20. Ans. (b) Hydrocortisone

[Ref. Intensive Care Unit Manual by Lanken, 2/ e p425]

21. Ans. (b) Psoriasis

[Ref. Comprehensive Dermatologic Drug Therapy by Wolverton, 3/e p281]

- The combination of psoralens and ultraviolet light (UVA, 320-400 nm), referred to as PUVA, inhibits proliferation of a variety of cell types
- Psoralen intercalates into the DNA double helix where it is ideally positioned to form adduct(s) with adjacent pyrimidine bases, preferentially thymine, upon excitation by an ultraviolet photon
- PUVA treatment produces both DNA interstrand crosslinks (ICLs) and monoadducts
- The ICLs introduced by psoralen are highly genotoxic to actively replicating cells

22. Ans. (e) Mepacrine

[Ref. Neena Khanna, 5/e p223]

Drugs Implicated in Fixed Drug Eruption (FDE)

- Sulphonamide antibiotics: Cotrimoxazole, Sulfasalazine, Dapsone.
- Tetracycline antibiotics: Doxycycline, Minocycline, Panmycin
- Acetylsalicylic acid/ Aspirin
- Nonsteroidal anti-inflammatories (NSAIDs): Ibuprofen, Paracetamol /Phenacetin
- Sedatives: Barbiturates, Benzodiazepines, Chlordiazepoxide
- Hyoscine butylbromide
- Phenolphthalein

23. Ans. (d) 120-150 mg/kg

[Ref. The 5-Minute Clinical Consult Premium 2015 by Domino,23/ep15; Systemic Drug Treatment in Dermatology by Wakelin, 1/e p164]

Isotretinoin

- 0.5-1mg/kg/d divided b.i.d (Maximum 2 mg/kg/d divided b.i.d for very severe disease)
- 60-90% cure rate
- Usually given for 12-20 weeks: Clinical improvement may only be evident after 6-8 weeks
- Maximum cumulative dose = 120-150 mg/kg
- A cumulative dose of 120-150 mg/kg associated with reduced relapse rate than lower doses: 20% patient relapse and require retreatment

24. Ans. (d) All of the above
[Ref. Neena Khanna, 5/e p223]

25. Ans. (d) Chloroquine

Drug-Induced Photosensitivity

- Photosensitivity may be due to toxic or immunological mechanisms or both, from systemic or topical exposure to the medication
- The rash affects sites of light exposure (UVA), but may spare habitually exposed areas such as the face and hands

Phototoxic reactions	Photoallergic reactions
Antimicrobials: Quinolones, Doxycycline, Nalidixic Acid, Sulphonamides, Tetracyclines	**Antimicrobials:** Sulfonamides, Tetracycline, Quinolones, Griseofulvin
NSAIDs: Naproxen, Piroxicam	
Others: Frusemide, Griseofulvin, Psoralens, Chlorpromazine	Phenothiazines, Psoralens, Quinine, Antihistaminics (Promethazine)

26. Ans. (a) Tines versicolor
[Ref. Neena Khanna, 5/e p311-312]

Treatment of Pityriasis Versicolor/ Tinea Versicolor

- Topical agent
  - Ketokonazole 2%
  - 2.5% selenium sulphide
- Systemic agent
  - Fluconazole- 300 mg once wkly X 2 week
  - Itraconazole – 200 mg, OD X 5 days
  - Ketokonazole- 400 mg SOD

27. Ans. (a) Acne vulgaris
[Ref. Neena Khanna, 5/e p448]

Systematic Therapy of Retinoid

- Nodulocystic acne including acne conglobata
- Moderately severe acne
- Acne excoriee

28. Ans. (a) Hydroxychloroquine
[Ref. Modern Pharmacology by Craig, 6/e p619]

29. Ans. (d) 450 nm
[Ref. Neonatology and Blood Transfusion by Smit-Sibinga, p121; Neena Khanna, 5/e p433]

- For unconjugated hyperbilirubinemia, wavelength of phototherapy most effective is 450 nm
- For treating skin diseases, wavelength of phototherapy most effective is 311±2 nm

30. Ans. (b) Useful for drugs with high molecular weights
[Ref. Pharmaceutical Systems by Marcos, 1/e p163]

Transdermal Drug Delivery

- Advantages:
  - Useful for drugs with poor bioavailability
  - Useful for drugs with short half lives
  - Useful for drugs with narrow therapeutic window
  - Steady drug serum concentration
  - Minimal side effects
  - Minimal gastric discomfort
  - Increased patient compliance
- Disadvantages:
  - Not useful for drugs with high molecular weights
  - Not suitable if drug need high blood levels
  - Skin irritation
  - Expensive
  - Not useful for all skin types

31. Ans. (c) 1, 2 and 4
[Ref. Photosensitizing Compounds Symposium, 1/e p131]

- PUVA is an ultraviolet light therapy treatment using the sensitizing effects of the drug psoralen for:
  - Eczema/ Atopic dermatitis
  - Psoriasis
  - Graft-versus-host disease
  - Vitiligo
  - Mycosis fungoides
  - Large-plaque parapsoriasis
  - Cutaneous T-cell lymphoma Alopecia areata
  - *Lichen planus*

32. Ans. (a) Methoxsalen
[Ref. Pharmacology and Pharmacotherapeutics by Satoskar, 24/e p1032]

Methoxsalen (Oxsoralen)

- Topical application (0.1-1.0%) is followed by exposure to Sunlight/ UV light
  - Leads to erythematous reaction and activation of melanocytes
- In the presence of UVA, methoxsalen bonds with DNA inhibiting DNA synthesis and cell division, and can lead to cell injury
  - Recovery from the cell injury may be followed by increased melanisation of the epidermis.

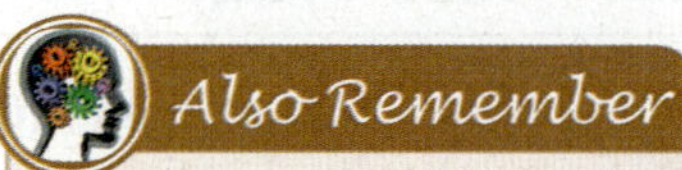

- Melanising agents include Trioxsalen, Methoxsalen
- Demelanising agents include Hydroquinone, Monobenzone

33. Ans. (c) Postinflammatory hypomelanosis
[Ref. Dermatology Secrets Plus by Fitzpatrick, 5/e p552]

- Drug-induced hypopigmentation refers to pigment dilution caused by or associated with the use of a medication

34. Ans. (a) Retinoic acid
[Ref. Neena Khanna, 4/e p50]

Types of Retinoids

- First generation retinoids: Retinol, Retinal, Tretinoin (Retinoic acid), Isotretinoin, Alitretinoin
- Second generation retinoids: Etretinate, Acitretin
- Third generation retinoids: Tazarotene, Bexarotene, Adapelene

35. Ans. (b) Acne
[Ref. DVL by Thappa, 4/e p.156,157]

Local or Topical Treatment Options for Acne Vulgaris

- Benzoyl peroxide 2.5-5% (Comedolytic)
- Antibiotics: Clindamycin (1%), Erythromycin (2-3%), Sodium sulfacetamide, Tetracycline
- Sulphur & Resorcinol
- Tretinoine (0.025-0.1% cream/ gel), Adapalene (0.1% gel), Tazarotene (0.05% - 0.1%)

36. Ans. (d) Nystatin
[Ref. Remington and Klein's Infectious Diseases, 8/e p1031]

- Topical antifungal agents are indicated for Thrush, Diaper dermatitis, and Uncomplicated Congenital candidiasis in the term infant
- Nystatin, the most commonly used topical therapy, is a polyene drug that is not absorbed by the gastrointestinal tract, making it a topical agent in any of the three common formulations: oral suspension, ointment, or powder
- Nystatin is antifungal by interfering with fungal cell membranes: It binds to ergosterol, an essential component of fungal cell membranes, disrupting the cell membrane and leading to potassium leakage and fungal inhibition

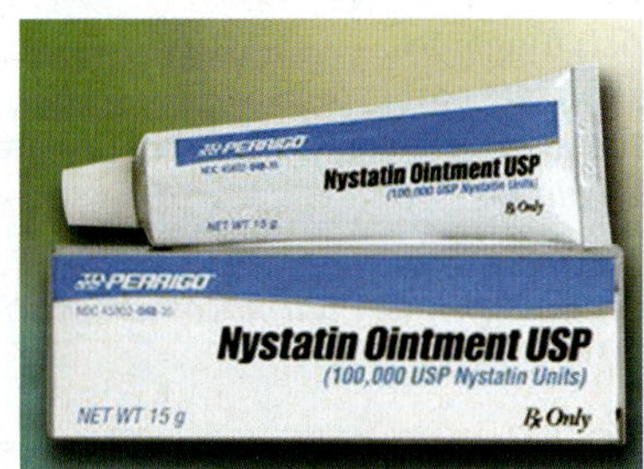

Fig. Topical nystatin

37. Ans. (a) Melanising agent
[Ref. Pharmacology and Pharmacotherapeutics by Satoskar, 24/e p1032]

Melanising Agents

- Trioxsalen (Trisoralen)
- Methoxsalen (Oxsoralen)

38. Ans. (b) Betamethasone propionate cream 0.1%
[Ref. Applied Pharmacology by Bardal, 1/e p138]

Topical Steroids Potency Chart

- Class 1 (Superpotent): 0.05% Clobetasol propionate, 0.05% Flurandrenolide, 0.05% Clobetasol propionate, 0.05% Betamethasone dipropionate, 0.05% Clobetasol propionate, 0.05% Clobetasol propionate, 0.05% Diflorasone diacetate, 0.05% Diflorasone diacetate, 0.05% Clobetasol propionate, 0.25% Desoximetasone, 0.05% Halobetasol propionate, 0.05% Halobetasol propionate, 0.1% Fluocinonide
- Class 2 (Potent): 0.05% Betamethasone dipropionate, 0.1% Mometasone furoate, 0.05% Diflorasone diacetate, 0.1% Halcinonide, 0.05% Fluocinonide, 0.05% Diflorasone diacetate, 0.25% Desoximetasone, 0.05% Desoximetasone
- Class 3 (Upper Mid-Strength): 0.005% Fluticasone propionate, 0.05% Fluocinonide, 0.12% Betamethasone valerate
- Class 4 (Mid-Strength): 0.05% Flurandrenolide, 0.1% Mometasone furoate, 0.1% Triamcinolone acetonide, 0.03% Fluocinolone acetonide, 0.05% Desoximetasone, 0.05% Desoximetasone, 0.2% Hydrocortisone valerate
- Class 5 (Lower Mid-Strength): 0.01% Fluocinolone acetonide, 0.05% Flurandrenolide, 0.05% Fluticasone propionate, 0.1% Prednicarbate, 0.05% Desonide, 0.1% Hydrocortisone, 0.03%/ 0.01% Fluocinolone acetonide, 0.2% Hydrocortisone valerate 
- Class 6 (Mild): 0.05% Alclometasone dipropionate, 0.01% Fluocinolone acetonide, 0.05% Desonide, 0.01% Fluocinolone acetonide, 0.05% Desonide
- Class 7 (Least Potent): 0.5%/1% Hydrocortisone, 1%/2.5% Hydrocortisone, 2%/2.5% Hydrocortisone, 1%/2.5% Hydrocortisone, 1%/2.5% Hydrocortisone

HIGH YIELD MCQs ANSWERS WITH EXPLANATIONS

1. Ans. (b) Phenytoin; (c) Isoniazid; (d) Steroid; (e) Potassium iodide
[Ref. Clinical Dermatology by Habif, 6/e p571]

- Lithium, Iodides, Bromides, Oral contraceptives, Androgens or Glucocorticosteroids, Antituberculosis and Anticonvulsant therapy may cause an Acneiform rash

2. Ans. (b) 280-320 nm
[Ref. DVL by Thappa, 4/e p431]

Name	Wave length	Common use
UVA	400-320 nm	Tanning solutions, black lights
UVB	320-280 nm	Medical treatment
UVC	280-100 nm	Germicidal , irradiation

3. Ans. (a) Retinoids
[Ref. Neena Khanna, 5/e p440, 448]

Uses of Retinoids

- Topical use of retinoids
  - Acne vulgaris
  - Acne rosacea
  - Acanthosis nigricans
  - Keratinopathic ichthyosis
  - Plane warts
  - Palmoplantar psoriasis
- Systematic therapy of retinoid
  - Nodulocystic acne including acne conglobata
  - Moderately severe acne
  - Acne excoriee

4. Ans. (b) Vitiligo
[Ref. Neena Khanna, 5/e p165]

- Psoralens: Naturally occurring tricyclic furocoumarins derived from plants

- Most frequently used psoralen for vitiligo: 8-methoxypsoralen (8-MOP)

5. Ans. (d) Para tetra butyl phenol
[Ref. Pigmentary Disorders by Lahiri, 1/e p66]
- Hypopigmentation occurs in women at an extremely prominent site (center of the forehead)
- Moreover, the pressure to conform to religious and social norms makes many women continue to use the offending article even when the damage caused by it is clearly evident
- The sticker type of bindi is the main cause
- Causative agent is Para Tertiary Butyl Phenol (PTBP) present in high concentration in the glue: This chemical is a known melanocytotoxic agent and hypopigmentation in workers exposed to it during its manufacture

6. Ans. (c) Azathioprine

7. Ans. (a) Drug may be the cause and discontinuation may improve the skin condition

8. Ans. (b) Steroid
[Ref. Pharmacology by Bhattacharya, 2/e p275]

Gold Poisoning
- Dermatitis and stomatitis are the most common toxic manifestations of Gold therapy
- Continuation of gold may lead to a Generalized exfoliative dermatitis
- A mild rash may be treated with local steroid preparations; however, Systemic steroids may be necessary for severe disease.

9. Ans. (a) Genital warts
[Ref. Neena Khanna, 5/e p292]
- Podophyllin & Podophylotoxin is used in Anogenital warts

10. Ans. (a) Pigmented purpuric lesion; (c) Mycosis fungoides; (e) Lichenoid dermatitits of Gougerot & Blum
[Ref. Neena Khanna, 5/e p433]

Indications of Puva
- Psoriasis
- Vitiligo
- Atopic dermatitis
- Alopecia totalis & universalis
- Lichen planus
- Pityriasis lichenoides chronic
- Pityriasisrosea
- Morphea and patch/ plaque stage of mycosis fungoides

11. Ans. (d) Psoriasis
[Ref. Neena Khanna, 5/e p433]

12. Ans. (c) UV-C
[Ref. Photoimmunology by Parrish, 1/e p208]
- Human T lymphocytes were reported to be more sensitive to UV-C and UV-B radiation than were B lymphocytes

13. Ans. (a) Ultraviolet light
[Ref. Primary Care Medicine by Allan H. 6/e p1244]
- Ultraviolet radiation (narrow-band ultraviolet B, psoralens with ultraviolet A) can be used for renal and biliary pruritus.

14. Ans. (a) Derived from plant source; (c) Teratogenic; (d) High recurrence rate of wart after podophyllin resin treatment; (e) Individual variation in response rate
[Ref. Textbook of Therapeutics by Helms, 8/e p2086]

Podophyllin Resin
- Podophyllotoxin is a non-alkaloid toxin lignan extracted from the roots and rhizomes of Podophyllum species
- As a solution or cream, it is used on the skin as a topical treatment of external genital warts, caused by some types of the human papillomavirus (HPV) and other warts
- Its synthetic derivatives (Etoposide and Teniposide) display a wide selection in medical applications such as purgative, vesicant, antirheumatic, antiviral, and antitumor agents
- Anticancer activity has been heavily under study and used in various chemotherapies, including lung cancer, lymphomas, and genital tumors
- Contraindications: Diabetes mellitus, poor circulation, corticosteroid therapy, pregnancy, breast-feeding, and application to bleeding warts, moles, birthmarks, or unusual warts with hair growing from them

15. Ans. (a) Steroids
[Ref. Harrison's, 18/e p1366; Pharmacological Classification of Drugs with Doses and Preparations by KDT, 5/e p714; Neena Khanna, 5/e p285]

16. Ans. (a) Phenytoin; (b) Penicillin
[Ref. Porth Pathophysiology by Pooler, 1/e p1505]

Toxic Epidermal Necrolysis
- Drug reactions have been reported to cause 80-95% of TEN cases
- Drugs most often implicated in TEN:
  - Antibiotics
  - Sulfonamides (Sulfamethoxazole, Sulfadiazine, Sulfapyridine)
  - Beta-Lactams (Cephalosporins, Penicillins, Carbapenems)
  - Non Steroidal Anti-Inflammatory Drugs
  - Allopurinol
  - Antimetabolites (Methotrexate)
  - Antiretroviral drugs (Nevirapine)
  - Corticosteroids
  - Anxiolytics (Chlormezanone)
  - Anticonvulsants (Phenobarbital, Phenytoin, Carbamazepine, and Valproic Acid)

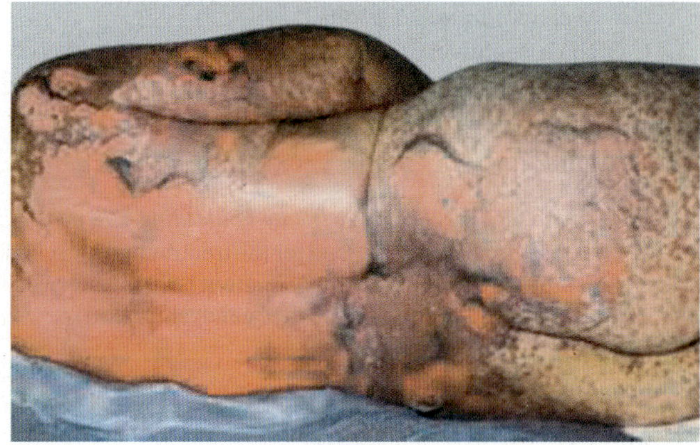

Fig. TEN

17. Ans. (b) Sulfonyl urea; (c) Aspirin
[Ref. Porth Pathophysiology by Pooler, 1/e p1505]

18. Ans. (b) Staphylococcal scalded skin syndrome
[Ref. Neena Khanna, 5/e p433]

Staphylococcal Scalded Skin Syndrome

- Aetiology: Staphylococcus aureus infections at distant site like Middle ear (otitis media), Lungs (pneumonia), Skin (trivial wounds and rarely bullous impetigo)
- Produces exotoxin (exfoliative toxin) which spreads haematogenously and causes a split in the upper layers
- Generally seen in Infants
- Erythema and tenderness: Superficial peeling of skin.
- Absence of mucosal lesion
- Good prognosis with low mortality.

19. Ans. (b) Thiacetazone
[Ref. Neena Khanna, 5/e p433]

Drugs Used in Treatment of Leprosy

- Rifampicin
- Dapsone
- Clofazimine
- Ofloxacin
- Sparfloxacin
- Minocycline
- Clarithromycin

20. Ans. (b) Lepra II reaction
[Ref. Harrison's, 18/e p1366; Pharmacological Classification of Drugs with Doses and Preparations by KDT, 5/e p714; Neena Khanna, 5/e p285]

21. Ans. (c) Fixed drug eruption
[Ref. Neena Khanna, 5/e p223]

22. Ans. (a) Dermatophytosis
[Ref. Infectious Diseases by Bennett, 8/e p2991]

- Potent topical antifungal agents used in the treatment of dermatophytosis:
  - Ciclopirox olamine
  - Terbinafine
  - Butenafine
  - Naftifine

23. Ans. (b) Itraconazole; (d) Terbinafine
[Ref. Neena Khanna, 5/e p309]

24. Ans. (d) 3 months
[Ref. Neena Khanna, 5/e p309]

- Oral Griseofulvin for Finger nail Dermatophytosis: 3-9 months therapy
  - 24 weeks for finger nail
  - 36 weeks for toe nail

25. Ans. (a) Foscarnet
[Ref. Sande's HIV/AIDS Medicine by Volberding, 2/e p447]

- The dosage of Foscarnet used for the treatment of acyclovir-resistant HSV infection in AIDS patient is 40 mg/kg every 8 hour (with reduction of dose in renal dysfunction)

26. Ans. (a) 1-2 mg/kg
[Ref. Neena Khanna, 5/e p449]

27. Ans. (c) Salmon rash
[Ref. Neena Khanna, 5/e p242-243]

Clinical Features of Dermatomyositis

- Itichy lesion
- Facial lesion's- heliotrope erythema, malar erythema, oedema
- Gottron's papule-violaceous, atrophic papules over knuckles and pressure points
- Gottron's sign- symmetrical, somewhat linear, lilac papulosquamous plaques
- Telangiectasia and ragged cuticles
- Poikiloderma- hyperpigmentation, hypopigmentation, telangiectasia and atrophy
- Mechanic's hand- confluent symmetric hyperkeratosis along ulnar aspect of thumb and radial aspect of fingers
- Calcinosis cutis
- Shawl sign- symmetrical confluent violaceous erythema extend ing from dorsolateral aspect of forearms and arms to deltoid region, shoulder and neck

28. Ans. (b) 200-300 mg
[Ref. Clinical Leprosy by Sehgal, 4/e p91]

29. Ans. (b) Dermatomyositis
[Ref. Neena Khanna, 5/e p242-243]

30. Ans. (a) Anti-jo 1
[Ref. Autoantibodies by Shoenfeld, 2/e p578; Lange U1, Piegsa M, Müller-Ladner U, Strunk J. Anti-Jo-1 antibody positive polymyositis- Successful therapy with leflunomide. Autoimmunity. 2006 May;39(3):261-4]

Antibodies In Polymyositis

- Idiopathic inflammatory myopathies (IM), including Dermatomyositis (DM) and Polymyositis (PM), are a groupof systemic rheumatologic diseases of unknown etiology characterized by chronic myositis
- Antisynthetase antibodies such as the Anti-Jo-1 antibody are known to be highly specific for inflammatory myopathies
- Patients with this antibody frequently show a combination of symptoms including Interstitial lung disease, fever, polyarthritis, myositis, Raynaud's phenomenon and "mechanic's hands"
- In the management of PM with Anti-Jo-1 antibody, immunosuppressive agents are used to control the disease
- Leflunomide is a new immunosuppressive drug recently introduced in the treatment of Rheumatoid and Psoriatic arthritis
- Here, we report two cases of female patients with PM and anti-Jo-1 antibodies, who were successfully treated with Leflunomide

31. Ans. (a) Chloroquine
[Ref. Skin Disease In Old Age by Ronald Mark, 2/e p99]

Drug-Induced Lupus

- Most common medicines:
  - Isoniazid
  - Hydralazine
  - Procainamide
- Less common drugs:
  - Anti-seizure medications
  - Capoten
  - Chlorpromazine

- Etanercept
- Infliximab
- Methyldopa
- Minocycline
- Penicillamine
- Quinidine
- Sulfasalazine

32. Ans. (d) Lichen Planus
[Ref. Neena Khanna, 5/e p62]

33. Ans. (b) Fixed Drug Eruption
[Ref. Neena Khanna, 5/e p223]

34. Ans. (c) Disinfection of all clothes and beddings
[Ref. Neena Khanna, 5/e p365]

- General measure: Disinfection of all clothes and beddings
- Definitive measure: Permethrin 1% cream applied for 8-10 hours

35. Ans. (c) Comdylomata accuminata
[Ref. Neena Khanna, 5/e p292]

36. Ans. (d) HIV associated neuropathy
[Ref. The Skin in Systemic Autoimmune Diseases by Sarzi-Puttini. Vol 5 p79]

37. Ans. (b) Skin rashes
[Ref. Neena Khanna, 5/e p440]

- MC frequent adverse effect of topical retinoids are known as 'Retinoid reaction', characterized by pruritus, burning sensation at the sites of application, erythema, peeling
- Most common side effect is skin irritation
- Other common side effects are photosensitivity and dryness

38. Ans. (b) Minocycline
[Ref. Tavares J, Leung WWS. Discoloration of nail beds and skin from minocycline. CMAJ : Canadian Medical Association Journal. 2011;183(2):224]

- Nail bed discoloration is an uncommon side effect of Minocycline therapy but often accompanies discoloration at other sites (Skin, sclera, palate, teeth, thyroid and bone)
- Three patterns of Minocycline-induced pigmentation:
  - Type I results in blue-black macules localized to areas of active inflammation or scarring: Dose-independent and results from local pigment deposition by macrophages
  - Type II pigmentation most commonly presents as blue-grey or brown patches on the shins, ankles and arms: Pigment complexes in dermal macrophages or scattered freely within dermal collagen
  - Type III pigmentation is a symmetric and generalized pigmentation on sun-exposed areas: Caused by increased melanin or melanin–minocycline complexes at the dermal–epidermal interface
- The patient's discoloration was thought to be most consistent with type II pigmentation of the nail beds and type III pigmentation of the face.

39. Ans. (d) Busulphan
[Ref. Dermatology Secrets Plus by Fitzpatrick, 5/e p167]

- Arsenicals, busulfan, 5-Fluorouracil, Cyclophosphamide, Topical nitrogen mustard (mechlorethamine), and Bleomycin most commonly cause increased skin pigmentation

40. Ans. (d) Thiacetazone

41. Ans. (c) Gold
[Ref. Fitzpatrick's Dermatology in General Medicine, 7/e p164]

42. Ans. (b) Psoriasis
[Ref. An Atlas of Psoriasis by Lionel Fry, 2/e p80]

- Calcipotriol, Calcitriol, Maxacalcitol and Tacalcitol are the various vitamin D analogs useful in the treatment of psoriasis
- When combined with Betamethasone the effect is better than either agent used alone

43. Ans. (b) Psoriasis
[Ref. Neena Khanna, 5/e p45]

44. Ans. (b) Methotrexate
[Ref. Neena Khanna, 5/e p57]

Indications of Methotrexate in Psoriasis

- Generalized pustular psoriasis
- Erythrodermic psoriasis
- Debilitating palmoplantar psoriasis
- Debilitating psoriatic arthritis

45. Ans. (d) Exfoliative
[Ref. Neena Khanna, 5/e p58]

Adverse Effect of PUVA

- Nausea & giddiness- Commonest
- Premature ageing of skin
- Photo toxicity
- Cutaneous malignancies (controversial)
- Cataract

46. Ans. (a) Psoriasis; (e) Vitiligo
[Ref. Neena Khanna, 5/e p433]

Indications of Puva

- Psoriasis
- Vitiligo
- Atopic dermatitis
- Alopecia totalis & universalis
- Lichen planus
- Pityriasis lichenoides chronic
- Pityriasisrosea
- Morphea and patch/ plaque stage of mycosis fungoides

47. Ans. (b) Lyell's syndrome
[Ref. Dermatology by Otto Braun-Falco, 1/e p282]

48. Ans. (a) Psoriasis
[Ref. Neena Khanna, 5/e p58]

49. Ans. (c) Antihistone antibodies are found
[Ref. Adverse Cutaneous Drug Reactions to Cardiovascular Drugs by Özkaya, 1/e p41]

- Classical Drug-induced lupus is characterized by the presence of Antinuclear antibodies (ANA) and Antihistone antibodies

50. Ans. (c) Cyclosporine
[Ref. Harrison's, 18/e p1366; Pharmacological Classification of Drugs with Doses and Preparations by KDT, 5/e p714; Neena Khanna, 5/e p285]

51. Ans. (d) Thalidomide
[Ref. Andrews' Diseases of the Skin by James, 12/e p338

52. Ans. (d) Clofazimine
[Ref. Comprehensive Dermatologic Drug Therapy by Wolverton, 3/e p428]

Clofazimine

- Clofazimine is a fat-soluble iminophenazine dye used in combination with rifampicin and dapsone as multidrug therapy (MDT) for the treatment of leprosy
- Clofazimine works by binding to the guanine bases of bacterial DNA, thereby blocking the template function of the DNA and inhibiting bacterial proliferation
- It also increases activity of bacterial phospholipase A2, leading to release and accumulation of lysophospholipids, which are toxic and inhibit bacterial proliferation
- Clofazimine is also a FIASMA (Functional inhibitor of acid sphingomyelinase)

53. Ans. (c) Griseofulvin
[Ref. Evidence-Based Dermatology by Williams, 2/e p388]

- Griseofulvin is an orally administered antifungal drug

54. Ans. (c) Tinea versicolor
[Ref. Evidence-Based Dermatology by Williams, 2/e p388]

- Griseofulvin is not used in Tinea versicolor and Candida infection

55. Ans. (a) Amphotericin
[Ref. Lehne's Pharmacology for Nursing Care by Burchum, 8/e p1093]

- Amphotericin B is active against a broad spectrum of pathogenic fungi and is a drug of choice for most systemic mycoses

56. Ans. (b) UV-B
[Ref. Neena Khanna, 5/e p433]

- Wavelength found most effective in treating skin diseases with phototherapy is UVB with wave length of 311±2 nm (narrow band UVB; NBUVB)

57. Ans. (b) 290-360 nm

58. Ans. (b) Tinea Versicolor & Candida
[Ref. Evidence-Based Dermatology by Williams, 2/e p388]

59. Ans. (b) Scabies
[Ref. Neena Khanna, 5/e p370]

60. Ans. (c) Herpes
[Ref. Sexually Transmitted Infections by Bhushan Kumar, 2/e p1138]

61. Ans. (c) Fixed drug eruption
[Ref. Neena Khanna, 4/e p209]

Fixed Drug Eruptions (FDE)

- Lesions occur within 8-16 hours of drug intake
- Lesion recur at same sites
- Well-defined, circular, erythematous plaques
- Slate-grey hyperpigmentation
- MC sites: Mucocutaneous junctions (Lips, Glans)
- Diagnosis: Provocative test
- Common drugs implicated: Sulphonamides, Tetracyclines, NSAIDs, Fluoroquinolones, Barbiturates, Metronidazole

62. Ans. (b) TEN
[Ref. Neena Khanna, 4/e p174]

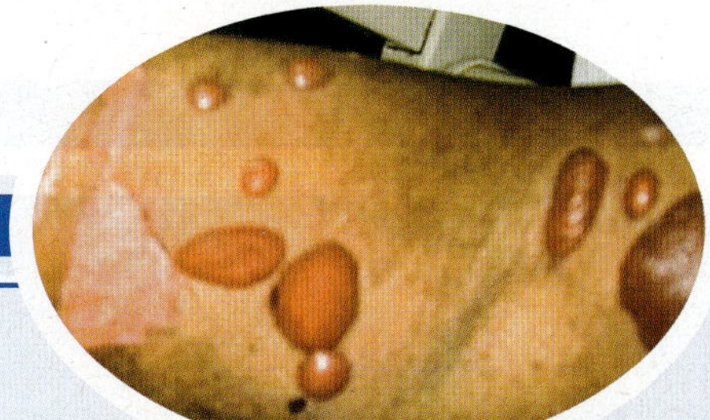

Chapter 8

Vesiculobullous Diseases

THEORETICAL CONCEPTS

Vesiculobullous/Blistering Disorders

INTRAEPIDERMAL			
Granular layer • Pemphigus foliaceous^Q^ • Bullous impetigo^Q^ • SSSS^Q^ • Miliaria crystallina	**Spinous layer** • Familial benign pemphigus^Q^ • Molluscum contagiosum^Q^ • Atopic dermatitis^Q^ • Herpes/Varicella infection	**Suprabasal layer** • Pemphigus vulgaris^Q^ • Darier's disease^Q^	**Basal layer** • Erythema multiforme^Q^ • Epidermolysis bullosa simplex^Q^
SUBEPIDERMAL			
Junctional/Basal lamina • Toxic epidermolysis necrolysis (TEN ^Q^) • Bullous pemphigoid ^Q^ • Junctional epidermolysis bullosa ^Q^		**Dermolytic/Below basal lamina** • Dermatitis herpetiformis^Q^ • Epidermolysis bullosa acquisita^Q^ • Epidermolysis bullosa atrophicans • Porphyria cutaneatarda^Q^ • Deep burns	

(SSSS: Staphylococcal scalded skin syndrome)

VIII A. PEMPHIGUS—INTRAEPIDERMAL BULLOUS DISORDERS

- *Definition*: Intraepidermal bullous disorder characterised clinically by blisters and histologically by acantholysis (separation of viable epidermal cells)
- *Underlying cause*:
  - IgG antibodies: Against Desmoglobins^Q^
  - Neoplasms: Thymoma, lymphoma
  - Drugs:
    - **Penicillamine (Most common)** ^Q^
    - Rifampicin
    - Captopril
- *Clinical types of Pemphigus*: Acantholytic bullae^Q^
  - ***Pemphigus vulgaris*: Suprabasal split**^Q^
    - **Nikolsky sign**^Q^
    - Bulla-spread sign
    - Scalp, face, trunk, mucosal lesions
    - Sepsis and electrolyte imbalance
  - ***Pemphigus vegetans*: Suprabasal split**^Q^
    - Heaped-up vegetating lesions
    - Groins, axilla, angles of mouth, mucosal

- ***Pemphigus foliaceus***: Split in granular layer or just below horny layer
  - Transient superficial bullae rupture to form crusts/scales
- ***Pemphigus erythematosus***: Split in granular layer or just below stratum corneum
  - Less severe form of P. foliaceus[Q]
  - Dry, hyperkeratotic lesions on face (malar region)

- *Diagnostic tests*:
  - **Tzanck smear: Show acantholytic cells**[Q]
  - Biopsy of edge of bulla:
  - Split in supra-basal layer
  - Presence of acantholytic cells[Q]
  - Direct immunofluorescence of perilesional skin: *'Fishnet appearance'* due to IgG intercellular deposits[Q]
  - ELISA/IIF: Circulating antibodies to desmoglobins[Q]
- *Treatment*:
  - Corticosteroids
  - Immunosuppressants
  - Azathioprine
  - Methotrexate
  - Cyclophosphamide
  - Other drugs: Mycophenolate mofetil, I/v IgG, Plasmapheresis

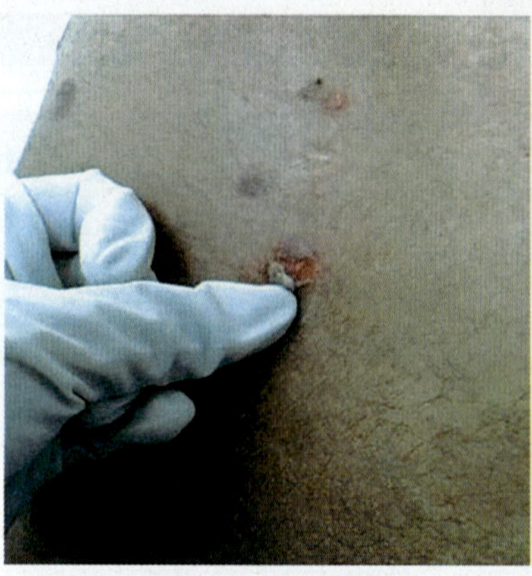
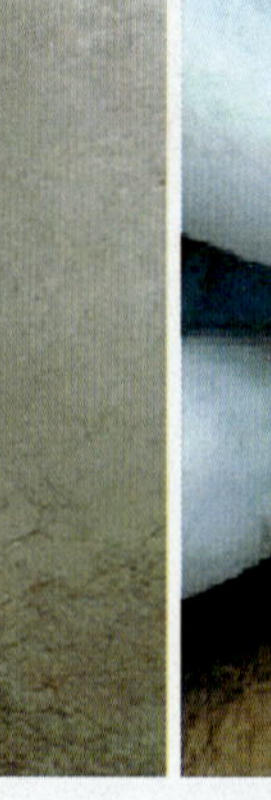

Fig. Nikolsky sign

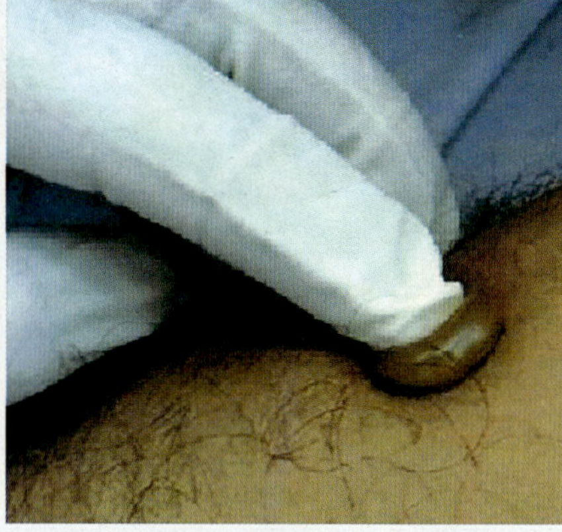

Fig. Bulla spread sign

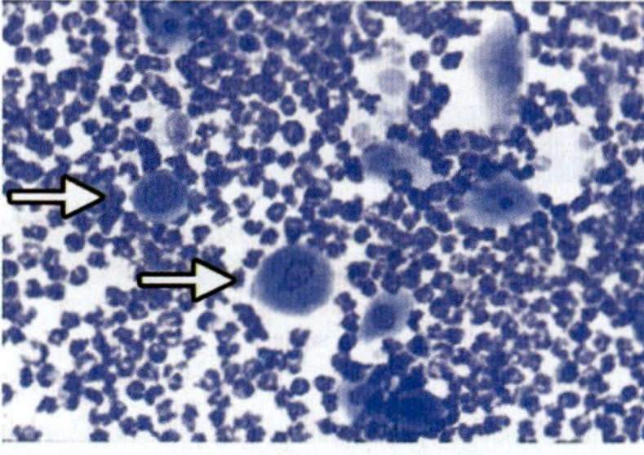

Fig. Acantholytic cells

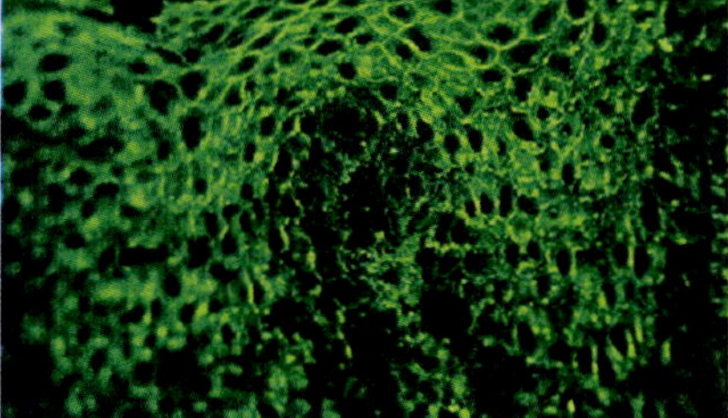

Fig. Fish-net pattern

VIII B. BULLOUS PEMPHIGOID—DERMO-EPIDERMAL BULLOUS DISORDERS

- *Definition*: Bullous disorder characterised deposition of IgG and C3 at **dermo-epidermal junction**
- *Underlying cause*: IgG antibodies: **Against IgG and C3**[Q]
- *Clinical presentation*:
  - *Itchy, large, haemorrhagic bullae*[Q]
  - **Nikolsky sign** NEGATIVE[Q]
  - **Bulla-spread sign** NEGATIVE[Q]
  - Lesions heal with Milia formation (Interepidermal cysts)
  - Sites: Thighs, groin, flexures, oro-mucosal
  - Secondary infections
  - Associated malignancies: Breasts, Lungs, Stomach
- *Diagnostic tests*:
  - Biopsy: Dermo-epidermal bullae with neutrophils and eosinophils[Q]
  - Direct immunofluorescence: IgG and C3 deposits along dermo-epidermal junction[Q]
- *Treatment*:
  - Corticosteroids
  - Immunosuppressants: Azathioprine[Q]

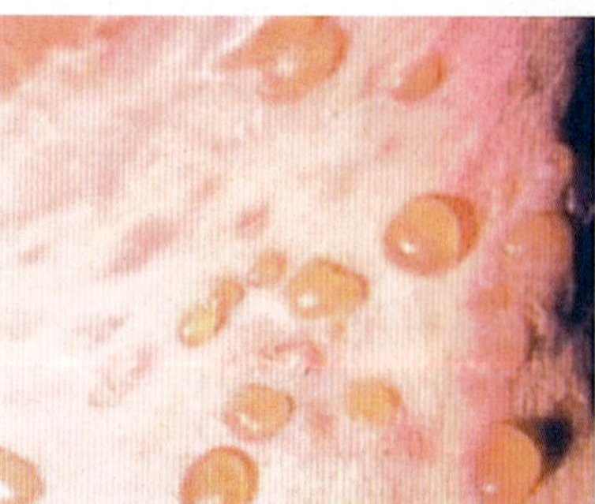

Fig. Large bullae

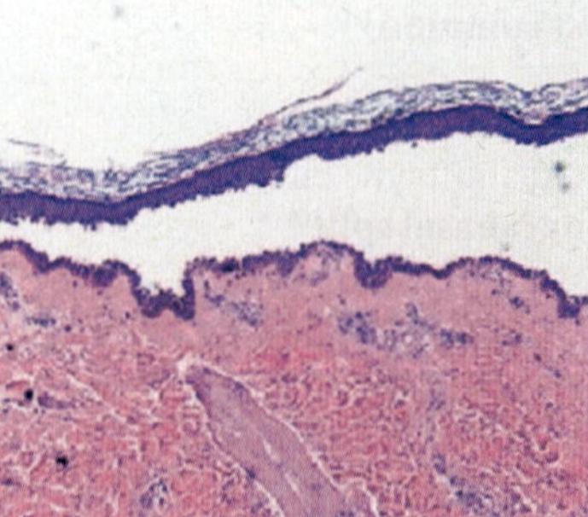

Fig. Subepidermal blister

VIII C. DERMATITIS HERPETIFORMIS—DERMO-EPIDERMAL BULLOUS DISORDERS

- *Underlying cause*: **Gluten sensitive enteropathy (GSE)**[Q]
- *Clinical presentation*: Associated 100% with GSE
  - Itchy grouped papules or vesicles
  - Eczematous changes and secondary infection
  - Most frequent on extensor surfaces[Q]
- *Diagnostic tests*:
  - **Biopsy**: Dermo-epidermal split with microabscesses at tip of dermal papillae
  - **Direct immunoflorescence**: IgA deposits in dermal papillae
- *Treatment*:
  - Gluten-free diet
  - **Dapsone (Drug of choice)**[Q]
  - Sulphapyridine

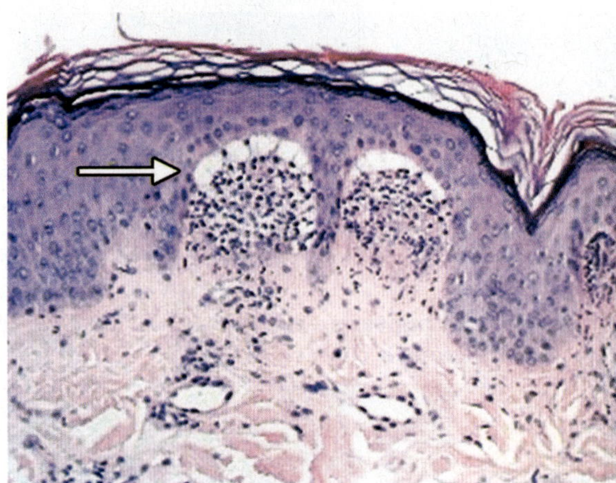

Fig. Subepidermal cleft

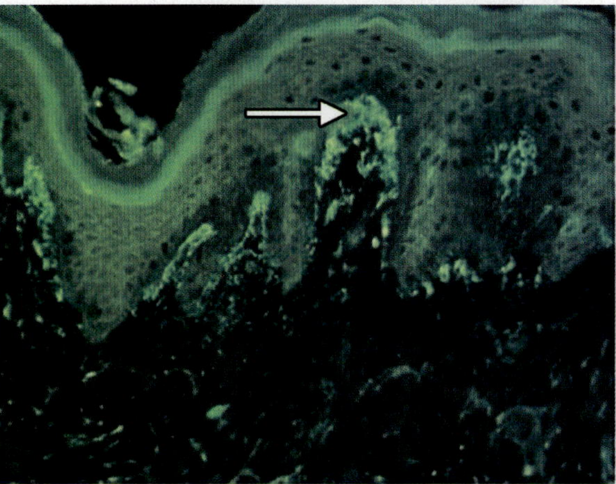

Fig. IgA granular deposits

VIII D. IMMUNOFLUORESCENCE IN VESICULOBULLOUS DISORDERS

Key Immunofluorescence Findings in Vesiculobullous Disorders
Dermatitis herpetiformis [Q] • IgA granular band at Dermoepidermal junction/ Basement membrane
Pemphigus vulgaris [Q] • Fish-net pattern Intercellular IgG in epidermis
Bullous pemphigoid [Q] • C3, IgG linear band at Dermoepidermal junction/ Basement membrane
Linear Ig A disease [Q] • IgA linear band at dermal papillary tip
Epidermolysis bullosa acquisita [Q] • C3, IgG linear band at Dermoepidermal junction/ Basement membrane

Direct Immunofluorescence in Vesiculobullous Disorders	
POSITIVE	***NEGATIVE***
• Dermatitis herpetiformis [Q] • Pemphigus vulgaris [Q] • Pemphigus foliaceous [Q] • Bullous pemphigoid [Q] • Linear IgA disease [Q] • Erythema multiforme • Epidermolysis bullosa acquisita	• Impetigo contagiosa [Q] • Darier disease [Q] • Hailey-Hailey disease [Q] • Staphylococcal scalded skin syndrome (SSSS) • Porphyria cutanea tarda • Herpes/ Varicella infection

IMAGE-BASED QUESTIONS

1. **A girl presents with painful blisters in mouth, on genitals and other parts of body. Flaccid bullae rupture easily. Following pattern (Photograph) as seen on Direct fluorescence. Diagnosis is** ***[AIIMS November 2016]***

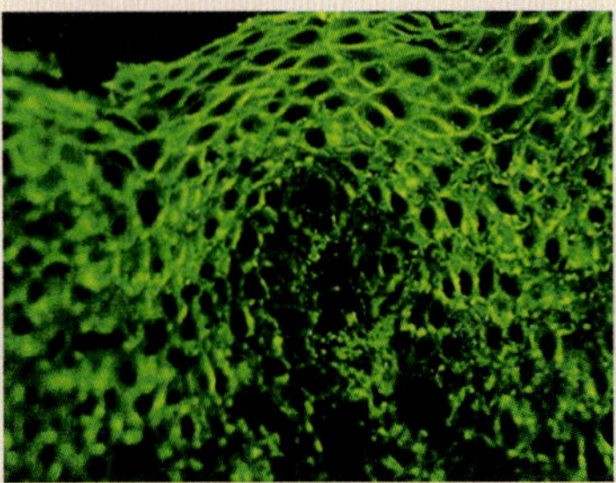

a. Pemphigus
b. Bullous pemphigoid
c. Dermatitis herpetiformis
d. Staphylococcal scalded skin syndrome

2. **Identify the Bullous skin disorder in an Infant (Photograph)**

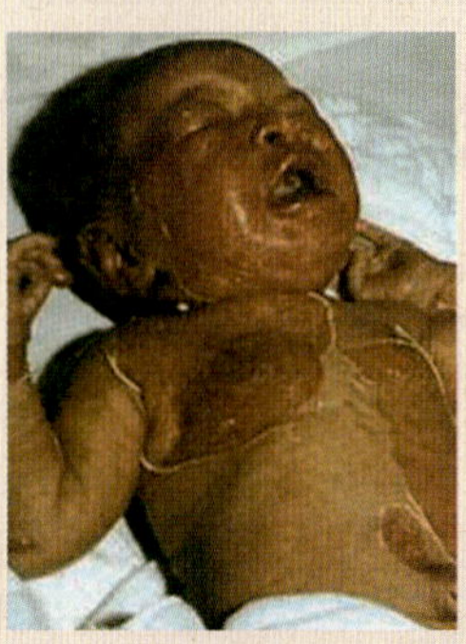

a. Pemphigus
b. Bullous pemphigoid
c. Dermatitis herpetiformis
d. Staphylococcal scalded skin syndrome

3. **Sign (Arrow) shown in Photograph is positive in all except** ***[Recent Question 2012]***

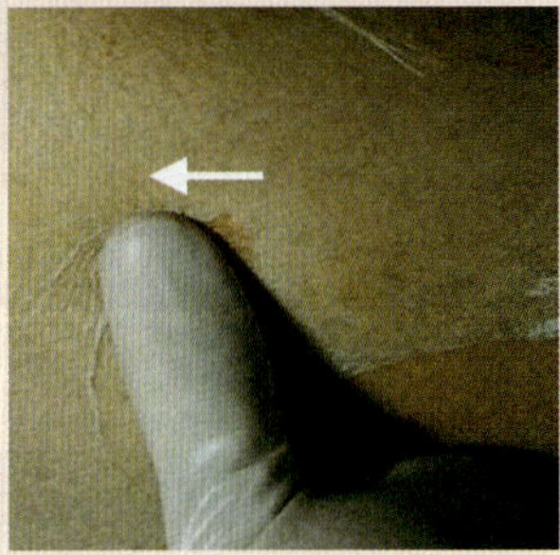

a. Staphylococcal scalded skin syndrome
b. Bullous pemphigoid
c. Pemphigus vulgaris
d. Toxic epidermal necrolysis

4. **Typical appearance (Arrows) of lesions shown in Photograph is characteristic of**

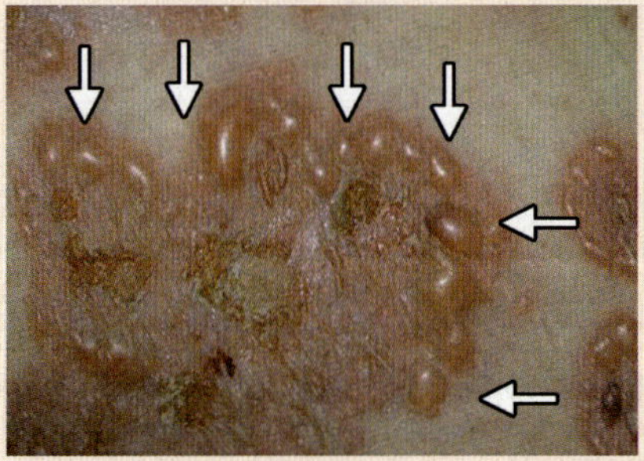

a. SSSS
b. Pemphigus vulgaris
c. Bullous pemphigoid
d. Chronic bullous disease

5. **Smear (Photograph) used for identification of Pemphigus is**

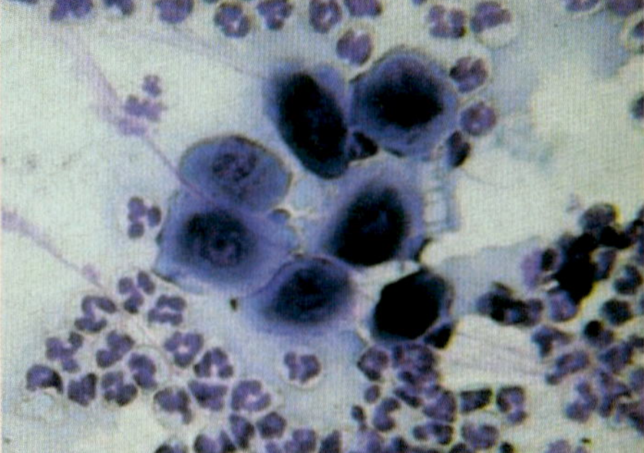

a. KOH mount
b. Albert stain
c. Tzanck smear
d. None of the above

6. **Typical deposits on Direct Immunofluorescence (Photograph) is seen in**

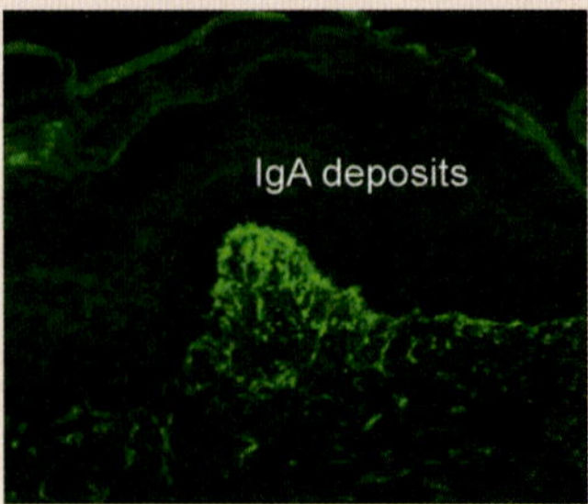

a. Dermatitis herpetiformis
b. Bullous pemphogoid
c. Pemphigus vulgaris
d. Chronic bullous disease

7. **Dermatological sign shown in Photograph is known as**

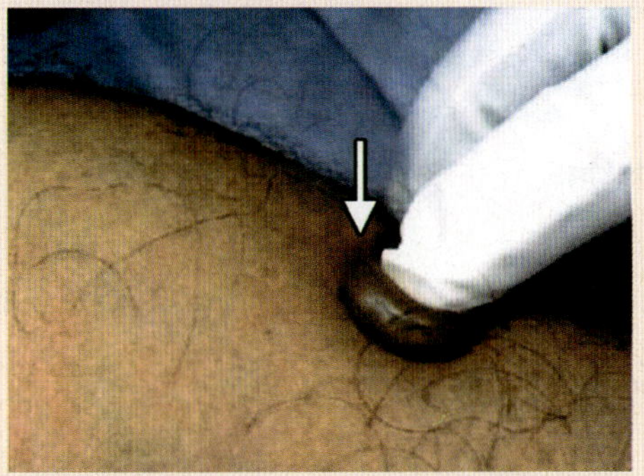

a. Auspitz sign
b. Nikolsky sign
c. Bulla spread sign
d. Hutchinson's sign

8. **Identify the skin disorder in a 60 years old person (Photograph)**

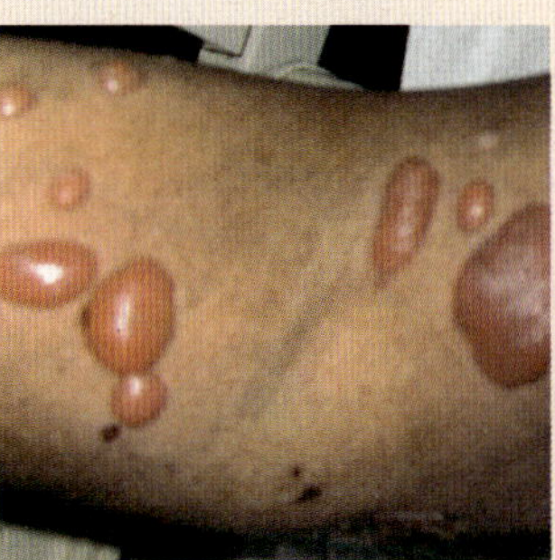

a. SSSS
b. Pemphigus vulgaris
c. Pemphigus foliaceous
d. Bullous pemphigoid

9. **Typical pattern on Direct Immunofluorescence (Photograph) is seen in**

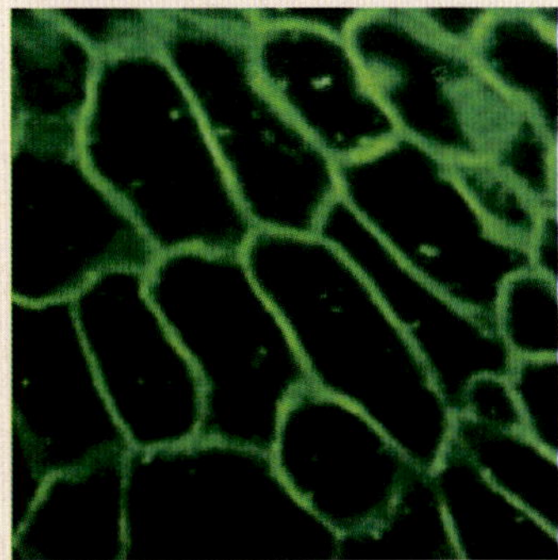

a. Lichen planus
b. Staphylococcal scalded skin syndrome
c. Pemphigus
d. Leprosy

10. **A patient presents with history of bullae involving >30% of body surface area and erosions of lips for past 7 days. Most probable etiology is** ***[AIIMS PG May 2015]***

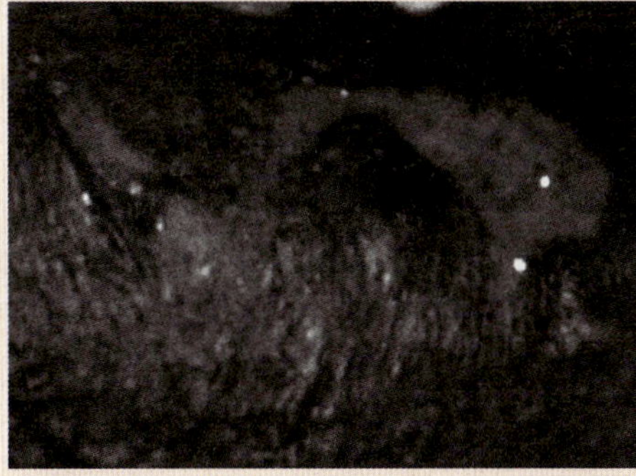

a. Viral infection
b. Bacterial infection
c. Drugs
d. Malignancy

11. **A patient comes with itchy tense blisters whose roof settled on normal shin as well as urticarial plaques (See Photograph). Diagnose the condition** ***[AIIMS PG May 2015]***

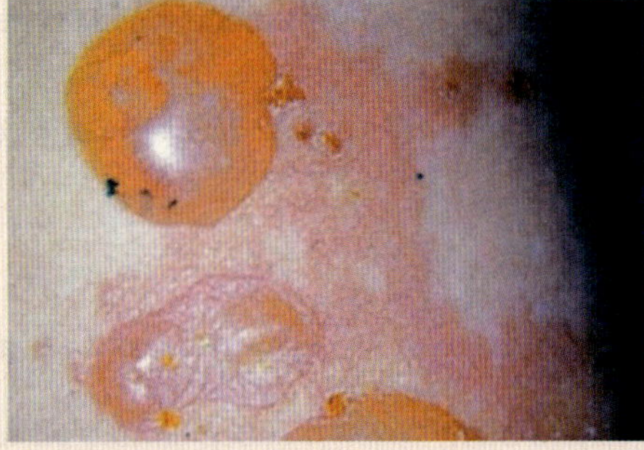

a. Pemphigus vulgaris
b. Bullous pemphigoid
c. Linear IgA
d. Dermatitis herpetiformis

ANSWERS WITH EXPLANATIONS OF IBQs

1. Ans. (a) Pemphigus vulgaris *[Ref. Neena Khanna, 3/e p63]*

Diagnosis of Pemphigus Vulgaris

- Patients with persistent blisters and erosions of mucous membranes and skin
- Positive Nikolsky sign
- Histology:
- Suprabasal acantholysis and detection of tissue-bound IgG with an intercellular ("cobblestone", "fishnet") pattern by direct IF microscopy **(Photograph)**
- Circulating IgG autoantibodies binding to the intercellular junctions of epithelial cells by indirect IF microscopy
- ELISA: Recognizing desmoglein 3

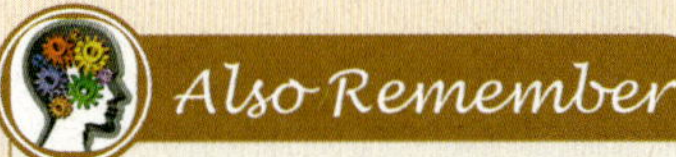

Key Immunofluorescence Findings in Vesiculobullous Disorders

- Dermatitis herpetiformis: IgA granular band at Dermoepidermal junction/ Basement membrane
- Pemphigus vulgaris: Fish-net pattern Intercellular IgG in epidermis
- Bullous pemphigoid: C3, IgG linear band at Dermoepidermal junction/ Basement membrane
- Linear Ig A disease: IgA linear band at dermal papillary tip
- Epidermolysis bullosa acquisita: C3, IgG linear band at Dermoepidermal junction/ Basement membrane

2. Ans. (d) Staphylococcal scalded skin syndrome *[Ref. Neena Khanna, 4/e p71]*

Staphylococcus Scalded Skin Syndrome (SSSS)

- Causative agent: Staphylococcus aureus
- Characteristic feature:
  - Begin as diffuse painful erythema with wrinkled appearance
  - Peeling of skin in sheets leaving an erythematous surface
  - Peeling occur due to Exfoliative toxin

3. Ans. (b) Bullous pemphigoid *[Ref. Neena Khanna, 4/e p73]*

- In contrast to pemphigus, the Nikolsky s sign and bulla-spread sign are usually negative in Bullous pemphigoid

4. Ans. (d) Chronic bullous disease *[Ref. Pediatric Secrets by Ditmar, 5/e p152]*

- Appearance of new vesicles or bullae in a 'String-of-pearls' or 'Cluster-of-jewels' appearance around crusted/erythematous plaques is seen in Chronic bullous disease

5. Ans. (c) Tzanck smear *[Ref. Neena Khanna, 4/e p15]*

Tzanck Smear

- Use: Cytological examination of skin blisters
- Method:
  - Rupture roof of blister, scrape floor with surgical blade and transfer material to slide
  - Stain with Giemsa/ Wright/ Toluidine blue stain and observe under microscope

6. Ans. (a) Dermatitis herpetiformis *[Ref. Neena Khanna, 4/e p81]*

- Granular deposits of IgA in tips of Dermal papillae, and Dermo-epidermal junction on Direct Immunofluorescence is characteristic of Dermatitis herpetiformis

7. Ans. (c) Bulla spread sign *[Ref. Neena Khanna, 4/e p73]*

Bulla Spread Sign (Asboe-Hansen Sign/Lutz Sign):

- Description: Marking the boundary of bulla and then applying pressure with a finger on the edge of the bulla (Lutz sign) or center of the bulla (Asboe-Hansen sign)
- Positive sign: All varieties of pemphigus and many cases of subepidermal blisters, including bullous pemphigoid, dermatitis herpetiformis, epidermolysis bullosa acquisita, cicatricial pemphigoid, dystrophic epidermolysis bullosa, Stevens-Johnson syndrome and toxic epidermal necrolysis
- Negative sign: Due to fragility of the roof of the blister it is usually negative in Hailey-Hailey disease and staphylococcal scalded skin syndrome

8. Ans. (d) Bullous pemphigoid *[Ref. Neena Khanna, 4/e p77]*

Bullous Pemphigoid

- Itchy, large, haemorrhagic bullae
- Nikolsky sign NEGATIVE
- Bulla-spread sign NEGATIVE
- Lesions heal with Milia formation (Interepidermal cysts)
- Sites: Thighs, groin, flexures, oro-mucosal
- Secondary infections
- Associated malignancies: Breasts, Lungs, Stomach

9. Ans. (c) Pemphigus

Direct Immunofluorescence Patterns

- Dermatitis herpetiformis: Granular deposits of IgA in tips of Dermal papillae, and Dermo-epidermal junction on Direct Immunofluorescence
- Bullous pemphigoid: IgG and C3 deposition at basement membrane zone in a linear pattern
- IgA disease: Linear deposition of IgA at basement membrane zone
- Pemphigus vulgaris: Fish net pattern deposition of IgG between cells of epidermis
- Lichen planus:
  - IgM Colloid bodies, Linear/ shaggy fibrinogen deposition at dermo-epidermal junction
  - Granular IgM, Linear C3 deposits (with/ without IgG) at basement membrane

10. Ans. (c) Drugs *[Ref. Emergency Medicine by Wolfson, 5/e p825]*

Stevens-Johnson Syndrome (SJS)

- An immune-complex–mediated hypersensitivity complex that typically involves the skin and the mucous membranes
  - SJS: A minor form of toxic epidermal necrolysis, with less than 10% body surface area (BSA) detachment
  - Overlapping SJS/ Toxic epidermal necrolysis (TEN): Detachment of 10-30% of the BSA
  - Toxic epidermal necrolysis (TEN): Detachment of more than 30% of the BSA
- Etiology:
  - Infectious
  - Drug-induced (Most common; Photograph)
  - Malignancy-related
  - Idiopathic

11. Ans. (b) Bullous pemphigoid *[Ref. Oral Pathology by Lewis, 4/e p152]*

Bullous Pemphigoid (Photograph)

- MC autoimmune subepidermal blistering disease
- Acute or chronic skin disease, involving the formation of blisters, known as 'bullae', at the space between the skin layers epidermis and dermis
- Blisters develop on flexural areas, i.e. lower abdomen, upper thighs or armpits
- Type II hypersensitivity reaction
- Formation of anti-hemidesmosome antibodies

 NEET/NBE PATTERN MCQs 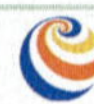

1. **Senear-Usher syndrome is associated with?** *[Recent Question 2016]*
   a. Pemphigus vulgaris
   b. Pemphigus foliaceous
   c. Pemphigus erythematous
   d. Paraneoplastic pemphigus
2. **Rarest variety of Pemphigus** *[Recent Question 2016]*
   a. P. vulgaris b. P. foliaceus
   c. P. vegetans d. P. neoplastic
3. **Tzanck smear in a case of pemphigus vulgaris show** *[Recent Question 2016]*
   a. Acantholytic cells b. Macrophages
   c. Fibroblasts d. Neutrophils
4. **Congenital dystrophic epidermolysis bullosa, defect is in** *[Recent Question 2016]*
   a. Laminin 4 b. Collagen 4
   c. Collagen 7 d. Collagen 3
5. **Row of tombstones is seen in** *[Recent Question 2016]*
   a. Irritant dermatitis b. Pemphigus
   c. Pemphigoid d. Herpes zoster
6. **Pemphigus neonatorum is a variety of** *[Recent Question 2016]*
   a. Bullous impetigo b. Epidermolysis bullosa
   c. Congenital syphilis d. Pemphigus
7. **Photosensitive rash in common in** *[Recent Question 2016]*
   a. Acute intermittent porphyria
   b. Erythropoietic porphyria
   c. Leprosy
   d. Lichen planus
8. **Flaccid bullae with mucosal involvement and intra-epidermal acantholysis are characteristic of** *[Recent Question 2016]*
   a. Pemphigus vulgaris b. Pemphigus foliaceous
   c. Psoriasis d. Vitiligo
9. **Antigen defect in Pemphigus vulgaris** *[Recent Question 2016]*
   a. Desmoglein-1 b. Desmoglein-3
   c. Desmocollin-3 d. Desmocollin-2
10. **30 years old male presents with painful flaccid bullae on right face and oral mucosa without evidence of inflammation or redness; what is the most probable diagnosis?** *[Recent Question 2016]*
    a. Pemphigus vulgaris b. Pemphigus foliaceous
    c. Bullous pemphoid d. Dermatitis herpetiformis
11. **Mutation in which collagen is present in Epidermolysis bullosa** *[Recent Question 2016]*
    a. II b. IV
    c. V d. VII
12. **Which of the following is a subepidermal vesiculobullous disorder?** *[Recent Question 2016]*
    a. Pemphigus vulgaris
    b. Bullous pemphigoid
    c. Pemphigus vegetans
    d. Pemphigus erythematosus
13. **Tense itching bulla is seen in** *[Recent Question 2016]*
    a. Bullous pemphigoid b. Dermatitis herpetiformis
    c. Pemphigus vulgaris d. Erythema multiforme
14. **Immunofluorescence pattern in Pemphigus vulgaris is suggestive of** *[Recent Question 2016]*
    a. Intercellular IgG deposition
    b. C3 and IgG deposition at dermo-epidermal junction
    c. IgA deposition at dermo-epidermal junction
    d. IgA at papillary tip
15. **Most common cause of Pemphigus in India is** *[NBE FMGE March 2010]*
    a. Pemphigus vulgaris
    b. Pemphigus foliaceus
    c. Pemphigus erythematosus
    d. Pemphigus vegetans
16. **Chronic Familial benign pemphigus is also known as** *[NBE DNB 2011]*
    a. Hailey-Hailey disease
    b. Fogo Selvagem
    c. Darner's disease
    d. Chronic bullous disorder of childhood
17. **Characteristic microscopic feature of Pemphigus vulgaris is** *[NBE FMGE March 2009]*
    a. Subepidermal acantholytic blister
    b. Subcorneal non-acantholytic blister
    c. Suprabasal acantholytic blister
    d. Sub-epidermal non-acantholytic blister
18. **In pemphigus vulgaris blisters are located in?** *[Recent Question 2012]*
    a. Subepidermal b. Intraepidermal
    c. Subdermal d. Subfascial
19. **Drug of choice in dermatitis herpetiformis is** *[NBE DNB 2002, 2011, NBE FMGE September 2012]* *[Recent Question 2014]*
    a. Corticosteroids b. Colchicine
    c. Dapsone d. Chloroquine
20. **Dermatitis herpetiformis is associated with** *[NBE FMGE September 2008, Recent Question 2014, 2016]*
    a. Ulcerative colitis
    b. Crohn's disease
    c. Irritable bowel disease
    d. Gluten-sensitive enteropathy
21. **In pemphigus vulgaris blisters are located in** *[Recent Question 2012]*
    a. Subepidermal b. Suprabasal
    c. Subdermal d. Intrafascial
22. **Intra-epidermal bullae is the feature of** *[NBE DNB 1994]*
    a. Pemphigoid
    b. Pemphigus
    c. Dermatitis herpetiformis
    d. Polymorphous light eruption
23. **Intrapidermal IgG deposition is seen in** *[NBE DNB 2009]*
    a. Pemphigus
    b. Bullous pemphigoid
    c. Herpes genitalis
    d. None of the above
24. **In Pemphigus vulgaris, Tzanck smear shows** *[Recent Question 2012]*
    a. Acantholytic cells b. Macrophages
    c. Fibroblasts d. Neutrophils

25. Tzanck test is positive in the following, except *[NBE DNB 1998, 1999, 2001, 2004, 2007]*
 a. Pemphigus foliaceous and pemphigus vegetans
 b. Pemphigus vulgaris
 c. Senear Usher's syndrome
 d. Bullous pemphigoid

26. Diagnosis of a 6-year-old girl child with bullous lesions over palate and trunk is *[NBE FMGE September 2008]*
 a. Pemphigus vulgaris
 b. Bullous pemphigoid
 c. Dermatitis herpetiformis
 d. Pemphigus foliaceous

27. Acantholytic bullae are found in *[NBE DNB 1993]*
 a. Eczema b. Impetigo
 c. Pemphigoid d. Pemphigus vulgaris
 e. Burns

28. Diseases characterised by Bullous eruptions include all except *[UPSC 2009]*
 a. Porphyria cutanea tarda b. Variegate porphyria
 c. Dermatitis herpetiformis
 d. Lichen planus

29. Mucosal involvement is seen in all except *[NBE FMGE September 2005]*
 a. Pemphigus vulgaris b. Bullous pemphigoid
 c. Pemphigus foliaceous d. Epidermolysis bullosa

30. 'Bulla spread sign' is seen in *[NBE DNB 1996, 1999, 2001, 2003, 2004, 2006]*
 a. Herpes gestationis b. Bullous pemphigoid
 c. Pemphigus vulgaris d. D. herpetiformis

31. All of the following are histological features of Pemphigus except *[NBE FMGE March 2010]*
 a. Acanthosis b. Acantholysis
 c. Fish-net appearance d. Basal cell degeneration

32. Drug of choice for dermatitis herpetiformis is *[NBE FMGE March 2010]*
 a. Thalidomide b. Rifampicin
 c. Dapsone d. Clofazimine

33. Acantholytic cells are seen in *[NBE FMGE March 2012]*
 a. Pemphigus vulgaris b. Bullous Pemphigoid
 c. Cicatricial Pemphigoid d. Dermatitis herpetiformis

34. Intercellular antibodies deposition on immunofluorescence is seen in *[NBE FMGE March 2012]*
 a. Psoriasis b. Pemphigus
 c. Pemphigoid d. Prophyria

35. Level of split in Pemphigus foliaceus is at the level of? *[Recent Question 2017]*
 a. Stratum corneum b. Stratum spinosum
 c. Stratum granulosum d. Stratum basale

36. Which of the following disease is closely related to Enteropathy? *[Recent Question 2017]*
 a. Linear Ig A disease
 b. Pemphigus foliaceous
 c. Dermatitis herpetiformis
 d. Erythema multiforme

37. HLA DR3 is associated with? *[Recent Question 2017]*
 a. Dermatitis herpetiformis
 b. Pemphigus vulgaris
 c. Behcet disease
 d. Psoriasis vulgaris

38. Female with tense bullae over erythematous base. Diagnosis is? *[Recent Question 2017]*
 a. Pemphigus erythematosus
 b. Bullous Pemphigoid
 c. Pemphigus vulgaris
 d. Pemphigus vegetans

39. Which of the following drug is used for the treatment of Dermatitis herpetiformis? *[Recent Question 2017]*
 a. Acitretin b. Methotrexate
 c. Cyclophosphamide d. Sulphapyridine

40. A patient presenting with tense bullae on erythematous base. On histopathological examination following can be seen? *[Recent Question 2017]*
 a. Subcorneal split
 b. Subepidermal split
 c. Fishnet pattern
 d. Raw of tomb stones appearance

41. Pemphigus vulgaris is caused due to which type of hypersensitivity reaction? *[Recent Question 2017]*
 a. I b. II
 c. III d. IV

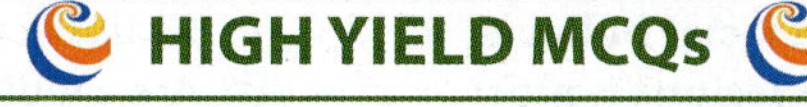

HIGH YIELD MCQs

1. Hailey-Hailey disease is *[Jharkhand PGMEE 2003]*
 a. Benign familial chronic pemphigus
 b. Pemphigus acutus
 c. Pemphigus
 d. Lyell's syndrome

2. Intra-epidermal lesions seen in *[PGI 2008]*
 a. Pemphigus vulgaris
 b. Epidermolysis bullosa acquisita
 c. Dermatitis Herpetiformis
 d. Bullous pemphigoid
 e. Paraneoplastic pemphigus

3. Sub-epidermal splitting is not found in *[PGI 1999]*
 a. Bullous pemphigoid
 b. Pemphigus foliaceus
 c. Dermatitis herpetiformis
 d. Burns

4. Acantholytic cell in pemphigus is derived from *[AIIMS PGMEE 1993]*
 a. Stratum granulosum b. Stratum basale
 c. Stratum spinosum d. Langerhans cell

5. Subepidermal blistreing is seen in all except *[JIPMER PGMEE 1991, AMU PGMEE 1996]*
 a. Pemphigus vulgaris
 b. Dermatitis herpetiformis
 c. Toxic epidermal necrolysis
 d. Bullous pemphigoid
 e. Hailey-Hailey disease

6. Subepidermal lesion are *[PGI 2009]*
a. Bullous pemphigoid b. Pemphigus vulgaris
c. Hailey-Hailey disease d. Darier's disease
e. Acanthosis nigricans

7. Intra epithelial bulla is seen in *[All India PGMEE 1991]*
a. Pemphigus
b. Pemphigoid
c. Dermatitis herpetiformis
d. Light eruption

8. Subepidermal bulla are seen in *[AIIMS PGMEE 1991]*
a. Pemphigoid b. Pemphigus
c. Pityriasis rosea d. Psoriasis

9. Intraepidermal vesicles are seen in *[PGI 2004]*
a. Pemphigus vulgaris
b. Carcinomatous pemphigus
c. Dermatitis herpetiformis
d. Congenital epidermolysis bullosa
e. Trauma

10. Intradermal acantholytic blister is seen in *[PGI 2006]*
a. Pemphigus vulgaris
b. Bullous pemphigoid
c. Dermatitis herpetiformis
d. Epidermolysis bullosa

11. Intraepidermal Bullae are seen in *[AIIMS PGMEE 1995]*
a. Pemphigoid
b. Pemphigus
c. D. Herpetiformis
d. Light reaction

12. Acantholytic cells in pemphigus is *[PGI 1996]*
a. Cell with hyperchromatic nuclei and perinuclear halo
b. Cell with hypochromatic nuclei and perinuclear halo
c. Multinucleated cells
d. None of the above

13. A 40 years old male reported with recurrent episodes of oral ulcers, large areas of denuded skin and flaccid vesiculo-bullous eruptions. Which is the most important bed-side investigation helpful in establishing the diagnosis? *[Karnataka PGMEE 1994]*
a. Gram staining of the blister fluid
b. Culture and sensitivity
c. Skin biopsy and immunofluorescence
d. Tzanck smear from the floor of bulla

14. A 50 years old man has a 2 years history of facial bullae & oral ulcers. A microscopic smear from skin lesions is most likely to disclose *[All India PGMEE 1996]*
a. Tzanck cells b. Acantholytic cells
c. Necrosis d. Koilogytosis

15. Acantholysis is seen in *[AIIMS PGMEE 1991]*
a. Pemphigoid b. Pemphigus vulgaris
c. Erythema multiforme d. Dermatitis herpetiformis

16. A middle aged female has flaccid bullae in the skin and oral erosion. Histopathology shows intraepidermal acantholytic blisters. The most likely diagnosis is *[PGI 2005]*
a. Pemphigus vulgaris
b. Paraneoplastic pemphigus
c. Bullous pemphigoid
d. Dermatitis herpetiformis
e. Epidermolysis bullosa acquisita

17. Acantholysis is seen in all of the following except *[MP PGMEE 2006]*
a. Pemphigus
b. Bullous pemphigoid
c. Steven-Johnson syndrome
d. Toxic epidermonecrolysis

18. Nikolsky sign is positive in all except *[AIIMS PGMEE 2000]*
a. Pemphigus
b. Bullous pemphigoid
c. Toxic epidermal Necrolysis
d. Staphylococcal skin scaled syndrome

19. Nikolsky sign not present in *[BIHAR PGMEE 2006]*
a. Pemphigus b. Pemphigoid
c. Vitiligo
d. Staphylococcal scalded syndrome

20. A patient developed bullae without erythema on elbows, knee & sacral area f/b crust formation, scarring & milia. He had no photo sensitivity and negative family history for bullous diseases. On DIF IgG deposition at DEJ with no blood vessel involvement is seen probable diagnosis is *[AIIMS PGMEE 2007]*
a. EB dystrophic b. EB acquisita
c. Porphyria CT d. Pemphigoid bullous

21. In a 8 days old child with no history of consanguinity in the parents. The mother reports blisters and peeling off of skin at the site of handling and pressure. There was a similar history in previous child which proved to be fatal. The diagnosis *[AIIMS PGMEE 2001]*
a. Bullous pemphigoid b. Congenital Syphilis
c. Congenital Epidermolysis bullosa
d. Litterer-Siwe disease

22. Etiology of Epidermolysis bullosa is *[Rohtak PGMEE 1997]*
a. Genetic b. Infections
c. Senile d. Malignant
e. Metabolic

23. In congenital dystrophic epidermolysis bullosa defect is seen in *[AIIMS PGMEE 2008]*
a. Laminin 4 b. Collagen type 7
c. Collagen 4 d. Collagen 3

24. All are true about linear IgA disease except *[PGI 2001]*
a. Subepidermal involvement
b. Severe itching
c. Granular deposition of IgA
d. Are candidates for gluten free diet
e. A variant of dermatitis herpetiformis

25. A 24 years old female has flaccid bullae in the skin and oral erosions. Histopathology shows intraepidermal acantholytic blister. The most likely diagnosis is *[AIIMS PGMEE 2003]*
a. Pemphigoid b. Erythema multiforme
c. Pemphigus vulgaris d. Dermatitis herpetiformis

26. A 50 years old male known case of myasthenia with erythematic shallow erosions with few blisters and scales. Oral mucosa is not involved Immunopathology demonstrates IgG deposition on keratinocytes and auto antibodies against Dsg-1. The diagnosis is *[PGI 1998]*
a. Pemphigus vulgaris b. Bullous pemphigoid
c. Pemphigus foliaceus d. Dermatitis herpetiformis

27. Rarest variety of pemphigus is *[JIPMER PGMEE 1980, AMU PGMEE 1984]*
a. P. vulgaris b. P. foliaceus
c. P. vegetans d. P. erythematosis

28. A 30 years old male had severely itchy papula-vesicular lesions on extremities, knees, elbows and buttocks for one year. Direct immunofluorescence staining of the lesions showed IgA deposition at dermoepidermal junction. The most probable diagnosis is *[Recent Question 2016, All India PGMEE 2004]*
a. Pemphigus vulagris b. Bullous pemphigoid
c. Dermatitis herpetiformis d. Nummular eczema

29. A 40-year-old male developed persistent oral ulcers followed by multiple flaccid bullae on trunk and extremities. Direct examination of a skin biopsy immunofluorescence showed intercellular IgG deposits in the epidermis. The most probable diagnosis is *[All India PGMEE 2003]*
a. Pemphigus vulgaris
b. Bullous Pemphigoid
c. Bullous Lupus erythematosus
d. Epidermolysis bullosa acquisita

30. Extremely pruritic excoriation & papules on buttocks with autoantibodies against epidermal transglutaminase and IgA deposition in dermis on immuno-histological examination of normal perilesional skin. Diagnosis is *[SGPGI 2001]*
a. Pemphigus vulgaris b. Pemphigoid
c. Linear IgA disease d. Dermatitis herpetiformis

31. A patient with Bullous eruption on lower limb and trunk, biopsy show epidermal bullae. The correct diagnosis is *[All India PGMEE 2000]*
a. Pemphigoid b. Pemphigus vulgaris
c. Impetigo d. Internal Malignancy

32. A 56 years old male lallu presents with painful bullous lesion in lower extremity, the most likely diagnosis is *[AIIMS PGMEE 1997]*
a. Pemphigus Vulgaris b. Bullous pemphigoid
c. Necrotic Pemphigus d. Contact eczema

33. A 85 years old woman with Nikolsky sign-ve, blisters on thigh & trunk, lesions come on & off. What is the cause *[PGI 2000]*
a. Pemphigus vulgaris b. Pemphigoid
c. Lichen planus d. Dermatitis herpetiformis
e. Leprosy

34. A young boy with multiple flaccid bullous lesions over trunk with oral mucosal lesions. Most likely finding on biopsy would be *[AIIMS PGMEE 2009]*
a. 'Fishnet' IgG deposits in epidermis
b. Linear IgG in Deposits
c. Linear IgA in dermal papillae
d. Granular IgA in reticular dermis

35. A female presents with persistent painful oral lesions, with acantholytic cells. Most likely diagnosis is *[All India PGMEE 2008]*
a. Pemphigus vulgaris b. Dermatitis herpetiformis
c. Epidermolysis bullosa d. Bullous pemphigoid

36. A 40 years old male had multiple blisters over the trunk & Extremities. Direct Immunofluoresce studies showed linear IgG deposits along the Basement membrane, which of the following is the most likely diagnosis. *[AIIMS PGMEE 2004]*
a. Pemphigus vulgaris b. Bullous pemphigoid
c. Pemphigus foliaceous d. Dermatitis herpetiformis

37. Spontaneous remission is most frequent with *[SGPGI 2004]*
a. Herpes labialis b. Herpes genitalis
c. Herpetic chancroid d. Herpes gestationis

38. Commonest site of Herpes Gestationalis is *[AIIMS PGMEE 1993, Delhi PGMEE 2002]*
a. Periumbilical region b. Flanks of abdomen
c. Vulva d. Infraorbital

39. A 28 years old patient has multiple grouped papulo-vesicular lesions on both elbows, knees buttocks and upper back associated with severe itching. The most likely diagnosis is *[AIIMS PGMEE 2002]*
a. Pemphigus vulgaris
b. Bullous pemphigoid
c. Dermatitis Herpetiformis
d. Herpes Zoster

40. A 25 years old female has palatal ulcer (vesicular lesion in buccal mucosa) and skin blister most likely diagnosis is *[All India PGMEE 1997]*
a. Pemphigus vulgaris b. Pemphigus Foliaceous
c. Dermatitis herpetiformisd. Pemphigoid

41. The treatment of Dermatitis herpetiformis is *[All India PGMEE 2002]*
a. Gluten free diet with minerals and vitamins
b. Carbamazepine
c. Acyclovir
d. Corticosteroids

42. A 60-year-old patient presented with several bullous lesions for the last 3 days; each bulla was surrounded by an erythematous halo. There were multiple target lesions. Patient also had oral erosions. The most likely diagnosis is *[SGPGI 2004]*
a. Chicken pox b. Herpes simplex
c. Herpes zoster d. Steven-Johnson syndrome

43. An eight years old boy presents with multiple umbilicated pearly white papules on trunk & face. Diagnosis is *[AIIMS PGMEE 1998]*
a. Molluscum contagiosum b. Chicken Pox
c. Herpes zoster d. Dermatophytosis

44. A 45 years old male has multiple grouped vesicular lesions present on the T10 segment dermatome associated with pain. The most likely diagnosis is *[AIIMS PGMEE 2002]*
a. Herpes zoster b. Dermatitis herpetiformis
c. Herpes simplex d. Scabies

45. Inter cellular IgG deposition in epidermis is seen in *[AIIMS PGMEE 2009]*
a. Pemphigus
b. Sub corneal pustular dermatosis
c. Bullous pemphigoid
d. Dermatitis herpetiformis

46. Intra epidermal blisters are seen in *[PGI 2009]*
a. Bullous pemphigoid
b. Pemphigus folliaceous
c. Dermatitis herpetiformis

d. Bullous impetigo
e. Pemphigus vulgaris

47. All are Vesiculo-bullous lesions except *[Kerala PGMEE 1996]*
a. Dermatitis Herpetiformis
b. Scabies
c. Pemphigus
d. Pemphigoid

48. Subepithelial Bullae are seen in *[AIIMS PGMEE 1991]*
a. Dermatitis herpetiformis b. Molluscumcontagiosum
c. Pemphigus d. Pemphigoid

49. All of the following are bullous lesions except *[SGPGI 2003]*
a. Pemphigus vulgaris b. Dermatitis herpetiformis
c. Atopic dermatitis d. Pemphigoid

50. Nikolsky sign is positive in all of the following except *[MP PGMEE 2006]*
a. Staphylococcal scalded skin syndrome
b. Toxic epidermonecrolysis
c. Bullous pemphigoid
d. Pemphigus

51. Nikolsky sign is seen in *[PGI 1986]*
a. Pemphigus vulgaris b. Herpes zoster
c. Herpes simplex d. Leukemia
e. All of the above

52. True about pemphigus vulgaris all except *[PGI 2009]*
a. Subepidermal
b. Autoimmune disease
c. Tzanck smear shows acantholytic cells
d. Antibody are formed against desmogleins
e. Blister on skin & mucosa

53. 'Row of tombstones' appearance is seen in *[JIPMER PGMEE 1998, PGI 2002]*
a. Irritant dermatitis b. Pemphigus
c. Pemphigoid d. Herpes zoster

54. Commonest variety of Pemphigus *[Kerala PGMEE 1987]*
a. Pemphigus vulgaris b. Pemphigus vegetans
c. Pemphigus foliaceus d. Pemphigus erythematosis

55. Granular IgA deposits at dermal papilla are found in *[AIIMS PGMEE 2009]*
a. Dermatitis herpetiformis b. IgA disease of childhood
c. Herpetic gestation d. Bullous pemphigoid

56. DOC for Dermatitis herpetiformis is *[AIIMS PGMEE 1991, 1992, 1997, 2005]*
a. Steroids b. Dapsone
c. PUVA d. Antihistaminic

57. All are associated with pemphigus except *[SGPGI 2002, PGI 1998]*
a. Thymoma b. CLL
c. Myasthenia gravis d. Non-Hodgkins lymphoma
e. Atrophic gastritis

58. Drug induced pemphigus is seen in all except *[All India PGMEE 1994]*
a. Penicillin b. Phenolphtha
c. Iodine d. Frusemide

59. HLA associated with Dermatitis herpetiformis *[All India PGMEE 1998]*
a. HLA A5 b. HLB B8
c. HLA B27 d. HLA A28

60. In pemphigus vulgaris, antibodies are present against *[PGI 2000]*
a. Basement membrane b. Intercellular substance
c. Cell nucleus d. Keratin
e. Cell membrane

61. All are true about Dermatitis herpetiformis except *[Jharkhand PGME 2005]*
a. More common in young adult
b. Intense pruritus
c. Deposits of IgG at the epidermodermal lesion
d. None

62. Blister formation in burn case is in *[Bihar PGMEE 2006]*
a. Intraepidermal b. Subepidermal
c. Subdermal d. Subfascial

63. Acantholysis is characteristic of *[All India PGMEE 2003, AIIMS PGMEE 1991]*
a. Pemphigus vulgaris b. Pemphigoid
c. Erythema multiforme d. Dermatitis herpetiformis

64. Ballooning is characteristic of *[JIPMER PGMEE 1992]*
a. Herpes zoster b. Pemphigus
c. Pemphigoid d. Insect bite

65. In pemphigus vulgaris, antibodies are present against *[SGPGI 2000]*
a. Basement membrane b. Intercellular substance
c. Keratin d. Cell nucleus

66. Correct regarding Hailey-Hailey disease is/are *[PGI November 2014]*
a. Steroid no use b. ATP2C1 impairment
c. Autosomal recessive d. Flexural distribution
e. Benign pemphigus

67. A 20 years old patient with Neurocysticercosis develops Generalised peeling of skin (Except palms and soles) starting one month after taking medications for seizures. Most probable diagnosis is *[AIIMS November 2015]*
a. Stevens Johnson syndrome
b. TEN
c. Pemphigus vulgaris
d. Fixed drug eruption

68. Pemphigus neonatorum is a variety of *[PGMCET 2015]*
a. Bullous impetigo
b. Epidermolysis Bullosa
c. Congenital syphilis
d. Pemphigus

NEET/NBE PATTERN MCQs ANSWERS WITH EXPLANATIONS

1. **Ans. (c) Pemphigus erythematous**
[Ref. Clinical Dermatology by Habif, 6/e p669]

Pemphigus Erythematosus/ Senear-Usher Syndrome
- May be a combination of localized pemphigus foliaceus and systemic lupus erythematosus, because many of these patients have a positive antinuclear antibody
- If the eruption becomes more diffuse or generalized, the term pemphigus foliaceus is used

2. **Ans. (d) P. neoplastic**
[Ref. Clinical Eye Atlas by Gold, 2/e p59]

Paraneoplastic Pemphigus
- Paraneoplastic autoimmune multi-organ syndrome
- Least common and most severe form of pemphigus
- Shares clinical features of both Pemphigus and Severe erythema multiforme
- Shows cutaneous and systemic involvement
- Autoimmune disease of the skin and oral mucosa that develops in patients with an underlying neoplasm, most typically non-Hodgkins lymphoma
- Erosions of the oral cavity, and large, tense bullae

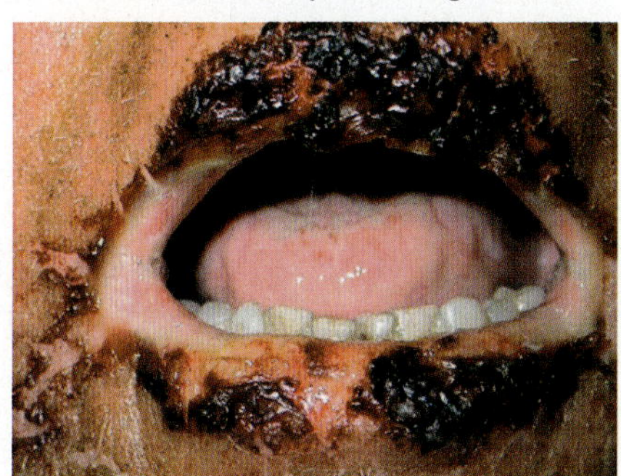

Fig. Paraneoplastic pemphigus

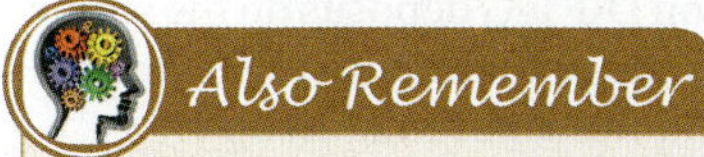

Also Remember
- Pemphigus vulgaris is MC type of Pemphigus

3. **Ans. (a) Acantholytic cells**
[Ref. DVL by Thappa, 4/e p36, 37]
- Tzanck smear is used to diagnose various skin disorders characterized by vesicles, pustules, bullae, erosion & in particular viral infections like HSV, herpes zoster, & varicella infection

Disease	Interpretation of Tzanck smear
Viral infections: HSV, varicella, Herpes zoster	Multinucleated gaint cells
Pemphigus	Acantholytic epidermal cells
SSSS & Bullous impetigo	Dyskeratotic acantholytic cells
Mollusca contagiosum	Intracytoplasmic inclusion bodies Henderson- Paterson bodies
Spongiotic vascular dementia	> 10 tadpole cells at X100 magnification is an indicator

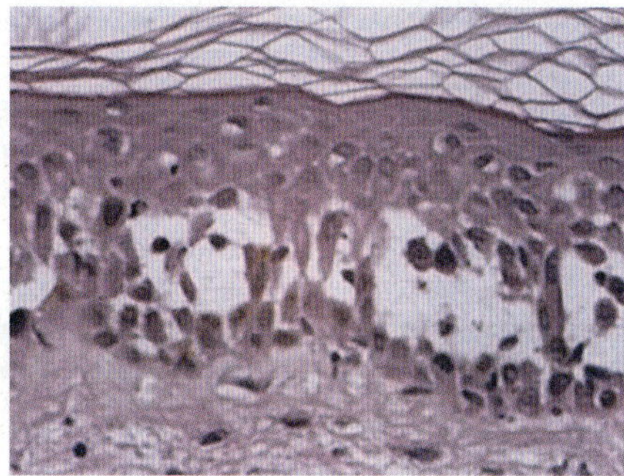

Fig. Pemphigus—Acantholytic cells

4. **Ans. (c) Collagen 7**
[Ref. Clinical dermatology by Habif, 6/e p666]

Dystrophic Epidermolysis Bullosa
- Blistering in response to the slightest trauma
- Repetitive trauma leads to a mitten-like deformity with digits encased in an epidermal "cocoon"
- This is due to defect in collagen 7

5. **Ans. (b) Pemphigus**
[Ref. DVL by Thappa, 4/e p167]

Pemphigus
- Auto immune intra-epidermal blistering disorder of skin & mucosa
- Signs positive: Nikolsky's sign positive, Bullae spread sign may or may not be positive
- HPE findings: Supra-basal clefting with blister cavity containing acantholytic cells & loss of intracellular attachment in basal layer giving a "row of tomb stone appearance"

6. **Ans. (a) Bullous impetigo**
[Ref. Tropical Dermatology and Venereology by Schaller, 1/e Fig. 3.56]
- Severe highly contagious Bullous impetigo in infants 4–10 days old used to be called Pemphigus neonatorum or Ritter's disease

7. **Ans. (b) Erythropoietic porphyria**
[Ref. Paediatric Emergency Medicine by Cameron, 1/e p332]

Erythropoietic protoporphyria
- MC childhood porphyria
- Congenital erythropoietic porphyria is rare and presents in early childhood with extreme photosensitivity leading to painful blisters
- As with other photosensitivity syndromes, the rash can occur rapidly or days after the sun exposure

8. **Ans. (a) Pemphigus vulgaris**
[Ref. Clinical Dermatology by Habif, 6/e p667,669]

Pemphigus Vulgaris
- MC form of pemphigus
- Non-pruritic acid blisters varying in size from 1 cm to several centimetres appear gradually on normal or erythematous skin and may be localized for a considerable time

- MC sites are the scalp, face, axillae, and oral cavity
- Blisters invariably become generalized if left untreated
- Blisters rupture easily because the vesicle roof, which consists of only a thin portion of the upper epidermis, is fragile
- Application of pressure to small intact bullae causes the fluid to dissect laterally into the mid-epidermal areas altered by bound IgG (Nikolsky's sign)

9. Ans. (b) Desmoglein-3
[Ref. Clinical Dermatology by Habif, 6/e p638, 647]

Pemphigus Type	Target Desmosomal Protein
Pemphigus vulgaris	Desmoglein 3
Pemphigus foliceus	Desmoglein 1
Paraneoplastic pemphigus	DS 3, desmoplakin 1 & 2, envoplakin, periplakin, BP230
IgA pemphigus	Desmocolin 1

10. Ans. (a) Pemphigus vulgaris
[Ref. Dermatology by Bolognia, 1/e p216]

Pemphigus Vulgaris
- MC form of pemphigus
- MC sites are the scalp, face, axillae, and oral cavity
- Additional clinical clues for the diagnosis include the development of hemorrhagic crusts of the vermilion lips and a positive Nikolsky sign in areas of active disease - the epidermis can be easily moved laterally with rubbing (due to reduction in intercellular adhesion)

11. Ans. (d) VII
[Ref. Clinical Dermatology by Habif, 6/e p638]

Bullous disease	Target molecule
Bullous pemphigoid (BP)	BP180, BP230 (hemidesmosome and lamina lucida)
Herpes gestations	BP180, BP230 (hemidesmosome and lamina lucida)
Cicatricial pemphigoid	BP180, laminin V (hemidesmosome and lamina lucida
Epidermolysis bullosa acquisita	Type VII collagen (anchoring fibrils)
Bullous SLE	Type VII collagen (anchoring fibrils)
Linear IgA disease	LAD antigen (BP180) (hemidesmosome and lamina lucida)
Dermatitis herpetiformis	Unknown

12. Ans. (b) Bullous pemphigoid
[Ref. Clinical Dermatology by Habif, 6/e p655]

Subepidermal Vesiculobullous disorders
- Bullous pemphigoid
- Pemphigoid gestationis
- Mucus membrane/Cicatricial pemphigoid
- Dermatitis herpetiformis
- Linear IgA disease and Chronic bullous disease of childhood
- Bullous lupus erythematosus
- Epidermolysis bullosa acquisita
- Junctional epidermolysis bullosa
- Dystrophic epidermolysis bullosa
- Bullous drug eruption
- Porphyria & Pseudoporphyria

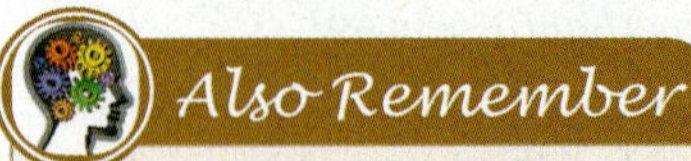

Bullous Pemphigoid
- Most common autoimmune blistering skin disease and is associated with an increased mortality.
- Bullous pemphigoid, herpes gestationis, and cicatricial pemphigoid are autoimmune subepidermal vesiculobullous diseases with circulating IgG and basement membrane zone-bound IgG antibodies and C3

13. Ans. (a) Bullous pemphigoid
[Ref. Clinical Dermatology by Habif, 6/e 655]

Bullous pemphigoid
- Presence of Oral blisters
- Pemphigoid begins with a localized area of erythema or with pruritic urticarial plaques that gradually become more edematous and extensive
- MC sites: Lower part of the abdomen, the groin, and the flexor surfaces of the arms and legs

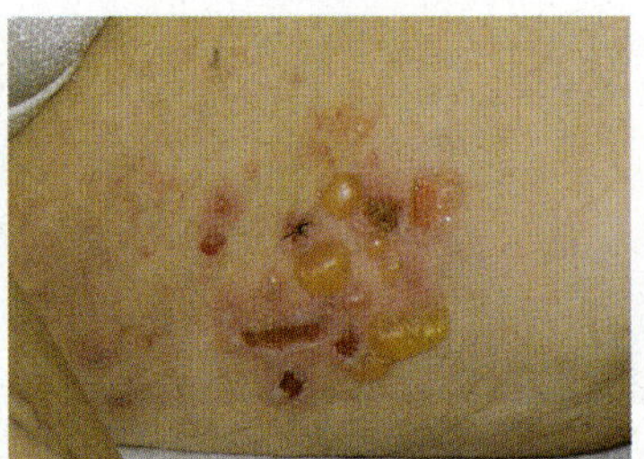

Fig. Bullous pemphigoid

14. Ans. (a) Intercellular IgG deposition
[Ref. DVL by Thappa, 4/e p167]
- In pemphigus vulagaris on DIF IgG deposits on the surface of keratinocytes through the epidermis giving a "Fish net appearance" under the fluorescence microscope
- Less frequently C3, IgM, IgA can also be deposited

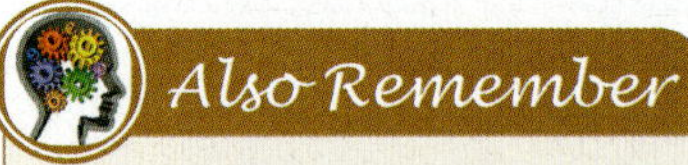

- In contrast Bullous Pemphigoid has linear deposits of C3 or C3 IgG deposit along basement membrane zone

15. Ans. (a) Pemphigus vulgaris
[Ref. Pemphigus in India by Kanwar, IJDVL, 77(4) Pg. 439-449]
- *MC Pemphigus in India*: Pemphigus vulgaris [> Pemphigus foliaceus> Pemphigus erythematosus> Pemphigus vegetans]

16. Ans. (a) Hailey-Hailey disease
[Ref. Dermatology and Sexually Transmitted Diseases by Neena Khanna, 5/e p 84]
- Familial benign pemphigus is also known as Hailey-Hailey disease

17. Ans. (c) Suprabasal acantholytic blister
[Ref. Neena Khanna, 4/e p71-73]

Clinical Presentation of Pemphigus: Acantholytic Bullae

- *Pemphigus vulgaris*: Suprabasal split
  - Nikolsky sign
  - Bulla-spread sign
  - Scalp, face, trunk, mucosal lesions
  - Sepsis and electrolyte imbalance
- *Pemphigus vegetans*: Suprabasal split
  - Heaped-up vegetating lesions
  - Groins, axilla, angles of mouth, mucosal
- *Pemphigus foliaceus*: Split in granular layer or just below horny layer
  - Transient superficial bullae rupture to form crusts/ scales
- *Pemphigus erythematosus*: Split in granular layer or just below stratum corneum
  - Less severe form of P. foliaceus
  - Dry, hyperkeratotic lesions on face (malar region)

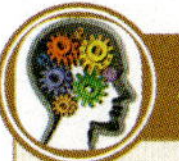

Also Remember

Uses of Azelaic Acid

- Acne
- Rosacea
- Pigment disorders: Melasma, Post-inflammatory Hyperpigmentation
- Hair growth stimulant

18. Ans. (b) Intraepidermal

[Ref. Dermatology by Braun-Falco, 1/e p12]

Blisters

- Subcorneal (impetigo)
- Intraepidermal (pemphigus vulgaris)
- Subepidermal (bullous pemphigoid)
- Dermal (dystrophic epidermolysis bullosa)

19. Ans. (c) Dapsone

[Ref. Neena Khanna, 5/e p 449]

- **Dapsone is drug of choice:**
  - Dermatitis herpetiformis
  - Erythema elevatumdiutinum

20. Ans. (d) Gluten sensitive enteropathy

[Ref. Neena Khanna, 4/e p80]

Dermatitis Herpetiformis

- Type of disorder: Dermo-epidermal bullous disorder
- *Underlying cause*: Gluten sensitive enteropathy (GSE)
- *Clinical presentation*: Associated 100% with GSE
  - Itchy grouped papules or vesicles
  - Eczematous changes and secondary infection
  - Most frequent on extensor surfaces

Also Remember

Skin Manifestations associated with Ulcerative Colitis and Crohn's Disease

- Erythema nodosum
- Pyoderma gangrenosum
- Aphthous stomatitis
- Mucosal nodularity (Cobblestoning): Crohn's disease mainly
- Pyostomatitis vegetans: Ulcerative colitis mainly
- Perianal ulcers/ fistulae: Crohn's disease mainly

21. Ans. (b) Suprabasal

[Ref. Neena Khanna, 5/e p 79]

Pemphigus is classified based on level of split:

Pemphigus vulgaris	Split is suprabarsal
Pemphigus vegetans	Split is suprabarsal
Pemphigus foliaceus	Split is either in granulosa layer or just below horny layer

22. Ans. (b) Pemphigus

[Ref. Dermatology by Braun-Falco, 1/e p12]

23. Ans. (a) Pemphigus

[Ref. Neena Khanna, 5/e p 79]

- Pemphigus is an autoimmune disorder characterized by presence of IgG autoantibodies against desmogleins (Dsg)

24. Ans. (a) Acantholytic cells

[Ref. Neena Khanna, 5/e p 79 & Figure 5.5]

- Acantholytic cells (Tzanck cell) appear as round cells with perinuclear halo in Tzanck smear, and characteristic of Pemphigus.

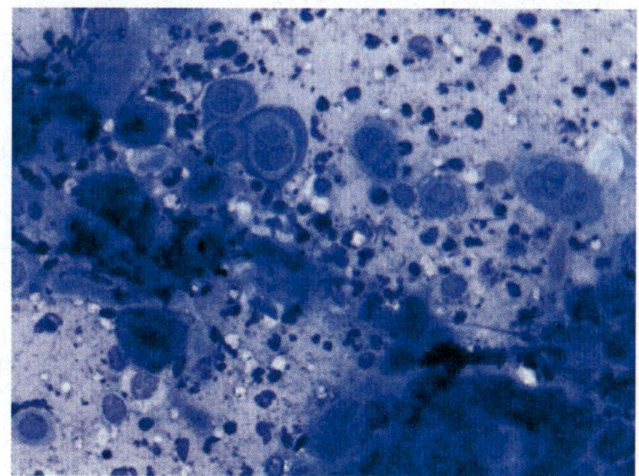

Fig. Acantholytic cells

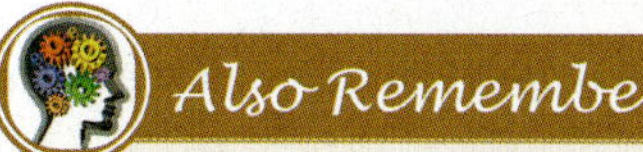

Also Remember

- Key Tzanck Smear Features in Bullous Disorders
  - Pemphigus: Acantholytic cells
  - Bullous pemphigoid: Eosinophilic predominance
  - Herpes simplex/ Varicella zoster: Multinucleate giant cells
  - Toxic epidermal necrolysis (TEN): Necrotic ells

25. Ans. (d) Bullous phemphigoid

[Ref. Neena Khanna, 5/e p78,79,85]

26. Ans. (a) Pemphigus vulgaris

[Ref. Neena Khanna, 4/e p73]

27. Ans. (a) Eczema; (b) Impetigo; (d) Pemphigus vulgaris; (e) Burns

[A Manual of Dermatology by Zohra Zaidi, 2/e p335]

- Some causes of Acantholytic bullae are eczema, impetigo, fungal infections (zoophilic), superficial burns, viral infections and pemphigus

28. Ans. (d) Lichen planus

[Ref. Neena Khanna, 5/e p 62]

29. Ans. (c) Pemphigus foliaceous

[Ref. Neena Khanna, 4/e p253]

- *Mucosal involvement is seen in*:
  - Pemphigus vulgaris
  - Pemphigus vegetans
  - Paraneoplastic Pemphigus
  - Bullous pemphigoid
  - Epidermolysis bullosa
- *Mucosal involvement is NOT seen in*:
  - Pemphigus foliaceous
  - Pemphigus erythematosus

30. Ans. (c) Pemphigus vulgaris

[Ref. Neena Khanna, 5/e p 79]

- In pemphigus vulgaris, when tangential pressure is applied over pre-existing bulla, it results in spread of bulla which is known as 'bulla spread sign' or 'Asboe-Hansen sign'

31. Ans. (a) Acanthosis

[Ref. Neena Khanna, 4/e p74]

Diagnostic tests of pemphigus:

- Tzanck smear: Show acantholytic cells
- Biopsy of edge of bulla:
  - **Split in supra-basal layer**
  - **Presence of acantholytic cells**
- Direct immunofluorescence of peri-lesional skin: ***'Fishnet appearance'*** due to IgG intercellular deposits
- ELISA/ IIF: Circulating antibodies to desmoglobins

32. Ans. (c) Dapsone

[Ref. Neena Khanna, 4/e p82]

Dermatitis Herpetiformis

- *Type of disorder*: Dermo-epidermal bullous disorders
- *Underlying cause*: Gluten sensitive enteropathy (GSE)
- *Clinical presentation*: Associated 100% with GSE
  - Itchy grouped papules or vesicles
  - Eczematous changes and secondary infection
  - Most frequent on extensor surfaces
- *Diagnostic tests*:
  - Biopsy: Dermo-epidermal split with microabscesses at tip of dermal papillae
  - Direct immunoflorescence: IgA deposits in dermal papillae
- *Treatment*:
  - Gluten-free diet
  - Dapsone (Drug of choice)
  - Sulphapyridine

33. Ans. (a) Pemphigus vulgaris

[Ref. Neena Khanna, 4/e p74]

Pemphigus – Intraepidermal Bullous Disorders

- *Definition*: Intra-epidermal bullous disorder characterised clinically by blisters and histologically by acantholysis (separation of viable epidermal cells)
- *Underlying cause*:
  - IgG antibodies: Against Desmoglobins
  - Neoplasms: Thymoma, lymphoma
  - Drugs: Penicillamine (Most common), Rifampicin, Captopril
- *Clinical types of Pemphigus*:
  - Pemphigus vulgaris
  - Pemphigus vegetans
  - Pemphigus foliaceus
  - Pemphigus erythematosus
- *Diagnostic tests*:
  - Tzanck smear: Show acantholytic cells
  - Biopsy of edge of bulla:
  - Split in supra-basal layer
  - Presence of acantholytic cells
  - Direct immunofluorescence: *'Fishnet appearance'* due to intercellular deposit of IgG throughout epidermis
  - ELISA/ IIF: Circulating antibodies to desmoglobins
- *Treatment*:
  - Corticosteroids
  - Immunosuppressants: Azathioprine, Methotrexate, Cyclophosphamide
  - Other drugs: Mycophenolate mofetil, I/V IgG, Plasmapheresis

34. Ans. (b) Pemphigus

[Ref. Neena Khanna, 4/e p75]

35. Ans. (c) Stratum granulosum

[Ref. Robbins Basic Pathology, 9/e p859]

Pemphigus foliaceus (PF)

- Generally a benign variety of Pemphigus
- An autoimmune skin disorder characterized by the loss of intercellular adhesion of keratinocytes in the upper parts of the epidermis (acantholysis), resulting in the formation of superficial blisters
- Acantholysis selectively involves the superficial epidermis at the level of the stratum granulosum
- Typified by clinical involvement of healthy-appearing skin that blisters when rubbed (the Nikolsky sign)

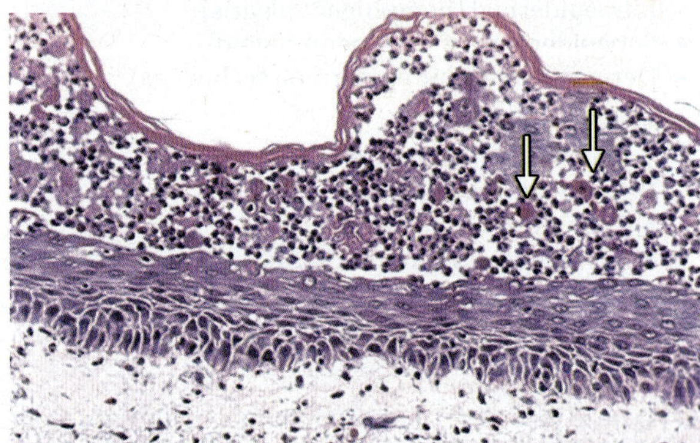

Fig. Pemphigus foliaceus (with Acantholysis – Arrows)

36. Ans. (c) Dermatitis herpetiformis

[Ref. Oral Pathology by Regezi, 6/e p18]

- Dermatitis herpetiformis is strongly associated with Celiac disease (Gluten-sensitive enteropathy)
- Approximately, 70% of patients with dermatitis herpetiformis show evidence of villous atrophy on small bowel biopsy

37. Ans. (a) Dermatitis herpetiformis

[Ref. Ferri's Clinical Advisor 2015, p365]

Dermatitis Herpetiformis

- An immunologically mediated blistering disease
- Strong association of with HLA-B8, HLA-DR3
- Gluten-sensitive enteropathy is a common association

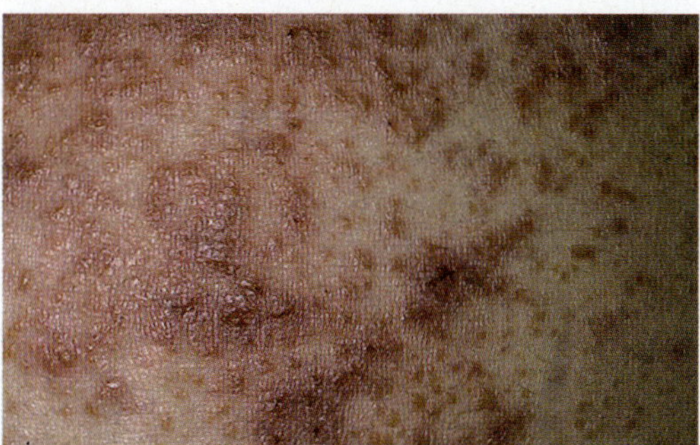

Fig. Dermatitis herpetiformis

38. Ans. (b) Bullous Pemphigoid
[Ref. Hurwitz Clinical Pediatric Dermatology, 5/e p330]

Bullous Pemphigoid

- Blistering disorder characterized by large, tense, subepidermal bullae that appear on normal-appearing or erythematous skin
- Itchy, large, haemorrhagic bullae
- Nikolsky sign NEGATIVE
- Bulla-spread sign NEGATIVE
- Lesions heal with Milia formation (Interepidermal cysts)
- Sites: Thighs, groin, flexures, oro-mucosal
- Secondary infections
- Associated malignancies: Breasts, Lungs, Stomach

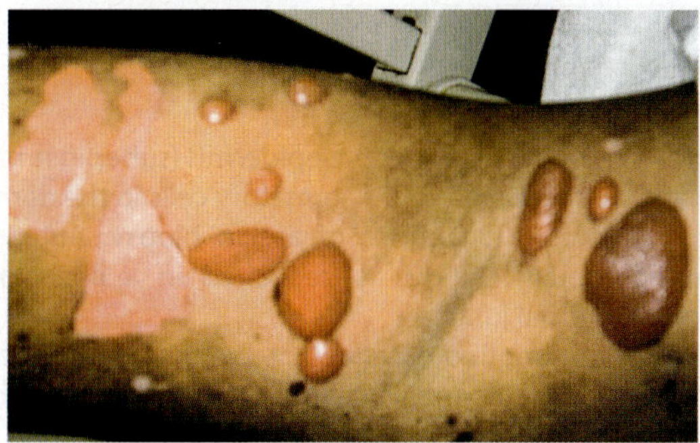

Fig. Bullous Pemphigoid

39. Ans. (d) Sulphapyridine
[Ref. Neena Khanna, 4/e p82]

Treatment of Dermatitis Herpetiformis

- Gluten-free diet
- Dapsone (Drug of choice)
- Sulphapyridine

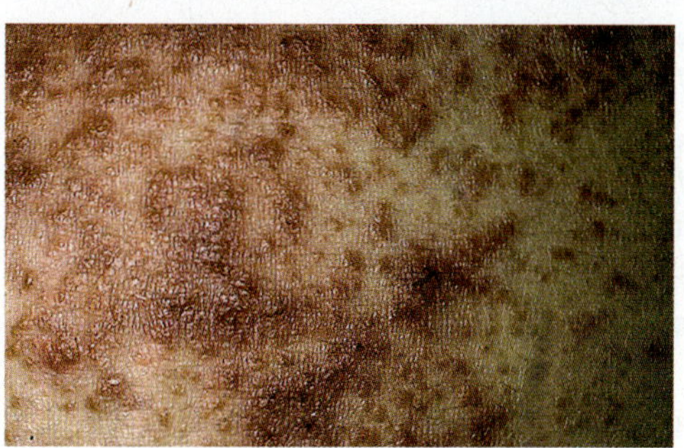

Fig. Dermatitis Herpetiformis

40. Ans. (b) Subepidermal split
[Ref. Hurwitz Clinical Pediatric Dermatology, 5/e p330]

Bullous Pemphigoid

- Blistering disorder characterized by large, tense, subepidermal bullae that appear on normal-appearing or erythematous skin
- Skin biopsy of pemphigoid reveals a subepidermal split, non-necrotic epidermis, and variable inflammation, often with prominent eosinophils
- Pemphigoid group of autoimmune bullous disorders is characterized by subepidermal blister formation due to the loss of adhesion between the basal layer keratinocytes and the underlying basement membrane

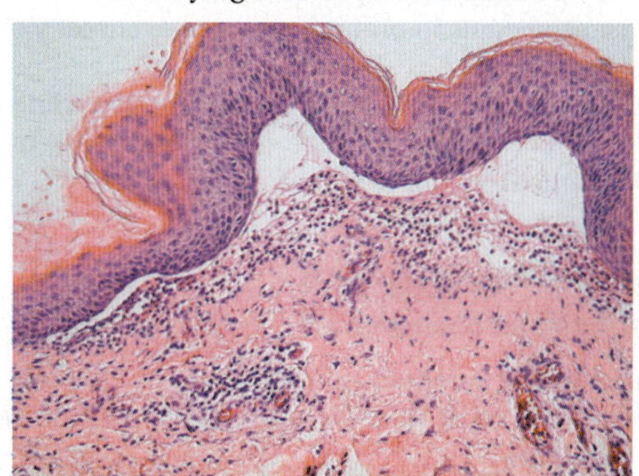

Fig. Subepidermal Split

41. Ans. (b) II
[Ref. Hardcore Pathology by Wahl, 1/e p26]

- Type II hypersensitivity reactions include blood transfusion reactions, Erythroblastosis fetalis, Autoimmune hemolytic anemia, Pemphigus vulgaris, Good pasture syndrome and Graves disease

 HIGH YIELD MCQs ANSWERS WITH EXPLANATIONS 

1. Ans. (a) Benign Familial chronic pemphigus
[Ref. Neena Khanna, 5/e p84]

2. Ans. (a) Pempigus vulgaris; (e) Paraneoplastic pemphigus
[Ref. Dermatology by Otto Braun-Falco, 1/e p12]

3. Ans. (b) Pemphigus foliaceus
[Ref. Neena Khanna, 5/e p79]

4. Ans. (c) Stratum spinosum
[Ref. Neena Khanna, 5/e p79 & Figure 5.5]

5. Ans. (a) Pemphigul vulgaris; (c) Toxic epidermal necrolysis; (e) Hailey-Hailey disease
[Ref. Neena Khanna, 5/e p79]

6. Ans. (a) Bullous pemphigoid
[Ref. Neena Khanna, 5/e p79]

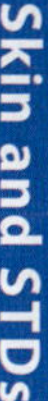

7. Ans. (a) Pemphigus
[Ref. Neena Khanna, 5/e p79]

8. Ans. (a) Pemphigoid
[Ref. Neena Khanna, 5/e p86]
- In pemphigoid, a dermoepidermal bulla with neutrophils and eosinophils both in the bulla and dermis

9. Ans. (a) Pemphigus vulgaris; (b) Carcinomatous pemphigus

10. Ans. (a) Pemphigus vulgaris
[Ref. Neena Khanna, 5/e p79]

11. Ans. (b) Pemphigus
[Ref. Neena Khanna, 5/e p79]

12. Ans. (a) Cell with hyperchromatic nuclei and perinuclear halo
[Ref. Neena Khanna, 5/e p79, Fig. 5.5]
- Acantholytic cells appear as round cells with perinuclear halo in Tzanck smear: Characteristic of Pemphigus

13. Ans. (d) Tzanck smear from the floor of bulla
[Ref. Neena Khanna, 5/e p79]

Characteristics of Pemphigus
- Disease of middle age
- MC cause of autoimmune blistering in India
- Flaccid bullae developed on normal skin
- Disease begins in oral mucosa and eventually oral lesions are universal
- Other mucosa like genitalia & eye are sometime involved
- Scalp, face, flexures (axillae, groins) and trunk are involved
- Periungual lesions frequent
- Oral lesion universal

Also Remember
- Bedside tests of Pemphigus:
  - Demonstration of Nikolsky sign & Bulla spread sign/Asboe-Hansen sign
  - Tzanck smear from the floor of bulla

14. Ans. (b) Acantholytic cells
[Ref. Neena Khanna, 5/e p79]

15. Ans. (b) Pemphigus vulgaris
[Ref. Neena Khanna, 5/e p79 & Fig. 5.5]

16. Ans. (a) Pemphigus vulgaris
[Ref. Neena Khanna, 5/e p79 & Fig. 5.5]

17. Ans. (b) Bullous pemphigoid
[Ref. Neena Khanna, 5/e p78]

18. Ans. (b) Bullous pemphigoid
[Ref. Neena Khanna, 5/e p79]

Nikoklsy's Sign
- Description: Application of tangential pressure on normal skin (usually in peritibial area) results in formation of new bulla
- It is seen in:
  - Pemphigus vulgaris
  - Staphylococcal scalded skin syndrome
  - Epidermal necrolysis

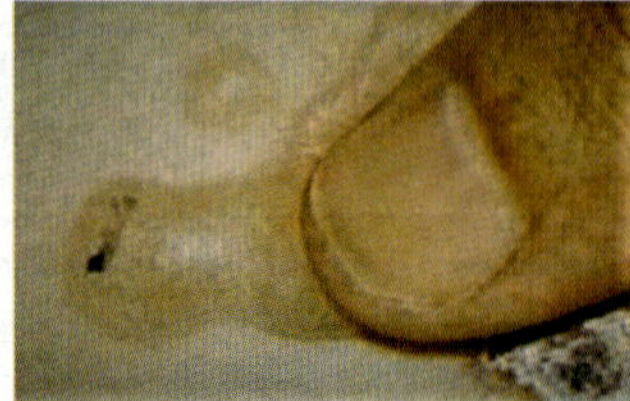

Fig. Nikolsky's sign

19. Ans. (b) Pemphigoid; (c) Vitiligo
[Ref. Neena Khanna, 5/e p79]

20. Ans. (b) EB acquisita
[Ref. Practical Dermatopathology by Ronald P. Rapini, 1/e p99]

Epidermolysis Bullosa Acquisita (EBA)
- Epidermolysis bullosa (EB) are a group of inherited blistering diseases that are present from birth BUT EBA is not inherited and usually presents in adult life
- EBA MC presents as an acquired form of mechanobullous disorder
- EBA is a rare disease in which tense blisters appear at sites of trauma
  - EBA blisters tend to be localized to areas that are easily injured such as the hands, feet, knees, elbows, and buttocks
  - Sometimes there is mucosal involvement with blisters forming in mouth, nose and eyes
- EBA may mimic other inflammatory blistering diseases, most often Bullous pemphigoid

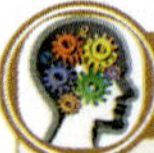

Also Remember
Tests to Establish a Diagnosis of EBA
- Skin biopsy: A blister under the epidermis (subepidermal bulla) and an infiltrate of mixed inflammatory cells in the dermis
- Direct immunofluorescence of a skin biopsy: Autoantibody immunoglobulin G (IgG) is deposited in a line along the dermoepidermal junction
- Indirect immunofluorescence of serum (a blood test): Circulating IgG autoantibodies that target the skin basement membrane and type VII collagen
- Other tests:
  - Skin biopsy for direct and indirect immunoelectron microscopy
  - Blood tests for immunoblotting, enzyme-linked immunosorbent assay (ELISA) and immunoprecipitation

21. Ans. (c) Congenital Epidermolysis bullosa

22. Ans. (a) Genetic
[Ref. Neena Khanna, 5/e p31]
- Epidermolysis bullosa is genetic, inherited as both dominant & recessive forms

23. Ans. (b) Collagen type 7
[Ref. Varki R, Sadowski S, Uitto J, Pfendner E. Epidermolysis bullosa II. Type VII collagen mutations and phenotype-genotype correlations in the dystrophic subtypes. J. Med Genet. 2007;44(3): 181–92]

Dystrophic Epidermolysis Bullosa
- An inherited variant affecting the skin and other organs
- "Butterfly children": Skin is seen to be as delicate and fragile as a butterfly's wings

- Caused by genetic defects (or mutations) within the human COL7A1 gene encoding the protein type VII collagen (collagen VII)

24. Ans. (c) Granular deposition of Ig A; (d) Are candidates for gluten free diet; (e) A variant of dermatitis herpetiformis
[Ref. Clinical Oral Medicine and Pathology by Jean M. Bruch, 1/e p68]

Linear IgA Bullous Disease/Chronic Bullous Disease of Childhood

- An autoimmune skin disorder in which blisters form in the skin and mucous membranes
- Characteristic findings on direct immunofluorescence of a skin biopsy: A line of IgA antibodies just below the epidermis
- Prolonged period of prodromal itching or transient pruritus or burning before lesions appear
- Patients with ocular manifestations may complain of pain, grittiness, or discharge

25. Ans. (c) Pemphigous vulgaris
[Ref. Neena Khanna, 5/e p79]

26. Ans. (c) Pemphigus foliaceus
[Ref. Neena Khanna, 5/e p79, 80]

- In pemphigus foliaceus transient superficial bullae ruptures rapidly to form extensive areas of scaling and crusting
- Most important differentiating feature (Pathognomonic):
  - Pemphigus vulgaris: Antibodies to Dsg 3 & 1
  - Pemphigus foliaceus: Antibodies to Dsg 1

27. Ans. (c) P. vegetans
[Ref. Almeida et al. Pemphigus vegetans associated with verrucous lesions: expanding a phenotype. Clinics, 2006;61(3):279-82]

Fig. Pemphigus vegetans

Pemphigus Vegetans (PV)

- A variant of pemphigus vulgaris
- Autoimmune disease
- Rarest form of pemphigus: 2-5.7% of patients with this class of disease
- Faccid bullae or pustules that erode to form hypertrophic papillated plaques involving predominantly skin folds, scalp, face, and mucous membranes

28. Ans. (c) Dermatitis herpetiformis
[Ref. Neena Khanna, 5/e p90]

Dermatitis Herpetiformis

- Itchy, grouped, erythematous, papulovesicular lesions, frequently manifesting as grouped excoriations
- Extensor and pressure points of trunk and extremities
- Histology: Dermoepidermal split
- DIF findings: Granular IgA deposit at dermal papillary tips
- Dramatic response to Dapsone

29. Ans. (a) Pemphigus vulgaris
[Ref. Neena Khanna, 5/e p79]

30. Ans. (d) Dermatitis herpetiformis
[Ref. Neena Khanna, 5/e p90]

31. Ans. (b) Pemphigus vulgaris
[Ref. Neena Khanna, 5/e p79]

32. Ans. (b) Bullous pemphigoid
[Ref. Neena Khanna, 5/e p85]

- Bullous pemphigoid is to be suspected when elderly patient present with itchy, tense hemorrhagic blisters in lower abdomen, inner thigh, groins, flexures and intertriginous areas
- Lesions heal with milia formation
- Bulla spread sign or Nikolsky's sign negative

33. Ans. (b) Pemphigoid
[Ref. Neena Khanna, 5/e p85]

34. Ans. (a) Fishnet Ig G deposits in epidermis
[Ref. Neena Khanna, 5/e p79, 83]

- Multiple bullous lesion over trunk with oral mucosa involvement hints towards Pemphigus vulgaris
- Though a disease of middle age, may occur in children
- DIF: Deposition of IgG in intecellular spaces throughout the epidermis, giving a *'fishnet appearance'*

35. Ans. (a) Pemphigus vulgaris
[Ref. Neena Khanna, 5/e p79]

36. Ans. (b) Bullous pemphigoid
[Ref. Neena Khanna, 5/e p85]

37. Ans. (d) Herpes gestationis
[Ref. Thomas S, Rajan U, George S, George M. Postpartum Pemphigoid Gestationis. Indian Journal of Dermatology. 2012;57(2):146-48 & Neena Khanna, 5/e p91]

Pemphigoid Gestationis (PG) or Herpes Gestationis

- Description: A rare autoimmune subepidermal blistering disorder associated with pregnancy targeting the hemidesmosomal proteins BP180 and less commonly BP230
- Clinical presentation:
  - Starts as intensely pruritic, erythematous annular urticarial plaques on which blisters develop
  - Lesions are described more frequently on the abdomen, with extension to flexural areas
  - Face, mucus membranes, palms and soles are usually spared
  - Typically develops during the second or third trimester of pregnancy, but has been rarely reported in the first trimester and postpartum period: Disease often resolves during the latter part of gestation and flares at the time of delivery, and then usually resolves within 3 months after delivery
- Histopathology: Subepidermal bulla containing numerous eosinophils
- DIF:
  - C3 with or without IgG in a linear band along the BMZ of perilesional skin
  - C3 and IgG deposits are seen in the placenta and fetal skin also

38. Ans. (a) Periumbilical region
[Ref. Thomas S, Rajan U, George S, George M. Postpartum Pemphigoid Gestationis. Indian Journal of Dermatology. 2012;57(2):146-148]

39. Ans. (c) Dermatitis Herpetiformis
[Ref. Neena Khanna, 5/e p90]

40. Ans. (a) Pemphigus vulgaris
[Ref. Neena Khanna, 5/e p79]

41. Ans. (a) Gluten free diet with minerals and vitamins
[Ref. Neena Khanna, 5/e p91]

- Two pronged approach brings quick and lasting response in Dermatitis herpetiformis:
  - Gluten free diet with minerals and vitamins.
  - Dapsone 100-200 mg, daily & Sulfapyridine 1-1.5 g, daily work dramatically

42. Ans. (d) Steven–Johnson syndrome
[Ref. Neena Khanna, 5/e p91-93]

Important Points of Steven–Johnson Syndrome

- Acute onse, usually in adults
- Tender erythematous sin lesion
- Nikolsky sign positive
- Atypical target lesion seen
- Mucous membrane of mouth and eyes are frequently involved
- High fever, pain and weakness
- Biopsy shows subepidermal split with apoptotic keratinocyte necrosis.

43. Ans. (a) Molluscum contagiosum
[Ref. Neena Khanna, 5/e p292]

Morphology of Molluscum Contagiosum

- Multiple, pearly white, dome-shaped papules which are umbilicated
- Under a hand lens, may have a mosaic appearance
- On piercing the umbilicated center, a white cheesy material can be extruded

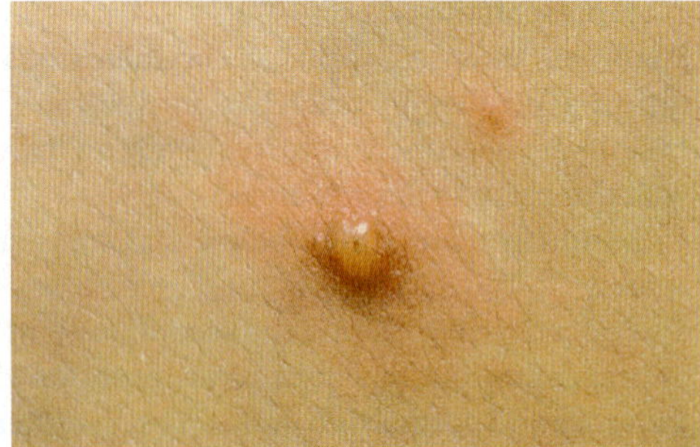

Fig. Molluscum contagiosum

44. Ans. (b) Dermatitis herpetiformis
[Ref. Neena Khanna, 5/e p90]

45. Ans. (a) Pemphigus
[Ref. Neena Khanna, 5/e p79]

46. Ans. (b) Pemphigus folliaceous; (d) Bullous impetigo; (e) Pemphigus vulgaris
[Ref. Neena Khanna, 5/e p79]

47. Ans. (b) Scabies
[Ref. Neena Khanna, 5/e p166]

- Lesion of scabies is in form of papules, papulovesicles and nodules

48. Ans. (a) Dermatitis herpetiformis; (d) Pemphigoid
[Ref. Neena Khanna, 5/e p85, 90]

49. Ans. (c) Atopic dermatitis
[Ref. Neena Khanna, 5/e p102]

- Lesion of Atopic dermatitis is in form of papules and vesicles

50. Ans. (c) Bullous pemphigoid
[Ref. Neena Khanna, 5/e p79]

51. Ans. (e) All of the above
[Ref. Neena Khanna, 5/e p79]

52. Ans. (a) Subepidermal
[Ref. Neena Khanna, 5/e p79]

53. Ans. (b) Pemphigus
[Ref. Madke B, Doshi B, Khopkar U, Dongre A. Appearances in dermatopathology: The diagnostic and the deceptive. Indian J DermatolVenereolLeprol 2013;79:338-48]

Tombstone Appearance

- Occurrence: Fresh blister of Pemphigus vulgaris or drug-induced pemphigus
- Description: Suprabasal splitting of the epidermis leads to blister formation, with the basal layer still remaining adherent to the basement membrane, and gives the resemblance to the row of the tomb stone
- Classification of Tomb-stoning **(Ackerman and colleagues)**:
  - Decorated tomb stone (Discrete dermal papillae covered by a single row of basal keratinocytes that project into an intraepidermal blister): Decorated tombstones have been described apart from pemphigus in Grover's disease, Darier's disease, Hailey-Hailey disease, Warty dyskeratoma and Solar keratosis
  - Undecorated tomb stone (discrete, well-preserved dermal papillae beneath a subepidermal blister): Undecorated tomb stone has been described in Suction blister, Porphyria, Pseudoporphyria, Bullous pemphigoid, Herpes gestationis and Epidermolysis bullosa junctional and dystrophic variant

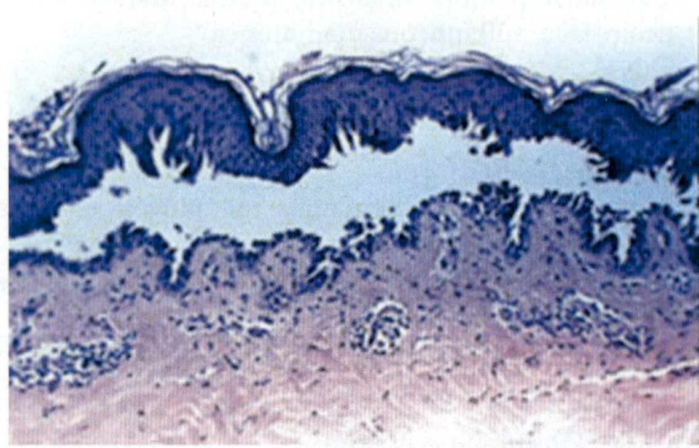

Fig. Tombstone appearance

54. Ans. (a) Phempigus vulgaris
[Ref. Neena Khanna, 5/e p79]
- Pemphigus is MC cause of autoimmune blistering in India
- Pemphigus vulgaris is the commonest type
- Pemphigus vegetans is rarest

55. Ans. (a) Dermatitis herpetiformis
[Ref. Neena Khanna, 5/e p90]
- Characteristic histology Dermoepidermal split
- DIF findings: Granular IgA deposit at dermal papillary tips

56. Ans. (b) Dapsone
[Ref. Neena Khanna, 5/e p449]

Dapsone is Drug of Choice
- Dermatitis herpetiformis
- Erythema elevatum diutinum

57. Ans. (d) Non Hodgkin lymphoma

58. Ans. (d) Frusemide
[Ref. Neena Khanna, 5/e p81]

Drugs causing Pemphigus-Like Eruptions
- Captopril, Enalapril
- Flupenthixol
- Frusemide
- Interleukin-2
- Penicillamine
- Penicillins
- Sulphasalazine

59. Ans. (b) HLA B8
[Ref. Dermatalogical Diseases by Venkataram Mysore, p15]

HLA-associated Dermatological Disorders

HLA	Associated disease
HLA B8	Oral lichen planus, Dermatitis herpetiformis
HLA B13	Guttate psoriasis, Erythrodermic psoriasis
HLA B17	Guttate psoriasis, Erythrodermic psoriasis
HLA B27	Psoriasis vulgaris, Psoriatic arthritis, Ankylosing spondylitis, Reactive arthritis, Acrodermatitis of Hallopeau, Lichen planus
HLA B51	Bechet's disease, lichen planus
HLA Cw6	Early onset psoriasis
HLA DR 1	Lichen planus (Oral and cutaneous)
HLA DR 2	Lupus
HLA DR 3	Guttate dermatitis herpetiformis, Pemphigus gestationis, Lupus erythematosus, Lichen planus
HLA DR 4	Psoriasis vulgaris, Idiopathic chronic urticaria, Pemphigoid gestations
HLA DR 6	Pemphigus vulgaris
HLA DR 10	Lichen planus
HLA DQ 2	Dermatitis herpetiformis
HLA DQ 8	Dermatitis herpetiformis, chronic urticaria

60. Ans. (b) Intercellular substance
[Ref. Neena Khanna, 5/e p79]

61. Ans. (c) Deposits of IgG at the epidermodermal lesion
[Ref. Neena Khanna, 5/e p90]

62. Ans. (b) Subepidermal
[Ref. Forensic Medicine by Jason Payne-James, 1/e p189]
- First degree burns show epidermal necrosis, subepidermal blister formation and perivascular inflammatory cells

63. Ans. (a) Pemphigus vulgaris
[Ref. Neena Khanna, 5/e p78]

64. Ans. (a) Herpes zoster
[Ref. Herpes Zoster: Recent Aspects of Diagnosis and Control edited by Gerd Gross, p29]
- Diagnosis of zoster is exceptionally done by histo-pathological means
- Histopathological features:
  - Focal intercellular oedema
  - Ballooning degeneration of keratinocytes
  - Multinucleated giant cells
  - Intranuclear inclusions

65. Ans. (b) Intercellular substance

66. Ans. (b) ATP2C1 impairment; (d) Flexural distribution; (e) Benign pemphigus
[Ref. Dermatology in General Medicine, 3/e p1247]

Hailey-Hailey Disease
- Synonym: Benign familial pemphigus
- Genetics: Autosomal dominant inheritance, ATP2C1 enzyme haplo-insufficiency
- Flexural distribution: Painful erosions, vesico-pustules and scaly erythematous plaques appear at sites of friction such as the sides of the neck, the axillae, the groins and the perineum
- Treatment: Not available

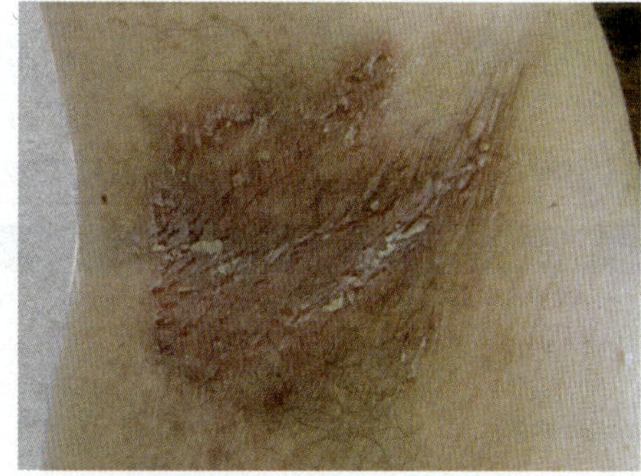

Fig. Hailey-Hailey disease

67. Ans. (b) TEN
[Ref. Neena Khanna, 4/e p174]

Body Surface Area (BSA) Involvement
- SJS: <10% of BSA
- SJS-TEN overlap: 10-30% of BSA
- TEN: >30% of BSA

68. Ans. (a) Bullous impetigo
[Ref. Diseases of Skin by Sequiera, 1/e p177]

Pemphigus Neonatorum
- Bullous impetigo of infants
- Occurs in the first week after birth

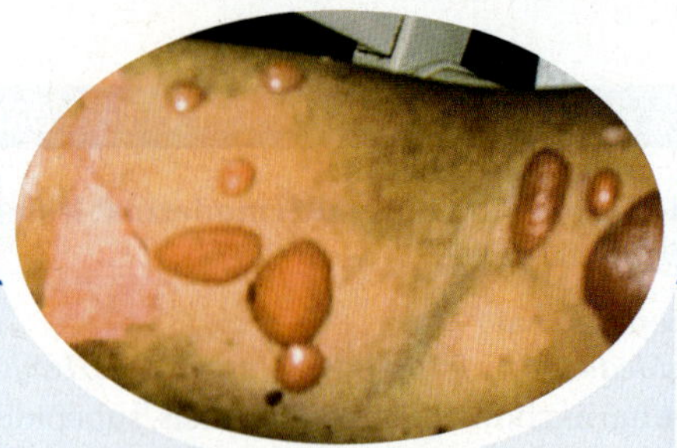

Chapter 9

Hair, Alopecia, Hirsutism

THEORETICAL CONCEPTS

IX A. TYPES OF ALOPECIA

Scarring/Cicatricial alopecia[Q]	Non-scarring/Non-cicatricial alopecia[Q]
• **B**asal cell carcinoma • **L**ichen planus, lichen planopilaris • **F**olliculitis decalvans • **C**utaneous lupus • **H**erpes zoster • **D**iscoid lupus erythematosus • **C**utaneous metastasis • **L**inear scleroderma (Morphea) • **S**arcoidosis	• **H**IV • **H**ypo/hyperthyroidism • **H**ypopituitarism • **D**eficiency of Iron, Zinc, Protein, Biotin • **S**econdary syphilis • **A**ndrogenic alopecia • **A**lopecia areata • **L**upus erythematosus • **T**raumatic alopecia (Trichotillomania) • **T**inea capitis • **T**elogen effluvium
[Mnemonic: **B**y **L**owering **F**at **C**oronary **H**eart **D**isease **C**hances **L**essen **S**ignificantly**]**	**[Mnemonic: H**igh **D**ensity **SALT]**

IX B. SCARRING/CICATRICIAL ALOPECIA

Primary skin disorders	Systemic disorders[Q]
• Lichen planus • Discoid lupus erythematosus • Lupus vulgaris • Linear scleroderma • Leprosy • Alopecia cutis • Burns, Radiation, Injury	• Sarcoidosis • Systematic lupus erythematosus • Cutaneous metastases

IX C. NON-SCARRING/NON-CICATRICIAL ALOPECIA

Primary skin disorders	Systemic disorders[Q]
• Alopecia areata • Tinea capitis • Traumatic alopecia • Androgenic alopecia • Telogen effluvium • Anagen effluvium	• Systematic lupus erythematosus • Secondary syphilis • Hypopituitarism • Hypothyroidism • Hyperthyroidism • Zinc/Iron/Biotin/Protein deficiency
Drugs[Q] Heparin, Warfarin, Lithium, Vitamin A, Colchicine, Amphetamines, Beta-blockers, PTU, Vitamin A	

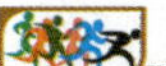
Topper's Edge

Cicatricial vs Non-cicatricial Alopecia[Q]

	Cicatricial alopecia	Non-cicatricial alopecia
Skin	Shiny with no follicular openings	Visible follicular openings
Hair follicles	Irreversible destruction	No destruction, reversible
Inflammation	Present	Absent
Scarring	Present	Absent

IX D. ALOPECIA AREATA

- MC age group: Young adults
- Subtypes:
  - Ophiasis: Alopecia along margin of scalp
  - Alopecia totalis: Loss of hair on total scalp[Q]
  - Alopecia universalis: Loss of hair on whole body
- Features:
  - Sharply defined alopecia
  - ***'Exclamation mark hair'***[Q]
  - Sparing of grey/ white hair
  - *'Going white over-night'* phenomenon[Q]
  - First site affected: Scalp
  - Nails: 'Hammered brass' (Fine stippled pitting[Q])
- Treatment:
  - Few lesions: Topical Minoxidil[Q], Topical Corticosteroids, Topical Psoralen + UVA
  - Extensive lesions: Oral Corticosteroids, Oral Psoralen + UVA

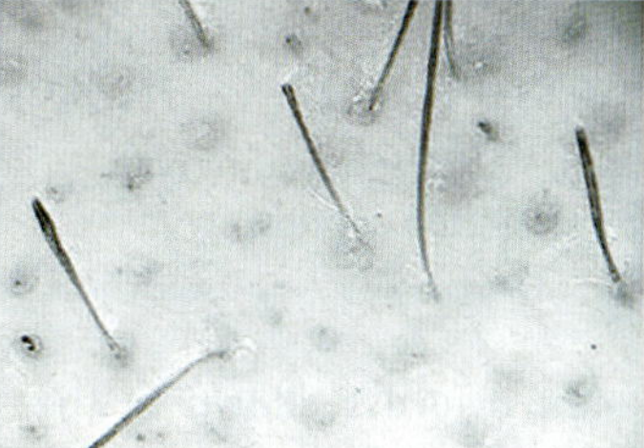
Fig. Exclamation hair

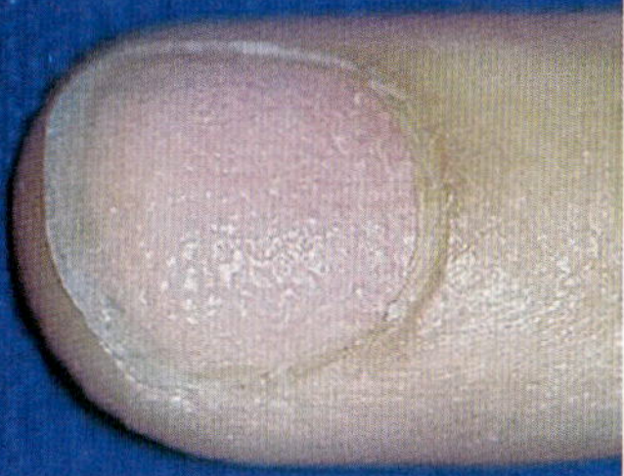
Fig. Hammered brass

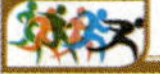
Topper's Edge

ALOPECIA

Androgenetic alopecia

- Male pattern alopecia
- Basic pathology: Miniaturization of hair follicles[Q]
- Types/patterns of hair loss: Hamilton Norwood grading[Q]

Telogen effluvium

- Infections[Q]: Typhoid, Malaria, Dengue, Chikungunya
- Prolonged difficult childbirth
- Surgical trauma
- Hemorrhage
- Emotional stress

Trichotillomania

- Hair pulling tic[Q]

Pseudopelade of Brocq

- Scarring alopecia with unknown cause[Q]
- Cicatricial alopecia
- 'Foot prints in snow' appearance[Q]

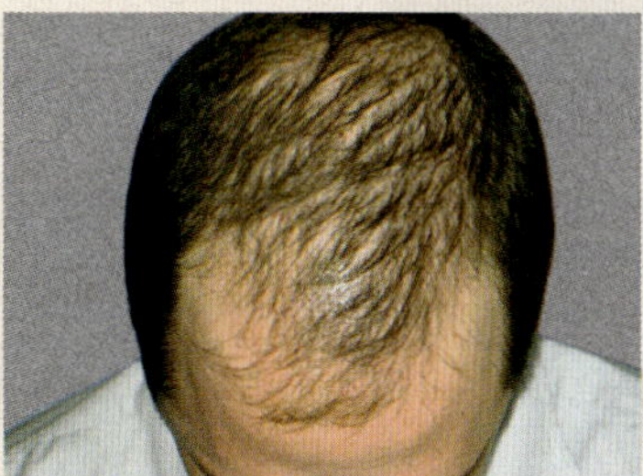
Fig. Androgenetic alopecia

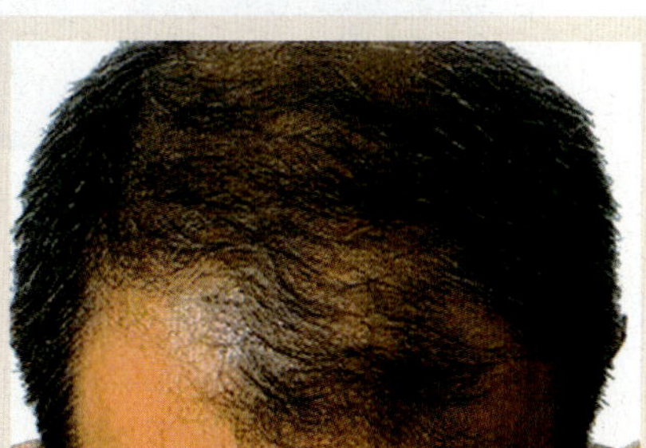
Fig. Telogen effluvium

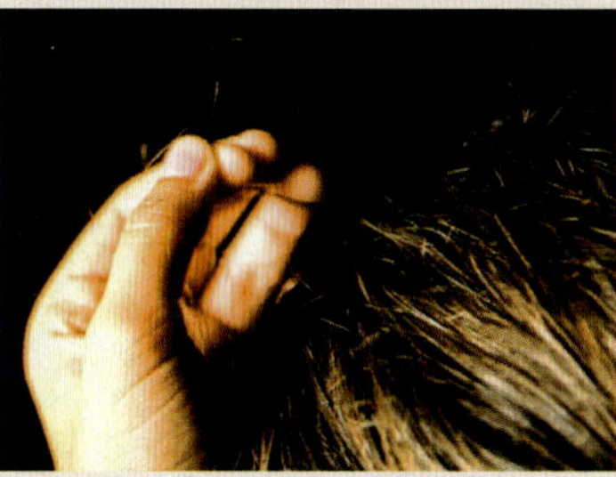
Fig. Trichotillomania

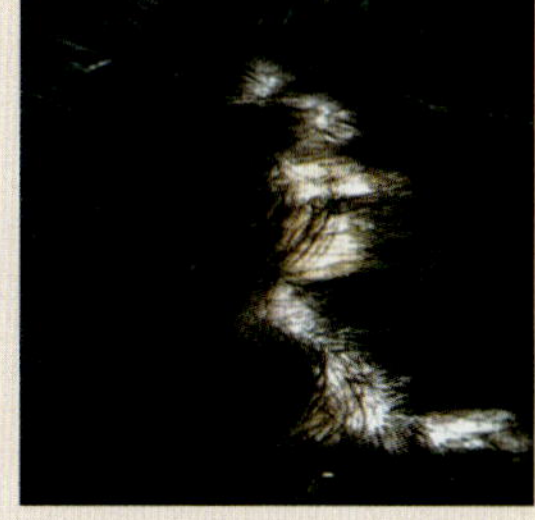
Fig. Pseudopelade of Brocq

IMAGE-BASED QUESTIONS

1. What is the likely diagnosis of the disorder as shown in the photograph? ***[Recent Question 2016]***

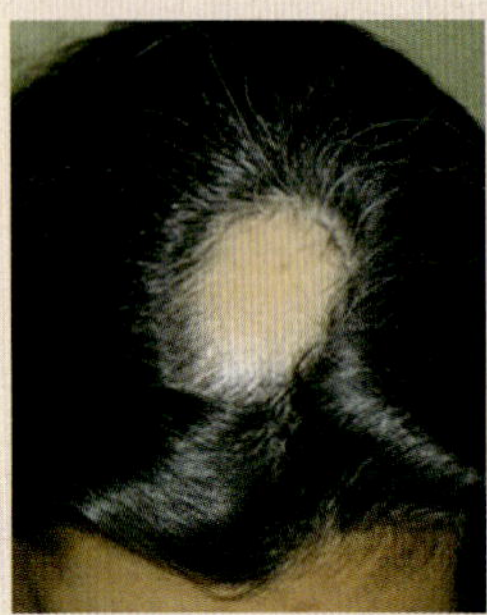

a. Alopecia areata
b. Androgenic alopecia
c. Telogen effluvium
d. Tinea capitis

2. Diagnose the skin appendage disorder shown in the photograph

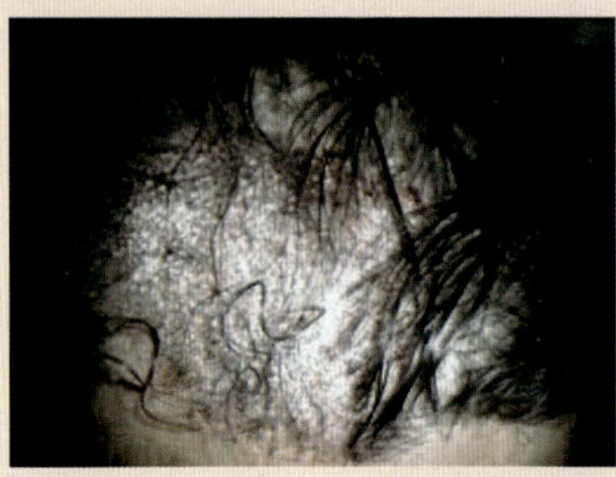

a. Alopecia areata
b. Telogen effluvium
c. Cicatricial alopecia
d. Alopecia totalis

3. Diagnose the underlying skin disorder shown in the photograph

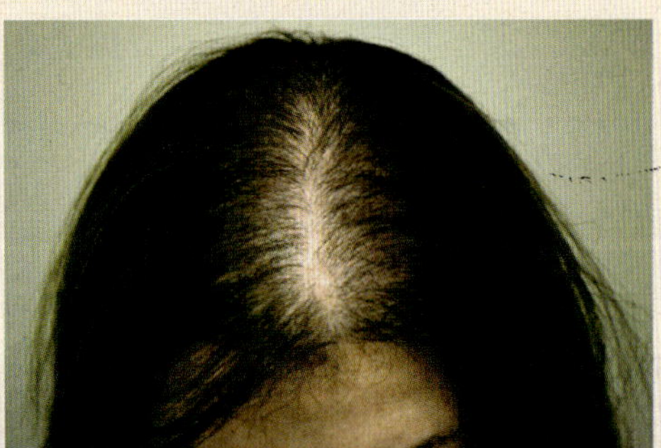

a. Alopecia totalis
b. Alopecia universalis
c. Telogen effluvium
d. Androgenetic alopecia

4. Diagnose the underlying skin disorder shown in the photograph

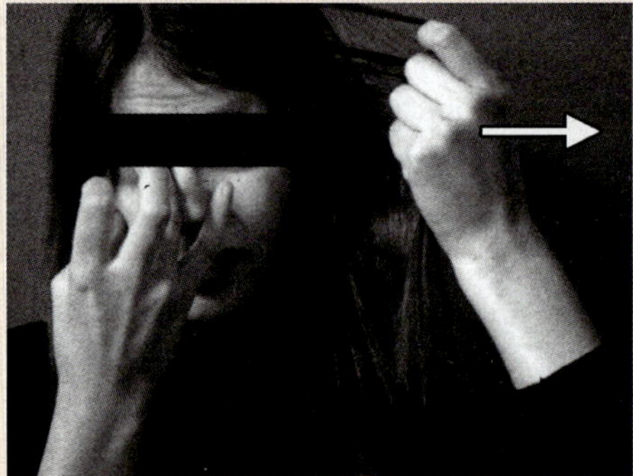

a. Traction alopecia
b. Trichotillomania
c. Telogen effluvium
d. Hirsutism

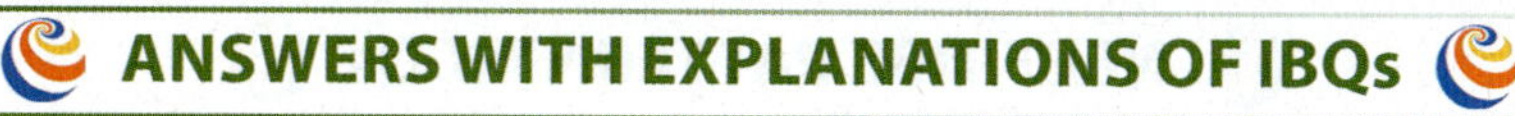

1. Ans. (a) Alopecia areata *Ref. DVL by Thappa, 4/e p261,262]*

Alopecia Areata

- Patchy alopecia with exclamation mark hair **(Photograph)**
- Circular to oval areas of alopecia that may progress to total scalp hair loss (Alopecia totalis) or total body hair loss (Alopecia universalis)
- Positive pull test (easily extractable telogen hairs at periphery of oval areas of loss) correlates with active disease.
- Ophiasis pattern is a band-like pattern of loss along the temporal/occipital scalp that may be less responsive to therapy
- Associated nail findings: Nail pitting, trachyonychia, brittle nails, onycholysis, koilonychia, onychomadesis

2. Ans. (c) Cicatricial alopecia *[Ref. Neena Khanna, 4/e p137]*

Cicatricial Alopecia

- Permanent hair loss due to irreversible destruction of hair follicles
- Pseudopelade of Brocq/Footprints in snow appearance
- Shiny skin and follicular opening absent
- Visible signs of inflammation
- Scarring alopecia

3. Ans. (d) Androgenetic alopecia *[Ref. Neena Khanna, 4/e p133]*

Androgenetic Alopecia in Women

- Terminal hair replaced by fine vellus hair
- Diffuse hair loss initially
- Widening of central parting

4. Ans. (b) Trichotillomania *[Ref. Neena Khanna, 4/e p136]*

Trichotillomania

- Hair pulling tic
- Young women pull hair to relieve pain
- Alopecia patch with hair of different length in different directions

Skin and STDs

 NEET/NBE PATTERN MCQs 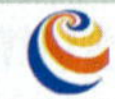

1. **Nonscarring loss of hair is seen in** *[Recent Question 2016]*
   a. Alopecia areata b. Lichen planus
   c. SLE d. Dissecting folliculitis
2. **Pseudopelade is** *[Recent Question 2016]*
   a. Premature alopecia b. Traction
   c. Cicatricial alopecia d. Alopecia steatoides
3. **Alopecia areata is a/an** *[Recent Question 2016]*
   a. Autoimmune disorder b. Allergic disorder
   c. Anaphylactic disorder d. Bacterial infection
4. **Which of the following can cause both cicatricial as well as noncicatricial alopecia?** *[Recent Question 2016]*
   a. Alopecia areata b. Telogen effluvium
   c. SLE d. Hypothyroidism
5. **Nonscarring alopecia is seen in all except** *[NBE FMGE September 2005]*
   a. Telogen effluvium b. Tinea capitis
   c. Alopecia areata d. Lichen planus
6. **Scarring alopecia may be caused by** *[NBE DNB 1994]*
   a. Secondary syphilis b. Lichen planus
   c. Psoriasis d. Cyclophosphamide
7. **Noncicatricial alopecia is present in** *[NBE DNB 1993]*
   a. Scleroderma b. Lichen planus
   c. Psoriasis d. Discoid lupus
8. **Most common type of nonscarring alopecia is** *[NBE DNB 2008,2010]*
   a. Androgenic b. Areata
   c. Tinea capitis d. Traction
9. **Following conditions cause nonscarring alopecia except** *[UPSC 2012]*
   a. Alopecia areata b. Tinea capitis
   c. Secondary syphilis d. Sarcoidosis
10. **Nonscarring loss of hair** *[Recent Question 2012]*
    a. Alopecia areata
    b. Lichen planus
    c. SLE
    d. Dissecting folliculitis
11. **A cystic boggy inflammatory swelling over scalp in a child with partial or complete alopecia is** *[UPSC 2010]*
    a. Folliculitis decalvans b. Hematoma
    c. Kerion d. Congenital syphilis
12. **A 23-year-old female patient presented with severe diffuse hair fall for last 1 month. She had a major accident with severe blood loss 5 months back for which she had to be hospitalized for 1 month. She very anxious that all her hair will fall. Most likely diagnosis is?** *[Recent Question 2017]*
    a. Alopecia areata b. Telogen effluvium
    c. Anagen effluvium d. Androgenetic alopecia
13. **Preferred concentration of Minoxidil for female androgenetic alopecia is?** *[Recent Question 2017]*
    a. 2% b. 5%
    c. 8% d. 10%
14. **Alopecia universalis is?** *[Recent Question 2017]*
    a. Loss of all the scalp hair
    b. Loss of all body hair
    c. Loss hair at the scalp margin
    d. Male pattern hair loss
15. **A female patient presents with patchy hair loss with normal looking skin on scalp. Diagnosis is?** *[Recent Question 2017]*
    a. Tinea capitis
    b. Cicatricial alopecia
    c. Alopecia areata
    d. Telogen effluvium
16. **Pseudopelade of Brocq shows following feature on histopathology** *[Recent Question 2017]*
    a. Clutching the ball appearance
    b. Church spire appearance
    c. Concentric perifollicular lamellar fibrosis
    d. Saw tooth appearance

HIGH YIELD MCQs

1. **Cicatricial alopecia is/are seen in** *[PGI November 2016]*
   a. Lichen planopilaris
   b. Discoid lupus erythematous
   c. Androgen effluvium
   d. Lichen planus
   e. Trichotillomania
2. **A 35-year-old male presents with bald patches and with no scars. The patches are well-demarcated with broken hair at the edges. Diagnosis is** *[AIIMS May 2016]*
   a. Alopecia areata b. Androgenic alopecia
   c. DLE d. Telogen effluvium
3. **A patient presents with several patches of nonscarring alopecia on occipital and temporal regions. Histopathology shows several empty follicles with perifollicular infiltrates as well as pieces of broken hair with few hemorrhages. Diagnosis is** *[AIIMS November 2016]*
   a. Alopecia areata b. Lichen planus
   c. Trichotillomania d. Loose anagen syndrome
4. **The time period that elapses between the physic emotional stress and the hair loss is about** *[JIPMER PGMEE 1999, NBE DNB 2001]*
   a. 21 days b. 30 days
   c. 3 months d. 6 months
5. **A 30-year-old female developed diffuse hair loss 3 months after delivery of her first. The probable diagnosis is** *[PGI 2001, SGPGI 2003]*
   a. Androgenic alopecia b. Endocrinal alopecia
   c. Telogen effluvium d. SLE

6. All of the following are causes of cicatrizing alopecia except *[AIIMS PGMEE 2007]*
a. Lichen planus
b. Discoid lupus erythematosus
c. Alopecia areata
d. Lupus vulgaris

7. Cicatricial alopecia is seen in *[All India PGMEE 1999]*
a. Tinea capitis b. Psoriasis
c. DLE d. Alopecia areata

8. Pseudopelade is synonym of *[AIIMS PGMEE 1991, PGI 1994]*
a. Alopecia steatoides b. Premature alopecia
c. Traction d. Cicatricial alopecia

9. Cicatricial alopecia is seen in *[PGI 2004, 2007]*
a. DLE b. SLE
c. Secondary syphilis d. Psoriasis
e. Lichen planus

10. Exclamation mark hairs is seen in *[BIHAR PGMEE 2006)*
a. Alopecia areata b. Traumatic alopecia
c. Lichen planus d. All

11. In alopecia areata, seen is *[PGI 1997]*
a. Exclamatory mark hair b. Scaring
c. Fungal infection d. Traumatic

12. Male with patchy loss of scalp hair and grey hair in the eyebrows and beard diagnosis is *[All India PGMEE 2008]*
a. Anagen effluvium b. Alopecia areata
c. Telogen effluvium d. Androgenic alopecia

13. Diagnosis of a man with diffuse hair loss involving crown and frontal scalp with maintenance of frontal hair line *[JIPMER PGMEE 1998]*
a. Alopecia areata b. Anagen effluvium
c. Male pattern baldness d. Female pattern baldness

14. Exclamation mark alopecia is a feature of *[AIIMS PGMEE 2005]*
a. Telogen effluvium b. Androgenic alopecia
c. Alopecia areata d. Alopecia mucinosa

15. Contraindicated in androgenic alopecia *[All India PGMEE 2000)*
a. Testosterone b. Minoxidil
c. Cyproterone d. Finasteride

16. Anagen phase of the hair indicates *[AIIMS PGMEE 2006]*
a. The phase of activity and growth
b. The phase of transition
c. The phase of resting
d. The phase of degeneration

17. A female patient presents with diffuse alopecia to you. She had suffered from typhoid fever 4 months back. Most probable diagnosis is *[AIIMS PGMEE 2007]*
a. Androgenetic alopecia b. Telogen effluvium
c. Anagen effluvium d. Alopecia areata

18. Scarring alopecia is seen in *[All India PGMEE 2009]*
a. T. capitis b. Androgenic alopecia
c. Alopecia areata d. Lichen planus

19. Exclamation mark hairs are seen in *[Kerala PGMEE 2001]*
a. Syphilis b. Alopecia areata
c. Psoriasis d. Dermatophytosis

20. Alopecia areata is treated by *[JIPMER PGMEE 1992]*
a. Minoxidil
b. Tranquilizers
c. Whitfield's ointment
d. Parental penicillin

21. Non cicatricial alopecia is present in *[AIIMS PGMEE 1998]*
a. Scleroderma b. Lichen planus
c. Psoriasis d. Parvovirus

22. Alopecia areata is *[SGPGI 2004]*
a. Cicatricial scar
b. Non cicatricial scar
c. Fungal infection
d. None

23. All of the following are stages of hair except *[PGMCET 2015]*
a. Catagen b. Telogen
c. Anagen d. Metagen

24. Endothrix is caused by *[Recent Question 2016, 2015]*
a. Pityrosporum
b. Trichophyton tonsurans
c. Corynebacterium minutissimum
d. Staphylococcus aureus

25. A patient presented with itching and mild discharge and hair loss as shown below. Which of the following is useful for diagnosis? *[AIIMS May 2017]*
a. Gram stain
b. Slit skin smear
c. KOH mount
d. Tzanck smear

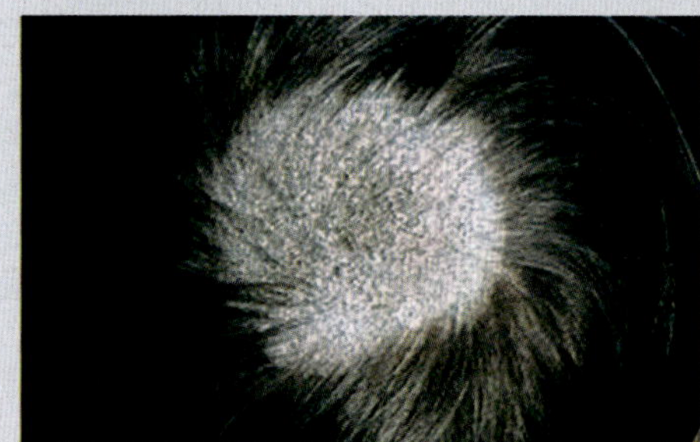

Fig. Tinea capitis

NEET/NBE PATTERN MCQs ANSWERS WITH EXPLANATIONS

1. Ans. (a) Alopecia areata

[Ref. DVL by Thappa, 4/e p261]

Alopecia Areata

- An example of patchy nonscarring alopecia
- Characteristic initial lesion is a circumscribed bald smooth patch
- Exclamation point may be seen at periphery of the patch
- **MC site is scalp** but may involve any site

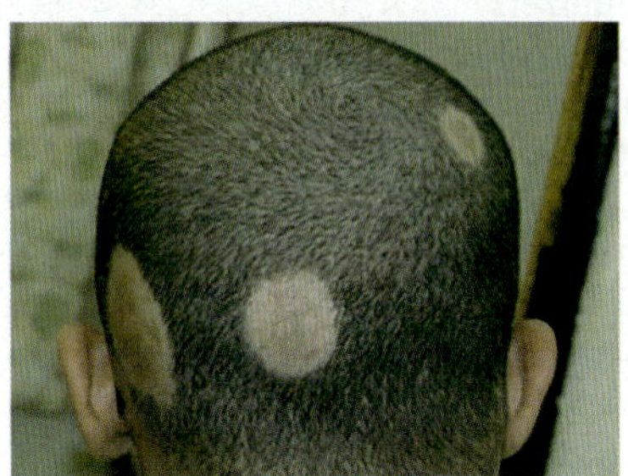

Fig. Alopecia areata

2. Ans. (c) Cicatricial alopecia

[Ref. DVL by Thappa, 4/e p260,261]

Pseudopelade

- First described by Neumann in 1869
- Classic pseudopelade is characterized as a non-inflammatory, intermittently progressive scarring alopecia of unknown origin

3. Ans. (a) Autoimmune disorder

[Ref. Clinical Dermatology by Habif, 6/e p949]

- **Alopecia areata**, also known as **spot baldness**, is an autoimmune disease in which hair is lost from some or all areas of the body, usually from the scalp due to the body's failure to recognize its own body cells and subsequent destruction of its own tissue

4. Ans. (c) SLE

[Ref. Clinical Dermatology by Habif, 6/e p630]

- Alopecia is one of the major features of SLE
- Both scarring and nonscarring types of alopecia occur
- Nonscarring hair loss occurs more frequently in SLE, and scarring alopecia is more common in DLE

5. Ans. (d) Lichen planus

[Ref. Sure Success in PGMEE by Ramgopal, 1/e p194]

6. Ans. (b) Lichen planus

[Ref. Neena Khanna, 5/e p65]

- Scalp lesions in Lichen planus: Follicular lesions of LP on the scalp result in Cicatricial (Scarring) alopecia

7. Ans. (c) Psoriasis

[Ref. Neena Khanna, 5/e p49]

8. Ans. (a) Androgenic

[Ref. Neena Khanna, 5/e p141]

- **MC cause of scarring alopecia**: Lichen planopilaris, DLE
- **MC cause of Nonscarring alopecia**: Androgenetic alopecia

9. Ans. (d) Sarcoidosis

[Ref. Andrews' Diseases of the Skin by James, p709]

- Sarcoidosis causes scarring alopecia

10. Ans. (a) Alopecia areata

[Ref. Neena Khanna, 5/e p141]

Alopecia

Noncicatricial alopecia	Cicatricial alopecia
Localized	• Aplasia cutis
• Alopecia areata	• Lichen planopilaris
• Androgenetic alopecia	• DLE
• Traction alopecia	• Favus
• Tinea capitis	• Kerion
Generalized	• Nevus sebaceous
• Alopecia universalis	• Physical or chemical trauma
• Ectodermal dysplasia	• Basal cell carcinoma
• Shaft abnormalities	• Pseudopelade of Brocq

11. Ans. (c) Kerion

[Ref. Neena Khanna, 5/e p303]

Kerion

- A type of inflammatory tinea capitis
- Boggy swelling, studded with pustules present on scalp
- There may be pus discharge from multiple orifices
- May develop in beard region of the face in adult males

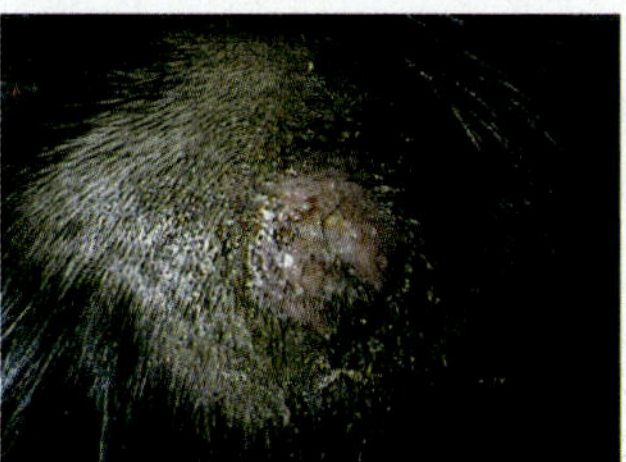

Fig. Kerion

12. Ans. (B) Telogen effluvium

[Ref. Lookingbill and Marks' Principles of Dermatology, 5/e p247]

Telogen Effluvium

- Severe physical stress, such as going through childbirth, surgery, or suffering a serious illness may precipitate a type of hair loss
- Stress induced alopecia: Stress forces large numbers of follicles to enter the resting phase, and after a few months, hair will fall out
- Acute telogen effluvium is related do stressful events, chronic telogen effluvium is rather accompanying chronic illnesses

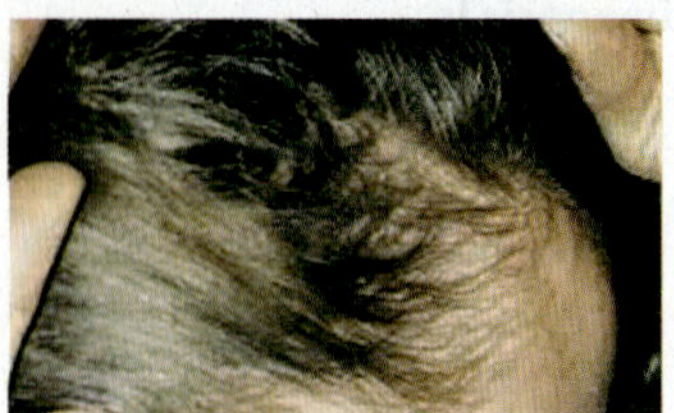

Fig. Telogen effluvium

13. Ans. (a) 2%

[Ref. Clinical Dermatology by Habif, 5/e p923]

- In women with androgenetic alopecia, 2% topical Minoxidil has good results in increasing hair growth
- In men with androgenetic alopecia, 5% topical Minoxidil was clearly superior to 2% topical Minoxidil in increasing hair growth

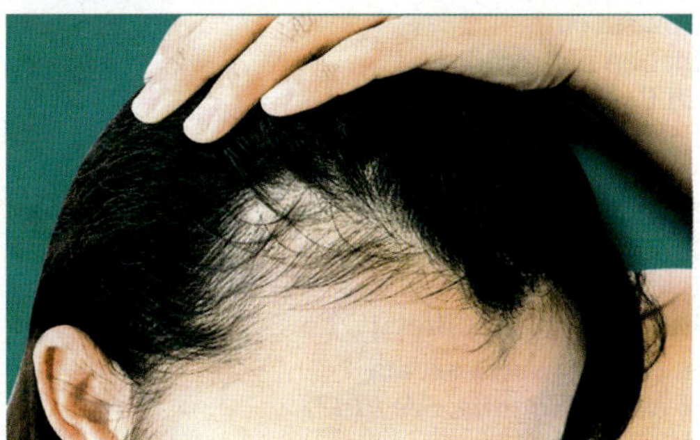

Fig. Female androgenetic alopecia

14. Ans. (b) Loss of all body hair

[Ref. Diseases of the Skin by Mahmoudi, 1/e p329]

- Alopecia areata is an autoimmune condition causing nonscarring hair loss, usually in circular areas on the scalp
- It can progress to the complete loss of scalp hair (Alopecia totalis) or loss of all body hair (Alopecia universalis)

15. Ans. (c) Alopecia areata

[Ref. Clinical Dermatology by Habif, 5/e p932]

- Alopecia areata is the consequence of an immune reaction in the skin, leading to patches of total hair loss that expose a normal-appearing, rounded area of scalp skin
- Most patches regrow after a few weeks, but not always

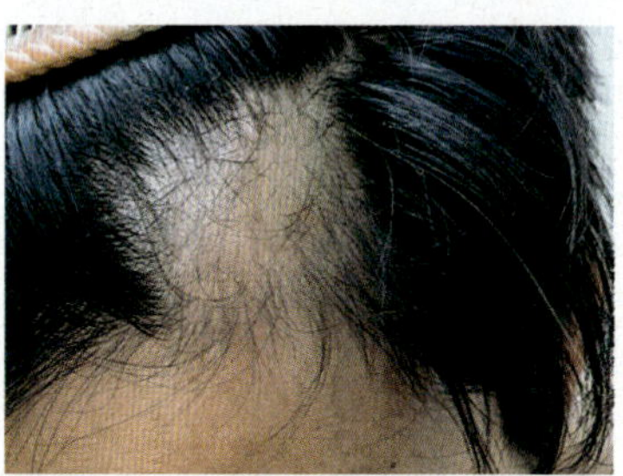

Fig. Alopecia areata

16. Ans. (c) Concentric perifollicular lamellar fibrosis

[Ref. Fitzpatrick's Clinical Dermatology, 8/e p802]

Pseudopelade of Brocq

- Destructive, fibrosing lymphocytic folliculitis seen in Cicatricial alopecia
- No associated epidermal change is present
- Dense peri-infundibular lymphocytic infiltrates are present in early lesions at the periphery of prominent concentric lamellar fibroplasia that encompasses the infundibulum
- Perivascular lymphocytic infiltrates are variably prominent

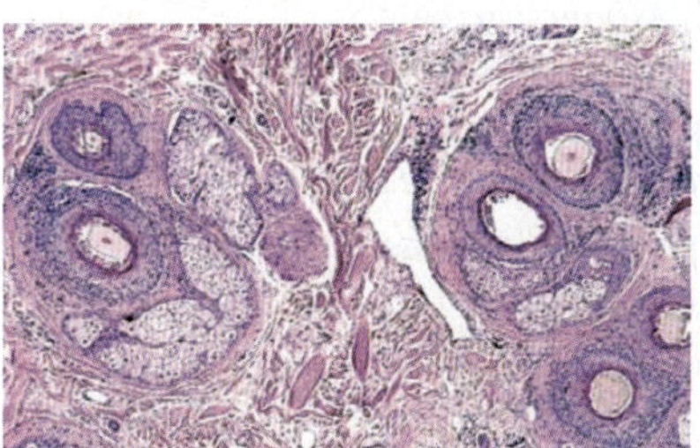

Fig. Pseudopelade of Brocq

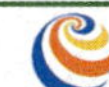 HIGH YIELD MCQs ANSWERS WITH EXPLANATIONS 

1. Ans. (a) Lichen planopilaris; (b) Discoid lupus erythematous; (d) Lichen planus

[Ref. DVL by Thappa, 4/e p260,261]

Scarring/Cicatricial alopecia	Nonscarring/Noncicatricial alopecia
Basal cell carcinoma Lichen planus/ planopilaris Folliculitis decalvans Cutaneous lupus Herpes zoster Discoid lupus erythematosus Cutaneous metastasis Linear scleroderma (Morphea) Sarcoidosis	HIV Hypo/hyperthyroidism Hypopituitarism Deficiency of Iron, Zinc, Protein, Biotin Secondary syphilis Androgenic alopecia Alopecia areata Lupus erythematosus Traumatic alopecia (Trichotilomania) Tinea capitis Telogen effluvium
[Mnemonic: By **L**owering **F**at **C**oronary **H**eart **D**isease **C**hances **L**essen **S**ignificantly**]**	[Mnemonic: High Density SALT]

2. Ans. (a) Alopecia areata

[Ref. DVT by Thappa, 4/e p261]

Alopecia Areata

- Alopecia areata is a form of nonscarring alopecia
- Characteristic initial lesion is a circumscribed bald smooth patch
- Exclamation point may be seen at periphery of the patch
- MC site is scalp but may involve any site

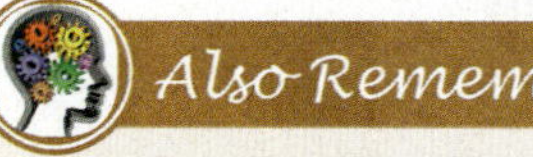

Also Remember

- Androgenic alopecia presents with diffuse involvement of frontotemporal regions and vertex, sparing occiput
- **Telogen effluvium** presents with diffuse involvement of scalp, with a history of a precipitating factor 3–4 months earlier, e.g. severe febrile illness, crash dieting, mental stress

3. Ans. (c) Trichotillomania

[Ref. Neena Khanna, 4/e p136]

Trichotillomania

- **Hair pulling tic**
- Young women pull hair to relieve pain

- Defined as the irresistible urge to pull out hair, accompanied by a sense of relief after it has been plucked
- Alopecia patch with hair of different length in different directions

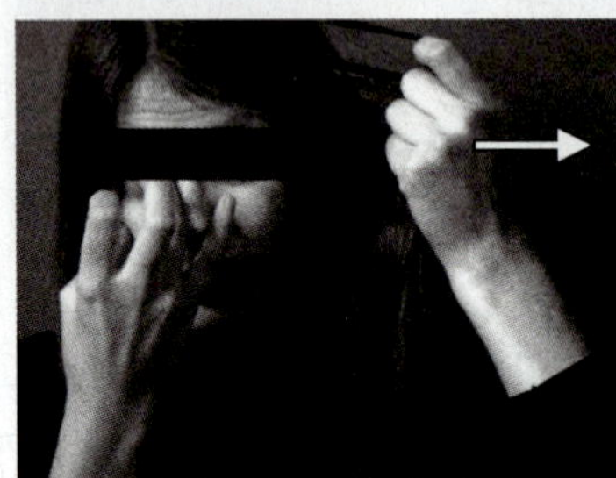

Fig. Trichotillomania

4. Ans. (c) 3 months
[Ref. Hair Care by Draelos, 1/e p18]
- Telogen effluvium usually occurs 2-3 months after significant physical or emotional stress

5. Ans. (c) Telogen effluvium
[Ref. Hair Care by Draelos, 1/e p18]

6. Ans. (c) Alopecia areata
[Ref. Neena Khanna, 5/e p141]

7. Ans. (c) DLE
[Ref. Neena Khanna, 5/e p141]

8. Ans. (d) Cicatricial alopecia
[Ref. Neena Khanna, 5/e p148]

Pseudopelade of Brocq
- A scarring alopecia for which no cause identified
- Presents as patches of Cicatricial alopecia with 'foot prints in snow' appearance

9. Ans. (a) DLE; (b) SLE; (e) Lichen planus
[Ref. Neena Khanna, 5/e p141]

10. Ans. (a) Alopecia areata
[Ref. Neena Khanna, 5/e p142]
- Presence of exclamation mark hairs at the periphery of the lesion is pathognomonic of alopecia areata
- Hair is broken off about 4 mm from the scalp due to constriction in the shaft

11. Ans. (a) Exclamatory mark hair
[Ref. Neena Khanna, 5/e p142]

12. Ans. (b) Alopecia areata
[Ref. Neena Khanna, 5/e p142]

13. Ans. (d) Female pattern baldness

14. Ans. (c) Alopecia areata
[Ref. Neena Khanna, 5/e p142]

15. Ans. (a) Testosterone
[Ref. Neena Khanna, 5/e p146]
- Anti androgen is therapy hence testosterone is contraindicated

16. Ans. (a) The phase of activity and growth
[Ref. Neena Khanna, 5/e p140]
- Anagen: Phase of activity and growth, Hair shows pigmented angulated bulb
- Catagen: Phase of involution
- Telogen: Phase of resting, Hair shows depigmented club shaped bulb

17. Ans. (b) Telogen effluvium
[Ref. Hair Care by Draelos, 1/e p18]
- Telogen effluvium usually occurs 2-3 months after significant physical or emotional stress

18. Ans. (d) Lichen planus
[Ref. Neena Khanna, 5/e p141]

Cicatricial Alopecia
- Aplasia cutis
- Lichen planopilaris
- DLE
- Favus
- Kerion
- Nevus sebaceous
- Physical or chemical trauma
- Basal cell carcinoma
- Pseudopelade of Brocq

19. Ans. (b) Alopecia areata
[Ref. Neena Khanna, 5/e p142]

20. Ans. (a) Minoxidil
[Ref. Neena Khanna, 5/e p144]
- Treatment for few lesions of more than 6 months duration:
  - Topical steroids
  - Minoxidil
  - PUVA/ PUVA sol

21. Ans. (c) Psoriasis
[Ref. Neena Khanna, 5/e p141]

22. Ans. (b) Noncicatricial scar
[Ref. Neena Khanna, 5/e p141]

23. Ans. (d) Metagen
[Ref. Dermatology by Wolff, 2/e p1101]

Hair Passes through Four Stages
- Anagen: Growing phase (Lasts years)
- Catagen: Transitional phase (Lasts 2 weeks)
- Telogen: Resting phase (3-4 months)
- Exogen: Shedding phase

24. Ans. (b) Trichophyton tonsurans
[Ref. Clinical Dermatology by Habif, 6/e p505]
- T. tonsurans/ T. violaceum causes endothrix hair invasion often referred to as "black-dot"
- Hair cortex is almost completely replaced by spores.

25. Ans. (c) KOH mount
[Ref. Fitzpatrick's Dermatology, 8/e p2284-85]

Tinea Capitis
- Dermatophyte infection of hair and scalp, typically caused by Trichophyton and Microsporum species
- Ectothrix infections: Using KOH examination, in, only the arthroconidia on the surface of the hair shaft may be visualized, although hyphae are also present within the hair shaft
  - Cuticle is destroyed
  - Circumscribed erythematous scaly patches of nonscarring alopecia with breakage of hairs: "Gray patch" type
  - On Wood's lamp examination, a yellow-green fluorescence may be detected, depending on the causative organism
- Endothrix infections: Arthroconidia and hyphae remain within the hair shaft and leave the cortex and cuticle intact
  - Appearance of "black dots" which represent broken hairs at the surface
- Favus: Longitudinally arranged hyphae and air spaces within the hair shaft
  - Arthroconidia are not usually noted in infected hairs

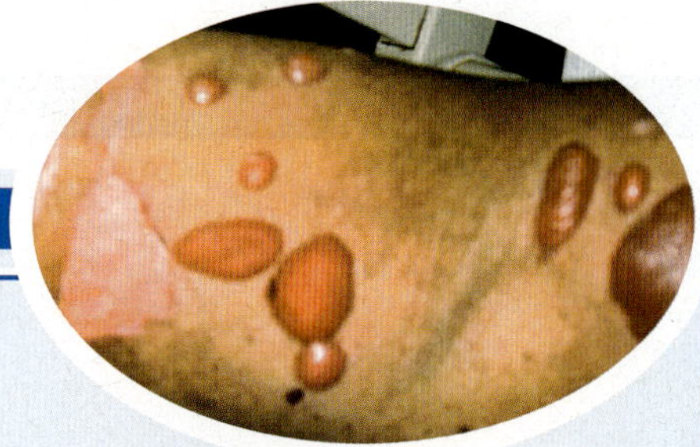

Chapter 10

Sweat, Sebaceous and Other Glands and Diseases

THEORETICAL CONCEPTS

X A. ACNE VULGARIS

- Underlying cause:
  - *Organisms*:[Q]
    - **Propionibacterium acnes**[Q]
    - Malassezia furfur
    - Staphylococcus epidermidis
  - *Other factors associated*:
    - Familial predisposition
    - High glycaemic diet[Q]
    - Oil-based cosmetics
    - Facial massage
    - Premenstrual oedema of pilosebaceous duct
    - Increased anger and anxiety
  - *Pathogenesis*: Type IV inflammatory response
- Associated risk factors:
  - Hormonal: Androgens[Q], Glucocorticoids
  - Infections[Q]: Staphylococcus epidermidis, Pityrosporum, Propionibacterium
  - Hyperkeratosis of Pilosebaceous ostia[Q]
  - Premenstrual part of cycle
  - High temperature, High humidity
  - Drugs: Phenytoin, Phenobarbitone, Carbamazepine, Isoniazid, Rifampicin, Ethionamide, Vitamin B12, Antidepressants, Cyclosporine
- Clinical presentation:
  - Sites: Face, shoulders, upper trunk
  - *Polymorphic eruption*:[Q] Comedones, papules, nodules, cysts
  - ***Comedones***: Pathognomonic lesions of acne vulgaris[Q]
    - **Open comedones (Black heads)**: Block on skin surface
    - **Closed comedones (White heads)**: Block below skin surface
  - *Scars*:
    - Depressed scars: Ice pick scars, Box car scars
    - Hypertrophic, keloid scars
- Treatment:[Q]
  - *Topical Retinoids*:
    - **Retinoic acid**
    - Adapalene
    - Isotretinoin
    - Tazarotene

- *Topical Benzoyl peroxide*
- *Topical antibiotics*: Clindamycin, Eryhtromycin
- *Other topical agents*: Glycolic acid, Azelaic acid
- *Systemic antibiotics*: Doxycycline, Minocycline, Eryhtromycin, Azithromycin
- *Anti-androgenic hormones*: Cyproterone acetate, Spironolactone
- *Isotretinoin*

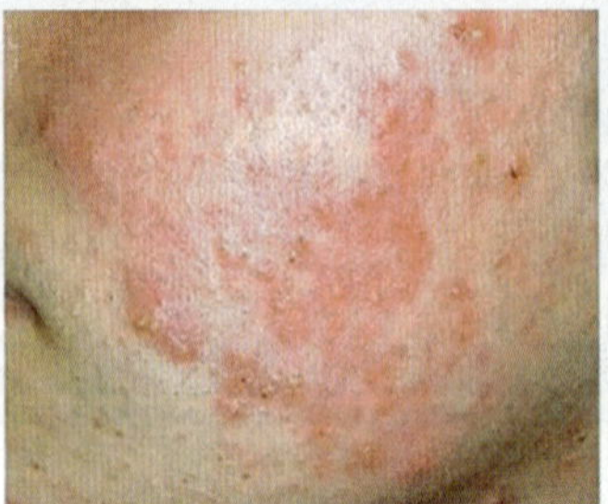

Fig. Acne vulgaris

Fig. Open comedones

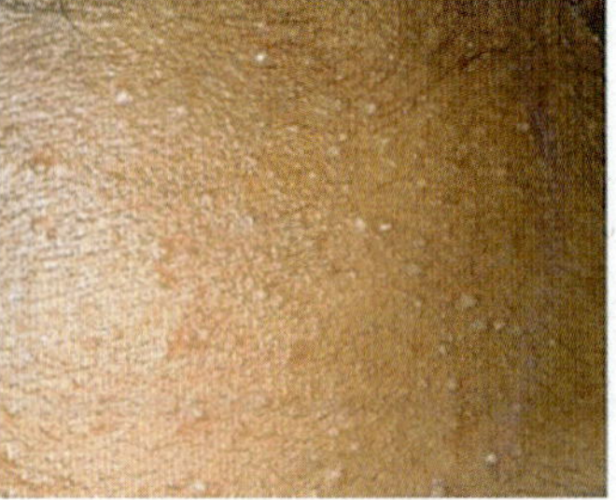

Fig. Closed comedones

X B. ROSACEA

- *Underlying cause*: Unknown
- *Clinical presentation*:
  - Erythema
  - Telangiectasia
  - Papules and pustules
  - Sites: Cheeks, forehead, chin, nose
- *Treatment*:[Q]
  - Topical Metronidazole
  - Tetracyclines

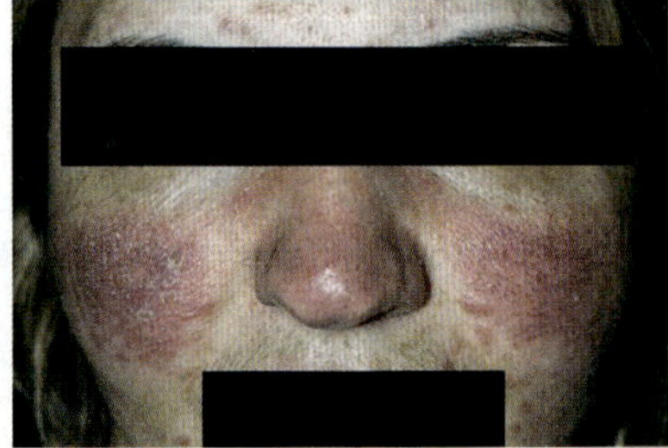

Fig. Acne rosacea

Topper's Edge

Acne Vulgaris Vs Acne Rosacea[Q]

	Acne Vulgaris	Acne Rosacea
Age group affected	Adolescents	Middle aged women
Distribution	Face, upper trunk	Cheeks, Nose, Forehead
Morphology	Typical comedones	Papules, nodules, pustules
Other features	Greasy skin	Erythema, telangiectasia

X C. OTHER DISORDERS OF GLANDS IN SKIN

- **Fordyce disease** (Fordyce spot): Benign hamartoma of Ectopic sebaceous glands[Q]
  - Common sites[Q]: Lips (MC site[Q]), Oral mucosa
  - Tyson's glands[Q]: Penis, Vulva
  - MC age group: Pubertal males
- **Fox-Fordyce disease** (Apocrine Miliaria[Q]): Chronic blockade of ducts of Apocrine sweat glands[Q]
  - MC site: Axilla[Q]
  - MC age group: 13-35 years women
- **Miliaria** (Sweat rash): Obstruction of ducts of Eccrine sweat glands[Q]
  - MC type: Miliaria rubra (Prickly heat)

IMAGE-BASED QUESTIONS

1. **Diagnose the Skin appendage disorder shown in the Photograph** ***[Recent Question 2016]***

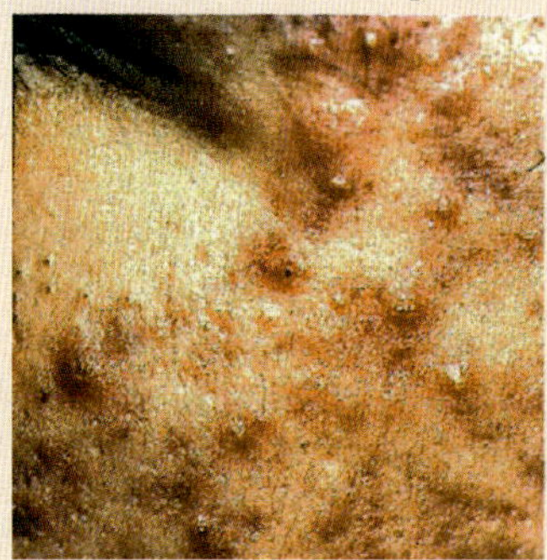

a. Acne vulgaris b. Hyperhidrosis
c. Miliaria d. Alopecia areata

2. **Diagnose the Skin appendage disorder shown in the Photograph**

a. Hidradenitis suppurativa b. Miliaria
c. Acne conglobata d. Acne vulgaris

3. **Identify the Type of skin lesion from a case of Acne vulgaris (Photograph)**

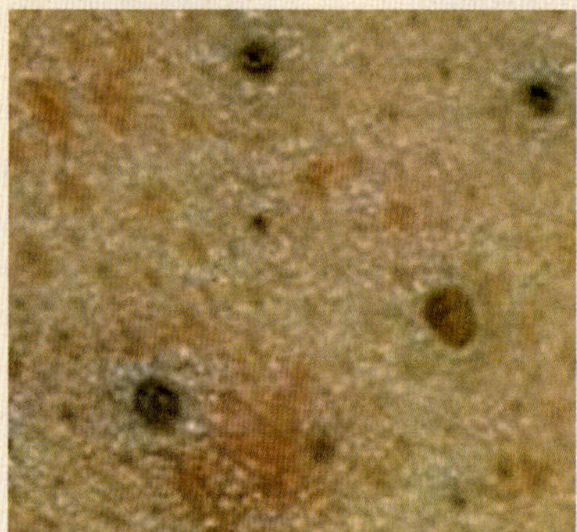

a. Open comedone b. Closed comedone
c. Submarine comedone d. None of the above

4. **A young boy with Oily skin presents to Dermatology OPD with condition as shown in Photograph. Treatment of choice** ***[AIIMS November 2015]***

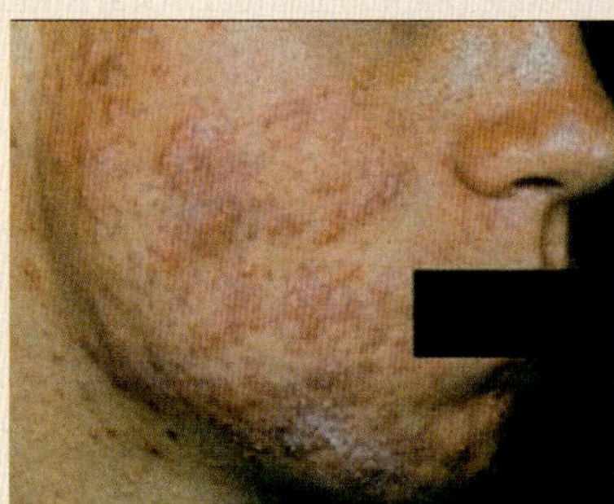

a. Oral Steroids b. Oral Isotretinoin
c. Topical Retinoic acid d. Topical Steroids

5. **A woman presented with Red macular lesions on central part of face and chin (See Photograph) with flushing on sun exposure and increasing with emotional disturbance. Diagnosis is** ***[AIIMS PG May 2015]***

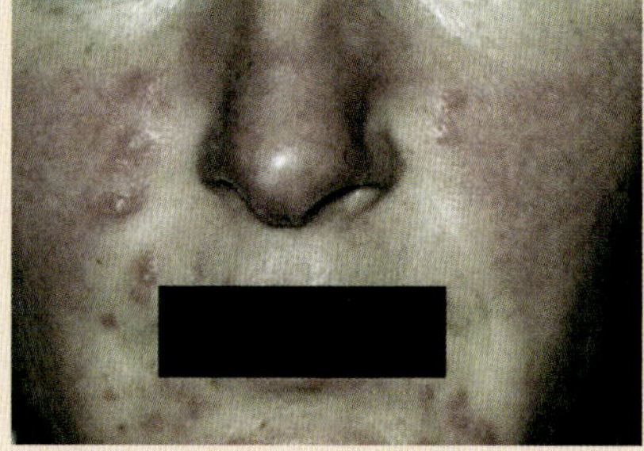

a. SLE b. DLE
c. Acne rosacea d. Acne vulgaris

ANSWERS WITH EXPLANATIONS OF IBQs 

1. Ans. (a) Acne vulgaris *[Ref. Neena Khanna, 4/e p111]*

Clinical Presentation of Acne

- *Sites*: Face, shoulders, upper trunk
- *Polymorphic eruption*: Comedones, papules, nodules, cysts
- *Comedones*: Pathognomonic lesions of acne vulgaris
  - Open comedones (Black heads): Block on skin surface
  - Closed comedones (White heads): Block below skin surface
- *Scars*:
  - Depressed scars: Ice pick scars, Box car scars
  - Hypertrophic, keloid scars

2. Ans. (b) Miliaria *[Ref. Neena Khanna, 4/e p126]*

- Miliaria crystallina: Tiny, clear, non-inflamed (crystalline) vesicles occurring during episodes of lysis of fever

3. Ans. (a) Open comedone *[Ref. Neena Khanna, 4/e p111]*

- *Comedones*: Pathognomonic lesions of acne vulgaris
  - Open comedones (Black heads): Block on skin surface
  - Closed comedones (White heads): Block below skin surface

4. Ans. (b) Oral Isotretinoin *[Ref. Neena Khanna, 4/e p120]*

Treatment of Choice in Acne

- Mild acne (Comedonal): Topical Retinoids
- Mild acne (Papulopustular): Topical Retinoids + Topical Antibiotics/ Benzoyl peroxide
- Moderate acne (Papulopustular): Oral Antibiotics + Topical Retinoids + Benzoyl peroxide
- Severe acne (Nodular) [Photograph]: Oral Retinoids

5. Ans. (c) Acne rosacea *[Ref. Clinical Neuropathic Medicine by Hechtman, 1/e p661]*

Acne Rosacea (Photograph)

- Acne-like bumps may appear, often in the redder area of the central face
- Flushing that brings on rosacea's redness can be associated with a build-up of fluid in the tissues of the face; It often occurs above the nasolabial folds and cause a "baggy cheek" appearance
- Common triggers: Sun exposure, Emotional stress, Hot/ Cold weather, Wind, Alcohol, Spicy foods, Heavy exercise, Hot baths, Heated beverages and Certain skin-care products

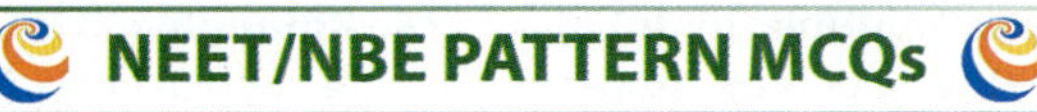

1. **Eccrine glands are involved in** *[Recent Question 2016]*
   a. Bromhidrosis
   b. Miliaria
   c. Hidradenitis suppurativa
   d. Fox-Fordyce disease
2. **Fordyce disease most commonly involves** *[Recent Question 2016, 2017]*
   a. Lips b. Neck
   c. Buccal mucosa d. Trunk
3. **Treatment options for Acne vulgaris is /are** *[Recent Question 2016]*
   a. Topical erythromycin b. Oral minocycline
   c. Isotretinoin d. All the above
4. **Comedones are characteristic of** *[NBE FMGE September 2004]*
   a. Psoriasis b. Acne vulgaris
   c. Lichen planus d. Pemphigus
5. **Hidradenitis suppurativa is a disease of?** *[Recent Question 2012, 2013]*
   a. Apocrine glands b. Eccrine glands
   c. Holocrine glands d. None of the above
6. **In sebaceous glands accumulation of sebum leads to** *[Recent Question 2012, 2013]*
   a. Milia b. Acne
   c. Epidermoid cyst d. Miliaria
7. **Acne is a chronic inflammatory disease of** *[NBE DNB 2011]*
   a. Sweat unit b. Pilosebaceous unit
   c. Hair follicle d. Dennis
8. **Eccrine glands are involved in** *[Recent Question 2012, 2013]*
   a. Bromhidrosis
   b. Miliaria
   c. Hidradenitis suppurativa
   d. Fox - Fordyce disease
9. **Long term tetracycline therapy helps in Acne rosacea by** *[NBE DNB 1992]*
   a. Preventing fibrosis
   b. Suppressing the papulopustular
   c. Preventing auto sensitization
   d. Decreasing serum cholesterol
10. **Fordyce spots involve?** *[Recent Question 2017]*
    a. Penis b. Tongue
    c. Fingers d. Nails
11. **Fox-Fordyce disease is a disease of?** *[Recent Question 2017]*
    a. Eccrine glands
    b. Apocrine glands
    c. Holocrine glands
    d. Endocrine glands
12. **Differential diagnosis of Rosacea includes all of the following except?** *[Recent Question 2017]*
    a. Acne vulgaris
    b. Lupus erythematosus
    c. BCC
    d. Melasma
13. **Best treatment for Nodulocystic acne** *[Recent Question 2017]*
    a. Azithromycin
    b. Adapalene
    c. Clindamycin
    d. Dapsone
14. **A female presented with erythematous lesions on face with intolerance to spicy food is. Most likely diagnosis is** *[Recent Question 2017]*
    a. Acne rosacea
    b. SLE
    c. Chloasma
    d. LPP

HIGH YIELD MCQs

1. **Comedones are seen in** *[AIIMS PGMEE 1998]*
   a. Acne vulgaris b. Lichen planus
   c. Adenoma sebaceum d. Pityriasis
2. **Treatment of acne vulgaris may include all except** *[PGI 1996, AIIMS PGMEE 2003]*
   a. Cryotherapy b. Oestrogens
   c. UV light d. Androgens
3. **Treatment of nodulocystic acne is** *[AIIMS PGMEE 1995]*
   a. Erythromycin b. Tertacycline
   c. Isotretinoin d. Steroids
4. **Recalcitrant Pustular Acne is treated by** *[AIIMS PGMEE 1992]*
   a. Oral erythromycin
   b. Oral tetracycline
   c. Steroid
   d. Retinoid
5. **Rhinophyma complicates** *[Recent Question 2016, All India PGMEE 1997, UP PGMEE 2004, AP PGMEE 1998]*
   a. Acne vulgaris b. Acne rosacea
   c. Psoriasis d. Pemphigus
6. **Treatment of choice for Acne vulgaris** *[PGI 2005]*
   a. Minocycline for inflammatory acne
   b. Retinoids for comedonal acne
   c. Etretinate
   d. Rifampicin
   e. Dapsone
7. **Treatment of choice in nodulocystic acne is** *[All India PGMEE 1994]*
   a. Systemic steroid b. Retinoic acid
   c. Benzoyl peroxide d. Estrogen

8. A 24-year-old unmarried woman has multiple nodular, cystic, pustular and comadonic lesions on face, upper back and shoulders for 2 years. The drug of choice for her treatment would be *[All India PGMEE 2006]*
a. Acitretin b. Isotretinoin
c. Doxycycline d. Azithromycin

9. A 40-year-old woman presents with a 2 year old history of erythematous papulo-pustular lesions on convexities of the face. There is a background of erythema & telangiectasia. The most likely diagnosis is *[All India PGMEE 2005]*
a. Acne vulgaris
b. Rosacea
c. SLE
d. Polymorphic light eruption

10. Acne vulgaris is due to involvement of *[AIIMS PGMEE 2001]*
a. Sebaceous gland b. Pilosebaceous glands
c. Eccrine gland d. Apocrine gland

11. Sweat glands of palm can be differentiated from others by the following *[JIPMER PGMEE 1991, Delhi PGMEE 1993]*
a. Apocrine glands
b. High chloride content
c. Secretion stimulated by emotional stimuli
d. Chemical mediators control the secretion

12. Sebaceous cysts are seen in *[AIPGMEE 2011]*
a. Turcot's syndrome b. Gardener's syndrome
c. Cowden syndrome d. Muir Torre syndrome

13. Acne vulgaris is due to involvement of *[PGI 2006]*
a. Sebaceous glands b. Eccrine glands
c. Pilosebaceous glands d. Apocrine glands
e. Sweat glands

14. All are false except *[PGI 2008]*
a. Sweat glands are most numerous on back & least on sole
b. Palm & sole sweat glands are last to appear
c. Sweat duct produce isotonic sweat
d. Gonadectomy of adults impair apocrine sweat secretion
e. Apocrine glands are under cholinergic control

15. True about apocrine gland is all except *[PGI 2009]*
a. Modified sweat gland
b. Modified sebaceous gland
c. Present in groin & axilla
d. Infection is known as hydradenitis suppurative

16. Miliaria is a disorder of *[PGI 2007]*
a. Sebaceous glands
b. Apocrine glands
c. Merocrine glands
d. Holocrine glands
e. Eccrine glands

17. In Fox-Fordyce disease, true is/are *[PGI 2002]*
a. Common in adult woman
b. Bullous lesions are common
c. Common in areola and axilla
d. Associated with other malignancies

18. Rhinophyma is *[PGI 1996]*
a. Glandular form of acne rosacea
b. Form of acne vulgaris
c. Affects the scalp
d. A form of dermatofibroma

19. Rhinophyma is (Potato nose) *[AP PGMEE 1996]*
a. Septal deviation of nose
b. Sweat gland hypertrophy
c. Mucous gland hypertrophy
d. Sebaceous gland hypertrophy

20. Bromhidrosis may be produced by intake of the following except *[JIPMER PGMEE 1993, Rohtak PGMEE 1996]*
a. Asafoetida b. Ginger
c. Onions d. Garlic

21. Crystalline miliaria is due to obstruction to *[JIPMER PGMEE 1993]*
a. Sebaceous glands b. Sweat glands
c. Hair roots d. Accessory sweat glands

22. Causative factor for acne are all except *[PGI 2000]*
a. Androgen
b. Only food
c. Bacterial contamination
d. Hypercornification of duct
e. Lipophilic yeast

23. Fordyce's disease mainly involves *[PGI 1997, AIIMS PGMEE 2000]*
a. Lips b. Buccal mucosa
c. Neck d. Trunk

24. Comedones are characteristics of *[Kerala PGMEE 1994]*
a. Acne vulgaris b. Acne rosacea
c. SLE d. Adenoma sebaceum

25. Treatment of acne *[PGI 2005]*
a. 13 cis-retinol b. Minocycline
c. Erythromycin d. Dapsone
e. Rifampicin

26. Causative factor for acne are following except *[SGPGI 2000]*
a. Androgen b. Only food
c. Keratin d. Cell nucleus

27. A 19 years old girl has multiple papulopustular erythematous lesions on face and neck, the likely diagnosis is *[AIIMS PGMEE 1994]*
a. Acne rosacea b. Acne vulgaris
c. Pityriasis versicolor d. Lupus vulgaris

28. Regarding Fordyce spots *[PGI 2002]*
a. Represent internal malignancy
b. Ectopic sebaceous glands
c. Present in axillae
d. Found in healthy people
e. Are erythematous

29. Acne vulgaris is caused by *[JIPMER PGMEE 1991]*
a. Staph aureus
b. Diphtheroids
c. Sweat gland hyperplasia
d. Obstruction to pilosebaceous duct

30. Drug treatment of acne vulgaris *[PGI 2005]*
a. Minocycline b. Penicillin
c. Cotrimoxazole d. Gentamycin
e. Tetracycline

31. A 16 years old girl with nodular and cystic acne, treatment is *[AIIMS November 2014]*
a. Azelaic acid b. Benzoyl peroxide
c. Acitretin d. Isotretinoin

 NEET/NBE PATTERN MCQs ANSWERS WITH EXPLANATIONS 

1. Ans. (b) Miliaria

[Ref. DVL by Thappa, 4/e p258]

Miliaria

- Occurs due to obstruction of free flow of eccrine sweat to the skin surrounding face, sweat is retained resulting in signs and symptoms
- Based on HPE and clinical examination Miliaria is divided into
  - Miliaria crystalline (sudamina): Superficial, subcorneal, non-inflammatory vesicles easy to rupture and follow by high grade fever
  - Miliaria rubra (prickly heat) is the commonest type of miliaria
  - Miliaria profunda results when the sweat leaks into dermis

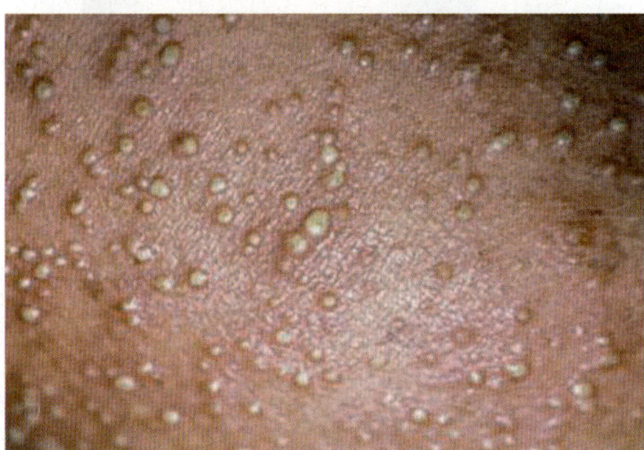

Fig. Miliaria

2. Ans. (a) Lips

[Ref. Diseases of the Skin with Illustrations by Dearborn, 1/e p526]

Fordyce's Disease (Pseudo-colloid of Lips)

- Involves Vermilion of the lips and mucous membranes of mouth
- Congenital ectopic sebaceous glands seen mainly in the buccal mucosa or lips

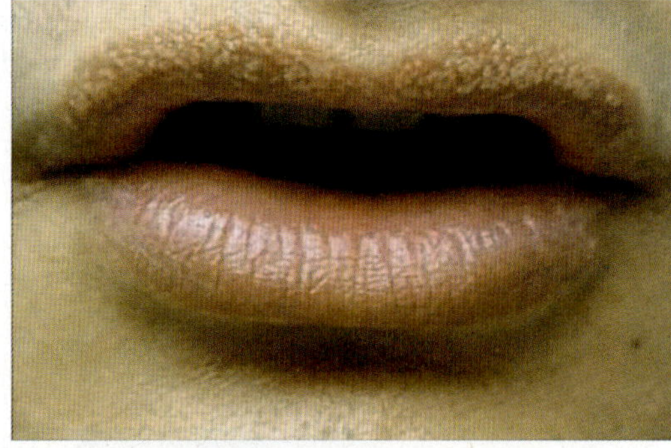

Fig. Fordyce's disease

3. Ans. (d) All of the above

[Ref. DVL by Thappa, 4/e p.156,157]

Treatment Options for Acne Vulgaris

Local or topical therapy	Systemic therapy
Benzoyl peroxide 2.5-5% acts as comedolytic	Antibiotics: Tetracycline, minocycline, azithromycin, clarithromycin
Antibiotics: Clindamycin (1%), erythromycin (2-3%), sodium sulfacetamide & tetracycline	Dapsone: Severe acne conglobates (rarely used today)
Sulphur & resorcinol eg., Sulphur calamine lotion	Corticosteroids (Prednisolone 2.5-7.5 mg)
Tretinoine (0.025-0.1% cream or gel) Adapalene (0.1% gel) Tazarotene (0.05% - 0.1%)	Oral retinoids: Isotretinoin (0.5-1 mg/ kg/ day)

4. Ans. (b) Acne vulgaris

[Ref. Neena Khanna, 4/e p111]

Clinical Presentation of Acne

- *Sites*: Face, shoulders, upper trunk
- *Polymorphic eruption*: Comedones, papules, nodules, cysts
- *Comedones*: **Pathognomonic lesions of acne vulgaris**
  - Open comedones (Black heads): Block on skin surface
  - Closed comedones (White heads): Block below skin surface
- *Scars*:
  - Depressed scars: Ice pick scars, Box car scars
  - Hypertrophic, keloid scars

5. Ans. (a) Apocrine glands

[Ref. Neena Khanna, 5/e p139]

Hidradentis Suppurativa/ Apocrine Acne

- Aetiology: Follicular occlusion, a consistent early finding
- Features: Occlusion of apocrine gland
  - Follicular rupture
  - Perifollicular rupture
  - Perifollicular inflammation
  - Secondary inflammation

6. Ans. (b) Acne

[Ref. Neena Khanna, 5/e p121]

Pathogenesis of Acne Vulgaris

- Induces follicular epidermal hyperproliferation
- Microbial colonization
- Increased sebum production
- And release of inflammatory mediators

7. Ans. (b) Pilosebaceous unit

[Ref. Neena Khanna, 5/e p120]

- Acne vulgaris: A disorder of pilosebaceous unit which predominantly affects the peripubertal population

8. Ans. (b) Miliaria

[Ref. Neena Khanna, 5/e p137]

- Etiology of Miliaria: Obstruction and rupture of eccrine sweat ducts, leading to spillage of sweat into adjoining tissues

9. Ans. (b) Suppressing the papulo pustular

[Ref. Neena Khanna, 5/e p129]

10. Ans. (a) Penis

[Ref. Hurwitz Clinical Pediatric Dermatology, 5/e p189]

Fordyce Disease (Fordyce Spot)

- Benign hamartoma of Ectopic sebaceous glands; composed of 'free' (not associated with hair follicles) sebaceous glands, and they probably represent a normal anatomic variant
- Common sites: Lips (MC site), Oral mucosa
- Tyson's glands: Penis, Vulva
- MC age group: Pubertal males
- Asymptomatic, and treatment is unnecessary

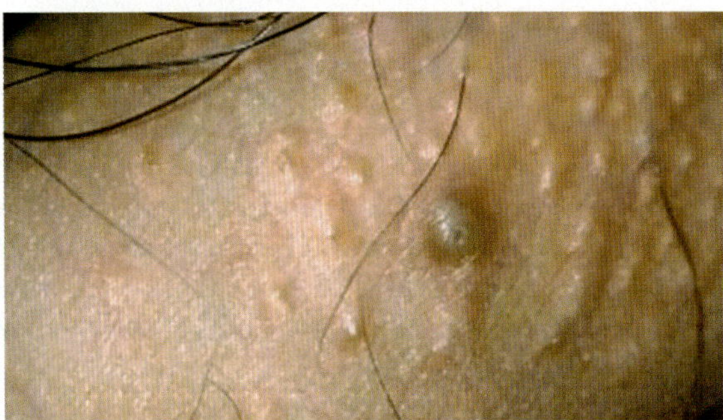

Fig. Fordyce spots (Penis)

11. Ans. (b) Apocrine glands

[Ref. Liposuction by Shiffman, 1/e p502; Neena Khanna, 5/e p120]

Fox-Fordyce Disease

- A rare, chronic, pruritic disorder characterized by small perifollicular papules localized to the apocrine gland bearing regions of the skin: Very common mainly due to ectopic sebaceous gland.
- Axillae, periareolar region, lips, buccal mucosa, vulva and penile shaft are most commonly involved

12. Ans. (d) Melasma

[Ref. Dermatology by Bolognia, 3/e p565]

- Differential diagnosis of Rosacea includes Acne vulgaris, Seborrhoeic dermatitis, Perioral dermatitis, Carcinoid syndrome, Lupus erythematosus, Basal cell carcinoma
- Most common potential diagnostic confusion is between rosacea and acne vulgaris, owing to the presence of pustules and papules

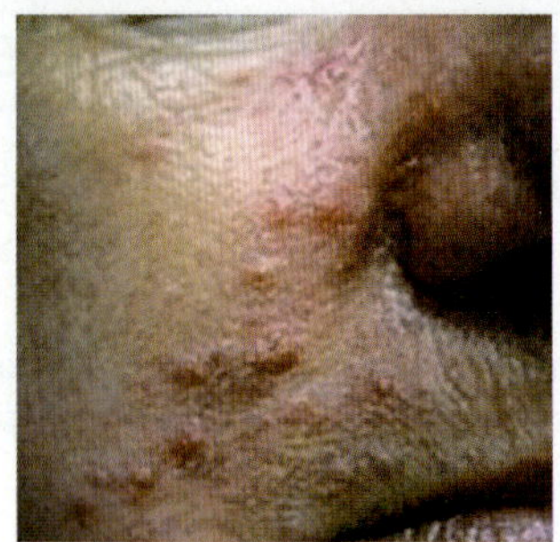

Fig. Rosacea

13. Ans. (d) Dapsone

[Ref. Pediatric Dermatology by Teng, 1/e p116]

- In patients with recalcitrant nodular acne, or with contraindications to Isotretinoin, oral dapsone is sometimes used at a dose of 100 mg daily

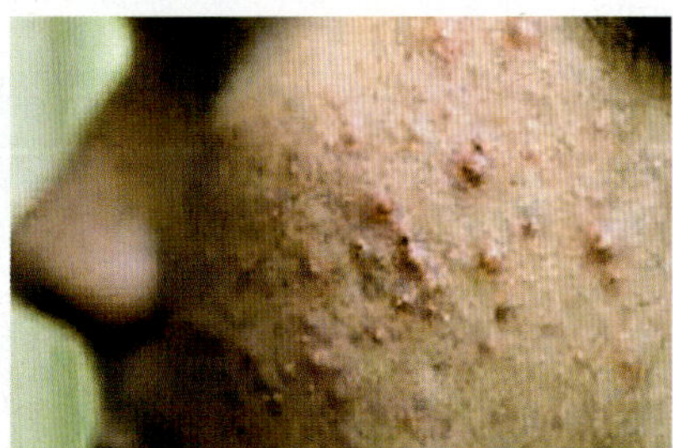

Fig. Nodulocystic acne

14. Ans. (a) Acne rosacea

[Ref. Neena Khanna, 4/e p122]

Acne Rosacea

- Diagnostic points:
  - Middle aged women
  - Episodes of flushing and intolerance to heat and spicy foods
  - Background erythema and telangiectasia with episodes of papules and pustules
  - Absence of comedones
  - Convexities of the face involved - forehead, nose, cheeks, and chin
  - Characteristic sparing of periorbital and perioral area
- Hot or cold temperature, sunlight, alcohol, exercise, spicy foods, emotional stress, topical irritants, and medications are triggers of Rosacea

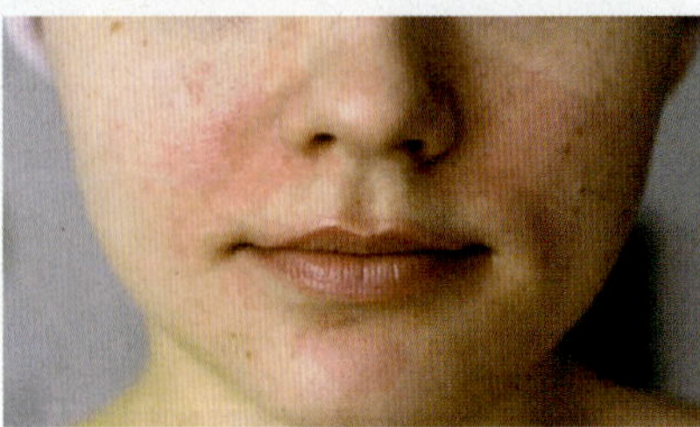

Fig. Acne rosacea

HIGH YIELD MCQs ANSWERS WITH EXPLANATIONS

1. **Ans. (a) Acne vulgaris**
   [Ref. Neena Khanna, 5/e p123]
   - Comedones are pathognomonic lesion of acne vulgaris
   - Two types: Open (Black headed), Closed (White headed)

2. **Ans. (d) Androgens**
   [Ref. Neena Khanna, 5/e p146]

3. **Ans. (c) Isotretinoin**
   [Ref. Neena Khanna, 5/e p129]

4. **Ans. (d) Retinoid**
   [Ref. Neena Khanna, 5/e p129]

5. **Ans. (b) Acne rosacea**
   [Ref. Neoplasms with Sebaceous Differentiation by Charles Steffen, 1/e p270]
   - Rhinophyma may be complicated by features of rosacea

6. **Ans. (a) Minocycline for inflammatory acne; (b) Retinoids for comedonal acne**
   [Ref. Neena Khanna, 5/e p128-129]

7. **Ans. (b) Retinoic acid**
   [Ref. Neena Khanna, 5/e p129]

8. **Ans. (b) Isoretinoin**
   [Ref. Neena Khanna, 5/e p129]

9. **Ans. (b) Rosacea**
   [Ref. Neena Khanna, 5/e p126]

   Diagnostic Features of Rosacea
   - Middle aged women
   - Comedones absent. Papules, nodules & pustules present
   - Lesions on convexities of face (cheeks, nose & forehead)
   - Spares periorificial area
   - Background erythema and telangiectasia prominent

10. **Ans. (b) Pilosebaceous glands**
    [Ref. Neena Khanna, 5/e p120]

11. **Ans. (c) Secretion stimulated by emotional stimuli**
    [Ref. Neena Khanna, 5/e p135]
    - Emotional sweating, provoked by fear, anxiety and worry are mainly seen on palms, soles and axillae

12. **Ans. (b) Gardener's syndrome**
    [Ref. SRB's Surgery for Dental Students by Sriram M Bhat, 2/e p68]
    - Multiple sebaceous cysts may be associated with syndromes like Gardner's syndrome

13. **Ans. (c) Pilosebaceous glands**
    [Ref. Neena Khanna, 5/e p120]

14. **Ans. (d) Gonadectomy of adults impair apocrine sweat secretion**

15. **Ans. (b) Modified sebaceous gland**
    [Ref. Neena Khanna, 5/e p120]

16. **Ans. (e) Eccrine glands**
    [Ref. Neena Khanna, 5/e p137]

17. **Ans. (a) Common in adult woman; (c) Common in areola and axilla**
    [Ref. Liposuction: Principles and Practice by Shiffman, 1/e p502; Neena Khanna, 5/e p120]

    Fox–Fordyce Disease
    - A rare, chronic, pruritic disorder characterized by small perifollicular papules localized to the apocrine gland-bearing regions of the skin: Very common mainly due to ectopic sebaceous gland.
    - Appear as symmetric, multiple, yellow, flat topped papules.
    - The disorder affects women more commonly than men (90% women in age group 15–35 years) during the second to fourth decade
    - Axillae, periareolar region, lips, buccal mucosa, vulva and penile shaft are most commonly involved

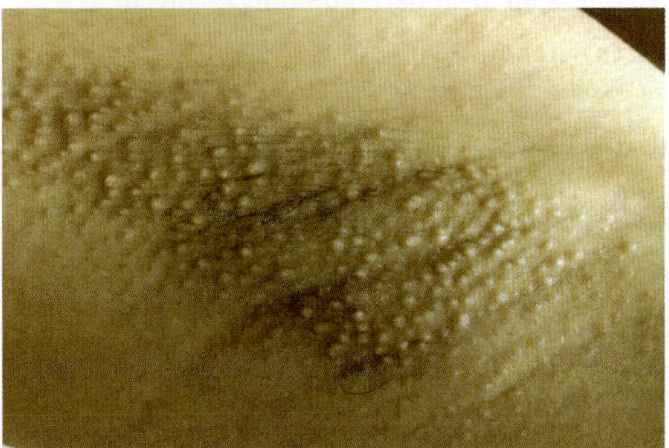

Fig. Fox-Fordyce disease

18. **Ans. (a) Glandular form of acne rosacea**
    [Ref. Neena Khanna, 5/e p132]

    Rhinophyma
    - Potato disease is seen in males mainly due to rosacea mainly and sometime by acne vulgaris
    - Begins as patulous follicles and telangiectasia on the distal portion of the nose, followed by development of a bulbous nose due to hyperplasia of sebaceous glands and connective tissue of the nose

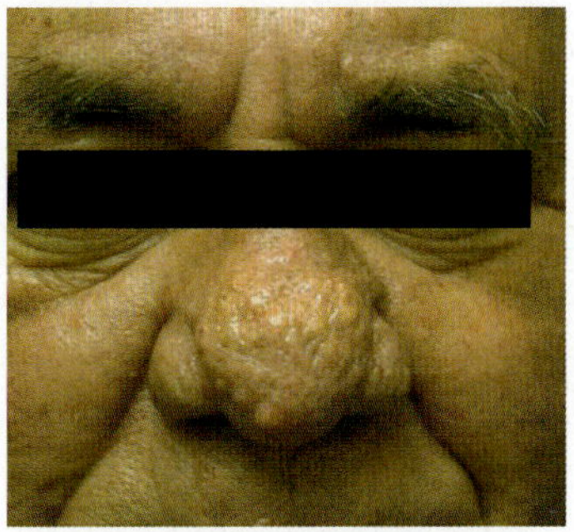

Fig. Rhinophyma

19. **Ans. (d) Sebaceous gland hypertrophy**
    [Ref. Neena Khanna, 5/e p132]

20. Ans. (b) Ginger
[Ref. Beauty Therapy Fact File by Susan Cressy, p368]

21. Ans. (b) Sweat glands
[Ref. Neena Khanna, 5/e p137]
- Crystalline miliaria is due to pillage of sweat into dermis due to obstruction of sweat duct

22. Ans. (b) Only food
[Ref. Neena Khanna, 5/e p121]
- Recently dermatologist believes that diet plays very little role
- Some paper shows association with high glycemic diet and rich in dairy products
- There is no conclusive evidence to restrict oily foods, chocolates and aerated drinks

23. Ans. (a) Lips; (b) Buccal mucosa
[Ref. Neena Khanna, 5/e p120]
- Axillae, periareolar region, lips, buccal mucosa, vulva and penile shaft are most commonly involved

24. Ans. (a) Acne vulgaris
[Ref. Neena Khanna, 5/e p123]

25. Ans. (a) 13 cis-retinol; (b) Minocycline; (c) Erythromycin
[Ref. Neena Khanna, 5/e p127-130]

26. Ans. (b) Only food
[Ref. Neena Khanna, 5/e p121]

27. Ans. (b) Acne vulgaris
[Ref. Neena Khanna, 5/e p126]
- Papulopastular erythematous lesion is seen both in rosea and vulgaris
- Age point for identification: Rosea is common in middle age whereas acne vulgaris in adolescent age group

28. Ans. (b) Ectopic sebaceous glands; (d) Found in healthy people
[Ref. Liposuction: Principles and Practice by Shiffman, 1/e p502; Neena Khanna, 5/e p120]

29. Ans. (d) Obstruction to pilosebaceous duct
[Ref. Neena Khanna, 5/e p120]

30. Ans. (a) Minocycline; (e) Tetracycline
[Ref. Neena Khanna, 5/e p129]
- Acne vulgaris treatment:
  - Doxycycline and minocycline are most commonly used
  - Less frequently, erythromycin and azithromycin is used

31. Ans. (d) Isotretinoin
[Ref. Pediatric Dermatology by Raghunatha, 2/e p349]

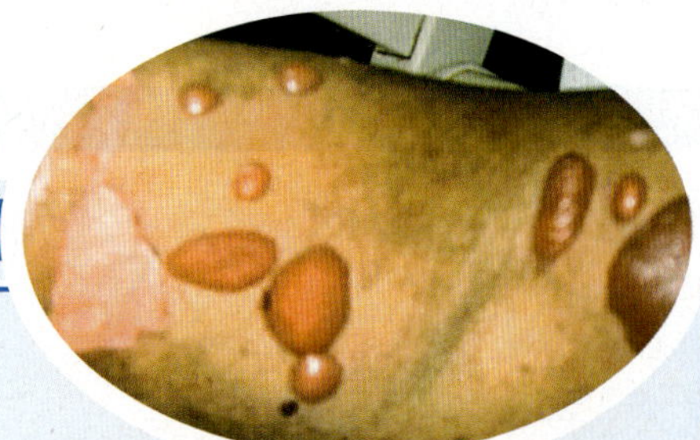

Chapter 11

Leprosy/Hansen's Disease

THEORETICAL CONCEPTS

XI A. DEFINITION

- Chronic infectious disease caused by mycobacterium leprae and affecting mainly peripheral nerves
- *Leprosy is a disease of 'high infectivity but low pathogenicity'*
- *Classification of leprosy:*[Q]

Ridley Jopling Classification	Indian Classification	Madrid Classification
• TT (Tuberculoid) • BT (Borderline tuberculoid) • BB (Borderline borderline) • BL(Borderline lepromatous) • LL (Lepromatous leprosy)	• Indeterminate • Tuberculoid • Borderline • Lepromatous • Pure neuritic	• Indeterminate • Tuberculoid • Borderline • Lepromatous

- Pure neuritic type leprosy (Indian classification): No skin lesions (Slit skin smears negative) [Q]
- ***Operational Classification of Leprosy*** *(according to skin smear positivity) to serve as a basis for chemotherapy*:
  - Paucibacillary leprosy (5 or less skin lesions)
  - Multibacillary leprosy (More than 5 skin lesions)

XI B. MODE OF TRANSMISSION OF LEPROSY

- Droplet infection (Aerosols)
- Contact transmission(Infectious patient and healthy susceptible)
- Direct contact (Skin to skin)
- Indirect contact (Soil, fomites, clothes and linen)
- Breast milk from lepromatous mothers
- Insect vectors
- Tattoo needles

XI C. CLINICAL PRESENTATION IN LEPROSY[Q]

- ***Lepromatous leprosy***:
  - Innumerable small, normoesthetic, symmetrical skin lesions [Q]
  - **Subepidermal free zones** [Q]
  - **Virchow/Lepra cells** (Macrophages with AFB) [Q]
  - Superciliary madarosis [Q]
  - **Globi** [Q]

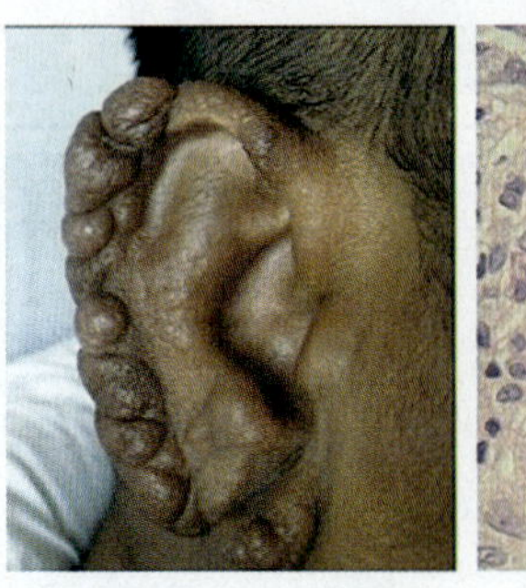

Fig. Lepromatous leprosy

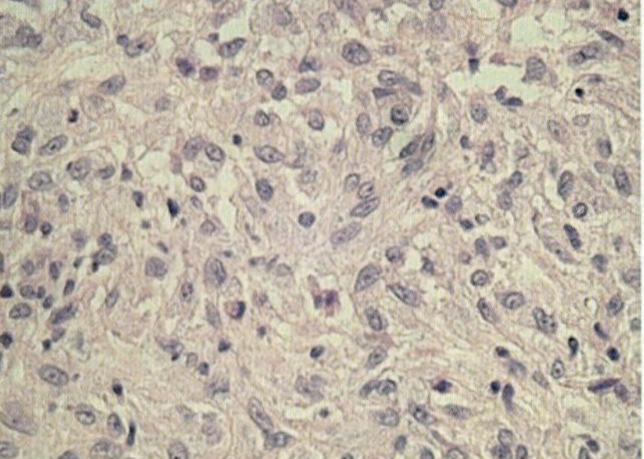

Fig. Virchow cells

- ***Tuberculoid leprosy***:
  - Noncaseating granulomas [Q]
  - Giant cells and epithelioid cells [Q]

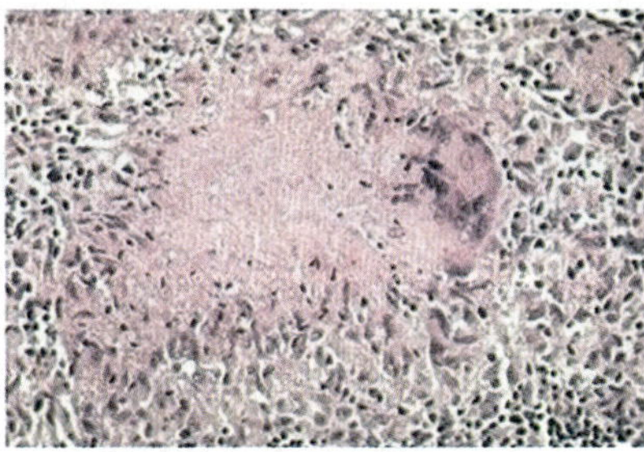

Fig. Noncaseating granulomas

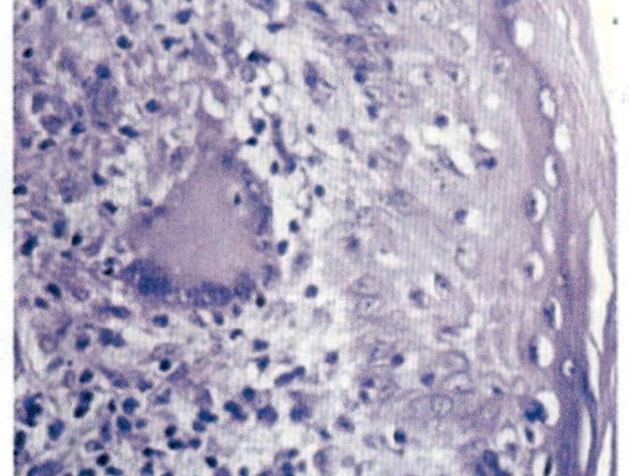

Fig. Multinucleated giant cells

- ***Indeterminate leprosy***:
  - Sensory loss absent
  - Always macule
- ***Borderline tuberculoid leprosy***:
  - **Satellite lesions** [Q]

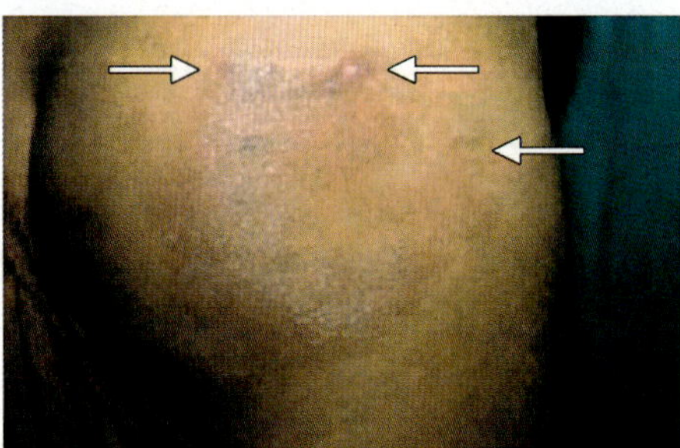

Fig. Satellite lesions

- ***Borderline borderline leprosy***:[Q]
  - **Inverted saucer-shaped lesions** [Q]
  - Hypoanaesthetic lesion
  - Multiple asymmetric nerve involvement

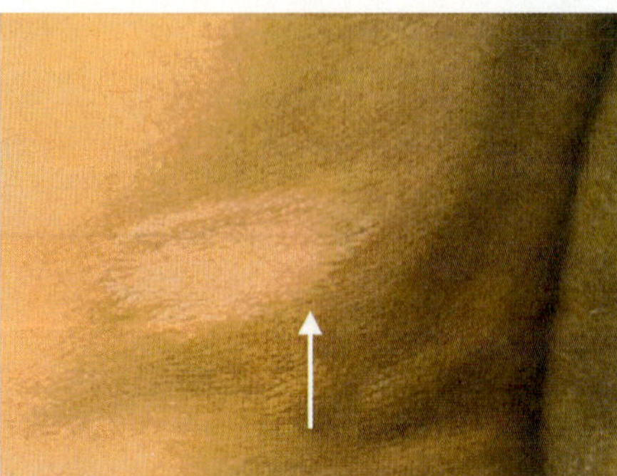

Fig. Saucer lesions

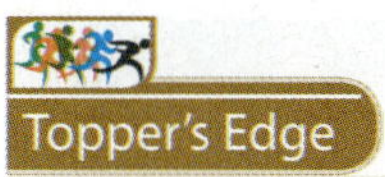

Topper's Edge

Types of Leprosy[Q]

	Number	Size	Sensation[Q]	Symmetry	Morphology	Reactions[Q]	Lepromin[Q]	Granuloma	Grenz zone[Q]	AFB
TT	Single	Variable	Anesthetic	No	Macule, papule	Stable	++++	Epithelioid cell granuloma	-	-
BT	Few	Large	Hypoaesthetic	No	Plaque Satellite lesions[Q]	Type 1	+/-	Epithelioid cell granuloma	+	-
BB	Several	Variable	Hypoaesthetic	No	Plaque Inverted saucer lesions[Q]	Type 1	-		++	-/+
BL	Numerous	Small	Hypoaesthetic	Yes	Macule, papule	Type 1/ 2	-	Macrophage granuloma	++	+
LL	Innumerable	Small	Normoesthetic	Yes	Macule, papule	Type 2	-	Macrophage granuloma	++	++

XI D. HISTOLOGY ON BIOPSY[Q]

- *Noncaseating granulomas in tuberculoid leprosy*: Epithelioid cells, giant cells, lymphocytes
- *Granulomas in lepromatous leprosy*: Foamy macrophages laden with AFB (acid fast bacilli)

XI E. TESTS FOR DETECTING IMMUNITY IN LEPROSY

Tests of Cell Mediated Immunity[Q]	Tests of Humoral Immunity
• Lepromin test • Lymphocyte transformation test • Leucocyte migration inhibition test	• FLA – ABS test • Monoclonal antibodies test • ELISA tests • Radioimmunoassay

XI F. LEPROMIN TEST

- *Definition*: Test of CMI in Leprosy[Q]
- *Antigens used in Lepromin test*:
  - **Dharmendra antigen** (extensively used in India)
  - Mitsuda antigen
- ***Readings*: After 48 hours and after 21 days**
- *Reactions in Lepromin test*:

Early Reaction (Fernandez Reaction)[Q]	Late Reaction (Mitsuda Reaction)[Q]
• Read at 48 hours • Redness > 10 mm indicates +ve test • **Delayed type of hypersensitivity** • Induced by soluble components of bacilli • Corresponds to Mantoux reaction (TB)	• Read at 21 days • Nodule > 5 mm diameter is +ve • **Indicates cell mediated immunity** • Induced by bacillary component of antigen • BCG vaccine can convert it from –ve to +ve

- *Uses of Lepromin test*:
  - Evaluation of CMI status of patients
  - Aid to confirm the classification of Leprosy
  - Estimation of prognosis of cases
- *Drawbacks of Lepromin test as a diagnostic test*:
  - Positive in non-cases
  - Negative in lepromatous and near-lepromatous cases
- *Interpretation of Lepromin Test*: [Q]

Reaction	Interpretation
++ to +++	Tuberculoid Leprosy (TT)[Q]
+ to ++	Maculo-anaesthetic Leprosy (MA)
– or ± or +	Intermediate Leprosy (I)
+ to ++	Borderline Tuberculoid Leprosy (BT)
± or +	Borderline Borderline Leprosy (BB)
– or ±	Borderline Lepromatous Leprosy (BL)
–	Lepromatous Leprosy (LL)

XI G. TREATMENT OF LEPROSY[Q]

	Paucibacillary Leprosy (PBL)	Multibacillary Leprosy (MBL)
	BI < 2	**BI ≥ 2**
Included types	• Indeterminate • Polar tuberculoid (TT) • Border tuberculoid (BT)	• Polar lepromatous (LL) • Borderline lepromatous (BL) • Mid-borderline (BB)
Multidrug therapy (MDT)	• Rifampicin 600 mg OAMS • Dapsone 100 mg daily	• Rifampicin 600 mg OAMS • Dapsone 100 mg daily • Clofazimine 300 mg OAMS + 50 mg OD
Treatment duration	**6 months** [Q]	**12 months** [Q]
Follow up later[Q]	**Annually for 2 yrs**	**Annually for 5 yrs**

(BI: Bacteriological index; OAMS: Once a month supervised)

XI H. LEPRA REACTIONS

- *Definition*: Is an inflammation that can affect skin patches, nerves, eyes and in few case, internal organs. They can occur anytime in a leprosy patient
  - Before diagnosis
  - At time of diagnosis
  - During treatment
  - After treatment has finished
- *Types of Lepra Reactions*:

Type I: Lepra Reactions *Reversal reactions*	Type II: Lepra Reactions Erythema Nodosum Leprosum (ENL)
More common in Borderline leprosy[Q]	More common in LL and BL leprosy[Q]
• Reddish & swollen skin lesions • Painful, tender, swollen nerves • Signs of nerve damage • Fever & malaise • Swollen hands & feet • New skin lesions (rare)	• Tender, reddish & transient skin nodules • Occasionally painful & swollen nerves • Fever, joint pains & malaise • Eye involvement

- *Treatment of Lepra Reactions*:
  - *Type I (Reversal) Reactions*: **Prednisolone (steroid)**
  - *Type II (ENL) Reactions*:
    - Mild cases: Analgesics or antipyretics like aspirin
    - Severe cases: **Prednisolone (steroid)**
    - During steroid withdrawal: Clofazimine

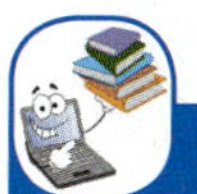

IMAGE-BASED QUESTIONS

1. Identify the Leprosy subtype of skin as shown in photograph

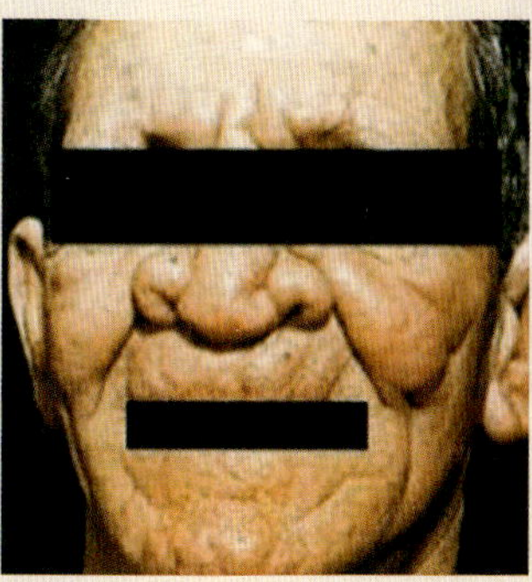

a. Tuberculoid
b. Lepromatous
c. Borderline
d. Indeterminate

2. A case of Leprosy on multidrug therapy develop lesions (photograph). Treatment is

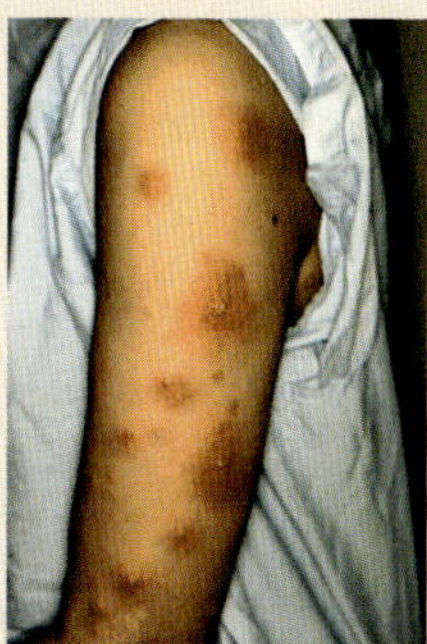

a. Thalidomide
b. Rifampicin
c. Dapsone
d. Prednisolone

3. Identify the Leprosy subtype of skin as shown in photograph

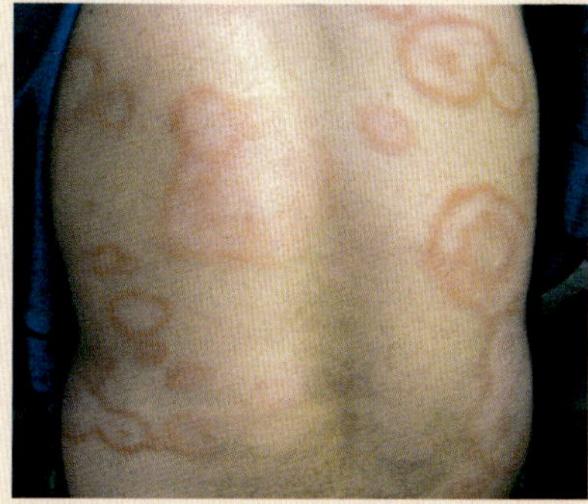

a. Borderline tuberculoid
b. Lepromatous
c. Borderline lepromatous
d. Indeterminate

4. Identify the Leprosy subtype of skin as shown in photograph

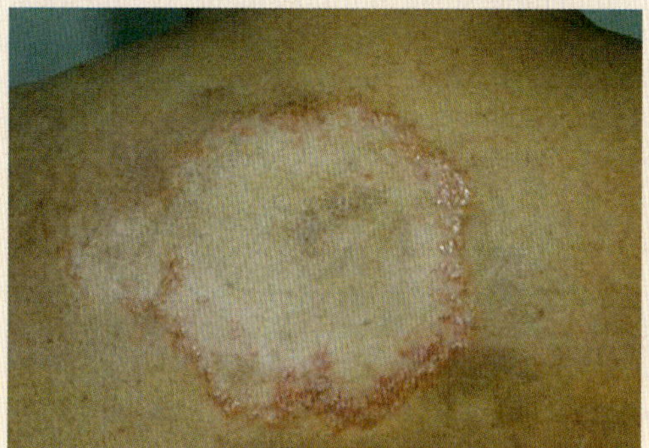

a. Tuberculoid
b. Lepromatous
c. Borderline
d. Indeterminate

5. A young male presents with a hypoanesthetic patch on right forearm. On examination a thickened nerve is palpable. Histopathology is given in photograph. Diagnosis is ***[AIIMS November 2015]***

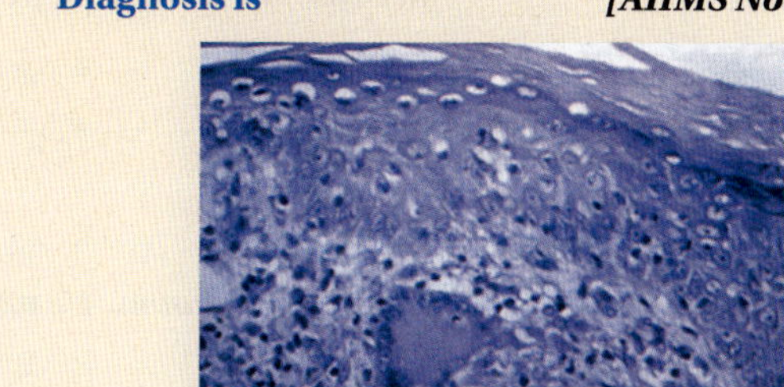

a. Tuberculoid leprosy
b. Lepromatous leprosy
c. Lymphoma
d. Histiocytosis

6. Multidrug therapy as treatment shown in the figure is used for ***[AIIMS November 2015]***

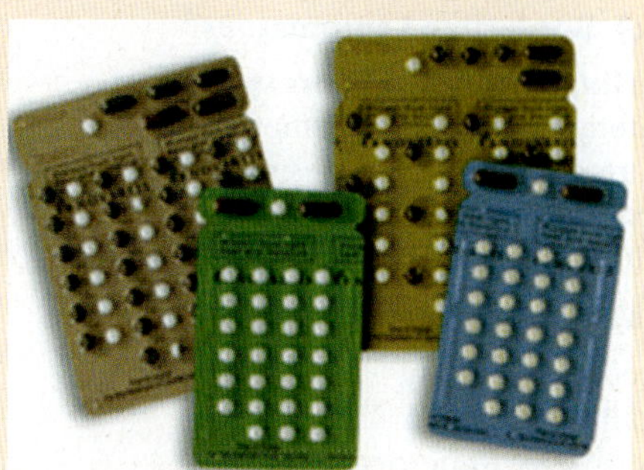

a. HIV/AIDS
b. Leprosy
c. Urethral discharge
d. Vaginal discharge

7. A man presented with a lesion having hypopigmented margins with 'Punched out' appearance. Diagnose the skin lesion shown in photograph. ***[AIIMS PG May 2015]***

a. BB
b. BL
c. LL
d. Histoid leprosy

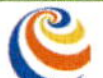 ANSWERS WITH EXPLANATIONS OF IBQs 

1. Ans. (b) Lepromatous *[Ref. Neena Khanna, 4/e p259]*

Lepromatous Leprosy

- Innumerable small, normoesthetic, symmetrical skin lesions
- Face: Diffuse infiltration of face/ ear lobules/ alae nasi
- Subepidermal free zones
- Virchow/Lepra cells (Macrophages with AFB)
- Superciliary madarosis
- Globi

2. Ans. (d) Prednisolone *[Ref. Neena Khanna, 4/e p263]*

Erythema Nodosum Leprosum

- Features:
  - Tender, reddish & transient skin nodules
  - Occasionally painful & swollen nerves
  - Fever, joint pains & malaise
  - Eye involvement
- Treatment of Lepra Reactions:
  - Type I (Reversal) reactions: Prednisolone (Steroid)
  - Type II (ENL) reactions (Photograph):
    1. Mild cases: Analgesics or antipyretics like aspirin
    2. Severe cases: Prednisolone (steroid)
    3. During steroid withdrawal: Clofazimine

3. Ans. (c) Borderline Lepromatous *[Ref. Neena Khanna, 4/e p261]*

Borderline Borderline Leprosy

- Bilateral lesions, less symmetrical
- Inverted saucer-shaped lesions
- Hypoanaesthetic lesion
- Multiple asymmetric nerve involvement

4. Ans. (a) Tuberculoid *[Ref. Neena Khanna, 4/e p259]*

Tuberculoid Leprosy

- Localized infection
- One/two asymmetrical lesion(s)
- Well-defined hypopigmented hypoanesthetic macules/ plaques with an active border
- Noncaseating granulomas
- Giant cells and epithelioid cells

5. Ans. (a) Tuberculoid Leprosy *[Ref. Neena Khanna, 4/e p266]*

- Hypoanesthetic patch on right forearm with a thickened nerve palpable indicated Leprosy
- Histology of Tuberculoid Leprosy:
  - Well-defined epithelioid cell granuloma
  - Absence of clear zone separating dermis and epidermis (Grenz zone)
  - Absence of bacilli

6. Ans. (b) Leprosy *[Ref. Neena Khanna, 4/e p267]*

Multidrug Therapy (MDT) for Leprosy

- Paucibacillary Leprosy (PBL):
  - Day 1 (Supervised monthly treatment): Rifampicin 600 mg + Clofazimine 300 mg + Dapsone 100 mg
  - Day 2-28 (Daily): Clofazimine 50 mg + Dapsone 100 mg
- Multibacillary Leprosy (MBL):
  - Day 1 (Supervised monthly treatment): Rifampicin 600 mg + Dapsone 100 mg
  - Day 2-28 (Daily): Dapsone 100 mg

7. Ans. (a) BB *[Ref. Manson's Tropical Diseases, 23/e p510]*

Borderline Borderline Leprosy

- Macular/ Papular/ Plaque like skin lesions
- Larger lesions may have a geographic appearance and some lesions have an ill-defined outer margin with a well-defined ('Punched-out') anesthetic margin
- Characteristic feature: Annular lesions

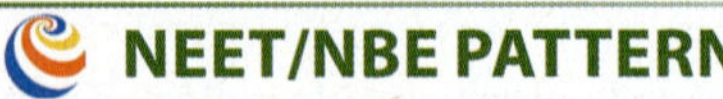

NEET/NBE PATTERN MCQs

1. **Most important in the diagnosis of leprosy is** *[Recent Question 2016]*
   a. Evidence of neural involvement
   b. Hypopigmented patch
   c. Slit skin smears
   d. Positive lepromin test
2. **True about lepromatous leprosy is** *[Recent Question 2016]*
   a. Only 3 cutaneous lesions are seen
   b. Lepromin test is highly positive
   c. Thickened nerve roots
   d. ENL > 50% cases
3. **Earliest sensation lost in leprosy is** *[Recent Question 2016]*
   a. Thermal b. Tactile
   c. Pain d. Vibration
4. **Which of the following is not approved for treatment of leprosy?** *[Recent Question 2016]*
   a. Ofloxacin b. Minocycline
   c. Azathioprine d. Clarithromycin
5. **Antileprosy drug causing Ichthyoses is** *[Recent Question 2016]*
   a. Dapsone b. Clofazimine
   c. Rifampicin d. Clarithromycin
6. **Slit skin smear is negative in** *[NBE FMGE September 2008]*
   a. Tuberculoid leprosy b. Borderline leprosy
   c. Neuritic leprosy d. Indeterminate leprosy
7. **Satellite lesions around large macules or plaques are characteristic of** *[Recent Question 2016, NBE DNB 2011]*
   a. Tuberculoid leprosy
   b. Borderline tuberculoid leprosy
   c. Borderline leprosy
   d. Borderline lepromatous leprosy
8. **Seen associated with leprosy is**
   a. Epithelioid cells *[NBE FMGE September 2005]*
   b. Foamy histiocytes/macrophages
   c. Noncaseating granulomas
   d. All of the above
9. **Leprosy will affect all organs except** *[NBE DNB 2009]*
   a. Ovary b. Uterus
   c. Nerves d. Eye
10. **Earliest sensation to be lost in leprosy is** *[UPSC 2010]*
    a. Thermal b. Tactile
    c. Pain d. Vibration
11. **Asymmetrical multiple nerve thickening with hypo-anaesthetic macules on skin is seen in** *[NBE FMGE March 2009]*
    a. Tuberculoid leprosy
    b. Borderline borderline leprosy
    c. Borderline tuberculoid leprosy
    d. Borderline lepromatous leprosy
12. **Drugs used in lepra reaction is** *[NBE DNB 2002]*
    a. Thalidomide
    b. Clofazimine
    c. Chloroquine
    d. All of the above
13. **True about multibacillary leprosy is** *[NBE FMGE September 2006]*
    a. More than 5 skin lesions
    b. Clofazimine is used in therapy
    c. Total treatment duration is 12 months
    d. All of the above
14. **Most effective drug for type 2 Lepra reaction is** *[NBE DNB 1992]*
    a. Systemic steroid b. Clofazimine
    c. Colchicine d. Thalidomide
15. **Which of the following features differentiate lepromatous leprosy from tuberculoid leprosy?** *[UPSC 2009]*
    a. Absence of infectivity of affected patients
    b. Organisms are scanty in number
    c. Blood-borne spread from dermis throughout the body
    d. Anesthetic hypopigmented skin macules and plaques
16. **Innumerable small, normoesthetic, symmetrical skin lesions are seen in** *[NBE FMGE September 2009]*
    a. Tuberculoid leprosy
    b. Borderline borderline leprosy
    c. Borderline tuberculoid leprosy
    d. Lepromatous leprosy
17. **True about lepromatous leprosy** *[Recent Question 2012, 2013]*
    a. Only 3 cutaneous lesions
    b. Lepromin test highly positive
    c. Thickened nerve roots d. ENL in > 50% cases
18. **Type-II Lepra reaction is found in** *[NBE DNB 2001, 2005]*
    a. BL b. LL
    c. BT d. None of the above
19. **Drug of choice in ENL is** *[NBE DNB 1998]*
    a. Steroids b. Chloroquine
    c. Thalidomide d. Dapsone
20. **As per WHO guidelines, minimum duration of treatment for Multibacillary leprosy is** *[NBE FMGE September 2009]*
    a. 3 months b. 6 months
    c. 9 months d. 12 months
21. **A young boy, single hypoanaesthetic patch over hand + thickened ulnar nerve, diagnosis is** *[NBE DNB 2002]*
    a. Tuberculoid leprosy b. Lepromatous leprosy
    c. Indeterminate d. Borderline
22. **Treatment of lepra type-II reaction are following except** *[NBE DNB 1995]*
    a. Clofazimine b. Thalidomide
    c. Corticosteroids d. Antileprosy treatment
    e. Cessation of antileprosy treatment
23. **Most important in diagnosis of leprosy is** *[NBE FMGE March 2010]*
    a. Evidence of neural involvement
    b. Hypopigmented patches
    c. Slit skin smears for AFB d. Positive lepromin test
24. **Lucio's phenomenon is seen in?** *[Recent Question 2017]*
    a. Tuberculoid leprosy
    b. Lepromatous leprosy
    c. Borderline leprosy
    d. Borderline tuberculoid leprosy

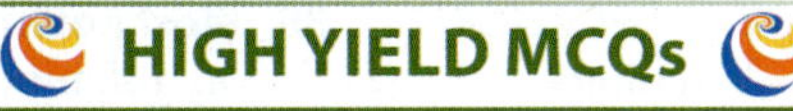

HIGH YIELD MCQs

1. **A 45-year-old patient had multiple hypoaesthetic and mildly erythematous patches on his trunk. His both ulnar and lateral popliteal nerves were thickened. The most probable diagnosis is** *[AIIMS May 2016]*
   a. Borderline lepromatous leprosy
   b. Borderline tuberculoid leprosy
   c. Borderline leprosy
   d. Lepromatous leprosy
2. **Manifestation of ENL includes all of the following except** *[PGI 2005]*
   a. Pancreatistis b. Fever
   c. Hepatitis d. Arthritis
   e. Cutaneous nodules
3. **A 27-year-old patient was diagnosed to have borderline leprosy and started on multibacillary multidrug therapy. Six weeks later, he developed pain in the nerves and redness and swelling of the skin lesions. The management of his illness should include all of the following except** *[AIIMS PGMEE 2004]*
   a. Stop antileprosy drugs
   b. Systemic corticosteroids
   c. Rest to the limbs affected
   d. Analgesics
4. **A 16-year-old student reported for the evaluation of multiple hypopigmented macules on the trunk and limbs. All of the following tests are useful in making a diagnosis of leprosy, except** *[AIIMS PGMEE 2003]*
   a. Sensation testing b. Lepromin test
   c. Slit smears d. Skin biopsy
5. **A 45-year-old male had multiple hypoaesthetic mildly erythematous large plaques with elevated margins on trunk and extremities. His ulnar and lateral popliteal nerves on both sides were enlarged. The most probable diagnosis is** *[AIIMS PGMEE 2003]*
   a. Lepromatous leprosy
   b. Borderline leprosy
   c. Borderline tuberculoid leprosy
   d. Borderline lepromatous leprosy
6. **All are true Lepromatous leprosy except** *[TN PGMEE 1996]*
   a. Presence of globin
   b. Subepidermal free zone
   c. Decreased cell mediated immunity
   d. Presence of granulomas subdermally
7. **A single hypopigmented anesthetic patch with satellite lesion on forearm, likely diagnosis is** *[AIIMS PGMEE 1994]*
   a. Indeterminate leprosy b. Tuberculoid leprosy
   c. Neuritic leprosy d. Lupus vulgaris
8. **In Leprosy which of the following is not seen** *[PGI 2000]*
   a. Abnormal EMG
   b. Voluntary muscle wasting
   c. Decreased proprioception
   d. Decreased response to tactile sensation
   e. Increased response to tactile sensation
9. **Cell mediated immunity is maximum suppressed in** *[AIIMS PGMEE 1993]*
   a. BT b. LL
   c. TT d. Indeterminate
10. **Erythema nodosum leprosum is seen in** *[AIIMS PGMEE 1992]*
    a. TT b. BT
    c. Lepromatous leprosy d. Indeterminate leprosy
11. **Drug of choice in Erythema Nodosum Leprosum** *[AIIMS PGMEE 1992]*
    a. Steroid b. Thalidomide
    c. Clofazimine d. Aspirin
12. **Most effective drug against M. Leprae is** *[All India PGMEE 2003]*
    a. Dapsone b. Rifampicin
    c. Clofazimine d. Prothionamide
13. **A 8-year-old boy from Tamil Nadu presents with a white, non anaesthetic, non scaly hypopigmented macule on his face, likely diagnosis is** *[All India PGMEE 2001]*
    a. Pityriasis alba b. Pityriasis versicolour
    c. Indeterminate leprosy d. Neuritic leprosy
14. **Satellite Lesion are seen in** *[All India PGMEE 1999]*
    a. Tuberculoid leprosy
    b. Lepromatous leprosy
    c. Borderline tuberculoid leprosy
    d. Histoid leprosy
15. **Skin biopsy in leprosy is characterized by**
    a. Pariappendiceal bacilli *[All India PGMEE 1997]*
    b. Pariappendiceal lymphocytosis
    c. Perivascular lymphocytosis
    d. All of the above
16. **All lesions are seen in leprosy except** *[All India PGMEE 1997]*
    a. Erythematous macule b. Hypopigmented patch
    c. Vesicles d. Flat & raised patches
17. **WHO regime for paucibacillary leprosy** *[All India PGMEE 1996]*
    a. 100 mg Dapsone daily + Rifampicin monthly (600 mg)
    b. Dapsone daily + Rifampicin daily
    c. Dapsone + Rifampicin + Clofazimine daily
    d. Rifampicin + Clofazimine daily
18. **First line antileprosy drugs include all except** *[PGI 1978, Delhi PGMEE 1983]*
    a. Dapsone b. Thiacetazone
    c. Clofazimine d. Rifampicin
19. **Skin pigmentation & ichthyosis like side effects are seen in** *[All India PGMEE 1996]*
    a. Rifampicin b. Clofazimine
    c. Dapsone d. Steroid
20. **DOC in type I lepra reaction with severe neuritis** *[All India PGMEE 1995]*
    a. Thalidomide b. Clofazimine
    c. Dapsone d. Systemic corticosteroid
21. **Treatment of acute neuritis in Lepra I reaction is A/E** *[All India PGMEE 1994]*
    a. Dapsone b. Steroid
    c. Thalidomide d. Incision and drainage
22. **Single lesion in skin is seen in which type of leprosy** *[All India PGMEE 1993]*
    a. TT b. BT
    c. BL d. LL

23. Erythema leprosum nodosum is seen in *[PGI 2004]*
a. Lepromatous leprosy b. Borderline tuberculoid
c. Borderline lepromatous d. Tuberculoid

24. Tuberculid are seen in *[AIIMS PGMEE 2007]*
a. Lupus vulgaris b. Scrofuloderma
c. Lichen scrofulosorum d. Erythema nodosum

25. A boy comes from Bihar with nonanesthetic hypopigmented atrophic patch over face, diagnosis is *[AIIMS PGMEE 1999]*
a. P. alba b. P. versicolour
c. Indeterminate leprosy d. Borderline leprosy

26. Satellite lesions are seen in *[AIIMS PGMEE 1999]*
a. Indeterminate leprosy
b. Borderline leprosy
c. Borderline tuberculoid leprosy
d. Tuberculoid leprosy

27. Tuberculoid leprosy is characterised by *[JIPMER PGMEE 1992]*
a. Noncaseating granuloma in nerve
b. Subepidermal free zone
c. Bacilli in skin
d. Skin caseation

28. Commonest nerve involved in leprosy is *[AIIMS PGMEE 1994]*
a. Ulnar b. Median
c. Radial d. Sciatic

29. ENL is seen in which form of leprosy *[PGI 2005]*
a. Indeterminate b. BT
c. LL d. BL
e. TT

30. Lepromin test is used for *[AIIMS PGMEE 2008]*
a. Diagnosis
b. Treatment
c. Prognosis
d. Epidemiological investigation

31. Virchow's cells are seen in *[UP PGMEE 1995]*
a. Henoch schonlein purpura
b. Toxic epidermal necrolysis
c. Congenital syphilis
d. Leprosy

32. The following test is not used for diagnosis of leprosy *[AIIMS PGMEE 2006]*
a. Lepromin test
b. Slit skin smear
c. Fine needle aspiration cytology
d. Skin biopsy

33. Not true about Lepromin test is *[AIIMS PGMEE 2010]*
a. It is diagnostic
b. Negative in infants < 6 months
c. Used to classify
d. BCG vaccination may convert negative to positive

34. All are features of lepromatous leprosy except *[Recent Question 2016]* *[TN PGME 1996, AIIMS PGMEE 1994]*
a. Gynaecomastia b. Madarosis
c. Saddle nose d. Perforating ulcer

35. Lepromin test is positive in which leprosy *[AIIMS PGMEE 2000]*
a. Lepromatous b. Indeterminate
c. Histoid d. Tuberculoid

36. Most potent antileprotic drug is *[AIIMS PGMEE 1997]*
a. Rifampicin b. Dapsone
c. Clofazimine d. Norflox

37. Best method of treatment of ulna never abscess in case of leprosy is *[AIIMS PGMEE 1996]*
a. High does of steroid b. Incision and drainage
c. Thalidomide d. High does of clofazimine

38. Inverted saucer shaped lesion is found in *[Recent Question 2016, AIIMS PGMEE 1995]*
a. Lepromatous leprosy b. Tuberculoid leprosy
c. Borderline leprosy d. Indeterminate leprosy

39. Average duration of treatment in multibacillary leprosy is *[AIIMS PGMEE 1993]*
a. 1 year b. 2 year
c. 3 year d. Life long

40. Skin smear is negative in which leprosy *[DPG 2008]*
a. Indeterminate b. Neuritic
c. Lepromatous d. Borderline

41. Earliest sensation to be lost in Hansen's disease is *[UP PGMEE 1998]*
a. Pain b. Touch
c. Vibration d. Temperature

42. Leprosy do not involve *[PGI 1998]*
a. CNS b. Testis
c. Skin d. Cornea

43. Leprosy affects all organs except *[AIIMS PGMEE 2010]*
a. Eyes b. Nerves
c. Uterus d. Ovary

44. Duration of treatment in paucibacillary leprosy is *[JIPMER PGMEE 1993]*
a. 6 months b. 9 months
c. 2 years d. Till symptoms subside

45. One of the following is a side effect of clofazimine used in leprosy therapy *[All India PGMEE 1996]*
a. Hyperpigmentation
b. Erythema
c. Discoloration of body secretions
d. Macular rash

46. In leprosy nerves commonly involved are *[PGI 1997]*
a. High ulnar, low median
b. High median, low ulnar
c. Triple nerve palsy
d. High radial, low median

47. Most common type of leprosy in India *[PGI 1997]*
a. BT b. TT
c. LL d. BL

48. Antileprotic drug also used in lepra reaction is *[AIIMS PGMEE 1997]*
a. Rifampicin b. Dapsone
c. Ciprofloxacin d. Clofazimine

49. Multidrug therapy is given for *[All India PGMEE 1994]*
a. Syphilis b. Leprosy
c. Herpetiformis d. Ichthyosis vulgaris

50. Nerve biopsy in leprosy is usually taken from *[PGMCET 2015]*
a. Ulnar b. Median
c. Lateral popliteal d. Sural

51. Newer drugs which can be used for the treatment of Leprosy consists of the following drugs, except *[PGMCET 2015]*
a. Ofloxacin b. Minocycline
c. Azathioprine d. Clarithromycin

 **NEET/NBE PATTERN MCQs ANSWERS WITH EXPLANATIONS** 

1. **Ans. (b) Hypopigmented patch**
   [Ref. DVL by Thappa, 4/e p338,339]
   - Awareness is the most important factor for the diagnosis of Leprosy
   - When a patient lives or has lived in a leprosy endemic country, leprosy must always be considered in the differential diagnosis of a hypopigmented or erythematous patch or a popular or nodular patch
   - Most important diagnostic finding of borderline tuberculoid leprosy, presence of hypopigmented patch with central clearing and peripheral irregular borders

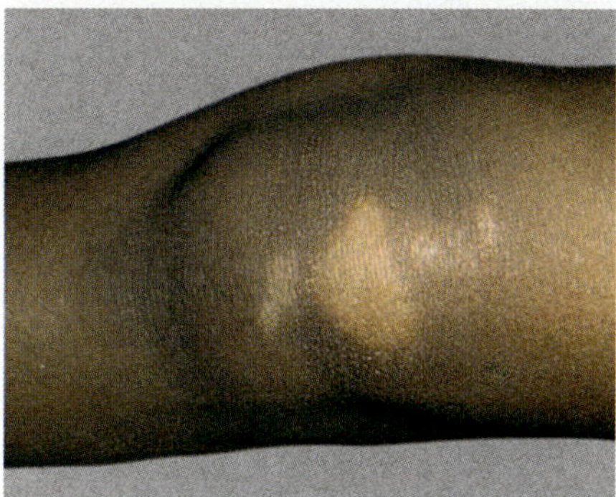

Fig. Hypopigmented patch

2. **Ans. (c) Thickened nerve roots**
   [Ref. DVL by Thappa, 4/e p341]

   Lepromatous Leprosy
   - Multibacillary type leprosy: >5 skin lesions
   - Low cell mediated immunity: Lepromin test negative
   - Insidious in onset and steady progression
   - Early lesions are macules
   - Later these lesions give way to diffuse infiltration of skin, which manifest most often over cooler areas of body like face, especially forehead, ear lobes, eyebrows, nose & malar surfaces
   - Skin at this stage looks shiny & thickened & margins of lesions cannot be made out
   - As infiltration of face becomes marked skin is thrown into folds over forehead giving appearance of "Leonine facies"
   - Symmetrical polyneuropathy, which occurs late in the disease
   - Peripheral nerves become thickened but reflexes are retained, often until the neuropathy is advanced

3. **Ans. (a) Thermal**
   [Ref. Conn's Current Therapy 2006, 1/e p118]
   - Thermal sensations arc probably the first to be affected in several cases of leprosy
   - Touch sensation is the last to be affected
   - Touch and pain sensations are tested with a pointed pin, whereas thermal sensation is tested with a test tube containing hot and cold water

4. **Ans. (c) Azathioprine**
   [Ref. DVL by Thappa, 4/e p415]

   Agents Used in Treatment of Leprosy
   - Commonly used: Rifampicin, Clofazimine, Dapsone
   - Other agents: Ofloxacin/Moxifloxacin/Perfloxacin/Sparfloxacin, Minocycline, Clarithromycin, Streptomycin, Rifabutin/Rifapentine, Bromopropane, Fusidic acid, Amoxicillin + Clavulanic acid

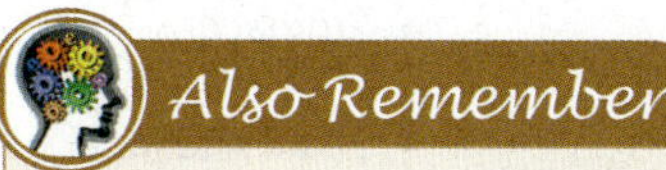

Minocycline
- Used earlier as a drug effective in leprosy
- Within 1 month it completely kills bacteria & within 3 months of administration complete clearance of erythema & induration of leprosy can be noticed
- Earlier it was included In ROM regimen, which acts in conjunction with Ofloxacin by preventing Rifampicin resistance

Indications of Azathioprine
- Vasculitis
- Autoimmune bullous disorders
- Auto immune connective tissue disorders
- Contact dermatitis & papulosquamous dermatoses
- Photodermatoses

5. **Ans. (b) Clofazimine**
   [Ref. DVL by Thappa 4/e p409]

   Side effects of Clofazimine
   - Conjunctival pigmentation
   - Eosinophilic enteropathy
   - Photo toxicity, nonspecific skin rash, acneiform eruption
   - Ichthyosis
   - Reversible, dose-related, reddish-brownish black discoloration of hair, sweat , urine , sputum & feces

6. **Ans. (c) Neuritic leprosy**
   [Ref. Neena Khanna, 4/e p175]
   - Pure neuritic type Leprosy (Indian classification): No skin lesions therefore slit skin smears are negative

7. **Ans. (b) Borderline tuberculoid leprosy**
   [Ref. Neena Khanna, 5/e p276]

   Lesion Characteristic of BT Leprosy
   - Initially small , but may attain large size
   - More in number (2-15)
   - Less asymmetrical
   - Less sharply demarcated, with 'Satellite lesions'
   - Less hypoesthetic

8. **Ans. (d) All of the above**
   [Ref. Neena Khanna, 4/e p265]

   Histology on Biopsy in Leprosy
   - *Noncaseating granulomas in Tuberculoid leprosy*: Epitheloid cells, giant cells, lymphocytes
   - *Granulomas in Lepromatous leprosy*: Foamy macrophages laden with AFB (acid fast bacilli)

9. **Ans. (b) Uterus**
   [Ref. Klioze AM, Ramos-Caro FA. Visceral leprosy. Int J Dermatol. 200;39:641-58; Blaustein's Pathology of the Female Genital Tract, 4/e p602]

Organs affected by Leprosy

Significant Infiltration/ Dysfunction	None/Minimal Infiltration/Dysfunction	
• Skin • Eyes • Peripheral nerves • Nasopharynx • Kidney • Larynx • Liver • Testicles	• Brain • Striated muscle • Cerebellum • Ureter • Leptomeninges • Bladder • Spinal cord • Urethra • Pancreas • Prostate • Lungs • Seminal vesicles • Heart • External genitalia • Great vessels	• Breasts • Gallbladder • Vagina • Pancreas • Uterus • Esophagus • Ovaries • Stomach • Thyroid gland • Small intestine • Parathyroid gland • Large intestine • Pituitary gland • Striated muscle • Pineal gland
Mild-moderate Infiltration/ Dysfunction • Tongue • Autonomic nervous system • Spleen • Bone marrow • Adrenals • Bone • Lymph nodes • Joints • Peripheral vasculature		

- Although Leprosy rarely involves the female genital tract, the ovary is the most commonly involved gynecological site

10. Ans. (a) Thermal

[Ref. Textbook of Pathology by V Krishna, 1/e p350]

- Sensation loss in leprosy:
  - Temperature is the first sensation that is lost
  - Next sensation lost is light touch then pain
  - Deep pressure is lost finally

11. Ans. (b) Borderline borderline leprosy

[Ref. Neena Khanna, 4/e p262]

Clinical Presentation in Leprosy Types

- *Lepromatous leprosy*:
  - Innumerable small, normoesthetic, symmetrical skin lesions
  - Subepidermal free zones
  - Virchow/Lepra cells (Macrophages with AFB)
  - Superciliary madarosis
  - Globi
- *Tuberculoid leprosy*:
  - Noncaseating granulomas
  - Giant cells and epithelioid cells
- *Indeterminate leprosy*:
  - Sensory loss absent
  - Always macule
- *Borderline tuberculoid leprosy*:
  - Satellite lesions
- *Borderline borderline leprosy*:
  - Inverted saucer-shaped lesions
  - Hypoanaesthetic lesion
  - Multiple asymmetric nerve involvement

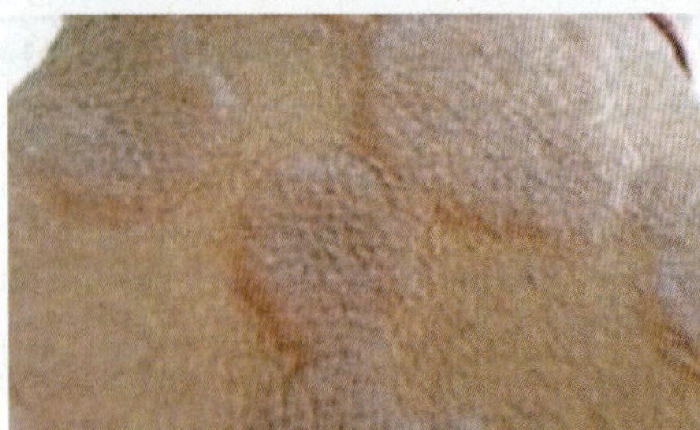

Fig. Satellite lesions

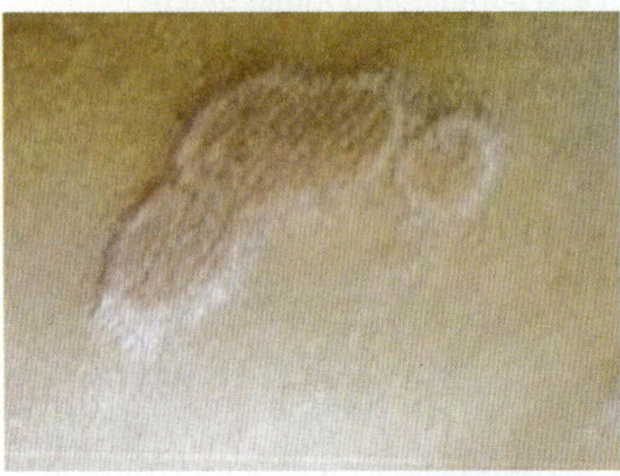

Fig. Inverted saucer lesions

12. Ans. (d) All of the above

[Ref. Harrison's, 18/e p1366; Pharmacological Classification of Drugs with Doses and Preparations by KDT, 5/e p714; Neena Khanna, 5/e p285]

Treatment of Lepra Reaction

Type I	Type II
• Mild: Antipyretics (NSAIDs) • Glucocorticoids (DOC) • Clofazimine: Less efficacious	• Mild: Antipyretics (NSAIDs) • Severe: Glucocorticoids (DOC) • Thalidomide: If 2 courses of glucocorticoids fail • Clofazimine • Chloroquine

13. Ans. (d) All of the above

[Ref. Neena Khanna, 4/e p267]

Treatment of Leprosy (MDT – Multidrug Therapy)

	Paucibacillary Leprosy (PBL)	Multibacillary Leprosy (MBL)
Types	Indeterminate Polar tuberculoid (TT) Border tuberculoid (BT)	Polar lepromatous (LL) Borderline lepromatous (BL) Midborderline (BB)
MDT	Rifampicin 600 mg OAMS Dapsone 100 mg daily	Rifampicin 600 mg OAMS Dapsone 100 mg daily Clofazimine 300 mg OAMS + 50 mg OD
Duration	6 months	12 months
Follow up	Annually for 2 yrs	Annually for 5 yrs

14. Ans. (d) Thalidomide
[Ref. Neena Khanna, 5/e p285]
- Thalidomide is the 'most effective drug' for treatment of Lepra reaction II
- But corticosteroids are considered drug of choice for type II reaction: As Thalidomide is absolutely contraindicated in females in the reproductive age group (Due to its teratogenic effect: Phocomelia 'Seal limbs')

15. Ans. (c) Blood-borne spread from dermis throughout the body
[Ref. Neena Khanna, 5/e p275-276]

16. Ans. (d) Lepromatous leprosy
[Ref. Neena Khanna, 4/e p260]

17. Ans. (c) Thickened nerve roots
[Ref. Neena Khanna, 5/e p276]
- Nerve involvement in Lepromatous leprosy: Bilaterally symmetrical peripheral nerve thickening

18. Ans. (b) LL
[Ref. Neena Khanna, 5/e p278]
- Type II Lepra reaction/ Erythema Nodosum Leprosum: MC occur in LL (Sometimes in BL leprosy)

19. Ans. (a) Steroids
[Ref. Neena Khanna, 5/e p285]

20. Ans. (d) 12 months
[Ref. Dermatology and Sexually Transmitted Infections by Neena Khanna, 4th Ed., p. 267]

21. Ans. (a) Tuberculoid leprosy
[Ref. Neena Khanna, 5/e p274-275]

Features of Tuberculoid Leprosy
- One/two lesion
- Asymmetrical
- Well defined, hypopigmented/erythematous, anaesthetic macule/plaque, often with an active border
- Lesions show hair loss and impairment of sweating
- A superficial feeder nerve or a single regional nerve is often thickened

22. Ans. (e) Cessation of antileprosy treatment
[Ref. Harrison's, 18/e p1366; KDT, 5/e p714; Neena Khanna, 5/e p285]
- As per Guidelines of National Leprosy Elimination Program (Government of India), Antileprosy treatment is never stopped (unless absolutely necessary) after starting
- Side effects (including Lepra reactions) must be treatment simultaneously

23. Ans. (c) Slit skin smears for AFB
[Ref. Neena Khanna, 4/e p265]
- *Evidence of neural involvement, hypopigmented patches*: Are nonspecific features
  - *Slit skin smears for AFB*: Is diagnostic of Leprosy even in absence of sensory loss
  - *Lepromin test*: Is used for evaluation of immunity status, predicting prognosis or confirmation of classification
  - Lepromin test is not useful for diagnosis.

24. Ans. (b) Lepromatous leprosy
[Ref. Andrew's Diseases of the Skin, 11/e p341]

Lucio's Phenomenon
- An uncommon and unusual reaction that occurs in patients with diffuse Lepromatous leprosy of the 'la bonita' type
- Characterised by recurrent crops of large, sharply demarcated, ulcerative lesions, affecting mainly the lower extremities, but may generalise and become fatal as a result of secondary bacterial infection and sepsis
- Patient develops a striking, diffuse skin edema, which tends to efface the age-related wrinkles on the face and gave rise to the historic term, "la belle femme"
- Hemorrhagic plaques can occur suddenly on the arms, legs, and buttocks, and these eventually lead to widespread severe ulcerations

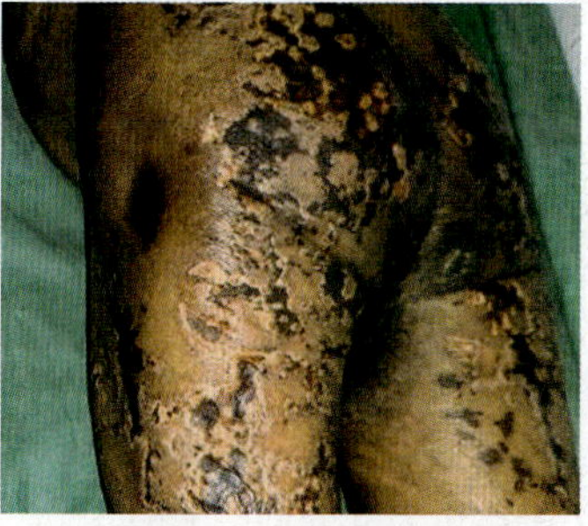

Fig. Lucio phenomenon

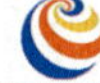 HIGH YIELD MCQs ANSWERS WITH EXPLANATIONS 

1. Ans. (a) Borderline lepromatous leprosy
[Ref. DVT by Thappa, 4/e p340]

Borderline Lepromatous Leprosy
- Disease classically starts as macules, evolve into plaque & nodular lesions.
- Inverted saucer shaped lesions
- Peripheral nerves become thickened in borderline lepromatous leprosy

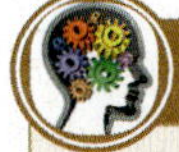

Also Remember
- Borderline tuberculoid leprosy: Few skin lesions with satellite lesions and fewer involvement of nerves
- Lepromatous leprosy: Nerve involvement and skin lesions are usually more widely distributed and there will also be involvement of earlobes with infiltration and other deformities of leprosy will usually be present

2. Ans. (a) Pancreatistis; (c) Hepatitis
[Ref. Neena Khanna, 5/e p279] & [Ref. Conn's Current Therapy 2014 by Edward T. Bope, p130]

Disease associated with ENL

- Fever
- Arthralgia, Orchitis, Iridocyclitis
- Neuritis
- Cutaneous ulcer
- Hand foot syndrome

3. Ans. (a) Stop antileprosy drugs
[Ref. Neena Khanna, 5/e p285]

4. Ans. (b) Lepromin test
[Ref. Neena Khanna, 5/e p282]

- Lepromin test is NOT a diagnostic test
- Lepromin test is used for:
  - Prognosis
  - Confirmation of classification
  - Assesssment of CMI status

5. Ans. (d) Borderline lepromatous leprosy
[Ref. Neena Khanna, 5/e p277]

- Bilateral nerve involvement, hypoasthetic lesion, multiple small cutaneous lesion hints towards diagnosis of BL Leprosy

6. Ans. (d) Presence of granulomas subdermally
[Ref. Neena Khanna, 5/e p283]

Lepromatous Leprosy

- Diffuse macrophage infiltration loaded with bacilli in form of cigar bundles called globi
- 'Subepidermal zone of Grenz' is free of infiltrate
- Maximally depressed cell mediated immunity

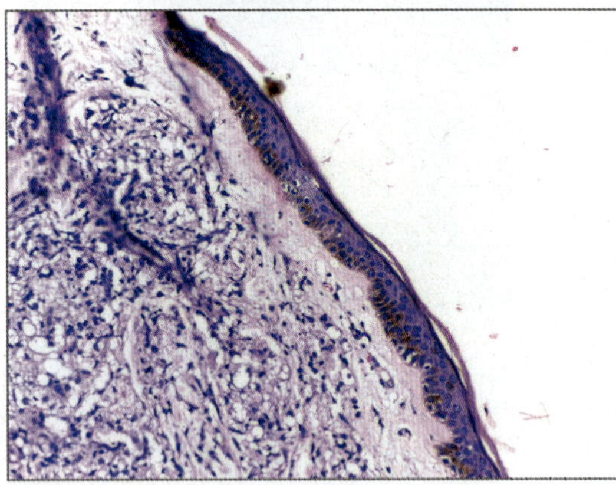

Fig. Grenz zone in leprosy

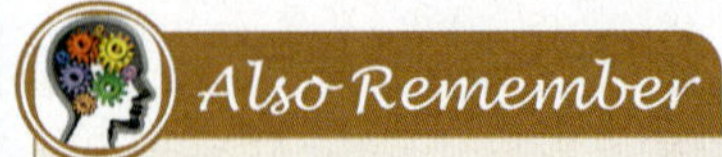

- Granuloma is seen in TT and BT

7. Ans. (b) Tuberculoid leprosy
[Ref. Neena Khanna, 5/e p276]

8. Ans. (e) Increased response to tactile sensation
[Ref. Leprosy by Nunzi, p167]

9. Ans. (b) LL
[Ref. Illustrated Dictionary of Immunology by Julius M. Cruse, 3/e p517]

- In lepromatous leprosy, T cell-mediated immunity is depressed

10. Ans. (c) Lepromatous leprosy
[Ref. Neena Khanna, 5/e p278]

11. Ans. (a) Steroid
[Ref. Neena Khanna, 5/e p285]

12. Ans. (b) Rifampicin
[Ref. Park Textbook of Preventive and Social Medicine by K Park, 20/e p284]

- Rifampicin is the only drug that is highly bactericidal against M. leprae

13. Ans. (c) Indeterminate leprosy
[Ref. Neena Khanna, 5/e p274]

Indeterminate Leprosy

- Seen on face of children, in endemic areas
- Always a macule
- Ill-defined, atrophic, hypoesthetic/normoaesthetic, hypopigmented or slightly erythematous lesion with or without nerve thickening

14. Ans. (c) Borderline tuberculoid leprosy
[Ref. Neena Khanna, 5/e p276]

15. Ans. (d) All of the above
[Ref. Neena Khanna, 5/e p283]

16. Ans. (c) Vesicles
[Ref. Neena Khanna, 5/e p272]

- Macules/ plaques/ papules are seen in leprosy, not vesicles

17. Ans. (a) 100 mg Dapsone daily + Rifampicin monthly (600 mg)
[Ref. Neena Khanna, 5/e p284]

- **Adult Paucibacillary pack** is Green in colour and contains 600 mg and Dapsone 100 mg taken under supervision on Day 1 followed by Dapsone, 100 mg daily for 27 days

18. Ans. (b) Thiacetazone
[Ref. Neena Khanna, 5/e p284-285]

19. Ans. (b) Clofazimine
[Ref. Neena Khanna, 5/e p285]

- Ichthyosis, pigmentation and gastrointestinal are side effects of Clofazimine

20. Ans. (d) Systemic corticosteroid
[Ref. Harrison's, 18/e p1366; KDT, 5/e p714; Neena Khanna, 5/e p285]

21. Ans. (d) Incision and drainage
[Ref. Harrison's Principles of Internal Medicine by Dan Longo, 18/e p1366]

22. Ans. (a) TT
[Ref. Neena Khanna, 5/e p274-275]

23. Ans. (a) Lepromatous leprosy; (c) Borderline lepromatous
[Ref. Neena Khanna, 5/e p278]

24. Ans. (c) Lichen scrofulosorum
[Ref. Neena Khanna, 5/e p270]

Well-established Tuberculids

- **Lichen scrofulosorum**: characterized by grouped popular lesion on trunk
- **Papulonecrotic tuberculid**: characterized by papules surmounted with pustules/crusts and healing with scarring

25. Ans. (c) Indeterminate leprosy
[Ref. Neena Khanna, 5/e p274]

26. Ans. (c) Borderline tuberculoid leprosy
[Ref. Neena Khanna, 5/e p276]

27. Ans. (a) Noncaseating granuloma in nerve
[Ref. Neena Khanna, 5/e p283]

28. Ans. (a) Ulnar
[Ref. Manson's Tropical Diseases by Jeremy Farrar, 23/e p511]

- **MC peripheral nerve involved: Ulnar nerve** > Posterior tibial nerve > Median nerve > Lateral popliteal nerve
- **MC nerve affected in hand: Ulnar nerve**> Median nerve > Radial nerve

29. Ans. (c) LL; (d) BL
[Ref. Neena Khanna, 5/e p278]

30. Ans. (c) Prognosis
[Ref. Neena Khanna, 5/e p282]

31. Ans. (d) Leprosy
[Ref. Dermatopathology by Busam, p138]

- Foamy histiocytes of leprosy resemble those seen in xanthoma; they are called Lepra/ Virchow cells

32. Ans. (a) Lepromin test
[Ref. Neena Khanna, 5/e p282]

33. Ans. (a) It is diagnostic
[Ref. Neena Khanna, 5/e p282]

34. Ans. (d) Perforating ulcer
[Ref. Neena Khanna, 5/e p275-276]

35. Ans. (d) Tuberculoid
[Ref. Neena Khanna, 5/e p282]

- Lepromin positivity indicates good immunity to M. leprae and that the patient has been able to contain the infection, i.e. he has Tuberculoid or Borderline tuberculoid leprosy

36. Ans. (a) Rifampicin
[Ref. Park, 20/e p284]

37. Ans. (b) Incision and drainage
[Ref. Neurology, India, Volume 20, p102]

- Nerve abscesses are seen in tuberculoid leprosy and may be solitary or multiple, in the cutaneous nerves draining a patch or in a major nerve trunk
- A nerve abscess should be treated by surgical release of the nerve
- Skin incision should be closed without drainage
- Ulnar nerve is the most commonly involved nerve in leprosy

38. Ans. (c) Borderline leprosy
[Ref. Textbook of Pediatric Dermatology by Inamadar, 2/e p176]

- Punched out or **'Inverted saucer' shaped lesion**: Mid borderline leprosy and Borderline lepromatous leprosy
- Clinical features of Midborderline (BB) leprosy : Very unstable type of leprosy, seldom seen
  - Multiple irregular inverted saucer or ring-shaped skin lesions are observed
  - Moderate sensory loss.

39. Ans. (a) 1 year
[Ref. Neena Khanna, 5/e p284]

- Duration of multidrug therapy (MDT):
  - Paucibacillary leprosy: **6 months** (Can be completed in 9 months)
  - Multibacillary leprosy: **12 months** (Can be completed in 18 months)

40. Ans. (b) Neuritic
[Ref. Textbook of Pediatric Dermatology by Arun C Inamadar, 2/e p175]

- Pure neuritic' leprosy: No characteristic skin lesions and the skin smear is negative

41. Ans. (d) Temperature
[Ref. Textbook of Pathology by V. Krishna, 1/e p350]

42. Ans. (a) CNS
[Ref. Klioze AM, Ramos-Caro FA. Visceral leprosy. Int J Dermatol. 200;39:641-58]

Organs with Significant Infiltration/ Dysfunction

- Skin
- Eyes
- Peripheral nerves
- Nasopharynx
- Kidney
- Larynx
- Liver
- Testicles

43. Ans. (c) Uterus
[Ref. Klioze, A. M. and Ramos-Caro, F. A. Visceral leprosy. International Journal of Dermatology, 200;39: 641–58; Blaustein's Pathology of the Female Genital Tract, 4/e p602]

44. Ans. (a) 6 months
[Ref. Neena Khanna, 5/e p284]

45. Ans. (a) Hyperpigmentation; (c) Discoloration of body secretions
[Ref. Neena Khanna, 5/e p285]

46. Ans. (a) High ulnar, low median
[Ref. Manson's Tropical Diseases by Jeremy Farrar, 23/e p511]

47. Ans. (a) BT
[Ref. Textbook of Pediatric Dermatology by Arun C Inamadar, 2/e p180]

- Single lesion leprosy is MC presentation: BT is MC clinical type
- MC leprosy type is Borderline (47.7%), Least common is Lepromatous (24.4%) with Tuberculoid group in between (27.9%)

48. Ans. (d) Clofazimine
[Ref. Neena Khanna, 5/e p285]

49. Ans. (b) Leprosy
[Ref. Neena Khanna, 5/e p284]

50. Ans. (d) Sural
[Ref. Pathology of Infectious Diseases by Pritt, 1/e p438]

51. Ans. (c) Azathioprine
[Ref. Handbook of Dermatological Drug Therapy by Khopkar, 1/e p100]

Newer Drugs in Leprosy

- Pefloxacin, Ofloxacin, Sparfloxacin
- Minocycline
- Clarithromycin
- Streptomycin
- Rifabutin, Rifapentine
- Fusidic acid
- Amoxycillin-Clavulanic acid
- PH22, PQ22 (Thiacetazone)
- Desoxyfructo-Serotonin
- Diuciphone

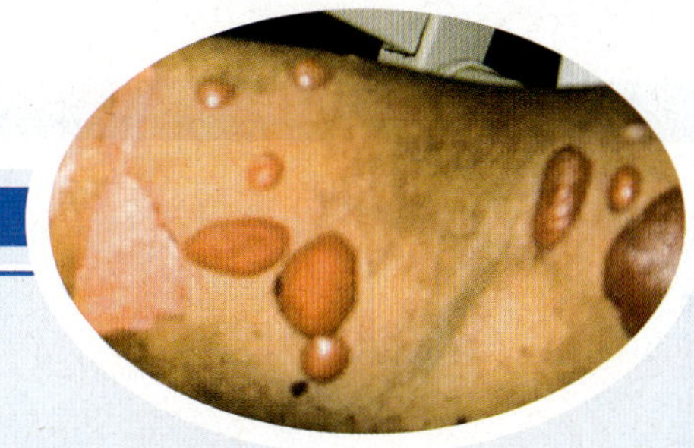

Chapter 12

Psoriasis and Papulosquamous Disorders

THEORETICAL CONCEPTS

XII A. PAPULOSQUAMOUS LESIONS

Primary skin disorders	Systemic disorders
• Psoriasis[Q] • Lichen planus[Q] • Pityriasis rosea[Q] • Pityriasis rubra pilaris • Mycosis fungoides[Q] • Secondary syphilis • Bowen's disease[Q] • Drug rash • Seborrheic dermatitis[Q]	• Systemic lupus erythematosus[Q] • Reiter's disease[Q] • Sarcoidosis[Q] • Drugs

XII B. PSORIASIS

XII B1. Definition

- Chronic dermatosis with unpredictable remissions and relapses, and presence of erythematous plaques/ papules with **silvery-scales**[Q]
- Increased epidermal cell proliferation[Q]

XII B2. Underlying Cause and Pathogenesis

- *Increased association with*: **HLA-CW6**[Q]
- *Physical trauma*: Isomorphic/ Koebner's phenomenon[Q]
- *Infections*: Beta-hemolytic streptococci (Guttate psoriasis), HIV (Explosive psoriasis) [Q]
- *Drugs*: Antimalarials, Lithium, Beta-adrenergic blockers, Corticosteroid withdrawal[Q]

XII B3. Histological Presentation [Mnemonic: SPASM][Q]

- **S**pongiform pustules
- **P**arakeratosis[Q]
- **A**canthosis
- **S**quirting papillae (thinned)
- ***M**unro's microabscesses* (Neutrophils in stratum corneum) [Q]

XII B4. Types of Psoriasis

Psoriasis Vulgaris/Chronic Plaque Psoriasis/Stable Plaque Psoriasis

- **Most common type of Psoriasis**[Q]
- *Clinical presentation*:
  - Well-demarcated, indurated, scaly, silvery[Q], discoid lesions
  - Erythematous **(*Ring of Woronoff*)**
  - ***Koebner's/Isomorphic phenomenon*** (lesions at site of trauma)[Q]
  - *Sites*:Extensor surfaces[Q], Pressure points (elbows, knees)[Q], Scalp
  - *Bed-side tests*:
    - ***Grattage test***: Accentuation of scales with glass-slide[Q]
    - ***Auspitz sign***: Bleeding points on removing membrane[Q]

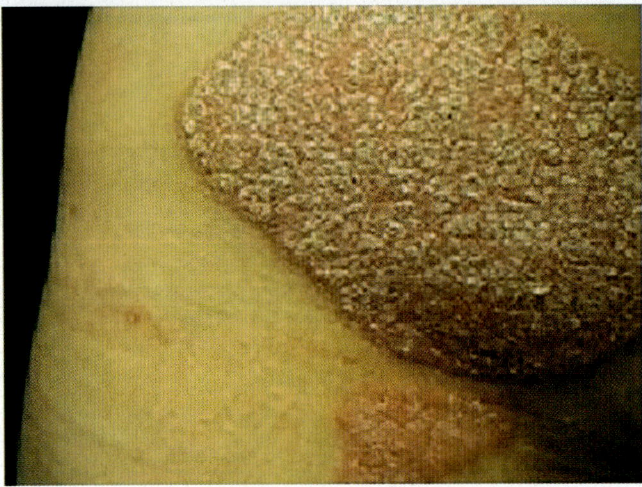

Fig. Psoriasis vulgaris

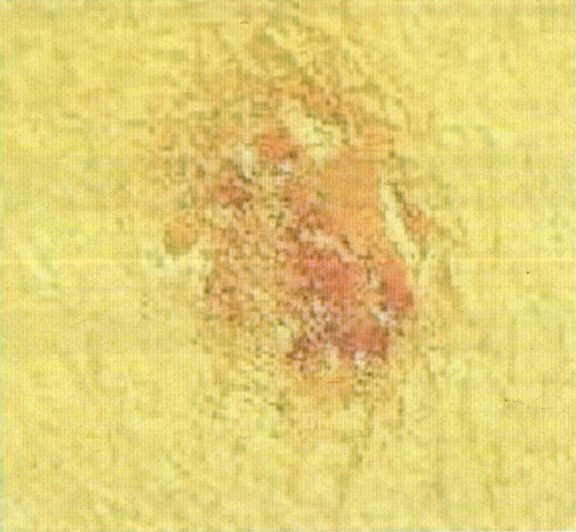

Fig. Auspitz sign

Guttate/Eruptive/Rain-drop Psoriasis

- Common on trunk in children and adolescents[Q]
- Frequent preceded by: Streptococcal sore throat/tonsillitis

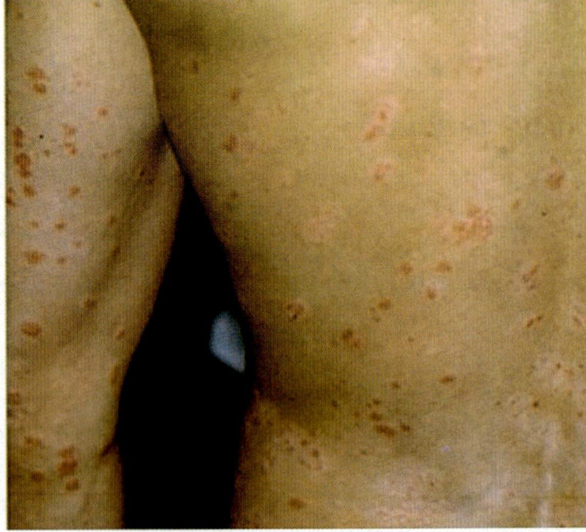

Fig. Guttate psoriasis

Rupioid Psoriasis

- *Limpet-like scales* (heaped and adherent)
- Seen in: Reiter's syndrome **(HLA-B27)**[Q]

Flexural Psoriasis

- Well-defined, salmon-pink lesions[Q]
- Seen in elderly females

Scalp Psoriasis

- Demarcated, indurated, scaly plaques
- *Pityriasis amiantacea*: Asbestos-like scales adherent to scalp

Erythrodermic Psoriasis

- Merging of psoriatic plaques
- Red-skin with marked scaling

Von Zumbusch Psoriasis

- Erythrodermic and pustular psoriasis

XII B5. Other System Involvement in Psoriasis

- **Nails [Mnemonic: The Only Drug Of Psoriasis is Topical Steroids]** Q
  - **T**hickened nail-plates
  - **O**il-spots/Oil-drop sign Q
  - **D**ystrophy, **D**iscolouration
  - **O**nycholysis Q
  - **P**itting
  - **T**himble-pitting Q
  - **S**ubungual hyperkeratosis Q
- **Joints**
  - Oligoarticular arthritis
  - DIP joint arthritis
  - Rheumatoid arthritis like
  - Arthritis mutilans

XII B6. Treatment of Psoriasis Q

Topical agents	*Biological response modifiers*
• Coal tar • Dithranol • Calcipotriol • Tazarotene	• Etanercept • Alafacept • Infliximab • Efalizumab
Systemic agents • Methotrexate • Acitretin • Cyclosporine	***Phytochemotherapy*** • 8-methoxy psoralen • Petrolatum • PUVA
Phototherapy • UVB	

XII C. PITYRIASIS ROSEA

- *Definition*: Self-limiting papulo-squamous skin disorder
- *Age group*: 10-35 years
- *Underlying cause*: HHV7 (or HHV6) Q
- *Clinical presentation*: Flexures in trunks
  - ***Herald/Mother patch***: Q
    - Central clearing with peripheral ***'Cigarette papery scales'*** Q
    - *Trailing/**Collarette of scales*** Q
  - Secondary lesions: (Lesions resemble secondary syphilis)
    - ***Fir-tree/Christmas-tree appearance of scales*** Q
- *Treatment*: Symptomatic

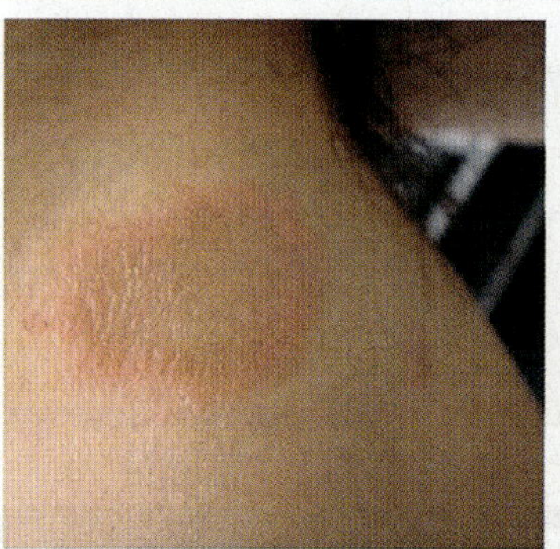
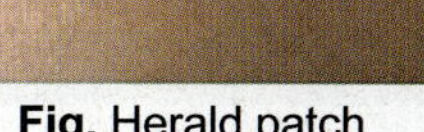

Fig. Herald patch

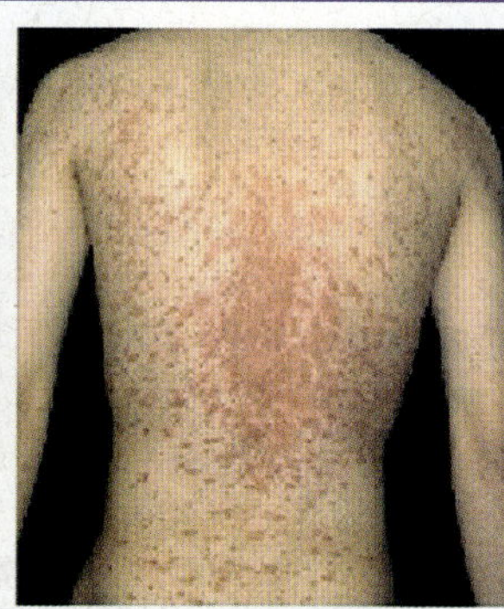

Fig. Fir-tree appearance

XII D. PITYRIASIS RUBRA PILARIS

- *Definition*: Inherited or acquired papulo-squamous skin disorder
- *Age group*:
  - Juvenile form: 5–10 years
  - Adult form: 40–60 years
- *Underlying cause*: Unknown
- *Clinical presentation*: Trunks, dorsal aspects of digits
  - Erythroderma with islands of normal skin
  - Orange-pink follicular papules
  - ***Keratodermic sandals*** Q (Orangish thickening of palms/ soles)
  - Yellow-brown nails with thick nail-plates

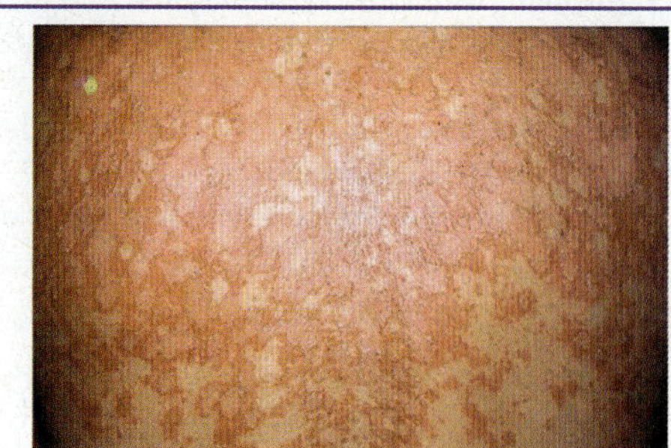

Fig. Pityriasis rubra pilaris

- *Treatment*:
  - Corticosteroids
  - Keratolytics
  - Acitretin
  - Methotrexate

XII E. PITYRIASIS SIMPLEX CAPILLITII: DANDRUFF

- *Definition*: Common disorder of scalp characterised by shedding of dead skin cells
- *Underlying cause*: ***'Hyper-proliferation of keratinocytes'***[Q]
  - *Organism*: Malassezia furfur[Q]
  - *Other factors*:
    - Sebaceous secretions, Metabolic products of skin organisms, Individual susceptibility
    - Allergic reaction
    - Perspiration, climate
- *Treatment*: [Q]
  - Keratinization regulators: Zinc pyrithione
  - Corticosteroids
  - Selenium sulphide[Q]
  - Imidazole topical antifungals: Ketoconazole[Q]
  - Hydroxypyridones: Ciclopirox[Q]

Differential diagnosis of scales in papulosquamous disorders	
Psoriasis • Silvery scales [Q] **Seborrheic dermatitis** • Stuck-on appearance [Q]of Greasy-yellow scales [Q]on erythematous papules	**Pityriasis rosea** • Collarette of scales [Q] • Central clearing with peripheral *'Cigarette papery scales'*[Q] **Pityriasis lichenoid chronica** • Adherent scales • Mica-like appearance

Differential diagnosis of lesions in papulosquamous disorders	
Lichen planus • Flat violaceous papules [Q] with Wickham's striae [Q] • Flexural surface **Psoriasis** • Erythematous papules/ plaques • Extensor surfaces[Q] **Seborrheic dermatitis** • Yellow follicular papules • Scalp and face [Q]	**Pityriasis rosea** • Annular plaques • Trunk **Pityriasis rubra pilaris** • Erythematous follicular papules • Trunk, Dorsum of hand

Differential diagnosis of pityriasis	
Pityriasis rosea • Annular plaques – Erythematous: *'Herald/ Mother patch'*[Q] • *'Christmas tree appearance* [Q]*'*, Collarette scales [Q] • Trunk **Pityriasis alba** • Children (6–12 years old) • Hypopigmented macule with fine scales on face	**Pityriasis versicolor** • Young adults • Hypopigmented macule with fine *'Furfuraceous/ Rice-powdery'*scales [Q] • Trunk, Shoulders **Pityriasis rubra pilaris** • Children, Adults • Erythematous follicular papules • Trunk, Dorsum of hand • Nutmeg papules on knuckles [Q]

IMAGE-BASED QUESTIONS

1. **What is the diagnosis of the given image?** ***[Recent Question 2016]***

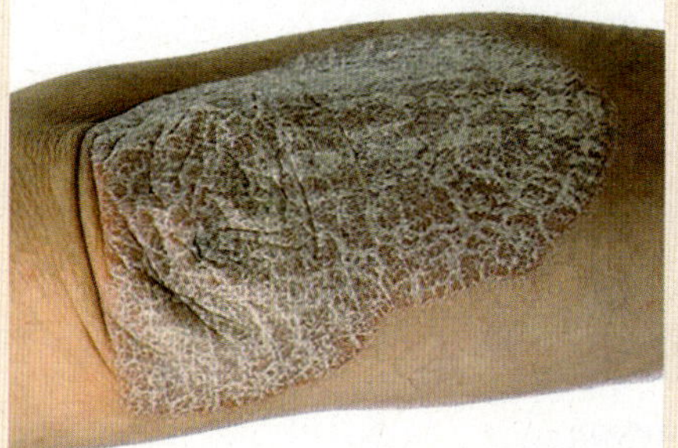

a. Lichen planus b. Lichenoid dermatitis
c. Psoriasis d. Pityriasis rosea

2. **On membrane removal of a lesion, Sign (Arrows) seen in Psoriasis**

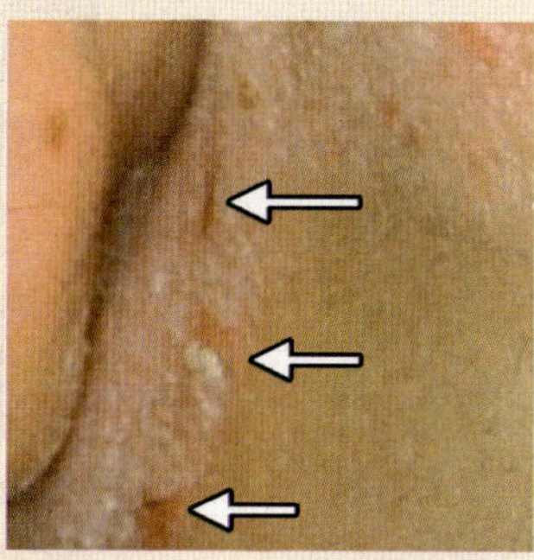

a. Gottron's sign b. Darier's sign
c. Auspitz sign d. Crowe's sign

3. **Identify the Lesion of a case of Pityriasis rosea as shown in Photograph**

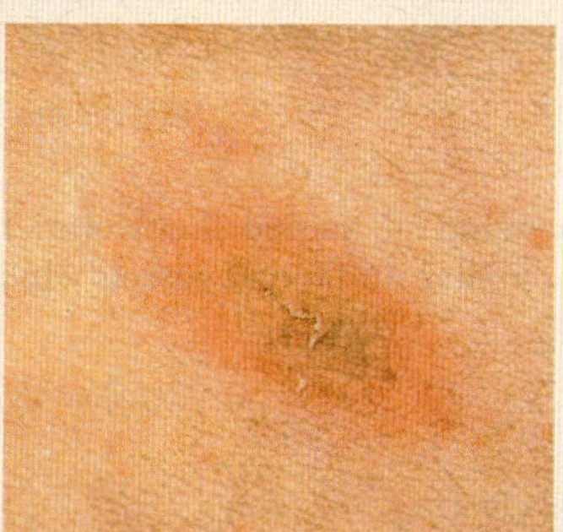

a. Herald patch b. Target lesion
c. Ash leaf macule d. Shagreen patch

4. **Diagnose the Skin disorder shown in the Photograph** ***[Recent Question 2013, Recent Question 2014]***

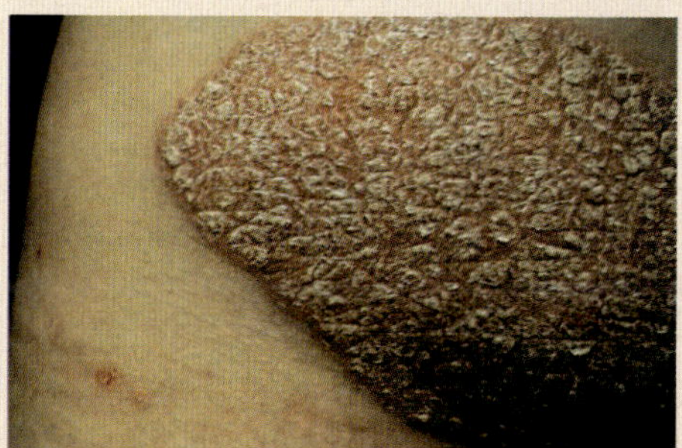

a. Guttate psoriasis b. Psoriasis vulgaris
c. Penile psoriasis d. Flexural psoriasis

5. **Skin disorder shown in Photograph based on its distribution in body** ***[Recent Question 2014]***

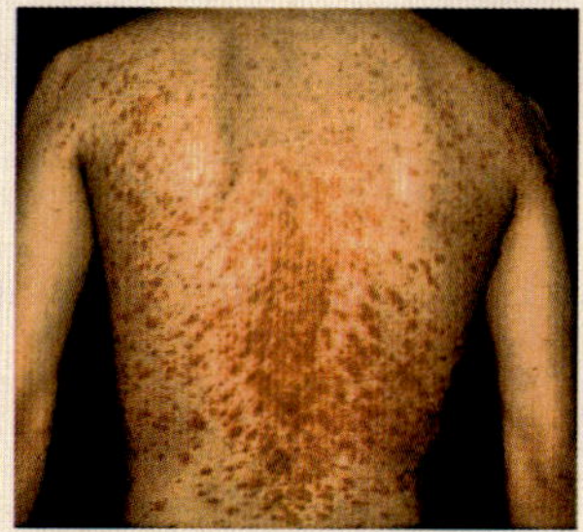

a. Psoriasis b. Tuberous sclerosis
c. Seborrhoeic dermatitis d. Pityriasis rosea

6. **Identify the test shown in Photograph performed on a suspected case of Psoriasis**

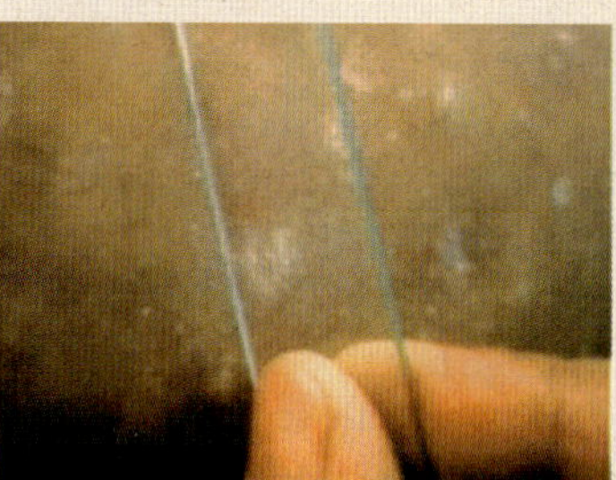

a. Auspitz sign b. Diascopy test
c. Dermoscopy d. Grattage test

7. A 7-month pregnant woman presented with lesions all over the body (See Photograph), showing multiple small pustules over skin. Most appropriate drug treatment is ***[AIIMS PG May 2015]***

a. Retinoids
b. Methotrexate
c. Azathioprine
d. Cyclosporine

 ANSWERS WITH EXPLANATIONS OF IBQs 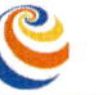

1. Ans. (c) Psoriasis *[Ref. DVL by Thappa, 4/e p120]*

- Psoriasis is a chronic papulo squamous disorder of unknown aetiology characterized by well-defined erythematous papular and plaque lesions with silvery white micaceous scales **(Photograph)**

2. Ans. (c) Auspitz sign *[Ref. Neena Khanna, 4/e p42]*

Auspitz's Sign

- Description: Appearance of punctate bleeding spots when psoriasis scales are scraped off, named after Heinrich Auspitz
- Underlying basis: Thinning of the epidermal layer overlying the tips of dermal papillae and blood vessels which are dilated and tortuous

3. Ans. (a) Herald patch *[Ref. Neena Khanna, 4/e p54]*

Herald Patch

- Salmon-colored wrinkled patch with Colarette of scales at periphery and central clearing
- First lesion to appear in Pityriasis rosea
- Seen in 80% of patients

4. Ans. (b) Psoriasis vulgaris *[Ref. Neena Khanna, 4/e p41]*

Psoriasis Vulgaris

- Clinical presentation:
  - Well-demarcated, indurated, scaly, silvery, discoid lesions
  - Erythematous (Ring of Woronoff)
- Sites: Extensor surfaces, Pressure points (elbows, knees), Scalp

5. Ans. (d) Pityriasis rosea *[Ref. Neena Khanna, 4/e p55]*

Secondary Lesions of Pityriasis Rosea

- Scaly papules enlarge forming oval annular patches
- Smaller and less erythematous, less scaly than Herald patch
- Christmas/Fir tree appearance: Long axis of patches run downwards and outwards from spine, lining along the ribs

6. Ans. (d) Grattage test *[Ref. Neena Khanna, 4/e p42]*

- Grattage test: On gentle scraping of lesions of Psoriasis with a glass slide, accentuation of Silvery scales occur

7. Ans. (d) Cyclosporine *[Ref. Psoriasis by Leon, 4/e p284]*

- For management of Generalized pustular psoriasis (Photograph) or erythrodermic psoriasis in pregnancy, cyclosporine, infliximab, and oral steroids are the first-line agents recommended
- Despite being Category C drug, Cyclosporine use during pregnancy is safe, and is not associated with birth defects.

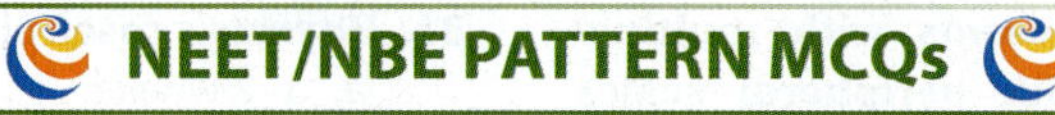

NEET/NBE PATTERN MCQs

1. **Nappes claires is seen in** *[Recent Question 2016]*
   a. Pityriasis. versicolor b. P. alba
   c. P. rubra d. P. rosea
2. **Keratodermic sandals is a feature of** *[Recent Question 2016]*
   a Pityriasis rosacea b. Lichen planus
   c. Psoriasis d. Pityriasis rubra pilaris
3. **Effective topical agents for treatment of dandruff include all except** *[NBE FMGE March 2010]*
   a. Azelaic acid b. Ciclopiroxalamine
   c. Ketoconazole d. Selenium sulphide
4. **A topical retinoid recently introduced for the treatment of psoriasis is** *[NBE DNB 2011]*
   a. Adapalene b. Tazarotene
   c. Alitretinoin d. Bexarotene
5. **Isomorphic-phenomenon is caused by all except** *[Recent Question 2016, NBE FMGE September 2007]*
   a. Psoriasis b. Vitiligo
   c. Lichen planus d. Lichen sclerosus
6. **In the management of psoriasis, false is** *[NBE DNB 1994]*
   a. Steroid creams are completely safe
   b. Dithranol therapy always produce staining and this is sign of effectiveness
   c. Natural sunlight is helpful in 75% of cases
   d. Systemic steroids should be avoided if possible
7. **Spaghetti and meatball appearance is seen in** *[Recent Question 2012]*
   a. Dermatophytes b. Aspergillus
   c. Pityriasis versicolor d. Candida
8. **Recently introduced treatment for psoriasis is** *[NBE FMGE September 2007]*
   a. Adapalene b. Tazarotene
   c. Alitretinoin d. Bexarotene
9. **Psoriasis may present with all of the following clinical features, except** *[NBE DNB 1993]*
   a. Pitting of nails
   b. Extensive large plaques
   c. Drop shaped lesions
   d. Progression of lesions unless therapy applied
10. **Munro's microabscesses are seen in** *[NBE FMGE March 2007]*
    a. Lichen planus b. Psoriasis
    c. Mycosis fungoides d. All of the above
11. **Koebner's phenomenon is seen in** *[Recent Question 2016, NBE DNB 1994]*
    a. Lichen planus b. Psoriasis
    c. Ichthyosis d. Leprosy
    e. Pemphigus
12. **A 40 years old male has rah over his groins with demarcated peripheral scaling and central clearing. He is a case of** *[NBE FMGE September 2005]*
    a. Candidiasis b. Aspergillosis
    c. Malassezia furfur d. Human herpes virus
13. **Auspitz sign is seen in** *[Recent Question 2016, NBE DNB 2009]*
    a. Pustular psoriasis b. Plaque type psoriasis
    c. Lichen planus d. Pityriasis rubra pilaris
14. **Silver plaques are seen in** *[NBE FMGE September 2006]*
    a. Psoriasis b. Vitiligo
    c. Albinism d. Lichen sclerosis
15. **Nail changes in psoriasis include following, except** *[NBE DNB 1998, 1999]*
    a. Onycholysis b. Discolouration
    c. Pitting d. Subungual hyperkeratosis
16. **Auspitz sign is found in** *[NBE FMGE March 2007, September 2010]*
    a. Psoriasis b. Vitiligo
    c. Fungal infections d. Melasma
17. **Lesions of pityriasis rosea are distributed mostly on the** *[NBE DNB 1995, 1999, 2003]*
    a. Face b. Trunk
    c. Scalp d. Palms and soleus
18. **Important feature of Psoriasis is** *[NBE FMGE September 2009]*
    a. Coarse bleeing b. Silver scales
    c. Crusting d. Erythematous macules
19. **Drug of choice for pustular psoriasis is** *[NBE DNB 1998, 1999]*
    a. Methotrexate b. PUVA
    c. Coal tar d. Steroids
20. **'*Fir-tree pattern*' lesions on trunk are seen in** *[Recent Question 2016, NBE FMGE September 2009]*
    a. Psoriasis b. Pityriasis rosea
    c. Pityriasis versicolor d. Pemphigoid
21. **Photosensitive rash is common in** *[NBE DNB 1996, 2003]*
    a. Acute intermittent porphyria
    b. Erythropoietic protoporphyria
    c. Leprosy
    d. Lichen planus
22. **Triad of Psoriasis include** *[NBE FMGE September 2009]*
    a. Munro's microabscesses, Parakeratosis, Epidermal hyperplasia
    b. Munro's microabscesses, Satellite pustules, Epidermal hyperplasia
    c. Munro's microabscesses, Fir-tree appearance, Epidermal hyperplasia
    d. Munro's microabscesses, Wickham's striae, Epidermal hyperplasia
23. **The microorganism most intimately associated with Seborrheic dermatitis is** *[NBE FMGE September 2011]*
    a. *Microsporum* b. *Streptococcus*
    c. *Corynebacterium* d. Pityrosporum
24. **Ingram regimen is used in treatment of** *[Recent Question 2016, 2015]*
    a. Vitiligo b. Psoriasis
    c. Lichen planus d. Lichen nitidus
25. **Palmoplantar keratoderma is a feature of?** *[Recent Question 2017]*
    a. Pemphigus b. Verruca plana
    c. Psoriasis d. Pityriasis rubra pilaris

26. A 40 years old male patient presents with multiple erythematous annular lesions with peripheral scales arranged predominantly on trunk. Treatment of choice is *[Recent Question 2017]*
a. Topical steroids b. Systemic steroids
c. Systemic Azathioprine d. Topical antifungal

27. Woronoff's ring is a feature of? *[Recent Question 2017]*
a. Psoriasis b. Lichen planus
c. Pityriasis rosea d. Pemphigus

28. Koebner's phenomenon is seen in? *[Recent Question 2017]*
a. Leprosy b. Pemphigus
c. Lichen nitidus d. Scabies

29. Best treatment option for Psoriasis is pregnancy among the following is? *[Recent Question 2017]*
a. Systemic cyclosporine b. Topical steroids
c. PUVA therapy d. Infliximab

30. Only definitive indication of Systemic steroids in Psoriasis is? *[Recent Question 2017]*
a. Pustular psoriasis
b. Pregnancy associated pustular psoriasis
c. Chronic plaque psoriasis
d. Erythroderma

31. Pityriasis rosea clears with in? *[Recent Question 2017]*
a. 1–2 weeks b. 2–4 weeks
c. 4–8 weeks d. 6–12 weeks

32. Treatment of choice for Erythrodermic psoriasis is? *[Recent Question 2017]*
a. Prednisolone b. Hydroxyurea
c. Acitretin d. Ciclosporin

33. Multiple psoriatic lesions on hands. Treatment of choice is? *[Recent Question 2017]*
a. NBUVB
b. Systemic methotrexate
c. Topical steroids and salicylic acid
d. Systemic steroids

34. A known case of diabetes develops annular orange skin lesions, which disappear after biopsy. This phenomenon is known as? *[Recent Question 2017]*
a. Koebner's phenomenon
b. Reverse Koebner's Phenomenon
c. Asboe Hansen sign
d. Isotopic Phenomenon

35. Kogoj's pustules are seen in? *[Recent Question 2017]*
a. Lichen planus b. Pemphigus vulgaris
c. Mycosis fungoides d. Psoriasis vulgaris

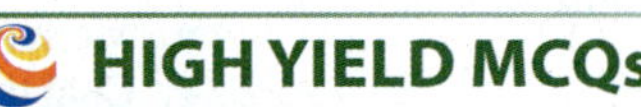

HIGH YIELD MCQs

1. Which of the following is/are used in treatment of Psoriasis? *[PGI June 2016]*
a. High dose oral dexamethasone
b. Methotrexate
c. TNF-alpha inhibitor
d. Acitretin
e. Narrow band UVB

2. Annular herald patch is seen in *[Recent Question 2016, AIIMS PGMEE 1990, 1997, PGI 1996, AP PGMEE 1996, TN PGMEE 1998, Kerala PGMEE 1998, SGPGI 2003, Jharkhand PGMEE 2005]*
a. Pityriasis versicolour b. Pityriasis alba
c. Pityriasis rosea d. Psoriasis

3. A 24-year-old woman with multiple erythematous annular lesions with peripheral collarette of scales arranged predominantly on trunk are seen in *[All India PGMEE 2002]*
a. Pityriasis vesicular
b. Pityriasis rubra pilaris
c. Pityriasis rosea
d. Pityriasis lichenoides chronica

4. A 7-year-old boy presents with recurrent, scaly, hypopigmented patch on face, diagnosis is *[AIIMS PGMEE 1996]*
a. Vitiligo b. Indeterminate leprosy
c. Pityriasis alba d. Pityriasis rosea

5. A 5-year-old boy has multiple asymptomatic oval and circular faintly hypopigmented macules with fine scaling on his face. The most probable clinical diagnosis is *[All India PGMEE 2003]*
a. Ptyriasis versicolor b. Indeterminate leprosy
c. Ptyriasis alba d. Acrofacial vitiligo

6. Pitting nail dystrophy seen in *[PGI 2008]*
a. Dermatophytic infection b. Psoriasis
c. Lichen planus d. Seborrheic dermatitis

7. Pityriasis rosea in a *[All India PGMEE 2007]*
a. Chronic relapsing disease
b. It is an autoimmune disease
c. Caused by dermatophytes
d. Self resolving

8. True about Pityriasis alba *[PGI 2001]*
a. No active treatment required
b. Common in elderly
c. Variant of vitiligo
d. Common over the face
e. Presents as scaly, whitish macules

9. Which of the following statements is true regarding Pityriasis Rubra Pilaris *[PGI 2001]*
a. Isolated patches of normal skin are found
b. Cephalocaudal distribution
c. I.V. Cyclosporine is effective
d. More common in females
e. Oral cyclosporine is effective

10. All are causes of papulosquamous lesions except *[PGI 2000, SGPGI 2002]*
a. Psoriasis
b. Para psoriasis
c. Squamous cell carcinoma d. Mycosis fungoides
e. Congenital syphilis

11. About micro-munro abscesses which of the following statements are true *[PGI 2009]*

a. Seen in stratum corneum
b. Seen in psoriasis
c. Contain neutrophils and lymphocyte
d. Contain neutrophils only
e. Associated pustules are normally seen

12. Treatment of psoriasis *[PGI 2005]*
a. PUVA b. Methotrexate
c. Systemic steroids d. Femicycline
e. Terbinafine

13. All are true about Psoriasis except *[PGI 2000]*
a. Very pruritic
b. Pitting of nails
c. Joint involvement in 5–10%
d. Parakeratosis and acanthosis
e. Munro abscess

14. A 30 years old male presented with silvery scales on elbow and knee that bleed on removal. The probable diagnosis is *[Recent Question 2017, AIIMS PGMEE 1999]*
a. Pityriasis b. Seborrheic dermatitis
c. Psoriasis d. Secondary syphilis

15. HPR finding in psoriasis *[PGI 2006, PGI 2009]*
a. Micro-Munro abscess b. Suprapapillary thinning
c. Grenz zone present d. Pautrier's abscess
e. Hyperkeratosis

16. Fir-tree type distribution is seen in *[Recent Question 2016, AIIMS PGMEE 2006]*
a. Pityriasis Rosea b. Psoriasis
c. Measles d. Secondary syphilis

17. All are common of psoriasis except *[AIIMS PGMEE 1996, AP PGMEE 1999, UP PGMEE 2003]*
a. Nail changes
b. Extensor distribution
c. Arthritis
d. Erythematuous squamous-lesions

18. The important feature of psoriasis is *[Bihar PGMEE 2004, AMU PGMEE 1999]*
a. Crusting
b. Scaling
c. Oozing
d. Erythema

19. Psoriasis is characterized by all except *[All India PGMEE 1992, AP PGMEE 1998]*
a. Definite pink plaque with clear margin
b. In children disappears in 2 weeks to reappear again
c. Always associated with nail infection
d. Involves knees and elbow

20. All of the following are seen in psoriasis except
a. Auspitz sign present *[SGPGI 2003]*
b. 10% associated with arthritis
c. It is premalignant disease
d. Worsening of disease during winter

21. Which viral association is found in Pityriasis rosea? *[Jharkhand PGMEE 2004]*
a. HHV 7 b. CMV
c. Vericella Zoster d. E.B.V

22. All are presentation in psoriasis except *[SGPGI 2001]*
a. Nail changes b. CNS involvement
c. Arthritis d. Skin involvement

23. Munro micro abscess is seen in *[Recent Question 2016, PGI 1999]*
a. Dermal tissue b. Stratum basale
c. Stratum corneum d. Stratum malpighi

24. A patient with psoriasis was started on systemic steroids. After stopping the treatment, patient developed universally red scaly skin with plaques losing their margins all over his body. Most likely cause is *[AIIMS PGMEE 2001]*
a. Drug induced reaction b. Pustular psoriasis
c. Bacterial infection d. Erythrodermic Psoriasis

25. Mother patch is seen in *[AIIMS PGMEE 1991]*
a. Lichen planus b. Pityriasis rosea
c. P. alba d. Pemphigus

26. All are true regarding Psoriasis except
a. Arthritis in 5% *[All India PGMEE 2000]*
b. Abscess is seen
c. Head, neck and face are not involved
d. No scaly, red lesions are seen in inframammary and natal area

27. Least common site involvement in psoriasis is *[All India PGMEE 1998]*
a. Scalp b. Nail Involvement
c. CNS involvement d. Arthritis

28. A 16-year-old boy presented with asymptomatic multiple erythematous annular lesions with a collarette of scales at periphery of the lesions present on the trunk. The most likely diagnosis is *[All India PGMEE 2005]*
a. Pityriasis versicolor
b. Pityriasis alba
c. Pityriasis rosacea
d. Pityriasis rubra pilaris

29. A patient presents with erythematous scaly lesions on extensor aspect of elbows and knee. The clinical diagnosis is got by *[AIIMS PGMEE 2002]*
a. Auspitz sign b. KOH smear
c. Tzanck smear d. Skin biopsy

30. Koebner's phenomenon is seen typically with *[Recent Question 2016, PGI 1997]*
a. Psoriasis b. Eczema
c. Scabies d. Lupus vulgaris

31. Koebner's phenomenon is seen in *[All India PGMEE 1992]*
a. Pemphigus b. Darier's Disease
c. Lichen Planus d. Tinea

32. Kobner's phenomenon is seen in *[All India PGMEE 1991]*
a. Lupus erythematous b. Syphilis
c. Lupus Vulgaris d. Psoriasis

33. An adult presents with oval scaly hypopigmented macules over chest and back. The diagnosis is *[AIIMS PGMEE 2001]*
a. Leprosy b. Lupus vulgaris
c. Pityriasis versicolour d. Lichen planus

34. Koebner's phenomenon is seen in *[PGI 2004]*
a. Lichen planus b. Warts
c. Bechet syndrome d. Psoriasis
e. Vitiligo

35. The treatment of Pustular psoriasis is *[SGPGI 2002]*
a. Retinoids b. Steroids
c. Thalidomide d. Hydroxyurea

36. The treatment of psoriatic erythroderma is *[PGI 1996]*
a. Methotrexate b. Retinols
c. Diethrenol d. Corticosteroid

37. The treatment of choice for erythrodermic psoriasis is *[SGPGI 2004]*
a. Corticosteriods b. Methotrexate
c. Coal tar topically d. Topical corticosteroids

38. All of the following is given for the treatment for Pityriasis versicolor except *[All India PGMEE 2002]*
a. Ketoconazole b. Griseofulvin
c. Clotrimazole d. Selenium sulphate

39. Treatment of erythematous skin rash with multiple pus lakes in a pregnant woman is *[All India PGMEE 2010]*
a. Corticosteroids b. Retinoids
c. Methotrexate d. Psoralen with PUVA

40. A 10-year-old child Kallu has hypopigmented multiple scaly patch over face. The likely diagnosis is *[AIIMS PGMEE 1995, 1998, 1999, 2001]*
a. Tinea versicolor b. Pityriasis alba
c. Indeterminate leprosy d. Lupus vulgaris

41. "Auspitz" sign is characteristically seen in *[Bihar PGMEE 2005, AIIMS PGMEE 2008]*
a. Plaque Psoriasis b. Pustular Psoriasis
c. Licken Planus d. Inverse Psoriasis

42. Koebner's phenomenon is characteristic of *[PGI 1999]*
a. Psoriasis b. Pemphigus vulgaris
c. Pityriasis rosea d. Lupus vulgaris

43. The only indication of giving corticosteroids in pustular psoriasis is *[All India PGMEE 2005]*
a. Psoriatic erythroderma with pregnancy
b. Psoriasis in a patient with alcoholic cirrhosis
c. Moderate arthritis
d. Extensive lesions

44. Treatment of choice in Pustular psoriasis *[All India PGMEE 1994]*
a. Psoralen + UV therapy b. Systemic steroid
c. Methotrexate d. Estrogen

45. The mechanism of action of psoralen is *[PGI 1996, JIPMER PGMEE 1998]*
a. Binding to DNA
b. Inhibiting protein synthesis
c. Inhibiting angiogenesis d. Inhibiting keratinization

46. Which of the following seen in Psoriasis? *[PGI 2007]*
a. Pautrier's micro abscess b. Micro-Munro abscess
c. Grenz zone d. Hyperkeratosis
e. Suprapapillary thinning

47. Psoralen + ultraviolet light (PUVA) therapy is useful in the treatment of *[Karnataka PGMEE 1994]*
a. Psoriasis b. Vitiligo
c. Mycosis fungoides d. All of the above

48. Treatment of pustular psoriasis is *[AIIMS PGMEE 2002]*
a. Thalidomide b. Retinoids
c. Hydroxyurea d. Methotrexate

49. Photo-chemotherapy is indicated which of the following *[SGPGI 2003]*
a. Erythema nodosum b. Psoriasis
c. Lichen planus d. Pemphigus

50. Psoriasis is exacerbated by *[Recent Question 2016, All India PGMEE 1998]*
a. Lithium b. β-blockers
c. Antimalarials d. All of the above

51. DOC for a pregnant woman in 2nd trimester with pustular psoriasis is *[All India PGMEE 2008]*
a. Prednisolone b. Dapsone
c. Acitretin d. Methotrexate

52. Psoralen with UV-A is used for treating *[All India PGMEE 1991]*
a. Porphyria b. Psoriasis
c. Pemphigus d. Tinea versicolor

53. Psoralen-A is used in the treatment of *[JIPMER PGMEE 1996]*
a. Pemphigus b. Vitiligo
c. Pityriasis alba d. Icthyosis

54. In psoriatic arthropathy TOC is *[AIIMS PGMEE 1993]*
a. Methotrexate b. 5FU
c. PUVA d. Steroid

55. A patient with psoriasis was started on systemic steroids. After stopping treatment, the patient developed generalized pustules all over the body. The cause is most likely to be *[All India PGMEE 2002]*
a. Drug induced reaction b. Pustular psoriasis
c. Bacterial infections d. Septicemia

56. Tinea versicolor is caused by *[PGI 1998]*
a. *Malassezia furfur*
b. *Candida*
c. *Trichophyton rubrum*
d. *Trichophyton mentagrophyte*

57. Treatment of tinea versicolor *[Kerala PGMEE 1997]*
a. Clotrimazole b. Sod thiosulphate
c. Selenium sulphide d. Miconazole
e. All of the above

58. All of the following drugs are effective in treatment of Pityriasis versicolor except *[All India PGMEE 2005]*
a. Selenium sulphide b. Ketoconazole
c. Griseofulvin d. Clotrimazole

59. Bulkeley membrane is seen in *[PGI 2002]*
a. Psoriasis b. Pemphigus
c. Tinea d. Pityriasis

60. A 6-year-old child from Tamil Nadu presents with a solitary nonanaesthetic patch on face, the possible diagnosis is *[AIIMS PGMEE 1998]*
a. Pityriasis alba b. Indeterminate leprosy
c. Pityriasis versicolor d. Tinea infection

 NEET/NBE PATTERN MCQs ANSWERS WITH EXPLANATIONS 

1. Ans. (c) P. Rubra
[Ref. Dermatology by Bolognia, 1/e Fig11.6]

Pityriasis rubra pilaris

- Large thin scales
- Characteristic orange-red color, papules on the knees, elbows and dorsal aspects of the fingers
- Nappes claires: Islands of uninvolved skin within the erythroderma

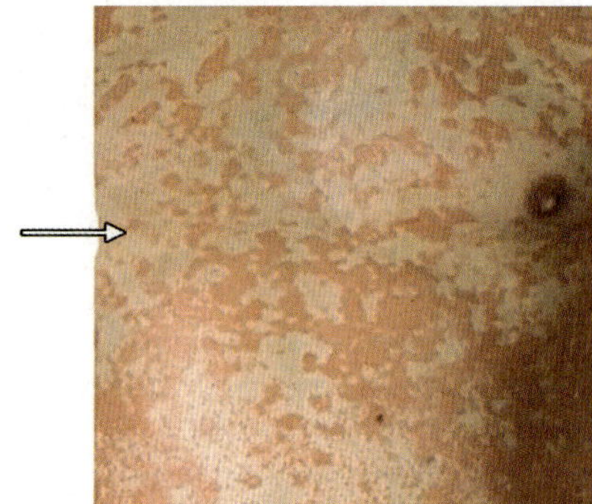

Fig. Nappes claires

2. Ans. (d) Pityriasis rubra pilaris
[Ref. Clinical Dermatology by Habif, 6/e p299-301]

- Classic adult PRP begins insidiously, usually in the fifth or sixth decade of life, with a small, indolent, red scaling plaque on the face or upper body
- Features:
  - Erythroderma; islands of sparing, salmon-colored palmoplantar keratoderma
  - Follicular hyperkeratosis, cephalocaudal spread

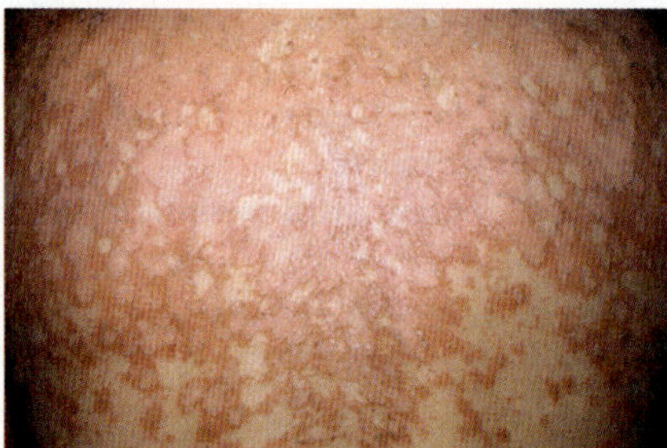

Fig. Pityriasis rubra pilaris (PRP)

3. Ans. (a) Azelaic acid
[Ref. Wikipedia]

Pityriasis Simplex Capillitii: Dandruff

- Definition: Common disorder of scalp characterised by shedding of dead skin cells
- Underlying cause: 'Hyper-proliferation of keratinocytes'
  - Organism: *Malassezia furfur*
  - Other factors:
    1. **Sebaceous secretions, Metabolic products of skin organisms, Individual susceptibility**
    2. **Allergic reaction**
    3. **Perspiration, climate**
- Treatment:
  - Keratinization regulators: Zinc pyrithione
  - Corticosteroids
  - Selenium sulphide
  - Imidazole topical antifungals: Ketoconazole
  - Hydroxypyridones: Ciclopirox

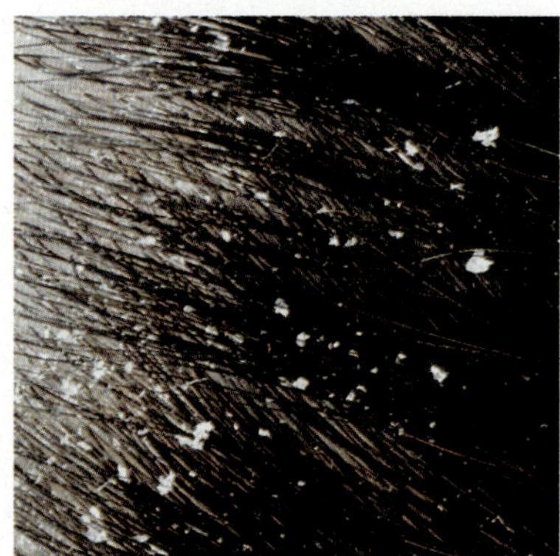

Fig. Pityriasis simplex capillitii (PSC)

4. Ans. (b) Tazarotene
[Ref. Neena Khanna, 5/e p56]

- Newer topical retinoid used in Psoriasis is Tazarotene (0.05-0.1% formulation)
- Keratolytic, Keratoplastic agent

5. Ans. (d) Lichen sclerosus
[Ref. Neena Khanna, 4/e p41, 57, 153, 236; Isomorphic Phenomenon of Koebner by DM Thappa, IJDVL 2004, 70(3), Pg 187-189]

Isomorphic/ Koebner Phenomenon

- *Definition*: Are skin lesions appearing on lines of trauma
- *Underlying causes*:
  - Thermal trauma
  - Dermatoses
  - Allergic reactions
  - Therapy
- *Types of Koebner phenomena*: **[Mnemonic: Left Ventricular Pulsations Will Make Blood Pressure HELP Decrease Creatinine Kinase]**

True isomorphic phenomena • Lichen planus • Vitiligo • Psoriasis	***Occasional isomorphic phenomena*** (Localised to trauma-site) • Hailey-Hailey disease • Erythema multiforme • Lichen sclerosus et atrophicus • Pellagra • Darier's disease • Cancers • Kaposi's sarcoma
Pseudo-isomorphic phenomena (In infectious diseases) • Warts • Molluscum contagiosum • Behcet's syndrome • Pyoderma gangrenosum	

  - Rare Isomorphic phenomenon: Kyrle disease, Morphoea, Necrobiosis lipoidica, Perforating folliculitis, Reactive perforating collagenosis

6. Ans. (a) Steroid creams are completely safe
[Ref. Neena Khanna, 5/e p56]

Side Effects of Topical Corticosteroid in Psoriasis

- Dermal atrophy and tachyphylaxis
- Early relapse
- Precipitation of unstable psoriasis

7. Ans. (c) Pityriasis versicolor
[Ref. Neena Khanna, 5/e p311]

Pityriasis Versicolor

- Adolescent or young adult
- Hypopigmented (sometimes hyperpigmented), perifollicular macules that become confluent
- Lesions appear to be sitting on neck
- Branny scales, accentuated by scratching with glass slide
- Upper trunk and neck

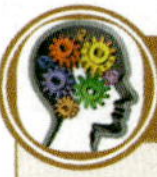

Also Remember

- KOH mount is confirmatory for P. versicolor: Mixture of short, branched hyphae and spores ("Spaghetti and meatball" appearance)

8. Ans. (b) Tazarotene
[Ref. Neena Khanna, 4/e p50]

Retinoids

- *Definition*: Chemical compounds related chemically to Vitamin A
- *Types of Retinoids*:

Retinoids	Use(s)
First generation retinoids	
Retinol	Vision, bone/tooth/ reproductive system development
Retinal	
Tretinoin (Retinoic acid)	Acne vulgaris
Isotretinoin	Nodulocystic acne, Acne rosacea
Alitretinoin	Kaposi sarcoma, Chronic hand eczema/ dermatitis
Second generation retinoids	
Etretinate	Psoriasis
Acitretin	Psoriasis
Third generation retinoids	
Tazarotene	Psoriasis, Breast/Lung carcinoma
Bexarotene	Cutaneous T cell lymphoma, Breast/Lung carcinoma
Adapalene	Acne vulgaris

(Tazarotene is a new topical retinoid recommended for Psoriasis treatment)

9. Ans. (d) Progression of lesions unless therapy applied
[Ref. Neena Khanna, 5/e p55]

10. Ans. (b) Psoriasis
[Ref. Neena Khanna, 4/e p48]

Histological Presentation of Psoriasis

[Mnemonic: SPASM]

- **S**pongiform pustules
- **P**arakeratosis
- **A**canthosis
- **S**quirting papillae (thinned)
- **M**unro's microabscesses (Neutrophils in stratum corneum)

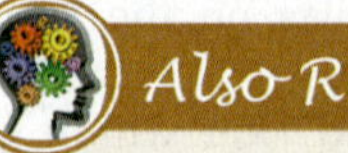

Also Remember

- *Dermatological conditions showing Munro's microabscesses*:
  - Psoriasis
  - Seborrheic dermatitis
- *Dermatological conditions showing Pautrier's microabscesses*:
  - T-cell lymphomas
  - Mycosis fungoides
- *Dermatological conditions showing Papillary microabscesses*:
  - Bullous pemphigoid

11. Ans. (a) Lichen planus; (b) Psoriasis
[Ref. Neena Khanna, 5/e p45; Differential Diagnosis in Dermatology by Ashton, 3/e p179]

- Koebner's phenomenon/Isomorphic phenomenon: New lesions of the original disease develop at sites of trauma (scratches, surgical incisions, and injury) and indicates active disease
  - Psoriasis
  - Lichen planus
  - Vitiligo
  - Plane warts

12. Ans. (d) Human herpes virus
[Ref. Neena Khanna, 4/e p54]

Pityriasis Rosea

- *Definition*: Self-limiting papulosquamous skin disorder
- *Age group*: 10–35 years
- *Underlying cause*: HHV7 (or HHV6)
- *Clinical presentation*: Flexures in trunks
  - *Herald/ Mother patch*:
    1. Central clearing with peripheral *'Cigarette papery scales'*
    2. *Trailing/ Collarette of scales*
  - Secondary lesions: (Lesions resemble secondary syphilis)
    1. *Fir-tree/ Christmas-tree appearance of scales*
    2. *Treatment*: Symptomatic

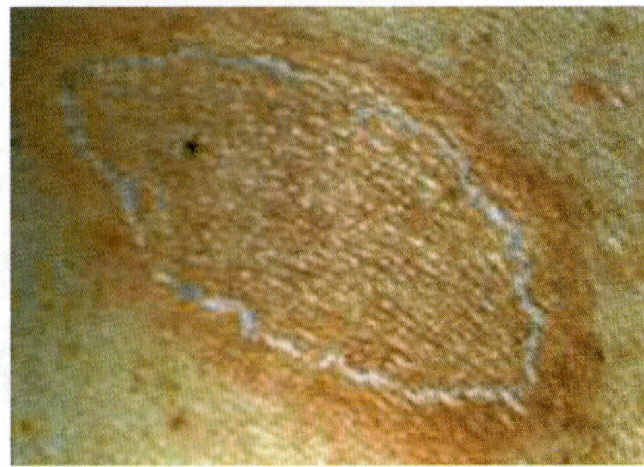

Fig. Pityriasis rosea: Collarette

13. Ans. (b) Plaque type psoriasis
[Ref. Neena Khanna, 5/e p46]
- Positive Auspitz sign: On removing the membrane, punctuate bleeding points become visible

14. Ans. (a) Psoriasis
[Ref. Neena Khanna, 4/e p40]

Clinical Presentation of Psoriasis: Extensor, pressure points
- Well-demarcated, indurated, scaly, silvery, discoid lesions
- Erythematous (***Ring of Woronoff***)
- *Koebner's/Isomorphic phenomenon* (lesions at site of trauma)
- Nail changes: Thickened nail-plates, Oil-spots/Oil-drop sign, Dystrophy, Discolouration, Onycholysis, Thimble-pitting, Subungual hyperkeratosis
- *Bedside tests*:
  - *Grattage test*: Accentuation of scales with glass-slide
  - *Auspitz sign*: Bleeding points on removing membrane

15. Ans. NONE
[Ref. Neena Khanna, 5/e p50]

Nail Changes in Psoriasis (10–50% patients)
- Pitting-deep, irregular
- Onycholysis
- Nail plate thickening
- Subungual hyperkeratosis
- Discolouration and dystrophy of nail plate: Nail plate becomes yellow or brown or dysmorphic
- Oil spots (oil-drop discoloration): Yellow red discoloration in center of nail.

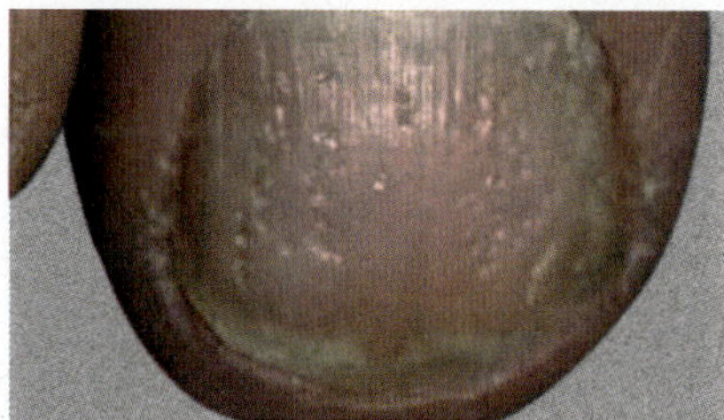

Fig. Psoriatic nails

16. Ans. (a) Psoriasis
[Ref. Neena Khanna, 4/e p42]

Auspitz Sign is seen in
- Psoriasis
- Darier's disease
- Actinic keratosis

17. Ans. (b) Trunk
[Ref. Neena Khanna, 5/e p60]
- Trunk, along the lines of cleavage in a typical 'Fir tree appearance' is involved in Pityriasis rosea

18. Ans. (b) Silver scales
[Ref. Neena Khanna, 4/e p40]

19. Ans. (a) Methotrexate
[Ref. Neena Khanna, 5/e p59]

20. Ans. (b) Pityriasis rosea
[Ref. Neena Khanna, 4/e p55]

21. Ans. (b) Erythropoietic photoporphyria
[Ref. Neena Khanna, 5/e p415-416]
- Manifest as burning, oedema and urticaria on sun exposure

22. Ans. (a) Munro's microabscesses, Parakeratosis, Epidermal hyperplasia
[Ref. Neena Khanna, 4/e p40]
- *Psoriasis*: Chronic dermatosis with unpredictable remissions and relapses, and presence of erythematous plaques/ papules with silvery-scales
  - Increased epidermal cell proliferation
- *Histological presentation* **[Mnemonic: SPASM]**
  - **S**pongiform pustules
  - **P**arakeratosis
  - **A**canthosis
  - **S**quirting papillae (thinned)
  - **M**unro's microabscesses (Neutrophils in stratum corneum)

23. Ans. (d) Pityrosporum
[Ref. Neena Khanna, 4/e p97]

Seborrhoeic Dermatitis
- *Cause*: *Malassezia furfur* (Pityrosporum ovale)
- *Clinical presentation*:
  - Usually on face, upper trunk, upper extremities
  - Multiple brown-black papules with *'Stuck-on' appearance*
  - *Currant bun appearance*: Scattered keratin plugs on greasy skin
  - Hyperkeratosis, Papillomatosis, Horn cysts
  - Is MC dermatosis in AIDS patients
- *Treatment*:
  - Topical antifungals: Ketoconazole, Ciclopirox, Selenium sulphide
  - Topical steroids
  - Topical immunomodulators: Tacrolimus, Pimecrolimus

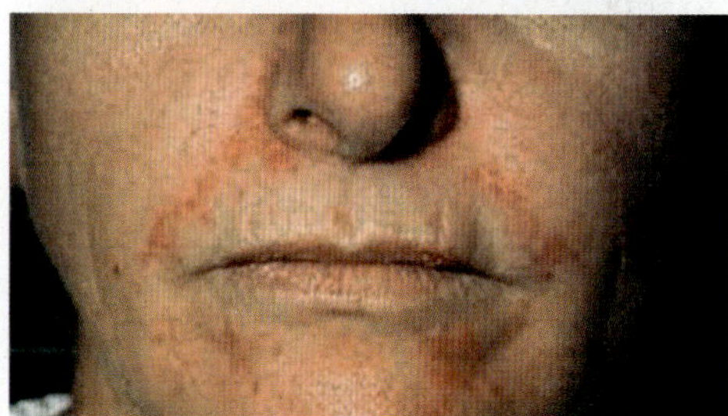

Fig. Seborrheic dermatitis

24. Ans. (b) Psoriasis
[Ref. Psoriasis by Kirby, 1/e p50]

Inpatient Daycare Treatment of Psoriasis
- Goeckerman Regimen: Coal tar + UVB phototherapy
- Ingram Regimen: Dithranol + UVB phototherapy

25. Ans. (d) Pityriasis rubra pilaris
[Ref. PG Textbook of Pediatrics - Volume 3 by Gupta, 1/e p2702]

Griffiths Classification of Pityriasis Rubra Pilaris
- Type I: Classical Adult PRP
  - MC type
  - Present with Erythroderma with islands of sparing, Palmoplantar keratoderma, Follicular hyperkeratosis

- Type II: Atypical PRP
- Type III: Classic Juvenile PRP
- Type IV: Circumscribed Juvenile PRP
- Type V: Atypical Juvenile PRP
- Type VI: HIV-associated PRP

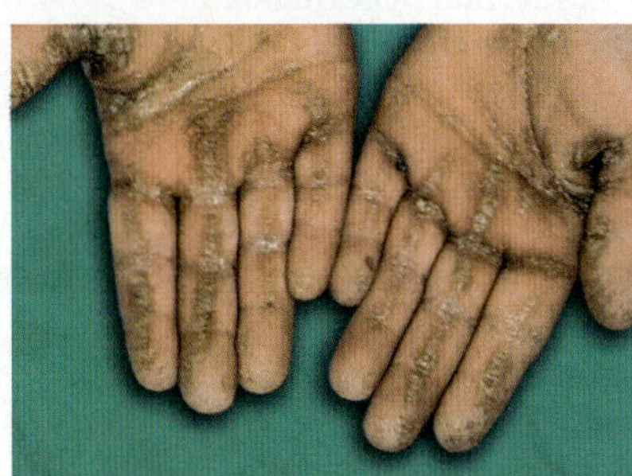

Fig. Palmar keratoderma

26. Ans. (a) Topical steroids

[Ref. The Washington Manual of Outpatient Internal Medicine, 1/e p841]

Pityriasis Rosea (PR)

- Self-limited disease; treatment is supportive
- Herald/Mother patch: Central clearing with peripheral 'Cigarette papery scales' with Trailing/ Collarette of scales
- Drug therapy for pityriasis rosea primarily consists of symptomatic treatment of pruritus
- Topical zinc oxide and calamine lotion may be helpful
- Oral antihistamines and topical corticosteroids can be used as needed

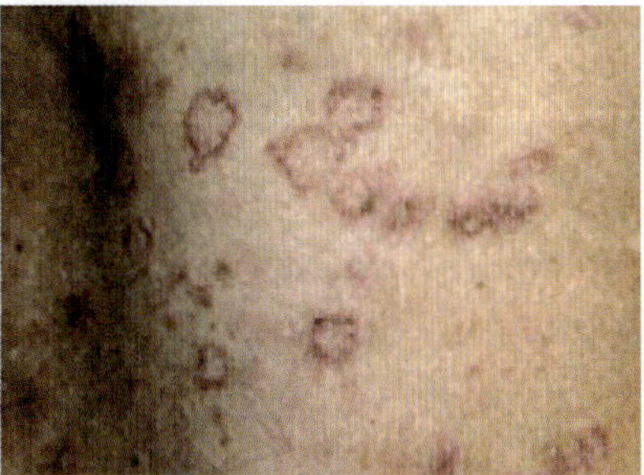

Fig. Pityriasis rosea

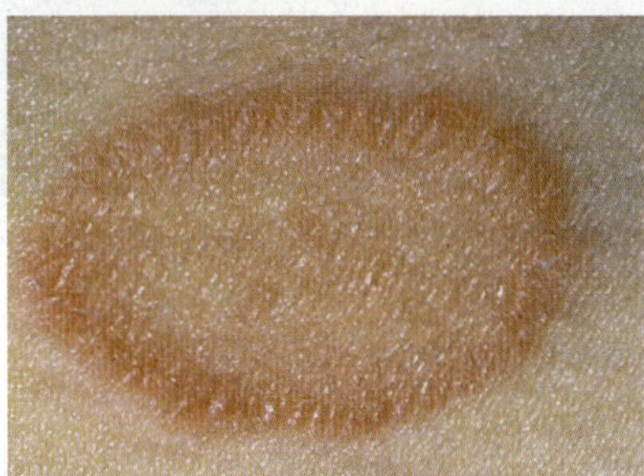

Fig. Herald patch

27. Ans. (a) Psoriasis

[Ref. Immunodermatology by Safai, 1/e p171]

Woronoff Ring

- Woronoff's 1926 described a pale halo encircling a plaque of psoriasis
- Woronoff's ring is therefore not unique to Psoritic skin: Epidermal damage (Atopic dermatitis, Contact dermatitis, Cutaneous lupus erythematosus) consistently depress prostaglandin synthesis compared with homogenates of normal skin from the same patient; subsequent increased prostaglandin release and the presence of inhibitor probably reflect epidermal damage
- It also refers to the presence of a white ring around erythematous plaques undergoing topical treatment or phototherapy

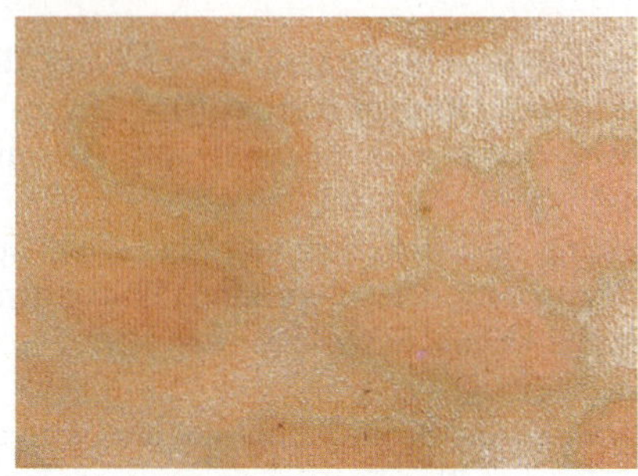

Fig. Woronoff ring

28. Ans. (c) Lichen nitidus

[Ref. Pediatric Emergency Medicine by Fleisher, 6/e p528]

- Lichen nitidus is a rarer condition than idiopathic Lichen planus
- Characterized clinically by the presence of pinpoint to pinhead-sized papules, which are usually asymptomatic and flesh-coloured, with a flat, shiny surface
- Early tiny LP papules may be clinically and histopathologically indistinguishable from Lichen nitidus
- Conditions that feature Koebner's Phenomenon: Lichen nitidus, Lichen planus, Psoriasis

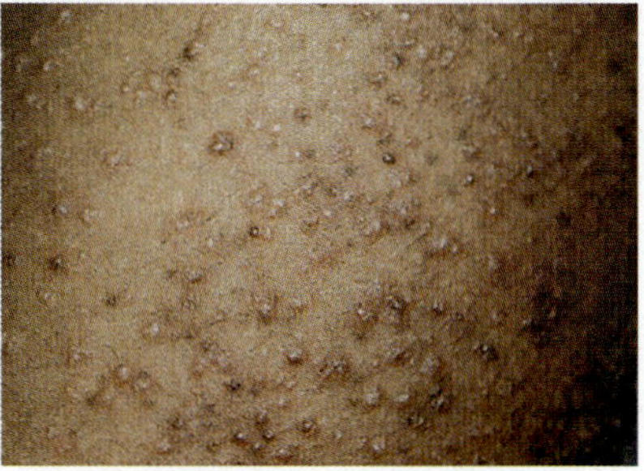

Fig. Lichen nitidus

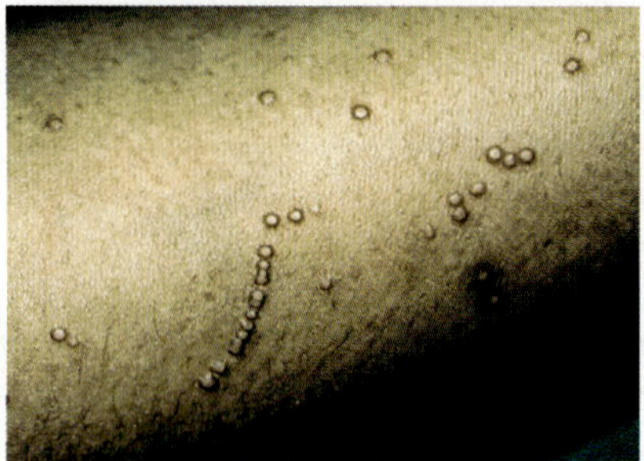

Fig. Koebner's phenomenon

29. Ans. (b) Topical steroids

[Ref. Creasy and Resnik's Maternal-Fetal Medicine, 6/e p1132]

- Psoriasis in pregnancy is commonly treated with topical corticosteroids (mostly category C agents)

30. Ans. (b) Pregnancy-associated pustular psoriasis
[Ref. Psoriasis by Van de Kerkhof, 2/e p165]

- Systemic corticosteroids are rarely used in the treatment of Psoriasis
- Very occasionally its use may be justified in the setting of Generalized psoriasis, Erythrodermic pustular psoriasis or Impetigo herpetiformis (Pustular psoriasis related to pregnancy or the OCP)
- They are only used for conditions where other treatment is unresponsive or contraindicated or severe enough to require therapeutic trial

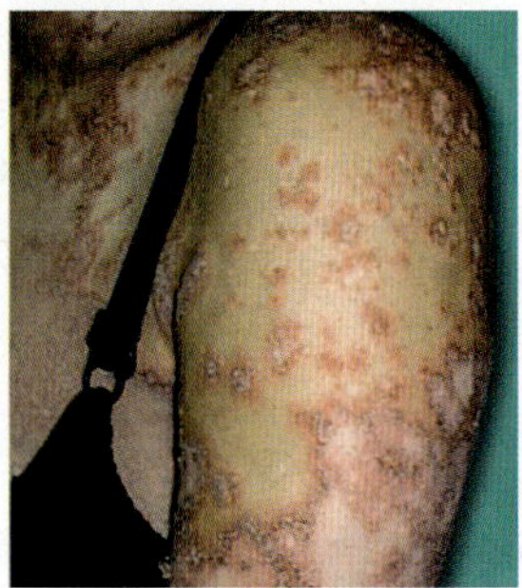

Fig. Pustular psoriasis of pregnancy

31. Ans. (d) 6–12 weeks
[Ref. Dermatology Made Easy by Oakley, 1/e p128]

- Pityriasis rosea clears up in about 6–12 weeks
- Post-inflammatory dyspigmentation may persist for a few months in dark-skinned people

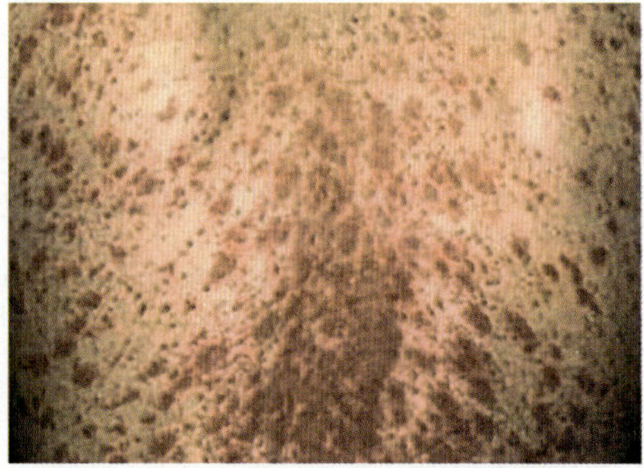

Fig. Pityriasis rosea (Fir-tree pattern)

32. Ans. (c) Acitretin
[Ref. Pediatric Dermatology by Schachner, 4/e p948]

- Retinoids such as Acitretin are particularly effective in Erythrodermic psoriasis and Palmoplantar pustulosis as well being the treatment of choice for Generalized pustular psoriasis and Severe psoriasis in HIV

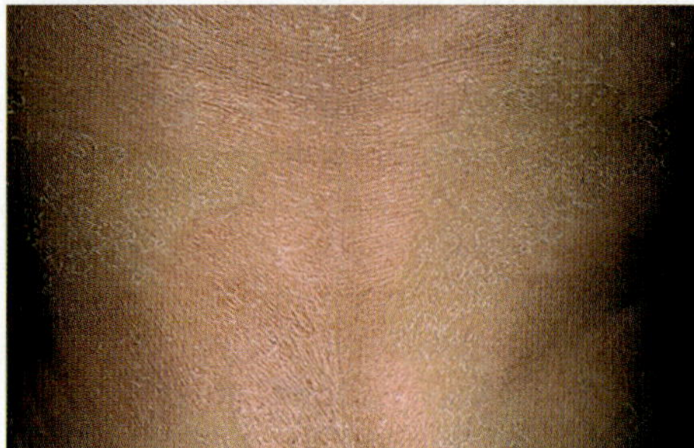

Fig. Erythrodermic psoriasis

33. Ans. (c) Topical steroids and salicylic acid
[Ref. Neena Khanna, 4/e p54]

Treatment of Pustular Psoriasis

- Hands and feet: Topical high potency steroids + Salicylic acid, Topical PUVA/ PUVA sol
- Generalised type: Methotrexate + Emollients

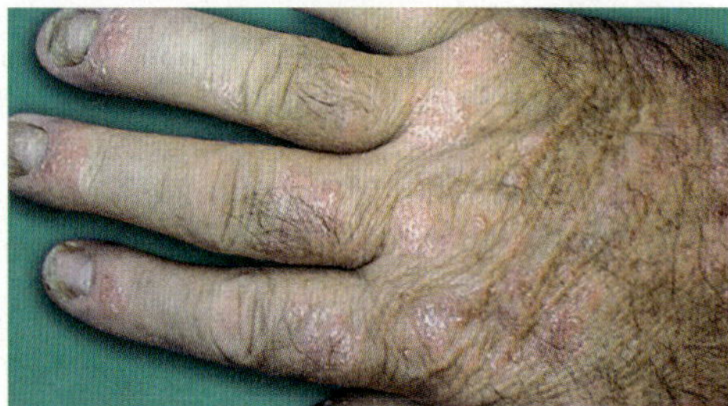

Fig. Psoriasis of hands

34. Ans. (b) Reverse Koebner's Phenomenon
[Ref. DVT by Thappa, 4/e Fig4.3]

Types of Koebner Phenomena

- Koebner/Isomorphic phenomena: Skin lesions appearing on lines of trauma; seen in Thermal trauma, Dermatoses, Allergic reactions, Therapy
  - True isomorphic phenomena: Lichen planus, Vitiligo, Psoriasis
  - Pseudo-isomorphic phenomena (Infections; due to inoculation of viruses): Warts, Molluscum contagiosum, Behcet's syndrome, Pyoderma gangrenosum
  - Occasional isomorphic phenomena (Localised to trauma-site): Hailey-Hailey disease, Erythema multiforme, Lichen sclerosus et atrophicus, Pellagra, Darier's disease, Cancers, Kaposi's sarcoma
- Reverse Koebner phenomena: Granuloma annulare clears off after biopsy
- Remote Koebner phenomena: Spontaneous repigmentation of patches distant from the autologous skin graft sites

35. Ans. (d) Psoriasis vulgaris
[Ref. Dermatopathology by Zappi, 1/e p76]

Pustule of Psoriasis (Clusters of neutrophils)

- In the spinous zone (Microabscess of Munro)
- Sponge-like array in the upper part of the epidermis (Spongiform pustule of Kogoj)
- Beneath the normal stratum corneum (Subcorneal pustule)
- Within parakeratosis (Intracorneal pustule)

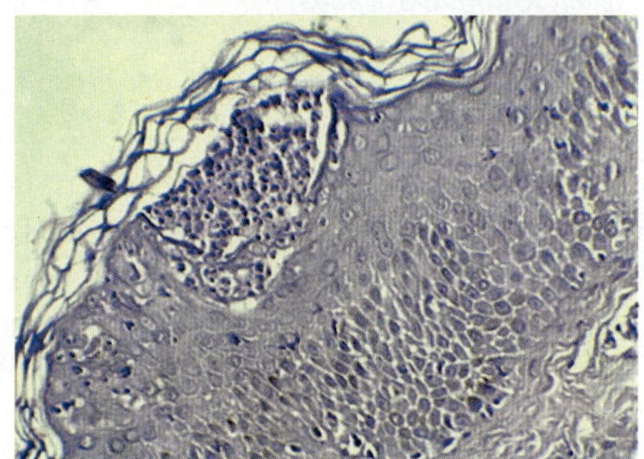

Fig. Pustules of Kogoj

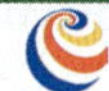

HIGH YIELD MCQs ANSWERS WITH EXPLANATIONS

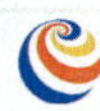

1. Ans. (b) Methotrexate; (c) TNF-alpha inhibitor; (d) Acitretin; (e) Narrow band UVB

[Ref. DVL by Thappa, 4/e p125,126]

Treatment of Psoriasis

- Topical therapy: Salicylic acid, Emollients for dryness, Tacrolimus and Pimecrolimus (effective in inverse and facial psoriasis), Topical steroids, Tazarotene (0.1–0.05% gel), Calcipotriol, Dithranol (anthralin) (0.1–1.0%), Ichthyol salicyclic ointment (6% Ichthyol and 3% Salicyclic acid)
- Phototherapy: Narrow band wavelength of 311 is used in psoriasis; An Excimer laser lamp with 380 nm UVB radiation can clear a plaque
- Systemic therapy: MTX, Retinoid, Cyclosporine, TNF-alpha blockers, Etanercept, Acitretin, Infliximab and Adalimumab

2. Ans. (c) Pityriasis rosea

[Ref. Neena Khanna, 5/e p60]

Herald Patch

- It is the 1st lesion of PR and is seen in about 80% of patient
- Characteristically an annular lesion with wrinkled, salmon pink center and collarette of scales at the periphery

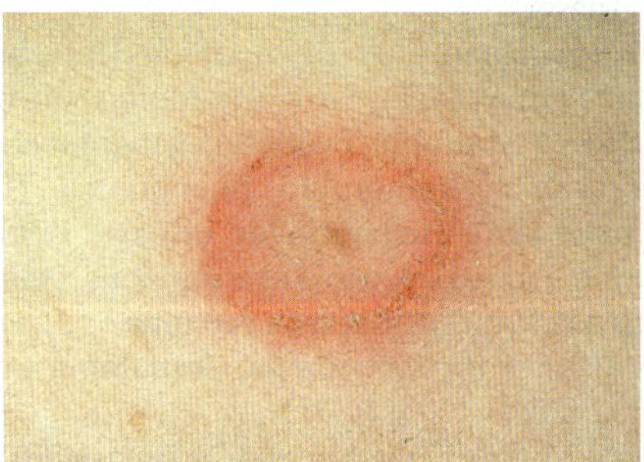

Fig. Herald patch

3. Ans. (c) Pityriasis rosea

[Ref. Neena Khanna, 5/e p60]

4. Ans. (c) Pityriasis alba

[Ref. Neena Khanna, 5/e p283]

- Scaly, hypopigmented macule on the face of children with normal sensation and no thickening of nerve hints toward Pityriasis alba

5. Ans. (c) Ptyriasis alba

[Ref. Neena Khanna, 5/e p283]

6. Ans. (b) Psoriasis

[Ref. Neena Khanna, 5/e p50]

7. Ans. (d) Self-resolving

[Ref. Neena Khanna, 5/e p62]

- Patient of Pityriasis rosea should be counseled about self-resolving nature of disease

8. Ans. (a) No active treatment required; (d) Common over the face; (e) Presents as scaly, whitish macules

[Ref. Neena Khanna, 5/e p283]

9. Ans. (a) Isolated patches of normal skin are found

[Ref. Neena Khanna, 5/e p69]

Pityriasis Rubra Pilaris

- Scaly (Pityriasis)
- Pink to orange (Rubra)
- Follicular papules (pilaris)
- Grouped papules frequently coalesce to form large plaques, typically with distinct islands of normal skin
- These islands of normal skin, are often studded with erythematous follicular scaly papules

10. Ans. (e) Congenital syphilis

[Ref. Harrison's, 18/e p405]

Selected Causes of Papulosquamous Skin Lesions

- Primary cutaneous disorders
  - Psoriasis
  - Tinea
  - Pityriasis rosea
  - Lichen planus
  - Parapsoriasis
  - Bowen's disease (squamous cell carcinoma in situ)
- Drugs
- Systemic diseases
  - Lupus erythematosus
  - Cutaneous T cell lymphoma/ Mycosis fungoides
  - Secondary syphilis
  - Reiter's disease
  - Sarcoidosis

11. Ans. (a) Seen in stratum corneum; (b) Seen in psoriasis; (d) Contain neutrophils only

[Ref. Neena Khanna, 5/e p53]

- Epidermal changes in skin biopsy of psoriasis patient:
  - Munro's microabscess: Collection of polyps in parakeratotic stratum corneum
  - Spongioform pustule of Kogog: Accumulation of neutrophils within a spongiotic pustule in spinous layer

12. Ans. (a) PUVA; (b) Methotrexate

[Ref. Neena Khanna, 5/e p59]

13. Ans. (a) Very pruritic

[Ref. Neena Khanna, 5/e p43-46, 51]

- Lesions of psoriasis are non-pruritic or mildly pruritic except Erythrodermic psoriasis

14. Ans. (c) Psoriasis

[Ref. Neena Khanna, 5/e p44-46]

Diagnostic Clue for Psoriasis

- Incidence in early 3rd decade or in 5th mid decade
- Silver white scales (due to air trapped)
- Demonstration of Auspitz sign

15. Ans. (a) Micro-Munro abscess; (b) Suprapapillary thinning; (e) Hyperkeratosis

[Ref. Neena Khanna, 5/e p53; Practice of Dermatology by Behal, 10/e p253-254]

HPR Findings in Psoriasis

- Parakeratosis: Nuclei retained in horny layer
- Loss of granular layer and regular acanthosis (thickening of viable epidermis)/Hyperkeratosis

- Increased mitotic figures in basal keratinocytes
- Suprapapillary thinning: Histological marker of Berkley's membrane when Auspitz sign is being elicited
- Collection of polymorphs in the epidermis to form spongiform pustule of Kogoj and Munro's microabscesses
- Dilatation and tortuosity of capillary loops in the dermal papillae
- Lymphocytic infiltrate in the upper dermis

16. Ans. (a) Pityriasis Rosea
[Ref. Neena Khanna, 5/e p60]

17. Ans. (c) Arthritis
[Ref. Neena Khanna, 5/e p48]
- Arthritis is not very common (10%) in Psoriasis

18. Ans. (b) Scaling
[Ref. Neena Khanna, 5/e p46]
- Scales are loose, lamellar, silvery white and are accentuated by grating with glass slides

19. Ans. (c) Always associated with nail infection
[Ref. Neena Khanna, 5/e p50]
- Nail is involved in 10–50% of patients

20. Ans. (c) It is premalignant disease
[Ref. Neena Khanna, 5/e p43-46]

21. Ans. (a) HHV 7
[Ref. Neena Khanna, 5/e p60]
- Though aetiology is unknown, Human Herpes Virus (HHV-7) more frequently and HHV-6 less frequently has been implicated for Pityriasis rosea

22. Ans. (b) CNS involvement
[Ref. Neena Khanna, 5/e p43-46]

23. Ans. (c) Stratum corneum
[Ref. Neena Khanna, 5/e p53]

24. Ans. (d) Erythrodermic Psoriasis
[Ref. Neena Khanna, 5/e p51]

Erythrodermic Psoriasis

- Precipitating factor:
  - Irritant effect of topical therapy
  - Withdraw of topical/ systemic steroids
- Clinical manifestation
  - Extremely itchy
  - Psoriatic plaques become ill defined and merge
  - Skin becomes uniformly red with marked fine scaling
- Complications
  - Temperature dysregulation—hypo/hyper thermia
  - Nutritional imbalance—water & electrolyte and hypoproteinemia

25. Ans. (b) Pityriasis rosea
[Ref. Dermatology by Otto Braun-Falco, 2/e p584]
- Initial lesion of Pityriasis rosea: A characteristic eruption seen on the trunk called the Herald/Mother patch

26. Ans. (c) Head, neck and face are not involved
[Ref. Neena Khanna, 5/e p47]
- Scalp psoriasis may spill onto forehead or neck
- Face is usually spared.

27. Ans. (c) CNS involvement
[Ref. Neena Khanna, 5/e p43-46]

28. Ans. (c) Pityriasis rosea
[Ref. Neena Khanna, 5/e p60-61]

29. Ans. (a) Auspitz sign
[Ref. Neena Khanna, 5/e p46]

Psoriasis Lesions

- Clinical diagnosis is got by Auspitz sign: Not performed generally now and considered a test of historical significance
- Skin biopsy is best investigation of choice

30. Ans. (a) Psoriasis
[Ref. Neena Khanna, 5/e p45]
- Koebner's phenomenon/Isomorphic phenomenon: New lesions of the original disease developat sites of trauma (scratches, surgical incisions and injury)
- Seen in Psoriasis, Lichen planus and Vitiligo
- It indicates active disease.

31. Ans. (c) Lichen Planus
[Ref. Neena Khanna, 5/e p45]

32. Ans. (d) Psoriasis
[Ref. Neena Khanna, 5/e p45]

33. Ans. (c) Pityriasis versicolour
[Ref. Neena Khanna, 5/e p60-61]

34. Ans. (a) Lichen planus; (d) Psoriasis; (e) Vitiligo
[Ref. Neena Khanna, 5/e p45; Koebner phenomenon. Clin Dermatol. 201;29(2):231-6; Clinical significance of Koebner phenomenon in vitiligo. Br J Dermatol. 2012;167(5): 1017-24]

35. Ans. (a) Retinoids
[Ref. Neena Khanna, 5/e p56]
- Tazarotene, a newer retinoid is used

36. Ans. (a) Methotrexate; (b) Retinols
[Ref. Neena Khanna, 5/e p57]

37. Ans. (b) Methotrexate
[Ref. Neena Khanna, 5/e p57]
- Methotrexate 7.5–25 mg weekly, orally (as Single dose/ in 3 divided doses at 12 hours interval)

38. Ans. (b) Griseofulvin
[Ref. Neena Khanna, 5/e p311-312]

Treatment of Pityriasis Versicolor

- Topical agents:
  - Ketoconazole 2%
  - 2.5% selenium sulphide
- Systemic agents:
  - Fluconazole—300 mg once wkly × 2 week
  - Itraconazole—200 mg, OD × 5 days
  - Ketoconazole—400 mg SOD

39. Ans. (a) Corticosteroids
[Ref. Rook's Textbook of Dermatology by Burns,7/e 68.5]
- Multiple pus lakes and erythematous skin changes in pregnancy suggests the diagnosis of Impetigo herpetiformis/

Generalized pustular psoriasis of pregnancy/Pastular dermatoses of pregnancy
- Treatment: Systemic and topical steroids

40. Ans. (b) Pityriasis alba
[Ref. Neena Khanna, 5/e p283]
- Scaly, hypopigmented macule on the face of children with normal sensation and no thickening of nerve hints toward Pityriasis alba

41. Ans. (a) Plaque Psoriasis
[Ref. Neena Khanna, 5/e p45-46]
- Auspitz sign is characteristic of Chronic Plaque psoriasis/ Psoriasis vulgaris

42. Ans. (a) Psoriasis
[Ref. Neena Khanna, 5/e p45-46]

43. Ans. (d) Extensive lesions
[Ref. DVL by Bansal, 1/e p186]
- Systemic corticosteroids are not recommended in treatment of pustular psoriasis: Disease can recur with increased severity once the treatment is stopped
- Steroids are very useful as a short-term life saving measure in severe disease when other drugs have failed
- Only indication for use of Systemic steroids is Generalized pustular psoriasis o Erythroderma in pregnancy (impetigo herpetiformis)

44. Ans. (c) Methotrexate
[Ref. Neena Khanna, 5/e p57]

45. Ans. (a) Binding to DNA
[Ref. Comprehensive Dermatologic Drug Therapy by Wolverton, 3/e p281]
- Combination of psoralens and ultraviolet light (UVA, 320-400 nm), referred to as PUVA, inhibits proliferation of a variety of cell types
- Psoralen intercalates into the DNA double helix where it is ideally positioned to form adduct(s) with adjacent pyrimidine bases, preferentially thymine, upon excitation by an ultraviolet photon
- PUVA treatment produces both DNA interstrand crosslinks (ICLs) and monoadducts
- The ICLs introduced by psoralen are highly genotoxic to actively replicating cells

46. Ans. (b) Micro-Munro abscess; (d) Hyperkeratosis; (e) Suprapapillary thinning
[Ref. Neena Khanna, 5/e p53; Practice of Dermatology by Behal, 10/e p253-254]

47. Ans. (d) All of the above
[Ref. Comprehensive Dermatologic Drug Therapy by Wolverton, 3/e p281]

48. Ans. (b) Retinoids; (d) Methotrexate
[Ref. Neena Khanna, 5/e p57]

49. Ans. (b) Psoriasis
[Ref. Comprehensive Dermatologic Drug Therapy by Wolverton, 3/e p281]

50. Ans. (d) All of the above
[Ref. Neena Khanna, 5/e p45]

Drugs that Exacerbate Psoriasis
- Antimalarials
- Lithium
- Beta adrenergic blockers
- NSAIDs
- Corticosteroid withdrawl (may aggravate or may precipitate pustular lesions)

51. Ans. (a) Prednisolone
[Ref. Rook's Textbook of Dermatology edited by Tony Burns, 7/e 68.5]

52. Ans. (b) Psoriasis
[Ref. Neena Khanna, 5/e p59]

53. Ans. (b) Vitiligo
[Ref. Neena Khanna, 5/e p165]

54. Ans. (a) Methotrexate
[Ref. Psoriasis and Psoriatic Arthritis by Gordon, 1/e p190]

55. Ans. (b) Pustular psoriasis
[Ref. Neena Khanna, 5/e p53]

Von Zumbusch's Pustular Psoriasis
- Serious condition
- High fever, chills and tachypnoea
- Generalized fiery red erythema followed by appearance of waves of tiny, superficial pustules, which become confluent to form circinate and lakes of pus
- Appearance of new pustules as the old ones are crusting

56. Ans. (a) *Malassezia furfur*
[Ref. Neena Khanna, 5/e p310]
- *Malassezia furfur* (earlier classified as *Pityrosporum ovale*), a commensal yeast is causative agent of Tinea versicolor

57. Ans. (e) All of the above
[Ref. Neena Khanna, 5/e p311-312]

58. Ans. (c) Griseofulvin
[Ref. Neena Khanna, 5/e p311-312]

59. Ans. (a) Psoriasis
[Ref. Neena Khanna, 5/e p53; Dermatology by Behal, 10/e p253-254]

60. Ans. (d) Tinea infection
[Ref. Neena Khanna, 5/e p301-302]

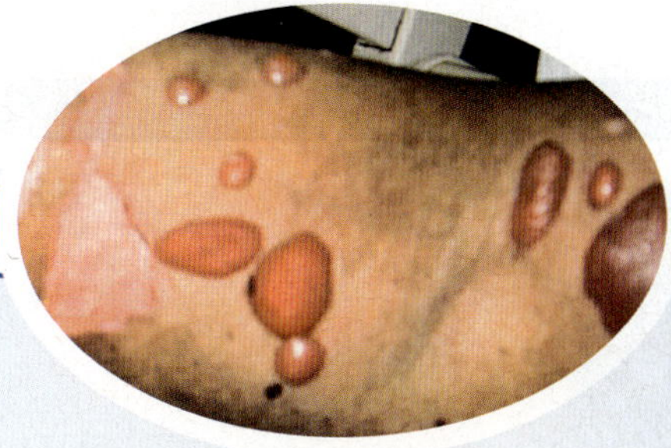

Chapter 13

STDs

THEORETICAL CONCEPTS

XIII A. SYPHILIS

- Underlying cause:
  - *Causative agent*: **Treponema pallidum**[Q]
    - ***'Cork-screw shaped'* spirochaete**[Q]
    - Angulation[Q] -rotatory-bending movements
- Transmission:
  - Sexual: Most common route[Q]
  - Blood
  - Needle prick injury
  - Mother to child (vertical) transmission
- Incubation period: 9-90 days[Q]
- Clinical presentation:
  - *Primary syphilis*:
    - ***Hunterian chancre***:[Q] Characteristic lesion in genitals of males (coronal sulcus, glans, prepuce, shaft of penis) and females (labia minora/ majora, mons pubis) or extra-genitally (lips, nipples, fingers)
    - *Inguinal lymphadenopathy*: Multiple, short, ***'Lead shots'***
  - *Secondary syphilis*:
    - Rash: Roseolar/papular/psoriasiform/malignant syphilides
    - *Coppery-red scaly lesions* on palms[Q]
    - ***Condylomata lata*** with split papules[Q]
    - Snail-track mucosal ulcers
    - Lymphadenopathy: Axillary, cervical, inguinal
    - Systemic involvement

System	Involvement
Musculoskeletal system	Periostitis, Osteoarthritis
Ocular system	Iridocyclitis, Uveitis[Q]
Renal system	Nephrotic syndrome[Q]
CNS	CSF abnormalities

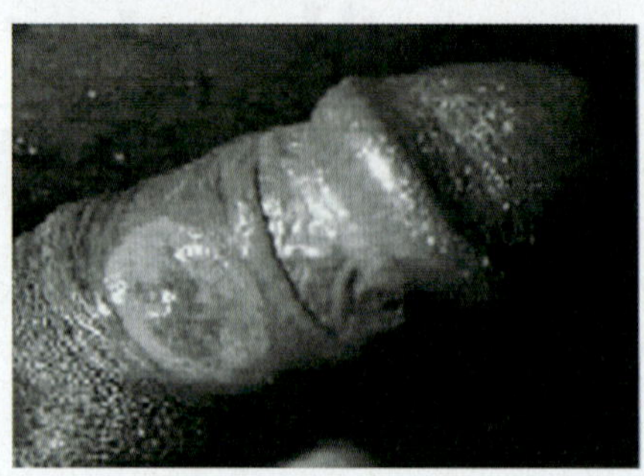
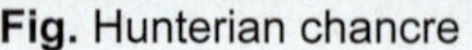

Fig. Hunterian chancre

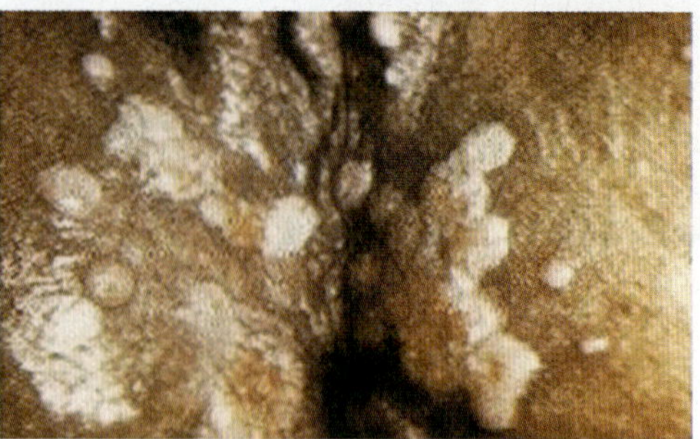

Fig. Condylomata lata

- *Tertiary syphilis*:

System	Involvement
Skin	Nodular/Noduloulcerative gummata
Mucosa	**Gummata**[Q]
Musculoskeletal system	Periostitis, Gummatous osteitis
CNS	Meningovascular syphilis
CVS	**Aortic insufficiency**[Q], Aneurysm
Liver	Hepatic gummata

- *Congenital syphilis*:

System	Involvement
General	Low birth weight, anaemia
Skin	Fissuring of lips/ angles of mouth
Mucosa	Snuffles (Syphilitic rhinitis)[Q]
Musculoskeletal system	Epiphysitis, Pseudoparalysis of parrot[Q]
Reticuloendothelial system	Hepatosplenomegaly

- Tests for diagnosis of Syphilis:
  - *Demonstration of Treponema pallidum*
    - **Dark ground microscopy**
    - Direct fluorescent antibody technique
    - PCR
  - *Serological tests*

Non-treponemal/Standard Tests	Treponemal Tests
Kahn's flocculation test	TPHA (Treponema pallidum hemagglutination)
VDRL flocculation test	FTA-Abs (Fluorescent treponemal antibody)
RPR flocculation test	RTCF (Reiter treponemal complement fixation)
Wasserman's complement fixation test	TPI (Treponema pallidum immobilization)

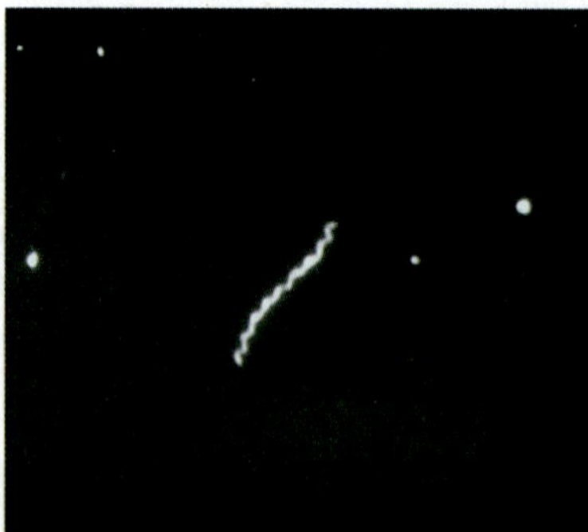

Fig. Treponema pallidum (Dark ground microscopy)

- *Treatment*:
  - **Benzathine penicillin (Drug of choice)**[Q]
  - Doxycycline (In penicillin-sensitive patients)
  - Erythromycin stearate (In penicillin-sensitive patients)
  - Crystalline penicillin (In Neurosyphilis)[Q]
  - Procaine penicillin (In Congenital syphilis)[Q]

XIII B. CHANCROID

- *Underlying cause*: Haemophilus ducreyi[Q]
- *Incubation period*: 3-5 days[Q]
- Clinical presentation:
  - ***Soft sore/Soft chancre***: Superficial, tender ulcers[Q]
  - ***Inguinal bubo***[Q]

- *Phagedenic ulcer*: Secondary infection with Vincent's spirochaetes
- *Gram smear*: Gram negative bacilli in *'school of fish/rail-track appearance'*[Q]

❑ *Treatment*:
- Azithromycin
- Ceftriaxone
- Ciprofloxacin
- Erythromycin

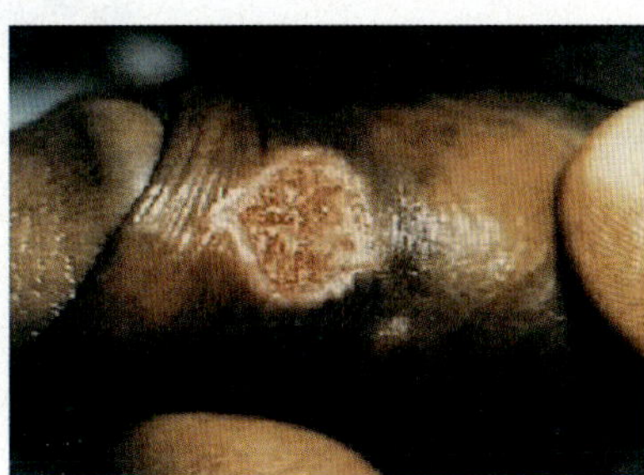

Fig. Soft chancre

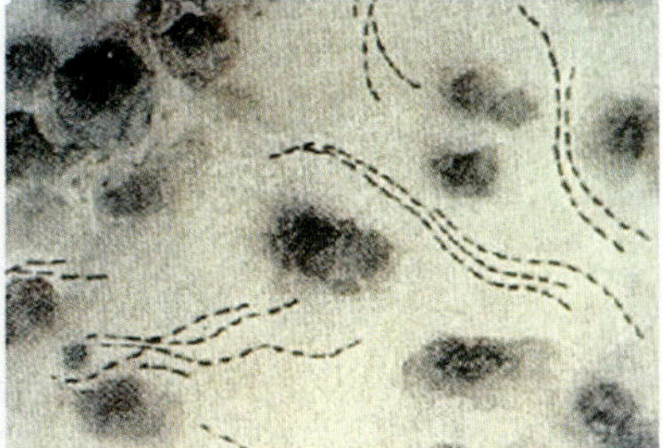

Fig. School-of-fish appearance

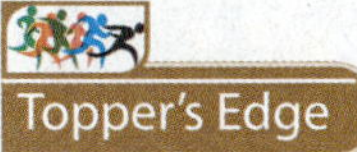

Topper's Edge

Chancre vs Chancroid[Q]

	Chancre	Chancroid
Incubation period	9-90 days	3-5 days
Number	Single	Multiple
Pain	Absent	Present
Margin	Regular	Irregular
Induration	Present	Absent
Application of pressure	Exudes serum	Bleeds
Lymphadenopathy	Shotty	Bubo
Darkground M/E	Positive	Negative
VDRL	+/-	-

XIII C. DONOVANOSIS/GRANULOMA VENERUM/GRANULOMA INGUINALE

❑ *Underlying cause*: Klebsiella **(Calymmatobacterium) granulomatis**[Q]

❑ *Clinical presentation*:
- Single asymptomatic ulcer
- *Pseudo-buboes*[Q]
- *Tissue smear*: Intracellular bipolar inclusion organisms—*'Safety-pin/Telephone handle appearance'*[Q]

❑ *Treatment*:
- Doxycycline
- Azithromycin
- Erythromycin

XIII D. LYMPHOGRANULOMA VENERUM (LGV)

❑ *Underlying cause*: **Chlamydia trachomatis (L1, L2 or L3)**[Q]

❑ *Incubation period*: 3-12 days

❑ *Clinical presentation*:
- *Primary stage*: Usually asymptomatic lesion
- *Inguinal syndrome*: Buboes, **Sign of groove**[Q]
- *Genito-anorectal syndrome*: Esthiomene in females

❑ *Treatment*:
- Doxycycline[Q]
- Erythromycin

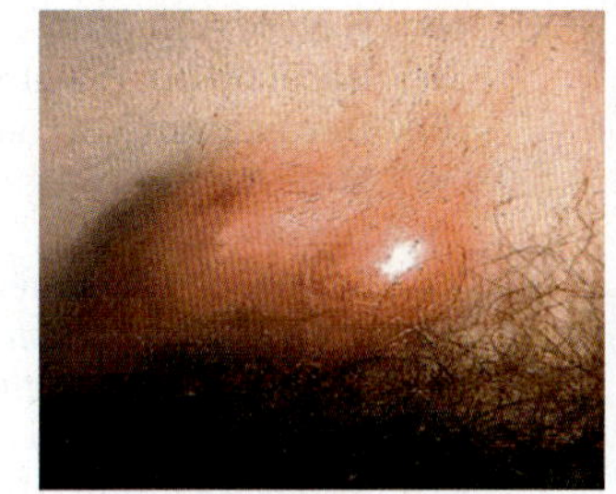

Fig. Groove sign

XIII E. GONOCOCCAL INFECTION

- *Underlying cause*: Neisseria gonorrhoeae[Q]
- *Incubation period*: 1-5 days
- *Clinical presentation*:
  - *Asymptomatic*
  - *Symptomatic males*: **Anterior urethritis (Most common)**[Q]
  - *Symptomatic females*: Endocervicitis with urethritis
  - *Metastatic*: Disseminated gonococcal infection in skin, joints, liver, heart, bones
  - *Gram's stain*: Gram negative *'kidney shaped'* extracellular/intracellular diplococci[Q]
- *Treatment*:
  - Uncomplicated infection
  - Cefixime
  - Ceftriaxone
  - Ciprofloxacin
  - Complicated infection
  - Cefixime
  - Ceftriaxone

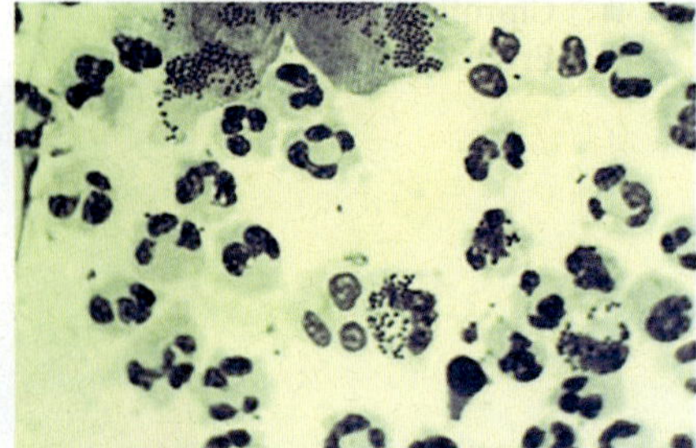

Fig. Neisseria gonorrhoeae

XIII F. ANOGENITAL WARTS

- *Underlying cause*: Human Papilloma virus (HPV 6, 11, 16, 18, 31, 33, 35, 39, 51-59)[Q]
  - *MC sub-types*: HPV 6, 11
- *Clinical presentation*:
  - ***Condylomata acuminata*** **(Most common type)**[Q]
  - Papular anogenital warts
  - Bowenoid papulosis
- *Treatment*:[Q]
  - Podophyllin
  - Imiquimod
  - 5-Fluorouracil

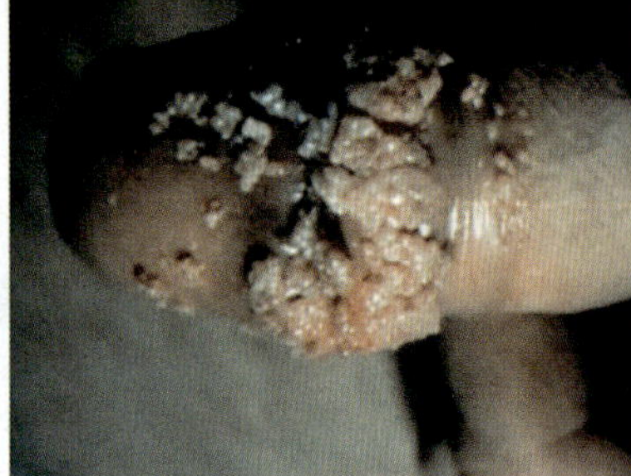

Fig. Anogenital warts

XIII G. MOLLUSCUM CONTAGIOSUM

- *Underlying cause*: Molluscum contagiosum virus
- *Clinical presentation*: Pearly-white ***'umbilicated'*** **papules**[Q]
- Treatment:
  - Cryotherapy
  - Mechanical removal with curette

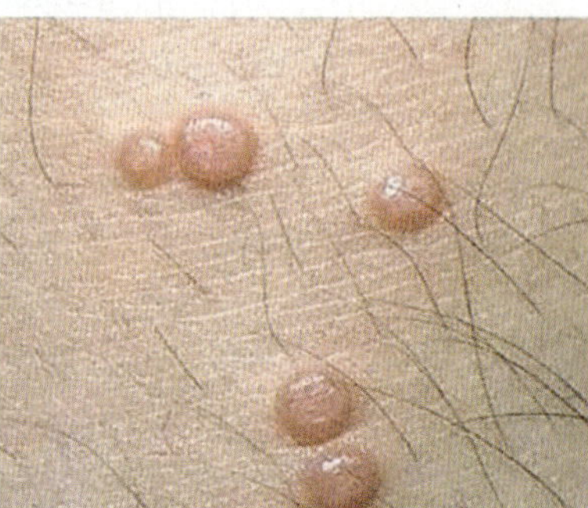

Fig. Molluscum contagiosum

XIII H. HUMAN IMMUNODEFICIENCY VIRUS (HIV) INFECTION

- *Underlying cause*: HIV virus
- *Routes of transmission*:[Q]
  - Sexual (Most common route of HIV transmission—**Heterosexual**)
  - Blood/blood products transfusion
  - Needle stick injuries
  - Mother to child (vertical) transmission
- *Clinical dermatological manifestations*:
  - *Infectious manifestations*: **[Mnemonic: H**IV **C**ausative **E**tiology **H**as **B**een **D**efined **M**ainly **H**etero **S**exual**]**[Q]
    - **H**uman papilloma virus
    - **C**andidiasis (Most common skin infection in HIV)[Q]
    - **E**bstein-Barr virus
    - **H**erpes genitalis
    - **B**acillary angiomatosis
    - **D**ermatophytosis (subungual onychomycosis)
    - **M**olluscum contagiosum
    - **H**erpes zoster
    - **S**taphylococcal infection
  - *Noninfectious manifestations*:
    - Seborrheic dermatitis (Most common dermatosis in AIDS)[Q]
    - Psoriasis
    - Kaposi sarcoma (HHV8)
- *Treatment*: Antiretroviral therapy (ART)

IMAGE-BASED QUESTIONS

1. **HPV subtype causing following penile lesion is** ***[AIIMS November 2016]***

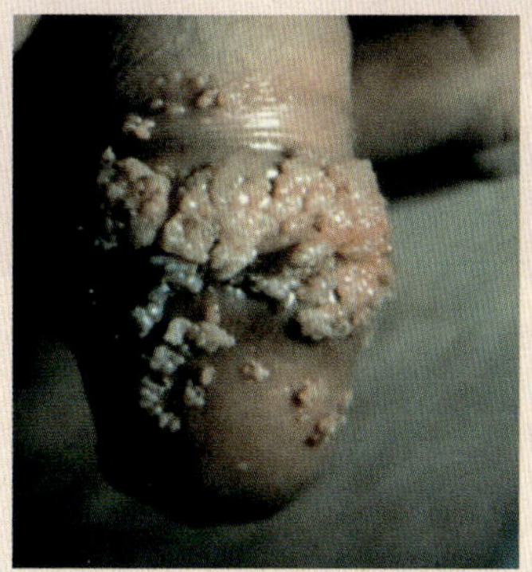

a. 3, 6 b. 6, 11
c. 34, 36 d. 50, 51

2. **Causative organism of disease shown in Photograph** ***[Recent Question 2013]***

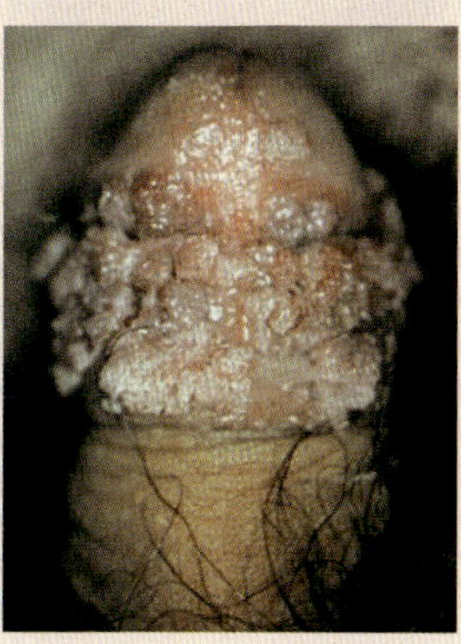

a. HIV b. HBV
c. Herpes d. HPV

3. **Diagnose the STD shown in the photograph** ***[Recent Question 2014]***

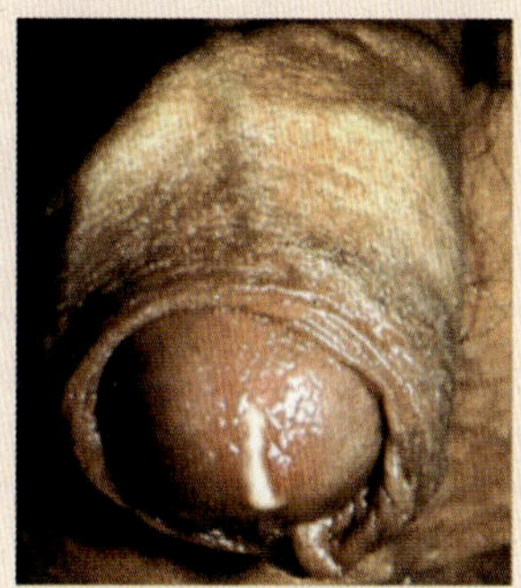

a. Syphilis b. Gonorrhoea
c. Herpes d. LGV

4. **Diagnose the STD based on Tzanck smear Photograph**

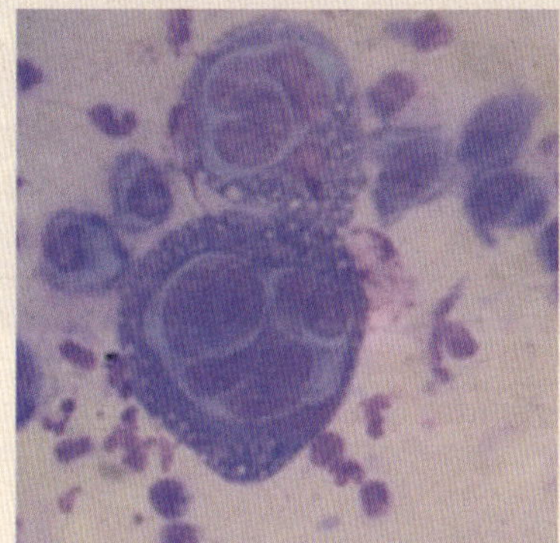

a. Chancroid b. Donovanosis
c. Herpes d. LGV

5. **Diagnose the STD shown in the photograph** ***[Recent Question 2012]***

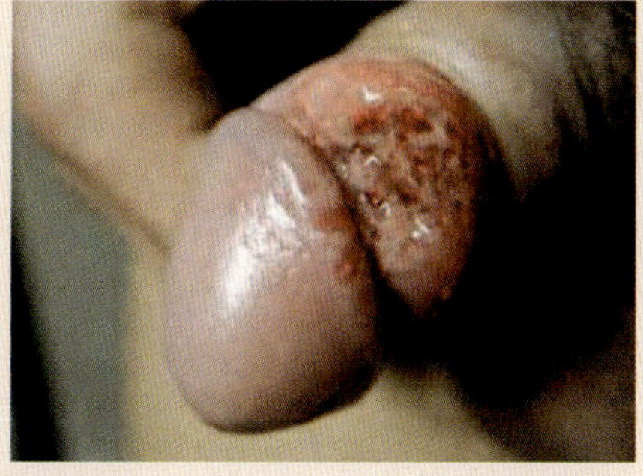

a. Chancroid b. Donovanosis
c. Hunterian chancre d. LGV

6. **Diagnose the STD shown in the photograph**

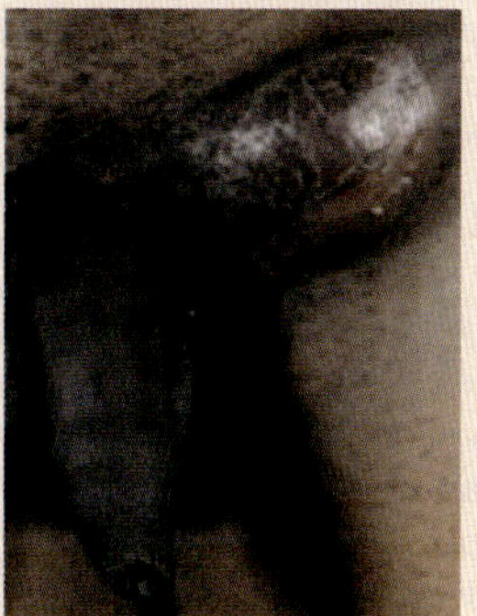

a. Chancroid b. Donovanosis
c. HIV d. LGV

7. Diagnose the STD shown in the photograph

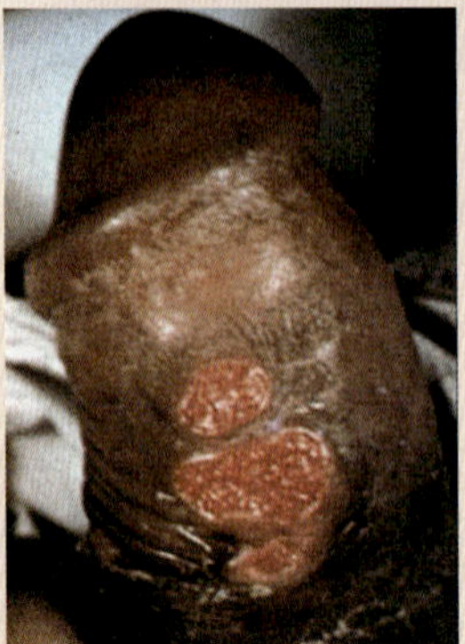

a. Chancroid
b. Donovanosis
c. HIV
d. LGV

8. Diagnose the STD shown in the photograph

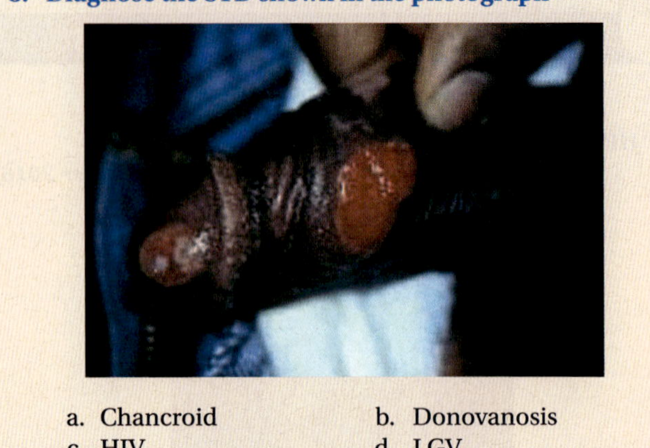

a. Chancroid
b. Donovanosis
c. HIV
d. LGV

9. STD shown in dark field microscopy photograph is *[Recent Question 2014]*

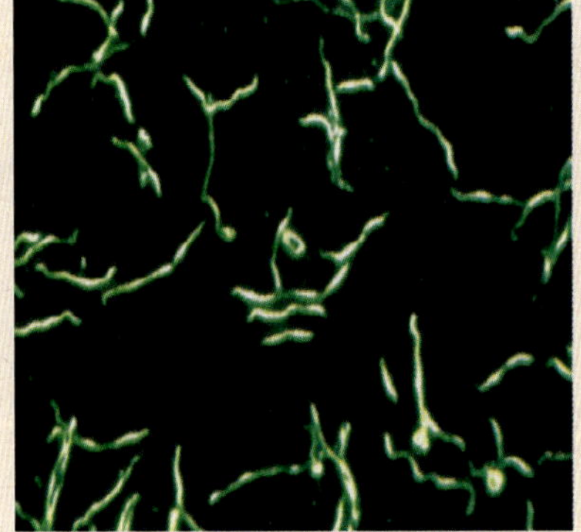

a. LGV
b. Chancroid
c. Donovanosis
d. Syphilis

10. A smear was prepared from genital ulcer. Identify the organism responsible *[AIIMS November 2015]*

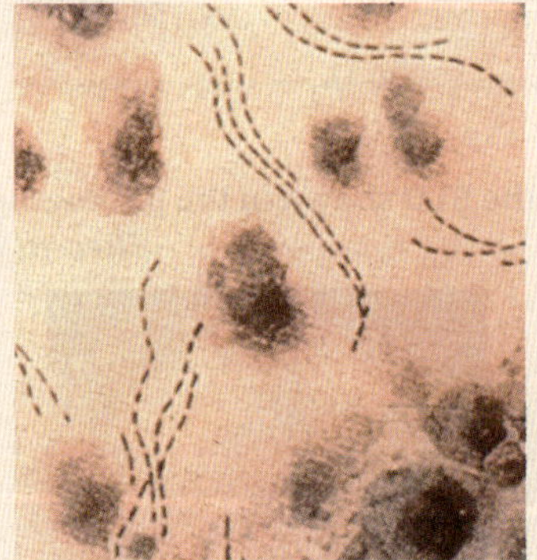

a. Chlamydia
b. H. ducreyi
c. Gonococcus
d. T. pallidum

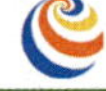 ANSWERS WITH EXPLANATIONS OF IBQs 

1. Ans. (b) 6, 11 *[Ref. Laboratory Diagnosis of Infectious Diseases by Lennette, 1/e p306]*

Condylomata Acuminata

- Occur on penis and vulva, in the urethra and vagina, at the uterine cervix, and in the perianal region
- Mainly induced by HPV 6 or 11
- May become large and invasive

2. Ans. (d) HPV *[Ref. Neena Khanna, 4/e p269]*

Warts

- Causative agent: Human papilloma virus
- Clinical types:
  - Verruca vulgaris (Common warts)
  - Palmoplantar warts
  - Verruca plana (Plane warts)
  - Filiform warts
  - Epidermodysplasia verruciformis
  - Anogenital warts (Photograph)

3. Ans. (b) Gonorrhoea *[Ref. Neena Khanna, 4/e p315]*

Gonococcal Infection

- Underlying cause: Neisseria gonorrhoeae
- Incubation period: 1-5 days
- Clinical presentation:
  - Asymptomatic
  - Symptomatic males: Anterior urethritis (Most common) [Photograph]
  - Symptomatic females: Endocervicitis with urethritis

4. Ans. (c) Herpes *[Ref. Microbiology and Immunology by Parija, 2/e p478]*

- Herpes on Tzanck smear: Multinucleate Giant cells with faceted nuclei and homogenously stained ground glass chromatin

5. Ans. (c) Hunterian chancre *[Ref. Neena Khanna, 4/e p301]*

Hunterian Chancre

- Typical lesion of primary syphilis
- Single, painless, irregular, indurated, reddish-brown plaque which ulcerates
- Ulcer has clean floor, oozes clear serum on pressure
- Heals spontaneously with slightly atrophic scar

6. Ans. (d) LGV *[Ref. Neena Khanna, 4/e p310]*

Lymphogranuloma Venereum (LGV)

- Underlying cause: Chlamydia trachomatis (L1, L2 or L3)
- Incubation period: 3-12 days
- Clinical presentation:
  - Primary stage: Usually asymptomatic lesion
  - Inguinal syndrome:
    - Buboes (Photograph): Painful swelling of Inguinal lymph nodes
    - Sign of groove: When both Inguinal and femoral LN are involved, they are separated by inguinal ligament
  - Genitoanorectal syndrome: Esthiomene in females

7. Ans. (a) Chancroid *[Ref. Neena Khanna, 4/e p306]*

Chancroid

- Soft sore/chancre: Multiple, dirty-looking, tender ulcers which bleed on pressure
- Irregular, ragged margins
- Induration absent
- Pain present
- Lymphadenopathy: Bubo present

8. Ans. (b) Donovanosis *[Ref. Neena Khanna, 4/e p309]*

Donovanosis/Granuloma Venereum/Granuloma Inguinale

- Underlying cause: Klebsiella (Calymmatobacterium) granulomatis
- Clinical presentation:
  - Single asymptomatic ulcer: Beefy-red ulcer with granulation tissue
  - Pseudobuboes

9. Ans. (d) Syphilis *[Ref. Neena Khanna, 4/e p305]*

Syphilis Dark Ground Microscopy

- Causative organism: Treponema pallidum
- Characteristic appearance: Cork-screw shaped organisms
- Characteristic movements: Angulation movements

10. Ans. (b) H. ducreyi *[Ref. Valvular Disease by Wilkinson, 3/e p130]*

Chancroid

- Organism: Hemophilus ducreyi
- Smear:
  - Granulomatous reaction without caseation
  - Lymphocytes and plasma cells predominance
  - Gram negative organism in large parallel chains

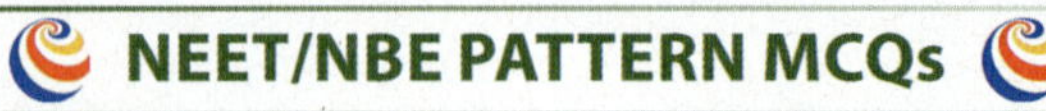

NEET/NBE PATTERN MCQs

1. **Patient presents with discharge per urethra and microscopy shows presence of intracytoplasmic gram negative cocci; what is the most probable diagnosis?** *[Recent Question 2016]*
   a. Gonorrhea b. Donovanosis
   c. Bacterial vaginosis d. Syphilis
2. **STD with pseudobubo formation** *[Recent Question 2016]*
   a. Granuloma inguinale
   b. LGV
   c. Chancroid
   d. Syphilis erode through skin to produce ulcer
3. **Groove sign of greenbelt is seen in** *[Recent Question 2016, 2017]*
   a. LGV b. Donovanosis
   c. Chancroid d. Genital herpes
4. **Donovan bodies are seen in** *[Recent Question 2016]*
   a. Leishmania donovani
   b. Chlamydia trachomatis
   c. Klebsiella
   d. Calymmatobacterium granulomatis
5. **Bilateral symmetrical maculopapular 4 rash on palms and soles is feature of** *[Recent Question 2016]*
   a. Primary syphilis b. Secondary syphilis
   c. Tertiary syphilis d. Congenital syphilis
6. **Recurrent genital ulcer is caused by** *[Recent Question 2016]*
   a. HSV 1 b. HSV 2
   c. HSV 3 d. HSV 4
7. **Genital ulcer with intracytoplasmic telephone-handle shapes are seen in** *[NBE FMGE September 2005]*
   a. Lymphogranuloma venereum
   b. Chancroid
   c. Syphilis
   d. Donovanosis
8. **Contraceptive protective against PID and STDs is which one of the following** *[NBE DNB 2011]*
   a. Condoms b. CuT
   c. Mala D d. All of the above
9. **Inguinal bubo is caused by all except** *[NBE DNB 1995]*
   a. Syphilis b. Chancroid
   c. Plague d. LGV
10. **Treatment of primary syphilis is** *[NBE FMGE September 2012]*
    a. Benzathine penicillin b. Procaine penicillin
    c. Procaine penicillin d. Tetracycline
11. **Causative agent of chancroid is** *[NBE FMGE September 2005]*
    a. Human papilloma virus b. Herpes simplex virus
    c. Treponema pallidum d. Hemophilus ducreyi
12. **Soft sore is caused by?** *[Recent Question 2016, 2012, 2013]*
    a. H ducreyi
    b. Calymmatobacterium granulomatis
    c. Chlamydia trachomatis
    d. T. Pallidum
13. **'Chancre redux' is a clinical feature on** *[Recent Question 2016, NBE DNB 2009]*
    a. Early relapsing syphilis
    b. Late syphilis
    c. Chancroid
    d. Recurrent herpes simplex infection
14. **The lesions not containing treponema are** *[NBE DNB 1998]*
    a. Chancre
    b. Condylomata
    c. Lesions of secondary syphilis
    d. Gumma
15. **STD with pseudobubo formation** *[Recent Question 2016]* *[Recent Question 2012]*
    a. Granuloma inguinale
    b. IGV
    c. Chancroid
    d. Syphilis erode through skin to produce ulcer.
16. **Commonest venereal disease in India is** *[NBE DNB 1997, 1999, 2000]*
    a. Gonorrhoea b. Syphilis
    c. Chancroid d. LGV
17. **In the first 8 weeks of syphilis the most specific test is** *[Recent Question 2016, NBE DNB 1992]*
    a. VDRL b. Kahn
    c. TPI d. FTA-ABS
18. **Frei's test is diagnostic of** *[NBE DNB 1994, 1999, 2004, 2007, 2008, 2010]*
    a. Lymphogranuloma venereum
    b. Lymphogranuloma inguinale
    c. Donovanosis d. Soft chancre
19. **Purulent genital discharge indicates which of the following infection** *[NBE FMGE September 2011]*
    a. Syphilis b. AIDS
    c. Gonorrhoea d. Donovanosis
20. **Most specific test for diagnosis of syphilis** *[NBE DNB 2009]*
    a. VDRL b. FTA-ABS
    c. RPR d. Kahn test
21. **Recurrent plaques on glans which heal with residual hyperpigmentation is suggestive of** *[NBE DNB 2010]*
    a. Aphthous ulcer
    b. Fixed drug eruption
    c. Herpes gestationis
    d. Chlamydial infection
22. **All of the following are the standard tests for syphilis except** *[NBE FMGE September 2011]*
    a. Wassermann test b. Kahn's test
    c. VDRL d. TPHA
23. **'Chancre redux' is a feature of** *[Recent Question 2015]*
    a. Early relapsing syphilis
    b. Late syphilis
    c. Recurrent herpes simplex
    d. Chancroid
24. **Multiple painful ulcers with lymphadenopathy. Diagnosis is?** *[Recent Question 2017]*
    a. Syphilis b. Chancroid
    c. LGV d. Donovanosis

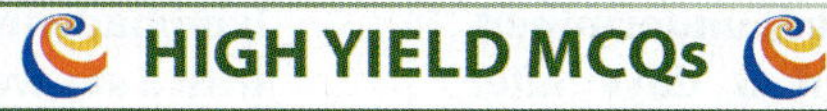

1. **A 20-year-old male developed multiple tender non-indurated bleeding ulcers over prepuce 4 days after sexual exposure. The most probable diagnosis in this patient is** *[Kerala PGMEE 1994]*
   a. Primary syphilis
   b. Lymphogranuloma venereum
   c. Chancroid
   d. Donovanosis
2. **Verruca vulgaris is caused by** *[BIHAR PGMEE 2004]*
   a. HPV b. EBV
   c. CMV d. HIV
3. **Myrmecia warts are** *[JIPMER PGMEE 1998]*
   a. Planer wart b. Plantar wart
   c. Verrucous wart d. Palmer wart
4. **Genital warts are most commonly caused by which of the following serotypes of HPV?** *[AIIMS PGMEE 2008]*
   a. HPV 6 b. HPV 16
   c. HPV 18 d. HPV 33
5. **All are true regarding viral warts except** *[PGI 1997]*
   a. Basophilic stippling
   b. Koilocytes are characteristic
   c. Spontaneous regression common in children
   d. Perinucear vacuolization
   e. Verruca vulgaris is associated with HPV7
6. **Treatment of choice for genital warts in pregnancy?** *[AIIMS PGMEE 2009]*
   a. Salicylic acid with Lactic acid solution
   b. Podophylin
   c. Imiquimod d. Cryotherapy
7. **Immunomodulator used in treatment of genital warts is** *[All India PGMEE 2008]*
   a. ATRA b. Podophyllin
   c. Imiquimod d. Prednisolone
8. **Secondary syphilis manifested by** *[PGI 2003]*
   a. Painless lymphadenopathy
   b. Pruritus rash c. Mucosal erosion
   d. Asymptomatic rash e. Mostly asymptomatic
9. **Most specific test for syphilis** *[AIIMS PGMEE 2010]*
   a. VDRL b. RPR
   c. FTA-ABS d. Kahn's test
10. **Commonest venereal disease in India is** *[AIIMS PGMEE 1998, TN PGMEE 1999]*
    a. Gonorrhoea b. Syphilis
    c. Chancroid d. LGV
11. **Main feature of gonorrhoea is** *[Karnataka PGMEE 1998]*
    a. Purulent discharge per urethra
    b. Inguinal adenitis
    c. Ulcer over glans penis
    d. Rashes
12. **TOC for penicillin resistant gonorrhoea** *[AIIMS PGMEE 1998]*
    a. Ciprofloxacin b. Ceftriaxone
    c. Streptomycin d. Erythromycin
13. **DOC in gonorrhoea is** *[AIIMS PGMEE 1992]*
    a. Benzathine penicillin b. Procaine penicillin
    c. Benzyl penicillin d. Phenoxymethyl penicillin
14. **School of fish appearance is shown by** *[All India PGMEE 1998]*
    a. Homophiles ducreyi b. Gonococcus
    c. Chlamydia d. Donovania granulomatis
15. **DOC in chancroid is** *[AIIMS PGMEE 1998]* *[AP PGMEE 1998, UP PGMEE 1999]*
    a. Tetracycline b. Doxycycline
    c. Erythromycin d. Streptomycin
16. **Genital ulcer is seen in all except** *[AIIMS PGMEE 1997]*
    a. Granuloma inguinale b. Syphilis *[PGI 1997]*
    c. LGV d. Donovanosis
17. **Drug of choice for lymphogranuloma venereum** *[AP PGMEE 1995]*
    a. Sulphonamides b. Streptomycin
    c. Penicillin d. Erythromycin
    e. Gentamycin
18. **Pseudobubo is seen in** *[All India PGMEE 1996]*
    a. Donovanosis b. LGV
    c. Chancroid d. Syphilis
19. **Esthiomene is seen in** *[AP PGMEE 1998]*
    a. Chancroid b. Syphilis
    c. LGV d. Gonorrhoea
20. **Bubos with multiple sinuses discharging into inguinal lymph nodes are seen in** *[All India PGMEE 1994]*
    a. Chancroid b. Granuloma inguinale
    c. LGV d. Syphilis
21. **Safety-pin appearance is shown by** *[All India PGMEE 1989]*
    a. Haemophilus ducreyi b. Chlamydia
    c. Donovanosis granulomatis
    d. Mycoplasma
22. **DOC for granuloma inguinale** *[AIIMS PGMEE 1993]*
    a. Streptomycin b. Tetracycline
    c. Sulfonamide d. Penicillin
23. **A 23-year-old male had unprotected sexual intercourse with a commercial sex worker. Two weeks later, he developed a painless, indurated ulcer on the glans which exuded clear serum on pressure. Inguinal lymph nodes in the groins were enlarged and not tender. The most appropriate diagnostic test is** *[AIIMS PGMEE 2004]*
    a. Gram's stain of ulcer discharge
    b. Darkfield microscopy of ulcer discharge
    c. Giemsa stain of lymph node aspirate
    d. ELISA for HIV infection
24. **Hutchison's syphilitic triad includes all except** *[All India PGMEE 1998]*
    a. Associated with congenital syphilis
    b. Notched incisor teeth
    c. Nerve deafness
    d. Interstitial keratitis
    e. Associated with CVS anomalies
25. **A 30-year-old male patient has a large, spreading and exuberant ulcer with bright red granulation tissue over the glands penis. There was no lymphadenopathy. The most likely causative organism is** *[AIIMS PGMEE 2003]*
    a. Treponema pallidum
    b. Herpes simplex virus type 1
    c. Herpes simplex virus type 2
    d. Calymmatobacterium granulomatis

26. A man having multiple, painful, indurated, undermined, sloughed edged glans which occurred 5 days after exposures; most likely diagnosis is *[All India PGMEE 2008]*
a. Chancroid b. Primary chancre
c. Herpes genitalis d. LGV

27. Streptomycin is useful in treatment of *[AIIMS PGMEE 1990]*
a. Granuloma venereum b. LGV
c. Syphilis d. Chancroid

28. Lymphadenopathy is seen is all except *[All India PGMEE 1995]*
a. Syphilis 1st stage b. Donovanosis
c. LGV d. Chancroid

29. Gonococcus resistant structure is *[All India PGMEE 1998, All India PGMEE 1996]*
a. Urethra b. Testis
c. Fallopian tube d. Ampulla of cervix

30. MC cause of Nongonococcal urethritis *[AIIMS PGMEE 1992]*
a. Chlamydia b. Mycoplasma
c. Trichomonas d. Gram negative rod

31. Syndromic management of urethral discharge includes treatment of *[All India PGMEE 2003]*
a. Neisseria gonorrhoeae and herpes genitalis
b. Chlamydia trachomatis and herpes genitalis
c. Neisseria gonorrhoeae and chlamydia trachomatis
d. Syphilis and chancroid

32. Lymphogranuloma venereum (LGV) is caused by *[AIIMS 1999, PGI 1998, Kerala PGMEE 1999 Bihar PGMEE 2008, Recent Question 2014]*
a. Chlamydia trachomatis
b. Haemophilus ducreyi
c. HTLV type II
d. Donovanosis granulomatis

33. Genital elephantiasis is caused by *[All India PGMEE 2002]*
a. Donovanosis b. Congenital syphilis
c. Herpes genitalis
d. Lymphogranuloma venereum

34. Sign of Groove is found in *[All India PGMEE 1998]*
a. Chancroid b. Granuloma inguinale
c. LGV d. Syphilis

35. Frie's test is done in *[All India PGMEE 1996]*
a. Donovanosis b. LGV
c. Syphilis d. Leprosy

36. DOC for LGV *[AIIMS 1993, Karnataka PGMEE 1994]*
a. Doxycycline b. Ampicillin
c. Erythromycin d. C eftriaxone

37. 'Pseudoisomorphic phenomenon' is shown by *[Recent Question 2016, All India PGMEE 2011]*
a. Psoriasis b. Warts
c. Lichen planus d. Vitiligo

38. Donovanosis is caused by *[All India PGMEE 1997]*
a. Calymmatobacterium granulomatis
b. T. pertenue
c. Chlamydia trachomatis
d. H. ducreyi

39. Pseudobubo is seen in *[AIIMS PGMEE 1995, All India PGMEE 1996]*
a. Chancroid b. LGV
c. Donovanosis d. Syphilis

40. 20-year-old male develops multiple ulcer over prepuce and glans which are painful along with suppurative lymphadenopathy, 5 days after having sexual intercourse with a sex worker, most probable disease is *[AIIMS PGMEE 1996]*
a. Herpes simplex b. Herpes genitalis
c. Molluscum contagiosum d. Chancroid

41. Reliable test for chancroid detection *[AP PGMEE 1988]*
a. Skin test b. Biopsy
c. Grams stained smear d. Clinical examination

42. Multiple painful ulcers over glans without induration is suggestive of *[AIIMS PGMEE 1993]*
a. LGV b. Granuloma inguinal
c. Chancroid d. Secondary syphilis

43. Chancroid is caused by *[AP PGMEE 1985]*
a. Haemophilus ducreyi b. Haemophilus vaginalis
c. Trachoma virus d. Treponema pallidum

44. Painful lymphadenopathy is seen in *[PGI 2002]*
a. Donovanosis b. Syphilis
c. Chancroid d. Herpes simplex
e. Gonorrhea

45. Discharging sinus is seen in *[All India PGMEE 1996]*
a. Syphilis b. Herpes
c. Actinomycosis d. Molluscum contagiosum

46. The most frequent cause of recurrent genital ulceration in a sexually active male is *[All India PGMEE 2003]*
a. Herpes genitalis b. Aphthous ulcer
c. Syphilis d. Chancroid

47. DOC for Herpes zoster is *[AIIMS PGMEE 1996, 1998]*
a. Vidarabine b. Acyclovir
c. Idoxuridine d. Aclidinium

48. A 24-year-old male presents to a STD clinic with a single painless ulcer on external genitalia. The choice of laboratory test to look for the etiological agent would be *[AIIMS PGMEE 2003]*
a. Scrapings from ulcer for culture on chocolate agar with antibiotic supplement
b. Serology for detection of specific IgM antibodies
c. Scrapings from ulcer for dark field microscopy
d. Scrapings from ulcer for tissue culture

49. Sabre tibia is seen in *[All India PGMEE 1993]*
a. Scurvy b. Rickets
c. Leprosy d. Syphilis

50. Recurrent balanoposthitis seen in *[PGI 2002]*
a. DM b. Herpes simplex
c. Smoking d. Alcohol
e. Bad hygiene

51. 'Chancre redux' is a clinical feature at *[AIIMS PGMEE 2006]*
a. Early relapsing syphilis
b. Late syphilis
c. Chancroid
d. Recurrent herpes simplex infection

52. Early eruption of secondary syphilis are all except *[All India PGMEE 1998]*
a. Intensely pruritic
b. Papular/maculo popular eruption
c. Symmetrical
d. Pleomorphic

53. Multiple necrotic ulcers in prepuce of penis with tender, suppurative inguinal nodes is caused by *[AIIMS PGMEE 1994]*
a. Chlamydia b. Hemophilus ducreyi
c. Herpes simplex d. Syphilis

54. Characteristic feature of early congenital syphilis is
a. Microcephaly *[PGI 1999]*
b. Saddle nose
c. Interstitial keratitis with saber skin
d. Vesicular rash with bulla over palms and soles

55. Gonococcus is *[PGI 1996, Kerala PGMEE 1998]*
a. Extracellular gram positive
b. Intracytoplasmic gram positive
c. Intracytoplasmic gram negative
d. Intra nuclear gram positive

56. Chancroid may be caused by *[All India PGMEE 1999]*
a. T. pallidum b. G. donovani
c. Chlamydia trachomatis d. Herpes hominis virus

57. In secondary syphilis all are seen except *[PGI 1998]*
a. Condyloma lata b. Interstitial keratitis
c. Arthritis d. Proteinuria

58. Condylomata lata are seen in *[AIIMS PGMEE 1998, 1999]*
a. Congenital syphilis b. Primary syphilis
c. Secondary syphilis d. Tertiary syphilis

59. Test not used for diagnosis of syphilis
a. VDRL b. TPI *[All India PGMEE 1993]*
c. Reagin test d. Frei test

60. DOC in primary syphilis is *[All India PGMEE 1992]*
a. Corticosteroids b. Oral penicillin
c. Benzathine penicillin d. Crystalline penicillin

61. Jarisch Herxheimer reaction is commonly seen in
a. Early syphilis *[SGPGI 2005]*
b. Late congenital syphilis
c. Latent syphilis
d. Syphilis of cardiovascular system

62. Not transmitted sexually *[All India PGMEE 1992]*
a. Syphilis b. T. pertenue
c. Candida d. Gonorrhoea

63. Primary bullous lesions is seen in which type of syphilis *[All India PGMEE 1994]*
a. Primary b. Secondary
c. Tertiary d. Congenital

64. A 23-yeard-old college student has asymptomatic and hyperpigmented macules on both palms for three weeks. The most appropriate diagnostic test is *[AIIMS PGMEE 2004]*
a. Venereal diseases research laboratory (VDRL) test
b. Skin biopsy
c. Serum cortisol levels
d. Assay for arsenic in skin, hair and nails

65. Granuloma venereum is caused by *[Bihar PGMEE 2006]*
a. Donovanosis granulomatis
b. Chlamydia
c. Haemophilus ducreyi
d. None of the above

66. Treatment of granuloma inguinale is *[All India PGMEE 1997]*
a. Tetracycline b. Sulphonamide
c. Streptomycin d. Penicillin

67. Not true of secondary syphilis *[All India PGMEE 1991]*
a. be asymptomatic
b. Usually involve palms and soles
c. Lymphadenopathy
d. Vesicular lesions

68. Not a manifestation of secondary syphilis *[AIIMS PGMEE 1996]*
a. Vesicles and bullae b. Nodule
c. Rash d. Hyperpigmented macule

69. All are features of secondary syphilis except *[AIIMS PGMEE 1997, AIIMS PGMEE 1998]*
a. Papulosquamous lesion b. Bullous lesion
c. Nodular lesion d. Lichenoid type lesion

70. In secondary syphilis, true about rash is *[PGI 1998]*
a. Pruritic b. Vesicular
c. Asymptomatic d. Tender

71. Treponema pallidum isolation from CSF is maximum in which stage of syphilis? *[AIIMS PGMEE 2009]*
a. Primary syphilis b. Secondary syphilis
c. Tertiary syphilis d. Tabes dorsalis

72. True about syphilis is all except *[All India PGMEE 1998]*
a. VDRL is sensitive but not specific
b. Infection leads to life long immunity
c. IgM and IgA
d. T. palladium when inoculated in rabbit produce progressive disease

73. A patient has syphilis since 2 year. CSF examination was done and treatment started. Which of the following test is most useful in monitoring treatment? *[AIIMS PGMEE 2009]*
a. TPI b. VDRL
c. FTA d. Dark ground microscopy

74. Genital ulcer is/are caused by *[PGI 2009]*
a. Human papilloma virus b. Herpes simplex virus
c. HIV d. Treponema pallidum
e. Lymphogranuloma venereum

75. A 30-year-old male presented with ulcerative lesion on glans penis. Wright-Giemsa stain showed 1-2 rounded structure in macrophage vacuoles. What is the etiology
a. Chlamydia trachomatis *[AIIMS PGMEE 2010]*
b. N. gonorrhoea
c. H. ducreyi
d. Calymmatobacterium granulomatis

76. A 19-year-male develops painless penile ulcers 8 days after sexual intercourse with a professional sex worker likely diagnosis is *[All India PGMEE 2001]*
a. Chancroid b. Herpes
c. Chancre d. Traumatic ulcer

77. Jarisch herxheimer reaction is seen in early cases of
a. Syphilis b. Gonorrhoea *[PGI 1998]*
c. LGV d. Granuloma inguinale

78. Incorrect statement is *[All India PGMEE 1992]*
a. VDRL titre decreases with treatment
b. VDRL becomes positive after 21 days of infection
c. FTA-ABS is earliest and most sensitive test
d. Yaws and Pinta can be differentiated by serological tests

79. Treatment in both Gonococcal and Nongonococcal urethritis is *[AIIMS November 2017]*
a. Cefixime 400 mg OD Single dose
b. Ciprofloxacin 500 mg Single dose
c. Azithromycin 2 gm Single dose
d. Ceftriaxone 250 IM Single dose

80. All the following features are associated chancroid except
a. Painful ulcer *[Recent Question 2017]*
b. Painless lymphadenopathy
c. School of fish appearance on staining
d. Azithromycin is useful in treatment

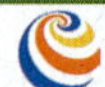 NEET/NBE PATTERN MCQs ANSWERS WITH EXPLANATIONS 

1. Ans. (a) Gonorrhea
[Ref. DVL by Thappa, 4/e p310, 311]

Gonorrhea

- Causative organism: Neisseria gonorrhoeae
- **MCC of Urethral discharge**
- Clinically it manifests usually in males and remain asymptomatic in females
- On examination:
- Mucoid or mucopurulent discharge is seen from the urethral meatus and the meatus is erythematous and edematous
- Gram stain of urethral or cervical discharge helps in diagnosis
  - 5 pus cells should be present in discharge
- Pus cells have gram negative diplococci

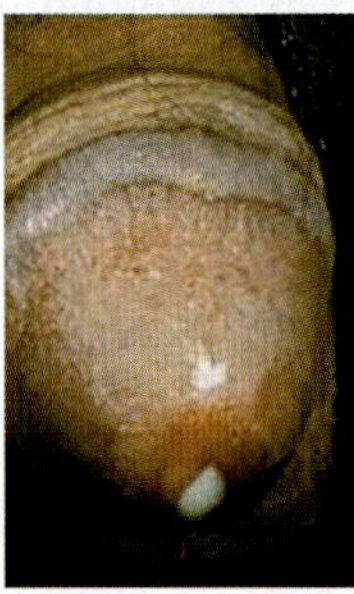
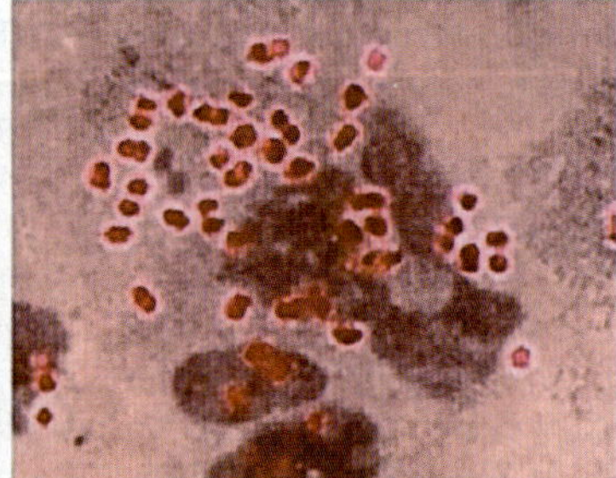

Fig. Gonorrhea

2. Ans. (a) Granuloma inguinale
[Ref. Clinical Dermatology by Habif, 6/e p408]

Granuloma Inguinale

- Genital ulcerative disease caused by the intracellular gram-negative bacterium *Klebsiella granulomatis* (formerly known as *Calymmatobacterium granulomatis*)
- Diagnosis: Visualization of dark-staining Donovan bodies on tissue crush preparation or biopsy
- Painless, slowly progressive ulcerative lesions on the genitals or perineum without regional lymphadenopathy; subcutaneous granulomas **(Pseudobuboes)**
- Lesions are highly vascular **(beefy red appearance)** and bleed
- Extragenital infection can occur with extension of infection to the pelvis, or it can disseminate to intra-abdominal organs, bones, or the mouth
- Lesions also can develop secondary bacterial infection and can coexist with other sexually transmitted pathogens

3. Ans. (a) LGV
[Ref. DVL by Thappa, 4/e p307,309]

Lymphogranuloma Venereum (LGV)

- Mainly a disease of lymphatic tissue that spreads to tissue surrounding lymphatics
- Lymphadenopathy: Painful inguinal bubo, Multilocular, when palpated groove is formed called as **GROOVE SIGN**
- Genitoanorectal syndrome is late stage occurs more often in women who were previously asymptomatic
- Enlargement, thickening, and fibrosis of the labia are termed esthiomene. Penile and/or scrotal edema and gross distortion of the penis are called "saxophone penis"

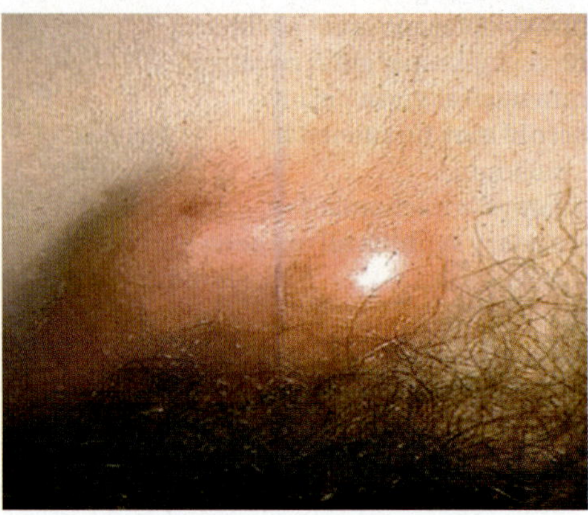

Fig. LGV—Groove sign

4. Ans. (d) Calymmatobacterium granulomatis
[Ref. DVL by Thappa, 4/e p303, 304]

- Calymmatobacterium granulomatis causes granuloma inguinale or donovanosis.
- Primary lesion: single bleeding ulcer, indurated
- Only STD in which there is no lymphadenopathy but at the site of lymph node formation of subcutaneous nodule **(PSEUDOBUBO formation)**
- Diagnosis: Giemsa stain (demonstration of Donovan bodies with in mononuclear cells)
- Microscopic examination: Safety pin appearance (also in Yersinia pestis)

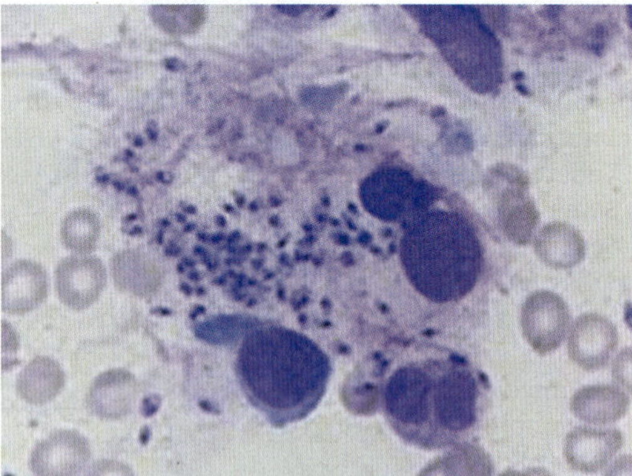

Fig. Safety pin appearance

5. Ans. (b) Secondary syphilis
[Ref. Clinical Dermatology by Habif, 6/e p414]

- Secondary syphilis is characterized by mucocutaneous lesions, a flulike syndrome, and generalized adenopathy
- Lesions of secondary syphilis have certain characteristics that differentiate them from other cutaneous diseases
- Types of lesions in approximate order of frequency are maculopapular, papular, macular, annular, papulopustular, psoriasiform, and follicular

- Temporary irregular **("moth eaten")** alopecia of the beard, scalp, or eyelashes may occur

6. Ans. (b) HSV2
[Ref. Nelson Textbook of Pediatrics, 20/e p988]

Genital herpes
- MC ulcerative STI among adolescents, is a chronic, lifelong viral infection
- Two sexually transmitted HSV types have been identified, HSV-1 and HSV-2
- Majority of cases of recurrent genital herpes are caused by HSV-2

7. Ans. (d) Donovanosis
[Ref. Neena Khanna, 4/e p309]

Donovanosis/Granuloma Venerum/Granuloma Inguinale
- *Underlying cause*: Klebsiella (Calymmatobacterium) granulomatis
- *Clinical presentation*:
  - Single asymptomatic ulcer
  - *Pseudobuboes*
  - *Tissue smear*: Intracellular bipolar inclusion organisms – *'Safety-pin/Telephone handle appearance'*
- *Treatment*: Doxycycline/Azithromycin/Erythromycin

8. Ans. (a) Condoms
[Ref. Health Counseling by Blonna, 1/e p232]

9. Ans. (a) Syphilis
[Ref. Sexually Transmitted Infections by Kumar, 2/e p683]
- Painful enlarged lymph nodes (buboes) are seen in TB, Gonorrhea, LGV, HSV, Plague, Chancroid

10. Ans. (a) Benzathine penicillin
[Ref. Neena Khanna, 5/e p60]
- Benzathine penicillin, 2.4 mega units, deep IM (in 2 equally divided doses, 1 in each buttock)

11. Ans. (d) Hemophilus ducreyi
[Ref. Neena Khanna, 4/e p307]

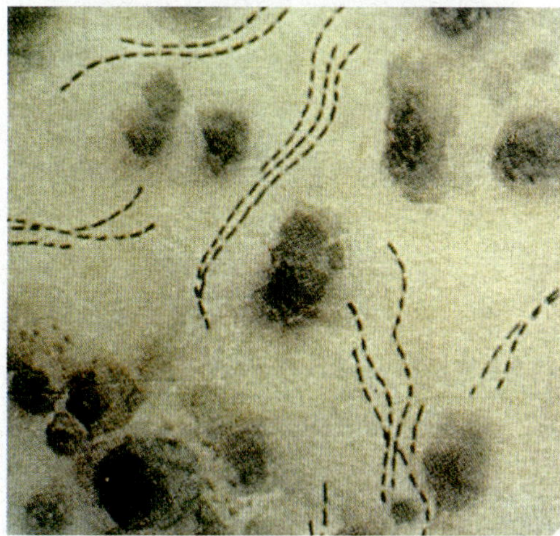

Fig. School of fish

Chancroid
- *Underlying cause*: Hemophilus ducreyi
- *Incubation period*: 3-5 days
- *Clinical presentation*:
  - *Soft sore/Soft chancre*: Superficial, tender ulcers
  - *Inguinal bubo*
  - *Phagedenic ulcer*: Secondary infection with Vincent's spirochetes
  - *Gram smear*: Gram negative bacilli in *'school of fish/ rail-track appearance'*
- *Treatment*:
  - Azithromycin
  - Ceftriaxone
  - Ciprofloxacin
  - Erythromycin

12. Ans. (a) H ducreyi
[Ref. Neena Khanna, 5/e p327]

13. Ans. (a) Early relapsing syphilis
[Ref. Sexually Transmitted Diseases by Sehgal, 4/e p54]
- Occasionally, a primary chancre may reappear on the original site and is known as Chancre redux or Monorecidive

14. Ans. (d) Gumma
[Ref. Sexually Transmitted Diseases by Sehgal, 4/e p321]
- Late syphilis not infective are Gumma, neurosyphilis, cardiovascular syphilis.

15. Ans. (a) Granuloma inguinale
[Ref. Johns Hopkins ABX Guide 2012 by Bartlett, 3/e p190]
- Granuloma inguinale **(Donovanosis)**: Painless, single or multiple ulcer(s) presenting 1-4 weeks after sexual contact with an infected person
- Not associated with true lymphadenopathy
- Instead there is subcutaneous spread of granulomata (hence the name granuloma inguinale) which leads to Pseudobubo formation.

16. Ans. NONE
[Ref. Thappa. Sexually Transmitted Infections in India. Indian J Dermatol 2007;52:78-82]
- Bacterial STDs like Chancroid and Gonorrhea are showing a declining trend in India
- Viral STDs like Herpes genitalis and Condylomata acuminata are showing upward trend
- Currently Herpes, Trichomonas are more common

17. Ans. (d) FTA-ABS
[Ref. Step-up to Medicine by Agabegi, 2/e p374]

Seroly in Syphilis
- Sensitivity of the VDRL and RPR tests:
  - 78-86% for detecting primary syphilis
  - 100% for detecting secondary syphilis
  - 95-98% for detecting tertiary syphilis
- Specificity ranges from 85-99% and may be reduced in individuals who have coexisting conditions (i.e, Collagen vascular disease, Pregnancy, Intravenous drug use, Advanced malignancy, Tuberculosis, Malaria, Viral and Rickettsial diseases)
- VDRL test results turn positive 1-2 weeks after chancre formation

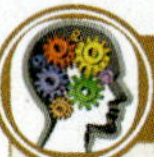

Also Remember

- Nontreponemal tests usually become nonreactive with time after treatment: However, in some patients, nontreponemal antibodies can persist, sometimes for the life of the patient
  - Because of the possibility of false-positive results, confirmation for any positive or equivocal non-treponemal test result should follow with a treponemal test, such as the fluorescent treponemal antibody-absorption (FTA-ABS), quantitative VDRL/RPR, microhemagglutination assay T pallidum (MHA-TP), T pallidum hemagglutination (TPHA), and T pallidum particle agglutination (TPPA) tests
  - Treponemal enzyme immunoassay (EIA) for immunoglobulin G (IgG) and immunoglobulin M (IgM) may be performed
- FTA-ABS is commonly used as a confirmatory test following positive VDRL or RPR test findings:
  - FTA-ABS has a sensitivity of 84% (For Primary syphilis) and 100% (For Syphilis infection in other stages); Its specificity is 96%

18. Ans. (a) Lymphogranuloma venereum
[Ref. Neena Khanna, 5/e p331]
- Frei test is a nonspecific intradermal test for Lymphogranuloma venereum
- It's now almost obsolete

19. Ans. (c) Gonorrhoea
[Ref. Neena Khanna, 4/e p315]
- *Urethral discharge in gonococcal infection in males*: Profuse, thick , purulent, creamy discharge
- *Discharge in gonococcal infection in females*: Scanty or profuse discharge

20. Ans. (b) FTA-ABS
[Ref. Step-up to Medicine by Agabegi, 2/e p374]

21. Ans. (c) Herpes gestationis
[Ref. Sexually Transmitted Infections by Zenilman, 1/e p100]

22. Ans. (d) TPHA
[Ref. Textbook of Microbiology by Ananthanarayan & Paniker, 7/e p387]
- Tests for diagnosis of Syphilis:
  - *Demonstration of Treponema pallidum*
    - Dark ground microscopy
    - Direct fluorescent antibody technique
    - PCR
  - *Serological tests*

Non-treponemal/ Standard tests	Treponemal tests
• Kahn's flocculation test • VDRL flocculation test • RPR flocculation test • Wasserman's Complement fixation test	• TPHA (Treponema pallidum hemagglutination) • FTA-Abs (Fluorescent treponemal antibody) • RTCF (Reiter treponemal complement fixation) • TPI (Treponema pallidum immobilization)

23. Ans. (a) Early relapsing syphilis
[Ref. Cutaneous Medicine by Provost, 1/e p566]

Chance Redux (Monorecidive Chance)
- With inadequate treatment of Syphilis majority of Treponemes die but few survive, multiply and reproduce the early lesions
- A new chancre appears at site of original chancre

24. Ans. (b) Chancroid
[Ref. Neena Khanna, 4/e p307]

Chancroid
- Underlying cause: Hemophilus ducreyi
- Incubation period: 3-5 days
- Clinical presentation: Soft sore/Soft chancre (superficial, tender ulcers), Inguinal bubo, Phagedenic ulcer (Secondary infection with Vincent's spirochetes)
- Gram smear: Gram negative bacilli in 'School of fish/railtrack appearance'
- Treatment: Azithromycin, Ceftriaxone, Ciprofloxacin, Erythromycin

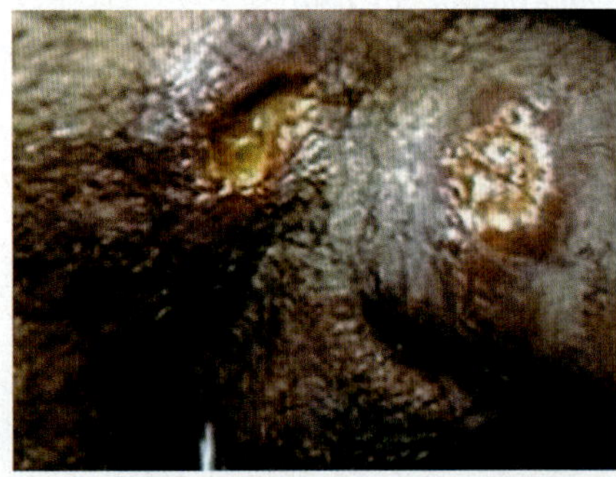

Fig. Chancroid

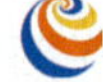 HIGH YIELD MCQs ANSWERS WITH EXPLANATIONS 

1. Ans. (c) Chancroid
[Ref. Neena Khanna, 5/e p327]

Chancroid
- Cause: Haemophilus ducreyi (Gram negative bacteria)
- Incubation period: 3-5 days
- Multiple, superficial, tender, nonindurated ulcers
- Floor covered with an exudates, which on removal reveals a bleeding surface
- In 50% of the patients, Inguinal bubo, usually unilateral, develops within a few days
- In males: Prepuce, frenulum and coronal sulcus is involved
- In female: Fourchette, vestibule and labia minora involved

2. Ans. (a) HPV
[Ref. Neena Khanna, 5/e p287]

Clinical Manifestations and HPV Type

Clinical manifestations	HPV type
Verruca vulgaris	1, 2, 27
Palmoplantar warts	1, 2, 57
Verruca plana	3, 10
Epidermodysplasia verruciformis	3, 5, 8
Anogenital wart	Low oncogenic- 6, 11 (MC in Anogenital wart)
	High oncogenic- 16, 18

3. Ans. (b) Plantar wart
[Ref. Medical Microbiology by Chamberlain, 1/e p47]
- Myrmecia warts that occur on the soles of the feet (plantar surface) are commonly found on weight-bearing areas (e.g. metatarsal head)

4. Ans. (a) HPV 6
[Ref. Neena Khanna, 5/e p287]
- Though HPV 6, 16, 18 are involved, most common among them is type 6.

5. Ans. (e) Verruca vulgaris is associated with HPV7
[Ref. Neena Khanna, 5/e p287]
- Verruca vulgaris is caused by HPV 1, 2, 27

6. Ans. (d) Cryotherapy
[Ref. Clinical Obstetrics by Reece, 3/e p917]
- During pregnancy, the best approach to treatment is removal of lesions by excision, electrocautery, or cryosurgery

7. Ans. (c) Imiquimod
[Ref. Neena Khanna, 5/e p340]
- Imiquimod 5% cream is an immunomodulator
- Applied OD for 6-10 hours at bed time, 3 times/week X 16 weeks

8. Ans. (a) Painless lymphadenopathy; (c) Mucosal erosion; (d) Asymptomatic rash
[Ref. Neena Khanna, 5/e p322]

9. Ans. (c) FTA-ABS
[Ref. Step-up to Medicine by Steven S. Agabegi, 2/e p374]

10. Ans. (a) Gonorrhoea
[Ref. Thappa. Current Status of STIs. Indian J Dermatol 2007;52:78-82]

11. Ans. (a) Purulent discharge per urethra
[Ref. Neena Khanna, 5/e p340]
- Gonococcal urethritis presents with urethral discharge, which is purulent, profuse, thick and creamy

12. Ans. (b) Ceftriaxone
[Ref. Neena Khanna, 5/e p338]

Treatment of gonococcal infection	
Uncomplicated infection	Cefixime, 400 mg SOD
	Ceftriaxone, 125 mg IM , SD
Complicated infection	Ceftriaxone, 1g IM , OD × 7d
	Cefixime, 400 mg BD × 7d

13. Ans. (b) Procaine penicillin
[Ref. Neena Khanna, 5/e p338]

14. Ans. (a) Homophiles ducreyi
[Ref. Neena Khanna, 5/e p328]
- Gram stain from floor of ulcer of Chancroid: Gram negative bacilli in Rail track/ School of fish formation appearance.

15. Ans. (c) Erythromycin
[Ref. Neena Khanna, 5/e p329]

Antibiotics in Chancroid
- Azithromycin , 1g SOD
- Ceftriaxone, 250 mg IM, SD
- Ciprofloxacin, 500 mg BD × 3 d
- Erythromycin base, 500 mg TDS × 7d

16. Ans. (c) LGV
[Ref. Neena Khanna, 5/e p330]
- Transient genital lesion is usually noticed in LGV

17. Ans. (d) Erythromycin
[Ref. Neena Khanna, 5/e p331]
- DOC for LGV:
  - Doxycycline l00 mg twice daily for 21 days
  - Erythromycin 500 mg four times a day for 21 days

18. Ans. (a) Donovanosis
[Ref. Neena Khanna, 5/e p329]

Swellings in Donovanosis
- Lymphadenopathy is not seen
- Sometime subcutaneous swellings appear in the inguinal region (Pseudobubobes) and these may ulcerate to form typical ulcers of Donovanosis

19. Ans. (c) LGV
[Ref. Neena Khanna, 5/e p331]
- Tertiary stage of LGV consist of lymphedema, hyperplastic and ulcerative changes on genitalia with typical manifestation being esthiomene
- Occurrence together of elephantiasis and chronic ulceration of the vulva

20. Ans. (c) LGV
[Ref. Neena Khanna, 5/e p330]
- Secondary stage of LGV: Nodes suppurate at many sites giving rising to multiple sinuses with undermined edge

21. Ans. (c) Donovanosis granulomatis
[Ref. Neena Khanna, 5/e p329]
- Smear finding of Donovanosis: Organisms appear as intracellular (in macrophages) bipolar inclusion (Safety pin or Telephone handle appearance)

22. Ans. (b) Tetracycline
[Ref. Neena Khanna, 5/e p330]

Doc Granuloma Venereum/Granuloma Inguinale/ Donovanosis
- Doxycycline 100 mg BD
- Azithromycin 1g once a week
- Erythromycin base 500 mg QDS

23. Ans. (b) Darkfield microscopy of ulcer discharge
[Ref. Neena Khanna, 5/e p324]

- The features described hints towards a diagnosis of syphilis
- Demonstration of T. palladium from lesion is the most specific diagnostic test for syphilis
- Dark ground microscopy is used to demonstrate that T. pallidum appears as a Corkscrew-shaped organism with characteristic movements (especially angulation)

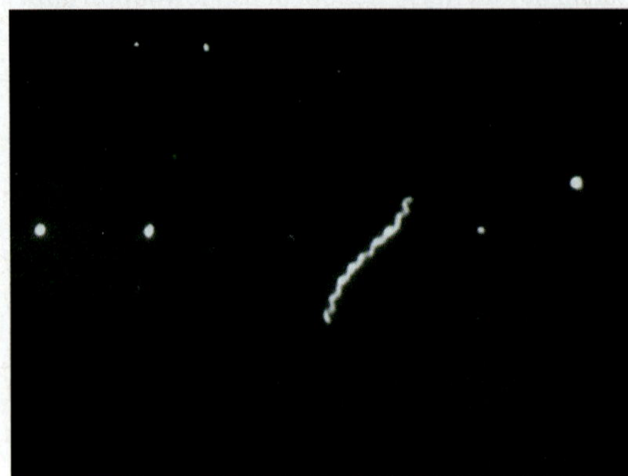

Fig. Dark ground microscopy

24. Ans. (e) Associated with CVS anomalies
[Ref. Neena Khanna, 5/e p324]
- Cardiovascular involvement is infrequent
- Hutchinson's triad (Sir Jonathan Hutchinson 1828–1913: Common pattern of presentation for congenital syphilis
  - Triad: Interstitial keratitis, Hutchinson incisors, and Eighth nerve deafness
  - Other features: Saddle nose and Saber shins

25. Ans. (d) Calymmatobacterium granulomatis
[Ref. Neena Khanna, 5/e p329]
- Exuberant granulation tissue and no lymphadenopathy leads to diagnosis of Granuloma venereum
- It is caused by Klebsiella granulomatis (earlier known as Calymmatobacterium)

26. Ans. (a) Chancroid
[Ref. Neena Khanna, 5/e p327]

27. Ans. (a) Granuloma venereum
[Ref. Sexually Transmitted Diseases by Parish, 1/e p117]
- Streptomycin is used for 10-20 days of total dose of 20-40 gm at daily 2 gm in two equal doses

28. Ans. (b) Donovanosis
[Ref. Neena Khanna, 5/e p327]

29. Ans. (b) Testis
[Ref. Neena Khanna, 5/e p336]
- Gonococcus infects columnar cells while stratified squamous epithelium and transition cells are usually resistant
- Following sites are infected:
  - Males: Urethra, Littre's/ Cowper's gland, Prostrate, Seminal vesicle, Epididymis
  - Female: Urethra, Bartholin's/ Skene's gland, Ampulla of cervix, Fallopian tube
  - Extragenital: Rectum, Pharynx

30. Ans. (a) Chlamydia
[Ref. Thappa. Sexually transmitted infections in India: Current status. Indian J Dermatol 2007;52:78-82]

31. Ans. (c) Neisseria gonorrhoeae and chlamydia trachomatis
[Ref. Neena Khanna, 5/e p340-341]

32. Ans. (a) Chlamydia trachomatis
[Ref. Neena Khanna, 5/e p330]
- Chlamydia trachomatis, serovars L1, L2, L3 causes LGV

33. Ans. (d) Lymphogranuloma venereum
[Ref. Neena Khanna, 5/e p331]
- Genital elephantiasis or Esthiomene is seen in LGV

34. Ans. (c) LGV
[Ref. Neena Khanna, 5/e p330]
- Sign of Groove/ Greenblatt: When both inguinal and femoral groups of lymph nodes are involved in LGV, they are separated by inguinal ligament producing the sign

35. Ans. (b) LGV
[Ref. Neena Khanna, 5/e p331]

36. Ans. (a) Doxycycline
[Ref. Neena Khanna, 5/e p331]

37. Ans. (b) Warts
[Ref. Neena Khanna, 5/e p45]
- Pseudoisomorphic phenomenon: Due to auto-inoculation and is seen in infections (like plane warts, Molluscum contagiosum) and Eczema

38. Ans. (a) Calymmatobacterium granulomatis
[Ref. Neena Khanna, 5/e p329]

39. Ans. (c) Donovanosis
[Ref. Neena Khanna, 5/e p329]

40. Ans. (d) Chancroid
[Ref. Neena Khanna, 5/e p327]

41. Ans. (c) Grams stained smear
[Ref. Neena Khanna, 5/e p328]

Detection of H. Ducreyi
- Gram staining- not very sensitive
- Detection of antigen by immunofluorescence technique- very sensitive, but not specific
- Culture- difficult
- PCR-rapid, sensitive and specific but costly; used in research
- Biopsy-usually not done

42. Ans. (c) Chancroid
[Ref. Neena Khanna, 5/e p327]

43. Ans. (a) Haemophilus ducreyi
[Ref. Neena Khanna, 5/e p327]

44. Ans. (c) Chancroid; (d) Herpes simplex
[Ref. Neena Khanna, 5/e p327]

45. Ans. (c) Actinomycosis
[Ref. Textbook of Microbiology & Immunology by Subhash Chandra Parija, 2/e p394]

46. Ans. (a) Herpes genitalis
[Ref. Neena Khanna, 5/e p332]

47. Ans. (b) Acyclovir
[Ref. Neena Khanna, 5/e p335]
- Acyclovir is the most frequently used antiviral agent

48. Ans. (c) Scrapings from ulcer for dark field microscopy
[Ref. Neena Khanna, 5/e p324]

49. Ans. (d) Syphilis
[Ref. Neena Khanna, 5/e p324]

50. Ans. (a) DM
[Ref. Oxford Handbook of General Practice by Chantal Simon, 4/e p464]

51. Ans. (a) Early relapsing syphilis
[Ref. Sexually Transmitted Diseases by Sehgal, 4/e p54]

52. Ans. (a) Intensely pruritic
[Ref. Neena Khanna, 5/e p321-333]

53. Ans. (b) Hemophilus ducreyi
[Ref. Neena Khanna, 5/e p327]

54. Ans. (d) Vesicular rash with bulla over palms and soles
[Ref. Neena Khanna, 5/e p324]

Features of Early Congenital Syphilis

- Children < 2 year
- Highly infectious
- Low birth weight and anemia
- Bullous lesion
- Fissuring of lips, angles of mouth and nasolabial folds
- Syphilitic rhinitis
- Pharyngitis and laryngitis
- Epiphysitis
  - Pain, swelling and tender of long bones
  - Pseudoparalysis of parrot
- Periostitis
- Dactylitis
- Hepatosplenomegaly
- Lymphadenopathy

55. Ans. (c) Intracytoplasmic gram negative
[Ref. Textbook of Microbiology & Immunology by Parija, 2/e p202]

56. Ans. (d) Herpes hominis virus
[Ref. Manson's Tropical Diseases, 22/e p422]

Causes of Chancroid

- Major cause: Hemophilus ducreyi
- Rare causes: Herpes virus hominis, Corynebacterium species, Staphylococcus epidermidis, Streptococci, B melaninogenicus, N. gonorrhea

57. Ans. (b) Interstitial keratitis
[Ref. Neena Khanna, 5/e p321-322]

58. Ans. (c) Secondary syphilis
[Ref. Neena Khanna, 5/e p322]

- Condyloma lata: In intertriginous area, the papules may erode superficially

59. Ans. (d) Frei test
[Ref. Neena Khanna, 5/e p331]

60. Ans. (c) Benzathine penicillin
[Ref. Neena Khanna, 5/e p60]

61. Ans. (a) Early syphilis
[Ref. Oxford Textbook of Medicine, Volume 1 by DA Warrell, p617]

- In some patients with early syphilis, a secondary rash may become visible which was absent before treatment
- Rarely, syphilis may be suspected by the appearance of the febrile reaction of the Jarisch-Herxheimer, perhaps with a fleeting rash, when treating another infection with a treponemocidal antibiotic

62. Ans. (b) T. pertenue
[Ref. Sexually Transmitted Infections by Bhushan Kumar, 2/e p468]

Yaws Transmission

- T. pertenue causes Yaws', which is similar to syphilis and follows the same phases, but it is not sexually transmitted
- Yaws is transmitted nonvenereally by direct skin-to-skin contact
- The infection spreads by close contact from an individual with an open lesion to an uninfected person with skin excoriations, scratches, bites, etc

63. Ans. (d) Congenital
[Ref. Neena Khanna, 5/e p324]

64. Ans. (a) Venereal diseases research laboratory (VDRL) test
[Ref. Neena Khanna, 5/e p322]

- Characteristic findings of palmoplantar lesions in syphilis: Hyperpigmented, coppery red, scaly lesions/ hyperkeratotic papules

65. Ans. (a) Donovanosis granulomatis
[Ref. Neena Khanna, 5/e p329]

66. Ans. (a) Tetracycline
[Ref. Neena Khanna, 5/e p330]

67. Ans. (d) Vesicular Lesions
[Ref. Neena Khanna, 5/e p322]

- Rash of secondary syphilis may have any morphology of macular, popular, papulosquamous and nodular BUT is never vesicular or bullous

68. Ans. (a) Vesicles and bullae
[Ref. Neena Khanna, 5/e p322]

69. Ans. (b) Bullous lesion
[Ref. Neena Khanna, 5/e p322]

70. Ans. (c) Asymptomatic; (d) Tender
[Ref. Neena Khanna, 5/e p322]

- Papular syphilide: MC rash of secondary syphilis is characterized by deep dermal tenderness on pressing the lesion with a pinhead (Buschke-Ollendorff sign)
- Rash is bilaterally symmetrical macule which is non-pruritic and asymptomatic

71. Ans. (a) Primary syphilis; (b) Secondary syphilis
[Ref. Neena Khanna, 5/e p321-322]

72. Ans. (b) Infection leads to lifelong immunity; (c) IgM & IgA
[Ref. Neena Khanna, 5/e p325]& Textbook of Microbiology by Ananthanarayan, 7/e p380-384]

73. Ans. (b) VDRL
[Ref. Textbook of Microbiology by Ananthanarayan & Paniker, 7/e p380-384]

- Specific treponemal test (FTA-ABS, TPHA, TPI) are of little value as indicators of clinical cure, as they tend to remain positive in spite of treatment
- Non treponemal test (e.g. VDRL) will become nonreactive or will be reactive at lower titers after therapy, so can be used for monitoring patient's response to treatment: Usually become negative 6-18 months after effective treatment of syphilis

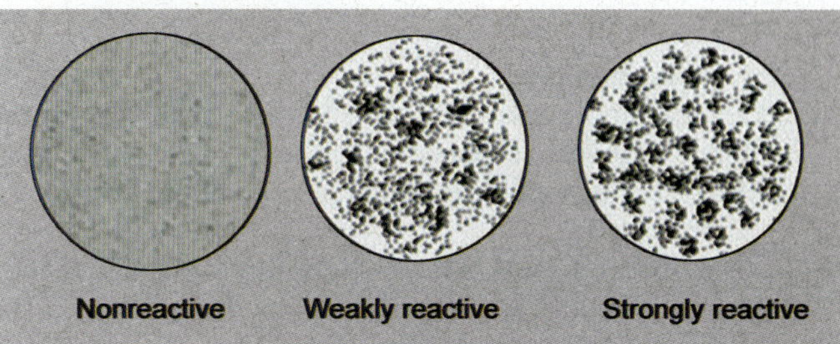

Fig. VDRL test

74. Ans. (b) Herpes simplex virus; (d) Treponema pallidum; (e) Lymphogranuloma venereum

[Ref. Neena Khanna, 5/e p287, 343-344]

- HPV causes warts; HIV does not causes ulcer

75. Ans. (d) Calymmatobacterium granulomatis

[Ref. Neena Khanna, 5/e p330]

Calymmatobacterium granulomatis in giemsa or Leishman's stain appear as intracellular (in macrophages) bipolar inclusions (safetypin or telephone handle appearance)

76. Ans. (c) Chancre

[Ref. Neena Khanna, 5/e p287, 320-321]

Chancre

- A painless ulceration most commonly formed during the primary stage of syphilis
- Lesion (infectious) forms approximately 21 days after the initial exposure to Treponema pallidum, the gram-negative spirochaete bacterium yielding syphilis
- Transmit the sexually transmissible disease of syphilis through direct physical contact
- Usually form on or around the anus, mouth, penis, and vagina
- May diminish between four to eight weeks without the application of medication

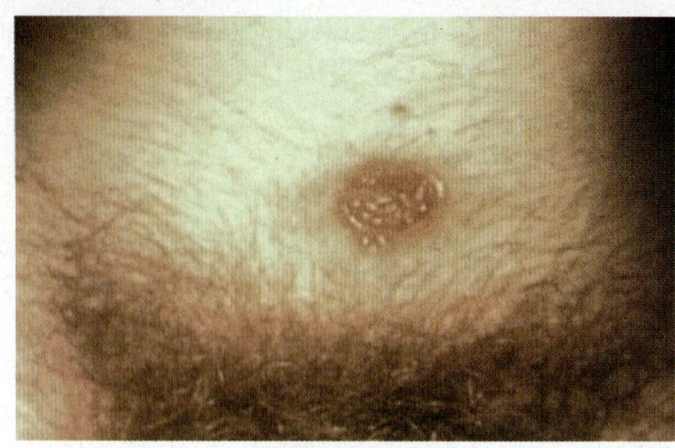

Fig. Chancre

77. Ans. (a) Syphilis

[Ref. Oxford Textbook of Medicine, Volume 1 by DA Warrell, p617]

78. Ans. (d) Yaws and Pinta can be differentiated by serological tests

[Ref. District Laboratory Practice in Tropical Countries, Part 2 by Cheesbrough, 2/e p224]

- Nonspecific and specific serological tests used in syphilis diagnosis are also positive in Yaws, Bejel, and Pinta
- Differentiation between the diseases is mainly based on the clinical appearance of lesions and areas of the body infected, differences in transmission and geographical distribution and the age of infected person

79. Ans. (c) Azithromycin 2 gm Single dose

[Ref. Emergency Medicine by Adams, 2/e p1107]

- In the emergency department, single-dose antibiotic therapy for urethritis is administered to cover both gonococcal urethritis (GCU) and nongonococcal urethritis (NGU)
- Azithromycin has shown equivalent cure rates when compared to conventional treatments for nongonococcal urethritis and gonorrhea

80. Ans. (b) Painless lymphadenopathy

[Ref. CURRENT Diagnosis and Treatment of Sexually Transmitted Diseases by Klausner, 1/e]

- Chancroid and lymphogranuloma venereum usually present with tender, fluctuant inguinal lymph nodes (Buboes)

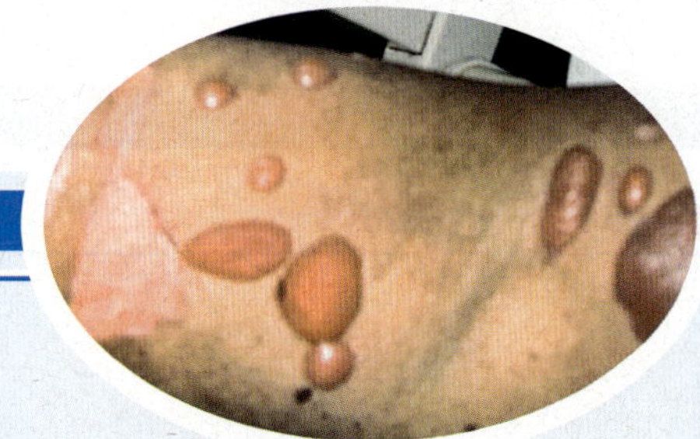

Chapter 14

Other Skin Disorders

THEORETICAL CONCEPTS

XIV A. WOOD'S LAMP EXAMINATION

- *Instrument*: A device which is made up of nickel-oxide and silica and emits ultraviolet rays **(wavelength: 360 nm – Black light)**
- *Clinical uses*:
  - Differentiate epidermal from dermal pigmentation
  - Enhance hypopigmented lesions
- *Interpretation of light colours emitted:*[Q]

Colour	Interpretation
Brilliant green[Q]	Tinea capitis
Dull yellow/Golden yellow[Q]	Pityriasis versicolor
Coral pink/ red[Q]	**Erythrasma**
White[Q]	**Vitiligo**
Blue-white[Q]	Tuberous sclerosis
Pale blue-green	Pseudomonas infection
Pinkish-red (Urine)	Porphyria cutanea tarda
Orange	Acne (Propionibacterium acne)

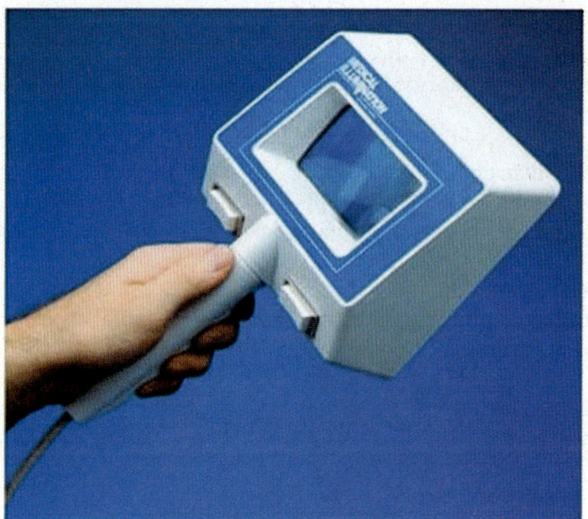

Fig. Wood's lamp

XIV B. ERYTHEMA MULTIFORME SYNDROME

XIV B1. Erythema Multiforme

- Underlying cause: Herpes simplex virus[Q]
- Clinical presentation: ***Target/Iris/Bull's-eye lesion*** *(Concentric three rings)*[Q]
- **Sites:** Face and acral parts
- Treatment: Acyclovir

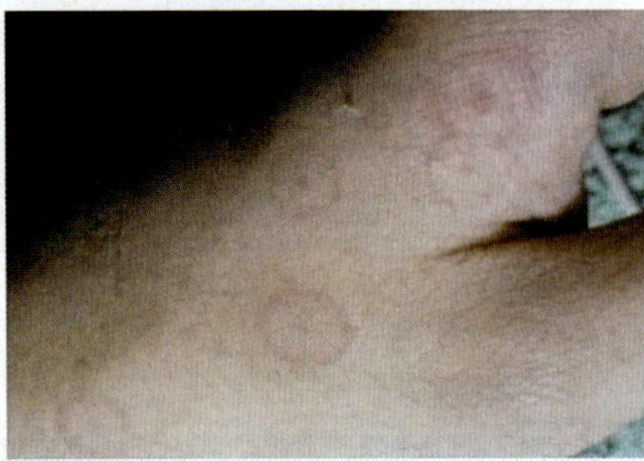

Fig. Target lesions

XIV B2. Stevens Johnson Syndrome

- *Underlying cause*: [**Mnemonic: H**is **S**everal **H**ealthy **P**atients **M**ade **N**urse **CLAP**] [Q]
  - **H**epatitis A
  - **S**LE
  - **H**istoplasmosis
  - **P**henytoin
  - **M**ycoplasma
  - **N**evirapine
  - **C**arbamazepine
  - **L**amotrigine
  - **A**llopurinol
  - **P**enicillin
- *Clinical presentation*:
  - Diffuse erythematous crinkled lesions
  - Hemorrhagic crusting of lips
  - Purulent conjunctivitis
- *Sites*: Extensively on body
- *Treatment*: Nursing care and cyclosporine

XIV C. DERMATOMYOSITIS

- *Definition*: Autoimmune disease with inflammatory injury to striated muscle and skin, causing itchy papules
- *Underlying cause*: Unknown
- *Clinical presentation*:
  - ***Heliotrope Erythema***[Q]: Periorbital lilac erythema
  - ***Gottron's papules***[Q]: Violaceous papules on knucles and pressure points
  - ***Gottron's sign***[Q]: Lilac erythema and edema over interphalangeal and Metacarpophalangeal joints
  - ***Poikiloderma***[Q]: Hyper/hypo-pigmentation, telangiectasia, atrophy
  - ***Shawl sign***[Q]: Symmetrical violaceous erythema
  - ***Mechanic's hand***[Q]: Hyperkeratosis on thumb (ulnar aspect) and fingers (radial aspect)
  - ***Calcinosis cutis***[Q]: Calcium deposits in skin
- *Systemic manifestations:*[Q]
  - Myositis (Weakness of proximal muscles)
  - Difficulty in speech and swallowing
  - Cardiomyopathy
  - Reynaud's phenomenon
  - Arthralgia
  - Carcinoma lungs/ ovaries/ breasts

- *Treatment*:
  - Antihistamines
  - Systemic steroids: Prednisolone
  - Immunosuppresive agents: Methotrexate, Azathioprine, Cyclosporine

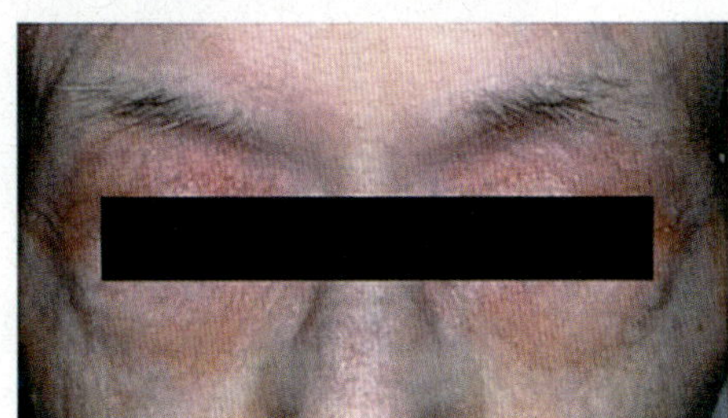

Fig. Heliotrope erythema

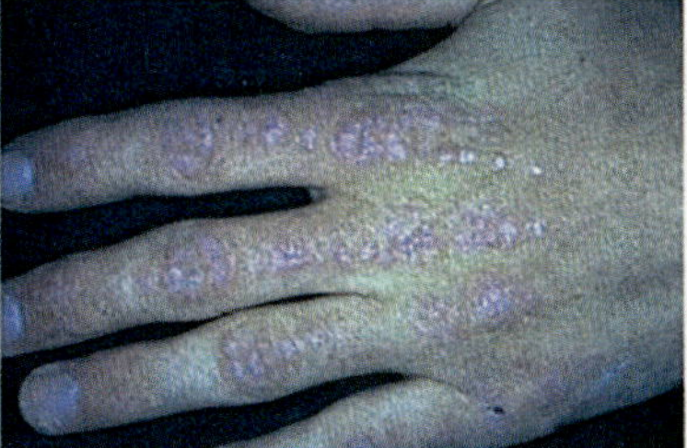

Fig. Gottron's papules

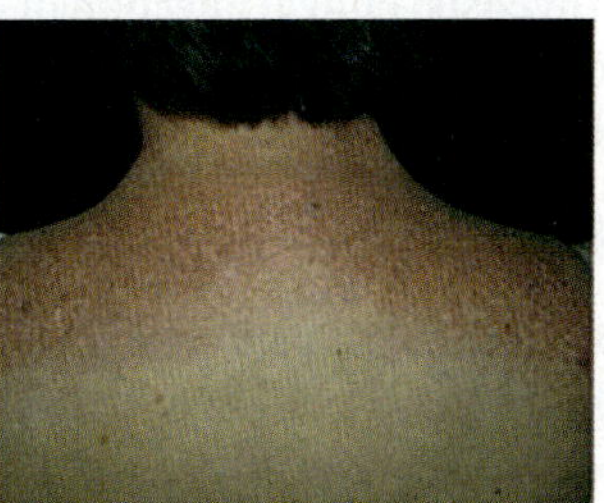

Fig. Shawl sign

XIV D. NAILS AND DISEASES

XIV D1. Common Nail Disorders

Disorders of nails	Disease condition(s) responsible
Onycholysis[Q]	Hyperthyroidism, Psoriasis, Fungal infections
Koilonychia[Q]	Iron deficiency anaemia, Syphilis, Ischaemic heart disease
Splinter haemorrhages[Q]	Trauma, Nail psoriasis, Subacute bacterial endocarditis
Pterygium of nails[Q]	Lichen planus, Idiopathic
Half-and-half nails	Chronic renal failure
Pitting of nails[Q]	Psoriasis, Alopecia areata, Hand eczema
Beau's lines[Q]	Acute systemic illnesses
Terry's nails	Cirrhosis
Hippocratic nails	Clubbing of nails
Mee's lines on nails[Q]	Chronic arsenic poisoning, Hypoalbuminemia
Hyperpigmentation of nails	Zidovudine, Mephalan, Daunorubicin, Bleomycin, Hydroxyurea
Blue nails	Chloroquine, Wilson's disease, Subungal hematoma
Yellow nail syndrome	Pleural effusion, Sinusitis, Ankle oedema
Nail fold telangeactasia[Q]	Dermatomyositis

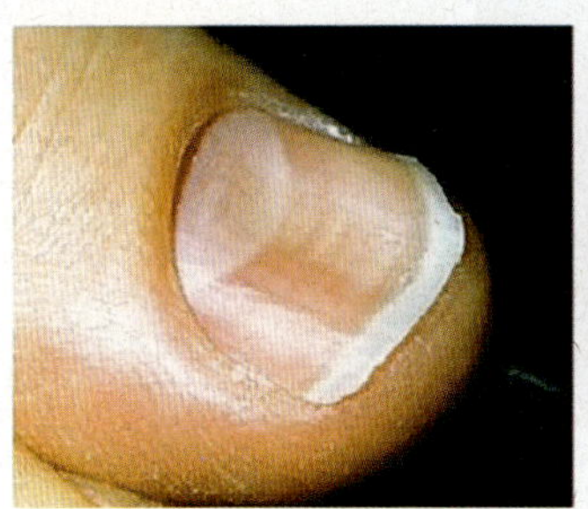

Fig. Koilonychia

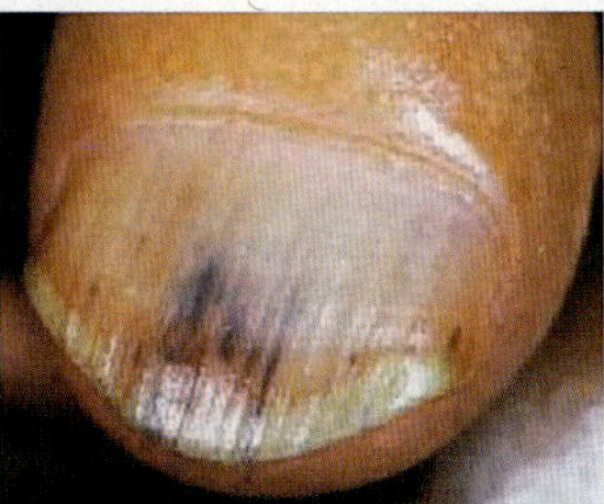

Fig. Splinter haem'ges

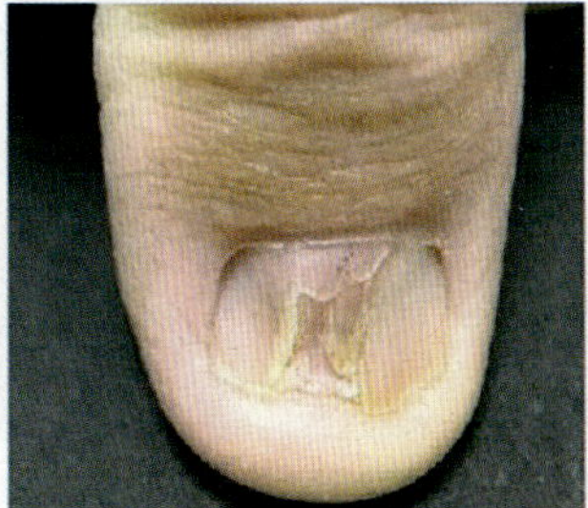

Fig. Pterygium of nails

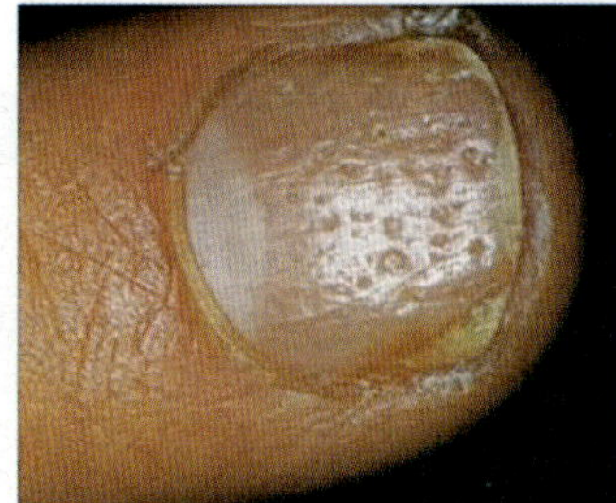

Fig. Pitting of nails

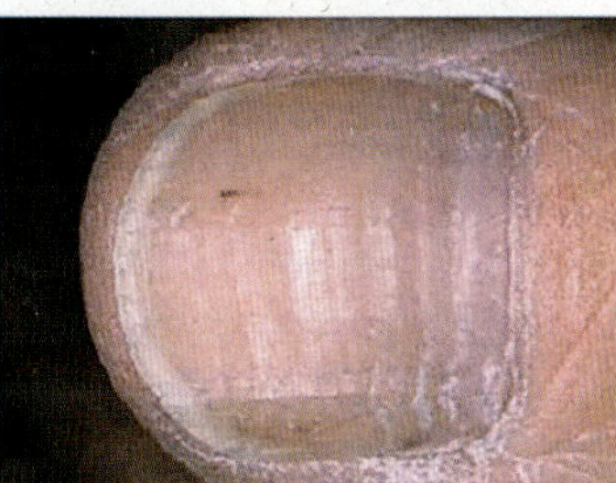

Fig. Beau's lines

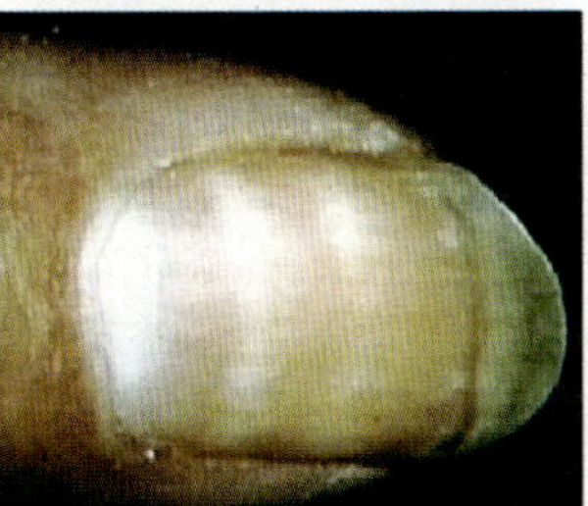

Fig. Mee's lines

XIV D2. Other Nail Disorders

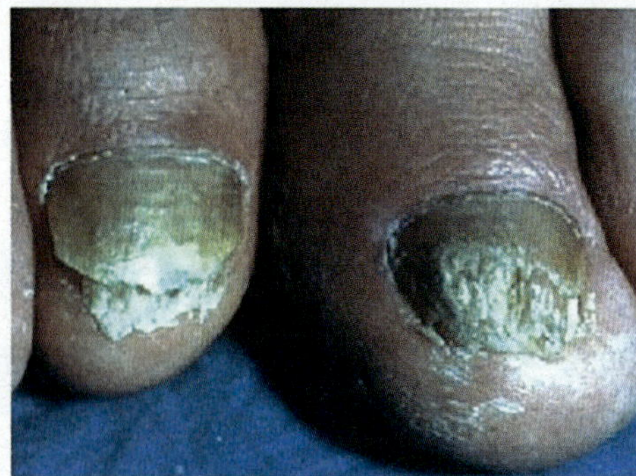
Fig. Subungual hyperkeratosis

- **Onychodystrophy:** Degeneration of nails
- **Onychorrhexis:** Splitting of nails
- **Onychomycosis:** Fungal infection of nails
- **Paronychia:** Bacterial/fungal infection of finger nail where it meets skin
- **Subungal hyperkeratosis:** Collection of keratotic debris under nail plate

XIV D3. Pitting of Nails[Q]

- **Skin disorders**[Q]: Alopecia areata, Psoriasis Lichen planus, Reiter's syndrome
- **Endocrinal causes**[Q]**:** Hypothyroidism, Hyperthyroidism, Hypoparathyroidism
- **Infectious causes**[Q]**:** Tinea unguium, Onychomycosis, Paronychia
- **Hereditary causes:** Nail patella syndrome, Ectodermal dysplasia

XIV E. CUTANEOUS MANIFESTATIONS OF TUBEROUS SCLEROSIS[Q]

- ***Angiofibroma***[Q]:
  - Most common manifestation[Q]
  - Dome shaped papules with telangiectasia
  - Nose, Nasolabial folds and cheeks
- ***Ash-leaf macules***[Q]:
  - Earliest manifestation[Q]
  - Hypopigmented macules on trunk
- ***Shagreen patch***[Q]:
  - Leathery pig-skin like plaques
  - Lumbosacral area[Q]
- ***Periungudal fibromas/Koenen's tumour***[Q]
  - Sausage type growth

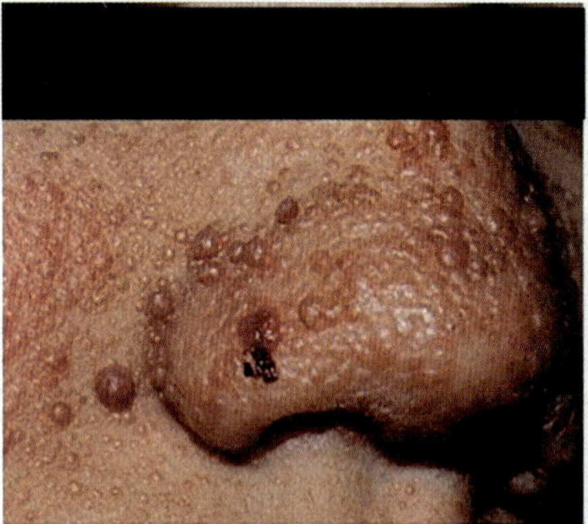
Fig. Angiofibroma

Fig. Ash-leaf macules

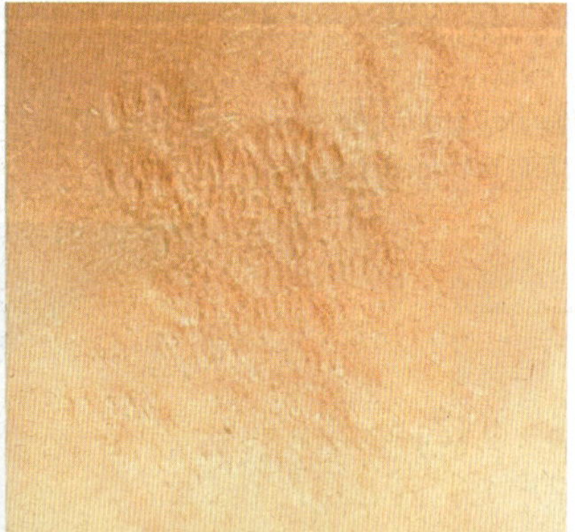
Fig. Shagreen patch

XIV F. ITCHING

DISEASES ASSOCIATED WITH ITCHING		
None/Mild Itching	**Moderate Itching**	**Severe Itching**
• Pemphigus[Q] • Psoriasis[Q] • Parapsoriasis • SLE • Pityriasis rosea[Q] • Secondary syphilis	• Bullous pemphigoid[Q] • Sun burn photosensitivity[Q] • Contact dermatitis[Q] • Dry skin	• Lichen planus[Q] • Lichen simplex chronicus[Q] • Scabies[Q] • Mastocytosis • Dermatitis herpetiformis

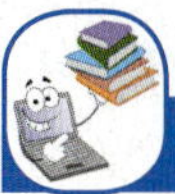

IMAGE-BASED QUESTIONS

1. **Patient present with Axillary freckling (Photograph). Diagnosis is** ***[Recent Question 2016]***

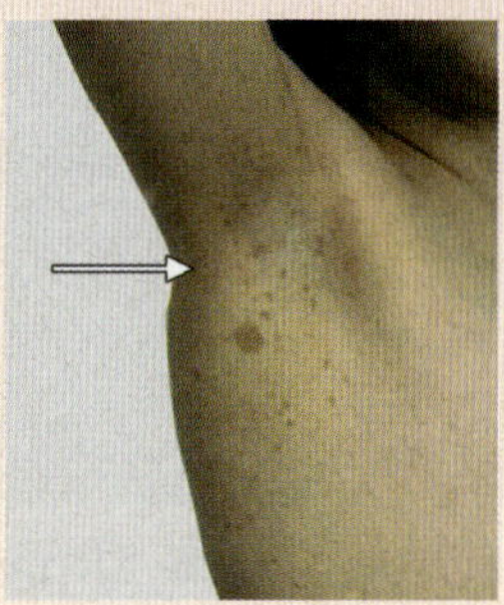

a. Neurofibromatosis b. Tuberous sclerosis
c. Ichthyosis Vulgaris
d. Von Hippel landau syndrome

2. **Dermatological test shown in the Photograph is**

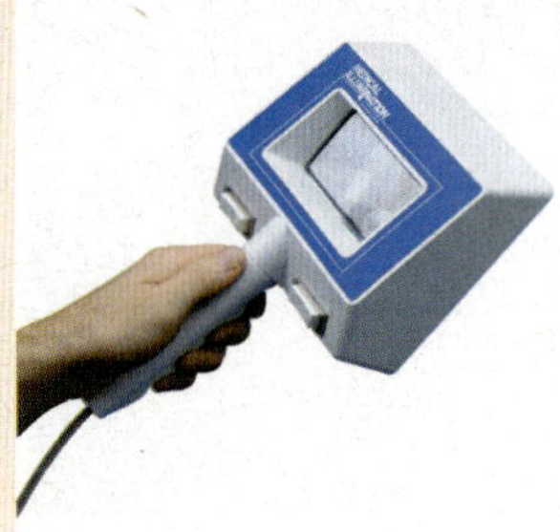

a. Wood lamp examination
b. Patch testing
c. Diascopy
d. Blanch test

3. **Fluorescence (Photograph) on Wood's lamp examination indicate** ***[Recent Question 2012]***

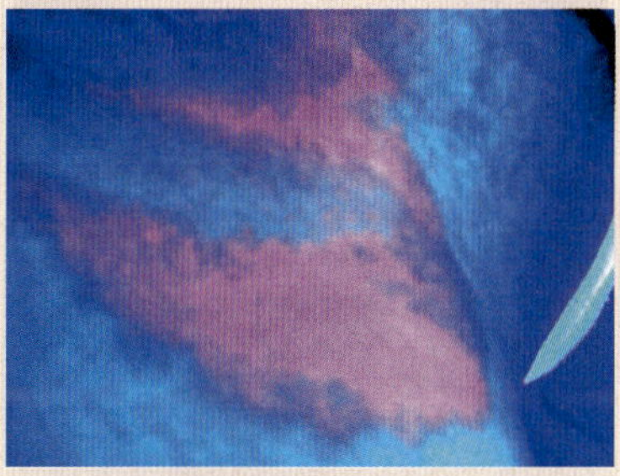

a. Pityrosporum
b. Microsporum
c. Trichophyton
d. Corynebacterium minutissimum

4. **Underlying Disorder based on Condition of nails shown in Photograph**

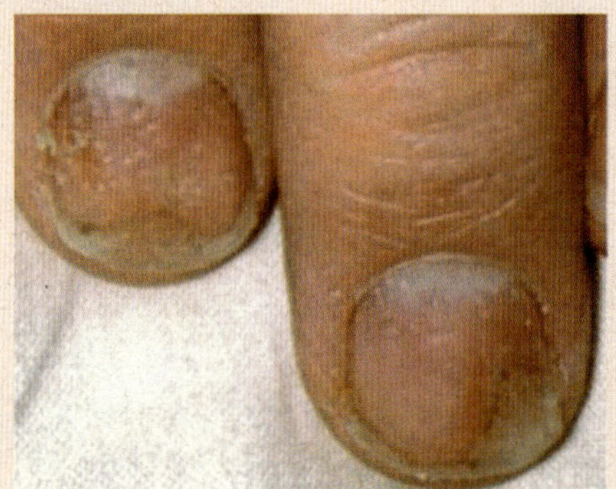

a. Lichen planus b. Dermatitis
c. Acute paronychia d. Psoriasis

5. **Most common cause of Nail disorder shown in the Photograph is**

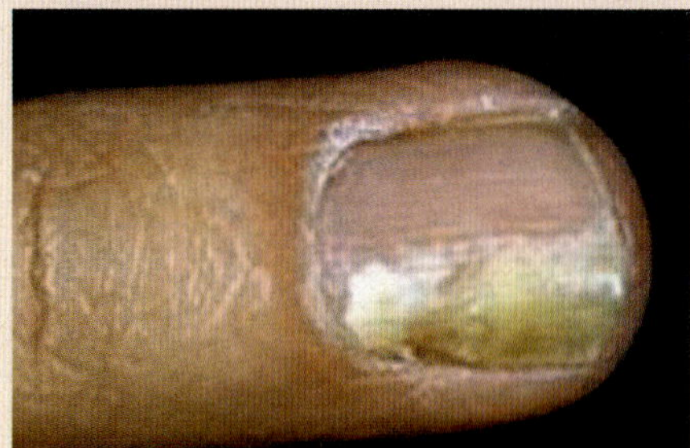

a. Epidermophyton flocculosum
b. Trichophyton mentagrophytes
c. Trichophyton rubrum
d. Tinea pedis

6. **Underlying Nail disorder shown in the Photograph is**

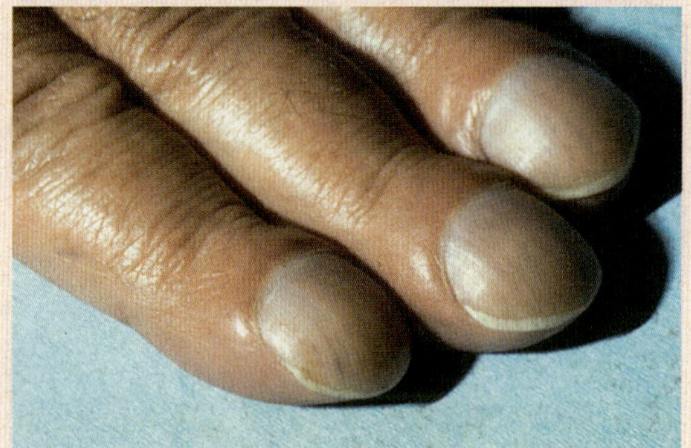

a. Leuconychia b. Melanonychia
c. Clubbing d. Koilonychia

7. **Underlying Nail disorder shown in the Photograph is**

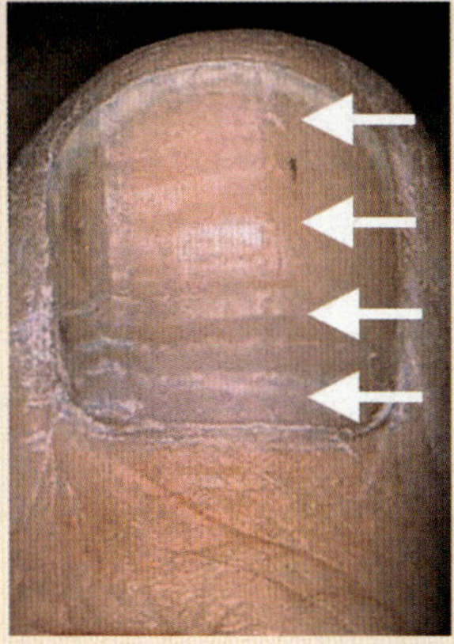

a. Leuconychia
b. Beau lines
c. Melanonychia
d. Koilonychia

8. **Underlying Disorder based on Condition of nails shown in Photograph**

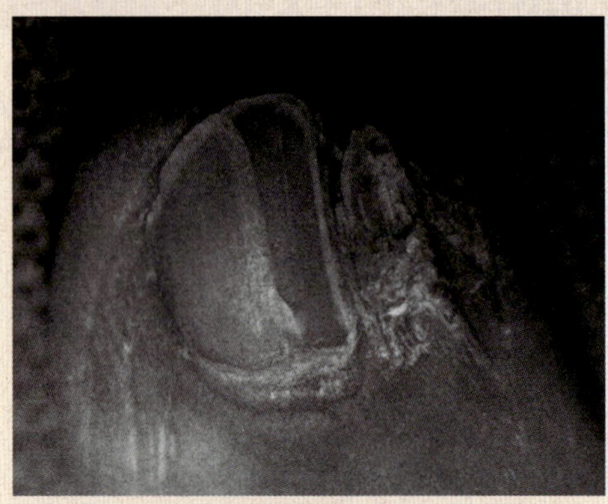

a. Lichen planus
b. Dermatitis
c. Acute paronychia
d. Psoriasis

9. **Skin disorder shown in the Photograph based on Skin lesions** ***[Recent Question 2014]***

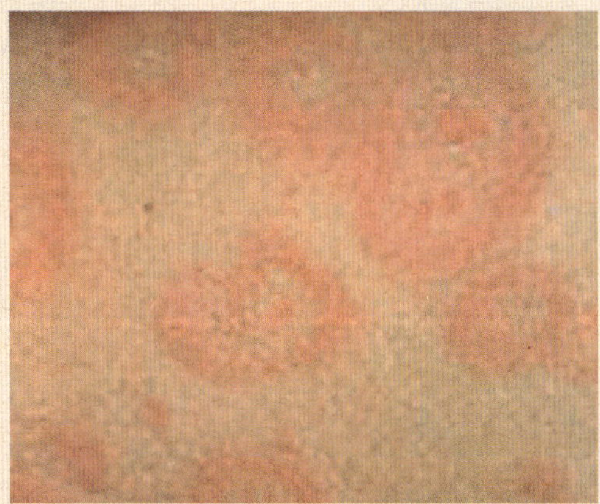

a. Polyarteritis nodosa
b. Lepromatous Leprosy
c. TB scrofuloderma
d. Erythema multiforme

10. **Identify sign of Dermatomyositis** ***[Recent Question 2014]***

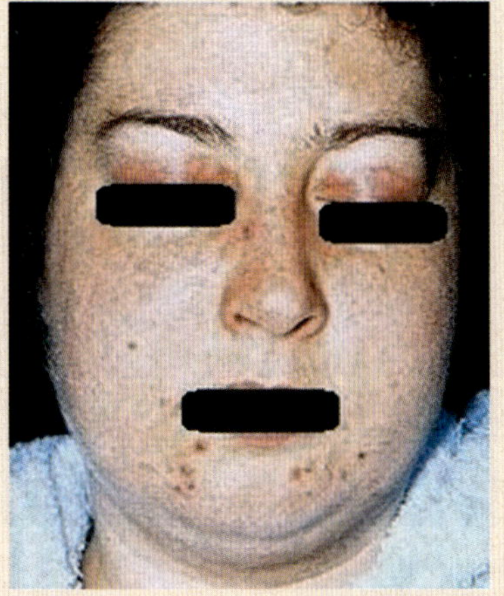

a. Shawl sign
b. Gottron's sign
c. Heliotrope erythema
d. Poikiloderma

11. **A child comes to Dermatology OPD with similar looking lesions over elbow and over shaft of penis (See Photograph). Diagnosis is** ***[AIIMS PG May 2015]***

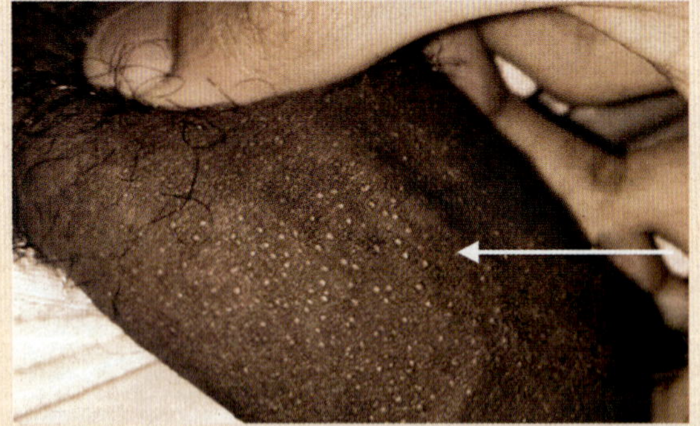

a. Lichen planus
b. Lichen scrofulosorum
c. Scabies
d. Lichen nitidus

12. **Skin condition shown in Photograph is associated with** ***[AIIMS November 2017]***

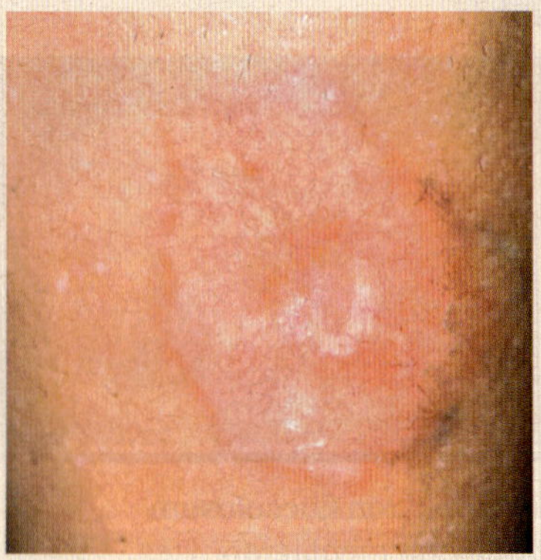

a. Hypothyroidism
b. Diabetes
c. Sarcoidosis
d. Hyperthyroidism

ANSWERS WITH EXPLANATIONS OF IBQs

1. Ans. (a) Neurofibromatosis *[Ref. DVL by Thappa, 4/e p238,239]*

Neurofibromatosis

- Genetic neuro-cutaneous disorder
- Café-au-lait spots or hyperpigmentation macules
- Multiple freckles [Crown sign] in axillary or inguinal region **(Photograph)**
- Typical neurofibroma's or plexiform neurofibroma
- Optic glioma
- Iris hamartomas (Lisch nodules)
- Sphenoid dysplasia
- First degree relative affected with NF-1

2. Ans. (a) Wood lamp examination *[Ref. Neena Khanna, 4/e p14]*

Wood Lamp Examination

- A diagnostic test in which the skin or hair is examined while exposed to the black light emitted by Wood lamp
- Black light is invisible to the naked eye because it is in the ultraviolet spectrum, with wavelength (360 nm) just shorter than the colour violet

3. Ans. (d) Corynebacterium minutissimum *[Ref. Neena Khanna, 4/e p15]*

Colours on Wood Lamp Examination

- Brilliant green: Tinea capitis
- Dull yellow: Pityriasis versicolor
- Coral pink/ red: Erythrasma (Corynebacterium minutissimum)
- White: Vitiligo
- Blue-white: Tuberous sclerosis
- Pale Blue-green: Pseudomonas
- Pinkish-red (Urine): Porphyria cutanea tarda
- Orange (Acne): Propionibacterium acne

4. Ans. (d) Psoriasis *[Ref. Neena Khanna, 4/e p45]*

Nails in Psoriasis

- Pitting of nails
- Nail plate thickening
- Subungual hyperkeratosis
- Discoloration, Dystrophy of nail plate
- Onycholysis
- Oil spots

5. Ans. (c) Trichophyton rubrum *[Ref. Neena Khanna, 4/e p287]*

Tinea Unguium

- Yellow brown discoloration
- Crumbling, Tunneling of nail plate
- Sunungual hyperkeratosis
- Onycholysis

6. Ans. (c) Clubbing *[Ref. Primary Care Medicine by Mulley, 6/e p370]*

- Clubbing: Enlargement and sponginess of the nail beds of the fingers and toes and reduction in the angle created by the nail and the dorsum of the distal phalanx
- It was described by Hippocrates

7. Ans. (b) Beau lines *[Ref. Neena Khanna, 4/e p144]*

- Beau lines: Transverse grooves on all nail plates simultaneously
- Grooves move distal with nail growth and disappear in 6 months

8. Ans. (a) Lichen planus *[Ref. Neena Khanna, 4/e p58]*

Nails in Lichen Planus

- Thinning, Distal splitting of nail plates
- Longitudinal ridges
- Pup-tent sign
- Trachonychia (Sand paper nails)
- Pterygium

9. Ans. (d) Erythema multiforme *[Ref. Neena Khanna, 4/e p174-175]*

Erythema Multiforme

- Cause: Herpes simplex virus
- Target lesions (Photograph): Central dusky erythema, Pale edematous ring, Erythematous halo

10. Ans. (c) Heliotrope erythema *[Ref. Neena Khanna, 4/e p228]*

- Heliotrope erythema: Faint lilac erythema peri-orbitally usually associated with edema in a case of Dermatomyositis

11. Ans. (d) Lichen nitidus *[Ref. Genitourinary Pain and Inflammation by Potts, 1/e p63]*

Lichen Nitidus (LN)

- An uncommon inflammatory disorder characterized by small, grouped, monomorphous, flesh-colored/shiny papules on the penis, arms, forearms, elbows, knees, and abdomen
- Pruritus is usually absent or mild
- Papules usually resolve within several months

12. Ans. (b) Diabetes *[Ref. Lookingbill and Marks' Principles of Dermatology, 5/e p230]*

Necrobiosis Lipoidica

- A necrotising skin condition that usually occurs in patients with Diabetes mellitus but can also be associated with Rheumatoid arthritis
- Disorder of collagen degeneration with a granulomatous response, thickening of blood vessel walls, and fat deposition
- Lesion of NL:
  - Brownish-red (early) papule that evolves into a plaque
  - With time, the center of the plaque becomes atrophic, takes on a yellowish hue, and develops prominent Telangiectasias
  - An elevated and sharply defined border is present
  - Lesion is firm to touch
  - Uncommonly ulcers and erosions develop within the plaques, often following trauma
- Commonly distributed symmetrically on the anterior shins
- Main complication is ulceration, usually occurring after trauma

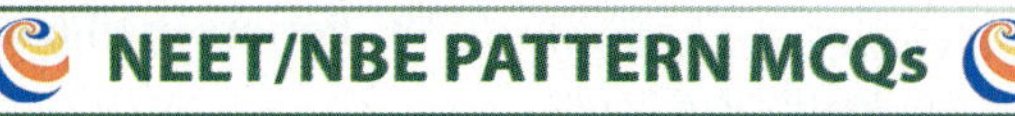

NEET/NBE PATTERN MCQs

1. **Erythema nodosum is seen in all except** *[Recent Question 2016]*
   a. Salicylate poisoning b. Typhoid
   c. Tuberculosis d. Leprosy
2. **True about Erythema toxicum neonatorum is** *[Recent Question 2016]*
   a. It is present in 3–5% of the newborns
   b. It is mostly present at birth
   c. It is called the flea-bitten rash of newborn
   d. Topical antibiotics is the treatment of choice
3. **Color of Tuberous sclerosis lesion on Wood's lamp examination** *[Recent Question 2016]*
   a. Bright green b. Milky white
   c. Golden yellow d. Blue white
4. **Patchy hair loss with velvety skin points to the diagnosis of** *[Recent Question 2016]*
   a. Alopecia aereata b. Trichotelomania
   c. Hyperthyroidism d. Adenoma sebaceum
5. **SAPHO Syndrome components are all except** *[Recent Question 2016]*
   a. Acne b. Hyperostosis
   c. Osteitis d. Acantholysis
6. **Thimble pitting of nails is seen in** *[Recent Question 2016]*
   a. Psoriasis b. Pemphigus
   c. Lichen planus d. Alopecia areata
7. **Wood's lamp examination is used in diagnosis of following conditions except** *[NBE FMGE September 2010]*
   a. Erythrasma b. Tinea capitis
   c. Pityriasis versicolor d. Psoriasis
8. **Munro microabscesses and positive Auspitz sign are seen in** *[NBE DNB 2011]*
   a. Erythema nodosum b. Malignant melanoma
   c. Psoriasis d. Keratoacanthoma
9. **All of the following are cause of acquired Ichthyosis, except** *[NBE DNB 1992]*
   a. AIDS b. Hypothyroidism
   c. Hyperthyroidism d. Leprosy
10. **Isomorphic phenomenon is seen in all of the following EXCEPT** *[NBE DNB 2011]*
    a. Lichen planus b. Psoriasis
    c. Vitiligo d. Lichen sclerosus
11. **Which of the following are known as *'gift spots'*?** *[NBE DNB 2007]*
    a. Paronychia b. Koilonychia
    c. Onycholysis d. Leuconychia
12. **Nikolsky's sign is positive in each of the following conditions, except** *[Recent Question 2016]* *[NBE DNB 1998, 2000, 2004, 2005, 2006, 2007]*
    a. Pemphigus
    b. Toxic epidermal necrolysis
    c. Epidermolysis bullosa
    d. Psoriasis
13. **Target/Iris lesions are seen in** *[NBE FMGE September 2008]*
    a. Urticaria b. Erythema multiforme
    c. Scabies d. Lichen planus
14. **Recurrent painful orogenital ulcers with arthritis is due to** *[UPSC 2009]*
    a. Gonorrhoea b. Syphilis
    c. Reiter's syndrome d. Behcet's syndrome
15. **Heliotype erythema is a feature of** *[Recent Question 2016, NBE DNB 1998, 1999, 2011]* *[NBE FMGE September 2006]*
    a. Lichen planus b. Dermatomyositis
    c. Psoriasis d. Scleroderma
16. **Onycholysis may be seen in all except** *[NBE DNB 1994]*
    a. Thyroid diseases b. Psoriasis
    c. Addison's disease d. Pityriasis rubra
17. **Increased level of IgE seen in** *[NBE DNB 2002, 2005]*
    a. Atopy b. Lepra reaction
    c. Cutaneous TB d. Lupus vulgaris
18. **Nail's involvement is not a feature of** *[NBE FMGE March 2003]*
    a. Psoriasis b. DLE
    c. Dermatomyositis d. Lichen planus
19. **Commonest cutaneous eruption in SLE is** *[NBE DNB 1995, 2000, 2001, 2005, 2006]*
    a. Palmar erythema
    b. Discoid lesions
    c. Erythema of light exposed area
    d. Diffuse morbiliform erythema
20. **Acantholysis is seen in** *[NBE DNB 1996]*
    a. Pemphigus b. Impetigo
    c. Herpes zoster d. All of the above
21. **Koebner's phenomenon is seen in** *[NBE DNB 2003]*
    a. Lichen planus b. Ichthyosis
    c. Psoriasis d. Pemphigus
22. **Earliest sign in tuberous sclerosis is** *[NBE DNB 2011]*
    a. Shagreen patch b. Subungual fibroma
    c. Angiofibromas d. Melanotic spots
23. **In American classification of SLE, the least important criteria is** *[NBE DNB 1997]*
    a. Convulsions b. Photosensitivity
    c. Malar rash over face d. Oral ulcers
24. **Butterfly rash is seen in** *[NBE FMGE September 2006, 2012]*
    a. SLE
    b. Rheumatoid arthritis
    c. DLE
    d. Reiter's syndrome
25. **Wood lamp wavelength** *[Recent Question 2016, 2012]*
    a. 360-385 b. 400-450
    c. 280-320 d. 450-500
26. **Nail involvement is not a feature of** *[NBE DNB 1996]*
    a. Psoriasis b. DLE
    c. Dermatophytosis d. Lichen planus
27. **Cafe au lait spots seen in?** *[Recent Question 2016, 2012, 2014]*
    a. NF b. Gardner syndrome
    c. Cockayne syndrome d. Down syndrome
28. **Berkeley membrane is seen in** *[NBE DNB 1996, 2004, 2006]*
    a. Psoriasis b. Pemphigus
    c. Tinea capitis d. Pityriasis rubra

29. Pitting of nails can be seen in *[Recent Question 2016]* *[NBE DNB 2008]*
a. Tinea unguium
b. Alopecia areata
c. Androgenic alopecia
d. Peripheral vascular disease

30. Wood's lamp is useful in recognition of 'Ash leaf spots' in patients with *[UPSC 2010]*
a. Atopic dermatitis
b. Lichen plannus
c. Nummular eczema
d. Tuberous sclerosis

31. In which of the following, Koebner phenomenon is NOT seen? *[Recent Question 2012, 2013]*
a. Lichen planus
b. Lichen sclerosis
c. Erythema multiforme
d. Lichen simplex chronicus

32. All are seen in Reiter's syndrome except
a. Subcutaneous nodules *[NBE DNB 2009]*
b. Oral ulcers
c. Keratoderma blenorrhagicum
d. Circinate balanitis

33. Patch test is done to document *[NBE DNB 2009]*
a. Type I hypersensitivity
b. Delayed type hypersensitivity
c. Autoimmune disease
d. Immunocomplex deposition

34. Leg ulcers are not seen in *[Recent Question 2012, 2013]*
a. TB b. Syphilis
c. Anemia d. Psoriasis

35. Mucosal lesion is common in *[NBE DNB 1993]*
a. Pemphigoid b. Psoriasis
c. Lichen planus d. Pityriasis rubra

36. A positive family history is a recognized feature of all except *[NBE DNB 1997]*
a. Psoriasis b. Bullous pemphigoid
c. Ichthyosis vulgaris d. Darrier's disease

37. Oculogenital ulcers are a feature of *[Recent Question 2012]*
a. Behcet disease b. Lichen planus
c. SIB d. Psoriasis

38. Ashleaf spots are characteristic of *[NBE FMGE March 2007]*
a. Psoriasis
b. Multiple sclerosis
c. Pemphigus vulgaris
d. Tuberous sclerosis

39. Prophyria cutanea tarda can be treated by *[NBE DNB 1994]*
a. Phlebotomy b. Heme
c. Low dose chloroquine d. Metronidazole

40. Dermatomyositis test of choice *[Recent Question 2012, 2013]*
a. CPK b. 24 hour urine creatinine
c. SOOT d. SGPT

41. Pitting of nails can be seen in *[NBE DNB 2010]*
a. Tinea unguium b. Alopecia areata
c. Androgenic alopecia d. Peripheral vascular disease

42. Immune reactants deposited at dermo-epidermal junction in positive lupus test *[Recent Question 2012, 2013]*
a. IgG only b. IgG with compliments
c. IgM only d. IgG and IgM only

43. Perioral pallor and Dennie's line are seen in *[NBE DNB 2010]*
a. Atopic dermatitis b. Chronic actinic dermatitis
c. Blood dyscrasia d. Perioral contact dermatitis

44. Dyskeratosis of dermo-epidermal junction and saw-tooth appearance of rete-ridges is seen in *[NBE FMGE September 2012]*
a. Vitiligo b. Lichen planus
c. Dermatomyositis d. Pityriasis rosea

45. What is not true about Erythema multiforme?
a. Associated with H simplex *[Recent Question 2012]*
b. Involves distal parts of extremities
c. No vesicle
d. Target lesions

46. Gumma are *[NBE DNB 1992]*
a. Highly infectious
b. Less infectious
c. Non-infectious
d. May or may not be infectious

47. Which of the following is not seen in Dermatomyositis?
a. Gottrons papules *[NBE DNB 2010]*
b. Mechanics Hand
c. Periungual telangiectasia
d. Salmon Rash

48. Pterygium of nail is seen in *[Recent Question 2016, 2012]*
a. Lichen planus b. Psoriasis
c. Tinea unguium d. Alopecia areata

49. Salt and pepper dyschromatosis is seen in *[NBE FMGE September 2009]*
a. SLE b. Psoriasis
c. Scleroderma d. Dermatofibrosis

50. Tzanck smear is positive in *[Recent Question 2012]*
a. Herpes simplex b. Psoriasis
c. LP d. Warts

51. Incidences of HIV infection is that every day .... people are affected in the world *[NBE DNB 1992]*
a. 1000 b. 2000
c. 5000 d. 15,000

52. Onycholysia is seen in all of the following, except *[NBE DNB 2002]*
a. Acute paronychia b. Psoriasis
c. Hyperthyroidism d. Nephrotic syndrome

53. Pterygium of nail is seen in *[Recent Question 2012]*
a. Lichen planus b. Psoriasis
c. Tinea unguium d. Alopecia aerata

54. The typical skin lesions seen in Erythema multiforme are *[NBE FMGE September 2011]*
a. Wheals b. Target lesions
c. Bullae d. Erosions

55. The target cell of rickettsial infections is mainly *[NBE DNB 1993]*
a. Platelets b. Endothelial cells
c. Mast cells d. Stem cells
e. Red blood cells

56. Itchy purple papule followed by hyperpigmentation on resolution, is seen in *[Recent Question 2012]*
a. Addison's disease b. DM
c. Hypothyroidism d. Lichen planus

57. Hidradenitis suppurativa is chronic infection is *[Recent Question 2016, NBE FMGE September 2011]*
a. Apocrine sweat gland b. Sebaceous gland
c. Lymph node d. Dermis

58. Tuberous sclerosis is characterized by all EXCEPT *[Recent Question 2014]*
a. Shagreen patch b. Ash leaf macules
c. Adenoma sebaceum d. Intertriginous freckling

59. Neurofibromatosis -1 is characterized by all except *[Recent Question 2014]*
a. Café au lait macules
b. Axillary freckling
c. Bilateral acoustic neuromas
d. Lisch nodules

60. Omenn Syndrome is a *[Recent Question 2016, 2015]*
a. Squamous cell carcinoma
b. Chronic Mucocutaneous Candidiasis
c. IgA deficiency d. SCID

61. Koenen's periungual fibroma is a feature of *[Recent Question 2017]*
a. Kawasaki's disease b. Refsum disease
c. Darrier's disease d. Bourneville's disease

62. Wood's lamp examination is useful in *[Recent Question 2017]*
a. Psoriasis b. Leprosy
c. Lichen planus d. Ichthyosis

63. Most common etiology of Erythema multiforme is *[Recent Question 2017]*
a. Idiopathic b. Drugs
c. HSV d. TB

64. Hypopigmented macules are found in *[Recent Question 2017]*
a. Addison's disease b. Porphyria
c. Cutaneous mastocytosis d. Tuberous sclerosis

65. Most common pattern of Onychomycosis is *[Recent Question 2017]*
a. Distal and lateral subungual
b. Proximal subungual
c. White superficial
d. Total dystrophic

66. Which of the following is not a feature of Dermatomyositis? *[Recent Question 2017]*
a. 'V' sign b. Holster sign
c. Poikiloderma d. Groove sign

67. Most important factor in causation of Ingrown toe nail is *[Recent Question 2017]*
a. Fungal infection b. Ill-fitting shoes
c. Genetic predisposition d. Nutritional deficiency

68. True about Dermatomyositis is? *[Recent Question 2017]*
a. Associated with HLA B27
b. Bimodal age distribution
c. No involvement of joints
d. Myopathy precedes skin lesions in most cases

69. Heliotrope rash is seen in? *[Recent Question 2017]*
a. SLE
b. Dermatomyositis
c. Scleroderma
d. Mixed connective tissue disorder

HIGH YIELD MCQs

1. Wrong statement is *[All India PGMEE 2000]*
a. Mees line in Arsenic poisoning
b. Pterygium of nails in Lichen Planus
c. Oncholysis in Psoriasis
d. Koilonychia in Megaloblastic Anemia (B12 deficiency)

2. Nail involvement is not a feature of *[AIIMS PGMEE 1994, SGPGI 2005]*
a. Psoriasis b. Lichen planus
c. Dermatophytosis d. DLE

3. All are true about erythema multiforme except *[Jharkhand PGMEE 2005]*
a. Due to herpes simplex
b. Due to sulphonamide
c. Lesion are symmetrical
d. Mucous membrane is usually involved

4. A 29-year-old male with a history of long leisure trip presented with right knee pain and swollen joint with foreign body sensation in eye. The most probable diagnosis is *[All India PGMEE 2009]*
a. Sarcoidosis b. Tuberculosis
c. Reiter's disease d. Behcet's disease

5. Koenen's periungal fibroma is seen in *[Recent Question 2016, PGI 1996, JIPMER PGMEE 2002]*
a. Tuberous sclerosis
b. Neurofibromatosis
c. Psoriasis
d. Alopecia aerate

6. A child presents with solitary white well defined patch on his right thigh. Diagnosis is *[AIIMS PGMEE 2000]*
a. Piebaldism b. Albinism
c. Nevus achromicus d. Acral vitiligo

7. A 27-year-old male had burning micturation & urethral discharge. After 4 weeks he developed joint pains involving both the knees & ankles, redness of the eyes & skin lesions. The most probable clinical diagnosis *[AIIMS PGMEE 2005]*
a. Psoriasis valgaris b. Reiter's syndrome
c. Behcet's syndrome d. Sarcoidosis

8. Hypopigmented patches can be seen in *[PGI 2005]*
a. Becker naevus b. Freckles
c. Nevus ITO d. Nevus Ota
e. Nevus anemicus

9. A patient had seven irregular hyperpigmented macules on the trunk and multiple small hyperpigmented macules in the axillae and groins since early childhood. There were no other skin lesions. Which is the most likely investigation to support the diagnosis? *[All India PGMEE 2006]*
a. Slit lamp examination of eye
b. Measurement of intraocular tension
c. Examination of fundus
d. Retinal artery angiography

10. In Tzank smear multinucleated cells are seen in *[PGI 1997]*
a. Chicken pox b. Psoriasis
c. Molluscum contagiosum d. Pemphigus vulgaris

11. Direct immunofluorescence is positive in *[PGI 2002]*
a. Atopic dermatitis b. SLE
c. Pemphigus d. Secondary syphilis

12. Commonest etiology of erythema multiforme is *[All India PGMEE 1995, UP PGMEE 2002]*
a. Viral b. Bacterial
c. Food d. Drugs

13. Adenoma sebaceum is a feature of *[AIIMS PGMEE 2005]*
a. Neurofibromatosis b. Tuberous sclerosis
c. Xanthomatosis d. Incontinentia pigmenti

14. A 45-year-old farmer has itchy erythematous popular lesions on face, neck, 'V' area of chest, dorsum of hands and forearms for 3 years. The lesions are more severe in summers and improve by 75% in winters. The most appropriate test to diagnose the condition would be
a. Skin biopsy *[All India PGMEE 2006]*
b. Estimation of IgE levels in blood
c. Patch test
d. Intradermal prick test

15. A 40-year-old farmer with history of recurrent attack of porphyria complains of itching when exposed to the sun and maculopapular rashes on sun exposed area. His symptoms are exaggerated in summer. The diagnosis is *[AIIMS PGMEE 2001]*
a. Seborrheic dermatitis b. Contact dermatitis
c. Psoriasis d. Porphyria cutanea tarda

16. A girl on sulphonamides developed abdominal pain and presented to emergency with seizure. What is the probable cause? *[AIIMS PGMEE 2008]*
a. Acute intermittent porphyria
b. Congenital erythropoietic porphyria
c. Infections mononucleosis
d. Kawasaki's disease

17. Babloo a 4 year male presents with history of seizures. On examination there is hypopigmented patches on face and mental retardation. Most probable diagnosis is *[AIIMS PGMEE 2000]*
a. Neurofibromatosis b. Tuberous sclerosis
c. Sturge Weber Syndrome d. Incontinentia Pigmenti

18. Treatment of choice in the cutaneous complication of porphyria is *[JIPMER PGMEE 1996, PGI 2001]*
a. IV dextrose b. I. V Haematin
c. Beta carotene d. Calamine

19. Porphyrins are synthesized mainly in *[AIIMS PGMEE 1995]*
a. Spleen b. Liver and spleen
c. Bone marrow and spleen d. Liver and Bone marrow

20. Palpable purpura is seen in all conditions except *[All India PGMEE 2000]*
a. Cryoglobulinuria b. H.S. Purpura
c. Giant cell arteritis d. Drug induced vasculitis

21. All are true regarding tuberous sclerosis except *[PGI 2008]*
a. Autosomal dominant sporadic transmission
b. Vogt triad of epiloia
c. Café au lait macules exclude the diagnosis
d. Fibrous facial plaque
e. Stippled confetti spots

22. Oil drop sign is seen in *[Recent Question 2016, AP PGMEE 1996]*
a. Psoriasis of nails b. Lichen planus of nails
c. Clubbing d. T Unguum

23. Tinea unguum effects *[All India PGMEE 1995]*
a. Nail fold b. Nail plate
c. Joints d. Inter digital space

24. A 42-year-old female has palpable purpura with rash over buttocks, pain in abdomen, and arthropathy diagnosis is *[All India PGMEE 2008]*
a. Sweet syndrome b. HSP
c. Purpura fulminans d. Meningococcemia

25. Morphea occurs usually in *[AIIMS PGMEE 1996, JIPMER PGMEE 1997]*
a. Forehead b. Sternum
c. Limbs d. Back

26. An 8-year-old boy from Bihar presents with a 6 month history of an ill defined hypopigmented slightly atrophic macule on the face. The most likely diagnosis is *[All India PGMEE 2005]*
a. Ptyriasis alba b. Indeterminate leprosy
c. Morphacea d. Calcium deficiency

27. Nail is involved in *[PGI 2007]*
a. Psoriasis b. Lichen planus
c. Fungal infection d. Alopecia
e. Viral infection

28. The main cytokine, involved in erythema nodosum leprosum (ENL) reaction is *[AIIMS PGMEE 2006]*
a. Interleukin-2
b. Interferon-gamma
c. Tumor necrosis factor-alpha
d. Macrophage colony stimulating factor

29. Pterygium of nail is characteristically seen in *[All India PGMEE 2006]*
a. Lichen planus b. Psoriasis
c. Tinea unguium d. Alopecia areata

30. A child develops non blanching macules and papules on lower extremities, mild abdominal pain, and skin biopsy showed IgA deposition and perivascular neutrophilic infiltrate. Most probably diagnosis is
a. Wegner's granulomatosis *[AIIMS PGMEE 2009]*
b. Poly arteritis nodosa
c. Henoch Schonlein purpura
d. Kawasaki disease

31. Which of following is/are not the feature of Henoch-Schonlein Purpura (HSP)? *[PGI 2008]*
a. Abdominal pain b. Splinter haemorrhage
c. Thrombocytopenia d. Epistaxis
e. Arthritis

32. All regarding HSP is true except *[PGI 2008]*
a. Hematuria resolve without treatment
b. Steroids best treat skin lesions
c. Self limiting arthralgia
d. Excellent prognosis
e. Purpura fulminans

33. Wood's lamp used in diagnosis of *[PGI 2006]*
a. P. versicolor b. Vitiligo
c. Porphyria d. Psoriasis
e. Lichen Planus

34. A 4-year-old child with high fever developed toxic look, eruptions of trunk & proximal extremities, bilateral bulbar conjunctivitis without discharge and fissuring-crusting-red lips. Due to limb edema walking became difficult. She also had desquamation in perineum & finger tips with cervical adenopathy. Diagnosis is *[UP PGMEE 2007, AIIMS PGMEE 2005]*
a. PAN b. HSP
c. Kawasaki syndrome d. Erythema infectiosum

35. Rain drop pigmentation is seen in *[AP PGMEE 1996]*
a. Chronic lead poisoning b. Chronic Arsenic poisoning
c. Chronic Mercury poisoning
d. All of the above

36. Uses of Woods' light includes *[All India PGMEE 1999]*
a. Urine examination in porphyria
b. Examination of hair in T. capitis
c. Sclerema d. All

37. Dyskeratosis is characteristic feature of *[PGI 2000]*
a. Darrier's disease b. Pemphigus vulgaris
c. Psoriasis d. Boweli's disease
e. Hailey-Hailey disease

38. Morbilliform eruptions is seen in *[PGI 2001]*
a. Scarlet fever b. Rubella
c. Toxic shock syndrome d. Measles
e. Mumps

39. Koebner phenomenon is present in all except *[Bihar PGMEE 2006]*
a. Psoriasis b. Lichen planus
c. Warts d. None

40. All the following are Primary cutaneous diseases except *[AIIMS PGMEE 2010, All India PGMEE 2009]*
a. Psoriasis b. Reiter's disease
c. Lichen planus
d. Icthiosis/Bowen's disease

41. Inheritance of Ichthyosis vulgaris is *[All India PGMEE 1993]*
a. X linked dominant b. X linked recessive
c. Autosomal dominant d. Autosomal recessive

42. Koebners phenomenon is seen in *[DPG 1998]*
a. Lichen Planus b. Psoriasis
c. Ichthyosis d. Pitriasis rubra
e. Phemphigus

43. A male child with cryptorchidism presents with large black scales on body flexures. Skin biopsy showed hyper granulosis & steroid sulfatase deficiency. Probable diagnosis is *[SGPGI 2008]*
a. Ichthyosis vulgaris
b. Ichthyosis-lamellar
c. X linked ichthyosis nigra
d. Nonullous ichthyosiform erythroderma

44. Granular layer is absent in *[Orissa PGMEE 1998]*
a. Ichthyosis vulgaris
b. X linked ichthyosis
c. Epidermolytic hyper keratosis
d. Lamellar ichthyosis

45. Acantholysis is seen in *[PGI 2009]*
a. Bullous pemphigoid b. Dermatitis herpetiformis
c. Hailey-Hailey disease d. Darrier's disease
e. Pemphigus vulgaris

46. The correct sequence of cell cycle is *[All India PGMEE 2003]*
a. G0-G1-S-G2-M b. G0-G1-G2-S-M
c. G0-M-G2-S-G1 d. G0-GI-S-M-G2

47. True about incontinentia pigmenti include the following except *[All India PGMEE 2009]*
a. X-linked dominant
b. Primary skin abnormality
c. Avascularity of peripheral retina
d. Ocular involvement is seen in almost 100% cases and is typically unilateral

48. Veldt sore is most common in *[JIPMER PGMEE 1998] [AMU PGMEE 1999]*
a. Hilly areas b. Tropical climate
c. Rainy areas d. Deserts

49. A patient has Bullous Lesion; on Tzank smear *[All India PGMEE 1996]*
a. Langerhans cells are seen
b. Acantholysis
c. Leucocytosis
d. Absence of melanin pigment

50. Tzank smear helps in the diagnosis of *[MP PGMEE 2005]*
a. Herpes viral infection b. Bullous pemphigoids
c. Carcinoma of cervix d. None

51. 'Cayenne pepper' stippling due to hemosiderin is found in *[All India PGMEE 1996]*
a. Erythroplasia of Queyrat
b. Pagets disease
c. Plasma cell balantitis of zoon
d. Metronidazole

52. Nails are involved in *[AIIMS PGMEE 1994]*
a. Pemphigus b. Pemphigoid
c. Psoriasis d. Dermatitis herpetiformis

53. Hyperpigmentation is not seen in *[All India PGMEE 1993]*
a. Addison's disease b. Cushing's disease
c. Graves disease d. Hypothyroidism

54. Pigmentation of the skin is seen in all of the following except *[All India PGMEE 1993]*
a. Myxedema b. Graves disease
c. Cushings syndrome d. Addisons disease

55. Mucous lesions are seen in *[PGI 2002, AIIMS PGMEE 1992]*
a. Sec syphilis b. Dermatitis herpetiformis
c. Psoriasis d. Pemphigus
e. Porphyria

56. Nail involvement is not a feature of *[AIIMS PGMEE 1992]*
a. Psoriasis
b. Drug induced lupus erythematous
c. Dermatophytosis/Taenia
d. Lichen Planus

57. 'Pinch purpura' is diagnostic of *[AIIMS PGMEE 2005]*
a. Systemic primary amyloidosis
b. Secondary systemic amyloidosis
c. ITP
d. Drug induced purpura

58. Pitting of nails is seen in *[AIIMS PGMEE 2001, JIPMER PGMEE 1990]*
a. Lichen planus b. Psoriasis
c. Phemphigus d. Arsenic poisoning
e. Leprosy

59. Regarding Erythema multiforme all are true except *[All India PGMEE 2000]*
a. No vesicles
b. Target lesions are seen
c. Involves face and neck regions
d. Sign of internal malignancy

60. Target or Iris lesion seen in *[Recent Question 2016] [All India PGMEE 1997, 1998]*
a. Urticaria b. Erythema multiforme
c. Scabies d. Lichen Planus

61. Riehl's melanosis mainly involves- *[Recent Question 2016, JIPMER PGMEE 1992] [AIIMS PGMEE 1992]*
a. Face and Neck b. Trunk
c. Extremities d. Palms only

62. True about dermatomyositis *[PGI 2009]*
a. Gottron papules
b. ANA associated with all cases
c. All associated with malignancy
d. Proximal muscle wasting

63. Control of TB and leprosy is by *[Kerala PGMEE 1994]*
a. Isolation of cases
b. Specific protection
c. Early diagnosis and treatment
d. Elimination of reservoirs

64. All are manifestations of SLE except *[PGI 1998]*
a. Lesions resembling Chronic DLE
b. Butterfly rash
c. Photosensitivity
d. Constitutional symptom
e. Sex ratio is nearly equal

65. Which of the following are photosensitive diseases? *[PGI 2001]*
a. SLE b. Liver spots
c. Calcinosis cutis d. Morphea
e. Prophyria cutanea tarda

66. Wood's lamp light is used in the diagnosis of *[AIIMS PGMEE 2002]*
a. Tinea capitis b. Candida albicans
c. Histoplasma d. Cryptococcus

67. Chandu 32 years male presents with abdominal pain and vomiting. He also complains of some psychiatric symptoms & visual hallucination. Most likely diagnosis is *[All India PGMEE 2001]*
a. Hypothyroidism b. Hyperthyroidism
c. Hysteria d. Intermittent porphyria

68. Porphyria cutanea tarda can be treated by *[All India PGMEE 1998]*
a. Phlebotomy b. Heme
c. Low dose chloroquine d. Metronidazole

69. Non palpable purpura is seen in all except *[AIIMS PGMEE 1994]*
a. H.S. Purpura
b. Drug unduced vasculitis
c. Idiopathic thrombocytopenic purpura
d. Amyloid

70. Palpable purpura is seen in all except *[PGI 1999]*
a. Wegeners GN b. ITP
c. HSP d. Serum sickness

71. Treatment of Kawasaki's disease is *[AIIMS PGMEE 1999]*
a. IVIg b. Steroids
c. Thalidomide d. Dapsone

72. Lisch nodule is seen in *[PGI 1999]*
a. Von Reclinghausens disease
b. Lupus vulgaris
c. Leprosy
d. LGV

73. Wood's lamp filter is made of *[AIIMS PGMEE 1999] [PGI 2000]*
a. Tin and chromium oxide
b. Nickel oxide and silica
c. Copper oxide and Barium oxide
d. Zinc oxide

74. Defective DNA repair is associated *[AIIMS PGMEE 2009]*
a. Albinism b. Xeroderma pigmentosa
c. Vitiligo d. Ichthyosis

75. Neurofibromatosis all is true except *[AIIMS PGMEE 2009]*
a. Autosomal recessive
b. Scoliosis
c. Neurofibroma
d. Association with cataract

76. Child with history of hypopigmented macule on back, infantile spasm and delayed milestone has *[AIIMS PGMEE 1993]*
a. Neurofibromatosis b. Sturge weber syndrome
c. Tuberous sclerosis d. Nevus anemicus

77. Koenen's periungual fibromas are seen in > 50% of cases with *[JIPMER PGMEE 2002]*
a. Tuberous sclerosis b. Sturge Weber syndrome
c. Alaxia telangiectasia d. Neurofibromatosis

78. Crocodile skin or Sauroderma is seen in *[AIIMS PGMEE 1996]*
a. Toxic epidermal necrolysis
b. Psoriasis
c. Darier's disease
d. Ichthyosis vulgaris

79. Ichthyosis is associated with *[UP PGMEE 2006] [Karnataka PGMEE 1996]*
a. Hodgkins disease b. AIDS
c. Hypothyroidism d. All

80. Ichthyosis is caused by *[Bihar PGMEE 2006] [NIMHANS 2001]*
a. Hemosiderosis
b. Refsum disease
c. Niacin deficiency
d. Steven Johnson syndrome

81. Recurrent oral ulcers with pain and erythematous halo around them, diagnosis is *[AIIMS PGMEE 1996]*
a. Apthous ulcer b. Herpes
c. Chicken pox d. Measels

82. Shagreen patch is usually found in *[DPG 2007]*
a. Face b. Cervical region
c. Limbs d. Lambosacral region

83. Commonest fungal infection of the female genitalia in diabetes is *[Karnataka PGMEE 1998]*
a. Cryptococcal b. Madura mycosis
c. Candida d. Aspergillosis

84. Erythema toxicum in a neonate indicates *[PGI 1996]*
a. Staphylococcal sepsis b. Pneumococcemia
c. Drug hypersensitivity d. Is not of any significance

85. Wavelength of light produced by wood's Lamp is *[PGI 1999, AIIMS PGMEE 2001]*
a. 320 nm b. 360 nm
c. 400 nm d. 480 nm
e. 760-800 nm

86. Coral red fluorescence wood's Lamp seen in *[PGI 1998] [AIIMS PGMEE 2000]*
a. Porphyria cutanea tarda b. Erythrasma
c. Livedo-reticularis d. Hypomelanosis

87. A pinkish red Fluorescence of urine with Wood's lamp is seen in *[JIPMER PGMEE 1999, PGI 2000]*
a. Lead poisoning b. Porphyria cutanea tarda
c. Erythromelagia d. Acrocyanosis

NEET/NBE PATTERN MCQs ANSWERS WITH EXPLANATIONS

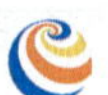

1. **Ans. (a) Salicylate Poisoning**
   [Ref. Clinical Dermatology by Habif, 6/e p714]

Erythema Nodosum

- MC panniculitis
- Raised, painful, bilateral, tender lesions located over both shins
- Lesions may coalesce and resemble cellulitis
- Causes:
  - Infections (Streptococci, Tuberculosis, Coccidioidomycosis)
  - Drugs (Sulfonamides, Oral contraceptives)
  - Systemic illness (Sarcoidosis, Ulcerative colitis, Crohn's disease, Lymphoma Leukemia)
  - Pregnancy

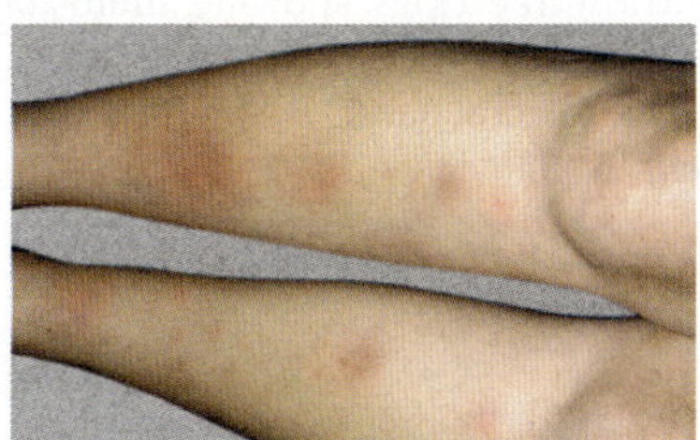

Fig. Erythema nodosum

2. **Ans. (c) It is called the flea-bitten rash of new born**
   [Ref. Clinical Dermatology by Habif, 6/e p672; Dermatology by Falco, 2/e p702]

Erythema Toxicum Neonatorum

- Common short-lived erythematous eruption of newborn in first 2 days of life; usually presents 24–48 hours
- Occurrence: 30–50% of newborns develop ETN
  - Flea bitten rash of newborn: Widespread erythematous macules, coalesce to become urticarial pustules
  - Rash often begins on the face; the trunk, proximal extremities, and buttocks are commonly involved
  - Palms and soles are not affected
  - Four types of lesions occur: Macules, Wheals, Papules, and Pustules
- Underlying cause: Transition from watery womb to dry external environment
- Treatment generally not required, Zinc oxide lotion may be used

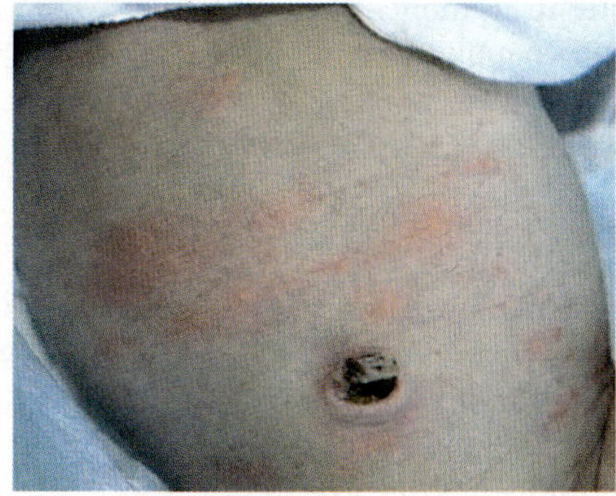

Fig. ETN

3. **Ans. (d) Blue white**
   [Ref. DVL by Thappa, 4/e p34,57]

Blue White Fluorescence on Wood's Lamp Examination

- Tuberous sclerosis
- Leprosy
- Albinism

4. **Ans. (c) Hyperthyroidism**
   [Ref. DVL by Thappa, 4/e p271,272]
   - Hyperthyroidism is a hypermetabolic state
   - Typical features include:
   - Pretibial myxedema, pink or skin colored nodules called as **"peau d' orange" appearance** with velvety skin appearance, hyperpigmentation
   - Other features include Plummer's nail, thinning of hair

5. **Ans. (d) Acantholysis**
   [Ref. Osteomyelitis of the Jaws by Baltensperger, 1/e p44]

SAPHO Syndrome

- Acronym for the combination of Synovitis, Acne, Pustulosis, Hyperostosis, and Osteitis
- Chronic disorder that involves the skin, bone, and joints
- Some researchers feel that the SAPHO syndrome is related to the group of arthritis conditions which typically affect the spine, called Spondyloarthropathies
- Treatment typically involves medications which reduce inflammation

6. **Ans. (a) Psoriasis**
   [Ref. Clinical Dermatology by Habif, 6/e p294]
   - **Nail pitting** is the best known and possibly the most frequent psoriatic nail abnormality.
   - Nail plate cells are shed in much the same way as psoriatic scale is shed, leaving a variable number of tiny, punched-out depressions on the nail plate surface
   - They emerge from under the cuticle and grow out with the nail
   - Many other cutaneous diseases may cause pitting (e.g., eczema, fungal infections, and alopecia areata), or it may occur as an isolated finding as a normal variation

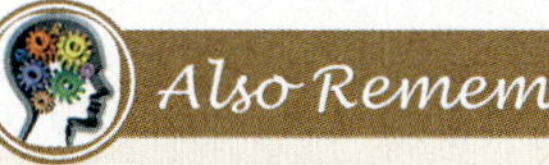

Nails [Mnemonic: The Only Drug Of Psoriasis is Topical Steroids]

- **T**hickened nail-plates
- **O**il-spots/ Oil-drop sign
- **D**ystrophy, **D**iscolouration
- **O**nycholysis
- **P**itting
- **T**himble-pitting
- **S**ubungual hyperkeratosis

7. **Ans. (d) Psoriasis**
   [Ref. Neena Khanna, 4/e p15]
   - *Interpretation of light colours emitted on Wood's Lamp examination*:

Colour	Interpretation
Brilliant green	Tinea capitis
Dull yellow	Pityriasis versicolor
Coral pink/ red	Erythrasma
White	Vitiligo
Blue-white	Tuberous sclerosis
Pale blue-green	Pseudomonas infection
Pinkish-red (Urine)	Porphyrea cutanea tarda
Orange	Acne (Propionibacterium acne)

8. Ans. (c) Psoriasis

[Ref. Neena Khanna, 5/e p53]

- Epidermal changes in skin biopsy of Psoriasis patient: Collection of polyps in parakeratotic Statum corneum (Munro's microabscess) and accumulation of neutrophils within a spongiotic pustule in spinous layer (Spongioform pustule of Kajog).
- Diagnostic clue for psoriasis:
  - Incidence in early 3rd decade or in 5th mid decade
  - **Silver white scales** (due to air trapped)
  - Demonstration of Auspitz sign

9. Ans. (c) Hyperthyroidism

[Ref. Skin Disease in Old Age by Marks, 2/e p230]

Ichthyosis

- Acquired ichthyosis appears in adult life
- Associated Systemic Diseases:
  - Underactive thyroid
  - Sarcoidosis
  - Hodgkin lymphoma
  - Cancer (ichthyosis may be a cutaneous marker of internal malignancy)
  - HIV infection
  - Leprosy
- Ichthyosis provoking medications:
  - Nicotinic acid
  - Kava
  - Targeted cancer therapy (e.g. vemurafenib, EGFR and protein kinase inhibitors)
  - Hydroxyurea

10. Ans. (d) Lichen sclerosus

[Ref. Neena Khanna, 5/e p45; Differential Diagnosis in Dermatology by Ashton,3/e p179]

- Koebner's phenomenon or Isomorphic phenomenon: New lesions of the original disease developing at sites of trauma (scratches, surgical incisions, & injury) and indicates active disease
  - Psoriasis
  - Lichen planus
  - Vitiligo
  - Plane warts

11. Ans. (d) Leuconychia

[Ref. Snapshots in Dermatology by Sacchidanand, 1/e p365]

- Total leukonychia may be due to hypoalbuminemia, familial or drug induced
- Subtotal leukonychia
  - Punctuate: MC type viz. alopecia, trauma
  - Striate: Due to manicure (gift spots)
  - Transverse: Arsenic and thallium poisoning

12. Ans. (d) Psoriasis

[Ref. Neena Khanna, 5/e p79]

- Nikolksy's sign: Application of tangential pressure on normal skin (usually in pretibial area) results in formation of new bulla.
  - Pemphigus vulgaris
  - Staphylococcal scalded skin syndrome
  - Epidermal necrolysis

13. Ans. (b) Erythema multiforme

[Ref. Neena Khanna, 4/e p175]

Erythema Multiforme

- *Underlying cause*: Herpes simplex virus
- *Clinical presentation*: *Target/ Iris/ Bull's-eye lesion* (Concentric three rings showing multi-forms - vesicles, macules, papules, bullae)
- *Sites*: Face and acral parts
- *Treatment*: Acyclovir

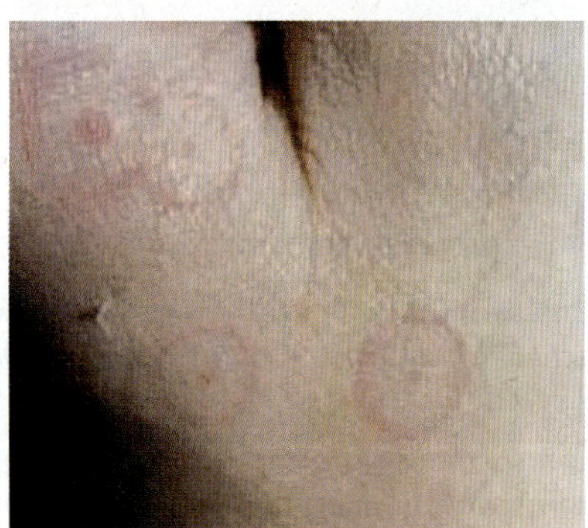

Fig. Target lesion

14. Ans. (d) Behcet's syndrome

[Ref. Neena Khanna, 5/e p203]

Behcet's Syndrome

- Mucocutaneous features: recurrent, persistant, extensive, oral & genital aphthae
- Systemic feature: arthritis, ophthalmological & neurological manifestation

15. Ans. (b) Dermatomyositis

[Ref. Neena Khanna, 4/e p228]

Clinical Presentation of Dermatomyositis

- Heliotrope Erythema
- Gottron's papules
- Gottron's sign
- Poikiloderma
- Shawl sign
- Mechanic's hand
- Cacinosis cutis
- Systemic manifestations: Myositis (Weakness of proximal muscles), Difficulty in speech and swallowing, Cardiomyopathy, Reynaud's phenomenon, Arthralgia, Carcinoma lungs/ ovaries/ breasts

16. Ans. (c) Addison's disease

[Ref. Nail Therapies by Baran, 1/e p69]

Onycholysis

- Psoriasis, Dermatitis, Pemphigus vulgaris, Porphyria cutanea tarda
- Dermatophyte fungus (i.e., Trichophyton rubrum, T. mentagrophytes infection), Yeast (Candida infection), Bacteria (Pseudomonas infection), Virus (Herpes simplex infection)
- Internal disease: Amyloid and multiple myeloma, Anaemia (iron deficiency), Diabetes mellitus, Erythropoietic porphyria, Hyperhidrosis, Hyperthyroidism, Hypothyroidism, Impaired peripheral circulation, Leprosy, Pellagra, Psoriatic arthritis, Reiter syndrome, Sarcoidosis, Scleroderma, Yellow nail syndrome due to chronic lung or sinus disease
- Drugs: Tetracyclines, Psoralens, Fluoroquinolone antibiotics, Chlorpromazine, Oral contraceptives
- Others: Congenital onycholysis, Hereditary partial onycholysis, Idiopathic acquired onycholysis, Hereditary distal onycholysis, Foreign body implantation, Contact allergy to nail glue (acrylate)

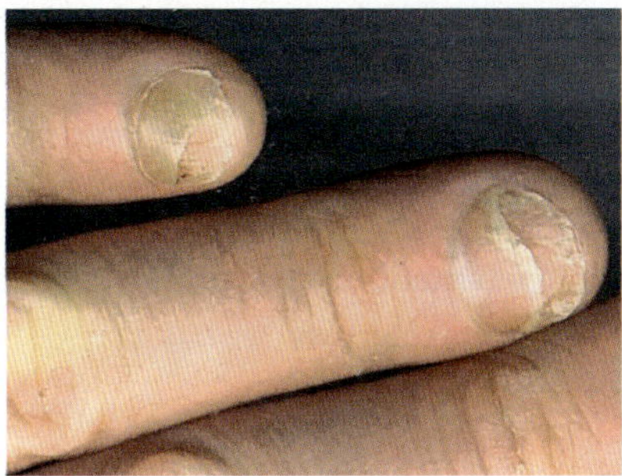

Fig. Onycholysis

17. Ans. (a) Atopy

[Ref. Skin Immune System (SIS) by Bos, 2/e p499]

- In atopic dermatitis, characteristic is the increased total serum IgE and the increased frequency of type I allergies to environmental allergens

18. Ans. (b) DLE

[Ref. Sure Success in PGMEE by Ramgopal, 1/e p181-182]

Disorders of nails	Disease condition(s) responsible
Onycholysis	Hyperthyroidism, Psoriasis, Fungal infections
Koilonychia	Iron deficiency anaemia, Syphilis, Ischaemic heart disease
Splinter haemorrhages	Trauma, Nail psoriasis, Subacute bacterial endocarditis
Pterygium of nails	Lichen planus, Idiopathic
Half-and-half nails	Chronic renal failure
Pitting of nails	Psoriasis, Alopecia areata, Hand eczema
Beau's lines	Acute systemic illnesses
Terry's nails	Cirrhosis
Hippocratic nails	Clubbing of nails
Mee's lines on nails	Chronic arsenic poisoning, Hypoalbuminemia
Hyperpigmentation of nails	Zidovudine, Mephalan, Daunorubicin, Bleomycin
Blue nails	Chloroquine, Wilson's disease, Subungal hematoma
Yellow nail syndrome	Pleural effusion, Sinusitis, Ankle oedema
Nail fold telangiectasia	Dermatomyositis

Contd...

Contd...

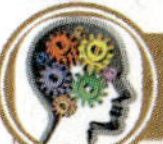

Also Remember

- DLE lesions are generally seen on sun-exposed areas of face and scalp especially near external ear

19. Ans. (c) Erythema of light exposed area

[Ref. Neena Khanna, 5/e p237]

- Malar rash/ butterfly rash (in the form of erythema and edema) with characteristic sparing of nasolabial folds & with photosensitivity is SLE specific lesion

20. Ans. (d) All of the above

[Ref. Neena Khanna, 5/e p79]

- **Acantholysis** is the loss of intercellular connections, such as desmosomes, resulting in loss of cohesion between keratinocytes, seen in diseases such as pemphigus vulgaris
- This histological feature is also seen in herpes simplex infections (HSV 1 and 2) and Vericella zoster infections (Chicken pox and Shingles) and Impetigo
- It is absent in bullous pemphigoid, making it useful for differential diagnosis

21. Ans. (a) Lichen planus (c) Psoriasis

[Ref. Neena Khanna, 5/e p45] & Differential Diagnosis in Dermatology by Richard Ashton,3/e p179]

22. Ans. (d) Melanotic spots

[Ref. Neena Khanna, 5/e p34; Harrison's, 17/e p325]

- Melanotic spots or Ash leaf macules is the earliest sign of tuberous sclerosis and often are present at birth

23. Ans. (a) Convulsions

24. Ans. (a) SLE

[Ref. Neena Khanna, 4/e p224]

Cutaneous Manifestations of SLE

- *Lupus erythematous specific lesions*:
  - *'Butterfly rash'* on malar area and nose
  - Papulo-squamous lesions of photo-exposed parts
  - Photosensitivity
- *Non-specific lesions*:
  - Vasculitis
  - Periungal telangiectasia
  - Reynaud's phenomena
  - Sclerodactyly
  - Oral ulcers
  - Alopecia (Lupus hair)

25. Ans. (a) 360–385

[Ref. Seidel's Guide to Physical Examination By Jane W. Ball, 8/e p48]

- The Wood's lamp contains a light source with a wavelength of 360 nm
- This is the black light that causes certain substances to fluoresce
- It is used primarily to determine the presence of fungi on skin lesions

26. Ans. (b) DLE

[Ref. Neena Khanna, 5/e p233]

- Lesions are seen predominantly on the sun-exposed areas of face, on scalp and characteristically in external ear
- In disseminated DLE, lesions occur below the neck (dorsolateral aspect of forearms, dorsae of hands, trunk and sometimes on the lower extremities)

27. Ans. (a) NF

[Ref. Neena Khanna, 5/e p36]

- Presence of ≥ 6 CALMs (Café-au-lait macules) is diagnostic of NF1
- CALMs: Oval, uniformly pigmented (light brown), macules with smooth margin

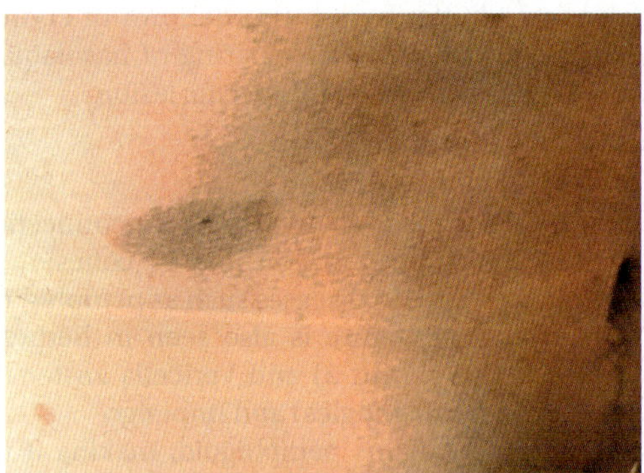

Fig. Cafe-au-lait

28. Ans. (a) Psoriasis

[Ref. Neena Khanna, 5/e p46]

- On scraping the psoriatic lesion, a glistening white adherent membrane appears (Berkley's membrane)

29. Ans. (b) Alopecia areata

[Ref. Neena Khanna, 5/e p143]

- Pitting and thinning of nail plates are seen associated in alopecia areata
- Lunula may be mottled
- Sometimes all 20 nails are affected (trachyonychia)

30. Ans. (d) Tuberous sclerosis

[Ref. Harrison's Principles of Internal Medicine by Anthony Fauci, 17/e p325]

- In tuberous sclerosis, the earliest cutaneous sign is an ash leaf spot
- These lesions are often present at birth and are usually multiple; however, detection may require Wood's lamp examination, especially in fair skinned individuals

31. Ans. (d) Lichen simplex chronicus

[Ref. Neena Khanna, 5/e p45; Differential Diagnosis in Dermatology by Ashton,3/e p179]

32. Ans. (a) Subcutaneous nodules

[Ref. Neena Khanna, 5/e p48]

Characteristic of Reiter's Syndrome

- HLA B27 positivity
- Sexually transmitted
- Arthritis
- Iridocyclitis & conjunctivitis
- Mucocutaneous lesions: Rupoid psoriasis, /Keratoderma blennorrhagicum (crusted, exudative plaques on palms and soles) and Circinate balanitis

33. Ans. (b) Delayed type hypersensitivity

[Ref. Neena Khanna, 5/e p15]

- Patch test detects antigens responsible for allergic contact dermatitis (type IV hypersensitivity/ delayed hypersensitivity)

34. Ans. (d) Psoriasis

[Ref. Neena Khanna, 5/e p45]

- Though leg is involved in psoriasis, ulcers are not seen

35. Ans. (c) Lichen planus

[Ref. Neena Khanna, 5/e p63]

- Both oral and genital mucosa are involved in Lichen planus

36. Ans. (b) Bullous pemphigoid

[Ref. Neena Khanna, 5/e p85]

37. Ans. (a) Behcet disease

[Ref. Neena Khanna, 5/e p203]

- Recurrent, persistent, extensive, oral & genital apthae

38. Ans. (d) Tuberous sclerosis

[Ref. Neena Khanna, 4/e p33]

Cutaneous Manifestations of Tuberous Sclerosis

- *Angiofibroma*:
  - Most common manifestation
  - Dome shaped papules with telangiectasia
  - Nose, Nasolabial folds and cheeks
- *Ash-leaf macules*:
  - Earliest manifestation
  - Hypopigmented macules on trunk
- *Shagreen patch*:
  - Leathery pig-skin like plaques
  - Lumbosacral area
- *Periungual fibromas/Koenen's tumour*:
  - Sausage type growth

Also Remember

- *Other systemic manifestations of Tuberous sclerosis*: Seizures, Hamartomas – Optic nerve/ retinal, Rhabdomyoma of heart, Angiomyolipomas of kidneys, Bony sclerosis (Skull, spine, pelvis), Mental retardation, Pigmentary anomalies in eyes

39. Ans. (a) Phlebotomy; (c) Low dose chloroquine

[Ref. Neena Khanna, 5/e p417]

Management of Porphyria Cutanea Tarda

- Avoidance of triggers like alcohol
- Treatment of HCV infection
- Venesection till Hb falls below 12 g/dL
- Low-dose therapy with hydroxychloroquine (100 mg twice a week)

40. Ans. (a) CPK
[Ref. Dubois' Lupus Erythematosus by Wallace, 7/e p651]

41. Ans. (b) Alopecia areata
[Ref. Neena Khanna, 5/e p143]

42. Ans. (b) IgG with compliments
[Ref. Neena Khanna, 5/e p240]

- In LE skin lesion , typically deposition of Ig G in a band like pattern at the dermoepidermal junction. IgM, IgA and C3 may also be found individually or together.

43. Ans. (a) Atopic dermatitis
[Ref. Lookingbill and Marks' Principles of Dermatology, 5/e p91]

- Atopic dermatitis have a characteristic expression
- The face has mild to moderate erythema, perioral pallor, and infraorbital folds (DennieMorgan lines) associated with dermatitis and hyperpigmentation

44. Ans. (b) Lichen planus
[Ref. Neena Khanna, 5/e p67]

Lichen Planus Histopathology

- Thickened granular layer
- Saw toothing of rete pegs
- Basal cell degeneration (leading to Max Joseph's spaces and colloid/Civatte body formation)
- Band like upper dermal infiltrate of lymphocytes

45. Ans. (c) No vesicle
[Ref. Neena Khanna, 5/e p187]

- In EM major, mucosal lesions consist of erythema and vesicles on buccal mucosa, plate and lips
- Vesicles rapidly evolve into painful erosions, which on lips are covered with haemorrhagic crusts

46. Ans. (c) Non-infectious
[Ref. Sexually Transmitted Diseases by Sehgal, 4/e p321]

- Late syphilis not infective are Gumma, neurosyphilis, cardiovascular syphilis.

47. Ans. (d) Salmon Rash
[Ref. Neena Khanna, 5/e p242-243]

Clinical Features of Dermatomyositis

- Itchy lesion
- Facial lesion's: Heliotrope erythema, malar erythema, oedema
- Gottron's papule: Violaceous, atrophic papules over knuckles and pressure points
- Gottron's sign: Symmetrical, somewhat linear, lilac papulosquamous plaques
- Telangiectasia and ragged cuticles
- Poikiloderma: Hyperpigmentation, hypopigmentation, telangiectasia and atrophy
- Mechanic's hand: Confluent symmetric hyperkeratosis along ulnar aspect of thumb and radial aspect of fingers
- Calcinosis cutis
- Shawl sign: Symmetrical confluent violaceous erythema extending from dorsolateral aspect of forearms and arms to deltoid region, shoulder and neck

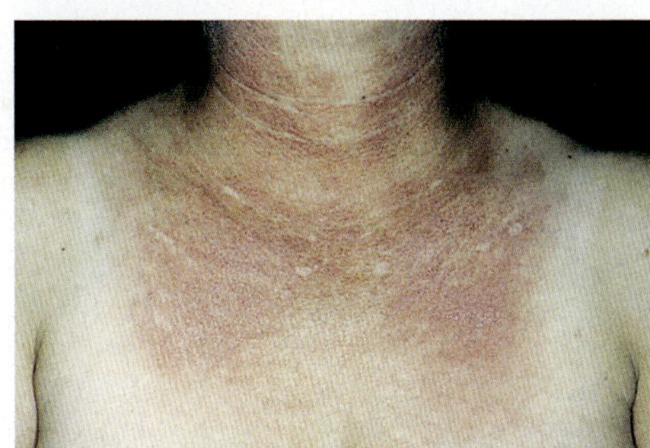

Fig. Dermatomyositis

48. Ans. (a) Lichen planus
[Ref. Neena Khanna, 5/e p65]

- Pterygium is diagnostic and is a manifestation of severe LP of nails
- The proximal fold is prolonged on to the nail bed, splitting and destroying nail plate

49. Ans. (c) Scleroderma
[Ref. Neena Khanna, 4/e p233]

Skin Manifestations of Scleroderma

- Raynaud's phenomenon (Most common and earliest symptom)
- Sclerodactyly and contractures in acral parts
- Mask-like features
- Beaking of nose
- Thinning of lips
- Radial furrowing around mouth
- Salt pepper dyschromatosis
- Calcinosis cutis
- Periungal telangiectasia

50. Ans. (a) Herpes simplex
[Ref. Andrews' Diseases of the Skin by James, 12/e p375]

- Up to 80% of varicella-zoster blistering lesions caused by herpes virus infections may be Tzanck smear positive

51. Ans. (c) 5000

52. Ans. (d) Nephrotic syndrome
[Ref. Nail Therapies by Robert Baran, 1/e p69]

53. Ans. (a) Lichen planus
[Ref. Neena Khanna, 5/e p65]

54. Ans. (b) Target lesions

55. Ans. (b) Endothelial cells
[Ref. Manson's Tropical Diseases by Jeremy Farrar, p280]

56. Ans. (d) Lichen planus
[Ref. Neena Khanna, 5/e p62]

Morphology of Lichen Planus

- Pruritic
- Polygonal
- Purple/ violaceous
- Plane (flat to plesion)
- Papules
- Wickham's stria on surface

57. Ans. (a) Apocrine sweat gland
[Ref. Neena Khanna, 4/e p127]

Disorders of Skin Appendages

Disorders of Sebaceous glands	Disorders of Nails
Acne vulgaris	Congenital disorders:
Rosacea	Paronychia congenital
Disorders of Eccrine sweat glands	Infective disorders
Hyperhidrosis	Onchomycosis
Hypohidrosis	Paronychia
Anhidrosis	Traumatic disorders
Miliaria	Splinter hemorrhages
Disorders of Apocrine glands	Subungal hematomas
Hidradentis suppurativa	Chronic injury
Disorders of Hair:	Nervous tics
Alopecia areata	Chemical injury
Androgenetic areata	Skin disorders
Miscellaneous alopecia	Psoriasis
Telogen effluvium	Lichen planus
Traction alopecia	Dermatitis
Cicatricial alopecia	Trachyonychia
Trichotillomania	Neoplastic disorders
Hirsutism	Systemic disorders
Hypertrichosis	

58. Ans. (d) Intertriginous freckling

[Ref. Goodheart's Photoguide to Common Skin Disorders, 3/e p493]

Tuberous Sclerosis

- *Classical triad of Tuberous sclerosis*:
  - Adenoma sebaceum
  - Epilepsy
  - Mental retardation
- *Classical skin lesions of Tuberous sclerosis*:
  - Shagreen patch
  - Ash leaf macules
  - Adenoma sebaceum
  - Koenen's tumors (Periungal fibromas)

59. Ans. (c) Bilateral acoustic neuromas

[Ref. Clinical Dermatology by Mann, 5/e p345]

Neurofibromatosis Type-1 (> 1 Criteria Required)

- Café au lait spots >5 mm in children, >15 mm in adults (Six or more)
- Cutaneous/ Subcutaneous neurofibroma (Six or more) OR Plexiform neurofibroma (One)
- Axillary/ groin freckling
- Optic pathway glioma
- Lisch nodules (Two or more)
- Bony dysplasia
- Relative (First degree) with NF-1

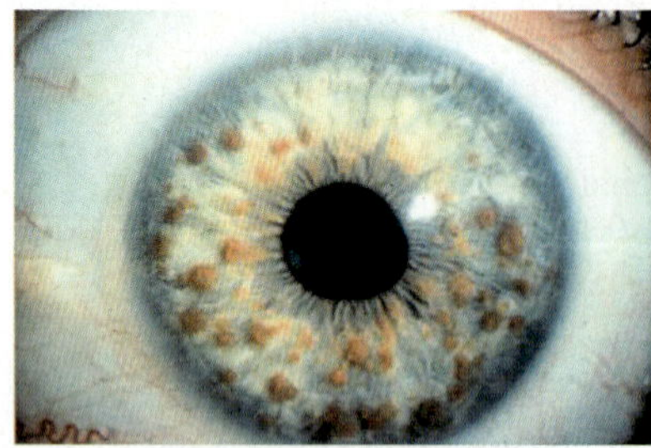

Fig. Lisch nodules

60. Ans. (d) SCID

[Ref. Surgical Pathology by Goldblum, 3/e p103]

Omenn Syndrome

- Autosomal recessive type of SCID with features of GVHD
- Hallmark: Expansion of Oligoclonal T-cells, Absence of B-cells
- Hypereosinophilia, Hypogammaglobulinemia
- Diffuse erythroderma, Diarrhoea, Hepatosplenomegaly, Lymphadenopathy, Alopecia, Failure to thrive

61. Ans. (d) Bourneville's disease

[Ref. Neale's Disorders of the Foot, 1/e p68]

Tuberous sclerosis complex (Epiloia, Bourneville disease)

- Cutaneous, mental retardation and epilepsy
- Skin problems: Facial angiofibromas (Adenoma sebaceum), Pigmented leathery lesions (Shagreen patches), Hypopigmented areas (Ash-leaf white macules) and Periungal fibromas (Koenen's tumours)
- Koenen's periungual fibromas are recurrent, friable, paronycnial lesions

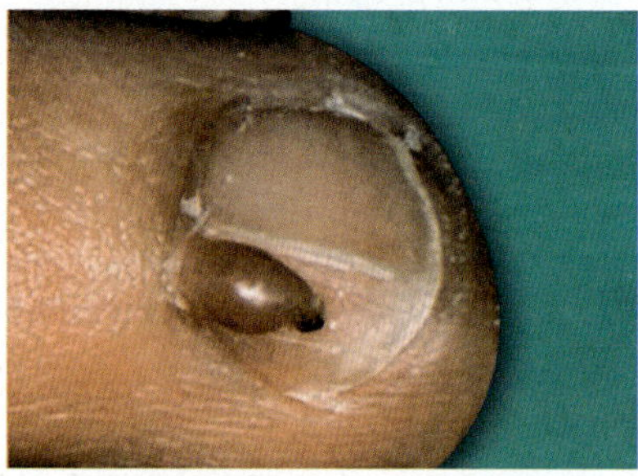

Fig. Koenen's tumor

62. Ans. (b) Leprosy

[Ref. Dermatologic Therapeutics by Arndt, 7/e p257]

- Wood's lamp examination for screening purposes
- Useful for Vitiligo, Albinism, Leprosy, and other disorders of hypopigmentation
- Also useful for Fungal infections, Bacterial infections, Scalp ringworm
- Wood's lamp can be helpful in demonstrating that the lesions in leprosy and tinea are hypopigmented and not depigmented as in vitiligo

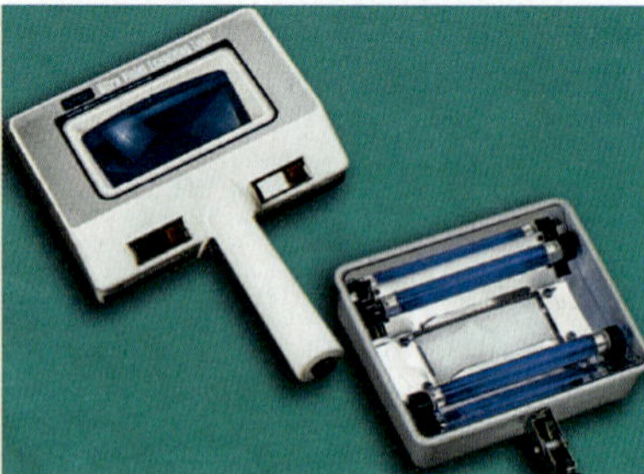

Fig. Wood's lamp

63. Ans. (a) Idiopathic

[Ref. NMS Medicine, 7/e p611]

Erythema Multiforme

- Approximately 50% of cases are idiopathic; no underlying cause is identified

- Infection: MCC infectious (viral, bacterial, and fungal); Herpes simplex virus (HSV) is MC infectious etiology

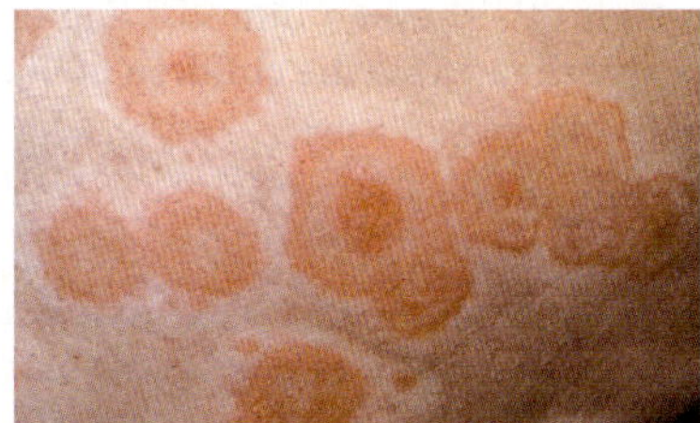

Fig. Erythema multiforme

64. Ans. (d) Tuberous sclerosis

[Ref. Retina E-Book by Ryan, 5/e p2161]

- Skin lesion formerly believed to be pathognomonic for Tuberous sclerosis is the hypopigmented macule or patch
- These lesions are variable in shape, with only an occasional one justifying the term Ash-leaf sign
- Often present at birth, this is the first clinical sign of disease

Fig. Ash-leaf spot

65. Ans. (a) Distal and lateral subungual

[Ref. Medical Mycology by Razzaghi-Abyaneh, 1/e p32]

- Main subtypes of Onychomycosis are Distal lateral subungual, Proximal subungual, Superficial, Endonyx, Mixed pattern, Totally dystrophic and Secondary onychomycosis
- Distal lateral subungual onychomycosis (DLSO) is the most common presentation
- DLSO commences when the organism infects the cornified layer of the hyponychium and distal or lateral nail bed
- This is followed by proximal invasion of the nail bed and ventral invasion of nail plate

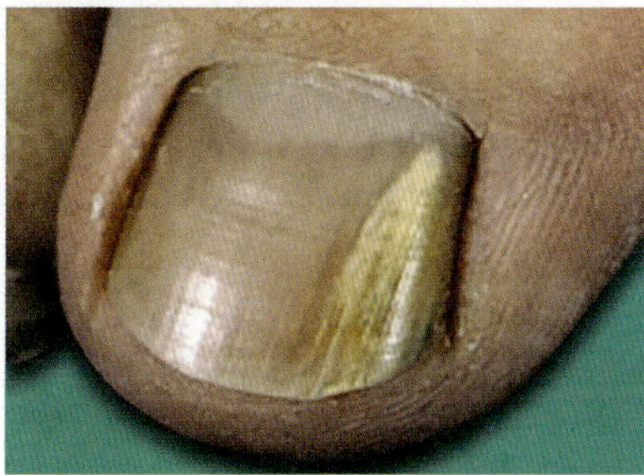

Fig. DLSO

66. Ans. (d) Groove sign

[Ref. Dermatology by Bolognia, 4/e fig42.5]

- Photodistributed poikiloderma is very characteristic of Dermatomyositis, often involving the upper chest **(V-neck sign)** and the upper back **(Shawl sign)**
- Poikiloderma can also affect photoprotected areas, such as the lateral thigh, referred to as the **Holster sign**

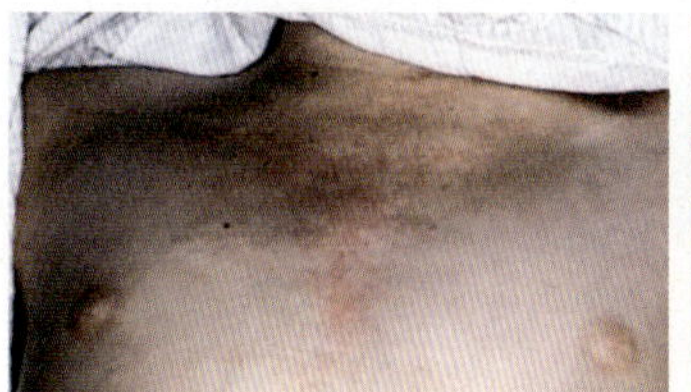

Fig. V-sign

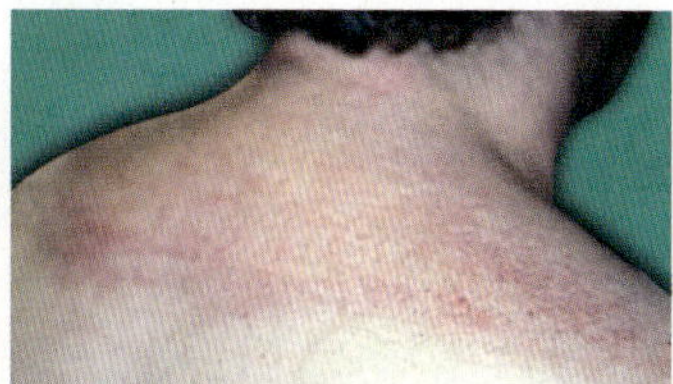

Fig. Shawl sign

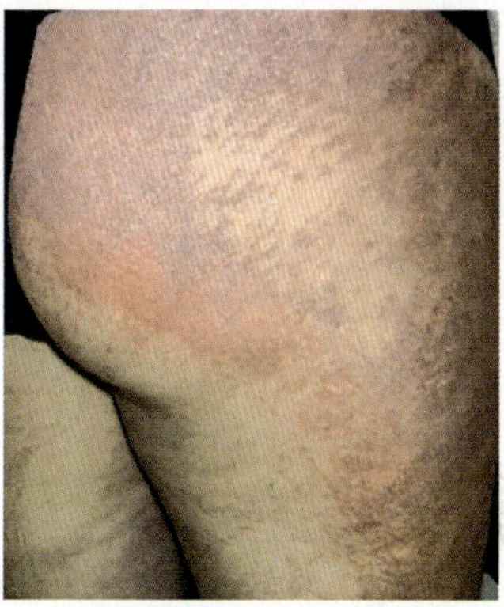

Fig. Holster sign

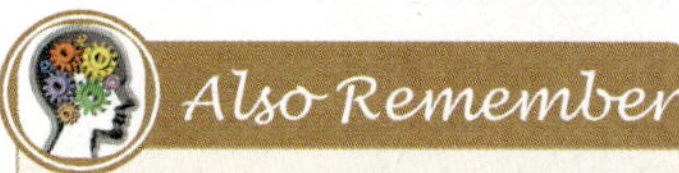

Also Remember

Groove Sign

- Lymphogranuloma Venerum (LGV) is mainly a disease of lymphatic tissue that spreads to tissue surrounding lymphatics
- Lymphadenopathy: Painful inguinal bubo, Multilocular, when palpated groove is formed called as Groove sign

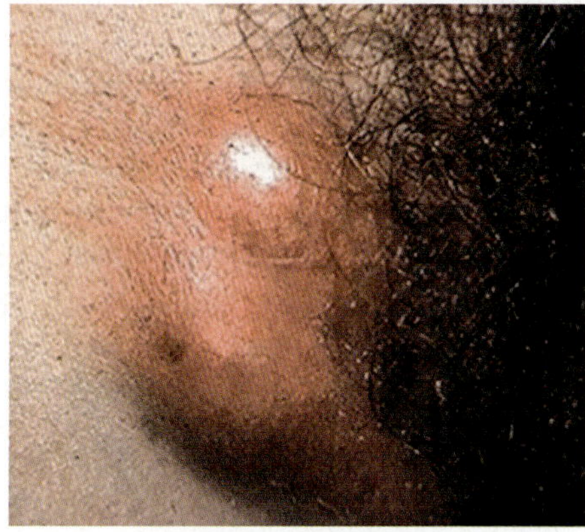

Fig. Groove sign

67. Ans. (b) Ill-fitting shoes

[Ref. Encyclopedia of Sports Medicine - Volume 1 by Micheli, 1/e p712]

Ingrown Toenails

- An ingrown toenail curves under on one or both sides and cuts into the surrounding skin, causing inflammation and sometimes infection
- Most commonly affects the big toe

- Causes: Poorly fitting shoes (MC reason), Hyperhidrosis (excessive sweating), Improper nail trimming, Nail shape and length

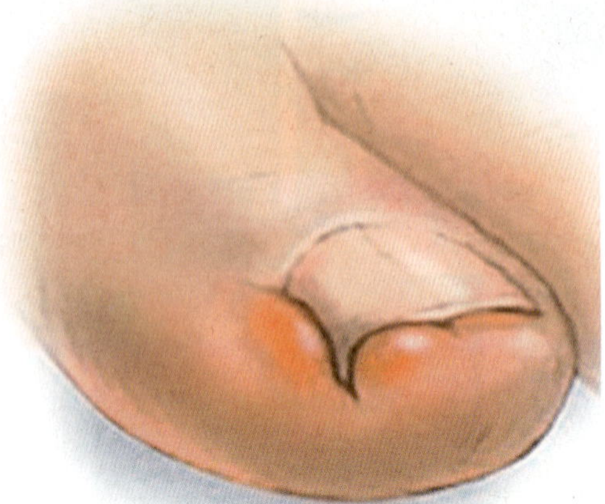

Fig. Ingrown toenail

68. Ans. (b) Bimodal age distribution

[Ref. Neuromuscular Diseases by Swash, 3/e p286]

- Dermatomyositis shows a bimodal age distribution, with peak incidence rates for the children at 5–14 years age and for adults at 45–64 years age

69. Ans. (b) Dermatomyositis

[Ref. Neena Khanna, 4/e p228]

- Heliotrope erythema: Faint lilac erythema peri-orbitally usually associated with edema in a case of Dermatomyositis

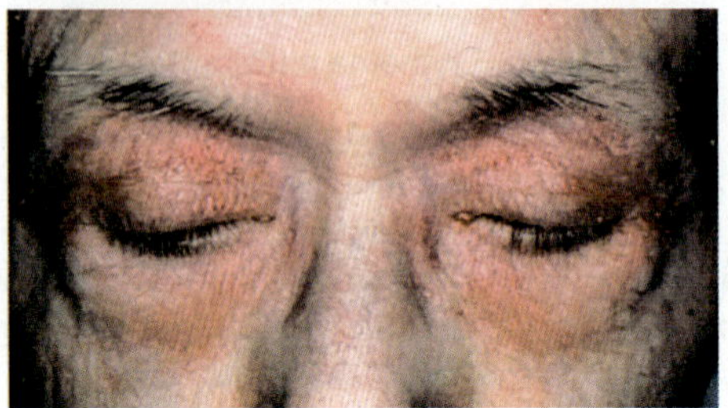

Fig. Dermatomyositis (Helitrope rash)

HIGH YIELD MCQs ANSWERS WITH EXPLANATIONS 

1. Ans. (d) Koilonychia in Megaloblastic Anemia (B12 deficiency)

[Ref. Illustrated Manual of Nursing Practice, 3/e p964]

- Koilonychia (spoon nail) is classically associated with Iron-deficiency hypochromic anemia or Plummer Vinson syndrome
- Platyonychia (abnormally broad or flat nails) may precede koilonychia development

2. Ans. (d) DLE

[Ref. Neena Khanna, 5/e p233]

- Lesions are seen predominantly on the sun-exposed areas of face, on scalp and characteristically in external ear
- In disseminated DLE, lesions occur below the neck (dorsolateral aspect of forearms, dorsae of hands, trunk and sometimes on the lower extremities)

3. Ans. (d) Mucous membrane is usually involved

[Ref. Neena Khanna, 5/e p187]

4. Ans. (c) Reiter's disease

[Ref. Neena Khanna, 5/e p48]

5. Ans. (a) Tuberous sclerosis

[Ref. Neena Khanna, 5/e p34]

Periungual Fibroma (Koenen's Tumor)

- Present in 20% of patient
- Develop in Adult life
- Small, sausage -shaped, pink growths arising from under the nail folds

6. Ans. (c) Nevus achromicus

[Ref. Neena Khanna, 5/e p164]

7. Ans. (b) Reiter's syndrome

[Ref. Neena Khanna, 5/e p48]

8. Ans. (e) Nevus anemicus

[Ref. Differential Diagnosis in Pediatric Dermatology by Ernesto Bonifazi, 1/e p26]

- Nevus anemicus manifests itself as a white spot from the earliest stages of life

9. Ans. (a) Slit lamp examination of eye

[Ref. Neena Khanna, 5/e p37]

Investigation Suggested for Neurofibromatosis 1

- Evaluation of IQ
- Ophthalmological examination of eyes for Lisch nodules (by slit lamp) and optic pathway tumors (visual acuity, colour vision, perimetry and fundoscopy)
- X-ray skull/ spine

10. Ans. (a) Chicken pox

[Ref. Weedon's Skin Pathology by Patterson, 1/e p727]

- A Tzanck smear of a vesicle scraping would show multinucleated cells if the rash is due to varicella or herpes simplex virus

11. Ans. (b) SLE; (c) Pemphigus

[Ref. The Washington Manual of Surgical Pathology by Humphrey, 1/e p689]

12. Ans. (a) Viral

[Ref. Neena Khanna, 5/e p186]

- Most commonly by HSV and less commonly by M. pneumonia (over all idiopathic MC)

13. Ans. (b) Tuberous sclerosis

[Ref. Neena Khanna, 5/e p34]

- Tuberous sclerosis complex: Classical triad of,
- Epilepsy
- Mental deficiency
- Adenoma sebaceum

14. Ans. (c) Patch test
[Ref. Neena Khanna, 5/e p99]
- The patient in suffering from photoallergic contact dermatitis
- Patient develops a reaction if exposed to antigen & ultraviolet rays and not when exposed to either
- Photopatch test is done to establish diagnosis and determine the cause

15. Ans. (d) Porphyria cutanea tarda
[Ref. Neena Khanna, 5/e p417]
- The farmer has porphyria, skin manifestations (photosensitivity) and no neurological component
- As mainly skin manifestation, the diagnosis will be porphyria cutanea tarda

16. Ans. (a) Acute intermittent porphyria
[Ref. Harrison's, 18/e p3177-3180]
- History of sulfonamides and acute presentation of abdominal pain and seizures hint towards Acute intermittent porphyria

17. Ans. (b) Tuberous sclerosis
[Ref. Neena Khanna, 5/e p34]

18. Ans. (c) Beta carotene
[Ref. Emery and Rimoin's Essential Medical Genetics, 1/e p391]
- Mainstay of management of cutaneous porphyrias: Avoiding sunlight exposure and use of protective clothing
- In erythropoietic protoporphyria (EPP), Oral beta-carotene may improve tolerance to sunlight in some patients
- Orally administered beta-carotene may improve symptoms when used over a period of 3-6 months by scavenging reactive oxygen species, but results are variable

19. Ans. (d) Liver and Bone marrow
[Ref. Neena Khanna, 5/e p415]

20. Ans. (c) Giant cell arteritis
[Ref. Textbook of Pathology by V. Krishna, 1/e p544]

Palpable Purpura
- Description: Purpura, which constitutes visible non-blanching hemorrhages, are raised and able to be touched or felt upon palpation
- Causes
  - Rocky mountain spotted fever
  - Acute meningococcemia
  - Disseminated gonococcal infection
  - Ecthyma gangrenosum
  - Henoch Schonlein purpura
  - Polyarteritis nodosa
  - Leucocytoclastic vasculitis
  - Microscopic polyangiitis
  - Mixed Essential Cryoglobulinemia
  - Drug induced allergic vasculitis

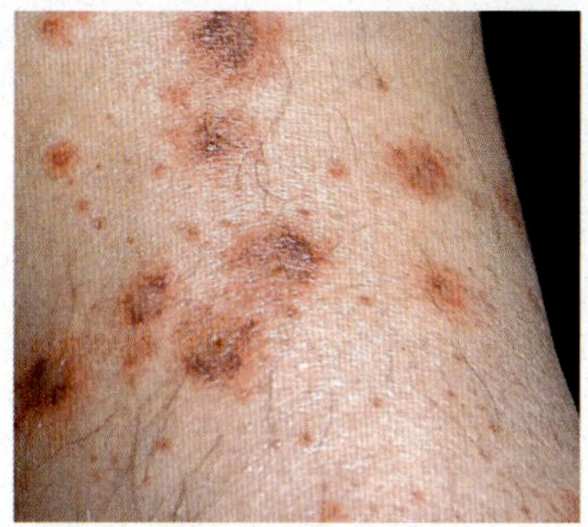

Fig. Palpable purpura

21. Ans. (c) Café au lait macules exclude the diagnosis
[Ref. Dermatology Essentials by Duncan, 1/e p444]
- Café au lait macules are seen in few cases of Tuberous sclerosis and usually is one if present

22. Ans. (a) Psoriasis of nails
[Ref. Neena Khanna, 5/e p50]

Nail Changes In Psoriasis
- 10–50% patient have nail involvement
- Pitting-deep, irregular
- Nail plate thickening
- Subungal hyperkeratosis
- Discolouration and dystrophy of nail plate—nail plate becomes yellow or brown or dysmorphic
- Oncholysis
- Oil spots: Yellow red discolouration in center of nail

23. Ans. (b) Nail plate
[Ref. Neena Khanna, 5/e p306]
- In tinea unguium, nail plate is involved
- Yellow brown discolouration and thickening of nail plate which crumbles easily and so appears tunneled

24. Ans. (b) HSP
[Ref. Neena Khanna, 5/e p196]

HSP is Characterized by Triad of
- Palpable purpura
- Arthritis
- Abdominal pain

25. Ans. (d) Back
[Ref. Neena Khanna, 5/e p251]
- Sites of morphea: Upper trunk (MC), buttocks & legs
- Linear lesions on extremities & face (en coupde sabre)

26. Ans. (b) Indeterminate leprosy
[Ref. Neena Khanna, 5/e p274]
- Indeterminate leprosy to be suspected if macule (ill defined, atrophic, hypoasthetic/normoanaesthetic, hypopigmented or slightly erythematous) seen on face of children from endemic areas

27. All choices

28. Ans. (c) Tumor necrosis factor-alpha
[Ref. Cecil Textbook of medicine, Volume 2, 21/e p1734]
- Both ENL and reversal reactions can occur before, during, and after the completion of antimycobacterial treatment for leprosy

- Tumor necrosis factor–alpha and other pro-inflammatory and anti- inflammatory cytokines are considered key mediators in these reactional states

29. Ans. (a) Lichen planus
[Ref. Neena Khanna, 5/e p64]

30. Ans. (c) Henoch Schonlein purpura
[Ref. Neena Khanna, 5/e p196]

31. Ans. (c) Thrombocytopenia
[Ref. Neena Khanna, 5/e p196]

32. Ans. (b) Steroids best treat skin lesions; (e) Purpura fulminans
[Ref. Neena Khanna, 5/e p196]

33. Ans. (a) P. versicolor; (b) Vitiligo; (c) Porphyria
[Ref. Neena Khanna, 5/e p13]

Wood Lamp is used in

- Disorders of epidermal pigmentation: Vitiligo, Ash leaf macule of TSC, Melasma, Post-inflammatory pigmentation
- Infections:
  - Tinea capitis: Green
  - Pityriasis versicolor: Yellow
  - Malassezia folliculitis: Bluish-white
  - Trichophyton schoenleinii: Dull blue
  - M canis, M audouinii, M ferrugineum, M distortum: Blue green
- Porphyria: Red-pink
- Others: Erythrasma Corynebacteria: Coral-pink color

34. Ans. (c) Kawasaki syndrome
[Ref. Neena Khanna, 5/e p300]

Kawasaki Syndrome

- Occurs in childhood
- Fever of 5 or more days without other explanation
- Plus 4 of 5 of the following criteria
  - Bilateral, painless, non-exudative conjunctival injection
  - Oropharyngeal lesions, fissured lips, red pharynx, strawberry tongue
  - Erythema and edema of acral parts and periungual desquamation
  - Polymorphous exanthem
  - Acute, nonsuppurative, large (>15 mm) cervical lymphadenopathy

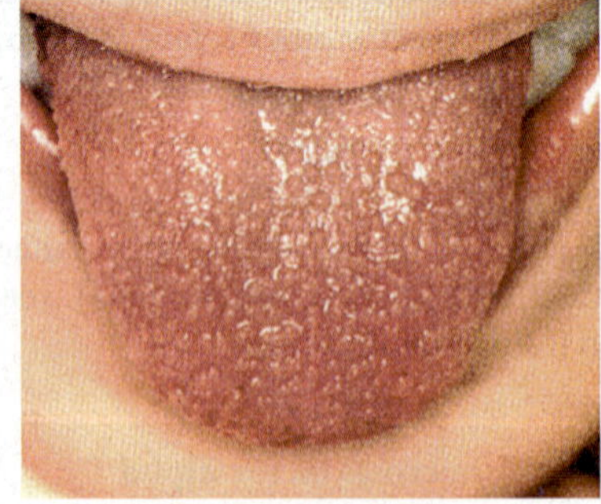

Fig. Strawberry tongue

35. Ans. (b) Chronic Arsenic poisoning
[Ref. Neena Khanna, 5/e p388]

Chronic arsenic poisoning as protean manifestation

- Arsenic keratoses
- Raindrop pigmentation
- Bowen's disease
- Mee's line in nail
- Visceral neoplasm

36. Ans. (d) All
[Ref. Neena Khanna, 5/e p13]

37. Ans. (a) Darrier's disease; (d) Boweli's disease; (e) Hailey-Hailey disease
[Ref. Weedon's Skin Pathology by James W Patterson, 1/e p310]

- Dyskeratosis is abnormal keratinization occurring prematurely within individual cells or groups of cells below the stratum granulosum

38. Ans. (b) Rubella; (d) Measles
[Ref. Cutaneous Drug Eruptions by Hall, 1/e p47]

39. Ans. (d) None
[Ref. Neena Khanna, 5/e p45; Differential Diagnosis in Dermatology by Ashton,3/e p179]

40. Ans. (b) Reiter's disease
[Ref. Neena Khanna, 5/e p48]

41. Ans. (c) Autosomal dominant
[Ref. Neena Khanna, 5/e p21]

- Ichthyosis vulgaris
  - Inheritance: AD
  - Molecular defect: reduced or absent filaggrin

42. Ans. (a) Lichen Planus; (b) Psoriasis
[Ref. Neena Khanna, 5/e p45; Differential Diagnosis in Dermatology by Ashton,3/e p179]

43. Ans. (c) X-linked ichthyosis nigra
[Ref. Neena Khanna, 5/e p23]

Characteristic of X-Linked Ichthyosis

- Affects male only
- X-linked RI
- Deficiency of steroid sulphatase
- Large geometrically shaped adherent dark brown black scales
- Generalized involvement, encroaches flexures

44. Ans. (a) Ichthyosis vulgaris
[Ref. Dermatopathology by Elston, 2/e p208]

- Ichthyosis vulgaris: There is little to no granular layer despite hyperkeratosis

45. Ans. (c) Hailey-Hailey disease; (d) Darrier's disease; (e) Pemphigus vulgaris
[Ref. Neena Khanna, 5/e p78]

46. Ans. (a) G0-G1-S-G2-M
[Ref. Cell Cycle Checkpoint Control Protocols by Lieberman, Vol/241 p22]

47. Ans. (d) Ocular involvement is seen in almost 100% cases and is typically unilateral
[Ref. Neena Khanna, 5/e p37]

- Ocular defect in a third of patients of Incontinenta pugmenti

48. **Ans. (d) Deserts**

49. **Ans. (b) Acantholysis**
[Ref. Neena Khanna, 5/e p78]

50. **Ans. (a) Herpes viral infection; (b) Bullous pemphigoids**
[Ref. Neena Khanna, 5/e p77]

Tzanck Smear Findings

Disorders	Findings
Pemphigus group	Acantholytic cells
VZ infection, HSV infection	Multinucleated giant cell
Epidermal necrolysis	Necrotic keratinocytes
Bullous pemphigoid	Predominantly eosinophils
Bullous impetigo Chronic bullous disease of childhood	Predominantly neutrophils

51. **Ans. (c) Plasma cell balantitis of zoon**
[Ref. DVL by Bansal. 1/e 0402]]

52. **Ans. (c) Psoriasis**
[Ref. Neena Khanna, 5/e p50]

53. **Ans. (d) Hypothyroidism**
[Ref. Cutaneous Medicine by Provost, 1/e p13]

54. **Ans. (a) Myxedema**
[Ref. Cutaneous Medicine by Provost, 1/e p13]

55. **Ans. (d) Pemphigus**
[Ref. Neena Khanna, 5/e p37]
- 50% cases mucosal lesion starts in oral region and then becomes universal

56. **Ans. (b) Drug induced lupus erythematous**
[Ref. Drug-induced and Iatrogenic Respiratory Disease by Camus, 1/e p293]

57. **Ans. (a) Systemic primary amyloidosis**
[Ref. Dermatology edited by Jean L. Bolognia, 3 /e p699]
- Systemic primary systemic (AL) amyloidosis include Waxy papulonodules and plaques, Ecchymoses, Pinch purpura, and Macroglossia

58. **Ans. (b) Psoriasis**
[Ref. Neena Khanna, 5/e p50]

59. **Ans. (a) No vesicles**
[Ref. Neena Khanna, 5/e p186-187]
- In EM major, large lesions have a central bulla and marginal ring of vesicles: Herpetic iris of Bateman

60. **Ans. (b) Erythema multiformae**
[Ref. Neena Khanna, 5/e p186-187]

61. **Ans. (a) Face and Neck**
[Ref. Unwanted Effects of Cosmetics and Drugs Used in Dermatology, Issue 282 by Anton C. de Groot, p41]
- Riehl's melanosis is a non-itching pigmented dermatosis localized on the face and neck

62. **Ans. (a) Gottron papules; (d) Proximal muscle wasting**
[Ref. Neena Khanna, 5/e p242-243]

63. **Ans. (c) Early diagnosis and treatment**
[Ref. Neena Khanna, 5/e p284]

64. **Ans. (a) Lesions resembling Chonic DLE**
[Ref. Neena Khanna, 5/e p237-239]

65. **Ans. (a) SLE; (b) Liver spots; (e) Prophyria cutanea tarda**
[Ref. Manual of Travel Medicine and Health by Steffen, 3/e p135]
- Photosensitivity and sunlight can provoke discoid and systemic lupus erythematosus, respectively
- Generally Porphyria cutanea tarda is a photosensitive disease with bullae formation on the light-exposed areas
- The same applies for chronic venous insufficiency, tinea pedis (athlete's foot), tinea versicolor (liver spots)

66. **Ans. (a) Tinea capitis**
[Ref. Seidel's Guide to Physical Examination by Ball, 8/e p48]
- Wood's lamp contains a light source with a wavelength of 360 nm
- This is the black light that causes certain substances to fluoresce
- It is used primarily to determine the presence of fungi on skin lesions

67. **Ans. (d) Intermittent porphyria**
[Ref. Hematology by Hoffman, 6/e p461]

68. **Ans. (a) Phlebotomy (c) Low dose chloroquine**
[Ref. Neena Khanna, 5/e p417]

Management
- Avoidance of triggers like alcohol
- Treatment of HCV infection
- Venesection till Hb falls below 12g/dL
- Low-dose therapy with hydroxychloroquine (100 mg twice a week)

69. **Ans. (a) HS Purpura**
[Ref. Neena Khanna, 5/e p196]
- Palpable purpura is characteristic of HSP

70. **Ans. (b) ITP**
[Ref. Textbook of Pathology by V. Krishna, 1/e p544]

71. **Ans. (a) IVIg**
[Ref. Oski's Pediatrics: Principles & Practice edited by Julia A. McMillan, 4/e p1019]
- The goals of therapy for Kawasaki disease are to decrease the inflammatory response and to reduce the severity of the cardiovascular complications
- Combination of IVIG and aspirin effectively remains the standard of care

72. **Ans. (a) Von Reclinghausens disease**
[Ref. Ophthalmology by Myron Yanoff, 3/e p937]
- Neurofibromatosis type 1 (peripheral NF, von Recklinghausen's disease) is characterized by cutaneous cafe-au-lait spots, axillary and inguinal freckling, Lisch nodules of the iris, several types of cutaneous neurofibromas, optic nerve gliomas

73. **Ans. (b) Nickel oxide and silica**
[Ref. Seidel's Guide to Physical Examination By Jane W. Ball, 8/e p48]

Wood's Lamp Examination

- Wood's lamp contains a light source with a wavelength of 360 nm
- Filter is made of nickel oxide and silica
- Black light causes certain substances to fluoresce
- It is used primarily to determine the presence of fungi on skin lesions

74. Ans. (b) Xeroderma pigmentosa
[Ref. DNA Repair and Human Disease by Balajee, 1/e p138]

- Xeroderma pigmentosum: A human disease in which an initial stage of DNA repair is defective

75. Ans. (a) Autosomal recessive
[Ref. Neena Khanna, 5/e p36]

- Neurofibromatosis has Autosomal dominant inheritance

76. Ans. (c) Tuberous sclerosis
[Ref. Neena Khanna, 5/e p34]

77. Ans. (a) Tuberous sclerosis
[Ref. Neena Khanna, 5/e p34]

Periungual Fibroma (Koenen's Tumor)

- Present in 20% of patient
- Develop in Adult life
- Small, sausage shaped, pink growths arising from under the nail folds

78. Ans. (d) Ichthyosis vulgaris
[Ref. Neena Khanna, 5/e p21-22]

79. Ans. (d) All
[Ref. Dermatology edited by Jean L. Bolognia, 3/e p842]

Ichthyosis

- Description:
  - Ichthyosis is a disorder of cornification, characterised by persistently dry, thickened, "fish scale" skin
  - At least 20 varieties of ichthyosis, including inherited and acquired forms.
- Ichthyosis vulgaris (1:250-1000): Autosomal dominant inheritance, meaning an abnormal gene is inherited from a parent, Penetrance is 90%, Onset is delayed until at least 3 months of age
- Recessive X-linked ichthyosis (1:2000-6000): Mainly affects males, who have a single X chromosome with the abnormal gene, Females are protected by usually having a normal second X chromosome, Onset may be congenital or delayed by up to 6 months.
- Autosomal recessive congenital ichthyosis (1:3-500,000): One abnormal gene is inherited from each parent
- Keratinopathic ichthyoses (1:200,000): Recessive and dominant forms and present at birth with a collodion membrane
- New spontaneous mutation
- Acquired ichthyosis: Acquired ichthyosis appears in adult life. People with ichthyosis may have systemic disease, such as:
  - Underactive thyroid
  - Sarcoidosis
  - Hodgkin lymphoma
  - Cancer (ichthyosis may be a cutaneous marker of internal malignancy)
  - HIV infection
  - Ichthyosis may be provoked by certain medications: Nicotinic acid, Targeted cancer therapy (e.g. Vemurafenib, EGFR and Protein kinase inhibitors), Hydroxyurea

80. Ans. (b) Refsum disease
[Ref. Dermatology edited by Jean L. Bolognia, 3/e p842]

81. Ans. (a) Apthous ulcer
[Ref. Neena Khanna, 5/e p203]

- Apthous ulcer: Extremely painful ulcer with a necrotic yellow floor surrounded by an erythematous halo

82. Ans. (d) Lambosacral region
[Ref. Neena Khanna, 5/e p34]

Shagreen Patch (Connective Tissue Naevus)

- Seen in Tuberous sclerosis
- 40% cases
- Leathery, cobble stoned, yellow brown plaque resembling shagreen skin
- Lumbosacral area, less frequently in face

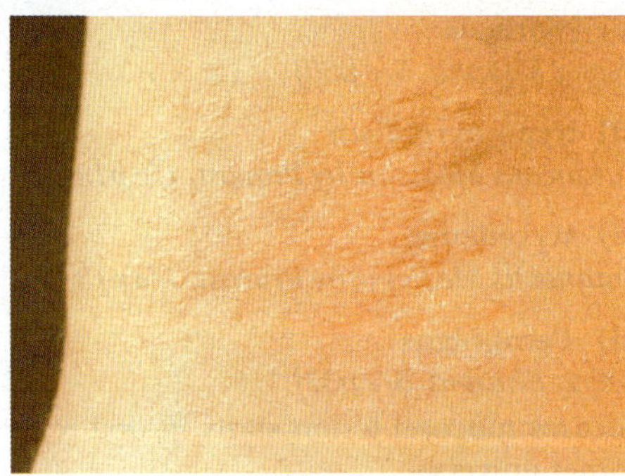

Fig. Shagreen patch

83. Ans. (c) Candida
[Ref. Primary Care for Women edited by Phyllis Carolyn Leppert, 2 /e p191]

- **Vulvovaginal candidiasis (VVC) is the most common infections of the female genital tract**
- About 75% of women at some time in their lives experience the discomfort of a vaginal yeast infection

84. Ans. (d) Is not of any significance
[Ref. Neonatal and Infant Dermatology by Lawrence F. Eichenfield, 3/e p126]

- Erythema toxicum neonatorum (toxic erythema of the newborn is a benign and self-limited condition that primarily affects term infants and is rare in preterm infants

85. Ans. (b) 360 nm
[Ref. Seidel's Guide to Physical Examination By Jane W. Ball, 8/e p48]

- Wood's lamp contains a light source with a wavelength of 360 nm.

86. Ans. (b) Erythrasma
[Ref. Neena Khanna, 5/e p13]

87. Ans. (b) Porphyria cutanea tarda
[Ref. Neena Khanna, 5/e p13]

- Porphyria: Red-pink fluorescence of urine

AIIMS PG 2018 MCQs

1. **Incubation period of LGV is** *[AIIMS May 2018]*
   a. 1-2 days
   b. 3-12 days
   c. 10-14 days
   d. 14-21 days
2. **Allergic contact dermatitis occurs due to exposure to cement. Agent responsible** *[AIIMS May 2018]*
   a. Aluminum
   b. Silica
   c. Asbestos fibre
   d. Potassium dichromate
3. **For diagnosis of Neuritic leprosy, which nerve is taken for test generally** *[AIIMS May 2018]*
   a. Radial cutaneous nerve
   b. Ulnar nerve
   c. Median nerve
   d. Any nerve
4. **A 50 years old woman has history of fever and joint pains. She was started on NSAIDS. After 8-10 days, she presented with the following skin lesions as shown in the Photograph. Diagnosis of underlying disorder is** *[AIIMS May 2018]*

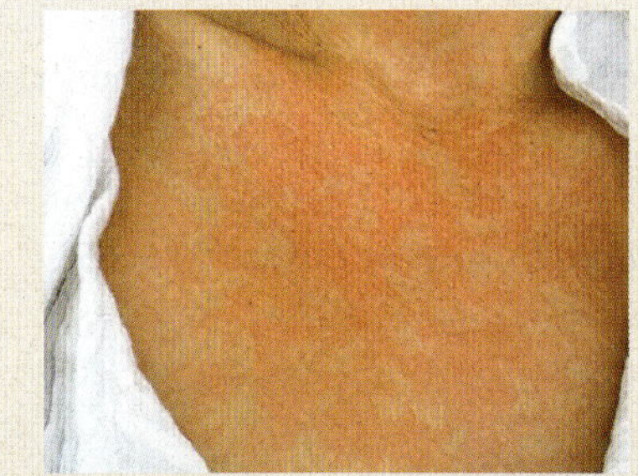

   a. Dengue b. Melasma
   c. Chikungunya fever d. Fixed drug eruption
5. **Cardiovascular Syphilis can be treated by** *[AIIMS May 2018]*
   a. Aqueous Crystalline Penicillin G 3-4 million units IV q4h for 10-14 days
   b. Benzathine Penicillin G 2.4 million Units IM one dose only
   c. Benzathine Penicillin G 2.4 million Units IM once every week for 3 weeks
   d. Procaine Penicillin 2.4 million units IM daily (with Probenecid) for 10-14 days

EXPLANATORY ANSWERS 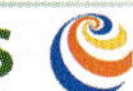

1. **Ans. (b) 3-12 days**
   [Ref. Neena Khanna, 4/e p310]

LYMPHOGRANULOMA VENERUM (LGV)

- Underlying cause: Chlamydia trachomatis (L1, L2 or L3)
- Incubation period: 3-12 days
- Clinical presentation: Primary stage (Usually asymptomatic lesion), Inguinal syndrome (Buboes, Sign of groove), Genito-anorectal syndrome (Esthiomene in females)
- Treatment: Doxycycline, Erythromycin

2. **Ans. (d) Potassium dichromate**
   [Ref. Contact Dermatitis by Johansen, 5/e p550]

Cement Dermatitis

- Cement has been considered as the main cause of Potassium dichromate allergy
- 1 Kg of normal cement dust contains 5-10 mg of water-soluble Chromium
- Cement dermatitis is decreasing in incidence, partly due to the introduction of Ferrous sulfate in cement in some countries in order to reduce the levels of hexavalent Chromium

3. **Ans. (a) Radial cutaneous nerve**
   [Ref. Procedural Dermatosurgery by Vasudevan, 1/e p281]

- Nerve biopsy is a key diagnostic procedure to definitely diagnose Pure neuritic leprosy
- MC performed on a pure cutaneous nerve like Sural nerve or Radial cutaneous nerve
- Biopsy of mixed or motors nerve is done very rarely in special circumstances

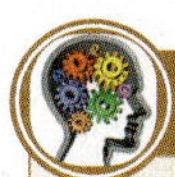

Also Remember

Gold Standard for Confirmation of Pure Neuritic Leprosy: Nerve Biopsy

- Although any nerve involved would show the pathology, it is prudent to biopsy a branch of a sensory nerve, rather than a mixed nerve or major nerve trunk
- Common nerves and sites where nerve biopsy is performed:
  - Superficial sensory radial nerve branch at the wrist
  - Ulnar cutaneous nerve near the ulnar border of base of the hand
  - Sural nerve near the ankle
- Proper processing of the nerve biopsy specimen and its staining with Hematoxylin and Eosin and modified Fite stains is required

4. **Ans. (c) Chikungunya fever**
   [Ref. Pediatric Dermatology by Inamadar, 1/e p188]

Cutaneous Lesions in Chikungunya

- Hyperpigmentation: Centrofacial/Generalized, Freckle/Melasma-like, Flagellate/Streaky, Addisonian type

- Maculopapular eruption, Transient/ generalized erythema
- Pruritis, Palmoplantar desquamation
- Vesiculobullous lesions, Aphthous like ulcers, Vasculitic lesions
- Lymphadenopathy, Ecchymosis, Hemorrhages

5. Ans. (c) Benzathine Penicillin G 2.4 million Units IM once every week for 3 weeks

[Ref. Infectious Diseases by Cohen, 4/e p565]

Treatment of Syphilis

- Early Syphilis (Primary, Secondary, Early latent syphilis of < 1-2 years duration): Benzathine Penicillin G 2.4 million Units IM one dose only
- Late Syphilis (Latent syphilis of > 1-2 years duration, Cardiovascular, Gummatous): Benzathine Penicillin G 2.4 million Units IM once every week for 3 weeks
- Neuro-syphilis: Procaine Penicillin 2.4 million units IM daily (with Probenecid) for 10-14 days

Anesthesiology

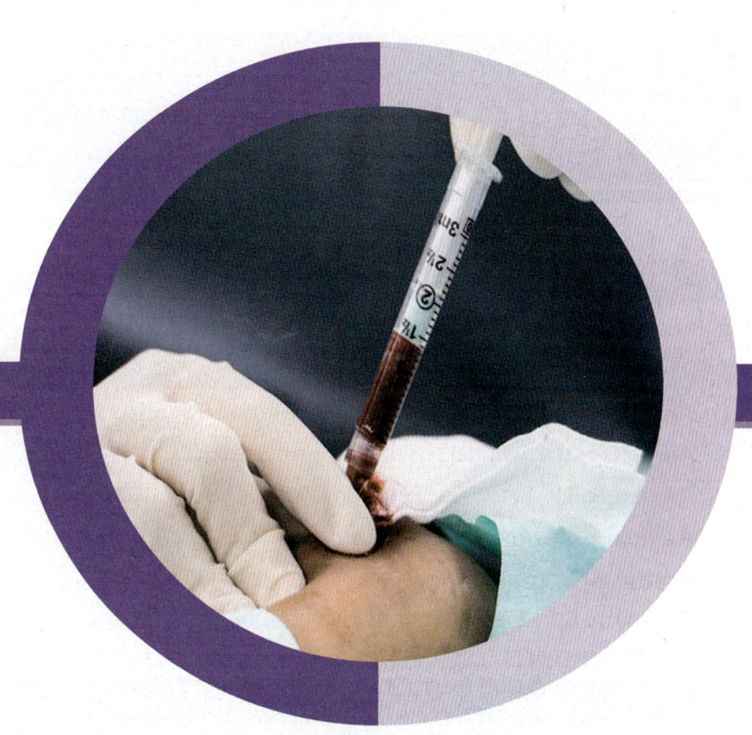

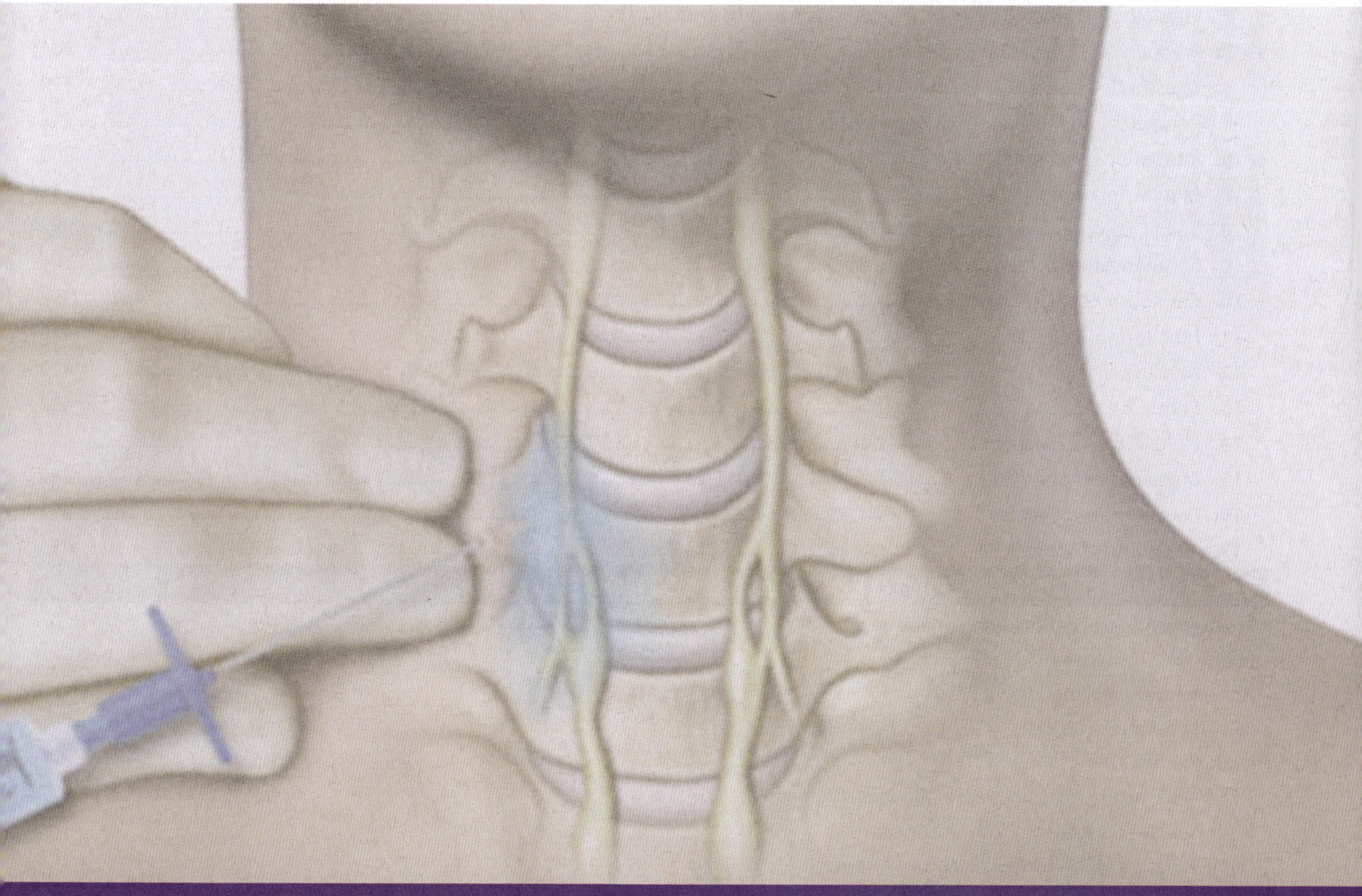

Contents

Anesthesiology

ANNEXURES

CHAPTERS

EACH CHAPTER DIVIDED INTO FOLLOWING SECTIONS

Theoretical Concepts (Including Images)
Image-Based Questions
Answers with Explanations of IBQs
NEET/NBE Pattern MCQs
High Yield MCQs
NEET/NBE Pattern MCQs Answers with Explanations
High Yield MCQs Answers with Explanations
AIIMS PG 2018 MCQs with Explanatory Answers

Annexures

ANNEXURE 1. FAMOUS ANESTHESIOLOGISTS AND SCIENTISTS

Anesthesiologists/Scientists	Contribution
Alfred Einhor	Developed procaine
Archie Brain	Developed laryngeal mask airway (LMA)
Arthur Ernest Guedel	Stages of general anesthesia; oropharyngeal airway
August Bier	First administration of spinal anesthetic; father of spinal anesthesia
Bain & Spoerel	Introduced coaxial anesthetic circuit
Bjorn Ibsen	Intermittent positive pressure ventilation (IPPV)
Brian Arthur Sellick	Sellick's (Cricoid pressure) maneuver
Carl Koller	First use of cocaine as local anesthetic
Cathelin & Sicard	Caudal analgesia; first epidural anesthesia
Collin Sullivan	Continuous positive airway pressure (CPAP)
Ephraim Cutter	Discovered laryngoscope
Friedrich Serturner	Discovered morphine
H JC Swan & William Ganz	Introduced pulmonary artery catheter
H Quincke	Technique of lumbar puncture
Henry Cocky Boyle	Developed first anesthetic machine
Humphry Davy	Discovered properties of chlorine
Ivan Magill	First endotracheal intubation
James Young Simpson	Discovered anesthetic properties of chloroform
John Lundy	Use of first intravenous anesthetic, Thiopentone
Joseph Priestly	Discovered nitrous oxide
Marshall Hall	Technique of resuscitation
Melzack & Wall	Gateway theory of pain
Paracelsus	First use of ether on animals
SR Mallampatti	Airway classification
William Mapleson	Semi-closed breathing systems
William Harvey	Systemic circulation
William TG Morton	First use of inhaled ether in surgical anesthesia

ANNEXURE 2. CYLINDERS USED IN ANESTHESIA

Colors of Cylinders	
Cylinder	**Color**
Oxygen	Black body with white shoulders
Nitrous oxide	Blue
Air	Grey body with black and white shoulders
Carbon dioxide	Gray

Contd...

Contd...

Cyclopropane	Orange
Helium	Brown
Entonox	Blue body with blue and white shoulders
Ethylene	Purple with red shoulders
Halothane bottle	Amber
Thiopentone	Yellow
Pin Indices of Cylinders	
Gas cylinder	**Pin index**
Oxygen	2, 5
Nitrous oxide	3, 5
Cyclopropane	3, 6
Air	1, 5
Nitrogen	1, 4
Entonox (50% O_2 + 50% NO)	7
Carbon dioxide (<7.5%)	2, 6
Carbon dioxide (>7.5%)	1, 6
Pressures of Cylinders	
Cylinder	**Pressure**
Oxygen	137 bar
Air	137 bar
Helium	137 bar
Nitrous oxide	40 bar
Carbon dioxide	50 bar
Cyclopropane	5 bar

ANNEXURE 3. BLOOD GAS PARTITION COEFFICIENTS

Agent	B/G partition coefficient
Desflurane	0.42
Cyclopropane	0.44
Nitrous oxide	0.47
Sevoflurane	0.69
Isoflurane	1.38
Enflurane	1.8
Halothane	2.4
Chloroform	8
Trielene	9
Ether	12
Methoxyflurane	15

ANNEXURE 4. ANESTHETICS OF CHOICE

Condition	Anesthetic of choice
Inhibiting stress response to laryngoscopy and intubation	Alfentanil
Muscle relaxant in hepatic failure	Atracurium
Muscle relaxant in renal failure	Atracurium

Contd...

Contd...

Muscle relaxant in myaesthenia gravis	Atracurium
Muscle relaxant in newborn age	Atracurium
Muscle relaxant in old age	Atracurium
Inhalational agent in shock	Cyclopropane
Induction in children	Desflurane
Reversal agent for Mivacurium	Edrophonium
Cardio-stable intravenous agent	Etomidate
Intravenous agent for aneurysm surgery	Etomidate
Inhibit stress response intubation or laryngoscopy	Fentanyl
Inhalational agent in asthmatics	Halothane
External versions, manual removal of placenta	Halothane
Maintenance agent in cardiac patients (except M. ischemia)	Isoflurane
Inhalational agent for neurosurgery	Isoflurane
Controlled hypotension	Isoflurane
Intravenous agent for shock	Ketamine
Intravenous agent for Asthmatics	Ketamine
Intramuscular agent for children	Ketamine
Induction in contractive pericarditis, cardiac tamponade, TOF	Ketamine
Patients with full stomach	Ketamine
Electroconvulsive therapy (ECT)	Methohexitone
Muscle relaxant for day care surgery	Mivacurium
Shivering	Pethidine
Local anesthetic in malignant hyperthermia	Procaine
Induction in those susceptible to malignant hyperthermia	Propofol
Combination in day care surgery	Propofol + Alfentanil
Total intravenous anesthesia	Propofol
Intravenous agent for day care surgery	Propofol
Reversal in renal failure patients	Pyridostigmine
Opioid for day care surgery	Remifentanil
Non-depolarizing agent for intubation	Rocuronium
Muscle relaxant for precurarization	Rocuronium
Inhalational method for induction in children	Sevoflurane
Depolarizing agent for Intubation	Succinycholine
MC used intravenous induction agent	Thiopentone
Cerebral protection	Thiopentone
Muscle relaxant for cardiac patients	Vecuronium

ANNEXURE 5. SPECIFIC SIDE-EFFECTS OF ANESTHETICS

Side Effects of Anesthesia	
Anesthetic	**Side-effect**
Alcuronium	Anaphylactic reactions, ganglionic blockade
Alfentanil	Muscle rigidity

Contd...

Contd...

Atracurium	Convulsions
Benzocaine	Methemoglobinemia
Chloroform	Maximum hyperglycemia
Enflurane	Maximum depression of respiration
Etomidate	Maximum nausea and vomiting
Halothane	Maximum inhibition to ventilatory response
Halothane	Inhibition of myocardial contractility
Halothane	Maximum sensitization of heart to adrenaline
Halothane	Maximum hepatocellular damage
Ketamine	Dissociative anesthesia
Ketamine	Raised intracranial tension
Ketamine	Hallucination, emergence reactions
Lignocaine	Malignant hyperthermia
Methoxyflurane	Maximum nephrotoxicity
Methoxyflurane	Slowest induction, slowest recovery with inhalational agents
Nitrous oxide	Megaloblastic anemia, aplastic anemia
Nitrous oxide	Subacute degeneration of spinal cord
Prilocaine	Methemoglobinemia
Isoflurane	Minimum nephrotoxicity
Isoflurane	Maximum hypotension
Pancuronium	Cardiac arrhythmias
Rapacuronium	Intense bronchospasm
Succinylcholine	Maximum malignant hyperthermia

ANNEXURE 6. SPECIFIC CONTRAINDICATIONS OF ANESTHETICS

Anesthetic	Contraindication(s)
Bupivacaine	Bier's block
Chloroform	Diabetes mellitus
Enflurane	Epilepsy, renal disease
Ether	Diabetes mellitus
Gallamine	Pregnancy, renal disease
Halothane	Caesarean section, abortions, intracranial lesions, aortic stenosis, pheochromocytoma
Isoflurane	Myocardial ischemia
Ketamine	Head injury, ICSOL, ophthalmic pathology, myocardial ischemia, vascular aneurysm, drug addiction, hypertension, psychiatric diseases
Lignocaine	Malignant hyperthermia
Methoxyflurane	Renal diseases, closed circuits
Metocurine	Allergy to iodine
Nitrous oxide	Middle ear surgeries, tympanoplasty, laparoscopic surgeries, acute intestinal obstruction, volvulus, microlaryngeal surgeries, pneumothorax, pneumoperitoneum, eye surgeries, pneumoencephalum
Pethidine	MAO therapy, myocardial ischemia
Rocuronium	Biliary obstruction
Succinylcholine	Hyperkalemia, head injury, glaucoma, ocular injuries, renal failure, Duchenne muscular dystrophy, tetanus, Guillain-Barre syndrome, Shock Spinal cord injury
Thiopentone	Acute intermittent prophyria, Variegate porphyria
Vecuronium	Biliary obstruction

Golden Points

Bones in children are break-resistant (only outer cortex breaks)	Greenstick fractures
Rate of axonal recovery/nerve regeneration	1 mm/day
Motor-march phenomenon is absent in	Neuropraxia
Tinel's percussion sign is used for	Nerve regeneration
Nerve grafting is done if nerve gap is more than	10 cm
Common donor nerve used for nerve grafting	Sural nerve
MCC of deformity of bone	Fractures
Joint most amenable to manipulation	Knee joint
MC donor site for bone grafts	Iliac crest
MC joint in human body to dislocate	Shoulder joint
MC dislocation at shoulder joint	Anterior
MC dislocation at elbow joint	Posterior
Radius head pulled out of annular ligament	Pulled elbow
Best treatment of fracture of forearm bones	Conservative
Fracture head of radius is a type of	Valgus injury
Type of injury causing Monteggia fracture-dislocation	Hyperpronation injury
Most characteristic displacement of Colles' fracture	Dorsal tilt
MC cause of Sudeck's dystrophy in upper limb	Colles' fracture
Glass holding position of cast	Scaphoid cast
Positioning of wrist in Scaphoid cast is reverse of	Colles' cast
Intraarticular fracture at base of 1st metacarpal	Bennet's fracture dislocation
Extraarticular fracture at base of 1st metacarpal	Rolando's fracture
MC pelvic fracture	Ischio-pubic rami fracture
Bilateral Ischio-pubic rami fracture is known as	Straddle fracture
Unsolved fracture (higher complications)	Fracture neck of femur
Prosthesis used in hemiarthroplasty (fracture neck of femur)	Austin-Moore prosthesis
K-nail is used for fracture of	Shaft of femur
Gallow's traction is used for fracture of	Shaft of femur (infants)
Most frequently injured joint	Knee joint
Comminuted fracture of patella is known as	Stellate fracture
Post fracture neck of talus, avascular necrosis occurs in	Body of talus
Jefferson's fracture is fracture of	Atlas
Clay shoveller's fracture is fracture of	Spinous process of D1 vertebra
Cord-hemisection (ipsilateral paralysis, c/l loss of pain)	Brown-Sequard syndrome
MC site of acute osteomyelitis (Hematogenous)	Lower femoral metaphysis
MC complication of acute osteomyelitis	Chronic osteomyelitis

Contd...

Contd...

MC cause for chronic osteomyelitis	Delayed/insufficient treatment
Dense sclerotic bone overlying a sequestrum is	Involucrum
MC clinical presentation of chronic osteomyelitis	Chronic discharging sinus
MC cause of septic arthritis	Staphylococcus aureus
Tom Smith arthritis is	Septic arthritis of infancy (hip)
MC site of gonococcal arthritis	Knee joint
Most common site of bone and joint tuberculosis	Spine (Pott's disease)
Most common site of spinal TB	Dorso-lumbar region
Investigation of choice for TB spine	MRI
MC cause of early onset Pott's paraplegia	Abscess
Besides spine, MC site of TB bones	Hip
MC cause of Hip-pain in children in India	TB hip
MC congenital foot deformity	CTEV
Most important muscle related to CTEV	Tibialis posterior
MC cause of cerebral palsy	Birth anoxia
MC type of Spina bifida	Spina bifida occulta
Most common primary bone malignancy	Multiple myeloma
Second most common primary bone malignancy	Osteosarcoma
Most common benign tumor of bone	Osteochondroma
Most common 'TRUE' benign tumor of bone	Osteoid osteoma
Most common malignant bone tumor	Secondaries to bone
Most common primary bone malignancy	Multiple myeloma
Second most common primary bone malignancy	Osteosarcoma
Most common benign tumor of bone	Osteochondroma
Most common 'TRUE' benign tumor of bone	Osteoid osteoma
Most common bone tumor in Hand	Enchondroma
MC site of vertebral disc prop lapse	L4-L5
MC joint affected in rheumatoid arthritis	MP joint (Index finger)
MC joint affected in gout	MP joint (Great toe)
Marie-Stumpell disease is	Ankylosing spondylitis
Squaring of patella is seen in	Hemophilic arthritis
MC site of cervical spondylosis	C5-C6
Dupuytren's contracture is contracture of	Palmar aponeurosis
Medial epicondylitis is	Golfer's elbow
Lateral epicondylitis	Tennis elbow
Pain over radial styloid process is	De Quervain's tenovaginitis
Constriction of fibrous digital sheath leads to	Trigger finger
Frozen shoulder is common among	Diabetics
Entrapment of lateral cutaneous nerve of thigh in fascia	Meralgia paresthetica
MC metabolic bone disease	Osteoporosis
MC site of fracture in osteoporosis	Dorso-lumbar spine
% bone-mass loss in osteoporosis for seen on X-rays	30%

Contd...

Contd...

MC cause of ricketsin children in India	Nutritional deficiency
Brown's tumor (Expansile bone lesion of osteoclasts) is in	Hyperparathyroidism
In fluorosis of bones, there is excess deposition of	Calcium
Earliest sign of dental fluorosis	Mottling
Best sign to see mottling of teeth due to fluorosis	Incisors (upper jaw)
Orthopedic disorders in dwarf circus jokers	Achondroplasia
Diaphysial achalasia (Multiple exostosis) is due to	Remodelling defect
Trumpet shaped metaphysic is in	Diaphysial achalasia
Dense brittle bones/Marble bones are in	Osteopetrosis
Paget's disease defect (Osteitis deformans)	Osteoclasts
MC osteochondritis	Perthes disease
MC Torticollis	Spasmodic
Infantile cortical hyperostosis is	Caffey's disease
Multiple enchondromatosis is	Ollier's disease
MC cause of congenital torticollis is	Sternocleidomastoid tumor
% population with cervical rib	0.5%
Trethovan's sign is seen in slipping of	Capital femoral epiphysis
MC cause of loose bodies in joints	Osteoarthritis
Blount's disease is a type of	Genu varum
MC cause of hallux valgus	Rheumatoid arthritis

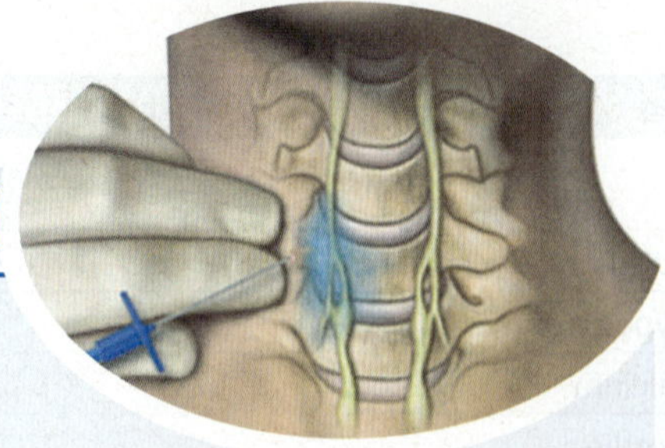

Chapter 1

Anatomy in Anesthesia and Historical Aspects

THEORETICAL CONCEPTS

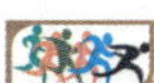

Topper's Edge

History of Anesthesia

- First IV injection was given by: Christopher Wren & Daniel Johann Major
- **Word 'anesthesia' was coined by[Q]: Oliver Wendell Holmes**
- Word anesthesiology & anaesthesiologist coined by: Mathias J. Seifert
- **Father of anesthesia[Q]: John Snow**
- **Father of modern anesthesia[Q]: WTG Mortem**
- Oxygen & nitrous oxide were synthesized by[Q]: Joseph Priestley
- Analgesic property of nitrous oxide was discovered by[Q]: Humphry Davy
- Public demonstration that nitrous oxide can provide pain relief: Horace Wells
- First public demonstration of ether anesthesia[Q]: WTG Morton (16 October 1846)
- First use of chloroform to women for pain during childbirth[Q]: James Y. Simpson
- **First Local anesthetic to be used[Q]: Cocaine**
- First introduction of cocaine as an anesthetic for eye surgery[Q]: Karl Koller
- **First spinal anesthesia was given by[Q]: August Bier**
- First description of Caudal epidural analgesia[Q]: Jean-Anthanase Sicard & Fernand Cathelin
- First to use curare products as muscle relaxant: Harold Griffith
- First endotracheal intubation done by: William Macewen
- Endotracheal intubation was made popular by: Evan Mcgill

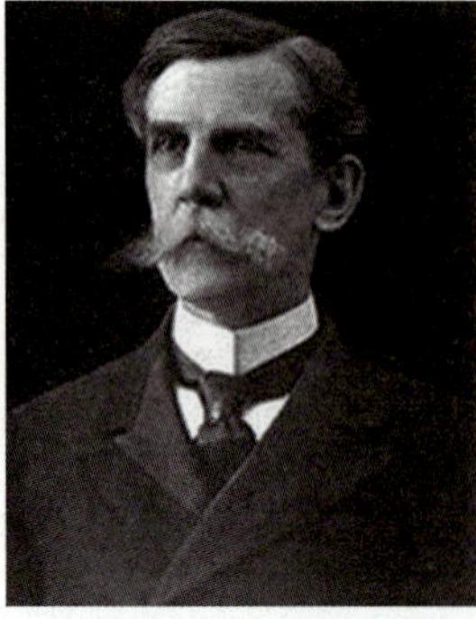

OW Holmes

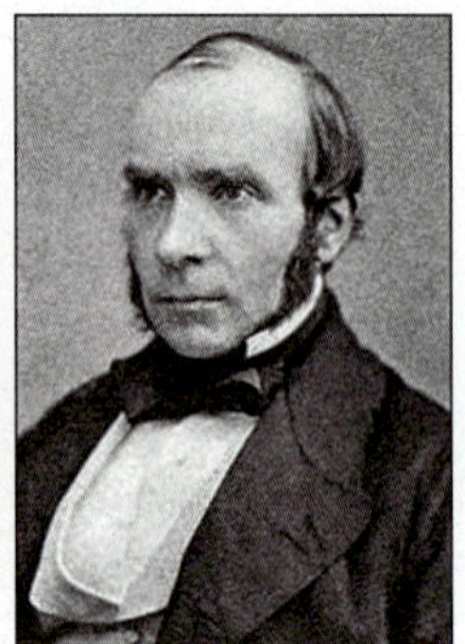

John Snow

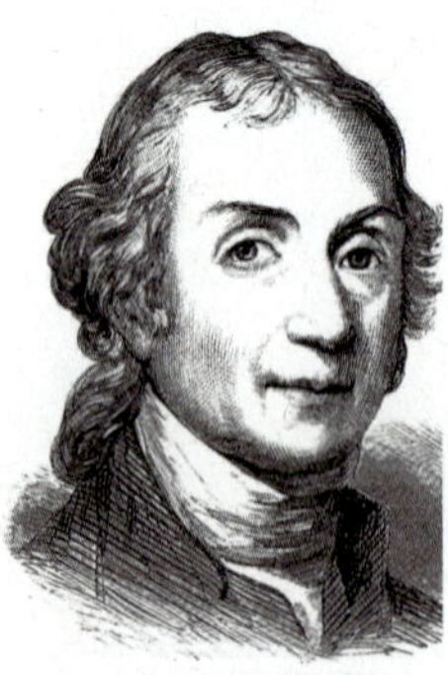

Joseph Priestley

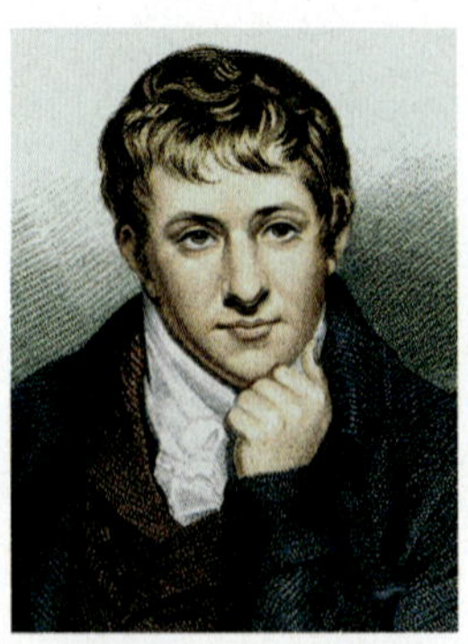

Sir Humphry Davy

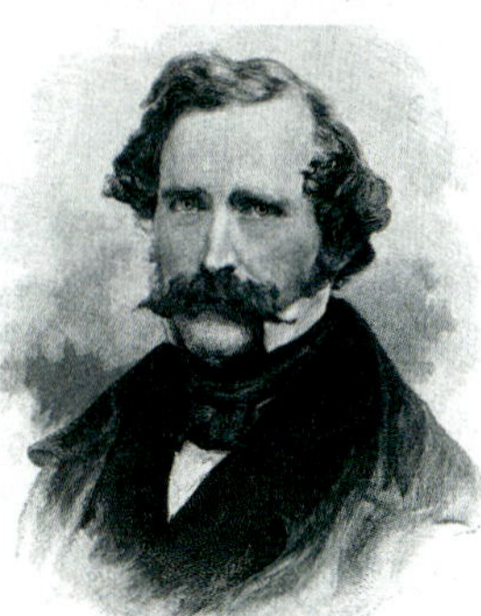

WTG Morton

I A. FACTS ABOUT ANATOMY

I B. DEAD SPACE

- Total physiological dead space: Anatomical dead space + Alveolar dead space

I B1. Anatomical Dead Space

- Constituted by: Air in nose, trachea, bronchial tree
- **Normal value: 150 ml**[Q] (30% of tidal volume)

Increased by[Q]	Decreased by
• Old age • Extension of neck • Jaw protrusion • Bronchodilators • Increasing lung volume • Atropine • Halothane • Anesthesia mask • IPPV • PEEP	• Supine position • Intubation[Q] • Tracheostomy[Q] • Hyperventilation • Flexion of neck • Bronchoconstriction

- Tracheostomy reduces dead space by: 70-100 ml[Q]
- Intubation reduce dead space by: 50-70 ml[Q]

I B2. Alveolar Dead Space

- Constituted by: Alveoli which are ventilated but not perfused
- **Normal value: 60–80 ml**

Increased by	Decreased by
• Lung pathologies • General anesthesia • Hypotension • IPPV • PEEP	• Lying down

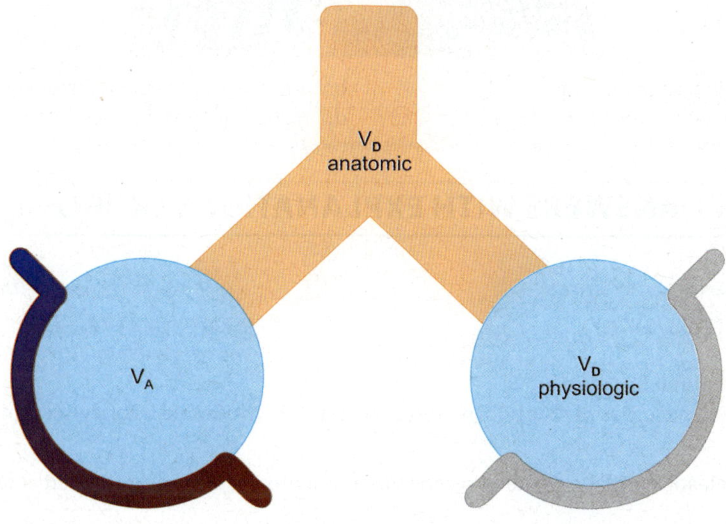

Fig. Dead space

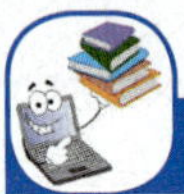

IMAGE-BASED QUESTIONS

1. Identify the contribution of Doctor in field of Anesthesia

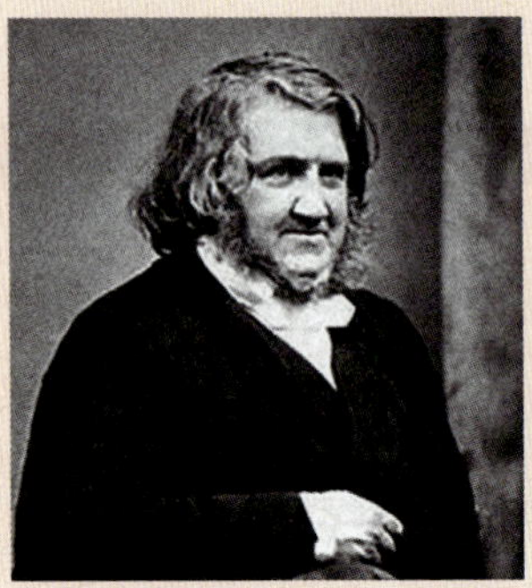

a. First use of ether
b. Stages of general anesthesia
c. Discovery of nitrous oxide
d. Use and properties of chloroform

2. Anatomical structure (Arrow) shown in laryngoscopic view (Photograph)

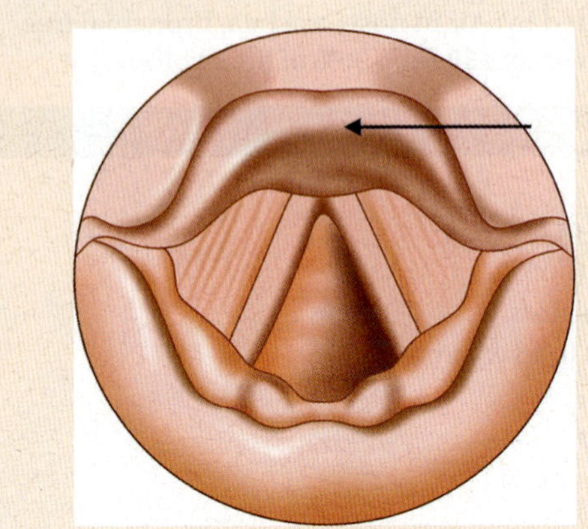

a. Aryepiglottic fold
b. Vocal cords
c. Epiglottis
d. Ventricular folds

3. Historical photograph shown depicts .... landmark in anesthesiology

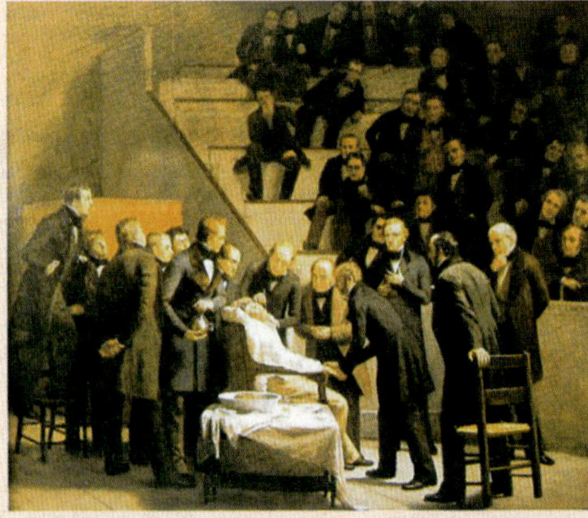

a. First ether anesthesia
b. First nitrous oxide anesthesia
c. First obstetric analgesia
d. Stages of general anesthesia

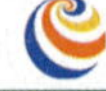

ANSWERS WITH EXPLANATIONS OF IBQs

1. Ans. (d) Use and properties of chloroform *[Ref. Clinical Anesthesia by Barash, 6/e p6]*

Sir James Young Simpson (1811-1870)
- Scottish obstetrician
- One of the first to use ether in labor pain
- Discovered the anesthetic properties of chloroform and successfully introduced it for general medical use

2. Ans. (c) Epiglottis *[Ref. Snell's Clinical Anatomy, 9/e p651]*
- Epiglottis: Flap made of elastic cartilage tissue covered with a mucous membrane, attached at laryngeal inlet

3. Ans. (a) First ether anesthesia *[Ref. Trauma by Wilson, 1/e p13]*
- Ether was first used in a surgical operation at the Massachusetts General Hospital on October 16, 1946
- It was demonstrated by Morton in front of Faculty and Students of Harvard Medical School.

NEET/NBE PATTERN MCQs

1. **Subarachnoid space ends at** *[Recent Question 2016]*
   a. T_{10-11} b. T_{11-12}
   c. S_{1-2} d. S_{2-3}
2. **Tracheostomy reduces dead space by** *[NBE FMGE September 2008]*
   a. 20-40 ml b. 30-50 ml
   c. 50-70 ml d. 70-100 ml
3. **Levels of ether anesthesia were demonstrated by whom** *[Recent Question 2012]*
   a. Morton b. Guedel
   c. Thompson d. None
4. **Narrowest part of trachea in a newborn is at the level of** *[NBE DNB 1995, 1999]*
   a. Cricoid b. Thyroid
   c. Vocal cords d. Subglottic
5. **First anesthetic used in clinical anesthesia** *[NBE DNB 2010, Recent Question 2014]*
   a. Bupivacaine b. Cocaine
   c. Lidocaine d. Procaine
6. **Epidural space is between** *[NBE DNB 1992]*
   a. Pia-arachnoid b. Spinal dura and arachnoid
   c. Arachnoid and cord
   d. Spinal dura and vertebral column
7. **Spinal cord ends at the level of lower border of** *[NBE DNB 1994, 1999]*
   a. T_{12} b. L_1
   c. L_2 d. L_3
8. **Mean distance from lips to carina in adults is approximately** *[NBE DNB 1992]*
   a. 20 cm
   b. 26 cm
   c. 32 cm
   d. 41.5 cm
9. **Cocaine was first used as local anesthetic by** *[Recent Question 2016, 2012]*
   a. Carl Kollar
   b. Holmer Wells
   c. Morton
   d. None
10. **Subarachnoid space is** *[NBE DNB 1996]*
    a. T_{10-11}
    b. T_{11-12}
    c. S_{1-2}
    d. S_{2-3}
11. **Dead space is increased by all, *except*** *[NBE DNB 2009]*
    a. Anticholinergic drugs
    b. Standing
    c. Hyperextension of neck
    d. Endotracheal intubation
12. **Term Anesthesia was coined by?** *[Recent Question 2017]*
    a. William Morton
    b. Wendell Holmes
    c. John Lundy
    d. Ralph Waters

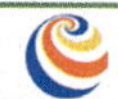

HIGH YIELD MCQs

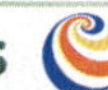

1. **Stages of anesthesia were established by** *[AIIMS PGMEE 1997]*
   a. Ether
   b. Nitrous oxide
   c. Halothane
   d. Chloroform
2. **Earliest (first) local anaesthetic used clinically** *[AIIMS PGMEE 1996, 2009]*
   a. Xylocaine/Lidocaine b. Morphine
   c. Cocaine d. Cannabis & Procaine
3. **High airway resistance is seen in** *[Kerala PGMEE 2006]*
   a. Respiratory bronchiole
   b. Terminal bronchiole
   c. Intermediate bronchiole
   d. Main bronchus
4. **Muscle most resistant to nondepolarizing block is** *[JIPMER PGMEE 2003]*
   a. Intercostal b. Abdominal
   c. Diaphragm d. Adductors
5. **Interscalene approach to brachial plexus block does not provide optimal surgical anesthesia in the area of distribution of which of the following nerve** *[All India PGMEE 2003]*
   a. Musculocutaneous b. Ulnar
   c. Radial d. Median
6. **Bethune and Brechner have developed** *[AIIMS November 2014]*
   a. Precordial Doppler
   b. Transesophageal echocardiography
   c. Plethysmography
   d. End tidal CO_2 monitoring

 NEET/NBE PATTERN MCQs ANSWERS WITH EXPLANATIONS

1. **Ans. (c)** S_{1-2}

[Ref. Clinical Anaesthesiology by Morgan, 5/e p955]

- Spinal subarachnoid space extends from the foramen magnum to S_2 in adults and S_3 in children
- Injection of local anesthetic below L_1 in adults and L_3 (below the termination of the conus medullaris) in children helps to avoid direct trauma to the spinal cord.

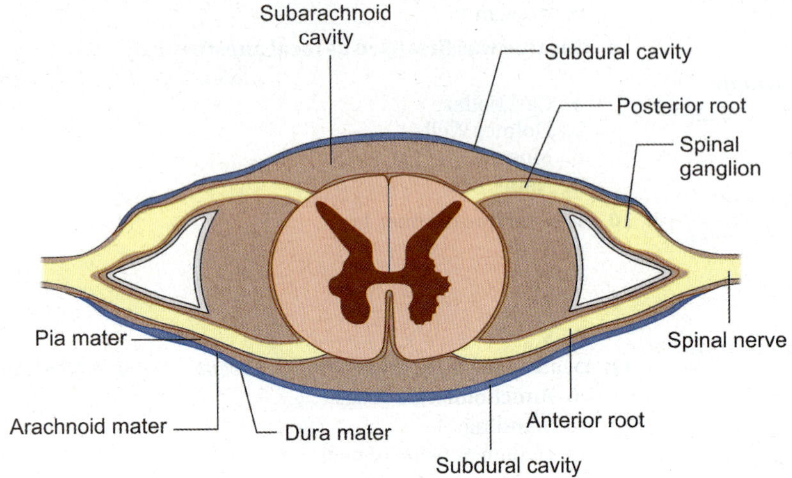

Fig. Subarachnoid space

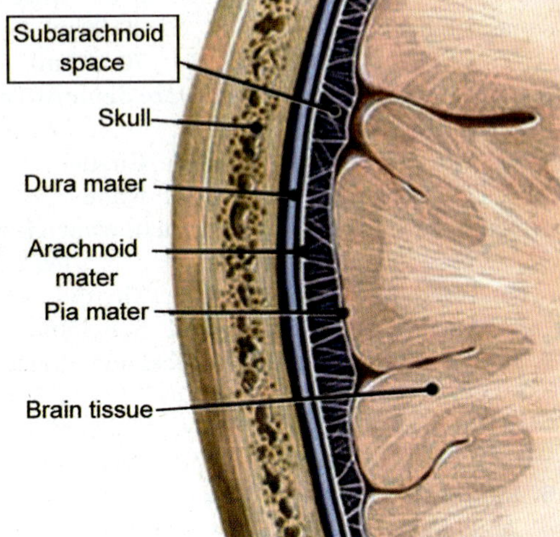

Fig. Subarachnoid space

2. **Ans. (d) 70–100 ml**

[Ref. Ref. Ajay Yadav, 4/e p4-5]

Dead Space

- Total physiological dead space: Anatomical dead space + Alveolar dead space
- Anatomical dead space:
  - Constituted by: Air in nose, trachea, bronchial tree
  - **Normal value: 150 ml** (30% of tidal volume)

Increased by	Decreased by
• Old age • Extension of neck • Jaw protrusion • Bronchodilators • Increasing lung volume • Atropine • Halothane • Anesthesia mask • IPPV • PEEP	• Supine position • Intubation • Tracheostomy • Hyperventilation • Flexion of neck • Bronchoconstriction

- Alveolar dead space:
  - Constituted by: Alveoli which are ventilated but not perfused
  - **Normal value: 60-80 ml**

Increased by	Decreased by
• Lung pathologies • General anesthesia • Hypotension • IPPV • PEEP	• Lying down

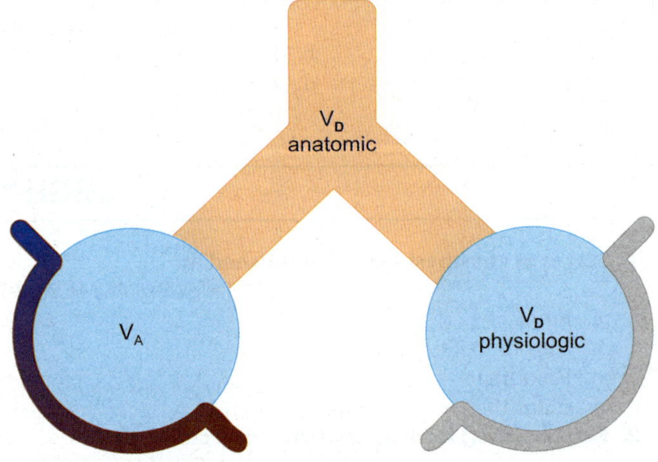

Fig. Dead space

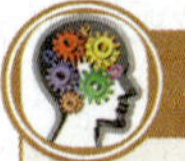

Also Remember

- Tracheostomy reduces dead space by: 70–100 ml
- Intubation reduces dead space by: 50–70 ml

3. **Ans. (b) Guedel**

[Ref. KDT, 6/e , p366-67]

- **Guedel**: Described four levels/ stages of ether anesthesia
- **Morton**: First to publicly demonstrate efficacy of ether as an anesthetic
- **Crawford W. Long**: First to use ether during a surgical operation

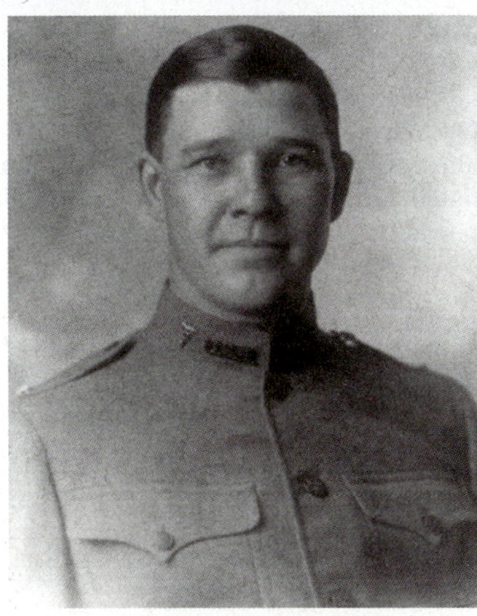

Arthur Guedel

4. **Ans. (a)** **Cricoid**

   [Ref. Principles of Airway Management by Brendan Finucane, 4/e p23]

   - Airway of the infant is narrowest at: Level of the cricoids cartilage
   - In adult airway it is narrowest at: Rima glottidis

5. **Ans. (b)** **Cocaine**

   [Ref. Short Textbook of Anaesthesia by Ajay Yadav, 4/e p118; The Practice of Medicinal Chemistry by Camille Georges Wermuth,2/e p11]

   - **Cocaine was the first local anaesthetic** used by Carl Koller and Sigmund Freud for anaesthetizing cornea before cataract surgery
     - They noticed that the drug was able to prevent oculomotor reflex in frog.

6. **Ans. (d)** **Spinal dura and vertebral column**

   [Ref. A Practical Approach to Regional Anaesthesia by Christopher M,4/e p103]

   - **Epidural space** is the space created between the spinal dura and the periosteum of the vertebral column and extends from foramen magnum to sacrococcygeal ligament
   - Epidural space is largest at the lumbar level

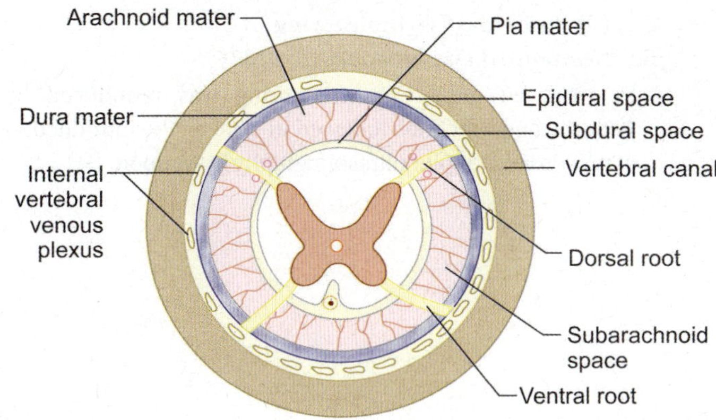

Fig. Epidural space

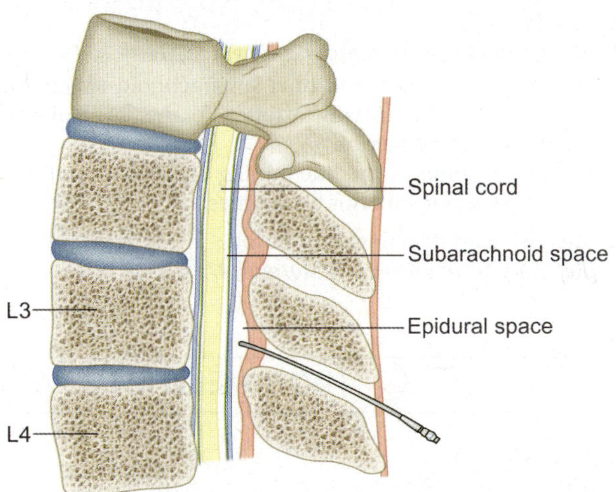

Fig. Epidural space

7. **Ans. (b)** L_1

   [Ref. Gray's Clinical Neuroanatomy,1/e p111]

   - At birth *spinal cord ends at the level* of third lumbar vertebra (or sometime at lower border of second lumbar vertebra) while in adult, it *terminates at the level of lower border of* L_1 (or the intervertebral disc between the L_1 and L_2)
   - It lies little above the level of the elbow joint when the arm is by the side and also lies approximately in the transpyloric plane

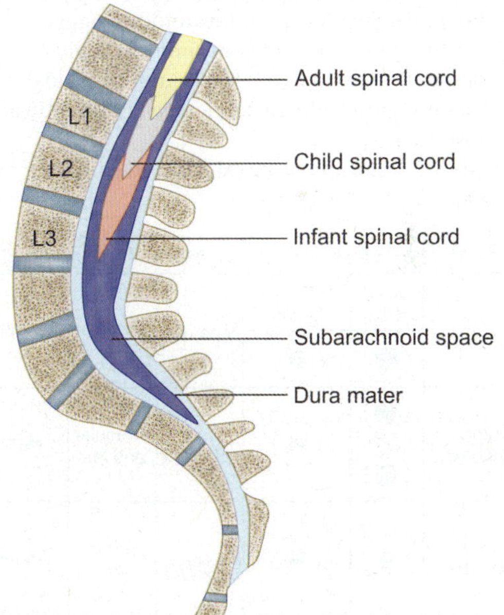

Fig. Termination of spinal cord

8. **Ans. (b)** **26 cm**

   [Ref. A Rational Basis for Anesthesiology by Gianfranco Dal Santo,1/e p336]

9. **Ans. (a)** **Carl Kollar**

   [Ref. Short Textbook of Anaesthesia by Ajay Yadav, 4/e p118; The Practice of Medicinal Chemistry by Camille Georges Wermuth 2/e p11]

10. Ans. (d) S_{2-3}

[Ref. Gray's Clinical Neuroanatomy, 1/e p111]

- Dural sac (theca), and thus subarachnoid space and its contained CSF, usually extends to the level of second segment of the sacrum
- It corresponds to the line joining dimples located in skin over posterior superior iliac spines.

11. Ans. (d) Endotracheal intubation

[Ref. Ajay Yadav, 4/e p4-5; Morgan, 4/e p 553]

12. Ans. (b) Wendell Holmes

[Ref. Wondrous Story of Anesthesia by Edmond, 1/e p618]

- Terms '**Anesthesia**' and '**Anesthetic**' were both introduced by Oliver Wendell Holmes
- Anaesthesia has precisely the same meaning as when it was first coined, i.e. the state in which an animal is insensible to pain resulting from the trauma of surgery.

HIGH YIELD MCQs ANSWERS WITH EXPLANATIONS

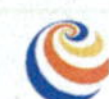

1. Ans. (a) Ether

[KDT, 6/e p366-67]

Guedel's Four Stages of Anesthesia (Ether)

- **Stage I (Analgesia)**: Extends till loss of consciousness
- **Stage II (Delirium or excitement)**: Extends till beginning of regular respiration
  - Maximum movement of eyeball takes place, pupil remains partially dilated and eyelash reflex is lost
- **Stage III (Surgical anesthesia)**: Extends till cessation of spontaneous breathing
  - Plane I: Eyeball become fixed, eyelid reflex lost and pupil size becomes normal (Regular respiration)
  - Plane II: Loss of corneal reflex and pupil starts dilating; Lacrimation is still present (Respiratory paresis)
  - Plane III: Swallowing reflex and laryngeal reflex is lost; Lacrimation is absent (Respiratory paralysis)
  - Plane IV: Carinal or cough reflex is lost with fully dilated pupil (Intercostal paralysis with only abdominal respiration)
- **Stage IV (medullary paralysis)**: Respiratory arrest and apnea.

Stage	Pupil		Resp.	Pulse	B.P
	Usual size	Reaction to light			
1st Induction				Irregular	Normal
2nd Excitement	OR			Irregular and fast	High
3rd Operative				Steady slow	Normal
4th Danger				Weak and thread	Low

Fig. Stages of ansthesia

Also Remember

- *Sequence of Reflexes loss/gain*:
  - First reflex to be lost is eyelash reflex and last reflex to lost is cough reflex
  - Return of reflexes is in opposite sequences

2. Ans. (c) Cocaine

[Ref. Short Textbook of Anaesthesia by Ajay Yadav, 4/e p118; The Practice of Medicinal Chemistry by Camille Georges Wermuth, 2/e p11]

3. Ans. (d) Main bronchus

[Ref. Ajay Yadav, 4/e p4]

- Maximum airway resistance to airflow: Trachea > Main bronchus

4. Ans. (c) Diaphragm

[Ref. Miller's Anaesthesia, 8/e p970]

- Diaphragm and laryngeal muscles are relatively resistant to nondepolarizing agents

5. Ans. (b) Ulnar

[Ref. Clinical Anaesthesiology by Morgan, 4/e p331]

- Interscalene brachial plexus block using ultrasound or electrical stimulation is ideally suited for shoulder procedures.

6. Ans. (d) End tidal CO_2 monitoring

[Ref. Neuroanesthesia by Stone, 1/e p123]

- In 1965, end-tidal CO_2 monitoring was introduced by Bethune and Brechner, followed in 1968 by the introduction of precordial Doppler ultrasonography by Maroon.

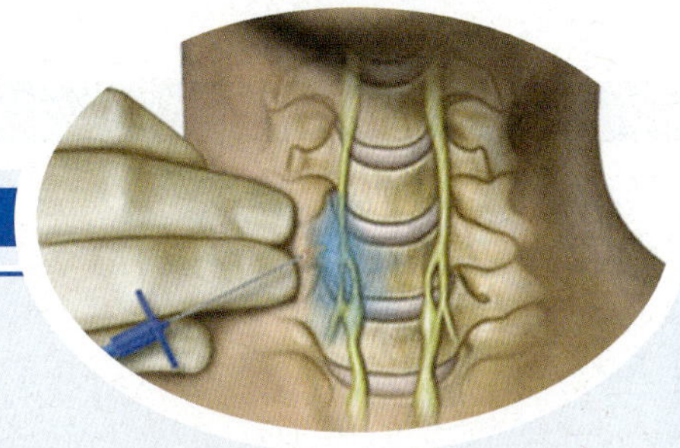

Chapter 2

Physiology, Oxygen Delivery, Cylinders, Instruments and Circuits

THEORETICAL CONCEPTS

II A. PULSE OXIMETRY

- *Definition*: Noninvasive method which **measures oxygen saturation in hemoglobin/blood (SpO_2)** [***Normal*** SpO_2**: 97–98%**[Q]]
- *Principle of pulse oximetry*:
  - Source of light emits at two wavelengths (660 nm and 940 nm) from a probe passes through tissue
  - Ratio of absorption by pulsatile arterial and capillary blood and nonpulsatile venous blood and tissue is calculated and converted to oxygen saturation
- *Application of probe*:
  - Finger nail bed
  - Toe nail bed
  - Ear lobule
  - Tip of nose
  - Foot (Infants)
- *Uses of pulse oximetry*: Detection of hypoxia in intraoperative and postoperative period (intensive care, critical care, surgery, emergency departments)
- ***Errors in pulse oximetry***:[Q]
  - Carboxyhemoglobinemia (shows 95% saturation always)
  - Methhemoglobinemia (shows 85% saturation always)
  - Cyanide poisoning (higher values)
  - Anemia (lower values)
  - Hypovolemia, vasoconstriction in cold (lower values)
  - Vasodilation (lower values)
  - Nail polish blue
  - Shivering (lower values)
  - SpO_2 less than 60% (lower values)
- *Newer technique for measurement of pulse co-oximetry*:
  - Oxygen saturation levels (SpO_2)
  - Hemoglobin level
  - Carboxyhemoglobin
  - Methhemoglobin
  - Pleth variability index

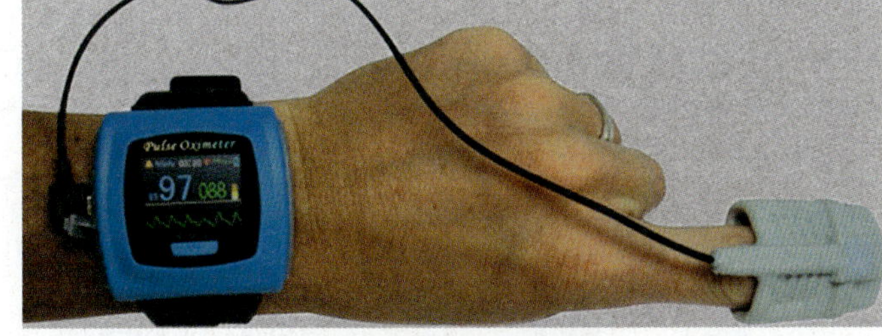

Fig. Pulse oximeter

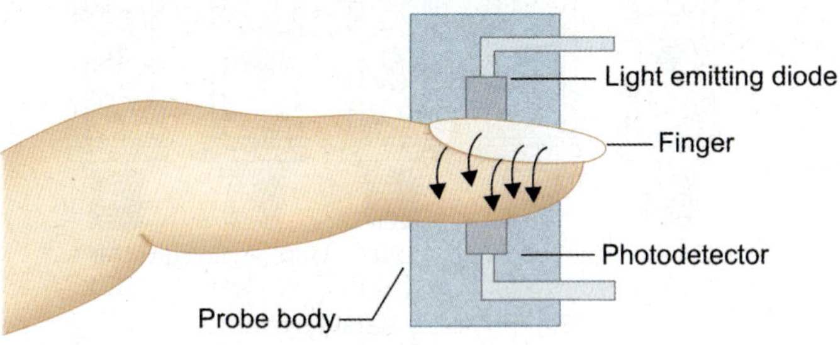

Fig. Pulse oximetry

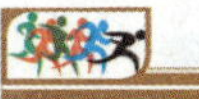

Topper's Edge

Pulse Oximetry

- Pulse oximetry:
  - Noninvasive method for monitoring a person's oxygen saturation (SO_2)
  - SpO_2 (Peripheral oxygen saturation) reading is not always identical to SaO_2 (Arterial oxygen saturation) from arterial blood gas analysis, but the two are correlated well enough that the safe, convenient, noninvasive, inexpensive pulse oximetry method is valuable for measuring oxygen saturation in clinical use
- TWO numerical values obtained from the pulse oximeter monitor[Q]:
  - **Oxygen saturation of hemoglobin in arterial blood**: Since oximeter detects saturation peripherally on a finger, toe or ear, the result is recorded as peripheral oxygen saturation (SpO_2[Q])
  - **Pulse rate in (beats per minute)**
- Pulse oximeter is an early-warning device:
  - It continuously measures the level of oxygen saturation of hemoglobin in the arterial blood
  - It can detect hypoxia much sooner than the anesthesia provider can see clinical signs of hypoxia such as cyanosis
  - This ability to provide an early warning has made the pulse oximeter essential for safe anesthesia
- Key facts:
  - In order to get a satisfactory reading the probe must be emitting a red light[Q] and must be correctly positioned to detect pulsatile blood flow
  - **During anesthesia the SpO_2 should be 95% or above**[Q]:
    1. If SpO_2 is 94% or below, the patient must be assessed quickly to identify and treat the cause[Q]
    2. SpO_2 of <90% is a clinical emergency and should be treated urgently[Q]
  - Hypovolemia is the MC cause of a weak pulse oximeter signal during anesthesia[Q]

II B. PIN INDEX SYSTEM

- *Definition*: Safety mechanism for gas cylinders used in anaesthesia so that one cannot be wrongly placed in another's position
- *Composition*: 2 pins - 4 mm and 6 mm long
- *Pin index for gases used in anesthesia*:

Gas	Pin index [Q]
Oxygen[Q]	**2, 5**
Nitrous oxide	3, 5
Cyclopropane	3, 6
Air	1, 5
Nitrogen	1, 4
Entonox (50% O_2 + 50% NO) [Q]	**7**
Carbon dioxide (<7.5%)	2, 6
Carbon dioxide (>7.5%)	1, 6

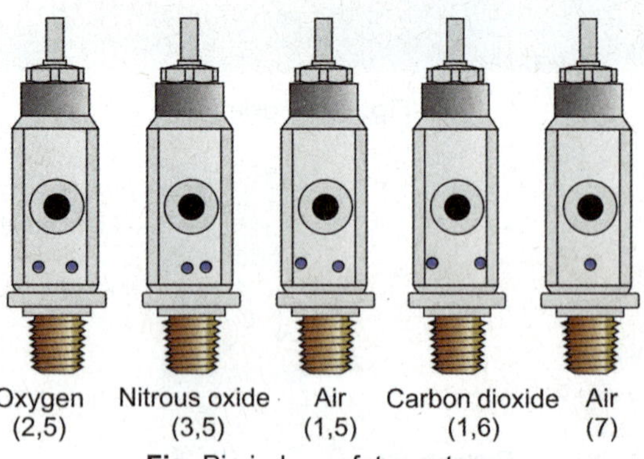

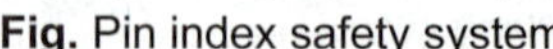

Fig. Pin index safety system

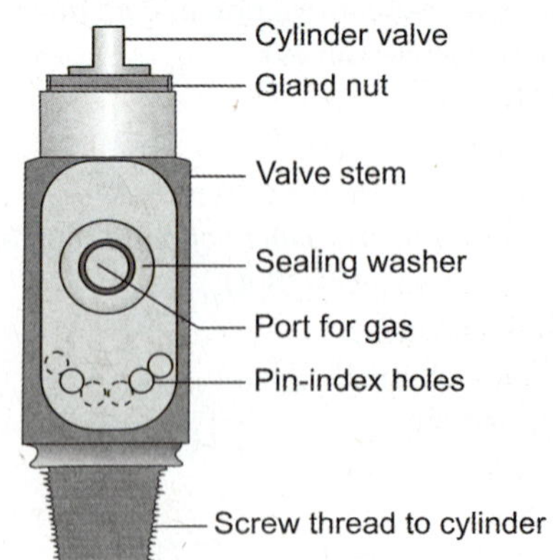

Fig. Cylinder valve

II C. CYLINDERS USED IN ANESTHESIA

II C1. Material Used in Cylinders

- *Material used*: Chromium molybedenum steel [Q]

II C2. Cylinder Pressures

Cylinder	Pressure
Oxygen [Q]	**137 bar**
Air	137 bar
Helium	137 bar
Nitrous oxide	40 bar
Carbon dioxide	50 bar
Cyclopropane	5 bar

II C3. Colors of Cylinders

Cylinder	Color [Q]
Oxygen[Q]	**Black body with white shoulders**
Nitrous oxide [Q]	**Blue**
Nitrogen	Black
Air [Q]	**Gray body with black and white shoulders**
Carbon dioxide[Q]	Brownish gray
Cyclopropane [Q]	**Orange**
Helium	Brown
Entonox [Q]	**Blue body with blue and white shoulders**
Ethylene	Purple with red shoulder
Halothane bottle	Amber
Thiopentone [Q]	**Yellow**

II D. OXYGEN CYLINDER

- *Cylinder colour*: **Black body with white shoulders**
- *Pressure recommended*: 2000 psi **(137 kg per cm square)**[Q]
- *Most commonly used cylinder type*: Type E
- *Acceptable purity*: 99%
- *Testing of cylinders*: Once every 5 years
- *Liquid oxygen*:
  - Storage temperature: Below minus 119°C
  - 1 ml liquid oxygen = 840 ml gas

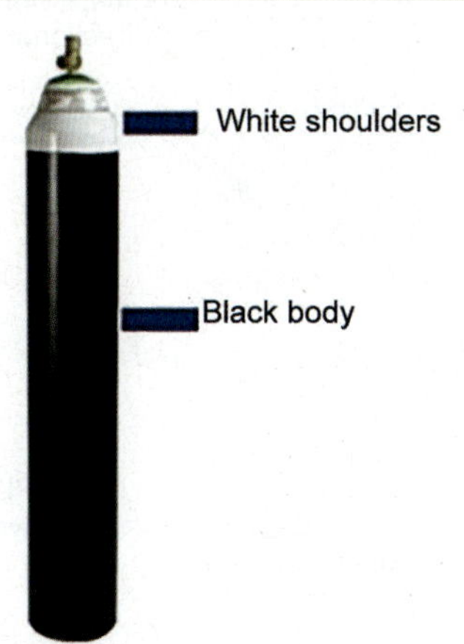

Fig. Oxygen cylinder

II E. BREATHING CIRCUITS

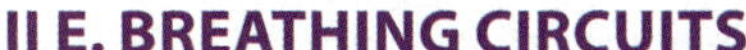

II E1. Open Circuits/Open Systems

- Underlying principle: Exhaled gases by patients are completely exhaled in atmosphere; Exhaled gases are NOT REUSED by the patients[Q]
- Examples:
  - Schimmelbusch mask (Open drop anaesthesia[Q])

II E2. Semi-closed Circuits/Mapleson Systems

- Underlying principle: Exhaled gases by patients are partially exhaled in atmosphere; Exhaled gases are PARTIALLY REUSED by the patients[Q]
- Examples:
  - **Type A (Magill circuit[Q]):**
    - Required fresh gas flow: Equal to minute volume[Q] (80 ml/kg/min[Q])
    - Circuit of choice for: Spontaneous ventilation[Q]
    - Not used for: Controlled ventilation[Q]
  - **Type B:**
    - Required fresh gas flow: Equal to Twice minute volume
  - **Type C (Waters' To and Fro[Q]):**
    - Required fresh gas flow: Equal to Twice minute volume
    - Coaxial system[Q]
  - **Type D (Bain's circuit[Q]):**
    - Required fresh gas flow: Equal to 2–3 times minute volume
    - Circuit of choice for: Controlled ventilation[Q]
    - May be used for: Spontaneous ventilation
    - MC used circuit[Q]
  - **Type E (Ayre's T-piece[Q]):**
    - Required fresh gas flow: Equal to 2–3 times minute volume
    - Circuit of 2nd choice for: Children
  - **Type F (Jackson Rees circuit[Q]):**
    - Required fresh gas flow: Equal to 2–3 times minute volume
    - Circuit of 1st choice for: Children[Q]

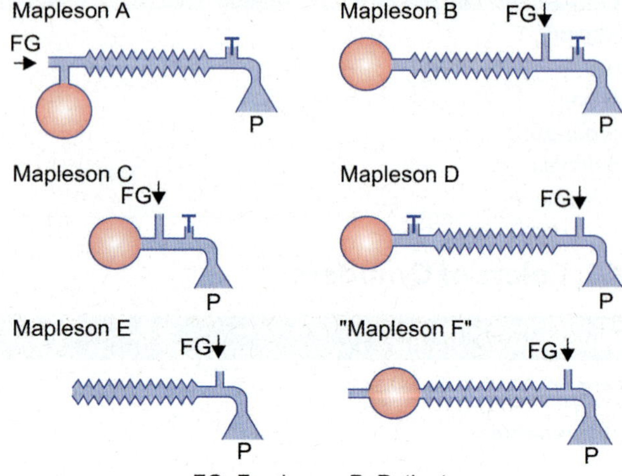

Fig. Mapleson systems

II E3. Closed Circuits/Rebreathing Systems

- Underlying principle: Nome of the exhaled gases by patients escape to atmosphere; Exhaled gases are COMPLETELY REUSED by the patients[Q]
- Examples:
  - Circle system (MC used[Q])
  - To and Fro (Water's/Mapleson's C system)[Q]

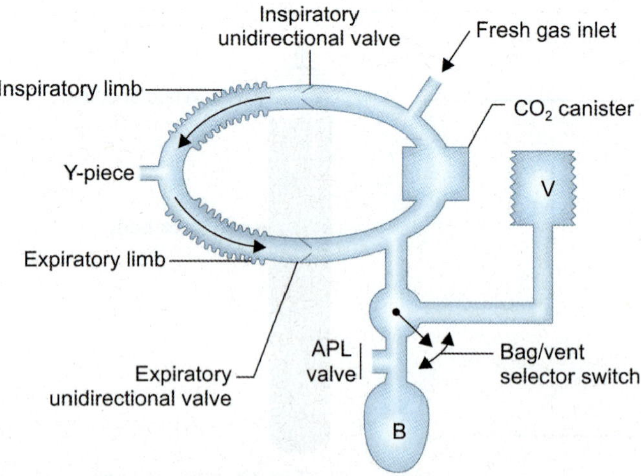

Fig. Circle Breathing System

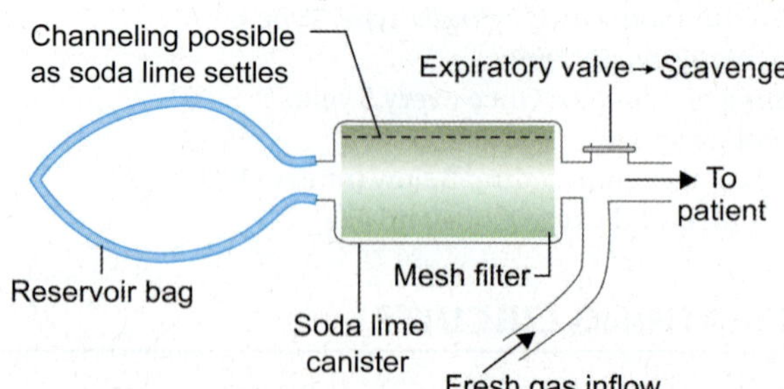

Fig. To-and-Fro system

Topper's Edge

Breathing Circuits

	Open drop	Mapleson	Circle
Complexity	Very simple	Simple	Complex
Control of anesthetic depth	Poor	Variable	Good
Ability to scavenge	Very poor	Variable	Good
Conservation of heat and humidity	No	No	Yes
Rebreathing of exhaled gases	No	No	Yes

Breathing Systems

- **Mapleson A design is the most efficient Mapleson circuit for spontaneous ventilation**: As fresh gas flow equal to minute ventilation is sufficient to prevent rebreathing
- Mapleson D circuit is efficient during controlled ventilation: As fresh gas flow forces alveolar air away from the patient and toward the APL valve
- Long breathing tubes with high compliance increase the difference between the volume of gas delivered to a circuit by a reservoir bag or ventilator and the volume actually delivered to the patient
- Adjustable pressure-limiting (APL) valve should be fully open during spontaneous ventilation so that circuit pressure remains negligible throughout inspiration and expiration
- Drier the soda lime, the more likely it will absorb and degrade volatile anesthetics
- Malfunction of either unidirectional valve in a circle system may allow rebreathing of carbon dioxide, resulting in hypercapnia.

IMAGE-BASED QUESTIONS

1. Identify the Law of Anesthesia shown in photograph

$$Q = \frac{\pi P r^4}{8 \eta l}$$

a. Boyle's law
b. Charles' law
c. Graham's law
d. Hagen Poiseuille law

2. Identify the gas cylinder shown in the photograph ***[Recent Question 2013]***

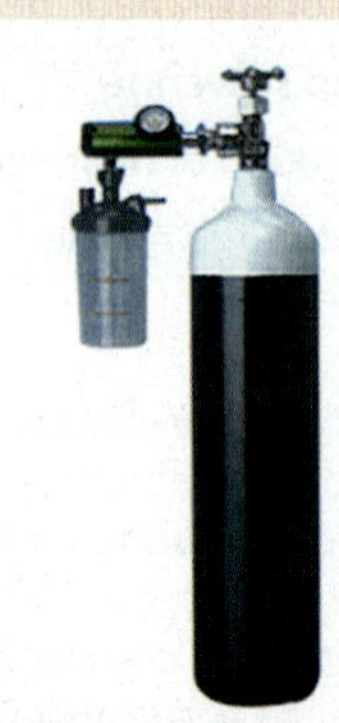

a. Oxygen
b. Cyclopropane
c. Nitrous oxide
d. Thiopentone

3. Type of Mapleson semi-closed circuit shown in photograph ***[Recent Question 2014]***

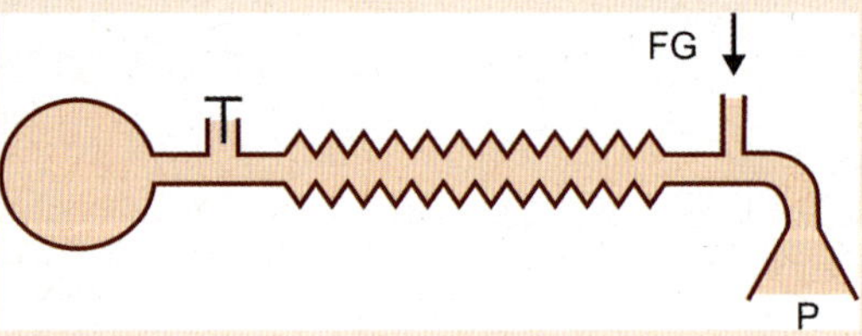

a. A
b. D
c. E
d. F

4. Identify the part of anaesthesia equipment shown in photograph

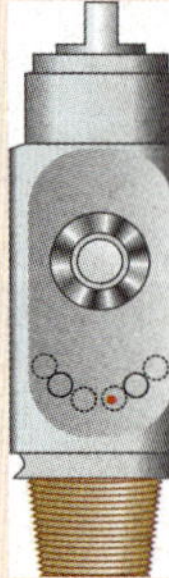

a. Yoke
b. Flowmeter
c. Vapouriser
d. Cylinder valve

ANSWERS WITH EXPLANATIONS OF IBQs 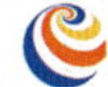

1. Ans. (d) Hagen Poiseuille law *[Ref. Ajay Yadav, 4/e p10]*

Hagen Poiseuille Law

- Equation: At a constant driving pressure the Flow rate (Q) of liquid through a capillary tube is
  - Directly proportional to the fourth power of the radius of the tube (r) and Pressure gradient (P)
  - Inversely proportional to viscosity (η) and length (l)

2. Ans. (a) Oxygen *[Ref. Ajay Yadav, 4/e p24]*

3. Ans. (b) D *[Ref. Ajay Yadav, 4/e p29]*

Mapleson Type D (Bain's Circuit)

- Required fresh gas flow: Equal to 2–3 times minute volume
- Circuit of choice for: Controlled ventilation
- May be used for: Spontaneous ventilation
- MC used circuit

4. Ans. (d) Cylinder valve *[Ref. Ajay Yadav, 4/e p25]*

- Cylinder valves ensure safety mechanism so that one cylinder is not fitted into another's place
- Holes on cylinder valves correspond to same pins at yolk of machine

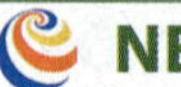 NEET/NBE PATTERN MCQs 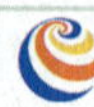

1. **What is pressure at which Oxygen in stored?** *[Recent Question 2016]*
   a. 75 psi b. 1600 psi
   c. 760 psi d. 2200 psi
2. **Henry law states that** *[Recent Question 2016]*
   a. At a constant temperature gas dissolves in solution in proportion to its partial pressure
   b. At a constant pressure gas dissolves in solution in proportion to its temperature
   c. At a constant temperature gas dissolves in solution in proportion to its fat solubility
   d. At a constant pressure gas dissolves in solution in proportion to its fat solubility
3. **Gas cylinder with single pin index** *[Recent Question 2016]*
   a. Oxygen
   b. Air
   c. Nitrogen
   d. Entonox
4. **Pulse oximetry monitors** *[NBE FMGE March 2010]*
   a. Oxygen content of blood
   b. Pulse pressure c. Oxygen partial pressure
   d. Oxygen saturation of hemoglobin
5. **Pin-index of oxygen is** *[NBE FMGE March 2007]*
   a. 5 b. 1,5
   c. 2,5 d. 3,5
6. **Which can replace N_2O as O_2 carrier?** *[Recent Question 2016, 2012]*
   a. Argon b. Xenon
   c. Helium d. None
7. **To counter central anticholinergic effect, drug used is** *[NBE DNB 2001]*
   a. Physostigmine
   b. Atropine
   c. Neostigmine
   d. Hyoscine
8. **Color of ethylene cylinder is** *[NBE DNB 1992, 2004]*
   a. Blue b. Grey
   c. Orange d. Purple
9. **Pin-index for Entonox is** *[NBE FMGE March 2005]*
   a. 1,4 b. 2,5
   c. 3,5 d. 7
10. **Pin code index of N_2O is** *[AIPGME 1997, AIIMS PG 2003, Recent Question 2012, 2013]*
    a. 1,6 b. 2,5
    c. 2,6 d. 3,5
11. **Pulse oximetry monitors** *[NBE DNB June 2011]*
    a. Oxygen saturation of hemoglobin
    b. Oxygen content of blood
    c. Pulse pressure
    d. Oxygen partial pressure
12. **DISS is used for** *[Recent Question 2016, 2013]*
    a. Correct application of cylinder to anaesthesia machine
    b. To provide analgesia
    c. To monitor BP
    d. To monitor CVP
13. **MAC stands for** *[Recent Question 2012, 2017]*
    a. Minimum alveolar concentration
    b. Minimal analgesic concentration
    c. Minimal anaesthetic concentration
    d. Maximum alveolar concentration
14. **Incorrect about oxygen storage is** *[NBE FMGE September 2006]*
    a. Pressure 2000 psi
    b. 99% acceptable purity
    c. Commonly used cylinders on anaesthesia machines is Type-E
    d. Blue cylinder with orange collar
15. **Ratio of $O_2 : N_2O$ in Entonox is** *[Recent Question 2016, 2012]*
    a. 50:50
    b. 60:40
    c. 40:60
    d. 25:75
16. **Which circuit is best for Controlled ventilation?** *[Recent Question 2017]*
    a. Jackson Rees modification of Ayre's T piece
    b. Mapleson A or Magill's circuit
    c. Mapleson C or water's to & fro canister
    d. Bain's circuit
17. **Blue cylinder with blue and white collar is for?** *[Recent Question 2017]*
    a. Oxygen
    b. Air
    c. Nitrogen
    d. Entonox
18. **Type E circuit is used for?** *[Recent Question 2017]*
    a. Spontaneous ventilation
    b. Controlled ventilation
    c. Children
    d. All of the above indications
19. **MAC of an anesthetic agent is the measure of its** *[Recent Question 2017]*
    a. Potency
    b. Speed of induction and recovery
    c. Lipid solubility
    d. Toxicity
20. **Use of Soda lime in anesthesia is?** *[Recent Question 2017]*
    a. As a hardner
    b. As an absorbent
    c. As a softner
    d. As an indicator
21. **Type of circuit use in a child of age 5 years for anesthesia is?** *[Recent Question 2017]*
    a. Jackson Rees modification of Ayre's T piece
    b. Mapleson A or Magill's circuit
    c. Mapleson C or Water's to & fro canister
    d. Bain's circuit

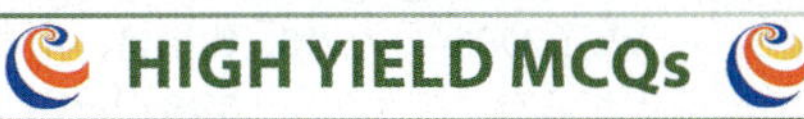

1. **Oxygen delivery is regulated by all except** *[AIIMS PGMEE 1994]*
   a. Oxygen tent b. Venti-mask
   c. Poly-mask d. Noval catheter
2. **Trendelenburg's position produces decrease in all of the following except** *[AIIMS PGMEE 2004]*
   a. Vital capacity
   b. Functional residual capacity
   c. Compliance
   d. Respiratory rate
3. **Maximum vital capacity decreased in** *[AIIMS PGMEE 1992]*
   a. Prone b. Supine
   c. Trendelenburg d. Left lateral
4. **Side effects of oxygen therapy are all except** *[AIIMS PGMEE 2007]*
   a. Absorption atelectasis
   b. Increased pulmonary compliance
   c. Decreased vital capacity
   d. Endothelial damage
5. **Pulse oximetry detects inaccurately in presence of** *[PGI 2005]*
   a. Hyperbilirubinemia b. Nail polish
   c. Methemoglobinemia d. Skin pigmentation
6. **True about N_2O cylinder** *[PGI 2004]*
   a. Pressure is 2200 PSI b. Blue in color
   c. Gas in liquid form d. Pin index 3, 5
   e. It is flammable
7. **Dead space is increased by all except** *[AIIMS PGMEE 2009]*
   a. Anticholinergic drugs b. Standing
   c. Hyperextension of neck d. Endotracheal intubation
8. **Hoffman's elimination is for** *[PGI 1998, 1999]*
   a. Atracurium b. Pancuronium
   c. Gallamine d. Ketamine
9. **For high pressure storage of compressed gases, cylinders are made up of** *[Delhi PGMEE 2008]*
   a. Molybdenum steel b. Iron and molybedenum
   c. Steel and copper d. Cast iron
10. **Partition coefficient of gas** *[PGI 1998]*
    a. Measure of potency
    b. Directly proportional to potency
    c. Measures solubility
    d. All of the above
11. **Anatomical dead space is increased by all except** *[All India PGMEE 1999]*
    a. Atropine b. Halothane
    c. Massive pleural effusion d. Inspiration
12. **Gas is filled as liquid in cylinder in** *[PGI 2007]*
    a. O_2 b. CO_2
    c. N_2O d. Cyclopropane
    e. Halothane
13. **The physiological dead space is decreased by** *[AIIMS PGMEE 2005]*
    a. Upright position
    b. Positive pressure ventilation
    c. Neck flexion
    d. Emphysema
14. **Pin index system is a safety feature adopted in anesthesia machines to prevent** *[Recent Question 2017, AIIMS PGMEE 2003]*
    a. Incorrect attachment of anaesthesia machines
    b. Incorrect attachment of anaesthesia face masks
    c. Incorrect inhalation agent delivery
    d. Incorrect gas cylinder attachment
15. **An anesthetist orders a new attendant to bring the oxygen cylinder. He will ask the attendant to identify the correct cylinder by following color code** *[All India PGMEE 2003, AIIMS November 2015]*
    a. Black cylinders with white shoulders
    b. Black cylinders with gray shoulders
    c. White cylinders with black shoulders
    d. Gray cylinder with white shoulders
16. **Color of oxygen cylinder is** *[All India PGMEE 1997, AIIMS 1992]*
    a. Gray
    b. Blue
    c. Black with white shoulder
    d. Orange
17. **True about N_2O** *[PGI 2008]*
    a. Pin index 3,5 b. Blue in color
    c. Stored as liquid d. MAC 105
18. **True about N_2O cylinder is/are all except** *[PGI 2000]*
    a. Blue color
    b. N_2O in liquid form in cylinder
    c. 2220 PSP is the pressure in cylinder
    d. Pin index 3,5
19. **All statements are true about gas cylinders except** *[MAHE PGMEE 2004 [JIPMER PGMEE 2002]*
    a. Pressure of N_2O is 745 psig at 20°C
    b. Higher pressure indicates impurity in N_2O
    c. N_2O is in liquid form
    d. Emergency oxygen 'E' cylinder has more gas than 'H' cylinder
20. **Regarding critical temperature which of following is true** *[PGI 2008]*
    a. TC of O_2 is – 119°C b. TC of O_2 is – 119°C
    c. TC of O_2 is – 36.5°C d. TC of N_2O is 36.5°C
    e. TC of air is – 140.6°C
21. **All of the following are suitable anaesthetic circuits for both controlled and assisted ventilation except** *[AIIMS PGMEE 2003]*
    a. Mapleson A b. Mapleson B & C
    c. Mapleson D d. Mapleson E
22. **Not true for Magills circuit** *[AIIMS PGMEE 1993]*
    a. Ideal for adults
    b. Ideal for infant
    c. Semiclosed
    d. Spontaneous breathing is a must
23. **A 25-year-old male is undergoing incision and drainage of abscess under general anesthesia with spontaneous respiration. The most efficient anaesthetic circuit is** *[Delhi PGMEE 2009]*
    a. Maplelson A b. Mapleson B
    c. Mapleson C d. Mapleson D

24. True about Bain circuit *[PGI 2009]*
a. Mapleson type B
b. Mapleson type D
c. Can be used for spontaneous respiration
d. Can be used for controlled ventilation
e. Coaxial

25. In Magill circuit airflow is *[All India PGMEE 1998, 2000]*
a. 1/2 of minute volume
b. Equal to M.V.
c. 2 X m.v.
d. 3 X m.v.

26. The most appropriate circuit for ventilating a spontaneously breathing infant during anesthesia is *[Recent Question 2016, 2017, All India PGMEE 2005]*
a. Jackson Rees' modification of Ayres' T Piece
b. Mapleson A or Magill's circuit
c. Mapleson C or Waters' to and fro canister
d. Bain's circuit

27. True about oxygen concentrator *[PGI 2005]*
a. Zeolite activation
b. Delivers O_2
c. Requires power supply
d. Gives O_2 at 100%

28. For rebreathing prevention valve incorrect is *[AIIMS PGMEE 1994]*
a. Should be as far as possible from the patient
b. Should be light
c. Well designed
d. Used at expiratory end of tube

29. All CO_2 absorption in circuit except *[PGI 2007]*
a. Resistance in circuit b. High flow
c. Small granule size d. Medium granule size
e. Chanelling

30. Reacts with sodalime *[Recent Question 2016, All India PGMEE 1993]*
a. Methoxyfluene b. Ketamine
c. Trilene d. SO_2

31. All decrease CO_2 absorption in circuit except *[AIIMS PGMEE 1993]*
a. Resistance in circuit b. Flow
c. Dead space d. Tidal volume

32. Water is used for hardening in *[PGI 1996, All India PGMEE 92)*
a. Sodalime b. Baralime
c. Both d. None

33. Clayton is used in a close breathing system for the purpose of *[PGI 1996, AMU 1998)*
a. As a hardner b. As an absorbent
c. As a softner d. As an indicator

34. Rebreathing systems are all except *[PGI 2005, SGPGI 2000, All India PGMEE 1991]*
a. To & fro system
b. Circle system
c. Water's system
d. Mapleson F

35. Which one of the following device provides fixed performance oxygen therapy? *[AIIMS PGMEE 2005]*
a. Nasal Cannula b. Venturi mask
c. O_2 by T-piece d. Edinburg mask

36. Which of the following does not represent a significant anesthetic problem in the morbidly obese patient? *[AIIMS PGMEE 2004]*
a. Difficulties in endotracheal intubation
b. Suboptimal arterial oxygen tension
c. Increased metabolism of volatile agents
d. Decreased cardiac output relative to total body mass

37. In venture mask maximum O_2 concentration attained is *[BIHAR PGMEE 2005]*
a. 90% b. 100%
c. 60% d. 80%

38. Which of the following produces the least damage to blood elements? *[AIIMS PGMEE 2004]*
a. Disc oxygenator b. Membrane oxygenator
c. Bubble oxygenator d. Screen oxygenator

39. End-tidal CO_2 is increased to maximum level in *[PGI 2000]*
a. Pul. embolism b. Malignant hyperthermia
c. Extubation d. Blockage of secretion

40. Characteristic of an ideal gas is *[PGI 1998]*
a. Volume is directly proportional to change in pressure
b. Volume is inversely proportional to change in temperature
c. At absolute temp. volume of gas is 1
d. Obeys Charles, Boyles and Avagadro' laws

41. Least blood gas partition coefficient anesthetic agent *[Jharkhand PGMEE 2005, WB PGMEE 2006]*
a. Desflurane b. Nitrous oxide
c. Halothane d. Ether

42. Least diffusion coefficient is for *[JIPMER PGMEE 2004, AMU PGMEE 2005]*
a. Isoflurane b. Enflurane
c. Halothane d. N_2O

43. Exception of Meyer overton rule are all except *[Recent Question 2016]* *[JIPMER PGMEE 2003, J&K PGMEE 2004]*
a. Nonanaesthetics b. Nonimmobilizer
c. Cut off effect d. Hydrophobic site

44. Pungent volatile anesthetic agents are *[PGI 2009]*
a. Halothane b. Isoflurane
c. Sevoflurane d. Desflurane
e. Nitrous oxide

45. Which of the following inhalational agents has the minimum blood gas solubility coefficient? *[AIIMS PGMEE 2006]*
a. Isoflurane b. Sevoflurane
c. Desflurane d. Nitrous oxide

46. Which of the following is not true about xenon anaesthesia? *[AIIMS PGMEE 2006]*
a. Non explosive
b. Minimal cardiovascular side effects
c. Slow induction and slow recovery
d. Minimal cardiovascular side effects

47. Diffusion hypoxia is seen during *[PGI 1998]*
a. Induction of anaesthesia
b. Recovering anaesthesia
c. Preoperatively
d. Postoperatively

48. At the end of anesthesia after discontinuation of nitrous oxide and removal of endotracheal tube, 100% oxygen is administered to the patient to prevent

[AIIMS PGMEE 2003]

a. Diffusion hypoxia
b. Second gas effect
c. Hyperoxia
d. Bronchospasm

49. After hyperventilation for some time holding the breath is dangerous since *[AIIMS PGMEE 2000]*

a. It can lead to CO_2 narcosis
b. Due to lack of stimulation by CO_2, anoxia can go into dangerous level
c. CO_2 shift O dissociation curve to left
d. Alkalosis can lead to tetany

50. Gas which produces systemic toxicity without causing local irritation is *[All India PGMEE 2002]*

a. Ammonium
b. Carbon monoxide
c. Hydrocyanic acid
d. Sulfur dioxide

51. In a patient with fixed respiratory obstruction Helium is used along with Oxygen instead of plain oxygen because

[All India PGMEE 2002]

a. It increases the absorption of oxygen
b. It decreases turbulence
c. It decreases the dead space
d. For analgesia

52. A 20 years old spontaneous breathing patient undergoing incision and drainage under general anesthesia, which is the breathing circuit of choice

[Recent Question 2018, AIIMS November 2014]

a. Mapleson A
b. Mapleson B
c. Mapleson C
d. Mapleson D

53. Abnormal sensation perceived without an apparent stimulus is called as *[PGMCET 2015]*

a. Hyperesthesia
b. Neuralgia
c. Paresthesia
d. Radiculopathy

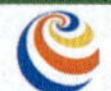 NEET/NBE PATTERN MCQs ANSWERS WITH EXPLANATIONS 

1. Ans. (d) 2200 psi

[Ref. McCurnin's Clinical Textbook, 9/e p1023]

- When full, a cylinder contains oxygen at a pressure of approximately 2200 pounds per square inch (psi)
- As oxygen is used, cylinder pressure gradually decreases
- Oxygen cylinder should be changed when pressure reaches 500 psi

2. Ans. (a) At a constant temperature gas dissolves in solution in proportion to its partial pressure

[Ref. Anaesthesia by Colin, 3/e p808]

- **Henry's law** is one of the gas laws formulated by William Henry states: At a constant temperature, the amount of a given gas that dissolves in a given type and volume of liquid is directly proportional to the partial pressure of that gas in equilibrium with that liquid

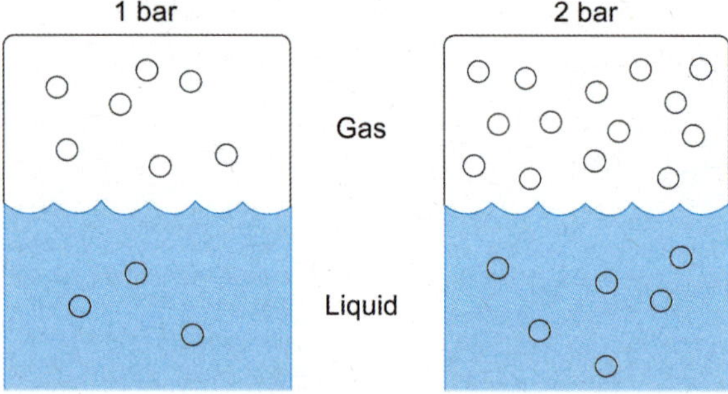

Fig. Henry's law

3. Ans. (d) Entonox

[Ref. Anaesthesia by Colin, 3/e p567]

Gas	Pin index
Oxygen	2,5
Nitrous oxide	3,5
Cyclopropane	3,6
Air	1,5
Nitrogen	1,4
Entonox	7

4. Ans. (d) Oxygen saturation of hemoglobin

[Ref. Ajay Yadav, 4/e p51]

Pulse Oximetry

- *Definition*: Non-invasive method which measures oxygen saturation in haemoglobin/ blood (SpO_2)
- *Application of probe*:
  - Finger nail bed
  - Toe nail bed
  - Ear lobule
  - Tip of nose
  - Foot (Infants)
- ***Normal SpO_2*: 97 – 98%**
- *Principle of Pulse oximetry*:
  - Source of light emits at two wavelengths (660 nm and 940 nm) from a probe passes through tissue
  - Ratio of absorption by pulsatile arterial & capillary blood and non-pulsatile venous blood & tissue is calculated and converted to oxygen saturation
- *Uses of Pulse oximetry*: Detection of hypoxia in intra-operative and post-operative period (intensive care, critical care, surgery, emergency departments)

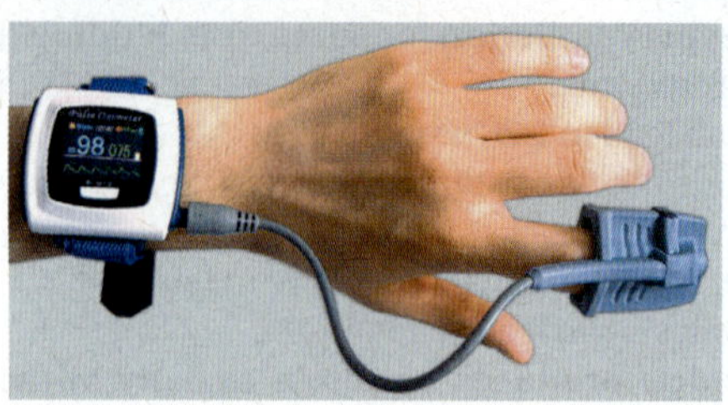

Fig. Pulse oximetry

5. Ans. (c) 2,5

[Ref. Ajay Yadav, 4/e p25]

PIN Index System

- Definition: Safety mechanism for gas cylinders used in anaesthesia so that one cannot be wrongly placed in another's position
- Composition: 2 pins – 4 mm and 6 mm long
- Pin index for gases used in anaesthesia:

Gas	Pin index
Oxygen	2, 5
Nitrous oxide	3, 5
Cyclopropane	3, 6
Air	1, 5
Nitrogen	1, 4
Entonox (50% O_2 + 50% NO)	7
Carbon dioxide (<7.5%)	2, 6
Carbon dioxide (>7.5%)	1, 6

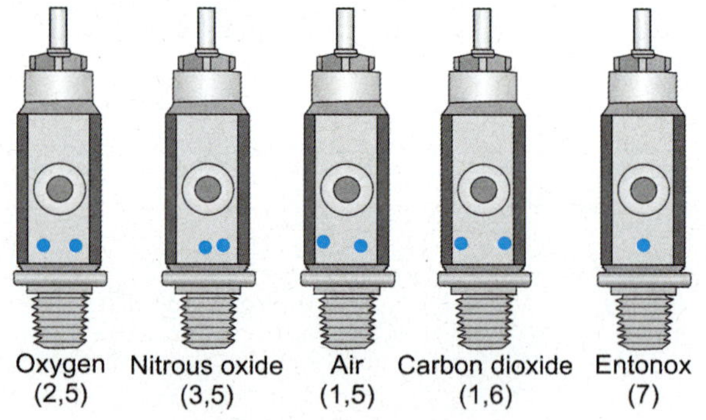

Fig. Pin index system

6. Ans. (c) Helium

[Ref. Pediatric Critical Care Study Guide: Text and Review by Lucking, 1/e p472]

- Helium can be used to replace nitrogen as carrier gas for oxygen (Heliox) to reduce the work of breathing in patients who have critical narrowing of the upper or lower airway

7. Ans. (a) Physostigmine

[Ref. Complications in Anaesthesia by Atlee, 2/e p686]

- Physostigmine 0.025 mg/kg is the treatment of choice to counter the central anticholinergic effects of atropine, scopolamine and other drugs with similar effects

8. Ans. (d) Purple

[Ref. Monheims Local Anaesthesia and Pain Control in Dental Practice, 7/e p278]

Gas cylinder	Colour code
Carbon dioxide	Brownish grey
Cyclopropane	Orange
Ethylene	Purple with red shoulder
Entonox ($O_2 + N_2$)	Blue body with white and blue quartered shoulder
Halothane	Amber (purple-red)
Nitrogen	Black
Nitrous oxide	Blue
Oxygen	Black body with white shoulder
Thiopentone	Yellow

9. Ans. (d) 7

[Ref Ajay Yadav, 4/e p25]

10. Ans. (d) 3,5

[Ref. Ajay Yadav, 4/e p25]

11. Ans. (a) Oxygen saturation of haemoglobin

[Ref. Ajay Yadav, 4/e p51]

12. Ans. (a) Correct application of cylinder to anaesthetic machine

[Ref. Respiratory Care: Principles and Practice by Dean R. Hess, 3/e p262]

Diameter Index Safety System (DISS)

- Gas enters the anaesthesia machine through the pipeline inlet connections
- Pipeline inlet fittings are gas specific Diameter Index Safety System body fittings which provides threaded, non-interchangeable connections for medical gas lines and thereby minimizes risk of misconnection
- A check valve is located downstream from inlet to prevent reverse flow of gases from the machine

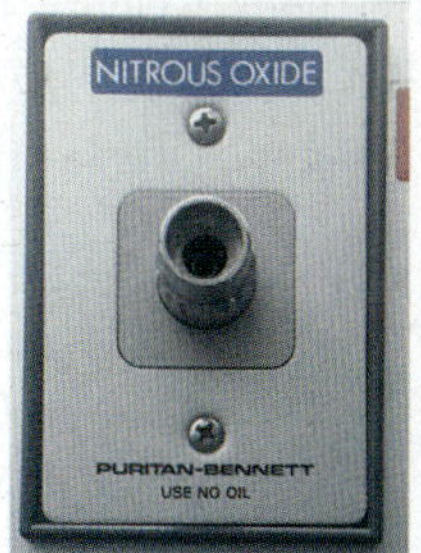

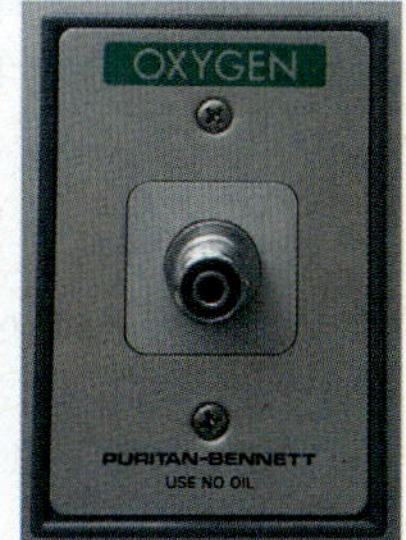

Fig. DISS

13. Ans. (a) Minimum alveolar concentration

[Ref. Anaesthesia Review by Michelle Bowman-Howard, 2/e p126]

- **MAC (Minimum alveolar concentration)**: Concentration of an inhaled anaesthetic at 1 atm required to prevent skeletal muscle movement in response to a noxious stimulant in 50% of patients

14. Ans. (d) Blue cylinder with orange collar

[Ref. Ajay Yadav, 4/e p23]

Oxygen Cylinder

- Cylinder colour: **Black body with white shoulders**
- Pressure recommended: **2000 psi (137 kg per cm square)**
- Most commonly used cylinder type: Type E
- Acceptable purity: 99%
- Testing of cylinders: Once every 5 years
- Liquid oxygen: Storage temperature: 119°C 1 ml liquid oxygen = 840 ml gas

15. Ans. (a) 50:50

[Ref. Textbook of Obstetric Anaesthesia by Rachel E. Collis, 1/e p65]

16. Ans. (d) Bain's circuit

[Ref. Ajay Yadav, 4/e p29]

Mapleson Type D (Bain's Circuit)

- Required fresh gas flow: Equal to 2–3 times minute volume
- Circuit of choice for: Controlled ventilation
- May be used for: Spontaneous ventilation
- MC used circuit

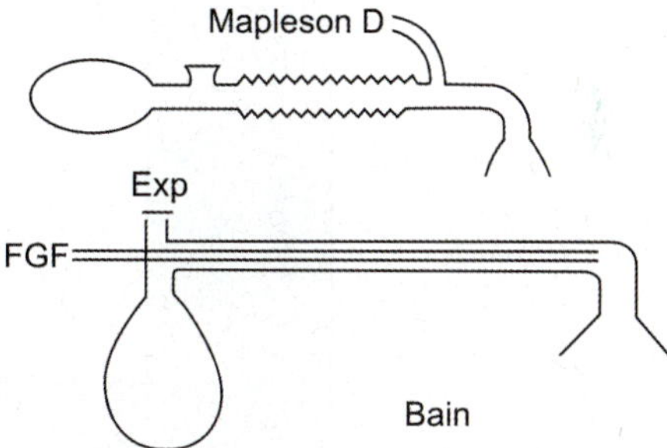

Fig. Mapleson type D (Bain's circuit)

17. Ans. (d) Entonox

[Ref. Ajay Yadav, 2/e p66]

Entonox

- Description: Mixture of 50% oxygen and 50% nitrous oxide
- Storage: Blue cylinders with blue and white shoulders. Above 10°C
- Used for: Painful dressings, changing thoracotomy drains

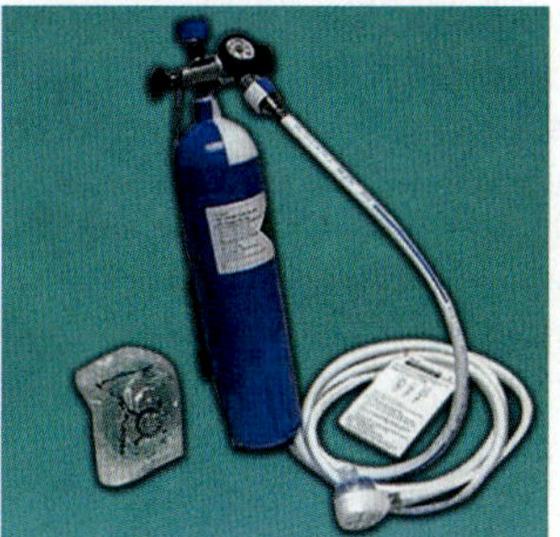

Fig. Entonox cylinder

18. Ans. (c) Children

[Ref. Smith's Anesthesia, 8/e p384]

- Type E (Ayre's T-piece) Mapleson's circuit:
  - Required fresh gas flow: Equal to 2–3 times minute volume
  - Circuit of 2nd choice for: Children

- Type F (Jackson Rees) Mapleson's circuit:
  - Required fresh gas flow: Equal to 2–3 times minute volume
  - Circuit of 1st choice for: Children

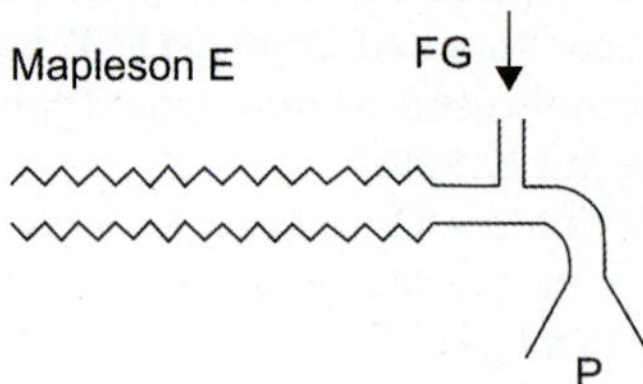

Fig. Mapleson E circuit

19. Ans. (a) Potency
[Ref. Ajay Yadav, 4/e p59]

Minimum Alveolar Concentration (MAC)

- MAC is minimum concentration of agent required to produce immobility in 50% of the subjects given noxious stimuli (which is surgical incision in human beings and tail clamping in rats)
- **MAC is best estimate for measuring potency**
- Agent with minimum MAC is most potent
  - Methoxyflurane with minimum MAC of 0.16% is most potent inhalational agent
  - Nitrous oxide with MAC of 104% is least potent

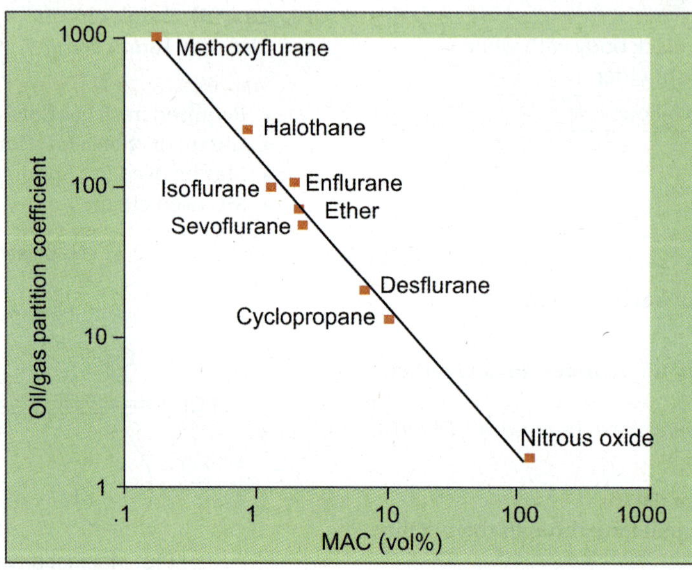

Fig. MAC (Potency) and OG partition coefficient (Lipid solubility)

20. Ans. (b) As an absorbent
[Ref. Clinical Anesthesia by Barash, 6/e p673]

CO_2 Absorbents

- Three formulations commonly available today in Anesthesia: Soda lime, Baralyme (a mixture of calcium hydroxide and barium hydroxide), and Calcium hydroxide lime (Amsorb)
- Of these agents, the **MC used is Soda lime**
- All serve to eliminate CO_2 from the breathing circuit with varying degrees of efficiency
- By weight, the approximate composition of "high moisture" Soda lime is 80% calcium hydroxide, 15% water, 4% sodium hydroxide, and 1% potassium hydroxide

21. Ans. (a) Jackson Rees modification of Ayre's T piece
[Ref. Anesthesia for Postgraduates By TK Agasti, 1/e p800]

- Anaesthetic circuit MC used in children under 5 years of age (or below 20 Kg of body weight): Jackson-Rees modification of Ayres T-piece (Mapleson F-system)

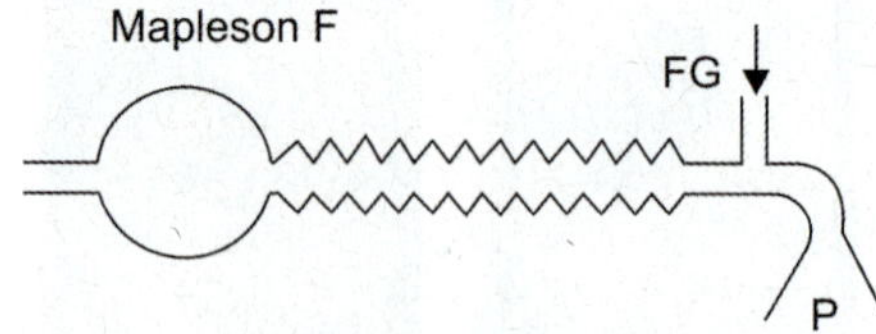

Fig. Mapleson F system

Anesthesiology

 HIGH YIELD MCQs ANSWERS WITH EXPLANATIONS 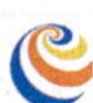

1. **Ans. (d)** **Noval catheter**
[Ref. Ajay Yadav, 4/e p42-43]

2. **Ans. (d)** **Respiratory rate**
[Ref. Pediatric Anaesthesia by Bruno Bissonnette 1/e, p1347]

Effect of Trendelenburg Position

Decreased parameters	Increased parameters
• Lung volume • Tidal volume • Lung compliance • Cerebral perfusion Pressure • Vital capacity • Functional residual capacity • Compliance	• Physiological dead space • Arterial to end tidal CO_2 gradient • Peak inspiratory pressure • Respiratory rate

3. **Ans. (c)** **Trendelenburg**
[Ref. Understanding Anaesthesiology by Ahanatha Pillai, 1/e p75]
   - Positions with maximum reduction in vital capacity:
     - Lithotomy position (18%)
     - Trendelenburg position (14.5%)

4. **Ans. (b)** **Increased pulmonary compliance**
[Ref. Morgans 4/e, p1028]

Side Effect of Oxygen Therapy
   - Acute oxygen toxicity/CNS toxicity/Bert effect: Nausea, Vertigo, Convulsion
   - Pulmonary toxicity/Smith effect: Pulmonary epithelium damage, Vascular endothelium damage, Decreased lung compliance, Decreased vital capacity, Absorption atelectasis, ARDS, Pulmonary interstitial fibrosis
   - Retrolental fibroplasias, Retinopathy of prematurity

5. **Ans. (b)** **Nail polish; (c) Methemoglobinemia; (d) Skin pigmentation**
[Ref. Ajay Yadav, 4/e p51]

Errors in Pulse Oximetry
   - Carboxyhemoglobinemia
   - Methemoglobinemia
   - Anemia
   - Hypovolemia, vasoconstriction
   - Vasodilatation
   - Nail polish (especially blue)
   - Shivering
   - SpO_2 below 60%

6. **Ans. (b)** **Blue in colour; (c) Gas in liquid form; (d) Pin index 3,5**
[Ref. Ajay Yadav, 4/e p24]

7. **Ans. (d)** **Endotracheal intubation**
[Ref. Ajay Yadav, 4/e p4-5; Morgan, 4/e p553]

8. **Ans. (a)** **Atracurium**
[Ref. Basic Clinical Anaesthesia by Paul, 1/e p154]
   - Hoffman elimination is an enzyme independent hydrolysis that relies on physiologic pH and temperature
   - Atracurium is metabolized by Hoffman elimination and plasma esterases

9. **Ans. (a)** **Molybdenum steel**
[Ref. Respiratory Care: Principles and Practice by Hess, 3/e p255]

Materials Used for Cylinders
   - Molybdenum steel
   - Chromium-molybdenum alloy
   - Aluminium alloy containing blend of magnesium and silic

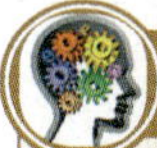
Also Remember
   - Composite cylinder material: Overwrapping a thin-walled aluminum cylinder with multiple layers of carbon/fiberglass/ Kevlar fibres in an epoxy resin wrap

10. **Ans. (a)** **Measure of potency; (c) Measures solubility**
[Ref. Rang & Dale's Pharmacology, 8/e p504]
   - Inhalation anesthetics can be regarded physiochemically as ideal gases; their solubility in different media is expressed as partition coefficient, defined as the ratio of the concentration of the agent in two phases at equilibrium
   - **Blood: gas partition coefficient**:
     - Definition: Ratio of the volume of gas that can dissolve in the same volume of a liquid phase, such as blood
     - Importance: Main factor that determines the rate of induction and recovery of an inhalation anesthetic
     - Interpretation: Higher the BG partition coefficient, the longer it takes to induce anaesthesia and the longer it takes to emerge from anaesthesia.

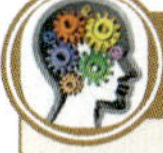
Also Remember
   - Oil: Gas partition coefficient: A measure of fat solubility, determines the potency of an anesthetic and also influences the kinetics of its distribution in the body

11. **Ans. (c)** **Massive pleural effusion**
[Ref. Morgan, 4/e p553]
   - Massive pleural effusion decreases the dead space

12. **Ans. (b)** **CO_2; (c) N_2O; (d) Cyclopropane**
[Ref. Lee's Synopsis of Anaesthesia, 13/e p85]
   - Stored in cylinder as gases:
     - Oxygen
     - Nitrogen
     - Air
     - Helium
   - Liquids in equilibrium with saturated vapour:
     - Nitrous oxide
     - Carbon dioxide
     - Cyclopropane

13. **Ans. (c)** **Neck flexion**
[Ref. Ajay Yadav, 4/e p4-5; Morgan, 4/e p553]

14. Ans. (d) Incorrect gas cylinder attachment
[Ref. Lee's Synopsis of Anaesthesia, 13/e p85]
- Cylinder outlet valves use the pin index system which makes it impossible to connect cylinders to the wrong yokes
- Yokes are connected to flowmeters via non-interchangaeable screw-threaded (NIST) connectors

15. Ans. (a) Black cylinder with white shoulders
[Ref. Monheims Local Anaesthesia and Pain Control in Dental Practice, 7/e p278]

16. Ans. (c) Black with white shoulder
[Ref. Monheims Local Anaesthesia and Pain Control in Dental Practice, 7/e p278]

17. Ans. All choices
[Ref. Ajay Yadav, 4/e p24]

18. Ans. (c) 2220 PSP is the pressure in cylinder
[Ref. Ajay Yadav, 4/e p24]

19. Ans. (d) Emergency oxygen "E" cylinder has more gas than "H" cylinder
[Ref. Ajay Yadav, 4/e p24]

20. Ans. (a) TC of O_2 is -119° C; (d) TC of N_2O is 36.5° C; (e) TC of air is -140.6° C
[Ref. Mosby's Respiratory Care Equipment, 1/e p8]
- Critical temperatures: Temperature and above which vapour of that substance cannot be liquefied
  - Oxygen: -119°C
  - Air: -140°C
  - Nitrogen: -146.9°C
  - Xenon: -16.6°C
  - Nitrous oxide: 36.5°C
  - Water: -374°C

21. Ans. (a) Mapleson A
[Ref. Ajay Yadav, 4/e p29]

22. Ans. (b) Ideal for infant
[Ref. Ajay Yadav, 4/e p29]

23. Ans. (a) Mapleson A
[Ref. Ajay Yadav, 4/e p29]

24. Ans. (b) Mapleson type D; (c) Can be used for spontaneous respiration; (d) Can be used for controlled ventilation; (e) Coaxial
[Ref. Ajay Yadav, 4/e p30]

25. Ans. (b) Equal to M.V.
[Ref. Ajay Yadav, 4/e p29]

26. Ans. (a) Jackson Ree's modification of Ayres' T piece
[Ref. Ajay Yadav, 4/e p30]

27. Ans. (a) Zeolite activation; (b) Delivers O_2; (c) Requires power supply
[Ref. Ajay Yadav, 4/e p75]
- Oxygen concentrators are portable electric run devices which can produce oxygen from ambient air by selective absorption of nitrogen on zeolites

28. Ans. (a) Should be as far as possible from the patient
[Ref. Ajay Yadav, 4/e p28]

29. Ans. (a) Resistance in circuit; (c) Small granule size
[Ref. Ajay Yadav, 4/e p32]

30. Ans. (c) Trilene
[Ref. Ajay Yadav, 4/e p33]

31. Ans. (a) Resistance in circuit
[Ref. Ajay Yadav, 4/e p32]

32. Ans. (b) Baralime
[Ref. Morgan's Anaesthesia, 4/e p38]
- Water of crystallization is used in baralime and silica is used in sodalime

33. Ans. (d) As an indicator
[Ref. Morgan's Anaesthesia, 4/e p38]
- **'Clayton'** when used as indicator, indicates red when sodalime is fresh and becomes yellow when sodalime is exhausted
- Nowadays good quality sodalime with prolonged life, **'Durasorb'** is used which is pink when fresh and becomes white when exhausted

34. Ans. (d) Mapleson F
[Ref. Ajay Yadav, 4/e p31]

35. Ans. (b) Venturi mask
[Ref. Ajay Yadav, 4/e p42]

36. Ans. (d) Decreased cardiac output relative to total body mass
[Ref. Ajay Yadav, 4/e p168]

37. Ans. (c) 60%
[Ref. Ajay Yadav, 4/e p43]

38. Ans. (b) Membrane oxygenator
[Ref. Morgan's Anaesthesia, 3/e p436]
- Advantages of Membrane oxygenator:
  - Less protein denaturation
  - Less trauma to RBCs, WBCs and platelets

39. Ans. (b) Malignant hyperthermia
[Ref. Ajay Yadav, 4/e p115]
- $ETCO_2$ may rise to more than 100 mm Hg (normal 32 to 42 mm Hg)
- Increased in $ETCO_2$ is most sensitive early sign of malignant hyperthermia

40. Ans. (d) Obeys Charles, Boyles and Avagadro' laws
[Ref. Ajay Yadav, 4/e p10]

41. Ans. (a) Desflurane
[Ref. Ajay Yadav, 4/e p61]

42. Ans. (d) N_2O
[Ref. Essential Clinical Anaesthesia by Vacanti, 1/e p213]

43. Ans. (d) Hydrophobic site
[Ref. Neural Mechanisms of Anaesthesia byAntognini, 1/e p375]

44. Ans. (b) Isoflurane; (d) Desflurane
[Ref. Ajay Yadav, 4/e p68,70]
- Pungent ethereal odour, hence induction is not pleasant

45. Ans. (c) Desflurane
[Ref. Ajay Yadav, 4/e p61]

46. Ans. (c) Slow induction and slow recovery
[Ref. Ajay Yadav, 4/e p66]
- For xenon, Blood gas coefficient is lowest (0.14) therefore induction and recovery is fastest (3 times faster than Desflurane)

47. Ans. (b) Recovering anesthesia
[Ref. Ajay Yadav, 4/e p62,65]

48. Ans. (a) Diffusion hypoxia
[Ref. Ajay Yadav, 4/e p65]

49. Ans. (b) Due to lack of stimulation by CO_2, anoxia can go into dangerous level
[Ref. Ajay Yadav, 4/e p112]

50. Ans. (b) Carbon monoxide
[Ref. Ajay Yadav, 4/e p214]

51. Ans. (b) It decreases turbulence
[Ref. Ajay Yadav, 4/e p10,77]

52. Ans. (a) Mapleson A
[Ref. Ajay Yadav, 4/e p29-30]

Semi-Closed Circuits/ Mapleson Systems
- Type A (Magill circuit):
  - Circuit of choice for: Spontaneous ventilation
  - Not used for: Controlled ventilation
- Type B
  - Not used nowadays
- Type C (Waters' To and Fro)
  - Not used nowadays
- Type D (Bain's circuit):
  - Circuit of choice for: Controlled ventilation
  - May be used for: Spontaneous ventilation
  - MC used circuit
- Type E (Ayre's T-piece):
  - Circuit of 2nd choice for: Children
- Type F (Jackson Rees circuit):
  - Circuit of 1st choice for: Children

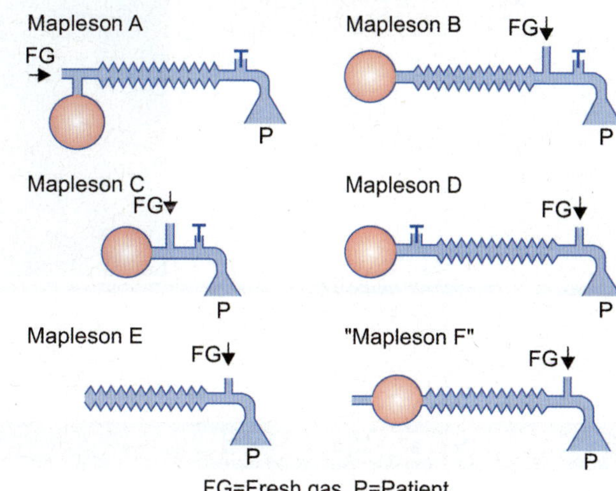

Fig. Mapleson Systems

53. Ans. (c) Paresthesia
[Ref. Nurse Anaesthesia by Burns, 1/e p187]
- Hyperesthesia: An abnormal increase in sensitivity to stimuli of the sense
- Paraesthesia: Abnormal sensation perceived without an apparent stimulus
- Neuralgia: Intense, typically intermittent pain along the course of a nerve, especially in the head or face
- Radiculopathy: Consequence of nerve root damage (from any cause)

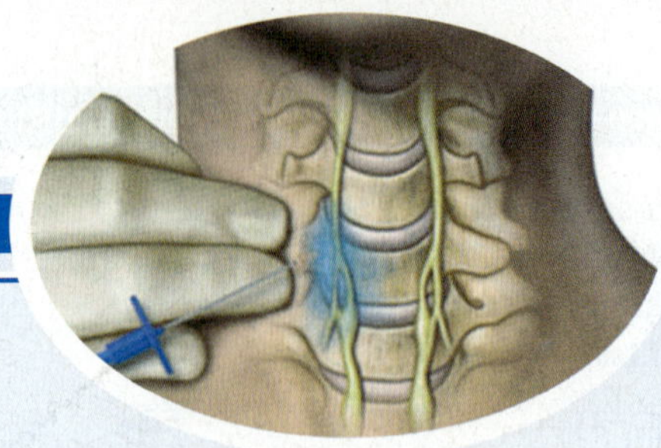

Chapter 3

Preoperative Evaluation and Premedication

THEORETICAL CONCEPTS

Topper's Edge

ASA Physical Status Classification System

- ASAPSCS: A system for assessing the fitness of patients before surgery[Q]

ASA	Definition	Characteristic
ASA I	Normal healthy patient	No chronic disease
ASA II	Mild systemic disease	Well controlled disease with no functional limitation[Q]
ASA III	Severe systemic disease	Functional limitations
ASA IV	Severe systemic disease that is a constant threat to life	Person is incapacitated
ASA V	Moribund patient who is not expected to survive without the operation	Survival not more than 24 hours[Q]
ASA VI	Declared brain-dead patient whose organs are being removed for donor purposes	

- Emergency in ASAPSCS:
  - If the surgery is an emergency, the physical status classification is followed by "E" (for emergency) for example "3E"[Q]
  - Class 5 is usually an emergency and is therefore usually "5E"
  - Class "6E" does not exist and is simply recorded as class "6", as all organ retrieval in brain-dead patients is done urgently
  - *Definition of emergency:* When delay in treatment would significantly increase the threat to the patient's life or body part

III. A. GOALS OF PREANAESTHETIC MEDICATION[Q]

- ❑ Decrease anxiety
- ❑ Produce hemodynamic stability
- ❑ Induce sedation
- ❑ Provide analgesia, amnesia
- ❑ Decrease chances of aspiration
- ❑ Decrease oral, respiratory secretions
- ❑ Decrease postoperative nausea and vomiting and other complications
- ❑ Decrease infections
- ❑ Decrease dose of anesthetic agents

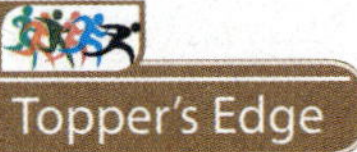

Topper's Edge

Preanaesthetic Medication

Medications that should be continued up to and including the day of surgery[Q]

- Alzheimer's medications
- Antianxiety, antidepressants and psychiatric medications (except MAO inhibitors[Q])
- Antihypertensive medications—Beta-blockers and others
- Anti-seizure medications
- Antivirals and antiretrovirals
- Asthma medications
- Birth control pills
- COX-2 inhibitors
- Eye drops
- Heartburn/Antireflux medications
- Immunosuppressants and rheumatologic medications
- Opioids
- Parkinson's medications
- Statins
- Steroids (oral and inhaled)
- Thyroid medications

Medications that Should be Discontinued Prior to Surgery[q]

- **ACE inhibitors** (Hold on day of surgery[Q])
- ARBs (Angiotensin II receptor blockers)
- Direct renin Inhibitor, Aliskiren
- Diuretics (Hold on day of surgery)
- **Antiplatelet agents** (Discontinue 7 days before surgery[Q])
- **Warfarin** (Discontinue 5 days before surgery[Q])
- **Heparin, low molecular weight heparins** (Doses held for 12 hours preoperatively, if prophylactic dosing and 24 hours, if therapeutic dosing[Q])
- NSAIDs (Discontinue 7 days prior to surgery)
- Herbal supplements and vitamin E-containing multivitamins (Discontinue 7 days prior to surgery)
- Bisphosphonates (Hold on day of surgery)
- Insulin
- Oral diabetic agents (Hold on day of surgery)
- Iron (Hold on day of surgery)
- Premarin (Hold on day of surgery)
- Sildenafil, Tadalafil, Vardenafil (Hold 24 hours preoperatively)
- MAO inhibitors
- *Other drugs:* Dabigatran, Rivaroxaban, Apixaban

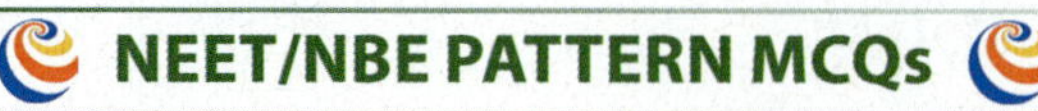

NEET/NBE PATTERN MCQs

1. **Warfarin to be stopped .... day before surgery** *[Recent Question 2016]*
   a. 2–3 days b. 4–5 days
   c. 6–7 days d. 8–9 days
2. **Preanaesthetic medication is given for all except** *[NBE FMGE March 2006]*
   a. Decrease secretions
   b. Decrease anxiety
   c. Decrease dose of anaesthetic agent
   d. Decrease aspiration
3. **A patient with sickle cell trait is posted for surgery in left arm. Which you will avoid?** *[NBE DNB 2009]*
   a. Intravenous regional anaesthesia
   b. Brachial plexus block through supraclavicular route
   c. Brachial plexus block through intraclavicular route
   d. Brachial plexus block through axillary route
4. **Preoxygenation is done to** *[Recent Question 2017]*
   a. Increase the oxygen content of FRC
   b. Decrease the nitrogen content of FRC
   c. Both
   d. None
5. **Preanesthetic medication is prescribed to** *[Recent Question 2017]*
   a. Decreasing the dose of anesthetic drugs
   b. Decreasing postoperative complications
   c. Relieving the anxiety
   d. All of the above
6. **American Anaesthetic Association says that clopidogrel should be withheld how many days before surgery?** *[Recent Question 2017]*
   a. 1 day b. 1 week
   c. 3 weeks d. 4 weeks
7. **Brain-dead patient comes under which category in ASA classification?** *[Recent Question 2017]*
   a. ASA 1 b. ASA 3
   c. ASA 4 d. ASA 6
8. **ASA grading is anesthesia is done for** *[Recent Question 2017]*
   a. Mental status b. Physical status
   c. Respiratory status d. Socioeconomic status
9. **ASA grading is to assess** *[Recent Question 2017]*
   a. Cardiac status b. Respiratory status
   c. Risk factors d. Mental status

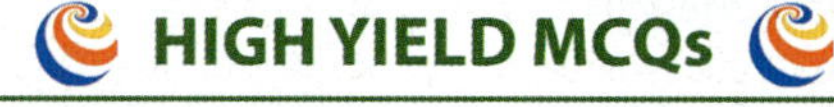

HIGH YIELD MCQs

1. **Most potent antiemetic agent used in preoperative period** *[AIIMS PGMEE 1996]*
   a. Glycopyrolate b. Hyoscine
   c. Atropine d. Metochlorpromide
2. **Atropine as preanaesthesia has all effects except** *[All India PGMEE 1996]*
   a. Decrease secretion b. Bronchoconstriction
   c. Prevent bradycardia d. Prevent hypotension
3. **Regarding preanesthethetic medication, all are true except** *[All India PGMEE 2002]*
   a. Secretions decrease b. Decrease anxiety
   c. Decrease dose of inducing agent
   d. Allay anxiety
4. **Drugs commonly used in preanaesthetic medication** *[PGI 2004]*
   a. Diazepam b. Scopolamine
   c. Morphine d. Succinylcholine
   e. Atracurium
5. **ASA classification is done for** *[Recent Question 2016, Rajasthan PGMEE 2001]*
   a. Status of patient b. Risk
   c. Pain d. Lung disease
6. **Anaesthesia used in microlaryngoscopy is** *[AIIMS PGMEE 1996]*
   a. Pollard tube of 10 mm diameter with heavy sedation
   b. Pollard tube of 15 mm diameter with topical sylocaine
   c. Pollard tube with infiltration block
   d. Heavy sedation on and endotracheal intubation
7. **A patient who was on aspirin for long period was selected for an elective surgery. What should be done?** *[AIIMS PGMEE 2001]*
   a. Stop aspirin for 7 days
   b. Infusion of fresh-frozen plasma
   c. Infusion of platelet concentration
   d. Go ahead with surgery maintaining adequate hemostatis
8. **During general anaesthesia shiverting is abolished by suppression of** *[All India PGMEE 1991]*
   a. Hypothalmus b. Thalmus
   c. Cerebral cortex d. Medulla
9. **Preanaesthetic medication is used for all except** *[PGI 2002]*
   a. Decrease of anaesthetic dose
   b. Decrease BP
   c. Prevent aspiration
   d. Produce amnesia for perioperative events
   e. Relieve anxiety
10. **A 5-year-old patient is scheduled for tonsillectomy. On the day of surgery, he had running nose, temperature 37.5°C and dry cough. Which of the following should be the most appropriate decision for surgery?** *[AIIMS PGMEE 1998]*
    a. Surgery should be cancelled
    b. Can proceed for surgery, if chest is clear and there is no history of asthma
    c. Should get X-ray chest before proceeding for surgery
    d. Cancel surgery for 3 weeks and patient to be on antibiotic
11. **Lithium therapy must be stopped .... prior to surgery** *[JIPMER PGMEE 2014]*
    a. 1 day b. 3–5 days
    c. 5–7 days d. 2 weeks
12. **To prevent aspiration under anaesthesia, for how many hours at least patients are kept nil by mouth for solid food preoperatively?** *[PGMCET 2015]*
    a. 2–4 hours b. 4–6 hours
    c. 6–8 hours d. 8–10 hours

Anesthesiology

 NEET/NBE PATTERN MCQs ANSWERS WITH EXPLANATIONS 

1. **Ans. (b)** **4–5 days**

   [Ref. Principles and Practice of Hematology Volume 1 by Handin, 2/e p1337]
   - Stop Warfarin 4–5 days before surgery
   - Start postoperative antithrombotic prophylaxis with low-dose unfractionated Heparin and Warfarin

2. **Ans. (c)** **Decrease dose of anaesthetic agent**

   [Ref. Ajay Yadav, 4/e p47-48]
   - *Goals of preanaesthetic medication*:
     - Decrease anxiety
     - Produce hemodynamic stability
     - Induce sedation
     - Provide analgesia, amnesia
     - Decrease chances of aspiration
     - Decrease oral, respiratory secretions
     - Decrease postoperative nausea and vomiting
     - Decrease infections

3. **Ans. (a)** **Intravenous regional anaesthesia**

   [Ref. Ajay Yadav,4/e p166]

   Intravenous Regional Anaesthesia (IVRA) or BIER Block Anaesthesia
   - *Importance:* A common anaesthetic technique for surgical procedures on the body's extremities where a local anaesthetic is injected intravenously
   - *Technique:* Involves exsanguination, which forces blood out of the extremity, followed by the application of pneumatic tourniquets to safely stop blood flow
   - *Contraindication:* Use of tourniquet and hence Bier's block is contraindicated in Sickle cell disease because blood stasis can cause local acidosis, hypoxia with sickling of cells.

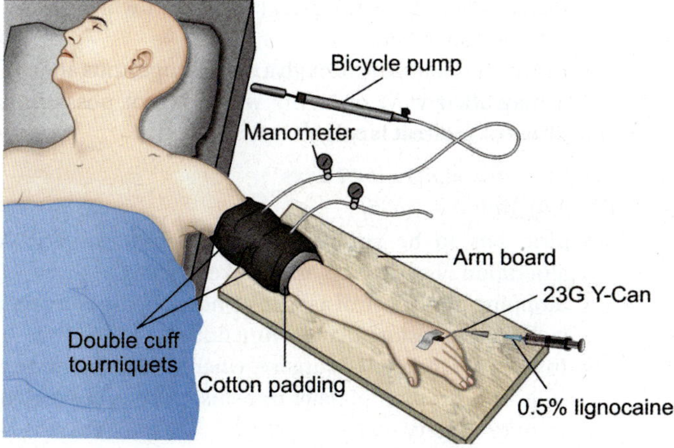

Fig. Bier's Block

4. **Ans. (c)** **Both**

   [Ref. Clinical Anaesthesia by Pollard, 3/e p673]
   - FRC is the most important store of oxygen in the body; greater the FRC, the longer apnoea can be tolerated before critical hypoxaemia develops.
   - Preoxygenation aims to replace nitrogen in the FRC with oxygen and hence is also referred to as 'Denitrogenation'
   - It causes a significant increase in body oxygen store and therefore increases tolerance to apnoea subsequently
   - Efficient preoxygenation (either for 3-5 min or with three VC breaths) will replace alveolar air with 100% oxygen
   - Allow complete washout of nitrogen, which allows the functional residual capacity (FRC) to serve as an oxygen reservoir

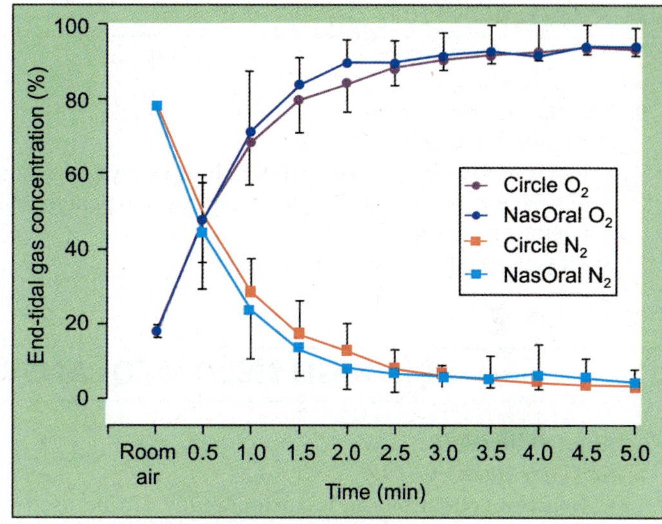

Fig. Preoxygenation

5. **Ans. (d)** **All of the above**

   [Ref. Practical Anesthesiology by Artusio, 1/e p89]

   Advantages of Preanaesthetic Agents
   - Relief of anxiety and apprehension
   - Amnesia
   - Supplement/augment analgesia
   - Decrease secretions (Prevents gastric aspiration)
   - Decrease vagal stimulation (Prevents cardiac arrest)
   - Anti-emetic effect
   - Decrease acidity (Avoid aspiration of gastric acids)
   - Reduce dose of general anesthetic required (for muscle relaxation, analgesia)

6. **Ans. (b)** **1 week**

   [Ref. Stoelting's Anesthesia by Hines, 6/e p14]
   - Clopidogrel, a thienopyridine derivative, inhibits ADP-induced platelet aggregation
   - In cases of neurosurgery, spinal cord decompression, aortic aneurysm surgery, and prostatectomy, and other surgeries, the risk of bleeding may outweigh the risk of thrombosis
   - So antiplatelet therapy should be stopped before these operations (at least 5-7 days before surgery for clopidogrel) and resumed as soon as feasible post-operatively

7. Ans. (d) ASA 6
[Ref. Miller's Anesthesia, 8/e p1144]

ASAPSCS: System for Assessing the Fitness of Patients Before Surgery

ASA	Definition	Characteristic
ASA I	Normal healthy patient	No chronic disease
ASA II	Mild systemic disease	Well-controlled disease with no functional limitation
ASA III	Severe systemic disease	Functional limitations
ASA IV	Severe systemic disease that is a constant threat to life	Person is incapacitated
ASA V	Moribund patient who is not expected to survive without the operation	Survival not more than 24 hours
ASA VI	Declared brain-dead patient whose organs are being removed for donor purposes	

8. Ans. (b) Physical status
[Ref. Miller's Anesthesia, 7/e p984]
- ASA uses a grading system to determine the physical status of a patient preoperatively and assess how the patient will tolerate the anesthesia
- This status rates patients in six classes

9. Ans. (c) Risk factors
[Ref. Clinical Anaesthesia by Pollard, 4/e p562]
American Society of Anesthesiologists (ASA) has developed a physical status classification system that has proved to be a valuable tool for Risk stratification

HIGH YIELD MCQs ANSWERS WITH EXPLANATIONS

1. Ans. (b) Hyoscine
[Ref. Ajay Yadav, 4/e p48]
- Hyoscine, ondansetron, metoclopramide can be used of which hyoscine is the most potent antiemetic as part of premedication
- Recommended for patients who have tendency for nausea and vomiting or in surgeries in which there are increased chances of postoperative nausea and vomiting like middle ear surgeries

2. Ans. (b) Bronchoconstriction
[Ref. Lee, 3/e p25]
- Atropine as preanaesthetic medication (Dose 0.01 mg/kg) prevents reflex bradycardia, hypotension, control secretion

Also Remember
- Choice of anticholinergic to decrease secretions:
  - *Antisialagouge*: Glycopyrrolate
  - *Antisialagouge plus sedation and amnesia*: Scopolamine
  - Preferred anticholinergic: Glycopyrrolate (Doesnot cross Blood-Brain-Barrier so no central side effect)

3. Ans. None of the choices
[Ref. KDT, 6/e p378]
Preanaesthetic medication is used for relief/allay of anxiety, decrease the dose of anaesthesia, prevent aspiration, perioperative amnesia, decrease secretion and preventing postoperative nausea

4. Ans. (a) Diazepam; (b) Scopolamine; (c) Morphine
[Ref. Ajay Yadav, 4/e p48]

5. Ans. (a) Status of patient
[Ref. Ajay Yadav, 4/e p48]
Based on the physical status, the patients are classified into 6 categories by AS(A). Mortality and morbidity are highest in grade V and minimum in grade I.

6. Ans. (c) Pollard tube with infiltration block
[Ref. Diseases of ENT by Scott-Brown, 1/e p733]
- *Microlaryngoscopy*:
  - Examination of your larynx (voice box) while under a general anaesthetic
  - Larynx is visualized through a microscope, thus allowing a magnified view of larynx which is not possible on direct or indirect laryngoscopy

7. Ans. (a) Stop aspirin for 7 days
[Ref. Ajay Yadav, 4/e p46]
- Aspirin has to be stopped 1 week before surgery: As regeneration of cyclo-oxygenase takes 1 week
  - Stopping mini-dose of aspirin 48 hours before surgery is sufficient to restore platelet function
  - In case of emergency surgery, when there is no time to stop aspirin, then platelet transfusion should be given prior to surgery.

8. Ans. (a) Hypothalmus
[Ref. Ajay Yadav, 4/e p114]

Shivering in General Anaesthesia
- *Physiological basis*: Shivering occurs a protective mechanism as inhalational agents/spinal-epidural block cause vasodilation leading to heat loss

- *MC agent causing shivering*: Halothane
- *Treatment*:
  - **Tramadol (Drug of choice)**
  - Pethidine, Pentazocine
  - Oxygen inhalation

9. Ans. (b) Decrease BP

[Ref. KDT, 6/e p378]

10. Ans. (d) Cancel surgery for 3 weeks and patient to be on antibiotic

[Ref. Practical Pediatrics by South, 6/e p802]

Contraindications for Tonsillectomy

- Poliomyelitis epidemic in vicinity (Absolute contraindication)
- Upper respiratory tract infection in preceding 2 weeks
- Acute tonsillar infection
- Systemic disorder (Diabetes mellitus)
- Bleeding disorder
- Very small tonsils

11. Ans. (a) 1 day

[Ref. Pass the PSA by Brown, 1/e p2]

Drugs to be Stopped Before Surgery

- *Combined OCPs*: 4 weeks before surgery
- *Hormone replacement therapy*: 4 weeks before surgery
- *Lithium*: 1 day before surgery
- *Potassium sparing diuretics*: Day of surgery
- *ACE inhibitors*: Day of surgery

12. Ans. (b) 4-6 hours

[Ref. Clinical Emergency Medicine by Mahadevan, 2/e p760]

- Preoperative NPO status for each patient must be regulated according to his/her age and timing of the surgery, the night before the operation
  - 2 hours for clear fluids
  - 4–6 hours for solid foods and milk

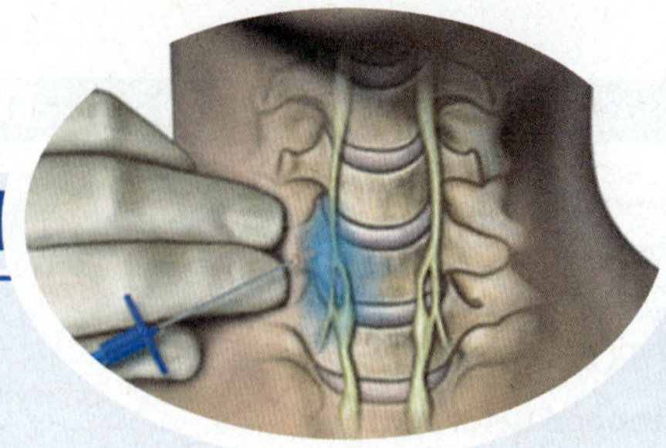

Chapter 4

Anesthetic Agents

THEORETICAL CONCEPTS

IV A. INDUCTION AND MAINTENANCE AGENTS

IV A1. Commonly used Induction Agents in Anesthesia

Intravenous induction agents[Q]	Inhalational induction agents[Q]
• Propofol • Thiopentone sodium • Etomidate • Ketamine • Methohexitone sodium	• Sevoflurane

IV A2. Commonly used Maintenance Agents in Anesthesia[Q]

- Benzodiazepines
  - Diazepam
  - Lorazepam
  - Midazolam
- Ketamine (causes **dissociative anesthesia**)
- Fentanyl
- Dexmedetomidine

IV A3. Intravenous Induction Agents

- Sodium thiopentone
- Propofol
- Etomidate
- Ketamine
- Methohexitone
- Midazolam

IV B. BLOOD GAS PARTITION COEFFICIENT

- Usefulness: Blood gas (B/G) coefficient is the most important factor in determination of speed of induction and recovery with a given anesthetic agent
- Interpretation: B/G coefficient implies percentage partial pressure in blood as compared to alveolar concentration
  - *Lesser B/G coefficient*: Faster induction and recovery[Q]
  - *Higher B/G coefficient*: Slower induction and recovery[Q]
- Blood gas partition coefficients of various agents: [**Mnemonic: D**octors **C**an **N**ever **S**ay **I**f **E**ther **H**as **C**aused **T**hem **E**asy **M**aintenance] [Q]

Agent	B/G partition coefficient
Desflurane[Q]	**0.42**
Cyclopropane[Q]	**0.44**
Nitrous oxide[Q]	**0.47**
Sevoflurane	0.69
Isoflurane	1.38
Enflurane	1.8
Halothane	2.4
Chloroform	8
Trielene	9
Ether[Q]	**12**
Methoxyflurane[Q]	**15**

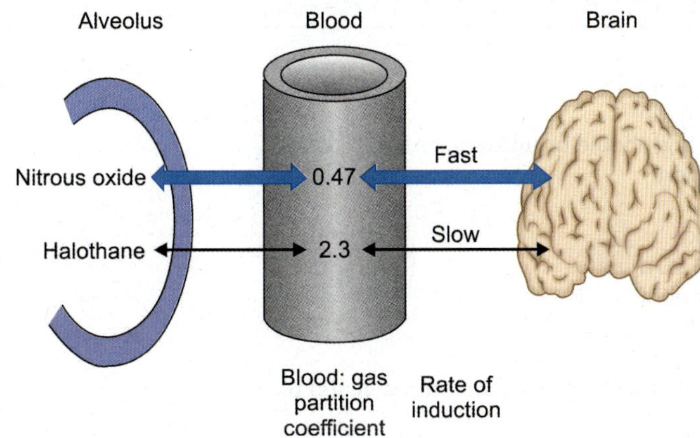

Fig. BG (Blood gas) partition coefficient

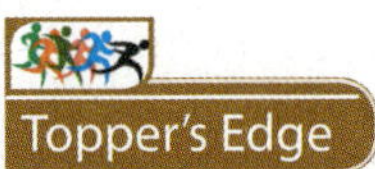

Topper's Edge

Blood Gas Partition Coefficient

- **Ostwald coefficient for blood gas**[Q]:
  - Describe the solubility of inhaled general anesthetics in blood
  - Coefficient is defined as the ratio of the concentration in blood to the concentration in gas that is in contact with that blood, when the partial pressure in both compartments is equal[Q]
  - Coefficient has no units[Q]
- Properties:
  - More soluble the inhaled anesthetic is in blood compared to in air, the more it binds to plasma proteins in the blood and the higher the blood gas partition coefficient[Q]
  - It is inversely related to induction rate
  - Potency of an anesthetic is associated with its lipid solubility which is measured by its oil/gas partition coefficient
- Low versus high coefficients:
  - Newer anesthetics (Desflurane) typically having smaller blood gas partition coefficients are preferred: They lead to faster onset of anesthesia and faster emergence from anesthesia once application of the anesthetic is stopped.
  - If an anesthetic has a high coefficient: A large amount of it will have to be taken up in the body's blood before being passed on to the fatty (lipid) tissues of the brain where it can exert its effect
- Minimum alveolar concentration (MAC): Concentration required to produce anesthetic effects[Q] **(An inverse indicator of anesthetic potency)**

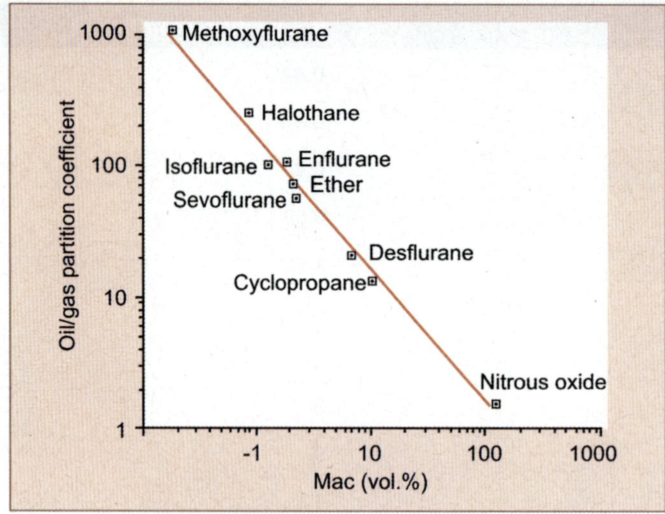

Fig. BGP coefficient versus MAC

IV C. METABOLISM AND RECOVERY WITH ANESTHETICS

- **Thiopentone:**
  - Regaining consciousness: 15 minutes
  - Half-life of elimination: 10.4 hours[Q]
  - No important work (e.g. driving) should be undertaken for 24 hours[Q]
  - Not suitable for day care surgery[Q]
- **Ketamine:**
  - Onset of action: 30-60 seconds
  - Regaining consciousness: 15-20 minutes
  - Half-life of elimination: 2-3 hours
  - Suitable for day care surgery[Q]
- **Nitrous oxide:**
  - Blood gas partition coefficient of 0.47 makes faster induction and recovery
  - Suitable for daycare surgery[Q]
- **Midazolam:**
  - Half-life of elimination: 2-3 hours
  - Suitable for daycare surgery[Q]

IV D. AGENTS USED IN DAY CARE SURGERIES[Q]

- **Desflurane**
- **Midazolam**
- **Mivacurium**
- **Sevoflurane**
- **Isoflurane**
- **Ketamine**
- **Alfentanil**
- **Nitrous oxide**
- **Propofol**

[Mnemonic: Dr. Man Mohan Singh Is Kind and Nice Politician]

IV E. NITROUS OXIDE

- Known as ***'Laughing gas'***: Produces euphoria after inhalation[Q]
- Is not a complete anesthetic: Is used as carrier to other inhalational agents
  - ***Second gas effect***: When given along with other inhalational agents it increases the alveolar concentration of that agent[Q]
  - *Concentration effect*: When given along with other inhalational agents, it increases the alveolar concentration of itself[Q]
  - Mixture of nitrous oxide (66%) and oxygen (33%) is generally given.
  - Can cause diffusion-hypoxia: So give 100% oxygen for 5–10 minutes

- Systemic actions and side-effects:
  - Safe in cardiac patients and patients in shock
  - Increases intracranial tension
  - Bone marrow depression: Aplastic anaemia, megaloblastic anaemia
  - Subacute combined degeneration of spinal cord
- Contraindications of nitrous oxide: **[Mnemonic: M**agic **LAMP E**mits **P**rosperity**]** [Q]
  - **M**iddle ear surgeries and tympanoplasty[Q]
  - **L**aparoscopic surgeries
  - **A**cute intestinal obstruction and volvulus[Q]
  - **M**icrolaryngeal surgeries
  - **P**neumothorax, pneumoperitoneum[q]
  - **E**ye surgeries
  - **P**neumoencephalum
- ***Entonox*: Mixture of 50% oxygen and 50% nitrous oxide**
  - Storage: Blue cylinders with blue and white shoulders
  - Used for: Painful dressings, changing thoracotomy drains

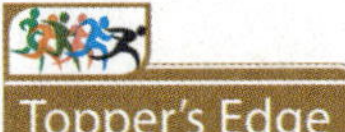

Topper's Edge

Nitrous Oxide

- Colorless and essentially odorless
- Non-explosive and non-flammable but supports combustion
- Gas at room temperature and ambient pressure[Q] (Can be kept as liquid under pressure)
- NMDA receptor antagonist[Q]
- Mechanism of action[Q]:
  - Anxiolytic effect: Enhanced activity of GABA-A receptors
  - Analgesic effect: Interaction between endogenous opioid system and descending noradrenergic system
  - Euphoric effect: Stimulates mesolimbic reward pathway via inducing dopamine release and activating dopaminergic neurons in the ventral tegmental area and nucleus accumbens, presumably through antagonisation of NMDA receptors
  - Neurotoxicity and neuroprotection: Due to hypoxia, depletion of Vitamin B_{12} levels
- Entonox: 50% nitrous oxide + 50% oxygen[Q]

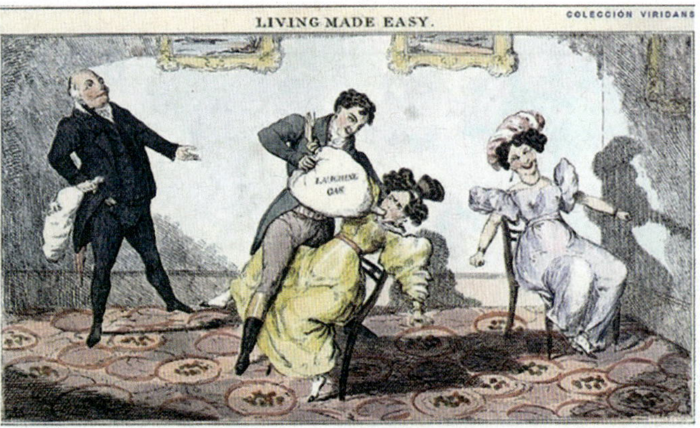

Fig. Prescription for scolding wives

Aquatint depiction of a laughing gas party

IV F. PROPOFOL

- Type of anesthetic: Phenol-based intravenous (parenteral) anesthetic
- Anesthetic properties:
  - Elimination half-life: 2–4 hours
  - Regaining of consciousness: 2-8 minutes
  - **No analgesia**[Q]
  - **No muscle relaxation**[Q]

- Systemic effects:
  - Hypotension[Q]
  - Apnoea
  - Bronchodilation in COPD patients[Q]
  - Cerebroprotective[Q]
  - Myoclonic
  - **Antiemetic[Q], antipruritic[Q]**
- Uses:
  - **Intravenous agent of choice for daycare surgery[Q]**
  - **Agent of choice for total intravenous anesthesia[Q]**
  - Sedative in ICU
  - **Agent of choice for induction in those susceptible to malignant hyperthermia[Q]**
- Advantages and disadvantages:

Advantages	Disadvantages
• Rapid smooth recovery • Early ambulation • Antiemetic • Antipruritic • Bronchodilator	• Apnoea • Hypotension • Painful injection • Allergic reactions, Infection (if used from vials) • Propofol infusion syndrome

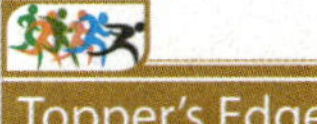

Topper's Edge

Uses of Propofol

- Anesthesia[Q]:
  - Induction and maintenance
  - Total intravenous anesthesia (Target controlled infusion, TCI)
  - Sedation of individuals who are receiving mechanical ventilation
- Procedural sedation
- Judicial executions
- Recreational use

Topper's Edge

HALOTHANE

Properties

- Stored in Amber-colored bottles[Q] (0.01% Thymol as preservative[Q])
- Smooth induction as non-irritant
- Highest fat-blood coefficient[Q]
- Potent anesthetic, moderate muscle relaxation, poor analgesic
- **Metabolic products[Q]: Trifluoroacetic acid, chloride, fluoride, bromide**

Systemic effects

- CVS: Reduce cardiac output and BP, sensitizes heart to adrenaline (ventricular arrhythmias[Q])
- Respiratory system: Bronchodilation, blunting of hypercarbic and hypoxic reflexes, reduction in tidal volume
- CNS: Marked increase in ICT[Q]
- Kidneys: GFR reduction
- Uterus: Uterine atony and PPH
- Thermoregulation: MC cause of postoperative shivering[Q] **(Halothane shakes[Q])** and hypothermia
- Liver: Halothane hepatitis[Q]
  - Multiple exposure is most important factor[Q]
  - Pathology: Centrilobar necrosis[Q]

Contd…

Contd...

OTHER INHALATIONAL AGENTS

Isoflurane

- Fluorinated methyl ether[Q]
- Isomer of enflurane[Q]
- Non-smooth induction: Due to pungent ethereal odour[Q]
- Moderate induction/recovery, moderate muscle relaxation
- Highest incidence of hypotension
- Best maintenance of cardiac output in inhalational agents[Q]
- **Inhalational agent of choice for controlled hypotension**[Q]
- **Agent of choice for cardiac patients**, except myocardial ischemia patients: Coronary steal in myocardial ischemia patients[Q]
- **Agent of choice for neurosurgical procedures**[Q]**:** Lowest rise in ICT

Enflurane

- Increase ICT, spike and wave pattern on EEG, tonic clonic seizures
- Contraindications[Q]: Epilepsy, renal disease
- Desflurane
- Fastest acting induction agent
- Coughing, breath-holding, laryngospasm during induction
- **Agent of choice for hepatic disease patients**[Q]
- **Agent of choice for renal disease patients**[Q]
- **Agent of choice for old age patients**
- **Agent of choice for prolonged duration surgeries**

Sevoflurane

- Smooth induction due to sweet odour
- Maintains hepatic blood flow
- Induces epilepsy
- Produce toxic metabolite (Compound A[Q]) when used with sodalime
- **Agent of choice for induction in children**[Q]
  - Recommended interval between two successive exposures: 3 months[Q]

OLDER INHALATIONAL AGENTS

Ether

- Pungent smelling, highly inflammable, explosive liquid[Q]
- Only complete anesthetic agent[Q]
- High chances of laryngospasm during induction[Q]
- Only inhalational agent which preserves ciliary activity[Q]
- Highest incidence of nausea and vomiting among inhalational agents
- Not used in diabetics[Q]: Can cause hypoglycemia

Chloroform

- Not used with adrenaline[Q]: Cause ventricular fibrillation leading to cardiac arrest and death
- Lead to hepatotoxicity, hyperglycemia[Q]

Cyclopropane

- Inhalational agent of choice in shock[Q]: Stimulates sympathetic system and maintains BP
- Cyclopropane shock[Q]: If cyclopropane is discontinued fast it can lead to sudden withdrawal of sympathetic stimulation

Trichloroethylene (Trilene)

- Most potent analgesic[Q]
- Neurotoxicity due to dichloroacetylene[Q] (Reaction with sodalime[Q]): MC nerve involved is CN V[Q]
- Pulmonary toxicity due to phosgene[Q] (Reaction with sodalime)
- Earlier used for labour analgesia

Methoxyflurane

- Highly soluble in rubber tubings of closed circuit[Q]
- Slowest induction and recovery
- **Most potent inhalational agent**[Q]
- Contraindicated in renal disease: Cause vasopressin-resistant high-output polyuric renal failure[Q]

Contd...

Contd...

Thiopentone

- Sodium ethyl thiobarbiturate, an ultrashort acting barbiturate
- Yellow amorphous powder[Q]: **Sulphur is added** to increase lipid-solubility[Q]
- Inhibits acetylcholine, facilitates GABA at synapses
- Cause Hypokalemia on induction[Q]
- Anticonvulsant action, antanalgesic action, laryngospasm, transient apnea
- High alkalinity lead to local complications: Tissue necrosis (Subcutaneous/Intramuscular injection), Gangrene (Intra-arterial injection)
- **Agent of choice for cerebral protection**[Q]: Decreases cerebral O_2 consumption, cerebral metabolic rate and ICT
- Absolute contraindication: Acute intermittent porphyria[Q], previous history of anaphylaxis with injection

Ketamine

- Phencyclidine derivative[Q]
- Strong analgesic, no muscle relaxation
- Mechanism of action:
  - Site: Thalamocortical projection (Inhibits cortex, stimulates limbic system)
  - Inhibits NMDA receptors[Q]
- Systemic effects:
  - **Dissociative anesthesia**[Q] (Catalepsy state)
  - Emergence reactions[Q]
  - MC side effect[Q]: Hallucinations
  - **Increase ICT, intraocular tension, intragastrical pressure**, muscle tone, tracheobronchial/salivary secretions[Q]
- **Intravenous agent of choice for shock**[Q]: Stimulate sympathetic system (Cause tachycardia, hypertension)
- **Intravenous agent of choice for asthmatics**[Q]: Potent bronchodilation

OTHER INTRAVENOUS AGENTS

Propofol

- Painful injection[Q]
- Use within 6 hours of opening the vial[Q]: Death occurs due to contamination (Egg lecithin media promotes bacterial growth)
- All metabolic products of propofol are inactive[Q]
- Anti-emetic, anti-pruritic[Q]
- Intravenous agent of choice for daycare surgery[Q]: Early induction/recovery, smooth induction, inactive metabolites, antiemetic effect
- Propofol infusion syndrome, if continued >48 hours[Q]

Etomidate

- Imidazole derivative[Q]
- **Most cardiostable intravenous agent**[Q]
- **Highest incidence of nausea and vomiting** among Intravenous anesthetics[Q]
- High incidence of vitamin C deficiency[Q], myoclonus, thrombophlebitis

Other Agents

- Lorazepam: Agent of choice for preoperative sedation[Q]
- Midozolam:
  - Used commonly during intraoperative period
  - Safely used in day care surgeries[Q]
- Alfentanil: MC associated with muscle rigidity among opioids[Q]
- Sulfentanil:
  - **Most potent opioid**[Q]
  - Agent of choice for inhibition of stress response to laryngoscopy and intubation[Q]
- Remifentanil:
  - Fastest onset and recovery among opioids[Q]
  - Opioid of choice in daycare surgeries[Q]
  - Not suitable for epidural analgesia[Q]: As it contains glycine causing motor weakness
- Pethidine: DOC for shivering[Q]
- Pentazocine:
  - Used for sequential analgesic anesthesia[Q]
  - Ceiling effect on respiratory depression[Q]

Contd...

Contd...

Neuroleptanalgesia

- Composition: Analgesia, sedation and variable amnesia[Q]
- Combination used: **Droperidol + Fentanyl**[Q]
  - Ratio: D 50: F 1[Q]
  - Droperidol produces: Hypnosis, detachment, catatonia, antiemetic effect, hypotension
  - Fentanyl produces: Analgesia, bradycardia, respiratory depression, muscle rigidity
- Uses of neuroleptanalgesia:
  - Induction agent
  - Premedication
  - Sedation for minor procedures
  - Surgeries with high incidence of nausea and vomiting
  - Neurosurgical procedures
- **Neuroleptanesthesia**[Q]:
  - Inhalational agent + Droperidol + Fentanyl
  - MC Inhalational agent used[Q]: Nitrous oxide

IV G. NEPHROTOXICITY DUE TO ANESTHETIC AGENTS

- Underlying cause: High fluoride content of several inhalational anesthetics raise fluoride ion concentrations resulting in nephrotoxicity
- Fluoride levels required to induce nephrotoxicity[Q]: More than 50 micromol per liter
- Chances of nephrotoxicity:

Highly nephrotoxic[Q]	Moderate nephrotoxic	Non-nephrotoxic[Q]
• Methoxyflurane	• Enflurane • Sevoflurane	• Halothane • Desflurane • Isoflurane

- *Highest fluoride content/nephrotoxic nature*: Methoxyflurane[Q]
- *Least fluoride content/nephrotoxic nature*: Isoflurane[Q]
- Methoxyflurane leads to *'Vasopressin-resistant high-output renal failure'*[Q]

IV H. FEW COMMONLY USED DRUGS CAUSING HEPATOTOXICITY

- Anesthetics (Methoxyflurane, Halothane) [Q]
- Allopurinol
- Amiodarone
- Azathioprine
- Hormonal contraceptivres
- Tuberculosis drugs (Rifampicin, Isoniazid, Pyrazinamide)
- NSAIDs (Ibuprofen, Indomethacin)
- Ketoconazole
- Methotrexate
- Methyldopa
- Minocycline
- Nifedipine
- Paracetamol
- Valproate
- Zidovudine

IV I. SYSTEMIC EFFECTS OF INHALATIONAL AGENTS

- *Maximum depression of respiration*: Enflurane[Q]
- *Maximum inhibition to ventilatory response*: Halothane
- *Maximum bronchodilation in asthmatics*: Halothane **(Agent of choice in asthmatics)**[Q]
- *Maximum bronchodilation in non-asthmatics*: Sevoflurane[Q]
- *Non-inhibitor of ciliary activity (reduced coughing out of secretions)*: Ether
- *Best maintenance of cardiac output*: Isoflurane **(Agent of choice in cardiac patients[Q])**

- *Maximum hypotension*: Isoflurane[Q]
- *Inhibition of myocardial contractility*: Halothane
- *Maximum sensitization of heart to adrenaline*: Halothane[Q]
- *Maximum hepatocellular damage*: Halothane[Q]
- *Maximum nephrotoxicity*: Methoxyflurane[Q]
- *Agent causing megaloblastic and aplastic anemia*: Nitrous oxide[Q]
- *Agent causing Subacute combined degeneration of spinal cord*: Nitrous oxide[Q]
- *Agent causing maximum muscle relaxation*: Desflurane
- *Agent causing maximum analgesia*: Trielene
- *Agent causing maximum hyperglycaemia*: Chloroform

IV J. COMMONLY USED DRUGS CAUSING HYPOTENSION[Q]

- **A**lpha blockers
- **B**eta blockers
- **C**alcium-channel blockers
- **A**nesthetic agents
  - Halothane
  - **Isoflurane (Most common inhalational anesthetic responsible)**
  - Enflurane
  - Desflurane
  - Methoxyflurane
  - Chloroform
- **P**arkinsonism drugs
- **D**iuretics, **D**igoxin, **D**epression drugs
- **P**otassium
- **A**lcohol
- **S**idenafil

[Mnemonic: A Big CAP Does Protect Against Sun]

IMAGE-BASED QUESTIONS

1. **Anesthetic agent shown in photograph is** *[Recent Question 2012]*

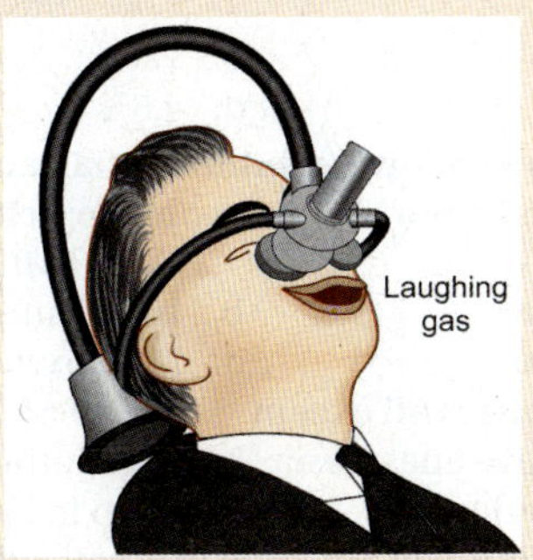

a. Desflurane
b. Nitrous oxide
c. Halothane
d. Enflurane

2. **Anesthetic agent shown in photograph comprise of** *[Recent Question 2012]*

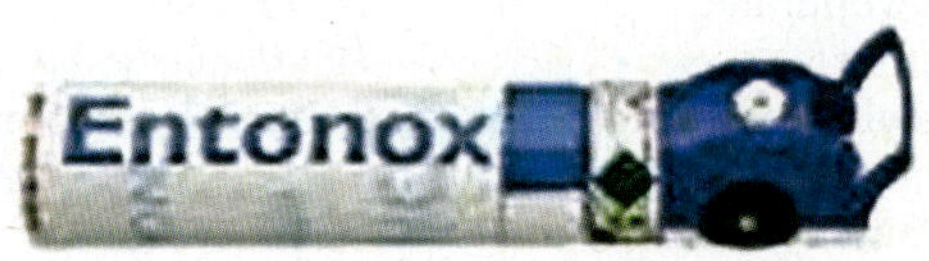

a. 20% oxygen + 80% nitrous oxide
b. 30% oxygen + 70% nitrous oxide
c. 70% oxygen + 30% nitrous oxide
d. 50% oxygen + 50% nitrous oxide

3. **Anesthetic agent shown in photograph is associated with deficiency of**

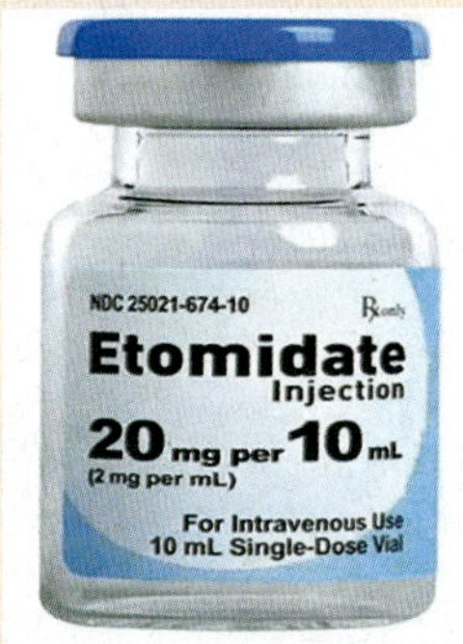

a. Vitamin A
b. Vitamin B_3
c. Vitamin C
d. Vitamin D

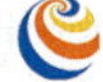

ANSWERS WITH EXPLANATIONS OF IBQs

1. **Ans. (b) Nitrous oxide** *[Ref. Ajay Yadav, 2/e p64]*

Nitrous Oxide
- Discovered by: Joseph Priestley
- Known as 'Laughing gas' (Name given by Humphry Davy): Produces euphoria after inhalation
- Is not a complete anesthetic: Is used as carrier to other inhalational agents
- Second gas effect: When given along with other inhalational agents, it increases the alveolar concentration of that agent
- Concentration effect: When given along with other inhalational agents, it increases the alveolar concentration of itself

2. **Ans. (d) 50% oxygen + 50% nitrous oxide** *[Ref. Ajay Yadav, 2/e p66]*

Entonox
- Description: Mixture of 50% oxygen and 50% nitrous oxide
- Storage: Blue cylinders with blue and white shoulders. Above 10°C
- Used for: Painful dressings, changing thoracotomy drains

3. **Ans. (c) Vitamin C** *[Ref. Ajay Yadav, 2/e p82]*
- Etomidate can cause vitamin C deficiency.

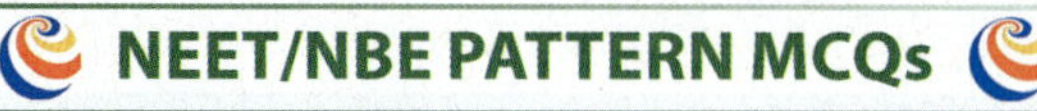

NEET/NBE PATTERN MCQs

1. **Which of the following anesthetic agent leads to increase in ICT?** *[Recent Question 2016]*
   a. Thiopentone b. Ketamine
   c. Propofol d. Sevoflurane
2. **Which of the following inhalational agent sensitizes myocardium to catecholamines?** *[Recent Question 2016]*
   a. Sevoflurane b. Isoflurane
   c. Ether d. Halothane
3. **Following are the features of persistent postoperative pain except** *[Recent Question 2016]*
   a. Pain the develops after surgical procedure
   b. Pain present for at least 3 months
   c. Pain where other causes are excluded
   d. Pain from presurgical problem is excluded
4. **Ketamine contraindicated in all except** *[Recent Question 2016]*
   a. Head injury b. Hypertension
   c. Asthma d. Glaucoma
5. **Bone marrow depression in seen with chronic administration of** *[Recent Question 2016, 2017]*
   a. Isoflurane b. Nitrous oxide
   c. Ether d. Halothane
6. **Thiopentone is not used in** *[Recent Question 2016]*
   a. Induction of anesthesia b. Medically induced coma
   c. As truth serum d. As antidepressant
7. **Drugs used for daycare surgery are all except** *[Recent Question 2016]*
   a. Propofol b. Sevoflurane
   c. Doxacurium d. Desflurane
8. **Propofol infusion syndrome all except** *[Recent Question 2016]*
   a. Occurs with infusion of propofol for 48 hours or longer
   b. Occurs in critically ill patients
   c. Features are nausea and vomiting
   d. Features are cardiomyopathy, hepatomegaly
9. **Anesthetic agents which have tocolytic effect are** *[Recent Question 2016]*
   a. Halothane b. Enflurane
   c. Isoflurane d. All the above
10. **Following are hepatotoxic anesthetic agent except** *[Recent Question 2016]*
    a. Halothane b. Chloroform
    c. Ether d. Propofol
11. **Action of which anesthetic agent is through NMDA** *[Recent Question 2016]*
    a. Xenon b. Succinylcholine
    c. Etomidate d. None
12. **Not as used as induction agent among the following is** *[Recent Question 2016]*
    a. Midazolam b. Etomidate
    c. Ketamine d. Propofol
13. **Halothane causes** *[Recent Question 2016]*
    a. Bradycardia b. Fall in BP
    c. Uterine relaxation d. All of the above
14. **Ketamine acts on which receptors** *[Recent Question 2016]*
    a. GABA b. Muscarinic
    c. 5-HT4 d. NMDA
15. **Benefit of ketamine is** *[Recent Question 2016]*
    a. Causes decrease in BP b. Good analgesic action
    c. Decrease ICT d. No change in ICT
16. **Percentage of thiopentone used for induction is** *[Recent Question 2016]*
    a. 0.5% b. 1.5%
    c. 2.5% d. 4.5%
17. **Which of the following inhalational anesthetics is most likely to cause fluoride ion nephrotoxicity?** *[NBE FMGE September 2009]*
    a. Halothane b. Isoflurane
    c. Enflurane d. Methoxyflurane
18. **Ketamine causes all except** *[NBE FMGE September 2012]*
    a. Dissociative anesthesia b. High intracranial tension
    c. Hallucinations d. Drop in blood pressure
19. **Fastest induction of anesthesia is caused by** *[NBE FMGE September 2008]*
    a. Chloroform
    b. Cyclopropane
    c. Halothane d. Equally with all of the above
20. **True about ketamine** *[Recent Question 2012]*
    a. Bronchodilator b. Depressed airway reflexes
    c. Causes hypotension d. Decreases ICT
21. **Fast induction and recovery is seen in** *[Recent Question 2012]*
    a. Methoxyflurane b. Ether
    c. Halothane d. N_2O
22. **High output renal failure may be caused by** *[NBE DNB 1995, 2000, 2005]*
    a. Methoxyflurane b. Diethyl ether
    c. Enflurane d. Halothane
23. **Preferred anesthetic agents in Daycare surgery include all except** *[NBE FMGE September 2008, September 2010]*
    a. Ketamine b. Isoflurane
    c. Midazolam d. Thiopentone
24. **Which is the critical temperature of N_2O?** *[Recent Question 2016, 2012]*
    a. 118°C b. 88°C
    c. 26°C d. 36.5°C
25. **'Laughing gas' is** *[Recent Question 2016]* *[NBE FMGE March 2007]*
    a. Nitrous oxide
    b. Halothane
    c. Chloroform
    d. Diethyl ether
26. **All are true about halothane except** *[Recent Question 2013]*
    a. Tachycardia b. Hepatitis
    c. Bronchodilatation d. Uterine relaxation
27. **Contraindicated in head injury** *[Recent Question 2012]*
    a. Halothane b. Ketamine
    c. N_2O d. Propofol
28. **Which of the following intravenous induction agent is the most suitable for daycare surgery?** *[Recent Question 2016, 2017, NBE DNB December 2011, AIIMS November 2014]*
    a. Morphine b. Propofol
    c. Ketamine d. Thiopentone

29. True about N_2O *[Recent Question 2012]*
a. Good muscle relaxant
b. Low potency and good analgesia
c. High potency and poor analgesia
d. None

30. Which of the following anesthetic is safe in heart failure? *[Recent Question 2012]*
a. Etomidate b. Propofol
c. Thiopentone d. Ketamine

31. Dissociative anesthesia is produced by *[NBE DNB 1994, 2003, 2006, 2007] [AIPGME 2006, AIIMS 1996]*
a. Ketamine b. Thiopentone
c. Suxamethonium d. Diazepam

32. True about midazolam as inducing agent *[Recent Question 2012, 2013]*
a. Increase in BP
b. Does not produce pain an IV injection
c. Increase cerebral oxygen consumption
d. Increase peripheral vascular resistance

33. All of the following are intravenous induction agents, except *[NBE FMGE March 2007]*
a. Ketamine b. Etomidate
c. Bupivacaine d. Thiopentone sodium

34. True about N_2O *[Recent Question 2012, 2013]*
a. Good muscle relaxant
b. Low potency and good analgesia
c. High potency and poor analgesia
d. None

35. Benefit of Ketamine *[Recent Question 2012, 2013]*
a. Causes decrease in BP
b. Good analgesic action
c. Decrease ICT
d. Decrease IOT

36. Following increases intra-ocular pressure *[NBE DNB 1995, 2000, 2005]*
a. Thiopentone b. Althesin
c. Ketamine d. Barbiturate

37. Postoperative nausea and vomiting are uncommon with *[NBE FMGE September 2012]*
a. Thiopentone
b. Propofol
c. Etomidate
d. All of the above

38. All are true about halothane, except *[Recent Question 2012]*
a. Tachycardia b. Hepatitis
c. Bronchodilatation d. Uterine relaxation

39. Which of the following drugs is contraindicated in a patient with raised intracranial pressure? *[Recent Question 2012, 2017]*
a. Thiopentone b. Propofol
c. Midazolam d. Ketamine

40. True about propofol is *[NBE FMGE September 2005]*
a. Causes analgesia b. Parenteral
c. Causes hypertension d. Is non-cerebroprotective

41. Which of the following inhalation anesthetics should be avoided in middle ear surgery when tympanic grafts are used? *[NBE DNB 2009]*
a. Halothane b. Nitrous oxide
c. Ether d. Isoflurane

42. Which does not cause malignant hyperthermia? *[Recent Question 2013]*
a. Isoflurane b. Desflurane
c. N_2O d. Enflurane

43. MAC of desflurane is *[Recent Question 2012]*
a. 1.15 b. 2
c. 4 d. 6

44. Anesthetic agent associated with hallucination is *[NBE DNB 1998, 1999, 2001, 2006]*
a. Ketamine b. Halothane
c. Ether d. Cyclopropane

45. Anesthetic agent with least effect on myocardial contractility is *[Recent Question 2016, NBE DNB 1998]*
a. Ether b. Halothane
c. Enflurane d. Isoflurane

46. Inducing agent of choice in DIC *[Recent Question 2012]*
a. Thiopentone b. Ketamine
c. Methohexitone d. Propofol

47. Cause of hepatitis include all, except *[NBE FMGE September 2005]*
a. Nitrous oxide b. Methoxyflurane
c. Halothane d. Pyrazinamide

48. Intravenous agent with best analgesic effect is *[NBE DNB 1992]*
a. Ketamine b. Minoxidil
c. Althesin d. Etomidate

49. Hypotension in anesthesia can be induced by all of the following agents, except *[NBE FMGE September 2008]*
a. Pancuronium b. Halothane
c. Hexamethonium d. Sodium nitroprusside

50. Which of the following increases cerebral oxygen consumption? *[NBE DNB 2009]*
a. Propofol b. Ketamine
c. Thiopentone d. Alfentantanil

51. Which one of the following is the fastest acting inhalational agent? *[Recent Question 2016, 2017, NBE DNB 2007]*
a. Halothane b. Isoflurane
c. Ether d. Sevoflurane

52. Hyperglycaemia is caused by *[NBE FMGE September 2008]*
a. Ether b. Trilene
c. Halothane d. Nitrous oxide

53. Safe inducing agent in malignant hyperpyrexia is *[NBE DNB 2007]*
a. Thiopentone b. Etomidate
c. Halothane d. Propofol

54. Nitrous oxide was first introduced by *[NBE DNB 1996]*
a. Davy b. Bernard
c. Andrews d. Wells
e. Priestley

55. Severe hypotension is caused by *[NBE FMGE September 2005]*
a. Ether b. Halothane
c. Cyclopropane d. Nitrous oxide

56. Ketamine causes all, except *[NBE FMGE September 2012]*
a. Dissociative anesthesia b. High intracranial tension
c. Hallucinations d. Drop in blood pressure

57. Raised intracranial tension is caused by *[NBE DNB 1992]*
a. Thiopentone b. Althesin
c. Ketamine d. Etomidate

58. Postoperative nausea and vomiting are uncommon with *[NBE FMGE September 2012]*
- a. Thiopentone
- b. Propofol
- c. Etomidate
- d. All of the above

59. Ketamine produces *[NBE FMGE September 2011]*
- a. Emergence delirium
- b. Pain on injection
- c. Bronchoconstriction
- d. Depression of cardiovascular system

60. Hepatotoxic anesthetic agent *[Recent Question 2016, 2015]*
- a. Chloroform
- b. Halothane
- c. Isoflurane
- d. Desflurane

61. Postoperative vomiting is most common with which of the following agent? *[Recent Question 2017]*
- a. Propofol
- b. Etomidate
- c. Ketamine
- d. Thiopentone

62. Anaesthetic agent contraindicated in Acute hepatitis is *[Recent Question 2017]*
- a. Sevoflurane
- b. Halothane
- c. Ketamine
- d. Isoflurane

63. Malignant hyperthermia is associated with all of the following, except *[Recent Question 2017]*
- a. Succinylcholine
- b. Dantrolene
- c. Halothane
- d. Methoxyflurane

64. Propofol vial, once opened, should be used within *[Recent Question 2017]*
- a. 2 hours
- b. 4 hours
- c. 6 hours
- d. 8 hours

65. Effect of Ketamine on IOP is *[Recent Question 2017]*
- a. Increases it
- b. Decreases it
- c. Does not affect
- d. First increases then decreases

66. Which of the following inhalational anesthetic agent most easily crosses blood brain barrier? *[Recent Question 2017]*
- a. Methoxyflurane
- b. Sevoflurane
- c. Desflurane
- d. Nitrous oxide

67. Thiopentone injection produces which effect at the injection site? *[Recent Question 2017]*
- a. Pain
- b. Vasodilatation
- c. Necrosis of vessel wall
- d. Hypotension

68. Etomidate is not used for long-term infusion because *[Recent Question 2017]*
- a. Results in adrenal suppression
- b. May cause vasospasm
- c. Results in cardiac arrhythmias
- d. May cause increase in ICT

69. Among the following agents, maximum boiling point is associated with *[Recent Question 2017]*
- a. Sevoflurane
- b. Isoflurane
- c. Methoxyflurane
- d. Desflurane

70. Safest anesthetic agent in Porphyria patient is *[Recent Question 2017]*
- a. Pentazocine
- b. Etomidate
- c. Propofol
- d. Thiopentone

71. Anesthetic agent leading to bradycardia is *[Recent Question 2017]*
- a. Pancuronium
- b. Vecuronium
- c. Atracurium
- d. Propofol

72. Which of the following anesthetic agent is most lipid soluble? *[Recent Question 2017]*
- a. Nitrous oxide
- b. Methoxyflurane
- c. Isoflurane
- d. Halothane

73. Ketamine is contraindicated in *[Recent Question 2017]*
- a. Status asthmaticus
- b. Obstetric hemorrhage
- c. Glaucoma
- d. Shock

74. Propofol shows following effect on EEG *[Recent Question 2017]*
- a. Activation
- b. Depression
- c. Depression in low doses and activation in high doses
- d. None of the above

75. Anesthetic agent causing bradycardia is *[Recent Question 2017]*
- a. Gallamine
- b. Vecuronium
- c. Ketamine
- d. Morphine

76. Ideal inhalational inducing agent of choice is *[Recent Question 2017]*
- a. Halothane
- b. Desflurane
- c. Sevoflurane
- d. Isoflurane

77. Preferred Mask induction drug is *[Recent Question 2017]*
- a. Halothane
- b. Sevoflurane
- c. Desflurane
- d. Ether

78. Which of the following is not a property of Propofol? *[Recent Question 2017]*
- a. Pain on injection
- b. Anticonvulsant effect
- c. Increase chances of infection
- d. No muscle relaxant property

79. Which side effect is associated with Halothane? *[Recent Question 2017]*
- a. Hypertension
- b. Malignant hyperthermia
- c. Tachycardia
- d. Uterine contraction

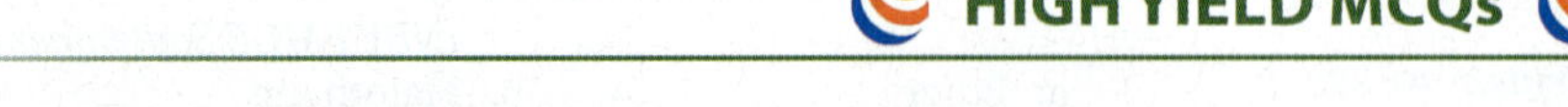
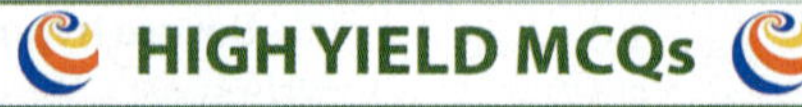

HIGH YIELD MCQs

1. True about Desflurane is/are *[PGI June 2016]*
- a. Boiling point is <23°C
- b. Chemically it is fluorinated methyl ethyl ether
- c. It increases the effect of muscle relaxant
- d. Can be given safely to patient susceptible to malignant hyperthermia
- e. More potent than isoflurane

2. Not intravenous anesthetic agent *[All India PGMEE 1995]*
- a. Ketamine
- b. Thiopentone
- c. Etomidate
- d. Cyclopropane

3. Induction agent for day care surgery *[AIIMS PGMEE 1998]*
a. Propofol b. Thiopentone
c. Diazepam d. Ketamine

4. All are true about Propofol, except *[PGI 1999, SGPGI 2002]*
a. Pleasant sedation and recovery
b. Safe in porphyria c. Antiemetic effect
d. Suppression of airway reflexes
e. Cardiac stimulant

5. Dose of Ketamine is *[AIIMS PGMEE 1993]*
a. 0.5 mg/kg i/m b. 2 mg/kg i/v
c. 5 mg/kg i/v d. 10 mg/kg i/m

6. Method of choice for induction in children is by *[AIIMS PGMEE 1993]*
a. I.M. b. Inhalation
c. I.V. d. O_2 tent

7. Least cardiotoxic agent *[All India PGMEE 1996, 1998]*
a. Isoflurane b. Enflurane
c. Sevoflurane d. Halothane

8. True about sevoflurane *[PGI 2004]*
a. Isopropyl ether b. MAC is 2%
c. Good to use in old age
d. Blood gas partition coefficient is more than halothane
e. Formation of compound A with baralyme

9. Delirium and hallucination is seen with *[All India PGMEE 1993]*
a. Halothane b. Ketamine
c. Ether d. N_2O

10. Intraocular tension increased in *[All India PGMEE 1993]*
a. Trilene b. Ketamine
c. Halothane d. Ether

11. Intraocular pressure is lowered by all, except *[All India PGMEE 1991]*
a. Ketamine b. Morphine
c. Halothane d. Thiopentone

12. Anesthetic agent safe to use in increased intracranial pressure *[PGI 2009]*
a. Halothane b. Thiopentone
c. Ketamine d. Ether

13. Intravenous thiopentone pentox, produces *[PGI 2003]*
a. Rash b. Pain
c. Spasm d. Hypotension
e. Muscular excitation (locally)

14. Drugs contraindicated in acute intermittent porphyria *[Recent Question 2017, PGI 2009, PGI 2004]*
a. Thiopentone b. Etomidate
c. Ketamine d. Propofol
e. Midazolam

15. Muscle rigidity is caused by which agent *[Recent Question 2016, All India PGMEE 1991]*
a. Fentanyl b. Halothane
c. Ketamine d. Droperidol

16. All of the following, cause myocardial depression, except *[PGI 2009]*
a. Halothane b. Etomidate
c. Thiopentone d. Ketamine
e. Propofol

17. Which anesthetic induction agent produces cardiac stability (Cardiostable anesthesia)? *[AIIMS PGMEE 2009]*
a. Ketamine b. Propofol
c. Thiopental d. Etomidate

18. Least soluble anesthetic agent is *[Jharkhand PGMEE 2005, TN PGMEE 2005]*
a. Desflurane b. Sevoflurane
c. Halothane d. Methoxyflurane

19. Fastest acting agent *[Recent Question 2017]* *[J&K PGMEE 2006, Jharkhand PGMEE 2004]*
a. Sevoflurane b. Desflurane
c. Isoflurane d. None of the above

20. Which one of the following is the fastest acting inhalational agent? *[All India PGMEE 2005]*
a. Halothane b. Isoflurane
c. Ether d. Sevoflurane

21. True about nitric oxide *[PGI 2007]*
a. Formed from L-Arginine by NO synthase
b. Causes vasodilation in all vessels
c. Used in portal hypertension
d. Interacts with Hemoglobin
e. Used in erectile dysfunction

22. Bone marrow depression is seen with *[AIIMS PGMEE 1996]*
a. Halothane b. Nitrous oxide
c. Ether d. Isoflurane

23. True about halothane *[PGI 2003]*
a. 1% Thymol is used as preservative
b. It senitizes heart to catecholamines at 1 MAC
c. 20% metabolized
d. It is not usually given in same patient within 3 months
e. It forms compound-A with soda lime

24. True about halothane *[PGI 2002]*
a. Causes bronchodilation
b. Antiarrhythmic
c. Can be used in hepatitis
d. Uterine contraction occurs
e. Causes hepatitis

25. Hepatitis is caused by *[PGI 1997]*
a. Cyclopropane
b. Halothane
c. Isoflurane
d. Enflurane

26. Hepatotoxic agent is *[AIIMS PGMEE 1997, Recent Question 2015]*
a. Ketamine b. Ether
c. Nitrous oxide d. Halothane

27. Bronchospasm is not caused by *[AIIMS PGMEE 1994]*
a. Regurgitation b. Aspiration
c. Intubation d. Halothane

28. Nephrotoxic agent is *[AIIMS PGMEE 1997]*
a. Methoxyflurane b. Isoflurane
c. Halothane d. N_2O

29. Inhalational agent of choice in children *[Recent Question 2017, PGI 2005, 2008]* *[AIPGME 2004, 2006]*
a. Sevoflurane b. Isoflurane
c. Desflurane d. Halothane
e. Nitrous oxide

30. Which of the following have analgesic property? *[PGI 2008]*
a. Nitrous oxide b. Ketamine
c. Thiopentone d. Etomidate

31. Ketamine can be used in all of the situations, except *[All India PGMEE 1992, SGPGI 2000]*
- a. Status asthmaticus
- b. For analgesia & sedation
- c. Obstetric haemorrhage
- d. Ischemic heart disease
- e. Aortic aneurysm

32. Contraindicated in epilepsy *[WB PGMEE 2006]*
- a. Isoflurane
- b. Halothane
- c. Enflurane
- d. Ether

33. Following will be the choice of anesthesia in an infected tooth posted for extraction *[MP PGMEE 2006]*
- a. Local block with lignocaine
- b. Local block with lignocaine and adrenaline
- c. Isoflurane
- d. Enflurane

34. Least effect on myocardial contractility *[AIIMS PGMEE 1993]*
- a. Ether
- b. Halothane
- c. Trilene
- d. Isoflurane

35. Anesthesia of choice for manual removal of placenta *[AIIMS PGMEE 1993]*
- a. General anesthesia
- b. Spinal anesthesia
- c. Epidural anesthesia
- d. Para-cervical anesthesia

36. A patient of alcoholic liver failure requires general anesthesia. Agent of choice *[All India PGMEE 2001]*
- a. Ether
- b. Halothane
- c. Isoflurane
- d. Methoxyflurane

37. Anesthesia of choice in renal disease *[PGI 2008, PGI 2009]*
- a. Atracurium
- b. Cisatracurium
- c. Vecuronium
- d. Rocuronium
- e. Mivacurium

38. Anesthesia of choice in renal failure *[All India PGMEE 2001, Jharkhand PGMEE 2006]*
- a. Methoxyflurane
- b. Isoflurane
- c. Enflurane
- d. None

39. Best anesthesia for status asthmaticus *[Recent Question 2017, AIIMS PGMEE 1997]*
- a. Thiopentone
- b. Ketamine
- c. Ether
- d. Nitrous oxide

40. Inducing agent contraindicated in asthma is *[AIIMS PGMEE 1993]*
- a. Ketamine
- b. Thiopentone
- c. Propofol
- d. Althesin

41. Which of the following anesthetic agents cause a rise in the Intracranial pressure? *[All India PGMEE 2005]*
- a. Sevoflurane
- b. Thiopentone sodium
- c. Lignocaine
- d. Propofol

42. Induction agent that may cause adrenal cortex suppression is *[All India PGMEE 2003]*
- a. Ketamine
- b. Etomidate
- c. Propofol
- d. Thiopentone

43. Coronary steal is caused by *[AIIMS PGMEE 1993]*
- a. Halothane
- b. Isoflurane
- c. Enflurane
- d. Ether

44. Least analgesic *[Kerala PGMEE 2007]*
- a. N_2O
- b. Ether
- c. Halothane
- d. Cyclopropane

45. Which of the following anesthetic agents have analgesic property? *[PGI 2001]*
- a. Ketamine
- b. Nitrous oxide
- c. Thiopentone
- d. Propofol
- e. Midazolam

46. The following anesthetic drug causes pain on intravenous administration *[AIIMS PGMEE 2006]*
- a. Midazolam
- b. Propofol
- c. Ketamine
- d. Thiopentone sodium

47. A 20-year-old patient presented with early pregnancy for Medical Termination of Pregnancy (MTP) in day-care facility. What will be the anesthetic induction agent of choice? *[AIIMS PGMEE 2006]*
- a. Thiopentone
- b. Ketamine
- c. Propofol
- d. Diazepam

48. Regarding features of propofol, which of the following statement is correct *[PGI 2005]*
- a. It suppresses adrenocortical hormone secretion
- b. I.M.inj. is painful
- c. Undergoes hepatic metabolism
- d. Chemically it is derivative of D-isopropyl phenol
- e. Cerebral protector action

49. A severely ill patient was maintained on an infusional anesthetic agent. On the 2nd day he started deteriorating. The probable culprit may be *[PGI 1999, JIPMER PGMEE 2004]*
- a. Etomidate
- b. Propofol
- c. Opioid
- d. Barbiturate

50. Which of the following is NOT TRUE regarding PROPOFOL? *[All India PGMEE 2008]*
- a. It is used in day-care anesthesia
- b. It is contraindicated in porphyria
- c. Commercial preparation contains egg extract
- d. It does not cause airway irritation

51. All statements regarding ketamine are true, except *[PGI 2002, SGPGI 2004]*
- a. Can be arrhythmogenic
- b. Raised ICT do not respond to CO_2 level
- c. Vasodilator and negative ionotropic effect
- d. Psychomimetic emergence
- e. Indirectly sympathetic action

52. Ketamine is safe in *[AIIMS PGMEE 1991, SGPGI 2002]*
- a. Raised ICT
- b. Open eye injury
- c. Ischemic heart disease
- d. Severe shock

53. Which of the following drugs is contraindicated in a patient with raised intracranial pressure? *[All India PGMEE 1998, AIIMS PGMEE 2006]*
- a. Thiopentone
- b. Propofol
- c. Midazolam
- d. Ketamine

54. Cerebral metabolism and O_2 consumption are increased by *[AIIMS PGMEE 2007]*
- a. Propofol
- b. Ketamine
- c. Atracurium
- d. Fentanyl

55. With regard to ketamine, all of the following are true, except *[AIIMS PGMEE 2005]*
- a. It is a direct myocardial depressant
- b. Emergence phenomenon are more likely if anticholinergic premedication is used
- c. It may induce cardiac dysrhythmia in patients receiving tricyclic antidepressants
- d. Has no effect on intracranial pressure

56. Increased cardiac oxygen demand is caused by *[AIIMS PGMEE 1993]*
a. Halothane b. Thiopentone
c. N_2O d. Ketamine

57. ICT caused by *[PGI 1997, All India PGMEE 2000]*
a. Ketamine b. Thiopentone
c. Halothane d. Propofol

58. Which of the following anaesthetic agents have good analgesic property? *[PGI 2006]*
a. Ketamine b. Nitrous oxide
c. Thiopentone d. Propofol
e. Midazolam

59. Which drug of anesthetics causes hallucination? *[All India PGMEE 1998]*
a. Ketamine b. Trilene
c. Halothane d. Trichloroethylene

60. Maximum analgesic action found in *[All India PGMEE 1997]*
a. Catecholamine b. Propofol
c. Ketamine d. Thiopentone

61. An unconscious patient of head injury comes in casualty. On examination shows raised intracranial pressure. Which anesthetic agent is contraindicated? *[AIIMS PGMEE 1999]*
a. Thiopentone b. Propofol
c. Ketamine d. Etomidate

62. Sodium Thiopentone is ultra short acting due to *[All India PGMEE 1996]*
a. Rapid absorption b. Rapid metabolism
c. Rapid redistribution d. Rapid excretion

63. Which of the following anesthetic agent lacks analgesic effect? *[PGI 2005]*
a. N_2O b. Thiopentone
c. Methohexitone d. Ketamine
e. Fentanyl

64. Intra-arterial injection of thiopentone causes *[Recent Question 2017, AIIMS PGMEE 1995]*
a. Vasospasm b. Vasodilation
c. Necrosis of vessel wall d. Hypotension

65. If thiopentone is injected accidentally into an artery the first symptom is *[All India PGMEE 1997]*
a. Analgesia b. Paralysis
c. Skin ulceration d. Pain

66. Use of thiopentone *[PGI 2004]*
a. Seizure
b. Truth spell
c. Reduction of ICP
d. Cerebral protection
e. Maintenance of an anesthesia

67. Dose of thiopentone used for induction is *[Recent Question 2017, JIPMER PGMEE 1996]*
a. 1 mg/kg b. 2 mg/kg
c. 5 mg/kg d. 10 mg/kg
e. 15 mg/kg

68. All are true about thiopentone, except *[AIIMS PGMEE 2007]*
a. $NaHCO_3$ is a preservative
b. Contraindicated in Porphyria
c. Agent of choice in shock
d. Has cerebroprotective action

69. Thiopentone is contraindicated in *[AIIMS PGMEE 1997]*
a. Acute intermittent porphyria
b. Bronchial asthma
c. Both d. None

70. Induction agent that may cause adrenal cortex suppression is *[PGI 2006]*
a. Ketamine b. Etomidate
c. Propofol d. Thiopentone
e. Fentanyl

71. An intravenous anesthetic agent that is associated with hemodynamic stability, maintenance of CPP with post-operative nausea, vomiting and myoclonus *[PGI 2002, SGPGI 2004]*
a. Ketamine b. Etomidate
c. Propofol d. Opioids

72. True about inhaled nitric oxide *[PGI 2007, 2009]*
a. Causes generalized vasodilation
b. Dilates pulmonary arteries
c. Causes hypotension d. Least systemic effects
e. Better ventilation perfusion match

73. Which of the following inhaled gas is used to decrease pulmonary artery pressure in adults and infants? *[AIIMS PGMEE 2002]*
a. Nitrous oxide b. Nitrogen dioxide
c. Nitric oxide d. Nitrogen

74. Which of the following statements is true regarding Nitric oxide? *[PGI 2001]*
a. Used in pulmonary hypertension
b. Decreases the dose of anesthetics
c. Sympathomimetic action
d. Causes systemic hypotension
e. Used as a vasoconstrictor

75. Use of nitrous oxide is contraindicated in all of the following surgeries, except *[AIIMS PGMEE 2008]*
a. Cochlear implant b. Microlaryngeal surgery
c. Vitreoretinal surgery d. Exenteration operation

76. Soda lime circuit is not used with *[Recent Question 2017, AIIMS PGMEE 1993]*
a. Enflurane b. Isoflurane
c. Methoxyflurane d. Trilene

77. Inhalation agent incompatible with soda lime *[AIIMS PGMEE 1992]* *[NBE DNB 1998, 1999, 2001, 2005, 2006]*
a. Isoflurane b. Trichloro ethylene
c. Methoxyflurane d. Enflurane

78. No effect on heart *[AIIMS PGMEE 1992]*
a. Chloroform b. Ether
c. Methoxyflurane d. Halothane

79. All of the following are the disadvantages of anesthetic ether, except *[All India PGMEE 2005]*
a. Induction is slow
b. Irritant nature of ether increases salivary and bronchial secretions
c. Cautery cannot be used
d. Affects blood pressure and is liable to produce arrhythmias

80. True about halothane *[PGI 2006]*
a. Non irritant
b. Antiarrhythmic
c. It antagonizes bronchospasm
d. Vasodilator

81. Which of the following is contraindication for halothane used? *[PGI 2001]*

a. Male sex b. Middle age
c. Recent halothane use d. Associated liver pathology
e. Obesity

82. Postoperative jaundice is because of use of *[PGI 1999]*

a. Isoflurane b. NO
c. Methoxyflurane d. Halothane

83. Repeated use of halothane causes *[All India PGMEE 1999]*

a. Hepatitis b. Pancreatitis
c. Encephalitis d. Meningitis

84. Anesthesia agent with least analgesic property *[All India PGMEE 1994]*

a. N_2O b. Halothane
c. Ether d. Propane

85. Agent which dissolves rubber *[Recent Question 2016, AIIMS PGMEE 1993]*

a. Halothane b. Enflurane
c. Cyclopropane d. Ether

86. Maximum uterine relaxation *[AIIMS PGMEE 1992]*

a. Ether b. N_2O
c. Halothane d. Chloroform

87. All are true, except *[All India PGMEE 2001]*

a. Halothane is good analgesic agent
b. Halothane sensitize heart to catecholamine
c. Halothane relaxes bronchi
d. Halothane causes hepatitis and liver cell necrosis

88. Which of the following fluorinated anesthetics corrodes metal in vaporizers and breathing systems? *[AIIMS PGMEE 2006]*

a. Sevoflurane b. Enflurane
c. Isoflurane d. Halothane

89. Nephrotoxicity is caused by *[All India PGMEE 1998]*

a. Sevoflurane b. Isoflurane
c. Methoxyflurane d. Halothane

90. Fluoride content is least *[Recent Question 2016] [PGI 1997]*

a. Methoxyflurane b. Enflurane
c. Isoflurane d. Sevoflurane

91. Which of the following inhalational agent is contraindicated in a patient with history of epilepsy? *[AIIMS PGMEE 2003]*

a. Isoflurane b. Enflurane
c. Halothane d. Sevoflurane

92. In increased ICT, agent used for anesthesia *[AIIMS PGMEE 1994]*

a. N_2O b. Trilene
c. Ether d. Isoflurane

93. Which of the following statements regarding desflurane is correct? *[AIIMS PGMEE 2004]*

a. It causes severe myocardial depression
b. It is a structural analogue of isoflurane
c. It has very high blood and tissue gas partition coefficients
d. It is metabolically unstable

94. A 70-year-old patient is posted for a surgery which is likely to last 4–6 hours. The best inhalational agent of choice for maintenance of anesthesia in such a case is *[AIIMS PGMEE 2004]*

a. Methoxyflurane b. Ether
c. Trichloroethylene d. Desflurane

95. Rapid induction of anesthesia occurs with which of the following inhalation anesthetics? *[AIIMS PGMEE 2002]*

a. Isoflurane b. Halothane
c. Desflurane d. Sevoflurane

96. A 6-year-old child is posted for elective urology surgery under general anesthesia. He refuses to allow the anaesthesiologist an I.V. access. The best inhalational agent of choice for induction of anesthesia is *[AIIMS PGMEE 2004]*

a. Sevoflurane
b. Methoxyflurane
c. Desflurane
d. Isoflurane

97. Which is contraindicated in closed system anesthesiology? *[BIHAR PGMEE 2005]*

a. Methoxyflurane
b. Isoflurane
c. Sevoflurane
d. Desflurane

98. NOT TRUE regarding sevoflurane *[All India PGMEE 2008]*

a. MAC is higher than isoflurane
b. Blood gas coefficient is higher than desflurane
c. Potency more than cardiodepressant than isoflurane
d. Sevoflurane is less cardiodepressant than isoflurane

99. Which of the following is the best indication for propofol as an intravenous induction agent?

a. Neurosurgery *[All India PGMEE 2004]*
b. Day care surgery
c. Patients with coronary artery disease
d. In neonates

100. A 38-year-old man is posted for extraction of last molar tooth under general anesthesia as a day care case. He wishes to resume his work after 6 hours. Which one of the following induction agents is preferred? *[All India PGMEE 2003]*

a. Thiopentone sodium b. Ketamine
c. Diazepam d. Propofol

101. The induction agent of choice in day care anesthesia is *[All India PGMEE 2003]*

a. Sevoflurane b. Ketamine
c. Propofol d. Methohexitone

102. In a 2 months old infant undergoing surgery for biliary atresia, you would avoid one of the following anesthetic *[AIIMS PGMEE 2003]*

a. Thiopentone b. Halothane
c. Propofol d. Sevoflurane

103. In a child with intestinal obstruction with deranged liver function test, the anesthetic of choice is *[PGI 2006]*

a. Enflurane b. Isoflurane
c. Halothane d. Sevoflurane
e. Ether

104. The following are used for treatment of postoperative nausea and vomiting, following squint surgery in children except *[All India PGMEE 2005]*

a. Ketamine b. Ondansetron
c. Propofol d. Dexamethasone

105. All agents can be given for induction of anesthesia in children, except *[All India PGMEE 2001]*

a. Halothane b. Sevoflurane
c. Morphine d. N_2O

Anesthesiology

106. A child is posted for operative repair of exstrophy of bladder with renal failure. Which anesthetic should be preferred? *[Recent Question 2016, AIIMS PGMEE 2009]*
   a. Pancuronium
   b. Vecuronium
   c. Atracurium
   d. Rocuronium

107. All anesthetic agents decrease portal vein flow. Portal flow is maximally reduced by *[AIIMS PGMEE 2010]*
   a. Ether
   b. Halothane
   c. Isoflurane
   d. Enflurane

108. Agent causing malignant hyperthermia *[All India PGMEE 1995]*
   a. Succinylcholine
   b. Pantroline
   c. Gallamine
   d. Ketamine

109. Cerebral blood flow is increased by *[JIPMER PGMEE 2014]*
   a. Barbiturates
   b. Benzodiazepines
   c. Ketamine
   d. Propofol

110. Hyperkalemia may occur due to *[JIPMER PGMEE 2014]*
   a. Succinylcholine
   b. Nitrous oxide
   c. Sevoflurane
   d. Desflurane

111. True about Sevoflurane *[PGI November 2014]*
   a. Nephrotoxic
   b. Decrease hepatic blood flow
   c. Anti-seizure activity
   d. Decrease intracranial tension
   e. Useful for induction in children

112. A 55-year-old overweight female was given Fentanyl-Pancuronium-Midazolam anesthesia for a surgery. After surgery she was extubated and on examination, her chest wall respiratory motion was slow and she was unable to move her upper body. She was conscious and able to understand what was said, but was lacking respiratory effort. Her blood pressure was normal and heart rate was also normal. What is the diagnosis? *[ESI IMO 2014]*
   a. Pulmonary embolism
   b. Fentanyl-induced chest wall rigidity
   c. Respiratory depression
   d. Recovery phase

113. Which of the following combinations can be used for day-care surgery? *[AIIMS PG May 2015]*
   a. Morphine, Midazolam, Propofol
   b. Morphine, Ketamine, Diazepam
   c. Fentanyl, Midazolam, Thiopentone sodium
   d. Remifentanil, Midazolam, Propofol

114. Anesthetic that causes pain on intravenous administration is *[AIIMS PG May 2015]*
   a. Thiopentone
   b. Propofol
   c. Ketamine
   d. Midazolam

115. In a patient with coronary artery disease having pulse rate 48/minute and low BP, Anesthetic contraindicated is *[AIIMS PG May 2015]*
   a. Ketamine
   b. Etomidate
   c. Dexmedetomidine
   d. Fentanyl

116. Following can be used as an Induction agent *[AIIMS November 2017]*
   a. Bupivacaine
   b. Lorazepam
   c. Neostigmine
   d. Dexmedetomidine

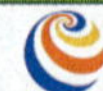 NEET/NBE PATTERN MCQs ANSWERS WITH EXPLANATIONS 

1. Ans. (b) Ketamine
[Ref. KDT, 7/e p384]

Ketamine and CNS
- Potent cerebral vasodilator
  - Increase cerebral blood flow
  - Increase intracranial pressure
  - Increase cerebrospinal pressure
- Underlying mechanism: Increased arterial carbondioxide tension

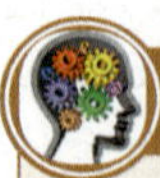

Also Remember

Ketamine
- Cyclohexanone derivative used for induction of anesthesia related to hallucinogen phencyclidine
- Indicated as sole anesthetic agent for diagnostic and surgical procedures that do not require skeletal muscle relaxation
- Anesthetic state produced by ketamine has been termed **"Dissociative anesthesia"** characterized by profound analgesia, immobility, amnesia with light sleep
- Respiration is not depressed
- Adverse effects: Poor muscle relaxation, increased salivation, tachycardia, increase in BP, increase in muscle tone, increased ICT, delirium, hallucination

2. Ans. (d) Halothane
[Ref. KDT, 7/e p379]
- Halothane causes a dose-related depression of the cardiovascular system and sensitizes the myocardium to catecholamine-induced premature ventricular contractions

3. Ans. (b) Pain present for at least 3 months
[Ref. Clinical Anaesthesiology by Morgan, 5/e p1089]
- Persistent postsurgical pain, defined as chronic pain that continues beyond the typical healing period of 1–2 months following surgery or well past the normal period for postoperative, follow-up by anesthesia providers is increasingly acknowledged as a common and significant issue following surgery
- The incidence of persistent postsurgical pain may exceed 30% after some operations, especially amputations, thoracotomy, mastectomy, and inguinal herniorrhaphy
- Although the cause is unclear, several risk factors have been identified, and aggressive, multimodal perioperative pain control is often suggested as a fundamental preemptive strategy

4. Ans. (c) Asthma
[Ref. KDT, 7/e p384]

Ketamine Contraindications
- Hypertension
- Head injury
- Psychiatric problems
- Glaucoma
- Open globe injury

5. Ans. (b) Nitrous oxide
[Ref. Pfenninger and Fowler's Procedures for Primary Care, 3/e p32]
- Chronic effects of N_2O exposure can include bone marrow suppression, mainly through inhibiting enzymes that depend on vitamin B_{12}
- Myelin formation and DNA synthesis are affected

6. Ans. (d) As antidepressant
[Ref. Katzung, 11/e p434]

Thiopentone
- Very short and very fast acting barbiturate
- **Most common intravenous agent**
- Termination of action is too fast due to quick redistribution
- It has an anticonvulsant action but no antidepressant
- Can cause hypotension (depress CVS)
- **Contraindicated in acute intermittent porphyria**
- Can lead to thrombosis, vasoconstriction, ischemia and gangrene if injected into arteries
- **Agent of choice for cerebral protection** because it decreases cerebral metabolic rate

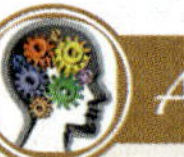

Also Remember
- Two common barbiturates used for the purpose of inducing a coma are pentobarbital and thiopental; this type of coma is referred to as a drug-induced coma or medically-induced coma
- Thiopental may be used as a hypnotic agent for narcoanalysis (the drug historically **misnomered as "truth serum'**) and narcosynthesis in psychiatric disorders

7. Ans. (c) Doxacurium
[Ref. Katzung, 11/e p350]

Agents Used in Day-Care Surgeries
- Desflurane
- Sevoflurane
- Midazolam
- Mivacurium
- Alfentanil
- Nitrous oxide
- Propofol
- Ketamine
- Isoflurane

8. Ans. (c) Features are nausea and vomiting
[Ref. Katzung, 11/e p375]

Propofol Infusion Syndrome
- Associated with high doses and long-term use of Propofol (>4 mg/kg/h for more than 24–48 hours)
- MC in children, and critically ill patients receiving catecholamines and glucocorticoids are at high risk
- Associated with cardiomyopathy, metabolic acidosis, skeletal myopathy, hyperkalemia, hepatomegaly, and lipemia
- High blood potassium, high blood triglycerides, and liver enlargement, proposed to be caused by either

"a direct mitochondrial respiratory chain inhibition or impaired mitochondrial fatty acid metabolism" are also key features

- Treatment is supportive
- Early recognition of the syndrome and discontinuation of the propofol infusion reduces morbidity and mortality

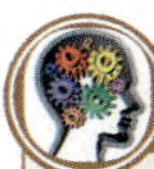

Also Remember

- The incidence of nausea and vomiting when propofol is used for induction also is markedly less than after the use of other IV anesthetics

9. Ans. (d) All the above

[Ref. KDT, 6/e p372]

- Inhalation agents halothane, enflurane, and isoflurane produce a dose-dependent reduction in uterine tone

10. Ans. (d) Propofol

[Ref. Essentials of Pharmacology by Kaye, 1/e p731]

- Older anesthetic agents chloroform, trichloroethylene, divinyl ether, tribromoethanol, and methoxyflurane all caused direct hepatotoxicity that resulted in centrilobular liver necrosis
- The introduction of halothane in 1956 marked a milestone in anesthesia but found later to be hepatotoxic too

11. Ans. (a) Xenon

[Ref. Rang & Dale's Pharmacology, 8/e p500]

- NMDA receptors are an important site of action for anesthetics such as nitrous oxide, xenon and ketamine

12. Ans. (a) Midazolam

[Ref. KDT, 6/e p376]

Inductions Agents

- Thiopentone
- Etomidate
- Propofol
- Ketamine
- Methohexitone

13. Ans. (d) Halothane

[Ref. KDT, 7/e p379]

Halothane

- Power tocolytic preferred during manual removal of placenta
- Halothane and sevoflurane preferred in children
- **Postoperative shivering and hypothermia is maximum**
- Direct depression of myocardial contractility by reducing intracellular ca2+ concentration.
- Sympathetic activity fails to increase reflex
- Cardiac output is reduced with deepening anesthesia
- BP starts falling early and parallels the depth

14. Ans. (d) NMDA

[Ref. KDT, 7/e p384]

- Ketamine is an NMDA **(N-methyl-D-aspartate)** receptor antagonist, with additional weak actions at Sigma1 receptors, the norepinephrine transporter

15. Ans. (b) Good analgesic action

[Ref. KDT, 7/e p384]

Ketamine

- Strong analgesia
- Bronchodilator and so is not contraindicated in patients suffering from asthma
- Tachycardia
- Hypertension
- **Intravenous agent of choice**
- **Produces dissociative anesthesia**
- **Preferred in patients with full stomach**
- **MC side effect is hallucination**

16. Ans. (c) 2.5%

[Ref. Clinical Anaesthesiology by Morgan, 5/e p178]

Drug	Purpose	Dose (mg/kg)
Thiopental	Induction (2.5%)	3–6
Ketamine	Induction Sedation	1–2 mg/kg (IV) 2.5–15 mcg/kg/min
Etomidate	Induction	0.2–0.5 mg/kg
Propofol	Induction Maintenance infusion Sedation infusion	1–2.5 mg/kg (I.V) 50–200 mcg/kg/min 25–100 mcg/kg/min

17. Ans. (d) Methoxyflurane

[Ref. Anaesthesia by Lee, 12/e p328]

Nephrotoxicity due to Anesthetic Agents

- Underlying cause: High fluoride content of several inhalational anesthetics raise fluoride ion concentrations resulting in nephrotoxicity
- Fluoride levels required to induce nephrotoxicity: More than 50 micro mol per liter
- Chances of nephrotoxicity:

Highly nephrotoxic	Moderate nephrotoxic	Non-nephrotoxic
Methoxyflurane	Enflurane Sevoflurane	Halothane Desflurane Isoflurane

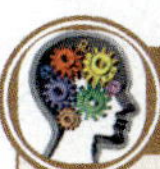

Also Remember

- *Highest fluoride content/nephrotoxic nature*: Methoxyflurane
- *Least fluoride content/nephrotoxic nature*: Isoflurane
- Methoxyflurane leads to *'Vasopressin-resistant high-output renal failure'*

18. Ans. (d) Drop in blood pressure

[Ref. Ajay Yadav, 4/e p77-78]

Effects of Ketamine

- Dissociative anesthesia **(Cataleptic state)**
- Raised intracranial tension, raised intraocular tension
- Emergence reaction (Vivid dreaming, illusions, extracorporeal experience like floating out of body, excitement, confusion, euphoria, fear)

- Hallucinations: Auditory hallucination > Visual hallucination (**Most common side effect** of ketamine; Reduced by giving benzodiazepines)
- Tachycardia, hypertension (Therefore, anesthetic of choice for Shock)
- Respiratory stimulant (Adult), respiratory depressant (Children)
- Bronchodilator (Therefore, anesthetic of choice for asthmatics)
- Increased tracheobronchial and salivary secretion
- Increased intragastric pressure
- Increased muscular tone (Non-purposeful movement)
- Nystagmus and dilated pupil

19. Ans. (b) Cyclopropane

[Ref. Ajay Yadav, 4/e p60-61]

- Blood : Gas Partition Coefficient Interpretation:
  - Lesser B/G coefficient: Faster induction and recovery
  - Higher B/G coefficient: Slower induction and recovery
- Blood gas partition coefficients of various agents: **[Mnemonic: D**octors **C**an **N**ever **S**ay **I**f **E**ther **H**as **C**aused **T**hem **E**asy **M**aintenance**]**

Agent	B/G partition coefficient
Desflurane	0.42
Cyclopropane	0.44
Nitrous oxide	0.47
Sevoflurane	0.69
Isoflurane	1.38
Enflurane	1.8
Halothane	2.4
Chloroform	8
Trilene	9
Ether	12
Methoxyflurane	15

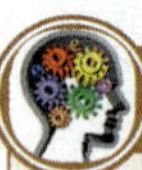

Also Remember

- In shock, agents with low blood gas partition coefficients are safe

20. Ans. (a) Bronchodilator

[Ref. Ajay Yadav, 4/e p77-78]

21. Ans. (d) N_2O

[Ref. Ajay Yadav, 4/e p59]

- Blood gas coefficient of N_2O is 0.47: Faster induction and recovery
- Methoxyflurane blood gas coefficient is 15: Slowest induction and recovery

22. Ans. (a) Methoxyflurane

[Ref. Ajay Yadav, 4/e p65]

- Methoxyflurane yields highest concentration of fluoride: Can damage the tubules, and cause Vasopressin-resistant High output (polyuric) renal failure

23. Ans. (d) Thiopentone

[Ref. Ajay Yadav, 4/e p79]

Agents used in Day-Care Surgeries

[Mnemonic: Dr. **M**an **M**ohan **S**ingh **I**s **K**ind **A**nd **N**ice **P**olitician**]**

- **D**esflurane
- **M**idazolam
- **M**ivacurium
- **S**evoflurane
- **I**soflurane
- **K**etamine
- **A**lfentanil
- **N**itrous oxide
- **P**ropofol

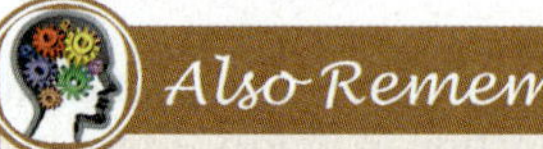

Also Remember

- Thiopentone:
  - Regaining consciousness: 15 minutes
  - Half-life of elimination: 10.4 hours
  - No important work (e.g. driving) should be undertaken for 24 hours
  - Not suitable for day-care surgery

24. Ans. (d) 36.5°C

[Ref. Ajay Yadav, 4/e p59]

- As critical temperature is above room temperature, N_2O can be kept in liquefied state

25. Ans. (a) Nitrous oxide

[Ref. Short Textbook of Anaesthesia by Ajay Yadav, 4th Ed., P64]

Nitrous Oxide

- Known as 'Laughing gas': Produces euphoria after inhalation

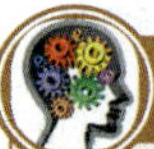

Also Remember

- Is not a complete anesthetic: Is used as carrier to other inhalational agents
- **Second gas effect**: When given along with other inhalational agents it increases the alveolar concentration of that agent
- **Concentration effect**: When given along with other inhalational agents, it increases the alveolar concentration of itself
- Systemic actions and side-effects:
  - Safe in cardiac patients and patients in shock
  - Increases intracranial tension
  - Bone marrow depression: Aplastic anaemia, megaloblastic anaemia
  - Subacute combined degeneration of spinal cord

26. Ans. (a) Tachycardia

[Ref. Ajay Yadav, 4/e p61]

Effects of Halothane

- Bradycardia
- Hypotension
- Severe ventricular arrhythmia
- Blunts baroreceptor reflex
- Hypercarbic and hypoxic reflexes are blunted
- Bronchodilator

- Raised intracranial tension
- GFR and urinary flow is decreased
- Moderate muscle relaxation
- Uterine atony/relaxation and postpartum haemorrhage (used for external version and manual removal of placenta; contraindicated in cesarean and abortion)
- Post-operative shivering
- Halothane hepatitis (Centrilobular necrosis)

27. Ans. (b) Ketamine
[Ref. Ajay Yadav, 4/e p87]
- Ketamine is contraindicated in Head injury as it raises Intracranial tension

28. Ans. (b) Propofol
[Ref. Ajay Yadav, 4/e p74]
- Propofol is the agent of choice: Because of its early induction and early and smooth recovery

29. Ans. (b) Low potency and good analgesia
[Ref. Ajay Yadav, 4/e p81]

30. Ans. (a) Etomidate
[Ref. Ajay Yadav, 4/e p82]
- Etomidate is Intravenous Anesthetic of choice for,
  - Aneurysm surgery
  - Patient with heart disease

31. Ans. (a) Ketamine
[Ref. Ajay Yadav, 4/e p77-78]
- **Ketamine produces dissociative anesthesia**: A stage which dissociates the individual from surroundings and himself, i.e. individuals is in cataleptic state

32. Ans. (b) Does not produce pain an IV injection
[Ref. Ajay Yadav, 2/e p77]
- Midazolam is a Water-based preparation, hence painless

33. Ans. (c) Bupivacaine
[Ref. Ajay Yadav, 4/e p78]

Intravenous Induction Agents
- Sodium thiopentone
- Propofol
- Etomidate
- Ketamine
- Methohexitone
- Midazolam

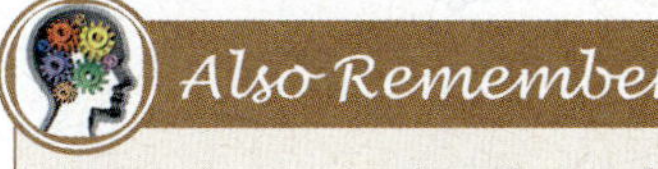

- Bupivacaine is a **local anesthetic having high cardiotoxicity**

34. Ans. (b) Low potency and good analgesia
[Ref. Ajay Yadav, 2/e p59]

35. Ans. (b) Good analgesic action
[Ref. Ajay Yadav, 2/e p77]

36. Ans. (c) Ketamine
[Ref. Ajay Yadav, 2/e p77]

37. Ans. (b) Propofol
[Ref. Ajay Yadav, 2/e p74]
- Propofol is an antiemetic so postoperative nausea, vomiting is uncommon

38. Ans. (a) Tachycardia
[Ref. Ajay Yadav, 2/e p61]

39. Ans. (d) Ketamine
[Ref. Ajay Yadav, 2/e p77]

40. Ans. (b) Parenteral
[Ref. Ajay Yadav, 4/e p81-82]

Propofol
- Type of anesthetic: Phenol-based intravenous (parenteral) anesthetic
- Anesthetic properties:
  - Elimination half-life: 2–4 hours
  - Regaining of consciousness: 2–8 minutes
  - No analgesia
  - No muscle relaxation
- Systemic effects:
  - Hypotension
  - Apnoea
  - Bronchodilation in COPD patients
  - Cerebroprotective
  - Myoclonic
  - Antiemetic, antipruritic
- Uses:
  - **Intravenous agent of choice for day-care surgery**
  - Agent of choice for **total intravenous anesthesia**
  - Agent of choice for **induction in those susceptible to malignant hyperthermia**
  - Sedative in ICU

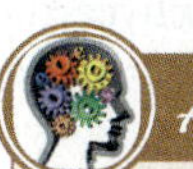

- Advantages and disadvantages of Propofol:

Advantages	Disadvantages
• Rapid smooth recovery • Early ambulation • Antiemetic • Antipruritic • Bronchodilator	• Apnoea • Hypotension • Painful injection • Allergic reactions • Propofol infusion syndrome

41. Ans. (b) Nitrous oxide
[Ref. Ajay Yadav, 2/e p59]

42. Ans. (c) N_2O
[Ref. Ajay Yadav, 2/e p59]

43. Ans. (d) 6
[Ref. Ajay Yadav, 2/e p63]

44. Ans. (a) Ketamine
[Ref. Ajay Yadav, 2/e p77]

45. Ans. (d) Isoflurane
[Ref. Ajay Yadav, 2/e p62]
- **Isoflurane:**
  - Does not depress myocardium
  - Does not cause bradycardia
  - Baroreceptor reflex is preserved or minimally depressed
  - Cardiac output is best maintained among all inhalational agents

46. Ans. (b) Ketamine

[Ref. A Practical Approach to Obstetric Anesthesia by Brenda, 1/e p125]

47. Ans. (a) Nitrous oxide

[Ref. Ajay Yadav, 4/e p65]

- Few commonly used drugs causing hepatotoxicity:
  - Anesthetics (Methoxyflurane, halothane)
  - Allopurinol
  - Amiodarone
  - Azathioprine
  - Hormonal contraceptives
  - Tuberculosis drugs (Rifampicin, isoniazid, pyrazinamide)
  - NSAIDs (Ibuprofen, Indomethacin)
  - Ketoconazole
  - Methotrexate
  - Methyl dopa
  - Minocycline
  - Nifedipine
  - Paracetamol
  - Valproate
  - Zidovudine

48. Ans. (a) Ketamine

[Ref. Ajay Yadav, 2/e p77]

49. Ans. (a) Pancuronium

[Ref. Ajay Yadav,4/e p100]

- *Pancuronium use increases chances of cardiac arrhythmias with Halothane*: Due to vagal block leading to tachycardia and hypertension

50. Ans. (b) Ketamine

[Ref. Ajay Yadav, 2/e p77]

51. Ans. (d) Sevoflurane

[Ref. Ajay Yadav, 2/e p63]

- **Sevoflurane**:
  - Faster, pleasant and smooth induction with no systemic toxicity
  - **Agent of choice for induction in children**
- Induction and recovery will be fast with agent with less B/G coefficient and slower with agents with high B/G Coefficient
  - Induction will be fastest with desflurane
  - Induction is slowest with methoxyflurane

52. Ans. (a) Ether

[Ref. Ajay Yadav, 4/e p64]

- *Hyperglycaemia is seen with*:
  - Ether
  - Chloroform **(Causes most profound hyperglycaemia)**
  - Cyclopropane

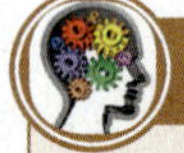

Also Remember

Systemic Effects of Inhalational Agents

- *Maximum depression of respiration*: Enflurane
- *Maximum inhibition to ventilatory response*: Halothane
- *Maximum bronchodilation in asthmatics*: Halothane (Agent of choice in asthmatics)
- *Maximum bronchodilation in non-asthmatics*: Sevoflurane

Contd...

Contd...

- *Non-inhibitor of ciliary activity (reduced coughing out of secretions)*: Ether
- *Best maintenance of cardiac output*: Isoflurane (Agent of choice in cardiac patients)
- *Maximum hypotension*: Isoflurane
- *Inhibition of myocardial contractility*: Halothane
- *Maximum sensitization of heart to adrenaline*: Halothane
- *Maximum hepatocellular damage*: Halothane
- *Maximum nephrotoxicity*: Methoxyflurane
- *Agent causing megaloblastic and aplastic anemia*: Nitrous oxide
- *Agent causing subacute combined degeneration of spinal cord*: Nitrous oxide
- *Agent causing maximum muscle relaxation*: Desflurane
- *Agent causing maximum analgesia*: Trilene
- *Agent causing maximum hyperglycaemia*: Chloroform

53. Ans. (d) Propofol

[Ref. Ajay Yadav, 2/e p74]

54. Ans. (d) Wells

[Ref. Nitrous Oxide and Oxygen Saturation by Clark, 1/e p11]

Nitrous Oxide

- **Joseph Priestley**: First discovered Nitrous oxide (1773–74)
- **Humphry Davy**: Discovered analgesic properties of Nitrous oxide, Called it 'Laughing gas' (1800)
- Horace Wells: Introduced its use as an Inhalational agent in dental extraction (1844)

55. Ans. (b) Halothane

[Ref. Ajay Yadav, 4/e p67]

Commonly used Drugs causing Hypotension

[Mnemonic: A Big CAP Does Protect Against Sun]

- **A**lpha blockers
- **B**eta blockers
- **C**alcium channel blockers
- **A**nesthetic agents
- Halothane
- Isoflurane (Most common inhalational anesthetic responsible)
- Enflurane
- Desflurane
- Methoxyflurane
- Chloroform
- **P**arkinsonism drugs
- **D**iuretics, **D**igoxin, **D**epression drugs
- **P**otassium
- **A**lcohol
- **S**ildenafil

56. Ans. (d) Drop in blood pressure

[Ref. Ajay Yadav, 2/e p77]

57. Ans. (c) Ketamine

[Ref. Ajay Yadav, 2/e p77]

58. Ans. (b) Propofol

[Ref. Ajay Yadav, 2/e p74]

59. Ans. (a) Emergence delirium

[Ref. Ajay Yadav, 4/e p86]

Ketamine

- Pharmacokinetics:
  - Phencyclidine derivative
  - Onset of action: 30–60 seconds

  - Regaining consciousness: 15–20 minutes
  - Half-life of elimination: 2–3 hours
- **Mechanism of action: Inhibits NMDA receptors**
- Systemic effects: Dissociative anesthesia
- CNS effects:
  - Emergence delirium
  - **Hallucinations (MC side effect)**
  - Raised intracranial tension
  - Strong analgesic
- CVS effects:
  - Tachycardia
  - Hypertension
- Respiratory system effects: Bronchodilator
- Other effects:
  - Raised intraocular tension
  - Raised intragastric pressure
  - Raised muscle tone
- Dose of Ketamine: 2 mg/kg (IV) or 5–10 mg/kg (IM)

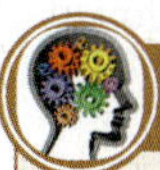

Also Remember

Ketamine Properties
- Intravenous agent of choice for **shock**
- Agent producing **dissociative anesthesia**
- Preferred agent for patients with **full stomach**
- Intravenous agent (and overall) of choice for **asthmatics**

60. Ans. (b) Halothane
[Ref. Anaesthesia by Yadav, 4/e p66]

Halothane Hepatitis
- Risk factors: Multiple exposures, Hypoxia, Middle age, Obesity, Females, Autoimmune diseases
- Pathology: **Centrilobular necrosis**
- Etiology: Reductive metabolites, Reduced cardiac output, Immunological injury

61. Ans. (b) Etomidate
[Ref. Pharmacology for Anesthetists by Current, 1/e p250]

Etomidate
- Consistently increases the amplitude of somatosensory-evoked potentials (in contrast to most anaesthetic agents)
- Etomidate in the propylene glycol formulation may produce pain on injection, a side effect which is less likely with the lipid formulation
- There is a 30-fold difference between the effective dose and the lethal dose of Etomidate, making it an extremely safe agent
- Postoperative vomiting is more common than with other induction agents (30–40% incidence)

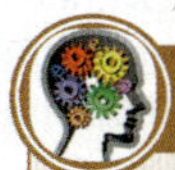

Also Remember

- Anesthesia-related risk factors for PONV include use of Volatile anesthetics, Nitrous oxide, Intravenous opioids, Ketamine, and Etomidate

62. Ans. (b) Halothane
[Ref. Anaesthesia by Fleisher, 6/e p197]

Halothane and Hepatitis
- Halothane decreases total hepatic blood flow by decreasing both portal venous and hepatic arterial blood flow
- Halothane hepatitis lead to gastrointestinal upset, jaundice, fever, rash, eosinophilia, and serum autoantibodies
- Halothane-induced hepatitis usually occurs in a patient who has been exposed previously to the same agent

63. Ans. (b) Dantrolene
[Ref. Ajay Yadav, 4/e p115]

Malignant Hyperthermia Causative Agents
- Halothane
- Isoflurane
- Enflurane
- Desflurane
- Sevoflurane
- Methoxyflurane
- Cyclopropane
- Ether
- Succinylcholine

64. Ans. (c) 6 hours
[Ref. A Practice of Anesthesia by Coté, 5/e p116]
- Propofol poses a high risk of bacterial infection
  - Propofol is not water soluble, and hence must be formulated in a lipid based medium, which is ideal for bacterial growth
  - In surgical patients, use of preparations that have become contaminated after opening has caused sepsis and death
- **To minimize the risk of infection, propofol solutions and opened vials should be discarded within 6 hours**
  - Unused Propofol in syringes, vials or administration tubing should be discarded at end of procedure or within 6 hours after opening an ampoule
  - Intravenous line administering Propofol should be flushed every 6 hours and at end of procedure to remove residual Propofol

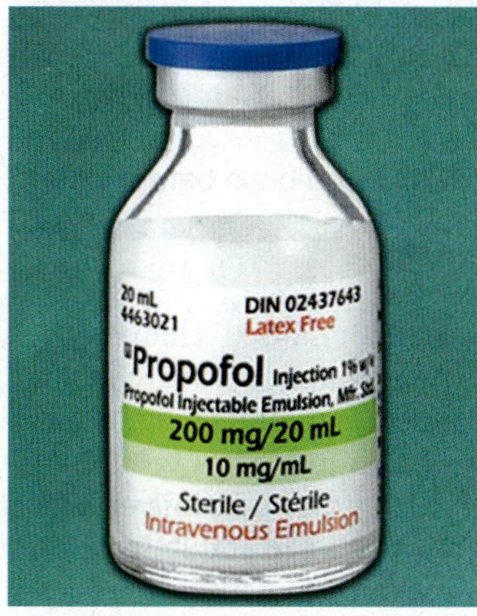

Fig. Propofol vial

65. Ans. (a) Increases it
[Ref. KDT, 7/e p384]

Ketamine
- Increase cerebral blood flow, Increase intracranial pressure, Increase cerebrospinal pressure
- Increased intraocular pressure, even when the depth of anesthesia was adequate

- Increased incidence of Emergence delirium and nausea and vomiting

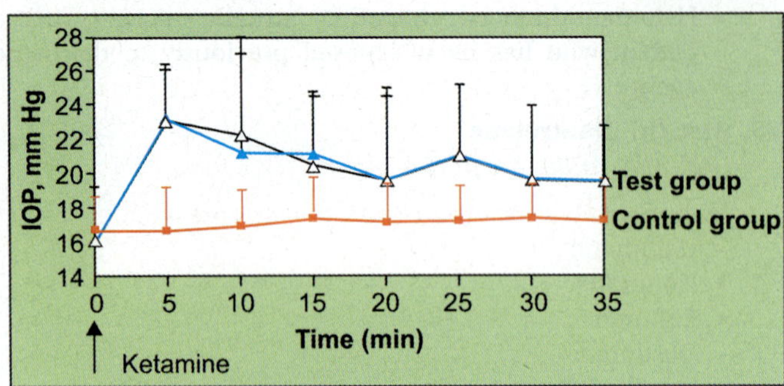

66. **Ans. (a) Methoxyflurane**
[Ref. Pharmacology by Rock, 1/e p208]
- Upon delivery to the brain, the anaesthetic agent has to additionally cross the blood brain barrier before a central effect (i.e. unconsciousness) can occur
- Alveolar pulmonary membrane and blood-brain barrier pose little problem as most of the agents are lipid soluble
- **Methoxyflurane is the most lipophilic of all the inhalational agents** and is also the most potent (greater the lipid solubility, greater is the potency of the inhalational anesthetic agent)

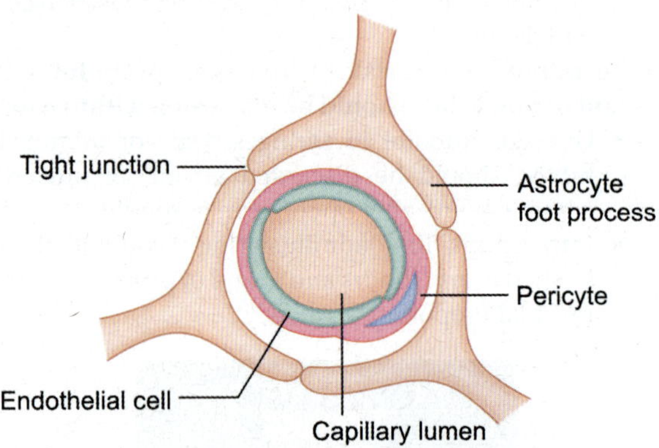

Fig. Blood-brain barrier (BBB)

67. **Ans. (a) Pain**
[Ref. Ajay Yadav, 2/e p72]
- At sub-anesthetic dose, Thiopentone is Antanalgesic: Severe burning pain down the injection site
- To decrease pain at the injection site, administer Thiopental by slow injection into large veins (rather than into small hand veins); may also administer a local anesthetic or an opiate agonist prior to induction to minimize pain, and avoid extravasation and intra-arterial administration

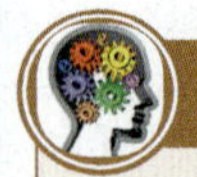

Also Remember

- Anesthetics causing pain at Injection site: Propofol, Etomidate, Methohexital, Thiopentone
- Propofol is the MCC of Injection site pain and Hypotension

68. **Ans. (a) Results in adrenal suppression**
[Ref. Faust's Anesthesiology, 4/e p165]
- Induction dose of Etomidate suppresses cortisol and aldosterone synthesis for up to 5–8 hours, which probably does not have significant clinical consequence
- However, long-term infusion of Etomidate may causes prolonged adrenal suppression and should be avoided

69. **Ans. (c) Methoxyflurane**
[Ref. Anaesthetic drugs by Thornton, 1/e p120]
- Methoxyflurane has the highest boiling point of any inhalation anaesthetic, coupled with the lowest vapour pressure
- Since its boiling point (about 104°C at standard atmospheric pressure) is higher than that of water, Methoxyflurane might be thought difficult to vaporise
- But, Methoxyflurane has low latent heat of vaporisation (about 58 cal/g, compared with 540 cal/g for water); this means only one-tenth as many calories are needed
- Methoxyflurane is completely stable in the presence of alkali, air, light or moisture and can be safely employed in a closed circuit

70. **Ans. (c) Propofol**
[Ref. Ajay Yadav, 2/e p73; Harrison's 17/e, Tab352-4]

Anesthetics in Porphyria
- Unsafe anesthetic which should be avoided in porphyria: Thiopentone, Pentazocine, Ropivacaine, Enflurane, Etomidate
- Relatively safe in porphyria: Propofol

71. **Ans. (d) Propofol**
[Ref. Shnider and Levinson's Anesthesia, 4/e p220]

Propofol
- A non-barbiturate induction agent
- Rapid onset of action which is within one arm-brain circulation time and clinical recovery occurs within 10–15 minutes even after prolonged infusion
- Causes fall in systemic vascular resistance leading to hypotension that is greater than one seen with Thiopentone
- Causes mild bradycardia probably due to central vagal activity
- Attenuates pressor response to laryngoscopy and intubation
- An antiemetic
- Depresses laryngeal/pharyngeal reflexes (Laryngospasm/bronchospasm not seen)
- Reduces intracranial pressure

72. **Ans. (b) Methoxyflurane**
[Ref. Pharmacology by Rock, 1/e p208]
- Methoxyflurane is the most lipophilic of all the inhalational agents and is also the most potent (greater the lipid solubility, greater is the potency of the inhalational anesthetic agent)
- Highly lipid-soluble agent with very high oil-water solubility, which is around 970 (i.e., the agent is 970 times as soluble in oil as in water); this lipid solubility makes Methoxyflurane the most potent inhalational agent

73. **Ans. (c) Glaucoma**
[Ref. Clinical Anesthesia by Barash, 6/e p824]
- Ketamine contraindications include Hypertension, Head injury, Psychiatric problems, Glaucoma, Open globe injury

- Ketamine can elevate intracranial and intraocular pressure and is thus relatively contraindicated in patients with increased intracranial pressure and with glaucoma or open-globe injuries

74. Ans. (b) Depression

[Ref. Miller's Anesthesia, 8/e p929]

- Propofol produces the typical EEG anesthetic depression, including burst suppression and electrical silence at higher doses
- Most benzodiazepines produce the typical EEG anesthetic depression pattern but have a less profound effect on the EEG, usually generalized slowing into the theta and delta range at high doses without progressing to burst suppression

75. Ans. (d) Morphine

[Ref. Surgical Intensive Care Medicine by Merritt, 1/e p149]

- Administration of morphine can cause hypotension as the result of either drug-induced bradycardia or histamine release
- Morphine-induced bradycardia occurs as a result of stimulation of the vagal nucleus in the medulla

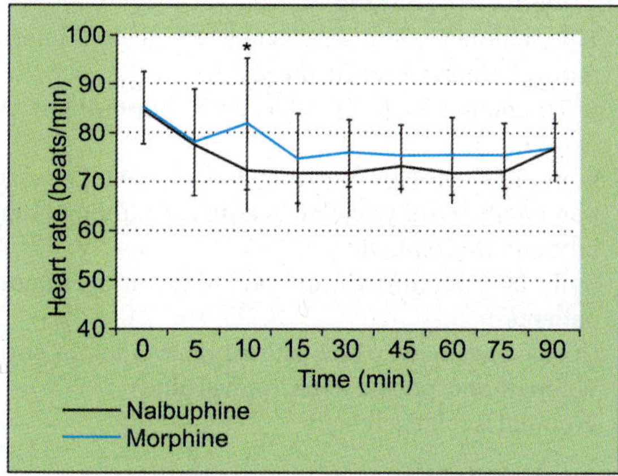

Fig. Morphine effect on heart rate

76. Ans (c) Sevoflurane

[Ref. Anesthesia for Infants and Children by Cote, 4/e p337]

- MC inhalational induction agent is Sevoflurane
- **Sevoflurane has replaced halothane as the Induction agent of choice**
- However, despite Sevoflurane's apparent better safety profile compared with halothane, it is still easy to overdose the child with CHD and produce bradycardia, hypotension, and apnea
- Sevoflurane should be carefully titrated and that the concentrations are rapidly reduced when an adequate level of anesthesia is achieved

77. Ans. (b) Sevoflurane

[Ref. Nurse Anesthesia by Nagelhout, 4/e p1195]

- Both Isoflurane and Desflurane have a 'pungent' odor that can cause breath holding and limit the usefulness of these gases for Mask and chamber induction
- Sevoflurane is preferred for Mask induction because of its **'pleasant' odour and less airway irritation**

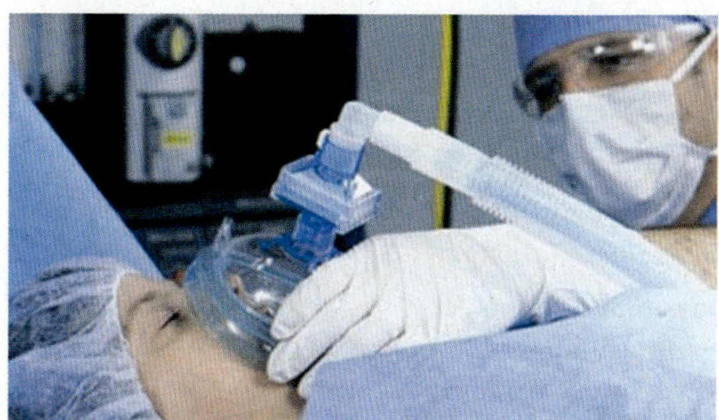

Fig. Mask induction

78. Ans. (b) Anticonvulsant effect

[Ref. Clinical Cases in Anesthesia by Reed, 4/e p383]

Properties of Propofol

- Anesthetic properties: Elimination half-life 2-4 hours, Regaining of consciousness 2-8 minutes, No analgesia, No muscle relaxation
- Systemic effects: Hypotension, Apnoea, Bronchodilation in COPD patients, Cerebroprotective, Myoclonic, Antiemetic, Antipruritic
- Advantages: Rapid smooth recovery, Early ambulation, Antiemetic, Antipruritic, Bronchodilator
- Disadvantages: Apnoea, Hypotension, Painful injection, Allergic reactions, Propofol infusion syndrome, Infection (if used from vials)

79. Ans. (b) Malignant hyperthermia

[Ref. Ajay Yadav, 2/e p101]

- Malignant hyperthermia causing Inhalation agents: Halothane >>Isoflurane, Enflurane, Desflurane, Sevoflurane, Methoxyflurane, Cyclopropane, Ether

HIGH YIELD MCQs ANSWERS WITH EXPLANATIONS 

1. Ans. (a) Boiling point is <23°C; (b) Chemically it is fluorinated methyl ethyl ether; (c) It increases the effect of muscle relaxant

[Ref. Anaesthesia for Postgraduates by Agasti, 1/e p422-424]

Desflurane

- Halogenated (fluorine only) methyl-ethyl-ether
- Peculiar vapour pressure is very close to the atmospheric pressure at room temperature. This is because the boiling point of desflurane is 23.5° C which is near about to the room temperature
- Direct coronary vasodilator
- Decreases the cerebrovascular resistance: Increases cerebral blood flow and intracranial pressure

- Like other inhaled anesthetic agents, desflurane depresses the neuromuscular function and augments the action of both non-depolarizing and depolarizing muscle relaxants
- Desflurane is a trigger of malignant hyperthermia in susceptible persons
- Isoflurane (MAC 1.1) is more potent than sevoflurane (MAC 2.0), and both are more potent than desflurane (MAC 6.35)

2. **Ans. (d) Cyclopropane**
[Ref. Ajay Yadav, 2/e p65]
   - Cyclopropane is Inhalation agent

3. **Ans. (a) Propofol.**
[Ref. Ajay Yadav, 2/e p74]

4. **Ans. (e) Cardiac stimulant**
[Ref. Ajay Yadav, 2/e p74]

5. **Ans. (b) 2 mg/kg i/v; (c) 5 mg/kg i/v**
[Ref. Miller,2/e p60]

Dose of Ketamine
- Intravenous: 1–2 mg/ kg
- Intramuscular: 5–10 mg/ kg

6. **Ans. (b) Inhalation**
[Ref. Ajay Yadav, 2/e p74]
   - **Inhalation induction** is the method of choice for induction in children
     - **Sevoflurane is the agent of choice**
     - Due to high cost of it, halothane is still most commonly used agent

7. **Ans. (a) Isoflurane**
[Ref. Ajay Yadav, 2/e p62]

Isoflurane
- Does not depress myocardium
- Does not cause bradycardia
- Baroreceptor reflex is preserved or minimally depressed
- Cardiac output is best maintained among all inhalational agents

8. **Ans. (a) Isopropyl ether; (b) MAC is 2%; (e) Formation of compound A with baralyme**
[Ref. Ajay Yadav, 2/e p74]

9. **Ans. (b) Ketamine**
[Ref. Ajay Yadav, 2/e p77-78]

10. **Ans. (b) Ketamine**
[Ref. Ajay Yadav, 2/e p78]

11. **Ans. (a) Ketamine**
[Ref. Ajay Yadav, 2/e p77-78]

12. **Ans. (b) Thiopentone**
[Ref. Ajay Yadav, 2/e p72]
   - **Thiopentone is the Agent of choice for cerebral protection**:
     - Decrease Cerebral oxygen consumption (CMO_2)
     - Decrease Cerebral metabolic rate (CMR)
     - Decrease Intracranial tension

13. **Ans. All choices**
[Ref. Ajay Yadav, 2/e p72]

Complications of Thiopentone
- Respiratory and cardiovascular depressant
- Severe laryngospasm and bronchospasm
- Transient apnea
- Hiccups and coughing
- Allergic manifestation (Cutaneous rash, pruritus, vertigo, euphoria, delirium)
- Postoperative vertigo, euphoria, delirium
- At sub-anesthetic dose, it is Antanalgesic: Severe burning pain down the injection site
- Hypotension (Venodilation & direct depression of vaso-motor center)
- Antithyroid activity
- Muscular excitation

14. **Ans. (a) Thiopentone; (b) Etomidate; (c) Ketamine**
[Ref. Ajay Yadav, 2/e p73; Harrison's Principles of Internal Medicine 17/e, Chapter 352, Table 352-4]

Anesthetics in Porphyria
- Thiopentone: Contraindicated in acute intermittent porphyria and variegate porphyria
  - Thiopentone can be safely given in porphyria cutanea tarda
- Etomidate should probably be avoided because it is potentially porphyrogenic in animals, although reports in humans are conflicting
- Enflurane, pentazocine are said to be unsafe in porphyric patients
- Unsafe anesthetic which should be avoided in porphyria: Thiopentone, pentazocine, ropivacaine
- Propofol is relatively safe

15. **Ans. (a) Fentanyl**
[Ref. Ajay Yadav, 2/e p81]
   - Fentanyl can produce significant muscle rigidity commonly known as **"Wooden Chest Syndrome"**

16. **Ans. (b) Etomidate**
[Ref. Ajay Yadav, 2/e p74]
   - Etomidate is a cardiovascular stable agent

17. **Ans. (d) Etomidate**
[Ref. Ajay Yadav, 2/e p74]

18. **Ans. (a) Desflurane**
[Ref. Ajay Yadav, 2/e p56]
   - Desflurane has least Blood-gas partition coefficient, hence least soluble anesthetic agent

19. **Ans. (b) Desflurane**
[Ref. Ajay Yadav, 2/e p63]
   - Induction and recovery will be fast with agent with less B/G coefficient and slower with agents with high B/G Coefficient
     - Induction will be fastest with Desflurane
     - Induction will be slowest with Methoxyflurane

20. Ans. (d) Sevoflurane
[Ref. Ajay Yadav, 2/e p56]
- Among the options, sevoflurane has least B/G coefficient (0.69)

21. Ans. All choices
[Ref. Lee, 13/e p51]

22. Ans. (b) Nitrous oxide
[Ref. Ajay Yadav, 2/e p60]

Nitrous Oxide in Body
- Nitrous oxide when used for more than 6 hours inactivates Vitamin B_{12}
- Impaired Methionine and Deoxythymidine synthesis lead to defect in folate metabolism
- Bone marrow depression cause aplastic anemia and Megaloblastic anemia

23. Ans. (d) It is not usually given in same patient within 3 months
[Ref. Ajay Yadav, 2/e p68]

24. Ans. (a) Causes bronchodilatation; (e) Causes hepatitis
[Ref. Ajay Yadav, 2/e p61]

25. Ans. (b) Halothane
[Ref. Ajay Yadav, 2/e p61]

26. Ans. (d) Halothane
[Ref. Ajay Yadav, 2/e p61]

27. Ans. (d) Halothane
[Ref. Ajay Yadav, 2/e p61]

28. Ans. (a) Methoxyflurane
[Ref. Ajay Yadav, 2/e p65]

Methoxyflurane
- Yields highest concentration of fluoride (F^-) which can damage the tubules and can cause vasopressin resistant High output (polyuric) renal failure (Not to be used in Renal disease)
- Hepatotoxic
- Bradycardia
- Decreased cardiac output

29. Ans. (a) Sevoflurane
[Ref. Ajay Yadav, 2/e p63]

30. Ans. (a) Nitrous oxide; (b) Ketamine
[Ref. Ajay Yadav, 2/e p59,77]

31. Ans. (d) Ischaemic heart disease; (e) Aortic aneurysm
[Ref. Ajay Yadav, 2/e p78]

Contraindication of Ketamine
- Head injury (raises intracranial pressure)
- Intracranial space occupying lesion
- Eye injury or ophthalmologic problem
- Ischemic heart disease (increases myocardial oxygen demand)
- Vascular aneurysm (causes hypertension)
- Hypertensive
- Psychiatric disease and drug addicts (increased hallucinations and emergence reaction)

32. Ans. (c) Enflurane
[Ref. Ajay Yadav, 2/e p63]
- **Enflurane is Contraindicated in:**
  - Epilepsy (It increases intracranial pressure; At high dose it produces spike and wave pattern EEG which culminate into frank Tonic-clonic seizures)
  - Renal disease (Depresses renal function due to decreased renal flow)

33. Ans. (d) Enflurane

34. Ans. (d) Isoflurane
[Ref. Ajay Yadav, 2/e p63]

35. Ans. (a) General anesthesia
[Ref. Manual of Obstetrics by Daftary, 3/e p391]

36. Ans. (c) Isoflurane
[Ref. Ajay Yadav, 2/e p58]

Anesthesia and Liver Damage
- Direct hepatocellular damage is seen with halothane, chloroform, fluroxene, methoxyflurane
- Isoflurane is the volatile agent of choice for maintenance in liver disease
- Desflurane and sevoflurane can also be used
- Hepatic functions are well preserved with ether
- Propofol is good choice among IV agents for liver disease

37. Ans. (a) Atracurium; (b) Cisatracurium
[Ref. Ajay Yadav, 2/e p90]
- Atracurium is relaxant of choice in:
  - Hepatic failure
  - Renal failure
  - Myasthenia gravis
  - Extreme of ages (Newborn & old age)

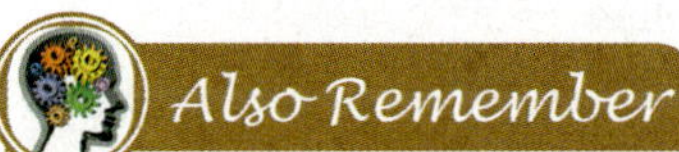

- Cisatracurium is a derivative of Atracurium

38. Ans. (b) Isoflurane
[Ref. Ajay Yadav, 2/e p58]

Renal Toxicity in Anesthesia
- Direct renal toxicity has been attributed to inorganic fluoride (F^-)
- Renal threshold beyond which fluoride levels are toxic is 50 µm

Agent	F^- level after 2.5 to 3 MAC hours
Methoxyflurane	50–80 µm
Sevoflurane	30–50 µm
Enflurane	20–25 µm
Isoflurane	4–8 µm
Halothane	Only in anaerobic condition
Desflurane	Does not produce

- Nephrotoxicity produced by fluorinated agent: Vasopressin resistant polyuric renal failure
- **Safety in Renal disease:** Desflurane > isoflurane > enflurane > sevoflurane > methoxyflurane

39. Ans. (b) Ketamine
[Ref. Ajay Yadav,2/e p78]

40. Ans. (d) Althesin
[Ref. Ajay Yadav,2/e p78]
- Althesin is a combination of two steroid, alfaxalone and alphadon
- Althesin causes hypersensitivity reaction and raised intracranial tension

41. Ans. (a) Sevoflurane
[Ref. Ajay Yadav,2/e p63]

42. Ans. (b) Etomidate
[Ref. Ajay Yadav,2/e p75]
- Because of its severe adrenocortical suppression (on long-term infusion) and high incidence of nausea and vomiting, Etomidate is no more used nowadays

43. Ans. (b) Isoflurane
[Ref. Ajay Yadav,2/e p62]
- Isoflurane increases the coronary blood flow to non-ischaemic area which in patients of myocardial ischaemia can cause coronary steal

44. Ans. (c) Halothane
[Ref. Ajay Yadav,2/e p58,84]

Analgesia in Anesthesia
- Maximum: Trilene
- Good: Ether, Nitrous oxide, Methoxyflurane, Ketamine
- Not good analgesics: Cyclopropane, Enflurane, Sevoflurane, Desflurane, Isoflurane
- Least: Halothane
- Lacking analgesic effect: Methohexital, Propofol, Etomidate, Benzodiazepines
- Antanalgesic: Thiopentone

45. Ans. (a) Ketamine; (b) Nitrous oxide
[Ref. Ajay Yadav,2/e p58,84]

46. Ans. (b) Propofol
[Ref. Ajay Yadav,2/e p74]

Propofol Painful Injection
- Propofol is oil-based preparation containing Soyabean oil, Egg lecithin and Glycerol
- Injection should be preceded by lignocaine injection

47. Ans. (c) Propofol
[Ref. Ajay Yadav,2/e p74]
- Because of its early induction and early and smooth recovery, Propofol is now the agent of choice for day-care surgery

48. Ans. (c) Undergoes hepatic metabolism; (d) Chemically its derivative of D-isopropyl phenol; (e) Cerebral protector action
[Ref. Ajay Yadav,2/e p74]

49. Ans. (a) Etomidate
[Ref. Ajay Yadav,2/e p75]
- On long-term infusion of etomidate, there is adrenocortical suppression leading to deterioration of patient with increased chance of mortality

50. Ans. (b) It contraindicated in porphyria
[Ref. Ajay Yadav,2/e p74]
- Propofol is relatively safe in porphyria

51. Ans. (c) Vasodilator and negative ionotropic effect
[Ref. Ajay Yadav,2/e p77]

52. Ans. (d) Severe shock
[Ref. Ajay Yadav,2/e p78]

53. Ans. (d) Ketamine
[Ref. Ajay Yadav,2/e p77]

54. Ans. (b) Ketamine
[Ref. Ajay Yadav,2/e p77]

55. Ans. (d) Has no effect on intracranial pressure
[Ref. Ajay Yadav,2/e p77]

56. Ans. (d) Ketamine
[Ref. Ajay Yadav,2/e p77]

57. Ans. (a) Ketamine
[Ref. Ajay Yadav,2/e p77]

58. Ans. (a) Ketamine; (b) Nitrous oxide
[Ref. Ajay Yadav,2/e p58]

59. Ans. (a) Ketamine
[Ref. Ajay Yadav,2/e p77]

60. Ans. (c) Ketamine
[Ref. Ajay Yadav,2/e p84]

61. Ans. (c) Ketamine
[Ref. Ajay Yadav,2/e p77]

62. Ans. (c) Rapid redistribution
[Ref. Ajay Yadav,2/e p71]
- Elimination half-line of thiopentone is 10.4 hours but consciousness is regained after 15–20 minutes which is because of rapid redistribution
- Drug is redistributed from brain to tissues with less vascularity like muscle or fat but repeated doses saturates these tissues, and regaining of consciousness after repeated doses depends on its metabolism and elimination

63. Ans. (b) Thiopentone; (c) Methohexitone
[Ref. Ajay Yadav,2/e p58, 84]

64. Ans. (a) Vasospasm
[Ref. Ajay Yadav,2/e p73]
- Because of high alkalinity of Thiopentone, it gets precipitated in acidic pH of the blood forming crystals leading to thrombus formation which blocks the micro-circulation
- It also causes endothelial damage
- Both these process produce vasospasm leading to ischaemia and gangrene of limb

65. Ans. (d) Pain
[Ref. Ajay Yadav,2/e p72]
- With injection patient complains of severe burning pain down the injection site which is followed by pallor, cyanosis, edema and finally gangrene of limb

66. Ans. All choices
[Ref. Ajay Yadav,4/e p78-80]
- ***Thiopental is known as Truth-serum***: Suppression of higher cortical functions lead to uncovering of truth

67. Ans. (c) 5 mg/kg
[Ref. Ajay Yadav,2/e p72]

68. Ans. (c) Agent of choice in shock
[Ref. Ajay Yadav,2/e p72]

69. Ans. (c) Both
[Ref. Ajay Yadav,2/e p73]

Contraindications for Thiopentone
- Absolute contraindications:
  - Porphyria: Acute intermittent & variegate (not cutanea tarda)
  - History of previous anaphylaxis to thiopentone
- Relative contraindications:
  - Shock & hypotension
  - Fixed cardiac output lesion (aortic stenosis)
  - Heart block
  - On beta blocker drug
  - Uncontrolled hypertensives
  - Asthmatics
  - Inflammatory condition of oral cavity, jaw, neck where airway management is difficult
  - Dystrophia myotonica
  - Familial hypokalemic periodic paralysis
  - Hepatic disease
  - Renal disease

70. Ans. (b) Etomidate
[Ref. Ajay Yadav,2/e p75]

71. Ans. (b) Etomidate
[Ref. Ajay Yadav,2/e p75]

72. Ans. (b) Dilated pulmonary arteries; **(d)** Least systemic effects; **(e)** Better ventilation perfusion match
[Ref. Ajay Yadav,2/e p190]

73. Ans. (c) Nitric oxide
[Ref. Ajay Yadav,2/e p190]

74. Ans. (a) Used in pulmonary hypertension; **(d)** Causes systemic hypotension
[Ref. Ajay Yadav,2/e p190]

75. Ans. (d) Exenteration operation
[Ref. Ajay Yadav, 2/e p60]

Contraindications for Nitrous Oxide
- Pneumothorax
- Pneumoperitoneum
- Pneumoencephalus
- Middle ear surgery and tympanoplasties
- Posterior fossa surgeries
- Laparoscopic surgeries
- Acute intestinal obstruction and volvulus of gut
- Eye surgery

76. Ans. (d) Trilene
[Ref. Ajay Yadav,2/e p59]

Reaction of Inhalational Agents with Soda lime
- Trilene: Dichloroacetylene (Neurotoxicity) and Phosgene (Pulmonary Toxicity)
- Sevoflurane: Compound A (Toxicity)
- Desflurane, Isoflurane and Enflurane:Carbon monoxide

77. Ans. (b) Trichloroethylene
[Ref. Ajay Yadav,2/e p63]

78. Ans. (b) Ether
[Ref. Ajay Yadav, 2/e p63]

79. Ans. (d) Affects blood pressure and is liable to produce arrhythmia
[Ref. Ajay Yadav, 2/e p64-65]
- Disadvantages of Ether:
  - Highly inflammable and explosive
  - Induction is slow, irritating and unpleasant
  - Tracheobronchial secretion increased
  - Delayed recovery
  - Postoperative nausea and vomiting

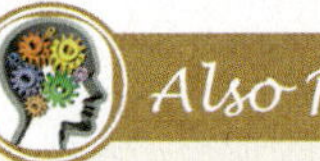

Also Remember

Ether
- Stimulates sympathetic system causing tachycardia and hypertension
- Does not depress myocardium
- Baroreceptor reflex is preserved

80. Ans. (a) Non irritant; **(c)** It antagonizes bronchospasm; **(d)** Vasodilator
[Ref. Ajay Yadav,2/e p60-61]

81. Ans. (c) Recent halothane use; **(d)** Associated liver pathology
[Ref. Ajay Yadav,2/e p61]

82. Ans. (d) Halothane
[Ref. Ajay Yadav,2/e p61]

83. Ans. (a) Hepatitis
[Ref. Ajay Yadav,2/e p61]

84. Ans. (b) Halothane
[Ref. Ajay Yadav,2/e p58]

85. Ans. (a) Halothane
[Ref. Ajay Yadav,2/e p59]
- Methoxyflurane and ether can react with rubber tubing (not with plastic tubing)

86. Ans. (c) Halothane
[Ref. Ajay Yadav,2/e p61]

87. Ans. (a) Halothane is a good analgesic agent
[Ref. Ajay Yadav,2/e p61]

88. Ans. (d) Halothane
[Ref. Ajay Yadav,2/e p24]
- Halothane is delivered through Goldman vaporizer (simple glass bottle)

89. Ans. (c) Methoxyflurane
[Ref. Ajay Yadav,2/e p58]

90. Ans. (c) Isoflurane
[Ref. Ajay Yadav,2/e p58]

91. Ans. (b) Enflurane
[Ref. Ajay Yadav,2/e p62]

92. Ans. (d) Isoflurane
[Ref. Ajay Yadav,2/e p62]

93. Ans. (b) It is a structural analogue to isoflurane
[Ref. Ajay Yadav,2/e p63]

- Desflurane is similar to isoflurane except that chlorine atom (of Isoflurane) is replaced by chlorine atom

94. Ans. (d) Desflurane
[Ref. Ajay Yadav,2/e p 63]

- **Desflurane is the agent of choice for**:
  - Prolonged duration surgeries
  - Old age patients
  - Hepatic and renal disease patients

95. Ans. (c) Desflurane
[Ref. Ajay Yadav,2/e p63]

96. Ans. (a) Sevoflurane
[Ref. Ajay Yadav,2/e p63]

97. Ans. (c) Sevoflurane
[Ref. Ajay Yadav,2/e p64]

98. Ans. (d) Sevoflurane is less cardio depressant than isoflurane
[Ref. Ajay Yadav,2/e p64]

99. Ans. (b) Day-care surgery
[Ref. Ajay Yadav,2/e p74]

100. Ans. (d) Propofol
[Ref. Ajay Yadav,2/e p74]

101. Ans. (c) Propofol
[Ref. Ajay Yadav,2/e p74]

102. Ans. (b) Halothane
[Ref. Ajay Yadav,2/e p61]

103. Ans. (d) Sevoflurane
[Ref. Ajay Yadav,2/e p63]

104. Ans. (a) Ketamine
[Ref. Ajay Yadav,2/e p74]

105. Ans. (c) Morphine
[Ref. Nelson's Pediatrics, 20/e p422]

106. Ans. (c) Atracurium
[Ref. Ajay Yadav,2/e p90]

107. Ans. (b) Halothane
[Ref. Cardiovascular Research by Gross, 3/e p136]

108. Ans. (a) Succinylcholine
[Ref. Ajay Yadav,2/e p101]

- Malignant hyperthermia:

Group	Drugs
Muscle relaxant	Succinylcholine
Inhalation	Halothane >>Isoflurane, Enflurane, Desflurane, Sevoflurane, Methoxyflurane, Cyclopropane, Ether
Local anesthetic	Lignocaine
Others	Tricyclic antidepressants, MAO inhibitors, Phenothiazines

109. Ans. (c) Ketamine
[Ref. Ajay Yadav,2/e p74]

110. Ans. (a) Succinylcholine
[Ref. Ajay Yadav,2/e p146]

- Succinylcholine is contraindicated in hyperkalemia

111. Ans. (a) Nephrotoxic; (e) Useful for induction in children
[Ref. Ajay Yadav,2/e p70-71]

Sevoflurane

- Induction agent of choice in children:
  - Smooth induction
  - No significant toxicity
  - B/G coefficient 0.69
- Systemic effects:
  - Depress respiratory system
  - Nephrotoxicity
  - Increase intracranial tension
  - Maintain hepatic blood flow
  - Epileptogenic

112. Ans. (b) Fentanyl-induced chest wall rigidity
[Ref. Clinical Anaesthesia by Barash, 6/e p478]

- Fentanyl may cause muscle rigidity, particularly involving the muscles of respiration; Occur or recur infrequently in the extended postoperative period usually following high dose administration
- Skeletal muscle movements of various groups in the extremities, neck and external eye have been reported during induction of anesthesia with fentanyl; these reported movements have, on rare occasions, been strong enough to pose patient management problems

113. Ans. (d) Remifentanil, midazolam, propofol
[Ref. Anaesthesia by Yadav, 4/e]

Agents of Choice in Day-Care Surgery

- Combination in day care surgery: Propofol + Alfentanil
- Intravenous agent for Day-care surgery: Propofol
- Muscle relaxant for Day-care surgery: Mivacurium
- Opioid for Day-care surgery: Remifentanil

Also Remember

Agents Used in Day-Care Surgeries

- **D**esflurane
- **M**idazolam
- **M**ivacurium
- **S**evoflurane
- **I**soflurane
- **K**etamine
- **A**lfentanil
- **N**itrous oxide
- **P**ropofol

[Mnemonic: Dr. Man Mohan Singh Is Kind And Nice Politician]

114. Ans. (b) Propofol

[Ref. Anaesthesiology Review by Murray, 4/e p163]

- Compared with the other intravenously administered anesthetic agents, propofol causes the most injection site pain and hypotension
- IV administration of Propofol often causes pain during the injection, especially if it is given via a small vein

115. Ans. (c) Dexmedetomidine

[Ref. Cardiology by Sleeper, 5/e p357]

Dexmedetomidine

- A potent Respiratory and Cardiac depressant
- Causes Intense vasoconstriction and reduced Cardiac output
- Increase PR interval

116. Ans. (d) Dexmedetomidine

[Ref. Benumof's Airway Management, 2/e p260]

- Dexmedetomidine
- A highly selective $\alpha 2$ adrenoceptor agonist that has sedative and analgesic properties with associated reduction in opioid and anesthetic requirements
- One significant advantage is that in the clinical dose range there is no respiratory depression: Highly specific $\alpha 2$-adrenoreceptor agonist with sedative, analgesic, and anesthetic-sparing effects that causes sedation without a change in ventilatory status
- Agonistic action on the $\alpha 2$ adrenoceptors in the sympathetic ganglia modulates the release of catecholamines, resulting in a sympatholytic effect and reports of bradycardia and hypotension

Anesthesiology

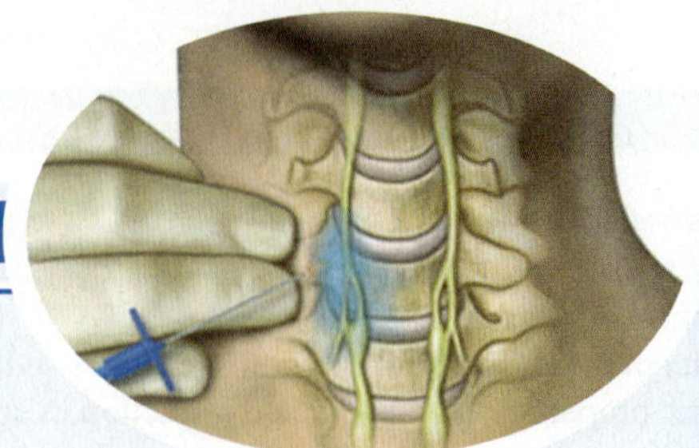

Chapter 5

Principles and Mechanism of Anesthesia

THEORETICAL CONCEPTS

V A. STAGES OF ANESTHESIA

	Respiration	Tidal volume	Pupils	Eyes position (Movement)	Reflexes abolished
Analgesia	Irregular	Small	Constricted	Divergent (Normal)	Nil
Excitement	Irregular	Large	Dilated	Divergent (Roving)	Eyelash
Surgical anesthesia					
Plane-1	Regular	Large	Constricted	Divergent (Roving initially, fixed end)	Conjunctival, Pharyngeal, Skin
Plane-2	Regular	Medium	½ Dilated	Fixed centrally	Corneal
Plane-3	Regular	Small	¾ Dilated	Fixed centrally	Laryngeal
Plane-4	Jerky	Small	Full Dilated	Fixed centrally	Carinal, Anal sphincter
Medullary paralysis	–	–	–	–	–

Stage	Pupil		Resp.	Pulse	B.P
	Usual size	Reaction to light			
1st Induction				Irregular	Normal
2nd Excitement	OR			Irregular and fast	High
3rd Operative				Steady slow	Normal
4th Danger				Weak and thread	Low

Fig. Stages of anesthesia

Topper's Edge

Stages of General Anesthesia

- In 1954, **Joseph F. Artusio** further divided the first stage in Guedel's classification into three planes
  - 1st plane : Patient does not experience amnesia or analgesia
  - 2nd plane: Patient is completely amnesic but experiences only partial analgesia
  - 3rd plane: Patient has complete analgesia and amnesia
- Stages of General Anesthesia classification was designed for use of a sole inhalational anesthetic agent, **Diethyl ether**, in patients who were usually premedicated with morphine and atropine
  - Introduction of neuromuscular blocking agents (such as succinylcholine and tubocurarine) changed the concept of general anesthesia as it could produce temporary paralysis without deep anesthesia
  - Most of the signs of Guedel's classification depend upon the muscular movements (including respiratory muscles), and paralyzed patients' traditional clinical signs were no longer detectable when such drugs were used
  - Now due to discontinuation of Ether, Guedel's classification is regarded as obsolete[Q]

V B. INFLAMMABLE INHALATIONAL ANESTHETICS[Q]

- Ether
- Ethylene
- Ethyl chloride
- Cyclopropane

V C. FEW IMPORTANT FACTS ABOUT ANESTHETICS

- *Most commonly used intravenous induction agent*: Thiopentone[Q]
- *Agent of choice for cerebral protection*: Thiopentone[Q]
- *Intravenous agent of choice for day care surgery*: Propofol[Q]
- *Combination of choice in day care surgery*: Propofol + Alfentanil
- *Agent of choice for total intravenous anesthesia*: Propofol[Q]
- *Agent of choice for induction of malignant hyperthermia susceptible*: Propofol[Q]
- *Agent of choice for Electroconvulsive therapy (ECT)*: Methohexitone
- *Most cardio-stable intravenous agent*: Etomidate[Q]
- *Intravenous agent causing maximum nausea and vomiting*: Etomidate
- *Intravenous agent of choice for shock*: Ketamine[Q]
- *Agent producing dissociative anesthesia*: Ketamine
- *Preferred agent for patients with full stomach*: Ketamine[Q]
- *Intravenous agent (and overall) of choice for asthmatics*: Ketamine[Q]
- *Drug of choice for shivering*: Pethidine
- *Agent of choice to inhibit stress response to intubation or laryngoscopy*: Fentanyl
- *Most common inhalational method for induction in children*: Sevoflurane[Q]
- *Earliest recovery with inhalational agents*: Desflurane[Q]
- *Last recovery with inhalational agents*: Methoxyflurane
- *Inhalational agent with maximum depression to respiration*: Enflurane
- *Inhalational agent with maximum inhibition to ventilatory response*: Halothane
- *Inhalational agent of choice for cardiac patients*: Isoflurane[Q]
- *Inhalational agent causing maximum hypotension*: Isoflurane
- *Inhalational agent of choice for neurosurgery*: Isoflurane[Q]
- *Inhalational agent causing megaloblastic and aplastic anaemia*: Nitrous oxide[Q]
- *Inhalational agent causing Subacute degeneration of spinal cord*: Nitrous oxide[Q]
- *Inhalational agent of choice for asthmatic patients*: Halothane[Q]
- *Most common drug implicated in Malignant hyperthermia*: Succinylcholine (SCh)[Q]

V D. ANESTHESIA IN SPECIAL CONDITIONS (SYSTEM-WISE)

- **Liver/ Hepatic disease**:
  - Muscle relaxants of choice: Cis-atracurium / Atracurium[Q]
  - Intravenous Induction agents used: Thiopentone, Propofol[Q]
  - Inhalational agent of choice for maintenance: Isoflurane[Q]
- **Kidney/ Renal disease**:
  - Muscle relaxants of choice: Atracurium/ Cis-atracurium[Q]
  - Muscle relaxants contraindicated: Gallamine, Metocurine[Q]
  - Intravenous Induction agents used: Propofol, Etomidate[Q]
  - Inhalational agent of choice: Desflurane[Q]
  - Inhalational agents contraindicated: Methoxyflurane[Q]
- **Asthma**:
  - Intravenous Induction agent of choice: Ketamine[Q]
  - Inhalational agent of choice: Halothane[Q]
  - Inhalational agent of choice in Children: Halothane/ Sevoflurane[Q]
  - Contraindicated in Status asthmaticus: Thiopentone[Q] (But used in Asthma[Q])
- **Dental procedures**:
  - Induction agent of choice in Children: Sevoflurane[Q]
  - Inhalational agent of choice for maintenance: Enflurane[Q]
- **Cardiovascular disease**:
  - Muscle relaxant of choice in CABG: Vecuronium[Q]
  - Muscle relaxant of choice in IHD: Vecuronium[Q]
  - Muscle relaxant of choice in Cyanotic heart disease: Pancuronium[Q]
  - Anesthetic of choice in Cyanotic heart disease: Ketamine[Q]
  - Induction agent of choice in Children with Acyanotic heart disease: Sevoflurane[Q]
- **Neurophysiological disease**:
  - Intravenous agent of choice for Neurosurgery: Thiopentone[Q]
  - Inhalational agent of choice for Neurosurgery: Isoflurane[Q]

IMAGE-BASED QUESTIONS

1. Identify the Famous Anaesthesiologist in Photograph ***[Recent Question 2014]***

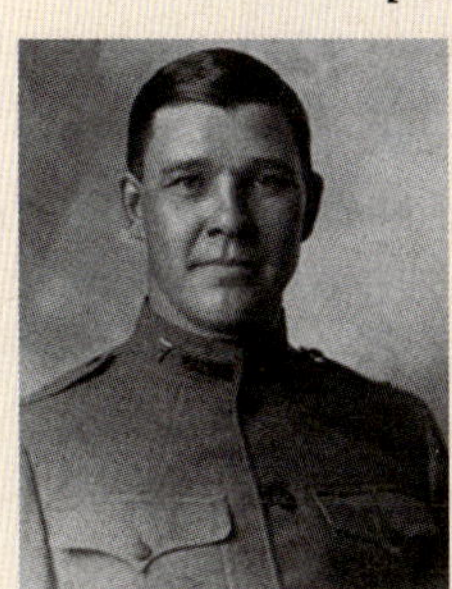

a. Humphry Davy
b. Arther Guedel
c. Macintosh
d. V Apgar

2. Identify the Use of diagram shown in Photograph

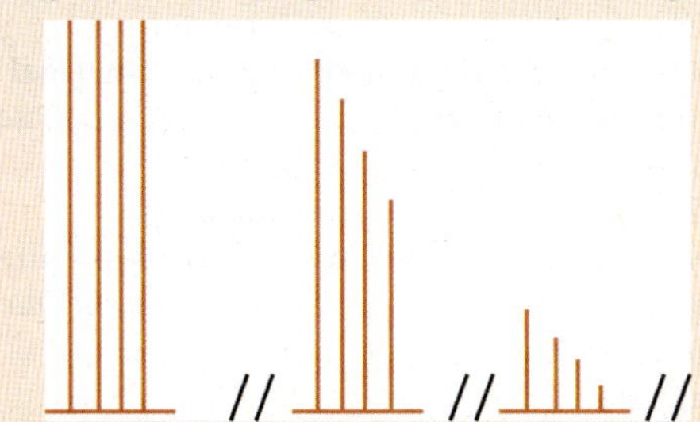

a. Obstetric Anesthesia monitoring
b. Neuromuscular monitoring
c. Pain alleviation monitoring
d. CVP monitoring

3. Stage of Excitement occurs during .... as shown in Photograph ***[Recent Question 2012]***

Stage	Pupil		Resp.	Pulse	B.P.
	Usual size	Reaction to light			
1st Induction				Irregular	Normal
2nd Excitement				Irregular and fast	High
3rd Operative				Steady slow	Normal
4th Danger				Weak and thready	Low

a. Stage 1
b. Stage 2
c. Stage 3
d. Stage 4

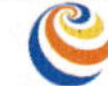 ANSWERS WITH EXPLANATIONS OF IBQs 

1. Ans. (b) Arther Guedel *[Ref. Ajay Yadav, 4/e p57-58]*

Aurther Guedel (1883-1956)

- Stages of General anesthesia
- Uptake and distribution of Inhalational anesthetics
- Guedel airway

2. Ans. (b) Neuromuscular monitoring *[Ref. Ajay Yadav, 4/e p53]*

Train of Four Monitoring

- Description: Neuromuscular monitoring is a technique used during recovery from the application of general anesthesia to objectively determine how well a patient's muscles are able to function
- Principle:
  - Application of electrical stimulation to nerves and recording of muscle response
  - When train of four monitoring is "used continuously, each set (train) of stimuli normally is repeated every 10th to 12th second
  - Each stimulus in the train causes the muscle to contract, and 'fade' in the response provides the basis for evaluation"

3. Ans. (b) Stage 2 *[Ref. Ajay Yadav, 4/e p57]*

- Stage 2 of Anesthesia: Irregular respiration, Large tidal volume, Dilated pupils, Divergent roving eyes, Eyelash reflex abolished

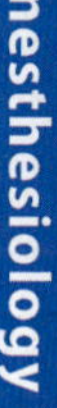

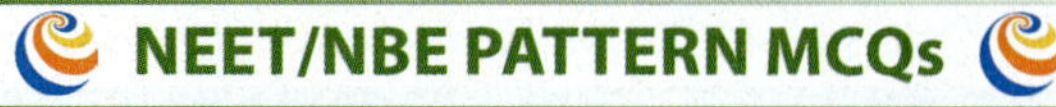

NEET/NBE PATTERN MCQs

1. **Which of the following is contraindicated in Head injury?** *[Recent Question 2016]*
   a. Ketamine b. Halothane
   c. N_2O d. Propofol
2. **Characteristic EEG pattern seen in Surgical tolerance stage of anesthesia is** *[Recent Question 2016]*
   a. Alpha b. Beta
   c. Delta d. Theta
3. **Elderly patient with fracture right hip, anesthetic of choice** *[Recent Question 2016]*
   a. Spinal/epidural
   b. General
   c. Local infiltration
   d. None of the above
4. **During General anesthesia, Shivering is abolished by suppression of** *[Recent Question 2016]*
   a. Hypothalamus b. Thalamus
   c. Cerebral cortex d. Medulla
5. **Which of the following is safe in heart failure?** *[Recent Question 2016]*
   a. Etomidate b. Propofol
   c. Thiopentone d. Ketamine
6. **All of the following are contraindicated in presence of cautery except** *[NBE FMGE September 2008]*
   a. Ether b. Ethylene
   c. Halothane d. Cyclopropane
7. **Anesthetic effects of chloroform were discovered by**
   a. Priestley b. Guedel *[NBE DNB 1992]*
   c. 36 years old medico d. A nurse
8. **Best induction agent is** *[NBE FMGE September 2009]*
   a. Ketamine b. Diazepam
   c. Nitrous oxide d. Thiopentone
9. **Guedel's classification of stages of anesthesia is usually seen with** *[NBE DNB 1992, 1993, 1996]*
   a. Ether b. Halothane
   c. Thiopentone d. Ethylchloride
10. **Tachypnoea is seen with** *[NBE DNB 1992, 1993, 1999, 2001, 2003, 2004, 2006]*
    a. Ether b. Halothane
    c. Trilene d. Cyclopropane
11. **Composition of soda lime is** *[NBE DNB 1998, 2000]*
    NaOH/ $Ca(OH)_2$/KOH
    a. 4%/ 95%/ 1% b. 20%/ 80%/ -
    c. 80%/ 20%/ - d. 15%/ 84%/ 1%
12. **All are stages of anesthesia except** *[Recent Question 2013, 2017]*
    a. Analgesia b. Allodynia
    c. Delirium d. Surgical anesthesia
13. **Which of the following is a sympathomimetic?** *[Recent Questions 2012, 2013]*
    a. Propofol b. Etomidate
    c. Ketamine d. N_2O
14. **Anesthetic of choice in asthma patients is** *[NBE FMGE March 2007]*
    a. Halothane b. Ketamine
    c. Thiopentone d. Fentanyl
15. **During rapid induction of anesthesia** *[Recent Questions 2012, 2013]*
    a. Sellick's maneuver is not required
    b. Pre-oxygenation is mandatory
    c. Suxamethonium is contraindicated
    d. Patient is mechanically ventilated before endotracheal intubation
16. **Onset of surgical anesthesia with diethyl ether is best indicated by** *[NBE DNB 1992]*
    a. Absent eyelash reflex
    b. Absent corneal reflex
    c. Size of pupil
    d. Onset of regular respiration

Match the following (Questions 17–20) Anesthetic contraindications *[NBE DNB 1994, 2000]*
   a. Intermittent porphyria
   b. Myasthenia gravis
   c. Previous CNS disease
   d. Obese patient with renal damage

17. **Muscle relaxants**
18. **Pentothal sodium**
19. **Spinal anesthesia**
20. **Methoxyflurane**
21. **All of the following are factors which slow the speed of induction, except** *[NBE DNB 1995]*
    a. Respiratory depression
    b. Laryngospasm
    c. Breath holding
    d. Presence at poor circulation to non-vital organs
    e. Bronchial secretions
22. **Anesthetic agent with anti-emetic property also is** *[NBE FMGE September 2006]*
    a. Ketamine b. Thiopentone
    c. Propofol d. Nitrous oxide
23. **Which of the following intravenous induction agent is the most suitable for day care surgery?** *[NBE DNB December 2011]*
    a. Morphine b. Propofol
    c. Ketamine d. Thiopentone
24. **All of the following are characteristics of reaction following a blood transfusion in a patient under general anesthesia, except** *[NBE DNB 2003]*
    a. Tachycardia
    b. Increase in cyanosis
    c. Increase in oozing from the wound
    d. Severe hypotension
25. **Infant circuit for anesthesia** *[Recent Questions 2012, 2016]*
    a. Bains circuit
    b. Magill circuit
    c. Ayres T piece
    d. Water's circuit
26. **Most harmful anesthetic for a diabetic patient is** *[NBE DNB 1993]*
    a. Nitrous oxide b. Cyclopropane
    c. Thiopentone sedium d. Ether

27. Depth of anesthesia can be best assessed by *[Recent Questions 2012, 2013, 2017]*
a. Pulse oximeter b. End-tidal pCO_2
c. Acid blood gas analysis d. Bispectral index

28. Nitrous oxide is contraindicated in all except *[NBE FMGE September 2006]*
a. Pneumothorax b. Shock
c. Tympanoplasty d. Volvulus surgery

29. Ayre's T-piece is which type of circuit *[Recent Question 2012]*
a. Type A z b. Type B
c. Type E d. Type D

30. Inducing agent of choice in asthma *[Recent Question 2012, 2013, 2016]*
a. Thiopentone b. Methhexitone
c. Ketamine d. Propofol

31. Bandle's contraction ring is most readily treated by *[Recent Question 2016, NBE DNB 1992]*
a. Chloroform b. TCE
c. Halothane d. Cyclopropane

32. Pudendal block is indicated in *[Recent Question 2016]* *[NBE FMGE March 2012]*
a. Manual removal of placenta
b. Forceps delivery c. IUCD insertion
d. Internal podalic version

33. Anesthesia used during Coronary angiography technique is *[Recent Questions 2015, 2016]*
a. Local anesthesia
b. High thoracic epidural block
c. Caudal anesthesia
d. General anesthesia

34. Anesthetic agent of choice in Asthma patient is? *[Recent Question 2017]*
a. Thiopentone b. Methexitone
c. Ketamine d. Propofol

35. Anesthetic agent of choice in a patient of Liver disease among the following is? *[Recent Question 2017]*
a. Ether b. Halothane
c. Propofol d. Methoxyflurane

36. Anesthesia that can be given on full stomach is? *[Recent Question 2017]*
a. Thiopentone
b. Methohexitone
c. Etomidate
d. Ketamine

37. Most surgeries are performed in which stage of General anesthesia? *[Recent Question 2017]*
a. 1 b. 2
c. 3 d. 4

HIGH YIELD MCQs

1. Drug(s) not given as Transdermal patch *[PGI November 2016]*
a. Fentanyl b. Diclofenac
c. Morphine d. Clonidine
e. Buprenorphine

2. 100% Oxygen is given to patient after Nitrous oxide anesthesia is for *[AIIMS November 2016]*
a. Second gas effect b. Barotrauma
c. Diffusion hypoxia d. Airway collapse

3. Primary action of NO in gut is *[All India PGMEE 2011]*
a. Vasodilator b. Vasoconstrictor
c. Secretomotor
d. GI smooth muscle inhibition

4. Which anesthetic modality is to be avoided in sickle cell disease? *[All India PGMEE 2011]*
a. General anesthesia b. IV regional anesthesia
c. Brachial plexus block d. Spinal anesthesia

5. Perception of ordinarily non-noxious stimuli as pain, is better known as *[PGI 2000, SGPGI 2003]*
a. Allodynia b. Huperalgesia
c. Hyperesthesia d. Radiculopathy

6. Which anti-anesthetic agent is contraindicated in hypertensive patient? *[All India PGMEE 2011]*
a. Ketamine b. Propofol
c. Etomidate d. Diazepam

7. Bradycardia during anesthesia seen in *[PGI 2004]*
a. Pancuronium b. Vecuronium
c. Atracurium d. Propofol
e. Succinylcholine

8. True about Boyle's apparatus *[PGI 2006]*
a. Continuous flow machine
b. Liquid anesthetic vapours not used
c. Resistance very high
d. Resistance low

9. Commonly used in narcoanalysis *[All India PGMEE 2010]*
a. Atropine b. Scopolamine
c. Opium d. Thiopentone

10. Hypothermia is used in all except *[PGI 1998]*
a. Neonatal asphyxia b. Cardiac surgery
c. Hyperthermia d. Arrhythmia

11. Index of potency of general anesthesia *[PGI 1997]*
a. Minimum alveolar concentration
b. Diffusion coefficient
c. Dead space concentration
d. Alveolar blood concentration

12. All are seen in malignant hyperthermia except *[AIIMS PGMEE 2007]*
a. Bradycardia b. Hyperkalemia
c. Metabolic acidosis d. Hypertension

13. In status epilepticus, drug of choice is *[PGI 1992]*
a. I/V diazepam b. I/M diazepam
c. Oral clonazepam d. I/M phenytoin

14. True about Rotameter *[MP PGMEE 2006]*
a. Rotameter reading may not get affected by dirt inside the tube
b. Rotameter reading may not get affected by static electricity
c. The height to which bobbin rises indicates the flow rate
d. A rotameter is a variable pressure flowmeter

15. True about anesthesia breathing circuit is *[PGI 2008]*
   a. Cylinder is a part of high pressure system
   b. O_2 flush delivers <35 lts
   c. O_2 flush delivers >35.00 lts
   d. Pipelines is a part low pressure system

16. Position with least vital capacity in G.A. *[All India PGMEE 1991]*
   a. Trendelenburg   b. Lithotomy
   c. Prone   d. Lateral

17. Train of four' is characteristically used in concern with
   a. Malignant hyperthermia *[All India PGMEE 2008]*
   b. Non-depolarizing neuromuscular blockers
   c. Mechanical ventilation
   d. To check hemodynamic parameters

18. % Thiopentone used in induction *[AIIMS PGMEE 1995]*
   a. 0.5%   b. 1.5%
   c. 2.5%   d. 4.5%

19. Characteristics of Remifentanil *[PGI 2007]*
   a. Metabolised by plasma esterase
   b. Short half life
   c. More potent than Alfentanyl
   d. Dose reduced in hepatic and renal disease
   e. Duration of action more than Alfentanyl

20. Which one of the common side effects is seen with fentanyl? *[AIIMS PGMEE 2006]*
   a. Chest wall rigidly
   b. Tachycardia
   c. Pain in abdomen
   d. Hypertension

21. Hypotensive Anesthesia in nasopharyngeal angiofibroma is/are given by *[PGI 2009]*
   a. Propofol   b. Ketamine
   c. Phentolamine   d. Halothane
   e. Na Nitroprusside

22. Sodium nitroprusside infusion may result in *[Recent Question 2016, AIIMS PGMEE 2005]*
   a. Hypertension   b. Pulmonary oedema
   c. Cyanide toxicity   d. Heart block

23. Lowest concentration of anesthetic agent is alveoli needed to produce immobility in response to painful stimulus in 50% of individual is termed as *[AIIMS PGMEE 1998]*
   a. Minimum alveolar concentration
   b. Minimal analgesic concentration
   c. Minimal anesthetic concentration
   d. Maximum alveolar concentration

24. All of the following factors decrease the Minimum Alveolar Concentration (MAC) of an inhalation anesthetic agent except *[AIIMS PGMEE 2003]*
   a. Hypothermia   b. Hyponatremia
   c. Hypocalcemia   d. Anemia

25. The potency of an inhalational anesthetic depends on
   a. Blood gas partition coefficient *[PGI 1999]*
   b. Oil-gas partition coefficient
   c. Gas pressure   d. Blood pressure

26. Which of the following intravenous induction agent is the most suitable for day care surgery? *[All India PGMEE 2006]*
   a. Morphine   b. Ketamine
   c. Propofol   d. Diazepam

27. Regarding neonatal circumcision, which one of the following is true *[AIIMS PGMEE 2003]*
   a. It should be done without anesthesia, as it is hazardous to give anesthesia
   b. It should be done without anesthesia, as neonates do not perceive pain as adults
   c. It should be done under local anesthesia only
   d. General anesthesia should be given to neonate for circumcision as they also feel pain as adults

28. A five-year old child is scheduled for strabismus (squint) correction. Induction of anesthesia is uneventful. After conjunctival incision as the surgeon grasps the medial rectus, the anaesthesiologist looks at the cardiac monitor. Why do you think he did that? *[AIIMS PGMEE 2002]*
   a. He wanted to check the depth of anesthesia
   b. He wanted to be sure that the blood pressure did not fall
   c. He wanted to see if there was an oculocardiac reflex
   d. He wanted to make sure there were no ventricular dysarrhythmias which normally accompany incision

29. A six-year old boy is scheduled for examination of the eye under anesthesia. The father informed that for the past six months the child is developing progressive weakness of both legs. His elder sibling had died at the age of 14 years. Which drug would you definitely avoid during the anesthetic management? *[AIIMS PGMEE 2002]*
   a. Succinylcholine   b. Thiopentone
   c. Nitrous oxide   d. Vecuronium

30. A 5-year-old boy suffering from Duchenne Muscular dystrophy and polymyositis has been fasting for 8 hrs and has to undergo tendon lengthening. Which anesthesia should be used? *[AIIMS PGMEE 2000]*
   a. Induction by IV Thiopentone & maintenance by N_2O & halothane
   b. Induction by IV Propofol and maintenance by N_2O & O_2
   c. Induction by IV scoline and maintenance by N_2O & Halothane
   d. Inhalation N_2O, O_2 & halothane

31. A 5-year-old boy suffering from Duchenne muscular dystrophy has to undergo tendon lengthening procedure. The most appropriate anesthetic would be *[All India PGMEE 2003]*
   a. Induction with intravenous thiopentone and N_2O; and halothane for maintenance
   b. Induction with intravenous suxamethonium and N_2O; and oxygen for maintenance
   c. Induction with intravenous suxamethonium and N_2O; and halothane for maintenance
   d. Inhalation induction with inhalation halothane and N_2O; oxygen for maintenance

32. A six-year-old child is posted for elective urology surgery under general anesthesia. He refuses to allow the anaesthesiologist an I.V. access. The best inhalational agent of choice for induction of anesthesia is *[AIIMS PGMEE 2004]*
   a. Sevoflurane
   b. Methoxyflurane
   c. Desflurane
   d. Isoflurane

33. A 30-year-old woman with Coarctation of aorta is admitted to the labour room for elective caesarean section. Which of the following is the anesthesia technique of choice? *[AIIMS PGMEE 2005]*
   a. Spinal anesthesia
   b. Epidural anesthesia
   c. General anesthesia
   d. Local anesthesia with nerve block

34. A 5-year-old child is suffering from cyanotic heart disease. He is planned for corrective surgery. The induction agent of the choice would be *[Recent Question 2016, AIIMS PGMEE 2005]*
   a. Thiopentone
   b. Ketamine
   c. Halothane
   d. Midazolam

35. A 6-month-old child is suffering from patent ductus arteriosus (PDA) with congestive cardiac failure. Ligation of ductus arteriosus was decided for surgical management. The most appropriate inhalational anesthetic agent of choice with minimal haemodynamic alteration for induction of anesthesia is *[AIIMS PGMEE 2005]*
   a. Sevoflurane
   b. Isoflurane
   c. Enflurane
   d. Halothane

36. A 52-year-old male diagnosed as triple vessel coronary artery disease with poor left ventricular function. Coronary artery bypass grafting surgery was decided. During maintenance of anesthesia which one of the following agents should be preferred? *[AIIMS PGMEE 2004]*
   a. IV Opioids
   b. Isoflurane
   c. Halothane
   d. Nitrous oxide

37. During surgery for aortic arch aneurysm under deep hypothermic circulatory arrest, which of the following anesthetic agent administered prior to circulatory arrest that also provides cerebral protection? *[AIIMS PGMEE 2002]*
   a. Etomidate
   b. Thiopental sodium
   c. Propofol
   d. Ketamine

38. Which of the following in anesthesia will produce decreased EEG activities, *[AIIMS PGMEE 2006]*
   a. Hypothermia
   b. Early Hypoxia
   c. Ketamine
   d. N_2O

39. During rapid sequence induction of anesthesia *[All India PGMEE 2003]*
   a. Sellick's maneuver is not required
   b. Pre-oxygenation is mandatory
   c. Suxamethonium is contraindicated
   d. Patient is mechanically ventilated before endotracheal intubation

40. Which is safest to be used in asthmatic patients? *[PGI 2001]*
   a. Nitrazepam
   b. Phenobarbitone
   c. Chloral hydrate
   d. All hypnotics are safe
   e. Morphine

41. A 40-year-old male with controlled thyrotoxicosis and Carcinoma rectum was undergoing laparoscopic Abdomino-perineal resection, during which he was found to have decreased Blood Pressure and Heart Rate. On examination, a mill-wheal murmur was heard. The End tidal pCO_2 was observed found reducing from 40 to 10. What is the most likely diagnosis? *[AIIMS PGMEE 1996]*
   a. Air embolism
   b. Thyroid storm
   c. Blood loss
   d. Acute hypoxia

42. A 5-year-old child going to sitting craniotomy while positioning in O.T. developed End Tidal CO_2 0 mm Hg PO_2 80 mm Hg implies *[AIIMS PGMEE 2000]*
   a. Endotracheal tube in oesophagus
   b. E.T. blocked with secretion
   c. Venous air embolism
   d. Left lung collapse

43. Drugs contraindicated in AIP *[PGI 2007]*
   a. Thiopentone
   b. Etomidate
   c. Ketamine
   d. Propofol
   e. Midazolam

44. The drug which is not suitable for patients with acute porphyria for intravenous induction is *[AIIMS PGMEE 2005]*
   a. Thiopentone sodium
   b. Propofol
   c. Midazolam
   d. Etomidate

45. Which of the following anesthetic agents does not trigger malignant hyperthermia? *[Recent Question 2016, All India PGMEE 2006]*
   a. Halothane
   b. Isoflurane
   c. Suxamethonium
   d. Thiopentone

46. Drugs which interfere with anesthesia are *[PGI 2001]*
   a. Calcium channel blocker nifedipine
   b. Beta blockers
   c. Aminoglycosides
   d. Steroid administration
   e. D-tubocurar

47. Hypothermia is used in *[PGI 2000]*
   a. Hyperpyrexia
   b. Prolonged surgeries
   c. Massive blood transfusion
   d. Hypertension

48. Calcium channel blockers in anesthesia, True is *[PGI 2000]*
   a. Needs to be decreased as they augment hypotension & muscle relaxation
   b. Withheld because they lower LES pressure
   c. Should be given in normal doses as they prevent MI & angina
   d. All of the above

49. Anesthetic agent contraindicated in epilepsy is *[JIPMER PGMEE 2014]*
   a. Ketamine
   b. Desflurane
   c. Isoflurane
   d. None

50. Least sensitive to effect of muscle relaxants is *[JIPMER PGMEE 2014]*
   a. Upper limb muscles
   b. Lower muscle limbs
   c. Diaphragm
   d. None

51. Intraoperative wheezing can be managed by *[Recent Question 2016, JIPMER PGMEE 2014]*
   a. Thiopental
   b. Propofol
   c. Ketamine
   d. All of the above

52. Most metabolized inhalational anesthetic *[JIPMER PGMEE 2014]*
   a. Isoflurane
   b. Sevoflurane
   c. Desflurane
   d. Halothane

 NEET/NBE PATTERN MCQs ANSWERS WITH EXPLANATIONS 

1. **Ans. (a) Ketamine**
[Ref. KDT, 7/e p384]

Ketamine
- Mechanism of action: Inhibits NMDA receptors
- Effects on CNS:
  - Most common side effect is hallucination
  - **Emergence delirium**
  - Raise in intracranial tension and so is contraindicated in head injury.
  - Strong analgesia

2. **Ans. (c) Delta**
[Ref. Miller's Anaesthesia, 5/e p1947]

EEG Changes in Inhalational Anesthesia

Guedel Stage	Clinical Situation	Characteristic EEG
I	Awake	Posterior alpha
II	Excitation	Activation of beta, induction of theta
III-1	Early anesthesia	Dominant alpha-theta, Some delta
III-2	Surgical tolerance	Dominant delta, Some theta
III-3	Deep surgical tolerance	Continuous high amplitude delta
III-4	Early overdose	Isoelectric stretches, Burst suppression EEG
IV	Toxicity	Continuous isoelectricity

3. **Ans. (a) Spinal/epidural**
[Ref. Objective Anaesthesia Review by Kulkarni, 3/e p206]
- Spinal or Epidural anesthesia should be considered for all patients undergoing hip fracture repair, unless contraindicated

4. **Ans. (a) Hypothalamus**
[Ref. Clinical Anaesthesiology by Morgan, 5/e p1184]
- In the normal anaesthetized patient, the hypothalamus maintains core body temperature within very narrow tolerances, termed the *interthreshold range,* with the threshold for sweating and vasodilation at one extreme and the threshold for vasoconstriction and shivering at the other
- Increasing core temperature, a fraction of a degree induces sweating and vasodilation, whereas a minimally reduced core temperature triggers vasoconstriction and shivering
- Anesthetic agents inhibit central thermoregulation by interfering with these hypothalamic responses.

5. **Ans. (a) Etomidate**
[Ref. Clinical Anaesthesiology by Morgan, 5/e p185]
- Etomidate has minimal effects on the cardiovascular system
  - For arrhythmic patients and patients with severe cardiac disease, etomidate is perhaps the safest drug for inducing anesthesia
- Etomidate is a popular agent for the induction of anesthesia in hemodynamically unstable patients
- Etomidate decreases cerebral metabolic rate, cerebral blood flow, and intracranial pressure.

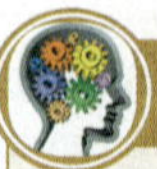

Also Remember
- **Major cardiovascular effect of propofol is a decrease in arterial blood pressure** due to a drop in systemic vascular resistance (inhibition of sympathetic vasoconstrictor activity), preload, and cardiac contractility
- Ketamine increases arterial blood pressure, heart rate, and cardiac output.

6. **Ans. (c) Halothane**
[Ref. Ajay Yadav, 4/e p60-61]

Inflammable Inhalational Anesthetics
- Ether
- Ethylene
- Ethyl chloride
- Cyclopropane

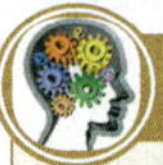

Also Remember
- **Anesthetics can be made non-inflammable by: Addition of fluorine**
- Cautery should not be used in vicinity of inflammable agents upto: 25 cms

7. **Ans. (c) 36 year old medico**
[Ref. Miller, 6/e p79]

Chloroform
- Discovered by: Liebig & Soubeiran
- Name given by: Duma
- Anesthetic effects discovered by **Dr James Simpson**, an Obstetrician: Relief of pain during labour and delivery

8. **Ans. (d) Thiopentone**
[Ref. Ajay Yadav, 4/e p78]

Key Facts of Thiopentone
- **Most commonly used intravenous induction agent**
- **Agent of choice for cerebral protection**
- Causes Mild hypokalemia, Hypotension, Laryngospasm, Transient apnoea
- Exhibits Antithyroid activity
- Tissue necrosis on injection

9. **Ans. (a) Ether**
[Ref. KDT, 6/e p366-67]
- Guedel described four levels/ stages of ether anesthesia

10. **Ans. (c) Trielene**
[Ref. Ajay Yadav, 4/e p73]
- Trielene stimulates respiration causing tachypnea

11. **Ans. (a) 4%/95%/1%**
[Ref. Ajay Yadav, 4/e p32]

Composition of Soda lime
- **$Ca(OH)_2$**: 94%
- **NaOH**: 5% (catalyses CO_2 absorption)

Anesthesiology

- **KOH**: 1%
- Silica (to prevent dust formation)
- Indicators: Phenolphthalein, Ethyl violet, Mimosa Z

12. Ans. (b) Allodynia
[Ref. KDT, 6/e , p 366-67]

Guedel's Four Stages of Anesthesia (Ether)

- Stage I **(Analgesia)**: Extends till loss of consciousness
- Stage II **(Delirium or excitement)**: Extends till beginning of regular respiration
  - Maximum movement of eyeball takes place, pupil remains partially dilated and eyelash reflex is lost
- Stage III **(Surgical anesthesia)**: Extends till cessation of spontaneous breathing
  - Plane I: Eyeball become fixed, eyelid reflex lost and pupil size becomes normal (Regular respiration)
  - Plane II: Loss of corneal reflex and pupil starts dilating; Lacrimation is still present (Respiratory paresis)
  - Plane III: swallowing reflex and laryngeal reflex is lost; Lacrimation is absent (Respiratory paralysis)
  - Plane IV: Carinal or cough reflex is lost with fully dilated pupil (Intercostal paralysis with only abdominal respiration)
- Stage IV **(medullary paralysis)**: Respiratory arrest and apnoea

13. Ans. (c) Ketamine
[Ref. Trauma: Critical Care Volume 2 by Wilson, 1/e p86]

- Analgesic and anesthetic effects of ketamine are achieved through several mechanisms:
  - Inhibition of cholinergic pathways
  - Strong sympathomimetic activity
  - Non-competitively inhibition of NMDA receptors

14. Ans. (b) Ketamine
[Ref. Ajay Yadav, 4/e p86]

15. Ans. (b) Preoxygenation is mandatory
[Ref. Ajay Yadav, 4/e p56]

Preoxygenation

- In rapid sequence intubation after preoxygenation for 4 to 5 minutes induction agent is given followed immediately by succinylcholine
  - Sellick's manoeuvre is carried out
  - Ventilation with bag and mask is not done
- Purpose: Increase oxygen reserve of body (Functional residual capacity)

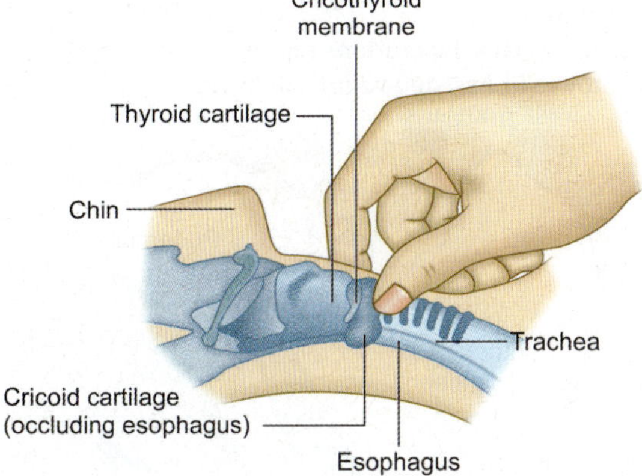

Fig. Sellick's maneuvre

16. Ans. (a) Absent eyelash reflex
[Ref. KDT, 6/e p366-67]

- First reflex to lost is eyelash reflex and last reflex to lost is cough reflex. Return of reflexes is in opposite sequences.

17. Ans. (b) Myasthenia gravis
[Ref. Ajay Yadav, 4/e p154]

- *Myasthenic syndrome/ Eaton-Lambert Syndrome*:
  - An autoimmune disease in which antibodies to presynaptic calcium channel are produced
  - Patients are sensitive to both depolarizing and non-depolarizing muscle relaxant

18. Ans. (a) Intermittent porphyria
[Ref. Ajay Yadav, 4/e p80]

19. Ans. (c) Previous CNS disease
[Ref. Ajay Yadav, 4/e p138]

Spinal Anesthesia Contraindications

Absolute Contraindications	Relative Contraindications
• Raised intracranial tension • Patient refusal • Severe hypovolemia • On anticoagulants • On thrombolytic/ fibrinolytic therapy • Bleeding/coagulation disorders • Septicemia • Infection at local site	• Fixed cardiac output lesions (AS, MS) • Mild to moderate hypotension/ hypovolemia • Uncontrolled hypertension • Myocardial infarction • Heart block • On Beta blocker, Aspirin, Mini-dose heparin • Spinal deformity • Psychiatric disorders • History of headache • GIT perforations • Neuropathies • Infective and degenerative CNS disorders

20. Ans. (d) Obese patients with renal damage
[Ref. Ajay Yadav, 4/e p72]

21. Ans. (d) Presence at poor circulation to non vital organs
[Ref. Trauma Management by Edwin, 1/e p238]

22. Ans. (c) Propofol
[Ref. Ajay Yadav, 4/e p82]

23. Ans. (b) Propofol
[Ref. Ajay Yadav, 4/e p82]

24. Ans. (b) Increase in cyanosis
[Ref. Ajay Yadav, 4/e p15]

Transfusion Reactions in Anesthetized Individual

- **Most common cause: Clerical errors**
- Presentation:
  - Tachycardia, hypotension (so minute to minute blood pressure monitoring during early transfusion is necessary)
  - Oozing from surgical site (Most specific feature)
  - Confirmed by haemoglobinuria

25. Ans. (c) Ayres T piece
[Ref. Ajay Yadav, 4/e p30]

- Pediatric circuit: Ayre's T piece
  - Jackson and Rees modification of Ayer's T piece/ Mapleson type F circuit
  - Ayre's T piece is type E semiclosed circuit

26. Ans. (d) Ether

[Ref. Ajay Yadav, 4/e p71]

- Ether releases catecholamines and can cause hyper-glycemia: Must not be used in diabetics

27. Ans. (d) Bispectral Index

[Ref. Anaesthesia Science by Webster, 1/e. p434]

Bispectral Index (BIS) Analysis

- Method of BIS:
  - Combines power spectral analysis of phase relationships with the component sine waves
  - EEG feature that best correlated with clinical depth of sedation and anesthesia fitted to a model
- Advantage: Agent (drug) independent and hence a good indicator of Depth of anesthesia.

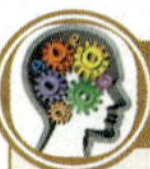

Also Remember

Assessing Depth of Anesthesia

- While variations in clinical observations may be associated with depth of anesthesia, they are not considered to be completely reliable
- End tidal agent monitoring is commonly used in clinical practice to assess anesthetic depth: Only possible when volatile anesthetic agents are used
- BIS offers a more effective method of assessing depth of anesthesia

28. Ans. (b) Shock

[Ref. Ajay Yadav, 4/e p65-66]

29. Ans. (c) Type E

[Ref. Ajay Yadav, 4/e p30]

30. Ans. (c) Ketamine

[Ref. Ajay Yadav, 4/e p86]

Ketamine

- **Dissociative anesthesia** (cataleptic state)
- Raised intracranial tension & raised intraocular tension
- **Emergence reaction** (vivid dreaming, illusions, extracorporeal experience like floating out of body, excitement, confusion, euphoria, fear)
- Hallucinations: Auditory hallucination>Visual hallucination (**MC side effect of ketamine**; decreased by giving benzodiazepines)
- Tachycardia, hypertension (hence Anesthetic of choice for shock)
- Respiratory stimulant (adult); respiratory depressant (children)
- Bronchodilator (hence Anesthetic of choice for asthmatics)
- Increased tracheobronchial and salivary secretion
- Increased intragastric pressure
- Increased muscular tone (non-purposeful movement)
- Nystagmus and dilated pupil

31. Ans. (c) Halothane

[Ref. Ajay Yadav, 4/e p67-68]

- ***Bandl's* ring** (also known as pathological *retraction ring*) is the abnormal junction between the two segments of the human uterus, which is a late sign associated with obstructed labor

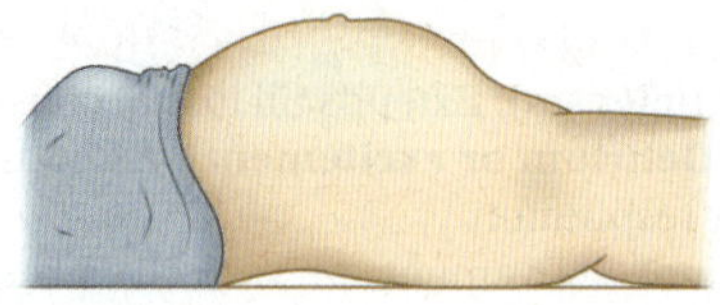

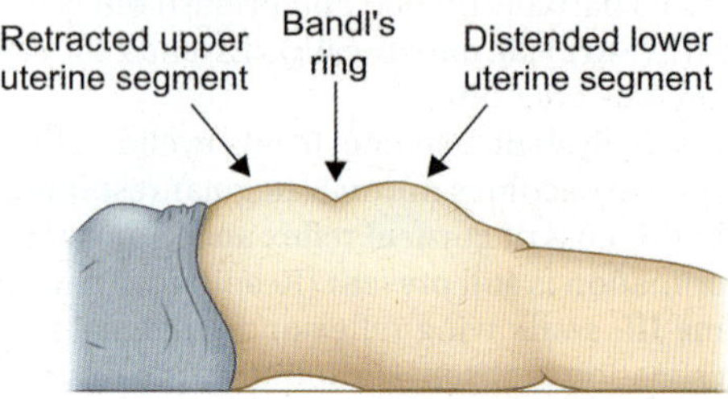

Fig. Bandl's ring

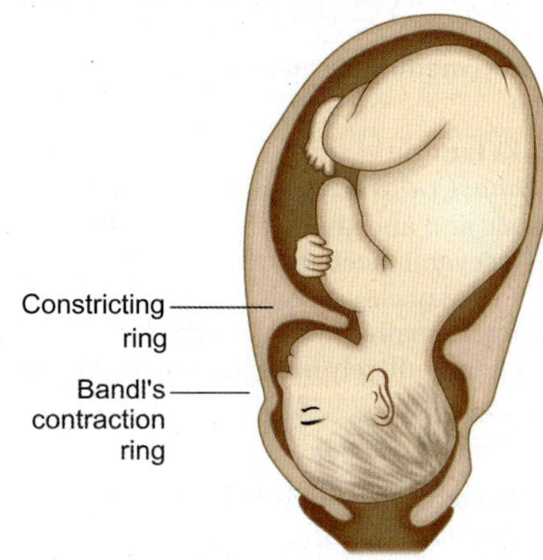

Fig. Bandl's ring

32. Ans. (b) Forceps delivery

[Ref. Manual of Obstetrics by Holland & Brews, 2/e p458]

Pudendal Block in Obstetrics

- Normal vaginal delivery with/ without episiotomy
- Forceps delivery
- Breech delivery
- Episiotomy repair
- Perineal tears/ lacerations repair
- Ventouse in Assisted vaginal delivery

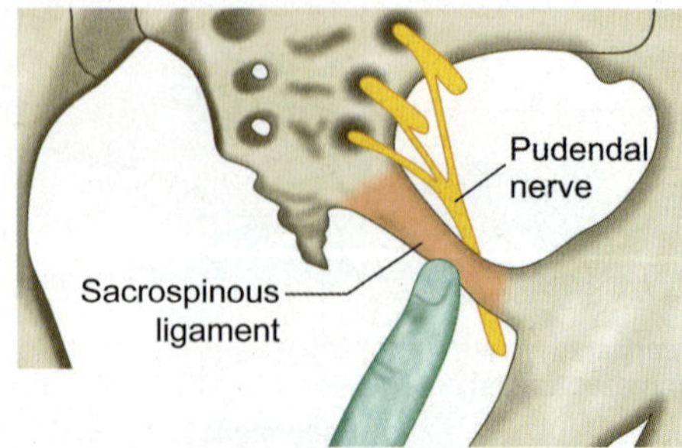

Fig. Pudendal nerve

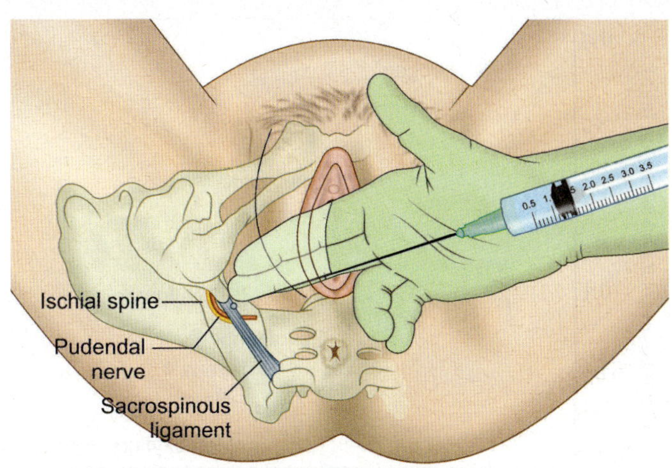

Fig. Pudendal block

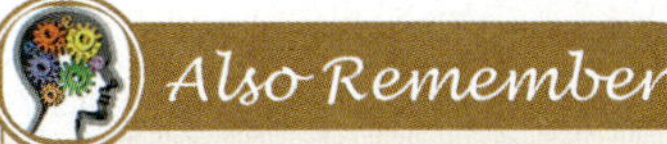

- *Paracervical block in Obstetrics*:
  - First stage of labour (analgesia)
- *Lumbar epidural block in Obstetrics*:
  - Labour (analgesia, anesthesia)
- *Saddle block in Obstetrics*:
  - Mid-cavity forceps delivery
  - Perineal tear (III degree) repair
- *Spinal block in Obstetrics*:
  - Labour
  - Caesarean section
- *General anesthesia in Obstetrics*:
  - Emergency situations

33. Ans. (a) Local anesthesia

[Ref. Anaesthesia by Agasti, 1/e p1127]

- During coronary angiography local anesthesia is provided at the site of the introduction of an arterial catheter which is either around Femoral artery or Brachial artery.

34. Ans. (c) Ketamine

[Ref. Chestnut's Obstetric Anesthesia, 5/e p451]

Anesthesia & Asthma

- Intravenous Induction agent of choice: Ketamine
- Inhalational agent of choice: Halothane
- Inhalational agent of choice in Children: Halothane/ Sevoflurane
- Contraindicated in Status asthmaticus: Thiopentone (But used in Asthma)

35. Ans. (c) Propofol

[Ref. Clinical Anesthesia by Barash, 6/e p453]

Propofol and Liver

- Propofol has a significant vasodilatory effect because it increases total hepatic blood flow in both hepatic arterial and portal venous circulation
- Among intravenous anesthetic agents, propofol is often a good choice in patients with liver disease
- Propofol has extrahepatic metabolism in addition to regular hepatic metabolism

36. Ans. (d) Ketamine

[Ref. Clinical Anesthesia by Barash, 6/e p456]

- In contrast to other IV anesthetics, airway reflexes are preserved more in Ketamine use
- Ketamine is the **Preferred agent for patients with full stomach**
- However, use of Ketamine does not obviate the need for tracheal intubation in the patient with a full stomach (because tracheal soiling has been reported in this situation)

37. Ans. (c) 3

[Ref. Pharmacology, Drug Therapy, and Nursing Considerations by Malseed, 1/e p144]

- Most surgery is performed at plane 2 or 3 of stage III, because muscle relaxation is usually optimal at this depth.

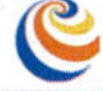 HIGH YIELD MCQs ANSWERS WITH EXPLANATIONS 

1. Ans. (c) Morphine

[Ref. Drug Delivery by Mitra, 1/e p294]

- Transdermal route is used only for the drugs which are highly lipid soluble and can be absorbed through intact skin
- Drugs used as transdermal patches: Buprenorpine, Capsaicin, Clonidine, Diclofenac, Estradiol, Estradiol levonorgestrel, Estradiol norethidrone acetate, Ethinyl estradiol norelgestromin, Fenatnyl, Granisetron, Lidocaine, Methylphenidate, Nicotine, Nitroglycerine, Oxybutynin, Rivastigmine, Selegiline, Scopalamine, Testosterone

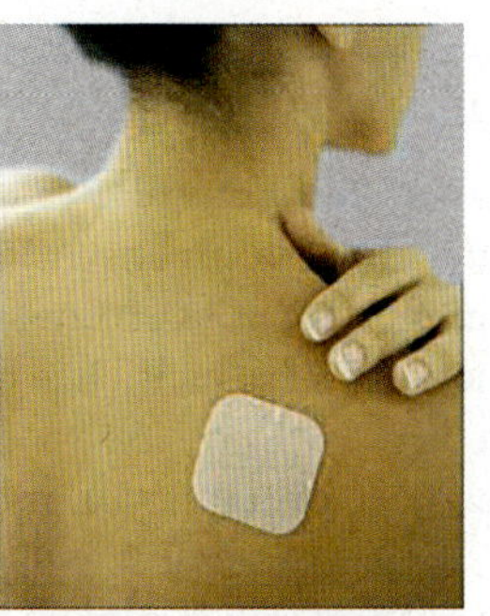

Fig. Transdermal patch

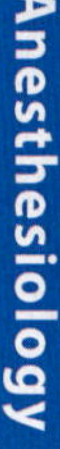

2. Ans. (c) Diffusion hypoxia
[Ref. Principles of Anaesthesia by Coetzee, 2/e p84]

Diffusion hypoxia/ Fink effect

- Reverse of Second Gas effect
- When administration of N_2O ceases, it rapidly washes out of blood and is exchanged with Nitrogen in alveolus
- Being 30 times more soluble, N_2O enters alveoli faster than Nitrogen leaving
- Alveolar dilution and expansion occurs leading to Diffusion hypoxia
- Hence, during recovery with N_2O anesthesia, 100% Oxygen administration is done to prevent it

3. Ans. (d) GI smooth muscle inhibition
[Ref. Pathophysiology of the Enteric Nervous System by Spiller, 1/e p6]

4. Ans. (b) IV regional anesthesia
[Ref. Ajay Yadav, 4/e p166]

- Use of Tourniquet/Bier's block (IV regional bock) is contraindicated in sickle cell disease: Blood stasis can cause local acidosis, hypoxia with sickling of cells

5. Ans. (a) Allodynia
[Ref. Ajay Yadav, 4/e p201]

6. Ans. (a) Ketamine
[Ref. Ajay Yadav, 4/e p86]

7. Ans. (c) Atracurium; (d) Propofol; (e) Succinylcholine
Ref. Ajay Yadav, 4/e Chapters 12,13]

8. Ans. (a) Continuous flow machine; (d) Resistance low
[Ref. A Practice of Anaesthesia for Infants and Children by Cote, 1/e, p1088]

9. Ans. (d) Thiopentone
[Ref. Textbook of Forensic Medicine & Toxicology by Vij, 5/e, p572]

10. Ans. (d) Arrhythmia
[Ref. Ajay Yadav, 4/e p53]

- Hypothermia causes ventricular arrhythmia if temperature is **less than 28°C**

11. Ans. (a) Minimum alveolar concentration
[Ref. Ajay Yadav, 4/e p59]

Minimum Alveolar Concentration

- Description: It is minimum concentration of agent required to produce immobility in 50% of the subjects given noxious stimuli (which is surgical incision in human beings and tail clamping in rats)
- Importance: **Best estimate for measuring potency is MAC**
- Interpretation: Agent with minimum MAC is most potent
  - Methoxyflurane with minimum MAC of 0.16% is most potent inhalational agent
  - Nitrous oxide with MAC of 104% is least potent

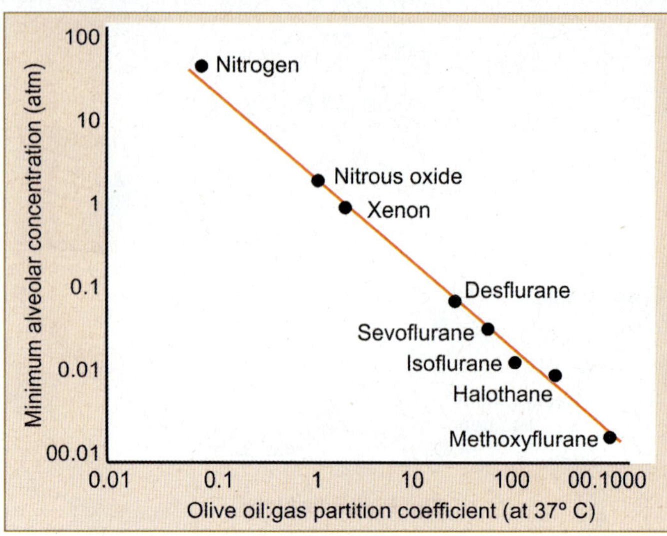

Fig. MAC

12. Ans. (a) Bradycardia
[Ref. Ajay Yadav, 4/e p115-116]

Clinical Features of Malignant Hyperthermia

- Hyperthermia
- **Increased end tidal CO_2 ($ETCO_2$) - most sensitive early sign of malignant hyperthermia**
- Hypoxia and cyanosis
- Tachycardia, arrhythmia, hypertension
- Severe metabolic acidosis
- Hyperkalemia, muscle rigidity, increased creatinine phosphokinase, increased myoglobin
- Renal failure, DIC, pulmonary and cerebral oedema
- Death

13. Ans. (a) I/V diazepam
[Ref. Basic & Clinical Pharmacology by Katzung, 11/e Chapter 24]

Status Epileptics

- Most common form of Status epilepticus: Generalized tonic-clonic status epilepticus
- **Diazepam is the most effective drug** in most patients for stopping the attacks
  - Given directly by intravenous push: Maximum total dose of 20–30 mg in adults
  - Effect of diazepam is not lasting, but the 30–40 minute seizure-free interval allows more definitive therapy to be initiated

14. Ans. (c) The height to which bobbin rises indicates the flow rate
[Ref. Ajay Yadav, 4/e p26]

- In each Thrope's tube of Rotameter, there is a float called bobbin (Indicator) which keeps on rotating by the gas stream passing all-round the bobbin and the upper end of bobbin determines the flow rate

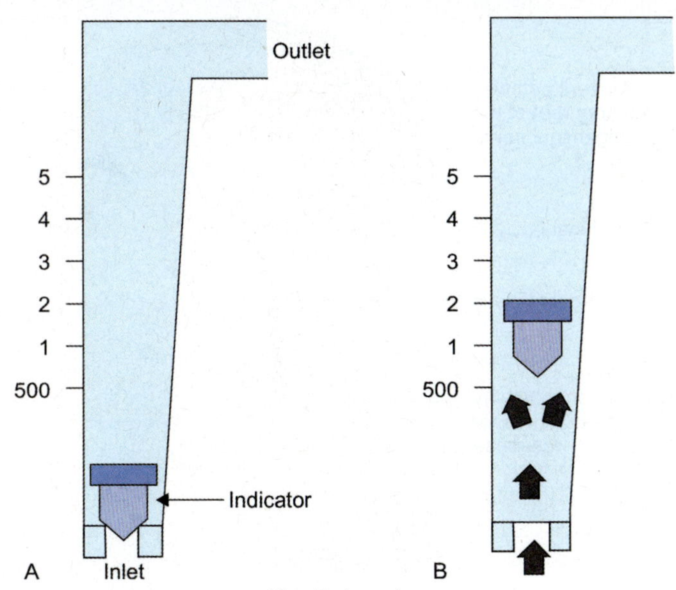

Fig. Rotameter

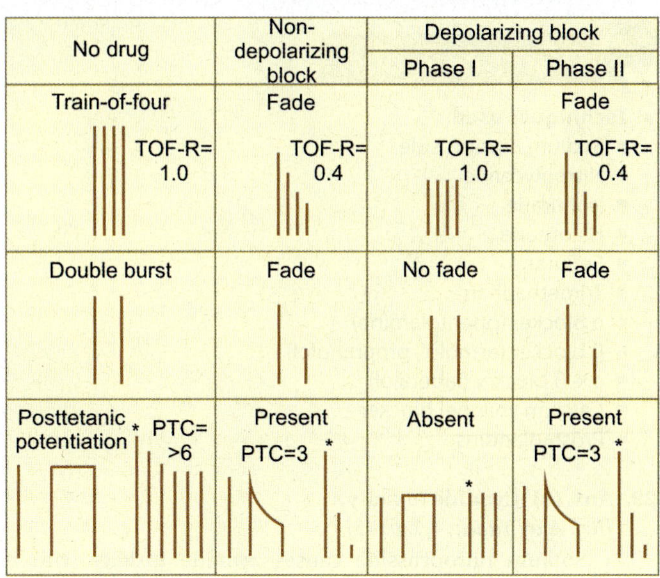

Fig. Train-of-Four

15. Ans. (a) **Cylinder is part of high pressure system**
[Ref. Ajay Yadav, 4/e p23]

16. Ans. (a) **Trendelenburg**
[Ref. Ajay Yadav, 4/e p116]

Complications of Trendelenburg Position
- Increased cardiac load
- Increased venous return
- Decreased vital capacity (15%)
- Decreased FRC (by 15 to 20%)
- Increased central venous pressure
- Increased intraocular and intracranial pressure
- Venous congestion of face
- Cerebral hemorrhage
- Lingual and buccal neuropathy

17. Ans. (b) **Non-depolarizing neuromuscular blockers**
[Ref. Ajay Yadav, 4/e p53-54]

Train of Four
- Description:
  - 4 stimuli each of 2Hz for 2 secs are given and recording are taken
  - Ratio of T_4 to T_1 is taken
  - Absence of T_4 response means 75% blockade of receptors which is sufficient for most surgeries
- **Importance**: Neuromuscular monitors deliver a number of stimuli among which train of four (TO_4) is most useful method of clinical monitoring
  - Best utilized for neuromuscular monitoring during maintenance of anesthesia
  - Best to differentiate between depolarizing and non-depolarizing block
    1. Nondepolarizing block: Show fading which means T_4 will go first and then T_3 and so on
    2. Depolarizing block: All four responses decrease simultaneously in amplitude.
  - Very useful in diagnosing phase II block: If a patient on succinylcholine starts showing fading it is pathognomonic of phase II block

18. Ans. (c) **2.5%**
[Ref. Ajay Yadav, 4/e p78]

19. Ans. (b) **Short half life; (c) More potent than Alfentanyl**
[Ref. Ajay Yadav, 4/e p91]

Remifentanil
- Ultrashort acting agent
- Metabolized by ester hydrolysis by non-specific esters in blood and tissues (Pseudo cholinesterases)
- Onset is fastest
- Recovery is most rapid
- As infusion, considered as opioid of choice for day care surgery
- Contains glycine which can cause motor weakness
- Not suitable for producing epidural analgesia
- Additional side effect is significant hypotension

20. Ans. (a) **Chest wall rigidity**
[Ref. Ajay Yadav, 4/e 91]
- Fentanyl can produce significant muscle rigidity **(Wooden chest syndrome)**

21. Ans. (c) **Phentolamine; (d) Halothane; (e) Na-nitropruside**
[Ref. Ajay Yadav, 4/e p144]

Indications of Hypotensive Anesthesia
- Neurosurgical operation for cerebral aneurysm/ arteriovenous malformations
- Cardiac surgery like coarctation of aorta and patent ductus repair
- Surgery for malignancy
- Vascular tumour resection
- Pheochromocytoma surgery
- Blood is not available or cannot be given due to religious reason **(Jehovah's convention)**

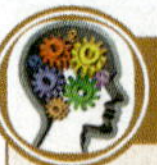

Also Remember

- **Techniques used**:
  - Sodium nitropruside
  - Nitroglycerine
  - Isoflurane
  - Halothane
  - Enflurane
  - Trimethaphan
  - α blocker (phentolamine)
  - β blocker (esmolol, propranolol)
  - α + β blocker (labetalol)
  - Calcium channel blocker
  - Prostaglandins

22. Ans. (c) Cyanide toxicity

[Ref. Ajay Yadav, 4/e p145]

- Sodium nitroprusside causes cyanide toxicity with its prolonged use which is diagnosed by continuous fall of oxygen saturation (histotoxic hypoxia) and cyanosis

23. Ans. (a) Minimum alveolar concentration

[Ref. Ajay Yadav, 4/e p59]

24. Ans. (c) Hypocalcemia

[Ref. Ajay Yadav, 4/e p59-60]

Factors Decreasing the MAC

- Maximum MAC is at age 6 month, thereafter decreasing (except a slight increase in puberty)
- Decreasing temperature; increasing temperature also (upto 42°C)
- Anaemia
- Hypoxia (PO_2 <40)
- Hypercarbia (PCO_2 > 95 mm Hg)
- Acute alcohol intoxication (chronic intoxication increases)
- Pregnancy
- Intravenous anesthesia
- Local anesthesia
- Hyponatremia, hypercalcemia, hypermagnesia [thyroid disease and sex has no effect]

25. Ans. (a) Blood gas partition coefficient

[Ref. Ajay Yadav, 4/e p60]

26. Ans. (c) Propofol

[Ref. Ajay Yadav, 4/e p82]

27. Ans. (d) General anesthesia should be given to neonate for circumcision as they also feel pain as adults

[Ref. Pediatric Urology by Jeffrey, 1/e p128]

28. Ans. (c) He wanted to see if there was an oculocardiac reflex

[Ref. Ajay Yadav, 4/e p184]

- **Oculocardiac reflex**: Triggered by pressure on globe or by traction on extraocular muscle (especially medial rectus)
  - Afferents are carried by Trigeminal and efferents by Vagus
  - It is manifested as bradycardia, AV block or even cardiac arrest

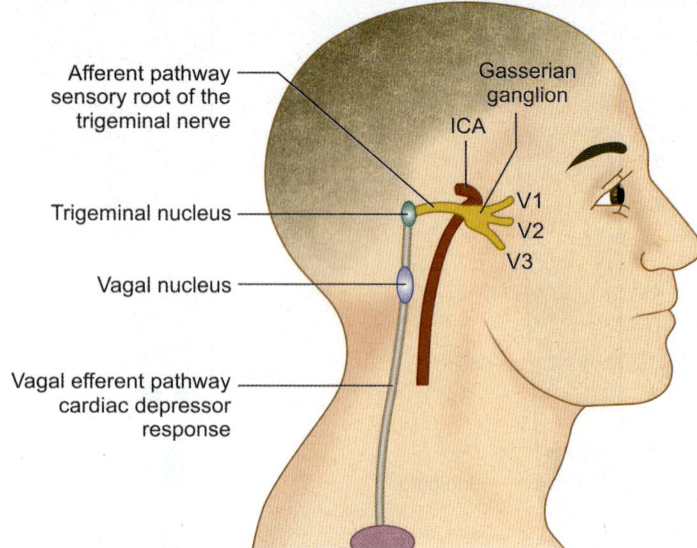

Fig. Oculocardiac reflex

29. Ans. (a) Succinylcholine

[Ref. Ajay Yadav, 4/e p98]

Contraindication of Succinylcholine

- Hyperkalemia or any condition that causes hyperkalemia
- Head injury
- Newborn and infant
- Glaucoma and eye injuries
- Upto 2-3 months after trauma
- Upto 6 months after hemiplegia
- Upto 1 year after burn
- Renal failure
- Prolonged intraabdominal infection
- Diagnosed case of atypical case pseudocholinesterase and low pseudocholinesterase
- Duchenne muscular dystrophy
- Tetanus
- Guillain-Barre syndrome
- Metabolic acidosis
- Shock
- Spinal cord injury

30. Ans. (b) Induction by IV Propofol and maintenance by N_2O & O_2

[Ref. Ajay Yadav, 4/e p155]

- If general anesthesia is to be given then if possible contemplate anesthesia with total intravenous anesthesia and maintenance by N_2O & O_2

Also Remember

- Anesthetic management in Duchenne's dystrophies/Pseudo-hypertrophic muscular dystrophy:
  - **Regional anesthesia is best** (Peripheral nerve blocks, Local and Central neuraxial block)
  - Any nondepolarizing agent should be given as per neuro-muscular monitoring response (Short-acting like Atracurium and Mivacurium are preferred)

Contd...

Contd...

- Opioids and sedatives should be avoided
- Cardiotoxic inhalational agents like Enflurane and Halothane should not be used
- **Succinylcholine/Suxamethonium is contraindicated** (Cardiac arrest due to hyperkalemia can occur and severe contracture can develop)
- Halothane should be avoided as patients are prone to for malignant hyperthermia
- Ketamine may increase muscle tone and so should be avoided

31. Ans. (a) Induction with IV thiopentone and N_2O; and halothane for maintenance
[Ref. Ajay Yadav, 4/e p155]
- **Please note**: Halothane, if possible, should also be avoided

32. Ans. (a) Sevoflurane
[Ref. Ajay Yadav, 4/e p70]

33. Ans. (c) General anesthesia
[Ref. Stoelting's Anaesthesia and Co-Existing Disease by Hines, 5/e p572]

34. Ans. (b) Ketamine
[Ref. Ajay Yadav, 4/e p148]
- **In cyanotic heart disease** (right to left shunt), induction agent of choice is ketamine as it increases the systemic vascular resistance (so afterload) thereby decreasing the shunt fraction
  - Maintenance of anesthesia is with Ketamine and Opioids
  - Nitrous oxide is avoided

Also Remember

- **In Acynotic heart disease** (left to right shunt), systemic vascular resistance should be decreased, hence volatile agent like isoflurane, sevoflurane or desflurane should be used.

35. Ans. (a) Sevoflurane
[Ref. Ajay Yadav, 4/e p70]

36. Ans. (a) IV Opioids
[Ref. Ajay Yadav, 4/e p148]
- Maintenance of anesthesia is with ketamine and opioids
- Nitrous oxide is avoided

37. Ans. (b) Thiopental sodium
[Ref. Ajay Yadav, 4/e p79]

38. Ans. (a) Hypothermia
[Ref. Cardiac Anaesthesia by Estafanous, 2/e. p427]

39. Ans. (b) Preoxygenation is mandatory
[Ref. Ajay Yadav, 4/e p70]

40. Ans. (c) Chloral hydrate
[Ref. Principles of Pediatric and Neonatal Emergencies by Panna Choudhury, 3/e p102]

41. Ans. (a) Air embolism
[Ref. Millers, 7/e Chapter 68]

Air Embolism
- The diagnosis of gas embolism depends on the detection of gas emboli in the right side of the heart or on recognition of the physiologic changes from embolization
- Early events, occurring with 0.5 mL/kg of air or less, include changes in Doppler sounds and increased mean pulmonary artery pressure
- When the size of the embolus increases (2 mL/kg of air), tachycardia, cardiac arrhythmias, hypotension, increased central venous pressure, alteration in heart tones (i.e., **millwheel murmur**), cyanosis, and electrocardiographic changes of right-sided heart strain can develop
- Pulmonary edema can also be an early sign of gas embolism
- Although pulse oximetry is helpful in recognizing hypoxemia, Capnometry and Capnography are more valuable in providing early diagnosis and extent

42. Ans. (c) Venous air embolism
[Ref. Millers Anesthesia, 7/e Chapter 68]

43. Ans. (a) Thiopentone; (b) Etomidate
[Ref. Harrison's Principles of Internal Medicine, 17/e T352-4]

44. Ans. (a) Thiopentone
[Ref. Harrison's Principles of Internal Medicine, 17/e T352-4]

45. Ans. (d) Thiopentone
[Ref. Ajay Yadav, 4/e p155]

46. Ans. (a) Calcium channel blocker nifedipine; (b) Beta blockers; (c) Aminoglycosides

47. Ans. (a) Hyperpyrexia; (b) Prolonged surgeries
[Ref. Ajay Yadav, 4/e p115]

48. Ans. (c) Should be given in normal doses as they prevent MI & angina

49. Ans. (a) Ketamine
[Ref. Ajay Yadav, 4/e p152]
- **Anesthetic drugs which have got epileptogenic potential** and should not be used are:
  - Induction agents: Methohexital, Ketamine, Propofol
  - Inhalation agent: Enflurane
  - Muscle relaxant: Atracurium

Also Remember

- Induction agent of choice in Epileptics: Thiopentone

50. Ans. (c) Diaphragm
[Ref. Ajay Yadav, 4/e p96]

51. Ans. (c) Ketamine
[Ref. Ajay Yadav, 4/e p86]

52. Ans. (d) Halothane
[Ref. Ajay Yadav, 4/e p67]

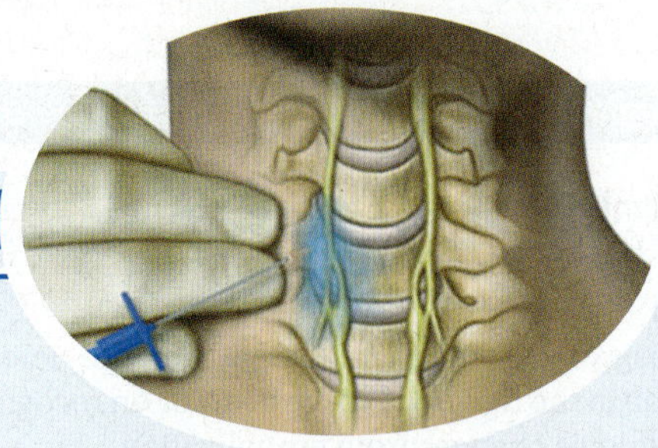

Chapter 6

Intubations and Ventilation

THEORETICAL CONCEPTS

VI A. COMPLICATIONS OF INTUBATION

- **Perioperative complications**:
  - Oesophageal intubation
  - Ischaemia, oedema, necrosis
  - Aspiration
  - Bronchial intubation and collapse of other lung
  - Accidental extubation
  - Trauma to gums, lips, nasal cavity, pharynx, larynx
  - Cardiac arrhythmias, hypertension
- **Postoperative complications**:
  - Sore throat: **Most common post-operative complication**[Q]
  - Laryngeal oedema
  - Laryngeal nerve palsies
  - Emphysema
  - Infections
  - Lung atelectasis
- **Delayed complications**:
  - Tracheal stenosis
  - Vocal cord granuloma
  - Tracheal collapse
  - Laryngeotracheal web

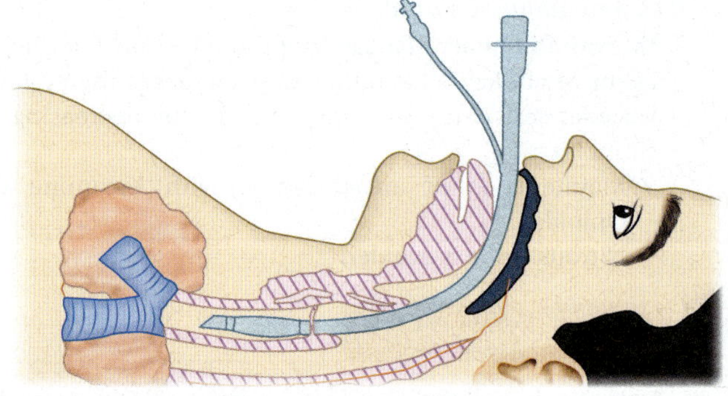

Fig. Tracheal Intubation

Topper's Edge

TRACHEAL INTUBATION

Procedure

- Placement of a flexible plastic tube into the trachea (windpipe) to maintain an open airway or to serve as a conduit through which to administer certain drugs
- Frequently performed in critically injured, ill, or anesthetized patients to facilitate ventilation of the lungs, including mechanical ventilation, and to prevent the possibility of asphyxiation or airway obstruction

Indications

- Depressed level of consciousness (MC Indication[Q]): Massive stroke, non-penetrating head injury, intoxication or poisoning
- Hypoxemia: Cervical spine injury, multiple rib fractures, severe pneumonia, acute respiratory distress syndrome, near-drowning
- Airway obstruction: Foreign body obstruction, expanding hematoma, smoke inhalation or burns within or near the airway or epiglottitis, sustained generalized seizure activity, angioedema
- Manipulation of the airway: Diagnostic or therapeutic manipulation of the airway (bronchoscopy, laser therapy or stenting of the bronchi)

Equipment[Q]

- Laryngoscopes
- Stylets
- Tracheal tubes

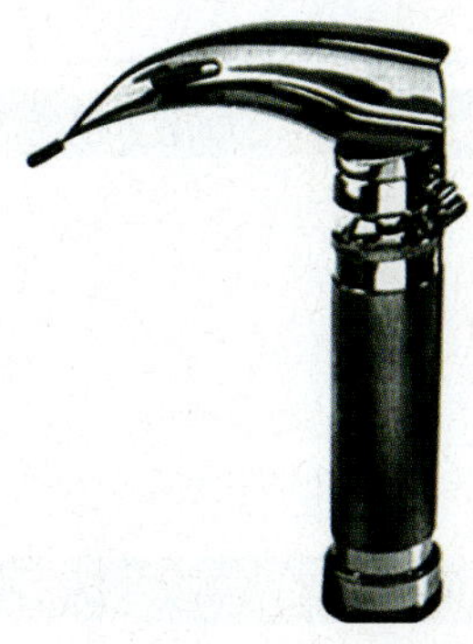
Fig. Laryngoscope

Fig. Stylets

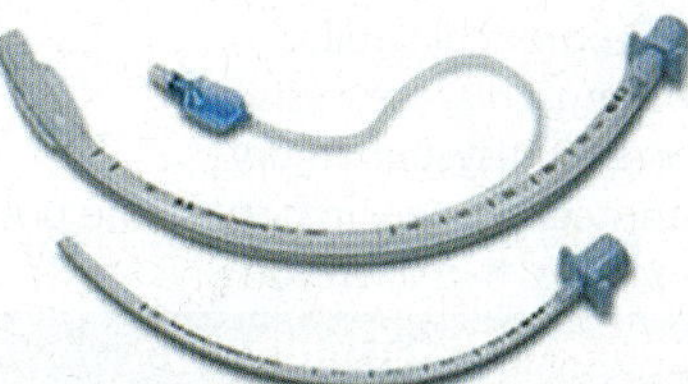
Fig. Endotracheal tube

VI B. LARYNGEAL MASK AIRWAY (LMA)

- Synonyms: Supraglottic airway/brain mask
- Principle: An effective gas tight seal around laryngeal inlet (nothing pass through vocal cords)
- **Indications**[Q]:
  - Difficult intubation/airway expected
  - Facilitation of endotracheal intubation in difficult airway
  - Secure airway in emergency situation (CPR)
  - Minor/short surgery
  - Extra or intraocular surgeries
- **Contraindications**[Q]:
  - High risk of aspiration patients (Full stomach, Pregnancy, Hiatus hernia)
  - Oropharyngeal mass/ tumor
  - Massive trauma (Thorax/ Maxillofacial)
- **Sizes of LMA**[Q]:

Mask size (Inflation volume)	Patients weight (Age)
1 (4 ml)	< 5 kg (Neonates/ Infants) [Q]
1.5 (7 ml)	5-10 kg (Infants)
2 (10 ml)	10-20 kg (Infants/ Children) [Q]
2.5 (14 ml)	20-30 kg (Children)
3 (14 ml)	30-50 kg (Children/ Small adults) [Q]
4 (30 ml)	50-70 kg (Adults) [Q]
5 (40 ml)	70-100 kg (Adults)
6	>100 kg (Adults)

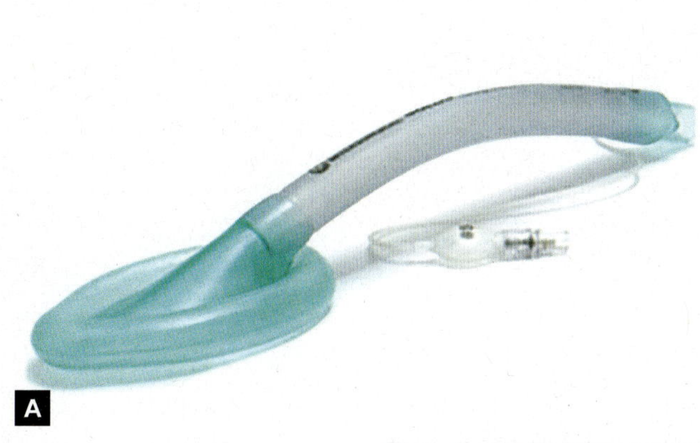
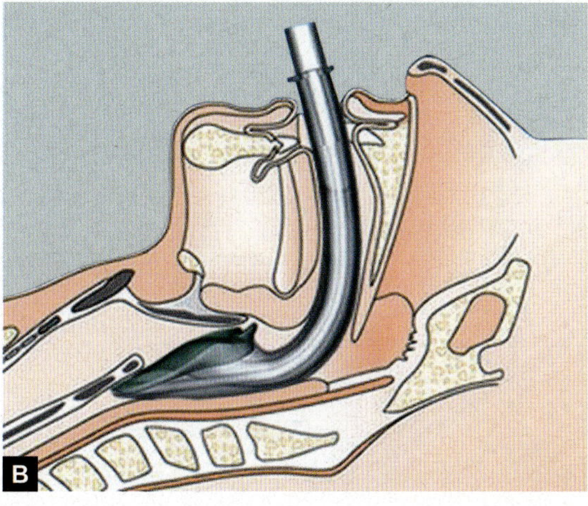
Figs. A and B: (A) Laryngeal mask airway (B) LMA

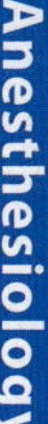

VI C. INTUBATIONS

Indications of Endotracheal intubation	Contraindications Oral and Nasal intubation[Q]
• Positive pressure ventilation[Q] • Protection of aspiration of gastric contents[Q] • Tracheobronchial toilet[Q] • Neuromuscular paralysis • Severe multisystem injury • Head/neck surgery in non-supine positions • Intracranial hypertension	• Laryngeal edema • Laryngotracheobronchitis • Epiglottitis
Indications of Nasal intubation	**Contraindications for Nasal intubation**
• Oral cavity obstruction (Neoplasm/ Abscess)[Q] • Improper mouth opening (Trismus, TMA, FM)[Q] • Cervical spine injury[Q] • Oral surgeries[Q]	• Basal skull fracture[Q] • Adenoids[Q] • Nasal polyp/Abscess/Foreign body[Q] • Coagulopathy/Bleeding disorders

(TMA: Temporomandibular joint ankylosis, FM: Fracture mandible)

IMAGE-BASED QUESTIONS

1. Classification showed in Photograph is used for Assessment of ***[Recent Question 2013]***

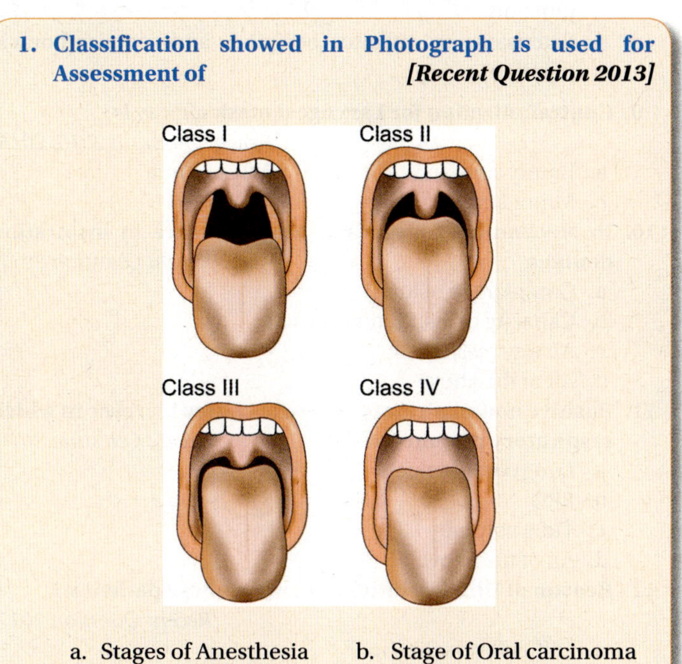

a. Stages of Anesthesia
b. Stage of Oral carcinoma
c. Grading of Trismus
d. Ease of Intubation

2. Identify the Mode of Ventilation shown in Photograph

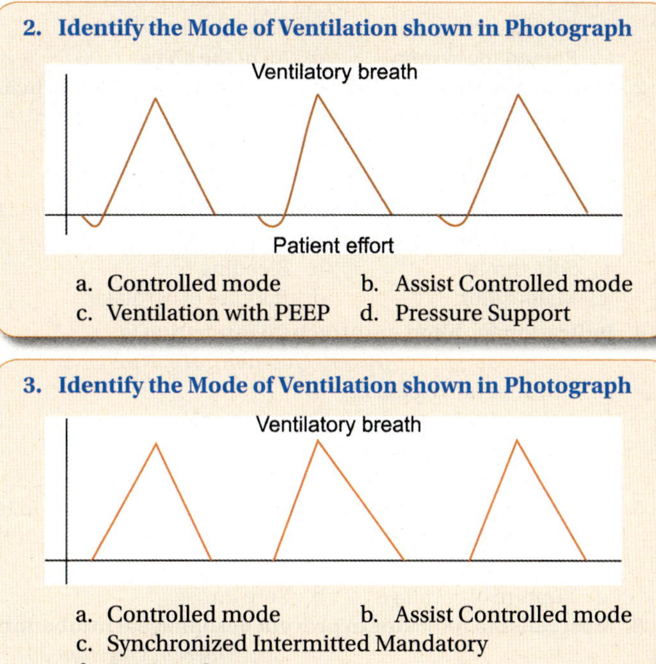

a. Controlled mode
b. Assist Controlled mode
c. Ventilation with PEEP
d. Pressure Support

3. Identify the Mode of Ventilation shown in Photograph

a. Controlled mode
b. Assist Controlled mode
c. Synchronized Intermitted Mandatory
d. Pressure Support

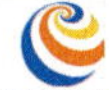

ANSWERS WITH EXPLANATIONS OF IBQs

1. Ans. (d) Ease of Intubation *[Ref. Nurse Anesthesia by Plauss, 5/e p431]*

Modified Mallampati Classification (MMC)

- Description: MMC is used to predict Ease of Endotracheal intubation
  - Class 0: Ability to see any part of the epiglottis upon mouth opening and tongue protrusion
  - Class I: Soft palate, fauces, uvula, pillars visible
  - Class II: Soft palate, fauces, uvula visible
  - Class III: Soft palate, base of uvula visible
  - Class IV: Soft palate not visible at all
- Method: Assessment is performed with the patient sitting up straight, mouth open and tongue maximally protruded, without speaking
- Clinical importance:
  - Mallampati classes I and II are associated with relatively easy intubation
  - Classes III and IV are associated with increased difficulty
  - MMC is a good predictor of difficult direct laryngoscopy and intubation, but poor at predicting difficult bag mask ventilation
  - MMC is not sufficiently accurate alone

2. Ans. (b) Assist Controlled mode *[Ref. Ajay Yadav, 4/e p205]*

- Assist control mode ventilation: Patients' spontaneous breath rate exceeds back-up rate

3. Ans. (a) Controlled mode *[Ref. Ajay Yadav, 4/e p38]*

- Intermittent Positive Pressure Ventilation (IPPV): Patients' own effort is absent, and only ventilator delivers preset tidal volume at preset frequency.

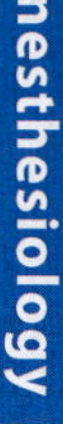

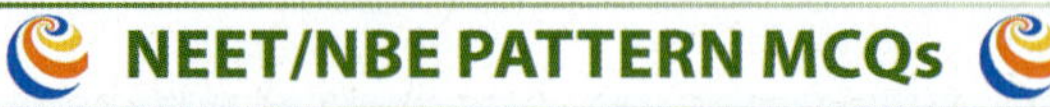

NEET/NBE PATTERN MCQs

1. **Which of the following systems can be used to produce PEEP?** *[Recent Question 2016]*
   a. Spring system b. Ball valve system
   c. Pneumatic system d. All of the above
2. **Standard method to differentiate between Endotracheal and Esophageal intubation is** *[Recent Question 2016]*
   a. End tidal CO_2 b. Chest x-ray
   c. Auscultation d. Partial pressure of o_2
3. **Most common complication of Endotracheal intubation is** *[NBE FMGE September 2009, NBE DNB June 2011]*
   a. Sore throat b. Bleeding
   c. Malposition d. Rupture of cartilage
4. **Indication for blind nasotracheal intubation is** *[Recent Question 2016, NBE DNB 1992]*
   a. Uncooperative patient
   b. Ankylosis of temporo-mandibular point
   c. Fracture mandible
   d. Cervical spondylosis
5. **Most common complication of Endotracheal intubation is which one of the following** *[NBE DNB June 2011]*
   a. Malposition b. Bleeding
   c. Rupture of cartilage d. Sore throat
6. **Most reliable indicator to prevent oesophageal intubation** *[Recent Question 2012]*
   a. Oxygen saturation on pulse oximeter
   b. Measurement of CO_2 in exhaled air ($EtCO_2$)
   c. Direct visualization of passing tube beneath vocal cords
   d. Auscultation over chest
7. **Heimlich valve is used for drainage of** *[NBE DNB 2009, 2010]*
   a. Pneumothorax b. Hemothorax
   c. Empyema d. Malignant pleural effusion
8. **Sniffing position for endotracheal intubations is achieved by** *[NBE FMGE March 2012]*
   a. Flexion at the atlanto occipital and extension at the cervicothoracic junctions
   b. Extension at atlanto occipital and flexion at cervico-thoracic junction
   c. Flexion at the atlanto occipital and cervicothoracic junction
   d. Extension at atlanto occipital and cervicothoracic junction
9. **Contraindication for Laryngeal mask airway is** *[Recent Question 2016, 2015]*
   a. Empty stomach b. Hiatus hernia
   c. Minor surgery d. Young age
10. **In Mechanical ventilation, peak pressure in inspiration denotes** *[Recent Question 2017]*
    a. Compliance of lung
    b. Capacity of inspiratory muscles
    c. Airway resistance
    d. All of the above
11. **Positive end-expiratory pressure causes increase in which respiratory parameter(s)?** *[Recent Question 2017]*
    a. Lung compliance
    b. FRC
    c. Tidal volume
    d. All of the above
12. **Reason of Difficult intubation in an obese patient is?** *[Recent Question 2017]*
    a. Difficult visualization
    b. Decreased safe apnea time
    c. Lower tidal volume
    d. All of the above
13. **Murphy's eye is seen in** *[Recent Question 2018]*
    a. Macintosh laryngoscope
    b. Endotracheal tube
    c. Flexible laryngoscope
    d. LMA
14. **Modified Mallampati grading is used in assessment of** *[Recent Question 2018]*
    a. Difficulty during intubation
    b. Airway obstruction
    c. Death due to aspiration
    d. Intubation

HIGH YIELD MCQs

1. **Endotracheal intubation is assessed by** *[PGI November 2016]*
   a. Mallampati grading
   b. ASA physical status grading
   c. Thyromental distance
   d. Teeth arrangement e. None
2. **Which of the following is not true regarding Rapid sequence intubation (RSI)?** *[AIIMS May 2016]*
   a. High volume low pressure cuffs are preferred
   b. Simultaneous administration of an induction and neuromuscular blocking agents
   c. Oxygenate the patient with 100% oxygen for 3 mins before intubation
   d. Preferred technique in cardiac arrest patients
3. **True about Laryngeal mask airway** *[PGI 1999]*
   a. More reliable than face mask
   b. Prevent aspiration
   c. Alternative to Endotracheal tube
   d. Does not require laryngoscope and visualization
   e. Can be used in full stomach
4. **Which of the following is not an indication for endotracheal intubation?** *[All India 2006]*
   a. Maintenance of a patent airway
   b. To provide positive pressure ventilation
   c. Pulmonary toilet
   d. Pneumothorax
   e. Equal volume, pressure

5. Sellick's manoeuvre is used to prevent
a. Alveolar collapse *[AIIMS 1997, PGI 2009]*
b. Hypertension
c. Aspiration of gastric content
d. Bradycardia
e. Glaucoma

6. Nasal intubation is contraindicated in *[AIIMS PGMEE 1995]*
a. CSF rhinorrhoea b. Fracture cervical spine
c. Fracture mandible d. Short neck

7. Both oral and nasal intubation are contraindicated *[Recent Question 2016, AIIMS PGMEE 1995]*
a. Laryngeal endema
b. CSF-Rhinorrhoea
c. Comastose patient
d. Acute Tracheolaryngobronchitis

8. Mendelson's syndrome is *[Recent Question 2016]*
a. Air leak *[AIIMS PGMEE 1994]*
b. Tracheal rupture during intubation
c. Oesophageal ruptures
d. Aspiration of gastric contents

9. Mallampatti grading is for *[Recent Question 2017, All India PGMEE 2000]*
a. Mobility of cervical spine
b. Mobility of atlanto axial joint
c. Assessment of free rotation of neck before intubation
d. Inspection of oral cavity before intubation

10. True about endotracheal cuff *[PGI 2004]*
a. Low volume, high pressure
b. Low volume, low pressure
c. High volume, low pressure
d. High volume, high pressure

11. True about endotracheal intubation is *[All India PGMEE 1999]*
a. It reduces normal anatomical dead space
b. It produces decrease in resistance to respiration
c. Subglottic edema is most common complication
d. All of the above

12. During laryngoscopy and endotracheal intubation, which of the maneuver is not performed?
a. Flexion of the neck *[AIIMS PGMEE 2003]*
b. Extension of Head at the atlanto-occipital joint
c. The laryngoscope is lifted upwards levering over the upper incisors
d. In a straight blade laryngoscope, the epiglottis is lifted by the tip

13. Size in <6 years old child, of endotracheal tube is *[Rajasthan PGMEE 2010]*
a. Age + 3.5/3.5 b. Age + 2.5/2.5
c. Age + 4.5/4.5 d. Age – 4.5/4.5

14. In infant (full term) diameter (mm) length (cm) of ETT used are *[AP PGMEE 2009]*
a. 3.5, 16 b. 7, 12
c. 3.5, 12 d. 7, 10

15. Merits of nasotracheal intubation is
a. Good oral hygiene *[AIIMS PGMEE 2007]*
b. Less infection
c. Less muscosal damage and bleeding
d. More movement or displacement of endotracheal tube

16. True about Laryngoscopy & intubation *[PGI 2004]*
a. Hypertension b. Tachycardia
c. ICT d. Intraocular pressure
e. Lower oesophageal sphincter tone

17. True about endotracheal intubation (during the process) is all except *[PGI 2001]*
a. Hypertension & tachycardia
b. Raised IOT
c. Raised ICT
d. Arrhythmias
e. Increased oesophageal peristalsis

18. In volume-cycled ventilation, the inspiratory flow rate is set at *[AIIMS PGMEE 2002]*
a. 140-160L/min b. 110-130L/min
c. 60-100L/min d. 30-50L/min

19. Not seen with controlled ventilation *[AIIMS PGMEE 1993]*
a. Barotrauma b. Alkalosis
c. Pulmonary embolism d. Cardiac temponade

20. The following modes of ventilation may be used for weaning off patients from mechanical ventilation except *[All India PGMEE 2005]*
a. Controlled Mechanical ventilation (CMV)
b. Synchronized intermittent mandatory ventilation (SIMV)
c. Pressure support ventilation (PSV)
d. Assist-control ventilation (ACV)

21. All are true about PEEP except *[PGI 1999]*
a. Useful in situations where PO_2 is low
b. CO
c. Impaired renal function
d. ICT

22. About CPAP all are true except *[AIIMS PGMEE 2009]*
a. Given prophylactically in all preterm with respiratory distress
b. Started with FiO2 50 to 60 percent
c. Given in infants less than 28 weeks and less than 1kg weight
d. Improves oxygenation and improves lung compliance

23. Placement of a double lumen tube (DLT) is best confirmed by *[AIIMS 2005, PGI 2008]*
a. Clinically by Auscultation b. Fibreoptic bronchoscopy
c. Capnography d. Chest radiography
e. Chest inflation on positive pressure

24. A 27 year old female was brought to emergency department for acute abdominal pain following which she was shifted to the operation theatre for Laparotomy. A speedy intubation was performed but after the intubation, breath sounds were observed to be decreased on the left side and a high end tidal CO_2 was recorded. The likely diagnosis is
a. Endotracheal tube blockage *[All India PGMEE 2010]*
b. Bronchospasm
c. Esophageal intubation
d. Endobronchial intubation

25. The narrowest part of larynx in infants is at the cricoid level. In administering anesthesia this may lead to all except *[AIIMS PGMEE 2003]*
a. Choosing a smaller size endotracheal tube
b. Trauma to the subglottic region
c. Post operative stridor
d. Laryngeal oedema

26. In a young patient who had extensive soft tissue and muscle injury, which of these muscle relaxants used for endotracheal intubation might lead to cardiac arrest *[AIIMS PGMEE 2003]*

a. Atracurium b. Suxamethonium
c. Vecuronium d. Pancuronium

27. 90% oxygen flow rate can be delivered by *[JIPMER PGMEE 2014]*

a. Simple breathing mask b. Partial rebreathing mask
c. Nonbreathing mask d. Venturi mask

28. Most important complication of effectively ventilating a patient with Positive pressure ventilation in Broncho-pleural fistula *[PGMCET 2015]*

a. Bronchiectasis b. Pulmonary cyst
c. Tension pneumothorax
d. Pulmonary hemorrhage

29. Maximum Oxygen concentration can be delivered by *[AIIMS November 2017]*

a. Venturi mask b. Nasal cannula
c. Face mask d. Face mask with reservoir

30. A patient on ventilator gets agitated and pulls out his ET tube. Patient's attendant rushes to Doctor-in-charge. Next step of management will be *[AIIMS November 2017]*

a. Sit the patient up and do chest physiotherapy
b. Give bag and mask ventilation and reassess spontaneous breathing
c. Apply face mask and give 100% oxygen
d. Reintubate the patient under sedation

31. Pre-oxygenation time necessary for ET tube insertion is *[AIIMS November 2017]*

NEET/NBE PATTERN MCQs ANSWERS WITH EXPLANATIONS

1. Ans. (d) All of the above

[Ref. Thoracic Anesthesia by Hartigan, 1/e p179]

Mechanisms Used to Generate PEEP

- Spring system
- Electronic system
- Pneumatic system
- Magnetic system
- Ball valve system

2. Ans. (a) End tidal CO_2

[Ref. Pediatric Emergency Medicine by Baren, 1/e p52]

- $ETCO_2$ measurement has been found to be the **most reliable method of confirming endotracheal tube position** and can distinguish between endotracheal and esophageal intubation

3. Ans. (a) Sore throat

[Ref. Ajay Yadav, 4/e p39]

Post-Operative Complications of Intubation

- Sore throat: **Most common post-operative complication**
- Laryngeal oedema
- Laryngeal nerve palsies
- Emphysema
- Infections
- Lung atelectasis

4. Ans. (b) Ankylosis of temppromandibular point

[Ref. Ajay Yadav, 4/e p39]

- Indications forBlind nasotracheal intubations:
  - Ankylosis of temppro-mandibular joint
  - Trismus because of quinsy, tetanus, etc
  - Neck contractures

5. Ans. (a) Malposition

[Ref. Ajay Yadav, 4/e p38]

- Complications are malposition of tube leading to hypoxia, trauma of larynx, bronchial rupture

6. Ans. (b) Measurement of CO_2 in exhaled air

[Ref. Ajay Yadav, 4/e p39]

7. Ans. (a) Pneumothorax

[Ref. Egan's Fundamentals of Respiratory Care, 1/e p575]

8. Ans. (b) Extension at atlanto-occipital and flexion at cervicothoracic junction

[Ref. Ajay Yadav, 4/e p35]

- **Sniffing position for Endotracheal intubation**: Extension of atlanto-occipital joint + Flexion at cervical spine

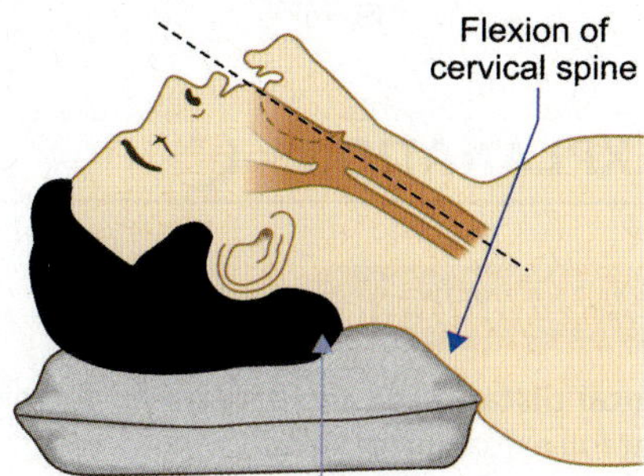

Fig. Sniffing Position

9. Ans. (b) Hiatus hernia

[Ref. Anesthesia by Yadav, 4/e p40]

Contraindications of LMA

- Full stomach patients
- Pregnancy
- Hiatus hernia
- Oropharyngeal abscess/ mass

10. Ans. (c) Airway resistance

[Ref. Mechanical Ventilation by Pupella, 1/e p42]

Peak Pressure

- Peak pressure applies when there is airflow in the circuit, i.e. during inspiration
- What determines the peak pressure is the airway resistance in the lungs
- So if there is a problem with the airways the peak pressure will rise
- **High peak pressure is an airway issue**, for example as in Bronchospasm, Retained secretions, Mucous plug, ETT tip occlusion

Plateau Pressure

- Plateau pressure applies when there is not airflow in the circuit, which is when inspiration is complete
- This pressure is determined by the lung compliance
- So if there is a problem with the compliance the plateau pressure will rise
- **High plateau pressure is a compliance issue**, for example as in Pneumothorax, Pulmonary oedema, ARDS, Pneumonia

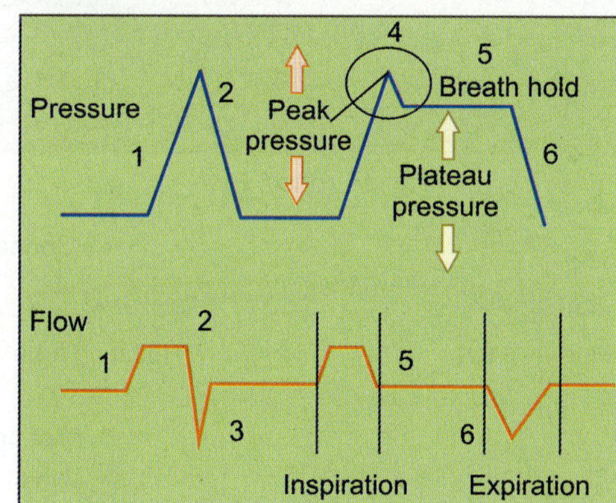

Fig. Peak pressure and plateau pressure

11. Ans. (d) All of the above

[Ref. Avoiding Common Anesthesia Errors by Marcucci, 1/e p10]

- PEEP is used to completely or partially replace the function of the respiratory muscles and therefore correct hypoxemia secondary to alveolar hypoventilation
- PEEP is effective in improving arterial oxygenation simply through increasing functional residual capacity (FRC), reducing venous admixture, shifting tidal volume, preventing loss of pulmonary compliance, and decreasing the work of breathing

12. Ans. (d) All of the above

[Ref. Hagberg and Benumof's Airway Management, 4/e p261]

Reasons of Difficult Intubation in Obese

- Difficult visualization (due to deposition of adipose tissue in pharyngeal tissues, uvula, tonsils, tongue, aryepiglottic folds, lateral pharyngeal walls)
- Decreased safe apnea time (decrease in FRC coupled with increased oxygen utilization shortens the safe apnea time after induction of anesthesia)
- Lower tidal volume

13. Ans. (b) Endotracheal tube

[Ref. Anesthesia for Infants and Children by Coté, 4/e p252]

Murphy Eye

- **It's the hole on the side of most endotracheal tubes** (ETTs), located at the distal end of the tube across from the bevel end, that functions as a vent
- It prevents the complete obstruction of the patient's airway (provides an alternate gas passage), should the primary distal opening of an ETT become occluded.

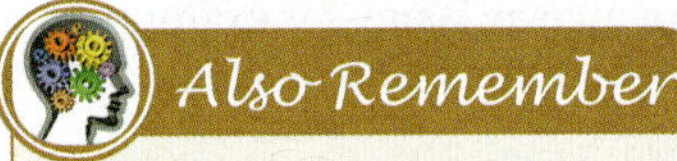

- Those endotracheal tubes without a Murphy eye are referred to as Magill-type tubes

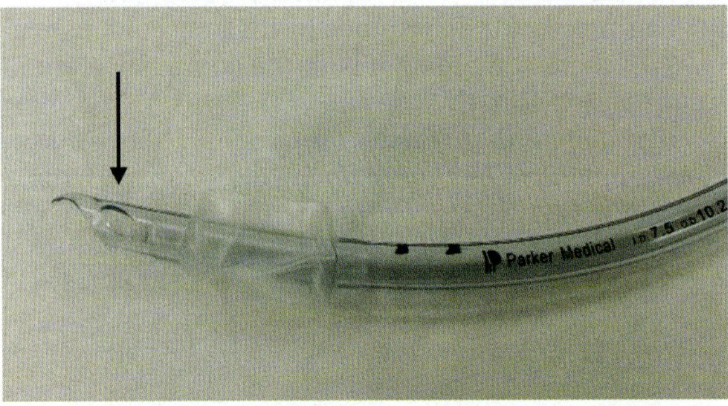

Fig. Murphy's Eye

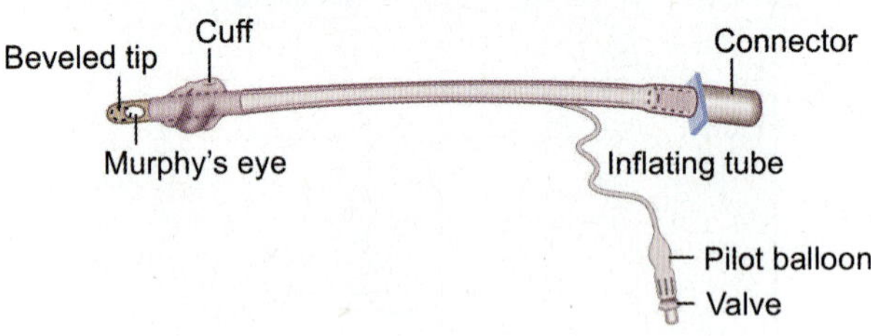

Fig. ET Tube

14. Ans. (a) Difficulty during intubation

[Ref. Nurse Anesthesia by Plauss, 5/e p431]

Modified Mallampati Classification (MMC)

- MMC remains a time-tested technique to date for recognizing an anticipated difficult tracheal intubation as assessed by Cormack-Lehane grade
  - It classifies the degree that the faucial pillars, soft palate, and uvula can be visualized
  - A higher score predicts a more difficult ET intubation
- Both Mallampati and its further modification by Samsoon and Young evaluate patients in the seated position
  - Mallampati classes I and II are associated with relatively easy intubation
  - Classes III and IV are associated with increased difficulty
  - MMC is a good predictor of difficult direct laryngoscopy and intubation, but poor at predicting difficult bag mask ventilation
  - MMC is not sufficiently accurate alone

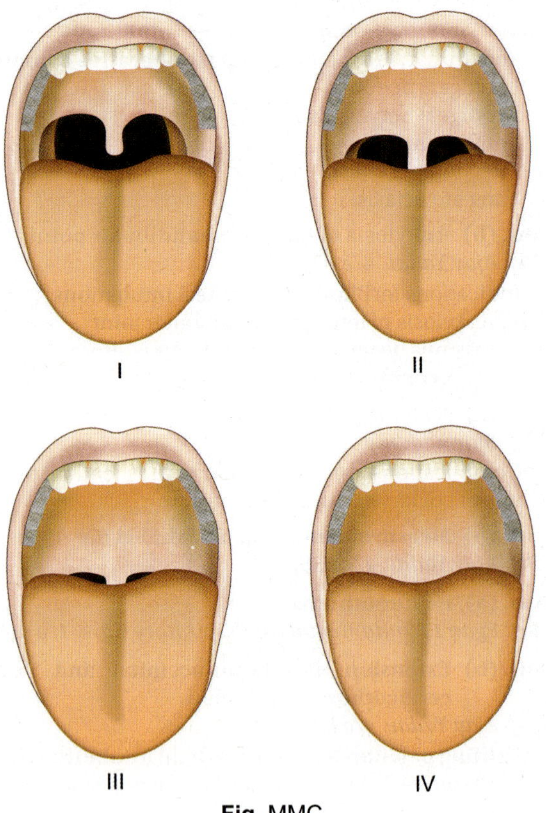

Fig. MMC

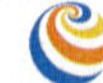 HIGH YIELD MCQs ANSWERS WITH EXPLANATIONS 

1. Ans. (a) Mallampati grading; (c) Thyromental distance; (d) Teeth arrangement

[Ref. Clinical Anaesthesia by Barash, 6/e p463]

- Mallampati's (modified) oropharyngeal classification for assessment of the relative difficulty of endotracheal intubation

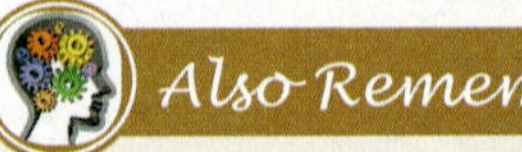

- **Thyromental distance**: Distance between thyroid notch and mentum at full extension of neck
  - 6.5 cms is normal intubation
  - 6.0–6.5 cms borderline (difficult laryngoscopy)
  - <6.0 cms almost impossible intubation

2. **Ans. (a) High volume low pressure cuffs are preferred**
[Ref. Tintinalli's Emergency Medicine, 8/e p184]

Rapid Sequence Intubation (RSI)

- Technique of RSI is performed to gain control of the airway in the shortest amount of time after the ablation of protective airway reflexes with the induction of anesthesia, to prevent regurgitation and aspiration
  - Administration of an intravenous anesthetic induction agent is immediately followed by a rapidly acting neuromuscular blocking drug
  - Laryngoscopy and intubation are performed as soon as muscle relaxation is confirmed
  - **Cricoid pressure (Sellick maneuver)** is applied by an assistant from the beginning of induction until confirmation of ETT placement
  - Cricoid pressure entails the downward displacement of the cricoid cartilage against the vertebral bodies
  - In this manner, the lumen of the esophagus is ablated, while the completely circular nature of the cricoid cartilage maintains the tracheal lumen.
- Two types of cuff systems used in endotracheal tube:
  - **High volume low pressure cuffs**:
    1. Advantages: Because of their large volume, they have a larger surface area in contact with the trachea causing a lower pressure against the tracheal wall and have a lower incidence of tracheal wall ischemia and necrosis
    2. Disadvantage: The seal is not as good as the seal in high pressure cuffs and because the large cuff may develop wrinkles that allow material to pass by the cuff; Does not protect against aspiration completely
  - **Low volume high pressure cuffs**:
    1. Advantage: High pressure seal that is more effective against aspiration
    2. Disadvantage: High pressure is more likely to cause tracheal ischaemia and necrosis if used for a prolonged period of time

3. **Ans. (a) More reliable than face mask; (c) Alternative to endotracheal tube; (d) Does not require laryngoscope & visualization**
[Ref. Ajay Yadav, 4/e p41]

4. **Ans. (d) Pneumothorax**
[Ref. Ajay Yadav, 4/e p41]

5. **Ans. (c) Aspiration of gastric content**
[Ref. Ajay Yadav, 4/e p111]

6. **Ans. (a) CSF rhinorrhoea**
[Ref. Ajay Yadav, 4/e p38]

7. **Ans. (d) Acute tracheolaryngobronchitis**
[Ref. Ajay Yadav, 4/e p38]

- Contraindications to both nasal and oral intubation:
  - Laryngeal oedema
  - Epiglotitis
  - Laryngotracheobronchitis

8. **Ans. (d) Aspiration of gastric content**
[Ref. Ajay Yadav, 4/e p110]

Mendelson Syndrome

- Description:
  - Acid aspiration in late pregnancy was described by Mendelson and called it as Mendelson syndrome
  - Chemical pneumonia within 30 minutes of aspiration of gastric juice
  - MCC of death in GA during Obstetric anesthesia
- Risk factors:
  - pH of aspirated fluid <2.5 (Critical pH)
  - Volume of aspirate > 0.4 ml/kg body weight (Critical volume: 25 ml in adults)
  - Induction phase
  - Full stomach (Most important single risk factor)

Prevention	Treatment
• Preoperative starvation • Prokinetic drugs (Metoclopramide) • H_2-antagonist (Ranitidine) • Regional block techniques • Rapid sequence anesthesia • Sellick's maneuvere • Awake intubation	• Head down position • Suctioning pharynx/trachea • Oxygen supplementation • Mechanical ventilation (Intubation, PEEP) • IV fluids

(Corticosteroids NOT recommended for treatment)

9. **Ans. (d) Inspection of oral cavity before intubation**
[Ref. Ajay Yadav, 4/e p45]

10. **Ans. (a) Low volume, high pressure; (c) High volume, low pressure**
[Ref. Ajay Yadav, 4/e p36]

11. **Ans. (a) It reduces normal anatomical dead space**
[Ref. Ajay Yadav, 4/e p35]

12. **Ans. (c) Laryngoscope is lifted upwards levering over the upper incisors**
[Ref. Ajay Yadav, 4/e p35]

13. **Ans. NONE**
[Ref. Ajay Yadav, 4/e p37]

Calculating Size of Endotracheal Tube

- Children 1-6 years age: (Age in years/3) + 3.5 ID
- Children >6 years age: (Age in years/4) + 4.5 ID

Calculating Length of Endotracheal Tube

- Children: (Age in years/2) + 12 cms

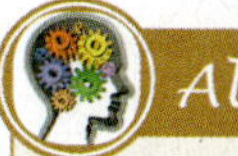

Also Remember

- Smallest size of ET tube available: 2.5 mm
- Largest size of ET tube available: 10.5 mm

14. **Ans. (c) 3.5, 12**
[Ref. Ajay Yadav, 4/e p37]

15. **Ans. (a) Good oral hygiene**
[Ref. Ajay Yadav, 4/e p38]

16. **Ans. ALL CHOICES**
[Ref. Ajay Yadav, 4/e p34-39]

17. Ans. (e) Increased oesophageal peristalsis
[Ref. Ajay Yadav, 4/e p37-38]

18. Ans. (c) 60-100 mL/min
[Ref. Ajay Yadav, 4/e p30]

19. Ans. (d) Cardiac temponade
[Ref. Ajay Yadav, 4/e p207]

20. Ans. (a) Controlled mechanical ventilation
[Ref. Ajay Yadav, 4/e p208]

21. Ans. (d) ICT
[Ref. Ajay Yadav, 4/e p206]

22. Ans. (b) Started with FiO_2 50 to 60%
[Ref. Ajay Yadav, 4/e p208]

23. Ans. (b) Fiberoptic bronchoscopy
[Ref. Ajay Yadav, 4/e p39]

24. Ans. (d) Endotracheal intubation
[Ref. Ajay Yadav, 4/e p39]

25. Ans. (a) Choosing a smaller size endotracheal tube
[Ref. Ajay Yadav, 4/e p179-180]

26. Ans. (b) Suxamethonium
[Ref. Ajay Yadav, 4/e p97]

27. Ans. (c) Nonbreathing mask
[Ref. Ajay Yadav, 4/e p43]

28. Ans. (c) Tension pneumothorax
[Ref. Critical Care Practice by Hoyt, 1/e p70]

- Bronchopleural fistula occurs when the air leak into the pleural space is continuous
- Tension pneumothorax arises when the site of the air leak into the pleural space acts as a unidirectional valve; Positive pressure ventilation may exacerbate this **'one-way-valve'** effect.

29. Ans. (d) Face mask with reservoir
[Ref. Emergency by American Academy of Orthopaedic Surgeons, 9/e p240]

- With an oxygen flow rate of 15 L/ min and an adequate bag-to-mask seal, Bag-valve-mask device with reservoir can deliver nearly 100% oxygen

Device	Flow rate	Oxygen delivered
Nasal canula	1-6 L/min	24-44%
Non-breathing mask	15 L/min	90-100%
Bag mask device with reservoir	15 L/min - Flush	Nearly 100%

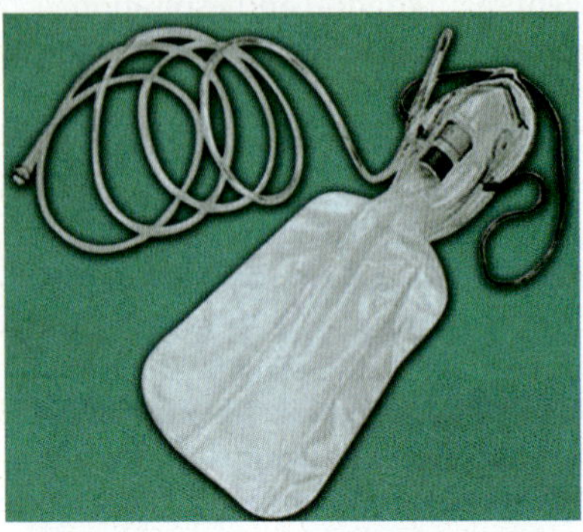

Fig. Oxygen Mask with Reservoir

30. Ans. (b) Give bag and mask ventilation and reassess spontaneous breathing
[Ref. Airway Management by Benumof, 1/e p826]

- Self-extubation often occurs in patients who are ready for elective extubation within the next few hours
- Patients who self-extubate within 72 hours of a planned extubation require re-intubation in only 14% of cases
- Therefore, in the majority of patients who do not require re-intubation, self-extubation can actually decrease the length of intubation and weaning

31. Ans. (b) 3 min
[Ref. Perioperative Medicine by Hudsmith, 1/e p51]

- Aim of Rapid sequence induction: To minimise the time between induction of anaesthesia, which abolishes protective airway reflexes and can lead to aspiration of acid passively regurgitated from the stomach, and the placement of a cuffed endotracheal tube that protects the airway
- Patient is 'pre-oxygenated' with 100% oxygen for 3 min, which aims to fully saturate haemoglobin and increase oxygen reserve in the lungs

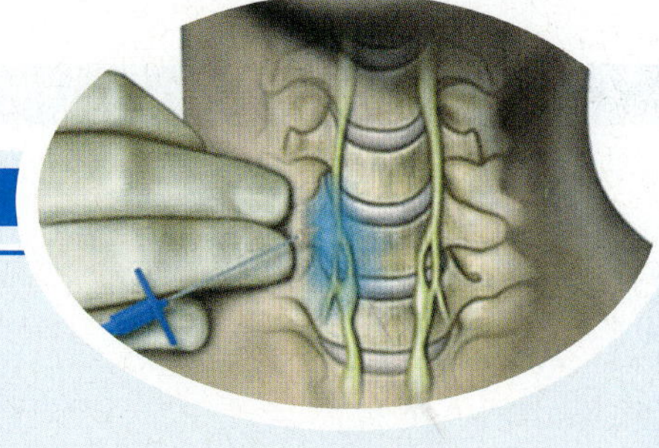

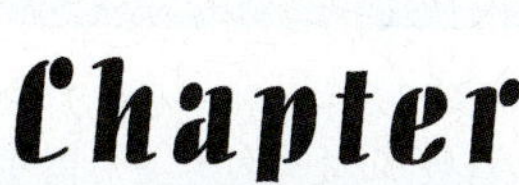

Chapter 7

Muscle Relaxants

THEORETICAL CONCEPTS

VII A. CLASSIFICATION OF MUSCLE RELAXANTS

- ***Centrally acting muscle relaxants:***[Q]
  - Chlorzoxazone
  - Diazepam
  - Baclofen
  - Tizanidine
  - Metaxalone
- ***Peripherally acting muscle relaxants***:
  - Neuromuscular blocking agents

Non-depolarising competitive blockers			Depolarizing blockers [Q]
Long-acting	***Intermediate-acting***	***Short-acting*** [Q]	
• d-Tubocuranine • Pancuronium • Doxacurium • Pipecuronium	• Vecuronium • Atracurium • Cis-atracurium • Rocuronium • Rapacuronium	• Mivacurium	• Succinylcholine • Decamethonium

  - **Directly acting agents** [Q]
    - Dantrolene sodium
    - Quinine

VII B. SUCCINYLCHOLINE (SCH)

- ***Anaesthetic of choice for intubation*** [Q]: Early onset and short duration of action
- **Metabolised by Pseudo-cholinesterase**[Q]
- *Mechanism of action*: Fasciculations
- *Systemic side effects* [Q]: **[Mnemonic: BHIMA]**
  - **B**radycardia
  - **H**yperkalemia (and paraplegias)
  - **I**ncreased intracranial tension
  - **I**ncreased intraocular tension
  - **I**ncreased salivation, gastric secretions, peristalsis
  - **M**uscle soreness
  - **M**alignant hyperthermia (Most commonly implicated drug)
  - **M**asseter spasm
  - **A**naphylaxis

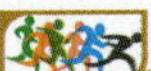

Topper's Edge

Contraindications to Succinylcholine[Q]

- **Hyperkalemia**[Q]
- Head injury
- Glaucoma, Eye injury
- Newborns, Infants
- Renal failure
- Duchenne muscular dystrophy
- Dystrophica myotonica
- Guillain Barre syndrome
- Tetanus
- Shock
- Metabolic acidosis
- Spinal cord injury
- Up to 2–3 months of trauma, Up to 6 month of hemiplegia/paraplegia, Up to 1 year after burns[Q]

VII C. PANCURONIUM

- *Avoided in Renal failure*: 80-90% excreted by kidneys
- ***Useful in asthma patients*** [Q]: Histamine release is rare
- ***Increased chances of cardiac arrhythmias with Halothane***[Q]: Due to vagal block leading to tachycardia, hypertension

VII D. PIPECURONIUM

- Is a long acting steroid analogue of Pancuronium
- *Cardiovascular stability*: No vagolytic activity

VII E. VECURONIUM

- ***Most commonly used muscle relaxant for routine surgery***[Q]
- ***Muscle relaxant of choice for cardiac patients***[Q]: Cardiovascular stability
- *Safe in hepatic failure*
- *Avoided in Biliary obstruction*: 40% excreted in bile
- *Causes polyneuropathy on long-term use*: Accumulation of 3-hydroxy metabolite
- *Reversal by Neostigmine required*: Only if repeated doses given

VII F. ROCURONIUM

- *Earliest onset of action among non-depolarising muscle relaxants*[Q]
- ***Muscle relaxant of choice for pre-curarisation***[Q]
- *Non-depolarising muscle relaxant of choice for intubation*[Q]

VII G. RAPACURONIUM

- *Causes intense brochospasm*

VII H. D-TUBOCURARE

- *Causes severe hypotension*[Q]
- *Causes asthma attacks, anaphylaxis*[Q]: Highest histamine release

VII I. METOCURINE

- Derivative of Tubocurare
- Contains iodine

VII J. ATRACURIUM

- Spontaneous degradation by ***'Hoffmann's elimination'***[Q]
- ***Relaxant of choice in:***[Q]
  - Hepatic failure
  - Renal failure
  - Myasthenia gravis
  - Newborns and old age

VII K. CIS-ATRACURIUM

- *Cardiovascular stability*[Q]: Does not release histamine

VII L. MIVACURIUM

- **Shortest acting** non-depolarising muscle relaxant[Q]
- ***Useful in day care surgery***: Due to short duration of action[Q]
- ***Reversal is done by Edrophonium***: Neostigmine may prolong effect

VII M. DOXACURIUM

- ***Most potent non-depolarizing muscle relaxant***[Q]

VII N. GALLAMINE

- *Cause severe tachycardia*: Maximum vagolytic
- ***Contraindicated in pregnancy***[Q]: As it crosses placenta
- ***Contraindicated in renal disease***: As 80% excreted by kidneys[Q]

Topper's Edge

Muscle Relaxants

- **Neurotransmitter responsible for neurotransmission at NM junction**: Acetylcholine[Q]
  - Acetylcholinesterase: Destroys Acetylcholine in <1 ms (Produced by underlying muscle)
  - Acetylcholine receptor: Most important subunit is Alpha where binding of SCh, ACh, non-depolarizing relaxants occur
- **MC muscle used for NM monitoring**: Adductor pollicis[Q]
  - First muscle to be blocked by both Depolarizing as well as Non-depolarizing relaxants: Central muscles (Face especially Eyelids[Q])
  - Sequence of blockade[Q]: Face > Jaw > Pharynx > Larynx > Respiratory muscles > Trunk muscles > Limb muscles
- Succinylcholine metabolism is done in plasma by Pseudocholinesterase (Butryl cholinesterase)[Q]
- Prolonged apnoea after Succinylcholine is due to:
  - Low pseudocholinesterase
  - Atypical pseudocholinesterase
  - Phase II block
- Non-depolarizing muscle relaxant of choice for Intubation when Sch is contraindicated: Rocuronium[Q]
- Metabolic product of Atracurium producing convulsions: Laundanosine[Q]
- Reversal agent of choice for Mivacurium: Edrophonium[Q]

Non-depolarizing Muscle Relaxants (NDMR)

- **NDMR of choice**:
  - For Cardiac patients[Q]: Vecuronium
  - For Rapid sequence intubation: Rapacuronium
  - For Hepatic & Renal disease[Q]: Atracurium
- **NDMR contraindicated**:
  - In Renal failure[Q]: Gallamine, Metocurine
  - In Biliary obstruction: Vecuronium, Rocuronium
  - In Pregnancy[Q]: Gallamine
- NDMR causing Ganglion blockade: d-TC, Metocurine, Alcuronium
- NDMR causing Vagal blockade: Gallamine, Pancuronium, Rocuronium

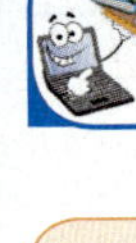

IMAGE-BASED QUESTIONS

1. Non-depolarising agent of choice for Maneuver shown in Photograph is

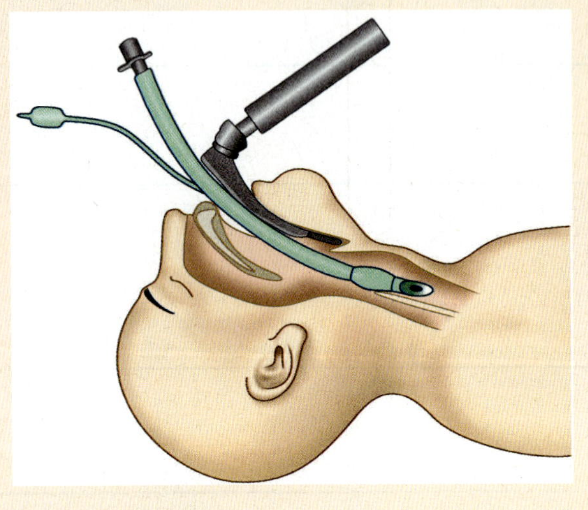

a. Pancuronium
b. Piperacuronium
c. Rocuronium
d. Rapacuronium

2. Non-depolarising Muscle relaxant Contraindicated in Person shown is

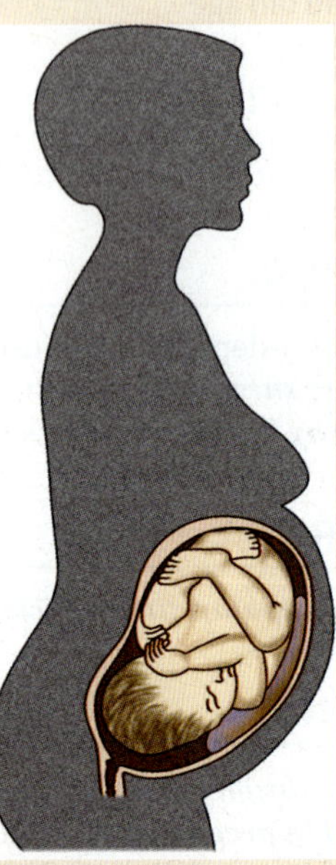

a. Pancuronium
b. Vacuronium
c. Rocuronium
d. Gallamine

 ANSWERS WITH EXPLANATIONS OF IBQs 

1. Ans. (c) Rocuronium *[Ref. Ajay Yadav, 4/e. p97]*

- Depolarising agent of choice for Intubation: Succinylcholine
- Non-depolarising agent of choice for Intubation: Rocuronium
  - Early onset (60 seconds)

2. Ans. (d) Gallamine *[Ref. Ajay Yadav, 4/e. p102]*

- Gallamine crosses placenta: Contraindicated in pregnancy
- More than 80% excreted in kidneys: Contraindicated in Renal disease

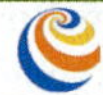 NEET/NBE PATTERN MCQs 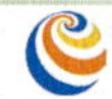

1. **Atracurium is excreted by** *[Recent Question 2016]*
   a. Renal excretion
   b. Hepatic elimination
   c. Non-enzymatic degradation
   d. All of the above
2. **Longest acting among muscle relaxant is** *[Recent Question 2016]*
   a. Doxacurium b. Rocuronium
   c. Vecuronium d. Atracurium
3. **Shortest acting Non-depolarizing muscle relaxant** *[Recent Question 2016]*
   a. Mivacurium b. Doxacuronium
   c. Pipecurium d. Vecuronium
4. **Alternative to Succinylcholine, which muscle relaxant can be used while Endotracheal intubation?** *[Recent Question 2016]*
   a. Atracurium b. Pancuronium
   c. Mivacurium d. Vecuronium
5. **Succinylcholine causes Hyperkalemia in patients with** *[Recent Question 2016]*
   a. Burn b. Severe infection
   c. High velocity trauma d. All of the above
6. **Regarding Mivacurium False is** *[Recent Question 2016]*
   a. Hypertension
   b. Increasing dose produces rapid onset of action
   c. Bronchospasm
   d. Flushing
7. **True statement about Muscle relaxants is** *[NBE FMGE September 2009]*
   a. Atracurium is contraindicated in Renal failure
   b. Pancuronium causes bradycardia
   c. Cis-atracurium is a depolarising muscle relaxant
   d. Vecuronium can be reversed by Neostigmine
8. **Postoperative pain is common with** *[NBE DNB 1994, 1995]*
   a. D-tubocurare b. Suxamethonium
   c. Alcuronium d. Pancuronium
9. **Drug causing anaphylactic reaction** *[NBE DNB 2007]*
   a. Propofol b. Alcuronium
   c. Thiopentone d. Glycopyrolate
10. **Muscle relaxant of choice in hepatic and renal failure** *[NBE DNB 2009]*
    a. Cis-atracurium b. Recuronium
    c. Vecuronium d. Rapacuronium
11. **Dibucaine number refers to** *[Recent Question 2016, 2012]*
    a. Ach cholinestrase activity derangement
    b. Potency of muscle relaxants
    c. Potency of general anaesthetics
    d. None
12. **Which of the following anaesthetic agent is contraindicated in renal failure?** *[NBE DNB 1997, 2000]*
    a. d-Tubocurarine b. Scoline
    c. Halothane d. Gallamine
13. **Use of Succinylcholine is not contraindicated in** *[NBE DNB 2007]*
    a. Tetanus b. Closed head injury
    c. Cerebral stroke d. Hepatic failure
14. **Suxamethonium can cause all except** *[NBE FMGE September 2012]*
    a. Hyperkalemia
    b. Tachycardia
    c. Raised intracranial tension
    d. Increased intraocular pressure
15. **Mivacurium false is** *[NBE DNB 2009]*
    a. Hypertension
    b. Increasing the dose produces rapid onset of action
    c. Bronchospasm
    d. Flushing
16. **Succinylcholine is used with caution in all except** *[Recent Question 2013]*
    a. Mysthenia gravis b. Burns
    c. Crush injury d. Tachycardia
17. **Train of fasciculations is seen in** *[NBE DNB 2008, 2010]*
    a. Mivacurium b. Succinylcholine
    c. Baclofen d. Gallamine
18. **Shortest acting Non-depolarizing muscle relaxant** *[NBE DNB 2009]*
    a. Succinyl choline b. Rapacuronium
    c. Atracurium d. Pancuronium
19. **Malignant hyperthermia is most commonly precipitated by** *[NBE DNB 1997, 2000, 2005, 2006, 2008]*
    a. Succinylcholine b. Dantrolene sodium
    c. Gallamine d. Pancuronium
20. **Agent causing malignant hyperthermia** *[Recent Question 2012]*
    a. Succinyl choline b. Dantrolene
    c. Gallamine d. Ketamine
21. **Regarding muscle relaxants which one of the following is true** *[NBE DNB June 2011]*
    a. Atracurium is contraindicated in renal failure
    b. Pancuronium causes bradycardia
    c. Cis-atracurium is a depolarizing muscle relaxant
    d. Vecuronium can be reversed by neostigmine
22. **Drug used to reverse the effect of d-tuborcurarine** *[NBE DNB 2001, 2005, 2007]*
    a. Neostigmine b. Physostigmine
    c. Dantrolene d. Scoline
23. **Which of the following skeletal muscle relaxants undergo Hoffman's elimination?** *[Recent Question 2016, 2012, 2013]*
    a. Atracurium b. Succinylcholine
    c. Mivacurium d. Vecuronium
24. **All are seen in Malignant hyperthermia except** *[NBE DNB 2009]*
    a. Bradycardia b. Hyperkalemia
    c. Metabolic acidosis d. Hypertension
25. **Which Anaesthetic agent is neither metabolized by liver nor by kidney?** *[Recent Question 2016, 2012]*
    a. Atracurium c. Pancuronium
    b. Vecuronium d. Rocuronium
26. **Which muscle relaxant increases intracranial pressure?** *[Recent Question 2017, NBE DNB 2007]*
    a. Mivacurium b. Atracurium
    c. Suxamethonium d. Vecuronium

27. Muscle relaxant used in renal failure *[Recent Question 2012]*
   a. Ketamine
   b. Atracurium
   c. Pancuronium
   d. Fentanyl

28. Regarding muscle relaxants which one of the following is true *[NBE DNB June 2011]*
   a. Atracurium is contraindicated in renal failure
   b. Pancuronium causes bradycardia
   c. Cis- atracurium is a depolarizing muscle relaxant
   d. Vecuronium can be reversed by neostigmine

29. Long acting Non-depolarizing competitive blocker is *[Recent Question 2016, 2015]*
   a. Doxacurium   b. Rocuronium
   c. Mivacurium   d. Atracurium

30. Muscle relaxant ideal for rapid intubation and short procedures is *[UPSC CMS 2015]*
   a. Vecuronium   b. Atracurium
   c. Rocuronium   d. Suxamethonium

31. Site of action of Vecuronium is? *[Recent Question 2017]*
   a. Cerebrum   b. Reticular formation
   c. Motor neuron   d. Neuro-muscular junction

32. Effects of d-Tubocurarine are reversed by? *[Recent Question 2017]*
   a. Atropine   b. Neostigmine
   c. Succinylcholine   d. Barbiturates

33. Which of the following agent is associated with maximum Histamine release? *[Recent Question 2017]*
   a. d-Tubocurarine   b. Cisatracurium
   c. Pancronium   d. Rocuronium

34. A patient with normal Succinylcholine metabolism will have Dibucaine number between *[Recent Question 2017]*
   a. 20-30   b. 40-45
   c. 50-60   d. 70-80

35. Succinylcholine is contraindicated in? *[Recent Question 2017]*
   a. Hyperkalemia   b. Hypokalemia
   c. Hypercalcemia   d. Hypocalcemia

36. True about Dibucaine number is? *[Recent Question 2017]*
   a. Used to measure the activity of normal psuedocholinesetrase
   b. Normal dibucaine number is 50
   c. Mivacurium inhibits pseudocholinesterase
   d. None of the above

37. What is mechanism of action of Curonium drugs as muscle relaxant? *[Recent Question 2018]*
   a. Persistently depolarizing at neuromuscular junction
   b. Act competitively on Ach receptors blocking post-synaptically
   c. Repetitive stimulation of Ach receptors on muscle end plate
   d. Inhibiting the calcium channel on presynaptic membrane

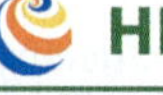 HIGH YIELD MCQs 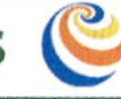

1. Muscle relaxant ideal for rapid intubation and short procedures is *[UPSC CMS 2016]*
   a. Vecuronium   b. Atracurium
   c. Rocuronium   d. Suxamethonium

2. All of the following act on Neuromuscular junction except? *[AIIMS May 2016]*
   a. Pipercurium   b. Dantrolene sodium
   c. Succinyl choline   d. Mivacurium

3. Which of the following skeletal muscle relaxants undergo Hoffman's elimination? *[PGI 2007, CGPG 2015]*
   a. Atracurium   b. Cis-atracurium
   c. Mivacurium   d. Vecuronium

4. Which of the following is the neuromuscular blocking agent with the shortest onset of action? *[AIIMS PGMEE 2006]*
   a. Mivocurium   b. Vecuronium
   c. Rapacuronium   d. Succinylcholine

5. Which ones are non-depolarising muscle relaxants? *[Recent Question 2016, PGI 2009]*
   a. Mivacurium   b. Halothane
   c. Desflurane   d. Isoflurane
   e. Ether

6. About malignant hyperthermia true *[PGI 2008]*
   a. Succinylcholine & Halothane predisposes
   b. Dantrolene useful in all cases
   c. Ketanserine can be used as an alternative o Dantrolene
   d. Propofol is safe
   e. Muscle biopsy is diagnostic

7. Treatment of malignant Hyperthermia includes *[PGI 2008]*
   a. Dantrolene
   b. Cooling
   c. Deepening plane of inhalational anaesthesia
   d. Discontinue inhalational anesthesia
   e. Give O_2 therapy with 100% O_2

8. Neostigmine is used for reversing the adverse effect of *[PGI 1997]*
   a. dTC and pancuronium   b. dTC only
   c. Alcuronium only   d. Ketamine complication

9. Site of action of Vecuronium is *[AIIMS PGMEE 1996]*
   a. Cerebrum   b. Ganglion
   c. Motor end plate   d. Myoneural

10. Muscle pain after anaesthesia is caused by *[PGI 1999]*
   a. Vecuronium   b. D-tubocurare
   c. Suxamethonium   d. All of the above

11. Bradycardia is common after injection of *[AIIMS PGMEE 2005]*
   a. Midazolam   b. Succinylcholine
   c. Dopamine   d. Isoprenaline

12. Which muscle relaxant increases intracranial pressure? *[AIIMS PGMEE 2002]*
   a. Mivacurium   b. Atracurium
   c. Suxamethonium   d. Vecuronium

13. Post-anaesthetic muscle soreness is caused by *[AIIMS PGMEE 1994]*
   a. Gallamine   b. d-TC
   c. Suxamethonium   d. Dantrolene

14. Fasciculation are caused by *[All India PGMEE 1997]*
a. Suxamethonium b. Pancuronium
c. d-TC d. Vecuronium

15. Hyperkalemia due to scoline is seen in all except
a. Crush injury b. Burn *[AIIMS PGMEE 2000]*
c. Abdominal sepsis d. Muscular dystrophy

16. Shortest acting muscle relaxant *[All India PGMEE 1997]*
a. Succinyl choline b. d-TC
c. Gallamine d. Ketamine

17. Cardiovascular side effects are minimal with *[PGI 2002, 2006]*
a. Pancuronium b. Rocuronium
c. Doxacurium d. Vecuronium
e. Mivacurium

18. Muscle relaxant of choice in hepatic and renal failure *[AIIMS PGMEE 2007]*
a. Cis-atracurium b. Rocuronium
c. Vecuronium d. Rapacuronium

19. Malignant hyperthermia is most common with *[AIIMS PGMEE 1993]*
a. Succinylcholine b. Gallamine
c. Dantrolene d. Ketamine

20. Drug causing anaphylactoid reaction *[PGI 1998]*
a. Propofol b. Alcuronium
c. Thiopentone d. Glycepyrrolate

21. Shortest acting non depolarizing muscle relaxant *[Recent Question 2016, All India PGMEE 2003, AIIMS 1998]*
a. Mivacurium b. Vercuronium
c. Atracurium d. Succinylcholine

22. Muscle relaxant contraindicated in Renal failure is *[All India PGMEE 1991, 1995, 1999]*
a. Gallamine b. d-TC
c. Vecuronism d. Atracurium

23. All of the following statements about neuromuscular blockage produced by succinylcholine are true, Except *[All India PGMEE 2010]*
a. No fade on Train of four stimulation
b. Fade on titanic stimulation
c. No post titanic facilitation
d. Train of four ratio >0.4

24. Features of depolarizing neuromuscular blocking agents are all/except *[PGI 2000, JIPMER PGMEE 1999]*
a. Cause muscle fasciculation
b. No fade c. No post titanic facilitation
d. Isoflurane potentiates e. Reversed by neostigmine

25. For non-depolarization block which of the following statement is correct *[AIIMS PGMEE 1993]*
a. Post titanic potentiation is seen
b. Tetanic fade is absent
c. Train of four is absent
d. Anticholinergic drugs potentiation of block

26. Phase II block is seen in *[AIIMS PGMEE 1998]*
a. Sexamethonium (Sch) b. d-TC
c. Ether d. N_2O

27. The administration of succinylocholine to a paraplegic patient led to the appearance of dysarrhythmias, conduction abnormalities and finally cardiac arrest. The most likely cause is *[AIIMS PGMEE 2003]*
a. Hypercalcemia b. Hyperkalemia
c. Anaphylaxis d. Hypermagnesemia

28. True about non-depolarizing muscle relaxants *[PGI 2005]*
a. Competitive inhibitor of acetylcholine
b. Metabolised by pseudocholinesterase
c. Mg^{2+} predisposes the block
d. Ca^{2+} antagonizes the block
e. Hypothermia prolongs the block

29. True about scoline are following except *[PGI 1997]*
a. Fasciculations
b. ICT increases
c. Non-depolarizing neuro muscular blocker
d. Short acting muscle relaxant

30. A 25 year old overweight female was given fentanyl-pancuronium anesthesia for surgery. After surgery and extubation she was observed to have limited movement of the upper body and chest wall in the recovery room. She was conscious and alert but voluntary respiratory effect was limited. Her blood pressure and heart rate were normal. The likely diagnosis is *[All India PGMEE 2010]*
a. Incomplete reversal of pancuronium
b. Pulmonary embolism
c. Fentanyl induced chest wall rigidity
d. Respiratory depression

31. Phase II blocker is *[PGI 1998]*
a. D-TC b. Cocaine
c. Scoline d. Vencuronium

32. All of the following statements are incorrect about the treatment of prolonged suxamethoniumapnoea due to plasma cholinesterase deficiency (after a single dose of suxamethonium) except- *[AIIMS PGMEE 2004]*
a. Reversal with incremental doses of neostigmine
b. Continue anaesthesia and mechanical ventilation till recovery
c. Transfussion of fresh frozen plasma
d. Plasmapheresis

33. Drugs metabolized by cholinesterase *[PGI 2004]*
a. Succinylcholine b. Mivacurium
c. Esmolol d. Remifentanyl
e. Ketamine

34. Myasthenics are resistant to following muscle relaxant *[PGI 2000]*
a. Suxamethonium b. Pancurium
c. Atracuronium d. Vecuronium

35. True about d-TC is all except *[PGI 1998]*
a. Excreted unchaged by kidney
b. Causes hypotension by ganglion blocking action
c. Vagolytic action
d. Effects lasts for 2-3 hours

36. The drug used for d-TC reversal is *[Recent Question 2016, All India PGMEE 1991]*
a. Atropine b. Atracurium
c. Diazepalm d. Neostigmine

37. Intubation dose of Pancuronium *[Recent Question 2017, AIIMS PGMEE 1993]*
a. 0.02 mg/Kg b. 0.04 mg/Kg
c. 0.06 mg/Kg d. 0.08 mg/Kg

38. Muscle Relaxant excreted exclusively by Kidney *[AIIMS PGMEE 1998]*
a. Gallamine b. Atracurium
c. Vercuronium d. SCh

39. Muscle relaxant most sensitive to patient of myasthenia gravis (MG) *[All India PGMEE 1993]*
a. Scoline b. Neostigmine
c. Gallamine d. Decamethonium

40. Mivacurium when given in high doses, all are true except *[AIIMS PGMEE 2007]*
a. Bronchospasm b. Hypertension
c. Flushing
d. Increase in dose increase the rapididity of onset

41. All of the following drugs are eliminated by kidney except *[AIIMS PGMEE 2004]*
a. Pancuronium bromide b. Atracuriumbesylate
c. Vecuronium bromide d. Pipecuronium

42. A 21 year old lady with a history of hypersensitivity to neostigmine is posted for an elective caesarean section under general anesthesia. The best muscle relaxant of choice in this patient should be *[AIIMS PGMEE 2004]*
a. Pancuronium b. Atracurium
c. Rocuronium d. Vecuronium

43. Ideal muscle relaxant used for a neonate undergoing porto-enterostomy for biliary atresia is *[AIIMS PGMEE 2003]*
a. Atracurium b. Vecuronium
c. Pancuronium d. Rocuronium

44. Which of the following statement is not correct for Vecuronium? *[AIIMS PGMEE 2002]*
a. It has high incidence of cardiovascular side effects
b. It has short duration of neuromuscular block
c. In usual doses the dose adjustment is not required in kidney disease
d. It has high liphophilic property

45. Muscle relaxant with ganglion blocker action are A/E *[Recent Question 2016, AIIMS PGMEE 1993]*
a. Pancuronium b. Trimethaphan
c. Curare d. Halothane

46. An ICU patient on atracurium infusion develops seizures after 2 days. The most probable cause is *[All India PGMEE 2006]*
a. Accumulation of landonosine
b. Allergy to drug c. Due to prolong infusion
d. None

47. A patient with bilirubin value of 8 mg/dl and serum creatinine of 1.9 mg/dl is planned for surgery. What is the muscle relaxant of choice in this patient *[All India PGMEE 2010]*
a. Vecuronium b. Pancuronium
c. Atracurium d. Rocuronium

48. At the end of a balanced anaesthesia technique with non-depolarizing muscle relaxant, a patient recovered spontaneously from the effect of muscle relaxant without any reversal. Which is the most probable relaxant the patient had received? *[All India PGMEE 2003]*
a. Pancuronium b. Gallamine
c. Atracurium d. Vecuronium

49. Muscle relaxant used in renal failure *[PGI 1997, 1999]*
a. Ketamine b. Atracurium
c. Pancuronium d. Fentanyl

50. Use of succinylcholine is not contraindicated in *[AIIMS PGMEE 2002]*
a. Tetanus b. Closed head injury
c. Cerebral stroke d. Hepatic failure

51. Adiminstration of Scoline (SCh) produces dangerous hyperkalemia in *[AIIMS PGMEE 1999]*
a. Acute Renal Failure (A.R.F.)
b. Raised ICT
c. Fracture femur d. Paraplegia

52. In myasthenia gravis, which drugs should not be used *[PGI 2002]*
a. Gallamine b. Neostigmine
c. Aminoglycosides d. Metronidazole
e. Ampiciliin

53. Shortest and fastest acting muscle relaxant is *[NIMHANS PGMEE 2014]*
a. Atracurium b. Pancuronium
c. Succinylcholine d. Decamethonium

54. A boy undergoes day care surgery with Propofol and Succinylcholine. After 8 hours, the boy experience pain on walking. Most probable cause is *[AIIMS November 2014]*
a. Propofol b. Succinylcholine
c. Early mobilisation d. Effect of eye surgery

55. Succinylcholine is not used in *[PGI November 2014]*
a. Renal failure b. Glaucoma
c. Tetanus d. CNS disease
e. Newborns

56. Long acting muscle relaxant is *[Recent Question 2014]*
a. Vecuronium b. Rocuronium
c. Atracurium d. Pancuronium

57. A 60 year old female was given anaesthesia for a prolonged surgery. After surgery she was extubated but was found to have poor respiration with BP of 100/80 mm of Hg. Blood analysis revealed PCO_2=200 and the blood pH was 7.42. What is the diagnosis? *[ESI IMO 2014]*
a. Respiratory failure
b. Intraoperative hypoxia
c. Incomplete recovery from muscle relaxants
d. None of these

58. Muscle relaxant that can be used in patient with high Serum bilirubin and Serum creatinine of 4.5 mg/dL is *[AIIMS PG May 2015]*
a. Atracurium b. Vecuronium
c. Pancuronium d. Mivacurium

59. Which Neuro-muscular blocking drug release Histamine? *[Recent Question 2016, PGMCET 2015]*
a. Pancuronium
b. Rocuronium
c. Vecuronium
d. Atracurium

 NEET/NBE PATTERN MCQs ANSWERS WITH EXPLANATIONS 

1. Ans. (c) Non-enzymatic degradation
[Ref. KDT, 6/e p345]

- Non-depolarising muscle relaxants atracurium and cisatracurium are broken down in plasma by enzymatic ester hydrolysis and by non-enzymatic alkaline degradation **(Hoffman elimination)** to their inactive products.
- Are not dependent on renal excretion for their termination of action, hence appear to be the agent of choice for renal failure patients

2. Ans. (a) Doxacurium
[Ref. Katzung, 11/e p348]

Doxacurium

- Benzyl-iso-quinolone derivative
- Release histamine
- **Most potent skeletal muscle relaxant**
- Elimination is through kidney
- **Longest acting nondepolarizing skeletal muscle relaxant**, which binds to cholinergic receptors on the motor end plate

3. Ans. (a) Mivacurium
[Ref. Katzung, 11/e p456]

- Mivacurium is another very short acting nondepolarizing muscle relaxant.
- Mivacurium has the **shortest duration of action** among all the non-depolarising drugs
- Action is same as succinylcholine terminated by Plasma pseudocholinesterase

4. Ans. (c) Mivacurium
[Ref. Katzung, 11/e p456]

Mivacurium

- Another very short acting nondepolarizing muscle relaxant
- Mivacurium has the shortest duration of action among all the non-depolarising drugs
- Action is same as succinylcholine and is used as an alternative
- Is a benzyl-iso-quinolone derivative
- Release histamine
- Terminated by Plasma pseudocholinesterase
- Its rapid onset allows it to be used as an alternative to succinylcholine in rapid-induction anaesthesia

5. Ans. (d) All of the above
[Ref. KDT, 7/e p344]

- **Succinylcholine (SCh)** is a depolarizing neuromuscular-blocking agent, which produce sustained opening of the nicotinic cholinergic receptor channel
  - Under normal conditions, post-junctional membrane depolarization results in leakage of potassium that produces an increase of 0.5–1.0 mEq/L in serum K+ concentration
  - When SCh depolarizes muscle that has been traumatized or denervated enough K+ may leak from cells to produce systemic hyperkalemia and cardiac arrest
  - This susceptibility to hyperkalemia is thought to be caused by proliferation of junctional and extrajunctional cholinergic receptors
- **Patient population at risk for SCh-induced hyperkalemia**:
  - Patients with upper motor neuron lesions resulting from stroke
  - Brain or spinal cord tumors
  - Intracerebral or spinal cord masses
  - Closed head injury, or encephalitis
  - Unhealed third-degree burns
  - Severe intra-abdominal infections
  - Severe metabolic acidosis with hypovolemia
  - Crush injuries
  - Prolonged nondepolarizing muscle blockade or immobility

6. Ans. (a) Hypertension
[Ref. KDT, 6/e p345]

Mivacurium

- Long acting non-depolarizing (competitive) NM blocking agents require reversal with neostigmine
- It has the potential to cause histamine release, causing facial erythema and reduce BP
- Shortest acting NDMR
- It does not require reversal due to its short duration of action
- Can be used in Day care surgery

7. Ans. (d) Vecuronium can be reversed by Neostigmine
[Ref. KDT, 6/e p339-345]

Vecuronium

- *Most commonly used muscle relaxant for routine surgery*
- *Muscle relaxant of choice for cardiac patients*: **Cardiovascular stability**
- *Safe in hepatic failure*
- *Avoided in Biliary obstruction*: 40% excreted in bile
- *Causes polyneuropathy on long term use*: Accumulation of 3-hydroxy metabolite
- *Reversal by Neostigmine required*: Only if repeated doses given

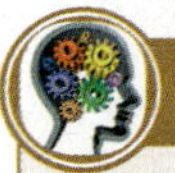

Also Remember

- **Pancuronium:**
  - *Avoided in Renal failure*: 80–90% excreted by kidneys
  - *Useful in asthma patients*: Histamine release is rare
  - *Increased chances of cardiac arrhythmias with Halothane*: Due to vagal block leading to tachycardia and hypertension
- **Atracurium:**
  - Spontaneous degradation by *'Hoffmann's elimination'*
  - *Relaxant of choice in*:
    1. Hepatic failure
    2. Renal failure
    3. Myasthenia gravis
    4. Newborns and old age
- Cis-atracurium (non-depolarising agent):
  - *Cardiovascular stability*: Does not release histamine

Anesthesiology

8. Ans. (b) Suxamethonium
[Ref. Ajay Yadav, 4/e. p97]
- Suxamethonium mainly muscle pain/ myalgia/ muscle soreness

9. Ans. (b) Alcuronium
[Ref. Ajay Yadav, 4/e. p102]
- **Alcuronium**: Anaphylactic reactions have been reported, hence not used nowadays

10. Ans. (a) Cis-atracurium
[Ref. Ajay Yadav, 4/e. p101]

11. Ans. (a) Ach cholinesterase activity derangement
[Ref. Ajay Yadav, 4/e. p98]
- **Dibucaine** is a local anaesthetic which can inhibit 80% of normal enzyme and 20% of abnormal enzyme
- **Normal dibucaine number** is homozygous typical (normal person) is 70 to 80%

12. Ans. (d) Gallamine
[Ref. Ajay Yadav, 4/e. p102]
- More than 80% is excreted by kidney, hence contraindicated in renal disease.

13. Ans. (c) Cerebral stroke
[Ref. Ajay Yadav, 4/e. p98]

14. Ans. (b) Tachycardia
[Ref. Ajay Yadav, 4/e. p97]
- Suxamethonium causes bradycardia, hyperkalemia, increased ICT, increased IOT, muscle pain, malignant hyperthermia, anaphylaxis, massester spasm

15. Ans. (a) Hypertension; (b) Increasing the dose produces rapid onset of action
[Ref. Ajay Yadav, 4/e. p101]

16. Ans. (d) Tachycardia
[Ref. Ajay Yadav, 4/e. p97]

17. Ans. (b) Succinylcholine
[Ref. Ajay Yadav, 4/e. p97]
- Excessive availability of SCh at NM junction produces repeated depolarization and contractions (fasciculations)

18. Ans. (b) Rapacuronium
[Ref. Ajay Yadav, 4/e. p103]
- Rapacuronium, Atracrium are short acting (10-15 mins)
- Mivacurium is shortest acting (5-10 mins)

19. Ans. (a) Succinylcholine
[Ref. Ajay Yadav, 4/e. p97]

20. Ans. (a) Succinylcholine
[Ref. Ajay Yadav, 4/e. p97]

21. Ans. (d) Vecuronium can be reversed by neostigmine
[Ref. Ajay Yadav, 4/e. p104]

22. Ans. (a) Neostigmine
[Ref. Ajay Yadav, 4/e. p104]

23. Ans. (a) Atracurium
[Ref. Ajay Yadav, 4/e. p101]
- Atracurium undergoes Hoffman degradation (95%) and ester hydrolysis (5%) in plasma

24. Ans. (a) Bradycardia
[Ref. Ajay Yadav, 4/e. p115]
- **Clinical features of Malignant Hypothermia**: Hyperthermia (> 109° F), Increased end tidal CO_2 **(Most sensitive early sign)**, Hypoxia, Cyanosis, Tachycardia, Hypertension, Cardiac arrhythmias, Severe metabolic acidosis, Hyperkalemia, Muscle rigidity, Increased creatinine phosphokinase, Increased myoglobin, Renal failure, DIC, Pulmonary and Cerebral oedema, DeatH

25. Ans. (a) Atracurium
[Ref. Ajay Yadav, 4/e. p101]

26. Ans. (c) Suxamethonium
[Ref. Ajay Yadav, 4/e. p97]

27. Ans. (b) Atracurium
[Ref. Ajay Yadav, 4/e. p101]

28. Ans. (d) Vecuronium can be reversed by neostigmine
[Ref. Ajay Yadav, 4/e. p104]

29. Ans. (a) Doxacurium
[Ref. Pharmacology by KDT, 7/e p347]
- Long acting nondepolarizing (Competitive) blockers: d-Tubocurarine, Pancuronium, Doxacurium, Pipecuronium

30. Ans. (d) Suxamethonium
[Ref. Baliey & Love, 26/e p241]

31. Ans. (d) Neuromuscular junction
[Ref. Clinical Anesthesia by Barash, 6/e p514]

Vecuronium–Mechanism of Action

- Bisquaternary nitrogen compound
- **Acts by competitively binding to Nicotinic cholinergic receptors**
- Binding of Vecuronium decreases the opportunity for Acetylcholine to bind to the Nicotinic receptor at the post-junctional membrane of the Myoneural junction

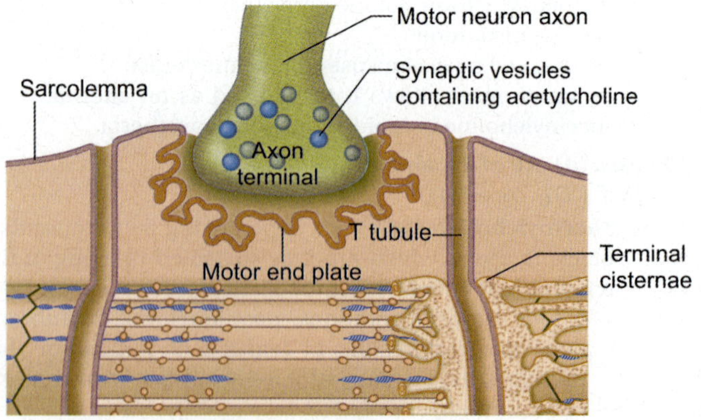

Fig. Neuromuscular Junction

32. Ans. (b) Neostigmine
[Ref. Clinical Anesthesia by Barash, 6/e p525]
- Tubocurarine is the prototype non-depolarizing skeletal muscle relaxants

- Because the binding of d-Tubocurarine is competitive, its effects can be rapidly reversed by administering a cholinesterase inhibitor (e.g. Neostigmine), which increase synaptic levels of acetylcholine

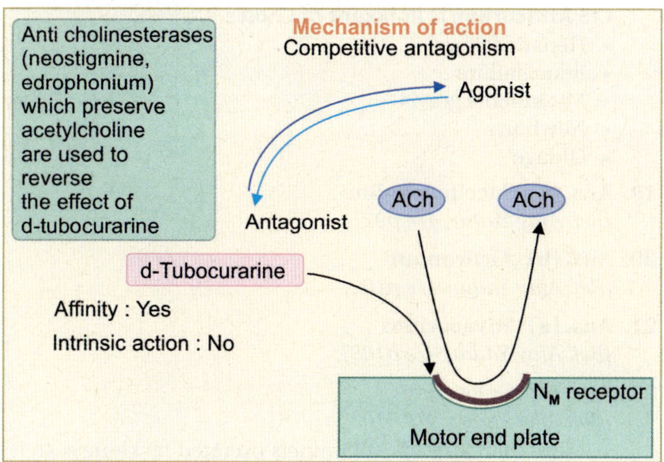

Fig. d-TC and neostigmine

33. Ans. (a) d-Tubocurarine

[Ref. Pharmacology by Seth, 3/e pIII.28]

- Benzylisoquinoline compounds have a tendency to cause histamine release
- Agents include d-Tubocurarine, Metocurine, Atracurium, cis-Atracurium, Doxacurium, Mivacurium
- Extent of this effect may vary with **maximum histamine release occurring with d-Tubocurarine and least with cis-Atracurium**

34. Ans. (d) 70-80

[Ref. Anesthesia by Stern, 1/e p456]

- Dibucaine number is the percentage inhibition of Cholinesterase enzyme by Dibucaine
- It inhibits normal enzyme to the extent of 80% and abnormal enzyme to the extent of 20%
- Patient having lesser Dibucaine number (decrease in plasma cholinesterase) will have a prolonged block
- A patient who is homozygous for the abnormal gene will have a Dibucaine number of 70-80 (representing the percentage inhibition by Dibucaine)
- Heterozygous individuals will have intermediate Dibucaine numbers (50-60)

35. Ans. (a) Hyperkalemia

[Ref. Ajay Yadav, 4/e p98]

- Contraindication of Succinylcholine include Hyperkalemia, Head injury, Newborn and infant, Glaucoma and eye injuries, Upto 2-3 months after trauma, Upto 6 months after hemiplegia, Upto 1 year after burn, Renal failure, Prolonged intraabdominal infection, Diagnosed case of atypical case pseudocholinesterase and low pseudocholinesterase, Duchenne muscular dystrophy, Tetanus, Guillain barre syndrome, Metabolic acidosis, Shock, Spinal cord injury

36. Ans. (c) Mivacurium inhibits pseudocholinesterase

[Ref. Anesthesia by Stern, 1/e p456]

- Dibucaine number is proportional to Pseudocholinesterase function and independent of the amount of enzyme
- Dibucaine number provides a qualitative estimate the adequacy of Pseudocholinesterase
- Mivacurium has spontaneous hydrolysis in plasma by Pseudocholinesterase like Succinylcholine, but slightly at slower rate (at about 80% of the rate of metabolism of succinylcholine)

37. Ans. (b) Act competitively on Ach receptors blocking post-synaptically

[Ref. Respiratory Care by Kacmarek, 4/e p317]

- Neuromuscular Blocking Agents (Curonium drugs) mechanism of action is Competitive inhibition of acetylcholine at muscle post- synaptic receptor sites
- Competitive inhibition ensures their effects are dose related
- The muscle tissue itself remains sensitive to external stimulus

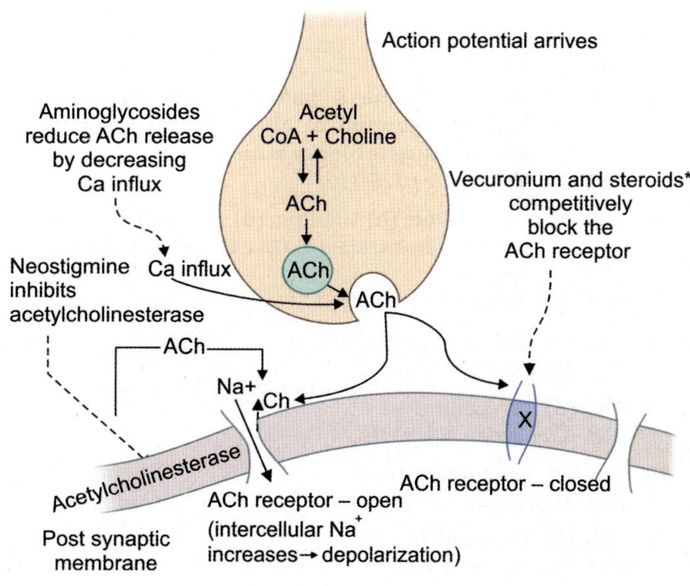

Fig. Mechanism of action—Curonium drugs

HIGH YIELD MCQs ANSWERS WITH EXPLANATIONS 

1. Ans. (d) Suxamethonium

[Ref. Anaesthesia for Postgraduates by Agasti, 1/e p449,450]

Suxamethonium/ Succinylcholine

- **MC used Depolarizing agent**
- **Shortest and fastest acting SMR**
- Due to its quick onset of action, very short duration and spontaneous recovery, it is the preferred SMR for Endotracheal intubation

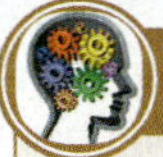

Also Remember

- **Suxamethonium is metabolized by pseudocholinesterase** that may be non-functioning (atypical pseudocholinesterase) in some individuals
  - This is a genetic condition and may result in prolonged apnea on SCh administration (due to decreased metabolism, action of SCh is prolonged)
- Activity of atypical enzyme can be assessed by Dibucaine number
- Adverse effects of Suxamethonium: Muscle pain, Hyperkalemia, Prolonged apnoea, Life threatening Malignant hyperthermia

2. Ans. (b) **Dantrolene sodium**
[Ref. Essentials of Medicinal Chemistry by Korolkovas, 2/e p236]

Dantrolene Sodium

- Is a hydantoin derivative that does not block neuromuscular transmission but causes muscle weakness by direct muscular action.
- Dantrolene is the **only drug that has been shown to be effective in reversing the symptoms of malignant hyperthermia**, with its ability to reduce efflux of Calcium from the sarcoplasmic reticulum, in the presence of abnormal Ryanodine receptor

3. Ans. (a) **Atracurium; (b) Cis atracurium**
[Ref. Ajay Yadav, 4/e p101]

4. Ans. (d) **Succinlycholine**
[Ref. Ajay Yadav, 4/e p97]
- Onset of action is 20-30 seconds

5. Ans. (a) **Mivacurium**
[Ref. Ajay Yadav, 4/e p101]

6. Ans. (a) **Succinylcholine & halothane predisposes; (b) Dantroleneusefull in all cases; (d) Propofol is safe; (e) Muscle biopsy is diagnostic**
[Ref. Ajay Yadav, 4/e p115-116]

7. Ans. (a) **Dantrolene; (b) Cooling; (d) Discontinue inhalational anaesthesia; (e) Give O_2 therapy with 100% oxygen**
[Ref. Ajay Yadav, 4/e p115-116]

8. Ans. (a) **dTC and pancuronium**
[Ref. Ajay Yadav, 4/e p104]

9. Ans. (d) **Myoneural**
[Ref. Ajay Yadav, 4/e p99]

10. Ans. (c) **Suxamethonium**
[Ref. Ajay Yadav, 4/e p97]

11. Ans. (b) **Succinylcholine**
[Ref. Ajay Yadav, 4/e p97]

12. Ans. (c) **Suxamethonium**
[Ref. Ajay Yadav, 4/e p97]

13. Ans. (c) **Suxamethonium**
[Ref. Ajay Yadav, 4/e p97]

14. Ans. (a) **Suxamethonium**
[Ref. Ajay Yadav, 4/e p97]

15. Ans. (c) **Abdominal sepsis**
[Ref. Pharmacology in Anesthesia Practice by Gupta, 1/e p25]

16. Ans. (a) **Succinylcholine**
[Ref. Ajay Yadav, 4/e p97]

17. Ans. (b) **Rocuronium; (c) Doxacurium; (d) Vecuronium**
[Ref. Ajay Yadav, 4/e p100]

18. Ans. (a) **Cis atracurium**
[Ref. Ajay Yadav, 4/e p101]

CIS Atracurium is Relaxant of Choice
- Hepatic failure
- Renal failure
- Myasthenia gravis
- Newborn
- Oldage

19. Ans. (a) **Succinylcholine**
[Ref. Ajay Yadav, 4/e p97]

20. Ans. (b) **Alcuronium**
[Ref. Ajay Yadav, 4/e p102]

21. Ans. (a) **Mivacurium**
[Ref. Ajay Yadav, 4/e p103]

22. Ans. (a) **Gallamine**
[Ref. Ajay Yadav, 4/e p102]
- More than 80% of Gallamineis excreted by kidneys so it is contraindicated in renal diseases.

23. Ans. (b) **Fade on titanic stimulation**
[Ref. Ajay Yadav, 4/e p54]

24. Ans. (e) **Reversed by neostigmine**
[Ref. Ajay Yadav, 4/e p54]

25. Ans. (a) **Post tetanic potential is seen**
[Ref. Ajay Yadav, 4/e p54]

26. Ans. (a) **Sch**
[Ref. Ajay Yadav, 4/e p99]
- Phase II Block: It is also called as **dual block**
- Succinylcholine showing fading on train of four response is pathognomic of phase II block

27. Ans. (b) **Hyperkalemia**
[Ref. Ajay Yadav, 4/e p97]

28. Ans. (a) **Competitive inhibitor of acetylcholine; (c) Mg^{2+} predisposes the block; (d) Ca^{2+} antagonizes the block; (e) Hypothermia prolongs the block**
[Ref. Ajay Yadav, 4/e p99-102]

29. Ans. (c) **Non depolarizing neuro muscular blockade**
[Ref. Ajay Yadav, 4/e p96]

30. Ans. (a) **Incomplete reversal of pancuronium**
[Ref. Ajay Yadav, 4/e p102]

31. Ans. (c) **Scoline**
[Ref. Ajay Yadav, 4/e p99]

32. Ans. (b) **Continue anaesthesia and mechanical ventilation till recovery**
[Ref. Ajay Yadav, 4/e p102]

33. Ans. (a) **Succinylcholine; (b)**
[Ref. Ajay Yadav, 4/e p101]

34. Ans. (a) **Suxamethonium**
[Ref. Ajay Yadav, 4/e p97]

35. Ans. (d) **Effects last for 2-3 hours**
[Ref. Ajay Yadav, 4/e p100]

36. Ans. (d) **Neostigmine**
[Ref. Ajay Yadav, 4/e p102]

37. Ans. (d) 0.08 mg/Kg
[Ref. Ajay Yadav, 4/e p99]

38. Ans. (a) Gallamine
[Ref. Ajay Yadav, 4/e p99]
- More than 80% of Gallamineis excreted through kidney, so contraindicated in renal diseases

39. Ans. (c) Gallamine
[Ref. Ajay Yadav, 4/e p154]
- Potent and longacting non-depolarizing agent like Tubocurae, Gallamine, Metocurine and Pancuronium are very sensitive to myasthenia gravis patients and should not be used

40. Ans. (b) Hypertension
[Ref. Ajay Yadav, 4/e p102]

41. Ans. (b) Atracuriumbesylate
[Ref. Ajay Yadav, 4/e p101]
- Atracurium metabolism is independent of renal and hepatic function.

42. Ans. (b) Atracurium
[Ref. Ajay Yadav, 4/e p101]

43. Ans. (a) Atracurium
[Ref. Ajay Yadav, 4/e p101]

44. Ans. (a) It has high incidence of cardiovascular side effects
[Ref. Ajay Yadav, 4/e p100]
- Vecuronium is muscle relaxant of choice for cardiac patient

45. Ans. (d) Halothane
[Ref. Ajay Yadav, 4/e p103]

46. Ans. (a) Accumulation of landonosine
[Ref. Ajay Yadav, 4/e p101]

47. Ans. (c) Atracurium
[Ref. Ajay Yadav, 4/e p101]
- Atracurium metabolism is independent of renal and hepatic function (undergoes Hoffman degradation)

48. Ans. (c) Atracurium
[Ref. Ajay Yadav, 4/e p101]

49. Ans. (b) Atracurium
[Ref. Ajay Yadav, 4/e p101]

50. Ans. (d) Hepatic failure
[Ref. Ajay Yadav, 4/e p97]

51. Ans. (d) Paraplegia
[Ref. Ajay Yadav, 4/e p98]
- **Succinylcholine is contraindicated**
  - Upto 2-3 months after trauma
  - Upto 6 months after hemiplegia/ paraplegi(a)
  - Upto 1 year after burns (the greatest risk is between 1 week to 2 months)

Also Remember

- In these conditions denervated/ regenerating nerve develops extrajunctional receptors which can produce hyperkalemia

52. Ans. (a) Gallamine; (c) Aminoglycosides
[Ref. Ajay Yadav, 4/e p154]

53. Ans. (c) Succinylcholine
[Ref. Ajay Yadav, 4/e p97]

54. Ans. (b) Succinylcholine
[Ref. Ajay Yadav, 4/e p97]
- **Post-operative Muscle soreness (Myalgia) after Succinylcholine**:
  - Common complication: Incidence 40-50%
  - Underlying cause: Excessive muscle contractions
  - Reduction modalities:
    1. Precurarization
    2. Self-taming (1/10th dose given 30-60 seconds prior to full dose)
    3. NSAIDs

55. Ans. ALL CHOICES
[Ref. Ajay Yadav, 4/e p98]

Contraindications to Succinylcholine
- **Hyperkalemia**
- Head injury (Increases ICT)
- Glaucoma, Eye injuries
- Newborns, Infants (Extrajunctional receptors produce Hyperkalemia)
- Post injury (2-3 months post-trauma, 0-6 months after hemiplegia/ paraplegia, 0-12 months after burns)
- Renal failure
- Abdominal infection (prolonged)
- Duchenne muscular dystrophy
- Dystrophicamyotonica
- Atypical/ low pseudocholinsterase
- Tetanus
- Guillain Barre syndrome
- Metabolic acidosis
- Shock
- Spina cord injury

56. Ans. (d) Pancuronium
[Ref. Ajay Yadav, 4/e p99]

Non-Depolarising Competitive Blockers

Long acting	Intermediate acting	Short acting
d-Tubocuranine Pancuronium Doxacurium Pipecuronium	Vecuronium Atracurium Cis-atracurium Rocuronium Rapacuronium	Mivacurium

57. Ans. (c) Incomplete recovery from muscle relaxants
[Ref. Pediatric Anesthesia by Paul, 2/e p87]

58. Ans. (a) Atracurium
[Ref. Anesthesia by Yadav, 4/e p101]
- Metabolism of Atracurium is independent of Renal and Hepatic functions
- **Atracurium is relaxant of choice in**:
  - Renal failure
  - Hepatic failure
  - Myasthenia gravis
  - Newborn
  - Old age

59. Ans. (d) Atracurium
[Ref. Anesthesia by Yadav, 4/e p101]
- Atracurium causes histamine release and may produce hypotension and tachycardia
- Cis-atracurium causes less histamine release

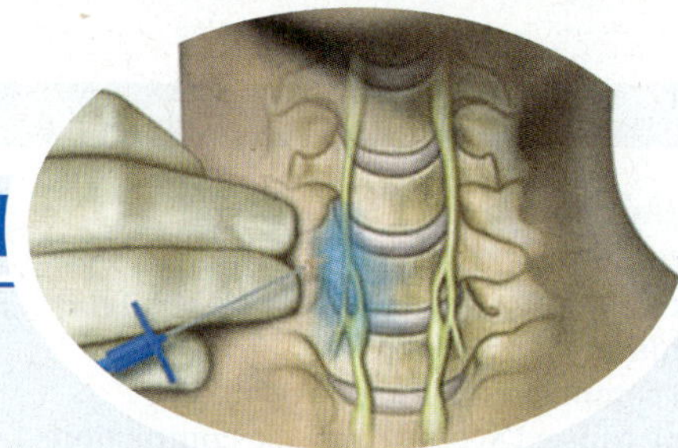

Chapter 8

Spinal, Epidural and Other Specific Anesthesia

THEORETICAL CONCEPTS

VIII A. EPIDURAL (EXTRADURAL/PERIDURAL) ANESTHESIA

- ***Indications***:
  - ***Postoperative pain control: Main indication***[Q]
  - Painless labour[Q]
  - All general surgeries
  - Chronic pain control in cancers and chronic conditions
  - Occlusive vascular conditions
  - Blood patch for post-spinal headache
- ***Needles***:
  - **Tuohy's needle (Most commonly used[Q])**
  - Weiss needle
  - Crawford needle
- ***Technique***:
  - **Loss of resistance technique (Most common technique[Q])**
  - Hanging drop technique
- ***Drugs used***:
  - Lignocaine 1–2%[Q]
  - Bupivacaine 0.25–0.5%[Q]
  - Fentanyl
  - Tramadol
- ***Most important factor affecting the level of spread***: Volume of drug
- ***Complications***:
  - Inadequate block
  - Hypotension[Q]

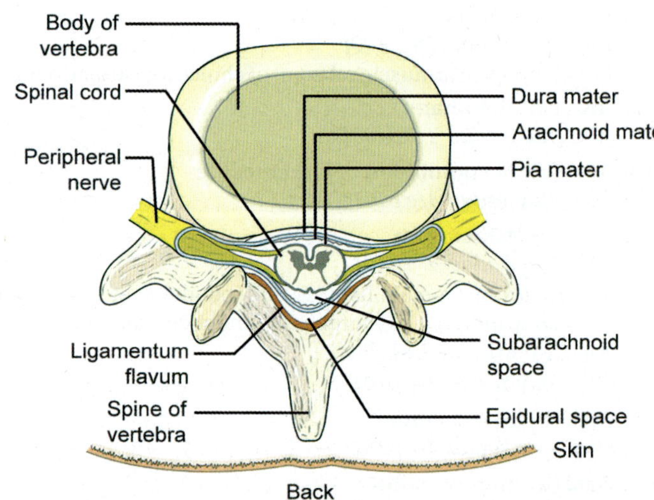

Fig. Epidural space

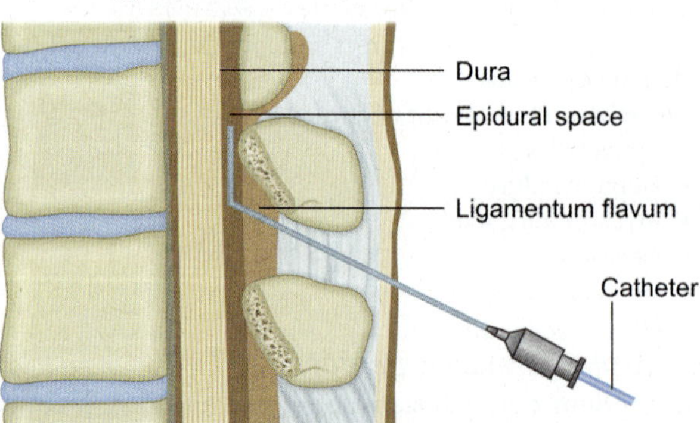

Fig. Epidural anesthesia

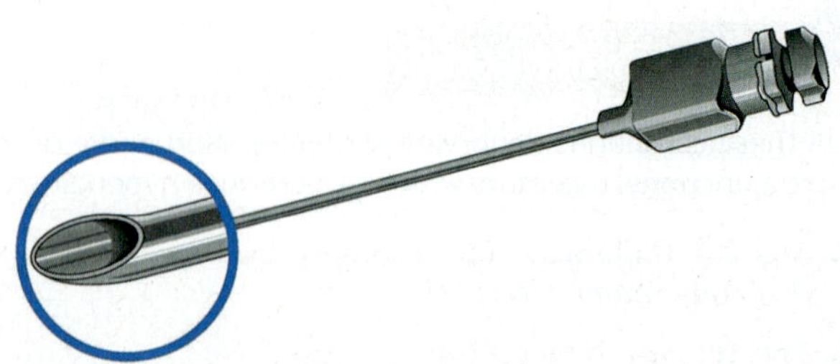

Fig. Tuohy needle

- Apnoea
- Total spinal/ Subdural puncture/ Dural puncture
- Intravascular injection[Q]
- Epidural hematoma, Epidural abscess[Q]
- Trigeminal nerve palsy

- ***Contraindications***:
  - Bleeding disorders[Q]
  - Raised intracranial tension[Q]
- ***Advantages***:
  - Lesser hypotension
  - No post-spinal headache
  - Level of block is changeable
  - Any duration of surgery can be performed
- ***Disadvantages***:
  - Expensive
  - Technical expertise required
  - High incidence of epidural hematoma

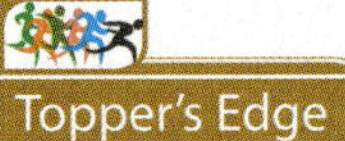

Topper's Edge

Contraindications to Neuraxial Blockade

Absolute C/I[Q]	Relative C/I	Controversial C/I
Infection at site of injection	Sepsis	Prior back surgery at site of injection
Patient refusal	Uncooperative patient	Complicated surgery
Coagulopathy/ bleeding diathesis	Preexisting neurological deficits	Prolonged operation
Severe hypovolemia	Demyelinating lesions	Major blood loss
Increased ICP	Stenotic valvular heart lesions	Maneuvers compromising respiration
Severe aortic stenosis	Left ventricular outflow obstruction	
Severe mitral stenosis	Severe spinal deformity	

VIII B. COMPARISON OF SPINAL AND EPIDURAL ANESTHESIA[Q]

Parameter	Spinal anesthesia	Epidural anesthesia
Level performed	Lumbar	Any level
Cost	Cheaper	Expensive
Onset of effect	2–3 minutes	15–20 minutes
Duration of effect[Q]	Lesser	Prolonged
Quality of block	Total	Patchy
Post spinal headache[Q]	**Present**	Absent
Epidural hematoma[Q]	Less common	**More common**
Total spinal[Q]	Rare	**High chances**
Intravascular injection[Q]	Rare	**High chances**
Drug toxicity	Less common	More common
Catheter complications	Absent	Present

Anesthesiology

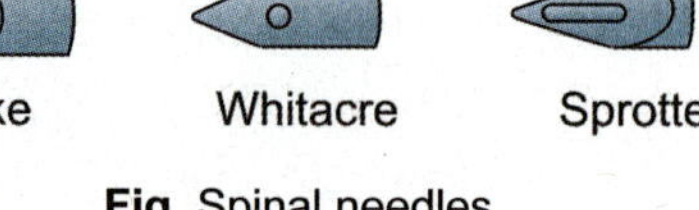

Fig. Spinal needles

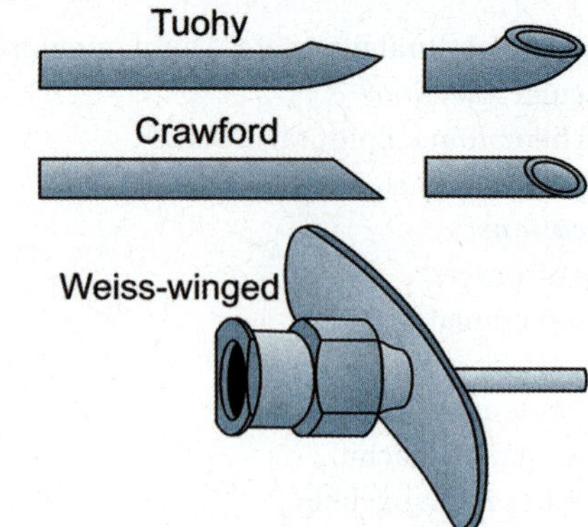

Fig. Epidural needles

VIII C. SPINAL EPIDURAL ABSCESS

- ***Causes of Spinal epidural abscess*:**
  - Hematogenous seeding: 50% cases[Q]
  - Direct extension of local infection: 10–30%
  - Invasive procedures: 15–20%
  - Unidentified causes: 10–30%
- ***Organisms causing Spinal epidural abscesses*:**
  - **Staphylococcus aureus (Most common cause)**
  - Streptococcus
  - Enterobacteriaceae
  - Coagulase negative staphylococci
  - Other causes
- ***Risk factors*:**
  - **Diabetes mellitus (Most common risk factor[Q])**
  - Trauma
  - Alcoholism
  - Pregnancy
  - Immunosuppression
- *Anatomy*: Mainly posterior location in thoracic or lumbar areas
- *Treatment*: Combined medical-surgical approach
- Urgent decompressive laminectomy[Q]

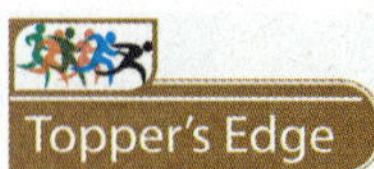
Topper's Edge

Peripheral Nerve Blocks

Techniques	**Upper Extremity Peripheral Nerve Blocks**
Field block technique Paresthesia technique Nerve stimulation technique Ultrasound technique Continuous peripheral nerve blocks	Interscalene block Supraclavicular block Infraclavicular block Axillary block Blocks of terminal nerves
Lower Extremity Peripheral Nerve Blocks	**Peripheral Nerve Blocks of Trunk**
Femoral nerve block Lateral femoral cutaneous nerve block Obturator nerve block Posterior lumbar plexus block Saphenous nerve block Sciatic nerve block Ankle block	Superficial cervical plexus block Intercostal block Paravertebral block Transversus abdominis plane block

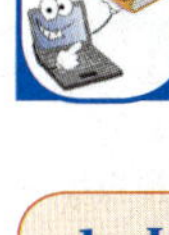

IMAGE-BASED QUESTIONS

1. Identify the Instrument/device shown in Photograph

a. Weiss needle
b. Hustead needle
c. Tuohy needle
d. Crawford needle

2. Which of the following is not true regarding the procedure done with the needle shown below? ***[AIIMS May 2017]***

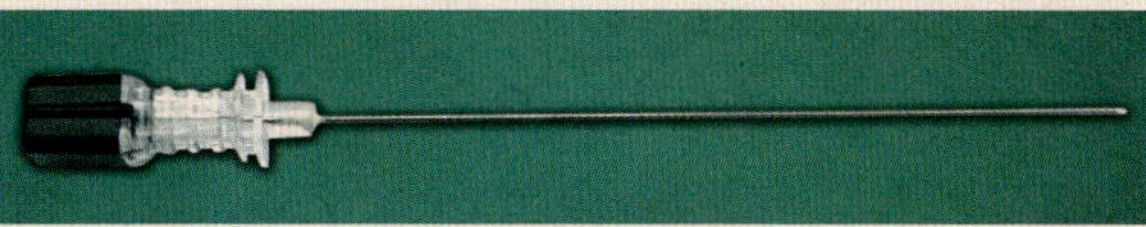

a. Breath holding is not necessary
b. Coagulopathy is not an absolute contraindication
c. Bevel should face upwards while inserting the needle
d. To be done in lateral recumbent position

 ANSWERS WITH EXPLANATIONS OF IBQs 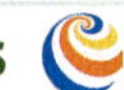

1. Ans. (c) Tuohy needle *[Ref. Ajay Yadav, 4/e p139]*

- Tuohy needle: Hollow hypodermic needle with slightly curved tip at end used for Epidural anesthesia.

2. Ans. (b) Coagulopathy is not an absolute contraindication *[Ref. Critical Care Study Guide by Criner, 1/e p122]*

Contraindications to Lumbar Puncture

Absolute contraindications	Relative contraindications
Patient refusal Sepsis at the site of injection Hypovolemia Coagulopathy Indeterminate neurologic disease Increased intracranial pressure	Infection distinct from the site of injection Unknown duration of surgery

- Absolute contraindication for Lumbar puncture include full anticoagulation or severe coagulopathy, because of the significantly increased risk of epidural hematoma formation with severe neurologic sequelae.

NEET/NBE PATTERN MCQs

1. **Post spinal headache lasts for** *[Recent Question 2016]*
   a. 10 min b. 1 hr
   c. 10 days d. 1 week
2. **Percentage of Lignocaine used in Spinal anesthesia is** *[Recent Question 2016]*
   a. 1% b. 2%
   c. 5% d. 10%
3. **True about post dural headache is all except** *[Recent Question 2016]*
   a. Orienting beveled edge needle parallel to long axis prevent it
   b. Thin bore needle prevents it
   c. It is more common in males
   d. Timing of ambulation has no effect over its incidence
4. **In epidural anesthesia drug is injected** *[Recent Question 2016]*
   a. Outside the dura b. Inside the dura mater
   c. Inside arachnoid mater d. Inside pia mater
5. **In Bier's block, anaesthetic agent given by which route?** *[Recent Question 2016]*
   a. Intravenous b. Peribulbar region
   c. Retrobulbar area d. Dermal
6. **Macintosh indicator is used for** *[Recent Question 2016]*
   a. To assess degree of nm blockade
   b. Localization of extradural space
   c. To assess level of gas
   d. To monitor respiratory depression
7. **Supraclavicular block is used for surgery of** *[Recent Question 2016]*
   a. Shoulder b. Neck
   c. Arm d. Forearm
8. **Onset of post spinal headache is usually at ..... hours after Spinal anesthesia** *[Recent Question 2016]*
   a. 0-6 b. 6-12
   c. 12-72 d. 72-96
9. **Treatment of choice for Post-spinal headache** *[Recent Question 2016]*
   a. Epidural blood patch b. Epidural fat patch
   c. IV fluid and analgesics d. IV antibiotics
10. **Which of the following cannot be given by Epidural anesthesia?** *[Recent Question 2016]*
    a. Morphine b. Remifentanil
    c. Alfentanil d. Fentanyl
11. **Commonest cranial nerve affected in Spinal anesthesia is** *[Recent Question 2016]*
    a. 2 b. 3
    c. 4 d. 6
12. **Used in Epidural anesthesia** *[NBE FMGE September 2005]*
    a. 0.5% lignocaine b. 2% lignocaine
    c. 4% lignocaine d. 5% lignocaine
13. **First fibers to be blocked in spinal anesthesia is** *[NBE DNB 1996, 1999, 2001, 2007]*
    a. Sympathetic preganglionic
    b. Afferent motor nerve
    c. Sensory fibers
    d. Efferent motor nerves
14. **Not a complication of epidural anesthesia** *[NBE DNB 2001]*
    a. Hypopnoea b. Total spinal analgesia
    c. Horner's syndrome d. Hypertension
15. **Commonest cranial nerve affected in spinal anesthesia is** *[NBE DNB 1993]*
    a. 2nd b. 3rd
    c. 4th d. 6th
    e. 10th
16. **In spinal anesthesia, the first nerve fibres to get blocked is** *[NBE DNB 2011]*
    a. Somatic motor fibres
    b. Sensory fibres
    c. Temperature fibres
    d. Sympathetic preganglionic
17. **For prevention of headache during spinal anesthesia** *[Recent Question 2012]*
    a. Diluted solution of local anaesthetic should be used
    b. Preloading with crystalloids
    c. Finer I.P. needle should be used
    d. Head end should be elevated
18. **All of the following are complications of epidural anesthesia except** *[NBE DNB 2011]*
    a. Headache b. Nausea
    c. Hypotension d. Bladder distension
19. **Maximum concentration for epidural block** *[Recent Question 2012]*
    a. Bupivacaine b. Lidocaine
    c. Ropivacaine d. Chlorprocaine
20. **Bupivacaine is used for spinal anesthesia is concentration (%) of** *[Recent Question 2016]* *[NBE DNB 1997]*
    a. 0.5% b. 2%
    c. 4% d. 5%
21. **Epidural anesthesia is preferred over spinal anesthesia because** *[NBE FMGE March 2006]*
    a. Prolonged duration of effect
    b. Cheaper
    c. Lesser chance of epidural hematoma
    d. Lesser chance of intravascular injection
22. **All are contraindications of spinal anesthesia except** *[Recent Question 2013]*
    a. Bleeding disorder b. Raised intracranial tension
    c. Hypertension d. Infection at injection site
23. **Percentage of xylocaine used in spinal anesthesia** *[Recent Question 2016, NBE DNB 1993]*
    a. 1% b. 2%
    c. 4% d. 5%
    e. 0.5%
24. **Spinal headache** *[NBE DNB 1995]*
    a. Is never associated with nuchal rigidity
    b. Is usually occipital
    c. Is completely relieved by aspirin
    d. May be relieved by an abnormal binder
25. **Not a complication of epidural anesthesia** *[NBE DNB 2005]*
    a. Hypopnea b. Total spinal analgesia
    c. Horner's syndrome d. Hypertension

26. In spinal anesthesia, drug is deposited between
a. Dura and arachnoid *[NBE DNB 2011]*
b. Pia and arachnoid
c. Ligamentum flavum and dura
d. Into the cord substance

27. Which can't be given by Epidural anesthesia? *[Recent Question 2013]*
a. Morphine b. Remifentanil
c. Alfentanil d. Fentanyl

28. Spinal epidural abscess is most commonly caused by *[NBE FMGE September 2004]*
a. Staphylococcus b. Pseudomonas
c. Meningococcus d. Escherichia coli

29. Benefits of Spinal anesthesia during LSCS include all except *[Recent Question 2015]*
a. Rapid onset
b. Minimal drug transfer to foetus
c. Less hypotension
d. Less failure

30. Anatomical landmark for Pudendal nerve block is *[Recent Question 2015, 2016]*
a. Iliac crest b. Iliac spine
c. Ischial spine d. Iliac tubercle

31. Which of the following is not included in Neuraxial anesthesia? *[Recent Question 2017]*
a. Spinal block b. Epidural block
c. Bier's block d. Caudal block

32. Relative contraindication of Neuraxial/Regional anesthesia is? *[Recent Question 2017]*
a. Hypertension b. Renal disease
c. Sepsis d. Diabetes

33. 'Triangle of Petit' is a landmark for which block? *[Recent Question 2017]*
a. Spinal block b. Bier's block
c. TAP block d. Epidural block

34. Hypotension following Spinal anesthesia can be best prevented by? *[Recent Question 2017]*
a. Preloading with colloids
b. Using small size needle
c. Preloading with crystalloids
d. All of the above

35. Complications of Stellate ganglion block are all except? *[Recent Question 2017]*
a. Cardiac arrest b. Pneumothorax
c. Hematoma d. Hoarseness of voice

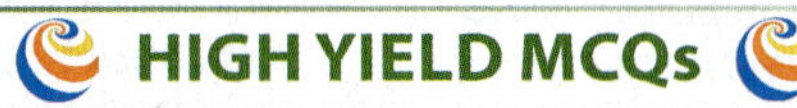

HIGH YIELD MCQs

1. On getting epidural anesthesia with 3% Xylocaine and Epinephrine, a patient develops Hypotension within 3 minutes. Most probable reason underlying is *[AIIMS November 2016]*
a. Systemic drug toxicity
b. Drug injected in Subarachnoid space
c. Vasovagal attack
d. Anaphylactic shock

2. Most common complication of celiac block
a. Pneumothorax *[Recent Question 2016]*
b. Postural hypotension *[AIIMS PGMEE 2009]*
c. Retroperitoneal hemorrhage
d. Intra-arterial injection

3. Most common complication of spinal anesthesia is *[AIIMS PGMEE 1994]*
a. Hypotension b. Headache
c. Meningitis d. Arrhythmia

4. In spinal anesthesia which fiber is lost first? *[AIIMS PGMEE 1992]*
a. Sympathetic b. Sensory
c. Motor d. Propioception

5. Post spinal headache is due to *[All India PGMEE 1995]*
a. Meningitis b. Encephalitis
c. CSF leak d. Increased ICT

6. In high spinal anesthesia what is seen *[AIIMS PGMEE 2001]*
a. Hypotension & Bradycardia
b. Hypotension & Tachycardia
c. Hypertension & Bradycardia
d. Hypertension & Tachycardia

7. Spinal anesthesia should be injected into the space between *[All India PGMEE 1997]*
a. T_{12}-L_1 b. L_1-L_2
c. L_3-L_4 d. L_5-S_1

8. Best way to prevent hypotension during spinal anesthesia *[AIPGME 1995]*
a. Preloading with crystalloids
b. Mephentermine
c. Dopamine
d. Trendelenburg's position

9. Complication of peribulbar block *[PGI 2004]*
a. Retrobulbar hemorrhage
b. Globe rupture
c. Optic neuritis
d. Local anaesthetic solution can migrate to brain
e. Vasovagal syncope

10. Structure(s) pierce in Lumbar spinal puncture is/are
a. Ligamentum flavum *[PGI 2009]*
b. Dura mater
c. Supraspinous ligament
d. Anterior longitudinal ligament
e. Posterior longitudinal ligament

11. Concentration of Lidocaine used in spinal anesthesia
a. 5% b. 3% *[AIPGME 1994]*
c. 2% d. 1%

12. Pudendal nerve block involve *[Recent Question 2016, All India PGMEE 1993]*
a. $L_1L_2L_3$ b. $L_2L_3L_4$
c. $S_1S_2S_3$ d. $S_2S_3S_4$

Anesthesiology

13. Pneumothorax is a complication of *[All India PGMEE 1992]*
a. Axillary block b. Brachial plexus block
c. Epidural block d. High spinal block

14. Post spinal headache can last for *[Recent Question 2016, All India PGMEE 1994]*
a. Upto 10 min b. Upto 10 hours
c. 7–10 days d. Upto 10 months

15. Site of action of epidural analgesia *[AIIMS PGMEE 1999]*
a. Sensory nerve endings b. Ventral horn
c. Substantia gelatinosa d. Cortex

16. Drug used for Epidural analgesia *[All India PGMEE 1993]*
a. Morphine b. Fentanyl
c. Piroxicam d. NSAIDs

17. True about epidural anesthesia in pregnancy
a. Given through subarachnoid space *[PGI 2003]*
b. Increases cardiac output
c. Decreases venous return
d. Venous pooling
e. Decreased placental circulation

18. Spinal anesthesia is given at which level? *[All India PGMEE 2011]*
a. L1-L2 b. L3-L4
c. S1 d. Thoracic segment

19. While receiving spinal anesthesia, a patient suddenly develops aphonia and loss of consciousness. Most probable diagnosis is *[All India PGMEE 2011]*
a. Intravessel injection b. Total spinal
c. Partial spinal d. Vasovagal attack

20. Neurolept analgesia all are true except *[PGI 1998]*
a. Can be used along with O_2& N_2O
b. Causes focal dystonia c. Fentanyl-droperidol
d. Cause hypotension e. None

21. A 30-year-old lady is to undergo surgery under intravenous regional anesthesia for her left 'trigger finger'. Which one of the following should not be used for patient? *[AIIMS PGMEE 2004]*
a. Lignocaine b. Bupivacaine
c. Prilocaine d. Lignocaine+ketorolac

22. A young boy has sickle cell trait. Which of the following anesthesia is contraindicated? *[AIIMS PGMEE 2010]*
a. IV regional anesthesia (IVRA)
b. Brachal plexus block by infraclavicular approach
c. Brachial plexus block by infraclavicular approach
d. Brachial plexus block by axillary approach

23. Correct statement regarding bupivacaine includes
a. Less carditoxic than prilocaine *[PGI 2005]*
b. It is an amide
c. The maximum tolerable dose is 8 mg/kg body wt
d. Duration more than 2 hrs

24. Levo-bupivacaine is administered by which of the following route *[PGI 2004]*
a. Nasogastric b. Epidural
c. Intravenous d. Intrathecal
e. Oral

25. In general, the last muscle to be rendered akinetic with a retrobulbar anesthetic block is *[AIIMS PGMEE 2006]*
a. Superior rectus b. Superior oblique
c. Inferior oblique d. Levator palpebral superioris

26. Which of the following is not a sign of successful stellate ganglion block? *[All India PGMEE 2009]*
a. Nasal stuffiness b. Guttman sign
c. Horner's syndrome d. Bradycardia

27. A patient in ICU was on invasive monitoring with intra arterial cannulation through right radial artery for last 3 days. Later he developed swelling and discolouration of right hand. The next line of management is *[AIIMS PGMEE 2001]*
a. Stellate ganglion block b. Brachial block
c. Radial Nerve block d. Celiac plexus block

28. The anesthetic drug injected for paravertebral block is least likely to diffuse to *[All India PGMEE 2009]*
a. Epidural space
b. Subarachnoid space
c. Intercostal space
d. Superior and inferior paravertebral spaces

29. Following spinal subarachnoid block a patient develops hypotension. This can be managed by the following means except *[AIIMS PGMEE 2003]*
a. Lowering the head end
b. Administration of 1000 ml of Ringer's lacate before the block
c. Vasopressor drug like methoxamine
d. Use of ionotrope like dopamine

30. In all of the following conditions neuraxial blockade is absolutely contraindicated, except
a. Patient refusal *[All India PGMEE 2003]*
b. Coagulopathy
c. Severe hypovolemia
d. Pre-existing neurological deficits

31. True about post spinal headache
a. Frontal *[All India PGMEE 1992]*
b. More in lying down
c. Low incidence with thin (25 G) needle
d. Increased by abdominal compression

32. Vasopressor of choice in hypotension produced during subarachnoid block *[PGI 2004]*
a. Ephedrine b. Mephentermine
c. Adrenaline d. Dopamine
e. Steroids

33. Post-dural puncture headache, true about *[PGI 2004]*
a. Common in elderly
b. Small bore needle prevents it
c. Early ambulation increases incidence
d. Occurs immediately after spinal anesthesia
e. Blood patch is the first line of treatment

34. Which is the true statement regarding post-dural anesthetic headache *[PGI 2001]*
a. Blood patch is the first line of treatment
b. Occurs due to low CSF pressure
c. Increased incidence with early mobilization of patient
d. Use of small gauge needle prevents headache
e. Common in old age

35. Centrineuraxial (spinal and epidural) anesthesia is not contraindicated in *[All India PGMEE 2007]*
a. Platelets <80,000 b. Patient on aspirin
c. Patient on oral anticoagulants
d. Patient on I.V.UFH

36. A patient was admitted epidural anesthesia with 15 ml of 1.5%. Lignocaine with adrenaline for hernia surgery. He developed hypotension and respiratory depression within 3 minutes after administration of block. The most common cause would be *[AIIMS PGMEE 2003, AIIMS PGMEE 2005]*

a. Allergy to drug administered
b. Systemic toxicity to drug administered
c. Patient got vasovagal shock
d. Drug has entered the subarachnoid space

37. Epidural narcotic is preferred over epidural LA because it causes *[Recent Question 2016, AIIMS PGMEE 1996]*

a. Less respiratory depression
b. Less dose is required
c. No motor paralysis
d. No retention of urine

38. A Lower Segment Caesarean section (LSCS) can be carried out under all the following techniques of anesthesia except *[All India PGMEE 2005]*

a. General anesthesia
b. Spinal anesthesia
c. Caudal anesthesia
d. Combined spinal epidural anesthesia

39. Contraindications to Spinal and Epidural anesthesia include all except *[JIPMER PGMEE 2014]*

a. Hypovolemia
b. Fever
c. Hypertension
d. Blood coagulation defects

40. A snap just before entering Epidural space, during Epidural anesthesia, is due to piercing of *[AIIMS November 2015]*

a. Supraspinous ligament
b. Posterior longitudinal ligament
c. Ligamentum flavum
d. Interspinous ligament

41. In spinal anesthesia, the drug is deposited between *[ESI IMO 2014]*

a. Dura and arachnoid
b. Pia and arachnoid
c. Dura and vertebra
d. Into the cord substance

42. To provide pain relief during First stage of Labour which sensory level should be blocked? *[PGMCET 2015]*

a. T8 to L1
b. T9 to L2
c. T10 to L1
d. T11 to L2

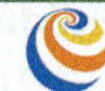 NEET/NBE PATTERN MCQs ANSWERS WITH EXPLANATIONS 

1. **Ans. (c) 10 days**
   [Ref. KDT, 6/e p359]
   - Onset of headache after lumbar puncture is **usually within 24–48 h after Dural puncture**, but contrary to the above definition, it could be delayed by up to 12 days
   - Headaches may develop within 1–3 days after the procedure and typically last 3–5 days, although in rare occasions can last for up to 10 days
   - It is **most probably related to the "hole" in the left dura** after the needle has been withdrawn, resulting in persistent leak of CSF from the subarachnoid space
   - This leakage results in a fall in intracranial CSF volume and CSF pressure
2. **Ans. (c) 5%**
   [Ref. Short Textbook of Surgery by Roy, 1/e p106]

   Lignocaine in Anesthesia
   - Local infiltration: 0.5%
   - Nerve blocks: 1.5%
   - Epidural anesthesia: 2.0%
   - Urethral dilation: 2.0% jelly
   - Tracheal intubation: 4% spray
   - Spinal bloc: 5.0%
3. **Ans. (c) It is common in males**
   [Ref. KDT, 6/e p359]

   Post-dural Puncture Headache
   - An unusual and specific kind of severe headache which can only happen after an epidural or spinal injection
   - It can be felt at the front or the back of the head. It is worse when sitting or standing and it gets better when lying down flat
   - **MCC: Leakage of CSF which can be prevented by using thin bore needle (25G)**
   - Relieved by raising the venous pressure by abdominal compression
   - First line treatment is IV fluids if not responding blood patch
4. **Ans. (a) Outside the dura**
   [Ref. Maternity and Pediatric Nursing by Ricci, 1/e p406]
   - **An epidural block** involves the injection of a drug into the epidural space, which is located outside the dura mater between the dura and the spinal canal
   - Epidural space is typically entered **thorough 3rd and 4th lumbar vertebrae**
5. **Ans. (a) Intravenous**
   [Ref. Anaesthesia by Colin, 3/e p132]
   - **Bier's block**: Intravenous regional anesthesia (IVRA) or bier block anesthesia is an anesthetic technique for surgical procedures on the body's extremities where a local anesthetic is injected intravenously
6. **Ans. (b) Localization of extradural space**
   [Ref. Final FRCA by Bahal, 1/e p155]

   Techniques to Localize Epidural Space
   - Negative pressure methods:
     - Hanging drop of Gutierrez
     - Odom capillary tube
     - Odom manometer indicator
   - Disappearance of resistance techniques:
     - Syringe technique of Sicard and Forestier
     - Modified pressure technique
     - Balloon technique of Macintosh
     - Mechanical devices like Ikle spring loaded syringe
     - Macintosh extradural space indicator
   - Drip infusion technique
7. **Ans. (a) Shoulder**
   [Ref. Anaesthesia by Colin, 3/e p127]
   - **Supraclavicular nerve block** is ideal for procedure of the upper arm, from the mid-humeral level down to the hand
   - Brachial plexus is most compact at the level of the trunks formed by the **c5–t1 nerve roots**, so blockade here has the greatest likelihood of blocking all of the branches of the brachial plexus
   - This results in rapid onset times and, ultimately, high success rates for surgery and analgesia of the upper extremity
8. **Ans. (c) 12-72**
   [Ref. Cousins and Bridenbaugh's Neural Blockade, 4/e p235]
   - Post spinal headache is usually at 12–72 hours after Spinal anesthesia
9. **Ans. (c) IV fluid and analgesics**
   [Ref. Anaesthesia by Colin, 3/e p120]
   - **Most common postoperative complication of spinal anesthesia** is post dural puncture headache
   - Majorly occurs after 12–24 hours.
   - Relieved raising the venous pressure by abdominal compression
   - Initial treatment consists of lying down and lots of IV fluids or a blood patch if not resolved by the primary measures taken
10. **Ans. (b) Remifentanil**
    [Ref. Duke's Anaesthesia Secrets, 5/e p371]
    - Remifentanil PCA is an intravenous form of opioid delivery and is especially useful if epidural anesthesia is contraindicated
11. **Ans. (d) 6**
    [Ref. Anaesthesia for Postgraduates by Agasti, 1/e p756]
    - Among all the cranial nerves sixth cranial nerve **(Abducens nerve) is more prone to injury** and it is due to its long and tortuous course
12. **Ans. (b) 2% lignocaine**
    [Ref. Ajay Yadav, 4/e p140]

    Epidural (Extradural/Peridural) Anesthesia
    - ***Indications***:
      - Postoperative pain control: Main indication
      - Painless labour
      - All general surgeries
      - Chronic pain control in cancers and chronic conditions
      - Occlusive vascular conditions
      - Blood patch for post-spinal headache

Anesthesiology

- ***Needles***:
  - Tuohy's needle (Most commonly used)
  - Weiss needle
  - Crawford needle
- ***Technique***:
  - Loss of resistance technique (Most common technique)
  - Hanging drop technique
- ***Drugs used***:
  - Lignocaine 1-2%
  - Bupivacaine 0.25-0.5%
  - Fentanyl
  - Tramadol

13. Ans. (a) Sympathetic preganglionic
[Ref. Ajay Yadav, 4/e p132]

14. Ans. (d) Hypertension
[Ref. Ajay Yadav, 4/e p141]

15. Ans. (d) 6th
[Ref. Ajay Yadav, 4/e p137]
- 6th cranial nerve is most involved (90%) in Spinal anesthesia because of its longest course
- Cranial nerves 1st, 9th and 10th are not involved

16. Ans. (d) Sympathetic preganglionic
[Ref. Ajay Yadav, 4/e p132]

17. Ans. (c) Finer I.P. needle should be used
[Ref. Ajay Yadav, 4/e p136]
- **Incidence of post spinal headache**:
  - With 16G needle: 75%
  - With 25G needle: <3%

18. Ans. (a) Headache
[Ref. Ajay Yadav, 4/e p141]

Complications of Epidural Anesthesia
- Inadequate (patchy) block
- Hypotension
- Apnoea
- Total spinal
- Distension of bladder (Urinary retention)

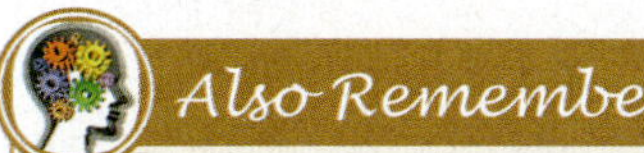

- Headache is more common with Spinal anesthesia as compared to Epidural anesthesia

19. Ans. (d) Chlorprocaine
[Ref. Ajay Yadav, 4/e p140]

Local Anesthetics in Epidural Anesthesia

Drugs	Concentration
Chloroprocaine	2–3%
Lignocaine	1–2%
Mepivacaine	1–2%
Prilocaine	2–3%
Bupivacaine	0.25–0.5%

20. Ans. (a) 0.5%
[Ref. Ajay Yadav, 4/e p140]

21. Ans. (a) Prolonged duration of effect
[Ref. Ajay Yadav, 4/e p140]
- *Comparison of spinal and epidural anesthesia*:

Parameter	Spinal anesthesia	Epidural anesthesia
Level performed	Lumbar	Any level
Cost	Cheaper	Expensive
Onset of effect	2–3 minutes	15–20 minutes
Duration of effect	Lesser	Prolonged
Quality of block	Total	Patchy
Post spinal headache	Present	Absent
Epidural hematoma	Less common	More common
Total spinal	Rare	High chances
Intravascular injection	Rare	High chances
Drug toxicity	Less common	More common
Catheter complications	Absent	Present

22. Ans. (c) Hypertension
[Ref. Ajay Yadav, 4/e p141]

23. Ans. (d) 5%
[Ref. Ajay Yadav, 4/e p134]
- In Spinal anesthesia, 5% lignocaine/xylocaine in 7.5% dextrose (Specific gravity 1.033)

24. Ans. (b) Is usually occipital
[Ref. Ajay Yadav, 4/e p136]

Post Spinal Headache
- Post spinal headache is usually occipital but can be frontal also
- May be associated with pain and stiffness in neck
- Pain increases on sitting and relieved on lying down
- Relieved in 3 weeks
- Analgesics, I/V fluids, abdominal binders, desmopressin, caffeine may help in reduction

25. Ans. (d) Hypertension
[Ref. Ajay Yadav, 4/e p141]

26. Ans. (b) Pia and arachnoid
[Ref. Ajay Yadav, 4/e p130]

27. Ans. (b) Remifentanil
[Ref. Ajay Yadav, 4/e p91]

Remifentanil
- Remifentanil contains glycine which can cause motor weakness: Not suitable for producing epidural analgesia
- Additional side effect is significant hypotension.

28. Ans. (a) Staphylococcus
[Ref. Infections of CNS by Scheld, 3/e p511]

Organisms causing Spinal Epidural Abscesses
- Staphylococcus aureus (**Most common cause**)
- Streptococcus

- Enterobacteriaceae
- Coagulase negative staphylococci
- Other causes

29. Ans. (c) Less hypotension

[Ref. Anesthesia by Kulkarni, 3/e p116]

Spinal Anesthesia in LSCS

Advantages	Disadvantages
• Rapid onset • Dense block • Infrequent failure • Minimal drug transfer to fetus • Reduced gastric content aspiration • Avoidance of depressant agents • Reduced risk of failure of intubation • Awake birthing experience by mother	• Higher chances of Hypotension • Finite duration of anesthesia • Post-dural puncture headache • Hematoma • Total spinal shock

30. Ans. (c) Ischial spine

[Ref. Snell's Clinical Anatomy, 9/e p326]

Bony Landmarks in Pudendal Nerve Block

- Transvaginal procedure: Ischial spine
- Perineal procedure: Ischial tuberosity

31. Ans. (c) Bier's block

[Ref. Anesthesiology by Modak, 2/e p382]

Neuraxial Anaesthesia

- Syn. Central neural blockade
- Pertains to local anesthetics placed around the nerves of the central nervous system
- Type of regional anesthesia that involves injection of anesthetic medication in the fatty tissue that surround the nerve roots as they exist the spine (Epidural) or into the cerebrospinal fluid which surrounds the spinal cord (Spinal)
- **NA includes Spinal, Epidural and Caudal administration** of local anaesthetic and opioid medications
- NA is most commonly used for lower abdominal and lower extremity surgery.

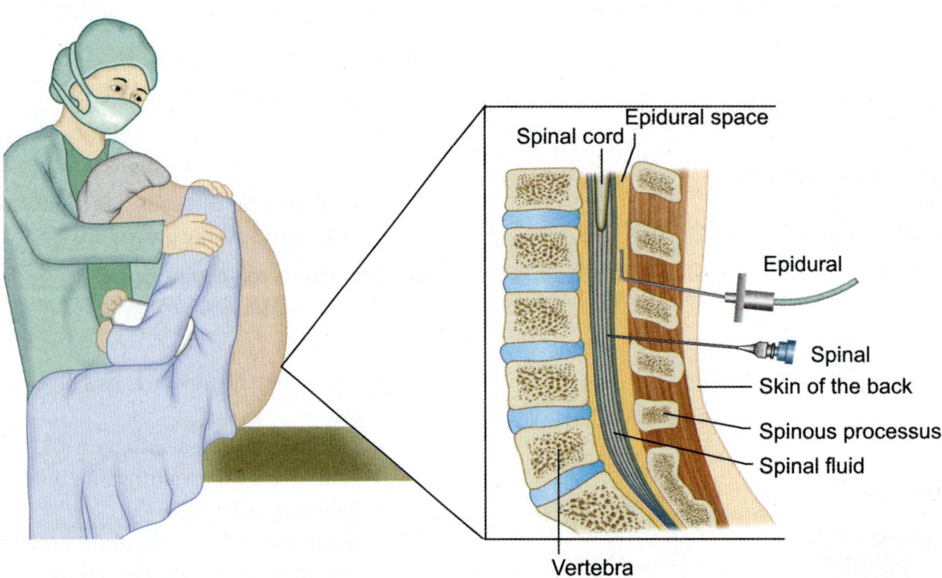

Fig. Neuraxial anesthesia

32. Ans. (c) Sepsis

[Ref. Regional Anesthesia by Kaye, 1/e p240]

Contraindications to Neuraxial Blockade

Absolute C/I	Relative C/I
• Infection at site of injection • Patient refusal • Coagulopathy/ bleeding diathesis • Severe hypovolemia • Increased ICP • Severe aortic stenosis • Severe mitral stenosis	• Sepsis • Uncooperative patient • Preexisting neurological deficits • Demyelinating lesions • Stenotic valvular heart lesions • Left ventricular outflow obstruction • Severe spinal deformity

33. Ans. (c) TAP block

[Ref. Clinical Cases in Anesthesia by Reed, 4/e p193]

Transversus Abdominis Plane (TAP) Block

- Traditionally known as a landmark-guided block performed at the Petit triangle
- Triangle landmarks include Iliac crest inferiorly, Latissimus dorsi muscle medially, and the External oblique muscle laterally
- This block is indicated for any lower abdominal surgery including Appendectomy, Hernia repair, Caesarean section, Abdominal hysterectomy, and Prostatectomy
- Aim of a TAP block is to deposit local anaesthetic in the plane between the internal oblique and transversus abdominis muscles targeting the spinal nerves in this plane

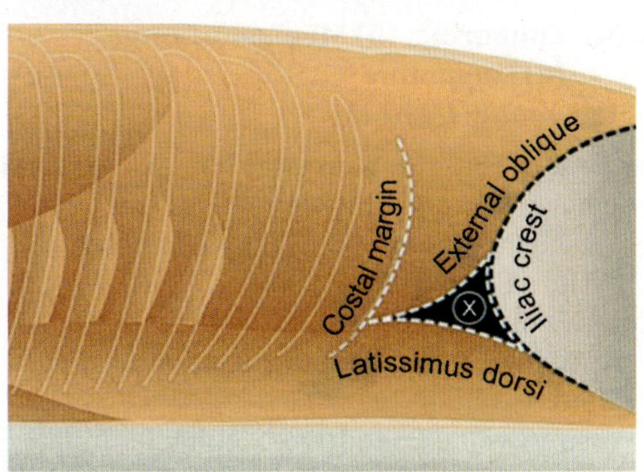

Fig. Triangle of petit

34. Ans. (a) Preloading with colloids

[Ref. Clinical Fluid Therapy by Hahn, 2/e p144]

- Colloids are more effective than crystalloids in preventing hypotension following Spinal anesthesia.

35. Ans. (a) Cardiac arrest

[Ref. Anesthesiology by Yao, 1/e p323]

Possible Complications of Stellate Ganglion Block

- Intraarterial injection: Toxic reaction, Hematoma
- Recurrent laryngeal nerve paralysis: Hoarseness of voice
- Brachial plexus block: Motor weakness
- Pneumothorax: Respiratory distress
- Rare complication: Accidental subarachnoid hemorrhage

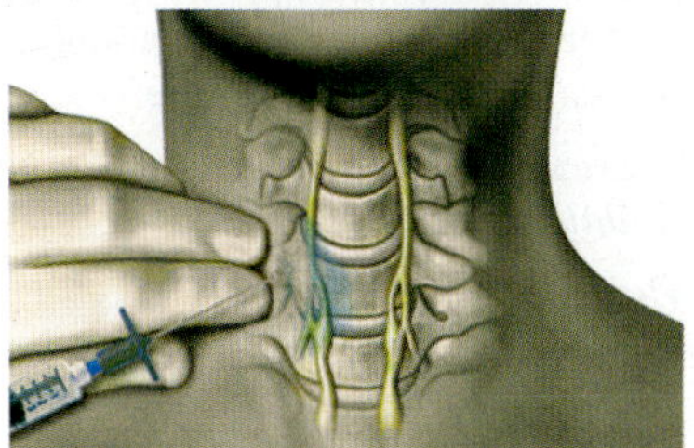

Fig. Stellate ganglion block

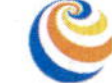 **HIGH YIELD MCQs ANSWERS WITH EXPLANATIONS** 

1. Ans. (b) Drug injected in Subarachnoid space

[Ref. Neurological Illness in Pregnancy by Klein, 1/e p75]

- Drug injected in Subarachnoid space, by mistake during epidural injection, can give rise to Total spinal block
  - Cardiovascular collapse with hypotension and bradycardia
  - Total sensory and motor block

Also Remember

- To identify Subarachnoid/intravascular placement of catheter, Epidural test dose should be given

2. Ans. (b) Postural hypotension

[Ref. Ajay Yadav, 4/e p132]

3. Ans. (a) Hypotension

[Ref. Ajay Yadav, 4/e p132]

4. Ans. (a) Sympathetic

[Ref. Ajay Yadav, 4/e p132]

5. Ans. (c) CSF leak

[Ref. Ajay Yadav, 4/e p136]

Post Spinal Headache

- Low pressure headache due to seepage of CSF fluid from dural rent created by spinal needle
- CSF leakage results in changes in hydrodynamics of brain causing traction of pain sensitive structure like dura, vessels and tentorium producing pain
- Loss is around 10 ml per hour

6. Ans. (a) Hypotension and bradycardia

[Ref. Ajay Yadav, 4/e p135]

7. Ans. (c) L3-L4

[Ref. Ajay Yadav, 4/e p131]

8. Ans. (a) Preloading with crystalloids

[Ref. Ajay Yadav, 4/e p135]

- Preloading with 1 to 1.5 l of crystalloids (RL) or 500 ml of colloid is best to prevent Hypotension in Spinal anesthesia

9. Ans. ALL CHOICES

[Ref. Ajay Yadav, 4/e p184]

10. Ans. (a) Ligamentum flavum; (b) Dura mater; (c) Supraspinous ligament

[Ref. Ajay Yadav, 4/e p130]

Structure Encountered in Lumbar Spinal Puncture

- Skin
- Subcutaneous tissue
- Supraspinous ligament
- Interspinous ligament
- Ligamentum flavum (yellow ligament)
- Dura
- Arachnoid

11. Ans. (a) 5%

[Ref. Ajay Yadav, 4/e p130]

12. Ans. (d) $S_2S_3S_4$

[Ref. Ajay Yadav, 4/e p177]

- Pudendal nerve block provides only perineal analgesia by blocking only sacral segments

13. Ans. (b) Brachial plexus block

[Ref. Ajay Yadav, 4/e p127]

14. Ans. (c) 7-10 days

[Ref. Ajay Yadav, 4/e p136]

15. Ans. (c) Substantia gelatinosa

[Ref. Epidural Analgesia in Acute Pain Management by Middleton, 1/e p56]

- Direct application of opioids to the spinal cord through the epidural route provides excellent analgesia at much lower doses

- Once in the CSF a part of the dose is taken by the spinal cord where it binds to the opioid receptors in the grey matter of the dorsal horn known as the substantia gelatinosa

16. Ans. (a) Morphine; (b) Fentanyl
[Ref. Ajay Yadav, 4/e p140; Anaesthesia by Sikka, 1/e p512]

Drugs used in Epidural Anesthesia
- Local anesthetics: Chlorprocaine, Lignocaine, Mepivacaine, Prilocaine, Bupivacaine, Ropivacaine
- Opioids: Morphine, Fentanyl, Sufentanil, Pethidine
- Other agents: Clonidone, Ketamine

17. Ans. (c) Decreases venous return; (d) Venous pooling
[Ref. Ajay Yadav, 4/e p140]

18. Ans. (b) L3-L4
[Ref. Ajay Yadav, 4/e p131]

19. Ans. (b) Total spinal
[Ref. Ajay Yadav, 4/e p135]

High/ Total Spinal
- **Mechanism**: Occur due to accidental subarachnoid puncture with local anesthetic intended for epidural
- **Features**: Hypotension, Complete sensory/ motor block, Bradycardia, Apnoea, Loss of protective airway reflexes, Unconsciousness Treatment: Establish airway, Oxygen, Endotracheal intubation, PPV, Vasopressors

20. Ans. (e) None
[Ref. Ajay Yadav, 4/e p83]

21. Ans. (b) Bupivucaine
[Ref. Ajay Yadav, 4/e p123]
It should not be used because of its carditoxic property

22. Ans. (a) IVRA
Ref. Ajay Yadav, 4/e p166]
- Use of tourniquet and hence Beir's block is contraindicated because blood stasis can cause local acidosis, hypoxia with sickling of cells

23. Ans. (b) It is an amide; (d) Duration is more than 2 hours
[Ref. Ajay Yadav, 4/e p123]

24. Ans. (b) Epidural; (d) Intrathecal
[Ref. Ajay Yadav, 4/e p124]

25. Ans. (b) Superior oblique
[Ref. Ajay Yadav, 4/e p184]

26. Ans. (d) Bradycardia
[Ref. Ajay Yadav, 4/e p126]

27. Ans. (a) Stellate ganglion block
[Ref. Ajay Yadav, 4/e p126]

28. Ans. (b) Subarachnoid space

29. Ans. (a) Lowering the head end
[Ref. Ajay Yadav, 4/e p135]
- Head low position specially below 15° increases the chance of high spinal and increased ICT

30. Ans. (d) Pre-existing neurological deficits
[Ref. Ajay Yadav, 4/e p138]

31. Ans. (c) Low incidence with thin (25G) needle
[Ref. Ajay Yadav, 4/e p136]

32. Ans. (a) Ephedrine; (b) Mephentermine; (d) Dopamine
[Ref. Ajay Yadav, 4/e p135]

Treatment of Hypotension after Spinal Anesthesia
- Prophylactic: Preloading
  - 1.0-1.5 litres Crystalloid (Ringer lactate)
  - 0.5 litre Colloid
- Curative approach:
  - Head low/ Trendelenburg position
  - Fluids (Colloids better)
  - Vasopressors: Ephedrine, Mephenteramine, Methoxamine
  - Inotropes: Dopamine, Dobutamine
  - Oxygen inhalation

33. Ans. (b) Small bore needle prevents it; (d) Occurs immediately after spinal anesthesia
[Ref. Ajay Yadav, 4/e p136]

34. Ans. (b) Occurs due to low CSF pressure; (d) Use of small gauze needle prevents headache
[Ref. Ajay Yadav, 4/e p136]

35. Ans. (b) Patient on aspirin
[Ref. Ajay Yadav, 4/e p138]

36. Ans. (d) Drug has entered the subarachnoid space
[Ref. Ajay Yadav, 4/e p132]

37. Ans. (c) No motor paralysis
[Ref. Ajay Yadav, 4/e p136]

38. Ans. (c) Caudal anesthesia
[Ref. Ajay Yadav, 4/e p143]

39. Ans. (c) Hypertension
[Ref. Ajay Yadav, 4/e p138]

Contraindications to Spinal/Epidural Anesthesia

Absolute Contraindications	Relative Contraindications
• Patient refusal • Raised intracranial tension • Severe hypovolemia (Shock) • Patient on Anticoagulants • Patients on Thrombolytics/ Fibrinolytics • Bleeding disorders/ Coagulopathy • Septicemia, Bacteremia • Infection at local site	• Fixed cardiac output lesions (AS, MS) • Hypotension, Hypovolemia • Fever • Uncontrolled hypertension • Severe Ischemic heart disease, Heart blocks • Patients on Beta-blockers • Patients on Aspirin, mini dose Heparin • Spinal deformity, Previous spinal surgery • GIT perforation • CNS disorders, Neuropathies

40. Ans. (c) Ligamentum flavum
[Ref. Grey's Anatomy, 3/e p82]

Epidural Anesthesia
- Spinal needle is inserted between Lumbar vertebrae L3/L4 or L4/L5 or L5/S1
- Needle is pushed until there is a **'give way'** indicating needle is just passed the Ligamentum flavum.

Anesthesiology

41. Ans. (b) Pia and arachnoid

[Ref. Anaesthesia and Analgesia by Thomas, 4/e p189]

- **Subarachnoid space**: Area between the arachnoid and the pia mater, filled with cerebrospinal fluid
- Spinal anesthesia involves deposition of a small mass or volume of drug around the nerve root in the subarachnoid space to induce profound, reproducible sensory analgesia, devoid of systemic pharmacologic effect.

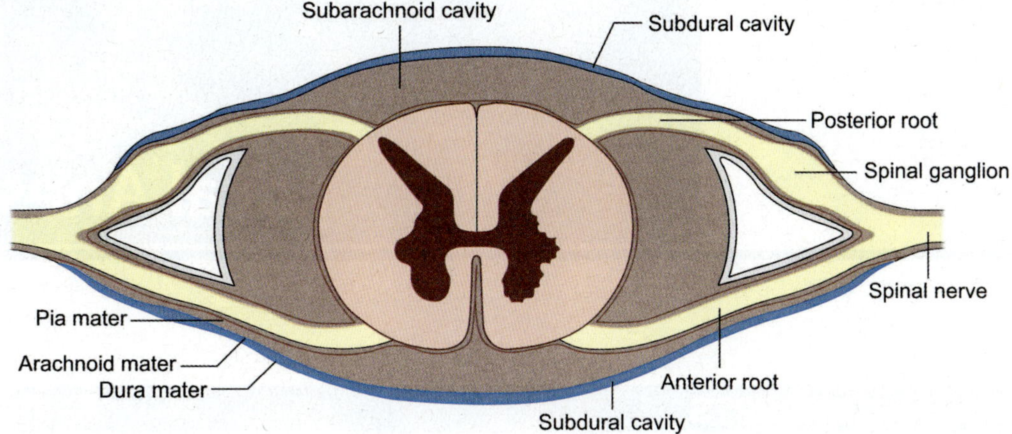

Fig. Subarachnoid space

42. Ans. (c) T10 to L1

[Ref. Anaesthesia in OBG by Tiwari, 1/e p86]

Pain Relief in Labour

- Pain relief for first stage requires block: T10 to L1 sensory level
- Pain relief for second stage requires block: T10 to S4 block sensory level

Anesthesiology

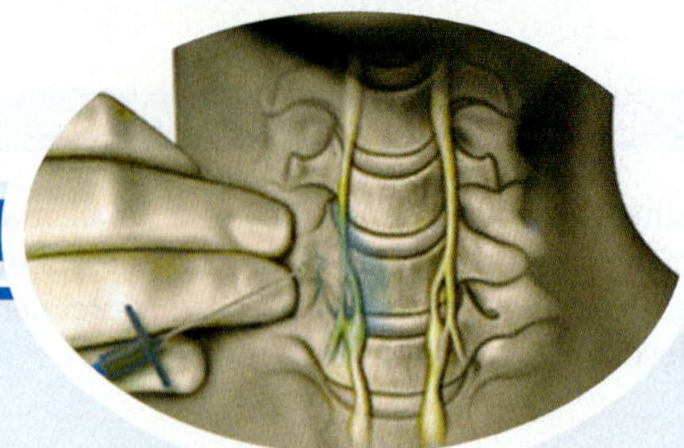

Chapter 9

Local Anesthesia

THEORETICAL CONCEPTS

IX A. LOCAL ANESTHETICS

Aminoesters	Aminoamides
• Procaine • Chlorprocaine • Cocaine • Benzocaine • Tetracaine	• Lignocaine • Mepivacaine • Prilocaine • Bupivacaine • Etidocaine • Ropivacaine • Dibucaine

Short duration [Q]	Intermediate duration	Long duration
Low potency	***Moderate potency***	***High potency***
• Procaine [Q] • Chlorprocaine (Shortest acting [Q])	• Lignocaine [Q] • Mepivacaine • Prilocaine [Qq] • Cocaine	• Bupivacaine [Q] • Etidocaine [Q] • Ropivacaine • Dibucaine [Q] • Tetracaine [Q]

IX B. MECHANISM OF ACTION OF LOCAL ANESTHETICS

- Undissociated (Non-ionised) form of anaesthetic molecules enter axonal membrane and gets dissociated (ionised)
- **Ionised form *'blocks sodium channel'***[Q], thus preventing depolarisation
- Some minor action is also present on potassium and calcium channels

IX C. METHODS OF LOCAL ANESTHESIA

- *Topical/ surface anesthesia*:

Use	Local anesthetic
Skin	**2.5% EMLA cream (2.5% Prilocaine + 2.5% Lignocaine)**
Mucous membranes (oropharynx)	4% Xylocaine spray, Tetracaine/ Benzocaine lozenges
Catheterization, Proctoscopy	2% Xylocaine (lignocaine) jelly
Eye	Cocaine drops, Tetracaine ointment
Anal canal, rectum	4% Lignocaine, 1% Dibucaine, 5% benzocaine ointment
Gastritis	0.2% Oxethazaine (mucaine) gel

- Infiltration anesthesia
- Nerve block
- Intravenous regional anesthesia (Bier's block)
- Central neuraxial blocks
- Refrigeration analgesia: CO_2 snow, Ice cooling, Ethyl chloride spray

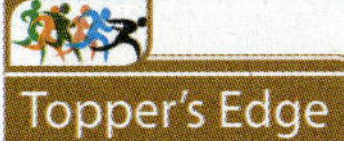

Topper's Edge

LOCAL ANESTHESIA (LA)

- **First local anesthetic used**[Q]: Cocaine (Carl Koller for Cornea[Q])
- **Cm**[Q]: Minimum concentration of Local anesthetic that will block nerve impulse conduction
- **Sequence of blockade (Fibre types**[Q]**)**: B > C > A
- Sequence of blockade (Functional terms[Q]): Autonomic > Sensory > Motor
- Sequence of blockade (Sensory fibres[Q]): Temperature (Cold > Hot) > Pain > Touch > Deep pressure > Proprioception
- Systemic absorption is highest after: Intercostal nerve block
- **Shortest acting LA**: Chlorprocaine[Q]
- All LAs are vasodilators except[Q]: Cocaine, Levobupivacaine, Ropivacaine
- First system involved in LA toxicity: CNS
- Metabolite of Cocaine causing CNS stimulation: Ecognine[Q]
- **Agent of choice in History of Malignant hyperthermia**[Q]: Procaine
- Agent of choice for **treating Ventricular tachycardia**[Q]: Lignocaine
- Agent of choice for **treating Ventricular tachycardia due to Bupivacaine**[Q]: Bretylium
- Bupivacaine is not used in Bier's block[Q]: As its cardiotoxic nature
- LA NOT to be used in History of Malignant hyperthermia[Q]: Lignocaine (As it releases Calcium from Endoplasmic reticulum)

IMAGE-BASED QUESTIONS

1. Composition of Cream shown in Photograph is ***[Recent Question 2014]***

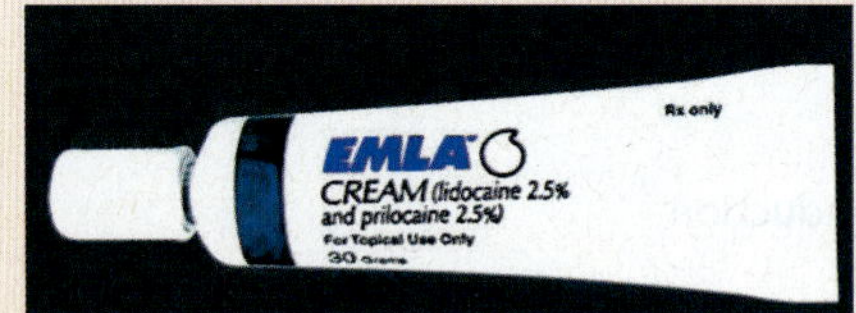

a. 2.5% Lignocaine + 2.5% Prilocaine
b. 5% Lignocaine + 2.5% Prilocaine
c. 2.5% Lignocaine + 5% Prilocaine
d. 5% Lignocaine + 7.5% Prilocaine

2. Concentration of Local anesthetic agent used for Bier's block is

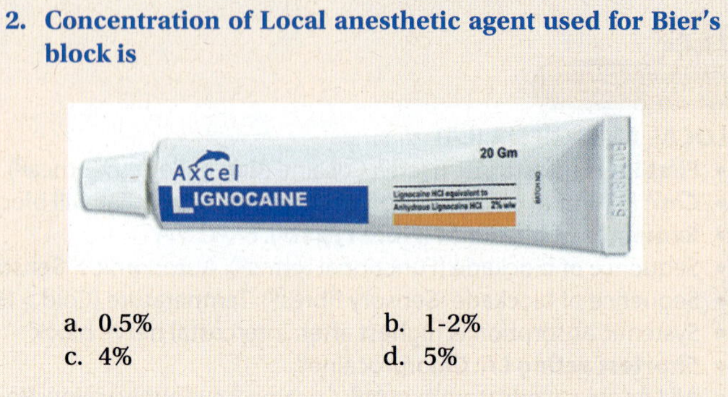

a. 0.5% b. 1-2%
c. 4% d. 5%

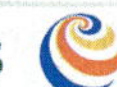

ANSWERS WITH EXPLANATIONS OF IBQs

1. Ans. (a) 2.5% Lignocaine + 2.5% Prilocaine *[Ref. Local Anesthesia by Dernetra, 1/e p99]*

- Most widely used Topical anesthetic: EMLA cream- 5% Eutectic mixture of 2.5% Lignocaine + 2.5% Prilocaine

2. Ans. (a) 0.5% *[Ref. Pharmacology by Shanbhag, 1/e p175]*

Local Anesthetic Techniques

- Surface topical anesthesia: Lignocaine (2-10%), Tetracaine (2%), Benzocaine
- Infiltration anesthesia: Lignocaine (0.5-1%), Procaine (0.5-1%), Bupivacaine (0.125-0.25%)
- Nerve block anesthesia: Most of the anesthetics
- Spinal anesthesia: Lignocaine (1.5-5%), Tetracaine (0.25-0.5%), Bupivacaine (0.5-0.75%)
- Epidural anesthesia: Lignocaine (2%), Bupivacaine (0.5-0.75%)
- Intravenous regional anesthesia (Bier's block): Lignocaine (0.5%), Prilocaine (0.5%)
- Anesthetizing Gastric mucosa: Oxethazine

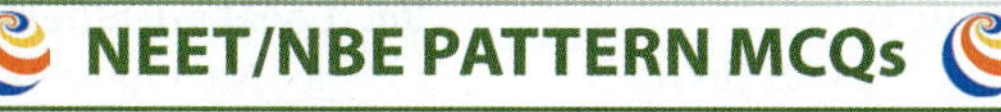

NEET/NBE PATTERN MCQs

1. Which of the following is not primarily used to anesthetize mucosa? *[Recent Question 2016]*
a. Benzocaine b. Lidocaine
c. Bupivacaine d. Tetracaine

2. Local anaesthetic causing Methemoglobinuria is *[Recent Question 2016]*
a. Dibucaine b. Chlorprocaine
c. Procaine d. Benzocaine

3. Percentage of Tetracaine used in Eye surgery *[Recent Question 2016]*
a. 0.5% b. 1%
c. 2% d. 4%

4. Drug used to prolong action of local anesthesia in hypertensive patients *[Recent Question 2016]*
a. Clonidine
b. Dexmedetomidine
c. Felypressine
d. Noradrenaline

5. False about Local anesthetics *[Recent Question 2016]*
a. Prilocaine is less toxic than lignocaine
b. Lignocaine is used as an antiarrhythmic
c. Mixture of Lignocaine + Prilocaine is known as Eutectic
d. Lidocaine is shorter acting than bupivacaine

6. About Lignocaine, all are true except *[Recent Question 2016]*
a. It is ester group of local anaesthetic
b. It has antiarrhythmic property
c. Can penetrate through mucous membrane
d. It can precipitate malignant hyperthermia

7. Local anaesthetic with maximum ionized form *[Recent Question 2016]*
a. Lignocaine b. Etidocaine
c. Bupivacaine d. Chloroprocaine

8. Local anesthesia acts by blockage of *[Recent Question 2016, 2017]*
a. Na^+ channel b. K^+ channel
c. Ca^{++} channel d. Mg^{++} channel

9. Speed of onset of action of Local anesthetics is indicated by *[Recent Question 2016]*
a. Minimum alveolar concentration
b. Blood: gas partition coefficient
c. Oil: gas partition coefficient
d. All of the above

10. Local anaesthetic in wound/ ulcer management *[Recent Question 2016]*
a. Prilocaine b. Chlorprocaine
c. Benzocaine d. Bupivacaine

11. Most commonly used Local anesthetics *[Recent Question 2016]*
a. Dibucaine
b. Bupivacaine
c. Prilocaine
d. Tetracaine

12. Long acting Local anaesthetic *[Recent Question 2016]*
a. Procaine b. Lignocaine
c. Prilocaine d. Dibucaine

13. Agent with short acting period *[Recent Question 2016]*
a. Procaine b. Lignocaine
c. Bupivacine d. Dibucaine

14. Local anesthetics act by inhibition of *[NBE FMGE September 2005, September 2012]*
a. Na^+ channels b. Mg^{++} channels
c. Ca^{++} channels d. K^+ channels

15. Dose of lignocaine when used as local anesthetic in mg/ kg is *[NBE DNB 2011]*
a. 1-3 b. 3-5
c. 5-7 d. 7-9

16. Local Anesthetic in wound/ ulcer management *[Recent Question 2012]*
a. Prilocaine b. Chlorprocaine
c. Benzocaine d. Bupivacaine

17. Shortest acting local anaesthetic is *[Recent Question 2016, NBE DNB 1993, 1997, 1999]*
a. Procaine b. Bupivacaine
c. Xylocaine d. Chlorprocaine

18. Maximum safe dose of lignocaine with adrenaline is *[NBE DNB 1992, 2004, 2008]*
a. 3 mg/kg wt b. 7 mg/kg wt
c. 10 mg/kg wt d. 15 mg/kg wt

19. Drug used to prolong action of LA in Hypertensive patients *[Recent Question 2012]*
a. Clonidine b. Felypressin
c. Dexeditomidate d. Noradrenaline

20. Vasoconstrictor adrenaline is used in local anaesthetic lidocaine in concentration of *[NBE DNB 2011]*
a. 1:200 b. 1:2000
c. 1:20000 d. 1:200000

21. Local anesthesia causing methemoglobinemia *[Recent Question 2012]*
a. Procaine b. Prilocaine
c. Etodicaine d. Ropivacaine

22. Local anaesthetic with prolonged action *[Recent Question 2012, 2013, 2016]*
a. Procaine b. Cocaine
c. Lidocaine d. Dibucaine

23. Earliest sign of systemic absorption of local anaesthetic is *[NBE DNB 1997]*
a. Convulsions
b. Circumoral numbness
c. Circulatory collapse
d. Respiratory arrest

24. Addition of epinephrine to lignocaine *[Recent Question 2013]*
a. Increaseses distribution of LA
b. Decreases absorption of LA
c. Decreases duration of LA
d. Increases metabolism of LA

25. Vasoconstrictor L.A. is *[Recent Question 2013, PGI 1997, AIPGME 1999]*
a. Cocaine b. Procaine
c. Lidocaine d. Chlorprocaine

26. Mechanism of action of local anaesthetic is *[NBE DNB 2001]*
a. Stabilization of membrane
b. Inhibition of Ca
c. Inhibition of Mg+ d. Increase dopamine

27. Local anaesthetic with maximum ionized form at physiological pH *[Recent Question 2012]*
a. Lignocaine b. Etidocaine
c. Bupivacaine d. Chloroprocaine

28. Eutectic mixture of local anaesthetic (EMLA) cream is *[Recent Question 2016, NBE FMGE September 2011]*
a. Bupivacaine 2.0% + Prilocaine 2.0%
b. Lidocaine 2.5% + Prilocaine 2.5%
c. Lidocaine 2.5% + Prilocaine 0.5%
d. Bupivacaine 0.5% + Lidocaine 2.5%

29. Agent with shortest acting period *[Recent Question 2013]*
a. Procaine b. Lignocaine
c. Bupivacaine d. Dibucaine

30. The sequence of recovery from local anesthesia is *[NBE DNB 1997]*
a. Presympathetic ganglionic, proprioception, motor
b. Motor, proprioception, presympathetic ganglionic
c. Presympathetic ganglionic, motor, proprioception
d. Proprioception, motor, presympathetic ganglionic

31. EMLA constituent is *[Recent Question 2012, 2013]*
a. Lidocaine + Cocaine b. Lidocaine + Prilocaine
c. Lidocaine + Bupivacaine d. Bupivacaine + Prilocaine

32. Bupivacaine toxicity causes *[Recent Question 2012, 2017]*
a. Renal toxicity b. Pulmonary toxicity
c. Cardiotoxicity d. None

33. Methemoglobinemia is caused by *[NBE DNB 1995, 1999, 2001, 2004, 2007, 2009]*
a. Procaine b. Bupivacaine
c. Prilocaine d. Lignocaine

34. Local anesthesia acts by *[Recent Question 2012, PGI 1997]*
a. Na^+ channel inhibition b. Ca^{++} channel inhibition
c. Mg^{++} channel inhibition d. K^+ channel inhibition

35. Among the following local anesthetics, the one that is associated with vasoconstriction and mydriasis is *[NBE DNB 2003]*
a. Cocaine b. Bupivacaine
c. Procaine d. Lignocaine

36. The best anaesthetic agent for acute paronychia is *[Recent Question 2016, NBE DNB 2002, 2008, 2010]*
a. 1% xylocaine b. 2% xylocaine
c. Ketamine d. Xylocaine + adrenaline

37. Fastest route of absorption of local anaesthetic is *[NBE DNB 2008, 2010]*
a. Intercostal b. Epidural
c. Brachial d. Caudal

38. All of the following are effective topically except *[Recent Question 2012, 2013]*
a. Procaine b. Cocaine
c. Lidocaine d. Amethocaine

39. CNS affection of a Local anaesthetic agent leads to *[Recent Question 2017]*
a. Convulsion b. Perioral numbness
c. Depression d. All of the above

40. Benzocaine is used in which type of anesthesia? *[Recent Question 2017]*
a. Topical b. Spinal
c. Epidural d. All of the above

41. Which of the following mixture of anaesthetics is applied on skin? *[Recent Question 2017]*
a. Lidocaine and Prilocaine
b. Bupivacaine and Prilocaine
c. Lidocaine and Bupivacaine
d. Lidocaine and Procaine

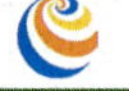 HIGH YIELD MCQs 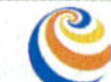

1. Which of the following is/are not local anesthesia? *[PGI 2009]*
a. Bupivacaine b. Mupivacaine
c. Mivacurium d. Butorphenol
e. Buprenorphine

2. From which of the following routes absorption of local anaesthetic is maximum? *[AIIMS PGMEE 2008]*
a. Intercostal b. Epidural
c. Brachial d. Caudal

3. Which one of the following is not an amide? *[All India PGMEE 2007]*
a. Lignocaine b. Procaine
c. Bupivacaine d. Dibucaine

4. All are vasodilators except *[All India PGMEE 1998]*
a. Procaine b. Lidocaine
c. Cocaine d. Chlorprocaine

5. Lignocaine in high dose produces *[PGI 2004]*
a. Convulsion b. Respiratory depression
c. Hypotension d. Cardiac arrest
e. Hypothermia

6. Which of the following local anesthetics is most likely to produce an allergic reaction? *[JIPMER PGMEE 2005]*
a. Prilocaine b. Ropivacaine
c. Etidocaine d. Benzocaine

7. A 25-year-old male with roadside accident underwent debridement and reduction of fractured both bones right forearm under axillary block. On the second postoperative day the patient complained of persistent numbness and paresthesia in the right forearm and the hand. The commonest cause of this neurological dysfunction could be all of the following except *[All India PGMEE 2004]*
a. Crush injury to the hand and lacerated nerves
b. A tight cast or dressing
c. Systemic toxicity of local anesthetics
d. Tourniquet pressure

8. Cardiac or central nervous system toxicity may result when standard lidocaine doses are administered to patients with circulatory failure. This may be due to the following reason *[All India PGMEE 2003]*
a. Lidocaine concentrations are initially higher in relatively well perfused tissues such as brain and heart

b. Histamine receptors in brain and heart gets suddenly activated in circulatory failure
c. There is a sudden out-burst of release of adrenaline, noradreneline and dopamine in brain and heart
d. Lidocaine is converted into a toxic metabolite due to its longer stay in liver

9. Shortest acting local anaesthetic agent is *[All India PGMEE 1997, PGI 2000]*
a. Procaine b. Lidocaine
c. Tetracaine d. Bupivacaine

10. Longest acting local anaesthetic agent *[All India PGMEE 1994]*
a. Bupivacaine b. Tetracaine
c. Xylocaine d. Procaine

11. About Lidocaine, all are true except *[PGI 1998]*
a. Local anaesthetic effect b. Cardiac arrhythmia
c. Ester d. Acts on mucous membranes

12. Local anaesthetic causing Methemoglobinemia *[AIIMS PGMEE 2010, All India PGMEE 1994]*
a. Procaine b. Prilocaine
c. Bupivacaine d. Cocaine

13. Which one of the following local anaesthetic is highly cardiotoxic? *[Recent Question 2016, AIIMS PGMEE 2005]*
a. Lignocaine b. Procaine
c. Mepivacaine d. Bupivacaine

14. True about local anaesthetic *[PGI 2001]*
a. Cocaine acts by decreasing norepinephrine
b. Act by decreasing sodium entry into cell
c. Lignocaine is an amide
d. Dibucaine is drug of choice for epidural anesthesia

15. True statements about local anesthesia *[PGI 2003]*
a. It inhibits the generation of action potential
b. Unmyelinated thin fibre are most susceptible than myelinated large fibers
c. Toxicity is reduced by addition of vasoconstrictor
d. Blocks all modalities of sensation at the same time

16. True about local anaesthetic agents *[PGI 2004]*
a. Duration depends on protein binding
b. Potency depends upon lipid solubility
c. LA with low PK is more active
d. Higher dose produces more block
e. Signal transduction blockade

17. Nerve fibre affected by local anesthesia first *[All India PGMEE 1995]*
a. Type A b. Type B
c. Type C d. Type II

18. Which of the following is not an amide? *[AIIMS PGMEE 2003]*
a. Lidocaine b. Procaine
c. Prilocaine d. Etidocaine

19. Cholinesterase metabolizes following except *[PGI 1997]*
a. Propanolol b. Procaine
c. Acetyl choline d. Bupivacaine

20. Concentration of lignocaine used *[PGI 2007]*
a. 2% b. 4%
c. 5% d. 10%
e. 1%

21. All are amide except *[All India PGMEE 1998]*
a. Lidocaine b. Procaine
c. Bupivacaine d. Mepivacaine

22. Topical use of following local anesthetic is not recommended? *[AIIMS PGMEE 2002]*
a. Ligocaine b. Bupivacaine
c. Cocaine d. Dibucaine

23. Sodium bicarbonate when given with local anesthetics has which of the following effect? *[All India PGMEE 2009]*
a. Increases speed and quality of anesthesia
b. Decreases diffusion of the anaesthetic drug
c. Causes rapid elimination of the local anaesthetic
d. Decreases speed and quality of anesthesia

24. True about EMLA *[PGI 2006]*
a. Can be used for intubation
b. Mixture of local anesthesia
c. Faster acting d. Used in children

25. Local anesthetic acting for more than 2 hours *[PGI 2000]*
a. Bupivaciane b. Etodocaine
c. Lignocaine d. Cholorprocaine

26. Which of the following is long acting local anesthetic >2 hours? *[PGI 2005]*
a. Bupivacaine b. Prilocaine
c. Etidocaine d. Dibucaine
e. Tetracaine

27. Xylocaine heavy in subarachnoid space has concentration of *[AIIMS PGMEE 1992]*
a. 1% b. 2%
c. 3% d. 5%

28. Maximum doses of lidocaine as local anesthesia is
a. 100 mg b. 200 mg *[AIIMS PGMEE 1992]*
c. 300 mg d. 500 mg

29. Maximum dose of lignocaine with adrenaline is *[All India PGMEE 1992]*
a. 3 mg/kg b. 4 mg/kg
c. 5 mg/kg d. 7 mg/kg

30. The afferent nerve fibres which are most sensitive to local anaesthetic belong to Group *[Recent Question 2016, AIIMS PGMEE 2004]*
a. A b. B
c. C d. D

31. Most potent Local anesthetic agent is *[JIPMER PGMEE 2014]*
a. Lidocaine b. Procaine
c. Ropivacaine d. Bupivacaine

32. Bier's block is *[Recent Question 2014]*
a. Topical anesthesia b. Tumescent anesthesia
c. Total intravenous regional anesthesia
d. Infiltrative anesthesia

33. Which among the following is exclusively used for Surface anesthesia? *[ESI IMO 2014]*
a. Lignocaine b. Procaine
c. Tetracaine d. Benzocaine

34. Amide type of Local Anaesthetic used to assess the possible presence of Atypical cholinesterase *[PGMCET 2015]*
a. Dibucaine b. Bupivacaine
c. Procaine d. Chlorprocaine

35. Addition of Adrenaline to Local anaesthetic results in all of the following effects, except *[PGMCET 2015]*
a. It makes the injection more painful
b. It decreases chances of subsequent local tissue edema
c. It provides a bloodless field for surgery
d. It reduces systemic toxicity of local anaesthetic

36. Nerve fibres least sensitive to the effect of Local anesthesia is *[AIIMS November 2017]*
a. A gamma b. A delta
c. B d. C

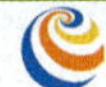 NEET/NBE PATTERN MCQs ANSWERS WITH EXPLANATIONS 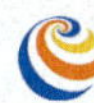

1. Ans. (c) Bupivacaine

[Ref. Anaesthesia for Postgraduates by Agasti, 1/e p384,385]

- Transmucosal route for drug delivery can be achieved through oral, lingual, oropharyngeal, nasopharyngeal, sublingual, rectal or tracheobronchial mucosa (by inhalation)
- Sublingual buprenorphine is a potent, synthetic, mixed agonist and antagonist opioid with long half-life and readily absorbed by sublingual route
- Buccal morphine for analgesia is not promising
- Oral transmucosal preparation of fentanyl is made of fentanyl citrate which is incorporated in a sweet lozenge
- Benzocaine, Tetracaine, Lidocaine is used primarily to anaesthetise mucosa

2. Ans. (d) Benzocaine

[Ref. Katzung, 11/e p449]

- Benzocaine is an ester which causes **Methemoglobinuria** as a side-effect
- Whereas Prilocaine has **Methemoglobinemia** as a side effect

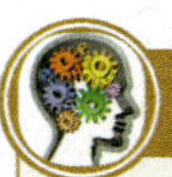

Also Remember

- Maximum nephrotoxicity shown by methoxyflurane
- Minimum nephrotoxicity is shown by isoflurane

3. Ans. (a) 0.5%

[Ref. Ophthalmology by Yanoff, 3/e p442]

Topical Anesthetics in Eye Surgeries

- 0.4% Benoxinate
- 0.5% Tetracaine
- 1% Amethocaine
- 1% Proparacaine

4. Ans. (b) Dexmedetomidine

[Ref. Miller's Anaesthesia, 7/e p753-757]

- Perioperative hemodynamic fluctuations are seen more often in hypertensive patients than in normotensive patients.
- In the hypertensive patients, dexmedetomidine premedication provides better hemodynamic stability compared with midazolam, and because it decreases the antihypertensive requirements, its use might be beneficial

5. Ans. NONE

[Ref. Katzung, 11/e p449]

- Prilocaine is approximately 40% less toxic than Lidocaine
- MC used antiarrhythmic agent in treatment of VT and VF is Lignocaine
- 2.5% Lidocaine + 2.5% Prilocaine Cream as an oil-in water emulsion is referred to as an EMLA (Eutectic mixtures of local anesthetics)
- Lidocaine and Mepivacaine are shorter acting than Bupivacaine due to their lower protein binding at the receptor, but faster in onset

6. Ans. (a) It is ester group of local anaesthetic

[Ref. KDT, 6/e p366]

Lignocaine

- **Lignocaine is the most common LA used**
- **Drug of choice for ventricular tachycardia**
- Choice of topical LA to mucous membrane, and is ineffective on intact skin
- Dose is limited to 7 mg/kg with adrenaline and 4 mg/kg without adrenaline
- Adrenaline is added to LA to make them long acting
- Sodium bicarbonate is added to LA to make them fast acting
- Lignocaine is the most commonly used for topical anesthesia of mucous membrane of ear, nose and throat
- Lignocaine and other class 1b drugs are avoided in arrhythmias
- And can precipitate to malignant hyperthermia due to release of calcium
- Lignocaine added with adrenaline should not be used in patients with:
  - Hyperthyroidism
  - Myocardial ischemia
  - Bier's block
  - With halothane

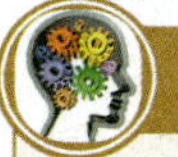

Also Remember

Amide class	Ester class
Lignocaine	Procaine
Prilocaine	Cocaine
Bupivacaine	Chlorprocaine
Dibucaine	Tetracaine
Etidocaine	Benzocaine
Ropivacaine	Amethocaine
Mepivacaine	

7. Ans. (d) Chlorprocaine

[Ref. Katzung, 11/e p449]

Chlorprocaine

- Shortest acting LA and with maximum ionized form
- Contraindicated in spinal anesthesia
- Neurotoxic

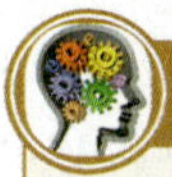

Also Remember

- Neutral (non-ionized) form of the molecule is able to pass through the lipid nerve cell membrane, whereas the ionized (protonated) form actually produces anesthesia
- Chloroprocaine has the highest pKa so exist in highest ionised form at any given pH

8. Ans. (a) Na channels

[Ref. Katzing, 12/e p453-457]

- Local anesthetics inhibit depolarization of the nerve membrane by interfering with both Na^+ and K^+ currents
- The action potential is not propagated because the threshold level is never attained

9. Ans. (b) Blood gas partition coefficient
[Ref. Anaesthesia by Colin, 3/e p558]

Blood Gas Partition Coefficient

- Factor that determines the speed of induction and recovery of the given anaesthetic agent
- It implies the percentage of partial pressure in the blood as compared to alveolar concentration
- Lesser blood gas partition coefficient indicates faster induction and recovery
- Higher blood gas partition coefficient indicates slower induction and recovery

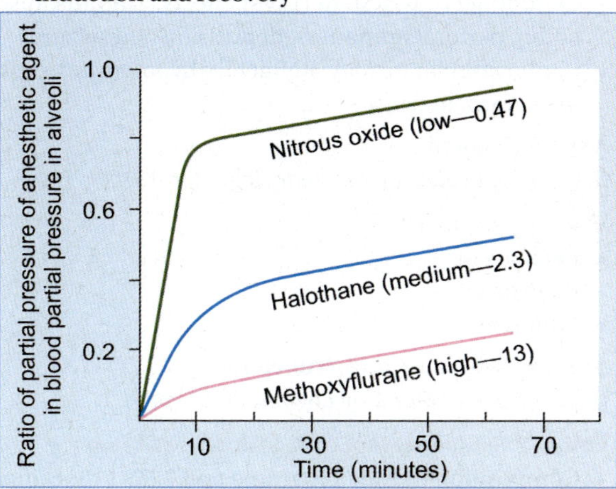

Fig. BG partition coefficient

10. Ans. (c) Benzocaine
[Ref. Acute and Chronic Wounds by Bryant, 5/e p535]

- Benzocaine, or ethyl amino benzoate, introduced under the trade name of **"Anesthesin"** has found wide usage as a local anesthetic in painful wounds, ulcers of the skin and accessible mucous surfaces because of its comparative insolubility

11. Ans. (b) Bupivacaine
[Ref. Katzung, 11/e p441]

- For many years, racemic bupivacaine was the only amide local anesthetic with long duration and therefore the most commonly used amide local anesthetic in children

12. Ans. (d) Dibucaine
[Ref. Anaesthesia by Colin, 3/e p611]

- Longest acting and most toxic and potent local anaesthetic is Dibucaine
- Chlorprocaine is the shortest acting LA

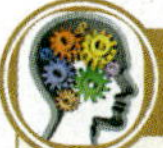

Also Remember

- Procaine is the local anaesthetic of choice in Malignant hyperthermia
- Cocaine is the only ester which is not metabolized by pseudocholinesterase, rather is metabolised by the liver
- Prilocaine produces a metabolite O-toludine an oxidizing agent which can oxidize haemoglobin to methemoglobin which can turn out to be a cause of methemoglobinemia
- Lignocaine is the most commonly used local anaesthetic and is drug of choice for ventricular tachycardia

13. Ans. (a) Procaine
[Ref. Anaesthesia for Postgraduates by Agasti, 1/e p336]

- Procaine is an ester with a rapid onset (3–5 minutes) and a short duration of action (60 minutes).
- **Procaine has several limitations:**
  - Short duration of action (<60 minutes)
  - Higher frequency of nausea and vomiting
  - Higher frequency of failed spinal anesthesia
  - Despite its short duration of action, it has a delayed time to full recovery

14. Ans. (a) Na^+ channels
[Ref. Ajay Yadav, 4/e p118]

Mechanism of Action of Local Anesthetics

- Undissociated (Non-ionised) form of anaesthetic molecules enter axonal membrane and gets dissociated (ionised)
- Ionised form blocks sodium channel, thus preventing depolarisation
- Some minor action is also present on potassium and calcium channels

15. Ans. (a) 1–3
[Ref. Ajay Yadav, 4/e p123]

16. Ans. (c) Benzocaine
[Ref. Ajay Yadav, 4/e p122]

- Used as lozenges for stomatitis, sore throat

17. Ans. (d) Chlorprocaine
[Ref. Ajay Yadav, 4/e p124]

- 15–25 minutes

18. Ans. (b) 7 mg/kg wt
[Ref. Ajay Yadav, 4/e p124]

- Without adrenaline it is 3 mg/ kg wt

19. Ans. (b) Felypressin
[Ref. Clinical Anaesthetic Pharmacology by Dundee, 1/e p574]

20. Ans. (d) 1:2,00,000
[Ref. Ajay Yadav, 4/e p120]

21. Ans. (b) Prilocaine
[Ref. Ajay Yadav, 4/e p123]

- Methaemoglobinemia occurs at high dose (>6 mg/kg) because of accumulation of metabolite Orthotoluidene which can convert Hb to metHb

22. Ans. (d) Dibucaine
[Ref. Ajay Yadav, 4/e p124]

- **Duration of action of Dibucaine**:
  - Without adrenaline: 2.5 to 3.5 hours
  - With adrenaline: 3.5-5.5 hours

23. Ans. (b) Circumoral numbness
[Ref. Ajay Yadav, 4/e p121]

Local Anesthetic Toxicity

- CNS is the first system involved in local anaesthetic toxicity
- Typical sequence: Excitation followed by depression of cerebral tissue

- Sign and symptoms: Circumoral numbness, dizziness, tongue paresthesia, visual and auditory disturbances, muscle twitching, tremors, convulsions followed by coma and death

24. Ans. (b) Decreases absorption of LA
[Ref. Ajay Yadav, 4/e p120]
- Addition of Epinephrine to Lignocaine increases the margin of safety by decreased absorption

25. Ans. (a) Cocaine
[Ref. Ajay Yadav, 4/e p122]
- Cocaine is a potent vasoconstrictor

26. Ans. (a) Stabilization of membrane
[Ref. Ajay Yadav, 4/e p119]

27. Ans. (d) Chloroprocaine
[Ref. Ajay Yadav, 4/e p124]
- pKa for chloroprocaine is 9 (max) and for mepivacaine is 7.6 (least)

28. Ans. (b) Lidocaine 2.5% + Prilocaine 2.5%
[Ref. Ajay Yadav, 4/e p121]

29. Ans. (a) Procaine
[Ref. Ajay Yadav, 4/e p124]

30. Ans. (b) Motor, pro, presymp ganglionic
[Ref. Ajay Yadav, 4/e p119]

31. Ans. (b) Lidocaine + prilocaine
[Ref. Ajay Yadav, 4/e p121]

32. Ans. (c) Cardiotoxicity
[Ref. Ajay Yadav, 4/e p123]
- Cardiotoxicity of Bupivacaine increases in pregnancy, hypoxia and acidosis

33. Ans. (c) Prilocaine
[Ref. Ajay Yadav, 4/e p123]

34. Ans. (a) Na^+ channel inhibition
[Ref. Ajay Yadav, 4/e p118-119]

35. Ans. (a) Cocaine
[Ref. Ajay Yadav, 4/e p122]

36. Ans. (a) 1% xylocaine
[Ref. Ajay Yadav, 4/e p123]

37. Ans. (a) Intercostal
[Ref. Ajay Yadav, 4/e p120]
- Systemic absorption is highest after intercostals nerve block

38. Ans. (a) Procaine
[Ref. Ajay Yadav, 4/e p122]

39. Ans. (d) All of the above
[Ref. Pain Medicine by Anitescu, 1/e p166]

Toxicity of Local Anesthetics

- Central nervous system (CNS) effects: Tinnitus, disorientation, perioral numbness, depression and seizures
- Cardiovascular toxicity: Refractory hypotension, dysrhythmias, cardiac arrest

40. Ans. (a) Topical
[Ref. Quick Review of Pharmacology, 1/e p207]

Used for Surface Anesthesia Only

- Benzocaine
- Benoxinate
- Butamben

41. Ans. (a) Lidocaine and Prilocaine
[Ref. Local Anesthesia by Logothetis, 2/e p85]

EMLA: 2.5% Lidocaine/2.5% Prilocaine Cream

- Composition of 2.5% Lidocaine and 2.5% Prilocaine as an oil-in water emulsion
- Eutectic mixtures of Local anesthetics
- First major breakthrough for Surface anaesthesia on intact skin

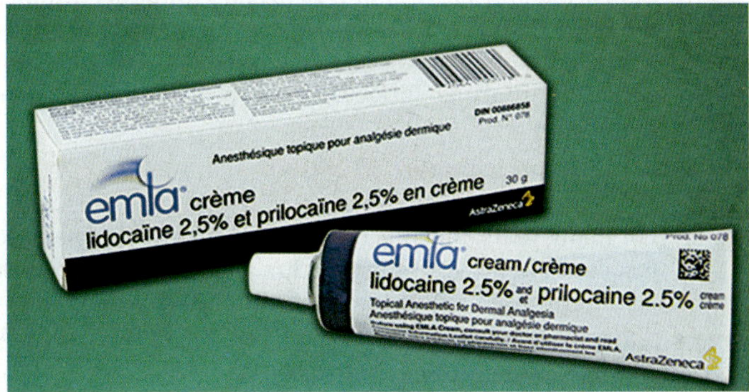

Fig. EMLA

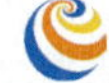 HIGH YIELD MCQs ANSWERS WITH EXPLANATIONS 

1. Ans. (c) Mivacurium; (d) Butorphenol; (e) Buprenorphine
[Ref. Ajay Yadav, 4/e p118]

2. Ans. (a) Intercostal
[Ref. Ajay Yadav, 4/e p120]

3. Ans. (b) Procaine
[Ref. Ajay Yadav, 4/e p122]

Commonly used Local Anesthetics

Esters	Amides
• Procaine • Tetracaine • 2-Chlorprocaine	• Lidocaine • Mepivacaine • Bupivacaine • Ropivacaine • Etidocaine

4. **Ans. (c) Cocaine**
[Ref. Ajay Yadav, 4/e p122]

5. **Ans. (a) Convulsion; (b) Respiratory depression; (c) Hypotension; (d) Cardiac arrest**
[Ref. Ajay Yadav, 4/e p123]

6. **Ans. (d) Benzocaine**
[Ref. Ajay Yadav, 4/e p122]

7. **Ans. (c) Systemic toxicity of local anesthetics**
[Ref. Ajay Yadav, 4/e p120-121]

8. **Ans. (a) Lidocaine concentration are initially higher in relatively well perfused tissues such as brain and heart**
[Ref. Ajay Yadav, 4/e p120-121]

9. **Ans. (a) Procaine**
[Ref. Ajay Yadav, 4/e p124]

10. **Ans. (b) Tetracaine**
[Ref. Ajay Yadav, 4/e p124]

11. **Ans. (c) Ester**
[Ref. Ajay Yadav, 4/e p122]

12. **Ans. (b) Prilocaine**
[Ref. Ajay Yadav, 4/e p123]

13. **Ans. (d) Bupivacaine**
[Ref. Ajay Yadav, 4/e p123]

14. **Ans. (b) Act by decreasing sodium entry into cell; (c) Ligocaine is an amide**
[Ref. Ajay Yadav, 4/e p118, 122]

15. **Ans. (a) It inhibits the generation of action potential (c) toxicity is reduced by addition of vasoconstrictor**
[Ref. Ajay Yadav, 4/e p118-120]

16. **Ans. ALL CHOICES**
[Ref. Ajay Yadav, 4/e p118-120]

17. **Ans. (b) Type B**
[Ref. Ajay Yadav, 4/e p119]
- Two factors which determine the sensitivity of nerve fibres to local anesthetics are fibre diameter and myelination
- Type B fibres (myelinated) are more readily blocked than type C (non-myelinated) inspite of being thinner diameter than B

18. **Ans. (b) Procaine**
[Ref. Ajay Yadav, 4/e p122]

19. **Ans. (d) Bupivacaine**
[Ref. Ajay Yadav, 4/ep123]
- Bupivacaine is metabolized in liver

20. **Ans. (a) 2%; (b) 4%; (c) 5%; (e) 1%**
[Ref. Ajay Yadav, 4/e p123]

21. **Ans. (b) Procaine**
[Ref. Ajay Yadav, 4/e p122]

22. **Ans. (b) Bupivacaine**
[Ref. Ajay Yadav, 4/e p122]
- Mepivacaine, bupivacaine and ropivacaine are not used as surface/topical analgesia

23. **Ans. (a) Increased speed and quality of anesthesia**
[Ref. Ajay Yadav, 4/e p120]
- **Addition of sodium bicarbonate** (1 ml of 8.4% to 10 ml of lignocaine) **increases both onset and duration of action**
- Sodium bicarbonate increases the onset by making the pH more alkaline so more drug is available in unionized form
- Later carbon dioxide released from sodium bicarbonate metabolism enters intracellularly making the pH more acidic making more drug to be available in ionized form, thereby increasing the duration of action also
- So it enhances the onset of action, increases the duration of action, improves the quality of block, decreases the pain of injection.

24. **Ans. (b) Mixture of local anesthesia; (d) Used in children**
[Ref. Ajay Yadav, 4/e p121]

25. **Ans. (a) Bupivacaine; (b) Etodocaine**
[Ref. Ajay Yadav, 4/e p124]
- Tetracaine, etidocaine, bupivacaine, ropivacaine and dibucaine can act more than 2 hours

26. **Ans. (a) Bupivacaine; (c) Etidocaine; (d) Dibucaine; (e) Tetracaine**
[Ref. Ajay Yadav, 4/e p124]

27. **Ans. (d) 5%**
[Ref. Ajay Yadav, 4/e p123]

28. **Ans. (d) 500 mg**
[Ref. Ajay Yadav, 4/e p123]
- Maximum dose of Lidocaine with Adrenaline: 500 mg
- Maximum dose of Lidocaine without adrenaline: 200 mg

29. **Ans. (d) 7 mg/kg**
[Ref. Ajay Yadav, 4/e p123]

30. **Ans. (b) Type B**
[Ref. Ajay Yadav, 4/e p119]

31. **Ans. (d) Bupivacaine**
[Ref. Ajay Yadav, 4/e p124]
- Potency of Local anesthetics: Bupivacaine>Ropivacaine>Lidocaine >Procaine

32. **Ans. (c) Total intravenous regional anesthesia**
[Ref. Miller's Anaesthesia, 2/e p182]

BIER'S Block
- Total intravenous regional anesthesia
- Anesthetics used: 0.5% Lidocaine/ Prilocaine
- **Indication**: Short surgical procedures on an extremity where postoperative pain is not expected to be significant
- **Contraindications**: Contraindications to tourniquet application-
  - Sickle cell disease
  - Infection
  - Ischemic vascular disease
- **Advantages**:
  - Easier, faster (than Brachial plexus/ Extremity block)
  - Useful in all age groups (including pediatric age group)

- **Disadvantages:**
  - Severe tourniquet pain
  - Limited postoperative analgesia

33. Ans. (d) Benzocaine

[Ref. Quick Review of Pharmacology, 1/e p207]

Used for Surface Anesthesia Only

- Benzocaine
- Benoxinate
- Butamben

34. Ans. (a) Dibucaine

[Ref. Ophthalmic Surgery by Krupin, 1/e p7]

- Dibucaine or Sodium fluoride are used as an inhibitor to measure the percentage inhibition of Serum cholinesterase
- By determining the Dibucaine number for a given patient the diagnosis of the presence of atypical plasma cholinesterase may be established

35. Ans. (b) It decreases chances of subsequent local tissue edema

[Ref. Clinical Skills by Patel, 1/e p266]

Addition of Adrenaline to LA

- Prolongs duration of action: Reducing rate of removal from the local site into circulation
- Reduces systemic toxicity
- Provides a more bloodless field for surgery
- Injection becomes more painful
- Increases chances of subsequent local tissue oedema and necrosis
- Delays the wound healing

36. Ans. (a) A gamma

[Ref. Clinical Anesthesia by Vacanti, 1/e p285]

- Order of susceptibility to blockade by Local anesthetic (Most susceptible to least susceptible): B < C < A-delta < A-gamma < A-beta < A-alpha

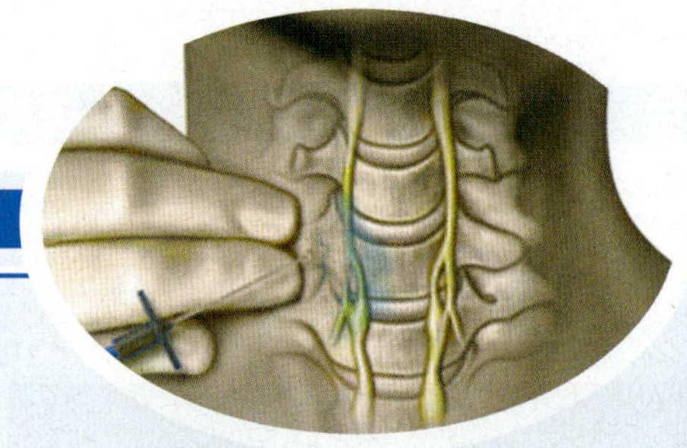

Chapter 10

Cardiopulmonary Resuscitation

THEORETICAL CONCEPTS

X A. CARDIOPULMONARY CEREBRAL RESUSCITATION (CPR/ CPCR)

- ***Sequence for maintenance of CPR*: [Mnemonic: ABC]**[Q]
  - **A**irway
  - **B**reathing
  - **C**irculation
- ***Components of CPR***:
  - Basic life support
  - Advanced life support
  - Post-resuscitation life support
- ***Four-link chain for survival***:
  - Early recognition and activation of emergency services
  - Immediate CPR
  - Early shock
  - Early advanced life support

X B. BASIC AND ADVANCED LIFE SUPPORT

	Basic life support	Advanced life support
	Primary A, B, C, D	Secondary A, B, C, D
Airway	Manual	Secondary equipments (Guedel's airway, LMA, Endotracheal tube, Tracheostomy tube)
Breathing	Mouth-to-mouth Mouth-to-nose Bag and mask	Advanced methods (LMA, Endotracheal tube, Tracheostomy tube, Combitube)
Circulation	Cardiac massage	Cardiac massage
Defibrillation	Automatic external defibrillator	Manual defibrillator
Drugs	–	+

(LMA: Laryngeal mask airway)*

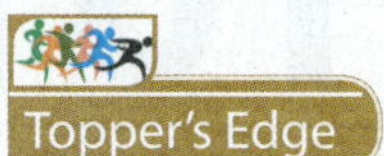

Topper's Edge

Summary of Recommended Basic Life Support Techniques

	Infant (1–12 months)	Child (>12 months)	Adult
Breathing rate	20 breaths/min	20 breaths/min	10–12 breaths/min
Pulse check	Brachial	Carotid	Carotid
Compression rate	>100/min	100/min	100/min
Compression method	Two or three fingers	Heel of one hand	Hands interlaced
Compression/ventilation ratio	**30:2**[Q]	**30:2**[Q]	**30:2**[Q]
Foreign body obstruction	Back blows, chest thrusts	Heimlich maneuver	Heimlich maneuver

X C. AIRWAY MANAGEMENT

X C1. Airway Maintenance in Life Supports

- *Airway maintenance in Basic life support*: No equipments
  - Manual
- *Airway maintenance in Advanced life support*: Secondary equipments [Q]
  - Guedel's airway
  - Laryngeal mask airway (LMA)
  - Endotracheal tube
  - Tracheostomy tube

X C2. Techniques of Airway Maintenance

- ***In cases of tongue fall***:
  - *Manual management*:
    - Open mouth, clear airway
    - Tilt head back and lift chin (hyperextension)
    - Jaw thrust forward
  - *Airway insertion*:
    - Guedel's airway
    - Safar airway
    - Nasophrayngeal airway
  - *Endotracheal tube*: Most definitive method
- ***In cases of foreign body obstruction***:
  - Infant chest thrusts
  - Back-blows
  - Heimlich manoeuvre
  - Chest thrust
  - Finger sweep method
  - Cricothyroidotomy
- ***In other cases of airway obstruction*** *(Laryngeal oedema, epiglottitis, laryngotracheobronchitis)*: [Q]
  - Tracheostomy

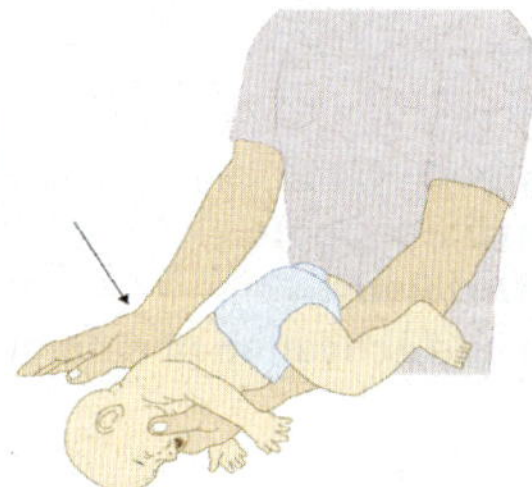

Fig. Infant chest thrusts **Fig.** Back blows

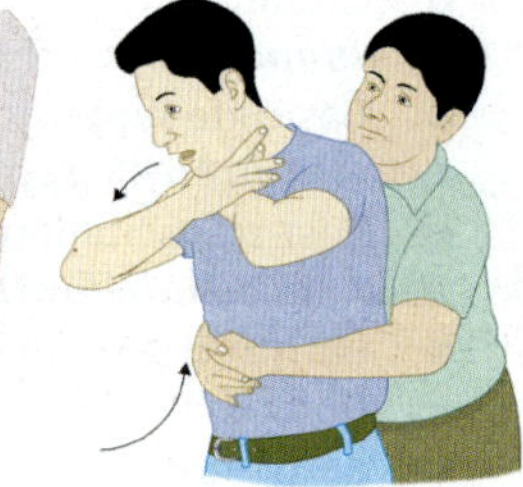

Fig. Heimlich maneuver

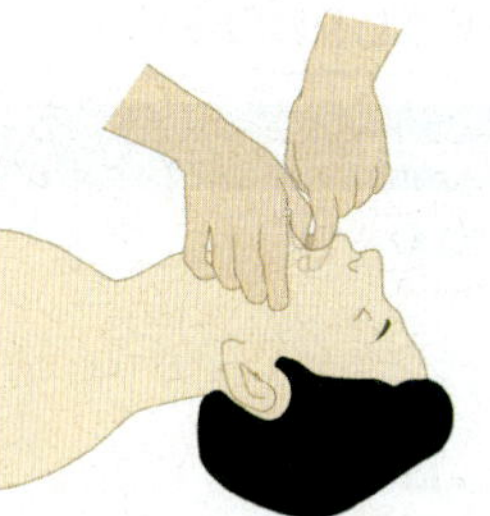

Fig. Finger sweep

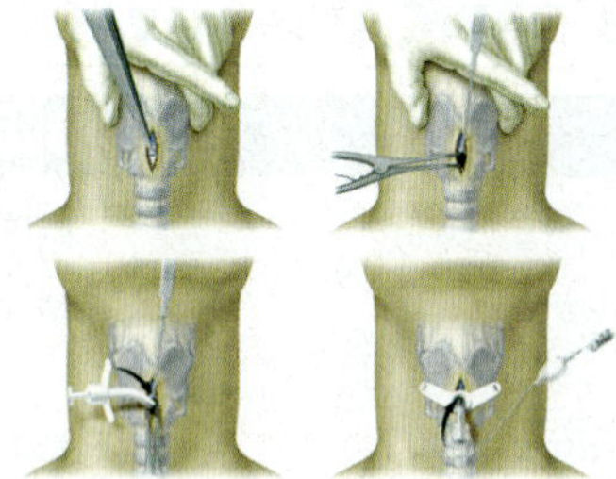

Fig. Cricothyroidotomy

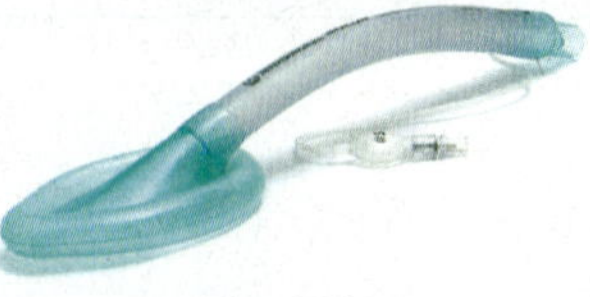

Fig. LMA

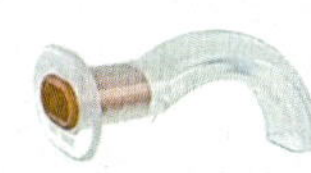

Fig. Guedel's airway

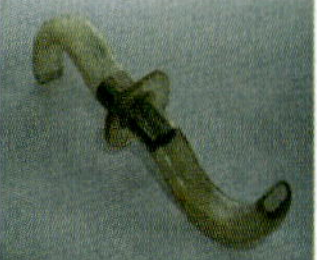

Fig. Safar airway

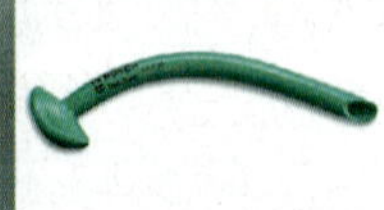

Fig. Nasophrayngeal airway

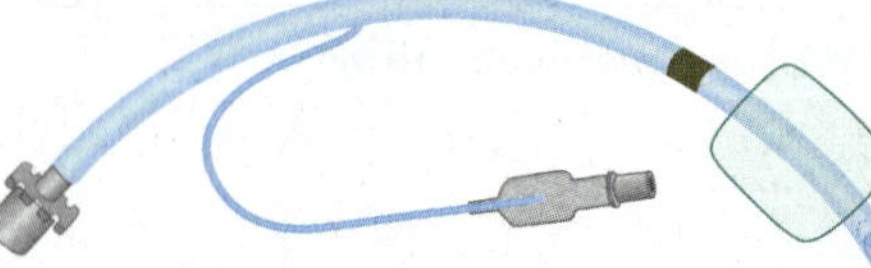

Fig. ET tube

Anesthesiology

X D. BREATHING/VENTILATION

- *Mouth-to-mouth*
- *Mouth-to-airway*: Safar or Brook airway
- *Bag-and-mask*: Increases aspiration, increases dead space, exhaustive
- *Advanced methods*:
  - **Endotracheal tube (Most definitive, best method)**
  - Laryngeal mask airway
  - Combitube
  - Tracheostomy tube
- *Automatic ventilators*

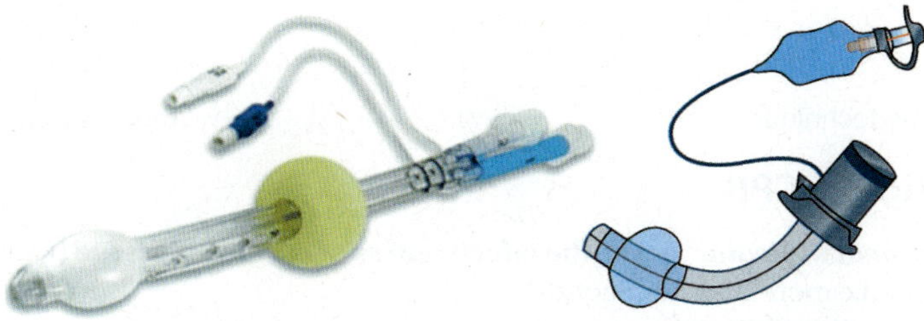

Fig. Combi-tube **Fig.** Tracheostomy tube

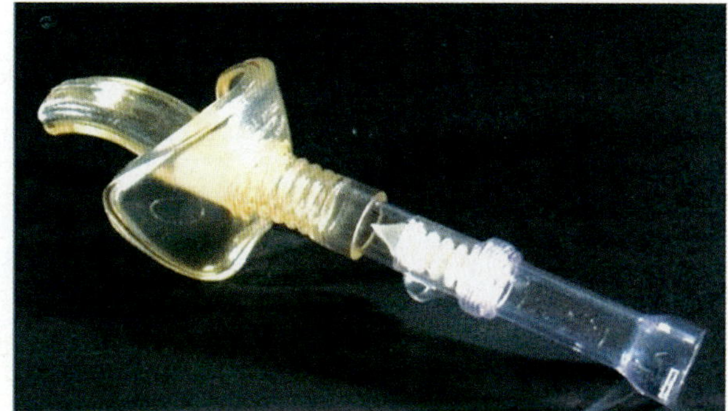

Fig. Brook airway

X E. CIRCULATION

- *Cardiac massage*

X E1. External Cardiac Massage

- *Cardiac massage in adults*:
  - Compressions: **Over lower third of sternum** (two fingers above Xiphoid process)[Q]
  - Depress sternum by: 1.5-2.0 inches
  - Effective cardiac output generated: 30% of normal
- *Cardiac massage in children*: **'Two thumbs technique'** for compressions [Q]
- *Cardiac massage in newborns*: 'Two thumbs with encircled chest technique' for compressions [Q]
- *Cardiac massage in pregnant*: External cardiac massage with lateral tilt
- ***Open chest massage indications***:
  - Cardiac tamponade
  - Blunt penetrating trauma
  - Air embolism
  - Chest deformities
  - Arrest during intrathoracic procedures

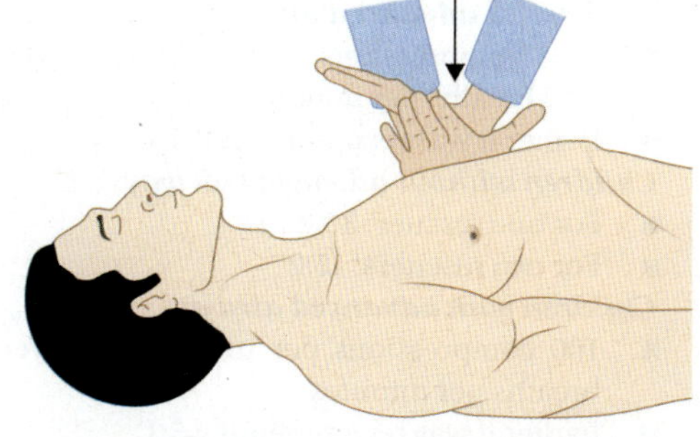

Fig. Cardiac massage (Compression)

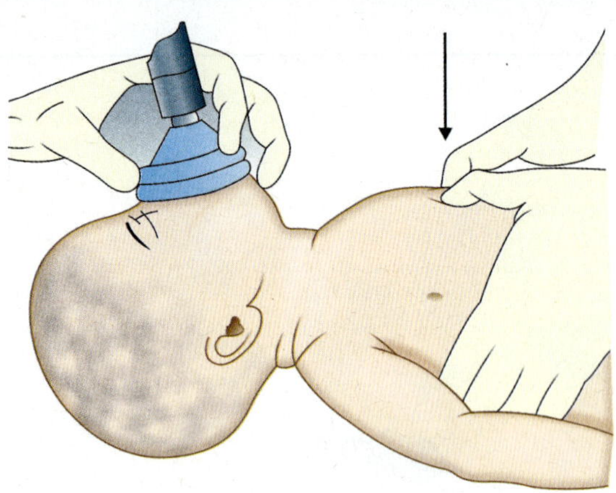

Fig. Two thumbs technique

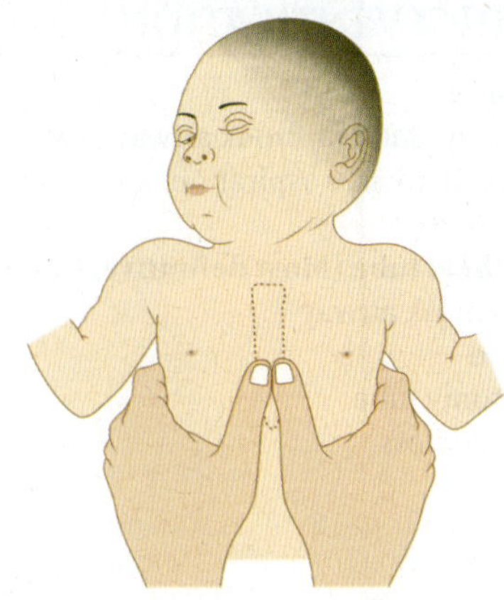

Fig. Two thumbs technique

X E2. Carotid Pulse Palpation in CPR

- Utility: Is the ***'most effective clinical indicator'* to see the effectiveness of cardiac massage** (Circulation component of ABC)[Q]
- *Carotid pulse check*: Should not take more than 10 seconds[Q]
- If not able to check pulse (Non-medicos): Treat it as no pulse
- Further management:
  - *If carotid pulse absent*:
    - Chest compressions (Compression: Ventilation ratio 3:2)
    - Defibrillator
  - *If carotid pulse present*:
    - Give breaths (rate 10-12 per minute)

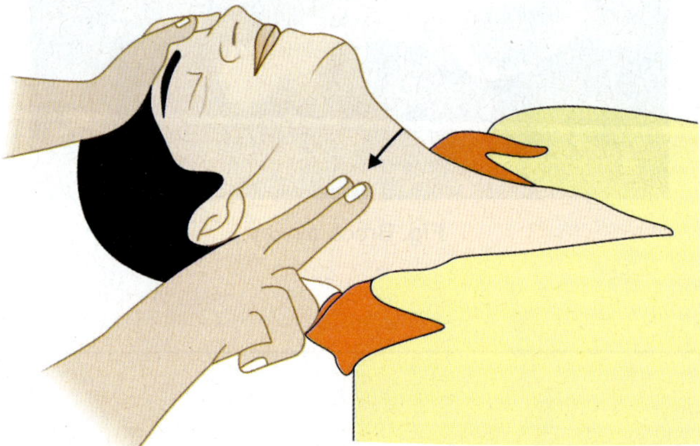

Fig. Carotid pulse check

X E3. Compression: Ventilation Ratios during CPR

- ***Adults without advanced airway*: 30:2**
- ***Adults with advanced airway***:
  - 100 compressions per minute AND Ventilation rate < 12 breaths per minutes
  - Earlier it was recommended 5:1
- ***Children without advanced airway***:
  - For one rescuer: **30:2**
  - For two rescuers: 15:2
- ***Children with advanced airway***:
  - 100 compressions per minute AND Ventilation rate 8–10 breaths per minutes
  - Earlier it was recommended 5:1
- ***Newborns*: 3:1**

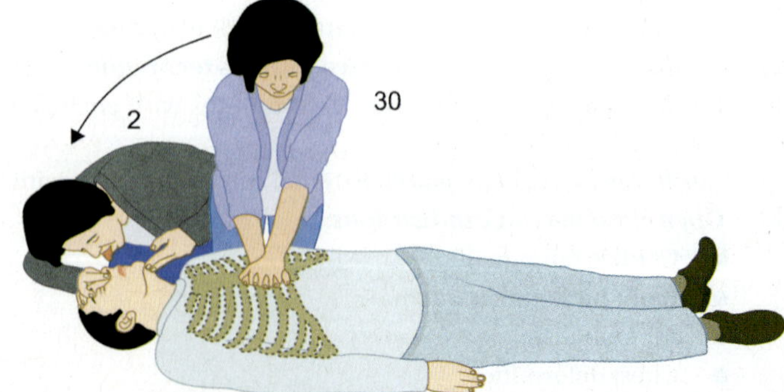

Fig. Compression ventilation ratio (adult)

Anesthesiology

X F. MONITORING OF CPR

- ***Capnography*: Most reliable, best indicator** [Q]
- ***Palpation of carotid pulse*: Most effective clinical indicator** [Q]
- *Coronary perfusion pressure*

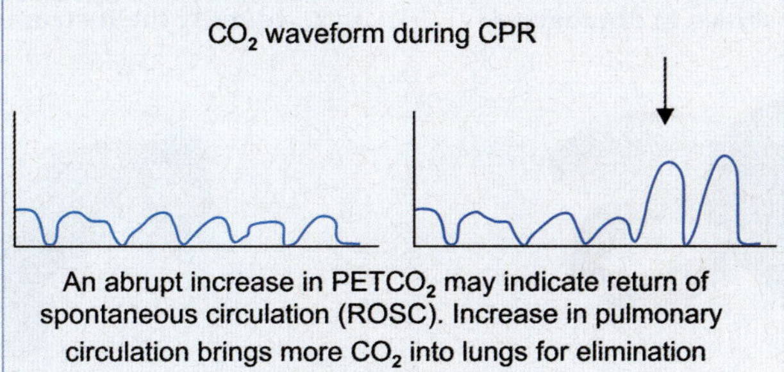

Fig. Capnography

X G. COMPLICATIONS OF CPR[Q]

- Rib fracture
- Pneumothroax
- Pneumomediastinum
- Pneumopericardium
- Injury to diaphragm
- Injury to stomach
- Injury to lungs
- Injury to major vessels
- Injury to abdominal organs (Spleen, liver)

X H. DRUGS USED IN CARDIOPULMONARY RESUSCITATION (CPR)

- ***Vasopressors***: [Q]
  - Adrenaline
  - Noradrenaline
  - Ephedrine
  - Mephenteramine
- ***Ionotropes***: [Q]
  - Dopamine
  - Dobutamine
- *Beta blockers*:
  - Propranolol
  - Esmolol
- *Anticholinergics*:
  - Atropine
  - Glycopyrrolate
- *Respiratory stimulants (Analeptics)*:
  - Doxapram
  - Ethamivan
- *Vasodilators*:
  - Sodium nitroprusside, Nitroglycerine
  - Nifedipine
  - Potassium chloride
- *Antiarrhythmics*:
  - Amiodarone
  - Xylocard
  - Bretyllium
  - Adenosine

IMAGE-BASED QUESTIONS

1. Identify the instrument/device shown in Photograph

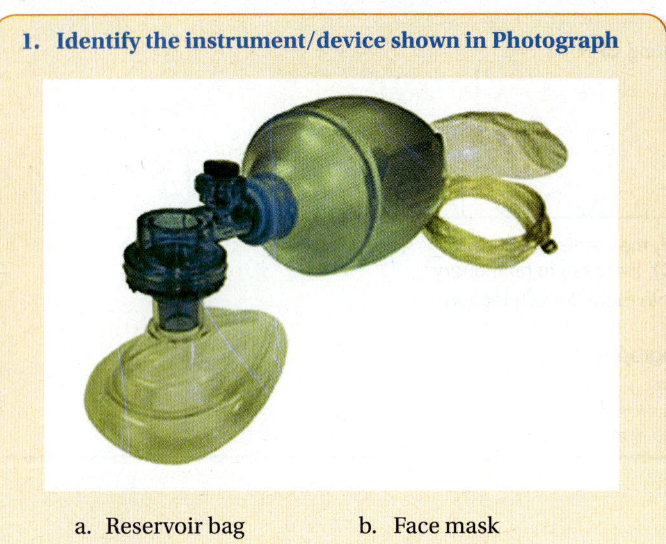

a. Reservoir bag
b. Face mask
c. LMA
d. Ambu bag

2. Identify the Instrument/ device shown in Photograph

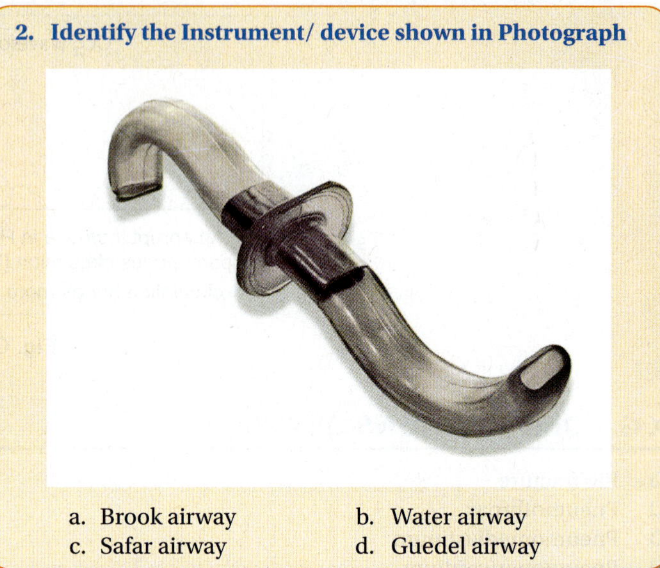

a. Brook airway
b. Water airway
c. Safar airway
d. Guedel airway

3. Identify the Instrument/ device shown in Photograph ***[Recent Question 2012]***

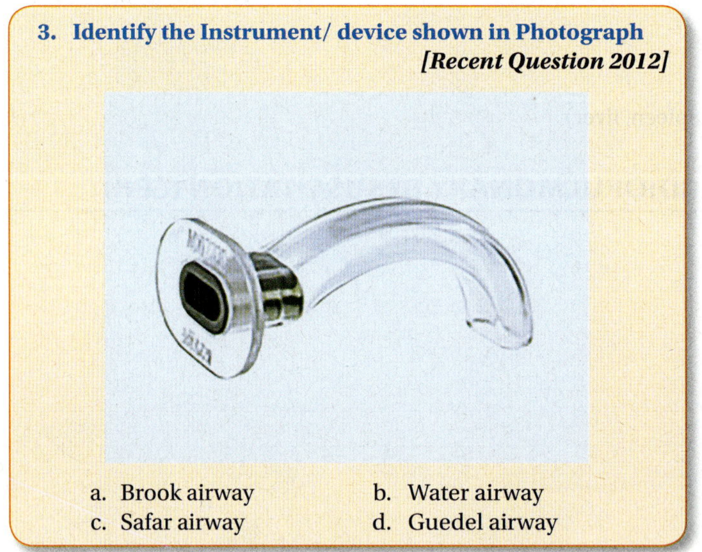

a. Brook airway
b. Water airway
c. Safar airway
d. Guedel airway

ANSWERS WITH EXPLANATIONS OF IBQs

1. Ans. (d) Ambu bag *[Ref. Ajay Yadav, 4/e p42]*

Artificial Manual Breathing Unit (AMBU)

- Can deliver 100% oxygen supply
- Maximum value of bag: 1200 ml

2. Ans. (c) Safar airway *[Ref. Ajay Yadav, 4/e p41]*

- Safar airway is used for Mouth-to-airway breathing during resuscitation while preventing tongue fall

3. Ans. (d) Guedel airway *[Ref. Ajay Yadav, 4/e p40]*

- Guedel airway is the MC type of airway used while also preventing tongue falling back on posterior pharyngeal wall

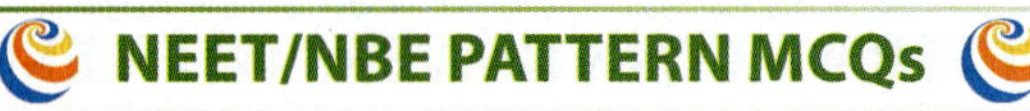

NEET/NBE PATTERN MCQs

1. **Machine used noninvasively to monitor a pulmonary chest compression during cardiopulmonary resuscitation is**
   a. Zoll aed-plus automatic external defibrillator
   b. Zoll depth synchronizer *[Recent Question 2016]*
   c. Zoll strength sensor d. Zoll PaO_2 monitor
2. **Ratio of Chest compression and Ventilation for all ages done by a Single rescuer is** *[AIIMS November 2016]*
   a. 30:1 b. 30:2
   c. 10:1 d. 15:1
3. **First priority in management of trauma patient is**
   a. Airway maintenance *[NBE FMGE September 2009]*
   b. Circulation management
   c. Maintain intravascular compartment
   d. Look at fractured bones
4. **In newborn, chest compression should be started if heart rate is** *[Recent Question 2012]*
   a. < l20/min b. < 100/min
   c. < 80/min d. < 60/min
5. **During basic life support, how much time should be spent looking for Carotid pulse** *[NBE FMGE September 2008]*
   a. Not more than 10 seconds
   b. Not more than 12 seconds
   c. Not more than 15 seconds
   d. Not more than 20 seconds
6. **Site for external cardiac massage is**
   a. Lower third sternum *[NBE FMGE March 2009]*
   b. Junction of body and manubrium sterni
   c. Xiphoid process
   d. Two fingers left of Xiphoid process
7. **Agent not widely used in Cardiopulmonary resuscitation is** *[NBE FMGE September 2006]*
   a. Adrenaline b. Calcium
   c. Atropine d. Vasopressin
8. **Recommended rate of chest compression during cardio-pulmonary resuscitation in adults is** *[NBE FMGE September 2011]*
   a. About 72 compressions per minute
   b. At least 72 compressions per minute
   c. About 100 compressions per minute
   d. At least 100 compressions per minute
9. **The ratio of chest compression to breathing in Pediatric life support is** *[NBE FMGE March 2012]*
   a. 3:1 b. 4:1
   c. 5:1 d. 6:1
10. **High quality CPR include all except** *[Recent Question 2015, 2016]*
   a. Chest compressions 200/minute
   b. Depth of 2 or more inches
   c. Complete recoil after compression
   d. Avoid excessive ventilation
11. **Not true about CPR?** *[Recent Question 2017]*
   a. Chest compressions at 100/min
   b. Ratio 30:2
   c. Chest compression >6 inches
   d. Breathing rate 8–10 breaths/min

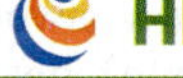
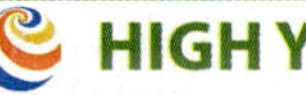

HIGH YIELD MCQs

1. **During cardiac resuscitation, the following can occur except**
   a. Rupture of lungs b. Rupture of liver *[PGI 2001]*
   c. Rupture of stomach d. Rupture of Spleen
   e. Disseminated intravascular coagulation
2. **First step in CPR (cardiopulmonary resuscitation) should be** *[PGI 2000]*
   a. IV adrenaline b. Intracardiac atropine
   c. Airway maintenance d. Hysterectomy
3. **The outcome following resuscitation of cardiac arrest is worsened if during resuscitation patient is given** *[AIIMS PGMEE 2005]*
   a. Ringer's lactate b. Colloids
   c. 5% Dextrose d. Whole blood transfusion
4. **True about adrenaline in CPR** *[PGI 2001]*
   a. Can be given intratracheally
   b. I.V. route better than intracardiac
   c. Intracardiac route better than IV
   d. Converts coarse fibrillation into fine ones
   e. The dose used in 2 ml containing 1 in 1000 concentration
5. **According to 2005 AHA guidelines true about number of chest compression in CPR** *[PGI 2007]*
   a. 80/min including neonate
   b. 90/min including neonate
   c. 100/min excluding neonate
   d. 120/min including neonate
   e. 120/min excluding
6. **In a patient with cardiorespiratory arrest, basic life support is given to support which of the following systems**
   a. Respiratory system *[PGI 2001]*
   b. Cardiovascular system c. Renal system
   d. Gastrointestinal system e. CNS
7. **During Adult Cardiopulmonary resuscitation, all the following drugs can be administered through a tracheal tube except** *[Recent Question 2016, PGMCET 2015]*
   a. Atropine b. Adrenaline
   c. Vasopressin d. Amiodarone
8. **Sequence of events according to BLS is** *[AIIMS November 2017]*
   a. Start CPR, Give 2 rescue breaths, Assess pulse
   b. Give rescue breaths, See pulse, Start CPR
   c. Assess patient, Activate emergency response team, Call for defibrillator, Start CPR
   d. Assess pulse, Defibrillate, Start CPR
9. **Balanced resuscitation means** *[AIIMS November 2017]*
   a. Maintaining acid base balance
   b. Equal use of colloids and crystalloids
   c. Permissive hypotension and limited crystalloid use
   d. Management of airway breathing and circulation

NEET/NBE PATTERN MCQs ANSWERS WITH EXPLANATIONS

1. **Ans. (a) Zoll aed-plus automatic external defibrillator**
[Ref. Cardiopulmonary Resuscitation by Ornato, 1/e p164]

Zoll aed-plus Automatic External Defibrillator

- Unique CPR feedback tool that is able to monitor CPR quality and provide real-time feedback for depth and rate of chest compressions
- Audio and visual prompts help you to rescue with a confidence and clarity unmatched by any other AED

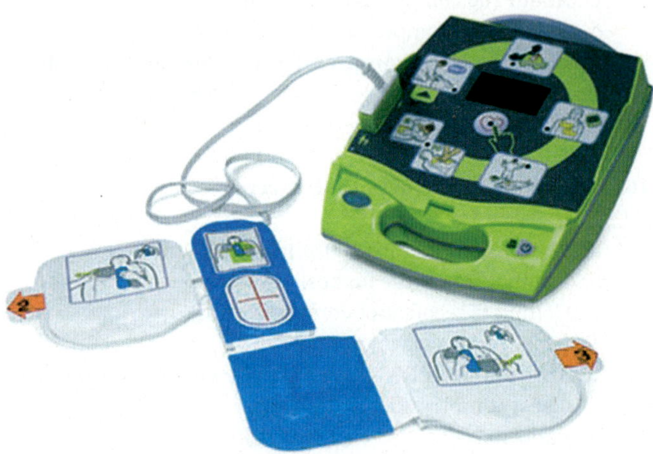

Fig. Zoll aed-plus automated external defibrillator

2. **Ans. (b) 30:2**
[Ref. Emergency Cardiovascular Care and CPR by Field, 1/e p236]

Chest compression: Ventilation Ratios

- **In adults**:
  - One rescuer = **30:2**
  - Two rescuers = 30:2
- **In children**:
  - One rescuer = **30:2**
  - Two rescuers = 15:2

3. **Ans. (a) Airway maintenance**
[Ref. Ajay Yadav, 4/e p220]

Cardiopulmonary Cerebral Resuscitation (CPR/ CPCR)

- *Sequence for maintenance of CPR*: **[Mnemonic: ABC]**
  - **A**irway
  - **B**reathing
  - **C**irculation
- *Airway maintenance in Basic life support*: No equipments
  - Manual
- *Airway maintenance in Advanced life support*: Secondary equipments
  - Guedel's airway
  - Laryngeal mask airway (LMA)
  - Endotracheal tube
  - Tracheostomy tube

Also Remember

- Most common cause of airway obstruction in unconscious patient: Tongue fall
- **Most definitive method to maintain airway in unconscious patient: Endotracheal tube (ET)**
- Airway management in cases of tongue fall:

Manual management	Open mouth, clear airway Tilt head back and lift chin (hyperextension) Jaw thrust forward
Airway insertion	Guedel's airway, Safar airway Nasophrayngeal airway Laryngeal mask airway (LMA)
Endotracheal tube	

- Airway management in cases of foreign body obstruction:
  - Infant chest thrusts
  - Back-blows
  - Heimlich manoeuvre
  - Chest thrust
  - Finger sweep method
  - Cricothyroidotomy
- Airway management in other cases of airway obstruction (Laryngeal oedema, epiglottitis, laryngotracheobronchitis): Tracheostomy

4. **Ans. (d) < 60/min**
[Ref. Hutchison's Paediatrics, 2/e p625; Ajay Yadav, 4/e p227]

- In a newborn, if the heart rate remains slow or absent (<60/min), despite adequate ventilation with chest movement for 30s, then chest compressions should be started
- **Most efficient way of delivering chest compressions** in the newborn is to encircle the chest with both hands, so that the fingers lie behind the baby and the thumbs are apposed on the sternum just below the inter-nipple line
- Once the heart rate is above 60 min/min and rising, chest compression should be discontinued

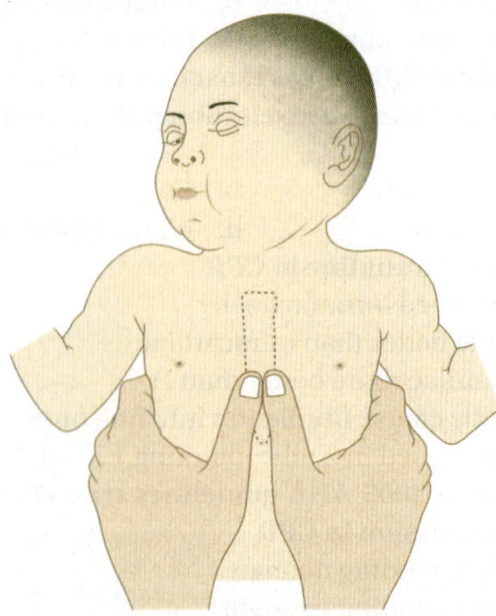

Fig. Chest compressions (Newborn)

5. Ans. (a) Not more than 10 seconds
[Ref. Ajay Yadav, 4/e p223]

Carotid Pulse Palpation in CPR

- Utility: Is the 'most effective clinical indicator' to see the effectiveness of cardiac massage (Circulation component of ABC)
- Carotid pulse check: Should not take more than 10 seconds

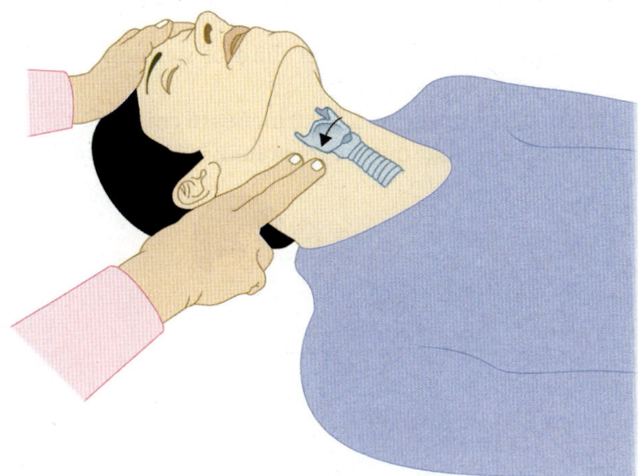

Fig. Carotid pulse check

6. Ans. (a) Lower third sternum
[Ref. Short Textbook of Anaesthesia by Ajay Yadav, 4th e p222]

External Cardiac Massage

- Cardiac massage in adults:
- Compressions: Over lower third of sternum (two fingers above Xiphoid process)
- **Depress sternum by: 1.5-2.0 inches**
- Effective cardiac output generated: 30% of normal
- Cardiac massage in children: **'Two thumbs technique'** for compressions
- Cardiac massage in newborns: 'Two thumbs with encircled chest technique' for compressions
- Cardiac massage in pregnant: External cardiac massage with lateral tilt

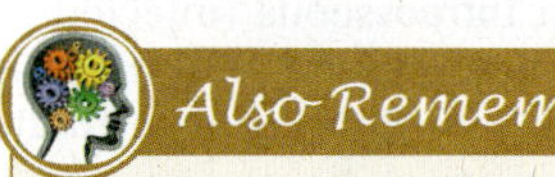

Also Remember

- ***Open chest massage indications***:
  - Cardiac tamponade
  - Blunt penetrating trauma
  - Air embolism
  - Chest deformities
  - Arrest during intrathoracic procedures

7. Ans. (b) Calcium
[Ref. Ajay Yadav, 4/e p230]

Drugs used in Cardiopulmonary Resuscitation (CPR)

Vasopressors	Adrenaline, Noradrenaline, Ephedrine, Mephentramine
Ionotropes	Dopamine, Dobutamine
Beta blockers	Propranolol, Esmolol
Anticholinergics	Atropine, Glycopyrrolate
Respiratory stimulants (Analeptics)	Doxapram, Ethamivan
Vasodilators	Sodium nitroprusside, Nitroglycerine, Nifedipine, Potassium chloride
Antiarrhythmics	Amiodarone, Xylocard, Bretylium, Adenosine

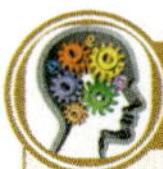

Also Remember

- *Calcium is contraindicated in CPR*: As excess calcium worsens cellular death
  - **Only indications of Calcium**:
    1. Hypocalcaemia
    2. Hyperkalemia
    3. Overdosage of calcium channel blockers
- *Sodium bicarbonate without blood gas analysis should be avoided in CPR*: As it worsens neuronal injury, increases intracranial tension, worsen intracellular acidosis, cause hypertonicity
  - **Only indications of Bicarbonates**:
    1. Metabolic acidosis
    2. Hyperkalemia
    3. CPR after blood gas reports

8. Ans. (c) About 100 compressions per minute
[Ref. Ajay Yadav, 4/e p223]

Compression to Ventilation (C:V) Ratio

- ***Before advanced airway***: Mouth-to-mouth/ Bag and mask ventilation
  - C:V ratio must be 30:2
- ***After advanced airway***: Endotracheal tube/ LMA/ Combitube
- Compressions at 100 compressions per minute
- Breathing rate at 8-10 breaths per minute
- Ventilation rate must be less than 12 breaths per minute
- Low tidal volume (6-7 ml per kg) preferred
- If there are 2 rescuers: Rotate after 2 minutes (or 5 cycles of 30:2)

Also Remember

- ***Key guidelines for CPR now-a-days***:
  - Push hard
  - Push fast
  - Allow full chest recoil
  - Minimize interruptions in chest compressions

9. Ans. (c) 5:1
[Ref. Ajay Yadav, 4/e p225]

Compression: Ventilation Ratios during CPR

- ***Adults without advanced airway***: 30:2
- ***Adults with advanced airway***:
  - 100 compressions per minute AND Ventilation rate < 12 breaths per minutes
  - Earlier it was recommended 5:1

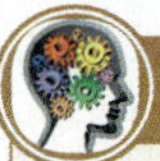

Also Remember

- ***Children without advanced airway***:
  - For one rescuer: 30:2
  - For two rescuers: 15:2
- ***Children with advanced airway***:
  - 100 compressions per minute AND Ventilation rate 8-10 breaths per minute
  - Earlier it was recommended 5:1
- ***Newborns***: 3:1

10. Ans. (a) Chest compressions 200/ minute
[Ref. Marino's The ICU Book, 4/e p328]

High-Quality Adult CPR Components

- Chest compressions at a rate of 100 per minute
- Depth of two or more inches (5 cms)
- Complete recoil after compression
- Minimal interruptions in compressions
- Avoidance of excessive ventilation

11. Ans. (c) Chest compression >6 inches
[Ref. Clinical Cases in Anesthesia by Reed, 4/e p456]

Compression: Ventilation Ratios during CPR

- Adults without advanced airway: 30:2
- Adults with advanced airway:
  - 100 compressions per minute
  - Ventilation rate < 12 breaths per minute
- Children without advanced airway:
  - For one rescuer: 30:2
  - For two rescuers: 15:2
- Children with advanced airway:
  - 100 compressions per minute
  - Ventilation rate 8–10 breaths per minute
- Newborns: 3:1

Cardiac Massage in Adults

- Compressions: Over lower third of sternum (two fingers above Xiphoid process)
- Depress sternum by: 1.5-2.0 inches (6 cms)
- Effective cardiac output generated: 30% of normal

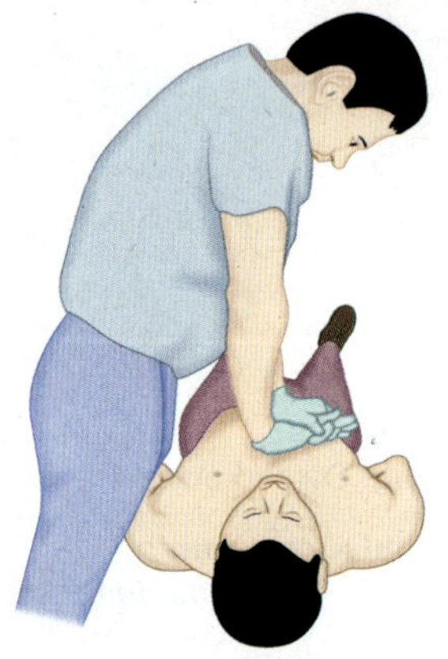

Fig. Chest compression (CPR)

HIGH YIELD MCQs ANSWERS WITH EXPLANATIONS

1. Ans. (e) Disseminated intravascular coagulation
[Ref. Ajay Yadav, 4/e p228]

Complications of CPR

- Rib fracture
- Injury to major vessels by rib fracture
- Pneumothorax
- Pneumopericardium
- Pneumomediastinum
- Injury to diaphragm
- Gastric injury
- Lung injury
- Injury to abdominal organs (liver, spleen and stomach)

2. Ans. (c) Airway maintenance
[Ref. Ajay Yadav, 4/e p225]

3. Ans. (c) 5% dextrose
[Ref. Ajay Yadav, 4/e p228]

- Glucose containing solutions should not be used as hyperglycemia increases cerebral oedema
- Ringer lactate should be avoided as calcium present in Ringer lactate can cause neuronal injury

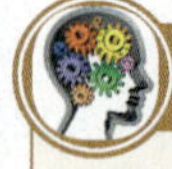

Also Remember

- **Fluid of choice in CPR**: Normal saline

4. Ans. (a) Can be given intrathecally; (b) IV route better than intracardiac
[Ref. Ajay Yadav, 4/e p228-230]

Adrenaline in CPR

- **Dose (1:10,000): 1 mg**
- Apart from IV, it can be given intraosseous (injected in medullary cavity for children) and endotracheal (dose is 2.5 times of IV route and diluted with 10ml saline in adults and 5 ml saline for children)
- Intracardiac route offer no advantage rather it can cause injury to myocardium

5. Ans. (b) 90/min including neonate
[Ref. Ajay Yadav, 4/e p227]

- Compression ventilation ratio is 3:1 (90 compression with 30 breaths) and syncronized

6. Ans. (a) Respiratory; (b) Cardiovascular; (e) CNS
[Ref. Ajay Yadav, 4/e p223]

7. Ans. (d) Amiodarone
[Ref. Miller, 6/e p722]

Drugs Used in Cardiopulmonary Resuscitation

- Effective even when administered through Endotracheal tube: Atropine, Epinephrine, Lidocaine, Vasopressin
- Not Effective when administered through Endotracheal tube: Adenosine, Amiodarone, Dopamine, Esmolol, Metoprolol, Procainamide, Verapamil

8. Ans. (c) Assess patient, Activate emergency response team, Call for defibrillator, Start CPR

[Ref. Obstetric and Gynecological Emergencies by Deepti, 1/e p195]

Basic Life Support (BLS)

- Determine if Patient is in Cardiac arrest:
  - Ensure if scene is safe to approach the patient (Wear gloves, etc)
  - Check for a response by tapping the shoulder and shouting
- Recognition of arrest and activation of emergency response:
  - If patient does not respond, activate the institutional emergency team, and call for a Defibrillator and Emergency cart
  - If patient is not breathing or gasping, assume he's in cardiac arrest
- Begin early CPR

9. Ans. (c) Permissive hypotension and limited crystalloid use

[Ref. Advances in Trauma by Napolitano, 1/e p73]

Balanced Resuscitation

- Includes Permissive hypotension, Limiting crystalloid use, and transfusion of blood products in ratios similar to whole blood
- Prompt initiation of massive transfusion and the protocolled use of 1:1:1 product ratios have improved the morbidity and mortality of patients with trauma in hemorrhagic shock
- It minimizes the impact of trauma-induced coagulopathy, limits blood product waste, and reduces the complications that occur with aggressive crystalloid resuscitation

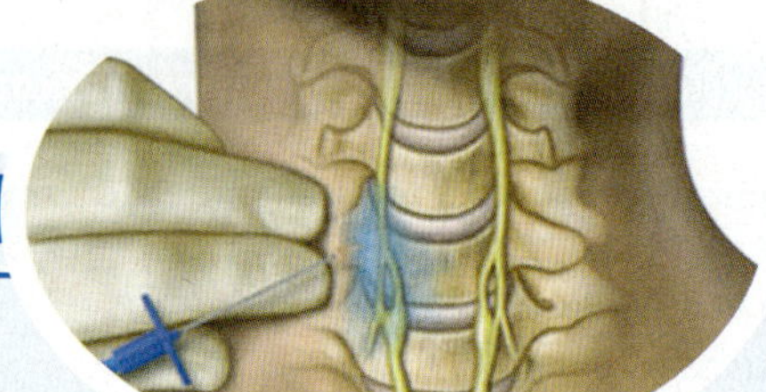

Chapter 11

Monitoring

THEORETICAL CONCEPTS

XI A. GLASGOW COMA SCALE (GCS)

- Definition: Neurological scale for 'assessment of conscious state' of a person[Q]
- Elements of GCS:

	Eye response	Verbal response[Q]	Motor response
Score 1	Do not open	No sounds	None
Score 2	To painful stimulus	Sounds only	Extension
Score 3	To verbal command	Inappropriate words	Abnormal flexion
Score 4	Spontaneously open	Confused	Withdrawal/ flexion
Score 5	–	Normal, oriented talk	Localises pain
Score 6	–	–	Obeys commands

- ***Interpretation of GCS scores***:
  - Lowest score 3: Deep coma or death
  - Highest score 15: Fully awake person
- ***Classification of brain injuries***:
  - Minor injury: GCS score ≥ 13
  - Moderate injury: GCS score 9–12
  - Severe injury: GCS score ≤ 8

Eye opening		Verbal response		Motor response	
Spontaneous	> 4	Orientated	> 5	Obey commands	> 6
To sound	> 3	Confused	> 4	Localising	> 5
To pressure	> 2	Words	> 3	Normal flexion	> 4
None	> 1	Sounds	> 2	Abnormal flexion	> 3
		None	> 1	Extension	> 2
				None	> 1

Fig. GCS

Topper's Edge

AVPU Scale

- **Acronym[Q]: "alert, voice, pain, unresponsive"**
  - A system by which a health care professional can measure and record a patient's responsiveness, indicating their level of consciousness
  - It is a simplification of the Glasgow Coma Scale, which assesses a patient response in three measures: Eyes, Voice and Motor skills
  - AVPU scale should be assessed using these three identifiable traits, looking for the best response of each
- AVPU scale has four possible outcomes for recording
  - **Alert**: Patient is fully awake (although not necessarily oriented)
    1. Spontaneously open eyes, will respond to voice (although may be confused) and will have bodily motor function
  - **Voice**: Patient makes some kind of response when you talk to them, which could be in any of the three component measures of eyes, voice or motor
    1. Response could be as little as a grunt, moan, or slight move of a limb when prompted by the voice of the rescuer
  - **Pain**: Patient makes a response on any of the three component measures on the application of pain stimulus, such as a central pain stimulus like a sternal rub or a peripheral stimulus such as squeezing the fingers
    1. Respond by using their voice, moving their eyes, or moving part of their body (including abnormal posturing).
  - **Unresponsive**: 'Unconscious' outcome is recorded if the patient does not give any eye, voice or motor response to voice or pain
- AVPU classification of alertness has been suggested to correspond in the following manner[Q]:
  - Alert: 15 GCS
  - Voice Responsive: 12 GCS
  - Pain Responsive: 8 GCS
  - Unconscious/ DOA: 3 GCS

XI B. CAPNOGRAPHY

- *Definition*: Continuous measurement of end tidal carbon dioxide
  - **Normal value: 32-42 mm Hg**
- *Principle*: Infrared light is absorbed by carbon dioxide
- ***Uses of Capnography***:
  - Surest confirmatory sign of correct intubation[Q]
  - Diagnosis of malignant hyperthermia[Q]
  - Detecting obstruction of Endotracheal tubes[Q]
  - Indicates cardiac output[Q]
  - Diagnoses pulmonary embolism[Q]

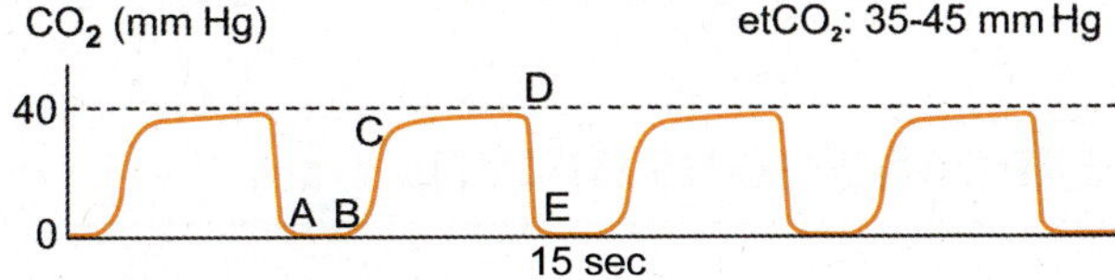

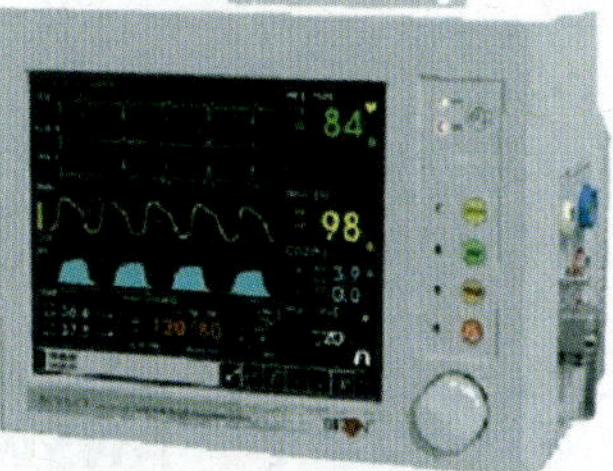

Fig. Capnograph meter

XI C. BLOOD GAS ANALYSIS

- *Normal values on room air*:
  - pH: 7.38-7.42[Q]
  - Partial pressure of air: 96-98 mm Hg
  - Partial pressure of carbon dioxide: 35-45 mm Hg
  - Bicarbonate: 24-28 mEq per litre[Q]
  - Oxygen saturation: 95-98%[Q]
  - Base deficit: – 3 to + 3

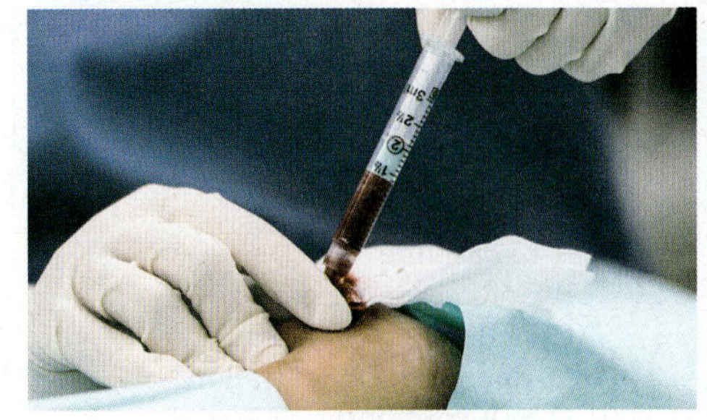

Fig. Blood gas analysis

IMAGE-BASED QUESTIONS

1. Capnograph shown in Photograph occur due to *[AIIMS November 2016]*

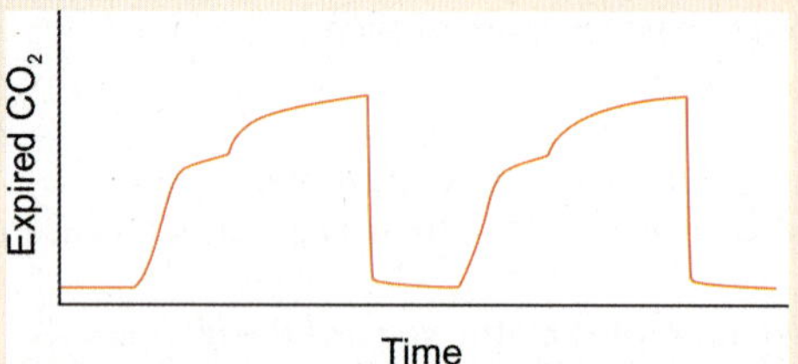

a. Leakage of gas from circuit
b. Obstruction of ET tube
c. Rebreathing
d. Intubation into bronchus

2. Identify the Machine used in Medicine as shown in Public Health

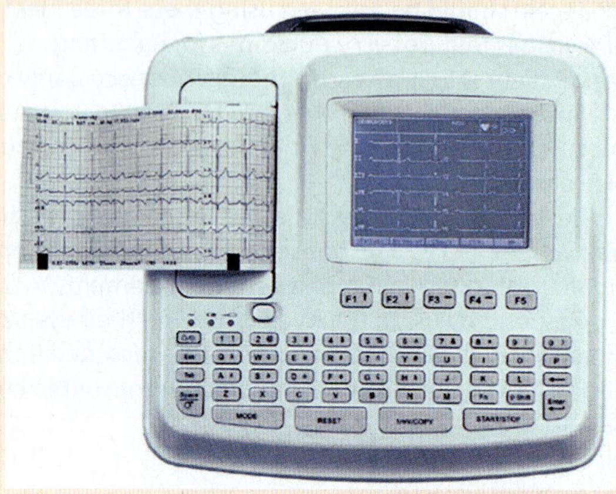

a. ECG machine
b. EEG machine
c. USG machine
d. CVP machine

3. Identify the Waveform shown in the Photograph

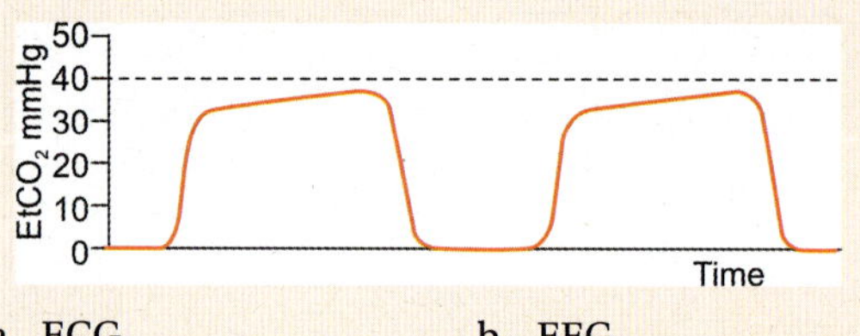

a. ECG
b. EEG
c. JVP
d. Capnograph

4. Next best appropriate step in Patient with Capnography tracing shown in Photograph is *[AIIMS November 2015]*

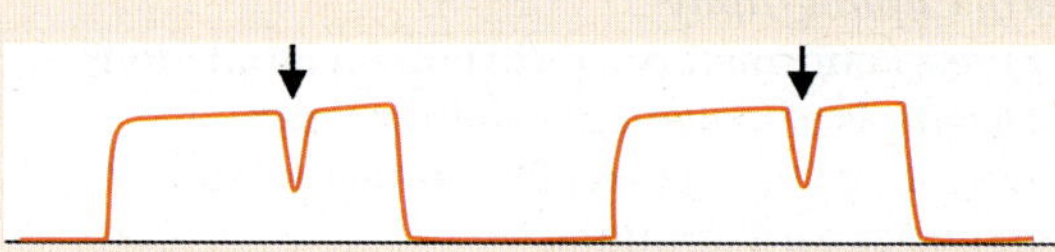

a. Check for Endotracheal tube position
b. Check Anesthesia machine connections
c. Change Sodalime canister
d. Administer Skeletal muscle relaxant

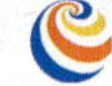

ANSWERS WITH EXPLANATIONS OF IBQs

1. Ans. (d) Intubation into bronchus *[Ref. Capnography by Gravenstein, 2/e p39]*

Normal Capnogram

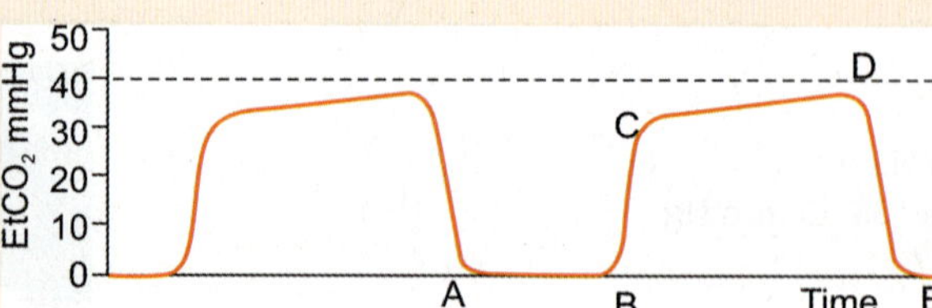

- A-B: Baseline
- B-C: Expiratory upstroke
- C-D: Expiratory plateau
- D: End tidal concentration
- D-E: Inspiration

Endotracheal intubation

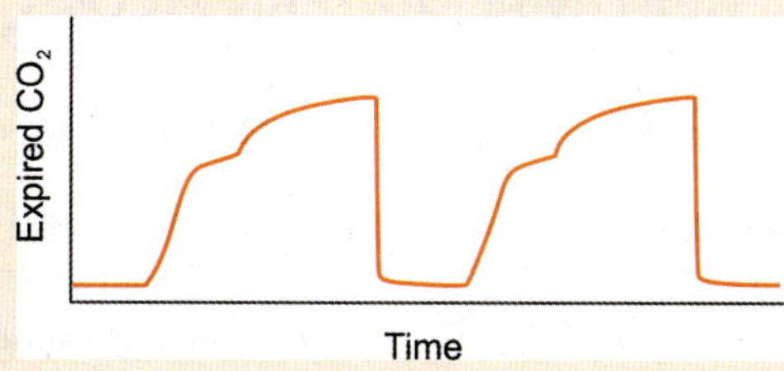

- Bifid waveform represents the differential ventilation of two lungs
- As the ETT is positioned mainly in the right main bronchus, the airflow through the right lung is the best, and right-sided gas forms the first (brisk and steep) part of the waveform
- Afterwards, one notices that there is a secondary transitional phase, which is the gas from the left lung escaping slowly up into the ETT

Also Remember

Important Capnograms

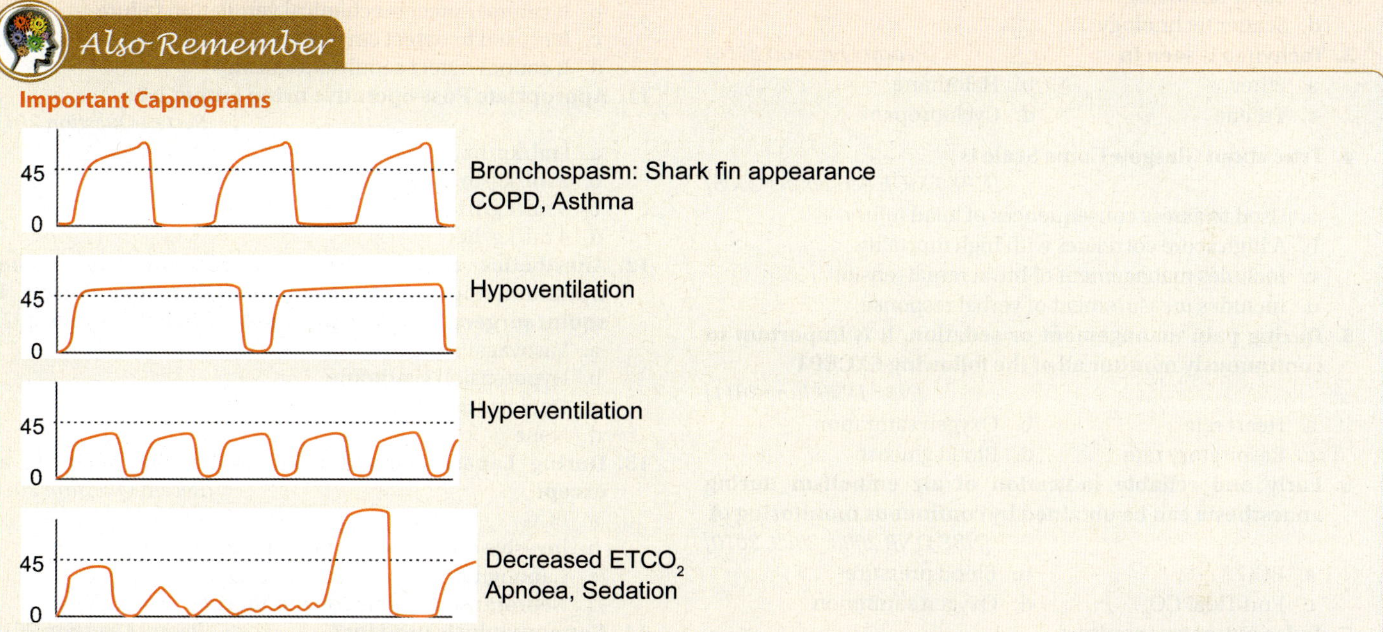

2. Ans. (a) ECG machine *[Ref. ECGs by Freed, 3/e p1]*

- Electrocardiogram (ECG/ EKG): Diagnostic tool that is routinely used to assess the electrical and muscular functions of the heart.

3. Ans. (d) Capnograph *[Ref. Ajay Yadav, 4/e p51]*

Capnography

- Description: Monitoring of the concentration or partial pressure of carbon dioxide in respiratory gases. Usually presented as a graph of End tidal CO_2
  - Normal $EtCO_2$: 32–42 mm Hg
- Uses of Capnography:
  - Monitoring tool for use during anesthesia and intensive care
  - Surest, confirmatory sign of correct intubation
  - Diagnose displacement of Endotracheal tube ($EtCO_2$ becomes Zero)
  - Diagnose Malignant hyperthermia ($EtCO_2$ >100)
  - Diagnose obstruction/ disconnections of endotracheal tube ($EtCO_2$ decrease)
  - Diagnose pulmonary embolism ($EtCO_2$ suddenly decrease)
  - Diagnose Cardiac arrest ($EtCO_2$ is Zero)

4. Ans. (d) Administer Skeletal muscle relaxant *[Ref. pediatric Surgery by Coran, 7/e p213]*

- Spontaneous respiratory efforts with patient-induced inhalation before mechanical ventilation-induced inhalation can cause a break or "cleft" in the alveolar plateau
- Clinical use: It indicates the patient has started to breathe; This can alert the anaesthesia provider that the muscle relaxant is wearing off

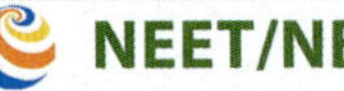 NEET/NBE PATTERN MCQs 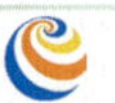

1. **Which of the following are features of Pulmonary oxygen toxicity?** *[Recent Question 2016]*
   a. Increased capillary endothelial permeability
   b. Decreased mucociliary transport in airways
   c. Inhibition of phagocytosis function of alveolar macrophages
   d. All the above
2. **Modern monitors to measure $ETCO_2$ make use of** *[Recent Question 2016]*
   a. Infrared absorption spectroscopy
   b. Ultra violet rays
   c. Laser technology
   d. Scatter technology
3. **Tachynea is seen in** *[Recent Question 2016]*
   a. Ether b. Halothane
   c. Trilene d. Cyclopropane
4. **True about Glasgow Coma Scale is** *[NBE FMGE September 2008]*
   a. Used to assess consequences of head injury
   b. A high score correlates with high mortality
   c. Includes management of Intracranial tension
   d. Includes measurement of verbal response
5. **During pain management or sedation, it is important to continuously monitor all of the following EXCEPT** *[NBE DNB June 2011]*
   a. Heart rate b. Oxygen saturation
   c. Respiratory rate d. Blood glucose
6. **Early and reliable indication of air embolism during anaesthesia can be obtained by continuous monitoring of** *[NBE DNB 2008, 2009, 2010]*
   a. ECG b. Blood pressure
   c. End Tidal CO_2 d. Oxygen saturation
7. **Pulse oximetry monitors** *[Recent Question 2016, NBE DNB June 2011]*
   a. Oxygen saturation of hemoglobin
   b. Oxygen content of blood c. Pulse pressure
   d. Oxygen partial pressure
8. **M.C. nerve used for monitoring during anaesthesia** *[Recent Question 2018, NBE DNB 2009]*
   a. Ulnar nerve b. Facial nerve
   c. Radial nerve d. Median nerve
9. **In the classification of head injury severity, moderate head injury has which of the following range of Glasgow Coma Scale score?** *[NBE FMGE September 2011]*
   a. 7-10 b. 8-11
   c. 9-12 d. 19-13
10. **True about Capnography is?** *[Recent Question 2017]*
    a. It cannot detect esophageal intubation
    b. It cannot detect mechanical ventilation failure
    c. It is used to detect correct intubation in patients
    d. It cannot detect saddle embolism
11. **Appropriate Post-operative urine output is?** *[Recent Question 2017]*
    a. 1 ml/kg/hr
    b. 2 ml/kg/hr
    c. 3 ml/kg/hr
    d. 4 ml/kg/hr
12. **Anesthetics usually check for BP and pulse when Ophthalmologist maneuvers Medial rectus muscle in squint surgery. This is to prevent?** *[Recent Question 2017]*
    a. Vasovagal attack
    b. Hypotension syndrome
    c. Oculocardiac reflex
    d. None
13. **During Laparoscopy, Routine monitoring includes all except** *[Recent Question 2017]*
    a. ECG
    b. Invasive arterial blood pressure monitoring
    c. Capnography
    d. Neuromuscular junction monitoring
14. **Capnography is used for?** *[Recent Question 2017]*
    a. Oxygen saturation of blood
    b. Amount of CO_2 transported in blood
    c. Diagnosing malignant hyperthermia
    d. Myocardial perfusion

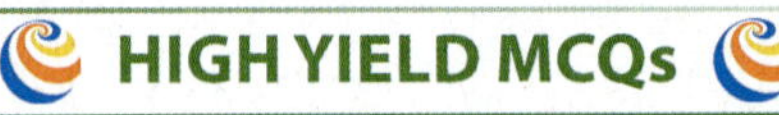

1. **Most common nerve used for monitoring during anaesthesia** *[AIIMS PGMEE 2007]*
   a. Ulnar nerve b. Facial nerve
   c. Radial nerve d. Median nerve
2. **Post-operative muscle ache is caused by** *[Recent Question 2016, All India PGMEE 1991]*
   a. D-Tubocurarine b. Suxamethonium
   c. Gallamine d. Poncuronium
3. **Criteria for brain death all except** *[PGI 2007]*
   a. ECG b. EEC
   c. Brain stem reflex
   d. Decreased body temperature
   e. Pupillary dilatation
4. **A 40 year old female underwent surgery. Post-operatively, she told anaesthetist that she was aware of intra-operative events. Such type of intra-operative awareness can be evaluated by (prevented by)** *[All India PGMEE 2011]*
   a. Pulse oximetry b. End tidal CO_2
   c. Colour Doppler d. Bispectral index
5. **Most common cause of morbidity and mortality in patients undergoing major vascular surgery is** *[AIIMS PGMEE 2005]*
   a. Renal complications
   b. Thromboembolic phenomenon
   c. Coagulopathies d. Cardiac complications

Anesthesiology

6. Which of the following is not used in controlling heart rate intraoperatively? *[All India PGMEE 2007]*
a. Propanolol/ Metoprolol
b. Verapamil
c. Esmolol
d. Procainamide

7. Which of the following is not a cardiovascular monitoring technique? *[AIIMS PGMEE 2005]*
a. Transesophageal echocardiography
b. Central venous pressure monitoring
c. Pulmonary artery catheterization
d. Capnography

8. Flat capnogram found in A/E *[AIIMS PGMEE 2009]*
a. Disconnection of anesthetic tubing
b. Accidental extubation
c. Mechanical ventilation failure
d. Bronchospasm

9. Most sensitive and practical technique for detection of myocardial ischemia in the perioperative period is *[AIIMS PGMEE 2005]*
a. Magnetic Resonance Spectroscopy
b. Radio-labeled lactate determination
c. Direct measurement of end diastolic pressure
d. Regional wall motion abnormality detected with the help of 2D transoephageal echocardiography

10. While introducing the Swan-Ganz catheter, its placement in the pulmonary artery can be identified by the following pressure tracing *[AIIMS PGMEE 2005]*
a. Diastolic pressure is lower in PA than in RV
b. Diatolic pressure is higher in PA than in RV
c. PA pressure tracing has diacritic notch from closure of pulmonary valve
d. RV pressure tracing for plateau and sharp drop in early diastole

11. Gas used to create pneumoperitoneum is *[PGI 2001]*
a. CO_2 b. N_2
c. O_2 d. Room air
e. N_2O

12. Which of following is used to monitor respiration in neonate (not intubated)? *[All India PGMEE 2007]*
a. Capnography b. Impedencepulmonometry
c. Chest movements d. Infrared end tidal CO_2

13. Which one of the following is the description used for the term allodynia during pain management? *[AIIMS PGMEE 2006]*
a. Absence of pain perception
b. Complete tack of pain sensation
c. Unpleasant sensation with or without a stimulus
d. Perception of an ordinarily non-noxious stimulus as severe pain

14. Pain rating index is provided by *[PGI 2002, JIPMER PGMEE 2000]*
a. Faces scale b. Visual analogue scale
c. McGill questionnaire d. CHEOP scale

15. Best Scale to measure pain in children of 5 years age *[SGPGI PGMEE 2002]*
a. VAS b. McGill Scale
c. Faces Scale d. CHEOPS

16. A children hospital Eastern Ontaria Pain Scale (CHEOPS) for rating postoperative pain in children includes all except *[AIIMS PGMEE 2008]*
a. Cry b. Touch
c. Torso d. Oxygen saturation

17. A two month old infant has undergone a major surgical procedure. Regarding postoperative pain relief which one of the following is recommended *[All India PGMEE 2006]*
a. No medication is needed as infant does not feel pain after surgery due to immaturity of nervous system
b. Only paracetamol suppository is adequate
c. Spinal narcotics via intrathecal route
d. Intravenous narcotic infusion in lower dosage

18. Most common rhythm disturbance during early post-operative period is *[AIIMS PGMEE 2005]*
a. Bradycardia b. Ventricular fibrillation
c. Tachycardia d. Complete heart block

19. A patient selected for surgery was induced with Thiopentoneiv through one of anticubital vein complains of severe pain of whole hand. The next line of management *[AIIMS PGMEE 2001]*
a. Give IV propofol through same needle
b. IV ketamine through same needle
c. IV lignocaine through same needle
d. Leave it done

20. ICT is treated by all except *[AIIMS PGMEE 1992]*
a. IV mannitol b. IV Frusemide
c. Controlled Hyperventilation
d. Addition of positive end respiratory pressure

21. Which of the following agents is not used to provide induced hypotension during surgery? *[All India PGMEE 2006]*
a. Sodium nitroprusside b. Hydralazine
c. Mephenteramine d. Esmolol

22. Which of the following agents is used for the treatment of postoperative shivering? *[Recent Question 2016, All India PGMEE 2006]*
a. Thiopentone b. Suxamethonium
c. Atropine d. Pethidine

23. Upper respiratory tract infection is a common problem in children. All of the following anesthetic complications can occur in children with respiratory infection except *[All India PGMEE 2002]*
a. Bacteremia b. Halothane granuloma
c. Increased mucosal bleeding
d. Laryngospasm

24. Which of the following is true about malignant hyperthermia? *[AIIMS PGMEE 2010]*
a. Hypernatremia b. Hypercalcemia
c. Hyperkalemia d. Hypothermia

25. All the following cause malignant hyperpyrexia except *[Karnataka PGMEE 2005]*
a. N_2O b. Halothane
c. Methoxyflurane d. Isoflurane

26. Cause of post operative hypertension *[PGI 2004]*
a. Pre-operative hypertension
b. Inadequate hypertension
c. Phaeochromocytoma
d. Hypoxemia e. Hypercarbia

27. True about aspiration pneumonia *[PGI 2004]*
a. Affected by volume of aspiration
b. Affected by pH of aspiration fluid
c. Incidence during induction
d. Inflammation
e. Infection

28. Hyperthermia is caused by *[PGI 2002]*
a. Anticholinergics b. MAO inhibitors
c. Lithium d. Chlorpromazine
e. Carbimazole

29. Factors favouring fat embolism in a patient with major trauma *[PGI 2001]*
a. Mobility of fracture b. Hypovolemic shock
c. Respiratory failure d. Diabetes

30. Use of Intra-arterial cannula in major surgery *[PGI 2005]*
a. Measurement of direct intra-arterial BP
b. Sample for ABG
c. Drug injection
d. BT

31. During intraoperative anaesthesia mismatch BT develops *[PGI 2007]*
a. Increased bleeding b. Hypotension
c. Bronchospasm d. Rash
e. Movements of limbs

32. Mismatched blood transfusion manifests intraoperatively as *[PGI 1999]*
a. Rise in B.P. b. Excessive bleeding
c. Dyspnoea d. Hematuria

33. Mendelson syndrome is due to *[PGI 1998]*
a. Aspiration pneumonitis
b. Chemical pneumonitis
c. Oesophagitis
d. Oesophageal spasm

34. True regarding Glasgow coma scale *[PGI November 2014]*
a. Best verbal response
b. Eye closure response
c. Best sensory response
d. Severity of head trauma
e. Limited use below 36 months of age

35. Which of the following does not increase ICT? *[PGI November 2014]*
a. Thiopentone b. Sevoflurane
c. Mannitol d. Ketamine
e. Succinylcholine

36. Ideal site for Internal temperature recording during Anesthesia is *[AIIMS November 2015]*
a. Pulmonary artery b. Distal esophagus
c. Tympanic membrane d. Nasopharynx

37. Glasgow Coma Score Scale pertains to *[Recent Question 2016, UPSC CMS 2015]*
a. Head injury only
b. Head and cervical injury
c. Chest injury
d. Level of consciousness

NEET/NBE PATTERN MCQs ANSWERS WITH EXPLANATIONS

1. Ans. (d) All of the above

[Ref. Anaesthesia for Postgraduates by Agasti, 1/e p74]

Pulmonary Oxygen Toxicity

- Increased capillary endothelial permeability causing accumulation of fluid in the interstitial space
- Depression of mucociliary transport function of airway
- Inhibition of phagocytosis of alveolar macrophages
- Changes in surfactant activity and its production

2. Ans. (a) Infrared absorption spectroscopy

[Ref. Pediatric Emergency Procedures by King, 2/e p755]

- Modern technology designed monitors that use infrared absorption spectroscopy to measure the amount of CO_2 in an exhaled breath

3. Ans. (a) Ether

[Ref. The Nervous System by Root, 1/e p72]

- Tachypnea during diethyl ether anesthesia is not abolished by bilateral vagotomy

4. Ans. (d) Includes measurement of verbal response

[Ref. Bailey and Love, 25/e p301-302]

Glasgow Coma Scale (GCS)

- *Definition*: Neurological scale for *'assessment of conscious state'* of a person
- *Elements of GCS*:

	Eye response	Verbal response	Motor response
Score 1	Do not open	No sounds	None
Score 2	To painful stimulus	Sounds only	Extension
Score 3	To verbal command	Inappropriate words	Abnormal flexion
Score 4	Spontaneously open	Confused	Withdrawal/ flexion
Score 5	–	Normal, oriented talk	Localises pain
Score 6	–	–	Obeys commands

5. Ans. (d) Blood glucose

[Ref. Ajay Yadav, 4/e p49-51]

6. Ans. (c) End tidal CO_2

[Ref. Ajay Yadav, 4/e p52]

- **Capnography is a sensitive tool for diagnosing pulmonary embolism** by air, fat or thrombus noted by sudden fall of $EtCO_2$
- It may become zero if embolus is large enough to block total pulmonary circulation.

7. Ans. (a) Oxygen saturation of haemoglobin

[Ref. Ajay Yadav, 4/e p51]

- It measures the saturation
- Pulse oxymeter is used for detection of hypoxia in intraoperative and postoperative period

8. Ans. (a) Ulnar nerve

[Ref. Ajay Yadav, 4/e p54]

- Most commonly used muscle for neuromascular monitoring is **adductor pollicis** supplied by Ulnar nerve

9. Ans. (c) 9-12

[Ref. Bailey and Love, 25/e p301-302]

10. Ans. (c) It is used to detect correct intubation in patients

[Ref. Clinical Anesthesiology by Benumof, 1/e p98]

Uses of Capnography

- Surest confirmatory sign of correct intubation
- Diagnosis of malignant hyperthermia
- Detecting obstruction of Endotracheal tubes
- Indicates cardiac output
- Diagnoses pulmonary embolism

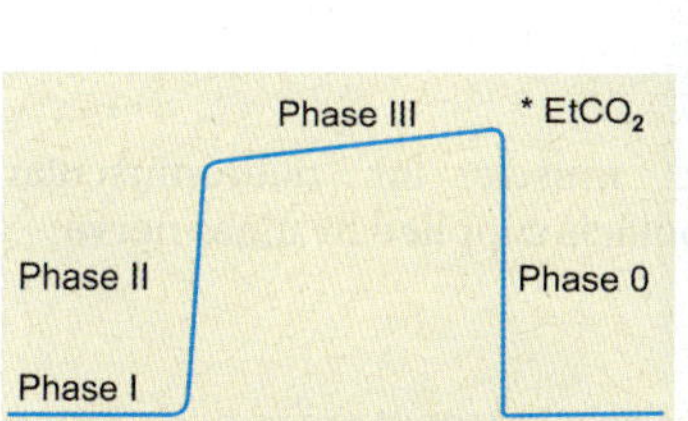

Fig. Normal capnogram

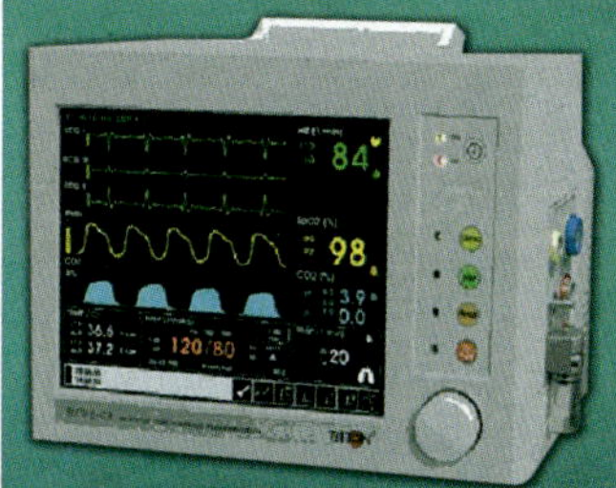

Fig. Capnography

11. Ans. (a) 1 ml/kg/hr

[Ref. Nurse Anesthesia by Nagelhout, 4/e p537]

- Urine Output Adequate: Urine output can be defined as at least 0.5–1 mL/kg/hr
- Inadequate urine output can be a sign of volume depletion and/or syndrome of inappropriate secretion of antidiuretic hormone (SIADH), both of which are commonly seen in postoperative patients

12. Ans. (c) Oculocardiac reflex

[Ref. Paediatric Anaesthesia by James, 1/e p269]

- Surgical handling of Extraocular muscles, Bronchi, Peritoneum, Scrotum, and Rectum can give rise to autonomic reflexes that include bronchospasm, bradycardia or tachycardia, hypotension or hypertension, and cardiac arrhythmias, especially in lightly anesthetized, hypoxic, or hypercapnic patients
- **Oculocardiac reflex (Aschner phenomenon/Aschner-Dagnini reflex)**: Decrease in pulse rate associated with traction applied to extraocular muscles and/or compression of the eyeball
- Reflex is mediated by nerve connections between the ophthalmic branch of the trigeminal cranial nerve via the ciliary ganglion, and the vagus nerve of the parasympathetic nervous system
- Strabismus surgery is also associated with the Oculocardiac reflex, a bradycardic response to extraocular muscle traction; it occurs most commonly when the medial rectus muscle is manipulated
- Also seen in Enucleation, Vitreoretinal surgery, Pressure on globe, and Surgery on maxilla

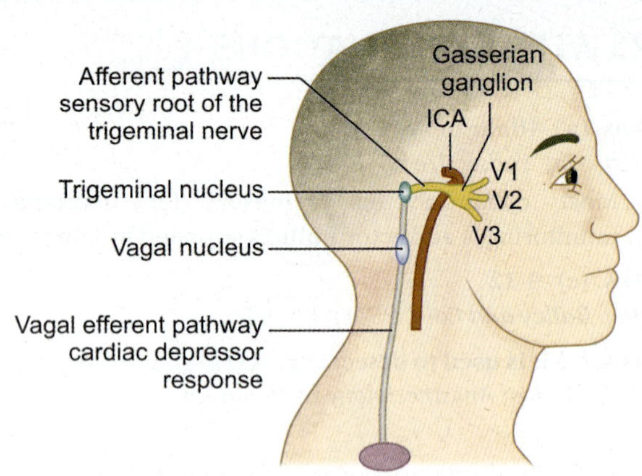

Fig. Oculocardiac reflex

13. Ans. (d) Neuromuscular junction monitoring
[Ref. Endoscopic Surgery by Bax, 1/e p231]

- Patient monitoring during laparoscopy using General anesthesia includes Electrocardiography, Pulse oximetry, Blood pressure, Precordial stethoscope, Airway pressure and Capnography
- Invasive monitoring with arterial lines and Swan-Ganz catheters may be indicated in selected high-risk individuals

14. Ans. (c) Diagnosing malignant hyperthermia
[Ref. Hemodynamic Monitoring by Lough, 1/e p244]

- Capnography plays an important role in the perioperative period because an increase in $PetCO_2$ ($EtCO_2$ >100) is one of the earliest signs of Malignant hyperthermia, and prompt diagnosis and treatment are critical

HIGH YIELD MCQs ANSWERS WITH EXPLANATIONS 

1. Ans. (a) Ulnar nerve
[Ref. Ajay Yadav, 4/e p54]

- Most commonly used muscle for neuromuscular monitoring is adductor pollicis supplied by ulnar nerve

2. Ans. (b) Suxamethonium
[Ref. Ajay Yadav, 4/e p97]

- Muscle pain/ myalgia/ muscle soreness are very common problem with suxamethonium in postoperative period, due to excessive muscle contraction (40-50%)
- It can be reduced by:
  - Precurarization
  - Self-taming (giving 1/10th dose of succinylcholine 30 to 60 secs prior to full dose)

3. Ans. (a) ECG; (d) Decreased body temperature
[Ref. Intensive Care Manual by Andrew, 6/e p576]

4. Ans. (d) Bispectral index
[Ref. Anaesthesia Science by Nigel Webster, 1/e p434]

Bispectral Index

- Bispectral Index (BIS) analysis combines power spectral analysis of phase relationships with the component sine waves
- EEG feature that best correlated with clinical depth of sedation and anaesthesia were then fitted to a model
- Resulting algorithm generates a bispectral index.

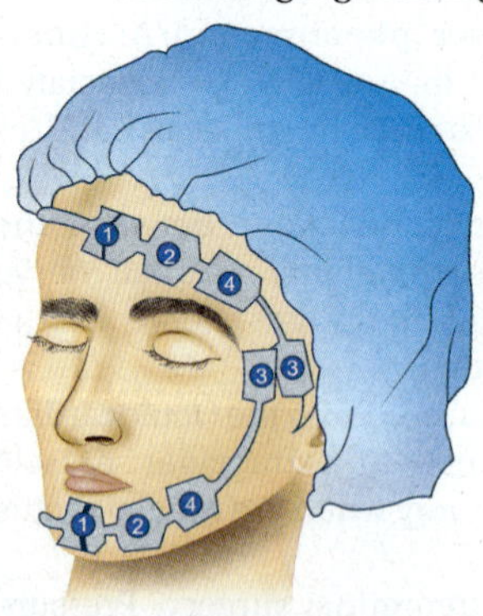

Fig. Bispectral index sensors

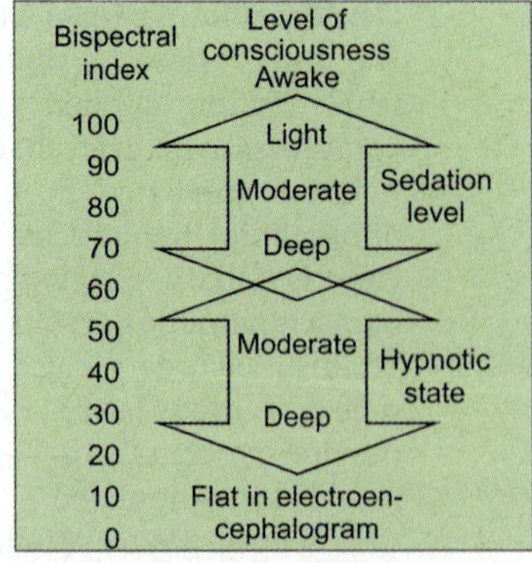

Fig. Bispectral index

5. Ans. (d) Cardiac complication
[Ref. European Manual of Medicine. Vascular Surgery by Christos, 1/ep85]

6. Ans. (d) Procainamide
[Ref. Ajay Yadav, 4/e p233]

- Propranolol, Esmolol are preferred agent for controlling heartbeat intraoperatively
- **Procainamide should only be used to treat life-threatening irregular heartbeat**: It has been associated with an increased risk of death when used to treat non-life-threatening irregular heartbeat

7. Ans. (d) Capnography
[Ref. Ajay Yadav, 4/e p51]

- Capnography is a respiratory monitoring technique

8. Ans. (d) Bronchospasm
[Ref. Ajay Yadav, 4/e p51]

- Bronchospasm produces the classic **"shark-fin"** wave form on the Capnogram

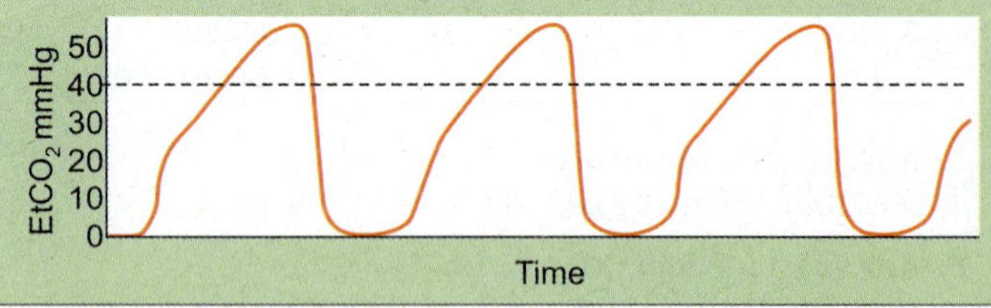

Fig. Shark-fin waves (Capnogram)

9. Ans. (d) Regional wall motion abnormality detected with the help of 2D transoesophagaeal echocardiography
[Ref. Ajay Yadav, 4/e p146]

- 2d TEE mainly monitors left ventricular function
- Abnormal regional wall motion is the earliest sign to detect infarction

10. Ans. (c) PA pressure tracing for diarcritic notch from closure of pulmonary valve

11. Ans. (a) CO_2; (c) O_2; (d) Room air; (e) N_2O
[Ref. Peritoneal Surgery by diZerega, 1/e. p175]

12. Ans. (b) Impedencepulmonometry

Monitoring Respiration

- **In incubated patients**: Capnography and Infrared end tidal CO_2 measurement
- **Non-intubated patients**: Impedance pulmonometry and Transcutaneous gas analysis

13. Ans. (d) Perception of an ordinarily non-noxious stimulus as severe pain
[Ref. Clinical Anesthesiology by Morgan, 3/e p361]

14. Ans. (c) McGill questionnaire
[Ref. Ajay Yadav, 4/e p200]

15. Ans. (d) CHEOPS
[Ref. Ajay Yadav, 4/e p200]

- CHEOPS is used for 1-7 years age
- CHEOPS includes cry, facial expression, verbal response, torso (body position), touch (touching wound), leg position

CHEOPS variables	Score 0	Score 1	Score 2
Cry	No	Crying, moaning	Scream
Facial	Smile	Neutral	Grimace
Verbal	Positive statement	Negative Statement	Suffering from pain
Torso	Neutral	Variable, upright	Stretched
Legs	Neutral	Continuous move kicking	Stretched

Fig. CHEOPS

16. Ans. (d) Oxygen saturation
[Ref. Ajay Yadav, 4/e p200]

17. Ans. (d) Intravenous narcotic infusion in lower dosage
[Ref. Ajay Yadav, 4/e p200]

18. Ans. (c) Tachycardia
[Ref. Cardiac Anesthesia by Fawzy G. Estafanous 2/e p530]

19. Ans. (c) IV lignocaine through same needle
[Ref. Ajay Yadav, 4/e p200]

- This type of complication is seen because in 10% of the cases brachial artery divides above elbow giving a very superficial abnormal ulnar artery which lies just deep to antecubital vein

Management

- Stop further injection
- Leave the needle at site for giving all therapeutic medication through same needle
- Inject 500 unit of heparin
- Inject papaverine 40 to 80 mg in 10 to 20 ml saline
- Tolazoline, phenoxybenzamine can also be used
- 10 ml of 1% xylocaine/ lignocaine
- Urokinase infusion
- Brachial plexus or stellate ganglion block should be given at the earliest (to relieve vasospasm)
- Defer elective surgery

20. Ans. (d) Addition of positive end respiratory pressure
[Ref. Ajay Yadav, 4/e p170-171]

Methods to Decrease ICT

- Hyperventilation
- Hyperosmotic drugs: mannitol, urea
- Diuretics : frusemide
- Steroids: dexamethasone, methylprednisolone
- Barbiturates: thiopentone
- Posture: head up

21. Ans. (c) Mephenteramine
[Ref. Ajay Yadav, 4/e p232]

- Mephenteramine is used to treat hypotension and not to provide induced hypotension

22. Ans. (d) Pethidine
[Ref. Ajay Yadav, 4/e p90]

- Pethidine abolishes shivering, so drug of choice for shivering

23. Ans. (b) Halothane granuloma
[Ref. Drug-Induced Pathology edited by E. Grundmann 1/e p102]

24. Ans. (c) Hyperkalemia
[Ref. Ajay Yadav, 4/e p115]

25. Ans. (a) N_2O
[Ref. Ajay Yadav, 4/e p115]

- **Malignant hyperthermia is caused by:**
  - Halothane
  - Isoflurane
  - Enflurane
  - Desflurane
  - Sevoflurane
  - Methoxyflurane
  - Cyclopropane
  - Ether
  - Succinylcholine

26. Ans. ALL CHOICES
[Ref. Ajay Yadav, 4/e p113, 148]

27. Ans. ALL CHOICES
[Ref. Ajay Yadav, 4/e p111]

28. Ans. (b) MAO inhibitors
[Ref. Ajay Yadav, 4/e p115]

29. Ans. (a) Mobility of fracture; (d) Diabetes
[Ref. Ajay Yadav, 4/e p194]

30. Ans. ALL CHOICES
[Ref. Ajay Yadav, 4/e p50]

31. Ans. (a) Increased bleeding; (b) Hypotension; (c) Bronchospasm; (d) Rash
[Ref. Ajay Yadav, 4/e. p15-16]

32. Ans. (b) Excessive bleeding
[Ref. Ajay Yadav, 4/e p15-16]

33. Ans. (a) Aspiration pneumonia
[Ref. Ajay Yadav, 4/e p110]

- Acid aspiration in late pregnancy was described by Mendelson and called it as Mendelson syndrome

34. Ans. (a) Best verbal response; (d) Severity of head trauma; (e) Limited use below 36 months of age

[Ref. Conn's Current Therapy 2013, p1901]

- Glasgow Coma Scale (GCS) is modified for use in infants under the age of 36 months

35. Ans. (a) Thiopentone; (c) Mannitol

[Ref. Ajay Yadav, 4/e p74]

Intracranial Tension (Pressure) Changes

ICT increased by	ICT decreased by
• Ether • Nitrous oxide • Trichloroethylene • Halothane, Isoflurane, Enflurane • Desflurane, Sevoflurane, Methoxyflurane • Cyclopropane • Chloroform • Ketamine • Pentazocine • Diazepam, Midazolam, Lorazepam • Succinylcholine	• Thiopentone • Methohexital • Propofol • Etomidate • Morphine • Fentanyl, Alfentanil, Sulfentanil • Mannitol, Glycerol

- Minimum rise in ICT by Inhalational agent: Isoflurane (Inhalational agent of choice for neurosurgical procedures)

36. Ans. (b) Distal esophagus

[Ref. Adult Perioperative Anesthesia by Michelle, 4/e p124]

Core Temperature Recording in Anesthesia

- Best site: Distal esophagus
- Good sites: pulmonary artery, Tympanic membrane
- Other sites: Brain (nasopharyngeal), Rectal, Axillary, Skin

37. Ans. (d) Level of consciousness

[Ref. Developmental Neuropsychology by Anderson, 1/e p146]

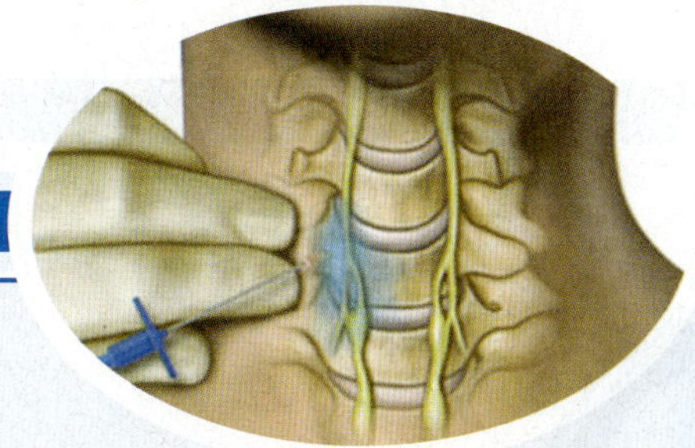

Chapter 12

Anesthesia in ICU

THEORETICAL CONCEPTS

XII A. TRACHEOSTOMY

XII A1. Indications of Tracheostomy

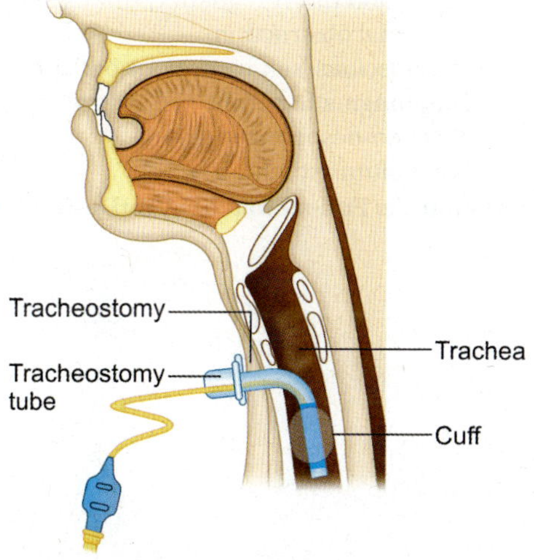

Fig. Tracheostomy

- *Elective procedure*: For prolonged ventilation
- *Switch-over procedure from intubation*: After 21 days
- Excessive secretions blocking Endotracheal tube
- If intubation is not possible
- Laryngeal surgeries
- *Upper airway obstruction*: **[Mnemonic:** **L**aryngeal **T**rauma **E**nhances **VITAL** **C**apacity**]**[Q]
  - **L**aryngitis
  - **T**rauma—facial/laryngeal
  - **E**dema—laryngeal
  - **V**ocal cord paralysis
  - **I**mpacted foreign bodies
  - **T**umours—congenital
  - **A**bscess—Peritonsillar (Quinsy)
  - **L**udwig's angina
  - **C**arcinoma head and neck

XII A2. Complications of Tracheostomy

Early complications	**Intermediate complications**
• Haemorrhage • Apnoea • Local damage • Cardiac arrest	• Displacement of tube • Surgical emphysema • Infection • Scabs • Pneumothorax • Tracheo-oesophageal fistula
Late complications • Difficult decannulation[Q] • Tracheal stenosis • Tracheo-oesophageal fistula	

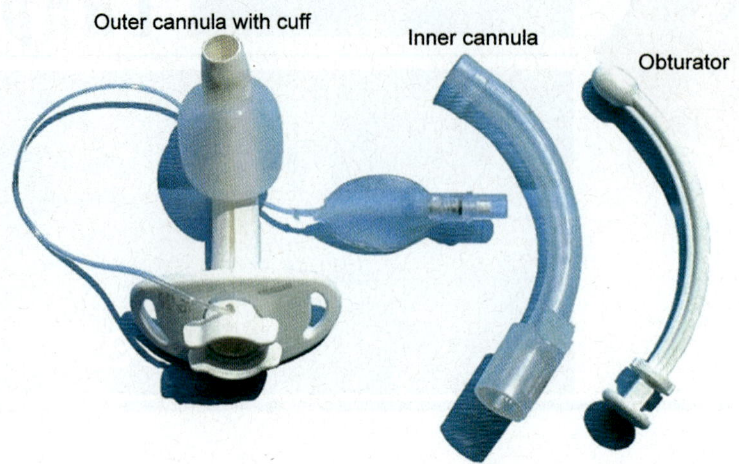

Fig. Tracheostomy tube with parts

XII B. BAG-AND-MASK VENTILATION

XII B1. Contraindications for Bag-and-Mask Ventilation[Q]

- **F**ull stomach
- **A**spiration risk (Pregnancy, Hiatus hernia)
- **I**ntestinal obstruction
- **U**nconscious/semiconscious patients
- **D**iaphragmatic hernia
- **T**racheo-oesophageal fistula
- **M**econium aspiration

[Mnemonic: Full-stomachIsA UnDesirableThing for Mask]

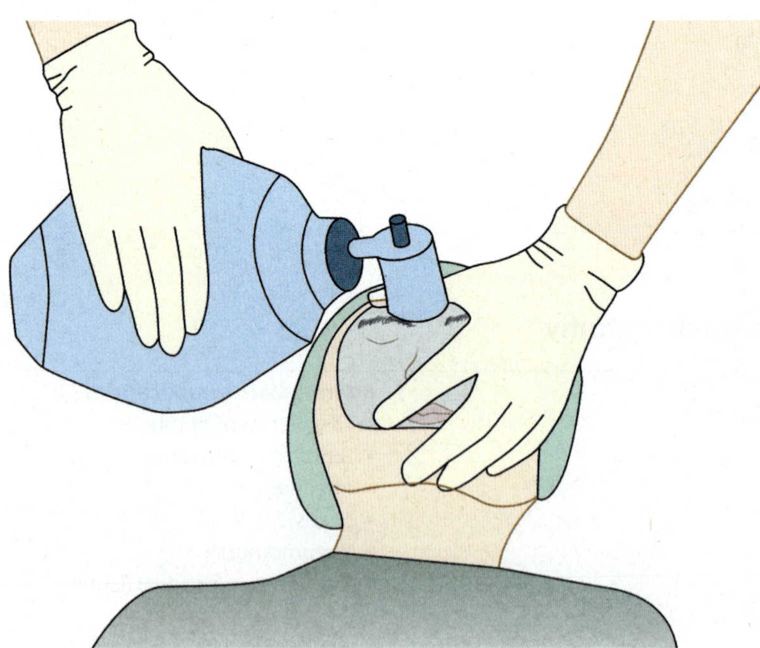

Fig. Bag-and-mask ventilation

IMAGE-BASED QUESTIONS

1. Identify the Instrument/device shown in Photograph
[Recent Question 2013]

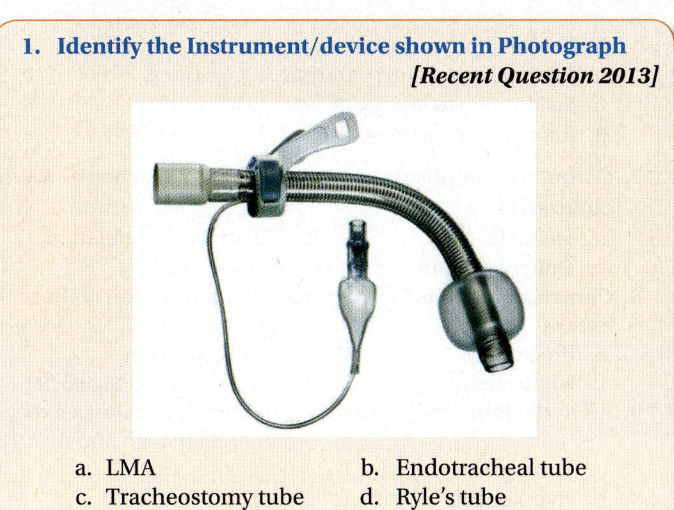

a. LMA
b. Endotracheal tube
c. Tracheostomy tube
d. Ryle's tube

2. Identify the Procedure performed on a Patient as shown in Photograph

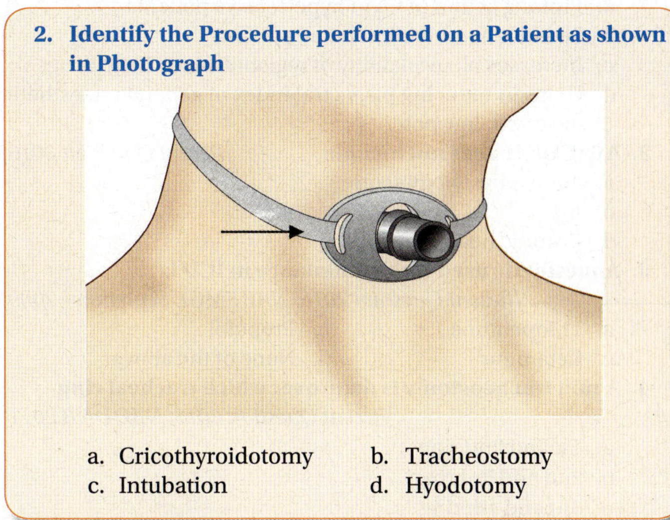

a. Cricothyroidotomy
b. Tracheostomy
c. Intubation
d. Hyodotomy

3. Identify the Procedure performed on a Patient as shown in Photograph

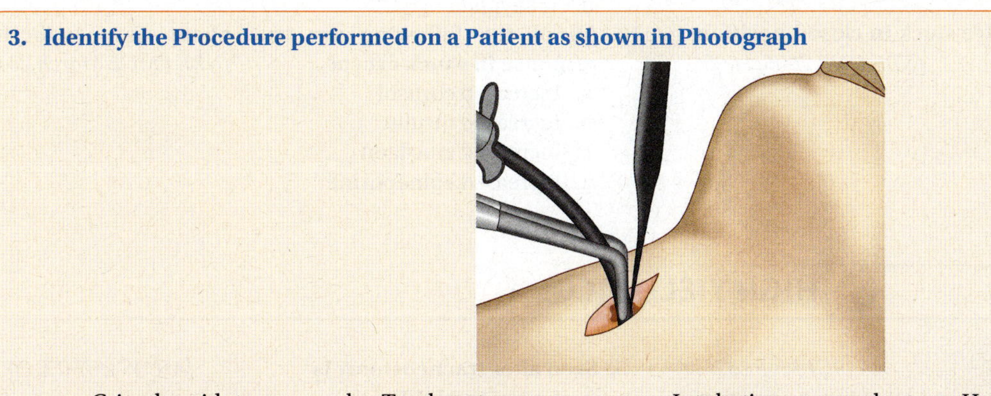

a. Cricothyroidotomy
b. Tracheostomy
c. Intubation
d Hyodotomy

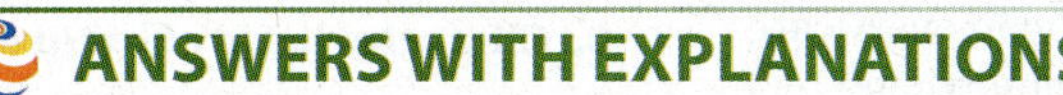

ANSWERS WITH EXPLANATIONS OF IBQs

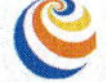

1 Ans. (c) Tracheostomy tube *[Ref. Ajay Yadav, 4/e p215]*

Indications of Tracheostomy
- Elective procedure: For prolonged ventilation
- Switch-over procedure from intubation: After 21 days
- Excessive secretions blocking Endotracheal tube
- If intubation is not possible
- Laryngeal surgeries
- Upper airway obstruction

2. Ans. (b) Tracheostomy *[Ref. Ajay Yadav, 4/e p215]*
- Tracheostomy: An incision in the trachea made to relieve an obstruction to breathing

3. Ans. (a) Cricothyroidotomy *[Ref. Ajay Yadav, 4/e p215]*
- Cricothyroidotomy/ Cricothyrotomy: Incision in Cricothyroid membrane
- Useful in life-threatening conditions
- Disadvantages: Injury to Cricoid cartilage, Larynx

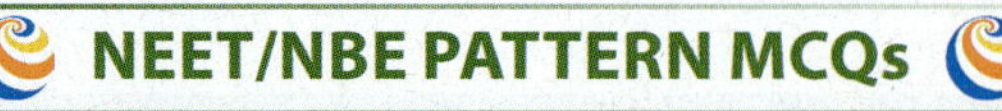

NEET/NBE PATTERN MCQs

1. **Use of Dexmedetomidine** *[Recent Question 2016]*
   a. Prolong action of LA in hypertensive patients
   b. Sedative agent for intubated patients
   c. Increases bioavailability of regional anaesthetic drugs
   d. Helps in reducing bispectral index of general anaesthetic drug with low potency
2. **APACHE II does not include** *[Recent Question 2016]*
   a. Acute physiology score
   b. Age c. Sex
   d. Chronic health evaluation
3. **Anaesthetic used for maintenance in ICU is** *[Recent Question 2016, NBE FMGE September 2009]*
   a. Thiopentone b. Propofol
   c. Ketamine d. None of the above
4. **A mid tracheostomy is done over which tracheal ring** *[Recent Question 2016, NBE DNB 2011]*
   a. 1st and 2nd ring
   b. 2nd and 3rd ring
   c. 3rd and 4th ring
   d. 5th and 6th ring
5. **A ventilator pressure relief valve stuck in closed position can result in** *[NBE DNB 2008, 2009]*
   a. Barotrauma
   b. Hypoventilation
   c. Hypoxia
   d. Hyperventilation
6. **Emergency tracheostomy is not indicated in** *[Recent Question 2016, NBE FMGE September 2008]*
   a. Foreign body in larynx
   b. Bilateral vocal cord paralysis
   c. Stridor due to laryngeal carcinoma
   d. Acute severe asthma
7. **Common complication occurring after tracheostomy in children is** *[NBE FMGE March 2004]*
   a. Stenosis b. Difficult decannulation
   c. Difficult weaning d. Infection
8. **Contraindications for Bag and mask ventilation include all except** *[NBE FMGE March 2009]*
   a. Pregnancy b. Empty stomach
   c. Hiatus hernia d. Tracheo-oesophageal fistula
9. **All of the following are signs of hemorrhagic shock except** *[NBE FMGE March 2012]*
   a. Tachycardia
   b. Hypotension
   c. Increased pulse pressure
   d. Tachypnea
10. **All of the following are true about neuroendocrine response in shock except** *[NBE FMGE March 2012]*
    a. Increased cortisol
    b. Increased insulin
    c. Increased glucagon
    d. Increased epinephrine

HIGH YIELD MCQs

1. **True about Tracheostomy** *[PGI June 2016]*
   a. Tracheostomy tube may be closed by mucous secretion and crust formation
   b. Copious secretion from tube is always due to pulmonary infection
   c. X-ray chest should be done for confirmation in every case
   d. Improper positioning may lead to fatal haemorrhage
   e. Displacing of tube after 2 weeks is medical emergency
2. **Most common cause of hypoxia during one lung ventilation is** *[AIIMS November 2005]*
   a. Malposition of the double lumen tube
   b. Increased shunt fraction
   c. Collapse of one lung
   d. Soiling of lung by secretions
3. **Incubator heat is delivered by all except** *[PGI 1998]*
   a. Conduction b. Convection
   c. Radiation d. Evaporation
4. **On examination, a patient with head injury eye opening in response to pain, inappropriate words and pain localisation. Calculate Glasgow Coma Scale score of the patient.** *[All India PGMEE 2011]*
   a. 8 b. 10
   c. 12 d. 14
5. **Seen after tracheostomy is** *[AIIMS PGMEE 2009]*
   a. Inversion of V/P ratio
   b. Increased V/P ratio
   c. Decrease in dead space
   d. Increased resistance to air, flow
6. **Clinical criteria of brain death is all except** *[JIPMER PGMEE 2005]*
   a. Coma
   b. Absent brainstem reflex
   c. Absent spinal cord reflex
   d. Absent motor activity
7. **Tracheostomy incision is made at** *[CGPG 2015]*
   a. Tracheal ring 1
   b. Tracheal ring 2–3
   c. Thyroid cartilage
   d. None of the above
8. **Time for which a Nurse should do suction in a Tracheotomised patient** *[AIIMS November 2017]*
   a. 10–15 seconds
   b. 30 seconds
   c. 45 seconds
   d. 60 seconds

 NEET/NBE PATTERN MCQs ANSWERS WITH EXPLANATIONS 

1. Ans. (b) Sedative agent for intubated patients
[Ref. Miller's Anesthesia, 7/e p756]

Dexmedetomidine

- Approved as a short-term sedative for adult intubated patients in the ICU
- A unique sedative agent for mechanically ventilated ICU patients and procedural sedation in nonintubated patients
- It is a selective alpha 2 receptor agonist, with mechanism of action similar to clonidine

2. Ans. (c) Sex
[Ref. Bailey & Love's, 26/e p1128]

Acute Physiologic Assessment and Chronic Health Evaluation II (APACHE II) Score

- Introduced in 1985
- Generates a point score ranging from 0-71 based on 12 physiologic variables, age, and underlying health
- Measurements APACHE II:
  - $AaDO_2$ or PaO_2 (depending on FiO_2)
  - Temperature (rectal)
  - Mean arterial pressure
  - pH arterial
  - Heart rate
  - Respiratory rate
  - Sodium (serum)
  - Potassium (serum)
  - Creatinine
  - Hematocrit
  - White blood cell count
  - Glasgow coma scale

3. Ans. (c) Ketamine
[Ref. KDT, 6/e p374-377]

- *Commonly used induction agents in anaesthesia*:

Intravenous induction agents	Inhalational induction agents
• Propofol • Thiopentone sodium • Etomidate • Ketamine • Methohexitone sodium	• Sevoflurane

- *Commonly used maintenance agents in anaesthesia*:
  - Benzodiazepines
  - Diazepam
  - Lorazepam
  - Midazolam
  - Ketamine (causes dissociative anaesthesia)
  - Fentanyl
  - Dexmedetomidine

4. Ans. (b) 2nd& 3rd ring
[Ref. SRB's Surgical Operations by Bhat M, 1/e p140]

Tracheostomy

- **High tracheostomy**: Above the level of isthmus
  - It can cause tracheal stenosis
  - It is above 2nd tracheal ring.
- **Mid-tracheostomy**: At level of Isthmus
  - Ideal and commonly used
  - It through 2nd and 3rd rings behind isthmus
  - It is approached by dividing thyroid isthmus
- **Low tracheostomy**: Below the isthmus level
  - It can cause torrential bleed which is difficult to control

5. Ans. (a) Barotrauma
[Ref. Miller's Anaesthesia, 7/e p702]

Ventilator Relief Valve Problems

- Hypoventilation occurs if the valve is incompetent because anesthetic gas is delivered to the scavenging system during the inspiratory phase instead of the patient
- Ventilator relief valve incompetency can result from a disconnected pilot line, a ruptured valve, or a damaged flapper valve
- A ventilator relief valve stuck in the closed or partially closed position can produce either barotrauma or undesired positive end-expiratory pressure (PEEP)

6. Ans. (d) Acute severe asthma
[Ref. Ajay Yadav, 4/e p215]

Indications of Tracheostomy

- Elective procedure: For prolonged ventilation
- Switch-over procedure from intubation: After 21 days
- Excessive secretions blocking Endotracheal tube
- If intubation is not possible
- Laryngeal surgeries
- *Upper airway obstruction*: **[Mnemonic: L**aryngeal **T**rauma **E**nhances **VITAL** Capacity**]**
  - **L**aryngitis
  - **T**rauma—facial/laryngeal
  - **E**dema—laryngeal
  - **V**ocal cord paralysis
  - **I**mpacted foreign bodies
  - **T**umours—congenital
  - **A**bscess—Peritonsillar (Quinsy)
  - **L**udwig's angina
  - **C**arcinoma head and neck

7. Ans. (b) Difficult decannulation
[Ref. Incidence of Complications of Tracheostomy and their Management, PJMS]

Complications of Tracheostomy

Early complications	Intermediate complications
• Haemorrhage • Apnoea • Local damage • Cardiac arrest **Late complications** • Difficult decannulation • Tracheal stenosis • Tracheo-oesophageal fistula	• Displacement of tube • Surgical emphysema • Infection • Scabs • Pneumothorax • Tracheo-oesophageal fistula

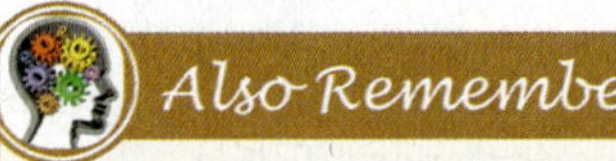

- *Most common presenting complaint in Tracheostomy patients*: Stridor

Anesthesiology

8. **Ans. (b) Empty stomach**
[Ref. Ajay Yadav, 4/e p235]

Contraindications for Bag-and-Mask Ventilation

[Mnemonic: Full-stomach **I**s **AU**n**D**esirable**T**hing for **M**ask]
- **F**ull stomach
- **A**spiration risk (Pregnancy, Hiatus hernia)
- **I**ntestinal obstruction
- **U**nconscious/semiconscious patients
- **D**iaphragmatic hernia
- **T**racheo-oesophageal fistula
- **M**econium aspiration

9. **Ans. (c) Increased pulse pressure**
[Ref. Lippincott's Nursing, 1/e p583]

Hemorrhagic Shock
- Tachycardia
- Tachypnoea
- Hypotension
- Narrow pulse pressure
- Restlessness, Thirst, Cold skin, Oliguria, Decreased body temperature

Also Remember

Neurogenic Shock
- Tachycardia/ Bradycardia
- Tachypnoea
- Apprehension
- Oliguria, Decreased body temperature, Warm dry skin

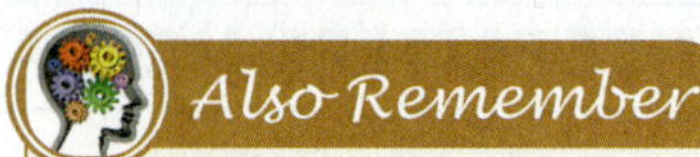

Cardiogenic Shock
- Tachycardia/ Bradycardia
- Tachypnoea
- Hypotension

10. **Ans. (b) Increased insulin**
[Ref. Surgery by Roshan Lall Gupta, 2/e p15]
- *Neuro-endocrine responses in shock:*

Neuro-endocrine parameter	Response to shock
ACTH and Cortisol	Increase
Catecholamines (Epinephrine, Norepinephrine)	Increase
Glucagon	Increase
Insulin	Decrease initially then increase
Insulin/ Glucagon ratio	Decrease
Growth hormone	Increase
Anti-diuretic hormone	Increase
Renin secretion	Increase
Cytokines	Increase
Acute phase reactants	Increase

HIGH YIELD MCQs ANSWERS WITH EXPLANATIONS

1. **Ans. (a) Tracheostomy tube may be closed by mucous secretion and crust formation; (d) Improper positioning may lead to fatal haemorrhage**
[Ref. Critical Care Medicine by Parrillo, 4/e p27]

Tracheostomy
- Nursing care is indispensable to the survival of the patient, as blockage of the tube by mucus or other secretions can lead to suffocation
- Causes of Copious secretions:
  - Presence of the tracheostomy tube: With the cuff inflated, excess secretions are expected because of poor pharyngeal and laryngeal sensation, and reduced subglottic pressure and cough strength
  - History of Chronic obstructive lung disease
  - Pulmonary infection
  - Low temperature in Oral/ laryngeal/ pharyngeal cavity
- Two ways to confirm correct tube placement:
  - Chest X-ray
  - Fibro-optic laryngoscopy
- Fatal complications of tracheostomy: Haemorrhage > Displaced tube > Infection > Obstruction > Aspiration > Tracheal erosion with resultant stenosis/fistula
- Displacement of Tracheostomy tube is medical emergency if placed less than 5–7 days

2. **Ans. (a) Malposition of the double lumen tube**
[Ref. Anesthesia Emergencies edited by Ruskin, 2/e p117]
- Most common cause of hypoxia/elevated airway pressure during one lung ventilation: Malposition of double lumen tube or lung isolation device

3. **Ans. (a) Conduction**
[Ref. Neonatal Nutrition and Metabolism by Thureen, 1/e p63]

4. **Ans. (b) 10**
[Ref. Ajay Yadav, 4/e p172]

Modified Glasgow Coma Scale

		Score
Eye opening	Nil	1
	To pain	2
	To speech	3
	Spontaneously	4
Best motor response	None	1
	Extension	2
	Decorticate flexion	3
	Withdrawal	4
	Localizes pain	5
	To verbal command	6

Contd...

Contd...

		Score
Best verbal response	Nil	1
	Incomprehensible sound	2
	Inappropriate words	3
	Confused	4
	Oriented	5

5. **Ans. (c) Decrease in dead space**
   [Ref. Ajay Yadav, 4/e p5]

6. **Ans. (c) Absent spinal cord reflex**
   [Ref. The Cambridge Textbook of Bioethics by Singer, 1/e p89]

7. **Ans. (b) Tracheal ring 2–3**
   [Ref. Head and Neck Surgery by Fliss, 1/e p211]

8. **Ans. (a) 10–15 seconds**
   [Ref. Tracheostomized and Ventilator Dependent Adults by Dikeman, 2/e p45]

Tracheal Suctioning

- Nasal/tracheal suctioning is performed by trained medical personnel when indicated
- Sterile technique is observed during tracheal suctioning
- Insert the flexible suction catheter gently with a slow rotational movement
- Negative pressure should never be applied for more than 10–15 seconds at a time to avoid deoxygenation of patient

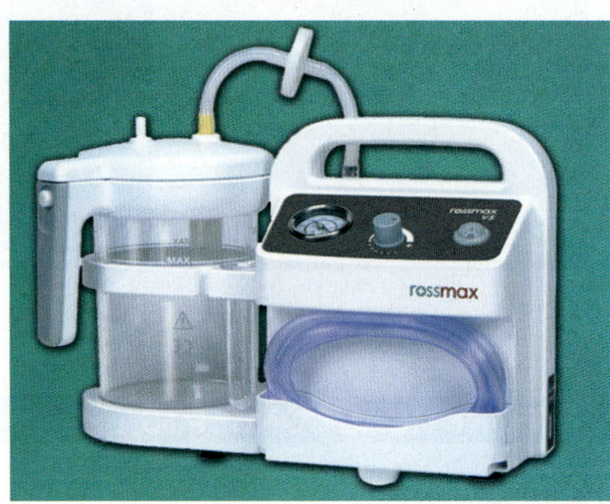

Fig. Suction machine

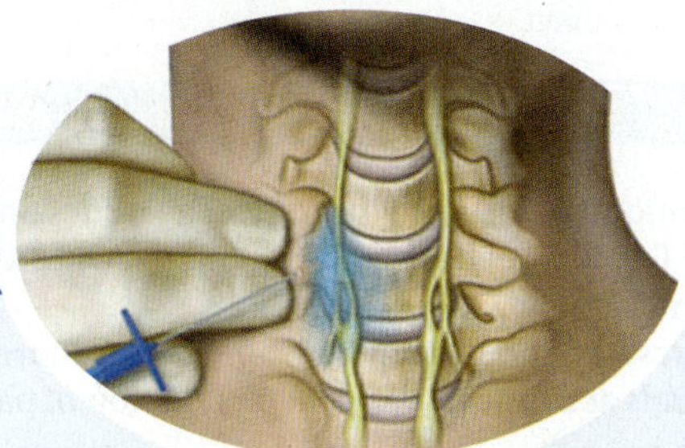

Chapter 13

Shock

THEORETICAL CONCEPTS

XIII A. DEFINITION

- *Definition*: State in which ineffective tissue perfusion leads to reversible (and then irreversible) cellular injury.

XIII B. CLASSIFICATION AND CAUSES[Q]

Hypovolemic shock	**Cardiogenic shock**
• Haemorrhage • Fluid loss (Diarrhoea, sweating) • Third space loss (Ascites) • Burns	• Left/right ventricular failure • Arrhythmias • Myocardial trauma • Regurgitant valvular disease
Distributive shock	**Obstructive shock**
• Neurogenic • Septic • Anaphylactic • Vasodilators • Adrenal insufficiency	• Cardiac tamponade, constrictive pericarditis • Pulmonary embolism/ hypertension • Tension pneumothorax • Obstructive valvular disease • Aortic dissection

XIII C. PARAMETERS IN SHOCK

XIII C1. Hemodynamic Parameters in Shock

	Hypovolemic	Cardiogenic	Distributive	Obstructive
Central venous pressure	Decrease	Increase	Decrease	Increase
Pul cap wedge pressure	Decrease	Increase	Decrease	Decrease
Cardiac output	Decrease	Decrease	Increase	Decrease
Blood pressure[Q]	Decrease	Decrease/N	Decrease	Decrease/N

XIII C2. Neuroendocrine Response in Shock

Neuroendocrine parameter	Response to shock
ACTH and Cortisol	Increase
Catecholamines (Epinephrine, Norepinephrine)	Increase
Glucagon	Increase
Insulin	Decrease initially then increase
Insulin/ Glucagon ratio	Decrease
Growth hormone	Increase
Antidiuretic hormone	Increase
Renin secretion	Increase
Cytokines	Increase
Acute phase reactants	Increase

XIII D. MANAGEMENT OF SHOCK

XIII D1. Aims of Management[Q]

- Mean arterial pressure > 60–65 mm Hg
- Pulmonary capillary wedge pressure 12–18 mm Hg
- Cardiac index > 3.5 (septicemic/ hypovolemic) or > 2.1 (Obstructive shock)
- Urine output > 0.5 mL/kg/hour
- Oxygen saturation > 90% (SVO_2 > 60%)

XIII D2. Treatment

- **Fluids**[Q]
  - *Fluids preferred in mild-moderate shock*: Crystalloids
  - *Fluids preferred in severe shock*: Colloids
- **Drugs**
  - *Vasopressors*: Phenylephrine, ephedrine, mephentramine, norepinephrine
  - *Inotropes*: Dopamine, dobutamine, dopexamine
  - *Vasodilators*: Nitroglycerine, Sodium nitroprusside, Hydralazine
- Steroids: useful in septicaemic shock only
- Acid-base management
- Nutritional support

XIII E. FEW FACTS ABOUT SHOCK

- *Drug of choice in neurogenic shock*: Phenylepherine[Q]

Anesthesiology

NEET/NBE PATTERN MCQs 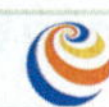

1. **Drug of choice in neurogenic shock is** *[NBE FMGE September 2008]*
   a. Ephedrine b. Phenylepherine
   c. Mephentramine d. Norepinephrine
2. **Drug of choice in Cardiogenic shock is** *[Recent Question 2016, NBE FMGE September 2012]*
   a. Dopamine b. Phenylephrine
   c. Noradrenaline d. Adrenaline
3. **Fluid status of patient in shock are best monitored with** *[NBE DNB 2011]*
   a. Arterial systolic pressure b. Arterial diastolic pressure
   c. Pulse pressure d. Central Venous pressure
4. **Dobutamine is preferred to Dopamine in the management of shock because** *[NBE DNB 2011]*
   a. It causes less arrhythmia
   b. It causes less renal vasodilation
   c. It causes more coronary vasoconstriction
   d. All of the above
5. **Pulmonary artery (Swan-Ganz) catheter can measure all except** *[UPSC 2012]*
   a. Cardiac output (CO)
   b. Pulmonary capillary wedge pressure (PCWP)
   c. Mixed venous oxygen saturation (SvO_2)
   d. Left ventricular end-diastolic volume
6. **In shock, Dopamine is used in the following dose** *[NBE DNB 2011]*
   a. 1-2 microgm/kg/min b. 1-2 mg/kg/min
   c. 5-10 microgm/kg/min d. 5-10 mg/kg/min
7. **Drug of choice in Cardiogenic shock is** *[NBE FMGE September 2012]*
   a. Dopamine b. Phenylephrine
   c. Noradrenaline d. Adrenaline
8. **Drug used for unresponsive shock with low BP and Warm peripheries** *[Recent Question 2015]*
   a. Adrenaline b. Noradrenaline
   c. Dopamine d. Beta blockers

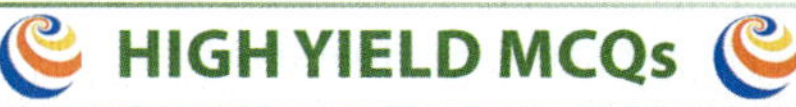

HIGH YIELD MCQs

1. **Complications of CVP line** *[PGI 2009]*
   a. Airway injury b. Haemothorax
   c. Septicaemia d. Air embolism
   e. Pseudoaneurysm
2. **Swan-Ganz catheter measure** *[PGI 2006]*
   a. PCWP
   b. CO
   c. Mixed venous oxygen saturation
   d. Right atrial pressure
3. **In a 10-year-old child presented with anaphylactic shock, drug of choice is** *[PGI 1997]*
   a. I/V adrenaline
   b. SC adrenaline
   c. Antihistamine
   d. Corticosteroids

 NEET/NBE PATTERN MCQs ANSWERS WITH EXPLANATIONS

1. **Ans. (b) Phenylepherine**
   [Ref. Ajay Yadav, 4/e p210]
   - Drug of choice in neurogenic shock: Phenylepherine

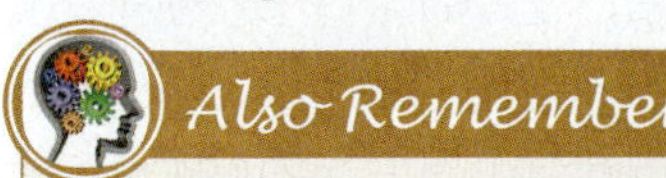

Also Remember

- Fluids preferred in mild-moderate shock: Crystalloids
- Fluids preferred in severe shock: Colloids

2. **Ans. (a) Dopamine**
   [Ref. Ajay Yadav, 4/e p210]
3. **Ans. (d) Central venous pressure**
   [Ref. Ajay Yadav, 4/e p210]
   - Central Venous Pressure (CVP) and Pulmonary capillary Wedge Pressure are good monitoring indicator for shock
   - Urine output is best clinical guide of tissue perfusion.
4. **Ans. (a) It causes less arrhythmia**
   [Ref. Ajay Yadav, 4/e p232]
   - Advantage of Dobutamine over Dopamine is that it does not causes tachycardia: Inotrope of choice in patients of myocardial ischaemia and in patients susceptible to develop arrhythmias
5. **Ans. (d) Left ventricular end-diastolic volume**
   [Ref. Ajay Yadav, 4/e p50-51]

   Swan-Ganz Catheter
   - **Swan-Ganz catheter is used for pulmonary artery catheterization**
   - It is done for:
     - Measuring cardiac chamber pressure (except left ventricle)
     - Cardiac output (by using ice cold saline: Thermodilution method)
     - Measuring Pulmonary Artery Occlusion Pressure (PAOP): Represents left atrial pressure
     - Taking sample for mixed venous blood
     - Titration of fluid infusion

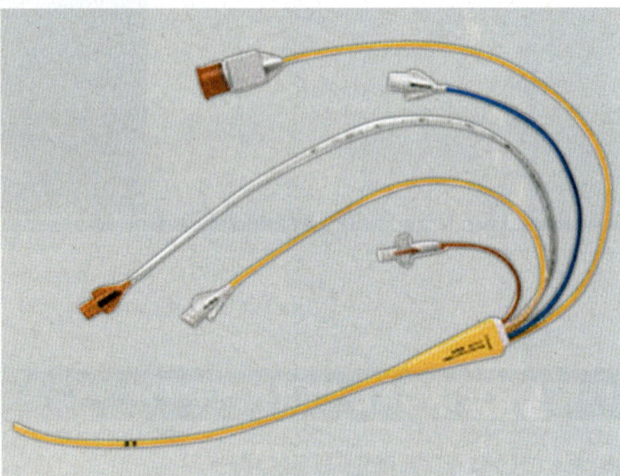

Fig. Swan-Ganz Catheter

6. **Ans. (c) 5-10 microgram/kg/min**
   [Ref. Ajay Yadav, 4/e p232]
7. **Ans. (a) Dopamine**
   [Ref. Ajay Yadav, 4/e p232]
8. **Ans. (c) Dopamine**
   [Ref. Emergency Medicine by Medzon, 1/e p30]
   - Neurogenic shock can occur with high cord lesions and manifests as hypotension unresponsive to aggressive volume resuscitation. There will usually be a bradycardia and warm, vasodilated peripheries
   - Ephedrine, Phenylephrine, Dopamine are used for their Vasoconstrictive effects

 HIGH YIELD MCQs ANSWERS WITH EXPLANATIONS 

1. **Ans. ALL OPTIONS**
   [Ref. Ajay Yadav, 4/e p50]

   Complications of CVP Catheterization
   - Air embolism
   - Thromboembolism
   - Cardiac arrhythmias
   - Pneumothorax/haemothorax/chylothorax
   - Cardiac perforation/cardiac tamponade.
   - Sepsis
   - Trauma to brachial plexus, carotid artery, phrenic nerve during insertion.
   - Pseudoaneurysm of left subclavian artery
2. **Ans. (b) ALL OPTIONS**
   [Ref. Ajay Yadav, 4/e p50-51
3. **Ans. (a) I/V adrenaline**
   [Ref. Ajay Yadav, 4/e p50-51]
   - Adrenaline (1: 10,000 concentration) 0.5 to 1 mg subcutaneously to be repeated every 3-5 mins in Anaphylaxis

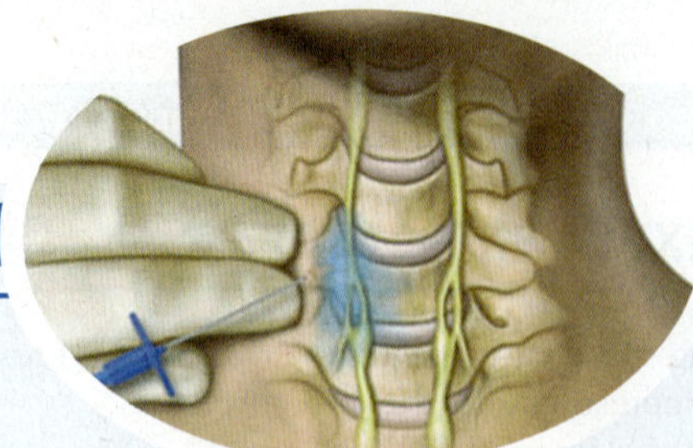

Chapter 14

Fluid Electoral Balance

THEORETICAL CONCEPTS

XIV A. BLOOD TRANSFUSION

- ***Whole blood***:
  - One unit: 500 ml anticoagulated blood (Hematocrit: 40%)[Q]
  - Contains normal concentration of albumin and clotting factors BUT low levels of factors V and VIII
- ***Packed red cells***:
  - One unit: 250 ml anticoagulated blood (Hematocrit: 60%)
  - Contains no platelets
  - One unit of packed cells increase haemoglobin by 1 gm% and Hematocrit by 3% [Q]
- ***Fresh frozen plasma***:
  - Frozen within 6 hours of donation
  - Contains all clotting factors, albumin, gammaglobulin
  - One unit: 150 ml anticoagulated blood
  - FFP does not transmit infections [Q]
- ***Cryoprecipitate***:
  - Obtained from FFP
  - Contains large quantities of Factor VIII, VWF, fibrinogen, fibrin, fibronectin, factor XIII [Q]
- ***Platelet concentrate***:
  - Contains 50-80% platelets in a unit of fresh whole blood
  - 1 unit PC increase platelet count by 5000–8000/ cu. mm [Q]

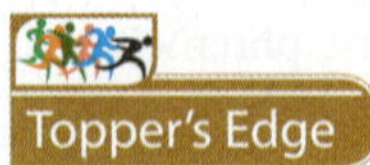

Topper's Edge

ADVERSE EFFECTS OF BLOOD TRANSFUSION

Immunologic Reactions

- **Acute hemolytic reactions**:
  - Fever and other symptoms/signs of haemolysis < 24 hours of transfusion[Q]
  - Fall of Hb, rise in LDH, positive direct antiglobulin test, positive crossmatch
- **Delayed hemolytic reactions**: Occur > 24 hours after a transfusion
- Febrile nonhemolytic reactions:
  - MC type of blood transfusion reaction[Q]
  - Occur due to the release of inflammatory chemical signals released by WBCs in stored donor blood
- Allergic reactions
- Post-transfusion purpura: Rare complication
- Transfusion-associated acute lung injury (TRALI): Syndrome of acute respiratory distress, often associated with fever, non-cardiogenic pulmonary edema, and hypotension

Contd…

Contd…

Infections

- HIV, Hepatitis C, Hepatitis B, Syphilis, Chagas disease, Cytomegalovirus infections (in immunocompromised recipients), HTLV, Malaria, Babesia

Other Adverse Reactions

- Transfusion-associated volume overload
- Hypothermia
- Inclination for bleeding due to disseminated intravascular coagulation
- Metabolic alkalosis
- Hypocalcemia
- Blood doping

XIV B. MASSIVE BLOOD TRANSFUSION

- ***Definition of Massive blood transfusion***:
  - Transfusion of blood more than patients blood volume (5 litres) in more than 24 hours [Q]
  - Transfusion of more than 10% blood volume in less than 10 minutes
- ***Complications of massive blood transfusion***: [Q]
  - Hypocalcemia
  - Hypothermia
  - Hyperkalemia
  - Hyperammonemia
  - Metabolic alkalosis
  - ARDS
  - Disseminated intravascular coagulation (DIC): Most common cause of death

XIV C. FLUIDS USEFUL IN COMMON CLINICAL SITUATIONS

Clinical situation	Resuscitation fluid
Burns	Ringer lactate
Renal failure	Crystalloids with low potassium
Liver failure	Albumin
Intestinal obstruction	Ringer lactate
Cerebral/pulmonary oedema (ARDS)	Colloids
Hypovolemic shock	Crystalloids (Ringer lactate)
Congestive heart failure	Colloids

IMAGE-BASED QUESTION

1. **False about composition of Fluid shown in Photograph**
[Recent Question 2012]

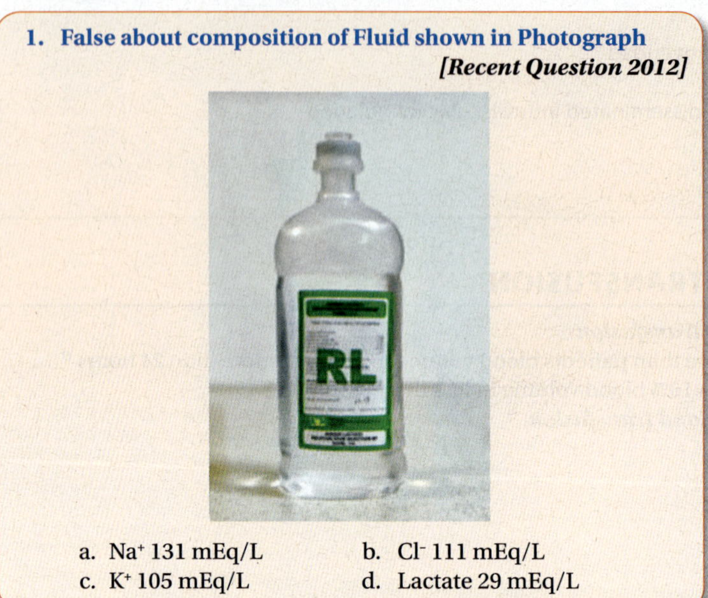

a. Na^+ 131 mEq/L
b. Cl^- 111 mEq/L
c. K^+ 105 mEq/L
d. Lactate 29 mEq/L

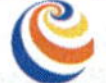

ANSWER WITH EXPLANATION OF IBQ

1. **Ans. (c)** K+ 105 mEq/L *[Ref. Ajay Yadav, 4/e p11]*

Ringer Lactate

- Crystalloid of choice for Blood-loss replacement
- Composition:
  - Na^+: 131 mEq/ L
  - Cl^-: 111 mEq/ L
  - K^+: 5 mEq/ L
  - Ca^{2+}: 2 mEq/ L
  - Lactate: 29 mEq/ L
  - pH: 6.5
- Total osmolarity: 273 mOsm/L (Slightly Hypotonic)

NEET/NBE PATTERN MCQs

1. **Most common cause of death after massive blood transfusion** *[NBE FMGE March 2008]*
   a. Hypocalcemia b. Hyperkalemia
   c. Hypothermia
   d. Disseminated intravascular coagulation
2. **Which of the following is NOT an Isotonic solution?** *[Recent Question 2016, 2014]*
   a. 0.5% Dextrose in water b. 0.9% Normal saline
   c. Lactated ringer d. 10% Dextrose in water
3. **In a normal child of weight 15 kg, the daily fluid maintenance requirement is** *[UPSC 2012]*
   a. 1000 ml b. 1250 ml
   c. 1500 ml d. 1750 ml
4. **The commonest fluid used for fluid resuscitation in burns is** *[NBE FMGE March 2012]*
   a. Normal saline b. Ringer lactate
   c. Human albumin d. Fresh frozen plasma
5. **0.9% Sodium chloride contains .... Sodium** *[Recent Question 2015]*
   a. 154 mmol/L b. 131 mmol/L
   c. 145 mmol/L d. 30 mmol/L
6. **Energy requirement of most patients post-surgery is** *[Recent Question 2016, 2015]*
   a. 10 kcal/kg/day b. 30 kcal/kg/day
   c. 50 kcal/kg/day d. 70 kcal/kg/day
7. **Most common complication of Central venous line insertion is?** *[Recent Question 2017]*
   a. Lung apex injury
   b. Infection at catheter site
   c. Cardiac tamponade
   d. Pneumothorax
8. **In Sepsis, management of fluid involves administration of** *[Recent Question 2017]*
   a. Colloids
   b. Crystalloids
   c. Hydroxyethyl starch
   d. None
9. **O_2 carrying capacity of Crystalloids and Colloids is?** *[Recent Question 2017]*
   a. More than whole blood
   b. Equivalent to whole blood
   c. More than packed RBCs
   d. None
10. **Complication of Massive blood transfusion?** *[Recent Question 2017]*
    a. Hypercalcemia
    b. Hypermagnesemia
    c. Hyperkalemia
    d. Hyperthermia

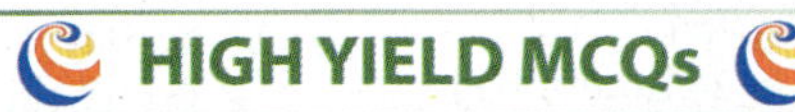

HIGH YIELD MCQs

1. **In an injured patient with hypovolemia, intravenous fluid administered is guided by** *[PGI 2003]*
   a. Central venous pressure b. Blood pressure
   c. Urine output d. Pulse rate
2. **Heparin interferes with which of the following results of ABG** *[PGI 2013]*
   a. PO_2 b. PCO_2
   c. pH d. HCO_3
   e. Anion gap
3. **Importance of CVP measurements is** *[PGI 2001]*
   a. Need for blood transfusion
   b. Assess amount of fluid to be given
   c. Need for inotropic support
   d. Rate of intravenous fluid replacement
   e. Assess need for plasma transfusion
4. **If we need to administer 180 mg of a drug available as 500 mg/5 ml via 2 ml syringe. Up to how many divisions will we fill the syringe?** *[AIIMS November 2017]*
   a. 1.8 divisions
   b. 8 divisions
   c. 18 divisions
   d. 12 divisions
5. **Which of the following is NOT considered as an indicator of adequate fluid resuscitation?** *[UPSC CMS 2017]*
   a. Urine output
   b. Respiratory rate
   c. Pulse
   d. Blood pressure

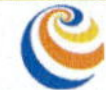 NEET/NBE PATTERN MCQs ANSWERS WITH EXPLANATIONS 

1. **Ans. (d) Disseminated intravascular coagulation**
   [Ref. Ajay Yadav, 4/e p17]
   - ***Massive blood transfusion***:
     - Transfusion of blood more than patients blood volume (5 litres) in more than 24 hours
     - Transfusion of more than 10% blood volume in less than 10 minutes
   - ***Complications of massive blood transfusion***:
     - Hypocalcemia
     - Hypothermia
     - Hyperkalemia
     - Hyperammonemia
     - Metabolic alkalosis
     - ARDS
     - Disseminated intravascular coagulation (DIC): Most common cause of death

2. **Ans. (d) 10% dextrose in water**
   [Ref. Ajay Yadav, 4/e p12]

3. **Ans. (b) 1250 ml**
   [Ref. Ajay Yadav, 4/e p12]
   - **Maintenance Fluid**: Hourly maintenance requirement is calculated by formula of 4-2-1
     - 0-10 kg = 4 ml/kg/hr
     - 10-20 kg = 2 ml/kg/hr
     - >20 kg = 1 ml/kg/hr

   In the given question, For a child of 15 kg, fluid requirement will be
   - For first 10 kg is 40 ml/hr (@ 4 ml/kg/hr)
   - For next 5 kg (10–25) is 10 ml/hr (@ 2 ml/kg/hr)
   - So, total in 1st hour it is 50ml (40+10), So in 24 hour it will be 1200 ml

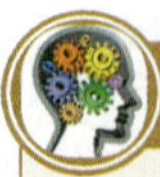

Also Remember

Another example: for an adult of 60 kg, replacement fluid will be
- For first 1 0kg is 40 ml/hr (@ 4 ml/kg/hr)
- For next 10 kg (20–10) is 20 ml/hr (@ 2 ml/kg/hr)
- For next 40 kg (60–20) is 40 ml/hr (@ 1 ml/kg/hr)
- So, total in 1st hour it is 100 ml (40+20+40), So in 24 hour it will be 2400 ml

4. **Ans. (b) Ringer lactate**
   [Ref. Ajay Yadav, 4/e p13]

Fluids useful in Common Clinical Situations

Clinical situation	Resuscitation fluid
Burns	Ringer lactate
Renal failure	Crystalloids with low potassium
Liver failure	Albumin
Intestinal obstruction	Ringer lactate
Cerebral/ pulmonary oedema (ARDS)	Colloids
Hypovolemic shock	Crystalloids (Ringer lactate)
Congestive heart failure	Colloids

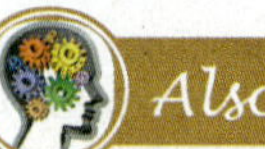

Also Remember

- Hypotonic solutions are contraindicated in cerebral and pulmonary oedema
- Glucose containing solutions are contraindicated in head injuries
- Colloids CAN BE GIVEN in acute phase of burns
- Colloids are preferable even in endothelial injury

5. **Ans. (a) 154 mmol/L**
   [Ref. How to Survive in Anesthesia by Robinson, 4/e p30]

Electrolyte Compostion of I/V Solutions (mmol/ Litre)

	Sodium	Potassium	Calcium	Chloride	Lactate
0.9% Sodium chloride	154	–	–	154	–
Hartmann's solution	131	5	2	111	29
5% Glucose	–	–	–	–	–
Haemaccel	145	5	6	145	–
Hydroxyethyl starch	154	–	–	154	–

6. **Ans. (b) 30 kcal/kg/day**
   [Ref. Schwartz Current Practice of Surgery, 9/e]
   - Energy requirement of most patient post-surgery: 30 Kcal/kg/day
   - Protein requirement of most patient post-surgery: 1.0-1.1 g/kg/day

7. **Ans. (d) Pneumothorax**
   [Ref. Pediatric Interventional Radiology by Towbin, 1/e p66]
   - MCC of Post-operative Pneumothorax is the insertion of a Central venous line, and a chest X-ray is necessary after this procedure to exclude this potential complication
   - An iatrogenic etiology underlies the majority of Pneumothoraces treated in most hospitals: Procedures such as percutaneous lung biopsy, transbronchial biopsy, and the insertion of central venous lines and pulmonary artery catheters are associated with increased rates

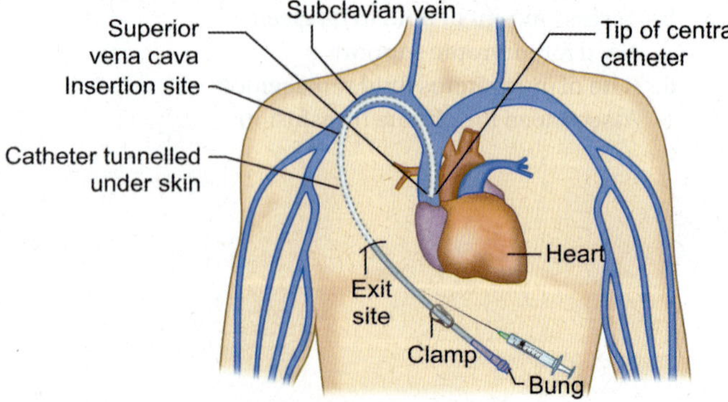

Fig. Central Venous Line

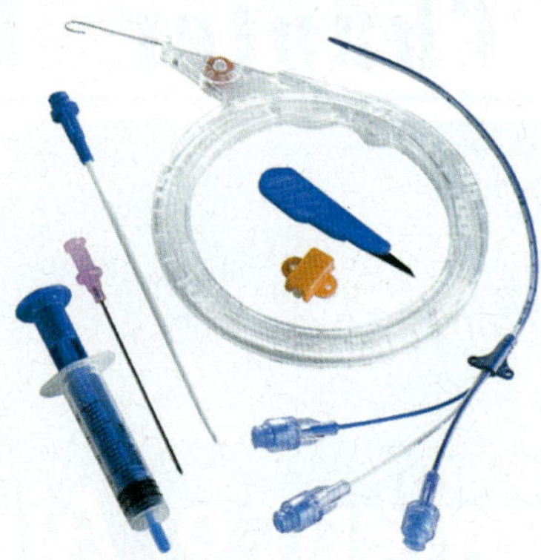

Fig. Central Venous Line Set

8. Ans. (b) Crystalloids

[Ref. Faust's Anesthesiology, 4/e p232]

- **Crystalloids should be the initial resuscitation fluid in Severe sepsis and Septic shock**
- Albumin should be added when substantial amounts of crystalloids are required
- Hydroxyethyl starches are not recommended
- A fluid bolus of 30 mL/kg should be administered in hypoperfusion states with presumed hypovolemia
- Fluid challenges should be repeated based on response

9. Ans. (d) None

[Ref. Nurse Anesthesia by Nagelhout, 4/e p411]

- Although both crystalloids and colloids can replace intravascular volume, neither product restores the oxygen-carrying capacity of the lost red blood cells or even coagulation factors

10. Ans. (c) Hyperkalemia

[Ref. Ajay Yadav, 4/e p17]

- Complications of massive blood transfusion: Hypocalcemia, Hypothermia, Hyperkalemia, Hyperammonemia, Metabolic alkalosis, ARDS, Disseminated intravascular coagulation (DIC - MCC of death)

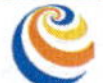 HIGH YIELD MCQs ANSWERS WITH EXPLANATIONS 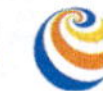

1. Ans. ALL CHOICES

[Ref. Ajay Yadav, 4/e p208]

2. Ans. (b) PCO_2; (c) pH; (d) HCO_3

[Ref. Pediatric Nephrology by Goodyer, 1/e p67]

- Excessive heparin (>10% of the sample volume) may decrease
  - pH
  - PCO_2
  - HCO_3

3. Ans. (a) Need for blood transfusion; (b) Access amount of fluid to be given; (c) Need for ionotropic support

[Ref. Ajay Yadav, 4/e p50]

4. Ans. (c) 18 divisions

[Ref. Math and Dosage Calculations for Medical Careers, 2/e p113]

In the given question,

- Drug strength 500 mg is present per 5 ml vial
- **So,** 180 mg will be present in $5/500 \times 180 = 1.8$ ml
- **Now,** a 2 ml syringe has 20 markings (divisions) of 0.1 ml each
- **So,** we'll need to fill syringe upto 1.8 ml/ 0.1 ml = 18 divisions

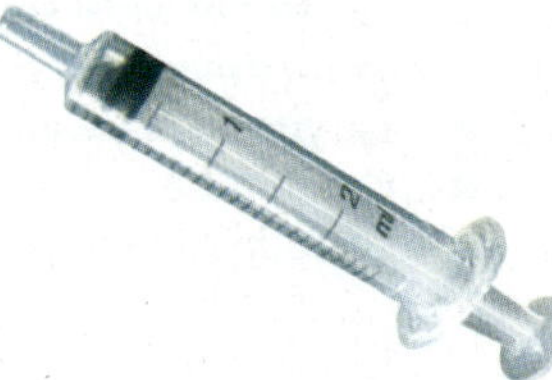

Fig. 2-ml syringe

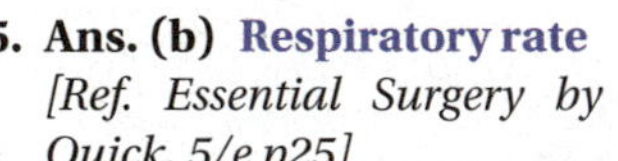

5. Ans. (b) Respiratory rate

[Ref. Essential Surgery by Quick, 5/e p25]

Indicators of Adequate Resuscitation

- MAP > 60
- HR < 100
- Urine output 0.5-1.0 ml/kg/hr (30 cc/hr) (Best/ Most reliable indicator)
- Serum lactate levels: Most sensitive indicator as to whether some circulatory beds remain inadequately perfused (normal < 2.5 mmol/L)
- Gastric mucosal pH
- Base deficit (Normal -2 to +2)

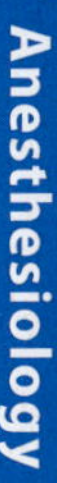

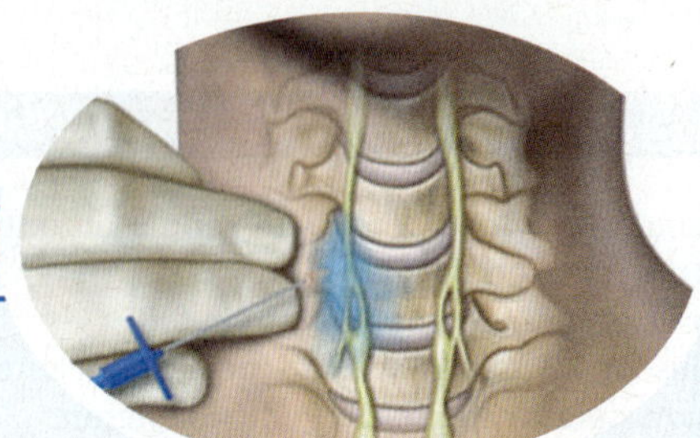

Chapter 15

Management of Airway

THEORETICAL CONCEPTS

XV A. AIRWAY MANAGEMENT FOR CERVICAL SPINE INJURY

- *Oral intubation with neck stabilisation*: Should be attempted first
- *Tracheostomy*: Most suitable method[Q]
- *Temporary measures if tracheostomy not available*:
  - Laryngeal mask airway
  - Combitube
  - Cricothyroidotomy

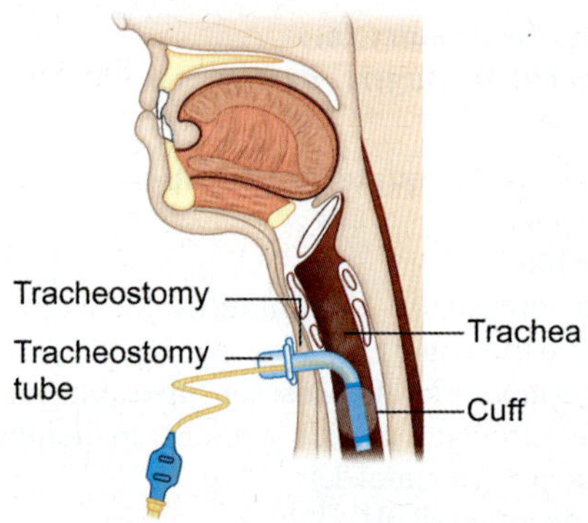

Fig. Tracheostomy

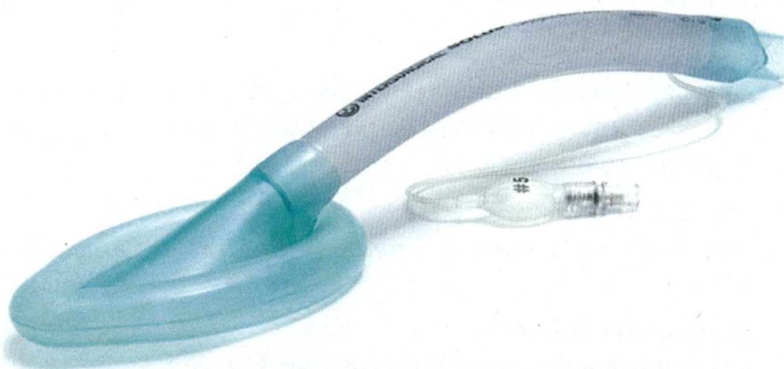

Fig. Laryngeal mask airway (LMA)

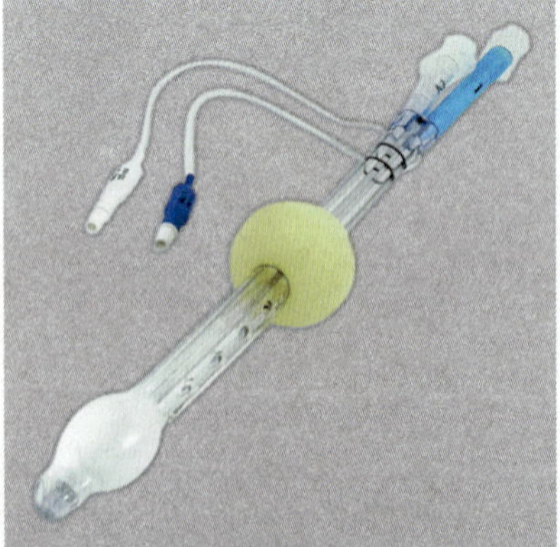

Fig. Combitube

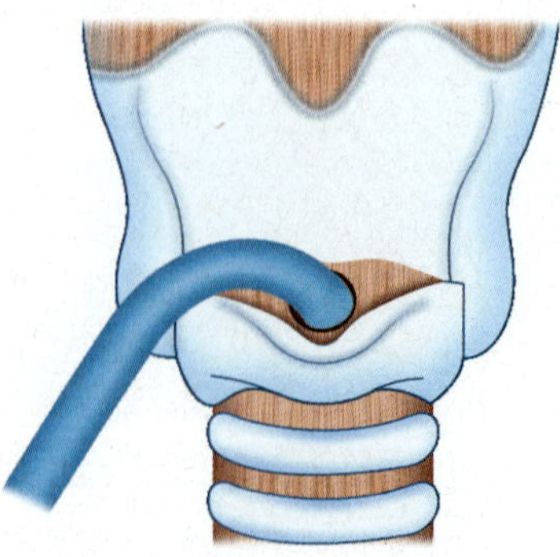

Fig. Cricothyroidotomy

XV B. AIRWAY ASSESSMENT

XV B1. Airway Assessment: Preliminary Assessment

- History of previous airway difficulty: Higher positive predictive value
- History of previous laryngoscopy
- Increased age
- Pathology

XV B2. Airway Tests to Assess Difficulty

- Mouth opening: Interincisor distance
  - 4 cm (2 fingerbreadths) is an indicator of probable difficult intubation
- Prognathic ability of the mandible: Depends on the size and shape of the mandible in relation to the maxilla and on TMJ function
- Head (Occipito-atlanto-axial) extension: Measured as the angle between the occlusal surface of the maxillary teeth and the horizontal
  - **Angles < 20 degrees suggesting difficult laryngoscopy**
- Mallampatti test (visibility of pharyngeal structures): Limited value
- Thyromental distance: Limited value
- Evaluation of dentition

XV C. LARYNGEAL MASK AIRWAY (BRAIN MASK)

- **Discoverer: Archie Bain**
- Principle: Places blindly in oropharynx and cuff is inflated; Cuff seals lateral and posterior pharyngeal walls to allow ventilation through ports

Indications	Contraindications
• Difficult intubation anticipated • Securing airway in emergency • Elective method for Minor surgery • Conduit for bronchoscopes, small tubes	• Full stomach patients • Hiatus hernia • Pregnancy • Oropharyngeal abscess/ mass
Advantages	**Disadvantages**
• Easy to insert • No need of muscle relaxants • Useful in Cervical injuries	• Does not prevent aspiration • High incidence of Laryngospasm

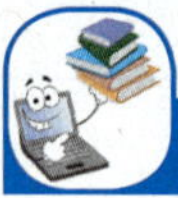

IMAGE-BASED QUESTIONS

1. Identify the Instrument/ device shown in Photograph ***[Recent Question 2013, 2014]***

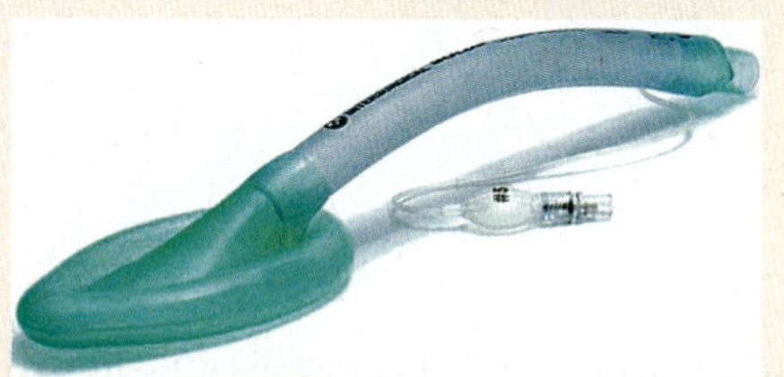

a. Brook airway
b. Endotracheal tube (Cuffed)
c. Laryngeal mask airway
d. Guedel airway

2. Identify the Type of laryngoscope shown in Photograph ***[Recent Question 2014]***

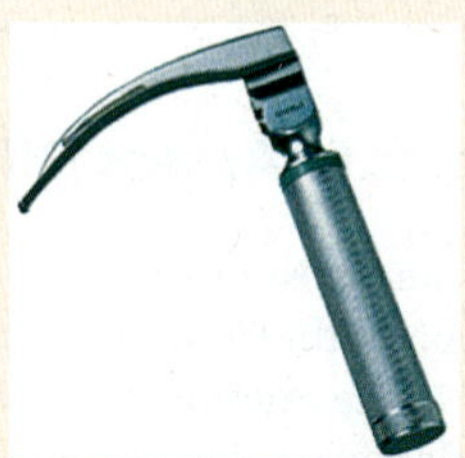

a. Macintosh
b. Miller
c. McCoy
d. Bullard

3. Identify the Instrument/device shown in Photograph ***[Recent Question 2012]***

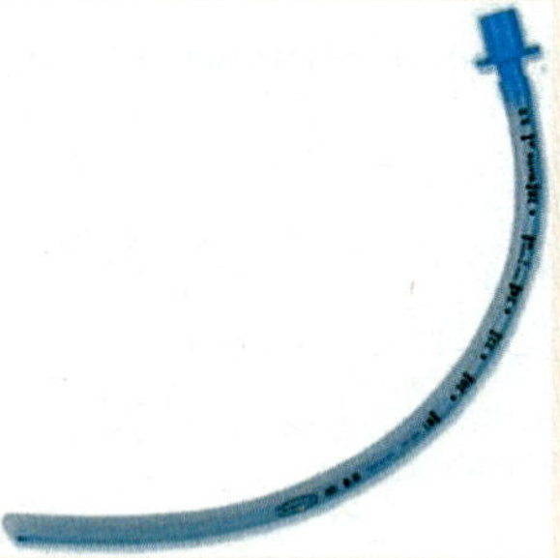

a. Uncuffed Endotracheal tube
b. Cuffed Endotracheal tube
c. Endotracheal tube Double lumen
d. Water's airway

4. In correct positioning, Tip of Instrument shown in Photograph lie at ***[AIIMS November 2015]***

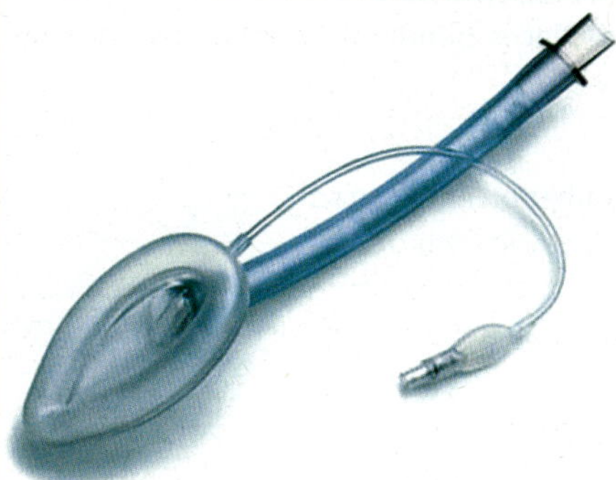

a. At Epiglottis
b. At level of Vocal cords
c. At Thyroid cartilage
d. Above esophagus

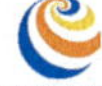

ANSWERS WITH EXPLANATIONS OF IBQs

1. Ans. (c) Laryngeal mask airway *[Ref. Ajay Yadav, 4/e p40]*

- LMA is placed blindly in oropharynx and cuff is inflated; Cuff seals lateral and posterior pharyngeal walls to allow ventilation through ports

2. Ans. (a) Macintosh *[Ref. Ajay Yadav, 4/e p34]*

Laryngoscopes

- Macintosh: MC used Laryngoscope; Curved blade
- Miller: Straight blade with Curve at tip
- Fibreoptic: Useful in Difficult intubation; Easy Nasal intubation
- Bullard: Fibreoptic channel to directly visualize laryngeal inlet
- McCoy: Movable tip

3. Ans. (a) Uncuffed Endotracheal tube *[Ref. Ajay Yadav, 4/e p35]*

- Technique of intubation: Extension at Atlanto-occipital joint and Flexion at Cervical spine

4. Ans. (d) Above esophagus *[Ref. Neurology of Breathing by Bolton, 1/e p138]*

- With correct positioning of Laryngeal mask airway (Photograph), Tip should rest at Base of Hypopharynx and against Upper Esophageal sphincter

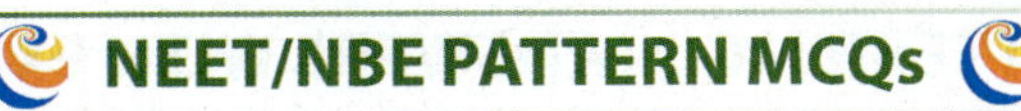

NEET/NBE PATTERN MCQs

1. **Gas used in Rapid airbag inflation** *[Recent Question 2016]*
   a. Sodium azide b. Nitrocellulose
   c. Mercuric nitrate d. Potassium nitrate
2. **Laryngeal mask airway not used in**
   a. Baby weighing <1500 gms *[Recent Question 2016]*
   b. Pregnant patients
   c. Ocular surgeries
   d. Difficult surgeries
3. **In Venturi mask oxygen concentration attained is** *[Recent Question 2016]*
   a. 90% b. 100%
   c. 60% d. 80%
4. **In patient with cervical cord injury best way to maintain airway is** *[NBE FMGE September 2009]*
   a. Bag and mask b. Tracheostomy
   c. Cricothyroidotomy d. Endotracheal tube
5. **A mid tracheostomy is done over which tracheal ring** *[NBE DNB 2011]*
   a. 1st and 2nd ring b. 2nd and 3rd ring
   c. 3rd and 4th ring d. 5th and 6th ring
6. **Laryngeal mask airway is used for** *[Recent Question 2016, NBE FMGE September 2012]*
   a. Airway maintenance
   b. Circulation maintenance
   c. Positive pressure ventilation
   d. All of the above
7. **All of the following are features of difficult airway EXCEPT** *[Recent Question 2016, NBE DNB 2011, 2012]*
   a. Miller's sign
   b. Micrognathia with macroglossia
   c. Temporo-mandibular joint ankylosis
   d. Increased thyromental distance
8. **In patient with suspected air embolism, patient should be placed in which of the following positions?** *[NBE FMGE September 2008]*
   a. Head-up and right side up
   b. Head-up and left side up
   c. Head-low and right side up
   d. Head-low and left side up
9. **Laryngeal mask airway is used for** *[NBE FMGE September 2012]*
   a. Airway maintenance
   b. Circulation maintenance
   c. Positive pressure ventilation
   d. All of the above
10. **Size of LMA for a 15 kg child is?** *[Recent Question 2017]*
    a. 1 b. 2
    c. 3 d. 4
11. **Which of the following prevents aspiration?** *[Recent Question 2017]*
    a. LMA b. Oropharyngeal airway
    c. Nasopharyngeal airway d. ProSeal LMA

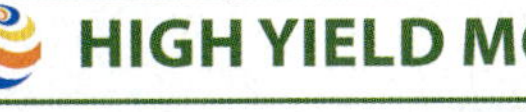

HIGH YIELD MCQs

1. **Which of the following are used to protect airways?** *[PGI 2009]*
   a. Laryngeal mask airway (LMA)
   b. Endotracheal tube
   c. Ryle's tube
   d. Combitube
   e. Sengstaken Blakemore tube
2. **Indications of tracheostomy are** *[PGI 2003]*
   a. Flail chest b. Head injury
   c. Tetanus d. Cardiac tamponade
   e. Foreign body
3. **In a patient with multiple injuries, first thing to be done is** *[PGI 1999]*
   a. Patency of airway
   b. Maintenance of BP
   c. Immobilize cervical spine
   d. Lateral position with mouth gag
4. **All of the following are Definitive Airway EXCEPT** *[All India PGMEE 2011]*
   a. Oro-tracheal tube b. Naso-tracheal tube
   c. Laryngeal mask airway d. Crico-thyroidectomy
5. **Laryngeal mask Airway (LMA) is used for** *[AIIMS PGMEE 2003]*
   a. Maintenance of the airway
   b. Facilitating laryngeal surgery
   c. Prevention of aspiration
   d. Removing oral secretions
6. **The laryngeal mask airway used for securing the airway of a patient in all of the following conditions except** *[All India PGMEE 2005]*
   a. In a difficult intubation
   b. In cardiopulmonary resuscitation
   c. In a child undergoing an elective/routine eye surgery
   d. In a patient with a large tumour in the oral cavity
7. **Laryngeal mask airway is indicated in** *[PGI 2001]*
   a. To prevent aspiration of stomach contents
   b. Short surgical procedure
   c. Where endotracheal intubation is contraindicated
   d. Difficult airway
   e. Facilitate endotracheal intubation
8. **True about LMA (Laryngeal Mask Airway)** *[PGI 2008]*
   a. Available in 8 sizes b. Intubation can be done
   c. Size 1 for neonates d. Size 3 for adults
   e. Full protection from aspiration
9. **All are features of difficult airway except** *[PGI 1999]*
   a. Miller's sign
   b. Micrognathia with macroglossia
   c. TMJ ankylosis
   d. Increased thyromental distance
10. **Plan C of anesthetic airway management is** *[MAHE PGMEE 2005]*
    a. Standard laryngoscopy and intubation
    b. Intubation catheter guided intubation
    c. Insertion of laryngeal mask airway and fiberoptic bronchoscopy
    d. Cancel the surgery or perform tracheostomy
11. **LMA used in a 25 kg child is** *[Recent Question 2016, JIPMER 2015]*
    a. 1 b. 1.5
    c. 2.5 d. 4

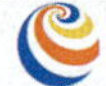 NEET/NBE PATTERN MCQs ANSWERS WITH EXPLANATIONS 

1. Ans. (a) Sodium azide

[Ref. Anaesthesia for Postgraduates by Agasti, 1/e p384,385]

- The chemical at the heart of the air bag reaction is called **sodium azide, or NaN_3**
- CRASHES trip sensors in cars that send an electric signal to an ignitor
- The heat generated causes sodium azide to decompose into sodium metal and nitrogen gas, which inflates the car's air bags

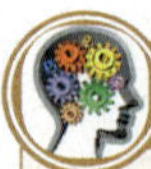

Also Remember

- Chemical reactions to generate the gas to fill an airbag
  - Decomposition of sodium azide (NaN_3)
  - Reactions to remove harmful products
  - Reaction stoichiometry

2. Ans. (b) Pregnant Patients

[Ref. Anaesthesia for Postgraduates by Agasti, 1/e p569]

Contraindications of LMA

- Full stomach (e.g. pregnancy, hiatal hernia, intestinal obstruction, etc.)
- Pharyngeal pathology (e.g. tumour, abscess, etc.), pharyngeal obstruction, low pulmonary compliance (e.g. asthma, COPD, etc.) requiring peak inspiratory pressure greater than 30 cm of H_2O, etc.

3. Ans. (c) 60%

[Ref. Anaesthesia for Postgraduates by Agasti, 1/e p75]

Delivery system	Flow rate (l/min)	FiO_2 (%)
Nasal cannula	2 4 6	25 30 40
Mask without reservoir	6 8	40 50
Mask with reservoir	4 6	40 50
Venturi mask	4 6 8 10 12	24 28 35 40 50

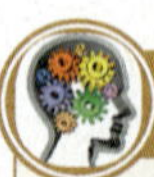

Also Remember

Venturi (Venti) Mask

- Delivers oxygen under pressure through various-sized orifices in the mask
- Entrains air into the mask at a specific ratio by passing oxygen through a calibrated opening under pressure
- Delivers oxygen 24–60%

4. Ans. (b) Tracheostomy

[Ref. Ajay Yadav, 4/e p108-109]

Airway Management for Cervical Spine Injury

- Oral intubation with neck stabilisation: Should be attempted first
- **Tracheostomy: Most suitable method**
- Temporary measures if tracheostomy not available:
  - Laryngeal mask airway
  - Combitube
  - Cricothyroidotomy

5. Ans. (b) 2nd and 3rd ring

[Ref. SRB's Surgical Operations by Bhat, 1/ep140]

Tracheostomy

- High tracheostomy: Above the level of isthmus
  - Can cause tracheal stenosis
  - Above 2nd tracheal ring
- Mid-tracheostomy: Ideal and commonly used
  - Through 2nd and 3rd rings behind isthmus
  - Approached by dividing thyroid isthmus
- Low tracheostomy: Below the isthmus level
  - Can cause torrential bleed which is difficult to control

6. Ans. (a) Airway maintenance

[Ref. Ajay Yadav, 4/e p40]

7. Ans. (d) Increased thyromental distance

[Ref. Ajay Yadav, 4/e p45]

- **Thyromental distance**: Distance between thyroid notch to mental prominence when the neck is fully extended
  - >6.5 cm: Normal
  - 6 to 6.5 cm: Difficult intubation
  - <6 cm: Laryngoscopy is impossible

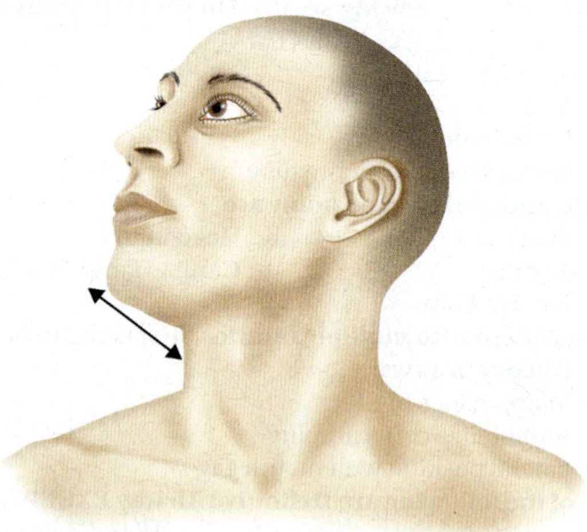

Fig. Thyromental (TM) distance

8. Ans. (c) Head-low and right side up

[Ref. Schwartz Principles of Surgery, 8th Ed., Pg 382]

- In cases of air embolism, positioning of patient's body: Trendelenburg's position
  - Head down, on left side down: lateral decubitus position
  - Lead to trapping of air in apex of ventricle and prevent it from reaching lung circulation

Anesthesiology

9. Ans. (a) Airway maintenance
[Ref. Ajay Yadav, 4/e p40]

10. Ans. (b) 2
[Ref. Pediatric Anesthesia by Bruno, 1/e p629]

LMA Sizes According to Weight

Mask size (Inflation volume)	Patients weight (Age)
1 (4 mL)	< 5kg (Neonates/Infants)
1.5 (7 mL)	5–10 kg (Infants)
2 (10 mL)	10–20 kg (Infants/Children)
2.5 (14 mL)	20–30 kg (Children)
3 (14 mL)	30–50 kg (Children/Small adults)
4 (30 mL)	50–70 kg (Adults)
5 (40 mL)	70–100 kg (Adults)
6	>100 kg (Adults)

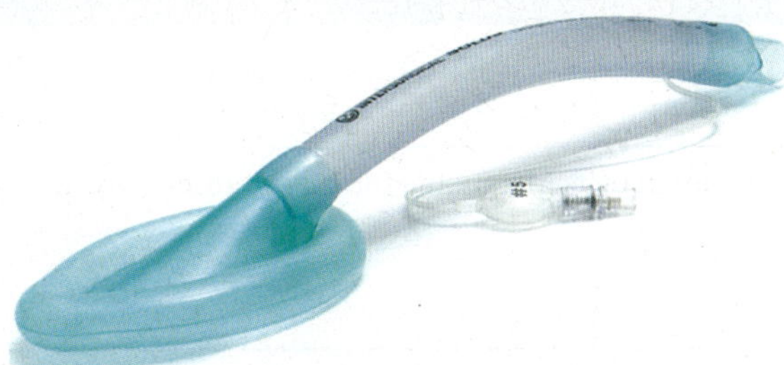

Fig. Laryngeal mask airway (LMA)

11. Ans. (d) ProSeal LMA
[Ref. Anesthesiology by Longnecker, 3/e p509]

ProSeal LMA

- Introduced in 2000, having double cuff, reinforced airway tube and an esophageal drainage tube offers several advantages over cLMA
- It forms a better seal than the cLMA without an increase in the mucosal pressure
- When correctly inserted and positioned the PLMA isolates the glottis from the upper esophagus thus protecting the lungs from possible aspiration making it useful for laparoscopic surgery too.
- PLMA is capable to protecting the airway in event of passive regurgitation intraoperatively by allowing the regurgitant fluid to pass up the drain tube and bypass the glottis

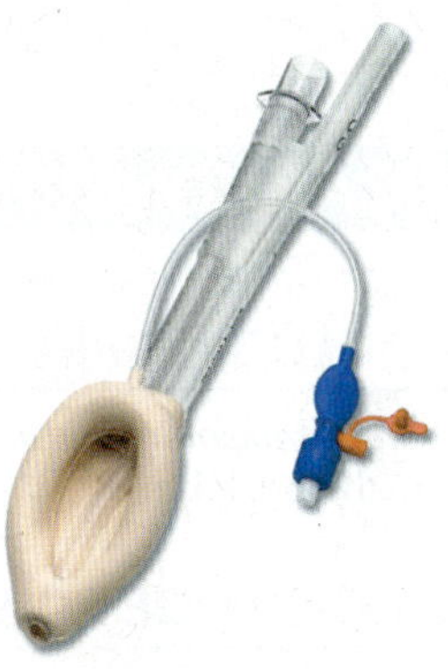

Fig. ProSeal LMA

HIGH YIELD MCQs ANSWERS WITH EXPLANATIONS 

1. Ans. (a) LMA; (b) Endotracheal tube; (d) Combitube
[Ref. Ajay Yadav, 4/e p40-41]

2. Ans. (a) Flail chest; (b) Head injury; (c) Tetanus; (e) Foreign body
[Ref. Ajay Yadav, 4/e p215]

3. Ans. (a) Patency of airways
[Ref. Ajay Yadav, 4/e p220]

Basic Life Support (Primary A, B, C, D)

- Airway management
- Breathing
- Circulation by cardiac massage
- Defibrillation by automatic external defibrillator

4. Ans. (c) Laryngeal mask airway
[Ref. Ajay Yadav, 4/e p40]

5. Ans. (a) Maintenance of airway
[Ref. Ajay Yadav, 4/e p40]

6. Ans. (d) In a patient with large tumour in the oral cavity
[Ref. Ajay Yadav, 4/e p40]

7. Ans. (d) Difficult airway; (e) Facilitate endotracheal intubation
[Ref. Ajay Yadav, 4/e p40]

8. Ans. (b) Intubation can be done; (c) Size 1 for neonates; (d) Size 3 for adults
[Ref. Ajay Yadav, 4/e p40; Miller's Anaesthesia, 7/e Chapter 50]

9. Ans. (d) Increased thyromental distance
[Ref. Ajay Yadav, 4/e p45]

10. Ans. (c) Insertion of laryngeal mask airway and fiberoptic bronchoscopy
[Ref. Pocket Anesthesia by Urman, 1/e p4-6]

Practical Approach to Unanticipated Airway Difficulty

- **Plan A**: Standard laryngoscopy with Blade of choice
  - If failure: Make another attempt with another sized blade
  - Make no more than 2 attempts
- **Plan B**: Direct laryngoscopy and Insertion of Bougie/Intubating catheter
- **Plan C**: Insertion of LMA with Fibro-optic assistance
- **Plan D**: Terminate anesthetic and Awaken the patient
  - Perform awake fibro-optic intubation
  - Perform surgical airway (Tracheostomy)

11. Ans. (c) 2.5
[Ref. Pediatric Anesthesia by Bruno, 1/e p629]

LMA Size according to Age

- <5 kg: Size 1
- 5–10 kg: Size 1.5
- 10–20 kg: Size 2
- 20–30 kg: Size 2.5
- >30 kg: Size 3
- Adult: Size 4
- Large adult: Size 5

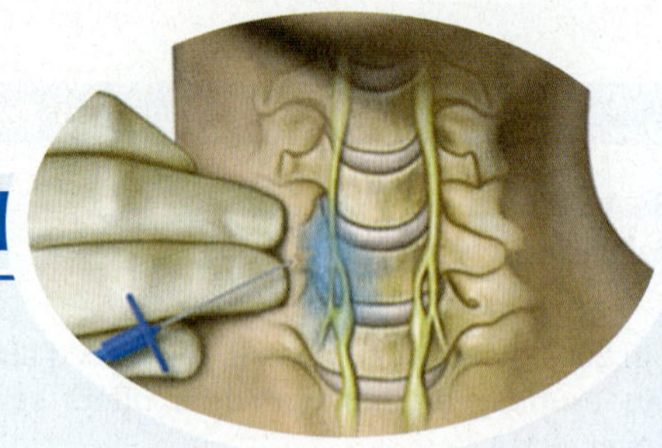

Chapter 16

Poisoning and Opioids in Anesthesia

THEORETICAL CONCEPTS

XVI A. METHEMOGLOBINEMIA

- *Prilocaine causes methemoglobinemia at higher doses (> 6 mg per kg)*: Accumulation of its metabolite (ortho-toulidine) which converts haemoglobin to methemoglobin[Q]

XVI B. CARBON MONOXIDE POISONING

- *Definition*: Carboxyhemoglobin > 20%[Q]
- *Treatment*: 100% oxygen or hyperbaric oxygen therapy[Q]

NEET/NBE PATTERN MCQs

1. **Which of the following agents cause methemoglobinemia?** *[Recent Question 2017, NBE FMGE March 2005]*
   a. Procaine b. Prilocaine
   c. Bupivacaine d. Cocaine
2. **Specific antagonist for benzodiazepines is** *[NBE DNB 1995]*
   a. Flumazenil b. Alprazolam
   c. Diisopropylphenol d. Cremopher EL
3. **Pure antagonist of morphine is** *[NBE DNB 1996]*
   a. Nalorphine
   b. Buprenorphine
   c. Naloxone
   d. Endorphine

HIGH YIELD MCQs

1. **Least sedative narcotic?** *[Recent Question 2016, AIIMS PGMEE 2009]*
   a. Morphine b. Codeine
   c. Papaverine d. Noscapine
2. **Best antagonist of morphine is** *[AIIMS PGMEE 1997]*
   a. Nalorphine b. Naloxone
   c. Buprenorphine d. Pentazocine
3. **Drug with Ceiling effect** *[All India PGMEE 1994]*
   a. Morphine b. Buprenorphine
   c. Fentanyl d. Alfentanil
4. **All are opioid agonist-antagonist compounds except** *[JIPMER PGMEE 2001, PGI 2002]*
   a. Buprenorphine b. Nalbuphine
   c. Pentazocine d. Nalmefene
   e. Papaverine
5. **In Belladonna poisoning antidote is** *[PGI 1997]*
   a. Physostigmine b. Neostigmine
   c. Anti histamine d. Atropine
6. **Atropine is used in following except** *[PGI 1997]*
   a. Glaucoma
   b. Mushroom poisoning
   c. Malathion poisoning
   d. Organophosphorus poisoning
7. **Bupivacaine toxicity treated with** *[PGI 2007]*
   a. Esmolol
   b. Epinephrine
   c. Lignocaine
   d. 5 percent dextrose
   e. Benzodiazepines
8. **True regarding morphine** *[PGI 2006]*
   a. Tolerance develops for all except miosis and constipation
   b. Tolerance to all effects develops with chronic usage
   c. Tolerance develops for all except euphoria and sedation
   d. Tolerance can develop to all effects in high doses

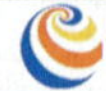 NEET/NBE PATTERN MCQs ANSWERS WITH EXPLANATIONS 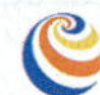

1. Ans. (b) Prilocaine
[Ref. Ajay Yadav, 4/e p123]

- **Prilocaine causes methemoglobinemia** at higher doses (> 6 mg per kg): Accumulation of its metabolite (ortho-touidine) which converts haemoglobin to methemoglobin

2. Ans. (a) Flumazenil
[Ref. Ajay Yadav, 4/e p85]

- Flumazenil is a competitive antagonist at BZ receptors
  - Antagonizes hypnosis, respiratory depression and sedation
  - Amnesia is minimally reversed

3. Ans. (c) Naloxone
[Ref. Ajay Yadav, 4/e p92]

- **Naloxone** is a pure opoid antagonist acting on all opoid receptors with maximum propensity for μ (mu) receptors
  - Reverses the actions of all opoids, with partial reversal of buprenorphine

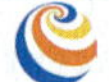 HIGH YIELD MCQs ANSWERS WITH EXPLANATIONS 

1. Ans. (c) Papaverine
[Ref. Katzung, 11/e p531]

2. Ans. (b) Naloxone
[Ref. Ajay Yadav, 4/e p92]

- Naloxone is a pure opioid antagonist acting on all opioid receptors with maximum propensity for μ receptors. It reverses the actions of all opioids, with partial reversal of buprenorphine.

3. Ans. (b) Buprenorphine
[Ref. Ajay Yadav, 4/e p92; Miller's Anaesthesia, 8/e p 904]

4. Ans. (d) Nalmefene; (e) Papaverine
[Ref. Ajay Yadav, 4/e p88]

- Based on Receptor interaction Opioids are classified as:

Pure Agonist	Agonist Antagonist	Pure Antagonist
• Morphine • Fentanyl • Alfentanil • Sufentanil • Remifentanil • Pethidine	• Pentazocine • Nalbuphine • Nalorphine • Butorphanol • Levallorphan • Dezocine • Meptazinol • Buprenorphine	• Naloxone • Naltrexone • Nalmefene • Diprenorphine • Methylnal-trexone

5. Ans. (a) Physostigmine
[Ref. Pharmacology & Toxicology by Yadav, 1/ep103]

6. Ans. (a) Glaucoma
[Ref. Clinical Ocular Pharmacology by Jimmy, 5/e p129]

- Systemically administered atropine may cause mydriasis and raise IOP in patients with open-angle glaucoma
- In acute or subacute narrow angle glaucoma, every form of atropine administration is contraindicated

7. Ans. (b) Epinephrine; (e) Benzodiazepines
[Ref. Morgans, 4/e p271]

8. Ans. (a) Tolerance develops for all except miosis and constipation
[Ref. Ajay Yadav, 4/e p90]

- **Tolerance** is seen to all actions of opioids except constipation and miosis and all tolerance is mainly pharmacodynamic.

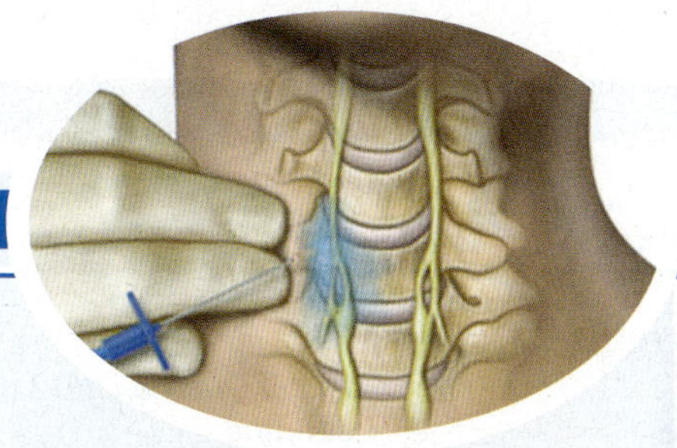

Chapter 17

Acute and Chronic Relief

THEORETICAL CONCEPTS

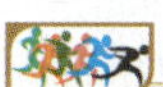

Topper's Edge

GLOSSARY—PAIN MANAGEMENT

- **Allodynia**[Q]: Perception of an ordinarily non-noxious stimulus as pain
- Analgesia: Absence of pain perception
- Anesthesia: Absence of all sensation
- Anesthesia dolorosa[Q]: Pain in an area that lacks sensation
- Dysesthesia: Unpleasant or abnormal sensation with or without a stimulus
- Hypalgesia (hypoalgesia): Diminished response to noxious stimulation (e.g. pinprick)
- Hyperalgesia: Increased response to noxious stimulation
- Hyperesthesi:a Increased response to mild stimulation
- Hyperpathia: Presence of hyperesthesia, allodynia, and hyperalgesia usually associated with overreaction, and persistence of the sensation after the stimulus
- Hypesthesia (hypoesthesia): Reduced cutaneous sensation (e.g. light touch, pressure, or temperature)
- Neuralgia: Pain in the distribution of a nerve or a group of nerves
- Paresthesia: Abnormal sensation perceived without an apparent stimulus
- Radiculopathy: Functional abnormality of one or more nerve roots

XVII A. LINGUAL NERVE BLOCK

- *Site for Lingual nerve block:* Near neck in ramus of mandible[Q]

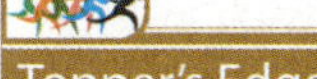

Topper's Edge

Patterns of Referred Pain (Location: Cutaneous Dermatome)

- Central diaphragm: C4
- Lungs: T2–T6
- Aorta: T1–L2
- Heart: T1–T4
- Esophagus: T3–T8
- Pancreas and spleen[Q]: T5–T10
- Stomach, liver, and gallbladder[Q]: T6–T9
- Adrenals: T8–L1
- Small intestine: T9–T11
- Colon: T10–L1
- Kidney, ovaries, and testes[Q]: T10–L1
- Ureters[Q]: T10–T12
- Uterus: T11–L2
- Bladder and prostate: S2–S4
- Urethra and rectum: S2–S4

NEET/NBE PATTERN MCQs

1. **Current mode of analgesia best for Intrapartum pain relief** *[Recent Question 2016]*
   a. Epidural analgesia b. Spinal anesthesia
   c. Inhalational d. Local analgesia
2. **Lingual nerve block is given in** *[NBE FMGE September 2005]*
   a. Upper molar b. Angle of mandible
   c. Base of mandible d. Neck of mandible
3. **During pain management or sedation, it is important to continuously monitor all of the following except** *[NBE DNB 2011]*
   a. Heart rate b. Oxygen saturation
   c. Respiratory rate d. Blood glucose
4. **The drug for OPD analgesia is** *[Recent Question 2012, 2017]*
   a. Morphine b. Pethidine
   c. Fentanyl d. Alfentanil
5. **Stellate ganglion block is characterized by following, except** *[Recent Question 2016, NBE DNB 1998]*
   a. Miosis b. Ptosis
   c. Flushing d. Sweating
6. **Transdermal patch for chronic pain contains which of the following opioid?** *[Recent Question 2017]*
   a. Fentanyl b. Morphine
   c. Pentazocine d. Alfentanil

HIGH YIELD MCQs

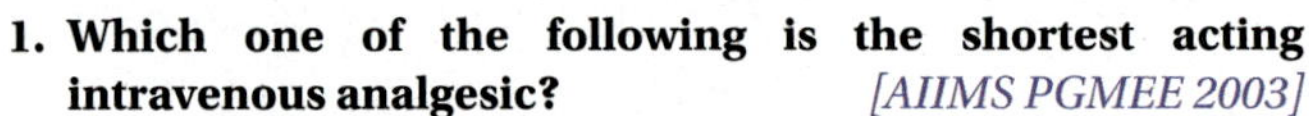

1. **Which one of the following is the shortest acting intravenous analgesic?** *[AIIMS PGMEE 2003]*
   a. Remifentanil b. Fentanyl
   c. Alfentanil d. Sufentanil
2. **Visual analogue scale (VAS) most widely used to measure** *[Recent Question 2016, Delhi PGMEE 2008]*
   a. Sleep b. Sedation
   c. Pain intensity d. Depth of anesthesia
3. **Best anaesthetic agent for out-patient anesthesia is** *[AIIMS PGMEE 1994]*
   a. Fentanyl b. Morphine
   c. Alfentanil d. Pethidine
4. **Following combination of agents are the most preferred for short day care surgeries** *[AIIMS PGMEE 2003]*
   a. Propofol, fentanyl, isoflurane
   b. Thiopentone sodium, morphine, halothane
   c. Ketamine, pethidine, halothane
   d. Propofol, morphine, halothane
5. **Narcotic of choice for out-patient anesthesia** *[AIIMS PGMEE 1994]*
   a. Morphine
   b. Alfentanil
   c. Fentanyl
   d. Pethidine

NEET/NBE PATTERN MCQs ANSWERS WITH EXPLANATIONS

1. Ans. (a) Epidural analgesia
[Ref. Anaesthesia by Colin, 3/e p81]

Advantages of Epidural Anesthesia in Labour

- Superior analgesia as compared to other methods
- Analgesia over prolonged periods of time
- Improves utero-placental perfusion
- Blunts hyperventilation-hypoventilation cycle
- Provides anesthesia for operative/instrumental delivery
- Low incidence of side effects
- Reduced need of General anesthesia for emergency CS

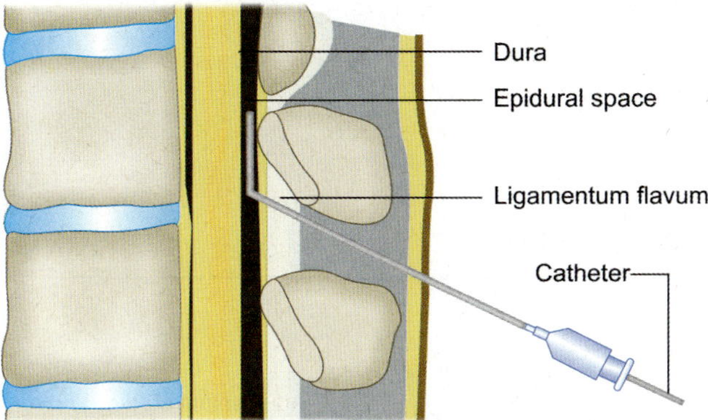

Fig. Epidural anesthesia

2. Ans. (d) Neck of mandible
[Ref. Neural blockade in Clinical Anaesthesia by Cousins and Bridenbough, 1/e p438]

- Site for Lingual nerve block: Near neck in ramus of mandible

3. Ans. (d) Blood glucose
[Ref. Ajay Yadav, 4/e. p49-55]

4. Ans. (d) Alfentanil
[Ref. Ajay Yadav, 4/e. p91]

- Alfentanil is twenty times more potent than morphine and superior to fentanyl because of rapid recovery and less chance of postoperative respiratory depression.

5. Ans. (d) Sweating
[Ref. Ajay Yadav, 4/e. p91]

Stellate Ganglion Block is characterized by

- Miosis
- Enophthalmos
- Ptosis
- Anhydrosis over the ipsilateral face and neck upto T3
- Absence of papillary dilatation on shading the eye
- Absence of ciliospinal reflex
- Flushing of face
- Conjunctival congestion
- Nasal stuffiness (guttman's sign)
- Injection of tympanic membrane (Mueller's syndrome)
- Increased skin temperature
- Lacrimation

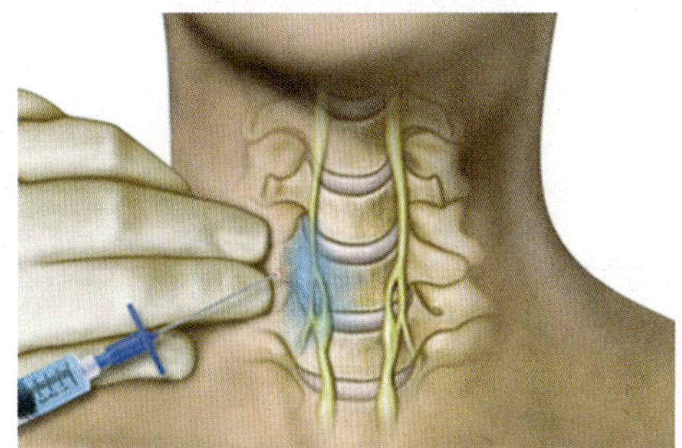

Fig. Stellate ganglion block

6. Ans. (a) Fentanyl
[Ref. Drug Delivery by Mitra, 1/e p294]

- Drugs used as transdermal patches: Buprenorphine, Capsaicin, Clonidine, Diclofenac, Estradiol, Estradiol levonorgestrel, Estradiol norethidrone acetate, Ethinyl estradiol norelgestromin, Fenatnyl, Granisetron, Lidocaine, Methylphenidate, Nicotine, Nitroglycerine, Oxybutynin, Rivastigmine, Selegiline, Scopalamine, Testosterone
- Fentanyl transdermal has the same properties as fentanyl citrate administered by IV, except in this formulation it is administered transdermally to produce pain relief and as an adjunct to other drugs in perioperative patients and in patients with chronic pain
- Fentanyl transdermal patch system delivers fentanyl through the skin at a constant rate to produce systemic effects

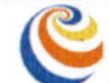

HIGH YIELD MCQs ANSWERS WITH EXPLANATIONS

1. Ans. (a) Remifentanil
[Ref. Ajay Yadav, 4/e. p91]

- Remifentanil is ultrashortacting
  - Duration 5–10 minutes

2. Ans. (c) Pain intensity
[Ref. Ajay Yadav, 4/e. p200]

Assessment of Pain

- Visual analogue scale
- McGill pain questionnaire (MPQ)
- Smiley scale or CHEOPS scale

3. Ans. (c) Alfentanil
[Ref. Ajay Yadav, 4/e p91]

4. Ans. (a) Propofol, fentanyl, isoflurane
[Ref. Ajay Yadav, 4/e p197]

5. Ans. (b) Alfentanil
[Ref. Ajay Yadav, 4/e. p91]

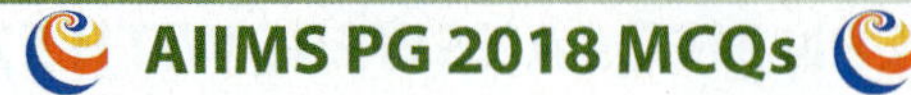

AIIMS PG 2018 MCQs

1. **Person intubated, abnormal flexion, eye opening on pain. GCS score is** *[AIIMS May 2018]*
   a. E3VntM3
   b. E2VntM3
   c. E2VtM4
   d. E3VtM4
2. **Spinal cord in Adult ends at ___ level** *[AIIMS May 2018]*
   a. T12
   b. L1
   c. L2
   d. L3
3. **Blood loss in Third degree hemorrhagic shock is** *[AIIMS May 2018]*
   a. <15%
   b. 15-30%
   c. 30-40%
   d. >40%
4. **Second phase of Damage Control is done at** *[AIIMS May 2018]*
   a. Emergency bay
   b. Operation theatre
   c. ICU
   d. Pre-hospital

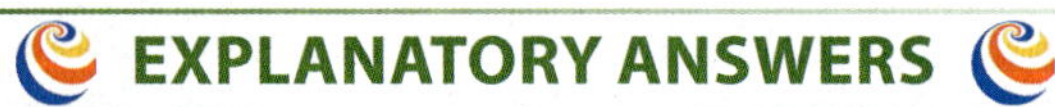

EXPLANATORY ANSWERS

1. Ans. (b) E2VntM3

[Ref. Bailey and Love, 25/e p301-302]

Glasgow coma scale (GCS)

- Definition: Neurological scale for 'assessment of conscious state' of a person

	Eye response	Verbal response	Motor response
Score 1	Do not open	No sounds	None
Score 2	To painful stimulus	Sounds only	Extension
Score 3	To verbal command	Inappropriate words	Abnormal flexion
Score 4	Spontaneously open	Confused	Withdrawal/ flexion
Score 5	-	Normal, oriented talk	Localises pain
Score 6	-	-	Obeys commands

- Tracheal intubation and severe facial/eye swelling or damage make it impossible to test the verbal and eye responses
- In these circumstances, the score is given as 1 with a modifier attached (e.g. "E1c", where "c" = closed, or "V1t" where t = tube); often the 1 is left out, so the scale reads Ec or Vt

2. Ans. (b) L1

[Ref. Gray's Clinical Neuroanatomy, 1/e p111]

- At birth spinal cord ends at the level of L3 vertebra (or sometime at lower border of L2 vertebra)
- In adult, it terminates at the level of lower border of L1 (or the intervertebral disc between the L1 and L2)

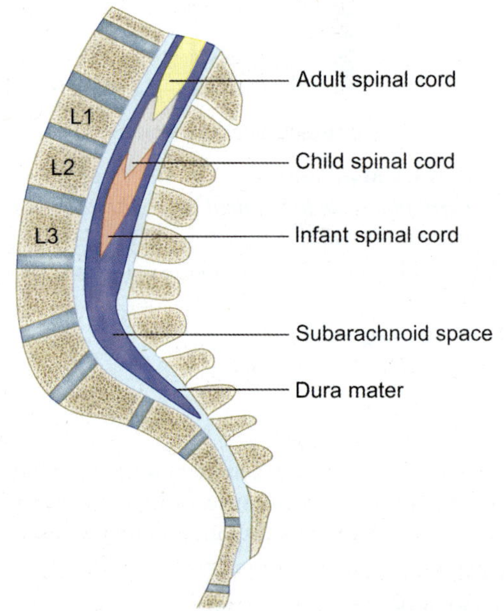

Fig. Termination of Spinal Cord

3. Ans. (c) 30-40%

[Ref. Trauma and Surgical Critical Care by Asensio, 1/e p64]

Classification of Hemorrhagic Shock

	Class 1	Class 2	Class 3	Class 4
Blood loss (%)	<15	15-30	30-40	>40
Blood loss (ml)	<750	750-1500	1500-2000	>2000
Systolic BP	Unchanged	Normal	Reduced	Very low
Diastolic BP	Unchanged	Raised	Reduced	Very low
Pulse	<100	>100	>120	>140

4. Ans. (b) **Operation theatre**

[Ref. Trauma Anesthesia by Smith, 2/e p330]

DAMAGE CONTROL RESUSCITATION (DCR) PROCESS

DCR is defined as a systemic approach to major trauma combining the <C>ABC (catastrophic bleeding, airway, breathing, circulation) paradigm with a series of clinical techniques from point of wounding to definitive treatment in order to minimise blood loss, maximise tissue oxygenation and optimise outcome

- **Phase 1: Rapid transfer to hospital**
  - Stop hemorrhage rather than over-resuscitate
  - Inform OT/ Anaesthetist/ Blood bank
  - Prevent hypothermia
  - ABG analysis
  - Rapid transfer to OT
- **Phase 2: Operating room (warmed)**
  - Prevent hypothermia
  - Control hemorrhage and contamination
  - Intra-abdominal packing, VAC pack dressing
  - Rapid temporary abdominal closure
  - Talk to anesthetist
  - Handover to Intensivist
- **Phase 3: Resuscitation in ICU**
  - Rewarming
  - Reverse coagulopathy
  - Optimize Ventilation and Perfusion
  - Correct acidosis and blood volume
- **Phase 4: Return to Operating room**
  - If major blood loss continues
  - For washout and further debridement
  - Planned second look after 12-48 hours post-stabilisation
  - Definitive surgery

Note

Radiodiagnosis and Radiotherapy

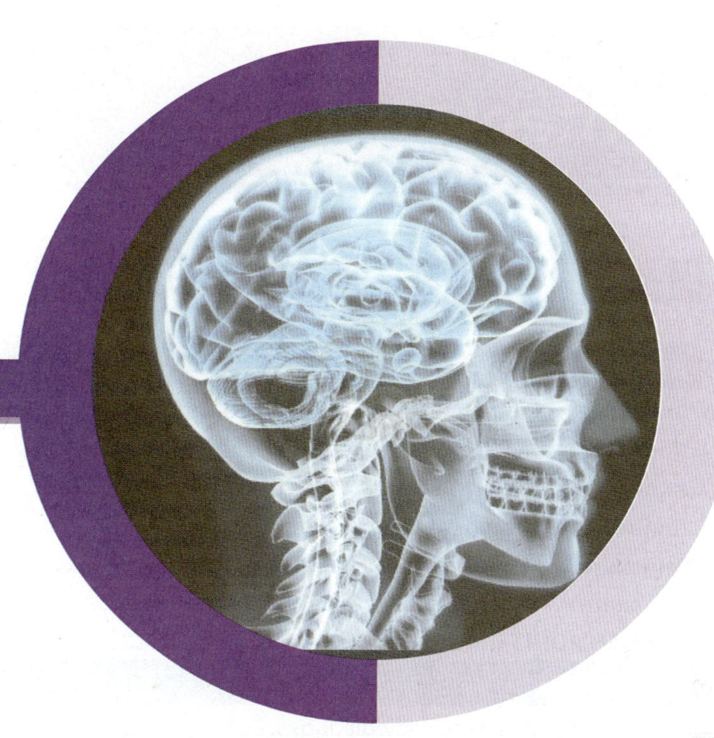

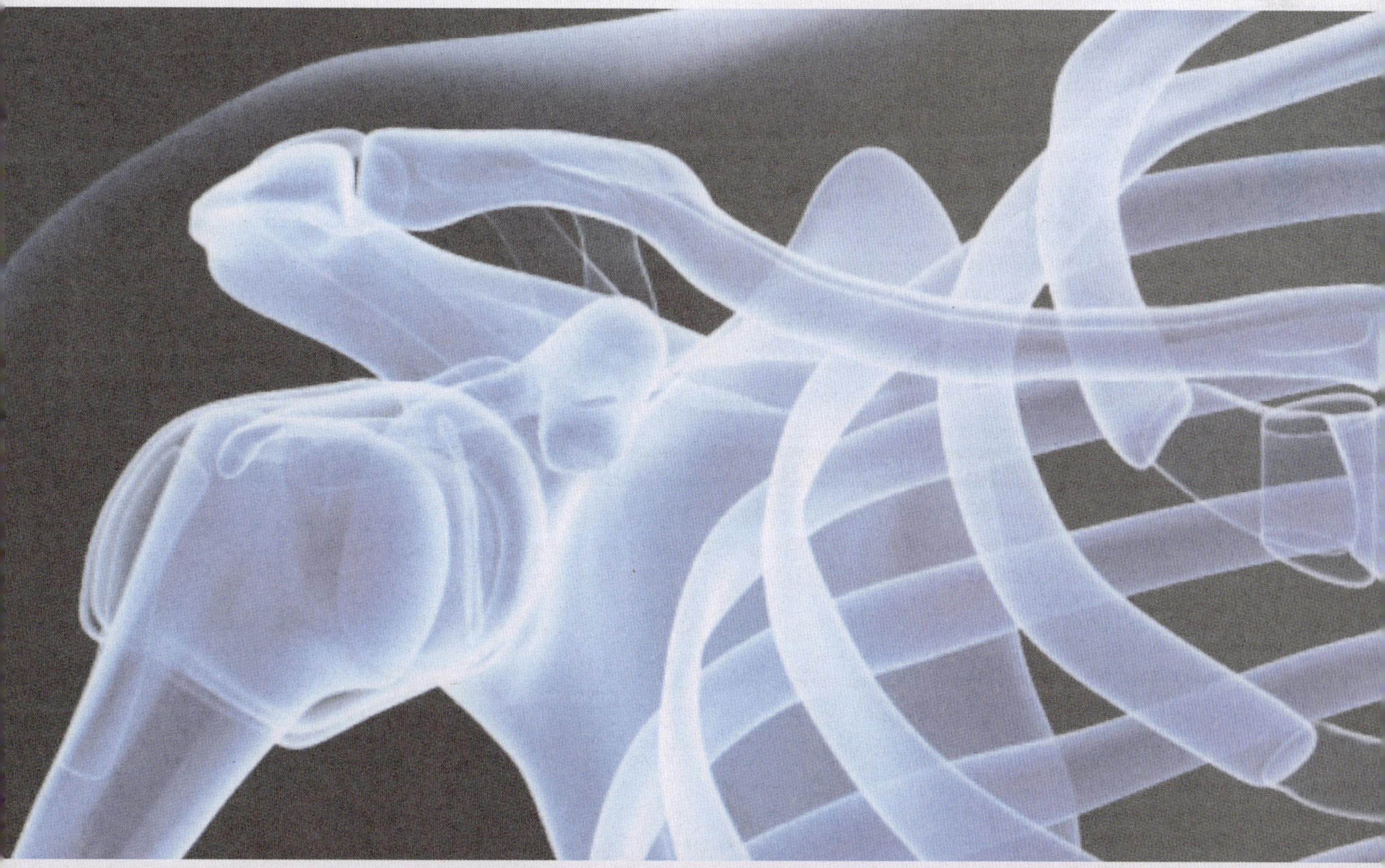

Contents

Radiodiagnosis and Radiotherapy

ANNEXURES

CHAPTERS

EACH CHAPTER DIVIDED INTO FOLLOWING SECTIONS

Theoretical Concepts (Including Images)
Image-Based Questions
Answers with Explanations of IBQs
NEET/NBE Pattern MCQs
High Yield MCQs
NEET/NBE Pattern MCQs Answers with Explanations
High Yield MCQs Answers with Explanations
AIIMS PG 2018 MCQs with Explanatory Answers

Annexures

ANNEXURE 1. SIGNS/APPEARANCES IN RADIODIAGNOSIS

Sign	Diagnosis
Air crescent sign	Aspergilloma/Hydatid cyst/Tumor in cavity/Pus in cavity
Antral pad sign	Carcinoma head of pancreas
Apple-core (Napkin-ring) sign (Bowel)	Colorectal carcinoma
Apple-core sign (Femur)	Synovial chondramatosis
Aneurysmal sign in spine	TB spine (anterior type)
Banana sign (Foetal posterior fossa)	Chiari II malformation
Bare orbit sign	Neurofibromatosis/Meningioma/Metastasis
Bat wing appearance (CxR)	Pulmonary oedema
Beheaded Scottish terrier sign	Spondylolisthesis
Bird-beak (Rat-tail) sign	Achalasia
Bird-of-prey sign	Sigmoid volvulus
Bulging fissure sign	Klebsiella pneumonia
Chain-of-lakes appearance (ERCP)	Chronic pancreatitis
Champagne pelvis	Achondroplasia
Clusters of Grapes appearance	Cystic bronchiectasis
Cobra-head/Adder-head (Spring-onion) sign	Ureterocoele
Coffee bean (Bent inner tube) sign	Sigmoid volvulus
Coiled spring appearance	Intussusception/Intramural duodenal hematoma
Continuous diaphragm sign	Pneumomediastinum (Air below pericardium)
Copper beaten appearance (Skull)	Raised intracranial tension
Cor-en-sabot/Boot shaped heart	Tetralogy of Fallot
Cottage loaf sign	Right sided diaphragmatic rupture with herniated liver
Cotton wool appearance (Skull)	Pagets disease of bone
Crazy pavement appearance	Alveolar proteinoses
CT angiogram sign	Bronchoalveolar carcinoma/Lymphoma/Pneumonias
Dagger sign	Ankylosing spondylitis
Deep sulcus sign (CxR)	Pneumothorax
Double bubble appearance	Annular pancreas
Double target sign	Intussusception
Driven snow appearance	Pindborg tumour
Egg-on-side appearance	Transposition of Great Arteries (Uncorrected TGA)
Figure-of-3 appearance of aortic knuckle	Coarctation of aorta
Figure-of-8/Snowman appearance	Total anomalous pulmonary venous drainage (TAPVC)
Finger-in-glove (Rabbit ear) sign (CxR)	Allergic bronchopulmonary aspergillosis (ABPA)
Frostberg Inverted-3 sign	Periampullary carcinoma pancreas

Contd...

Contd...

Sign	Diagnosis
Golden-S sign (CxR)	Bronchogenic carcinoma
Hair-on-end (Crew-cut) appearance	Thalassemia
Halo sign (CT scan)	Hemorrhagic pulmonary modules/Early invasive aspergillosis
Hampton's hump (CxR)	Pulmonary infarction/Pulmonary embolism
Hilar dance sign (Fluoroscopy)	Atrial septal defect (ASD)
Inverted Napoleon Hat Sign	Spondylolisthesis
Kidney bean sign	Caecal volvulus
Licked candy stick appearance	Psoriatic arthropathy/Leprosy/Rheumatoid arthritis/Neuropathic joints
Linguine sign	Intracapsular rupture of breast implant
Medusa-head appearance (CxR)	Ascariasis
Metacarpal (Archibald) sign	Turner's syndrome/Pseudohypoparathyroidism
Money-bag/Leather-bottle/Flask-shaped heart	Pericardial effusion
Onion-peel appearance	Ewing's sarcoma
Palla's sign (CxR)	Pulmonary embolism
Pencil-in-cup appearance	Psoriatic arthropathy
Polka-dot appearance (CT)	Hemangioma bone
Popcorn calcification	Pulmonary hamartoma
Pruned tree appearance	Pulmonary arterial hypertension (PAH)
Rim sign (Nephrogram)	Hydronephrosis (Severe) of kidneys
Rugger jersey spine appearance	Osteopetrosis/Renal osteodystrophy
Sagging rope sign	Perthe's disease
Salt and pepper appearance (Skull)	Hyperparathyroidism
Scottish terrier sign	Spondylolysis
Shepherd Crook deformity	Fibrous dysplasia
Sitting duck appearance	Normal jugular foramen
Snow-storm appearance (USG)	Hydatiform mole
Soap- bubble appearance	Osteoclastoma
Spinnaker sail sign	Pneumomediastinum (Air around thymus)
String-of-pearls (Beads) sign	Small bowel obstruction
String sign	Ileocaecal TB/Hypertrophic pyloric stenosis
String sign of Kantor	Crohn's disease
Sun-ray (Sun-burst) appearance	Osteosarcoma
Tag antlers' sign	Valvular heart disease
Tonguing of vertebra	Morquio-Brails disease
Tree-in-bud sign (CT)	Endobronchial TB
Trethowan's sign	Slipped capital femoral epiphysis
Trident hand	Achondroplasia
Water bottle sign	Pericardial effusion (large)
Water lily (Camalote) sign	Hydatid lung (Echinococcus)
Wave sign of Mulvey	Ribs-indentations on normal thymus
Westermark sign (CxR)	Pulmonary embolism
White pyramid sign	Medullary pyramids of normal kidney
Wimberger sign	Scurvy

ANNEXURE 2. RADIOLOGICAL INVESTIGATIONS OF CHOICE

Condition	Investigation of choice
Acute cholecystitis	Tc99 HIDA scan
Acute pancreatitis	Contrast enhanced CT scan
Acute subarachnoid hemorrhage (<48 hours)	CT scan
Asbestosis (Pleural plaques)	HRCT scan
Aortic dissection	MRI
Blunt trauma of abdomen	Diagnostic peritoneal lavage (DPL)
Bone density	DEXA scan
Bony metastasis (Except spine)	Bone scan
Bony metastasis (Spine)	MRI
Brain tumours	Contrast enhanced MRI
Breast implant evaluation	MRI
Bronchiectasis	HRCT scan
Bronchogenic carcinoma	CT scan
Bronchogenic carcinoma (Anterior chest wall involvement/Hilar LAP)	MRI
Chronic pancreatitis	ERCP
Chronic Subarachnoid hemorrhage (>48 hours)	MRI
Common bile duct stones	USG (Initial IOC)
Constrictive pericarditis	MRI (Echocardiography initial IOC)
Early TB of kidney	Intravenous pyelography (IVP)
Fallopian tube patency (Gold standard)	Laparoscopic chromotubation
Gallbladder pathology	USG
Gallbladder pathology (Acute cholecystitis)	Tc99 HIDA scan
Intra-abdominal mass in children	USG (Screening IOC)
Jaundice	USG (Initial IOC)
Lung imaging	CT scan
Lung imaging (Pancoast tumour/Superior sulcus tumour)	MRI
Lung Imaging (Posterior mediastinal mass)	MRI
Multiple sclerosis	MRI
Pancreatic imaging	CT scan
Pericardial effusion	Echocardiography
Perthes disease	MRI
Posterior fossa lesions	MRI
Pregnancy dating	USG
Pregnancy with upper abdominal mass	MRI
Renovascular hypertension (Screening)	Captopril DTPA scan
Renovascular hypertension (Gold standard)	Angiography
Sequestration of lung	Aortography
Small acoustic neuroma	High resolution MRI
Spinal cord tumour	MRI (Initial IOC)
Traumatic paraplegia	MRI
Uteteric colic/Flank pain	Spiral CT scan
Vestibular schwannoma	Gadolinium enhanced MRI

ANNEXURE 3. FAMOUS SCIENTISTS & RADIOLOGISTS

Scientist/Radiologist	Contribution/Remark
Antoine Henri Bacquerel	Radioactivity
Arthur Holly Compton	Compton effect
Charles Dotter	Image guided medical procedures; Father of Interventional Radiology
David E Kuhl	Positron Emission Tomography (PET)
Edmund Kells	Father of Dental Radiology
Enrico Fermi	Nobel Prize in Physics for work on Induced radioactivity
Ernest Lawrence	Cyclotron
Ernest Rutherford	Alpha/beta particles, neutrons; Father of Nuclear Physics
FJ Curie & IJ Curie	Radioactive isotopes (Radionuclides)
Gioacchino Failla	Work on radiation as a s cause of cancer and genetic mutation
Glenn T Seaborg	Ten Transuranium elements
Godfrey Hounsfield	Computed Tomography (CT) scan
Hermann Mueller	Father of Radiation Genetics
Ian Donald	Ultrasonography (USG); Father of Obstetric Ultrasound
James Chadwick	Discovery of neutron; Nobel prize in Physics
JJ Thomson	Electron; Mass spectrometer
John Caffey	Father of Pediatric Radiology
John Lawrence	Used Phosphorus-32 to treat Leukemia
Lauterbur & Mansfield	MRI (Nobel Prize in Medicine)
Niels Bohr	Bohr's effect
Otto Hahn	Nuclear Fission (Nobel Prize in Chemistry), Father of Nuclear Chemistry
Raymond Vahan Damadian	Magnetic Resonance Imaging (MRI)
Thomas Alva Edison	Fluoroscope (Vitascope)
Victor F Hess	Cosmic rays
Wilhelm Roentgen	X-rays (Nobel Prize in Physics); Father of Diagnostic Radiology
William David Coolidge	Ductile Tungsten

ANNEXURE 4. RECOMMENDED VIEWS IN RADIOLOGY

Condition	Recommended view
Acetabular fracture	Judet view
Ankle injuries	Mortise view
Congenital dislocation of hip	Von Rosen view
Head trauma	Lateral view skull (Horizontal beam)
Intervertebral foramina (Cervical)	Oblique view
Left atrial enlargement (Barium)	Right anterior oblique
Lung (Left)	Right anterior oblique
Lung (Right)	Left anterior oblique
Lung (Interlobar fissure effusion)	Lordotic view
Lung (Middle lobe pathology)	Lordotic view
Ocular orbit	Caldwell view
Optic canal	Rheese view
Paranasal sinus	Water's view
Patella femoral dysplasia	Sunset view
Patellofemoral articulation	Skyline view
Petrous bone	Townes/Stenvers view
Pituitary gland	Lateral view (Coned down)
Pleural effusion (Minimal)	Lateral decubitus (Same side)
Pneumothorax	PA view on expiration
Recurrent shoulder dislocation	Stryker's view
Sacroiliac joints	Oblique view
Scaphoid fracture	Oblique view of wrist
Subchondral erosions	Ball Catcher's view

ANNEXURE 5. HALF-LIVES OF RADIOACTIVE ISOTOPES

Substance	Half-life
Iodine-132	2.3 hours
Technetium-99	6 hours
Iodine-123	13 hours
Gold-198	2.7 days
Gallium-67	3.3 days
Iodine-131	8 days
Phosphorus-32	14.3 days
Iodine-125	59 days
Iridium-192	74 days
Cobalt-60	5.3 years
Strontium-90	29.1 years
Caesium-137	30 years
Radium-226	1600 years
Uranium-238	4.5 billion years

ANNEXURE 6. RADIOSENSITIVITY AND CHEMOSENSITIVITY

Radiosensitivity of body tissues	
Extremely radiosensitive • Bone marrow • Lymphoid tissues • Testes • Ovaries • Intestines	**Highly radiosensitive** • Skin • Cornea • Oral cavity, oesophagus • Rectum • Bladder, ureters • Vagina, uterine cervix
Moderately radiosensitive • Optic lens • Stomach • Growing cartilage/Bone • Fine vasculature	**Low radiosensitive** • Mature cartilage/bones • Salivary glands • Respiratory organs • Kidneys, adrenal, pancreas, liver • Thyroid, pituitary gland
Least radiosensitive • Muscle • Brain, spinal cord	
Radiosensitivity of tumours	
Highly radiosensitive • Lymphoma • Seminoma • Myeloma • Ewing's sarcoma • Wilm's tumour	**Moderately radiosensitive** • Small cell cancer lungs • Breast cancer • Basal cell carcinoma • Medulloblastoma • Teratoma • Ovarian cancer (Most: Dysgerminoma)
Relatively radioresistant • Squamous cell carcinoma lung • Hypernephroma • Rectal carcinoma • Bladder carcinoma • Soft tissue sarcoma • Soft tissue sarcoma • Cervical cancer	**Extremely radioresistant** • Melanoma • Osteosarcoma • Pancreatic carcinoma
Chemosensitivity of tumours	
Highly chemosensitive • Teratoma testis • Hodgkin's disease • Non-Hodgkin's disease (High grade) • Wilm's tumour • Choriocarcinoma • Acute lymphoblastic leukemia (ALL) • Ewing's sarcoma	**Moderately chemosensitive** • Ovarian cancer • Small cell carcinoma lungs • Non-Hodgkin's disease (Low grade) • Breast carcinoma • Myeloma • Acute myeloid leukemia (AML)
Relatively insensitive • Gastric carcinoma • Bladder carcinoma • Squamous cell carcinoma (Head, neck) • Soft tissue sarcoma • Cervical carcinoma	**Extremely resistant** • Melanoma • Squamous cell carcinoma lungs • Large bowel carcinoma

Golden Points

'Air crescent' sign on chest radiograph is seen in	Aspergilloma
'Figure of eight' of heart on skiagram	Total anomalous PV drainage
'Figure of 3' appearance of aortic knuckle	Coarctation of aorta
Hallmark feature of osteomalacia	Looser's zones/Pseudofractures
Earliest radiological change in thalassemia	Widening of short bones of hands
'Hair-on-end/Crew-cut/ Hair-brush' appearance is seen in	Thalassemia
Most characteristic radiologic finding in leukaemia	Metaphyseal translucencies
Golden-S/Reverse-S sign is characteristic of	Bronchogenic carcinoma
Right border of heart on chest X-ray is formed by	Right atrium, SVC, IVC
Wimberger's sign is found in	Scurvy
Earliest radiological change in rickets	Loss of provisional calcification zone
'Double-bubble' sign is characteristic of	Duodenal atresia
Radiological diagnosis of multiple sclerosis can be done by	MRI
Sentinel loops on X-ray are seen in	Acute pancreatitis
MC cause of pancreatic calcification	Chronic alcoholic pancreatitis
Gold standard test for pulmonary embolism	Pulmonary angiography
MC type of Langerhan's cells histiocytoma	Eosinophilic granuloma
'Rain-drop' multiple lytic lesions in skull is seen in	Letterer-Siwe disease
Diagnostic feature of hamartoma lung on chest X-ray is	Irregular calcification
Most common finding of Coccidioidomycosis on chest X-ray is	Parenchymal consolidation
White line of Frankel is generally seen in	Scurvy
Maximum permissible radiation exposure per person per year	5 rem
Best diagnostic test for best disease is	Electrooculography
Sun-ray appearance, Codman triangle in bone are seen in	Osteosarcoma
Onion-peel appearance in bones is seen in	Ewing's sarcoma
Tram-track appearance in skull radiograph is seen in	Sturge-weber syndrome
Cotton wool appearance in skull radiograph is seen in	Paget's disease of bone
Investigation of choice in traumatic paraplegia is	MRI
Most radiosensitive tissue of body	Bone marrow
Most radiosensitive blood cell of body	Lymphocyte
Most radiosensitive organ of body	Skin
Cells are most radiosensitive in	G2-M interphase
Most common malignant bone tumour post-irradiation	Osteosarcoma
'Crescent sign' on Intravenous urogram/pyelogram	Hydronephrosis
'Double barrel' sign on ultrasonography is seen in	Obstructive jaundice
'Saw-tooth' appearance is characteristic of	Diverticulosis
'Carman Meniscus sign' is seen in	Malignant gastric ulcer

Contd...

Contd...

'Thumb-printing sign' is seen in	Ischaemic colitis
'Chain of lakes' appearance on ERCP	Chronic pancreatitis
Best investigation for pleural effusion	USG
Best X-ray view for minimal pleural effusion	Lateral decubitus view
Investigation of choice for bronchiectasis	High resolution CT
Earliest congenital anomaly detectable on fetal USG	Anencephaly
'Snow-storm' appearance on obstetrical USG	Hydatiform mole
Investigation of choice for hydatid disease is	CT scan
Most useful investigation for lung sequestration is	Radionuclide angiography
'Water-lily' sign is seen in	Hydatid disease
'Westermark' sign is seen in	Pulmonary embolism
Pop-corn calcification is seen in	Pulmonary hamartoma
Box-shaped heart is found in	Ebstein's anomaly
Money-bag/Leather-bottle/Flask-shaped heart is seen in	Pericardial effusion
'Boot-shaped heart' or *'Cor-en sabot heart' is seen in*	Tetralogy of Fallot
'Egg-on-side' appearance is seen in	Transposition of great arteries (TGA)
Investigation of choice for most gallbladder pathologies	USG
Carman's meniscus sign is seen in	Malignant gastric ulcer
'String sign' in ileocaecal junction indicates	Tuberculosis
Pipe-stem colon is seen in	Ulcerative colitis
String sign of Kantor is found in	Crohn's disease
'Coiled spring' appearance is seen in	Intussusception
Investigation of choice for acute pancreatitis	CECT
Thimble bladder is seen in	Renal tuberculosis
'Golf-hole' ureters (on sigmoidoscopy) is seen in	Renal tuberculosis
'Cork-screw' oesophagus is seen in	Diffuse oesophageal spasm
Frostberg inverted 3 sign is seen in	Periampullary carcinoma pancreas
First investigation of choice in post-term pregnancy	USG
Champagne glass pelvis is seen in	Achondroplasia
'Punched-out lesions' in bones is seen in	Multiple myeloma
Pepper-pot skull is seen in	Multiple myeloma
Looser's zones/Pseudofractures are seen in	Osteomalacia
Rugger-jersey spine is seen in	Osteopetrosis
X-rays were discovered by	WC Roentgen
'Hair-on-end/ Crew-cut/ Hair-brush appearance' is seen in	Thalassemia
Cells are most radiosensitive in	G2-M interphase
Most sensitive and specific screening test for breast ca	Mammography
Maximum permissible radiation exposure per person per year	5 rem
Intracavitary radiotherapy in Ca-cervix is done by	Iridium-192
Most commonly used radio-isotope in imaging	Tecnetium-99

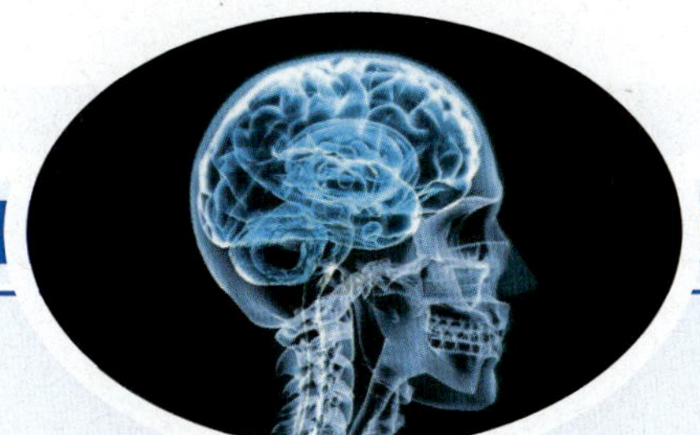

Chapter 1

Basic Concepts of Radiodiagnosis

THEORETICAL CONCEPTS

I A. IMPORTANT DISCOVERIES IN RADIOLOGY

Discovery	Scientist
X-rays[Q]	**WC Roentgen**
Computed tomography (CT)[Q]	**Godfrey Hounsfield**
Doppler	Christian Johann Doppler
Magnetic resonance imaging (MRI)	**Lauterbur & Mansfield**
SPECT, PET	Kuhl
Radioactivity[Q]	**Bacquerel**

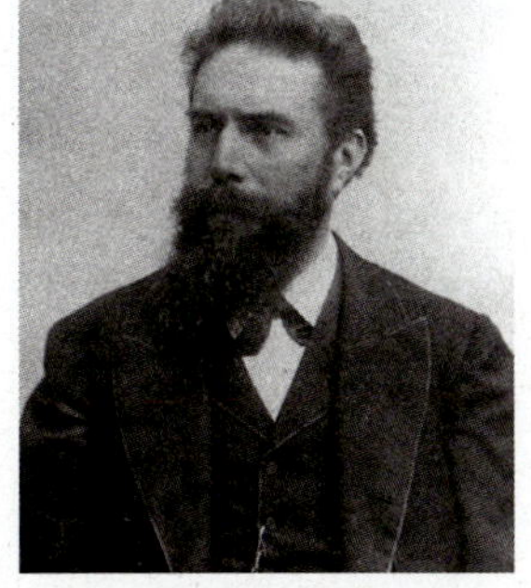

WC Roentgen

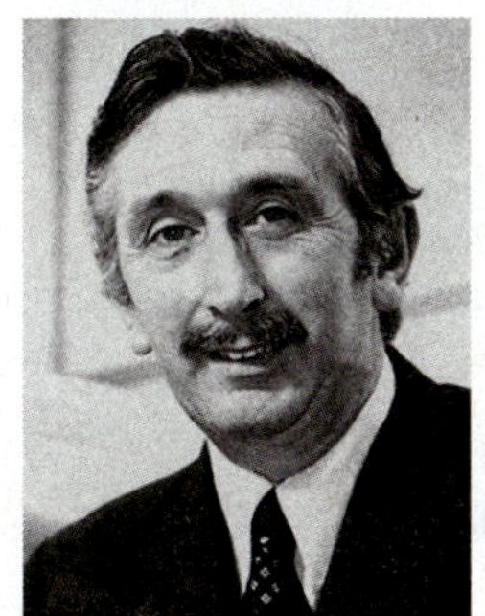

Godfrey N Hounsfield

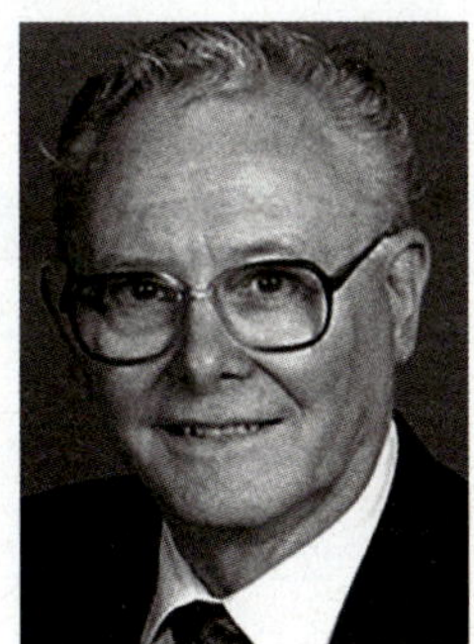

Peter Mansfield

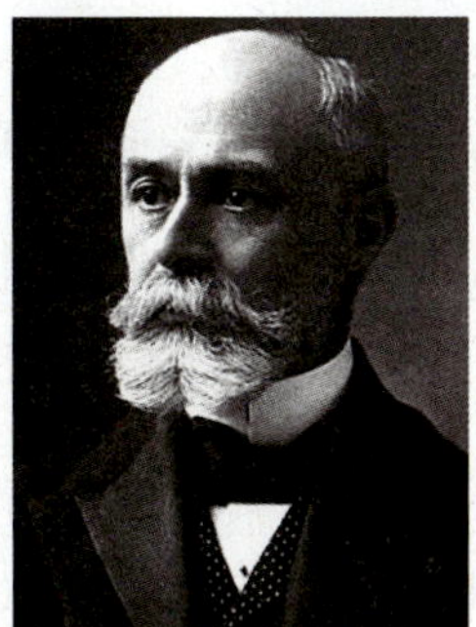

Antoine Henri Becquerel

Topper's Edge

Nobel Prize in Physics for Radiology

- **WC Roentgen (1901)**: Discovery of Roentgen rays (X-rays)[Q]
- **AH Bacquerel (1903)**: Discovery of spontaneous radioactivity[Q]
- Curie & Curie (1903): Joint researches on radiation phenomena[Q]
- Max Von Laue (1914): Discovery of diffraction of X-rays in crystals
- Compton (1927): Scattering of X-rays by electrons
- CV Raman (1930): Work on scattering of light and Raman effect[Q]
- Chadwick (1935): Discovery of Neutron[Q]
- Anderson (1936): Discovery of Positron
- Cormack and Hounsfield (1979): Computed axial tomography
- Siegbahn (1981): Development of high resolution electron spectroscopy

I B. UNITS POTENCY OF RADIATION[Q]

- **Roentgen**: Unit of exposure/radiation absorbed
- Coulomb per kg: New unit for exposure/radiation absorbed
- **Rem**: Unit of equivalent dose
- **Sievert** (Sv): New unit of equivalent dose (1 Sv = 100 rem)
- **Rad**: Product of absorbed dose and modifying factors (potential danger to health)
- **Gray** (Gy): Unit of absorbed dose (1 Gray = 100 rad)

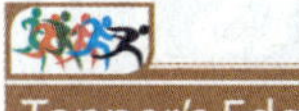

Topper's Edge

UNITS POTENCY OF RADIATION

- **Roentgen (R)** is a measure of exposure to X-ray or gamma ray radiation[Q]:
  - One roentgen is that amount of X-ray or gamma radiation that will deposit enough energy to strip about two billion electrons from their orbits (called one electrostatic unit) in one cubic centimeter of dry air
  - Roentgen technically applies only to ionization in dry air from X-ray or gamma radiation and does not apply to damage to body tissues
- **RAD (Radiation Absorbed Dose)** is a measure of the absorbed dose (energy deposited) in a material[Q]:
  - One RAD is the deposition of one hundred ergs of energy in one gram of any material (NRC regulations use per gram of body tissue) due to the ionization from any type of radiation
- **REM** is based on the biological damage caused by ionization in human body tissue[Q]:
  - It is a term for dose equivalence and equals the biological damage that would be caused by one RAD of dose
  - For Gamma and X-rays: 1 Roentgen = 1 RAD = 1 REM
- **Energy Deposition and Damage[Q]**:

Energy deposition	"Damage"
1 RAD Gamma	= 1 REM
1 RAD Beta	= 1 REM
1 RAD Neutron	= 10 REM
1 RAD Alpha	= 20 REM
REM = RAD × Quality factor	

- **International System of Units (SI)[Q]**:

Special units	SI units
Curie	Becquerel
RAD	Gray
REM	Sievert
Roentgen	Coulomb

Units Conversions

- 1 Curie = 3.7×10^{10} disintegrations/second[Q]
- 1 Becquerel = 1 disintegration/second
- 1 Becquerel = 2.7×10^{-11} Curie
- **1 RAD = 0.01 Gray**
- **1 Gray = 100 RADs[Q]**
- **1 REM = 0.01 Sievert[Q]**
- **1 Sievert = 100 REM**

I C. ROUTES FOR INVASIVE RADIOLOGICAL TECHNIQUES

- *Cerebral angiography*:[Q] **Transfemoral route** (*Seldinger technique*; Catheter introduced thorough a major vessel, threaded through circulatory system and dye injected into carotid artery)
- *Conventional 4-vessel angiography*: 2 internal carotids and 1 vertebral (fourth vessel fills by reflux)
- *Lymphangiography*: First web space of foot
- *Phlebography*: Dorsal metatarsal vein

I D. X-RAYS

I D1. X-rays Production

- *X-ray tube*: Cathode **(tungsten)** and Anode
- *Process*: Thermoionic emission (Electron beam from Tungsten cathode strike anode)[Q]

I D2. Factors in X-rays

- *Exposure factors*:
  - **KVP**: Determines beam penetration[Q]
    - **MAS**: Determines film blackening[Q]
- *Contrast factors*: Influenced by KVP
- *Body related factors*: Obese patients require higher KVP

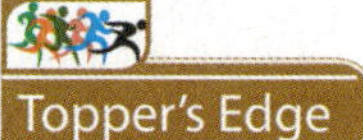

Topper's Edge

X-Rays

- Discovered by[Q]: **WC Roentgen** (Nobel Prize 1901[Q])
- Properties of X-rays:
  - **Wavelength: 0.1–1.0 Angstrom[Q]**
  - Electromagnetic radiation
  - Frequency: 30 petahertz to 30 exahertz
  - Energy: 100 eV to 100 KeV
  - Ionizing radiation: X-ray photons carry enough energy to ionize atoms and disrupt molecular bonds
- Used in medical radiography: Hard X-rays can traverse relatively thick objects without being much absorbed or scattered
- Types of X-rays:
  - Hard X-rays: Higher energy
  - Soft X-rays: Lower energy
- **X-rays interact with matter in three main ways[Q]:**
  - **Photoelectric absorption**
  - **Compton scattering**
  - **Rayleigh scattering**
- Production of X-rays[Q]: Occur when charged particles of sufficient energy hit a material
  - Production by electrons
  - Production by fast positive ions (Protons)

X-Rays Production

- Process of X-rays production:
  - Thermoionic emission
  - X-rays are produced when electron beams produced from cathode **(Tungsten filament)** strikes the anode[Q]
- X-ray tubes:
  - Conventional X-ray tube[Q]: Glass window and **aluminum filter**
  - Mammography tube[Q]: Molybdenum target, **molybdenum filter**, beryllium window
- Exposure factors:
  - kVP (Kilovolt peak): Determines beam penetration[Q]
  - mAS (Milliampere second): Determines amount of film blackening[Q]
- Intensifying screen:
  - Principle: Phosphorescence
  - Material: Calcium tungstate
- Other components:
  - Filter: Aluminum or aluminum-copper combination
  - Grid with radiolucent material: Absorb scatter radiation, improves contrast
  - Collimators and Cones: Restrict field size, decreases scatter radiation
  - Safe light used in dark rooms: Red light with 15 watt illumination[Q]
- X-ray films:
  - **Emulsion**[Q]: Silver halide (Photosensitive material)
  - **Development**: Hydroquinone + Metol/Phenindione
  - **Fixer**[Q]: Hypo Sodium thiosulfate

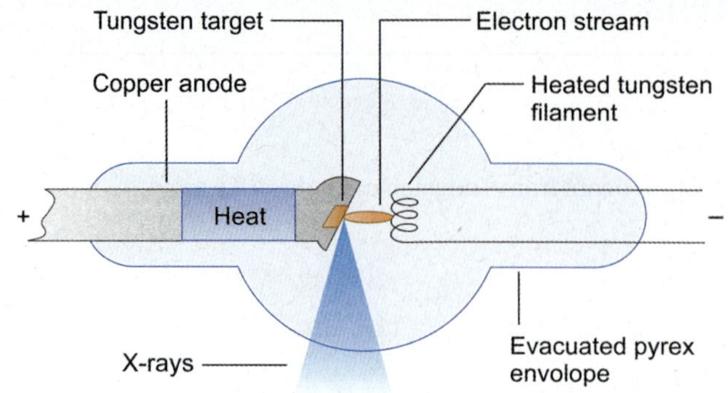

Fig. X-rays production

I E. MAGNETIC RESONANCE IMAGING (MRI)

I E1. MRI of Different Body Fluids and Tissues

Fluid/ Tissue	Example(s)	T1 weighted signal[Q]	T2 weighted signal[Q]
BODY FLUIDS			
Fluid	Bile, CSF[Q], Urine	Low	High
Hemorrhage	Acute hemorrhage	Low	Low
Hemorrhage	Chronic hemorrhage[Q]	High	High
High bound-water tissue	Adrenal, Liver, Pancreas, Muscle, Hyaline cartilage	Low	Low-to-intermediate
High free-water tissue	Gallbladder[Q], Kidney[Q], Spleen, Thyroid, Urinary bladder, Testes, Ovaries, Prostate gland, Penis	Low	High
Proteinaceous fluid	Abscess, Synovial fluid, Nucleus pulposus	Intermediate	High
BODY TISSUES			
Collagenous tissue	Tendons, Ligaments[Q], Scar, Fibrocartilage	Low	Low
Fat	**Adipose tissue, Fatty bone marrow**	**High**	**Intermediate-to-high**
Gas	Gas in bowel, Air in Lungs[Q]	Absent	Absent
Mineral rich tissue	Calculi, Cortical bone[Q]	Absent	Absent

I E2. MRI is the Investigation of Choice for

- Bony metastasis to spine (Bone scan for metastasis to other bones)
- Renal artery hypertension
- Posterior fossa tumour[Q]
- **Aortic dissection**[Q]
- Vestibular schwannoma (Gadolinium enhanced MRI)
- Ventricular function
- Perthes disease
- Pregnant lady with upper abdominal mass
- Spinal cord tumour[Q]
- **Multiple sclerosis**[Q]
- **Traumatic paraplegia**[Q]

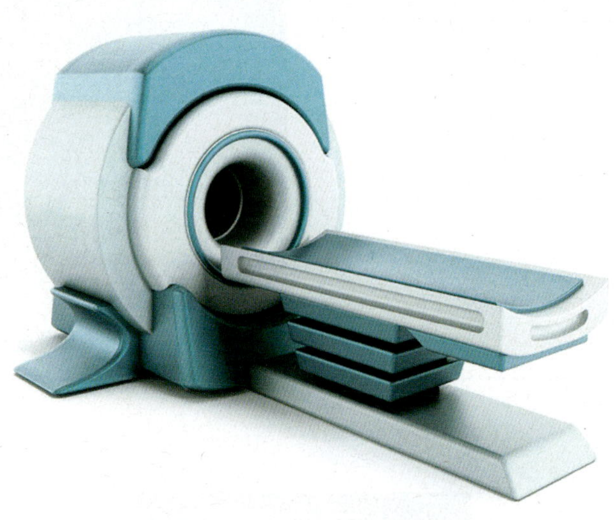

Fig. MRI machine

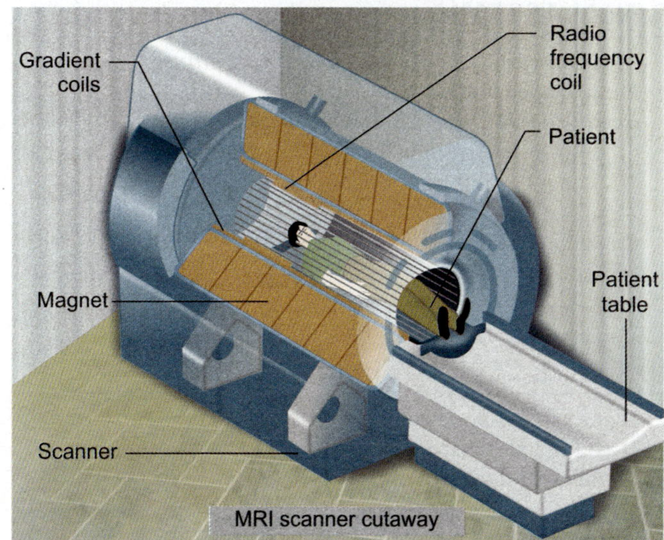

Fig. MRI scan procedure

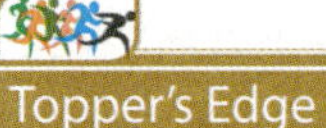

Topper's Edge

Magnetic Resonance Imaging (MRI)

- **Lauterbur and Mansfield** got Nobel Prize in Medicine (2003): MRI[Q]
- Principle[Q]:
  - **Proton (H^+) act as a dipole**
  - Magnetic dipole property and Gyromagnetic property
- Magnetic field is generated by:
  - Permanent magnets
  - Resistive air core
  - Super conductivity: Liquid helium bathed apparatus kept in liquid nitrogen
- Coils used in MRI:
  - Gradient coils: Vary strength of main magnetic field
  - Radiofrequency coils: Transmit and receive radiofrequency signals
- **Faraday's cage**:
  - Enclosure for entire MRI installation
  - Blocks local TV/radio signals that may interfere with MRI signals[Q]

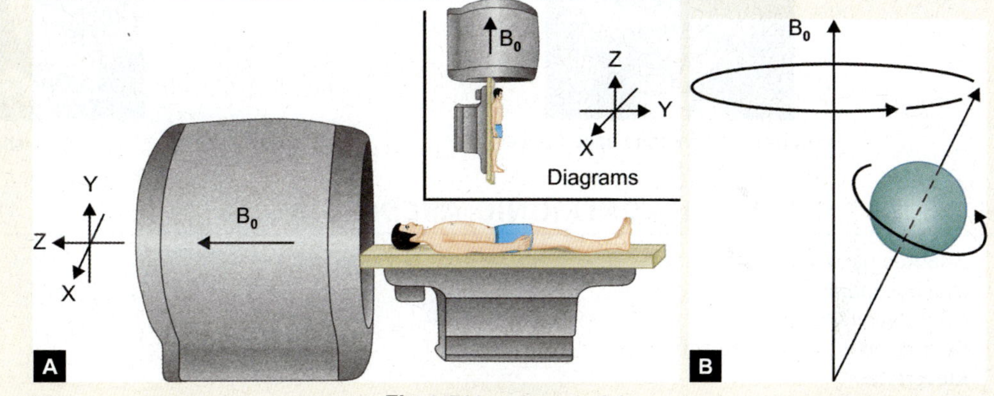

Fig. MRI imaging principle

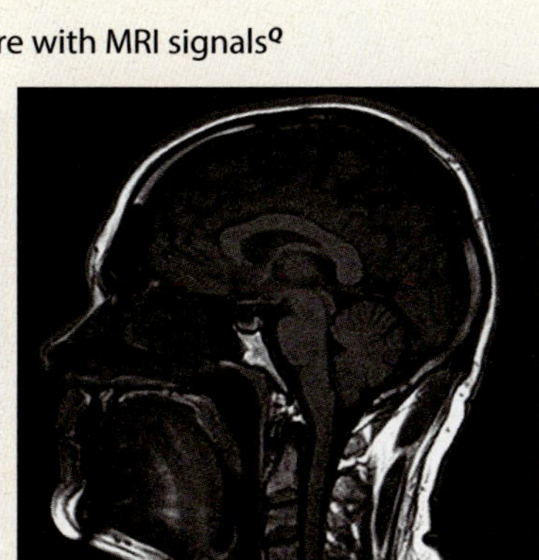

Fig. MRI scan (head)

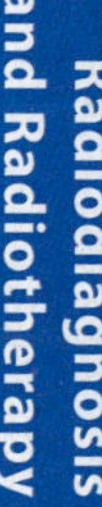

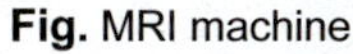

I F. THALASSEMIA

- ***'Hair-on-end**/Crew-cut/Hair-brush appearance'*[Q]
- Flask-shaped femora
- *Rodent facies*: Obliteration of paranasal sinuses

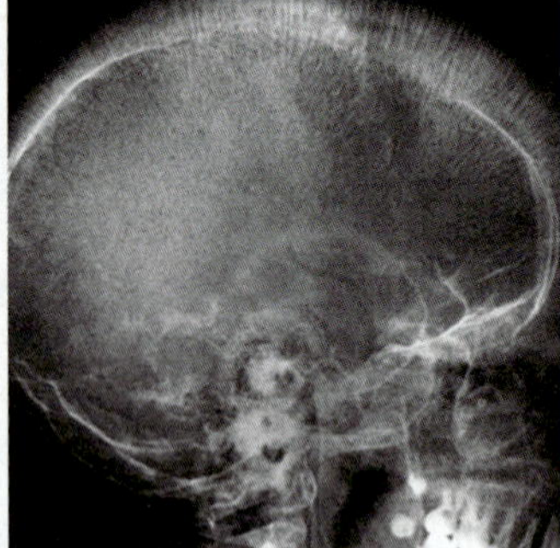

Fig. Hair-on-end appearance

I G. SICKLE CELL ANAEMIA

- ***'Bone-within-bone'* appearance**
- **H-shaped vertebrae**
- Medullary infarcts

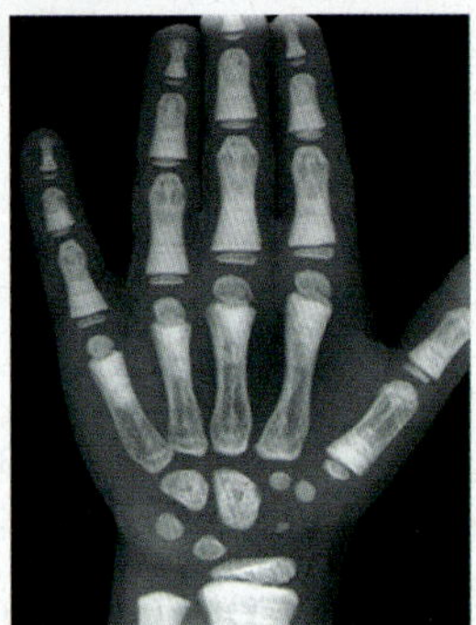

Fig. Bone-within-bone appearance

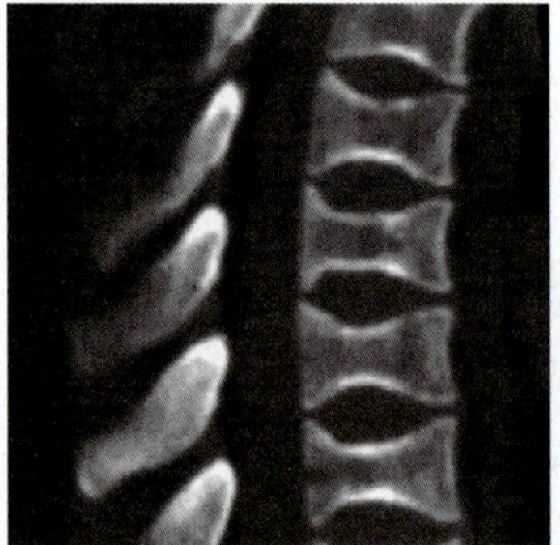

Fig. H-shaped vertebrae

I H. DOWN'S SYNDROME [MNEMONIC: ABCDEFGHI'S][Q]

- **A**tlantoaxial instability
- **B**rachycephaly
- **C**linodactyly
- **D**ecreased iliac index (less than 60)
- **E**leven ribs
- **F**rontal sinus absent
- **G**reater height of lumbar vertebrae
- **H**ydronephrosis
- **I**ncreased nuchal fold thickness (nuchal translucency)
- **S**ingle umbilical artery
- **S**hort femur/humerus
- **S**hort middle phalanx of little finger

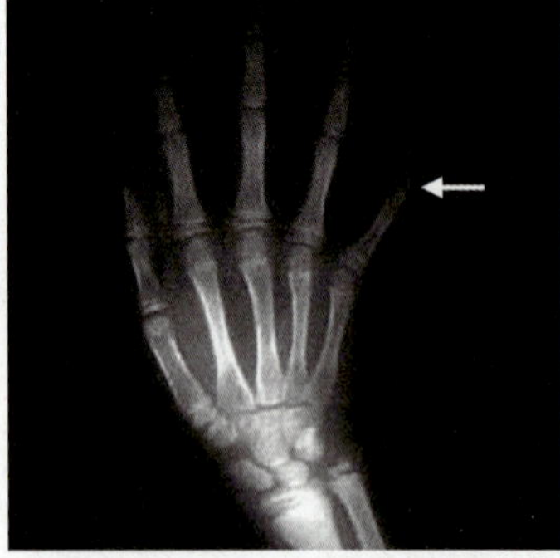

Fig. Clinodactyly

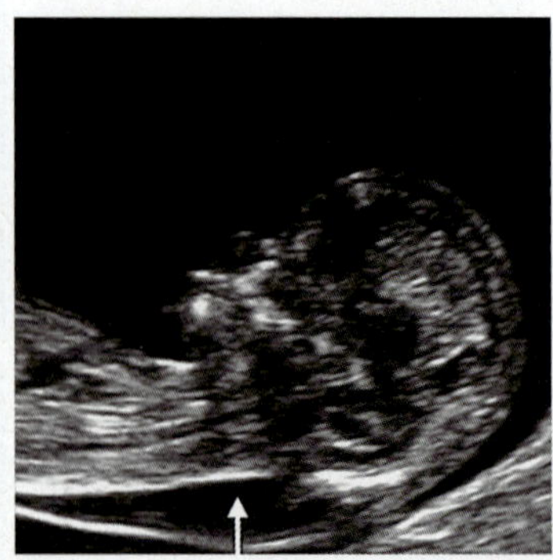

Fig. Increased nuchal translucency

I I. RADIATION TYPES IN RADIODIAGNOSIS

Types of radiation	Example(s) in radiodiagnosis
Ionizing radiation	• X-rays, fluoroscopy • Xeroradiography, mammography • Barium study, intravenous urography • CT scan • DEXA scan, PET scan
Non-ionizing radiation	• UV rays, infrared rays (thermography) • Ultrasonography • MRI • Microwaves, radiofrequency waves

Topper's Edge

KEY FACTS ABOUT RADIATION

Ionizing Radiation

- Directly ionizing radiation: Alpha particles and beta particles
  - They carry a charge and can, therefore, interact directly with atomic electrons through coulombic forces (i.e. like charges repel each other; opposite charges attract each other)
- Indirectly ionizing particle: Neutron
  - It does not carry an electrical charge
  - Ionization is caused by charged particles, which are produced during collisions with atomic nuclei.
- Electromagnetic, indirectly ionizing radiation: Gamma rays, X-rays
  - They are electrically neutral (as are all electromagnetic radiations) and do not interact with atomic electrons through coulombic forces

Key Points

- X-rays versus Gamma-rays:
  - X-rays are extranuclear in origin
  - **Gamma rays are intranuclear in origin (produced by isotopes)[Q]**
- Light versus X-rays:
  - Both are electromagnetic waves
  - Both have similar velocity
  - X-rays have high frequency, high energy (can penetrate human body[Q])
  - Light has low energy
- **Alpha particles**:
  - **Helium nuclei[Q]**
  - **Consist of 2 protons, 2 neutrons[Q]**
- Beta particles: Electrons
- Maximum penetrating power: Gamma rays[Q]
- Maximum biological damage is caused by: Alpha rays (maximum ionizing potential)[Q]

I J. DYES/CONTRAST USED IN RADIOLOGY

Radiological investigation	Contrast/Dye used
Angiography	**Urograffin**
Bronchography	Dianosil
Cholecystography	Iopanoic acid, Idopamide, Meglumineioglyconate
Foetography	Ethiodol
Hysterosalpingography (HSG)	**Dioden + Polyvinyl alcohol in water**
Intestinal obstruction	Gastrograffin
Intravenous Pyelography	**Sodium Diatrizoate**
Myelography, Ventriculography	Iohexol, Iopamidol, Metrizamide, Myodil

Contd...

Radiodiagnosis and Radiotherapy

Contd...

Radiological investigation	Contrast/Dye used
Oesophageal atresia, TrOF	Dianosil
Sialography	Neohydriol
Splenoportography	Sodium metrizoate
Urethrography	Umbradil viscous V

(TrOF: Tracheoesophageal fistula)

I K. ADVANTAGES AND DISADVANTAGES OF RADIODIAGNOSIS

Advantages	Disadvantages
Ultrasonography (USG)	
• Portability, Cheaper • Non-invasive • **Non-ionizing radiation**[Q] • Real time imaging	• Acoustic cavitation on small organism[Q] • No penetration through bone and air ▪ Limited depth penetration • Operator-dependent
Computerized tomography (CT scan)	
• Good sensitivity, Good specificity • Excellent spatial orientation • Multi-plane reconstruction • Good visualization of calcification[Q]	• Ionizing radiation • Expensive • Higher volume of imagery • Nephrotoxicity (contrast induced)
Magnetic Resonance Imaging (MRI)	
• **No ionizing radiation**[Q] • Multi-plane images[Q] • Good for soft tissue injuries • Excellent vascular structure visualization[Q] • Excellent soft tissue differentiation • Absence of health hazards	• Expensive than CT scan • Longer scan time • Limited availability • **Not useful for Bones**[Q] • Not good for calcified lesion[Q]

IMAGE-BASED QUESTIONS

1. Chest X-ray shown in photograph is .... view

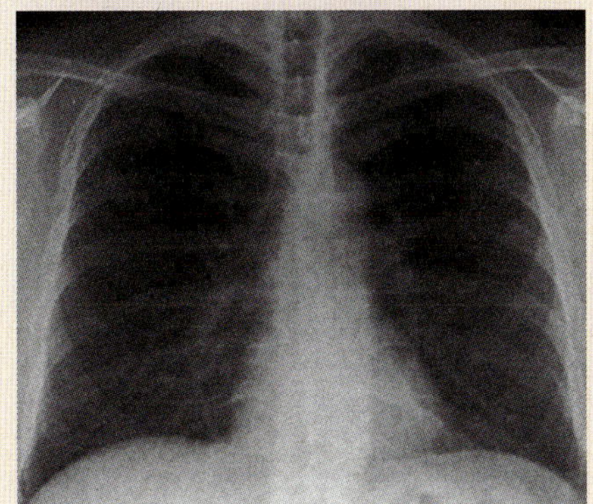

a. Anteroposterior
b. Posteroanterior
c. Oblique
d. Decubitus

2. Contribution of physicist (photograph) in field of radiology ***[Recent Question 2013]***

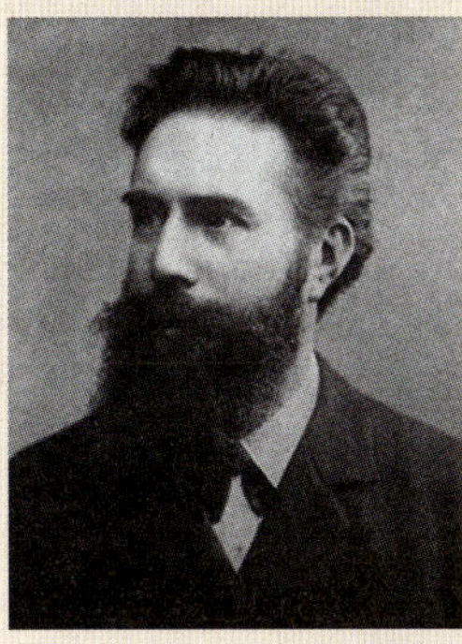

a. X-rays
b. CT scan
c. MRI
d. PET scan

3. Identify the scientist shown in photograph

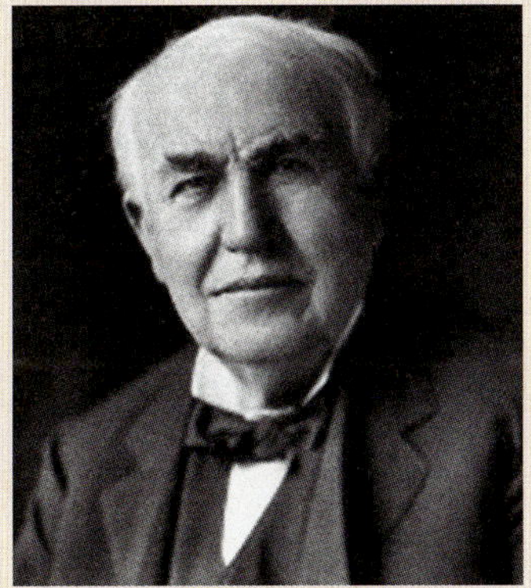

a. FJ Curie
b. TA Edison
c. Ian Donald
d. Charles Dotter

4. Machine shown in photograph is used for

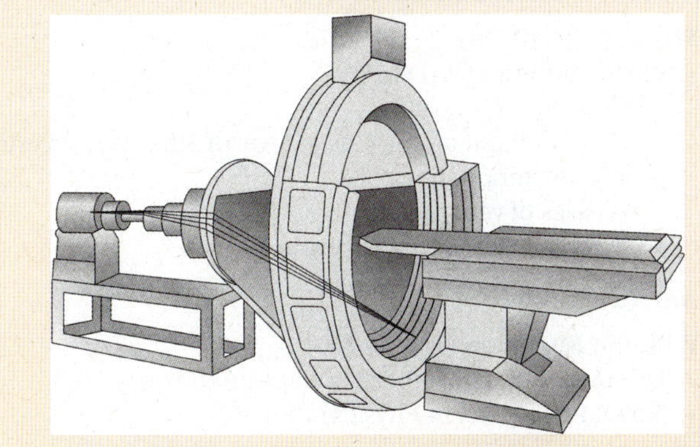

a. X-rays
b. CT scan
c. MRI
d. SPECT scan

5. Filament (encircled) shown in structure shown in photograph is generally composed of

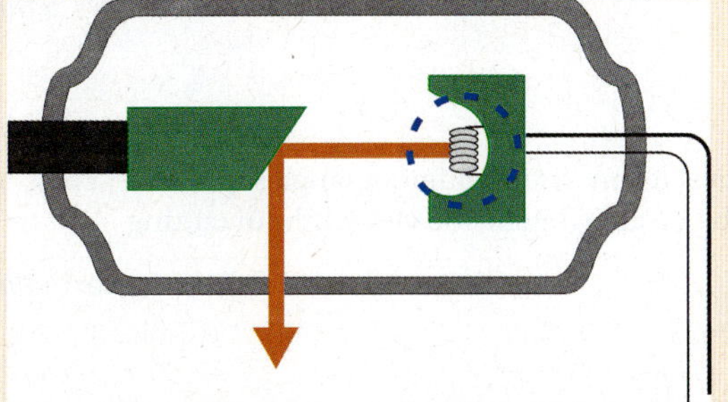

a. Molybdenum
b. Selenium
c. Tungsten
d. Gold

6. Identify the Nobel Laureate shown in photograph

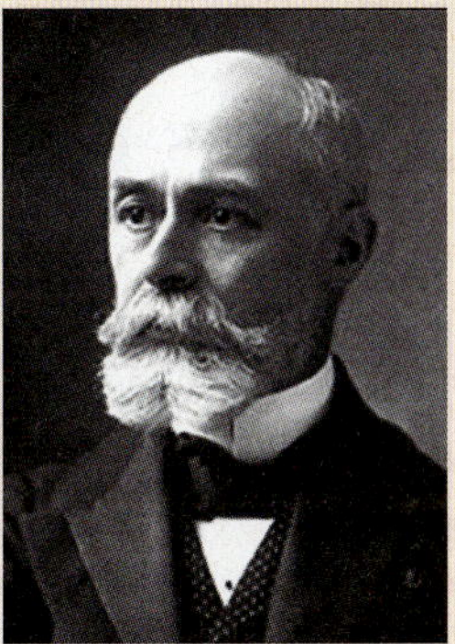

a. Wilhelm Roentgen
b. Hounsfield
c. Mansfield
d. Henri Bacquerel

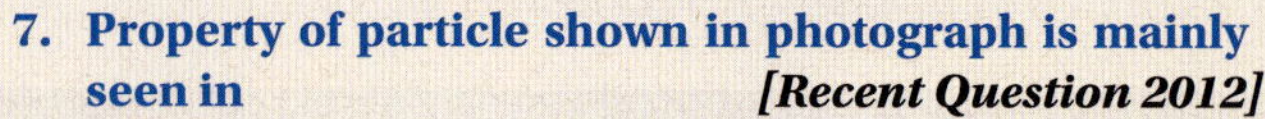

7. Property of particle shown in photograph is mainly seen in ***[Recent Question 2012]***

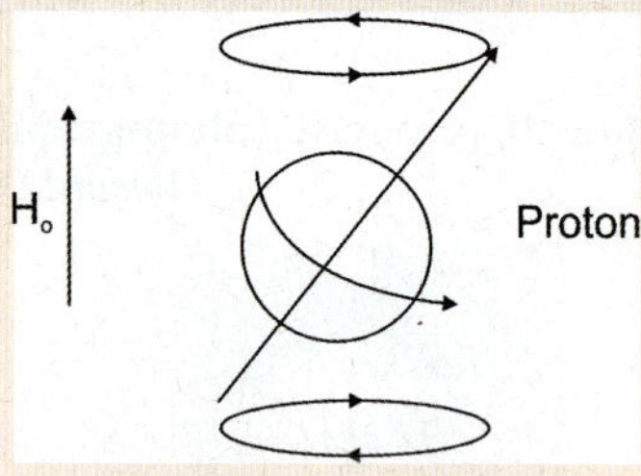

a. USG
b. CT scan
c. MRI scan
d. SPECT scan

8. Radiological modality shown in photograph is based on principle of

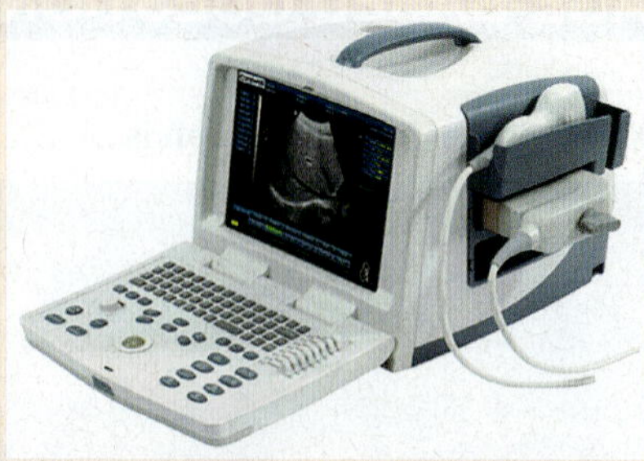

a. Electron beam strikes anode
b. Electron beam strikes cathode
c. Piezoelectric effect
d. Creation of axial sections of body

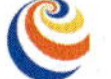 ANSWERS WITH EXPLANATIONS OF IBQs 

1. Ans. (b) Posteroanterior *[Ref. Chest X-ray Interpretation by Maskell, 1/e p5]*

Frontal Chest X-ray

- Posteroanterior (PA) view:
  - More common used
  - View centered on midline at level of 5th cervical vertebra
- Antero-posterior view:
  - In cases of very ill patient, unable to comply
  - Scapulae may obscure the lungs

2. Ans. (a) X-rays *[Ref. Nobel Prize Winners in Physics by Agarwal, 1/e p55]*

Wilhelm Roentgen (1845-1923)

- Discovered X-rays (1895; X means unknown)
- Nobel Prize (First in Physics) 1901

3. Ans. (b) TA Edison *[Ref. Thomas Edison by Linda, 1/e p118]*

Thomas Alva Edison (1847-1931) Discoveries/Inventions

- Phonograph
- Light bulb
- Motion picture
- Electrographic vote recorder
- Magnetic iron ore separator

4. Ans. (b) CT scan *[Ref. Sumer Sethi, 5/e p5]*

Computed Tomography

- Discovered by: Godfrey Hounsfield (1919-2004)
- Nobel Prize: 1979
- Principle: Computer-processed combinations of many X-ray images taken from different angles produce cross-sectional (tomographic) images (virtual 'slices') of specific areas of a scanned object, allowing inside view without cutting

5. Ans. (c) Tungsten *[Ref. Sumer Sethi, 5/e p2]*

X-rays Production

- Thermionic emission: Tungsten cathode produce electron beam
- X-rays are produced by interaction of accelerated electrons with Tungsten nuclei within the tube Anode
- When a high energy electron collides with an inner shell electron both are ejected from the tungsten atom leaving a 'hole' in the inner layer. This is filled by an outer shell electron with a loss of energy emitted as an X-ray photon

6. Ans. (d) Henri Bacquerel *[Ref. Century of X-rays and Radioactivity in Medicine by Mould, 1/e p10]*

Henri Bacquerel (1852-1908)
- Discovered radioactivity
- Nobel prize in Physics (1903)

7. Ans. (c) MRI scan *[Ref. Sumer Sethi, 5/e p8]*

MRI Scan
- Discovered by: Lauterbur
- Nobel Prize: Lauterbur and Mansfield
- Principle: Proton act as a dipole with magnetic dipole movement and gyromagnetic property

8. Ans. (c) Piezoelectric effect *[Ref. Ultrasonography by Bhargava, 1/e p1]*

Ultrasonography (USG)
- Principle: Piezoelectric effect (Pierre and Curie)
  - Ultrasound beam originates from mechanical oscillations of numerous crystals in a transducer, which are excited by electrical pulses
  - Transducer converts one type of energy into another (electrical to mechanical/sound)

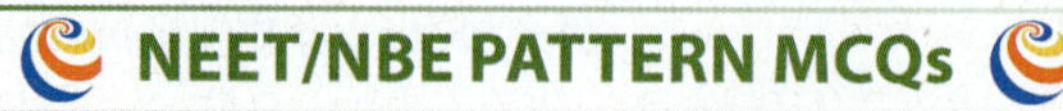

NEET/NBE PATTERN MCQs

1. **One Gray equals** *[Recent Question 2016]*
   a. 0.01 rad b. 1 rad
   c. 100 rad d. 10000 rad
2. **X-ray skull showing *'Crew-cut hair-on-end'* appearance is seen in** *[NBE FMGE March 2010, September 2010]*
   a. Sickle cell anaemia b. Thalassemia major
   c. Leukemia d. Down's syndrome
3. **Earliest detectable congenital malformation by USG is** *[NBE DNB 2009]*
   a. Spina bifida b. Cystic hygroma
   c. Anencephaly d. Encephalocele
4. **Which looks same on T_1 and T_2 on MRI?** *[Recent Question 2012]*
   a. Gallbladder b. Fat
   c. Kidney d. CSF
5. **Asymmetric growth on ultrasound imaging is seen in** *[NBE DNB 2002]*
   a. Anencephaly
   b. Trisomy 18
   c. Congenital rubella syndrome
   d. Renal anomalies
6. **Best diagnostic test for best disease is** *[NBE FMGE September 2008]*
   a. Electroretinography
   b. Electrooculography
   c. USG
   d. Fluorescence angiography
7. **X-rays were discovered by Wilhelm Roentgen in the year** *[NBE DNB 1993]*
   a. 1894 b. 1895
   c. 1896 d. 1897
8. **Capsule endoscopy is used for** *[Recent Question 2012, 2013]*
   a. GERD b. Motility disorder
   c. Bleeding d. None
9. **Investigation of choice for multiple sclerosis** *[Recent Question 2012]*
   a. CT b. MRI
   c. USG d. PET
10. **Gadolinium contrast is used in** *[NBE FMGE September 2012]*
    a. CT scan b. MRI
    c. USG d. MRCP
11. **True about MRI are all except** *[Recent Question 2012]*
    a. Not helpful in breast implant
    b. Not good for calcified lesions
    c. No radiation exposure
    d. Contraindicated in cardiac pacemaker
12. **Which view is used to visualize paranasal sinuses?** *[Recent Question 2018, NBE DNB 1993]*
    a. AP view b. Towne's view
    c. Water's view d. Submento vertical view
13. **Nonionic dye is** *[Recent Question 2012]*
    a. Ioxaglate c. Iothalamate
    b. Iohexol d. None
14. **Osteoblastic metastasis is seen** *[Recent Question 2013]*
    a. Prostate carcinoma b. Multiple myeloma
    c. Thyroid carcinoma d. Renal carcinoma
15. **CT scan was invented by** *[Recent Question 2017, NBE DNB 2003]*
    a. Godfrey Hounsfield b. Erik Storz
    c. John Snow d. Takeshita Koba
16. **X-rays were discovered by** *[NBE FMGE September 2007, September 2008]*
    a. Curie b. Gray
    c. Roentgen d. Maxwell
17. **CT scan was invented by** *[NBE DNB 1994]*
    a. Hounsfield b. Erik Storz
    c. John Snow d. Takeshita Koba
18. **Trident hand is seen in** *[Recent Question 2012]*
    a. Achondroplasia
    b. Mucopolysaccharide
    c. Diaphyseal achalasia
    d. Cleidocranial dysostosis
19. **HU is measure of** *[Recent Question 2012]*
    a. CT b. MRI
    c. PET d. USG
20. **Gray equals** *[Recent Question 2012, 2013]*
    a. 100 rad b. 1000 rad
    c. 10000 rad d. 100000 rad
21. **Investigation of choice in traumatic paraplegia is** *[NBE FMGE September 2007]*
    a. Plain X-ray b. CT scan
    c. MRI d. Myelography
22. **Which of the following techniques use piezoelectric crystals?** *[Recent Question 2012]*
    a. Ultrasonography c. NMR imaging
    b. X -ray diffraction d. Xeroradiography
23. **Lymphography in most commonly employed for** *[NBE DNB 1995]*
    a. Tuberculosis of spine
    b. Hodgkin's disease
    c. Cancers kidney
    d. Retroperitoneal liposarcoma
24. **Radiological appearance of Rickets include all except** *[Recent Question 2014]*
    a. Fraying b. Cupping
    c. Splaying d. Pelkan spur
25. **Von Rosen's view is for** *[Recent Question 2012]*
    a. CDH b. Perthe's disease
    c. CIEV d. None
26. **Amount of blackening is determined by** *[NBE FMGE September 2005]*
    a. KVP
    b. MAS
    c. Amount of X-rays
    d. Frequency or wavelength of X-rays

27. '*Central dot sign*' on CT scan is seen is *[Recent Question 2017, NBE DNB 2008]*
a. Caroli's disease
b. Primary sclerosing cholangitis
c. Polycystic liver disease
d. Liver hamartoma

28. Penetrating power of X-rays is due to *[NBE FMGE September 2005]*
a. KVP
b. MAS
c. Distance between source and patient
d. All of the above

29. CT or Hounsfield numbers depend upon *[NBE DNB 2009]*
a. Mass density b. Electron density
c. Atomic number d. Atomic mass

30. Filament in X-ray machine is composed of *[NBE FMGE March 2005]*
a. Silver b. Strontium
c. Molybdenum d. Tungsten

31. Sonographic finding of a solitary cyst containing clear fluid is *[UPSC 2011]*
a. Anechoic b. Hypoechoic
c. Isoechoic d. Hyperechoic

32. Roentgen is the unit of *[Recent Question 2017, NBE FMGE March 2010]*
a. Radiation exposure b. Radioactivity level
c. Absorbed dose d. None of the above

33. Dye used for myelography is *[NBE DNB 1995, 2000, 2003, 2005]*
a. Conray 320 b. Myodil
c. Dianosil d. Iopanoic acid

34. Gold standard for assessing pelvic pathology in infertility is *[NBE FMGE September 2011]*
a. Transvaginal sonography
b. Laparoscopy
c. Hysteroscopy
d. Magnetic resonance imaging

35. Tram-line calcification is seen in *[NBE DNB 1993, 2007, 2010]*
a. Ependymoma
b. Thrombosed cerebral vein
c. Meningioma
d. Sturge-Weber syndrome

36. An absolute contraindication of MRI is *[NBE DNB 2009]*
a. Pacemaker
b. Prosthetic cardiac valves
c. Insulin pump
d. Cochlear implants

37. Find out the wrong match *[NBE DNB 1999]*
a. Tetralogy of Fallot – Oligemic lungs
b. Rickets – Triradiate pelvis
c. Osteosarcoma – Sunray appearance
d. Osteoclastoma – Punched out lesions on skull

38. Iodipamide is best used for *[NBE DNB 1992]*
a. Splenoportography b. Angiography
c. Cholecystography d. Urethrography

39. Contrast used in barium enema study is *[NBE FMGE September 2011]*
a. Barium oxide b. Barium sulphide
c. Barium sulfate d. Lead sulfate

40. Magnetic field in a MRI machine is measured in *[Recent Question 2013]*
a. Hounsfield units b. Tesla
c. MHz d. None

41. Frequency of ultrasound waves in USG *[Recent Question 2013]*
a. 2000 Hz b. 5000 Hz
c. <2 MHz d. >2 MHz

42. PET stands for *[Recent Question 2013]*
a. Positive electron tomography
b. Proton-electron therapy
c. Positron emission tomography
d. Photon emitting tomography

43. Gyromagnetic property of proton is seen in *[Recent Question 2013]*
a. MRI b. CT
c. PET scan d. USG

44. Which delivers highest dose of radiation? *[Recent Question 2013]*
a. Cardiac perfusion scan b. CT chest
c. CT brain d. Mammogram

45. Maximum radiation dose tolerable tissue is *[Recent Question 2013]*
a. Hemopoietic tissue b. Testis
c. Ovary d. Bone

46. Enhancement in CT contrast is due to *[Recent Question 2013, 2015]*
a. Iodine b. Gadolinium
c. Silver d. Mercury

47. Osteolytic metastasis is seen with *[Recent Question 2013]*
a. Lung b. Kidney
c. Thyroid d. All of the above

48. Hounsfield unit is zero for which of the following? *[Recent Question 2017]*
a. Air b. Water
c. Fat d. Dense bone

49. Doppler effect results from change in *[Recent Question 2013]*
a. Amplitude of sound b. Frequency of sound
c. Direction of sound d. None of the above

50. Barium swallow is used for *[Recent Question 2013]*
a. Colon b. Esophagus
c. Duodenum d. Jejunum

51. Fluorescein angiography is used to examine *[Recent Question 2013]*
a. Ciliary vasculature b. Retinal vasculature
c. Corneal vasculature d. Conjunctival vasculature

52. Investigation of choice in whole body imaging in metastasis is *[Recent Question 2013, 2015]*
a. Magnetic resonance imaging
b. Angiography
c. Venography
d. CT scan

53. X-ray artifact is *[Recent Question 2013]*
a. A radiolucent area
b. Any abnormal opacity in the radiograph
c. Produced when patient moves while taking the shoot
d. All the above

54. Radiation dose is measured as *[Recent Question 2015]*
a. Roentgen b. Sievert
c. Rem d. Gray

55. Thickness of Lead apron is *[Recent Question 2017]*
a. 0.2 mm b. 0.3 mm
c. 0.5 mm d. 0.8 mm

56. Screen used for X-ray exposure prevention, is made of *[Recent Question 2017]*
a. Lead b. Tungsten
c. Manganese d. Titanium

57. T2 image in MRI is *[Recent Question 2017]*
a. Good to detect pathology b. Good to detect anatomy
c. Good for both d. Good for none

58. Photosensitive material used in X-ray film is *[Recent Question 2017]*
a. Silver chloride b. Silver bromide
c. Silver nitrate d. Gold chloride

59. CSF in TI weighted MRI gives following appearance *[Recent Question 2017]*
a. Hypointense b. Hyperintense
c. Isointense d. None

60. Least penetrating power among following mentioned rays is in *[Recent Question 2017]*
a. Alpha rays
b. Beta rays
c. Gamma rays
d. X-ray

61. SI unit of absorbed dose is *[Recent Question 2017]*
a. Becquerel b. Columb/cm
c. Gray d. Sievert [Sv]

62. Walls of CT scan rooms are coated with *[Recent Question 2017]*
a. Lead b. Glass
c. Tungsten d. Iron

63. Safe light in radiographic dark room is ideally should be of following color *[Recent Question 2017]*
a. Red b. Yellow
c. Purple d. Blue

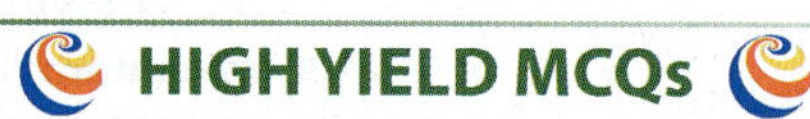

HIGH YIELD MCQs

1. After ingestion of Gastrografin when does the maximum concentration of contrast in the urine usually occur? *[Bihar PG 2016]*
a. <30 minutes after ingestion
b. 2–4 hours
c. 5–6 hours
d. 10–12 hours

2. True about contrast radiography is *[AIPGMEE 2011]*
a. 3 parts iodine + 2 parts solvent
b. Injection into artery associated with 1/3 times more complications than intravenous injection
c. Do a test dose, if hypersensitivity suspected
d. All of the above

3. In Cerebral angiography the dye is injected through *[All India PGMEE 1999]*
a. Femoral artery b. Brachial artery
c. Axillary artery d. Radial artery

4. Most common complication of myelography is *[All India PGMEE 1999]*
a. Allergic reaction
b. Headache
c. Focal neurological deficit
d. Arachnoiditis

5. Contrast used in CT *[PGI 2000]*
a. Gadolinium b. Technitium
c. Iodine d. Chromium

6. Which of the following is the most penetration beam? *[All India PGMEE 2004]*
a. Electron beam b. 8 MV photons
c. 18 MV photons d. Proton beam

7. X-rays are produced when *[AIIMS PGMEE 2002]*
a. Electron beam strike the nucleus of the atom
b. Electron beam strikes the anode
c. Electron beam reacts with the electromagnetic held
d. Electron beam strikes the cathode

8. The intensity of color in Doppler is determined by *[PGI 1998]*
a. Direction flow
b. Velocity of flow
c. Strength of returning echo
d. None of the above

9. Hounsfield units depends on *[AIIMS PGMEE 2009]*
a. Electron density
b. Mass density
c. Effective atomic number
d. Attenuation coefficient

10. Which one of the following imaging techniques gives maximum radiation exposure to the patient? *[All India PGMEE 2006]*
a. Chest X-ray b. MRI
c. CT scan d. Bone scan

11. Walls of CT scanner room are coated with *[All India PGMEE 2010]*
a. Lead b. Glass
c. Tungsten d. Iron

12. All of the following use non-ionizing radiation except *[All India PGMEE 2006]*
a. Ultrasonography b. Thermography
c. MRI d. Radiography

Radiodiagnosis and Radiotherapy

13. An absolute contraindication of MRI is *[AIIMS PGMEE 2008]*
a. Pacemaker wires b. Intravascular stents
c. Prosthetic cardiac valves d. Severe hypertension

14. Absolute contraindication of MRI is *[PGI 2005]*
a. Pacemaker b. Pregnancy at 1st trimester
c. Aneurysmal clip d. Phobia

15. Contrast used for MRI *[PGI 2000]*
a. Iodine b. Gadolinium
c. Metrizamide d. Omnipaque

16. Radiocontrast is contraindicated in all except *[All India PGMEE 2007]*
a. Renal failure b. Patient on metformin
c. Dehydration d. Obesity

17. Kerley B lines seen in *[PGI 2009]*
a. Pleural effusion b. Mitral stenosis
c. Pericardial effusion d. Interstitial edema
e. Lymphangitic carcinomatoses

18. '*Thumb print*' sign seen in *[PGI 2008]*
a. Candida b. Aspergillus
c. Thermomyces d. Epiglottitis

19. Which one is non-ionising radiation? *[PGI 1997]*
a. MRI b. CT scan
c. X-ray
d. Positron emission scintigraphy

20. In MRI the field used is *[All India PGMEE 1997]*
a. 0.05 tesla b. 100 tesla
c. 1.1 tesla d. 11 tesla

21. MR imaging in multiple sclerosis will show lesions in *[All India PGMEE 2006]*
a. White matter b. Grey matter
c. Thalamus d. Basal ganglia

22. Which one of the following is the earliest radiographic manifestation of childhood leukemia? *[AIIMS PGMEE 2004]*
a. Radiolucent transverse metaphyseal band
b. Diffuse demineralization of bones
c. Osteoblastic lesions in skull
d. Parenchymal pulmonary lesions on chest films

23. True about are MRCP *[PGI 2007]*
a. MRI is used to obtain the image
b. CT is used for the images
c. It shows the biliary tree
d. Dye has to be injected endoscopically
e. It is an invasive procedure

24. Drug used to perform stress ECHO *[AIIMS PGMEE 2008]*
a. Thallium b. Dobutamine
c. Adrenaline d. Adenosine

25. Caldwell Luc view (occipitofrontal) can visualise *[PGI 2002]*
a. Sphenoid sinus b. Nasal bone
c. Maxillary bone d. Ethmoid
e. Frontal sinus

26. Basal skull view (submentovertical view) X-ray is best to visualize *[PGI 2000]*
a. Ethmoid sinus b. Frontal sinus
c. Sphenoid sinus d. Maxillary sinus
e. Nasopharynx

27. Which of the following statements best describes '*Background radiation*'? *[All India PGMEE 2010]*
a. Radiation in the background of nuclear reactors
b. Radiation in the background during radiological investigations
c. Radiation present constantly from natural sources
d. Radiation from nuclear fall out

28. Major difference between X-rays and light is *[All India PGMEE 2010]*
a. Energy b. Mass
c. Speed d. Type of wave

29. In a Down's syndrome patient posted for surgery, the necessary preoperative investigation to be done is *[All India PGMEE 2009]*
a. CT brain b. Echocardiography
c. Ultrasound abdomen d. X-ray cervical spine

30. Invertogram to be done in a new born *[PGI 1998]*
a. Immediately b. After 2 hours
c. After 4 hours d. After 6 hours

31. First sign of hydrocephalus in children is *[PGI 1998]*
a. Post clinoid erosion b. Large head
c. Sutural diastasis d. Thinned out vault

32. Radiological findings of battered baby syndrome is *[AIIMS PGMEE 1994]*
a. Multiple Injuries not explained by one cause
b. Multiple fractures in different stage of healing
c. Excessive callus formation
d. All of the above

33. Contrasts used in USG *[PGI 2007]*
a. Urograffin b. Ultragraffin
c. Sonavist d. Conray
e. Barium

34. Which of the following techniques use '*Piezoelectric crystals*'? *[AIIMS PGMEE 2004]*
a. Ultrasonography b. X-ray diffraction
c. NMR imaging d. Xeroradiography

35. Acoustic shadow in USG is due to *[All India PGMEE 1994]*
a. Artefact b. Absorption
c. Reflection d. Refraction

36. Maximum scattering in X-ray plate occurs in *[All India PGMEE1996, 1997]*
a. Carbon b. Mercury
c. H^+ d. Ca^{++}

37. USG is sensitive in *[PGI 2004]*
a. Ureteric colic b. Gall stone
c. Blunt abdominal trauma d. Appendicitis
e. Pancreatic pathology

38. Piezoelectric crystals are made use of in which modality that is safe from radiation also *[PGI 1998]*
a. MRI b. USG
c. CT d. All

39. In computed tomography [CT], the attenuation value are measured in Hounsfield units [HU]. An attenuation value of '0' [zero] HV corresponds to *[AIIMS PGMEE 2004]*
a. Water b. Very dense bone structure
c. AIR d. Fat

40. Slice of tissue X-rays is *[PGI 1999]*
a. Tomography b. Mammography
c. Contrast studies d. All of the above

41. Radiation exposure occurs in all except *[All India PGMEE 1993]*
a. CT scan b. MRI
c. Fluoroscopy d. Plain X-ray

42. CT dose index, true is *[AIIMS PGMEE 2008]*
a. By reducing KVP by 5% radiation dose is reduced to
b. In pediatric patients dose should be reduced
c. CT dose index is not useful for control exposure in multi-slice CT
d. KV has no control over CT dose index

43. In MRI, images are produced due to *[AIIMS PGMEE 1993]*
a. H^+ [proton] b. CO_2
c. N_2O d. K^+

44. Patient with a metallic foreign body in eye, which investigation is not done *[PGI 2006]*
a. MRI b. USG
c. X-ray d. CT

45. The EEG cabins should be completely shielded by a continuous sheet of wire mesh of copper to avoid the picking of noise from external electromagnetic disturbances. Such a shielding is called as *[AIIMS PGMEE 2003, AIIMS PGMEE 2004]*
a. Maxwell cage b. Edison's cage
c. Faraday cage d. Ohm's cage

46. PACS in medical imaging stands for *[AIIMS PGMEE 2008]*
a. Portal archiving common system
b. Photo archiving computerized system
c. Picture archiving communication system
d. Planning archiving communication scheme

47. FAST Ultrasonography utilize following window(s) *[PGI May 2014]*
a. Perihepatic b. Perisplenic
c. Perirenal d. Pelvic
e. Pericardial

48. True regarding PET scan is *[PGI November 2014]*
a. Superior to CT scan
b. No radiation is used
c. Radionuclides with long half lives
d. Anatomy and physiology function test
e. Measures response to cancer therapy

49. Broken glass piece in left forefinger of a child, first investigation of choice is *[AIIMS November 2014, November 2015]*
a. X ray b. CT scan
c. MRI d. USG

50. Technique used to visualize biomolecules is *[AIIMS November 2014]*
a. MRI
b. CT scan
c. X-ray crystallography
d. USG

51. Following can be visualized on bronchoscopy except? *[ESI IMO 2014]*
a. Vocal cords
b. Trachea
c. Subcarinal nodes
d. First division of subsegmental bronchioles

52. Most definitive method of diagnosing pulmonary embolism is *[ESI IMO 2014]*
a. Pulmonary arteriography
b. Radioisotope perfusion pulmonary scintigraphy
c. EKG
d. Venography

53. Judet's view is used for *[AIIMS PG May 2015]*
a. Scaphoid b. Pelvis
c. Scaphoid d. Calcaneus

54. Tissue harmonic imaging involves use of *[PGMCET 2015]*
a. Radioisotope b. Sound waves
c. Intravenous contrast d. X-rays

55. One Gray is equivalent to *[CGPG 2015]*
a. 1 rad b. 100 rad
c. 1 million rad d. 0.1 rad

56. Which of the following may yield a negative test on FDG-PET scan? *[AIIMS November 2017]*
a. Atypical carcinoid
b. Small cell carcinoma
c. Typical carcinoid
d. Large cell neuroendocrine tumor

NEET/NBE PATTERN MCQs ANSWERS WITH EXPLANATIONS 

1. Ans. (c) 100 rad
[Ref. Patient Care in Radiography by Ehrlich, 9/e p34]

Radiation Units

- Roentgen: Unit of exposure/radiation absorbed
- Coulomb per kg: New unit for exposure/radiation absorbed
- Rem: Unit of equivalent dose
- Sievert (Sv): New unit of equivalent dose (1 Sv = 100 rem)
- Rad: Product of absorbed dose and modifying factors (potential danger to health)
- Gray (Gy): Unit of absorbed dose **(1 Gray = 100 rad)**

2. Ans. (b) Thalassemia major
[Ref. Sumer Sethi, 5/e p55]

Radiology in thalassemia

- *'Hair-on-end/ Crew-cut/ Hair-brush appearance'*
- Flask-shaped femora
- *Rodent facies*: Obliteration of paranasal sinuses

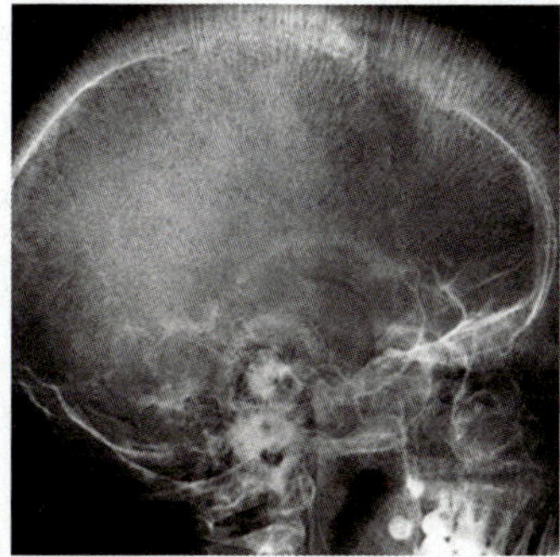

Fig. 'Crew-cut' Hair-on-end appearance

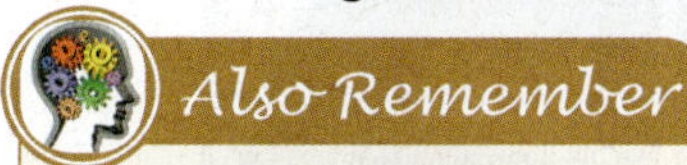

- *Sickle cell anaemia*:
  - *'Bone-within-bone'* appearance
  - H-shaped vertebrae
  - Medullary infarcts
- *Leukaemia*:
  - Metaphyseal translucencies (most characteristic)
- *Down's syndrome*: **[Mnemonic: ABCDEFGHI'S]**
  - **A**tlantoaxial instability
  - **B**rachycephaly
  - **C**linodactyly
  - **D**ecreased Iliac index (less than 60)
  - **E**leven ribs
  - **F**rontal sinus absent
  - **G**reater height of lumbar vertebrae
  - **H**ydronephrosis
  - **I**ncreased nuchal fold thickness (nuchal translucency)
  - **S**ingle umbilical artery
  - **S**hort femur/humerus
  - **S**hort middle phalanx of little finger

3. Ans. (c) Anencephaly
[Ref. Sumer K Sethi, 6/e p157]

- **Anencephaly:** Symmetric absence of cranial vault and brain structures above large and prominent orbits, diagnosis is suspected by 12-13 weeks and reliable around 15-16 weeks

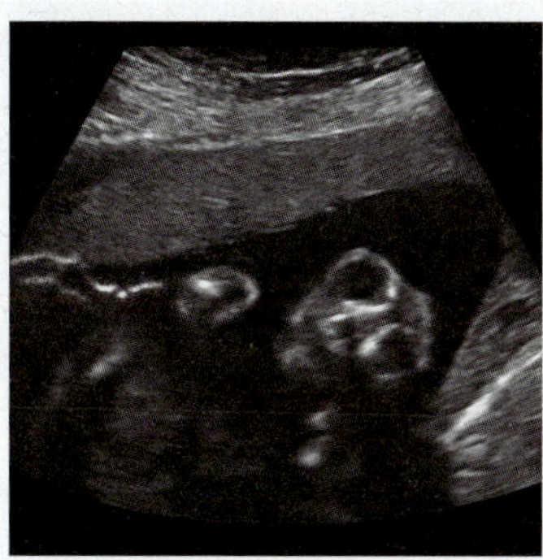

Fig. Anencephaly

4. Ans. (b) Fat
[Ref. Cardiovascular MRI by Lee, 1/e p167]

- Fat appears bright, both for T1- and T2-weighted imaging, because of J-decoupling

5. Ans. (a) Anencephaly
[Ref. David Sutton, 7/e p1051]

6. Ans. (b) Electrooculography
[Ref. Best Disease.net]

Best disease

- Disease type: Vitelliform macular dystrophy that cause progressive vision loss
- Underlying cause: Genetic affection of cells in macula leading to loss of central vision
- Tests of diagnosis:
  - *Electrooculogram*: Reduced light (peak): dark (trough) ratio
  - *Electroretinogram*: Usually turns out normal in best disease
  - *Optical coherence tomography*: Depends on stage of best disease

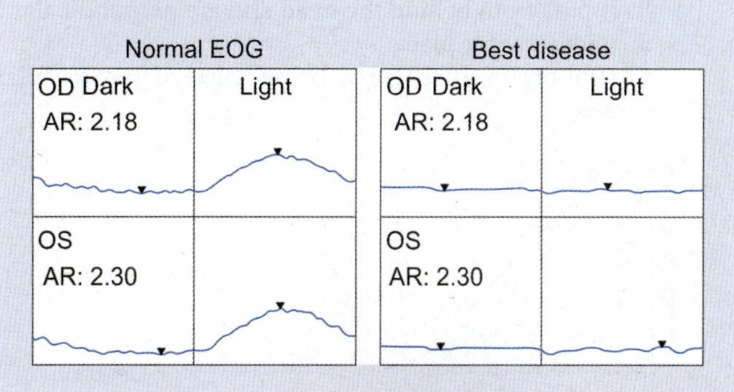

Fig. Electrooculogram

7. Ans. (b) 1895
[Ref. Sumer K Sethi, 6/e p1]

- X ray discovered on Nov 8, 1895 by Wilhelm Roentgen

8. Ans. (c) Bleeding

[Ref. Advanced Therapy in Gastroenterology and Liver Disease by Bayless, 5/e p587]

- Capsule endoscopy is a recent option for evaluating recurrent acute hemorrhage of possible small bowel origin

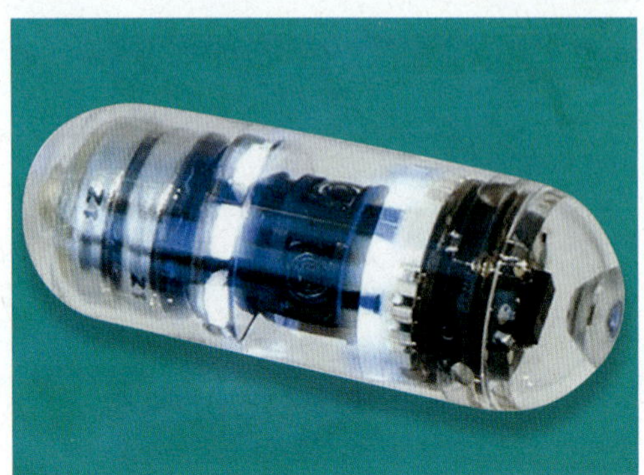

Fig. Capsule endoscopy

9. Ans. (b) MRI

[Ref. Diagnosis and Management of Multiple Sclerosis by Fleming, 1/e p51]

- MRI thus is the neuroimaging modality of choice in suspected and established multiple sclerosis

10. Ans. (b) MRI

[Ref. David Sutton, 7/e p75]

- The diagnosis is confirmed by MRI (or ("F), which shows a mass of intermediate signal intensity on T_1-weighted images and high signal intensity on T_2-weighted images with enhancement after gadolinium

11. Ans. (a) Not helpful in breast implant

[Ref. Breast MRI by Morris, 1/e p257]

- Saline-filled implants do not require special study with MRI

12. Ans. (c) Waters view

[Ref. Diseases of the Sinuses by Gershwin, 1/e p 64]

Waters' View

- Syn. Occipitomental view
- A radiographic view, where an X-ray beam is angled at 45° to the orbitomeatal line
- Rays pass from behind the head and are perpendicular to the radiographic plate
- Commonly used to get a better view of the maxillary sinuses

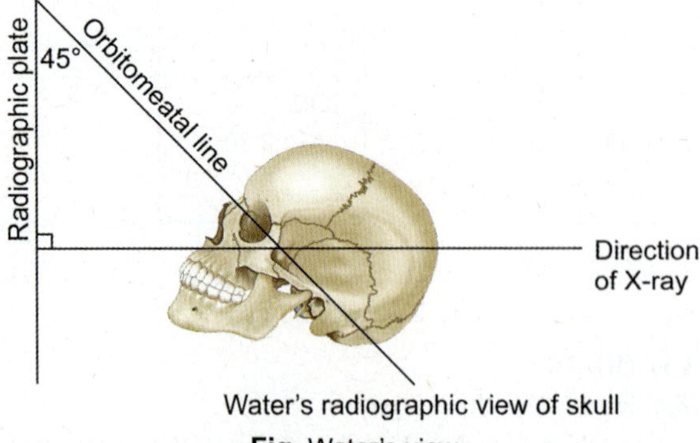

Fig. Water's view

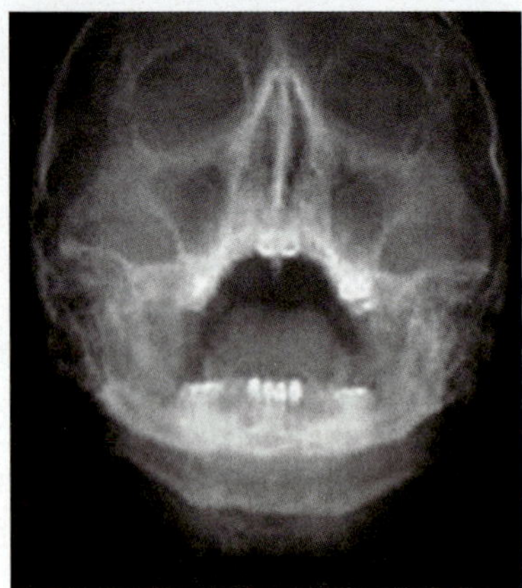

Fig. Water's view (normal skull)

13. Ans. (c) Iohexol

[Ref. The Adult and Pediatric Spine, Volume 1 by Frymoyer, 3/e p51]

- Iopamidol and iohexol are the agents of choice for myelography
- Iohexol (Omnipaque) is a non-ionic iodinated contrast agent that seems to be quite safe

14. Ans. (a) Prostate carcinoma

[Ref. The Pathophysiologic Basis of Nuclear Medicine by Elgazzar, 3/e p240]

15. Ans. (a) Godfrey Hounsfield

[Ref. Sumer K Sethi, 6/e p5]

- Nobel prize in Physiology or Medicine 1979 was awarded to A M Cormack & Godfrey N Hounsfield for development of computer assisted tomography

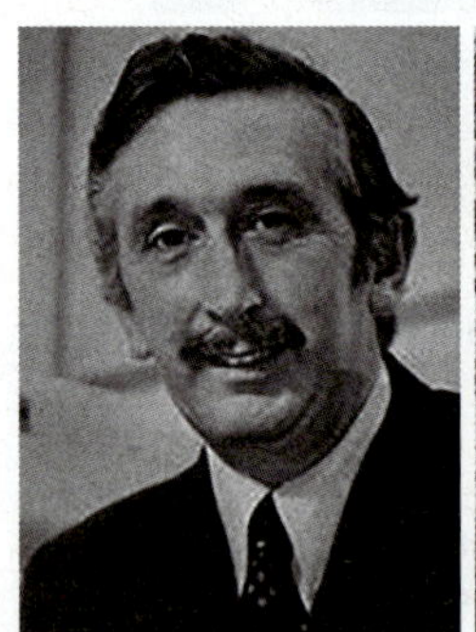
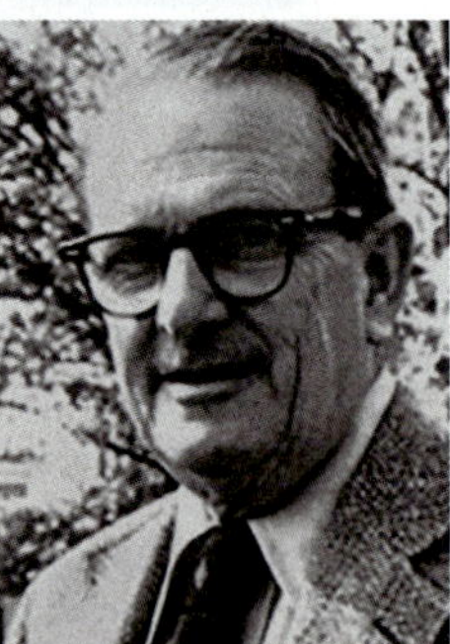

Fig. Hounsfield & Cormack

16. Ans. (c) Roentgen

[Ref. Sumer Sethi, 5/e p1]

Important Discoveries in Radiology

Discovery	Scientist
X-rays	WC Roentgen
Computed tomography (CT)	Godfrey Hounsfield
Doppler	Christian Johann Doppler
Magnetic resonance imaging (MRI)	Lauterbur & Mansfield
SPECT, PET	Kuhl
Radioactivity	Bacquerel

17. Ans. (a) Hounsfield

[Ref. Sumer K Sethi, 6/e p5]

18. Ans. (a) Achondroplasia

[Ref. Congenital Hand Anomalies and Associated Syndromes by Ghazi, 1/e p186]

- **Achondroplasia:** Dwarfism with short extremities, particularly in the proximal (rhizomelic) segments, large head with frontal bossing, hypoplasia of the midface, and trident hands

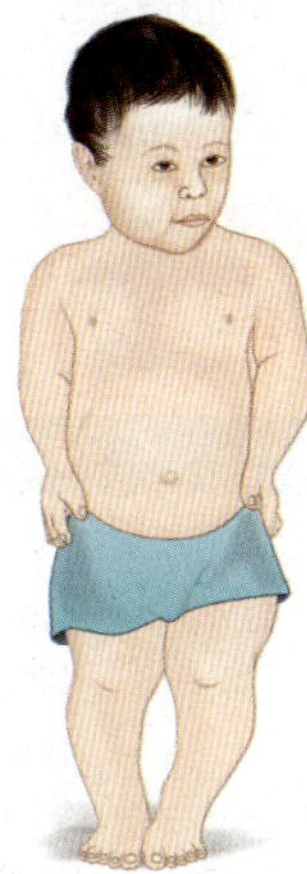

Fig. Achondroplasia

19. Ans. (a) CT

[Ref. Sumer K Sethi, 6/e p5]

- Attenuation of the X-ray beam is expressed as an absolute value measured in Hounsfield units (HU)
- HU is CT density scale

20. Ans. (a) 100 rad

[Ref. Patient Care in Radiography by Ehrlich, 8/e p37]

- One gray equals 100 rad
- 1 rad equals 1 centigray (cGy)

21. Ans. (c) MRI

[Ref. David Sutton, 6/e p236]

- *Investigation of choice in traumatic paraplegia*: MRI

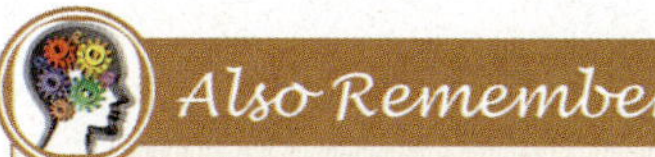

MRI as the investigation of choice

- Bony metastasis to spine (Bone scan for metastasis to other bones)
- Renal artery hypertension
- Posterior fossa tumour
- Aortic dissection
- Vestibular schwannoma (Gadolinium enhanced MRI)
- Ventricular function
- Perthes disease
- Pregnant lady with upper abdominal mass
- Spinal cord tumour
- Multiple sclerosis
- Traumatic paraplegia

22. Ans. (a) Ultrasonography

[Ref. Bipin Valchandji Daga, 1/e p30]

- US is produced by passing electric current through piezo-electric (PZE) crystals
- **Piezoelectric crystals** in the ultrasound probe: Innumerable dipoles arranged in geometric pattern

23. Ans. (b) Hodgkins disease

[Ref. Controversies in the Management of Lymphomas by Bennett, 1/e p121]

24. Ans. (d) Pelkan spur

[Ref. Sumer K Sethi, 6/e p96]

Rickets

- Saucer epiphysis
- Cupping, fraying, splaying
- Bowing of legs
- Rickety rosary
- Loss of provisional zone of calcification
- White line of healing
- Craniotabes

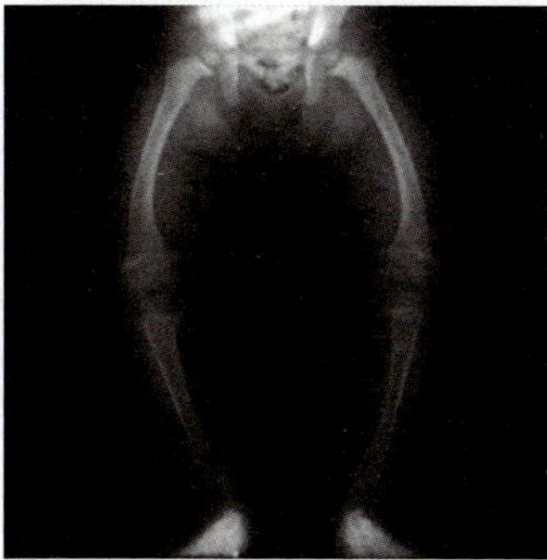

Fig 21. Bowing of legs

25. Ans. (a) CDH

[Ref. Short Textbook of Surgery by Roy, 1/e p400]

26. Ans. (b) MAS

[Ref. Sumer Sethi, 5/e p3]

Factors in X-rays

- *Exposure factors*:
  - KVP: Determines beam penetration
  - MAS: Determines film blackening
- *Contrast factors*: Influenced by KVP
- *Body related factors*: Obese patients require higher KVP

27. Ans. (a) Caroli's disease

[Ref. Metaphorical Signs in Computed Tomography of Chest and Abdomen by Yudin, 1/e p104]

- Central Dot Sign: On CT scan of liver in Caroli's disease, tiny dots with strong contrast enhancement within dilated intrahepatic bile ducts

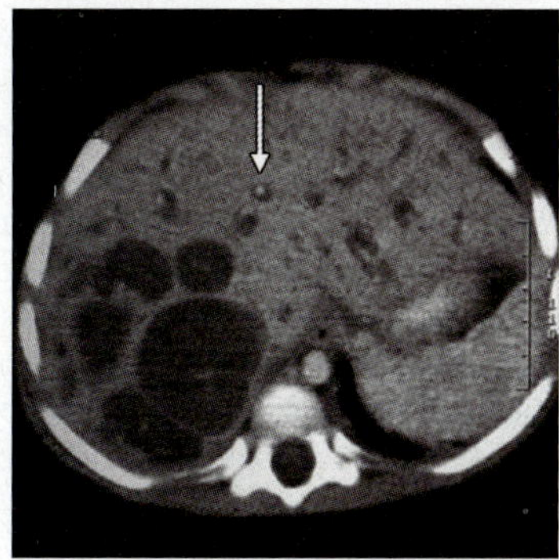

Fig. Central dot sign

28. Ans. (a) KVP

[Ref. Sumer Sethi, 5/e p3]

29. Ans. (a) Mass density

[Ref. Sumer K Sethi, 6/e p8]

30. Ans. (d) Tungsten

[Ref. Sumer Sethi, 5/e p2]

X-rays Production
- X-ray tube: Cathode (tungsten) and Anode
- Process: Thermoionic emission (Electron beam from Tungsten cathode strike anode)

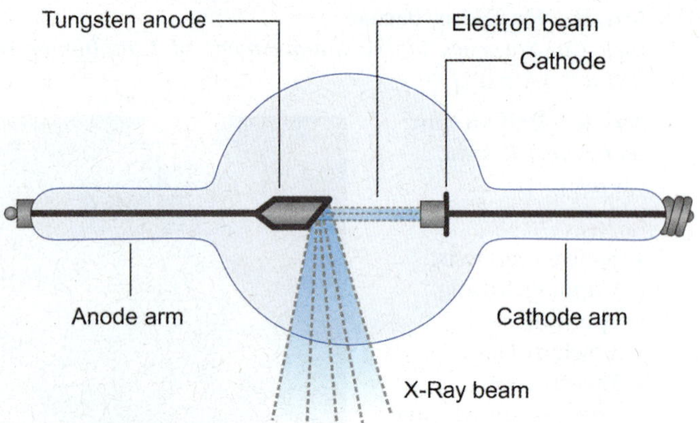

Fig. X-ray tube

31. **Ans. (a) Anechoic**
[Ref. David Sutton, 7/e p1057]

32. **Ans. (a) Radiation exposure**
[Ref. Park, 21/e p686]

Units potency of radiation
- Roentgen: Unit of exposure/radiation absorbed
- Coulomb per kg: New unit for exposure/radiation absorbed
- Rem: Unit of equivalent dose
- Sievert (Sv): New unit of equivalent dose (1 Sv = 100 rem)
- Rad: Product of absorbed dose and modifying factors (potential danger to health)
- Gray (Gy): Unit of absorbed dose (1 Gray = 100 rad)

33. **Ans. (b) Myodil**
[Ref. David Sutton, 7/e p1671]

34. **Ans. (b) Laparoscopy**
[Ref. Gynaecological Endoscopic Surgery by Desai, 1/e p1]

Radiological assessment of pelvic pathology in infertility
- *Laparoscopy*: Identifies tubal patency and pelvic pathology- **"Gold standard" for pelvic pathology**
- *Fertiloscopy*: New type of laparoscopy modified for trans-vaginal use - Recently found better than laparoscopy
- *Hysteroscopy*: Identifies intracavitary lesions
- *Salpingoscopy*: Transfimbrial approach to visualize from ampullary isthmic junction till fimbriae
- *Falloposcopy*: Trans-cervical approach to visualize from tubal ostium till fimbriae - Shows lesions of endosalpinx
- *Hydrolaparoscopy*: Trans-vaginal approach to see Pouch of Douglos

35. **Ans. (d) Sturge Weber syndrome**
[Ref. Sumer K Sethi, 6/e p140]

36. **Ans. (a) Pacemaker**
[Ref. MRI Handbook by Elmaoğlu, 1/e p97]

37. **Ans. (d) Osteoclastoma - Punched out lesion on skull**
[Ref. Sumer K Sethi, 6/e p110]
- Multiple Myeloma shows classical *'Rain drop appearance'* due to punched out lytic lesion in skull

38. **Ans. (c) Cholecystography**
[Ref. Radiocontrast Agents by Sovak, 1/e p407]

39. **Ans. (c) Barium sulfate**
[Ref. David Sutton, 6/e p7]

Contrast media used in radiology
- *Salts of heavy metals*: Heavy metal most widely used is Barium (Barium sulfate preparation)
- *Organic iodide preparations*: Used in pyelography, cholecystography, angiocardiography, arteriography, phlebography, myelography
- *Gas*: Used in double contrast studies

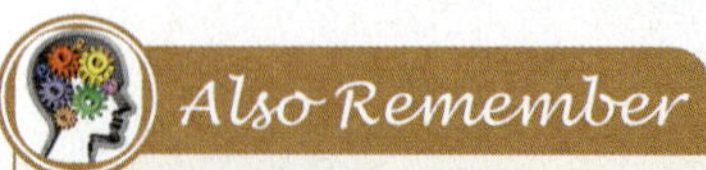

- *Barium imaging types*:

Type	Remark
Single contrast studies	Barium sulfate alone
Double contrast studies	Air + barium for small mucosal lesions
Barium meal	Barium paste for esophagus
Barium swallow	95% Barium sulfate for stomach/duodenum
Barium meal follow through	50% Barium sulfate for small bowel
Barium enema	25% Barium sulfate for large bowel

- *Barium sulfate contraindications*:
  - Tracheoesophageal fistula
  - Perforation peritonitis
  - Sensitivity to barium

40. **Ans. (b) Tesla**
[Ref. Sumer K Sethi, 6/e p5]

41. **Ans. (d) >2 MHz**
[Ref. Sumer K Sethi, 6/e p11]

42. **Ans. (c) Positron emission tomography**
[Ref. PET-CT by Peter, 1/e p291]

43. **Ans. (a) MRI**
[Ref. Sumer K Sethi, 6/e p14]
- Proton (H^+) acts as dipole with magnetic dipole movement and gyromagnetic property

44. **Ans. (a) Cardiac perfusion scan**
[Ref. Nuclear Cardiac Imaging by Crawford, 2/e p161]

45. **Ans. (d) Bone**
[Ref. Clinical Radiation Oncology by Leonard L. Gunderson, 1/e p437]

46. **Ans. (a) Iodine**
[Ref. Cardiovascular CT and MR Imaging by Catalano, 1/e p14]

47. **Ans. (d) All of the above**
[Ref. Orthopaedic Pathology by Vincent J, p529]

48. Ans. (b) **Water**

[Ref. Principles of Computerized Tomographic Imaging by Kak, 1/e p119]

- The values of the absorption coefficients are calculated on a standard scale, adopting zero as the value for water

49. Ans. (b) **Frequency of sound**

[Ref. Sumer K Sethi, 6/e p9]

50. Ans. (b) **Esophagus**

[Ref. David Sutton, 7/e p788]

51. Ans. (b) **Retinal vasculature**

[Ref. Atlas of Fundus Angiography, 1/e p 5]

- Fluorescein angiography documents retinal vascular anatomy in much better detail, as the fluorescein dye lights up the retinal vasculature

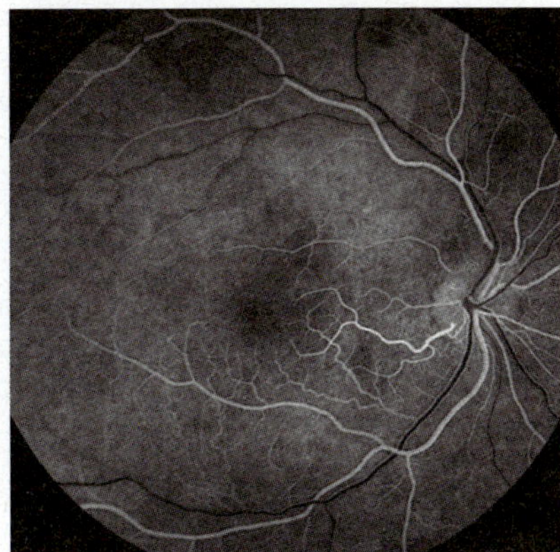

Fig. Fluorescein angiogram

52. Ans. (a) **MRI**

[Ref. Nuclear Oncology by CumaliAktolun, 1/e p65]

- In the assessment of skip lesions and metastases whole body MRI is ideal

53. Ans. (c) **Produced when patients move while taking the shoot**

[Ref. Medical Physics and Biomedical Engineering by Brown, 1/e p535]

54. Ans. (b) **Sievert**

[Ref. Molecular Imaging by Shankar, 1/e p340]

Units potency of radiation

- Roentgen: Unit of exposure/radiation absorbed
- Coulomb per kg: New unit for exposure/radiation absorbed
- Rem: Unit of equivalent dose
- Sievert (Sv): New unit of equivalent dose (1 Sv = 100 rem)
- Rad: Product of absorbed dose and modifying factors (potential danger to health)
- Gray (Gy): Unit of absorbed dose (1 Gray = 100 rad)

55. Ans. (c) **0.5 mm**

[Ref. ERCP E-Book by Baron, 2/e p20]

- Radiation protective apparel is available in 0.25–1.0 mm lead-equivalent thickness
- In most areas, regulations require that a **thickness of at least 0.5 mm lead-equivalent be used**, which attenuates more than 90% of scattered X-rays that strike it
- Different designs are available, including aprons with front coverage only, aprons that wrap around the body, and two-piece garments with vest and kilt

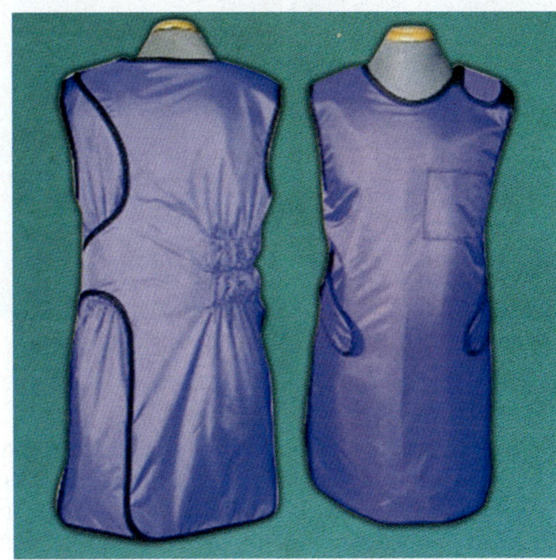

Fig. Lead apron

56. Ans. (a) **Lead**

[Ref. Surgical Technology for the Surgical Technologist, 4/e p90]

- Lead shielding refers to the use of lead as a form of radiation protection to shield people or objects from radiation, so as to reduce the effective dose
- Lead can effectively attenuate certain kinds of radiation because of its high density and high atomic number; principally, it is effective at stopping Gamma rays and X-rays
- Lead is used for shielding in X-ray machines, nuclear power plants, labs, military equipment
- Personal shielding includes lead aprons, thyroid shields, and lead gloves
- Shielding devices are also available for laboratory equipment, including lead castles, structures composed of lead bricks, and lead pigs, thick containers for storing and transporting radioactive samples

57. Ans. (a) **Good to detect pathology**

[Ref. Sports and Exercise Medicine by Narvani, 1/e p152]

T1 and T2 Images in MRI

- T2 is the time taken for hydrogen atoms to diphase
- T1 is the time taken for return to relaxed state (and release energy)

	T1 Image	T2 Image
Time to echo (TE)	40 ms	120 ms
Time to repetition (TR)	400 ms	1000 ms
Useful for	Demonstrating anatomy	Demonstrating pathology
Bright for	Fat, methaemoglobin, contrast, calcium, blood	Fluid (oedema), fat

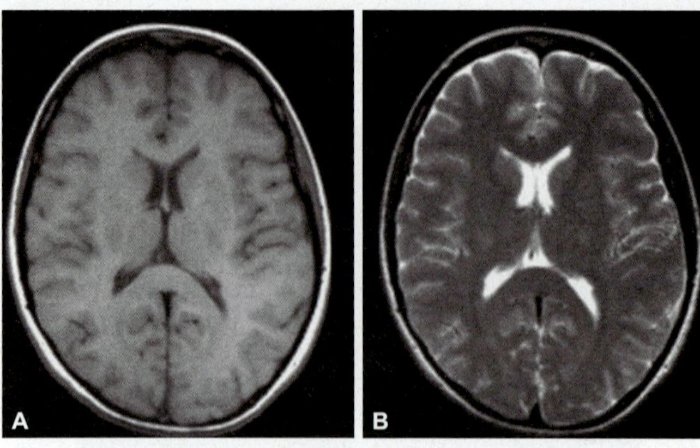

Figs. (A) T1-Weighted and (B) T2-Weighted Images

58. Ans. (b) Silver bromide
[Ref. X-ray Equipment by McClelland, 1/e p243]

- Standard X-ray film is photographic film, coated on both sides of a polyester film base, called 'double emulsion film'
- A variation 'Single emulsion film', is coated on one side only (Typical application is mammography, where maximum possible image sharpness is required)
- Photosensitive material is 'Silver halide', suspended in the form of small crystals in a gelatin solution; Silver halide consists of approximately 90-99% of Silver bromide and 1-10% Silver iodide

59. Ans. (a) Hypointense
[Ref. Inflammatory Diseases of the Brain by Hähnel, 1/e p114]

- MRI has unique potential to demonstrate fat as hyperintense material within the hypointense cerebrospinal fluid (CSF) on T1-weighted images

60. Ans. (a) Alpha rays
[Ref. Grainger & Allison's Diagnostic Radiology Essentials,4/e p39]

- Penetrating potential: Gamma rays > X-rays > Beta particle > Alpha article (helium ion)
- Gamma rays penetrate around 50 cm in tissue and 0.3 mm in Lead

61. Ans. (c) Gray
[Ref. Radiologic Technology by Gurley, 7/e p179]

Units Potency of Radiation

- Roentgen: Unit of exposure/radiation absorbed
- Coulomb per kg: New unit for exposure/radiation absorbed
- Rem: Unit of equivalent dose
- Sievert (Sv): New unit of equivalent dose (1 Sv = 100 rem)
- Rad: Product of absorbed dose and modifying factors (potential danger to health)
- Gray (Gy): Unit of absorbed dose (1 Gray = 100 rad)

Special units	SI units
Curie	Bacquerel
Rad	Gray
Rem	Sievert
Roentgen	Coulomb

62. Ans. (a) Lead
[Ref. Out of Operating Room Anesthesia by Goudra, 1/e p209]

- Both the CT scan rooms and hot lab and PET scanner room require radiation shielding, which is frequently achieved by installing lead at the wall stud surfaces

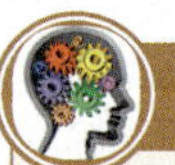

Also Remember

- Faraday cage, the walls of MRI scanner rooms are sheathed in metal (Copper or Aluminium) forming a complete box around the scanner, shielding it from external radiofrequency interference.

63. Ans. (a) Red
[Ref. RNA Methodologies by Farrell, 5/e p511]

Safelight

- Undeveloped X-ray films remain light sensitive until processed through the photographic fixer solution, though limited low-intensity illumination is permissible to allow movement and efficient handling in the darkroom
- A safelight typically consists of an ordinary 15 W frosted light bulb that shines through a filter, the color of which is compatible with the film being used
- Most commonly used films for chemiluminescence and autoradiography are blue-green sensitive, so the recommended setup is Red filter

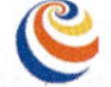 HIGH YIELD MCQs ANSWERS WITH EXPLANATIONS 

1. Ans. (b) 2–4 hours
[Ref. Nelson Textbook of Pediatrics, 18/e p1525]

Gastrograffin

- A Contrast medium for the radiological examination of gastrointestinal tract (also in combination with barium sulfate)
- It can be administered orally or as an enema and is primarily indicated in cases in which the use of barium sulfate is unsatisfactory, undesirable or contraindicated
- Contrast medium which has undergone renal excretion will appear within 2 hours

2. Ans. (c) Do a test dose, if hypersensitivity is suspected
[Ref. Grainger & Allison's Diagnostic Radiology Essentials by Lee, 5/e p39]

3. Ans. (a) Femoral artery
[Ref. Grainger & Allison's Diagnostic Radiology Essentials by Lee A Grant, 5/e p1256]

- For a cerebral arteriogram, a catheter is usually inserted into femoral artery. Sometimes, an artery in the arm is used
- Rarely, an artery in the neck may need to be used

- Femoral artery is most commonly used because it's easier to get to
- Once the catheter is inserted, the contrast dye is injected

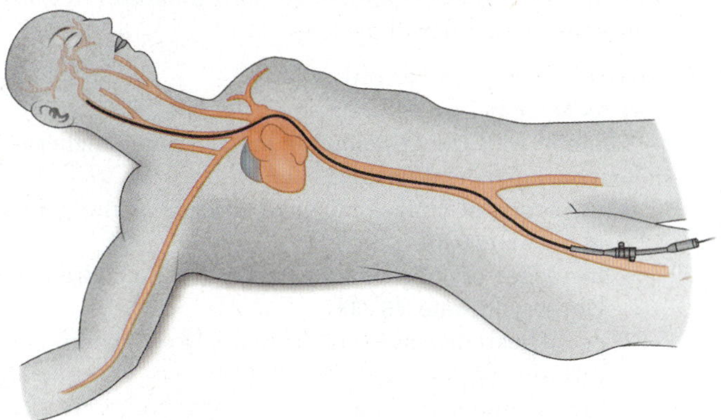

Fig. Cerebral angiogram (via femoral artery)

4. Ans. (b) Headache
[Ref. Grainger & Allison's Diagnostic Radiology Essentials by Lee, 5/e p1365]

Complications of myelography

- Most common complications: **Severe headache (20%)**, nausea, vomiting
- Meningeal irritation/changed CSF pressure after spinal tap may cause the development of a headache; fever; nausea; dizziness; stiff neck, shoulders, or back; and a sensitivity or aversion to light (photophobia)
- An infection of the membranes (meningitis), herniation of the brain, or seizures
- Mild to life-threatening allergic reaction to the dye used
- Anaphylactic shock

5. Ans. (c) Iodine
[Ref. Grainger & Allison's Diagnostic Radiology Essentials by Lee,5/e p1249]

6. Ans. (c) 18 MV photons
[Ref. Farr's Physics for Medical Imaging, 2/e p29]

- 18 mV photons have highest energy and that is why most penetrating beam

7. Ans. (b) Electron beam strikes the anode
[Ref. Christensen's Physics of Diagnostic Radiology,4/e p10]

- X-rays are produced by energy conversion when a fast moving stream of electrons is suddenly decelerated in the target anode of an X-ray tube

8. Ans. (b) Velocity of flow
[Ref. Clinical Doppler Ultrasound by Paul L Allan, 2/e p6]

9. Ans. (d) Attenuation coefficient
[Ref. Christensen's Physics of Diagnostic Radiology, 4/e p308]

10. Ans. (c) CT scan
[Ref. Medical Imaging in Clinical Trials by Miller, p57]

11. Ans. (a) Lead
[Ref. Christensen's Physics of Diagnostic Radiology, 4/e p379]

12. Ans. (d) Radiography
[Ref. Review of Radiology by Sumer Sethi,4/e p7]

13. Ans. (a) Pacemaker wires
[Ref. Review of Radiology by Sumer Sethi, 6/e p19]

- When suspecting a metallic foreign body in eye, MRI is contraindicated; also with pacemakers and cochlear implants because they experience a torque in the magnetic field

14. Ans. (a) Pacemaker; (c) Aneurysmal clip
[Ref. Sumer Sethi, 6/e p19]

15. Ans. (b) Gadolinium
[Ref. Sumer Sethi, 6/e p17]

- Contrast used in **MRI-Gadolinium DTPA**
- Gadolinium is a lanthanide
- Gd DTPA is classed as an acyclic, ionic gadolinium contrast medium, its paramagnetic property reduces the T1 relaxation time

16. Ans. (d) Obesity
[Ref. Sumer Sethi, 6/e p21]

- Patients with preexisting renal disease, particularly those with renal complication of diabetes mellitus, multiple myeloma, dehydration have an increased risk of an adverse reaction

17. Ans. (b) Mitral stenosis; (d) Interstitial edema; (e) Lymphangitis carcinomatosa
[Ref. Sumer K Sethi, 6/e p68]

Causes of kerley lines

- Left ventricular failure
- Mitral stenosis
- Pneumoconiosis
- Lymphangitis carcinomatosis
- Others: interstitial fibrosis, sarcoidosis, alveolar cell carcinoma, lymphoma, lymphatic obstruction, lymphangiectasia

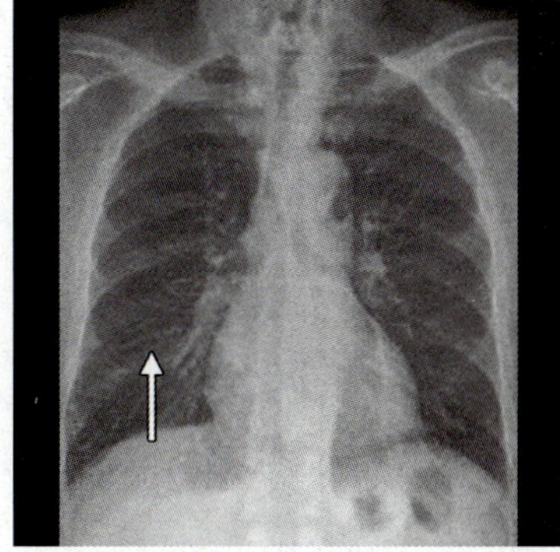

Fig. Kerley Lines

18. Ans. (d) Epiglottitis
[Ref. Diseases of Ear, Nose and Throat by Bansal, p 480]

- Epiglottitis may be seen radiographically on a lateral neck X-ray
- Epiglottic swelling (supraglottic) of three to four times normal is seen at the base of the tongue and appears as if someone left a thumb print

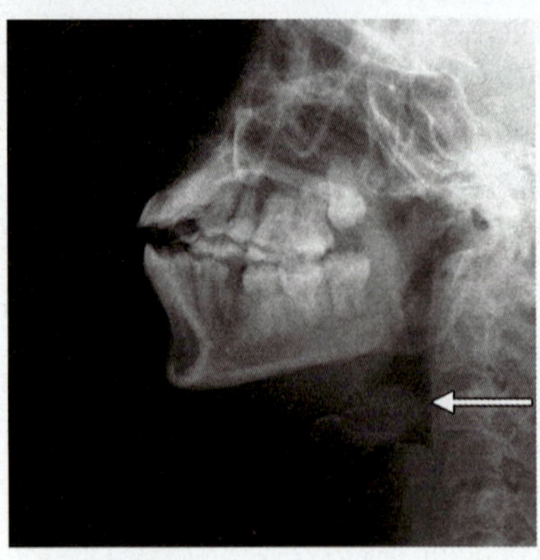

Fig. Thumb-print sign

19. Ans. (a) MRI

[Ref. Review of Radiology by Sumer Sethi, 6/e p19]

- No ionizing radiation, hence safe in pregnancy.

20. Ans. (c) 1.1 tesla

[Ref. Sumer Sethi, 6/e p15]

- Clinical imaging scanners have magnets with field strengths ranging from 0.02-1.5T, routinely used is 1.5 telsa

21. Ans. (a) White matter

[Ref. David Sutton, 7/e p11]

22. Ans. (a) Radiolucent transverse metaphyseal bands

[Ref. Comprehensive Radiographic Pathology by Ronald L, 1/e p 348]

- In childhood leukemia, radiographically detectable skeletal involvement is extremely common as a result of the infiltration.
- Earliest radiographic sign of disease is usually transverse radiolucent bands at the metaphyseal ends of the long bones
- Most characteristic sign is presence of metaphyseal translucencies (90%)

23. Ans. (a) MRI is used to obtain image; (c) It shows the biliary tree

[Ref. Review of Radiology Sumer Sethi, 6/e p19]

24. Ans. (b) Dobutamine

[Ref. Grainger & Allison's Diagnostic Radiology Essentials by Lee A Grant, 5/e p432]

- **Dobutamine Stress Echocardiogram** is a test used to assess the pumping function of heart in patients who are unable to exercise on a treadmill for a Stress Test

25. Ans. (b) Nasal bone; (c) Maxillary bone; (d) Ethmoid; (e) Frontal sinus

[Ref. Clark's Positioning in Radiography, 12/e p240]

26. Ans. (c) Sphenoid sinus

[Ref. Clark's Positioning in Radiography, 12/e p268]

27. Ans. (c) Radiation present constantly from natural sources

[Ref. Sumer Sethi, 4/e p99]

28. Ans. (a) Energy

[Ref. Limited Radiology by Campeau, 3/e p161]

- Major difference between X-ray and light is the energy in each photon
- An X-ray has about 5000 times the energy than an ordinary light photon
- X-ray have a shorter wavelength in comparison to visible light and hence a higher energy

29. Ans. (b) Echocardiography

[Ref. Sumer Sethi, 4/e p49]

- Children with Down syndrome are at a much higher risk for congenital heart disease
  - Incidence of congenital heart disease in the general population: 0.8%
  - Incidence of congenital heart disease in children with Down syndrome: 40–60%
- Types of heart defects in children with Down syndrome:
  - Atrioventricular Septal Defects (AVSDs) - These are the most common in children with Down syndrome.
  - ventricular septal defects (VSDs)
  - atrial septal defects
  - patent ductus arteriosus
  - tetralogy of fallot

30. Ans. (d) After 6 hours

[Ref. Gastrointestinal Radiology Ronald L.Eisenberg, 4/e p745]

- **Invertogram**: A coin/metal piece is placed over the expected anus and the baby is turned upside down (for a minimum 3 minutes)
- Distance of gas bubble in rectum from the metal piece is noted:
  - >2 cm: denotes high type
  - <2 cm: denotes low type

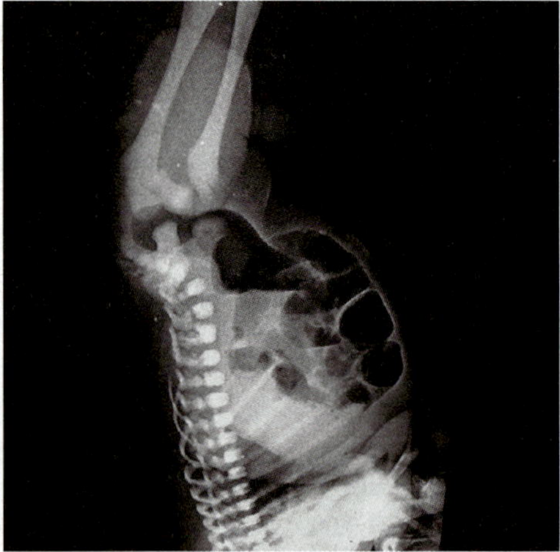

Fig. Invertogram

31. Ans. (c) Sutural diastasis

[Ref. David Sutton, 7/e p1626]

- Suture diastasis, the first and most important sign in small children, may be the only sign of raised pressure
- Sellar erosion may occur but is a late sign and implies longstanding chronic pressure
- In children under 10, Sellar erosion without suture diastasis is likely to be due to a local erosive lesion rather than raised pressure

- Above this age cellar changes are more likely to be due to raised pressure
- Sequence: Coronal > Sagittal > Lambdoid > Squamosal suture

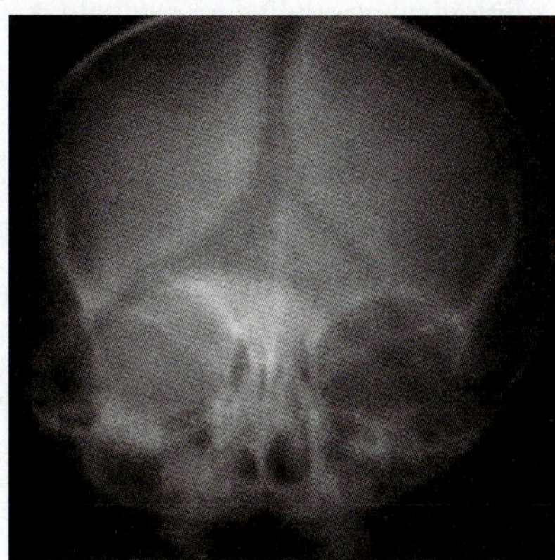

Fig. Sutural diastasis

32. Ans. (d) All of the above
[Ref. David Sutton, 7/e p1364-1385]

33. Ans. (c) Sonavist
[Ref. David Sutton, 7/e p763]

34. Ans. (a) Ultrasonography
[Ref. Sumer Sethi, 6/e p11]

USG

- Crystal: PZT Lead ZirconateTitanate
- Principle: Piezoelectric effect
- Advantage: no radiation; Portable

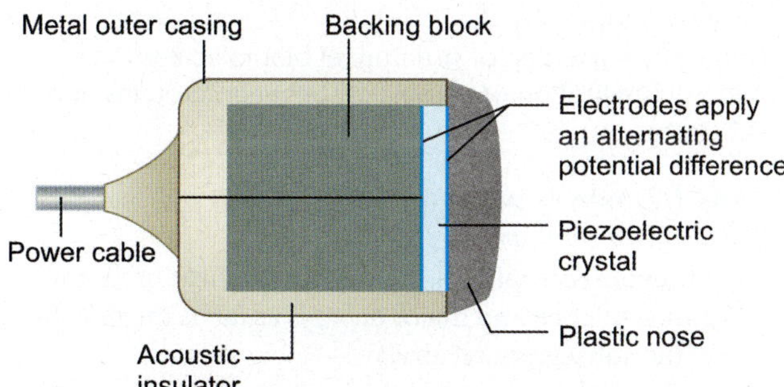

Fig. Principle of USG

35. Ans. (c) Reflection
[Ref. Christensen's Physics of Diagnostic Radiology, 4/e p334-35]

36. Ans. (c) H^+
[Ref. Christensen's Physics of Diagnostic Radiology, 4/e p63-64]

37. Ans. (b) Gallstone; (c) Blunt abdominal trauma; (d) Appendicitis
[Ref. Sumer Sethi, 6/e p10]

38. Ans. (b) USG
[Ref. Sumer Sethi, 6/e p11]

39. Ans. (a) Water
[Ref. Sumer Sethi, 4/e p6]

40. Ans. (a) Tomography
[Ref. Sumer Sethi, 6/e p5]

- Rotation of the X-ray tube allows calculation of the attenuation at every single point of the slice, which is used to produce a cross-sectional image of the body

41. Ans. (b) MRI
[Ref. Sumer Sethi, 6/e p19]

- No radiation exposure, hence safe in pregnancy

42. Ans. (b) In pediatric patients dose should be reduced
[Ref. Christensen's Physics of Diagnostic Radiology, 4/e p378-9]

- **CT dose index (CTDI)** provides a good approximation to the multiple scan average dose (MSAD) which is the average dose, at a particular depth from the surface, resulting from a large series of CT slices
- CTDI measurement protocol seeks to measure the scattered radiation dose from adjacent CT slices in a practical manner
- Best available risk estimates suggest that pediatric CT will result in significantly increased lifetime radiation risk over adult CT

43. Ans. (a) H^+ [proton]

44. Ans. (a) MRI
[Ref. Sumer Sethi, 6/e p19]

- When suspecting a metallic foreign body in eye, MRI is contraindicated; also with pacemakers and cochlear implants because they experience a torque in the magnetic field

45. Ans. (c) Faraday cage
[Ref. Sumer Sethi, 4/e p8]

Faraday cages

- Named after the English scientist Michael Faraday, who invented them in 1836
- Faraday cage/shield is an enclosure formed by conductive material or by a mesh of such material, used to block electric fields
- Operates because an external electrical field causes the electric charges within the cage's conducting material to be distributed, such that they cancel the field's effect in the cage's interior

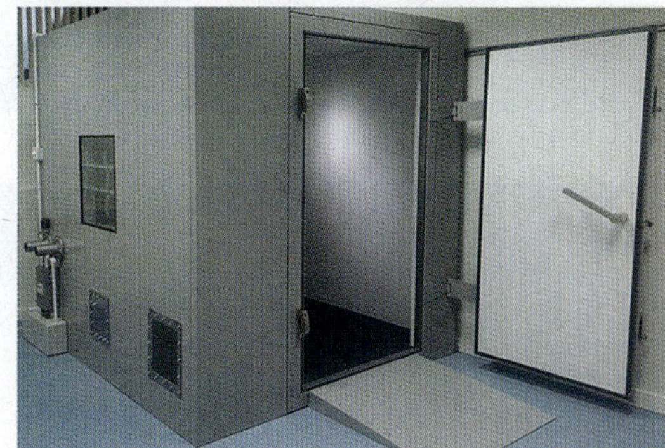

Fig. EEG room

46. Ans. (c) Picture archiving and communication system
[Ref. Grainger & Allison's Diagnostic Radiology Essentials by Grant, 5/e p185]

47. Ans. (a) Perihepatic; (b) Perisplenic; (d) Pelvic; (e) Pericardial

[Ref. Ultrasound in Emergency Care by Brooks, 1/e p 27-28]

- Guidelines for **FAST examination** have been published by the American Institute of Ultrasound in Medicine (AIUM) and the American College of Emergency Physicians (ACEP)
- Primary FAST examination classically includes the subxiphoid window of the heart to denote pericardial fluid
- Indications for FAST include evaluation of the torso for free fluid suggesting injury to the peritoneal, pericardial, and pleural cavities, particularly in cases of trauma
- FAST examination may be used to evaluate the lungs for pneumothorax

48. Ans. (a) Superior to CT scan; (d) Anatomy and physiology function test; (e) Measures response to cancer therapy

[Ref. Radiology by Bhargava, 4/e p452]

Positron emission tomography (PET)

- Agent used: **18-Fluorodeoxyglucose** (Half life 110 minutes)
- Uses:
  - Localization of cerebral tumors
  - Tumor classification as benign or malignant
  - Differentiate post-treatment recurrence and radiation necrosis
  - Evaluation of epileptic foci, dementia
  - Evaluation of cardiac function, tissue viability
- Disadvantage: Exposure to ionizing radiation

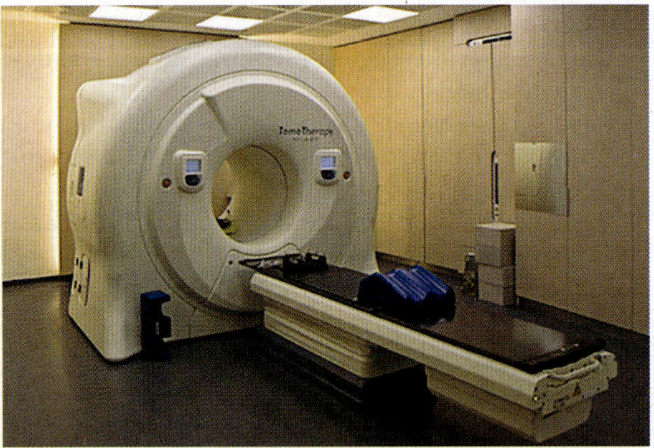

Fig. PET scan

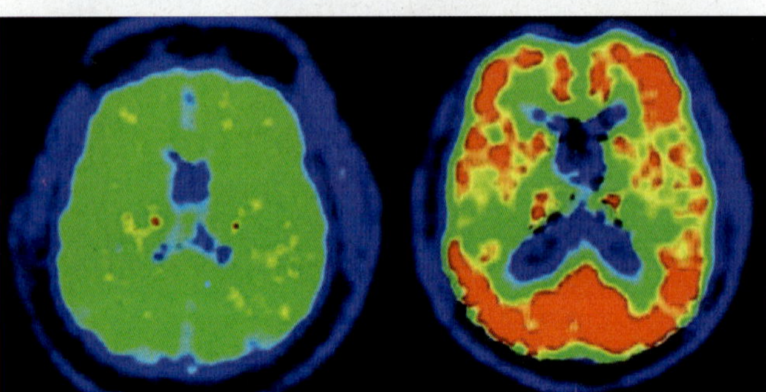

Fig. PET scan image

49. Ans. (a) X-rays

[Ref. Errors in Radiology by Pinto, 1/e p273]

- All glasses (irrespective of lead content) are visible on X-rays
- Best radiological modality to evaluate a glass splinter: X-rays

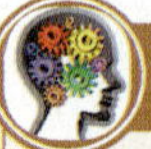

Also Remember

- Best modality to evaluate glass splinter in a child: Surgical exploration

50. Ans. (c) X-ray crystallography

[Ref. Crystallography, National Academy of Sciences, p6]

Evaluation of biomolecular structure

- X-ray crystallography (best modality)
- Nuclear magnetic resonance (NMR)
- Cryoelectron microscopy
- Electron tomography

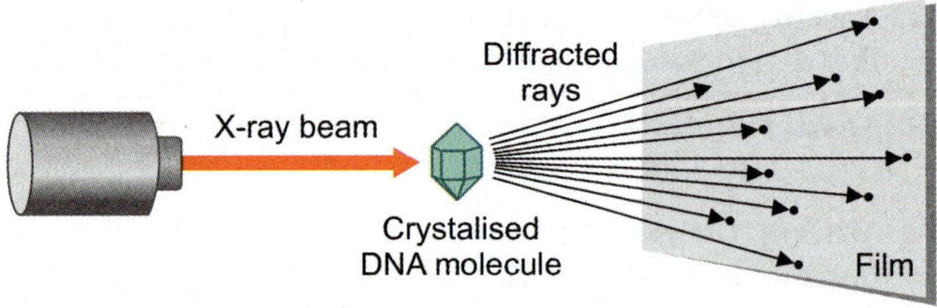

Fig. X-ray Crystallography

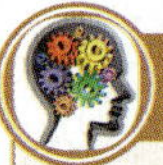

Also Remember

X-ray crystallography

- Unique in evaluation of structure of biomolecules
- Allows visualization of complexes between proteins and their substrates

51. Ans. (c) Subcarinal nodes

[Ref. Gray's Anatomy, 41/e p969]

- Bronchoscopy allows the direct visualization of the Vocal cords, trachea and major airways as far as the first division of the subsegmental airway

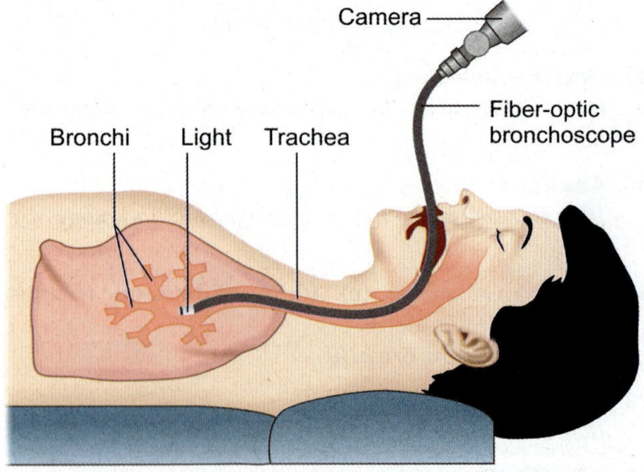

Fig. Bronchoscopy

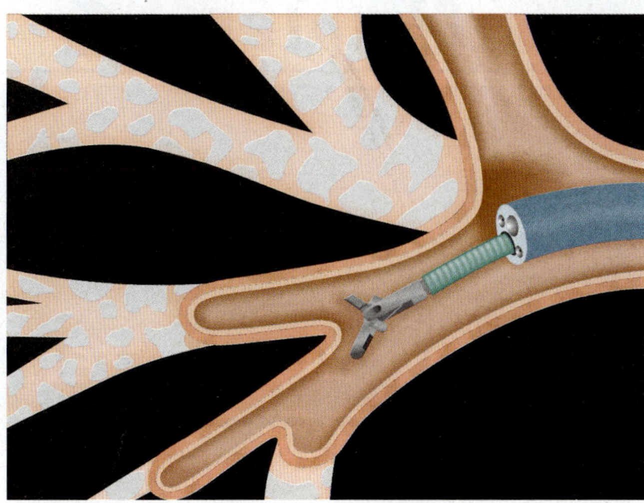

Fig. Flexible bronchoscopy

52. Ans. (a) Pulmonary arteriography
[Ref. Pleural Diseases by Lee, 2/e p401]

53. Ans. (b) Pelvis
[Ref. Musculoskeletal Imaging by Disler, 4/e p157]

Judet's View

- Judet's view: Centering the X-ray beam a little further downwards on the femoral head to obtain oblique views in Acetabular fractures
- Computed tomography (CT) is now used universally for detection and evaluation of pelvic fractures, and Judet's views are rarely requested

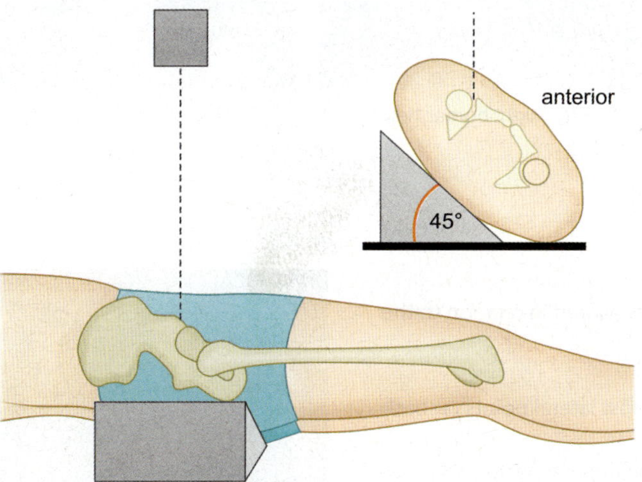

Fig. Judet's View

54. Ans. (b) Sound waves
[Ref. Color Doppler Sonography by Kurjak, 1/e Fig 1.3]

Harmonic Imaging

- Sound waves contain many competent sound frequencies
- Harmonics: Components whose frequencies are integral multiples of lowest frequency (fundamental or first-harmonic)
- Harmonic imaging: Transmitting at frequency 'f' and receiving at '2f' (second harmonic)
  - Use: Clearer artifact-free images in patients difficult to scan

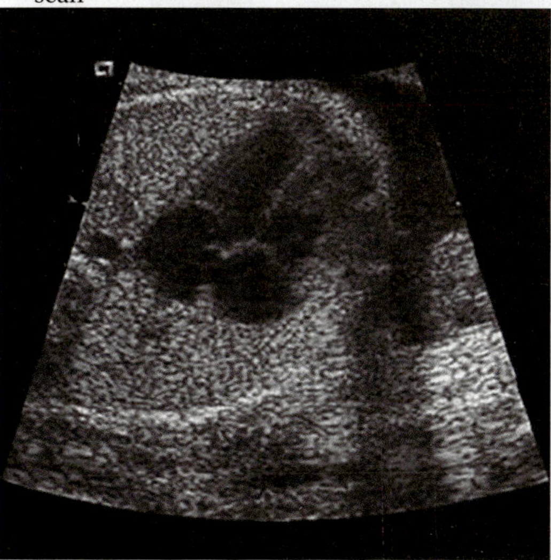

Fig. Tissue harmonic imaging

55. Ans. (b) 100 rad
[Ref. Dental Assistant by Anderson, 7/e p555]

Unit Conversions in Radiation

- 1 Roentgen = 1 rad = 1 rem
- 1 Gray = 100 rad
- 1 Sievert = 100 rem

56. Ans. (c) Typical carcinoid
[Ref. PET and PET-CT in Oncology by Oehr, 1/e p160]

False Positive Findings in FDG-PET scan

- Inflammatory cells, such as neutrophil and activated macrophages at the site of inflammation or infection show increased FDG accumulation
- Active granulomatous processes, other infectious conditions and active fibrotic lesions have also been reported to show increased FDG accumulation and cause false-positive PET scans for malignancy
  - Tuberculoma and tuberculous lymphadenopathy
  - Sarcoidosis
  - Cryptococcosis
  - Paragonimiasis
  - Other infectious conditions: abscesses, pneumocystis carinii infection
  - Radiation fibrosis
  - Sclerosing hemangioma
  - Granulation tissue around tumors

False Negative Findings in FDG-PET scan

- FDG PET is metabolic imaging using the activity of lesion; tumors with low activity are well-known major causes of false negative findings
  - Bronchioloalveolar carcinoma (BAC)
  - Small size lesion
  - Metastatic lung nodule of extrapulmonary neoplasm
  - Chemotherapy related factor
  - Carcinoid tumor
  - Hyperglycemia

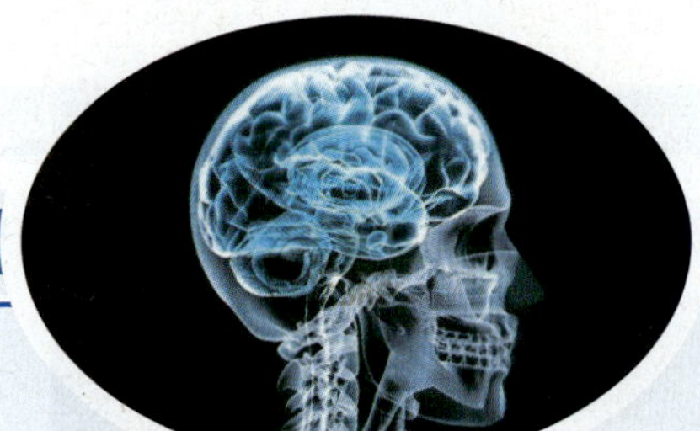

Chapter 2

Cardiovascular System

THEORETICAL CONCEPTS

II A. HEART BORDERS ON CHEST X-RAYS

- *Right border of heart (on Chest X-ray – PA View) is formed by:*[Q]
  - Right atrium
  - Superior vena cava
  - Inferior vena cava
- *Left border of heart (on Chest X-ray – PA View) is formed by:*
  - Subclavian artery
  - Aortic knuckle
  - Pulmonary artery segment
  - Left atrial appendage
  - Right ventricle
  - Left ventricle

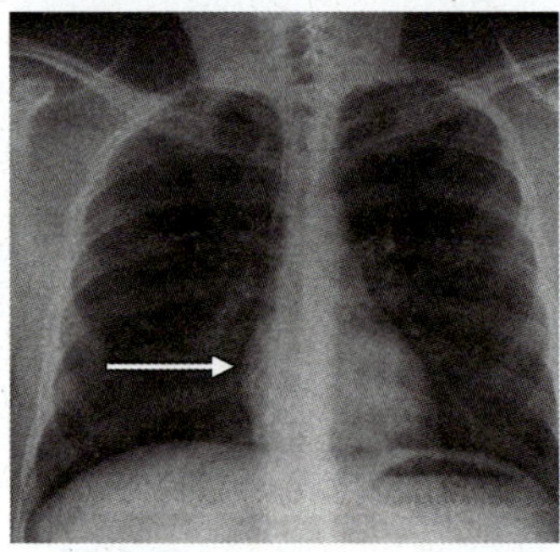

Fig. Right border heart

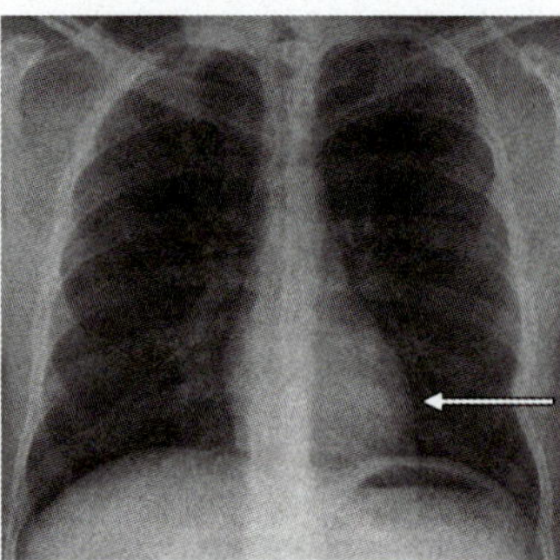

Fig. Left border heart

Topper's Edge

Cardiothoracic Ratio (CTR)

- Heart size is not assessed by an absolute measurement, but rather is measured in relation to the total thoracic width - the Cardiothoracic ratio (CTR)
- CTR = Cardiac Width: Thoracic Width
  - Cardiac size: Measured by drawing vertical parallel lines down the most lateral points on each side of the heart, and measuring between them
  - Thoracic width: Measured by drawing vertical parallel lines down the inner aspect of the widest points of the rib cage, and measuring between them
- **Normal CTR $\leq$ 0.5**[Q]
- CTR > 0.5 indicate Cardiac enlargement

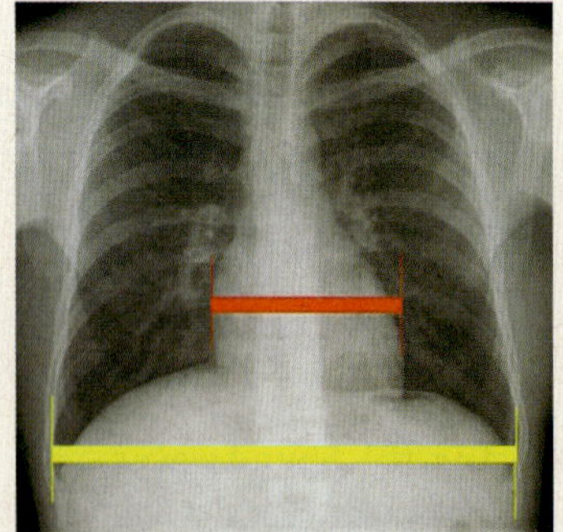

Fig. Cardiothoracic ratio

II B. COARCTATION OF AORTA

- *'Figure of 3 appearance'* of aortic knuckle[Q]
- **Inferior rib notching (3rd – 9th ribs)**

Topper's Edge

COARCTATION OF AORTA (COA)

Types of COA

- Infantile (Pre-ductal) form:
  - Diffuse hypoplasia/narrowing of aorta from just distal to the brachiocephalic artery to the level of ductus arteriosus
  - Blood supply to Descending aorta is via Patent ductus arteriosus.
- Adult (Juxta-ductal/Post-ductal/Middle aortic) form:
  - Short segment of abrupt stenosis of Post-ductal aorta
  - Due to thickening of Aortic media and typically occurs just distal to Ligamentum arteriosum (a remnant of the ductus arteriosus)

Associations of COA

- Cardiac associations: **Bicuspid aortic valve (MC association[Q])**, Ventricular septal defect, Truncus arteriosus, Transposition of the great arteries, Mitral valve defects (Hypoplastic valve, Parachute valve, Abnormal papillary muscles), Patent ductus arteriosus
- Non-cardiac associations: Intracranial berry aneurysms, Spinal scoliosis
- Recognized syndromic associations: Shone syndrome, PHACE syndrome, Turner syndrome

Plain Radiograph

- **Figure of 3 sign** (E-sign[Q]): Contour abnormality of the aorta
- **Inferior rib notching**: Roesler sign **(Single best sign[Q])**

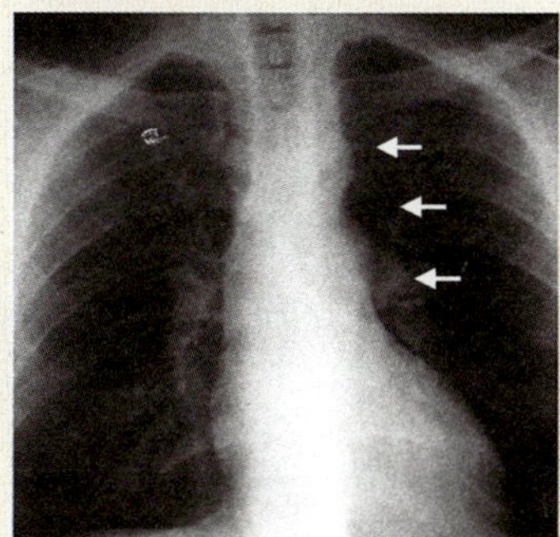

Fig. Reverse 3 sign

Fig. Inferior rib notching

II C. EBSTEIN'S ANOMALY

- ❑ Atrialisation of right ventricle
- ❑ ***'Box-shaped' heart*** [Q]

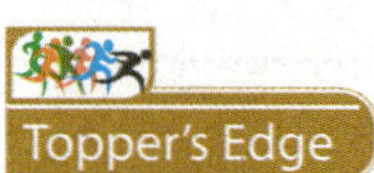

Topper's Edge

EBSTEIN'S ANOMALY (EA)

Description of EA

- An uncommon congenital cardiac anomaly
- Variable developmental anomaly of tricuspid valve[Q]
- **MC cause of congenital tricuspid regurgitation[Q]**

Main abnormality in EA[Q]

- Abnormal tricuspid valve (particularly septal and posterior leaflets), which is displaced apically into the right ventricle, resulting in '**Atrialisation of parts of ventricle**' above the valve
- Concurrent tricuspid regurgitation with/without stenosis

Associations of EA

- **Chromosomal anomalies: Trisomy 13, Trisomy 21, Turner syndrome**
- Congenital heart lesions (ASD)
- Wolff-Parkinson-White syndrome
- Maternal lithium carbonate ingestion

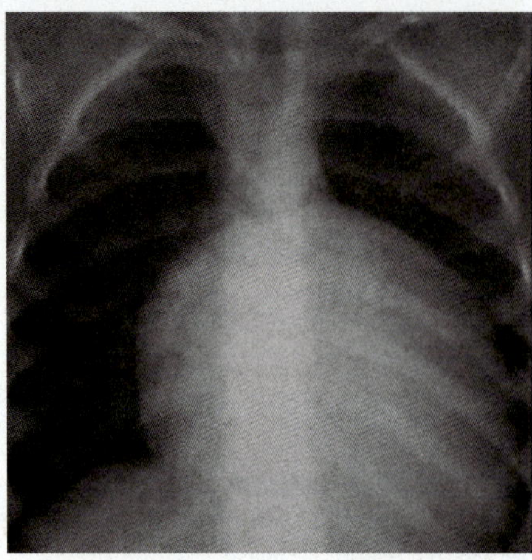

Fig. Box-shaped heart

II D. EISENMENGER'S COMPLEX

- Pulmonary plethora
- Normal sized heart

Topper's Edge

Eisenmenger's Syndrome

- A complication of an uncorrected high-flow, high-pressure congenital heart anomaly leading to chronic pulmonary arterial hypertension and shunt reversal
- Underlying causes[Q]:
  - **Ventricular septal defect (MC[Q])** (Known as **Eisenmenger complex 5**)
  - Atrioventricular septal defect
  - Patent ductus arteriosus
- Pathology:
  - Arteriolar medial hypertrophy
  - Intimal proliferation and fibrosis
  - Plexiform lesions and necrotising arteritis
  - Capillary and arteriolar occlusion

II E. EMPHYSEMA LUNGS

- **Barrel-shaped chest**
- Flattened diaphragm

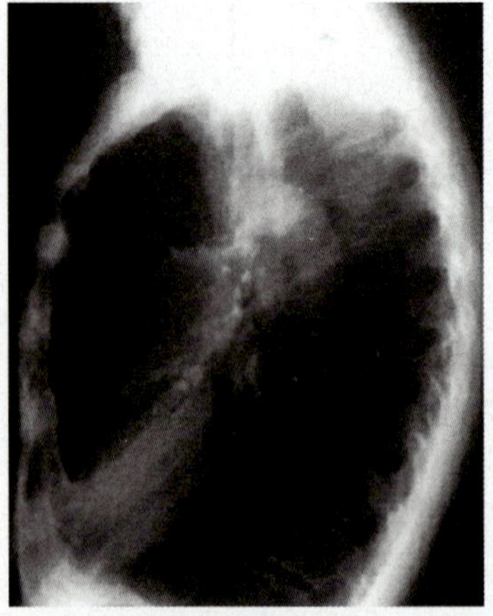

Fig. Barrel-chest

II F. PERICARDIAL EFFUSION

- Cardiomegaly with no particular chamber enlargement
- ***Money-bag/Leather-bottle/Flask-shaped heart*** [Q]
- Clear lung fields
- Investigation of choice: Echocardiography (Can detect less than 15 mL) [Q]

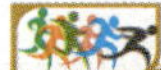

Topper's Edge

Pericardial Effusion

- Normal pericardial sac: **30–50 mL of fluid**[Q]
- Pericardial effusions: Excess fluid collects in the pericardial space
- Underlying causes:
  - Idiopathic
  - Inflammatory: Post myocardial infarction (Dressler syndrome), Connective tissue disorders
  - Infections: Viral, Bacterial (TB)
  - Other causes: Post-surgical, Trauma, Radiotherapy, Malignancy, Hyothyroidism
- Radiology:
  - Leather bottle/Water bottle heart[Q]: Globular enlargement of cardiac shadow
  - **Oreo cookie sign**[Q] (Appearance of pericardial effusion on lateral radiographs of chest): A vertical opaque line (pericardial fluid) separate a vertical lucent line directly behind sternum (pericardial fat) anteriorly from a similar lucent vertical lucent line (epicardial fat) posteriorly
  - Widening of the subcarinal angle

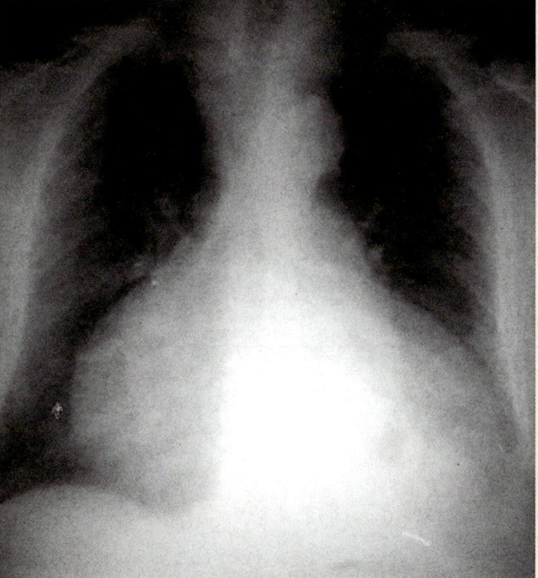

Fig. Leather bottle heart

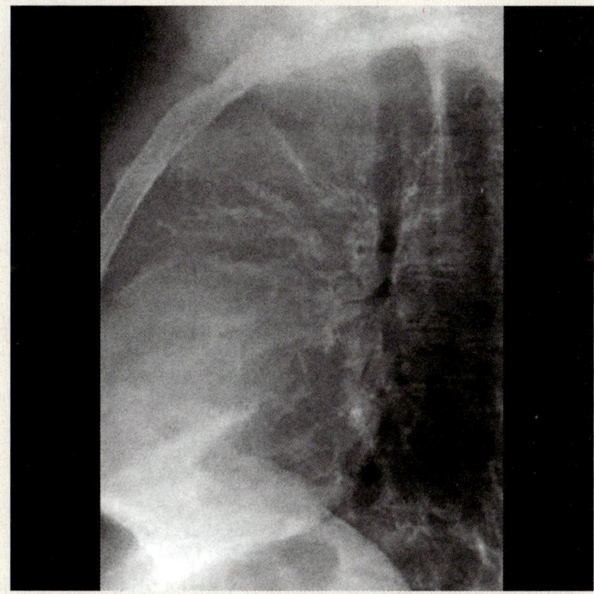

Fig. Oreo cookie sign

II G. TETRALOGY OF FALLOT

- Components:
  - Ventricular septal defect
  - Aortic root overrides VSD
  - Right ventricle hypertrophy
  - Infundibular stenosis
- ***'Boot-shaped heart'*** or ***'Cor-en-sabot heart'*** [Q]
  - Normal size heart
  - Pulmonary oligaemia

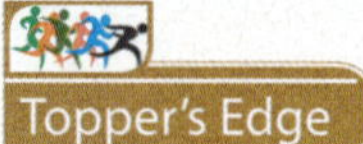

Topper's Edge

TETRALOGY OF FALLOT (TOF)

Components of TOF[Q]

- Second MC cyanotic congenital heart condition
  - Ventricular septal defect
  - Right ventricular outflow obstruction (Infundibular stenosis, Hypoplastic pulmonary valve annulus, Bicuspid pulmonary valve and/or Hypoplasia of pulmonary artery)
  - Overriding aorta
  - Right ventricular hypertrophy

Associations of TOF[Q]

Cardiovascular associations	Other associations
Right-sided aortic arch	Congenital lobar emphysema
Pulmonary hypoplasia, atresia	DiGeorge syndrome
Atrial septal defect	Fetal rubella syndrome
Patent ductus arteriosus	Prune-belly syndrome
Coronary artery anomalies	Tracheoesophageal fistula
Persistent left-sided SVC	VACTERL association

Chest Radiograph: Boot-shaped heart[Q]

- Upturned cardiac apex due to right ventricular hypertrophy and concave pulmonary arterial segment

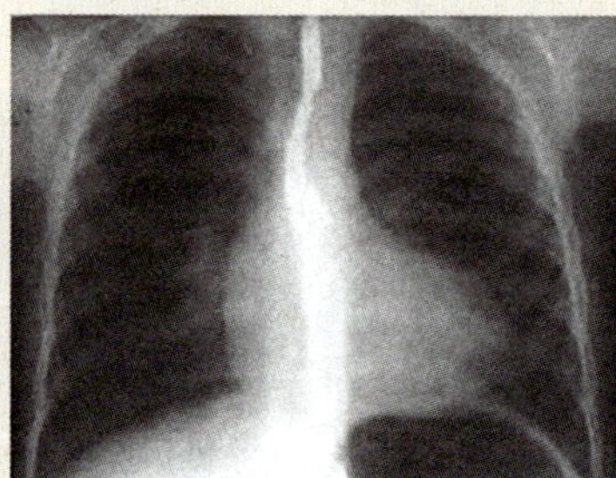

Fig. Boot-shaped heart

II H. TOTAL ANOMALOUS PULMONARY VENOUS DRAINAGE

- ***'Figure of 8 heart'*** or ***'Snowman heart'*** [Q]
- Normal to small heart with fluid in lungs

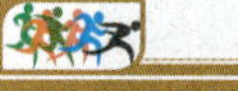

Topper's Edge

Total Anomalous Pulmonary Venous Return (TAPVR)

- Description of TAPVR:
  - Cyanotic congenital heart anomaly with an abnormal drainage anatomy of the entire pulmonary venous system
  - All systemic and pulmonary venous blood enters the right atrium and nothing drains into the left atrium
  - A right-to-left shunt is required for survival and is usually via Patent Foramen ovale (More commonly) or atrial septal defect
- Underlying pathology:
  - Embryological failure of pulmonary venous development
  - Persistent patency of primitive systemic veins
- Classification of TAVPR
  - **Type I: Supracardiac (MC type[Q])**
  - Type II: Cardiac
  - Type III: Infracardiac
  - Type IV: Mixed pattern
- Associations of TAPVR[Q]:
  - Asplenia
  - Thoracic lymphangiectasia

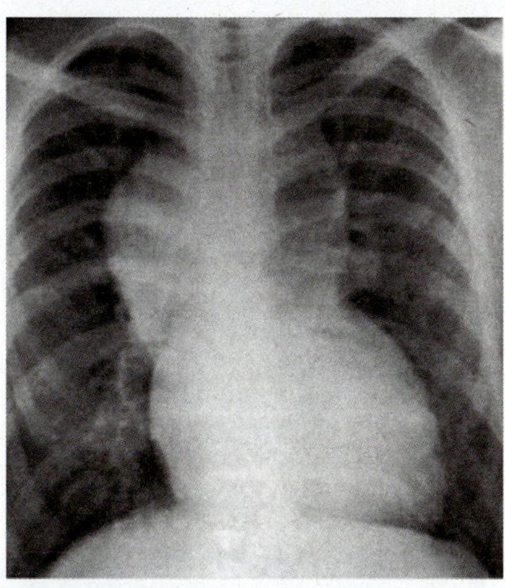

Figure of 8 heart
(Snowman heart)

II I. FEW IMPORTANT CARDIOVASCULAR SYSTEM RADIOLOGY FEATURES

- *Shoe-man Boot-shaped heart* ***(Cor-en sabot)***: Tetralogy of Fallot
- ***'Figure of 3'*** *appearance of aortic knuckle*: Coarctation of aorta
- ***Money-bag****/Leather-bottle/Flask-shaped heart*: Pericardial effusion[Q]
- *Banana-shaped left ventricle*: Hypertrophic cardiomyopathy
- ***'Egg-on-side' appearance***: Transposition of great arteries (TGA)[Q]
- *'Snowman'/* ***'Figure of 8'*** *appearance*: Total anomalous pulmonary venous drainage (TAPVC)
- *Hilar dance (Fluoroscopy)*: Atrial septal defect[Q]
- ***'Pruned-tree'*** *appearance*: Pulmonary arterial hypertension[Q]
- *Stag-antler's sign*: Mitral stenosis

II J. KEY SIGNS/FEATURES IN CARDIOVASCULAR SYSTEM RADIOLOGY

- **Box-shaped heart**[Q]: Tricuspid atresia, Ebstein anomaly
- Calcification of Ascending aorta [Q]: Aortitis
- **Cor-en-sabot**/Boot-shaped heart [Q]: Tetralogy of Fallot
- Cor-triatum [Q]: Pulmonary vein obstruction
- Dock's sign (Bilateral inferior notching of 3–8th ribs) [Q]: Coarctation of aorta
- Double atrial shadow [Q]: Left atrial enlargement
- **Egg in cup heart**[Q]: Constrictive pericarditis
- Egg-on-side heart[Q]: Transposition of Great arteries
- Ground glass ventricular septum [Q]: Hypertrophic obstructive cardiomyopathy
- Obliteration of Retrosternal clear space [Q]: Right atrial enlargement
- **Kerley B lines**[Q]: Pulmonary venous hypertension (19–24 mm Hg)
- Kerley B lines (Interlobar septal edema) [Q]: Congestive heart failure
- **Pruned-tree appearance** of pulmonary circulation [Q]: Pulmonary artery hypertension
- Pulmonary ossicles (Bone formation) [Q]: Pulmonary venous hypertension (Long standing)
- **Reverse figure-of-3**/Double bulge/ E-sign [Q]: Coarctation of aorta
- Small aortic knob [Q]: Atrial septal defect
- **Snowman/Figure-of-8**/Cottage loaf sign [Q]: Total anomalous pulmonary venous connection
- Spring water cyst [Q]: Pleuro-pericardial cyst
- Stag-antler/Inverted moustache/ Hands-up sign [Q]: Pulmonary venous hypertension (1st sign)
- Tear-drop heart [Q]: Chronic emphysema
- Triangular heart [Q]: Constrictive pericarditis
- Water-bottle/Flask-shaped heart [Q]: Pericardial effusion

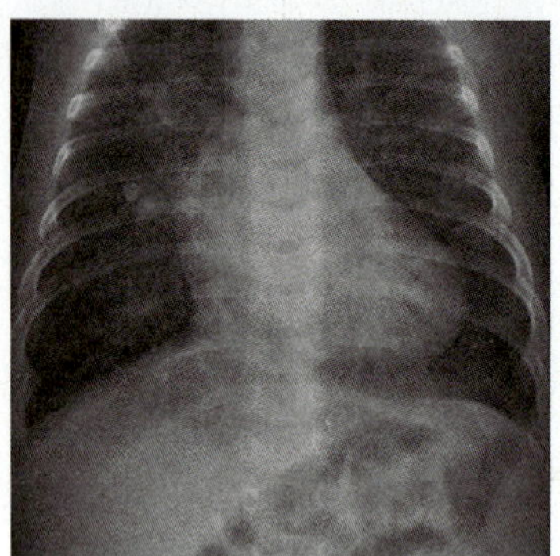

Fig. Egg on side appearance

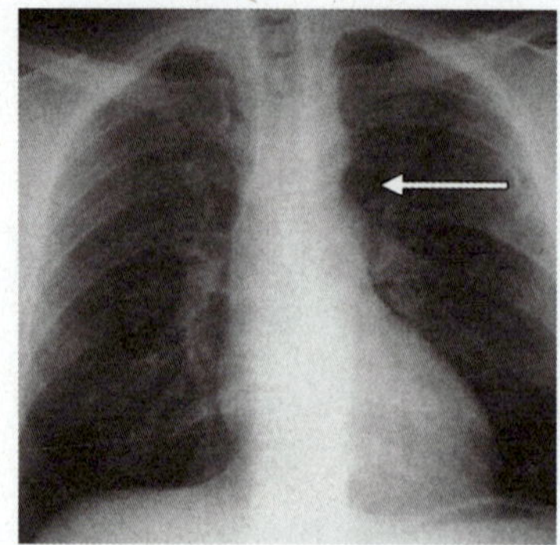

Fig. Figure of 3

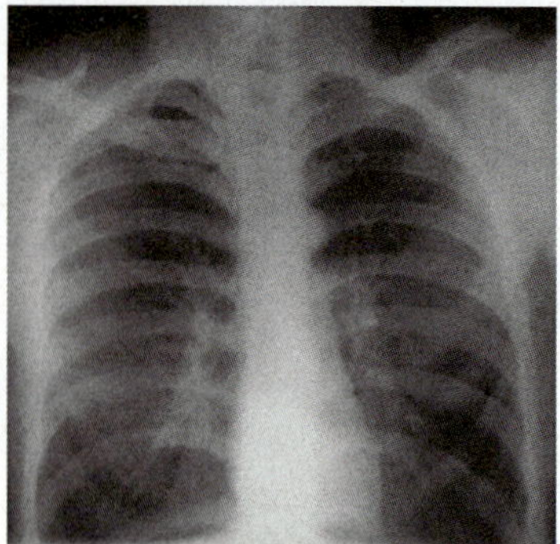

Fig. Tear drop heart

IMAGE-BASED QUESTIONS

1. Typical appearance of Ribs (Arrows) as shown in X-ray Photograph is due to ***[Recent Question 2012, 2014]***

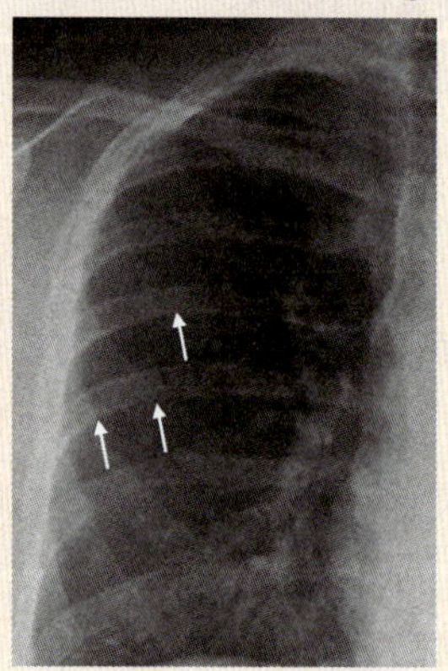

a. SLE b. Rheumatoid arthritis
c. Coarctation of aorta d. Scleroderma

2. Typical shape of heart (Arrows) is in ***[Recent Question 2013]***

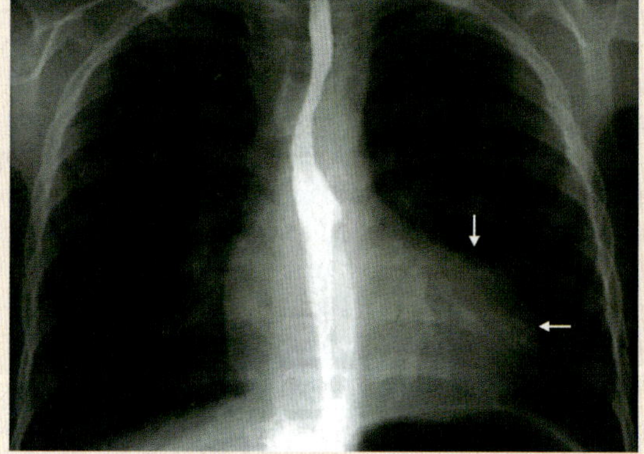

a. Ebstein's anomaly b. TAPVC
c. Tetralogy of Fallot d. Atrial septal defect

3. Condition (Arrows) shown in Photograph is characteristic of ***[Recent Question 2013]***

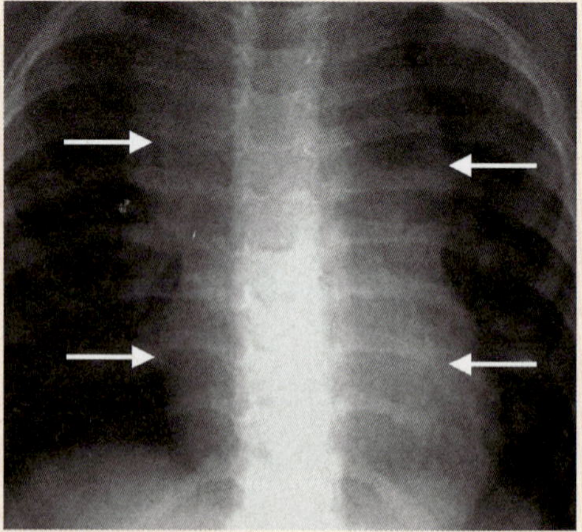

a. Pericardial effusion b. Ebstein's anomaly
c. Constrictive pericarditis d. TAPVC

4. Investigation of Choice for Condition (Arrow) shown in Photograph is

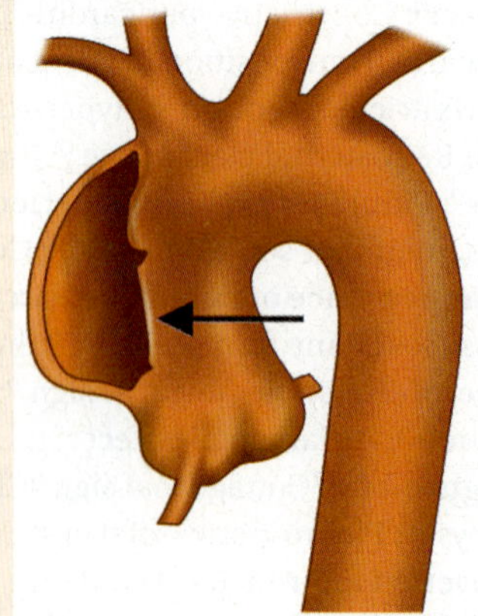

a. X-ray b. USG
c. CT scan d. MRI

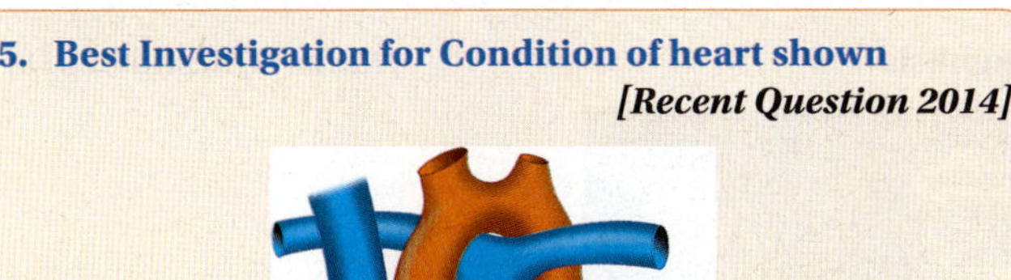

5. Best Investigation for Condition of heart shown ***[Recent Question 2014]***

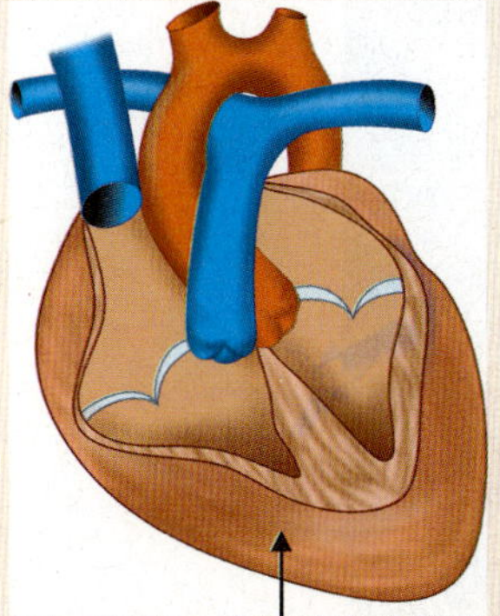

a. Plain X-ray b. CT scan
c. Echocardiography d. MRI scan

6. Condition shown in Photograph is due to ***[Recent Question 2012, 2013]***

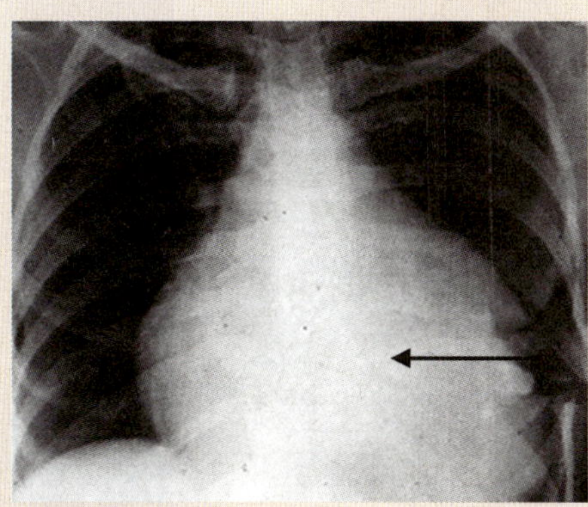

a. Patent ductus arteriosus b. Pericardial effusion
c. Constrictive pericarditis d. Chronic emphysema

7. Sign shown (Arrow) in Photograph is seen in

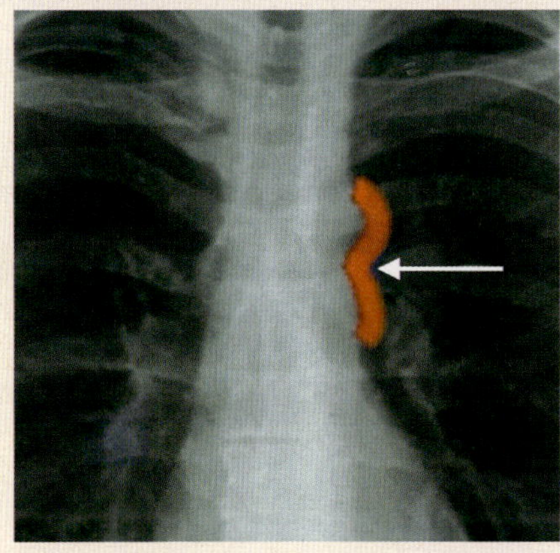

a. Tetralogy of Fallot b. Ebstein's anomaly
c. TAPVC d. Coarctation of Aorta

8. Condition (Arrow) shown in Photograph is best detected by ***[Recent Question 2012]***

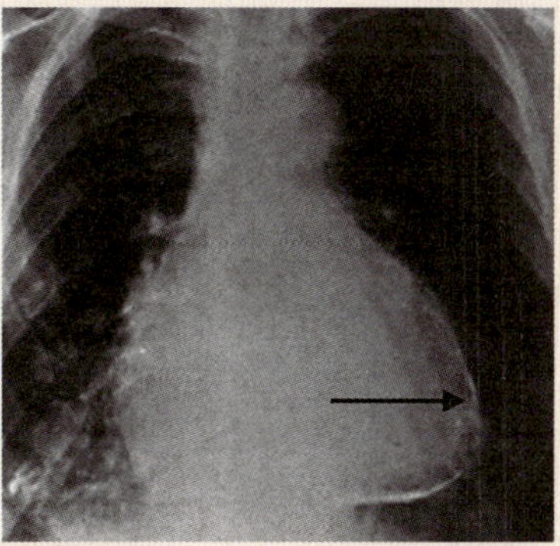

a. USG b. CT scan
c. MRI scan
d. Trans-esophageal cardiography

9. Structure (Arrow) shown in Normal X-ray Photograph is ***[Recent Question 2012]***

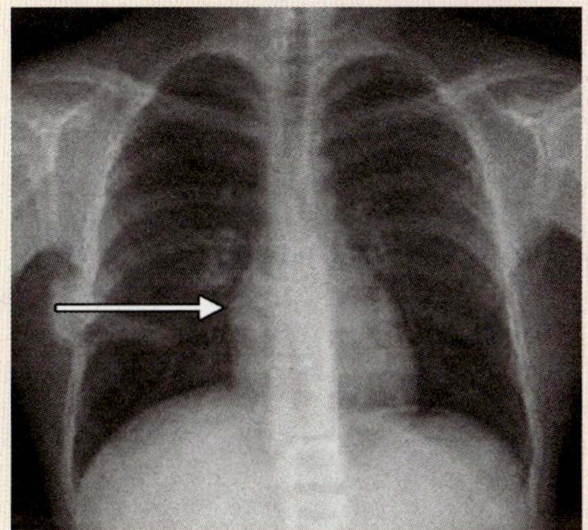

a. Right atrium b. Right ventricle
c. Left atrium d. Left ventricle

10. DSA Angiography was carried out on a patient in a Hospital. Image is given below. Make a diagnosis. ***[AIIMS November 2017]***

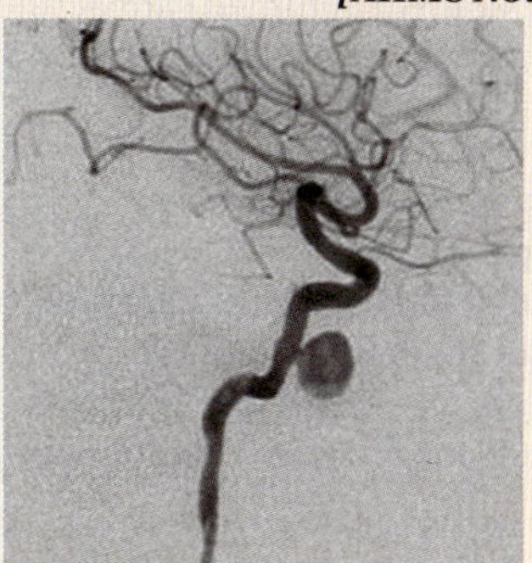

a. Angiofibroma tumor
b. Carotid cavernous fistula
c. Multiple hemangiomas
d. Pseudoaneurysm of Internal carotid artery

11. CT Thorax of a patient is given below. Make a most probable diagnosis ***[Recent Question 2018]***

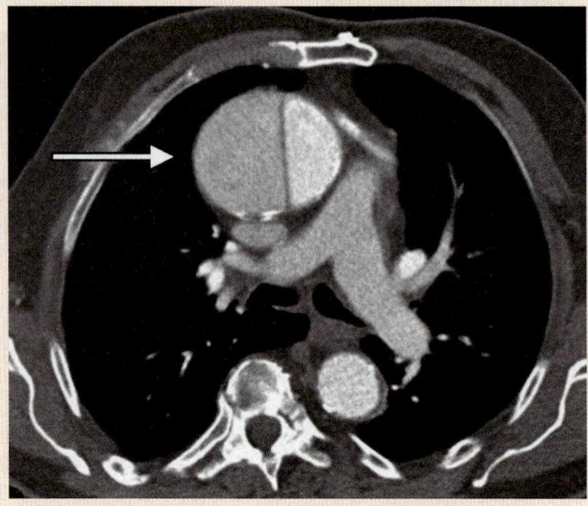

a. Atherosclerosis
b. Cystic fibrosis
c. Aortic aneurysm
d. Aortic dissection

ANSWERS WITH EXPLANATIONS OF IBQs

1. Ans. (c) Coarctation of aorta *[Ref. Sumer K Sethi, 5/e p42]*

Inferior Rib Notching

- Enlarged collateral vessels:
  - Coarctation of aorta
  - Takayasu disease
  - Blacock-Taussig shunt
  - SVC obstruction
  - AV malformation
  - Interrupted aortic arch
- Neurogenic tumors:
  - Schwannoma
  - Neurofibromtosis-1

2. Ans. (c) Tetralogy of Fallot *[Ref. Sumer K Sethi, 5/e p44]*

Boot-Shaped Heart (Cor-en-Sabot)

- Description: An upturned cardiac apex due to right ventricular hypertrophy and concave pulmonary arterial segment
- Seen in: Tetralogy of Fallot

3. Ans. (d) TAPVC *[Ref. Sumer K Sethi, 5/e p44]*

Snowman (Figure-of-8) Heart

- Description:
  - Head of the snowman: Paratracheal shadow on the right is the prominent SVC and on the left is the vertical vein, Innominate vessel lies in the midline above base of heart
  - Body of Snowman: Rest of the heart
- Seen in: Total anomalous pulmonary venous return/connection (TAPVC)

4. Ans. (d) MRI *[Ref. Sumer K Sethi, 5/e p46]*

- Investigation of choice for Aortic dissection: MRI

5. Ans. (c) Echocardiography *[Ref. Sumer K Sethi, 5/e p39]*

- Most sensitive investigation for Pleural effusion: Echocardiography
- It can detect even 15 mL of fluid

6. Ans. (b) Pericardial effusion *[Ref. Sumer K Sethi, 5/e p39]*

Money Bag/Leather Bottle/Flask-Shaped Heart

- Description:
  - Typically the effusion has accumulated over many weeks to months and the pericardium has gradually stretched
  - Fluid, often measuring a liter or more, causes the pericardium to sag, mimicking an old-fashioned water bottle sitting on the bench
- Seen in: Pericardial effusion

7. Ans. (d) Coarctation of Aorta *[Ref. Sumer K Sethi, 5/e p42]*

- Description: Formed by Pre-stenotic dilatation of the aortic arch and left subclavian artery, indentation at the Coarctation site (also known as the **"tuck"**), and Post-stenotic dilatation of the descending aorta
- Seen in: Coarctation of aorta

8. Ans. (b) CT scan *[Ref. MRI and CT of Cardiovascular System by Higgins, 2/e p137]*

- CT is the best method for depiction of pericardial calcification, a finding suggestive of constrictive pericarditis

9. Ans. (a) Right atrium *[Ref. Interpretation of Chest X-ray by Balachandran, 1/e p19]*

- Last contour on the right side of the heart is the right atrium.

10. Ans. (d) Pseudoaneurysm of Internal carotid artery *[Ref. Mastery of Surgery by Fischer, 5/e p1999]*

- Blunt trauma most often causes intimal tears and thrombosis with ensuing carotid occlusion
- If there is extensive disruption, it may lead to formation of a pseudoaneurysm; it occurs most commonly in Internal carotid artery
- More than 70% of these injuries are the result of motor vehicle collisions
- Penetrating injuries to the carotid artery disrupt all layers of the arterial wall and thus lead to late formation of a pseudoaneurysm

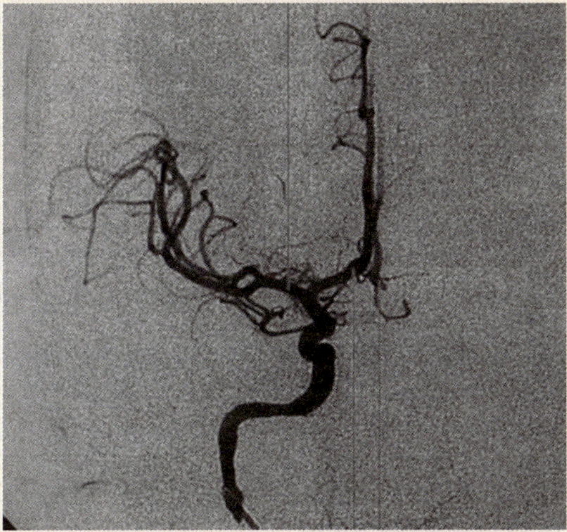

Fig. DSA Angiogram of ICA (Normal)

11. Ans. (d) Aortic dissection *[Ref. Computed Tomography of the Chest by Godwin, 1/e p27]*

CT findings in Aortic Dissection

- Splitting of the aorta into two or more contrast-filled channels with intervening intimal flaps
- Displaced intimal calcifications
- Irregular aortic enlargement and compression of the true lumen
- Variable thrombosis, particularly of the false lumen
- Pericardial, mediastinal, or pleural hematoma

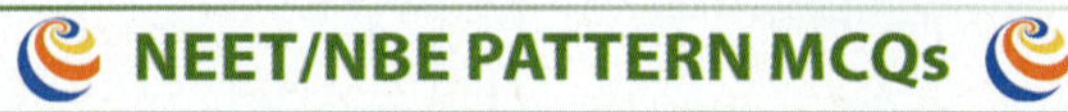

NEET/NBE PATTERN MCQs

1. ‘*Figure of eight*’ of heart on skiagram is representative of *[NBE FMGE September 2010]*
   a. Coarctation of aorta
   b. Total anomalous pulmonary venous drainage
   c. Emphysema lungs
   d. Eisenmenger's complex

2. Egg on side appearances is seen in *[Recent Question 2017, NBE DNB 2009]*
   a. TOF b. TAPVC
   c. Uncorrected TGA d. Truncus arteriosus

3. Following are radiological changes in Tetralogy of Fallot, except *[NBE DNB 1997]*
   a. Prominent cardiac apex
   b. Cardiomegaly
   c. Prominent pulmonary trunk
   d. Normal right atrial shadow

4. Right border of heart on a Chest X-ray is formed by *[NBE FMGE September 2010]*
   a. Right atrium
   b. Right atrium and right auricle
   c. Right atrium, Superior vena cava, Inferior vena cava
   d. Right atrium, Right ventricle, Superior vena cava, Inferior vena cava

5. X-ray findings of LVF are all except *[NBE DNB 2009]*
   a. Cardiomegaly
   b. Kerley B lines
   c. Diversion of blood to upper lobe
   d. Oligaemic lung fields

6. A vascular ring causing external airway compression can be diagnosed by *[NBE DNB 2010]*
   a. CT
   b. PET CT
   c. MRI
   d. Angiography of aortic and pulmonary circulation

7. Right margin of Cardiac silhouette on chest X-ray is not formed by *[Recent Question 2017, NBE FMGE September 2008, September 2010]*
   a. Right atrium b. Aorta
   c. Superior vena cava d. Inferior vena cava

8. Rib notching is seen in all, except *[NBE DNB 2009]*
   a. Blalock-Taussig shunt
   b. Pulmonary atresia with large VSD
   c. Waterston Cooley's shunt
   d. Aortic disruption

9. Carotid artery stenosis screening in-vivo choice *[Recent Question 2012]*
   a. USG b. CT
   c. MRI d. Doppler

10. Rib notching is a feature of *[NBE FMGE September 2012]*
    a. Tuberculosis b. Sarcoidosis
    c. Coarctation of aorta d. Osteomalacia

11. What is not seen on chest X-ray in pulmonary artery hypertension? *[Recent Question 2012, 2013]*
    a. Enlargement of central arteries
    b. Peripheral pruning
    c. Narrowing of central arteries
    d. None

12. Which view is taken for aortic window? *[Recent Question 2012]*
    a. AP b. LAO
    c. RAO d. LPO

13. Which test is performed to detect reversible myocardial ischemia? *[Recent Question 2012]*
    a. Coronary angiography b. MUGA scan
    c. Thallium scan d. Resting echocardiography

14. ‘Box-shaped heart’ is seen in *[NBE FMGE September 2005]*
    a. ASD b. PDA
    c. VSD d. Ebstein's anomaly

15. Flask-shaped heart is seen in *[Recent Question 2012, 2013]*
    a. Ebstein's anomaly b. Pericardial effusion
    c. TOF d. TAPVC

16. Gold-standard for diagnosis of arterial occlusive disease? *[UPSC 2009]*
    a. Duplex ultrasound blood flow detection
    b. Duplex imaging
    c. Treadmill
    d. Digital subtraction arteriography (DSA)

17. ‘Shoe-man’ shaped heart is seen in *[NBE FMGE September 2005]*
    a. ASD b. VSD
    c. TOF d. PDA

18. Snowman appearance on x-ray is seen in which cardiac pathology *[Recent Question 2012, 2013, 2017]*
    a. Fallot's tetralogy b. TAPVC
    c. TGA d. Ebstein's anomaly

19. Hilar dance on fluoroscopy is seen in *[NBE DNB 1997, 1999, 2004, 2005, 2007]*
    a. ASD b. TOF
    c. VSD d. TGV

20. Ground glass ventricular septum is seen in *[Recent Question 2012, 2013]*
    a. TOF b. HOCM
    c. TGA d. CHF

21. Right heart border is formed by all except *[Recent Question 2012, 2013]*
    a. SVC b. IVC
    c. Right atrium d. Left atrium

22. Pericardial effusion is best diagnosed by *[NBE FMGE September 2004, September 2011]*
    a. USG b. Angiography
    c. Gallium scan d. Echocardiography

23. Sign with patch of dullness beneath the angle of left scapula in a patient with pericardial effusion is named as *[Recent Question 2013]*
a. Carvallo's sign b. Ewart's sign
c. Homan's sign d. Hoffmann's sign

24. Best investigation for pericardial effusion is *[Recent Question 2013, 2015]*
a. MRI b. CT
c. X-ray d. Echocardiography

25. Which of the following causes rib notching on X-ray? *[Recent Question 2013]*
a. Coarctation of aorta
b. SVC occlusion
c. Modified Blalock-Taussing shunt
d. All of the above

26. Double shadow behind right atrium and straightening of left main bronchus indicates *[Recent Question 2013]*
a. Right atrium enlargement
b. Right ventricle enlargement
c. Left atrium enlargement
d. Left ventricle enlargement

27. Water bottle heart is seen in *[Recent Question 2013]*
a. PDA b. Chronic emphysema
c. Pericardial effusion d. Constrictive pericarditis

28. Snowman's heart is seen in *[Recent Question 2013]*
a. Pericardial effusion b. Ebstein's anomaly
c. TAPVC d. Constrictive pericarditis

29. Left atrial enlargement is seen in *[Recent Question 2013]*
a. Mitral stenosis b. Tricuspid regurgitation
c. AR d. None

30. For pericardial calcifications, which is the best investigation *[Recent Question 2013, 2015]*
a. MRI
b. Transesophageal echocardiography
c. USG
d. CT scan

31. Investigation of choice for DVT is *[Recent Question 2014, 2015]*
a. Doppler USG b. Angiography
c. CT scan d. MRI

32. First sign of Left atrial enlargement on Radiology is *[Recent Question 2015]*
a. Widening of carina
b. Double cardiac shadow
c. Displacement of left main bronchus
d. Pericardial effusion

33. Hockey-stick appearance in echocardiography is a feature of *[Recent Question 2016, UPSC CMS 2015]*
a. Mitral stenosis
b. Mitral incompetence
c. Aortic stenosis
d. Aortic regurgitation

HIGH YIELD MCQs

1. Hot spot in acute MI is seen in *[All India PGMEE 1998]*
a. Thallium b. Strontium
c. Tc99 Strontium Pyrophosphate
d. Gallium citrate

2. ASD is differentiated from VSD in an X-ray by *[All India PGMEE 2011]*
a. Normal left atrium b. Enlarged left atrium
c. Pulmonary congestion d. Aortic shadow

3. Most objective sign of identification of pulmonary plethora on a Chest X-ray is *[AIPGMEE 2011]*
a. Diameter of main pulmonary artery > 16 mm
b. Diameter of left pulmonary artery > 16 mm
c. Diameter of descending right pulmonary artery > 16 mm
d. Diameter of descending left pulmonary artery > 16 mm

4. Rib notching is found in *[PGI 2001]*
a. Neurofibromatosis b. Lymphangiomyomatosis
c. Aortic aneurysm d. Taussig-Bing operation
e. Aortic obstruction

5. True regarding radiological picture of Coarctation of aorta all except *[PGI 2004, WB PGMEE 2005]*
a. Involvement of upper two ribs
b. Bilateral
c. Inferior rib notching
d. Usually before 5 years of age
e. '3' sign

6. Inferior rib notching is seen in *[All India PGMEE 2008]*
a. Coarctation of aorta b. Rickets
c. ASD d. Multiple myeloma

7. In which of the following a 'Coeur en Sabot' shape of the heart is seen *[All India PGMEE 2000, All India PGMEE 2004]*
a. Tricuspid atresia
b. Ventricular septal defect
c. Transportation of great arteries
d. Tetralogy of Fallot

8. 'Snowman appearance' is seen in *[PGI 2009, AIIMS PGMEE 2008]*
a. Total anomalous pulmonary venous Connection
b. Ebstein's anomaly
c. Tetralogy of Fallot
d. VSD
e. Transposition of great vessel

9. 'Figure of 8' in chest X-ray is seen in *[Recent Question 2017, All India PGMEE 2000]*
a. Ebstein Anomaly
b. Total Anomalous pulmonary venous connection (TAPVC)
c. Tetralogy of Fallot
d. Transposition of great vessels

10. 'Flask shaped heart' is seen in following except *[PGI 1997]*
a. Ebstein's anomaly b. Pericardial effusion
c. TOF d. TAPVC

Radiodiagnosis and Radiotherapy

11. "Egg-on-side" appearance is seen in *[All India PGMEE 2010, AIIMS PGMEE 2008, PGI 2009]*
a. TOF b. Uncorrected TGV
c. TAPVC d. Constricted pericarditis

12. Left heart failure findings are all except *[AIIMS PGMEE 2009, AIIMS PGMEE 2010]*
a. Kerley B lines
b. Redistribution of blood vessels to apex (increased flow in upper lobe veins)
c. Oligaemic lung field (pulmonary oligaemia)
d. Cardiomegaly

13. All are seen on right side of cardiac shadow in X-ray chest PA view except *[AIIMS PGMEE 1991]*
a. Superior vena cava b. Right atrium
c. Ascending aorta d. Inferior vena cava

14. Base of heart is formed by *[PGI 2006]*
a. Right ventricle
b. Left ventricle
c. Left ventricle and right ventricle
d. Right atrium and right ventricle
e. Right atrium and left atrium

15. Left border of the heart in Chest X-ray is formed by *[PGI 2004]*
a. Pulmonary artery b. Pulmonary vein
c. Abdominal aorta d. Arch of aorta
e. Right ventricles

16. Right border of the heart in CXR is formed by *[PGI 2007]*
a. Pulmonary artery b. Superior vena cava
c. Right atrium d. Right ventricle

17. Pruning of Pulmonary arteries is seen in *[All India PGMEE 2009]*
a. Pulmonary hypertension
b. Chronic Bronchitis
c. Pulmonary infections
d. Pulmonary transplant

18. Earliest feature of pulmonary venous hypertension *[All India PGMEE 2008]*
a. Kerley B lines
b. Upper lobar diversion of vessels
c. Left atrial enlargement
d. Pleural effusion

19. Radiological features of Mitral stenosis are *[PGI 2009]*
a. Double contour of right heart border
b. Straightening of left heart border
c. Splaying of carinal angle
d. Prominent aortic knuckle
e. Kerley lines

20. Earliest Chest X-ray feature of left atrial enlargement is *[All India PGMEE 2008]*
a. Elevation of the left main bronchus
b. Double cardiac shadow
c. Widening of carina
d. Pericardial effusion

21. All are seen in congestive cardiac failure except *[All India PGMEE 2000]*
a. Kerley B lines
b. Prominent lower lobe vessel
c. Pleural Effusions
d. None

22. In all of the following increased cardiac silhouette sign is seen except *[MP PGMEE 2000]*
a. Tetralogy of Fallot b. Pericardial effusion
c. Aortic regurgitation d. Ebstein anomaly

23. If the Right cardiac silhouette is obliterated, it means the pathology involves *[AIIMS PGMEE 2008]*
a. Right lower lobe b. Right atrium
c. Right middle lobe d. Right ventricle

24. Investigation of choice for Pericardial effusion is *[AIIMS PGMEE 1993]*
a. CT scan b. MRI
c. Echocardiography d. X-ray Chest

25. Ground glass appearance is not seen in *[All India PGMEE 2001]*
a. Hyaline membrane disease
b. Left to right shunts
c. Pneumonia
d. Obstructive TAPVC

26. X-ray picture of VSD *[PGI 2004]*
a. Small Left ventricle b. Small Right ventricle
c. Dilated Left atrium d. Dilated pulmonary veins
e. Dilated pulmonary arteries

27. Investigation of choice in Aortic dissection is *[All India PGMEE 1996, AIIMS PGMEE 1997]*
a. USG
b. CT scan
c. MRI
d. Digital subtraction angiography

28. Best investigation for Cardiac tamponade is *[All India PGMEE 1994]*
a. 2-D Echocardiography
b. M-Mode Echocardiography
c. Real time Echocardiography
d. USG

29. Characteristic X-ray finding in ASD is *[AIIMS PGMEE 1993]*
a. Enlarged left ventricle b. Enlarged left atria
c. Pulmonary plethora d. PAH

30. Which of the following cause Rib-notching on Chest radiograph? *[All India PGMEE 2006]*
a. Bidirectional Glenn shunt
b. Modified Blalock-Taussing shunt
c. VC occlusion
d. Coarctation of aorta

31. Structure forming right border of heart *[Recent Question 2017, PGI 2006]*
a. SVC b. IVC
c. Right atrium d. Left atrium appendage
e. Pulmonary vessels

32. Obliteration of left cardiac shadow on PA view is due to *[AIIMS PGMEE 1991]*
a. Lingular lesion
b. Left hilar lymphadenopathy
c. Left lower lobe lesion
d. Left upper apical lobe lesion

33. Right side of mediastinum shadow is not formed by *[All India PGMEE 1995, All India PGMEE 1998]*
a. Superior vena cava b. Right innominates
c. Right atrium d. Right ventricle

34. Most recent advance in noninvasive cardiac output monitoring is use of *[AIIMS PGMEE 2002]*
a. PA catheter
b. Thermodilution technique
c. Echocardiography
d. Electrical impedance cardiography technology

35. About diagnosing air embolism with transesophageal echocardiography, which of the following is false? *[AIIMS PGMEE 2002]*
a. It can quantify the volume of air embolised
b. It is a very sensitive investigation
c. Continuous monitoring is needed to detect venous embolism
d. Interferes with Doppler when used together

36. Features of pulmonary venous hypertension are all except *[PGI 2006, JIPMER PGMEE 2005]*
a. Perihilar haze b. Peribronchial cuffing
c. Upper lobar diversion
d. Uniformly branching lines parallel to pleura
e. Pulmonary ossic1es and fine nodular pattern

37. A patient is having Mitral stenosis. His X-ray will show all of the following finding except *[AIIMS PGMEE 2002]*
a. Lifting up of left bronchus
b. Double atrial shadow
c. Obliteration of retrosternal shadow on lateral X-rays
d. Posterior displacement of esophagus on barium swallow

38. All are radiological features of Mitral stenosis except *[AIIMS PGMEE 2000]*
a. Straight left border of heart
b. Oligemia of upper lung fields
c. Pulmonary hemosiderosis
d. Lifting of left bronchus

39. Left cardiac border bulge can be seen in all, except *[All India PGMEE 2000]*
a. Enlarged azygous vein
b. Left appendicular overgrowth
c. Coronary artery aneurysm
d. Pericardial defect

40. Chest X-ray picture in CCF *[PGI 2004]*
a. Cardiomegaly
b. Thick interlobar septum
c. Superior mediastinal widening
d. Multinodular parenchymal lesion

41. Which of the following is virtually diagnostic of Aortitis on chest X-ray? *[All India PGMEE 2008]*
a. Calcification in descending aorta
b. Calcification of ascending aorta
c. Calcification of pulmonary artery
d. Focal oligemia

42. Posterior marking on Barium column in Barium swallow study is caused by? *[AIIMS PGMEE 2009]*
a. Aortic knuckle
b. Left atrium
c. Aberrant right subclavian artery
d. Pulmonary artery sling

43. William's syndrome is associated with *[AIIMS PGMEE 1997]*
a. Congenital Supravalvular Aortic stenosis
b. Congenital Subvalvular Aortic stenosis
c. VSD d. ASD

44. Most accurate investigation for assessing ventricular function is *[All India PGMEE 2006]*
a. Multislice CT b. Echocardiography
c. Nuclear scan d. MRI

45. Most important investigation for pericardial effusion *[All India PGMEE 1993, All India PGMEE 1997]*
a. Cardiac Catheterization
b. USG
c. Echocardiography
d. X-ray Chest

46. Highest sensitivity for detection of viability of myocardium post myocardial infarction is shown by *[JIPMER PGMEE 2014]*
a. Stress echocardiography
b. DSE
c. Tl-SPECT
d. FDG PET

47. In Chest X-ray of heart, right Cardiomediastinal contour is formed by *[PGI November 2014]*
a. Superior vena cava b. Inferior vena cava
c. Pulmonary artery d. Right atrium
e. Left atrium

48. In Coarctation of aorta, rib notching is seen in? *[AIIMS PG November 2015]*
a. 3rd to 9th ribs b. 1st to 9th ribs
c. 11th and 12th d. All ribs

49. Best diagnosis for Dissecting aorta is *[ESI IMO 2014]*
a. CT Scan b. MRI
c. Angiography d. X-ray

50. Egg on side appearance is seen in *[Recent Question 2017, ESI IMO 2014]*
a. TOF b. TAPVC
c. Uncorrected TGA d. Truncus arteriosus

51. Patient with history of tachycardia is put on Implantable cardioverter defibrillator. He develops shock. Best method to know the position and integrity of ICD is *[AIIMS PG May 2015]*
a. MRI b. CECT scan
c. USG d. Plain radiograph

52. In Coarctation of aorta, rib notching is seen in? *[AIIMS PG November 2015]*
a. 3rd to 9th ribs b. 1st to 9th ribs
c. 11th and 12th d. All ribs

53. Best non-invasive investigation to check for the viability of myocardium is *[AIIMS PG May 2015]*
a. Echocardiography b. FDG-18 PET CT
c. MIBG Scintigraphy d. Thallium Scintigraphy

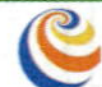

NEET/NBE PATTERN MCQs ANSWERS WITH EXPLANATIONS

1. **Ans. (b) Total anomalous pulmonary venous drainage**
   [Ref. Sure Success in PGMEE by B. Ramgopal, 1/e p130]
   - Radiography in Total anomalous pulmonary venous drainage:
     - *'Figure of 8 heart'* or *'Snowman heart'*
     - Normal to small heart with fluid in lungs

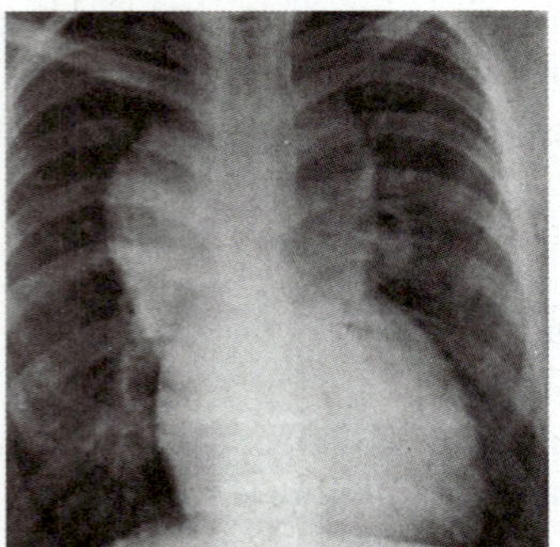

Fig. Figure of 8

Also Remember

- *Coarctation of aorta*:
  - *'Figure of 3 appearance'* of aortic knuckle
  - Inferior rib notching (3rd – 9th ribs)
- *Emphysema lungs*:
  - Barrel-shaped chest
  - Flattened diaphragm
- *Eisenmenger's complex*:
  - Pulmonary plethora
  - Normal sized heart

2. **Ans. (c) Uncorrected TGA**
   [Ref. Sumer K Sethi, 6/e p82]

D-TGA or Uncorrected TGA

- Egg on side appearance
- Enlarged, rounded heart with pulmonary plethora and a narrow pedicle

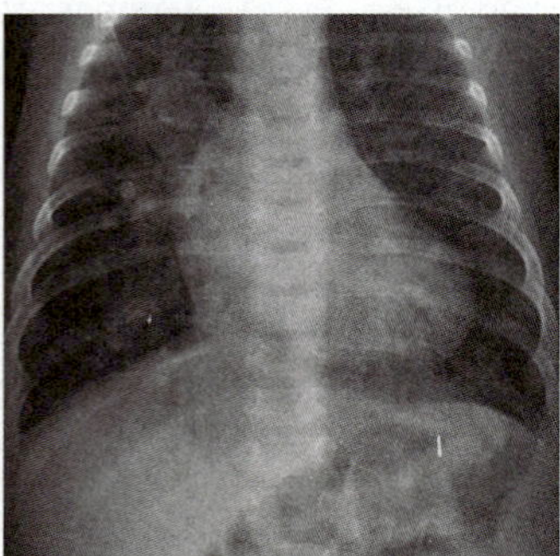

Fig. Egg on side appearance

3. **Ans. (b) Cardiomegaly**
   [Ref. David Sutton, 7/e p383]

4. **Ans. (c) Right atrium, Superior vena cava, Inferior vena cava**
   [Ref. Sumer K Sethi, 5/e p36]
   - *Right border of heart (on Chest X-ray – PA View) is formed by*:
     - Right atrium
     - Superior vena cava
     - Inferior vena cava

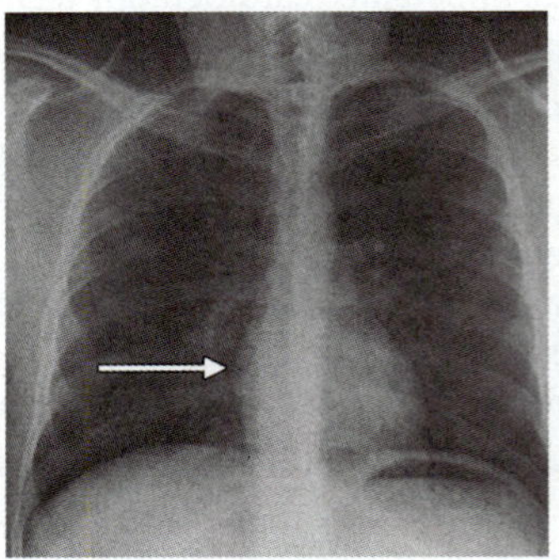

Fig. Right border of heart

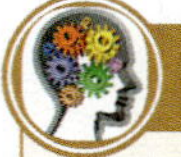

Also Remember

- *Left border of heart (on Chest X-ray – PA View) is formed by*:
  - Subclavian artery
  - Aortic knuckle
  - Pulmonary artery segment
  - Left atrial appendage
  - Right ventricle
  - Left ventricle

5. **Ans. (d) Oligaemic lung fields**
   [Ref. Radiology Review Manual by Dahnert, 6/e p645]

LVF Features

- Signs of pulmonary venous hypertension
- Progressive enlargement of heart
- Haziness + indistinctness of pulmonary arteries
- Increase in size of right descending pulmonary artery >17 mm
- Septal lines
- Peripheral ± peripheral parenchymal clouding
- Alveolar pulmonary oedema
- Indistinct vessel margins
- Karley B lines/ Karley A lines

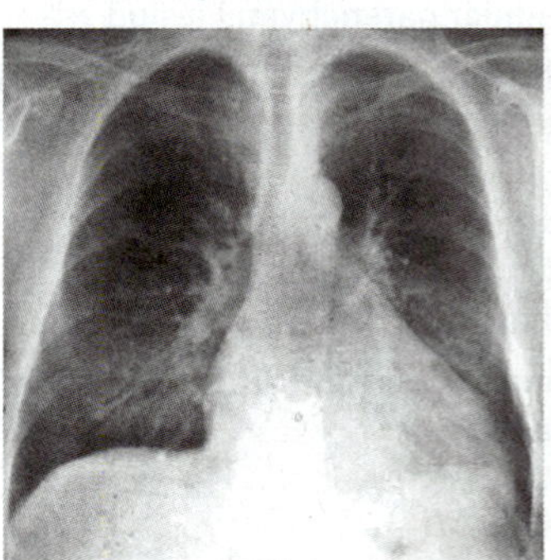

Fig. LVF

Radiodiagnosis and Radiotherapy

6. Ans. (d) Angiography of aortic and pulmonary circulation

7. Ans. (b) Aorta

[Ref. Sumer K Sethi, 5/e p36]

8. Ans. (c) Waterston's Cooley's shunt

[Ref. David Sutton, 7/e p48]

- **Superior rib notching**:
  - Normal elderly
  - Rheumatoid arthritis, SLE, Hyperparathyroidism, Marfan's syndrome, Neurofibromatosis, Paraplegics and Poliomyelitis
- **Inferior rib notching**:
  - Unilateral: Blalock-Taussig operation, Subclavian artery occlusion, Aortic Coarctation involving left subclavian artery or Anomalous right subclavian artery
  - Bilateral: Aorta (Coarctation, occlusion, aortitis), Subclavian (Takayasu's disease, atheroma), Pulmonary oligaemia (Fallot's tetralogy; pulmonary atresia, stenosis; truncus type IV), Venous (SVC, IVC obstruction), Shunts (intercostal-pulmonary fistula; pulmonary-intercostal arteriovenous fistula), Others (hyperparathyroidism; neurogenic; idiopathic)

9. Ans. (d) Doppler

[Ref. Duke Radiology Case Review: Imaging, Differential Diagnosis, and Discussion By James M. Provenzale, 1/e p519]

- Doppler screening helps in selecting appropriate patient for angiography before surgery
- Pulsed Doppler spectral analysis and Doppler ultrasound are nearly accurate (>90%)

10. Ans. (c) Coarctation of aorta

[Ref. David Sutton, 7/e p48]

11. Ans. (c) Narrowing of central arteries

[Ref. The Pulmonary Circulation in Health and Disease by James Wil, 1/e p502]

Primary Pulmonary Hypertension

- Element of the right descending pulmonary artery (remember its enlargement and not narrowing) and perhaps even bulging of the main pulmonary artery
- Varying degrees of cardiomegaly and clear lung fields

12. Ans. (b) LAO

[Ref. David Sutton, 7/e p377]

- LAO view will usually profile the duct well, but sometimes the superimposition of a large main pulmonary artery and the aorta can obscure detail
- Angiographers must be careful not to miss an aortopulmonary window, as it can often be out of profile if inappropriate projections are selected and may not be shown at all if the ascending aorta is not opacified

13. Ans. (c) Thallium scan

[Ref. David Sutton, 7/e p278, 317]

- Thallium scan is used for perfusion scan to see the viability (reversibility) of myocardium
- Advantage: A single study injected at stress, can be scanned immediately for stress abnormalities and after 4–6 hours a resting (redistribution) scan can be performed
- Newly launched Technetium agents (Sestamibi) allow higher image quality studies to be achieved but separate stress and rest studies must be performed on different days

See Figure on Next Page

14. Ans. (d) Ebstein's anomaly

[Ref. Sumer K Sethi, 5/e p44]

Ebstein Anomaly

- Atrialisation of right ventricle
- *'Box-shaped' heart*

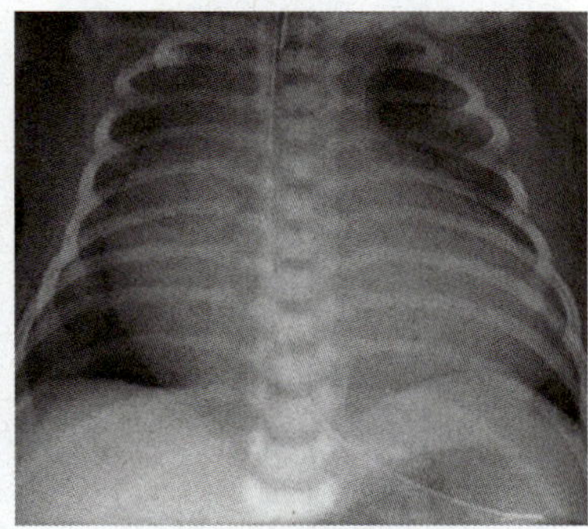

Fig. Box-shaped heart

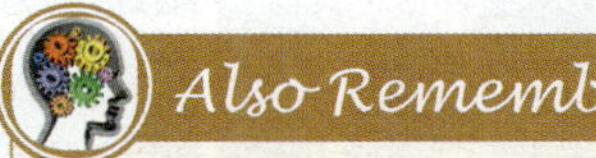

Other Important Cardiovascular System Radiology Features

- *Shoe-man Boot-shaped heart (Cor-en sabot)*: Tetralogy of Fallot
- *'Figure of 3' appearance of aortic knuckle*: Coarctation of aorta
- *Money-bag/Leather-bottle/Flask-shaped heart*: Pericardial effusion
- *Banana-shaped left ventricle*: Hypertrophic cardiomyopathy
- *'Egg-on-side' appearance*: Transposition of great arteries (TGA)
- *'Snowman'/'Figure of 8' appearance*: Total anomalous pulmonary venous drainage (TAPVC)
- *Hilar dance (Fluoroscopy)*: Atrial septal defect
- *'Pruned-tree' appearance*: Pulmonary arterial hypertension
- *Stag-antler's sign*: Mitral stenosis

15. Ans. (b) Pericardial effusion

[Ref. Bipin Valchandji Daga, 1/e p137]

- "Water-bottle" or "Flask-shaped" or **Money-bag" heart**: Pericardial effusion
- Scimitar sign/Scimitar vein/Turkish sword appearance: Congenital venolobar syndrome (TAPVC/PAPVC)
- "Stag -Antler" or "Hands up" sign: CCF
- **Boot shaped heart, Coren sabot**: TOF

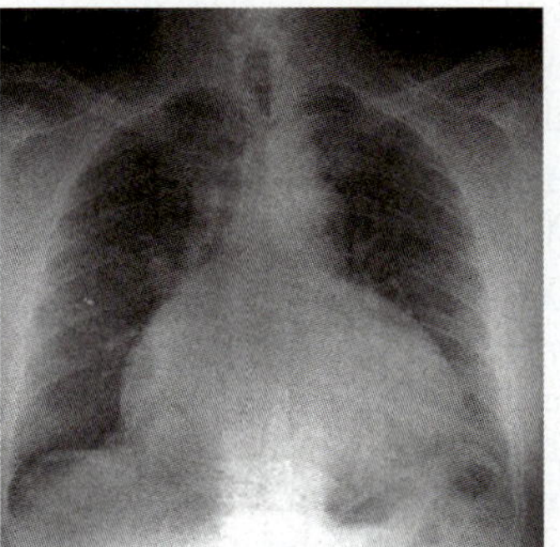

Fig. Water-bottle heart

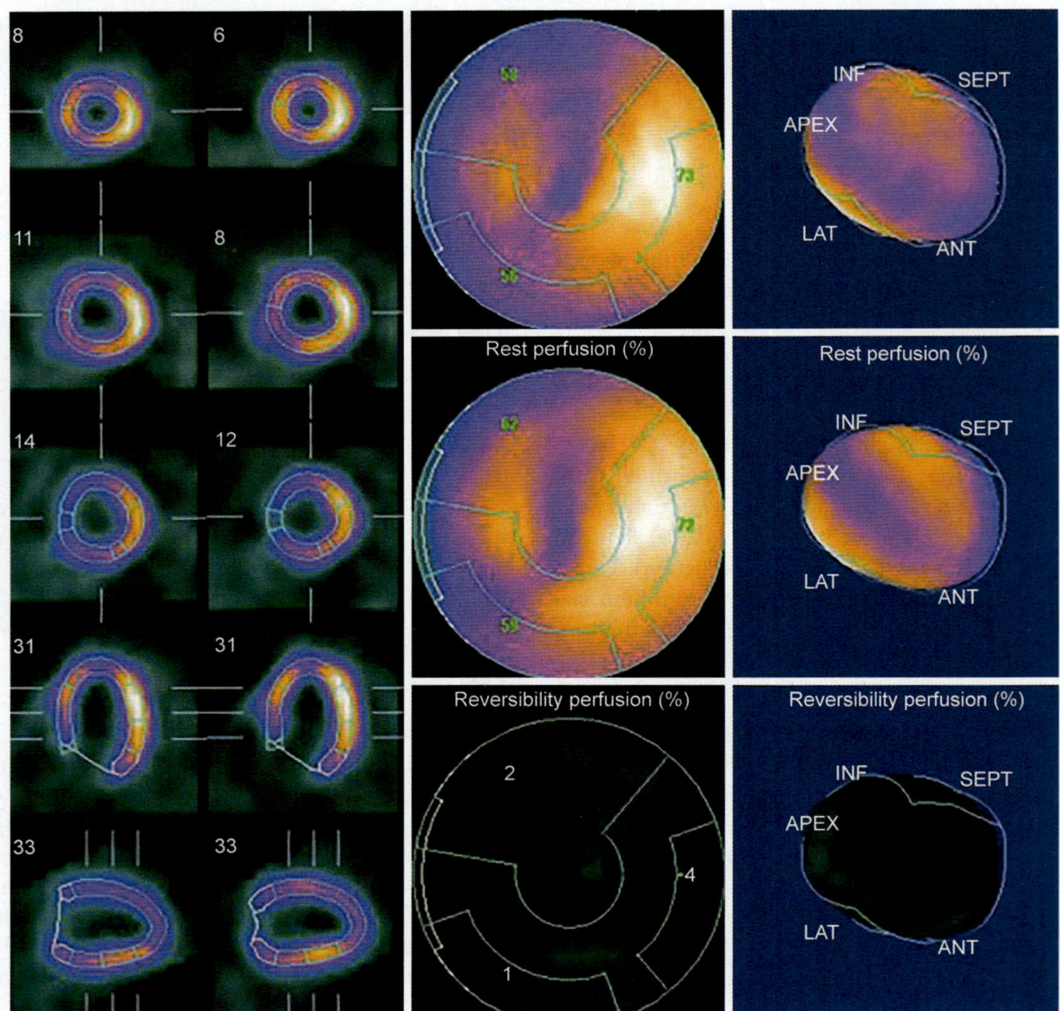

Fig. Thallium scan

16. Ans. (d) DSA
[Ref. David Sutton, 7/e p448]

17. Ans. (c) TOF
[Ref. Sumer K Sethi, 5/e p44]

18. Ans. (b) TAPVC
[Ref. BipinValchandji Daga, 1/e p137]
- Snowman heart (Figure of 8/2 Cottage loaf of bread) sign: Supracardiac TAPVC

19. Ans. (a) ASD
[Ref. BipinValchandji Daga, 1/e p139]
- "Great hilar dance" sign characterizes ASD on fluoroscopy.

20. Ans. (b) HOCM
[Ref. BipinValchandji Daga, 1/e p138]

21. Ans. (d) Left atrium
[Ref. Sumer K Sethi, 6/e p74]
- **Right border is formed**—from above downwards by SVC, Right atrium, IVC
- **Left border is formed**—from above downwards by Subclavian artery, aortic knuckle, pulmonary artery segment, left atrial appendages, left ventricle

22. Ans. (d) Echocardiography
[Ref. Sumer K Sethi, 5/e p15]

Pericardial Effusion

- Cardiomegaly with no particular chamber enlargement
- *Money-bag/Leather-bottle/Flask-shaped heart*
- Clear lung fields
- ***Investigation of choice***: Echocardiography (Can detect less than 15 mL)

23. Ans. (b) Ewart's sign
[Ref. Atlas of Adult Physical Diagnosis by Dale1 Berg, /e p79]
- The company a large pericardial effusion keeps includes an area of dullness to percussion over the medial aspect to the left scapula (Ewart's sign) and an associated decrease in tactile fremitus and decreased breath sounds over that are(a)

24. Ans. (d) Echocardiography
[Ref. David Sutton, 7/e p318-319]

25. Ans. (d) All of the above
[Ref. David Sutton, 7/e p48]

26. Ans. (c) Left atrium enlargement
[Ref. David Sutton, 7/e p318-319]

27. Ans. (c) Pericardial effusion
[Ref. BipinValchandji Daga, 1/e p137]

28. Ans. (c) TAPVC
[Ref. BipinValchandji Daga, 1/e p137]

29. Ans. (a) Mitral stenosis
[Ref. David Sutton, 7/e p301]

- In mitral stenosis, the chest radiograph demonstrates selective left atrial enlargement, which can vary from trivial to gross
- If the mitral stenosis is a result of rheumatic fever there is often marked enlargement of the left atrial appendage.

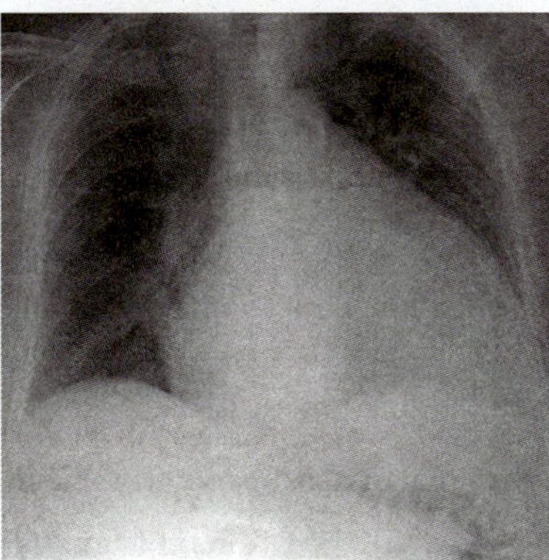

Fig. Mitral stenosis

30. Ans. (d) CT scan
[Ref. David Sutton, 7/e p333]

- CT can be used to demonstrate not only thickening of the pericardium by direct visualization, but also bilateral disproportionate dilatation of the atria, generated by the increase in atria pressure
- CT is the most accurate method of demonstrating the extent and distribution of pericardial calcification
- Pericardial calcification occurs in approximately one-third of cases of constrictive pericarditis, usually characterized as a fine irregular line of calcification
- CT will also demonstrate the presence of additional pleural effusions or ascites associated with.

31. Ans. (a) Doppler USG
[Ref. David Sutton, 7/e p503]

- Indications for venous ultrasound of the lower limb veins:
  - Diagnosis or exclusion of DVT
  - Assessment of chronic venous insufficiency
  - Mapping of veins

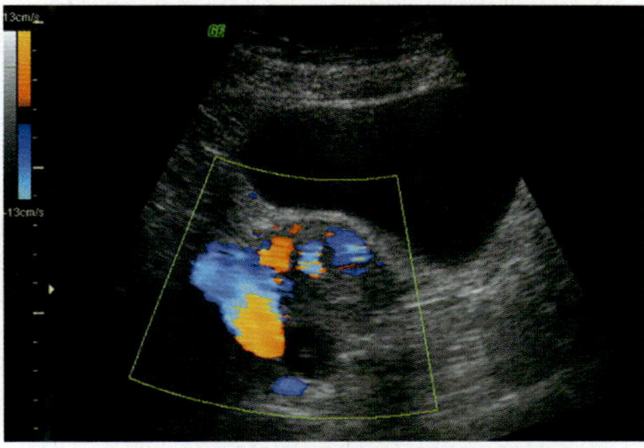

Fig. Doppler USG

32. Ans. (c) Displacement of left main bronchus
[Ref. Cardiology by Baliga, 1/e p509]

33. Ans. (a) Mitral stenosis
[Ref. Echo Manual by Tajik, 3/e p202]

Echo Features of Rheumatic Fever

- Thickened calcified mitral valve leaflets
- Decreased EF slope
- **'Hockey-stick appearance'** of Anterior mitral leaflet in diastole
- Immobility of Posterior mitral leaflet
- 'Fish-mouth orifice'
- Increased LA size

HIGH YIELD MCQs ANSWERS WITH EXPLANATIONS 

1. Ans. (c) Tc 99 Strontium Pyrophosphate
[Ref. Physical Therapist's Clinical Companion. 1/e p151]

- Tc 99 pyrophosphate screening is used to detect recent MI
- Isotope accumulates in damaged myocardial tissue, possibly by combining with calcium in the damaged myocardial cell, where it forms a hot spot on a scan made with a scintillation camera

2. Ans. (a) Normal left atrium
[Ref. Grainger & Allison's Diagnostic Radiology Essentials by Lee A Grant,5/e p160]

- Radiologically, In ASD left atrium is normal but in VSD left atrium is enlarged

3. Ans. (c) Diameter of the descending right pulmonary artery >16 mm
[Ref. Cardiothoracic Critical Care by David Sidebotham, 1/e p91]

4. Ans. (a) Neurofibromatosis; (c) Aortic aneurysm; (d) Taussig-Bing operation; (e) Aortic obstruction
[Ref. David Sutton, 7/e p48]

5. Ans. (a) Involvement of upper two ribs; (d) Usually before 5 years of age
[Ref. Radiology Review Manual by Dahnert, 6/e p630]

6. Ans. (a) Coarctation of aorta
[Ref. David Sutton, 7/e p48]

7. Ans. (d) Tetralogy of Fallot
[Ref. BipinValchandji Daga, 1/e p137]

8. Ans. (a) Total Anomalous Pulmonary Venous Connection
[Ref. BipinValchandji Daga, 1/e p137]

9. Ans. (b) Total Anomalous Pulmonary Venous Connection (TAPVC)
[Ref. BipinValchandji Daga, 1/e p137]

10. Ans. (b) Pericardial effusion
[Ref. BipinValchandji Daga, 1/e p137]

11. Ans. (b) Uncorrected TGV
[Ref. Sumer K Sethi, 6/e p82]

12. Ans. (c) Oligaemic lung field
[Ref. Radiology Review Manual by Dahnert, 6/e p645]

13. Ans. (c) Ascending aorta
[Ref. Sumer K Sethi, 6/e p74]
- Right border is formed by from above downwards by SVC, Right atrium, IVC.

14. Ans. (e) Right atrium and left atrium
[Ref. Textbook of Anesthesia for Postgraduates by TK Agasti]
- Base of heart is formed only by the two atria

15. Ans. (a) Pulmonary artery; (d) Arch of aorta
[Ref. Sumer K Sethi, 6/e p74]
- Left border is formed by (Above downwards): Subclavian artery, Aortic knuckle, Pulmonary artery segment, Left atrial appendages, Left ventricle

16. Ans. (b) SVC (c) Right atrium
[Ref. Sumer K Sethi, 6/e p74]

17. Ans. (a) Pulmonary hypertension
[Ref. Sumer K Sethi, 6/e p83]
- Pulmonary Arterial hypertension: Large main and large central pulmonary arteries which taper down rapidly to very small vessels over a few order of branches, giving a ***'pruned tree appearance'***
- Calcification may be seen in long standing pulmonary hypertension.

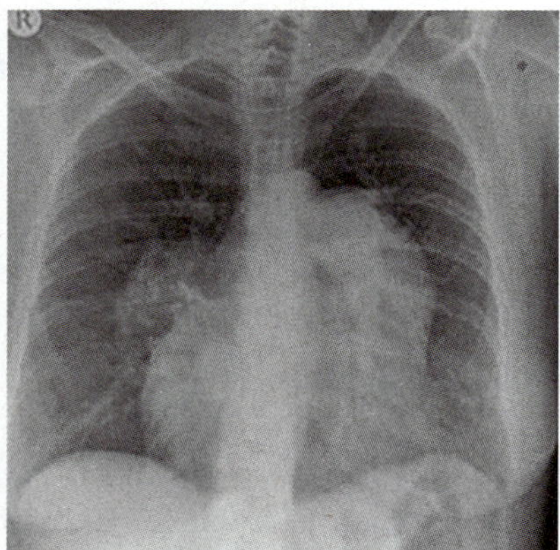

Fig. Pruned-tree appearance

18. Ans. (b) Upper lobar diversion of vessels
[Ref. David Sutton, 7/e p288]
- Changes in pulmonary venous hypertension are well-defined on the plain film and increase as the left atrial pressure increases, the first radiological feature being enlargement of the upper zone vessels

19. Ans. (a) Double contour of right heart border; (b) Straightening of left heart border; (c) Splaying of carinal angle; (e) Kerley lines
[Ref. Sumer K Sethi, 6/e p76]

Plain X-ray Features of MS

- Elevated left main bronchus
- Carinal widening (> 60°–75°)
- Double atrial shadow
- Upper lobe venous diversion with prominent upper lobe veins- Stag antler shadow
- Prominent left atrial appendage with straightening of left heart border
- Barium swallow-impression on oesophagus
- Lutembacher syndrome
- Long standing pulmonary venous hypertension leading to hemosiderosis
- Kerley B lines

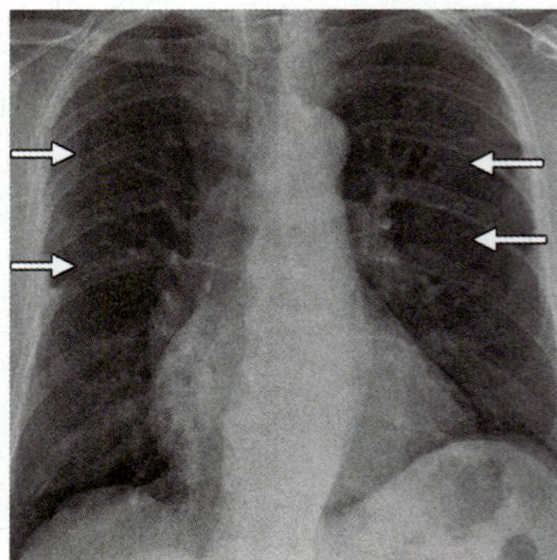

Fig. Stag Antler shadow

20. Ans. (a) Elevation of the left main bronchus
[Ref. BipinValchandji Daga, 1/e p137]
- Elevation of left main bronchus is the earliest sign on PA view which, if gross may lead to splaying of carina (second sign)

21. Ans. (b) Prominent lower lobe vessels
[Ref. Diagnostic imaging 5/e p117
- There are prominent upper lobe vessels and not lower lobe due to pulmonary venous hypertension

22. Ans. (a) Tetralogy of Fallot
[Ref. Sumer K Sethi, 6/e p49]
- In Tetralogy of Fallot there is normal size heart
- In other options there is increased cardiac silhouette

23. Ans. (c) Right middle lobe
[Ref. David Sutton, 7/e p175–179]
- Right middle lobe lesion causes obliteration of right cardiac border

24. Ans. (c) Echocardiography
[Ref. David Sutton, 7/e p318–319]

25. Ans. NONE
[Ref. BipinValchandji Daga, 1/e p97]

Differential Diagnosis of Ground Glass Haze on CXR

- Left to right shunt
- Hyaline membrane disease
- Staphylococcal pneumonia
- Infracardiac TAPVC
- Alveolar proteinosis
- Wegener's granulomatosis
- Diffuse pulmonary hemorrhage
- Eosinophilic pneumonia

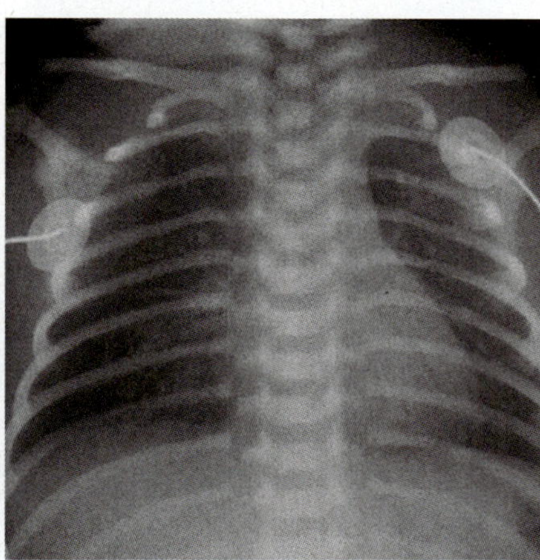

Fig. Ground glass appearance

26. Ans. (c) Dilated Left atrium; (e) Dilated pulmonary arteries
[Ref. Grainger & Allison's Diagnostic Radiology Essentials by Lee A Grant, 5/e p160]

Ventricular Septal Defect
- Small shunt: Normal CXR
- Large shunt: Enlargement of ventricles, Left atrium and Pulmonary vessels

27. Ans. (c) MRI
[Ref. BipinValchandji Daga, 1/e p58]

Chest MRI Indications
- Investigation of choice and best diagnosis for aortic dissection
- Demonstration of vascular sling
- Imaging of posterior mediastinal masses
- Imaging of Pancoast's tumor (superior sulcus tumor)

28. Ans. (a) 2D Echocardiography
[Ref. Perioperative Transesophageal Echocardiography by David L. Reich, 1/e p304]

29. Ans. (c) Pulmonary plethora
[Ref. Grainger & Allison's Diagnostic Radiology Essentials by Lee A Grant, 5/e p160]
- CXR features of ASD: Mild pulmonary plethora and cardiac enlargement (Left atrium though normal)

30. Ans. (d) Coarctation of Aorta
[Ref. David Sutton, 7/e p48]

31. Ans. (a) SVC; (b) IVC; (c) Right atrium
[Ref. Sumer K Sethi, 6/e p74]

32. Ans. (a) Lingular lesion

33. Ans. (d) Right ventricle
[Ref. Sumer K Sethi, 6/e p74]

34. Ans. (d) Electrical impedance cardiography technology
[Ref. BipinValchandji Daga, 1/e p131]

Non Invasive Cardiac Output Monitoring
- Pulmonary artery catheter (Swan-Ganz)
- Thermodilution technique
- Dynamic echocardiography
- Electrical impedance cardiography technology

35. Ans. (d) Interferes with Doppler when used together
[Ref. BipinValchandji Daga, 1/e p34]

36. Ans. (d) Uniformly branching lines parallel to pleura
[Ref. David Sutton, 7/e p288]

37. Ans. (c) Obliteration of retrosternal shadow on lateral X-rays
[Ref. Sumer K Sethi, 6/e p76]

38. Ans. (b) Oligemia of upper lung fields
[Ref. Sumer K Sethi, 6/e p76]

39. Ans. (a) Enlarged azygous vein
[Ref. Cardiac X-ray by Chockolingam, 1/e p30-40]

Bulging of Left Heart Border
- Left atrial appendage enlargement
- Left ventricular enlargement
- Right ventricular enlargement
- Left anterior descending coronary artery aneurysm
- Left sided pericardial defect

40. Ans. (a) Cardiomegaly
[Ref. David Sutton, 7/e p440]

41. Ans. (b) Calcification of ascending aorta
[Ref. David Sutton, 7/e p73]
- Calcification of ascending aorta aneurysm is diagnostic of Aortitis and is mainly due to syphilis or atherosclerosis

42. Ans. (c) Aberrant right subclavian artery
[Ref. Grainger & Allison's Diagnostic Radiology Essentials by Lee A Grant,4/e p1027]

Plain Radiograph with Barium Swallow
- Aberrant right subclavian artery:
  - Posterior impression on oesophagus
  - Left sided aortic arch impression
- Aberrant left subclavian artery:
  - Posterior impression on esophagus
  - Right sided aortic arch impression
  - Anterior displacement of esophagus
  - Compression of trachea

43. Ans. (a) Congenital supravalvular aortic stenosis
[Ref. BipinValchandji Daga, 1/e p138]
- **William's syndrome:** Supravalvular aortic stenosis and peripheral pulmonary artery stenosis

44. Ans. (b) Echocardiography
[Ref. David Sutton, 7/e p273]

45. Ans. (c) Echocardiography
[Ref. David Sutton, 7/e p273]

46. Ans. (c) TI-SPECT
[Ref. Cardiac SPECT Imaging edited by E. Gordon, 1/e p317]
- Both FDG and TI SPECT reinjection had a high sensitivity in predicting improvement of regional function (i.e. viability of myocardium post myocardial infarction)

47. Ans. (a) Superior vena cava; (b) Inferior vena cava; (d) Right atrium
[Ref. Sumer K Sethi, 5/e p36]

Borders of Heart on X-ray (Above downwards)

Right border	Left border
Superior vena cava Right atrium Left vena cava	Subclavian artery Aortic knuckle Pulmonary artery segment Left atrial appendage Left ventricle

48. Ans. (a) 3rd to 9th ribs
[Ref. Radiodiagnosis by Daga, 1/e p150]

Coarctation of Aorta

- *'Figure of 3 appearance'* of aortic knuckle
- Inferior rib notching (3rd – 9th ribs)

49. Ans. (b) MRI
[Ref. Radiodiagnosis by Daga, 1/e p58]

50. Ans. (c) Uncorrected TGA
[Ref. Radiodiagnosis by Daga, 1/e p137]

51. Ans. (d) Plain radiograph
[Ref. Critical Care Study Guide by Criner, 2/e p98]

- For implantable cardioverter-defibrillator (ICD), a chest X-ray should be obtained to confirm lead position and examine lead integrity
- Most pulse generators, both pacemakers and ICDs, can be identified from their appearance under radiography: Most helpful method of identifying unknown devices

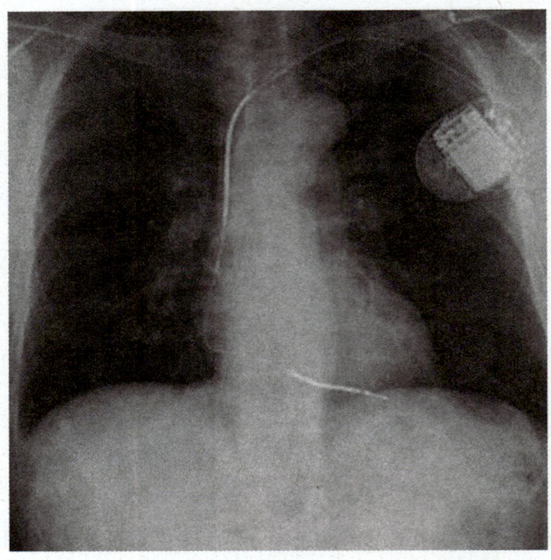

Fig. Implantable cardioverter-defibrillator (ICD)

52. Ans. (a) 3rd to 9th ribs
[Ref. Sutton, 6/e Vol 1 p309]

53. Ans. (b) FDG-18 PET CT
[Ref. Translational Cardiovascular Research by Dennis, 1/e p417]

- **18F-FDG PET** has been extensively used to assess myocardial viability and is still considered by some investigators as the Gold standard.

Chapter 3

Gastrointestinal System and Abdomen

THEORETICAL CONCEPTS

III A. FLUID LEVELS ON ABDOMINAL X-RAY

- *Number of physiologic fluid levels in abdomen on X-ray*: **Two**[Q]
  - Stomach fluid level
  - Caecum fluid level
- *Number of fluid levels* ***more than 5*** *in abdomen on X-ray*:
  - Obstruction
  - Ileus
  - Ischaemia
  - Gastroenteritis

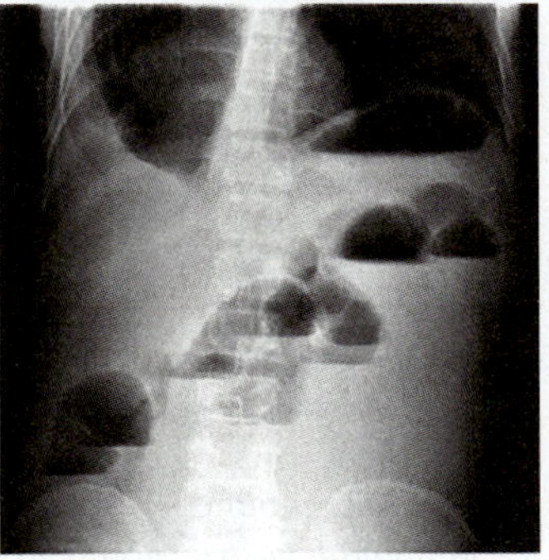

Fig. Multiple air-fluid levels

III B. ACHALASIA CARDIA

- Dilated sigmoid shaped oesophagus
- ***Rat-tail/Bird-beak appearance***[Q]

Topper's Edge

Achalasia

- Types of achalasia:
  - Primary achalasia: Failure of organised oesophageal peristalsis with an impaired relaxation of the lower oesophageal sphincter (LOS), resulting in often marked dilatation of the oesophagus and food stasis
  - Secondary achalasia (**Pseudoachalasia**[Q]): Obstruction of the distal oesophagus (often due to tumour)
- Clinical presentation of achalasia:
  - **MC**[Q]**: Dysphagia** (both for solids and liquids)
  - Complications: Oesophageal carcinoma, aspiration pneumonia, candida oesophagitis, acute airway obstruction
- Pathology of achalasia:
  - Abnormality of Auerbach plexus (Sometimes in vagus nerve)
  - Weak, uncoordinated, non-propulsive contractions
  - Loss of peristalsis in distal smooth muscle segment of oesophagus
  - Sphincter eventually fails to relax, partially/completely, with elevated pressures

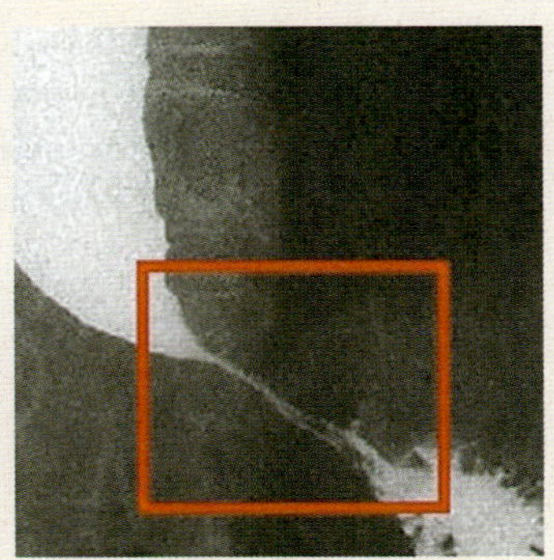

Fig. Bird-beak appearance

III C. BILIARY TRACT

- *Investigation of choice for* ***most gallsbladder pathologies***: USG[Q]
- *Investigation of choice for* ***Acute cholecystitis***: Tc-99 HIDA scan[Q]
- *Investigation of choice for* ***Low bile duct obstruction*** *(CBD obstruction)*: ERCP (Endoscopic cholangiopancreatography)
- *Investigation of choice for* ***High bile duct obstruction*** *(Klatskin tumour)*: PTC (Percutaneous transhepatic cholangiography)
- *Initial investigation of choice for surgical jaundice*: USG
- *Investigation of choice for Biliary atresia*: Peroperative cholangiography

III D. GASLESS ABDOMEN

Causes in infants[Q]	Causes in adults[Q]
• Oesophageal atresia • Duodenal atresia • Volvulus • Annular pancreas • Hypertrophic pyloric stenosis • Choledochal cyst • Excess vomiting • Fluid-filled bowel • Congenital diaphragmatic hernia	• High obstruction • Ascites • Acute pancreatitis • Fluid-filled bowel • Large abdominal mass • Normal

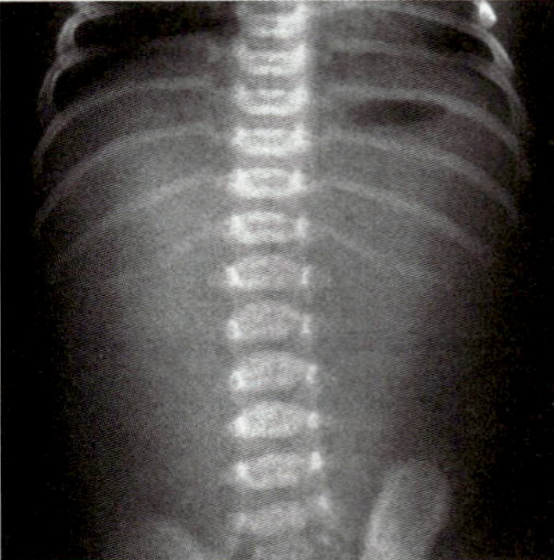

Fig. Gasless abdomen

III E. GIT ULCERS

- *Benign gastric ulcer*:
  - ***Hampton's line***[Q]
  - Ulcer collar
  - Ulcer mound
- *Malignant gastric ulcer*: ***Carman's meniscus sign***[Q]
- *Duodenal ulcer*: ***'Trapped air sign'*** **in upper abdomen**[Q]

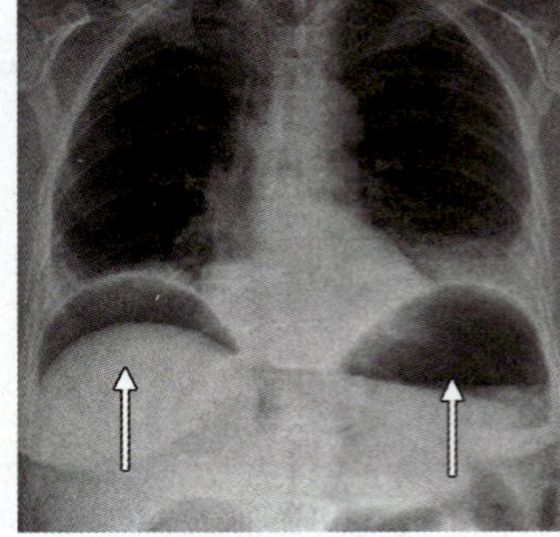

Fig. Trapped air sign

III F. ILEOCAECAL TUBERCULOSIS/KOCH'S

- ***'String sign'***[Q]
- Purse-string appearance
- Goose-neck appearance

Topper's Edge

Gastrointestinal Tuberculosis

- Organs affected:
  - **Ileocaecum (Terminal ileum and Caecum)**: MC due to abundance of lymphoid tissue[Q]
  - Other parts: Colon, Liver, Spleen, Peritoneum, Lymph nodes
- Pathological types:
  - Ulcerative
  - Hypertrophic
  - Ulcero-hypertrophic

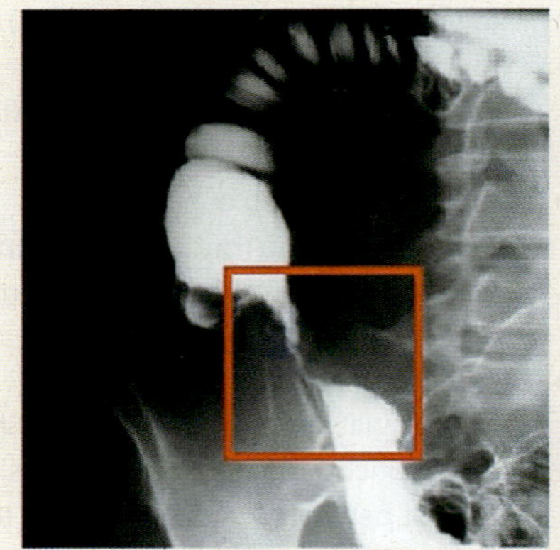

Fig. String sign

Radiodiagnosis and Radiotherapy

III G. INFLAMMATORY BOWEL DISEASE (IBD)

Ulcerative colitis[Q]	Crohn's disease[Q]
Pipe-stem colon[Q] **M**ucosal involvement (contiguous)[Q] **T**oxic megacolon[Q] **P**seudopolyps[Q] **S**tove pipe sign **B**lurred mucosal strips, granular appearance* **C**ollar-button ulcers[Q]	**T**ransmural involvement[Q] **S**kip lesions **C**obblestone colon[Q] **R**aspberry/ rose-thorn appearance[Q] **A**phthoid ulceration* **S**tring sign of Kantor[Q] **H**alo sign (CT)[Q] **R**ectal sparing[Q] **S**trictures/ fistulae[Q] **P**seudosacculations
[Mnemonic: PMT Process **S**elects **B**etter **C**andidates**]**	**[Mnemonic: T**raffic **S**ignal **CRASH R**esults in **S**erious **P**athology**]**

(Earliest sign)*

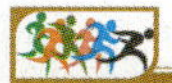

Topper's Edge

Ulcerative Colitis

- Ulcerative colitis: An inflammatory bowel disease that predominantly affects colon, along with extraintestinal manifestations
- Clinical presentation of UC:
  - Chronic diarrhea, Tenesmus, Pain, Fever
  - Extraintestinal manifestations: Uveitis and iritis, Erythema nodosum and pyoderma gangrenosum, Thrombotic complications, Fatty liver, Seronegative spondyloarthropathy
- **Associations of UC[Q]**:
  - Primary sclerosing cholangitis (PSC)
  - Ankylosing spondylitis
  - Colorectal carcinoma

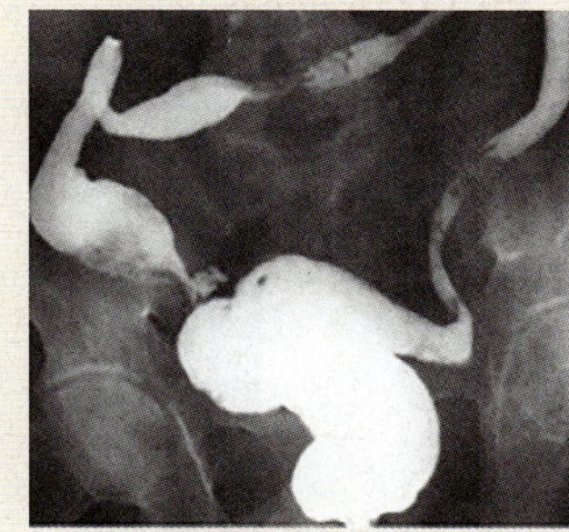

Fig. Pipe-stem colon

Crohn's Disease (CD)

- Description of CD:
  - Idiopathic inflammatory bowel disease
  - Widespread gastrointestinal tract involvement typically with skip lesions
  - Regional enteritis: Frequently has systemic involvement
- Clinical presentation of CD:
  - Chronic diarrhea, Recurrent abdominal pain
  - Complications: Linear longitudinal and circumferential ulcers, Fistulae, Fibrotic change, Stricture formation
- Extraintestinal manifestations of CD[Q]:
  - Digestive tract: Mucogingivitis, mucosal tags, deep ulceration, cobblestoning, lip swelling and pyostomatitis vegetans, esophageal ulcers and strictures
  - Skin: Erythema nodosum, Pyoderma gangrenosum
  - **Joints: Seronegative spondyloarthritis, Sacroiliitis[Q]**
  - **Eyes: Episcleritis, Iritis, Uveitis[Q]**
  - Liver and biliary system: Pericholangitis, Primary sclerosing cholangitis, Autoimmune hepatitis, Cirrhosis, Gallstones, Hepatic abscess, Pancreatitis
  - Renal tract: Renal calculi
  - Pulmonary and thoracic associations: Bronchiectasis, mosaic perfusion and air trapping

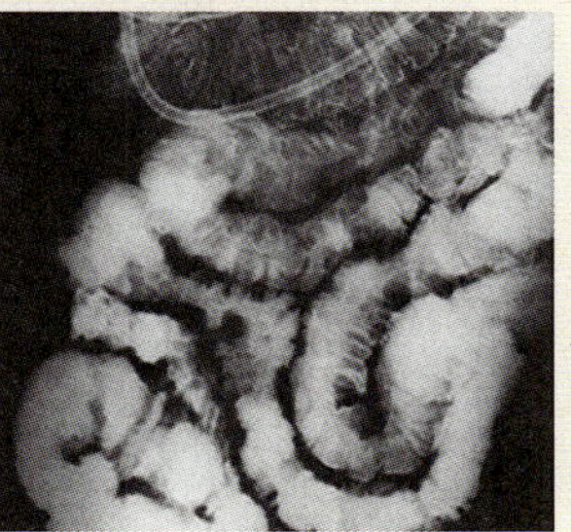

Fig. Cobblestone colon

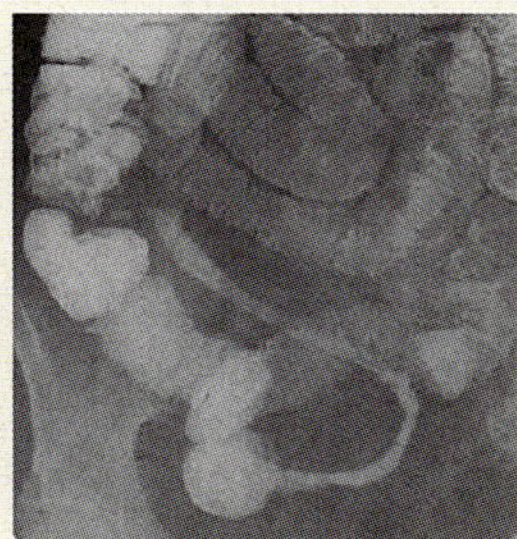

Fig. String sign

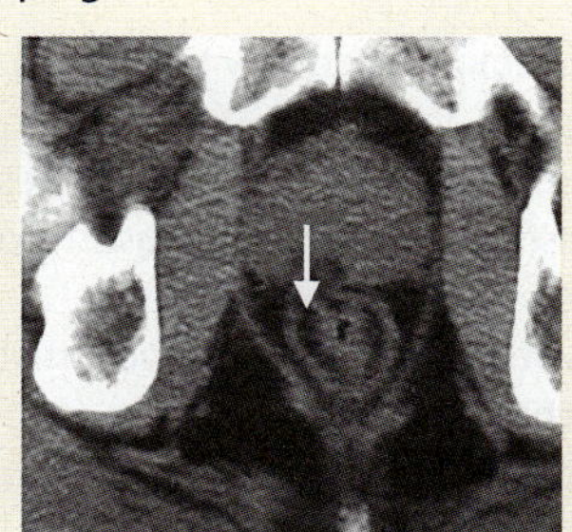

Fig. Halo sign (CT)

III H. INTUSSUSCEPTION

- *'Coiled spring' appearance*[Q]
- Claw sign
- **Double-target appearance**

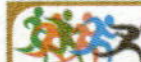

Topper's Edge

Intussusception

- Intussusception:
  - One segment of bowel is pulled into itself or a neighboring loop of bowel by peristalsis
  - Bowel telescoping into itself
  - Most cases occur in children (95%), usually after the first three months of life
  - **MC region affected[Q]: Ileocolic region (Children)**
- Clinical presentation:
  - Classic triad[Q]: Intermittent abdominal pain, vomiting, right upper quadrant mass
  - Occult blood on rectal examination
- Radiology:
  - Plain abdominal X-rays: Elongated soft tissue mass (upper right quadrant) with a bowel obstruction (air-fluid levels, bowel dilation) proximally
  - **Ultrasound: Reliable screening tool**
    1. Target/Doughnut sign[Q]
    2. Pseudo-kidney sign[Q]
    3. Crescent in a doughnut sign[Q]
  - Fluoroscopy[Q]: **"Coiled spring" appearance** (Barium in lumen of Intussusceptum and in Intraluminal space)
  - CT scan: Bowel-within-bowel configuration

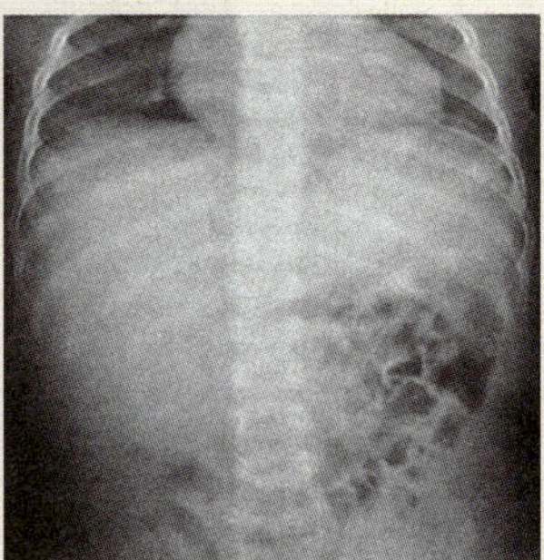

Fig. Mass + fluid levels

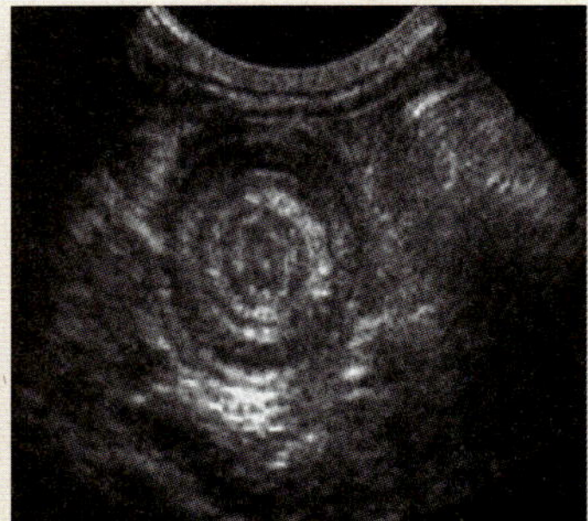

Fig. Target sign

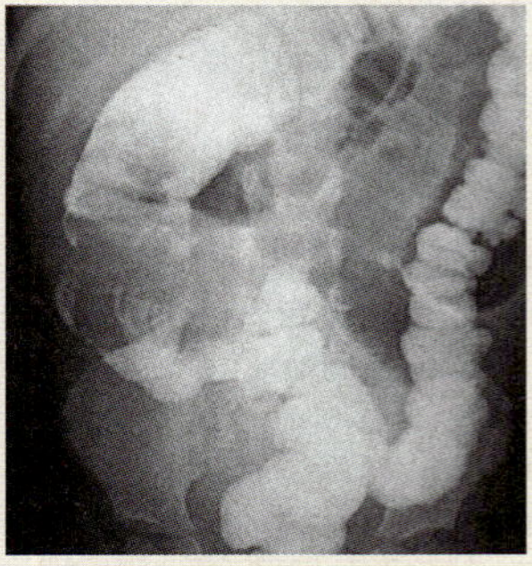

Fig. Coiled-spring appearance

III I. ISCHAEMIC COLITIS

- ***'Thumb-printing' sign***[Q]

Topper's Edge

Ischaemic Colitis

- Inflammation of the colon secondary to vascular insufficiency and ischaemia
- Underlying causes:
  - Arterial occlusion: Arteriosclerosis, vasculitides, arterial emboli
  - Venous thrombosis: Malignancy, OCP use, thrombosis
  - Primary mesenteric venous thrombosis
  - Other causes: Hypotension, CHF, cardiac arrhythmias, sickle cell disease
- **Location of the ischaemia**[Q]:
  - Superior mesenteric artery
  - Inferior mesenteric artery
  - Watershed areas: Splenic flexure (Griffiths' point), rectosigmoid junction (Sudeck's point)

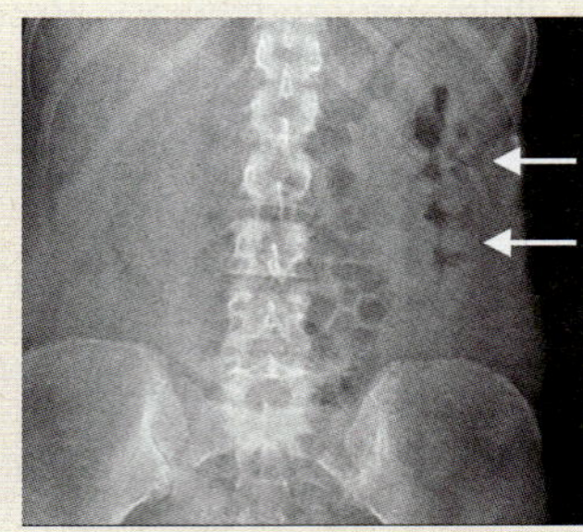

Fig. Thumb-printing

III J. NEUROBLASTOMA

- Calcification
- Vascular encasement
- Solid appearance (USG)
- Bony metastasis
- Secondaries in orbit

III K. PANCREATITIS

- *Investigation of choice*:
  - *Acute pancreatitis*: Contrast-enhanced CT (CECT) [Q]
  - *Chronic pancreatitis*: ERCP[Q]
- *X-rays abdomen*: Non-specific
  - **Sentinel loop**[Q]
  - **Colon cut-off sign**[Q]
  - **Renal halo sign**
- *Ultrasonography*:
  - Only useful for gall stones, cholecystitis and dilated bile duct
- *CT scan (CECT)/MRI*:
  - To establish diagnosis
  - Differentiate interstitial and necrotizing pancreatitis
  - Extent of necrosis (after 72 hours): Staging based on *'Balthazar criteria'*
- *EUS/MRCP*:
  - Stones in bile duct
  - Assessment of pancreatic parenchyma
- *ERCP*:
  - Identification and removal of gallstones
- *Key radiological findings of pancreatitis*:
  - ***Sentinel loop***[Q]
  - Gasless abdomen
  - **Colon cut-off**[Q]
  - Duodenal ileus
  - Mottled lucencies
  - ***Chain-of-lakes appearance*** **(ERCP in chronic pancreatitis)**[Q]
  - *Pancreatic calcification (Chronic alcoholism)* [Q]

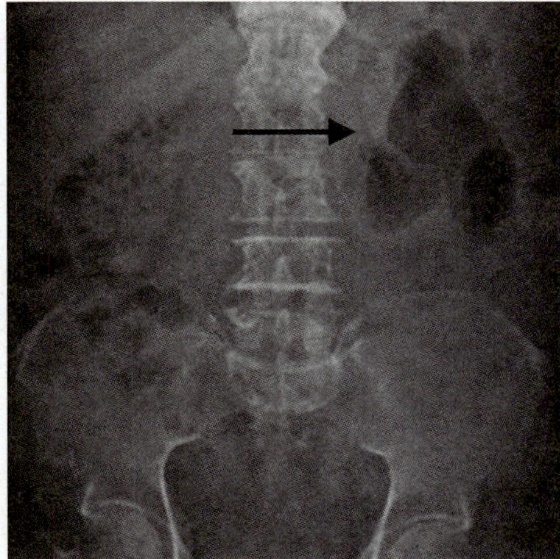

Fig. Sentinel loop sign

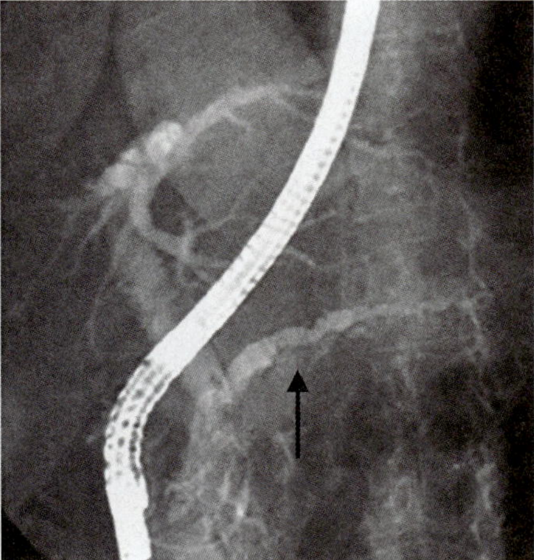

Fig. Chain-of-lakes (ERCP)

III L. RENAL CELL CARCINOMA

- Non-functioning kidney
- Bony metastasis: Lytic expansile lesions

III M. RENAL TUBERCULOSIS

- *Putty kidney* (Autonephrectomy)[Q]
- ***Thimble bladder***[Q]
- **Pipestem/Cork-screw ureters**[Q]
- *'Feathery appearance' of calyces* (Earliest sign on IVP)[Q]
- ***'Golf-hole' ureters*** (on Sigmoidoscopy)[Q]

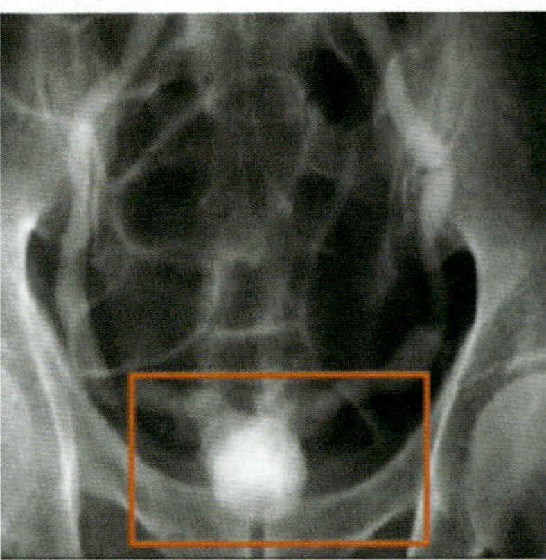

Fig. Thimble bladder

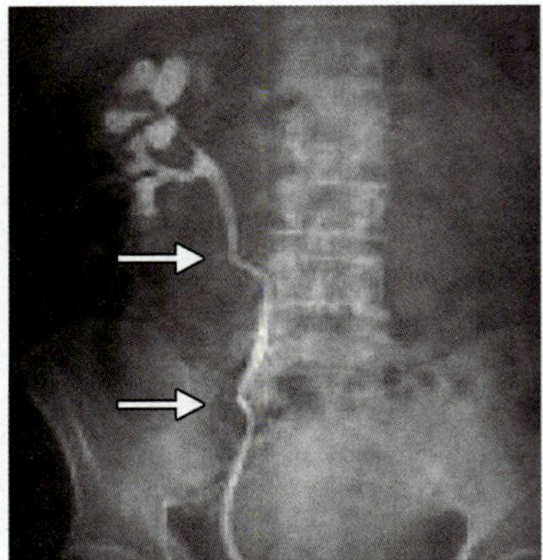

Fig. Cork-screw ureter

III N. VOLVULUS

- ***'Bird-of-prey' sign***
- Overlap sign

Topper's Edge

Intestinal Volvulus

- Volvulus:
  - Torsion of bowel around its mesentery
  - Torsion results in narrowing of lumen at the point of rotation and compromise of vessels that supply the torted gut
- 4 types of volvulus (4 main mesenteries):
  - Gastric volvulus
  - Midgut volvulus
  - Caecal volvulus
  - Sigmoid volvulus
- Radiology[Q]: ***'Bird's-beak/ Bird-of-prey sign'***
  - In single-contrast barium enema examination, barium readily enters the empty rectum and usually encounters a complete stenosis

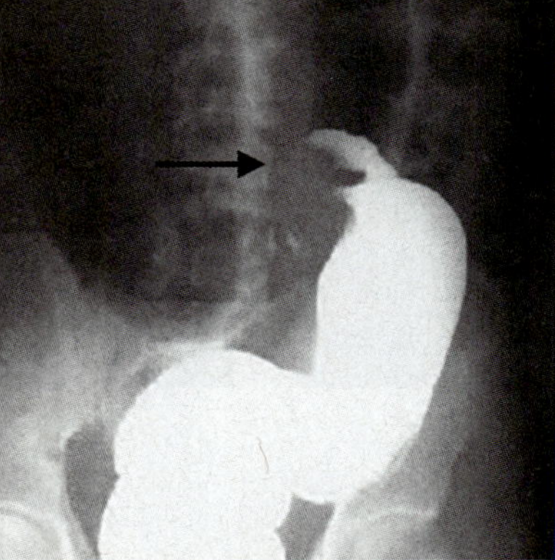

Fig. Bird-beak sign
(Bird-of-prey sign)

III O. FEW IMPORTANT SIGNS IN RADIOLOGY ABDOMEN

- Antral beaking sign: Congenital hypertrophic pyloric stenosis
- Antral pad sign[Q]: Pancreatic ductal adenocarcinoma
- **Bird-beak/Rat-tail sign**[Q]: Achalasia cardia
- **Bird-of-prey sign**[Q]: Sigmoid volvulus
- **Carman's meniscus sign**[Q]: Carcinoma stomach
- Chain of beads appearance[Q]: Diffuse esophageal spasm
- Coffee bean sign[Q]: Sigmoid volvulus
- Concertina pattern/Herringbone pattern: Jejunal obstruction
- **Cork-screw oesophagus**: Diffuse oesophageal spasm[Q]
- Creeping fat sign[Q]: Crohn's disease
- Crescentic shadow/Meniscus sign[Q]: Gallstone
- Cupola sign[Q]: Pneumoperitoneum (Gas under diaphragm)
- **Double-bubble sign**[Q]:Duodenal atresia (Most characteristic), Duodenal stenosis, Duodenal atresia, Annular pancreas, Malrotation of gut (Midgut volvulus), Pre-duodenal position of portal vein
- Double duct sign on USG: Pancreatic carcinoma[Q]
- Echogenic focus with posterior acoustic shadowing on USG: Gallstones
- Flower-vase kidney: Horseshoe-shaped kidney
- Football sign[Q]: Pneumoperitoneum
- **Frostberg inverted 3 sign**: Periampullary carcinoma Pancreas[Q]
- Inverted umbrella sign[Q]: Ileocaecal tuberculosis
- Lead-pipe/Pipe-stem colon[Q]: Ulcerative colon
- Meniscus sign on Cholangiogram: Common bile duct stones[Q]
- Mercedes Benz sign: Air in gallstones[Q]
- Pincer sign[Q]: Intussusception
- Pseudopolyps[Q]: Ulcerative polyps
- Purse ring/ Napkin ring stenosis[Q]: Ileocaecal stenosis
- **Reverse 3 sign of Frostburg**[Q]: Pancreatic ductal carcinoma
- Rigler's triad[Q] (Small bowel obstruction, Gall in gallbladder/bile ducts, Ectopic gallstone): Gallstone ileus
- Saw-tooth/Concertina/Serrated appearance: Diverticulosis **(MC: Sigmoid colon)**[Q]
- Scalloped edge of Sigmoid colon[Q]: Ulcerative colon
- **Sentinel loop sign**[Q]: Acute pancreatitis
- **Colon cut-off sign**[Q]: Acute pancreatitis
- Single bubble sign: Pyloric atresia[Q]
- Sonographic Murphy's sign: Acute cholecystitis
- Stack of coins appearance: Bowel wall bleeding (Regular thickening of small bowel folds)[Q]
- Sterlin sign[Q]: Ileocaecal tuberculosis
- String of beads sign[Q]: Small intestinal obstruction
- **String sign**[Q]: Congenital hypertrophic pyloric stenosis
- String of pearls/Chain of lakes/Hourglass appearance (ERCP) [Q]: Chronic pancreatitis
- Triple bubble sign: Jejunal atresia[Q]
- WES (Wall Echo/Double arc Shadow) sign[Q]: Cholelithiasis with Chronic cholecystitis
- Widening of Duodenal C loop[Q]: Pancreatic head carcinoma

III P. DIFFERENTIAL DIAGNOSIS IN ABDOMINAL RADIOLOGY

Pneumobilia[Q]	Central dot sign[Q]
• Gallstone ileus • Gallstone erosion • Emphysematous cholecystitis • Gallbladder carcinoma • Ascending cholangitis • Acute cholecystitis • Chronic cholecystitis	• Caroli's disease (MCC) • Obstructive jaundice • Periportal lymphedema • Prebiliary cyst

IMAGE-BASED QUESTIONS

1. Identify the Labelled structures in the CT Abdomen ***[APPG 2016]***

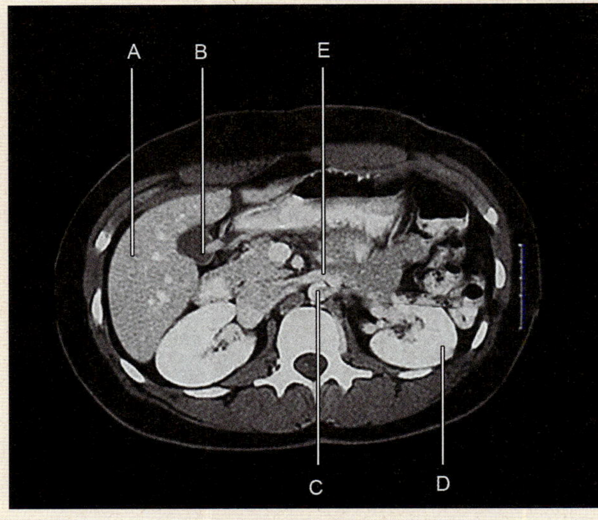

a. A = right kidney, B = inferior vena cava, C = head of pancreas, D = left psoas muscle, E = transverse colon
b. A = liver, B = inferior vena cava, C = head of pancreas, D = left kidney, E = transverse colon
c. A = right kidney, B = gall bladder, C = aorta, D = stomach, E = pancreas
d. A = liver, B = gall bladder, C = aorta, D = left kidney, E = pancreas

2. Most probable diagnosis shown in Photograph is ***[Recent Question 2013]***

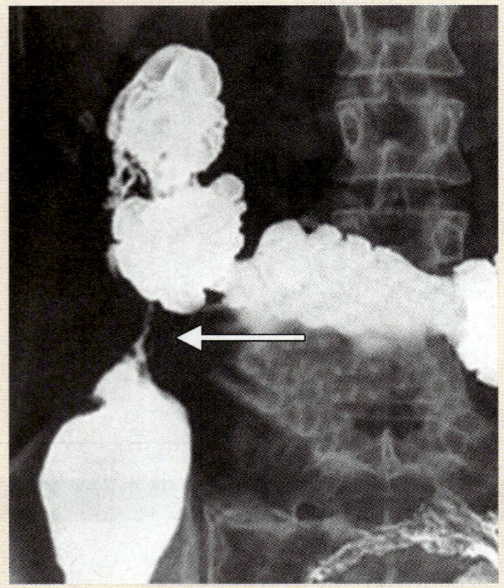

a. Lymphoma
b. Brucellosis
c. Tuberculosis
d. Caecal carcinoma

3. Bile ducts on Cholangiography (Photograph) is seen in

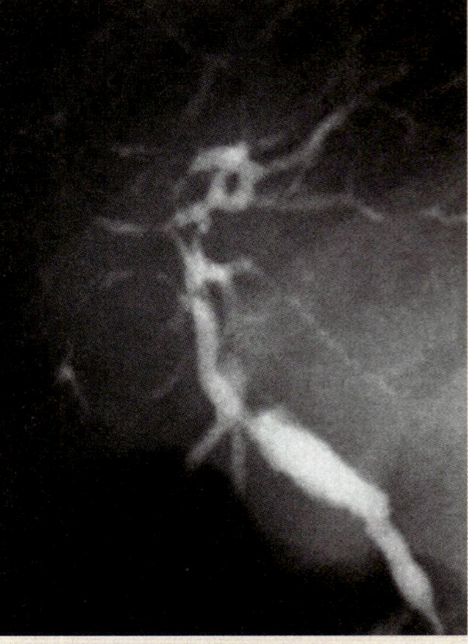

a. Choledochal cyst
b. Primary sclerosing cholangitis
c. Caroli's disease
d. Klatskin tumour

4. Diagnose the Oesophageal Condition (Photograph) based on Sign (Arrow)

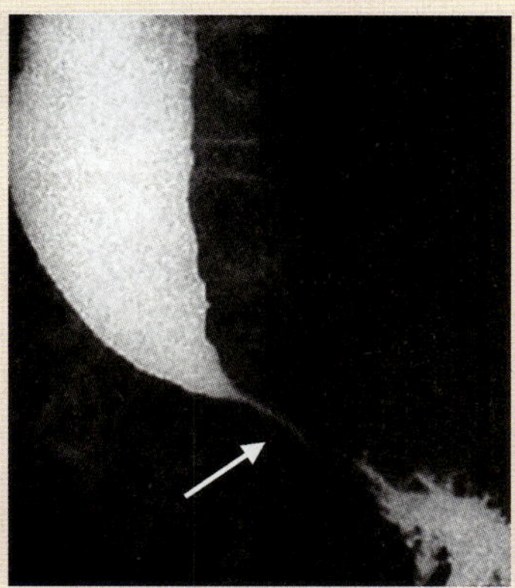

a. Carcinoma oesophagus
b. Traumatic injury
c. Achalasia cardia
d. Corkscrew oesophagus

5. Condition of Esophagus shown in Photograph is found in ***[Recent Question 2012]***

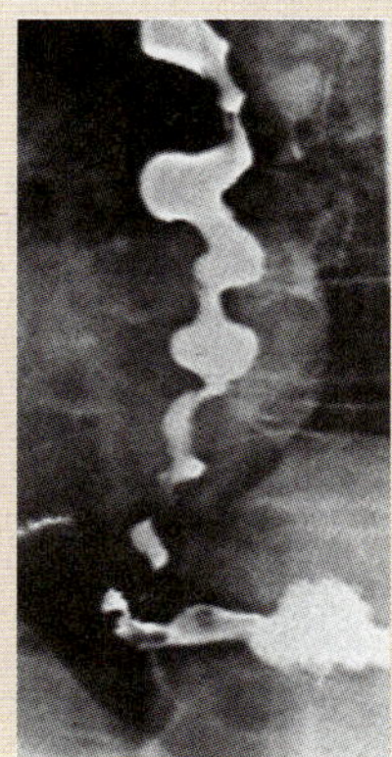

a. Carcinoma esophagus
b. Achalasia
c. Stricture esophagus
d. Diffuse esophageal spasm

6. Diagnose condition shown (Box) in the Photograph ***[Recent Question 2014]***

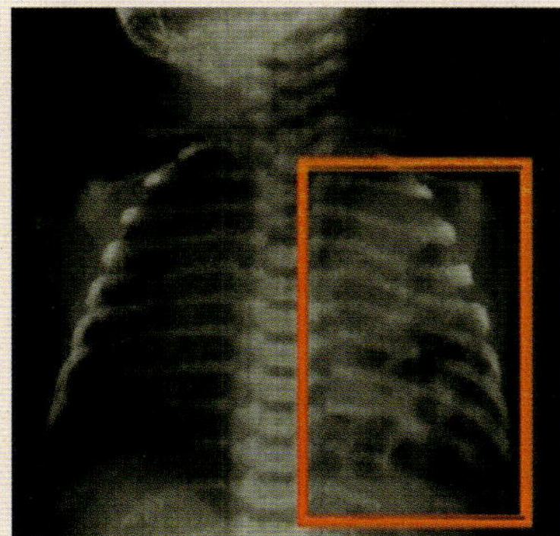

a. Diaphragmatic hernia
b. Bronchiectasis
c. Pneumatocoeles
d. Silicosis

7. Condition based on the Sign (Arrow) in Photograph ***[Recent Question 2012]***

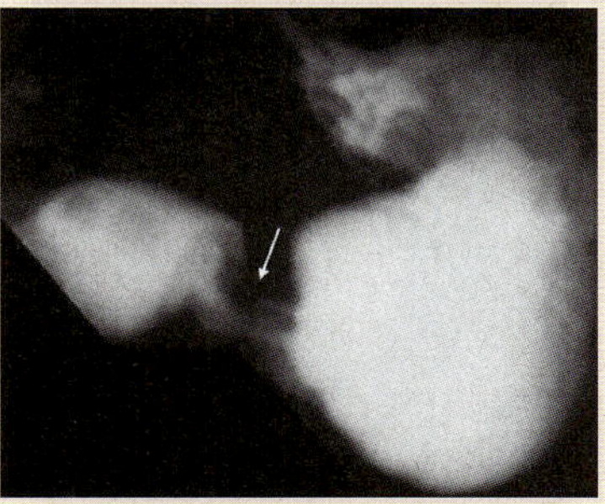

a. Stomach carcinoma
b. Ileocaecal TB
c. Ulcerative colitis
d. Hypertrophic pyloric Stenosis

8. Sign (Arrows) on Abdominal X-ray indicate ***[Recent Question 2014, 2015]***

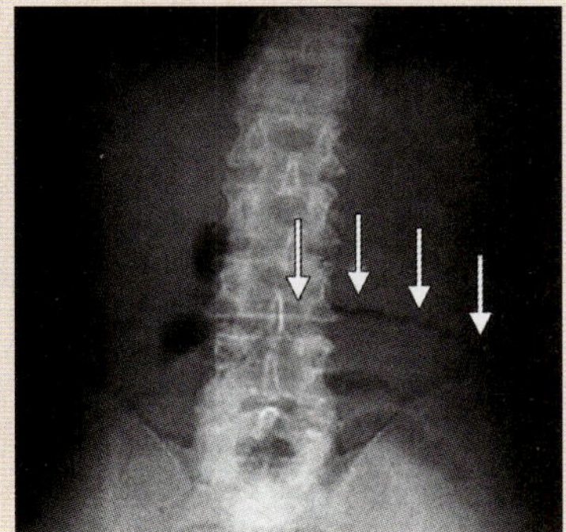

a. Crohn's disease
b. Ulcerative colitis
c. Small bowel obstruction
d. Ileocaecal Tuberculosis

9. Sign (Arrows) on Abdominal X-ray is seen in ***[Recent Question 2012, 2014]***

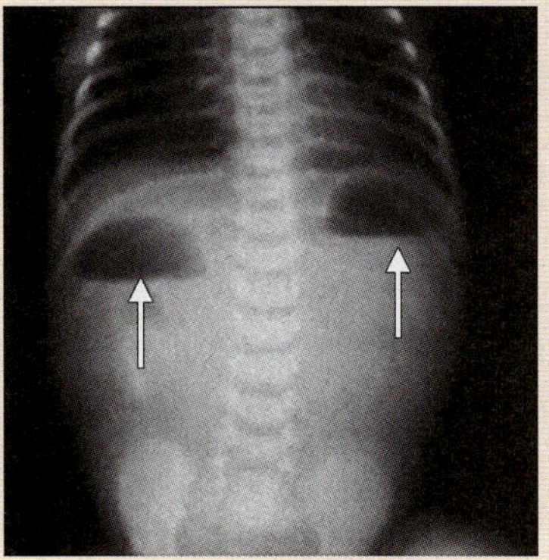

a. Duodenal atresia
b. Annular pancreas
c. Ladd's band
d. All of the above

10. Colonic Sign (Arrow) shown in Photograph is found in

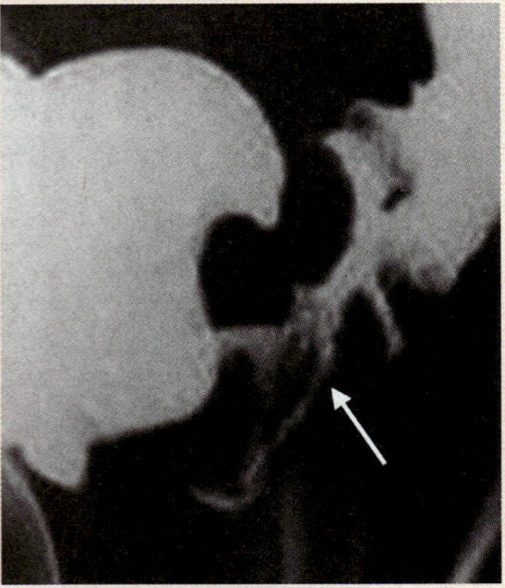

a. Colorectal carcinoma b. Ulcerative colitis
c. Crohn's disease d. All of the above

11. Appearance of Organ (Photograph) is seen in ***[Recent Question 2014]***

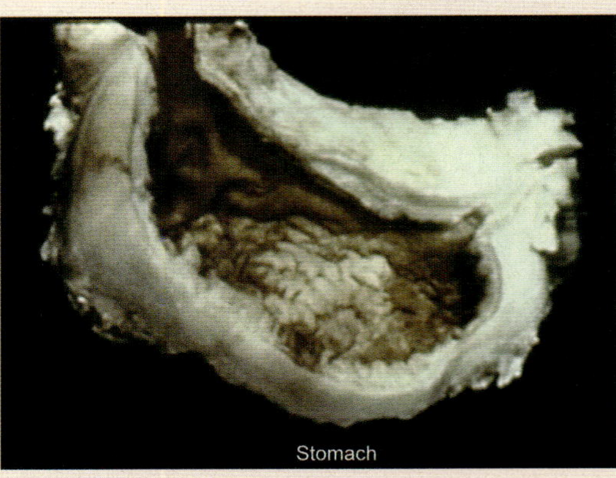

a. Gastric carcinoma b. Hodgkin's lymphoma
c. Kaposi sarcoma d. All of the above

12. Characteristic appearance (Arrows) of Colon in Photograph is in

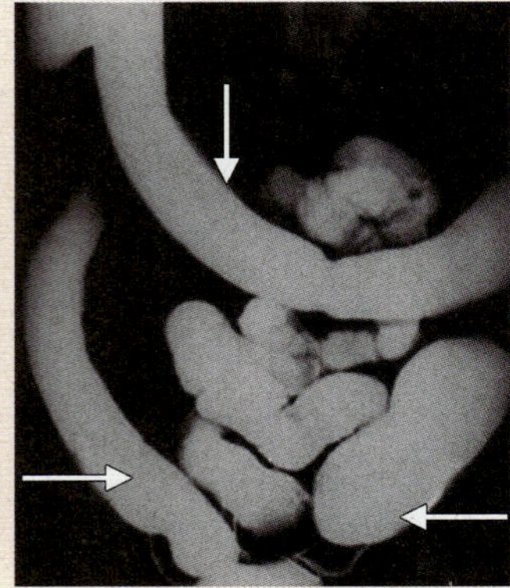

a. Crohn's disease b. Ulcerative colitis
c. Tuberculosis of colon d. Carcinoma colon

13. Sign shown in Abdominal X-ray (Photograph) is characteristic of

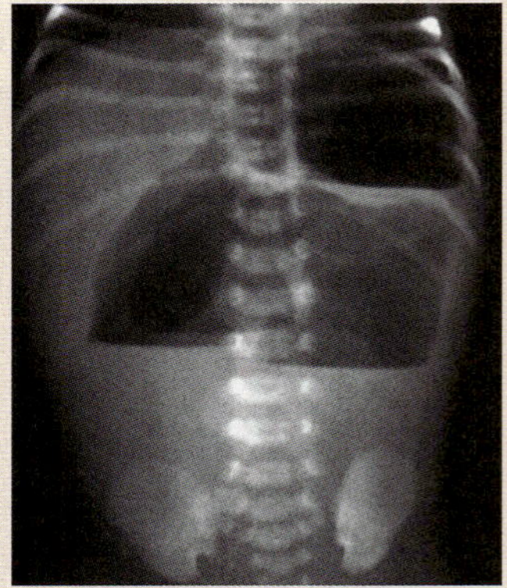

a. Pyloric obstruction b. Duodenal atresia
c. Jejunal atresia d. All of the above

14. Characteristic appearance of Bowel mucosa (Photograph) is seen in ***[Recent Question 2013]***

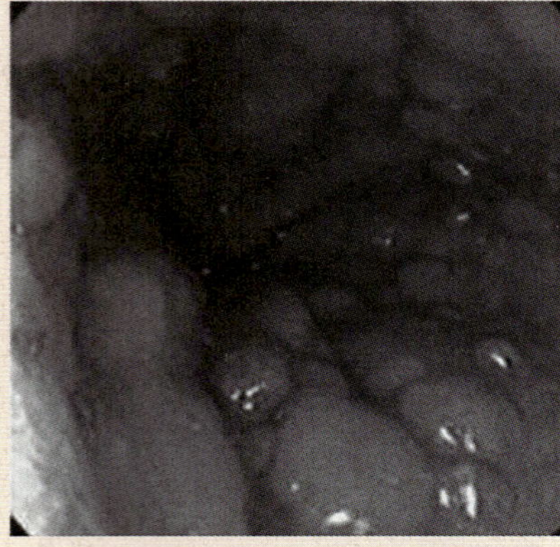

a. Tuberculosis b. Crohn's disease
c. Ulcerative colitis d. Carcinoma colon

15. Characteristic appearance of Colon in Photograph) is found in ***[Recent Question 2012]***

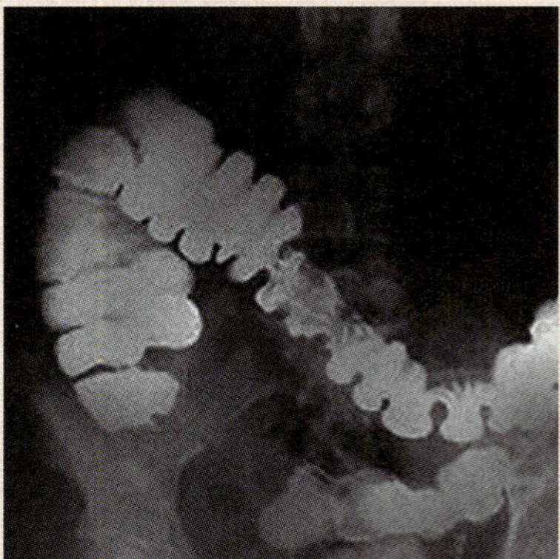

a. Tuberculosis b. Crohn's disease
c. Ulcerative colitis d. Diverticulitis

16. Typical appearance (Arrows) on ERCP is characteristic of ***[Recent Question 2014]***

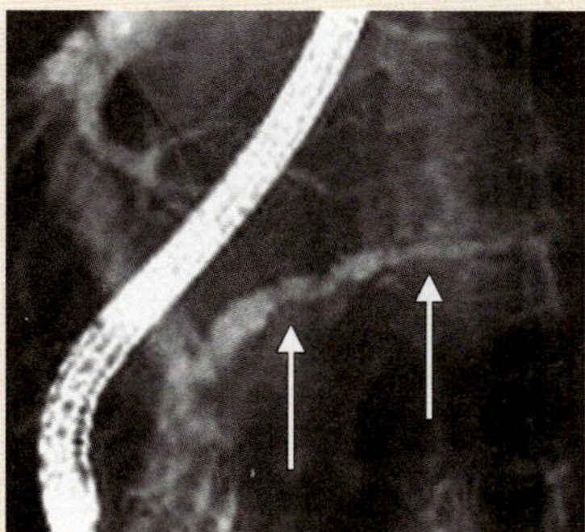

a. Annular pancreas
b. Pancreas divisum
c. Carcinoma head pancreas
d. Chronic pancreatitis

17. Typical sign of Duodenogram (Photograph) is characteristic of ***[Recent Question 2014]***

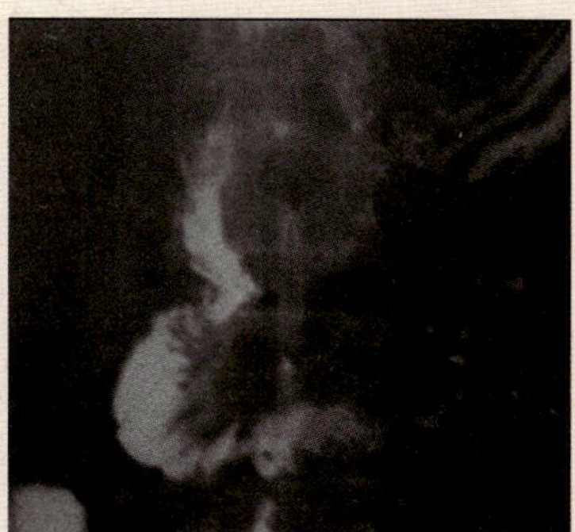

a. Annular pancreas
b. Pancreas divisum
c. Periampullary carcinoma
d. Chronic pancreatitis

18. Characteristic Sign of Colon on X-ray (Photograph) is seen in

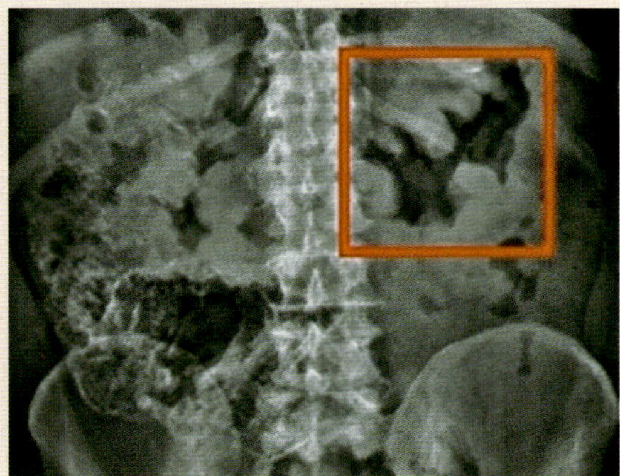

a. Ischemic colitis
b. Intussusception
c. Carcinoma pancreas
d. Carcinoma colon

19. A child has a history of not passing stool on first day of life. Radiological X-ray taken (Photograph) is ***[Recent Question 2015]***

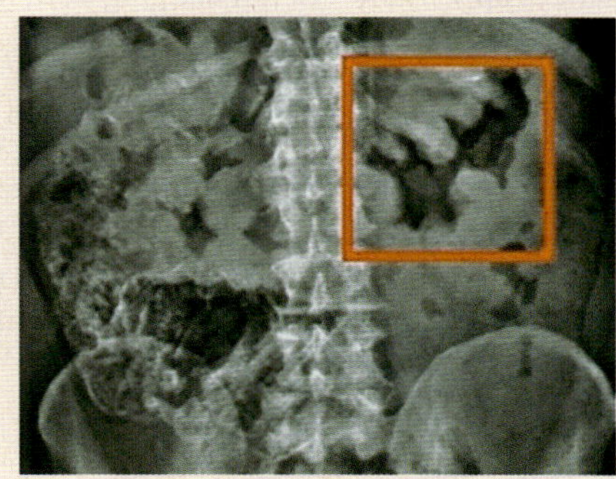

a. Barium meal follow through
b. X-ray abdomen supine
c. Invertogram
d. X-ray abdomen erect

20. CT scan of abdomen showing an area that branching into the liver. Identify the structure? ***[Recent Question 2018]***

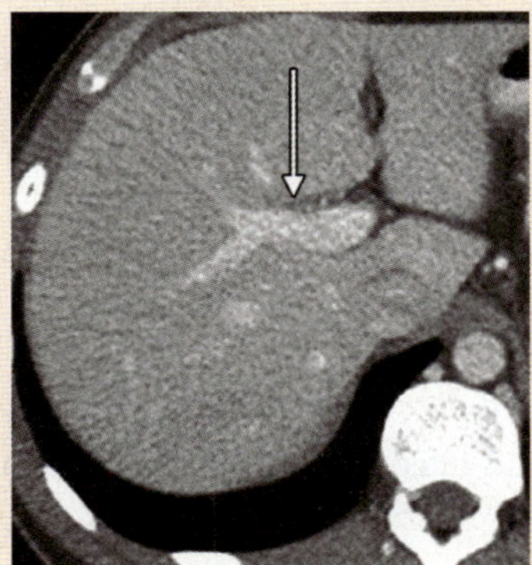

a. SVC
b. IVC
c. Portal vein
d. Splenic vein

21. Identify the marked vessel showing in Angiogram given below ***[Recent Question 2018]***

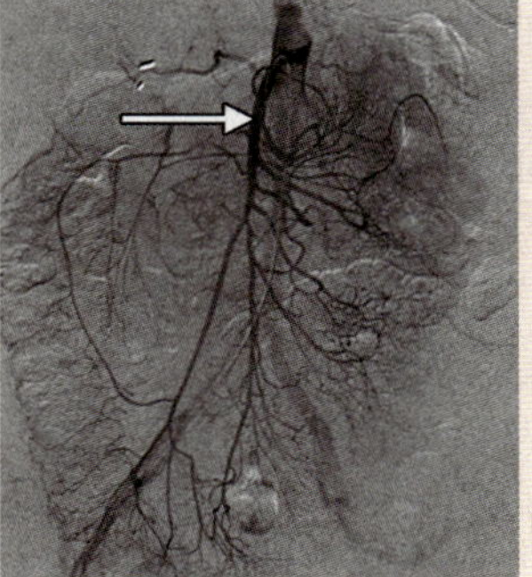

a. Superior mesenteric artery
b. Subclavian artery
c. Celiac artery
d. Brachiocephalic artery

 ANSWERS WITH EXPLANATIONS OF IBQs 

1. Ans. (d) **A = liver, B = gallbladder, C = aorta, D = left kidney, E = pancreas** *[Ref. CT Abdomen by Karthikeyan, 1/e p3]*

Normal Abdomen CT Scan

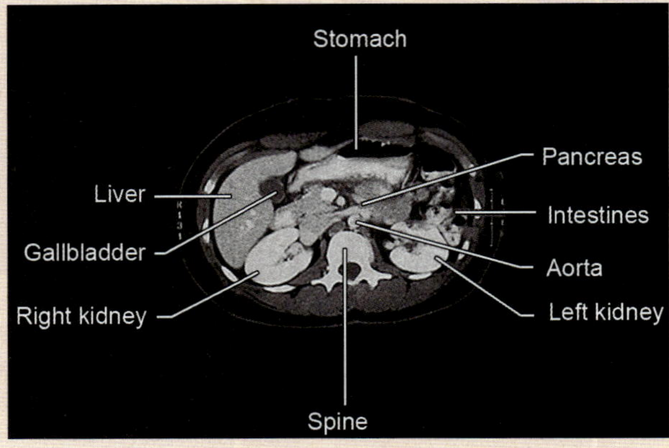

2. Ans. (c) **Tuberculosis** *[Ref. Sumer K Sethi, 5/e p69]*

GIT (Ileocaecal) Tuberculosis
- Pulled up caecum
- Gooseneck appearance: Ileum hanging from fibrosed pulled-up caecum
- Proximal ileal dilation
- String sign: Stricturous narrowing
- Purse-string appearance

3. Ans. (b) **Primary sclerosing cholangitis** *[Ref. Radiology Illustrated by Choi, 1/e p422]*

Primary Sclerosing Cholangitis
- Beading (Alternating pattern of strictures and normal/slightly dilated ducts)
- Pruned-tree appearance (Distal bile ducts are narrowed and difficult to see)
- Mural irregularity (Irregular luminal margin)
- Diverticula

4. Ans. (c) **Achalasia cardia** *[Ref. Sumer K Sethi, 5/e p65]*

Achalasia Cardia
- Rat-tail/Bird-beak tapering (Arrow in photograph)
- Dilated sigmoid esophagus

5. Ans. (d) **Diffuse esophageal spasm** *[Ref. Sumer K Sethi, 5/e p65]*
- Diffuse esophageal spasm shows Cork-screw/Rosary bead esophagus on Barium studies

6. Ans. (a) **Diaphragmatic hernia** *[Ref. Sumer K Sethi, 5/e p65-66]*
- Diaphragmatic hernia: Depending on the location and size of the defect retroperitoneal or intra-abdominal organs and tissues can prolapse into thoracic cavity due to negative intra-thoracic pressure

7. Ans. (d) **Hypertrophic pyloric Stenosis** *[Ref. Sumer K Sethi, 5/e p66]*

Hypertrophic Pyloric Stenosis
- String sign (Photograph)
- Apple core appearance
- Beak sign
- Shouldering
- Double track sign

8. Ans. (c) **Small bowel obstruction** *[Ref. Sumer K Sethi, 5/e p72]*
- String of beads appearance: Air trapped within valvulae and rest of loops are fluid-filled in small bowel obstruction

9. Ans. (d) **All of the above** *[Ref. Sumer K Sethi, 5/e p69]*

Double Bubble Sign
- Duodenal web
- Duodenal atresia

- Duodenal stenosis
- Annular pancreas
- Ladd's band
- Midgut volvulus
- Choledochal cyst
- Superior mesenteric artery syndrome

10. Ans. (d) All of the above *[Ref. Surgical Radiology by Banerjee, 1/e p65]*

Apple-Core (Napkin-Ring) Sign

- Colorectal carcinoma
- Ulcerative colitis
- Crohn's disease
- Ischemic colitis
- Infections (LGV, Tuberculosis, Amoeboma)
- Villous adenoma

11. Ans. (d) All of the above *[Ref. Sumer K Sethi, 5/e p68]*

Linitis Plastica of Stomach

- Gastric carcinoma
- Hodgkin's lymphoma
- Kaposi sarcoma
- Breast metastasis

12. Ans. (b) Ulcerative colitis *[Ref. Sumer K Sethi, 5/e p70]*

- Lead-pipe colon: Complete loss of haustral markings in the diseased section of colon, and the organ appears smooth walled and cylindrical seen in Ulcerative colitis

13. Ans. (c) Jejunal atresia *[Ref. NORD guide to Rare Disorders, 1/e p349]*

- Triple bubble sign: Dilation of proximal duodenum, stomach and jejunum

14. Ans. (b) Crohn's disease *[Ref. Sumer K Sethi, 5/e p70]*

Cobblestone Appearance

- Description: Longitudinal and circumferential fissures and ulcers separate islands of mucosa, giving it an appearance reminiscent of cobblestones
- Seen in:
  - Crohn's disease
  - Hirschsprung disease
  - Eosinophilic gastritis
  - Candida esophagitis
  - Duodenitis
  - Duodenal hamartoma

15. Ans. (d) Diverticulitis *[Ref. Sumer K Sethi, 5/e p70]*

Saw-Tooth Appearance

- Description: Serrated/ Concertina-like appearance
- MC Site: Sigmoid colon
- Seen in : Diverticulitis

16. Ans. (d) Chronic pancreatitis *[Ref. Sumer K Sethi, 5/e p74]*

- In Chronic Pancreatitis (ERCP), Main pancreatic duct may show a chain-of-lakes appearance due to alternating stenoses and dilatation

17. Ans. (c) Periampullary carcinoma *[Ref. Sumer K Sethi, 5/e p74]*

Frostburg Inverted 3 Sign

- Description: Effacement and distortion of the mucosal pattern on the medial wall of the second part of the duodenum due to focal mass and local oedema (Barium study)
- Seen in:
  - Carcinoma head of pancreas
  - Duodenal carcinoma
  - Pancreatitis

18. Ans. (a) Ischemic colitis *[Ref. Sumer K Sethi, 5/e p73]*

Thumbprinting Sign

- Description:
  - Large bowel wall thickening, usually caused by oedema, related to an infective or inflammatory process (colitis)
  - Normal haustrae become thickened at regular intervals appearing like thumbprints projecting into the aerated lumen
- Seen in:
  - Ischemic colitis
  - Ulcerative colitis
  - Crohn's disease
  - Diverticulitis
  - Pseudomembranous colitis
  - Lymphoma
  - Submucosal hemorrhage

19. Ans. (c) Invertogram *[Ref. Diagnostic Radiology by Berry, 2/e p90]*

Invertogram

- Description: An X-ray investigation in which a metal object is taped over the anal dimple, the child is held upside down (minimum 3 minutes) while an X-ray is made of the pelvis in a lateral projection
  - Only useful 12–24 hours or more after birth as gas needs to reach the distal rectum
- Uses:
  - Distance of gas bubble in rectum from the metal piece is noted:
    1. >2 cm: High Anal atresia type
    2. <2 cm: Low Anal atresia type
  - Imperforate anus
  - Surgical decisions

20. Ans. (c) Portal vein *[Ref. Grainger & Allison's Diagnostic Radiology, 6/e p756]*

Portal Vein (PV)

- Main vessel in the portal venous system and drains blood from the gastrointestinal tract and spleen to the liver
- Usually measures approximately 8 cm in length in adults (diameter 13 mm)
- Originates behind the neck of the pancreas, formed by the confluence of Superior mesenteric and Splenic veins and also receives blood from the inferior mesenteric, gastric, and cystic veins
- Immediately before reaching the liver, the portal vein divides in the porta hepatis into Left and Right portal veins

21. Ans. (a) Superior mesenteric artery *[Ref. Gray's Anatomy, 2/e p4]*

Superior Mesenteric Artery (SMA)

- Arises from the anterior surface of the abdominal aorta, just inferior to the origin of the celiac trunk
- Supplies the intestine from the lower part of the duodenum through two-thirds of the transverse colon, as well as the pancreas
- SMA Branches:
  - Inferior pancreaticoduodenal artery (Supplies Head of the pancreas, Ascending and inferior parts of the duodenum)
  - Intestinal arteries (Supplies Branches to ileum, jejunum)
  - Ileocolic artery (Supplies last part of ileum, cecum, and appendix)
  - Right colic artery (Supplies Ascending colon)
  - Middle colic artery (Supplies Transverse colon)

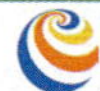 NEET/NBE PATTERN MCQs 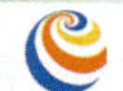

1. **A patient presents with abdominal distension and pain. What is the investigation you would like to do?** *[Recent Question 2016]*
   a. CT scan
   b. Barium enema
   c. X-ray with bowel preparation
   d. X-ray without bowel preparation
2. **'Double bubble sign' on X-ray abdomen is indicative of** *[NBE FMGE March 2005, September 2008, March 2010, NBE DNB 2001, 2005, 2006, AIIMS PGMEE 1999, Recent Question 2013]*
   a. Jejunal atresia b. Duodenal atresia
   c. Ileal atresia d. Ano-rectal malformation

PLEASE NOTE: Match the following (for Questions 3-4)
a. Frostburg sign b. Bird of prey sign
c. The pinwheel sign

3. **Appearance of gas pattern in volvulus of small bowel** *[NBE DNB 2005]*
4. **Inverted 3 or epsilon appearance of duodenal loop in lesions of head of pancreas** *[NBE DNB 2005]*
5. **'Sentinel loop' on X-ray is seen in** *[NBE FMGE September 2004, March 2010]*
   a. Splenomegaly b. Carcinoma colon
   c. Pancreatic mass d. Acute pancreatitis
6. **Consider the following radiological signs:**
   1. Claw-sign in barium enema
   2. Apple core sign in barium enema
   3. Multiple fluid levels with absent caecal gas in plain skiagram of abdomen
   4. Single large fluid and air level in plain skiagram of abdomen

   Which of these is/are suggestive of ileocaecal intussusception? *[UPSC 2010]*
   a. 1 and 2 b. 1 and 3
   c. 3 only d. 1, 2, 3 and 4
7. **"Rat-tail" appearance on barium swallow examination is seen in** *[Recent Question 2012]*
   a. Achalasia cardia b. Carcinoma esophagus
   c. Hiatus hernia d. Diffuse esophageal spasm
8. **"Spongy appearance" with central sunburst calcification is seen in** *[NBE DNB 2009]*
   a. Pancreatic adenocarcinoma
   b. Mucinous cyst adenocarcinoma
   c. Somatostatinoma
   d. Serous cyst adenoma
9. **Corkscrew appearance of esophagus is seen in** *[Recent Question 2012, 2017]*
   a. Carcinoma
   b. Achalasia
   c. Diffuse esophageal spasm
   d. Stricture
10. **Abdominal lump in a 6-month-old child with calcification on abdominal X-ray may be** *[NBE FMGE September 2008]*
    a. Lymphoma b. Leukemia
    c. Neuroblastoma d. Renal cell carcinoma
11. **Colon is identified on X-ray** *[Recent Question 2012]*
    a. Haustra
    b. Valvulae conniventes
    c. String of beads sign
    d. More number of loops Neonate triangular cord sign on
12. **Double track sign is seen in** *[Recent Question 2013]*
    a. Duodenal atresia b. CHPS
    c. Gastric ulcer d. Achalasia
13. **Inverted U-shaped grossly dilated loop of colon in straight X-ray abdomen is seen in** *[NBE DNB 1998]*
    a. Volvulus of colon
    b. Obstruction of descending colon
    c. Obstruction of ileocaecal junction
    d. Aganglionosis of sigmoid colon
14. **Severity of Pancreatitis can be assessed by** *[NBE FMGE September 2008]*
    a. Serum amylase levels
    b. Serum lipase levels
    c. Air-fluid levels on X-ray
    d. Extent of necrosis on CT scan
15. **Investigation of choice for evaluation of common bile duct is** *[UPSC 2011]*
    a. CECT scan b. Ultrasound
    c. HIDA scan d. MRCP
16. **Radio-opaque gallstones can be distinguished from renal stones by** *[NBE FMGE March 2007]*
    a. Anteroposterior view of X-ray abdomen
    b. Lateral view of X-ray abdomen
    c. IV cholecystography
    d. KUB X-ray abdomen
17. **Gold standard investigation for Recurrent gastrointestinal stromal tumor is** *[NBE DNB 2009]*
    a. MRI b. MIBG
    c. USG d. PET CT
18. **Congenital hypertrophic pyloric stenosis is diagnosed by** *[Recent Question 2012]*
    a. CT b. USG
    c. MRF d. X-ray
19. **Ideal investigation for evaluation of pathology in terminal common bile duct is** *[NBE FMGE March 2007]*
    a. USG b. CECT
    c. PTC d. ERCP
20. **Scan useful for imaging of pancreas is** *[NBE FMGE September 2006]*
    a. Gallium scan
    b. Technitium scan
    c. Seleno-methionine scan
    d. Rose Bengal scan
21. **A patients with progressive jaundice with clay coloured stool. The following investigations can be used, except** *[NBE DNB 2002]*
    a. Oral cholecystography b. Transhepatic biopsy
    c. ERCP d. USG

22. 'Cobblestoning' of colon is seen in *[NBE FMGE March 2006]*
a. Familial adenomatous polyposis
b. Ulcerative colitis
c. Crohn's disease
d. Amoebiasis

23. Best method of investigation is a case of acute cholecystitis is *[NBE DNB 2002]*
a. Ultrasound b. ERCP
c. OCG d. Radionuclide imaging

24. Investigation of choice in patient with blunt abdominal trauma and hematuria is *[UPSC 2009]*
a. Ultrasonography of abdomen
b. Contrast-enhanced computerized tomography
c. Intravenous urogram
d. Retrograde urogram

25. 'Double barrel' sign on Ultrasonography is indicative of *[NBE FMGE March 2006]*
a. Portal hypertension b. Portal vein cavernous
c. Portal vein thrombosis d. Obstructive jaundice

26. Meckel's diverticulum is best diagnosed by *[NBE DNB 1997, 2000, 2004, 2006]*
a. X-ray b. Ultrasound
c. CT scan d. Tc99 pertechnetium scan

27. 'Trapped air sign' in upper abdomen on plain X-ray is due to *[NBE FMGE March 2006]*
a. Splenic tumour b. Pancreatitis
c. Renal stones d. Chronic duodenal ulcer

28. Motility disorders of Esophagus are best diagnosed by *[UPSC 2009]*
a. Barium meal b. Manometry
c. Endoscopy d. Radiography

29. 'Stack of coins' appearance on plain X-ray in acute abdomen is found in *[NBE FMGE September 2003, NBE FMGE March 2006]*
a. Volvulus b. Mesenteric thrombus
c. Ischaemic colitis d. Intussusception

30. A patient presents to emergency department with pain and distension of abdomen and absolute constipation. What is the investigation of choice? *[UPSC 2009]*
a. Plain X-ray abdomen (erect)
b. Ultrasonography
c. Barium meal follow-through
d. Colonoscopy

31. 'Carman meniscus sign' in barium meal in pathognomonic of *[NBE FMGE March 2003, NBE FMGE March 2006]*
a. Malignant gastric ulcer b. Lipoma stomach
c. Gastric polyposis d. Lymphoma

32. "Bird of Prey" sign is seen in the radiographic barium examination of *[NBE DNB 2008, NBE DNB 2010]*
a. Gastric vulvulus b. Intussusception
c. Sigmoid vulvulus d. Caecal volvulus

33. 'Saw-tooth' appearance is characteristic of *[NBE FMGE September 2005]*
a. Crohn's disease b. Ischaemic colitis
c. Diverticulitis d. Bowel carcinoma

34. Widening of the C-loop in X-ray is diagnostic of *[NBE DNB 1997]*
a. Chronic pancreatitis
b. Carcinoma head of pancreas
c. Periampullary carcinoma
d. Calculi in the ampulla of water

35. Investigation of choice for Acute pancreatitis *[NBE FMGE September 2012]*
a. USG abdomen b. Contrast-enhanced CT
c. ERCP d. X-ray abdomen

36. Number of physiologic fluid levels in abdomen on X-ray should not be greater than *[NBE FMGE September 2003]*
a. 1 b. 2
c. 3 d. 4

37. Pain X-ray of an infant with abdominal pain show airless abdomen. Diagnosis is *[NBE FMGE March 2003]*
a. Necrotizing enterocolitis
b. Midgut volvulus
c. Worm colic
d. Intestinal pseudoobstruction

38. Gold standard test for diagnosis of Cystic Echinococcus is *[NBE FMGE September 2009]*
a. X-ray b. CT scan
c. USG d. ELISA

39. Initial investigation for amoebic liver abscess is *[NBE FMGE September 2009]*
a. Technetium-99 scan b. CT scan
c. Exploratory laparotomy d. USG

40. The gas used to create pneumoperitoneum during laparoscopy is *[NBE FMGE September 2011]*
a. O_2 b. NO_2
c. N d. CO_2

41. Pulled up caecum is seen in *[Recent Question 2013]*
a. Ileocecal TB b. Carcinoma cecum
c. Intussusception d. Carcinoma

42. Investigation of choice to see gallbladder *[Recent Question 2013]*
a. CT b. USG
c. Plain X-ray d. Oral cholecystogram

43. Investigation of choice in cholelithiasis is *[Recent Question 2013]*
a. MRI b. X-ray
c. CT d. USG

44. Investigation of choice in choledocholithiasis *[Recent Question 2013, 2015]*
a. CT b. PET scan
c. USG d. HIDA scan

45. Study using barium for small intestine is known as *[Recent Question 2013]*
a. Barium meal follow through
b. Barium swallow
c. Barium enema
d. None of the above

46. Corkscrew appearance of esophagus is seen in *[Recent Question 2013, 2015]*
a. Carcinoma
b. Achalasia
c. Diffuse esophageal spasm
d. Stricture

47. String of bead sign is seen in *[Recent Question 2013]*
a. Crohn's disease
b. Ulcerative colitis
c. Small intestine obstruction
d. Ileocaecal TB

48. Double bubble sign is seen in *[Recent Question 2013, 2015]*
a. Ladd's band b. Annular pancreas
c. Duodenal atresia d. All of the above

49. Investigation with least radiation dose in the diagnosis Meckel's diverticulum is *[Recent Question 2013]*
a. CT
b. MRI
c. Contrast radiography
d. Technetium - 99m scanning

50. CT, Balthazar grading is for *[Recent Question 2013]*
a. Acute pancreatitis b. Cholecystitis
c. Pancreatic carcinoma d. Chronic pancreatitis

51. Endoscopic USG criteria for Chronic pancreatitis, when echogenic lesion is *[Recent Question 2013]*
a. >1 mm b. 1.5 mm
c. >2 mm d. >3 mm

52. Use of water-soluble contrast medium is *[Recent Question 2013, 2014]*
a. Constipation b. Perforation
c. Ileocecal tuberculosis d. Gastroesophageal reflux

53. Hour-glass appearance of stomach is seen in *[Recent Question 2013]*
a. Linitis plastica b. Gastric ulcer
c. Duodenal ulcer d. Gastric carcinoma

54. Investigation of choice in a 65 years old male with occult blood in stools *[Recent Question 2014, 2015]*
a. X-ray b. Barium enema
c. Colonoscopy d. Intrarectal USG

55. Stepladder pattern is characteristic of *[Recent Question 2015]*
a. Acute appendicitis b. Diaphragmatic hernia
c. Intestinal perforation d. Small bowel obstruction

56. Barium meal follow through is helpful in diagnosing *[Recent Question 2017]*
a. Colonic stricture b. Ileal stricture
c. Rectal stricture d. Esophageal stricture

57. Bird beak appearance is seen in *[Recent Question 2017]*
a. Achlasia cardia b. Carcinoma esophagus
c. Hiatus hernia d. Diffuse esophageal spasm

58. Sonographic appearance of Hydatid cyst is *[Recent Question 2017]*
a. Hyperechoic aseptate lesion
b. Hypoechoic aseptate lesion
c. Hyperechoic septate lesion
d. Hypoechoic septate lesion

59. USG findings of focal anechoic lesion with floating membranes indicated toward which liver pathology? *[Recent Question 2017]*
a. Pyogenic abscess b. Hemangioma
c. Amoebic abscess d. Hydatid cyst

60. On barium swallow, Leiomyoma shows following characteristic appearance *[Recent Question 2017]*
a. Rat-tail appearance
b. Corkscrew appearance
c. Oval mass lined by barium
d. String sign

61. Best X-ray to diagnose Intraperitoneal air is? *[Recent Question 2017]*
a. Supine film of abdomen
b. Erect film of chest
c. Erect film of abdomen
d. Left lateral decubitus

62. Gold standard for detection of Gallstones is *[Recent Question 2017]*
a. CECT b. USG
c. X-ray d. Cholecystography

63. Dye used in diagnosis of Esophageal perforation is *[Recent Question 2018]*
a. Thorotrast b. Barium sulphate
c. Gadolinium d. Ioxaglate sodium

64. Diagnose the condition shown in the Double contrast esophagram radiograph given below. *[Recent Question 2018]*

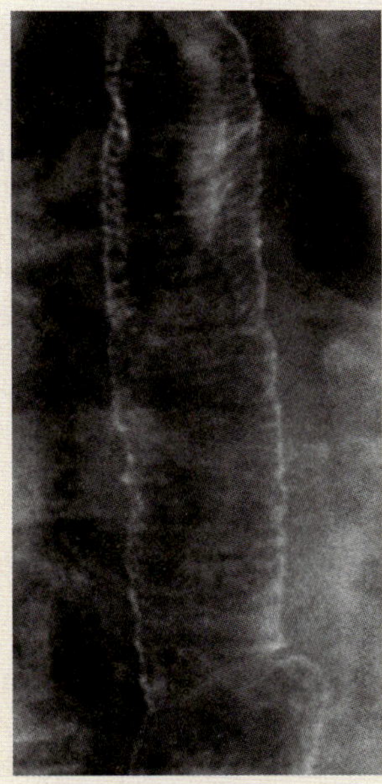

a. Esophageal atresia
b. Esophageal stenosis
c. Feline oesophagus
d. Tracheoesophageal fistula

HIGH YIELD MCQs

1. **Investigation of choice in upper GI bleeding is** *[Bihar PG 2016]*
   a. Ba swallow b. X-ray
   c. Endoscopy d. Ultrasound

2. **A newborn has not passed meconium since 48 hours. Investigation of choice is** *[AIIMS November 2014]*
   a. Anorectal manometry b. Rectal biopsy
   c. Contrast study d. Trypsin estimation

3. **Radiological signs of Crohn's disease** *[PGI 2008]*
   a. String sign of Kantor b. Pipe-stem appearance
   c. Pseudo polyp d. Backwash ileitis

4. **'Feathery appearance' in jejunum is due to** *[PGI 1999]*
   a. Valvulae conniventes b. Haustrations
   c. Luminal gas d. Vascular network

5. **X-ray appearance of CBD stone on Cholangiography is** *[AIIMS PGMEE 1998]*
   a. Meniscus appearance b. Sudden cut off
   c. Smooth tapering d. Eccentric occlusion

6. **'Double bubble sign' is seen in all except** *[PGI 2009]*
   a. Ladd's band
   b. Annular pancreas
   c. Pancreatic pseudocyst
   d. Duodenal atresia
   e. Diaphragmatic hernia

7. **'Lead pipe appearance' is seen in** *[PGI 1994, UP PGMEE 2002]*
   a. Crohn's disease b. Ulcerative colitis
   c. Schistosomiasis d. Carcinoma colon

8. **'Chain of lakes appearance' in ERCP is seen is** *[Recent Question 2017, All India PGMEE 1996]*
   a. Acute Pancreatitis b. Chronic Pancreatitis
   c. Carcinoma Pancreas d. Ductal Adenoma

9. **"Spongy appearance" with central sunburst calcification is seen in** *[AIIMS PGMEE 2007]*
   a. Pancreatic adenocarcinoma
   b. Mucinous cyst adenocarcinoma
   c. Somatostatinoma
   d. Serous cyst adenoma

10. **CT Scan is least accurate for** *[All India PGMEE 2011]*
    a. 1 cm gallstone
    b. 1 cm mass in pancreatic tail
    c. 1 cm lymph node in para-aortic region
    d. 1 cm aneurysm in hepatic artery

11. **Radiological feature of ischemic colitis is** *[PGI 1996, UP PGMEE 1999, Karnataka PGMEE 2001]*
    a. Saw toothing b. Craggy popcorn appearance
    c. Thumb printing d. Cobblestone appearance

12. **What is least useful as diagnostic procedure in case of acute haemetemesis?** *[AIIMS PGMEE 1991]*
    a. Barium meal
    b. Endoscopy
    c. Gastric content aspiration
    d. Angiography

13. **Diffuse esophageal dilatation on barium swallow is seen in** *[PGI 2005]*
    a. Achalasia b. Trypanosomiasis
    c. Etidronate therapy d. Scleroderma

14. **Radiological finding in Ileal atresia** *[PGI 2000]*
    a. Microcolon on the atresia
    b. Double bubble sign
    c. Coil spring appearance in Barium-Enema
    d. Obstruction in Barium meal

15. **All of the following are diagnostic barium follow through features of ileocecal tuberculosis except** *[All India PGMEE 2008]*
    a. Apple-core appearance
    b. Pulled up contracted caecum
    c. Widening of ileocaecal angle
    d. Strictures involving terminal ileum

16. **Investigation for small intestine includes all except** *[PGI 2005]*
    a. Enteroclysis b. Radionuclide enteroclysis
    c. MRI enteroclysis d. CT enteroclysis
    e. USG enteroclysis

17. **Gasless abdomen is a feature of** *[MP PGMEE 2001]*
    a. High obstruction
    b. Acute pancreatitis
    c. Congenital diaphragmatic hernia
    d. All

18. **Widening of C-loop of duodenum is a feature of** *[AIIMS PGMEE 1991]*
    a. Pancreatic head growth b. Carcinoma stomach
    c. Splenic involvement
    d. Involvement of upper right renal pole

19. **ERCP in pancreatitis is done to know about** *[PGI 2001]*
    a. Gallstones b. Associated cholangitis
    c. Ascites d. Pancreatic divisum
    e. Annular pancreas

20. **All of the following modalities can be used for in-situ ablation of liver secondaries, except** *[All India PGMEE 2006]*
    a. Ultrasonic waves b. Cryotherapy
    c. Alcohol d. Radio frequency

21. **X-ray appearance of CBD stone on cholangiography is** *[AIIMS PGMEE 1998]*
    a. Meniscus appearance b. Sudden cut off
    c. Smooth tapering d. Eccentric occlusion

22. **Thickened gallbladder wall in USG seen in** *[PGI 2004]*
    a. Acute cholecystitis b. Mucosal thickening
    c. Cholesterosis d. Ascites
    e. AIDS cholangitis

23. **True about features of cholecystitis on USG** *[PGI 2001]*
    a. Thick fibrosed gallbladder wall
    b. Stone impacted at neck of gallbladder
    c. Peri-gallbladder halo
    d. Increased vascularity

24. Investigation of choice in diffuse esophageal spasm is *[All India PGMEE 2008]*
a. Manometry
b. Esophagoscopy
c. Barium examination showing tertiary contractions
d. CT thorax

25. Splenic injury is diagnosed on X-ray by *[PGI 1997]*
a. Half stomach shadow
b. Obliteration of splenic shadow
c. Rib fracture
d. Gas under diaphragm

26. Investigation of choice for diagnosis of Splenic rupture is *[AIIMS PGMEE 1993]*
a. Peritoneal lavage
b. Ultrasound
c. CT scan
d. MRI

27. Minimal ascites can be best detected by *[AIIMS PGMEE 1998]*
a. USG
b. Plain X-ray abdomen
c. MRI
d. CT scan

28. Gastroesophageal reflux is best detected by *[AIIMS PGMEE 1992]*
a. Endoscopy
b. USG
c. Barium study
d. Isotope scan

29. Investigation of choice for gallstone *[DPG 2002]*
a. X-ray
b. USG
c. Cholecystography
d. CAT scan

30. Best investigation for acute cholecystitis is *[Maharashtra PGMEE 2002]*
a. FRCP
b. Oral cholecystography (OCG)
c. HIDA scan
d. IV cholangiography

31. Most common investigation done for obstructive jaundice *[AIIMS PGMEE 1999]*
a. CT scan
b. USG
c. X-ray
d. ERCP

32. True about OCG is *[PGI 2000]*
a. First done by Graham Cole in 1942
b. Dye ingested at rate of 1 ml/kg
c. Used for chronic gallbladder disease
d. Dye used is telepaque
e. Film taken is Right anterior oblique

33. Which is not required for visualization of gallbladder in oral cholecystography? *[AIIMS PGMEE 1995]*
a. Functioning liver
b. Motor mechanisms of gallbladder
c. Patency of cystic duct
d. Ability to absorb water

34. In a CT scan at the level of celiac trunk, following structures will be seen *[PGI 2002]*
a. Pancreas
b. Gallbladder
c. Inferior vena cava
d. Duodenum
e. Portal vein

35. Contrast material used in the diagnosis of esophageal atresia is *[PGI 1997]*
a. Gastrografin
b. Conray 42
c. Dianosil
d. Myodii

36. Double bubble sign is seen in *[PGI 2007, AIIMS PGMEE 2009]*
a. Duodenal atresia
b. Ileal atresia
c. Pyloric stenosis
d. Pancreatic divisum

37. String of Kantor is seen in *[AIIMS PGMEE 1996]*
a. Crohn's disease
b. Ulcerative colitis
c. TB
d. Carcinoma

38. X-ray feature of pyloric stenosis is *[AIIMS PGMEE 1997]*
a. Single bubble appearance
b. Double bubble appearance
c. Triple bubble appearance
d. Multiple air fluid levels

39. Soap Bubble appearance in X-ray is seen in *[AIIMS PGMEE 1999]*
a. Multiple cystic kidneys
b. Neuroblastoma
c. Cystic lymphangiectasia
d. Meconium ileus

40. Radiological sign of ischemic colitis is *[AIIMS PGMEE 1994]*
a. Popcorn appearance
b. Thumbprint appearance
c. Cobra-head appearance
d. Inverted 3 sign

41. String sign is suggestive of *[AIIMS PGMEE 1993]*
a. Toxic Megacolon
b. Hypertrophic Pyloric stenosis [HPS]
c. Ulcerative Colitis
d. IBS

42. A newborn presenting with intestinal obstruction showed on abdominal X-ray, multiple air fluid levels. The diagnosis is not likely to be *[All India PGMEE 2002]*
a. Pyloric obstruction
b. Duodenal atresia
c. Ileal atresia
d. Ladd's bands

43. Double bubble sign in children is seen in all except *[PGI 2004]*
a. Ladd's band
b. Annular pancreas
c. Pancreatic pseudocyst
d. Duodenal atresia
e. Diaphragmatic hernia

44. Central dot sign is seen in *[AIIMS PGMEE 2008]*
a. Caroli's disease
b. Primary sclerosing cholangitis
c. Polycystic liver disease
d. Liver hamartoma

45. Following are common features of malignant gastric ulcer on Barium meal, except *[AIIMS PGMEE 2004]*
a. Location on the greater curvature
b. Carman's meniscus sign
c. Radiating folds which do not reach the edge of the ulcer
d. Lesser curvature ulcer with a nodular rim

46. Ileocecal tuberculosis presents with all except *[PGI 2006, JIPMER PGMEE 2007]*
a. Rapid emptying of narrowed terminal ileum
b. Inverted umbrella sign
c. Stellate ulcer with elevated margins
d. Longitudinal ulcers are more common
e. Napkin ring stenosis

47. After taking a drug, a patient developed some abdominal problem for which he consulted a physician, who advised X-ray. X-ray showed radio-opacity in bowel. Probably he might have taken all except: *[AIIMS PGMEE 1995]*
a. Salicylate b. Iron
c. Phenothiazine d. Corticosteroid

48. According Couinaud's classification of functional segments of liver, which of the following is Segment IV of liver? *[AIIMS PGMEE 2007]*
a. Left lobe b. Right lobe
c. Caudate lobe d. Quadrate lobe

49. Differential diagnosis for Right upper quadrant calcification *[PGI 2006]*
a. Gallstone b. Renal stone
c. Calcification in vessels d. Hepatic hemangioma
e. None

50. Solitary hypoechoic lesion of the liver without septate or debris is most likely to be *[AIIMS PGMEE 2005]*
a. Hydatid cyst b. Caroli's disease
c. Liver abscess d. Simple cyst

51. Which one of the following hepatic lesions can be diagnosed with high accuracy by using nuclear imaging? *[AIIMS PGMEE 2004]*
a. Hepatocellular carcinoma
b. Hepatic adenoma
c. Focal nodular hyperplasia
d. Cholangiocarcinoma

52. A 22-year-old man presents with a solitary 2 cm space occupying lesion of mixed echogenicity in the right lobe of liver on ultrasound examination. The rest of the liver is normal. Which of the following tests should be done next? *[AIIMS PGMEE 2002]*
a. Ultrasound guided biopsy of the lesion
b. Hepatic Scintigraphy
c. Hepatic angiography
d. Contrast-enhanced CT scan of the liver

53. Air in biliary tract is seen in all except *[Delhi PGMEE 2007]*
a. Gallstone ileus
b. Sclerosing cholangitis
c. Carcinoma gallbladder
d. Endoscopic papillotomy

54. Focal and diffuse thickening of gallbladder wall with high amplitude reflections and 'comet tail' artifacts on USG suggest the diagnosis of *[All India PGMEE 2009]*
a. Xanthogranulomatous cholecysitis
b. Carcinoma of gallbladder
c. Adenomyomatosis
d. Cholesterolosis

55. A newborn baby has not passed meconium for 48 hours since birth, presents with vomiting and distension of abdomen. The most appropriate investigation for evaluation would be? *[AIIMS PGMEE 2007]*
a. Barium enema study
b. Manometry
c. Rectal biopsy
d. Fecal fat estimation

56. A newborn baby has not passed meconium for 48 hours since birth. She has vomiting and distension of abdomen. The most appropriate investigation for evaluation would be *[All India PGMEE 2008]*
a. Anorectal manometry b. Rectal biopsy
c. Lower GI contrast study d. Trypsin estimation

57. In a patient with abdominal trauma who is hemodynamically stable, what would be the investigation of choice? *[AIIMS PGMEE 2009]*
a. FAST b. DPL
c. Barium meal d. Erect X-ray abdomen

58. For the evaluation of blunt abdominal trauma, which of the following imaging modalities is ideal? *[AIIMS PGMEE 2004]*
a. Ultrasonography
b. Computed tomography
c. Nuclear scintigraphy
d. Magnetic resonance imaging

59. A patient complains of epigastric pain, radiating to back off and on. The investigation of choice is *[AIIMS PGMEE 1999]*
a. MRI b. CT scan
c. USG d. Radionucleotide scan

60. Investigation of choice for detection of minimal ascites *[AIIMS PGMEE 1992]*
a. Plain X-ray abdomen b. MRI
c. CT scan d. USG

61. Investigation of choice in obstructive jaundice is *[All India PGMEE 1997]*
a. ERCP b. USG
c. Cholecystography d. Laparoscopy

62. The investigation of choice for acute cholecystitis is *[PGI 2002]*
a. USG b. HIDA scan
c. CT scan d. OCG
e. X-ray

63. Investigation of choice for recurrent GIST *[AIIMS PGMEE 2008]*
a. MIBG b. PET
c. MRI d. CECT

64. For a child presenting with Appendicitis, investigation of choice is *[AIIMS November 2014]*
a. USG b. CT scan
c. MRI d. Barium study

65. A neonate having clay coloured stools was on Ursodeoxycholic acid. Eyes and urine show discolouration. Investigation of choice is *[AIIMS November 2014]*
a. USG b. HIDA
c. LFTs d. CT scan

66. Best investigation to diagnose Piles is *[ESI IMO 2014]*
a. Proctosigmoidoscopy b. Barium enema
c. Ultrasound d. Proctoscopy

67. Best investigation in Acute cholecystitis is *[ESI IMO 2014]*
a. Technetium scan b. HIDA scan
c. Pipida scan d. Plain X-ray abdomen

68. "Chain of lakes" is seen on ERCP in *[PGMCET 2015]*
a. Chronic pancreatitis b. Pancreatic divisum
c. Ileocecal TB d. Ca. head of pancreas

69. All the patients with proven Rectal cancer require staging by *[PGMCET 2015]*

a. Imaging of liver and chest, preferably by CT along with local petis imaging
b. Monoclonal antibodies
c. Colonography
d. PET scan

70. Gold standard for diagnosing Common Bile Duct Stones is *[PGMCET 2015]*

a. Plain X-ray abdomen
b. Oral cholecystography
c. Ultrasonography
d. Endoscopic cholangiography

71. Schatzki ring is demonstrated by *[PGMCET 2015]*

a. Barium meal
b. Barium enema
c. IVP
d. Barium Swallow

72. A 45 years old man, chronic smoker, progressive jaundice with pruritus and clay stools for 2 months, history of waxing and waning of jaundice. On CT common bile duct and main pancreatic duct dilated. What is the diagnosis? *[AIIMS PG November 2015]*

a. Ampullary Ca
b. Ca head pancreas
c. Pancreatitis
d. Cholangiocarcinoma

NEET/NBE PATTERN MCQs ANSWERS WITH EXPLANATIONS

1. Ans. (d) X-ray without bowel preparation

[Ref. SRB's Manual of Surgery, 5/e p927]

Intestinal Obstruction

- Conventional plain radiography: Investigation of choice for patients with suspected small-bowel obstructions
- Studies have shown the superiority of CT scanning in revealing not only the site of the obstruction but also its cause; CT scans may demonstrate signs of ischemia as well

2. Ans. (b) Duodenal atresia

[Ref. Sure Success in PGMEE by B. Ramgopal, 1/e p130]

'Double-Bubble Sign' (X-ray Abdomen)

- Duodenal atresia/ Severe stenosis (Most characteristic)
- Duodenal atresia
- Annular pancreas
- Malrotation of gut (Midgut volvulus)
- Pre-duodenal position of portal vein
- Duodenal web
- Ladd bands
- Duodenal duplication cyst

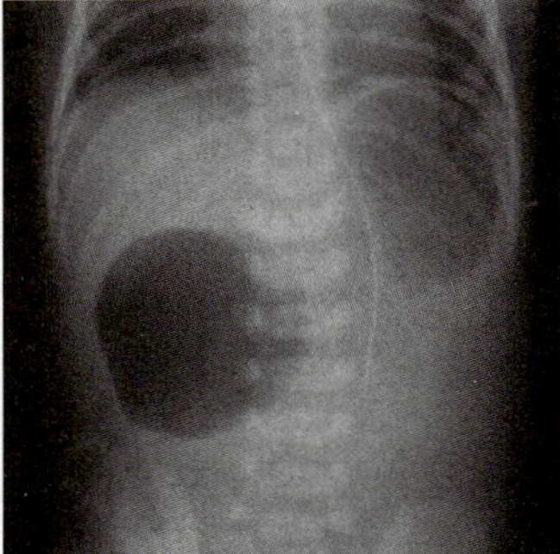

Fig. Double bubble sign

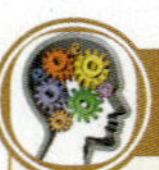

Also Remember

- *Single bubble sign*: Pyloric atresia
- *Triple bubble sign*: Jejunal atresia

3. Ans. (b) Bird of prey sign

[Ref. Bipin Valchandji Daga, 1/e p167]

- Sigmoid Volvulus: 'Bird of prey' sign, Liver overlap sign, Inverted U/V sign, Omega sign, Bent tyre tube sign and Coffee bean sign

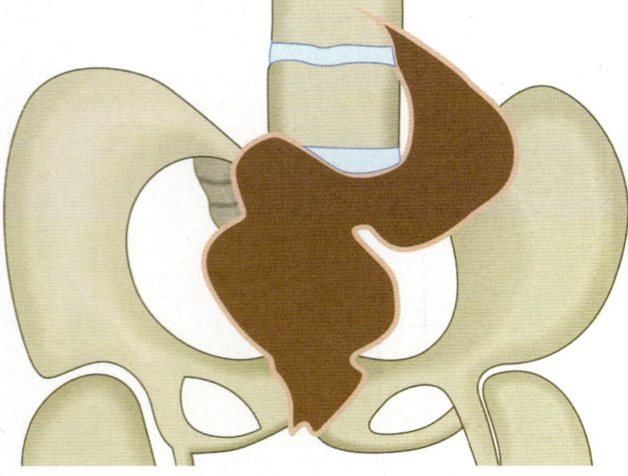

Fig. Bird of prey sign

4. Ans. (a) Frostburg sign

[Ref. Radiodiagnosis, Nuclear Medicine, Radiotherapy and Radiation oncology by Bipin Valchandji Daga, 1/e p167]

- Reverse '3' sign of Forstburg is for carcinoma head of pancreas.

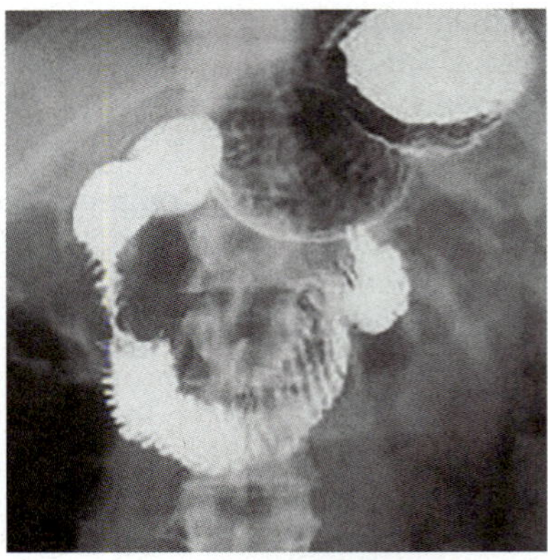

Fig. Reverse 3 sign

5. Ans. (d) Acute pancreatitis

[Ref. Sumer K Sethi, 5/e p74]

Radiology in Pancreatitis

- *Investigation of choice*:
  - Acute pancreatitis: Contrast-enhanced CT (CECT)
  - Chronic pancreatitis: ERCP
- *Findings of Pancreatitis*:
  - *Sentinel loop*
  - Gasless abdomen
  - Colon cut-off
  - Duodenal ileus
  - Mottled lucencies
  - *Chain of lakes appearance* (ERCP in Chronic pancreatitis)
  - *Pancreatic calcification (Chronic alcoholism)*

Also Remember

Causes of Pancreatic Calcification

- Chronic alcoholic pancreatitis (Most common cause)
- Hereditary pancreatitis
- Malnutrition
- Hyperparathyroidism

6. Ans. (b) 1 and 3

[Ref. Radiodiagnosis, Nuclear Medicine, Radiotherapy and Radiation oncology by Bipin Valchandji Daga, 1/e p167]

- 'Coiled spring' appearance and 'Claw' sign are indicative of intussusception

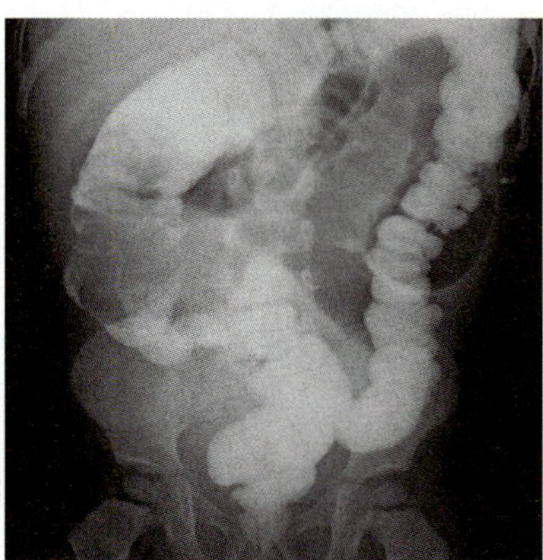

Fig. Coiled spring sign

7. Ans. (a) Achalasia cardia

[Ref. David Sutton, 7/e p552]

- Achalasia is a motor disorder of the oesophagus generally occurring in the 35–50 year age group. A barium swallow will show the gastro-oesophageal junction failing to open fully and tapering to a rat-tail or bird beak appearance.

8. Ans. (d) Serous cystadenoma

[Ref. Bipin Valchandji Daga, 1/e p225]

- Serous cystadenoma of pancreas: Sunburst calcification in a spongy mass
- Mucinous cystadenoma of pancreas: Eggshell calcification in a spongy mass

9. Ans. (c) Diffuse esophageal spasm

Ref. David Sutton, 7/e p549]

10. Ans. (c) Neuroblastoma

[Ref. Sumer K Sethi, 5/e p82]

Radiology in Neuroblastoma

- Calcification
- Vascular encasement
- Solid appearance (USG)
- Bony metastasis
- Secondaries in orbit

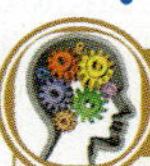

Also Remember

- *Renal cell carcinoma*:
  - Non-functioning kidney
  - Bony metastasis: Lytic expansile lesions
- *Lymphoma*: Thickened folds, nodularity, depressed lesions, ulcers, prominent area gastricae

11. Ans. (a) Haustra

[Ref. David Sutton, 7/e p618]

- It is occasionally difficult to distinguish distended small bowel from colon: Small bowel tends to lie centrally and the valvula conniventes are thinner than colonic haustra and also tend to cross the bowel diameter completely

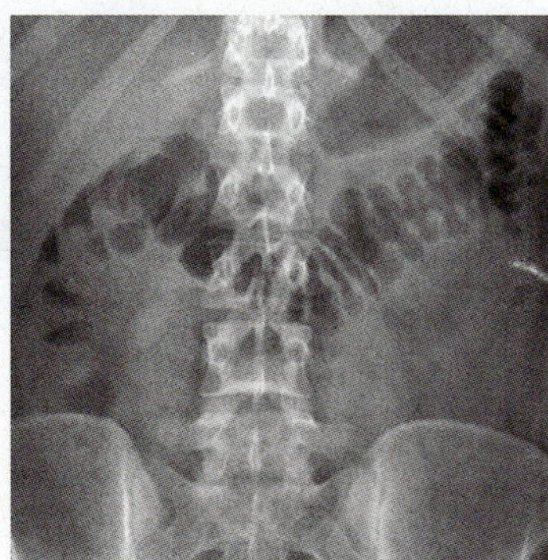

Fig. Colonic haustra

12. Ans. (b) CHPS

[Ref. David Sutton, 7/e p855]

- In Congenital Hypertrophic pyloric Stenosis (CHPS), hyper dynamic peristalsis in the antrum results in 'pyloric tit' and a 'double-track' appearance of the pyloric canal

13. Ans. (a) Volvulus of colon

[Ref. David Sutton, 7/e p677]

- When a sigmoid volvulus occurs, the inverted U-shaped loop is usually massively distended and it is commonly devoid of haustra (ahaustral)

14. Ans. (d) Extent of necrosis on CT scan

[Ref. Bailey and Love, 25/e p1141]

Radiology in Pancreatitis

- *X-rays abdomen*: Non-specific
  - Sentinel-loop
  - Colon cut-off sign
  - Renal halo sign
- *Ultrasonography*:
  - Only useful for gallstones, cholecystitis and dilated bile duct
- *CT scan (CECT)/MRI*:
  - To establish diagnosis
  - Differentiate interstitial and necrotizing pancreatitis
  - Extent of necrosis (after 72 hours): Staging based on *'Balthazar criteria'*
- *EUS/MRCP*:
  - Stones in bile duct
  - Assessment of pancreatic parenchyma
- *ERCP*:
  - Identification and removal of gallstones

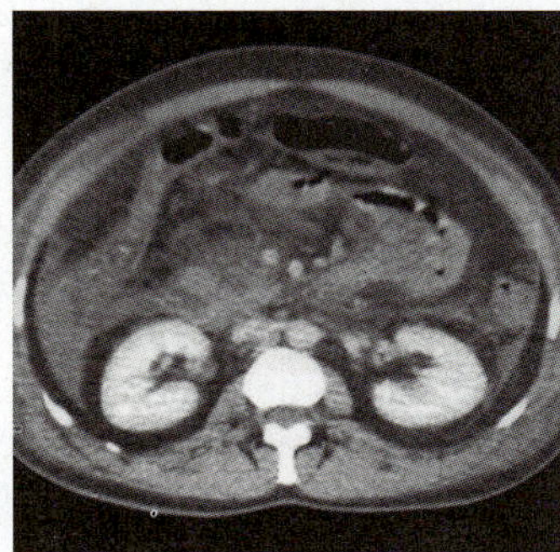

Fig. Renal halo sign

15. Ans. (b) Ultrasound

[Ref. David Sutton, 7/e p686, 714]

- The view of the pancreas at ultrasound may be poor in some patients, but ultrasound will provide valuable information regarding the biliary tree where common bile duct obstruction must be excluded
- Ultrasound is the technique which answers most of the clinical questions posed in patients with suspected biliary tract pathology

16. Ans. (b) Lateral view of X-ray abdomen

[Ref. Sumer K Sethi, 5/e p78]

- *On Lateral view of X-ray abdomen*:
  - Renal or ureteric calculus overlies the spine
  - Gallstone doesnot overlie the spine

17. Ans. (b) MIBG

[Ref. David Sutton, 7/e p832]

18. Ans. (b) USG

[Ref. David Sutton, 7/e p854]

- Ultrasound has now replaced the barium meal as the first-line investigation in the infant with non-bilious vomiting in whom HPS is the most likely diagnosis

- USG is a safe, non-ionising investigation which, with experience, is both highly sensitive and specific
- Infant is positioned in the left anterior oblique position and scanned over the right upper quadrant with a linear (>5 MHz) transducer
- Although overreliance on measurement criteria should be avoided, a muscle width measurement of >3.5 mm and a pyloric length of >16 mm in a term infant are usually taken as diagnostic of HPS

19. Ans. (d) ERCP

[Ref. Sumer K Sethi, 5/e p13]

Radiology of Biliary Tract

- ***Investigation of choice for most gallbladder pathologies*: USG**
- *Investigation of choice for Acute cholecystitis*: Tc-99 HIDA scan
- *Investigation of choice for Low bile duct obstruction (CBD obstruction)*: ERCP (Endoscopic cholangiopancreatography)
- *Investigation of choice for High bile duct obstruction (Klatskin tumour)*: PTC (Percutaneous transhepatic cholangiography)
- *Initial investigation of choice for surgical jaundine*: USG
- *Investigation of choice for Biliary atresia*: Peroperative cholangiography

20. Ans. (c) Selenomethionine scan

[Ref. Selenomethionine scanning in diagnosis of tumours of pancreas and other adjacent viscera, GUT 1975, 75-87]

- *Selenomethionine scan is useful for*:
  - Tumours of Pancreas and adjacent viscera
  - Assessment of pancreatic function
  - Differential diagnosis of cold thyroid nodule
  - Tumours of parathyroid

21. Ans. (a) Oral cholecystography

22. Ans. (c) Crohn's disease

[Ref. Sumer K Sethi, 5/e p70]

Radiology in Inflammatory Bowel Disease

Ulcerative colitis	Crohn's disease
Pipe-stem colon **M**ucosal involvement (contiguous) **T**oxic megacolon **P**seudopolyps **S**tove pipe sign **B**lurred mucosal strips, granular appearance* **C**ollar-button ulcers	**T**ransmural involvement **S**kip lesions **C**obblestone colon **R**aspberry/rose thorn appearance **A**phthoid ulceration* **S**tring sign of Kantor **H**alo-sign (CT) **R**ectal sparing **S**trictures/ fistulae **P**seudosacculations
[Mnemonic: PMT Process **S**elects **B**etter **C**andidates**]**	**[Mnemonic: T**raffic **S**ignal **CRASH R**esults in **S**erious **P**athology**]**

(Earliest sign)*

23. Ans. (d) Radionuclide imaging

[Ref. David Sutton, 7/e p759]

- If the gallbladder and bile ducts are demonstrated by 45 minutes but no tracer has passed into the bowel, a fatty meal or cholecystokinin (CCK) infusion may be used to provoke biliary drainage
- If the gallbladder is not demonstrated by 60 minutes and acute cholecystitis is suspected, imaging should be continued up to 4 hours, as some patients with chronic gallbladder disease show delayed filling
- Absence of filling at 4 hours is a good indication of acute cholecystitis with mechanical or functional obstruction of the cystic duct

24. Ans. (b) Contrast enhanced CT

[Ref. David Sutton, 7/e p700; Sumer K Sethi, 6/e p134]

- Rapid CT imaging has revolutionised the management of renal trauma
  - Helps in expedition of a further surgical procedure
- Intravenous urography can be negative in 21–34% of significant injuries and, even when positive, the findings are often non-specific and correlate poorly with renal injury severity
  - Excretory urography is screening procedure of choice in Blunt abdominal trauma without Renal injury and stable

25. Ans. (d) Obstructive jaundice

[Ref. Ultrasound in Emergency Care by Brroks, 1/e p53]

- *'Double barrel' sign on Ultrasonography*: Obstructive Jaundice

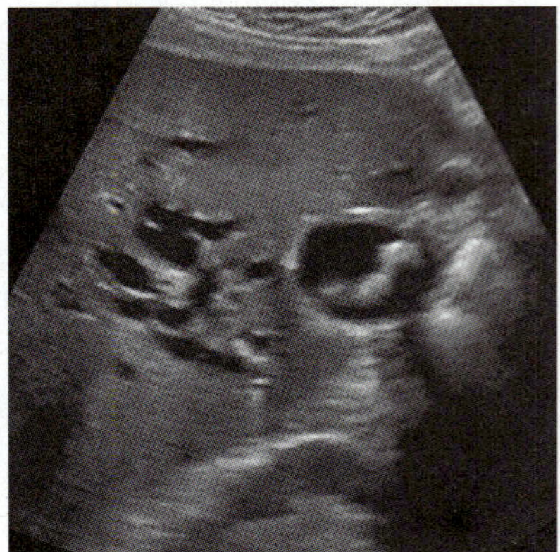

Fig. Double barrel sign

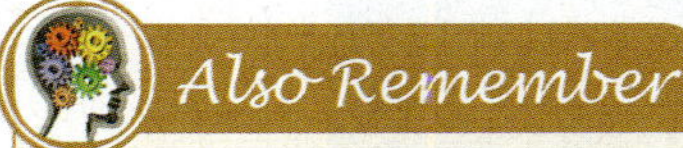

Few Signs on Hepato-Biliary-Pancreatic Imaging

- *'Double duct' sign on USG*: Pancreatic carcinoma
- *Echogenic focus with posterior acoustic shadowing on USG*: Gall-stones
- *Mercedes-Benz sign*: Air in gallstones
- *WES (Wall-Echo-Shadow) sign*: Cholelithiasis with Chronic cholecystitis
- *'Meniscus sign' on Cholangiogram*: Common bile duct stones
- *'Chain of lakes' appearance on ERCP*: Chronic pancreatitis
- *'Frostburg inverted 3 sign'*: Periampullary carcinoma Pancreas

26. Ans. (d) Tc 99 pertechnetium scan

[Ref. David Sutton, 7/e p851]

- Radionuclide imaging technique can provide functional information in a variety of specific applications
- More commonly encountered investigations include Meckel's (TcO4)

27. Ans. (d) Chronic duodenal ulcer

[Ref. MedScape]

Radiology in GIT Ulcers

- Benign gastric ulcer:
  - *Hampton's line*
  - Ulcer collar
  - Ulcer mound
- Malignant gastric ulcer:
  - *Carman's meniscus sign*
- Duodenal ulcer:
  - *'Trapped air sign'* in upper abdomen

28. Ans. (b) Manometry

[Ref. David Sutton, 7/e p549]

- Oesophageal manometry is used to evaluate motility, but when it is unavailable the barium swallow provides a useful alternative
- Motility often varies from one swallow to the next, so at least five single prone swallows should be recorded for proper evaluation
- Radionuclide imaging of the oesophagus is reserved for patients in whom the first-line tests of endoscopy and barium swallow produce unexpected or inconclusive results, and those in whom the initial tests are negative
- Scintigraphy has the advantages of using physiological fluids or solids, producing quantifiable results, and being highly sensitive in the early detection of motility disorders

29. Ans. (b) Mesenteric thrombus

[Ref. Gastrointestinal Radiology by Eisenberg, 4/e p453]

STACK OF COINS APPEARANCE (Bleeding into bowel wall leads to regular thickening of small bowel folds)

- *Ischaemia*:
  - Atherosclerosis
  - Thromboembolic disease
  - Mesenteric thrombosis
  - Hypotension, Congestive heart failure

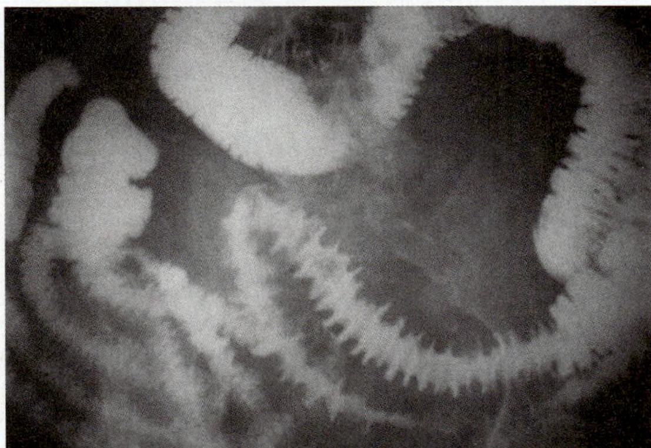

Fig. Stack of coins

- *Vasculitis*:
  - Henoch Schönlein Purpura
  - SLE
  - Polyarteritis nodosa
- *Radiation enteropathy*:
  - After radiotherapy for cervical cancer
  - After radiotherapy for prostate cancer
- *Intramural haemorrhage*:
  - Bleeding diathesis (Haemophilia)
  - Anticoagulation
  - Trauma

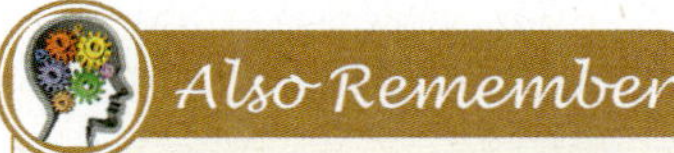

Also Remember

- ***Volvulus***:
  - *'Bird of prey' sign*
  - Overlap sign
- ***Ischaemic colitis***:
  - *'Thumbprinting' sign*
- ***Intussusception***:
  - *'Coiled spring' appearance*
  - Claw sign
  - Double-target appearance

30. Ans. (a) Plain X-ray abdomen (erect)

[Ref. David Sutton, 7/e p663]

- Patients with an acute abdomen comprise the largest group of people presenting as a general surgical emergency: Following the history and clinical examination, plain film radiographs have traditionally been one of the first and most useful methods of further investigation
- A supine abdomen and an erect chest can be regarded as the basic standard radiographs
- A horizontal-ray abdominal radiograph either erect or left lateral decubitus, is frequently taken to add more information and to demonstrate fluid levels

31. Ans. (a) Malignant gastric ulcer

[Ref. Sumer K Sethi, 5/e p67]

32. Ans. (c) Sigmoid volvulus

[Ref. Bipin Valchandji Daga, 1/e p167]

33. Ans. (c) Diverticulitis

[Ref. Sumer K Sethi, 5/e p70]

SAW-TOOTH APPEARANCE (Concertina/Serrated appearance)

- Diverticulosis
- ***Most common site*: Sigmoid colon**

34. Ans. (b) Carcinoma head of pancreas

[Ref. Sumer K Sethi, 6/e p126]

- Barium meal study shows widened duodenal 'C' loop -pad sign in carcinoma head of pancreas
- Reverse 3 sign is seen in carcinoma of periampullary region

35. Ans. (b) Contrast-enhanced CT

[Ref. Short Textbook of Surgery by Roy, 1/e p250]

- CT is best option: If there is any doubt with USG, CT scan gives correct diagnosis as in nearly 20% cases USG does not give correct diagnosis.

36. Ans. (b) 2

[Ref. Plain X-ray abdomen by M. Shuja Tahir, 1/e p01]

- *Number of physiologic fluid levels in abdomen on X-ray*: Two
  - Stomach fluid level
  - Caecum fluid level
- *Number of fluid levels more than 5 in abdomen on X-ray*:
  - Obstruction
  - Ileus
  - Ischaemia
  - Gastroenteritis

37. Ans. (b) Midgut volvulus

Ref. Sure Success in PGMEE by B. Ramgopal, 1/e p149]

Gasless Abdomen

Causes in infants	Causes in adults
• Oesophageal atresia • Duodenal atresia • Volvulus • Annular pancreas • Hypertrophic pyloric stenosis • Choledochal cyst • Excess vomiting • Fluid-filled bowel • Congenital diaphragmatic hernia	• High obstruction • Ascites • Acute pancreatitis • Fluid-filled bowel • Large abdominal mass • Normal

38. Ans. (b) CT scan

[Ref. Bailey and Love, 25/e p57]

39. Ans. (d) USG

[Ref. Amoebic liver abscess by MP Sharma, JIACM 2003, Pg 107–111]

- *Initial investigation for amoebic liver abscess*: Ultrasonography

40. Ans. (d) CO_2

[Ref. Bailey and Love, 25/e p246]

Laparoscopy

- *Principle*:
  - Rigid endoscope introduced through a sleeve into peritoneal cavity
  - Further sleeves and ports for instrument access and dissection
- *Gas used for pneumoperitoneum*: Carbon dioxide
- *Mainstay of management for*: Cholelithiasis

41. Ans. (a) Ileocaecal TB

[Ref. SRB's Manual of Surgery by Sriram Bhat, 1/e p617]

- In barium study pulled up caecum with obtuse ileocaecal angle is noted

42. Ans. (b) USG

[Ref. David Sutton, 7/e p722]

43. Ans. (d) USG

[Ref. David Sutton, 7/e p718]

- Now superseded by ultrasound as the primary investigation for suspected cholelithiasis, Oral Cholecystography still has a limited role in anatomical and functional assessment of the gallbladder

44. Ans. (c) USG

[Ref. David Sutton, 7/e p718]

45. Ans. (a) Barium meal follow through

[Ref. David Sutton, 7/e p577]

46. Ans. (c) Diffuse oesophageal spasm

[Ref. David Sutton, 7/e p549]

47. Ans. (c) Small intestine obstruction

[Ref. David Sutton, 7/e p618]

- Plain abdominal films are usually the primary investigation in suspected obstruction
- Diagnosis is by small-bowel distension down to the level of obstruction, with fluid levels and no distal gas
  - However, it may take several hours for bowel to dilate and a similar time for distal gas to be resorbed
  - Also, problems occur when only a few loops are dilated in high obstruction (where there is also vomiting) or if loops are completely fluid-filled (resulting in a 'grey' abdomen that is easily confused with ascites)
- A little residual gas may be trapped within adjacent valvulae; the `string of beads' sign.

48. Ans. (d) All of the above

[Ref. Radiology Review Manual by Dahnert, 6/e p772]

49. Ans. (c) Contrast radiography

[Ref. David Sutton, 7/e p657]

- Scintigraphic detection of Meckel's diverticulum depends upon the affinity of injected pertechnetate for the gastric mucosa contained in the diverticulum
- Technique requires only a single intravenous injection and carries a low radiation burden compared with enteroclysis or angiography

50. Ans. (a) Acute pancreatitis

[Ref. Bipin Valchandji Daga, 1/e p220]

- Scoring system for severity of acute pancreatitis is by CT **(Balthazar Grade)**:

Balthazar Grade 0	Normal gland
Balthazar Grade 1	Focal/diffuse enlargement
Balthazar Grade 2	Peripancreatic inflammatory changes
Balthazar Grade 3	Single peripancreatic fluid
Balthazar Grade 4	2 or more fluid collection or abscess

51. Ans. (d) >3 mm

[Ref. Endoscopic Ultrasonography edited by Frank Gress, 1/e Table 17.2]

- Endosonographic criteria for the diagnosis of chronic pancreatitis (Based on Ductal dilation)
  - >3 mm in head
  - >2 mm in body
  - >1 mm in tail

52. Ans. (b) Perforation

[Ref. David Sutton, 7/e p607]

- When duodenal stump rupture or an anastomotic leak is suspected, an urgent examination with a water-soluble contrast agent is indicated

53. Ans. (b) Gastric ulcer

[Ref. David Sutton, 7/e p583]

- If scarring has been pronounced, perhaps because of recurrent ulceration at the same site, gastric deformity may result and can lead to an hour-glass configuration to the stomach

54. Ans. (c) Colonoscopy

[Ref. Bailey & Love Surgery, 26/e p1165]

55. Ans. (d) Small bowel obstruction

[Ref. Clinical Imaging of Small Intestine by Birnbaum, 2/e p58]

- **Stepladder or hairpin loops** of small bowel without fluid levels in the colon is usually unequivocal for mechanical small bowel obstruction, usually high-grade and acute
- As additional bowel loops are affected, they appear to be placed one above the other, upward and to the left, producing a characteristic "stepladder" appearance.

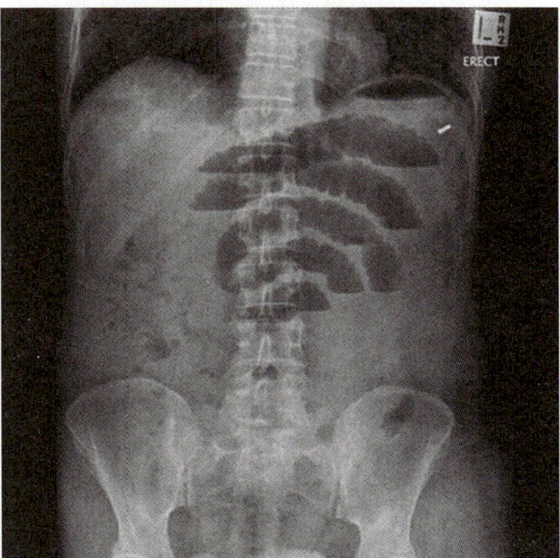

Fig. Step-ladder pattern

56. Ans. (b) Ileal stricture

[Ref. Geriatric Practice by Ratnaike, 1/e p67]

- Abnormalities seen on Barium meal follow through are anatomical lesions of the small bowel due to obstructions, perforations, previous resections, jejunal diverticulosis, stagnant loops, ileal strictures, fistulas and mixed lesions due to a combination of the above

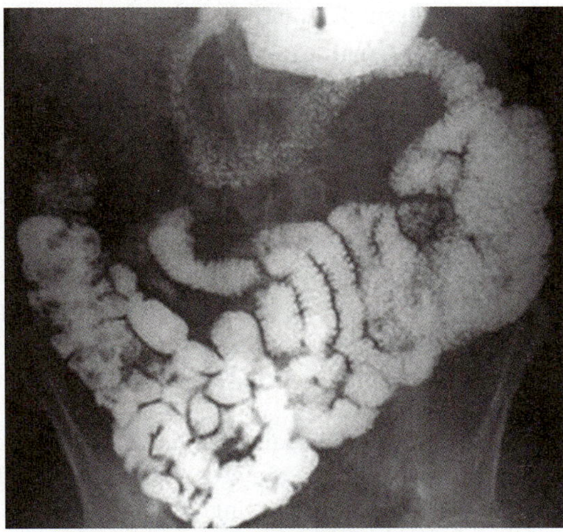

Fig. Barium meal follow through

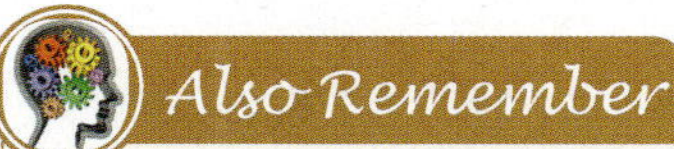

Barium Examinations in Radiology

- Barium swallow X-ray examinations are used to study the pharynx and esophagus
- Barium meal examinations are used to study the lower esophagus, stomach and duodenum
- Barium follow through examinations are used to study the small intestine

57. Ans. (a) Achhalasia cardia

[Ref. Sumer K Sethi, 5/e p65]

Achalasia Cardia

- Rat-tail/Bird beak tapering (Box in photograph): Dilated proximal segment representing the bird's head and the tapered lower end its beak
- Dilated sigmoid esophagus

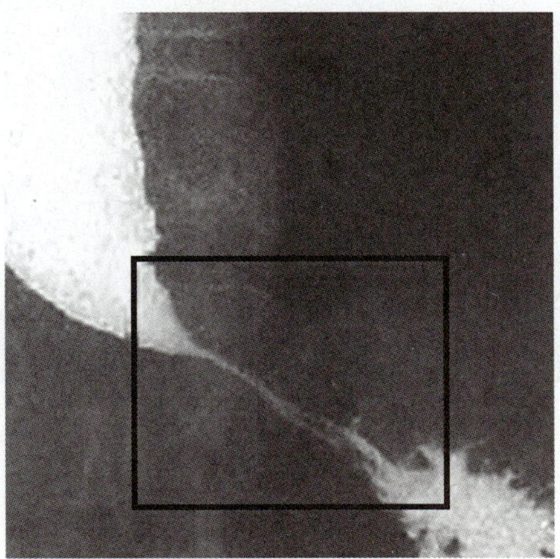

Fig. Bird beak appearance

58. Ans. (d) Hypoechoic septate lesion

[Ref. Focal Liver Lesions by Lencioni, 1/e p95]

- Sonographic appearance of Hydatid cysts is correlated with its evolution and six classes may be identified, namely, Type 1 (Simple cyst), Type 2 (Septate cyst), Type 3 (Cyst with membrane detachment), Type 4 (Cyst with mixed echo structure), Type 5 (Heterogeneous cyst), Type 6 (Calcified cyst)

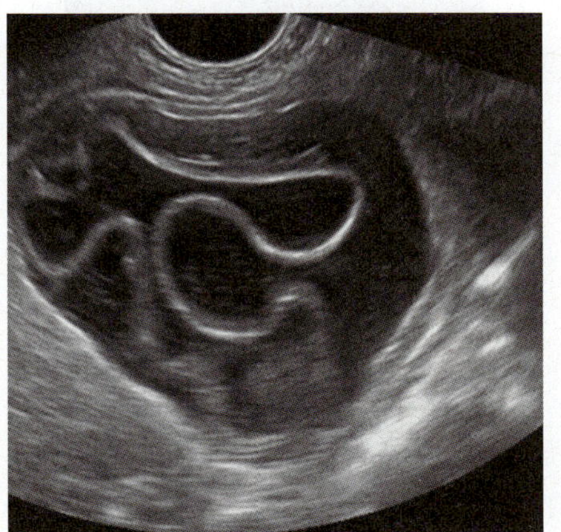

Fig. Septate cyst

59. Ans. (d) Hydatid cyst

[Ref. Genitourinary Radiology by Dogra, 1/e p87]

Sonographic appearance of Hydatid cysts in Gharbi classification

- Type I: Well-defined, purely anechoic lesions that may be indistinguishable from simple renal cysts; multiple echogenic foci due to Hydatid sands may be seen in the cyst
- Type II: A focal or diffuse detachment of the inner germinal layer results in a floating membrane inside the cyst
- Type III: Multiseptated cysts with multiple daughter cysts
- Type IV: Heterogeneous solid appearance with infolded membranes and internal echoes
- Type V: Solid appearance calcifications in cyst wall and germinative membranes

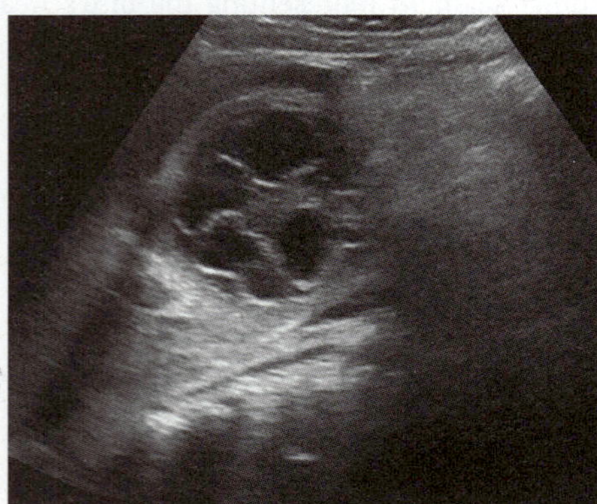

Fig. Hydatid cyst on USG

60. Ans. (c) Oval mass lined by barium

[Ref. Essential Practice of Surgery by Norton, 1/e p179]

Leiomyomas

- Typical solitary, although they can be multiple
- Typically, leiomyomas are oval, during their growth they remain intramural, having the bulk of their mass protruding toward the outer wall of the esophagus
- Barium swallow is the most useful method to demonstrate a leiomyoma of the esophagus
- Barium swallow reveals the classic smooth, oval-shaped filling defect of the esophageal lumen
- Endoscopy is necessary to rule out malignancy

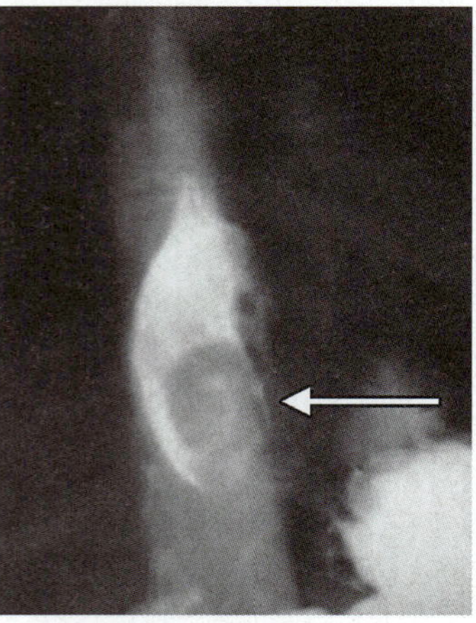

Fig. Leiomyoma esophagus

61. Ans. (d) Left lateral decubitus

[Ref. Diagnostic Imaging by Federle, 1/e p125]

- Left lateral decubitus radiograph of the abdomen can show small amounts of free air if the heavy exposure does not compromise the detection
- Plain radiographs may show evidence of free intraperitoneal gas (air); upright chest X-ray or left lateral decubitus position is most sensitive

62. Ans. (b) USG

[Ref. Clinical Hepatology by Dancygier, 1/e p1467]

- Gold standard in the diagnosis of gallbladder stones is Ultrasound: Repeatable, no side effects, provide useful information on the neighboring organs
- Limitations of sonography: Stones < 2 mm in diameter, small stones hiding in gallbladder sludge, the difficulty in determining the exact number of stones present, the detection of stones in cystic duct and diagnosis of bile duct concrements

63. Ans. (d) Ioxaglate sodium

[Ref. Pleural Diseases by Light, 5/e p259]

- Diagnosis of Esophageal rupture/ perforation is established when Esophageal disruption is confirmed by contrast studies of the esophagus
- Contrast agent of choice is probably Meglumine and Ioxaglate sodium (Hexabrix) as it does not elicit much of an inflammatory reaction or bronchospasm.

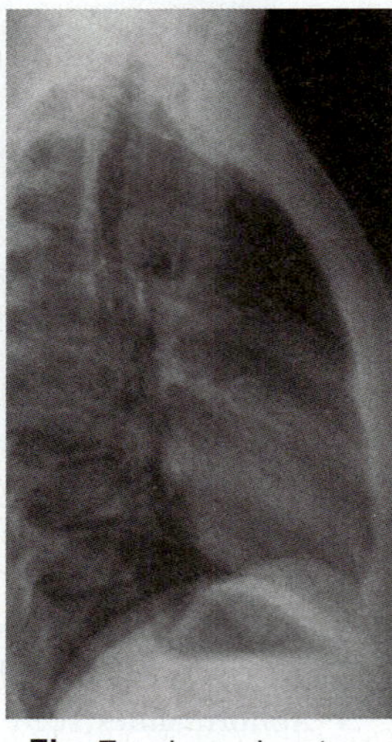

Fig. Esophageal rupture

- Barium has a greater radiographic density, better mucosal adherence, and causes minimal irritation to tracheobronchial tree but cause inflammatory repose once leaked into pleural, mediastinal or peritoneal cavities

64. Ans. (c) Feline oesophagus

[Ref. Radiology of the Stomach and Duodenum by Freeman, 1/e p78]

Feline Oesophagus/ Oesophageal Shiver

- Transient transverse bands seen in the mid and lower oesophagus on a double contrast barium swallow
- Occur due to contraction of the muscularis mucosae with resultant shortening of oesophagus and 'bunching up' of the mucosa in the lumen
- Appearance is almost always associated with active gastro-oesophageal reflux
- Folds are 1-2 mm thick and run horizontally around the entire circumference of the oesophageal lumen; findings are transient, seen following reflux and not during swallowing

 **HIGH YIELD MCQs ANSWERS WITH EXPLANATIONS** 

1. **Ans. (c) Endoscopy**
   [Ref. Oh's Intensive Care Manual, 7/e p487]
   - Endoscopy has replaced barium studies as investigation of choice in identifying the source of bleeding
   - Endoscopy should be offered within 24 hours of presentation

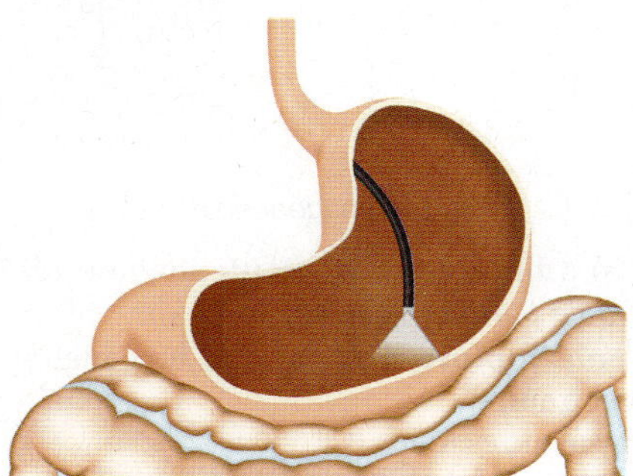

Fig. Endoscopy

2. **Ans. (c) Contrast study**
   [Ref. Pediatric Imaging by Newman, 1/e p207]
   - A newborn has not passed meconium since 48 hours indicate Intestinal obstruction
   - Investigation of choice for further evaluation: Lower GI contrast study
3. **Ans. (a) String sign of Kantor**
   [Ref. Bipin Valchandji Daga, 1/e p167]
4. **Ans. (a) Valvulae conniventes**
   [Ref. David Sutton, 7/e p615]
   - Small-bowel wall comprises mucosa, submucosa, muscularis propria and serosa, and should not measure more than 1–2 mm thick when distended
   - Great care should be taken when assessing mural thicskening or indeed any abnormal feature in underfilled, undistended loops
   - Normal undistended small bowel shows a 'feathery' pattern due to mucosal folds and the valvulae, although this may be absent in the distal ileum.

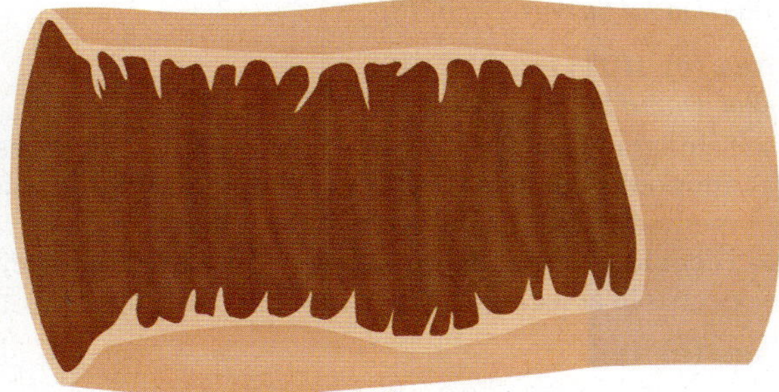

Fig. Valvulae conniventes

5. **Ans. (a) Meniscus appearance**
   [Ref. David Sutton, 7/e p726]
6. **Ans. (e) Diaphragmatic hernia**
   [Ref. Radiology Review Manual by Dahnert, 6/e p772]
7. **Ans. (b) Ulcerative colitis**
   [Ref. Bipin Valchandji Daga, 1/e p204]
   - Lead-pipe or pipe-stem colon is diagnostic of ulcerative colitis

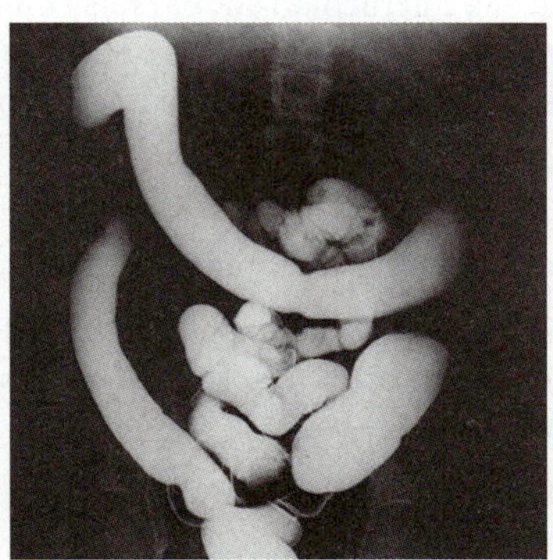

Fig. Lead-pipe colon

8. **Ans. (b) Chronic pancreatitis**
   [Ref. Bipin Valchandji Daga, 1/e p214]
   - In chronic pancreatitis, ERCP has advantage of providing details
   - Chain of lake appearance is characteristic of Chronic pancreatitis.
9. **Ans. (d) Serous cyst adenoma**
   [Ref. Bipin Valchandji Daga, 1/e p225]
   - Serous cystadenoma of pancreas: Sunburst calcification in a spongy mass
   - Mucinous cystadenoma of pancreas: Eggshell calcification in a spongy mass
10. **Ans. (a) 1 cm gallstone**
    [Ref. Hepatobiliary and Pancreatic Surgery: Imaging Strategies and Surgical Decision Making by Stephen R., 1/e p62]
11. **Ans. (c) Thumbprinting**
    [Ref. David Sutton, 7/e p680]
    - **Ischaemic colitis** most commonly occurs in middle-aged and elderly patients, and affects the splenic flexure and descending colon preferentially
    - Affected wall of the colon is greatly thickened due to submucosal haemorrhage and oedema: Thumbprinting on plain films/ barium studies

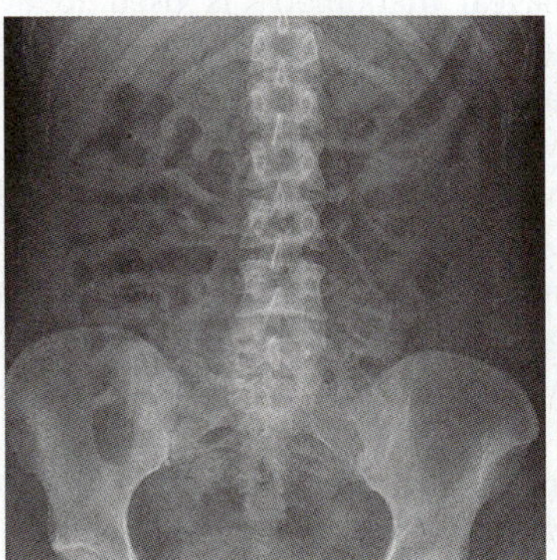

Fig. Thumbprinting

12. Ans. (c) Gastric content aspiration
[Ref. Oxford Handbook of Clinical Surgery, 4/e p294]

13. Ans. (a) Achalasia (b) Trypanosomiasis
[Ref. Oxford Handbook of Clinical Surgery, 4/e p274]

14. Ans. (a) Microcolon on the atresia
[Ref. David Sutton, 7/e p859]

- Presence of a microcolon should raise the suspicion of an earlier, more distal (ileal) atresia or the presence of further ileal atresias in addition to a proximal lesion

15. Ans. (a) Apple core appearance
[Ref. David Sutton, 7/e p641]

- Apple core appearance is frank feature of carcinoma

16. Ans. (b) Radionuclide enteroclysis; (c) MRI enteroclysis; (d) CT enteroclysis; (e) USG enteroclysis
[Ref. David Sutton, 7/e p617]

17. Ans. (d) ALL
[Ref. David Sutton, 7/e p791, 852]

- Gasless abdomen implies an isolated Oesophageal atresia, Acute pancreatitis

18. Ans. (a) Pancreatic head growth
[Ref. Sumer K Sethi, 6/e p126]

- Barium meal study shows widened duodenal 'C' loop -pad sign in carcinoma head of pancreas
- Reverse 3 sign is seen in carcinoma of periampullary region

19. Ans. (a) Gallstones; (d) Pancreatic divisum; (e) Annular pancreas
[Ref. David Sutton, 7/e p604,698, 719, 787]

20. Ans. (a) Ultrasonic waves
[Ref. David Sutton, 7/e p1446, 456]

21. Ans. (a) Meniscus appearance
[Ref. David Sutton, 7/e p726]

22. Ans. (b) Mucosal thickening; (c) Cholesterosis; (d) Ascites
[Ref. Bipin Valchandji Daga, 1/e p217]

23. Ans. (a) Thick fibrosed gallbladder; (b) Stone impacted at neck of gallbladder; (c) Peri Gallbladder halo
[Ref. Bipin Valchandji Daga, 1/e p217]

24. Ans. (a) Manometry
[Ref. David Sutton, 7/e p549]

- Oesophageal manometry is used to evaluate motility, but when it is unavailable the barium swallow provides a useful alternative
- Motility often varies from one swallow to the next, so at least five single prone swallows should be recorded for proper evaluation
- Radionuclide imaging of the oesophagus is reserved for patients in whom the first-line tests of endoscopy and barium swallow produce unexpected or inconclusive results, and those in whom the initial tests are negative
- Scintigraphy has the advantages of using physiological fluids or solids, producing quantifiable results, and being highly sensitive in the early detection of motility disorders

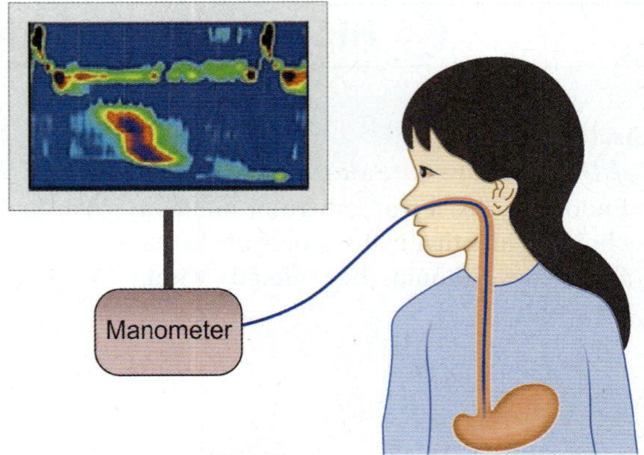

Fig. Esophageal manometry

25. Ans. (b) Obliteration of splenic shadow; (c) Rib fracture
[Ref. David Sutton, 7/e p749]

- **Splenic rupture** may be due to penetrating wound or direct trauma
- X-ray features are
  - Mass in left hypochondrium
  - Obliteration of splenic shadow
  - One or more lower rib fracture

26. Ans. (c) CT scan
[Ref. David Sutton, 7/e p749]

- Dynamic enhanced CT is important to show the extent of the tear and the remaining viable splenic tissue, which is much help to surgical management, as splenectomy is normally indicated if there is significant splenic haemorrhage

27. Ans. (a) USG
[Ref. API Textbook of Medicine (Volume I & II) by YP Munjal, 10/e p109]

- Ultrasound is the best modality for detection of minimal ascites and can also provide a clue to the aetiology, as well as provide information about liver

28. Ans. (a) Endoscopy
[Ref. Evidence-based Gastroenterology by E. Jan Irvine, 1/e p31]

- Upper GI endoscopy is the best test for the evaluation of patients with possible complications of GERD

29. Ans. (b) USG
[Ref. David Sutton, 7/e p718]

30. Ans. (c) HIDA scan
[Ref. David Sutton, 7/e p686]

- Scintigraphy, using 59 Tc-labelled derivatives of aminodiacetic acid (HIDA), is a simple and highly accurate method of diagnosing acute cholecystitis
- Technique depends on the fact that acute cholecystitis occurs in association with a blocked cystic duct

31. Ans. (b) USG
[Ref. David Sutton, 7/e p718]

32. Ans. (a) First done by Grahm Cole in 1942; (c) Used for chronic gallbladder disease; (d) Dye used is teleplaque; (e) Film taken in right anterior oblique
[Ref. Bipin Valchandji Daga, 1/e p215]

Radiodiagnosis and Radiotherapy

33. Ans. (b) Motor mechanism of gallbladder
[Ref. David Sutton, 7/e p718]
- The media in common use are sodium ipodate (Biloptin) and calcium ipodate (Solubiloptin): These are tri-iodinated benzene ring compounds whose concentration in the gallbladder is dependent upon ingestion and adequate absorption in the gut, take-up in the liver, excretion in the bile, enterohepatic recirculation and a patent cystic duct
- Any factor influencing this pathway will result in failure of opacification and a 'non-functioning gallbladder'

34. Ans. (a) Pancreas; (c) IVC; (e) Portal vein
[Ref. Fundamentals of Sectional Anatomy: An Imaging Approach by Denise Lazo, 2/e p 210]

35. Ans. (c) Dianosil
[Ref. SSS-Radiology 2]

Investigation	Dye used
Angiography	Urografin
Bronchography (esophageal atresia)	Dianosil
Sialography	Neohydiol
CT scan	Metrizamide
IV pyelography	Urograffin, Conray 420
Intestinal obstruction	Gastrografin
Hysterosalpingography	Conray 280
MRI	GDPA

36. Ans. (a) Duodenal atresia
[Ref. Radiology Review Manual by Dahnert, 6/e p772]

37. Ans. (a) Crohn's disease
[Ref. Bipin Valchandji Daga, 1/e p167]

38. Ans. (a) Single bubble appearance
[Ref. Pediatric Radiological Signs - Volume 1 p457]
- Sonographically, pyloric atresia and stenosis are associated with a single bubble

39. Ans. (d) Meconium ileus
[Ref. Bipin Valchandji Daga, 1/e p187]

40. Ans. (b) Thumbprint sign
[Ref. Bipin Valchandji Daga, 1/e p167]

41. Ans. (b) HPS
[Ref. Bipin Valchandji Daga, 1/e p167]

42. Ans. (a) Pyloric obstruction
[Ref. David Sutton, 7/e p849]
- Pyloric obstruction will produce single air shadow.

43. Ans. (e) Diaphragmatic hernia
[Ref. Radiology Review Manual by Dahnert, 6/e p772]

44. Ans. (a) Caroli's disease
[Ref. Bipin Valchandji Daga, 1/e p219]
- Portal radicals completely surrounded by ciliated bile ducts, called as **"central dot sign"** is diagnostic of Caroli's disease.

45. Ans. (d) Lesser curvature ulcer with a nodular rim
[Ref. David Sutton, 7/e p593]

46. Ans. (d) Longitudinal ulcers are most common
[Ref. David Sutton, 7/e p627]
- Ulcers tend to be discrete and transverse or star-shaped, in contrast to Crohn's disease (the major differential), where they are usually longitudinal.

47. Ans. (d) Corticosteroid
[Ref. Radiology Review Manual by Dahnert, 6/e p758]

Abdominal Calcifications and Opacities
[Mnemonic: CHIPS]
- **C**hloral hydrate
- **H**eavy metals (lead)
- **I**ron
- **P**henothiazines
- **S**alicylates

48. Ans. (d) Quadrate lobe
[Ref. David Sutton, 7/e p753]
- Physiological left lobe lies to the left of a line joining the inferior vena cava to the gallbladder fossa, and is divided into lateral and medial parts by the falciform ligament
- Medial part consists of segment II superiorly and III inferiorly, the lateral part being segment IV, known as the quadrate lobe
- Right lobe of liver has segment V anteroinferiorly, VI posteroinferiorly, VII posterosuperiorly, and VIII anterosuperiorly

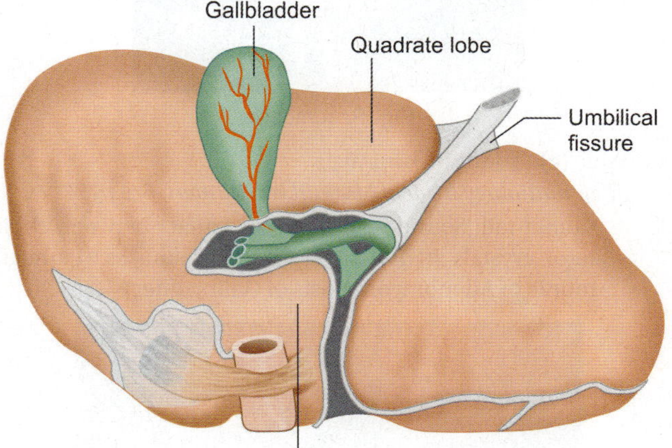

Fig. Quadrate lobe (liver)

49. Ans. (a) Gallstone; (b) Renal stone; (c) Calcification in vessels; (d) Hepatic hemangioma
[Ref. Radiology Review Manual by Dahnert, 6/e p758]

50. Ans. (d) Simple cyst
[Ref. David Sutton, 7/e p769]
- The cyst is usually single with a thin well-defined wall and anechoic contents with posterior acoustic enhancement
- Size is variable, Thin septations are common, Usually solitary
- Simple cysts may be simulated by Cystic metastases (Ovarian cancer), Treated liver abscesses/ hydatid cysts, Following trauma

51. Ans. (c) Focal nodular hyperplasia
[Ref. David Sutton, 7/e p778]

52. Ans. (b) Hepatic scintigraphy
[Ref. Diagnostic Radiology: Gastrointestinal and Hepatobiliary Imaging by Berry, 2/e p239]
- Mixed echogenicity in USG is suggestive of haemangioma

53. Ans. (b) Sclerosing cholangitis
[Ref. Radiology Review Manual by Dahnert, 6/e p673]

Gas in Biliary Tree (Pneumobilia)
- Incompetent sphincter of Oddi (after Sphincterotomy/ Passage of a gallstone)
- Gallstone ileus
- Carcinoma gallbladder
- Emphysematous cholecystitis (actually in gallbladder)
- Trauma
- Ulcer (duodenal ulcer perforating into CBD)
- Postoperative (eg, cholecystoenterostomy)
- Ascending cholangitis

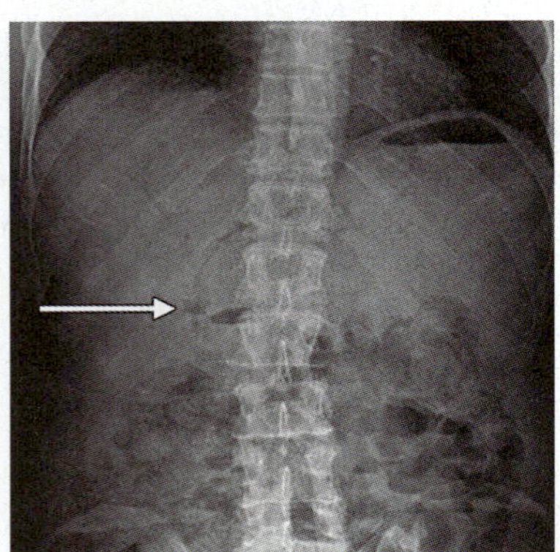

Fig. Pneumobilia

54. Ans. (c) Adenomyomatosis
[Ref. Radiology Review Manual by Dahnert, 6/e p727]
- Comet-tail: Sound reverberation artifact between cholesterol crystals in Rokitansky-Aschoff sinuses (Pathognomonic of Adenomyomatosis of Gallbladder)

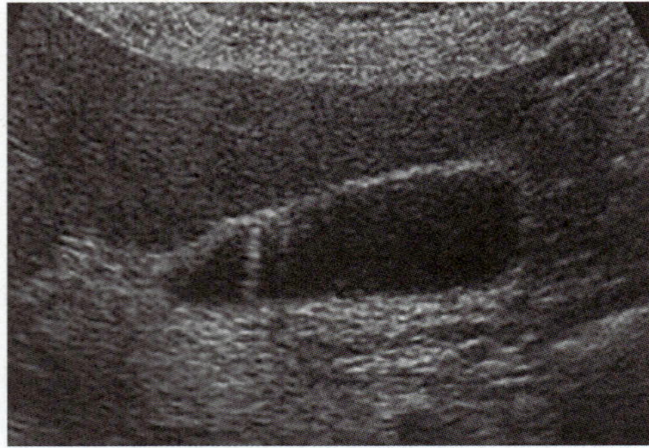

Fig. Comet-tail

55. Ans. (a) Barium enema study

56. Ans. (c) Lower GI contrast study

57. Ans. (a) FAST
[Ref. Bailey & Love's Short Practice of Surgery 26/e p359]
- **CT is the gold standard for intra-abdominal diagnosis of injury in stable patient**
- Focused abdominal sonar for trauma (FAST) is a technique whereby Ultrasound (sonar) imaging is used to assess the torso for the presence of free blood

58. Ans. (b) CT
[Ref. Bailey & Love's Short Practice of Surgery 26/e p359]
- CT is the gold standard for intraabdominal diagnosis of injury in stable patient

59. Ans. (b) CT scan
[Ref. Bailey & Love's Short Practice of Surgery 26/e p359]
- This is classical presentation of acute pancreatitis
- Pain is cardinal feature, characteristically develops quick, reaching maximum intensity within minutes, experienced first in epigastrium and there is radiation to the back in nearly 50% cases
- Contrast enhanced CT is best single imaging investigation.

60. Ans. (d) USG
[Ref. Bipin Valchandji Daga, 1/e p32]

USG as Investigation of Choice
- Hydrocephalus in infant
- Gallstone
- Obstructive jaundice
- Acute cholecystitis
- Renal colic in pregnancy
- Minimal ascites
- Obstetric indication
- Adenomyomatosis of gallbladder
- CPS
- Intussusception
- Hydronephrosis
- Popliteal cyst
- Retinal detachment

61. Ans. (b) USG
[Ref. Bipin Valchandji Daga, 1/e p32]

62. Ans. (a) USG
[Ref. Bipin Valchandji Daga, 1/e p32]

63. Ans. (b) PET
[Ref. Medical Imaging: Techniques, Reflection and Evaluation by Elizabeth Carver, 2/e p13]
- PET (Positron emission tomography) is highly sensitive in detecting early response and predicting long term response to Imatinib in patients with metastatic GIST

64. Ans. (a) USG
[Ref. Pediatric and Adolescent Gynecology by Sultan, 2/e p238]

Acute Appendicitis
- Investigation of choice in adults: CT scan
- Investigation of choice in children/adolescents: USG with graded compression (lack of ionizing radiation, high positive predictive accuracy)

65. Ans. (b) HIDA
[Ref. Pediatric Imaging by Newman, 1/e p207]
- Clay colored stools, discoloration of eyes/ urine and treatment with Ursodeoxycholic acid indicate it's a case of Biliary atresia
- Initial investigation of choice in newborn: USG
- Confirmatory investigation of choice: HIDA scan

66. Ans. (d) Proctoscopy
[Ref. Shackelford's Surgery of the Alimentary Tract, Volume 1 p1744]

67. Ans. (b) HIDA scan
[Ref. High Yield USMLE Step 1,2,3 by Patel, 478]

68. Ans. (a) Chronic pancreatitis
[Ref. SSS Radiology, 1/e p144]

ERCP in Chronic Pancreatitis
- Multifocal stricture with dilation
- Chain of lakes appearance
- Intraductal calculi

69. Ans. (a) Imaging of liver and chest, preferably by CT along with local PETIS imaging
[Ref. Multislice CT by Reiser, 2/e p245]
- Patients with endoscopically proven rectal tumors are examined by computed tomography (CT) for M-staging of liver and Local PETIS (Positron-Emitting Tracer Imaging System) Imaging

70. Ans. (d) Endoscopic cholangiography
[Ref. Greenfield's Surgery, 5/e]

71. Ans. (d) Barium Swallow
[Ref. Medicine by Tunkel, 1/e p309]

Schatzki Ring
- Description: A thin ring of tissue that is formed annular membranes of mucosa and submucosa
- Location: Level of Gastroeosophageal junction or just above it
- Importance: Associated with pathologic Gastroesophageal reflux
- Diagnosis: Barium swallow, Upper endoscopy
- Treatment : Balloon dilatation of rings

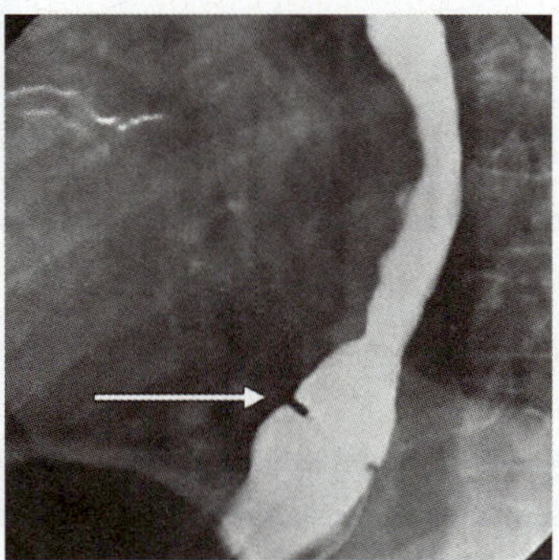

Fig. Schatzki ring

72. Ans. (b) Ca head pancreas
[Ref. Pancreatic Cancer by Cameron, 1/e p72]

Radiodiagnosis and Radiotherapy

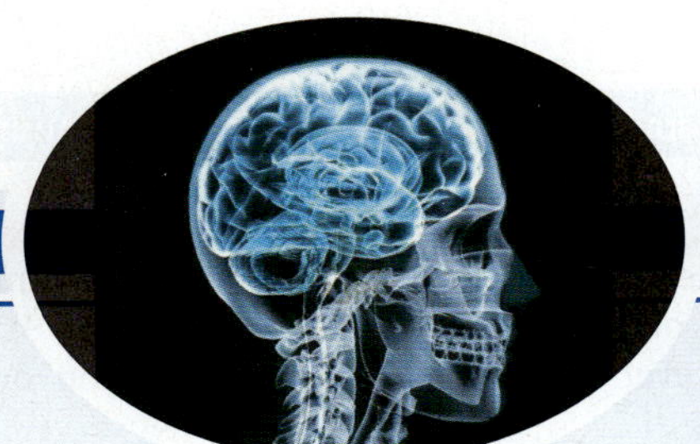

Chapter 4

Respiratory System

THEORETICAL CONCEPTS

IV A. ASPERGILLOSIS OF LUNG

- *Aspergilloma/Fungal ball*: *'**Air-crescent sign**'*[Q] (crescentic radiolucent lung cavity with air and radio-opaque mass)
- *Invasive aspergillosis*: *'Halo appearance'* (surrounding haemorrhagic inflammation)
- *Allergic bronchopulmonary aspergillosis*: ***'Gloved finger appearance'***

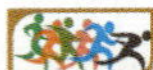

Topper's Edge

Air Crescent Sign (ACS)

- Meniscus/cap sign[Q]:
  - Air interposed between an intracavitary, ball-like mass and the cavity wall
  - Its shape ranges from crescent-like to total encapsulation
- Underlying causes:
  - **MC cause**[Q]: Fungus ball of angioinvasive aspergillosis
  - Other causes: Pulmonary hydatid cyst, blood clot, Rasmussen aneurysm in TB cavity, lung abscess with inspissated pus, staphylococcal pneumonia, nocardial infection, carcinoma of lung, pulmonary gangrene/hematoma

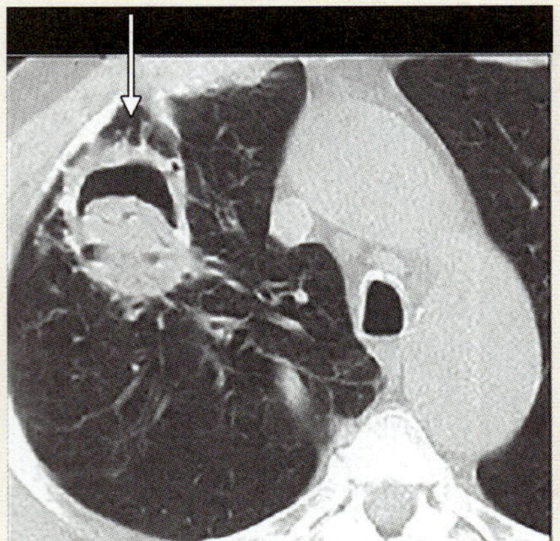

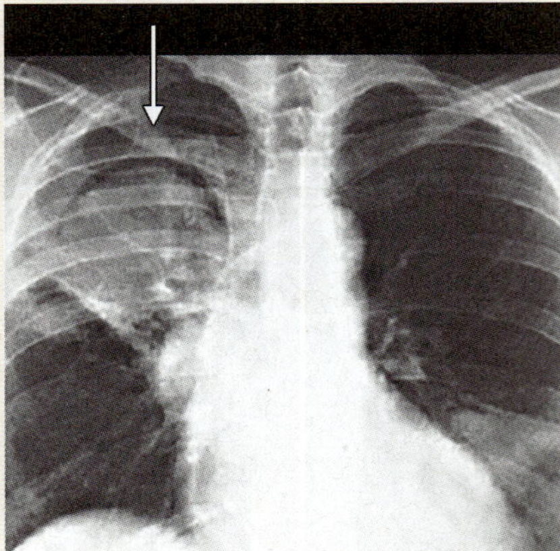

Fig. Air-crescent sign

IV B. BRONCHIECTASIS

- High resolution CT (HRCT) is **best investigation**

Feature^{Q}	Remark
Signet-ring sign	-
Cluster of grapes appearance	Cystic bronchiectasis
String of beads appearance	Varicose bronchiectasis
Tram track sign	Cylindrical bronchiectasis

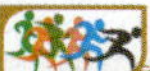

Topper's Edge

Bronchiectasis

- Bronchiectasis:
  - Abnormal dilatation of the bronchial tree
  - CT is the most accurate modality for diagnosis^{Q}
- Underlying causes:
  - **Post-infective (MC^{Q}):** Necrotising bacterial pneumonia, granulomatous disease (TB), allergic bronchopulmonary aspergillosis, measles
  - Congenital causes: Congenital cystic bronchiectasis, cystic fibrosis, Kartagener syndrome, pulmonary sequestration
  - Bronchial obstruction: Malignancy, Foreign body
  - Other causes: Rheumatoid arthritis, SLE, postradiotherapy, post-transplantation
- Subtypes of bronchiectasis:
  - **Cylindrical bronchiectasis (MC type^{Q})**
  - Varicose bronchiectasis
  - Cystic bronchiectasis

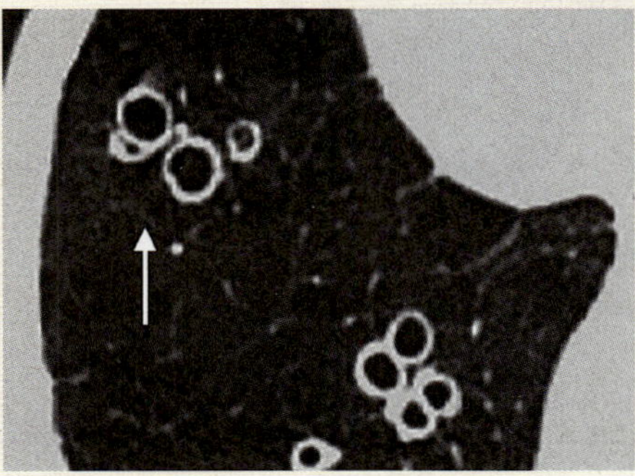

Fig. Signet-ring sign

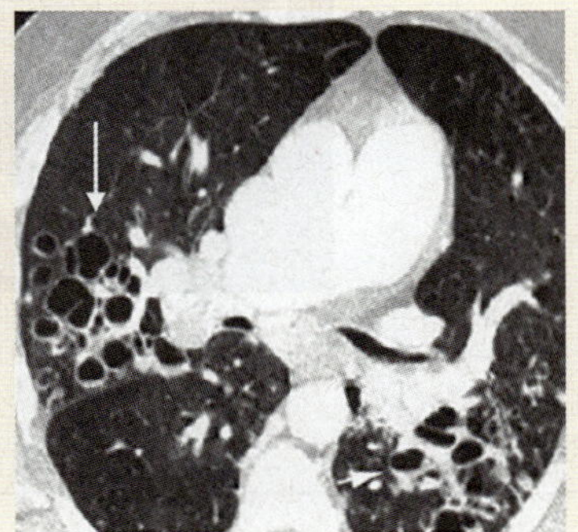

Fig. Cluster-of-grapes sign

IV C. BRONCHOGENIC CARCINOMA

❑ *Golden S-sign* ^{Q}

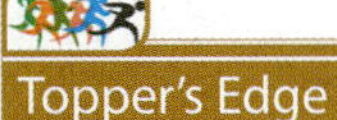

Topper's Edge

Golden S-sign

- Description: On chest radiograph, represents central lung mass or lung collapse
- Underlying causes^{Q}:
  - Bronchial carcinoma
  - Metastatic cancer
  - Enlarged lymph nodes
  - Collapse of the right upper lobe of lung
- Appearance:
  - Seen in right lung as a distorted minor fissure, whose lateral aspect is concave inferiorly and whose medial aspect is convex inferiorly
  - This produces a **"Reverse S" appearance**^{Q}

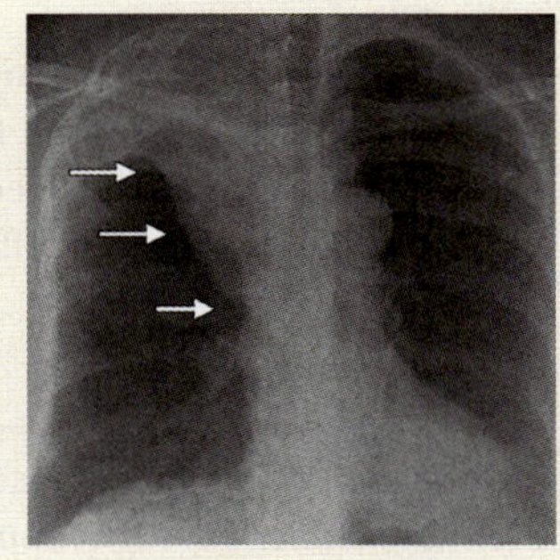

Fig. Reverse S-sign (Golden)

IV D. CHORIOCARCINOMA

- Multiple infiltrates of various shapes in both lungs

IV E. COCCIDIOMYCOSIS

- Parenchymal consolidation (Most common finding in acute form)
- Pulmonary nodules (Most common in chronic form)
- 'Grape-skin' thin-walled upper lobe cavities
- Ill-defined miliary pattern (Disseminated form)

IV F. HYDATID DISEASE

- CT scan is investigation of choice
- *'Floating membrane/Camalote* ***(Water-lily) sign'*** in liver [Q]
- Cysts, Hydatid sand, Cystic membranes, Septae

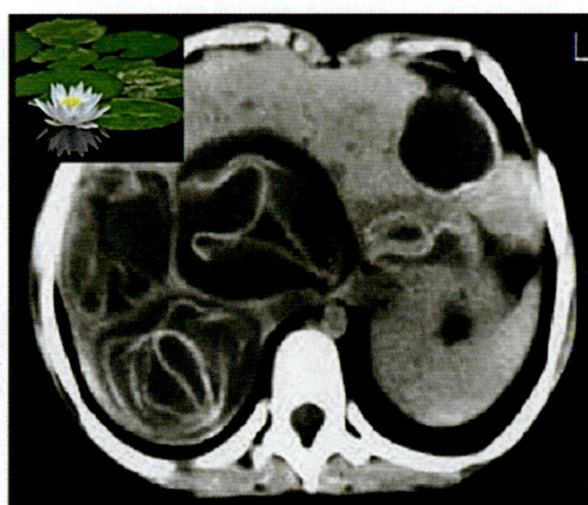

Fig. Water-lily sign

IV G. LUNG SEQUESTRATION

- *Angiography (especially radionuclide angiography)*: **Most useful investigation**[Q]
- Chest X-ray
- CT scans: 90% accuracy
- USG
- MRI

IV H. PLEURAL EFFUSION

- *Ultrasonography*: **Best investigation to detect minimal fluid**[Q]
- *Chest X-ray*:
  - *Lateral view*: Detects minimum 75 mL fluid
  - *PA view*: Detects minimum 100–200 mL fluid
  - *Lateral decubitus view*: Detects less than 10 mL fluid [Q] (Best view [Q])
  - *Lordotic view*: Inter-lobar effusion

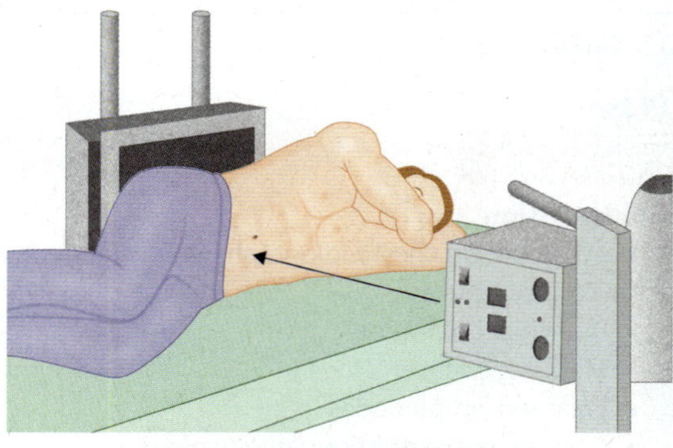

Fig. Left lateral decubitus view

IV I. PNEUMONIA

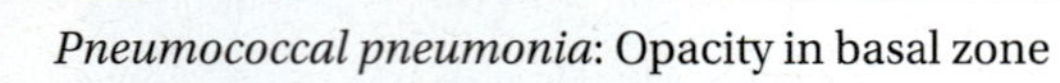

- *Pneumococcal pneumonia*: Opacity in basal zone
- *Klebsiella pneumonia*: Right upper lobe
- *Mycoplasma pneumonia*: Fine reticulo-nodular shadows followed by consolidation
- *Viral pneumonias*: Peribronchial shadowing, Fine reticulo-nodular shadows, consolidation

IV J. PULMONARY EDEMA

- Bat-wing appearance

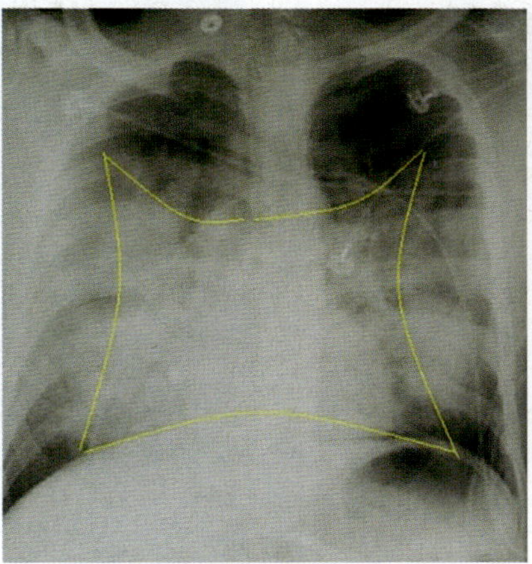

Fig. Bat-wing appearance

IV K. PULMONARY EMBOLISM

- *Chest X-ray*:
  - ***Westermark's sign***[Q] *(peripheral oligaemia)*
  - *Knuckle sign*
  - Hampton's hump
  - Melting sign
  - Fleischner's sign
- *Ventilation perfusion scan*: VP mismatch (Normal ventilation, defect in perfusion) [Q]

Ventilation agents	Perfusion agents
Xe-133 Kr-81 Technegas	Tc-99

- *Contrast-enhanced CT (CECT)*: Better than VP scan
- ***Pulmonary angiography*: Gold-standard test**[Q]

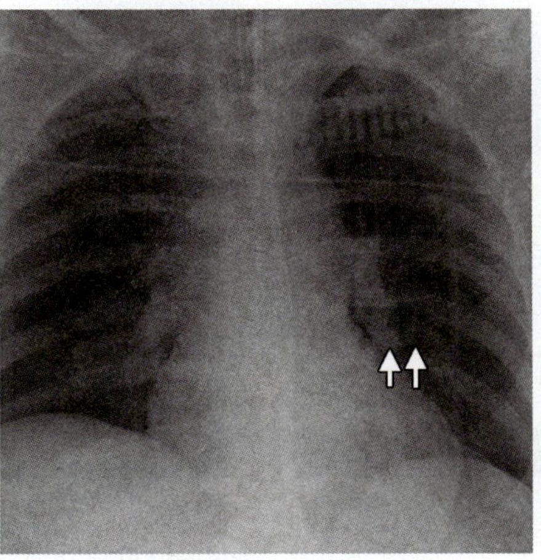

Fig. Westermark's sign

IV L. PULMONARY HAMARTOMA

- ***'Popcorn' calcification***[Q]
- *Irregular calcification* in lung (Diagnostic feature)

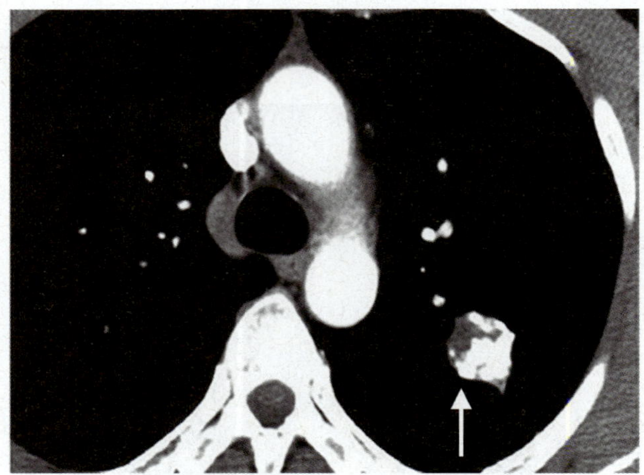

Fig. Popcorn calcification

IV M. PULMONARY TUBERCULOSIS

- *Primary TB*:
  - ***Ghon's lesion*[Q]**: Consolidation and enlarged lymph nodes
- *Secondary TB*:
  - Involves apical segments of upper/lower lobes
  - Cavitations, fibrosis
- *Miliary TB*: Pin-point mottling [Q] of millet seeds (Fine, uniform, 2–3 mm nodules in lung fields)
- *Endobronchial spread*: **Tree-in-bud appearance**

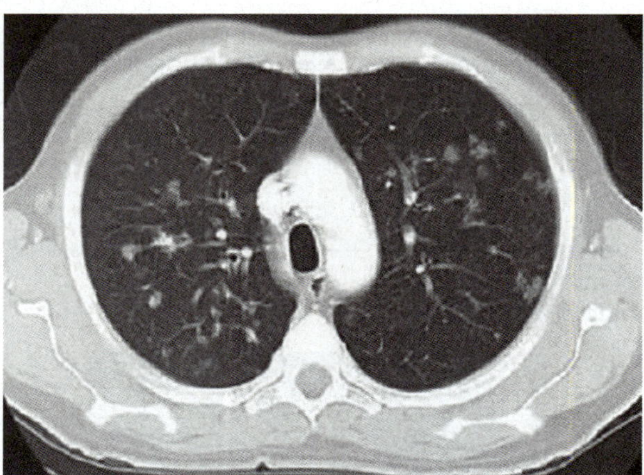

Fig. Tree-in-bud
(Linear branching opacities)

IV N. FEW IMPORTANT TOPICS IN CHEST RADIOLOGY

- *Recommended type of chest X-rays*:

Lung part/pathology	Recommended view
Right lung	Left anterior oblique view
Left lung	Right anterior oblique view
Apex of lung	Lordotic view
***Minimal pleural effusion*[Q]**	**Lateral decubitus view**
Middle lobe pathology	Lordotic view
Pneumothorax	Inspiratory erect PA view

IV O. USES OF COMPUTERIZED TOMOGRAPHY (CT) IN CHEST

- Mediastinal disease
- Staging lung cancer/malignant lesions
- Small pulmonary metastasis
- Pulmonary fibrosis
- Bronchiectasis
- **Interstitial lung disease (High-resolution CT)**

IV P. FEW IMPORTANT SIGNS IN CHEST RADIOLOGY

AIR CRESCENT SIGN[Q]
- **A**spergilloma
- **T**umour in cavity
- **P**us in cavity
- **C**lot in cavity
- **E**chinococcal cyst

[Mnemonic: A Teacher Puts Continuous Efforts]

HONEY-COMB LUNGS[Q]
- Rheumatoid arthritis
- Scleroderma
- Histiocytosis X
- Sarcoidosis
- Pneumoconiosis
- Interstitial lung disease
- Tuberculosis

REVERSE S-SIGN OF GOLDEN[Q]
- Bronchogenic carcinoma
- Metastatic cancer
- Enlarged lymph nodes
- Collapse of right upper lobe of lung

EGG-SHELL CALCIFICATION[Q]
- **Silicosis**
- Sarcoidosis
- Treated lymphoma

MILIARY SHADOWING[Q]
- **H**istoplasmosis
- **H**emosiderosis
- **P**neumoconioses
- **O**il embolism
- **S**arcoidosis
- **T**uberculosis
- **H**istiocytosis
- **C**hicken pox
- **M**etastasis

[Mnemonic: Heavy Heart POST Hypertrophic Cardio Myopathy]

CAVITATING LESIONS[Q]
- **H**istiocytosis
- **E**mbolism
- **W**egener's syndrome
- **C**ancers
- **R**heumatoid nodules
- **O**ccupational
- **S**equestrated cysts
- **S**arcoidosis
- **I**nfections (TB, Pneumocytis)
- **E**nvironmental

[Mnemonic: HE Will CROSS It Easily]

IV Q. KEY SIGNS/FEATURES IN RESPIRATORY SYSTEM RADIOLOGY

- Bilateral pleural thickening in lower/middle lungs[Q]: Asbestosis
- **Cluster of grapes** Bronchi on CT[Q]: Bronchiectasis
- Continuous diaphragm sign[Q]: Pneumomediastinum
- **Egg-shell calcification**[Q]: Silicosis
- Finger-in-glove sign[Q]: Allergic bronchopulmonary aspergillosis
- Flattened, depressed hemi-diaphragm (Terrace pattern[Q]): Emphysema
- **Golden 'S' sign**[Q]: Bronchogenic carcinoma
- Hampton hump sign[Q]: Pulmonary infarction secondary to pulmonary embolism
- Irregular central popcorn calcification[Q]: Hamartoma
- McConnell's sign on echocardiography[Q]: Pulmonary embolism
- **Meniscus sign**[Q]: Intracavitary body surrounded by air in aspergilloma
- Notch sign[Q]: Indentation at junction of thymus with heart
- **Palla's sign**[Q]: Enlarged right descending pulmonary artery in pulmonary embolism
- Sail sign[Q]: Thymic shadow
- **Signet-ring sign** on CT[Q]: Bronchiectasis

- Spinnaker sail sign[Q]: Pneumomediastinum
- **String of Pearls**[Q]: Bronchi: Bronchiectasis
- Stratosphere sign[Q]: Loss of Sea shore sign (Normal lung) in pneumothorax
- Tubular heart[Q]: Emphysema
- **Water-lily/Camalote sign**[Q]: Ruptured hydatid cyst
- Wave sign of Mulvey[Q]: Indentation of ribs on thymus
- **Westermark sign**[Q]: Oligemia of lung beyond occluded vessel in pulmonary embolism

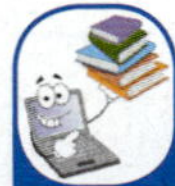

IMAGE-BASED QUESTIONS

1. Normal value of parameter calculated from the PA view chest X-ray (Photograph) is ***[Recent Question 2016]***

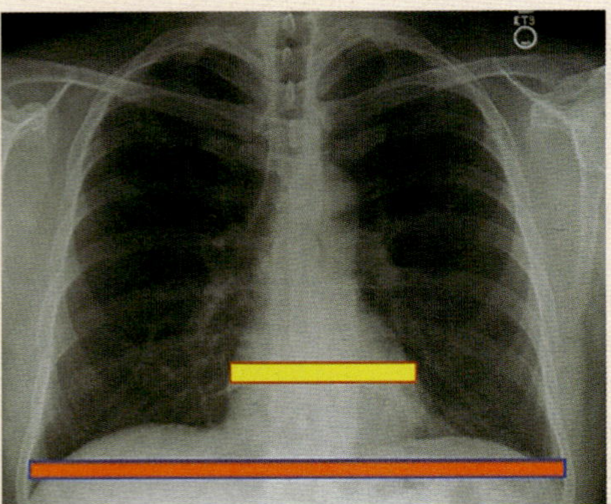

a. <1.5
b. <1.0
c. <0.5
d. <0.1

2. Sign (Arrow) shown in Photograph is due to

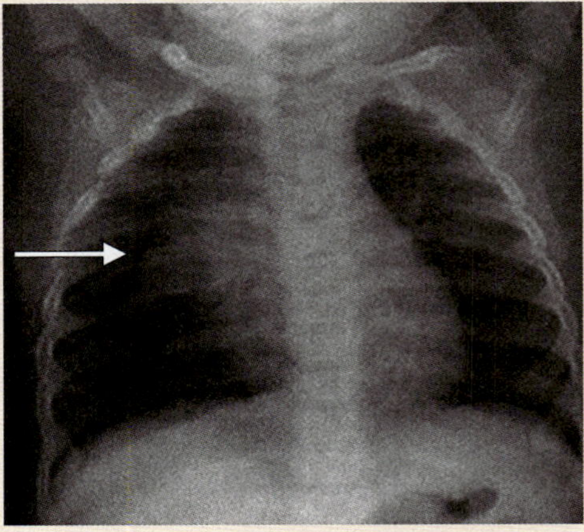

a. Peri-hilar lymphadenopathy
b. Aspergilloma
c. Bulging fissure
d. Thymus

3. Sign (Encircled) seen on HRCT scan (Photograph) is typical of ***[Recent Question 2015]***

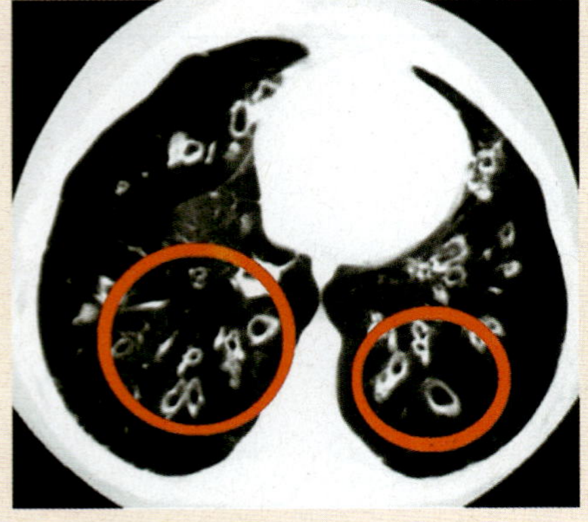

a. Pulmonary edema
b. Bronchogenic carcinoma
c. Bronchiectasis
d. Tuberculosis

4. Sign (Encircled) in Photograph is seen in all, except

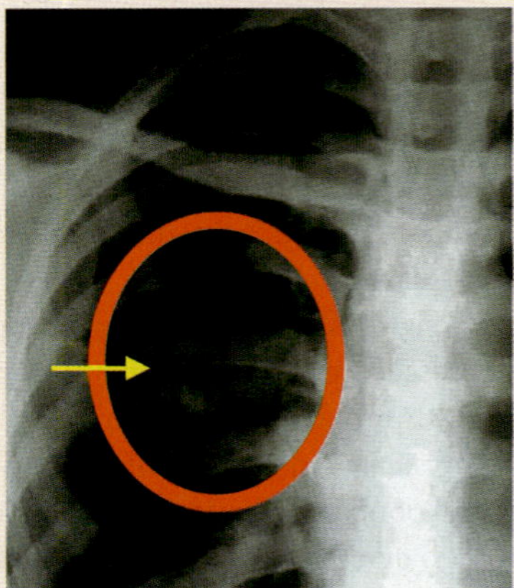

a. Allergic bronchopulmonary aspergillosis
b. Bronchogenic carcinoma
c. Sarcoidosis
d. Cystic fibrosis

5. Sign (Encircled) shown in X-ray Photograph is characteristic of

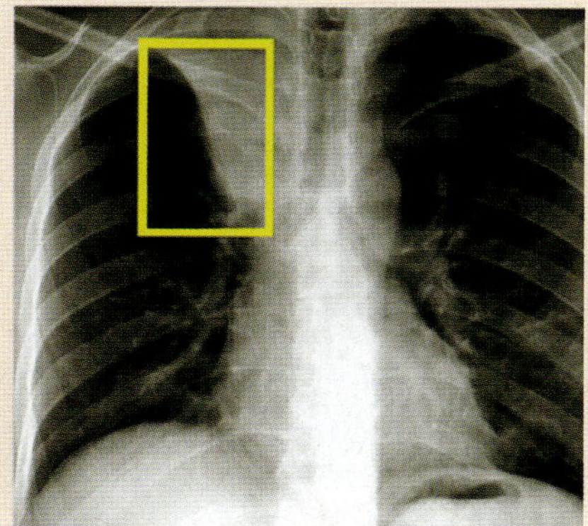

a. Bronchogenic carcinoma b. Bronchiectasis
c. Silicosis d. Aspergillosis

6. Appearance (Arrow) on axial CT scan is characteristic of

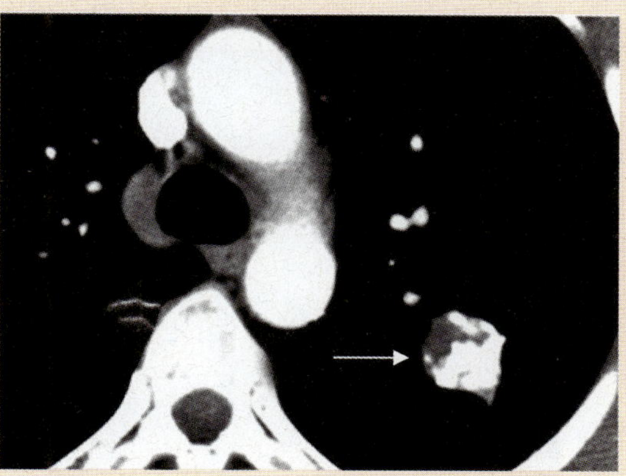

a. Bronchogenic carcinoma b. Bronchial atresia
c. Pulmonary hamartoma d. Silicosis

7. Sign (Arrow) seen in Photograph indicates
[Recent Question 2012, 2014]

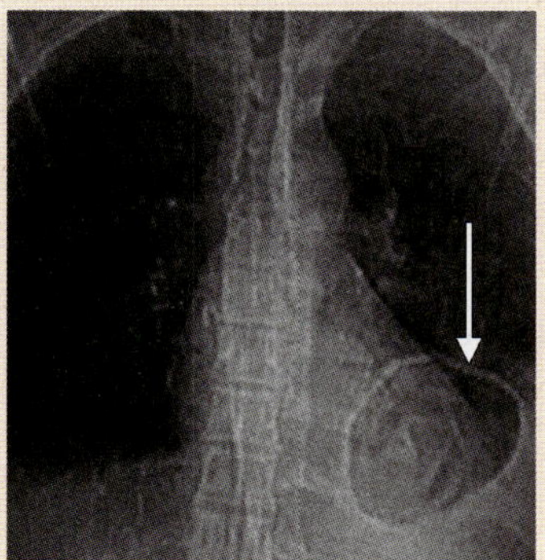

a. Tuberculosis b. Aspergillosis
c. Cryptococcosis d. Echinococcosis

8. Diagnose the disease shown in the Photograph on high-resolution CT scan ***[Recent Question 2015]***

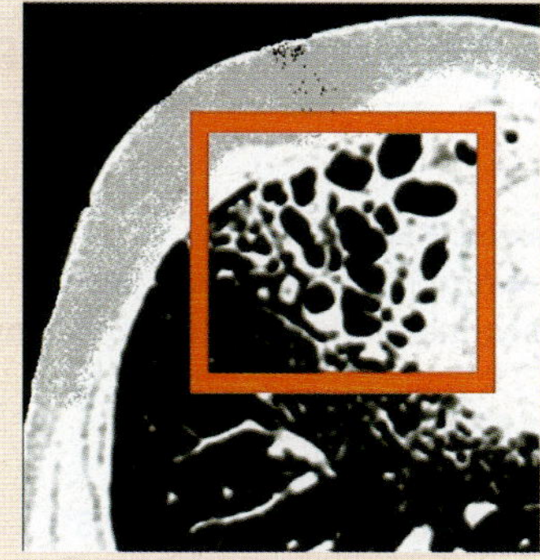

a. Pneumomediastinum b. Pulmonary hamartomas
c. Tuberculosis d. Bronchiectasis

9. Diagnose the disease shown in the Photograph
[Recent Question 2015]

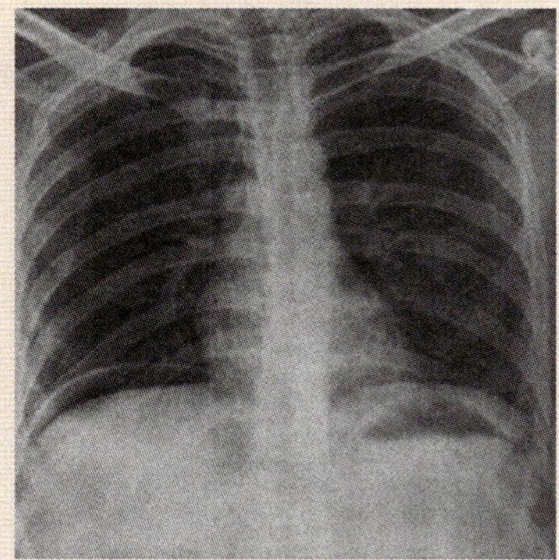

a. Pleural effusion
b. Bronchiectasis
c. Tuberculosis
d. Pneumoperitoneum

10. A 38 years old male, working in a glass factory, presents with fever and weight loss since last 2 months. AFB is negative. X-ray (Photograph) was taken. Diagnosis ***[Recent Question 2015]***

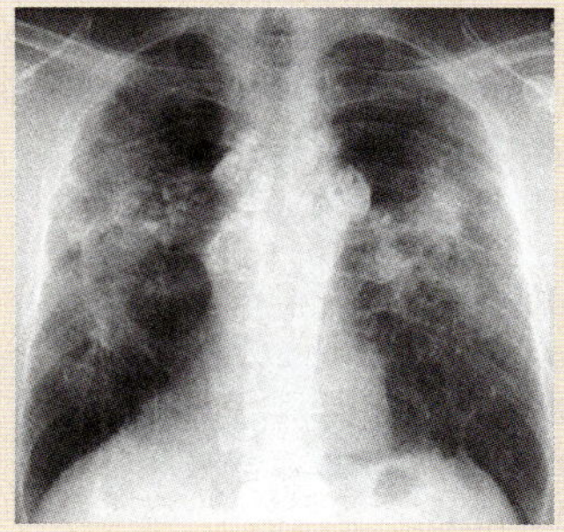

a. Tuberculosis
b. Pneumocystis carinii pneumonia
c. Sarcoidosis
d. Silicosis

Radiodiagnosis and Radiotherapy

11. A 38 years old male, presents with breathlessness. X-ray (Photograph) was taken. Diagnosis ***[Recent Question 2015]***

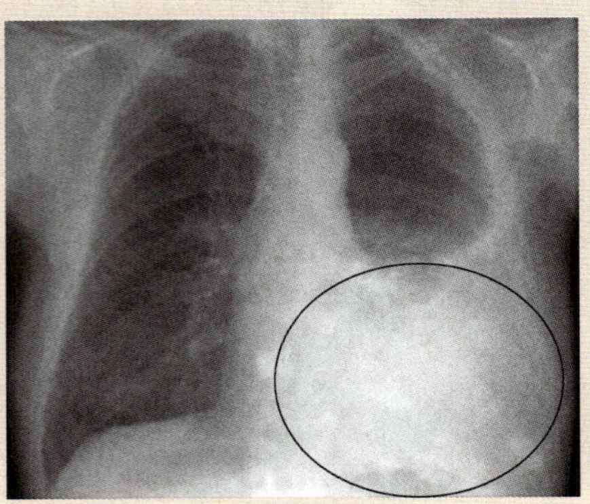

a. Tuberculosis
b. Pleural effusion
c. Pneumonia
d. Bronchogenic carcinoma

12. Which of the following is not a finding in the X-ray Photograph shown below? ***[AIIMS May 2017]***

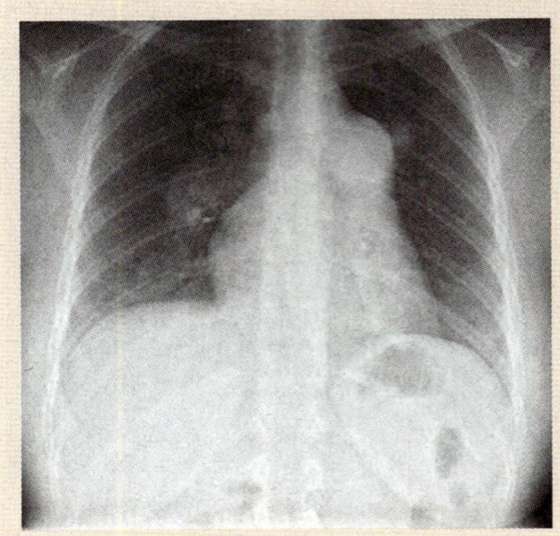

a. Right atrial enlargement
b. Pulmonary venous hypertension
c. Narrow vascular pedicle
d. Reduced pulmonary blood flow

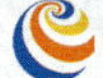 ANSWERS WITH EXPLANATIONS OF IBQs 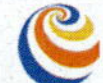

1. Ans. (c) < 0.5 *[Ref. Radiology for UGs & GPs by Singh, 1/e p40]*

Cardio Thoracic Ratio (CTR)

- CTR is measured on a PA chest X-ray
- Ratio of maximal horizontal cardiac diameter to maximal horizontal thoracic diameter (inner edge of ribs/edge of pleura)
- Normal CTR values:
  - Normal CTR (Adults): <0.5
  - Normal CTR (Newborns): <0.55
  - Normal CTR (1–6 years age): <0.45
  - Normal CTR (6–12 years age): <0.44

2. Ans. (d) Thymus *[Ref. Sumer K Sethi, 5/e p26]*

- Sail sign: Characteristic triangular shape of thymus on right side of mediastinum

3. Ans. (c) Bronchiectasis *[Ref. Sumer K Sethi, 5/e p28]*

Signet Ring Sign

- Dilated bronchus and accompanying pulmonary artery branch are seen in cross-section
- Characteristic of bronchiectasis

4. Ans. (c) Sarcoidosis *[Ref. Radiology Illustrated by Jeong, 1/e p77]*

Finger-in-Glove (Toothpaste) Appearance

- Allergic bronchopulmonary aspergillosis
- Bronchogenic carcinoma
- Cystic fibrosis
- Asthma
- Bronchial hamartoma
- Bronchial lipoma
- Bronchial carcinoid
- Bronchial tuberculosis
- Broncholithiasis
- Bronchial stricture

5. Ans. (a) Bronchogenic carcinoma *[Ref. Sumer K Sethi, 5/e p34]*

Golden-S-Sign

- Description: Reverse S-shape of a fissure involved when a lobe collapses around a large, central mass

- Conditions:
  - Bronchogenic carcinoma
  - Metastasis
  - Primary mediastinal tumor
  - Enlarged lymph nodes

6. Ans. (c) Pulmonary hamartoma *[Ref. Sumer K Sethi, 5/e p35]*

Popcorn Calcification
- Pulmonary hamartoma
- Fibroadenoma breast
- Uterine fibroid
- Fibrous dysplasia
- Enchondroma
- Chondrosarcoma

7. Ans. (d) Echinococcosis *[Ref. Sumer K Sethi, 5/e p27]*

Water-Lily/Camolote Sign
- Description: Detachment of the endocyst membrane results in floating membranes within pericyst that mimic the appearance of a water lily
- Seen in: *Echinococcus* (Hydatid cyst)

8. Ans. (d) Bronchiectasis *[Ref. Sumer K Sethi, 5/e p28]*

Cluster-of-Grapes Sign
- Bronchiectasis
- Hydatidiform mole (USG)
- Intraductal papillary mucinous neoplasm

9. Ans. (d) Pneumoperitoneum *[Ref. Emergency Radiology by Mirvis, 1/e p4]*

Pneumoperitoneum
- Description: Gas within the peritoneal cavity, and indicates a critical illness
- MC cause: perforation of hollow viscus
- Chest radiograph: An erect chest X-ray is probably the most sensitive plain radiograph for the detection of free intraperitoneal gas
- Sub-diaphragmatic free gas (Photograph)
- Cupola sign
- Abdominal radiograph: Free gas within the peritoneal cavity

10. Ans. (d) Silicosis *[Ref. Mechanical Ventilation by Lachmann, 1/e p6]*
- Glass factory worker with fever weight loss indicate Silicosis
- AFB negative rules out Tuberculosis
- X-ray/CT scan: Egg-shell calcification of Hilar lymph nodes (Photograph)

11. Ans. (b) Pleural effusion *[Ref. Sumer K Sethi, 5/e p24]*

Pleural Effusion Radiology
- Blunting of the costophrenic angle
- Blunting of the cardiophrenic angle
- Fluid within the horizontal or oblique fissures
- Eventually a meniscus will be seen, on frontal films seen laterally and gently sloping medially
- With large volume effusions, mediastinal shift occurs away from the effusion

12. Ans. (b) Pulmonary venous hypertension *[Ref. Principles and Interpretation of Chest X-rays by Mahesh, 1/e p145]*
- X-ray Photograph given in the question shows Cardiomegaly, Narrow vascular pedicles and Hyperlucent lung fields à suggestive of decreased pulmonary flow
- Pulmonary venous hypertension X-ray shows prominant hilar vessels with plethoric lung fields (See below)

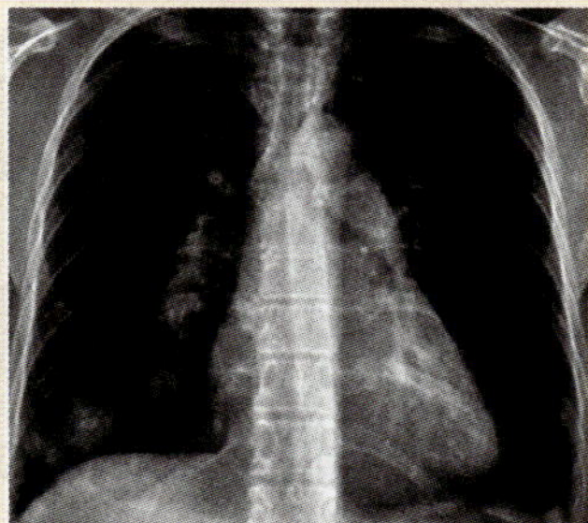

Fig. Pulmonary hypertension

Radiodiagnosis and Radiotherapy

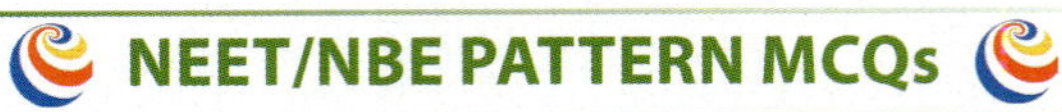

NEET/NBE PATTERN MCQs

1. **'Air crescent sign' on chest radiograph may be an indication of** *[NBE FMGE September 2010]*
   a. Aspergilloma
   b. Pneumococcal pneumonia
   c. Bronchiectasis
   d. Bronchogenic carcinoma
2. **'Kerley B lines' in chest X-ray is diagnostic of** *[UPSC 2009]*
   a. Respiratory failure b. Renal failure
   c. Heart failure d. Liver failure
3. **High-resolution CT scan is an ideal modality for evaluation of** *[NBE FMGE September 2007, September 2010]*
   a. Lung mass b. Pleural effusion
   c. Lymphadenopathy d. Interstitial lung disease
4. **H.R.C.T. of Thorax is indicated in all of the following conditions, except** *[NBE DNB December 2011]*
   a. Interstitial fibrosis b. Lung abscess
   c. Miliary tuberculosis d. Sarcoidosis
5. **Which of the following radiograph is best for diagnosis of pneumoperitoneum?** *[NBE DNB December 2011]*
   a. X-ray abdomen (erect)
   b. X-ray abdomen (supine)
   c. X-ray chest PA
   d. X-ray chest left lateral
6. **Water-lily appearance in chest X-ray suggestive of** *[NBE DNB 1995, 2004, 2007]*
   a. Bronchiectasis b. Bronchopleural fistula
   c. Hydatid cyst d. Sequestration cyst of lung
7. **Which of the following is the most reliable method for diagnosis of pulmonary embolism?** *[NBE FMGE March 2010, Recent Question 2015]*
   a. Plain X-ray b. Perfusion scan
   c. Angiography d. Electrocardiography
8. **Pleural effusion without evident lung infiltration is most often due to** *[NBE DNB 1996]*
   a. Viral pleurisy b. Carcinoma
   c. Lymphoma d. Tuberculosis
9. **Miliary shadow in chest X-ray is seen in A/E** *[Recent Question 2012]*
   a. 1B b. Sarcoidosis
   c. *Klebsiella* d. Metastasis
10. **'Exploded popcorn' appearance on chest X-ray is seen in** *[NBE FMGE March 2010]*
    a. Miliary tuberculosis b. Hamartoma
    c. Choriocarcinoma d. Coccidioidomycosis
11. **CAMALOTE sign appearance in chest X-ray suggestive of** *[NBE DNB 1999]*
    a. Bronchiectasis b. Hydatid cyst
    c. Bronchopleural fistula d. Sequestration cyst of lung
12. **Hypertranslucent chest X-ray is seen in all, except** *[Recent Question 2012]*
    a. Mcleod syndrome b. Emphysema
    c. Pneumonectomy d. Poland syndrome
13. **Kerley B-lines represent** *[NBE DNB 1995, 1999]*
    a. Linear fibrosis
    b. Haemosiderin deposits
    c. Small focal atelectasis
    d. Thickened interlobular septa
14. **Chest X-ray for Pneumothorax should be** *[NBE FMGE September 2008]*
    a. Inspiration in erect position
    b. Inspiration in supine position
    c. Inspiration in prone position
    d. Expiration in supine position
15. **Perihilar fluffy opacities on chest X-ray is seen** *[Recent Question 2012, 2013]*
    a. Sarcoidosis b. Pulmonary edema
    c. Silicosis d. Lung carcinoma
16. **Disseminated small nodules with calcification in chest suggest** *[NBE DNB 2000]*
    a. Histoplasmosis b. Aspergillosis
    c. Cryptococeosis d. Coccidioidomycosis
17. **Pleural effusion without evident lung infiltration is most often due to** *[NBE DNB 2004]*
    a. Viral pleurisy b. Carcinoma
    c. Lymphoma d. Tuberculosis
18. **'Water-lily' sign on chest X-ray is seen in** *[NBE FMGE September 2006]*
    a. Mycotic lung abscess b. Pleural effusion
    c. Hydatid disease d. All of the above
19. **Tracheal bifurcation is best visualized on which standard view of the chest** *[NBE DNB 1996, 2000, 2006]*
    a. Left anterior oblique b. Left posterior oblique
    c. Right anterior oblique d. Right posterior oblique
20. **Hypertranslucent chest X-ray is seen in all, except** *[Recent Question 2012, 2013]*
    a. Mcleod syndrome b. Emphysema
    c. Pneumonectomy d. Poland syndrome
21. **Atelectasis with positive 'Reverse-S' sign is seen in** *[NBE FMGE September 2006]*
    a. Asthma b. Tuberculosis
    c. Sarcoidosis d. Bronchogenic carcinoma
22. **"Egg-shell" calcification in hilar nodes suggest** *[NBE DNB 1994, 1999, 2007, 2010]*
    a. Asbestosis b. Silicosis
    c. Berylliosis d. Baritosis
23. **Golden-S sign is seen in** *[Recent Question 2014]*
    a. Bronchitis b. Bronchogenic carcinoma
    c. Metastasis to lungs d. Pleural hamartoma
24. **Investigation of choice for definitive diagnosis of Pulmonary embolism is** *[NBE FMGE March 2006]*
    a. Pulmonary angiography
    b. Ventilation perfusion scan
    c. Chest X-ray
    d. MRI pulmonary angiography

25. Nipple shadows on chest radiograph characteristically have a sharp *[NBE DNB 2008, 2009]*
a. Medial margin b. Lateral margin
c. Superior margin d. Inferior margin

26. Diagnostic investigation for Lung sequestration is *[NBE FMGE March 2006]*
a. Chest X-ray (PA view) b. CT scan
c. Angiography d. MRI

27. Finger-in-glove sign is seen in *[Recent Question 2014]*
a. Chronic bronchitis
b. Bronchocoele
c. Bronchogenic carcinoma
d. Pleuritis

28. Best investigation for Pleural effusion is *[NBE FMGE September 2005]*
a. X-ray b. CECT
c. MRI d. USG

29. H.R.C.T. of Thorax is indicated in all of the following conditions, except *[NBE DNB 2011]*
a. Interstitial fibrosis b. Lung abscess
c. Miliary tuberculosis d. Sarcoidosis

30. Most reliable method for diagnosis of Pulmonary embolism is *[NBE FMGE March 2004]*
a. Plain skiagram b. Angiography
c. Perfusion scan d. Electrocardiography

31. Interstitial lung disease diagnosis is done by *[NBE FMGE September 2012]*
a. High-resolution CT scan b. Pulmonary function tests
c. Bronchoscopic biopsy d. All of the above

32. Best view to detect minimal pleural effusion on chest X-ray is *[NBE FMGE March 2004]*
a. PA view b. Lateral decubitus view
c. Lordotic view d. Supine view

33. Investigation of choice for Bronchiectasis is *[Recent Question 2017, NBE FMGE September 2009]*
a. Chest X-ray b. CT scan
c. MRI d. Ventilation perfusion scan

34. Minimum amount of fluid collection sufficient for pleural effusion to be detected on X-ray in decubitus view is *[NBE FMGE September 2009]*
a. 15 mL b. 25 mL
c. 35 mL d. 45 mL

35. High-resolution CT is the ideal modality for evaluation of *[NBE FMGE September 2011]*
a. Pleural effusion b. Lung mass
c. Interstitial lung disease d. Lymphadenopathy

36. Investigation of choice for detecting minimal pleural effusion is *[NBE FMGE September 2011]*
a. Ultrasound b. CT scan
c. MRI d. Chest X-ray

37. Investigation of choice for detection & characterization of interstitial lung disease is *[NBE FMGE March 2012]*
a. MRI
b. Ventilation – Perfusion Scan
c. High-resolution CT scan
d. Chest X-ray

38. Miliary nodules are seen in all, except *[Recent Question 2013]*
a. Silicosis b. TB
c. Aspergillosis d. Anthracosis

39. Chest X-ray, most common view is *[Recent Question 2013]*
a. AP b. PA
c. RAO d. LAO

40. Best view for collapse of middle lobe lung is *[Recent Question 2013]*
a. Lateral b. AP
c. Oblique d. Lordotic

41. Gold standard to diagnose pulmonary thromboembolism *[Recent Question 2013]*
a. CT angiography b. USG
c. Plethysmography d. Ventilation perfusion scan

42. Differential diagnosis of solitary pulmonary nodule are all, except *[Recent Question 2013]*
a. Bronchogenic carcinoma
b. Mycetoma
c. Tuberculoma
d. Hamartoma

43. Air bronchogram on chest X-ray denotes *[Recent Question 2013, 2014]*
a. Intrapulmonary lesion b. Extrapulmonary lesion
c. Intrathoracic lesion d. Extrathoracic lesion

44. Calcified pulmonary metastasis is seen in which carcinoma *[Recent Question 2013]*
a. Pancreatic carcinoma b. Thyroid carcinoma
c. Endometrial carcinoma d. None

45. Water-lily sign on chest X-ray is seen in *[Recent Question 2013, 2014]*
a. TB b. Aspergillosis
c. Hydatid cyst d. Cryptococcosis

46. Most common radiological feature of sarcoidosis in India patients *[Recent Question 2013]*
a. Normal chest X-ray
b. Bilateral hilar lymphadenopathy
c. Bilateral hilar lymphadenopathy with parenchymal infiltrate
d. Only parenchymal infiltrate

47. Characteristic radiological finding in sarcoidosis *[Recent Question 2013]*
a. Parenchymal disease
b. Unilateral hilar lymphadenopathy
c. Bilateral hilar lymphadenopathy
d. Miliary shadow

48. Thick cavity in lung is caused by all, except *[Recent Question 2013, 2015]*
a. Lung abscess b. TB
c. Emphysematous bulla d. Hamartoma

49. Radiological feature of Sarcoidosis *[Recent Question 2013, 2015]*
a. Hilar lymphadenopathy
b. Hilar lymphadenopathy with parenchymal lung changes
c. No Hilar lymphadenopathy with parenchymal lung changes
d. All of the above

50. Necrotic nodules in lung are seen in *[Recent Question 2013, 2015]*
a. TB b. Sarcoidosis
c. RA d. All of the above

51. Currently high-resolution CT scanning is Investigation of choice for *[Recent Question 2015]*
a. Pulmonary embolism
b. Minimal pleural effusion
c. Bronchiectasis
d. Tuberculosis

52. Non-invasive method for investigation of Foreign body in bronchus *[Recent Question 2015]*
a. MDCT with VB
b. X-ray at height of inspiration
c. MRI scan
d. Clinical examination

53. Radiographic sign characteristic of Pulmonary edema is *[Recent Question 2017]*
a. Westermark's sign b. Hampton's hump
c. Palla sign d. Bat wing sign

54. Snow storm appearance on chest X-ray is seen in *[Recent Question 2017]*
a. Anthracosis b. Byssinosis
c. Silicosis d. Bagassosis

55. Tree in bud appearance on CT is seen in *[Recent Question 2017]*
a. Pulmonary tuberculosis b. Silicosis
c. Pulmonary hydatid cyst d. Small cell carcinoma

56. Which of the following is not an X-ray finding of Pulmonary embolism? *[Recent Question 2017]*
a. Westermark sign b. Palla sign
c. Felson sign d. Panda sign

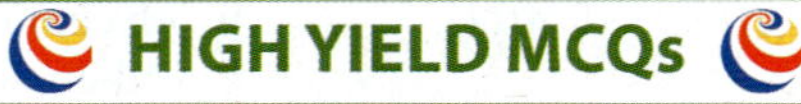

1. The best X-ray view for minimal pleural effusion *[All India PGMEE 1992]*
a. AP b. PA
c. Lateral d. Lateral decubitus

2. Decubitus view is useful in diagnosing *[PGI 2001]*
a. Pleural effusion
b. Pleural effusion with dependent hemithorax
c. Pericardial effusion
d. Middle lobe consolidation

3. Right anterior oblique view of chest X-ray true is/are *[PGI 1998]*
a. Cassette near right shoulder
b. Cassette near left shoulder
c. Arch of Aorta best seen
d. Left atrial enlargement can be diagnosed
e. Mitral & Tricuspid valves better seen

4. High-resolution computed tomography of the chest is the ideal modality for evaluating *[All India PGMEE 2003]*
a. Pleural effusion b. Interstitial lung disease
c. Lung mass d. Mediastinal adenopathy

5. Miliary shadow in chest X-ray is seen in all except *[PGI 1999]*
a. Tuberculosis b. Loeffler's pneumonia
c. *Klebsiella* d. Varicella pneumonia

6. Hyperinflation of lung in CXR is seen in *[PGI 2004]*
a. CCF
b. Congenital lobar emphysema
c. Diaphragmatic hernia
d. Foreign body
e. Mucoviscidosis

7. All are true regarding emphysema finding in X-ray, except *[AIIMS PGMEE 1992]*
a. Low flat diaphragm - Terrace pattern
b. Tubular heart
c. Decreased inter costal space
d. Increased radiolucence

8. True about chest X-ray *[PGI 2009]*
a. 40% lung tissue seen obscured by bony structure & mediastinum
b. 60% lung tissue seen obscured by bony structure & mediastinum
c. Right dome higher than left dome
d. Right dome pushed up by liver
e. Should be taken in expiration

9. On a chest X-ray (PA view), Aortic knuckle shadow is obliterated by consolidation of which portion of lung? *[All India PGMEE 2011]*
a. Lower lingual
b. Upper lingual
c. Apex of lower lobe
d. Posterior part of Upper lobe

10. Honeycombing of lung in CXR is seen in *[PGI 2003]*
a. Rheumatoid arthritis b. Tuberculosis
c. Scleroderma d. Carcinoma
e. Interstitial lung disease

11. 'Egg-shell calcification' is seen in all, except *[AIIMS PGMEE 1998]*
a. Sarcoidosis
b. Silicosis
c. Post irradiation lymphoma
d. Bronchogenic CA

12. Egg-shell calcification is seen in *[PGI 2009]*
a. Sarcoidosis b. Silicosis
c. Lung carcinoma d. Pneumoconiosis
e. Lymphoma following radiation treatment

13. 'Spring-water cyst' is another name for *[PGI 1997]*
a. Hydatid cyst of lung b. Lung amoebic cyst
c. Pleuro-pericardial cyst d. Enterogenous cyst

14. Normal hilar shadow in X-ray chest is produced by all except *[AIIMS PGMEE 1997]*
a. Pulmonary artery b. Bronchus
c. Lower lobe veins d. Upper lobe veins

Radiodiagnosis and Radiotherapy

15. All of the following produce cavitating nodules in the lung, except *[AIIMS PGMEE 1993]*
a. Squamous cell CA
b. Caplan's syndrome
c. Hamartoma
d. Silicosis

16. "Miliary shadow" on chest X-ray is seen in *[PGI 2003]*
a. Tuberculosis
b. Rheumatoid arthritis
c. Pneumoconiosis
d. COPD
e. Metastasis

17. Miliary mottling seen in *[PGI 2006]*
a. T.B.
b. Sarcoidosis
c. Silicosis
d. P. carinii pneumonia

18. Hampton hump is feature of? *[AIIMS PGMEE 2007]*
a. Pulmonary tuberculosis
b. Pulmonary embolism
c. Pulmonary haemorrhage
d. Bronchogenic carcinoma

19. Best method to diagnose pulmonary embolism *[PGI 1997]*
a. Pulmonary angiography
b. Scintillation perfusion scan
c. CT scan
d. X-ray chest

20. Gold standard for diagnosing pulmonary embolism *[Recent Question 2017, PGI 1997]*
a. X-ray chest
b. Ventilation perfusion scan
c. Blood gas analysis
d. Doppler

21. In lung X-ray, heterogeneous shadow is due to *[PGI 1997]*
a. Haemangioma
b. Pulmonary infarction
c. Metastatic lesion
d. TB

22. In pulmonary embolism, findings in perfusion scan is *[PGI 2000]*
a. Perfusion segmental defect
b. Perfusion defect with normal lung scan & radiography
c. Tenting of diaphragm
d. Normal chest scan

23. The following is not the differential diagnosis of an anterior mediastinal mass *[AIIMS PGMEE 2002]*
a. Teratoma
b. Neurogenic tumor
c. Thymoma
d. Lymphoma

24. Investigation of choice in bronchiectasis is *[AIIMS PGMEE 1994]*
a. X-ray
b. Bronchoscopy
c. Bronchography
d. USG

25. Most sensitive investigation for air embolism is *[All India PGMEE 1999]*
a. Decreased tidal volume of CO_2
b. Decreased tidal volume of NO_2
c. Doppler ultrasound
d. Central venous pressure

26. Investigation of choice for pulmonary embolism *[All India PGMEE 1998]*
a. CT scan
b. Contrast CT
c. Ventilation Perfusion Scan
d. MRI

27. Best view to diagnose pneumothorax *[PGI 1998]*
a. Lateral oblique
b. PA view in full expiration
c. PA view in full inspiration
d. AP view in full expiration

28. 'Floating water-lily sign' is feature of *[AIIMS PGMEE 2007]*
a. Hydatid disease of lungs
b. Bronchial adenoma
c. Lung abscess
d. Aspergilloma

29. 'Popcorn calcification' is characteristically seen in *[All India PGMEE 1997]*
a. TB
b. Metastasis
c. Pulmonary hamartoma
d. Fungal invagination

30. Plethoric lung fields are seen in all of the following conditions, except *[AIIMS PGMEE 2006]*
a. Atrial septal defect (ASD)
b. TAPVC (total anomalous pulmonary venous connection)
c. Ebstein's anomaly
d. Ventricular septal defect

31. Best view for right pleural effusion in X-ray chest *[All India PGMEE1993]*
a. Supine
b. Prone
c. Right lateral decubitus
d. Left lateral decubitus

32. Following will be most helpful radiological investigation in a patient suspected of left pleural effusion *[AIIMS PGMEE 1992]*
a. Right lateral decubitus
b. Left lateral decubitus
c. Left lateral erect
d. Right lateral erect

33. Inter lobar pleural effusion can be detected in best way in *[AIIMS PGMEE 1993]*
a. Lateral decubitus
b. Reverse lordotic
c. Lateral oblique
d. Posterior oblique

34. High-resolution CT of the lung is a specialized CT technique for greater detail of lung parenchyma and it utilizes *[AIIMS PGMEE 2002]*
a. Special lung filters
b. Thick collimation
c. Bone algorithm for image reconstruction
d. Large field of view

35. All are true about Kerley B line except *[AIIMS PGMEE 1997]*
a. Horizontal
b. Runs from hilar area to peripheral area
c. Due to thickening of septa
d. Due to pulmonary venous hypertension

36. Kerley's 'B' lines are found in *[PGI 2003]*
a. Interstitial edema
b. Pulmonary venous congestion
c. Pericardial effusion
d. Mitral stenosis

37. Water-lily sign is seen in chest X-ray of *[AIIMS PGMEE 1991]*
a. Pulmonary hypoplasia
b. *Echinococcus*
c. Pneumonia
d. Sarcoidosis

38. Egg-shell calcification is seen in *[PGI 2003]*
a. Silicosis
b. TB
c. Carcinoma metastatic to lymphnode
d. Lymphoma
e. Sarcoidosis

39. "Egg shell" calcification is seen in *[PGI 2001]*
a. Bronchiolitis b. Silicosis
c. Carcinoma bronchus d. Sarcoidosis
e. Histoplasmosis

40. Egg-shell calcification found in *[PGI 2006]*
a. Silicosis b. Sarcoidosis
c. Metastatic node d. Lymphoma
e. Tuberculosis

41. True about chest X-ray is all, except *[PGI 1997]*
a. Left hilum is higher
b. Left dome is higher
c. All fissures are clearly seen on lateral film
d. None

42. Which is the objective sign of identifying pulmonary plethora in a chest radiograph? *[All India PGMEE 2006]*
a. Diameter of the main pulmonary artery >16 mm
b. Diameter of the left pulmonary artery >16 mm
c. Diameter of the descending right pulmonary artery > 16 mm
d. Diameter of the descending left pulmonary artery > 16 mm

43. A young man with pulmonary tuberculosis presents with massive recurrent hemoptysis. For angiographic treatment, which vascular structure should be evaluated first? *[All India PGMEE 2004]*
a. Pulmonary artery b. Bronchial artery
c. Pulmonary vein d. Superior vena cava

44. A young man with tuberculosis presents with massive recurrent hemoptysis. Most probable cause would be *[AIIMS PGMEE 2002, 2003]*
a. Pulmonary artery b. Bronchial artery
c. Pulmonary vein d. Superior vena cava

45. A 40 years old man presents with a recurrent hemoptysis and purulent cough. X-ray was found to be normal. To next investigation done to aid in diagnosis is *[AIIMS PGMEE 2001, 2002]*
a. MRI b. Bronchoscopy
c. HRCT d. CT-guided biopsy

46. What does not make diagnosis of solitary pulmonary nodule? *[AIIMS PGMEE 1991]*
a. Tuberculoma b. Bronchial adenoma
c. Hamartoma d. Neurofibroma

47. A patient presents with a solitary pulmonary nodule [SPN] on X-ray. The best investigation to come to a diagnosis would be *[AIIMS PGMEE 2002]*
a. MID b. CT scan
c. USG d. Image-guided biopsy

48. Miliary mottling found in *[PGI 2006]*
a. Rheumatoid arthritis
b. TB
c. Pneumoucystis carinii pneumonia
d. Congestive heart failure
e. Pulmonary edema

49. Millary mottling on X-ray chest is seen in *[PGI 2000]*
a. Histoplasmosis b. Sarcoidosis
c. Secondaries from carcinoma colon
d. Gonococal pneumonia

50. Bulging fissures in lungs is seen in *[PGI 1999]*
a. Klebsiella pneumonia b. Staph pneumonia
c. Pulmonary oedema d. Pneumoconiosis

51. All show miliary shadow on chest X-ray except *[All India PGMEE 1991]*
a. Pneumoconiasis b. Sarcoidosis
c. MS d. Staphylococcal pneumonia

52. Increased radiolucency of one-sided hemithorax may be caused by all except *[All India PGMEE 1991]*
a. Obstructive emphysema b. Pneumothorax
c. Expiratory film d. Patient rotation

53. Hypertranslucency of lung unilaterally is seen on all except *[PGI 2000]*
a. Pneumothorax
b. Resection of mammary gland
c. Pulmonary artery obstruction
d. Pneumonectomy

54. In right-sided hemithorax on chest X-ray PA view what can be excluded *[PGI 1997]*
a. CCF b. TB
c. Pulmonary infarct d. None of the above

55. Uremic lung most often results due to *[PGI 1998]*
a. Pulmonary edema b. Fibrosis
c. Alveolar injury d. CVC liver

56. All of the following are true about loculated pleural effusion except *[All India PGMEE 2002]*
a. It makes an obtuse angle with the chest wall
b. The margins are diffuse when viewed end on
c. Not confined to any bronchopulmonary segment
d. Air bronchograms are seen within the opacity

57. A patient presented with minimal right-sided pleural effusion. The best method to detect this would be *[AIIMS PGMEE 2001]*
a. Right lateral b. Left lateral
c. Left lateral decubitus d. Right lateral decubitus

58. Extensive pleural thickening and calcification especially involving the diaphragmatic pleura are classical features of *[All India PGMEE 2003]*
a. Coal worker's pneumoconiosis
b. Asbestosis
c. Silicosis
d. Siderosis

59. Most likely diagnosis in a newborn who had a radiopaque shadow with an air fluid level in the chest along with hemivertebrae of the 6th thoracic vertebra on plain X-ray is *[AIIMS PGMEE 2002]*
a. Congenital diaphragmatic hernia
b. Oesophageal duplication cyst
c. Bronchogenic cyst
d. Staphylococcal pneumonia

60. A child has respiratory distress, chest X-ray shows multiple air filled space, the differential diagnosis is all except *[AIIMS PGMEE 1998]*

a. Congenital lung cyst
b. Congenital Diaphragmatic hernia
c. Congenital lobar aplasia of lung
d. Congenital adenomatous malformation

61. A new born baby with acute respiratory distress on day 1. X-ray chest PA view showed numerous gas lucencies in entire left hemithorax, most likely diagnosis is *[AIIMS PGMEE 1992]*

a. Congenital lobar emphysema
b. Pneumatocoele hernia
c. Congenital diaphragmatic hernia
d. Congenital lung cyst

62. Pappu 2 years old boy presents in the causality with history of sudden onset of respiratory difficulty & strider on auscultation, decreased breath sound & wheeze on the right side. The X-ray shows RT opaque hemithorax, what will be diagnosis? *[All India PGMEE 2002]*

a. Pneumothorax
b. Acute epiglottitis
c. Massive plural effusion
d. Foreign body aspiration

63. A child with acute respiratory distress showing hyperinflation of unilateral lung in X-ray is due to *[All India PGMEE 2002]*

a. Staphylococcal bronchopneumonia
b. Aspiration pneumonia
c. Congenital lobar emphysema
d. Foreign body aspiration

64. A neonate presents with respiratory distress, contra lateral meditational shift and multiple cystic air filled lesions in the chest. Most likely diagnosis is *[All India PGMEE 2001]*

a. Pneumonia
b. Congenital lung cyst
c. Congenital diaphragmatic hernia
d. Congenital lobar emphysema

65. Apgar scores were 3, and 6 at 1 and 5 minutes. At 10 minutes child shows features of breathlessness on CXR mediastinal shift was there, possible causes *[PGI 2000]*

a. Bilateral choanal atresia
b. Pneumothorax
c. Congenital diaphragmatic hernia
d. Hyaline Membrane disease.

66. In X-ray, loops of bowel on left side of hemithorax and shift of heart shadow is seen in *[PGI 1998]*

a. Eventration of diaphragm
b. Foramen of bochdalek hernia
c. Morgagnian hernia
d. Any of the above

67. A 3-year-old female child developed fever, cough and respiratory distress. On chest X-ray consolidation is seen in right lower lobe. She improved with antibiotics but on follow-up at 8 weeks was again found to have increasing consolidation in right lower lobe. Your next investigation would be *[AIIMS PGMEE 2007]*

a. Bronchoscopy
b. Bacterial culture of the nasopharynx
c. CT scan of the chest
d. Allergen sensitivity test

68. A 55-year-old man who has been on bed rest for the past 1 day, complains of breathlessness and chest pain. The chest X-ray is normal. The next step in investigation should be *[All India PGMEE 2004]*

a. Lung ventilation - perfusion scan
b. Pulmonary arteriography
c. Pulmonary venous wedge angiography
d. Echocardiography

69. A 55-year-old man who has been on bed rest for the past 1 day, complains of breathlessness. The chest X-ray shows Hampton's hump. The next investigation should be *[All India PGMEE 2003]*

a. Lung ventilation-perfusion scan
b. Pulmonary arteriography
c. Pulmonary venous angiography
d. Echocardiography

70. A 25-year-old man presented with fever, cough, expectoration and breathlessness of 2 months duration. Contrast-enhanced computed tomography of the chest showed bilateral upper lobe fibrotic lesions and mediastinum had enlarged necrotic nodes with peripheral rim enhancement. Which one of the following is the most probable diagnosis? *[All India PGMEE 2003, AIIMS PGMEE 2004]*

a. Sarcoidosis b. Tuberculosis
c. Lymphoma d. Silicosis

71. A patient suffering from AIDS presents with history of dyspnea and non-productive cough X-ray shows bilateral perihilar opacities without pleural effusion and lymphadenopathy. Most probable etiological agent is *[AIIMS PGMEE 2002]*

a. Tuberculosis b. CMV
c. Kaposi's sarcoma d. Pneumocystis carinii

72. A 48 years old man, resident of Baroda outskirts near a textile mill presents to his family physician with respiratory symptoms. Doctor advices X-ray chest which showed fine reticular & nodular pattern in lower zone with loss of clarity of diaphragm & cardiac shadows. He also doubts about the presence of small pleural effusion. The probable diagnosis is *[All India PGMEE 1993]*

a. Stannosis
b. Asbestosis
c. Silicosis
d. Coal worker's pneumoconiosis

73. Which of the following organs should always be imaged in a suspected case of bronchogenic carcinoma? *[AIIMS PGMEE 2004]*

a. Adrenals b. Spleen
c. Kidney d. Pancreas

74. All are true about thymus swelling except *[AIIMS PGMEE 1999]*

a. Widening of mediastinum on X-ray
b. Sharp border with sail like appearance
c. Steroid administration reduces size of swelling
d. Shift of trachea on X-ray

75. Soft tissue mass in chest with rib erosion in X-ray is seen in all except *[AIIMS PGMEE 1996]*

a. Leukemia
b. Ewing's sarcoma
c. Multiple myeloma
d. Osteosarcoma

76. To visualize vascular sling causing tracheal/external airway compression which of the following would you best prefer? *[AIIMS PGMEE 2009]*

a. Catheter angiography of aorta and pulmonary artery
b. MRI
c. CT
d. PET-CT

77. Investigation of choice for detection & characterization of interstitial lung disease is *[All India PGMEE 2008, AIIMS PGMEE 2005]*

a. MRI
b. Chest X-ray
c. High-resolution CT scan
d. Ventilation perfusion scan

78. Best diagnostic aid for bronchiectasis is *[AIIMS PGMEE 1992]*

a. Bronchoscopy
b. X- ray
c. Bronchography
d. CT scan

79. High-resolution computed tomography of the chest is the ideal modality for evaluating *[All India PGMEE 2003]*

a. Pleural effusion
b. Interstitial disease
c. Lung mass
d. Meditational adenopathy

80. In patient with high clinical suspicion of pulmonary thromboembolism, best investigation would be? *[AIIMS PGMEE 2007]*

a. D-dimer
b. CT angiography
c. Catheter angiography
d. Color Doppler

81. Pulmonary embolism is best diagnosed by *[All India PGMEE 1996]*

a. USG
b. X-ray Chest
c. Ventilation - Perfusion Scan
d. CT Scan

82. Best method for detecting minimal bronchiectasis *[All India PGMEE 1992]*

a. Bronchogram
b. CT Scan
c. Radio nucleotide scan
d. Chest X-ray

83. Stratosphere sign is seen in *[JIPMER PGMEE 2014]*

a. Pleural effusion
b. Pneumothorax
c. Rib fracture
d. Bronchogenic carcinoma

84. Gold standard for diagnosis of bronchiectasis *[AIIMS November 2014]*

a. MRI
b. Bronchography
c. HRCT chest
d. Chest X-ray

85. A neonate with bilious vomiting, investigation of choice is *[AIIMS November 2014]*

a. Upper GI contrast study
b. USG
c. CT scan
d. Baby gram

86. A patient presents with history of breathlessness, CXR shows right side air fluid level, CP angle is obliterated. What is your diagnosis? *[AIIMS PG November 2015]*

a. Pleural effusion
b. Lung abscess
c. Hydropneumothorax
d. Malignant infiltration

 **NEET/NBE PATTERN MCQs ANSWERS WITH EXPLANATIONS** 

1. **Ans. (a) Aspergilloma**
[Ref. Sumer K Sethi, 5/e p27-28]

Radiology in Aspergillosis of Lung
- *Aspergilloma/Fungal ball*: *'Air-crescent sign'* (crescentic radiolucent lung cavity with air and radio-opaque mass)
- *Invasive aspergillosis*: *'Halo appearance'* (surrounding haemorrhagic inflammation)
- *Allergic bronchopulmonary aspergillosis*: *'Gloved finger appearance'*

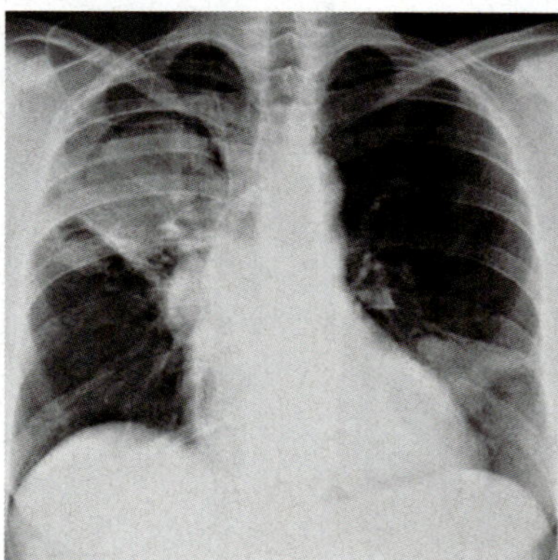

Fig. Air-crescent sign

Also Remember
- *Air crescent sign is shown by*: **[Mnemonic: A Teacher Puts Continuous Efforts]**
  - **A**spergilloma
  - **T**umour in cavity
  - **P**us in cavity
  - **C**lot in cavity
  - **E**chinococcal cyst
- *Pneumococcal pneumonia*: Opacity in basal zone
- *Bronchiectasis*: High-resolution CT (HRCT) is best investigation

Feature	Remark
Signet ring sign	–
Cluster of grapes appearance	Cystic bronchiectasis
String of beads appearance	Varicose bronchiectasis
Tram track sign	Cylindrical bronchiectasis

- *Bronchogenic carcinoma*: *Golden S-sign*

2. **Ans. (c) Heart failure**
[Ref. Sumer K Sethi, 6/e p68]

Causes of Kerley Lines
- Left ventricular failure
- Mitral stenosis
- Pneumoconiosis
- Lymphangitis carcinomatosis
- Others: Interstitial fibrosis, sarcoidosis, alveolar cell carcinoma, lymphoma, lymphatic obstruction, lymphangiectasia

3. **Ans. (d) Interstitial lung disease**
[Ref. David Sutton, 6/e p41]

Uses of Computerised Tomography in Chest
- Mediastinal disease
- Staging lung cancer/malignant lesions
- Small pulmonary metastasis
- Pulmonary fibrosis
- Bronchiectasis
- Interstitial lung disease (High-resolution CT)

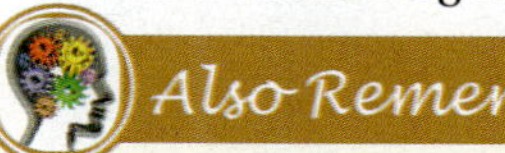

Also Remember
- Lung mass: Chest X-ray (PA view) + CT scan/MRI
- Pleural effusion: Chest X-ray (Lateral decubitus view)
- Lymphadenopathy: MRI

4. **Ans. (b) Lung abscess**
[Ref. Sumer K Sethi, 6/e p63-65]

5. **Ans. (b) X-ray abdomen (supine)**
[Ref. Sumer K Sethi, 6/e p122]

Important Signs of Pneumoperitoneum (Supine Film)
- **Football sign**: Collection of air in center of abdomen over a fluid collection
- **Rigler's sign**: Visualization of both aspects of bowel wall being outlined by air on either side
- Cupola sign: Large amount of gas under diaphragm
- Triangle sign: Air between bowel loop

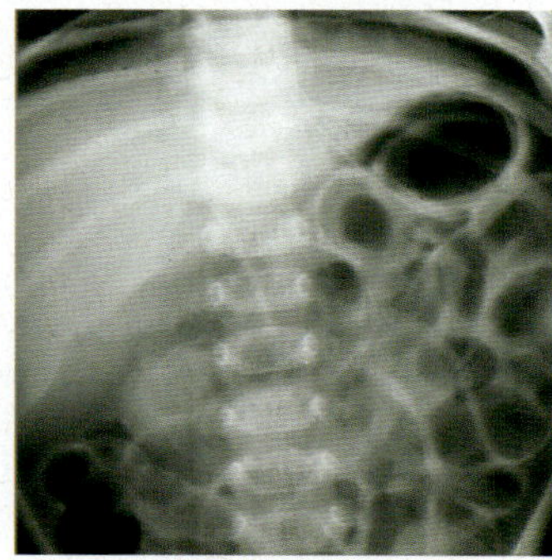

Fig. Rigler's sign

6. **Ans. (c) Hydatid cyst**
[Ref. Sumer K Sethi, 6/e p58]
- Water-lily sign is also known as Camalote sign

7. **Ans. (c) Angiography**
[Ref. David Sutton, 6/e p24; Sumer K Sethi, 5/e p34]

Pulmonary Embolism
- *Chest X-ray*:
  - *Westermark's sign (peripheral oligaemia)*
  - *Knuckle sign*
  - Hampton's hump
  - Melting sign
  - Fleischner's sign

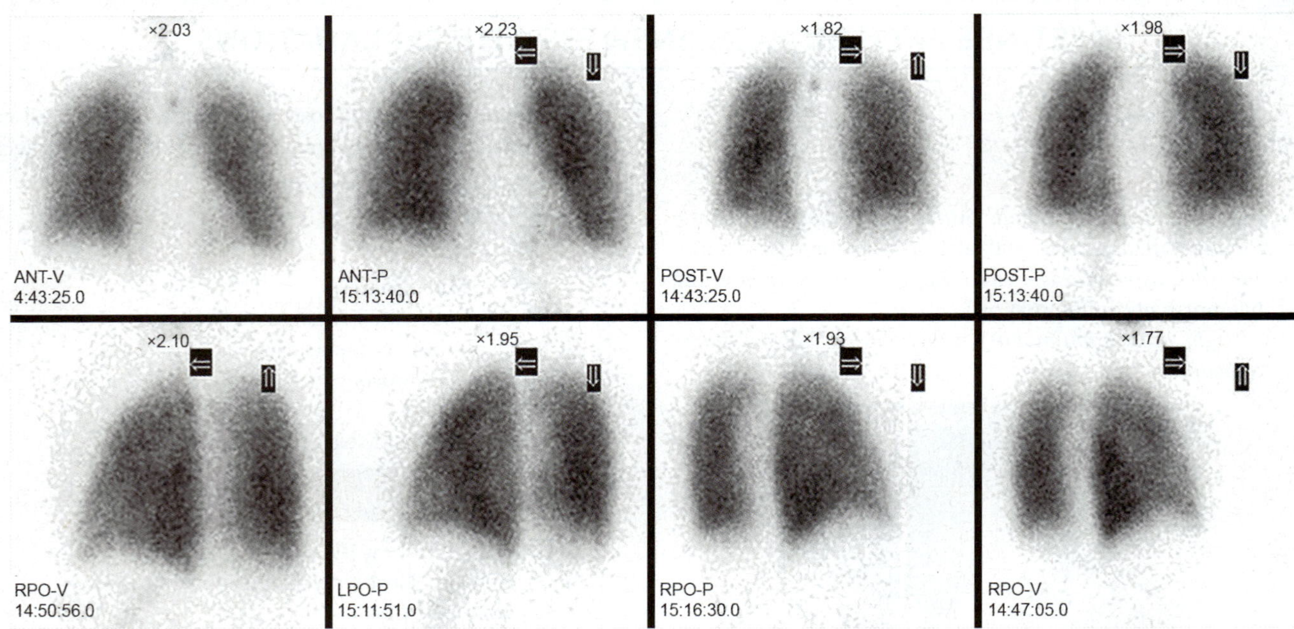

Fig. Ventilation perfusion scan

- *Ventilation perfusion (VP) scan*: VP mismatch (Normal ventilation, Defect in perfusion)

Ventilation agents	Perfusion agents
Xe-133 Kr-81 Technegas	Tc-99

- *Contrast-enhanced CT (CECT)*: Better than VP scan
- *Pulmonary angiography*: Gold-standard test

8. Ans. (d) Tuberculosis

[Ref. Sumer K Sethi, 6/e p56]

9. Ans. (c) Klebsiella

[Ref. Sumer K Sethi, 6/e p57, 65]

- **Bulging fissure**: Klebsiella
- **Miliary shadow**: TB, Sarcoidosis, Pneumoconiosis, Histoplasmosis, Chicken pox, Metastasis, Alveolar microlithiasis, Oil embolism, Hemosiderosis, Histiocytosis X

10. Ans. (b) Hamartoma

[Ref. Sumer K Sethi, 5/e p35]

Radiology in Pulmonary Hamartoma

- *'Popcorn' calcification*
- *Irregular calcification* in lung (Diagnostic feature)

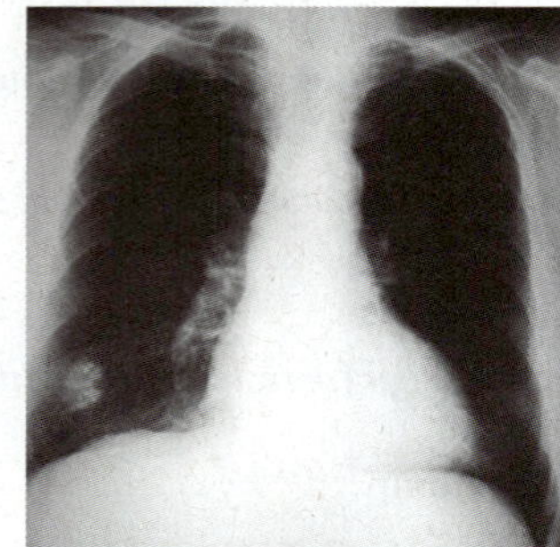

Fig. Pop-corn calcification

Also Remember

- *Miliary tuberculosis*: Pin-point mottling of millet seeds (Fine, uniform, 2–3 mm nodules in lung fields)
- *Choriocarcinoma*: Multiple infiltrates of various shapes in both lungs
- *Coccidioidomycosis*:
  - Parenchymal consolidation (Most common finding in acute form)
  - Pulmonary nodules (Most common in chronic form)
  - 'Grape-skin' thin-walled upper lobe cavities
  - Ill-defined miliary pattern (Disseminated form)

11. Ans. (b) Hydatid cyst

[Ref. Sumer K Sethi, 6/e p58]

12. Ans. (c) Pneumonectomy

[Ref. Excerpta medica Section 15; Chest diseases, Thoracic surgery, and Tuberculosis, Volume 39]

13. Ans. (d) Thickened interlobular septa

[Ref. Sumer K Sethi, 6/e p68]

- Kerley's B line: Transverse thin non branching lines, 1–3 cm long representing thick interlobular septa

14. Ans. (a) Inspiration in erect position

[Ref. Comparison of Inspiratory and Expiratory Chest X-rays for Pneumothoraces, American Journal of Roentgenology, A Seow, 1996]

- *Recommended type of Chest X-ray in Pneumothorax*: Inspiration in erect position (PA view)
- Expiratory film is equally sensitivity BUT creates more false-positive opacities and hinders interpretation of remainder of chest

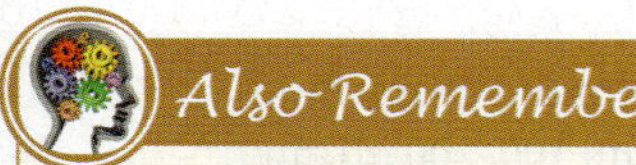

- *Recommended type of chest X-rays*:

Lung part/pathology	Recommended view
Right lung	Left anterior oblique view
Left lung	Right anterior oblique view
Apex of lung	Lordotic view
Minimal pleural effusion	Lateral decubitus view
Middle lobe pathology	Lordotic view

15. Ans. (b) Pulmonary oedema

[Ref. Radiology Review Manual by Dahnert, 6/e p416]

- Perihilar fluffy opacity/haze is sign of acute lung disorder
- Of the given choices, pulmonary oedema is of acute nature.

16. Ans. (a) Histoplasmosis

[Ref. Radiology Review Manual by Dahnert, 6/e p420]

Disseminated Small Nodules (<3 cm) with Calcification

- Granulomatous lung disease
  - Infections: Tuberculosis
  - Fungal disease: Histoplasmosis
  - Silicosis
  - Vasculitis: Wegener granulomatosis
- Neoplasm:
  - Metastatic lung diseases: Thyroid cancer
  - Lymphoma
  - Bronchoalveolar cell carcinoma
- Other diseases:
  - Drug-induced: Methotrexate
  - Non-granulomatous vasculitis
  - Sarcoidosis

17. Ans. (d) Tuberculosis

[Ref. Sumer K Sethi, 6/e p56]

18. Ans. (c) Hydatid disease

[Ref. Sumer K Sethi, 5/e p27]

- *Radiology in Hydatid disease*: CT scan is Investigation of choice
  - *'Floating membrane/Camalote (Water-lily) sign'* in liver
  - Cysts, Hydatid sand, Cystic membranes, Septae

19. Ans. (a) Left anterior oblique

[Ref. Surgery of the Esophagus by Raymond W. Postlethwait, 1/e p144]

20. Ans. (c) Pneumonectomy

[Ref. Sumer K Sethi, 6/e p58]

Hypertranslucent Chest X-rays

- Technical:
  - Rotation
  - Scoliosis
- Soft tissue:
  - Mastectomy
  - Poland syndrome (congenital absence of pectoralis muscle)
  - Poliomyelitis
- Emphysema:
  - Compensatory: Lobar collapse, lobectomy
  - Obstructive: Foreign body, tumour, Macleod's syndrome, congenital lobar emphysema
  - Bullous
- Vascular:
  - Absent/hypoplastic pulmonary artery
  - Obstructed pulmonary artery, e.g. by tumour, embolus
  - Mcleod syndrome/Swyer-James syndrome (Swyer-James-MacLeod syndrome or unilateral hyperlucent lung syndrome is a rare entity associated with postinfectious bronchiolitis obliterans occurring in childhood: It is characterized by hypoplasia and/or agenesis of the pulmonary arteries resulting in pulmonary parenchyma hypoperfusion)
- Pneumothorax

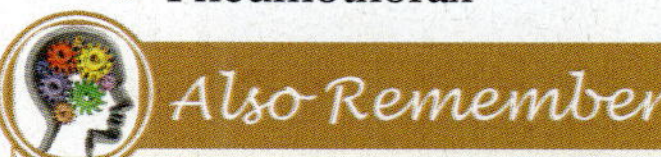

- In pneumothorax, there is hyper-translucency not in pneumonectomy.

21. Ans. (d) Bronchogenic carcinoma

[Ref. Sumer K Sethi, 5/e p34]

- ***Reverse S-sign of Golden*** *is seen in*:
  - Bronchogenic carcinoma
  - Metastatic cancer
  - Enlarged lymph nodes
  - Collapse of right upper lobe of lung

22. Ans. (b) Silicosis

[Ref. Sumer K Sethi, 6/e p64]

Egg-Shell Classification

- Silicosis (hilar nodes)
- Sarcoidosis
- Treated lymphoma

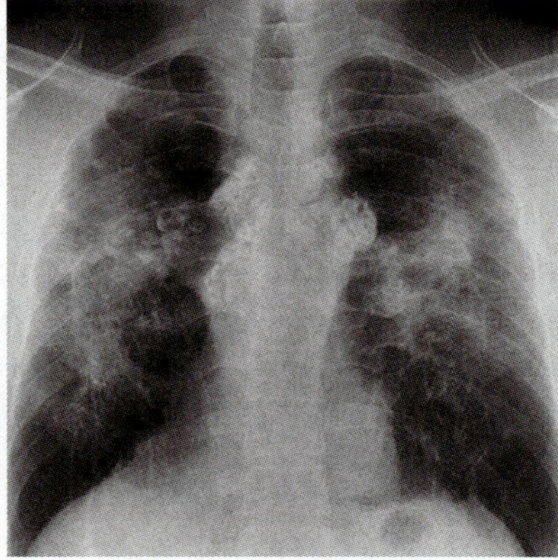

Fig. Egg-shell calcification

23. Ans. (b) Bronchogenic carcinoma

[Ref. Sumer K Sethi, 6/e p70]

- Bronchogenic carcinoma can be identified with Golden S-sign: Presence of a hilar mass with collapse can be identified by the 'Golden S-sign'
- Central mass gives a convexity to the concave displaced fissure (as described by Golden) forming the shape of an 'S'

24. Ans. (a) Pulmonary angiography
[Ref. David Sutton, 6/e p24; Sumer K Sethi, 5/e p34]

25. Ans. (b) Lateral margin
[Ref. David Sutton, 7/e p11]

- It is important to confirm the presence or absence of breast shadows: Breasts may partially obscure the lung bases
- Nipple shadows are variable in position, often asymmetrical, and frequently only one shadow is seen
- Nipple shadows are often well defined laterally and may have a lucent halo
- Care is necessary to avoid misinterpretation as a neoplasm or vice versa

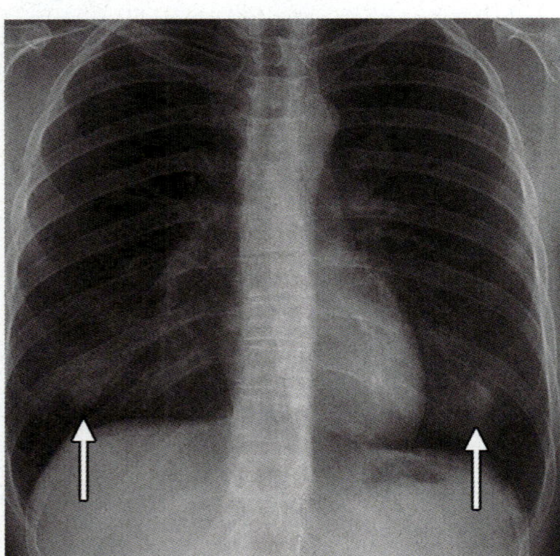

Fig. Nipple shadows

26. Ans. (c) Angiography
[Ref. Sumer K Sethi, 5/e p35-36]

Radiology in Lung Sequestration

- *Angiography (especially Radionuclide Angiography)*: Most useful investigation
- Chest X-ray
- CT scans: 90% accuracy
- USG
- MRI

27. Ans. (b) Bronchocoele
[Ref. David Sutton, 7/e p19]

- **Mucus-filled bronchi also known as bronchoceles,** which are bronchi distended with mucus or pus beyond an obstructing lesion but with aeration of the distal lung from collateral air flow
- Causes: Bronchopulmonary aspergillosis, Malignancy, Benign tumours, Foreign-body aspiration, Bronchial atresia
- Typically the bronchus has a gloved finger branching pattern with the fingers several millimeters wide

28. Ans. (d) USG
[Ref. Sumer K Sethi, 5/e p24]

Radiology in Pleural Effusion

- *Ultrasonography*: Best investigation to detect minimal fluid
- *Chest X-ray*:
  - *Lateral view*: Detects minimum 75 mL fluid
  - *PA view*: Detects minimum 100-200 mL fluid
  - *Lateral decubitus view*: Detects less than 10 mL fluid (Best view)
  - *Lordotic view*: Inter-lobar effusion

29. Ans. (b) Lung abscess
[Ref. Radiology Review Manual by Dahnert, 6/e p414]

HRCT is Useful In

- Interstitial fibrosis
- Miliary tuberculosis
- Industrial lung disease
- Idiopathic pulmonary fibrosis
- Collagen disorders/Connective tissue disease (rheumatoid lung, scleroderma, etc)
- Radiation-induced lung disease
- Diffuse metastatic disease (haematogenous, lymphangitis)
- Sarcoidosis (appearances may be diagnostic)
- Bronchio-alveolar carcinoma
- Mycobacterial infection (tuberculosis, non-tuberculous atypical)
- Hypersensitivity pneumonitides (appearances may be diagnostic)
- Interstitial pneumonitis (appearances may be diagnostic in usual interstitial pneumonitis)
- Histiocytosis X (appearances may be diagnostic)
- Lymphangiomyomatosis (appearances may be diagnostic)
- Cryptogenic organising pneumonia (COP)
- Bronchiolitis obliterans organising pneumonia (BOOP)
- Emphysema (appearances may be diagnostic)
- Bronchiectasis (appearances may be diagnostic)

30. Ans. (b) Angiography
[Ref. David Sutton, 6/e p24; Sumer K Sethi, 5/e p34]

31. Ans. (d) All of the above

32. Ans. (b) Lateral decubitus view
[Ref. Sumer K Sethi, 5/e p24]

33. Ans. (b) CT scan
[Ref. Sumer K Sethi, 5/e p28]

34. Ans. (a) 15 mL
[Ref. Sumer K Sethi, 5/e p24]

35. Ans. (c) Interstitial lung disease
[Ref. Sumer K Sethi, 5/e p29-30]

- *Interstitial lung shadows*:
  - Pneumoconioses
  - Sarcoidosis
  - Drugs
  - Collagen disorders
  - Idiopathic pulmonary fibrosis
- *Investigation of choice for ILD*: High-resolution CT scanning
  - 'Ground glass haze': Active reversible alveolitis

36. Ans. (a) Ultrasound
[Ref. Sumer K Sethi, 5/e p24]

Diagnostic Tests Used for Pleural Effusion

Test	Use(s) in pleural effusion
USG	Detect minimal effusion (Method of choice)
Lateral decubitus chest X-ray	Detect minimal effusion
CT scan	Differentiate pleural & parenchymal disease
Percutaneous pleural biopsy	Detects Granulomatous & malignant pleural disease
Thoracoscopy	Useful if less-invasive tests fail
Bronchoscopy	If features of hemoptysis/ obstruction

37. Ans. (c) High-resolution CT scan

[Ref. Sumer K Sethi, 5/e p30]

38. Ans. (c) Aspergillosis

[Ref. David Sutton, 7/e p18]

Causes of Miliary Shadowing

- Infections:
  - Tuberculosis
  - Coccidioidomycosis
  - Blastomycosis
  - Histoplasmosis
  - Chickenpox
- Dust inhalation:
  - Sarcoidosis
  - Tin
  - Barium
  - Beryllium
  - Silicosis
  - Anthracosis
  - Amyloidosis
- Metastases:
  - Hyaline membrane disease
  - Bronchiolitis obliterans
  - Alveolar microlithiasis
  - Secondary hyperparathyroidism
  - Histiocytosis X
  - Haemosiderosis

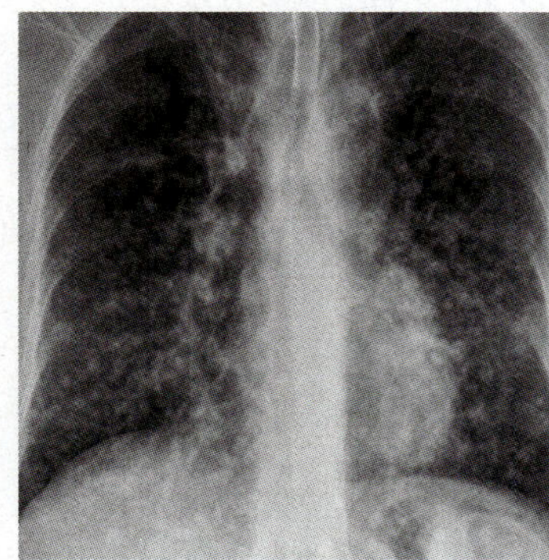

Fig. Miliary shadowing

39. Ans. (b) PA

[Ref. Sumer K Sethi, 6/e p48]

40. Ans. (d) Lordotic

[Ref. David Sutton, 7/e p177]

- In right middle lobe collapse the horizontal fissure and lower half of the oblique fissure move toward one another: Best be seen in lateral projection
- Horizontal fissure tends to be more mobile, and therefore usually shows greater displacement
- Signs of right middle lobe collapse are often subtle on the frontal projection, since the horizontal fissure may not be visible, and increased opacity does not become apparent until collapse is almost complete: Obscuration of the right heart border is often present, may be the only clue in this projection
- Lordotic AP projection brings the displaced fissure into the line of the X-ray beam, and may elegantly demonstrate right middle lobe collapse: Since the volume of this lobe is relatively small, indirect signs of volume loss are rarely present

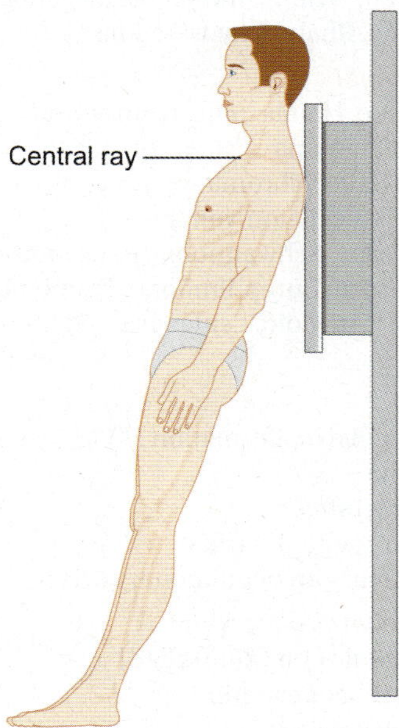

Fig. Lordotic view

41. Ans. (a) CT angiography

[Ref. David Sutton, 7/e p 238]

- An ideal test for PE would provide non-invasive direct visualization of thrombus within pulmonary arteries: CT pulmonary angiography (CTPA) comes close to fulfilling this description

42. Ans. (b) Mycetoma

[Ref. Radiology Review Manual by Dahnert, 6/e p425]

Solitary Pulmonary Nodules Differential Diagnosis

A. Inflammation/Infection

- Infectious
  - Granuloma (Most common lung mass): Sarcoidosis (MC), Tuberculosis, Histoplasmosis, Coccidioidomycosis, Nocardiosis, Cryptococcosis
  - Fluid-filled cavity: Abscess, Hydatid cyst, Bronchiectatic cyst, Bronchocele
  - Mass in preformed cavity: Fungus ball, Mucoid impaction

- Rounded atelectasis
- Inflammatory pseudotumor: Fibroxanthoma, Histiocytoma, Plasma cell granuloma, Sclerosing hemangioma
- Paraffinoma
- Focal organizing pneumonia
- Round pneumonia
- Noninfectious
- Rheumatoid arthritis
- Wegener granulomatosis

B. Malignant Tumors

- Malignant primaries of lung:
  - Bronchogenic carcinoma (2nd most common mass)
  - Primary pulmonary lymphoma
  - Primary sarcoma of lung
  - Plasmacytoma (primary/secondary)
  - Clear cell carcinoma, carcinoid, giant cell c(a)
- Metastases:
  - Adults: Kidney, Colon, Ovary, Testes
  - Children: Wilms tumor, Osteogenic sarcoma, Ewing sarcoma, Rhabdomyosarcoma

C. Benign Tumors

- Lung Tissue: Hamartoma, chondroma
- Fat Tissue: Lipoma
- Fibrous Tissue: Fibroma
- Muscle Tissue: Leiomyoma
- Neural Tissue: Schwannoma, neurofibroma
- Lymph Tissue: Intrapulmonary lymph node
- Deposits: Amyloid, splenosis, extramedullary hematopoiesis

D. Vascular

- Arteriovenous malformation (AVM), Hemangioma
- Hematoma
- Organizing infarct
- Pulmonary venous varix
- Pseudoaneurysm of pulmonary artery

E. Developmental/Congenital

- Bronchogenic cyst (fluid-filled)
- Pulmonary sequestration
- Bronchial atresia

F. Inhalational

- Silicosis
- Allergic aspergillosis

G. Mimicking Densities (20%)

- Pseudotumor:Fluid in fissure
- Mediastinal mass
- Chest wall lesion: Nipple, skin tumor (mole, neurofibroma, lipoma, keloid), rib fracture/osteophyte/osteochondroma, mesothelioma
- External object: ECG lead attachment, Buttons

43. Ans. (a) Intrapulmonary lesion

[Ref. David Sutton, 7/e p177]

- Originally described by I'Ieischner (1941), and named by Fclson (1973), the Air Bronchogram is an important sign showing that an opacity is intrapulmonary
- Bronchus, if air filled but not liquid filled, becomes visible when air is displaced from the surrounding parenchyma
- Frequently the Air Bronchogram is seen as scattered linear translucencies rather than continuous branching structures: Most commonly seen within pneumonic consolidation and pulmonary oedema

44. Ans. (b) Thyroid carcinoma

[Ref. Cardiopulmonary Imaging by Ella A. Kazerooni, 1/e p85]

- Calcified pulmonary metastasis though uncommon but does occur in breast, thyroid (papillary), testicular, ovarian cancers and in mucinous adenocarcinom(a)

45. Ans. (c) Hydatid cyst

[Ref. Sumer K Sethi, 6/e p58]

46. Ans. (c) Bilateral hilar lymphadenopathy with parenchymal infiltrate

[Ref. Sarcoidosis in North Indian population, Indian J Chest Dis Allied Sci. 2012, 54(2):99-104]

Sarcoidosis in Indian Population

- Age/Sex: Majority >40 years of age, Females
- Clinical presentation:
  - MC presenting symptom:Cough
  - Other salient manifestations: Joint symptoms, end inspiratory crepitations at lung bases, cutaneous involvement, digital clubbing
  - Pulmonary function testing: Restriction with impaired diffusion
- Radiology:
  - **MC radiological feature**: Bilaterally symmetrical hilar lymphadenopathy
  - Parenchymal infiltrates
  - Patterns: Reticular, reticulonodular, nodular, miliary, alveolar opacities
  - MC Radiological staging: Stage I disease
- Diagnosis: Transbronchial lung biopsy

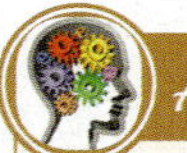

Also Remember

- Sarcoidosis has clinical, radiological and serological manifestations which vary according to race: In countries with high prevalence of TB, like India, sarcoidosis is often misdiagnosed as TB
- Patients having bilateral hilar lymphadenopathy with or without pulmonary infiltrates should be investigated for sarcoidosis.

47. Ans. (c) Bilateral hilar lymphadenopathy

[Ref. Sarcoidosis in North Indian population, Indian J Chest Dis Allied Sci. 2012; 54(2):99-104]

48. Ans. (d) Hamartoma

[Ref. Clinical Infectious Diseases by Richard K. Root, 1/e p539]

49. Ans. (d) All of the above

[Ref. Sarcoidosis in North Indian Population, Indian J Chest Dis Allied Sci. 2012;54(2):99-104]

50. Ans. (d) All of the above

[Ref. Medical Sciences by Jeannette Naish, 1/e p253]

51. Ans. (c) Bronchiectasis

[Ref. Tuberculosis by Madkour, 1/e p373]

- Bronchography was earlier the investigation of choice for the diagnosis of Bronchiectasis
- CT, particularly HRCT, has replaced Bronchography in the diagnosis of bronchiectasis in the recent years

52. Ans. (a) MDCT with VB

[Ref. Pediatric Bronchoscopy by Kostas, 1/e p104]

- Foreign-Body Aspiration: It has been proposed that low-dose MDCT (Multidetector CT scan) with VB (Virtual bronchoscopy) can serve as a first-line non-invasive technique for investigation.

53. Ans. (d) Bat wing sign

[Ref. Thoracic Imaging by Webb, 2/e p37]

Perihilar 'Bat-wing' Consolidation

- Central consolidation with sparing of the lung periphery
- Most typical of pulmonary edema (hydrostatic or permeability)
- Also may be seen with pulmonary hemorrhage, pneumonias (including bacteria and atypical pneumonias such as Pneumocystis jiroveci (*P. carinii*) pneumonia and viral pneumonia), hypoproteinemia, and inhalational lung injury

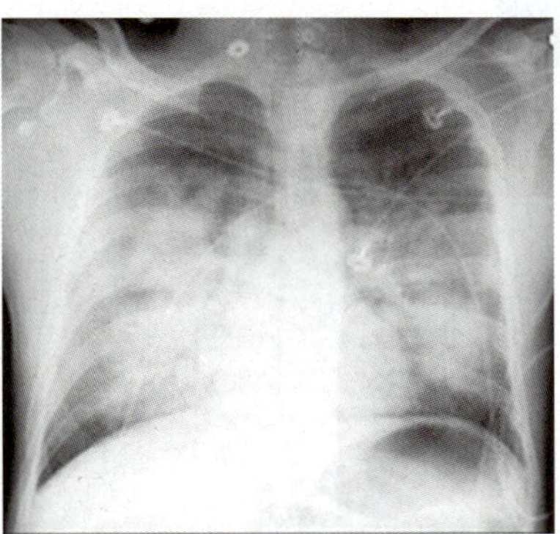

Fig. Bat-wing appearance

54. Ans. (c) Silicosis

[Ref. Radiology of Occupational Chest Disease by Solomon, 1/e p114]

- Calcification of Silicotic nodules may become very widespread and produce a 'Snow storm' effect on X-ray study

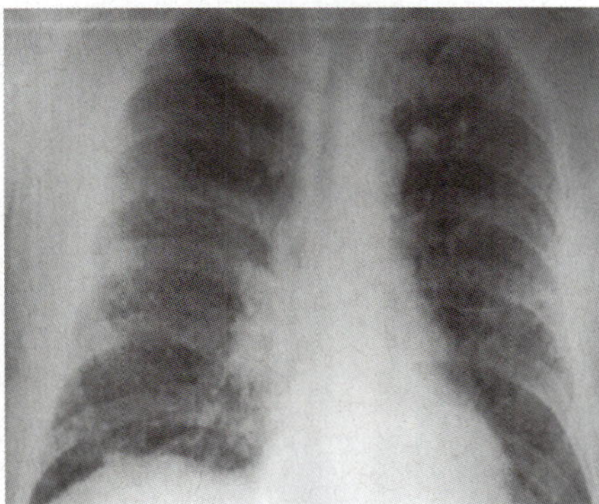

Fig. Snow storm chest X-ray

55. Ans. (a) Pulmonary tuberculosis

[Ref. Multi-Detector CT Imaging by Saba, 1/e p472]

- CT findings of pulmonary TB include tree-in-bud opacities, lung consolidation, septal thickening, bronchial wall thickening, and bronchial distortion
- Central opacities and Tree-in-bud appearance reflect inflammation and necrosis of distal small airways

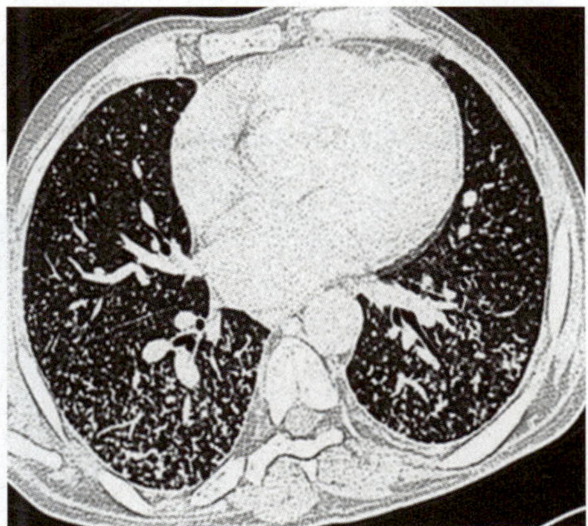

Fig. Tree-in-bud appearance

56. Ans. (d) Panda sign

[Ref. Magnetic Resonance Imaging of the Brain and Spine by Atlas, 4/e p1054]

X-ray in Pulmonary Embolism

- Westermark's sign: Focal peripheral lucency beyond an occluded vessel, often accompanied by mild dilation of the central pulmonary vessels
- Palla sign: An enlarged right descending pulmonary artery
- Felson silhouette sign: Loss of a normal lung-soft-tissue interface (loss of silhouette) caused by any pathologic mechanism that replaces or displaces air within the lung parenchyma

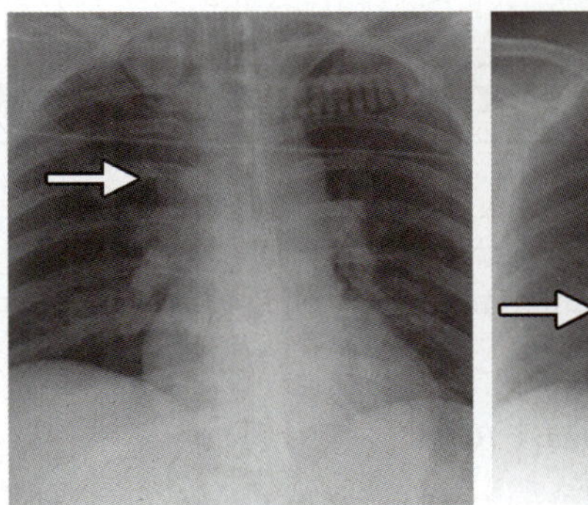

Fig. Westermark's sign

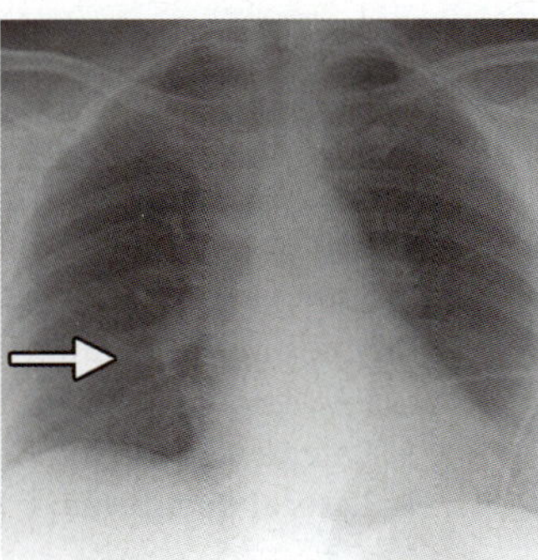

Fig. Palla's sign

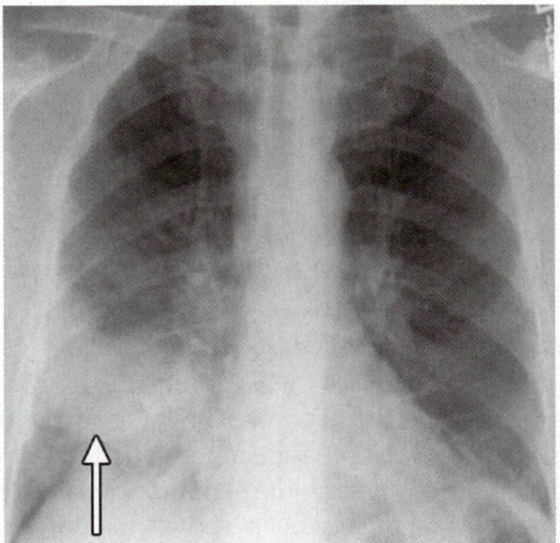

Fig. Felson's sign

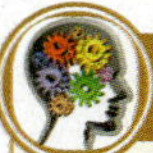

Also Remember

- Panda sign (Raccoon sign, Spectacle haematoma, Black eye): A characteristic panda's face appearance in MRI images of patients suffering from Wilson's Disease

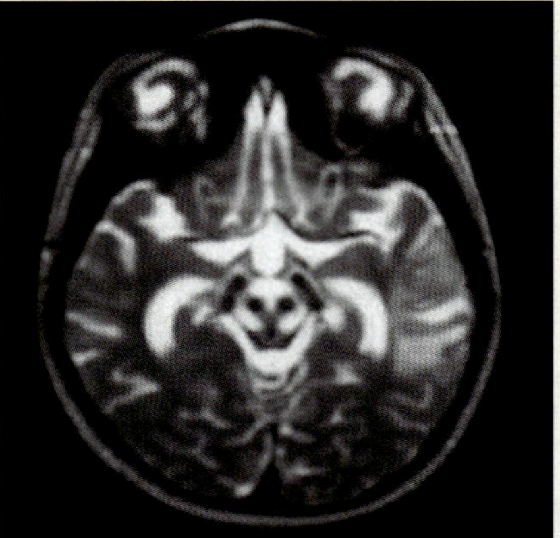

Fig. Panda's sign

HIGH YIELD MCQs ANSWERS WITH EXPLANATIONS

1. **Ans. (d) Lateral decubitus**

   [Ref. Sumer K Sethi, 6/e p49]

   - Pleural effusion: minimum amount required to be detected
     - PA view: 100 mL
     - Lateral view: 75 mL
     - **Lateral decubitus: < 10 mL**

2. **Ans. (a) Pleural effusion (b) Pleural effusion with dependent hemithorax**

   [Ref. Sumer K Sethi, 6/e p49; David Sutton, 7/e p5, 248 585]

   - Decubitus view is important in detecting small pleural fluid, pleural effusion with dependent hemithorax, pneumothorax especially in infant, pneumoperitoneum
   - Right lateral decubitus position best demonstrates leakage from duodenal and lesser curve gastric ulcers.

3. **Ans. (a) Cassette near right shoulder; (c) Arch of aorta best seen; (d) Left atrial enlargement can be diagnosed**

   [Ref. David Sutton, 7/e p284, 573]

   - Aortic arch and left main bronchus are two normal impressions on the left anterolateral aspect of the thoracic oesophagus: Best seen right anterior oblique view
   - A distance between middle of double density and left main bronchus >7 cm has been shown to indicate left atrial enlargement in over 90% of cases

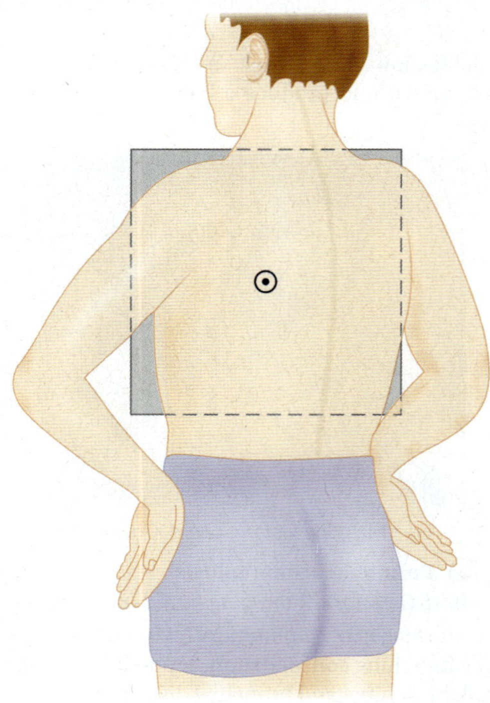

Fig. Right anterior oblique view

4. Ans. (b) Interstitial lung disease
[Ref. Sumer K Sethi, 6/e p63]
- HRCT is the investigation of choice for ILD

5. Ans. (c) Klebsiella
[Ref. Sumer K Sethi, 6/e p57, 65]

6. Ans. (b) Congenital lobar emphysema
[Ref. Textbook of Radiology and Imaging by David Sutton, 7/e p28]

Hyperinflated Image of Lung in CXR

- With conditions such as *Macleod's Syndrome*, congenital lobar emphysema, Inhaled foreign body, an expiratory film will demonstrate obstructive emphysema: There is displacement of the mediastinum away from the affected side with depression of the ipsilateral diaphragm

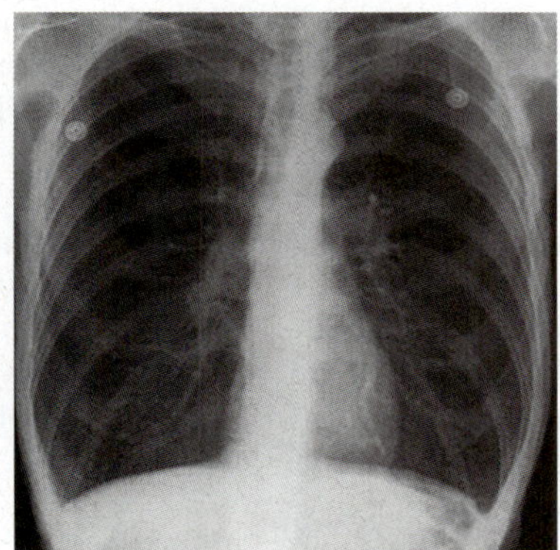

Fig. Hyperinflated lungs

7. Ans. (c) Decreased intercostals space
[Ref. David Sutton, 7/e p27]
- Increased transradiancy may be accompanied by signs of obstructive or compensatory emphysema such as Splaying of the ribs, Separation of the vascular markings, Mediastinal displacement and Depression of the hemidiaphragm

8. Ans. (a) 40% lung tissue seen obscured by bony structure & mediastinum; (c) Right dome is higher than left dome
[Ref. Sumer K Sethi, 6/e p52]
- Right dome is higher than left dome because heart pushes the left dome down.

9. Ans. (d) Posterior part of upper lobe
[Ref. Radiology In Medical Practice by Abdullah, 4/e p8]
- **Silhouette sign**: In CXR, intrathoracic lesion touching the border of either the heart, aorta or diaphragm may obliterate the border, thus helpful in localizing the disease
  - Apicoposterior segment of the left upper lobe lies adjacent to the aortic knuckle: Lesion here obliterates the aortic shadow.
  - Apical segments of the right upper lobe and middle lobe lie against the right aortic border: Lesion here obliterates the right aortic border
  - Obliteration of the diaphragm outline indicates diseases of pleura or of lesion in the lower lobe of the lung: Heart border remains visible
  - Obliteration of the heart border: Shadow lies in the anterior half of the chest

10. Ans. (a) Rheumatoid arthritis (c) Scleroderma (e) Interstitial lung disease
[Ref. Radiology Review Manual by Dahnert, 6/e p419]

Cause of Honey Combing

- Inhalational Disease:
  - Pneumoconioses: Asbestosis, Silicosis, Beryllíosis
- Chemical inhalation:
  - Silo-Filler's disease (nitrogen dioxide)
  - Sulfur dioxide, chlorine, phosgene, cadmium
  - Extrinsic allergic alveolitis
  - Oxygen toxicity: RDS therapy with oxygen
  - Chronic aspiration of mineral oil
- Granulomatous disease:
  - Sarcoidosis
  - Eosinophilic granuloma
- Collagen-vascular disease:
  - Rheumatoid lung
  - Scleroderma
  - Ankylosing spondylitis
  - SLE (rare)
- Iatrogenic:
  - Drug hypersensitivity
  - Radiotherapy
- Idiopathic:
  - Tuberous sclerosis
  - Neurofibromatosis
  - Pulmonary capillary hemangiomatosis

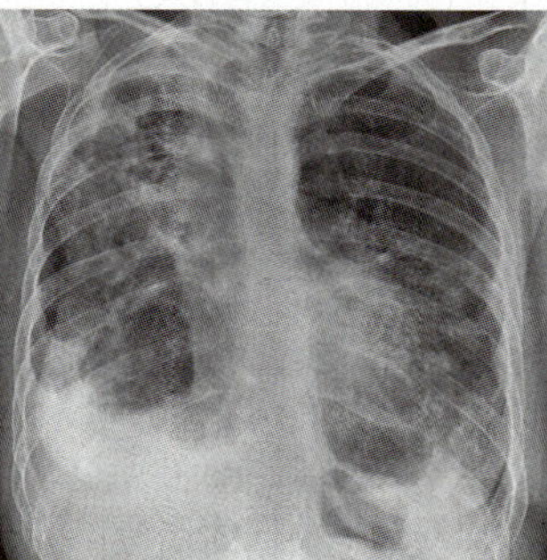

Fig. Honeycomb lungs

11. Ans. (d) Bronchogenic CA
[Ref. Radiology Review Manual by Dahnert, 6/e p446]

Eggshell Calcification of Nodes

- Pneumoconiosis:
  - Silicosis
  - Coal worker's pneumoconiosis
- Sarcoidosis
- Fungal + bacterial infection
  - Tuberculosis
  - Histoplasmosis
  - Coccidioidomycosis
- Fibrosing mediastinitis
- Lymphoma following radiation therapy

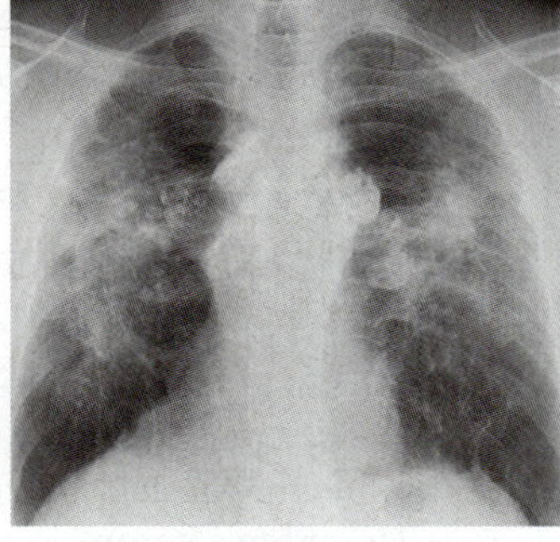

Fig. Egg-shell calcification

12. Ans. (a) Sarcoidosis (b) Silicosis (d) Pneumoconiosis
[Ref. Radiology Review Manual by Dahnert, 6/e p446]

13. Ans. (c) Pleuro-pericardial cyst
[Ref. David Sutton, 7/e p308]

Benign Pericardial/ Spring Water Cyst

- Unilocular and is intimately related to the pericardium: It does communicate with pericardial cavity
- Thin walled, seen in lower half of the mediastinum, and common on right side
- Diagnosis is usually straightforward on the plain radiograph: Cyst is rounded, sharply defined and is usually situated in the anterior cardiophrenic angle

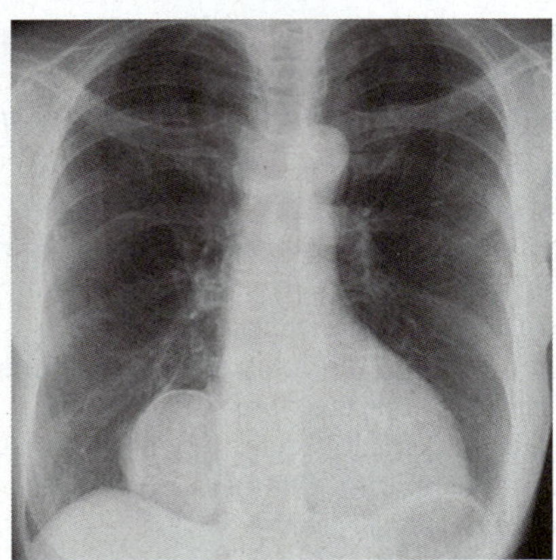

Fig. Pleuro-pericardial cyst

14. Ans. (c) Lower lobe veins
[Ref. Textbook of Radiology and Imaging by David Sutton, 7/e p8]
- Of all the structures in the hilum only the pulmonary arteries and upper lobe veins contribute significantly to the hilar shadows on the plain radiograph
- Normal lymph nodes are not seen
- Air can be identified within the proximal bronchi
- Anterior segment bronchus of the upper lobe is seen as a ring adjacent to the upper hilum and normally there is less than 5 mm of soft tissue lateral to this bronchus: Thickening of the sit tissues suggests the presence of abnormal pathology such as malignancy

15. Ans. (c) Hamartoma
[Ref. Sumer K Sethi, 6/e p65]

16. Ans. (a) Tuberculosis; (b) Rheumatoid Arthritis; (c) Pneumoconiosis; (e) Metastasis
[Ref. David Sutton, 7/e p18]

17. Ans. (a) TB
[Ref. Sumer K Sethi, 6/e p56]

18. Ans. (b) Pulmonary embolism
[Ref. David Sutton, 7/e p315]

Non-Acute Pulmonary Embolic Disease
- Classic triangular or wedge-shaped area of infarct can sometimes be detected but remains rare, this being termed **'Hampton's hump'**
- Often small areas of abnormality develop as linear shadows that are non-specific but often reversible
- Pleurae are invariably involved and often a small amount of pleural fluid will develop: This is sometimes large enough to be detected in the costophrenic angle

19. Ans. (a) Pulmonary angiography
[Ref. David Sutton, 7/e p 238]

20. Ans. NONE
[Ref. Sumer K Sethi, 6/e p56]
- **Gold standard** for diagnosis of pulmonary embolism is CT pulmonary angiography

21. Ans. (c) Metastatic lesion
[Ref. Radiology Review Manual by Dahnert, 6/e p536]

22. Ans. (a) Perfusion segmental defect; (b) Perfusion defect with normal lung scan & radiography
[Ref. Sumer K Sethi, 6/e p69]
- Ventilation/perfusion mismatch: A sign of Pulmonary infarct (Normal ventilation with a defect in perfusion)

23. Ans. (b) Neurogenic tumour
[Ref. Radiology Review Manual by Dahnert, 6/e p442]

Anterior Mediastinal Mass [Mnemonic: 4T's]
- Thymoma
- Teratoma
- Thyroid tumor/goiter
- Terrible lymphoma

24. Ans. NONE
[Ref. David Sutton, 7/e p 163]
- Bronchiectasis is the irreversible dilatation of one or more bronchi, and is usually the result of severe, recurrent or chronic infection: Childhood pneumonias (Pertussis and measles), Tuberculosis
- Other predisposing factors: Chronic sinusitis, bronchial obstruction and abnormalities of the cilia, nitrous and immune system (Kartagener syndrome, Cystic fibrosis and Agammaglobulinaemia)
- Bronchography was until relatively recently the definitive method of diagnosing bronchiectasis but has now been completely superseded by HRCT

25. Ans. (c) Doppler ultrasound
[Ref. Harrison's, 17/e p1653, 2517]

26. Ans. (b) Contrast CT
[Ref. David Sutton, 7/e p 238]

27. Ans. (b) PA view in full expiration
[Ref. David Sutton, 7/e p5]
- Traditionally it has been thought that small pneumothoraxes and interstitial shadowing may be more apparent on the expiratory film
- However, the inspiratory view is now considered to be as accurate as the expiratory view for diagnosing a pneumothorax

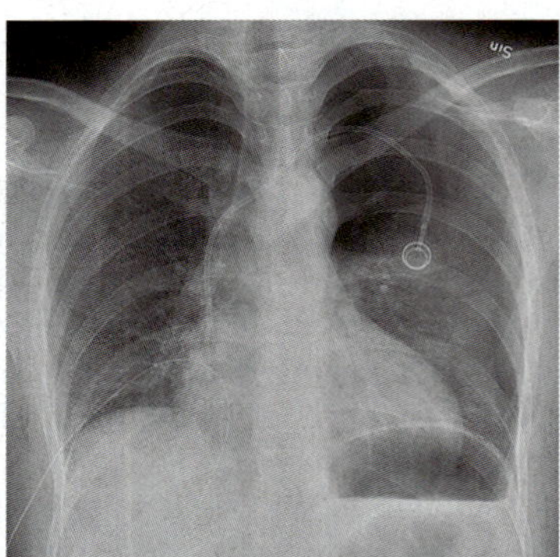

Fig. Pneumothorax

28. Ans. (a) Hydatid disease of lungs
[Ref. Sumer K Sethi, 6/e p58]

29. Ans. (c) Pulmonary hamartoma
[Ref. David Sutton, 7/e p21]

- Carcinomas often have irregular, spiculated or notched margins
- Calcification favours a benign lesion although a carcinoma may arise coincidentally at the site of an old calcified focus
- Popcorn calcification suggests a hamartoma

30. Ans. (c) Ebstein's anomaly

[Ref. David Sutton, 7/e p368-369]

31. Ans. (c) Right lateral decubitus

[Ref. Sumer K Sethi, 6/e p49]

- Lateral decubitus view of the same side is best view to detect minimum pleural effusion

32. Ans. (b) Left lateral decubitus

[Ref. Sumer K Sethi, 6/e p49]

- Lateral decubitus view of the same side is best view to detect minimum pleural effusion.

33. Ans. (b) Reverse lordotic

[Ref. Harrison's, 16/e Ch247]

- Lateral decubitus views are often useful for determining whether pleural abnormalities represent freely flowing fluid, whereas apical lordotic views can often visualize disease at the lung apices better than the standard posteroanterior view

34. Ans. (c) Bone algorithmic for image reconstruction

[Ref. Sumer K Sethi, 6/e p7]

Principle of HRCT

- Thin collimation (Process by which a beam of radiant electromagnetic energy is lined up to minimize divergence or convergence)
- High resolution bone algorithm for image reconstruction
- Small field of view

35. Ans. (b) Runs from hilar area to perihilar area

[Ref. Sumer K Sethi, 6/e p68]

- Kerley B lines: Short horizontally oriented peripheral lines extending + perpendicular to pleura in Costophrenic angles + Retrosternal clear space}

36. Ans. (a) Interstitial oedema (b) Pulmonary venous congestion (d) Mitral stenosis

[Ref. Sumer K Sethi, 6/e p68]

37. Ans. (b) Echinococcus

[Ref. Sumer K Sethi, 6/e p58]

38. Ans. (a) Silicosis; (b) TB; (e) Sarcoidosis

[Ref. Radiology Review Manual by Dahnert, 6/e p446]

39. Ans. (b) Silicosis; (d) Sarcoidosis; (e) Histoplasmosis

[Ref. Radiology Review Manual by Dahnert, 6/e p446]

40. Ans. (a) Silicosis; (b) Sarcoidosis; (e) Tuberculosis

[Ref. Radiology Review Manual by Dahnert, 6/e p446]

41. Ans. (b) Left dome is higher

[Ref. Sumer K Sethi, 6/e p52]

- Right dome is higher than left dome because heart pushes the left dome down

42. Ans. (c) Diameter of the descending right pulmonary artery >16 mm

[Ref. Cardiothoracic Critical Care by David Sidebotham, 1/e p91]

43. Ans. (b) Bronchial artery

[Ref. Synopsis of diseases of the chest by Richard S. Fraser, 2/e p416; Diagnosis and management of hemoptysis. Diagnostic and Interventional Radiology. 2014;20(4):299-309.]

- Bronchial arteries are the principal sources of hemoptysis amenable to treatment
- In cases of severe hemoptysis requiring treatment, the source of bleeding originates from bronchial and pulmonary arteries in 90% and 5% of cases, respectively
- Searching the bronchial arteries origin before treatment is helpful, because over 30% have an abnormal origin that may lead to endovascular treatment failure; Besides 90% of chance is that bleeding will be from bronchial artery, so it should be evaluated first
- In most cases, episodes of hemoptysis related to tuberculosis are mainly related to the systemic bronchial or non-bronchial arteries

44. Ans. (b) Bronchial artery

[Ref. Synopsis of diseases of the chest by Richard S. Fraser, 2/e p416]

45. Ans. (b) Bronchoscopy

[Ref. Synopsis of diseases of the chest by Richard S. Fraser, 2/e p416]

- If CXR is normal, next best step is bronchoscopy

46. Ans. ALL CHOICES

[Ref. Radiology Review Manual by Dahnert, 6/e p425]

47. Ans. (d) Image guided biopsy

[Ref. Radiology Review Manual by Dahnert, 6/e p427]

Solitary Pulmonary Nodule

- First investigation: CXR
- Investigation of choice: CT scan
- Most diagnostic: CT guided transthoracic biopsy

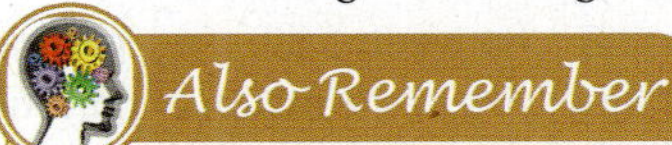

- Image guided biopsy: It is 100% sensitive for malignant lesion and upto 91% sensitive for benign disease.

48. Ans. (a) Rheumatoid arthritis; (b) TB; (e) Pulmonary oedema

[Ref. Radiology recall, 3/e p622]

49. Ans. (a) Histoplasmosis; (b) Sarcoidosis; (c) Secondaries from carcinoma colon

[Ref. Radiology recall, 3/e p622]

50. Ans. (a) Klebsiella pneumonia

[Ref. Textbook of Radiology and Imaging by David Sutton, 7/e p19]

- Bulging fissures indicate lobar expansion which may occur with an acute abscess, infections, large tumours
- Infections: Most commonly Klebsiella (But also *Pneumococcus, Staphylococcus* and tuberculosis)

51. Ans. (d) Staphylococcal pneumonia

[Ref. Radiology recall, 3/e p622]

52. Ans. (c) Expiratory film
[Ref. Sumer K Sethi, 6/e p58]

53. Ans. (d) Pneumonectomy
[Ref. Sumer K Sethi, 6/e p58]

54. Ans. (a) CCF
[Ref. Radiology Review Manual by Dahnert, 6/e p437]

- Congestive heart failure is usually bilateral
- TB and pulmonary infarct are usually unilateral

55. Ans. (a) Pulmonary oedema
[Ref. Replacement of Renal Function by Dialysis by Walter H. Hörl, 5 /e p849]

- Uremic lung is thus a form of pulmonary edema, which can eventually result in fibrotic interstitial changes
- In the early phase the alveoli fibrinous edema fluid and the interlobular septa are very edematous and swollen

56. Ans. (d) Air bronchograms are seen within the opacity
[Ref. Textbook of Radiology and Imaging by David Sutton, 7/e p91]

57. Ans. (d) Right lateral decubitus
[Ref. Sumer K Sethi, 6/e p49]

- Ipsilateral Decubitus view is important in detecting small pleural fluid, pleural effusion with dependent hemithorax

58. Ans. (b) Asbestosis
[Ref. Textbook of Radiology and Imaging by David Sutton, 7/e p194]

- **Diffuse pleural thickening** rarely calcifies and may be associated with short parenchymal lines extending into the adjacent lung: It is unclear if this appearance heralds asbestosis
- CT definition of diffuse pleural thickening, as suggested by Lynch and coworkers (1989), is a continuous sheet of pleural thickening greater than 5 cm by 8 cm and atleast 3 mm thick
- Importance in distinction between diffuse pleural thickening and pleural plaques lies in the fusion of parietal and visceral pleural layers in the former condition, with subsequent impairment in lung function
- By contrast, pleural plaques arc usually isolated discrete lesions that involve the parietal pleura

59. Ans. (b) Oesophageal duplication cyst
[Ref. David Sutton, 7/e p78]

60. Ans. (c) Congenital lobar aplasia of lung
[Ref. Pediatric Chest Imaging by Pilar,3/e p197]

- Congenital lobar aplasia does not produce air-filled spaces on CXR

61. Ans. (c) Congenital diaphragmatic hernia
[Ref. Textbook of Radiology and Imaging by David Sutton, 7/e p254, 255]

- Numerous lucencies in hemithorax are common feature observed in diaphragmatic hernia, other differential diagnosis in the newborn are, such as lobar emphysema, cystic adenomatoid malformations. Sequestration, bronchogenic cysts and other developmental abnormalities of the lung

62. Ans. (d) Foreign body aspiration
[Ref. Essentials of Pediatrics by OP Ghai, 7/e p367-368]

- Sudden onset of respiratory distress with hyperinflation of lung suggest the diagnosis of foreign body aspiration

63. Ans. (d) Foreign body aspiration
[Ref. Pediatrics by O P Ghai, 7/e p367-368]

64. Ans. (c) Congenital diaphragmatic hernia
[Ref. David Sutton, 7/e p254, 255]

65. Ans. (b) Pneumothorax (c) Congenital diaphragmatic hernia
[Ref. David Sutton, 7/e p94, 863]

- A large pneumothorax may lead to complete relaxation and retraction of the hang, with some mediastinal shift toward the normal side, which increases on expiration
- Congenital diaphragmatic hernia: Initial chest radiographs demonstrate an opaque hemithorax or soft tissue mass associated with mediastinal shift
  - **Abdomen is gasless with a scaphoid appearance** on the lateral film and on clinical examination
  - As air is swallowed, multiple lucencies due to air-filled bowel loops can he recognized
  - Tip of the nasogastric tube indicates the position of the stomach; an intrathoracic location is an adverse prognostic factor
  - Ultrasound can confirm the diagnosis, identifying bowel, stomach, liver or kidney within the hernia
  - All patients demonstrate malrotation or malfixation on contrast meal but volvulus is rare.

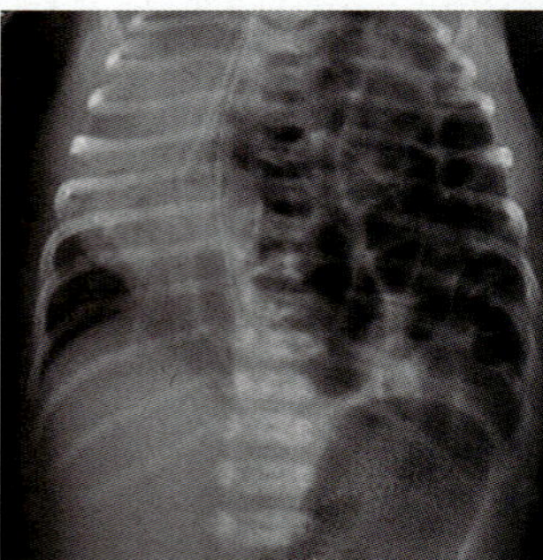

Fig. Congenital diaphragmatic hernia

66. Ans. (d) All of the above

67. Ans. (c) CT scan of chest

68. Ans. (a) Lung ventilation perfusion scan
[Ref. Harrison 17/e p1653-1654]

- Patient has high clinical likelihood of pulmonary embolism. CT contrast is the imaging of choice
- Ventilation perfusion scan could be carried out

69. Ans. (a) Lung ventilation perfusion scan
[Ref. Harrison 17/e p1653-1654]

70. Ans. (b) Tuberculosis
[Ref. David Sutton, 7/e p141]

- **Primary complex**: An area of peripheral consolidation **(Ghon focus)** spreading along draining lymphatics may lead to enlargement of regional lymph nodes
  - Subpleural infection may cause a serous effusion
  - Activation of the immune system usually leads to resolution, healing and fibrosis, dystrophic calcification
  - If the response to infection is weak the disease may progress and there is little difference between lesions

of primary and post-primary evolution: May manifest as further consolidation, possibly with cavitation, and bronchogenic spread of infection
  - Rupture of a cavity into the pleura may cause pneumothorax, pleural effusion or empyema, and erosion into a pulmonary vessel may lead to haematogenous spread
- Consolidation in post-primary infection: Usually appears in the apex of an upper or lower lobe, and almost never in the anterior segments of the upper lobes
  - Patchy and nodular and may be bilateral
  - Fibrosis and volume loss indicate healing
  - Cavities may be single or multiple, large or small and thin or thick walled
  - Fluid levels are sometimes visible within cavities
  - Areas of bronchiectasis and emphysema may develop
  - Healed lesions often calcify
  - Effects of fibrotic contraction are seen as the trachea being pulled away from the midline, elevation of the hila and distortion of the lung parenchyma

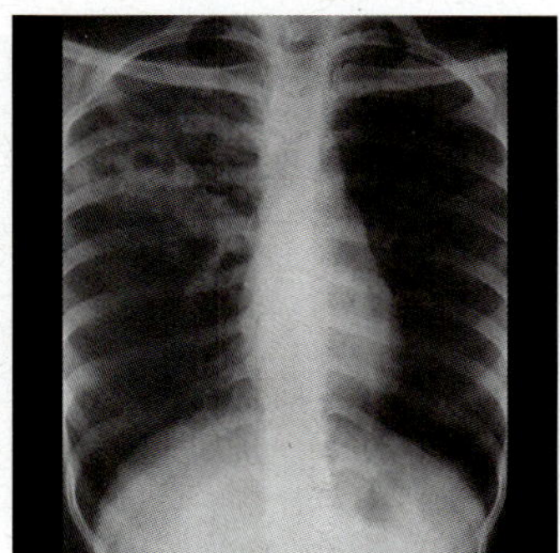

Fig. Ghon focus (right sided)

71. Ans. (d) Pneumocystis carinii

[Ref. David Sutton, 7/e p154, 155]

Pneumocystis Carinii Pneumonia (PCP)

- PCP: Protozoal infection occurs in all groups of immunocompromised patients with reduced cell-mediated immunity
  - AIDS population **(MC opportunistic infection)**
- Radiology: Perihilar and mid and lower zone bilateral interstitial or ground-glass infiltrate
- HRCT scanning: Ground-glass infiltrate extending from the hilar regions into the surrounding lung, occasionally demonstrating a geographical pattern
  - Cavities, usually thin walled, but occasionally with a wall up to several millimetres in thickness
- Complications:
  - Pneumothorax is a well-recognized complication
  - Miliary disease, discrete pulmonary nodules, pleural effusions and mediastinal lymphadenopathy
  - Mediastinal lymph nodes may become calcified and are particularly well seen on CT scanning.

72. Ans. (b) Asbestosis

[Ref. David Sutton, 7/e p192]

- Asbestos exposure may occur in asbestos mining and processing, in construction and demolition work, in shipbuilding and in the manufacture of some textiles
- Living near such workplaces, or with exposed workers, also carries some risk of exposure
- Manifestations of exposure may not become apparent for many years.

73. Ans. (a) Adrenal

[Ref. Radiology Review Manual by Dahnert, 6/e p477]

- Likelihood: Small cell > Adeno > Large cell > Squamous

74. Ans. (d) Shift of trachea on X-ray

[Ref. David Sutton, 7/e p248]

75. Ans. (a) Leukemia

76. Ans. (b) MRI

[Ref. David Sutton, 7/e p82]

- Mediastinal disease can involve the mediastinal great vessels. Vascular abnormalities can be assessed with MRI (without I/V contrast medium)
- MRI has significant advantages over CT: High intrinsic soft-tissue contrast due to the low signal from flowing blood compared with the intermediate signal from the vessel wall and high signal from adjacent fat

77. Ans. (c) High resolution CT

[Ref. Textbook of Radiology and Imaging by David Sutton, 7/e p187]

- There is no doubt that CT and, particularly, high-resolution CT (HRCT) can play a major role in the assessment of patients with chronic diffuse lung disease (CDLD)/ interstitial lung disease.
- HRCT has been shown to have a high sensitivity and specificity, and as a result there has been much recent interest in the role of this imaging technique in the diagnosis and management of many interstitial lung diseases.

78. Ans. (d) CT scan

[Ref. David Sutton, 7/e p162]

79. Ans. (b) Interstitial disease

[Ref. David Sutton, 7/e p187]

80. Ans. (b) CT angiography

[Ref. Sumer K Sethi, 6/e p56]

81. Ans. (d) CT scan

[Ref. Sumer K Sethi, 6/e p56]

82. Ans. (b) CT scan

[Ref. David Sutton, 7/e p162]

83. Ans. (b) Pneumothorax

[Ref. Pediatric Emergency Critical Care and Ultrasound edited by Stephanie J. Doniger, 1/e p79]

- Normal lung will exhibit a "seashore sign," while a pneumothorax will have a characteristic "stratosphere sign" or "barcode sign"

84. Ans. (c) HRCT chest

[Ref. Pediatric Respiratory Medicine by Eber, 1/e p255]

Bronchiectasis

- Before development of HRCT scans, diagnosis was made by Bronchograms using contrast material to map the airways

- Currently HRCT has replaced Bronchography as Gold Standard for diagnosis: Sensitivity of 97%

85. Ans. (a) Upper GI contrast study
[Ref. Pediatric Surgery by Puri, 1/e p197]

86. Ans. (c) Hydropneumothorax
[Ref. Radiology in Medical Practice by Abdullah, 4/e p32]

Hydropneumothorax

- Description: Presence of both air and fluid within pleural space surrounding the lung
- Causes: Iatrogenic, Trauma, Gas forming organisms, Bronchogenic fistula, Oesophageal rupture, Lung abscess fistula, Pulmonary tuberculosis, Erosion by Bronchogenic carcinoma, Thoracocentesis, Empyema
- Bed side test: Succussion splash
- Features on Radiology:
  - Increased translucency with Collapse lung margin
  - Horizontal fluid level
  - Obliteration of both Costophrenic and Cardiophrenic angles

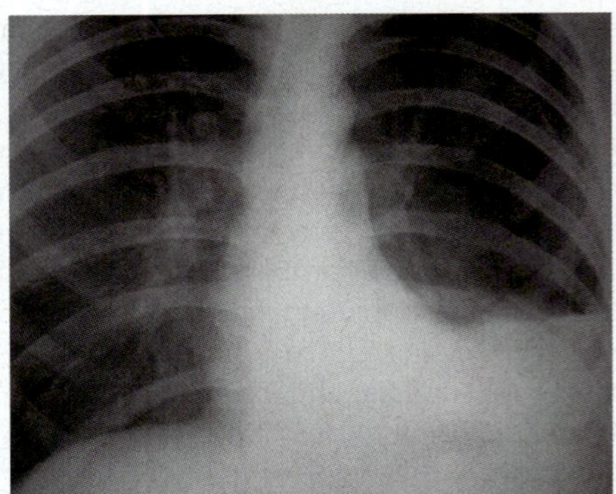

Fig. Hydropneumothorax

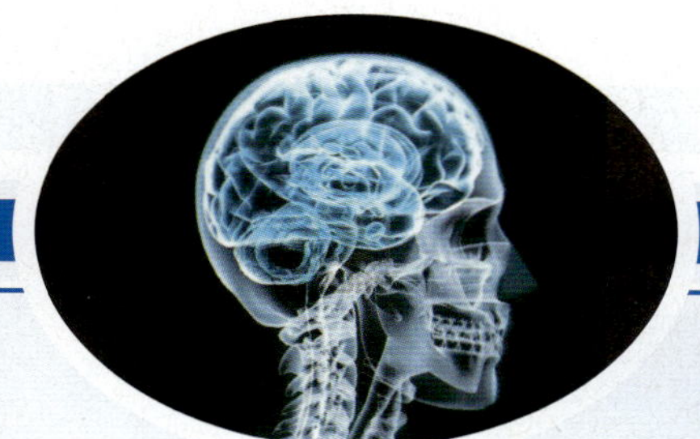

Chapter 5

Skeletal System, Bones and Traumatology

THEORETICAL CONCEPTS

V A. ACHONDROPLASIA

- ***'Champagne glass pelvis'***[Q]
- **Trident hand**[Q]
- Bullet-nose vertebrae
- Lumbar canal stenosis
- Posterior scalloping of vertebrae

Topper's Edge

Achondroplasia

- Congenital genetic disorder resulting in Rhizomelic dwarfism (Proximal limb shortening[Q])
- **MCC of Short limb dwarfism**[Q]
- **MC skeletal dysplasia**[Q]
- Normal intelligence with normal motor function
- SADDAN syndrome[Q]: Severe Achondroplasia with Developmental Delay and Acanthosis Nigricans

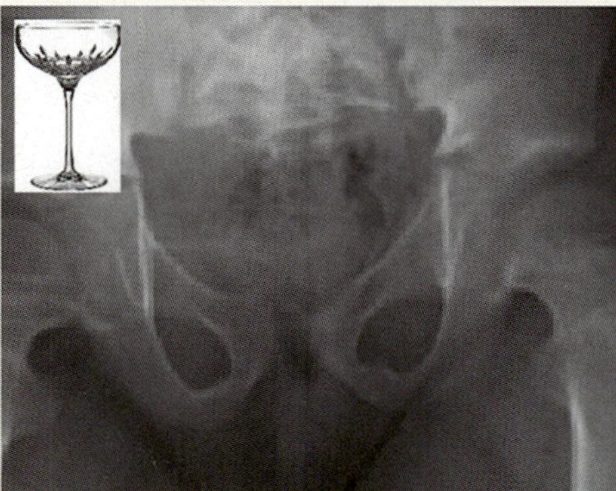

Fig. Champagne-glass pelvis

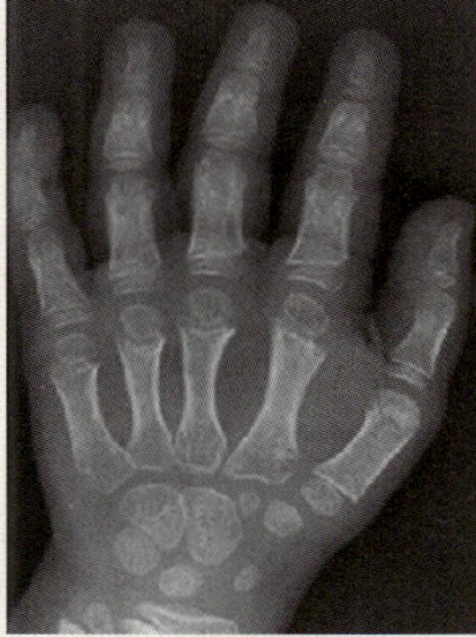

Fig. Trident hand

V B. HEMANGIOMA BONE

- X-rays:
  - *Spoke-wheel pattern/Sun-burst appearance* of calcification [Q]
  - ***Corduroy cloth appearance***: Vertical striations

- CT scan:
  - Polka-dot appearance

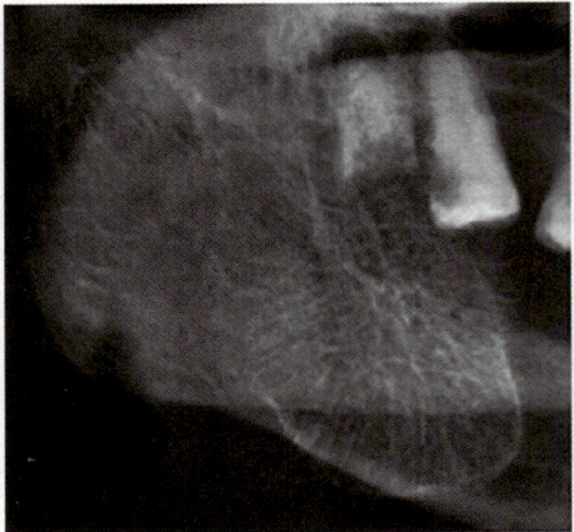
Fig. Sun-burst appearance

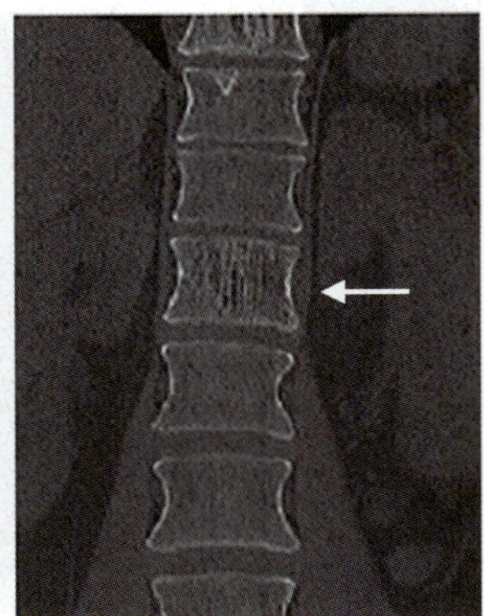
Fig. Corduroy cloth appearance

V C. HYDATID DISEASE

- CT scan is investigation of choice
- *'Floating membrane/Camalote* ***(Water-lily) sign****'* in liver [Q]
- Cysts, hydatid sand, cystic membranes, septae

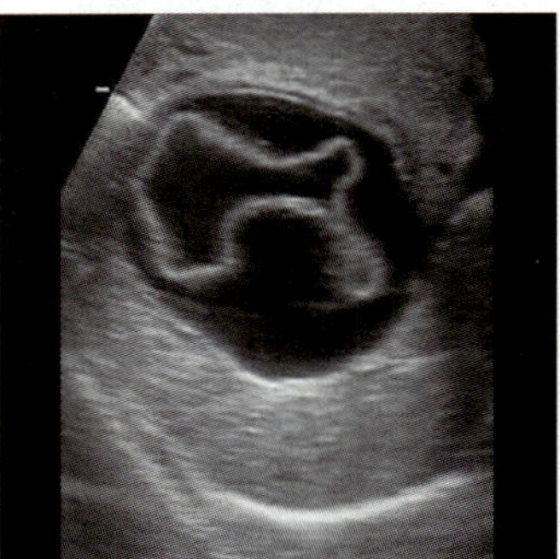
Fig. Water-lily sign

V D. LANGERHANS CELLS HISTIOCYTOSIS

- *Lesions seen*:
  - Lytic lesions in skull
  - 'Floating teeth' appearance of mandible
  - **Vertebra plana**
- *Clinical types*:
- *Eosinophilic granuloma*: *'Hole-in-bone'* (Solitary lytic lesion)
- *Hand-Schuller-Christian disease*: ***'Geographic skull'*** (large lytic skull lesions) [Q]
- *Letterer-Siwe disease*: Multiple, lytic, ***'rain-drop'* pattern lesions in skull** [Q]

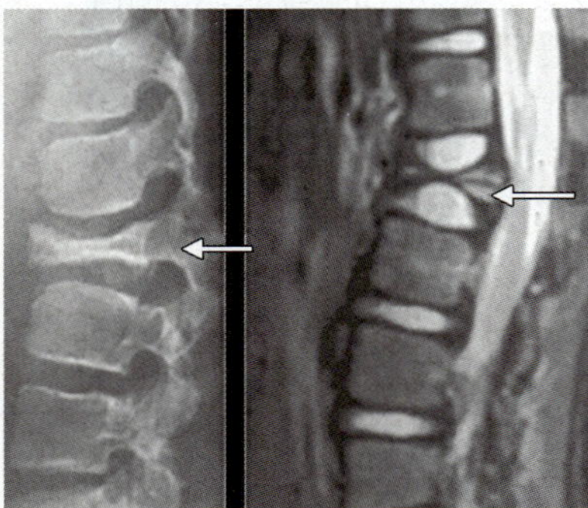
Fig. Vertebra plana

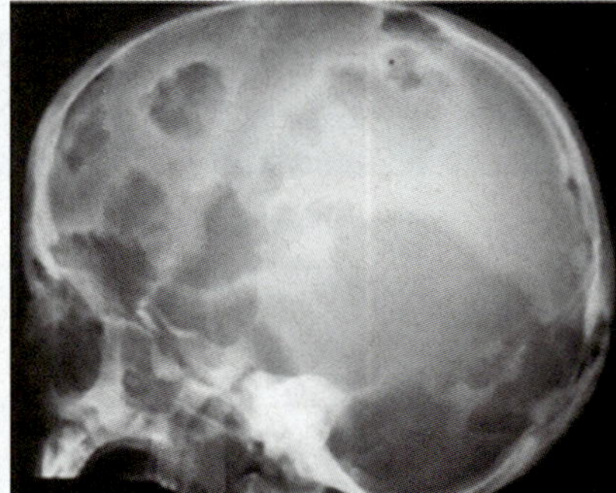
Fig. Geographic skull

V E. MULTIPLE MYELOMA

- ***'Punched-out lesions'* in bones** [Q]
- ***Pepper-pot skull***: Small punched out lesions in skull (Diagnostic feature) [Q]
- *Wedge collapse of vertebrae*
- Rarefaction of bones
- Erosion of ribs-borders

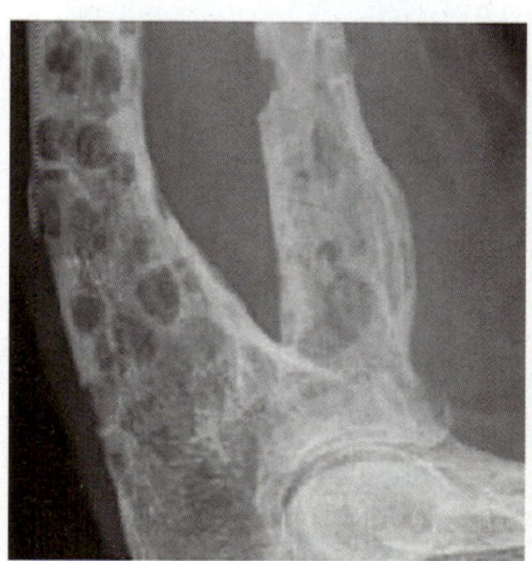

Fig. Punched-out lesions

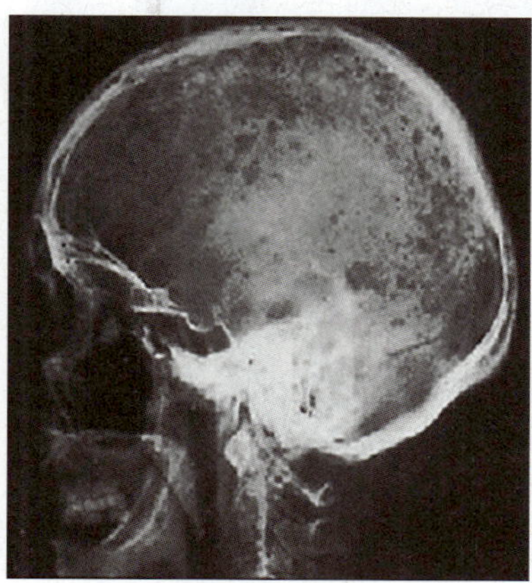

Fig. Pepper-pot skull

V F. NOTCHING OF RIBS

Unilateral Inferior notching	Bilateral Inferior notching	Superior notching
• Subclavian artery operation • Blalock-taussig operation	• Coarctation of aorta • Aortic thrombosis • Subclavian obstruction • SVC/IVC obstruction • Pulmonary AV malformation • Hyperparathyroidism • Neurogenic	• Rheumatoid arthritis • SLE • Scleroderma • Marfans syndrome • Poliomyelitis • Hyperparathyroidism

V G. OSTEOMALACIA

- ***Looser's zones/ Pseudofractures***: Hallmark feature [Q]
- ***Triradiate pelvis*** [Q]
- ***Cod-fish vertebrae***: Biconcave vertebrae [Q]

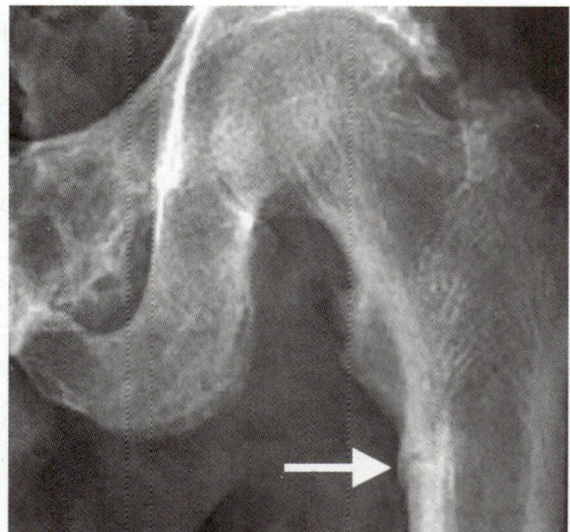

Fig. Looser's zones

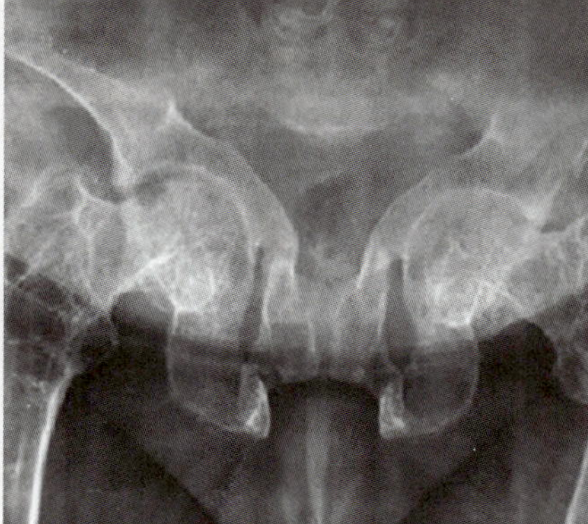

Fig. Triradiate pelvis

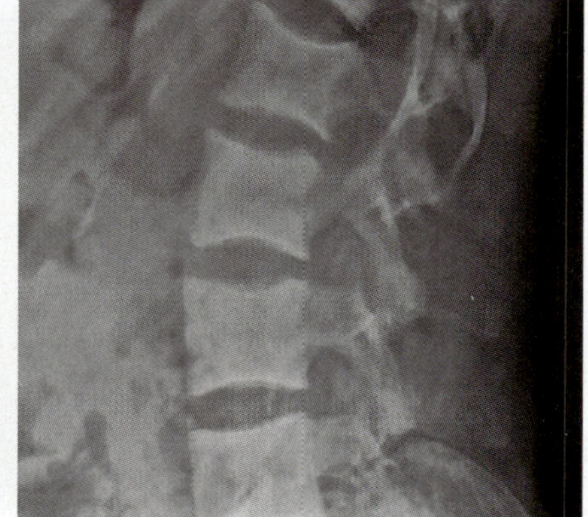

Fig. Cod-fish vertebrae

V H. OSTEOPETROSIS

- ***'Erlenmeyer flask' deformity*** [Q]
- ***Rugger-Jersey spine*** [Q]
- **Bone-within-bone appearance**

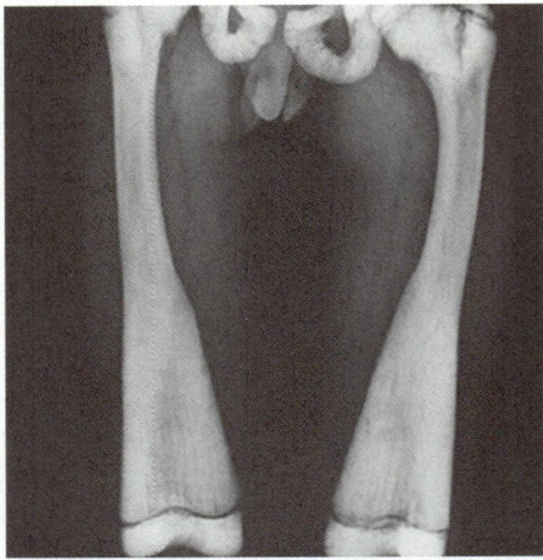

Fig. Erlenmeyer flask deformity

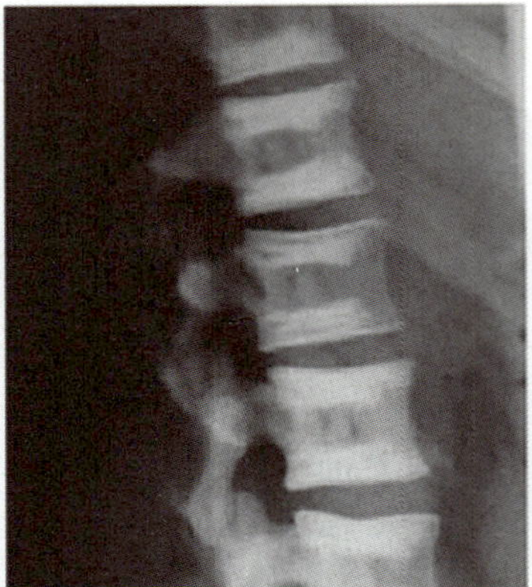

Fig. Rugger-Jersey spine

V I. OSTEOSARCOMA

- ***Sun-ray appearance*** [Q]
- ***Codman's triangle*** [Q]
- Periosteal reaction

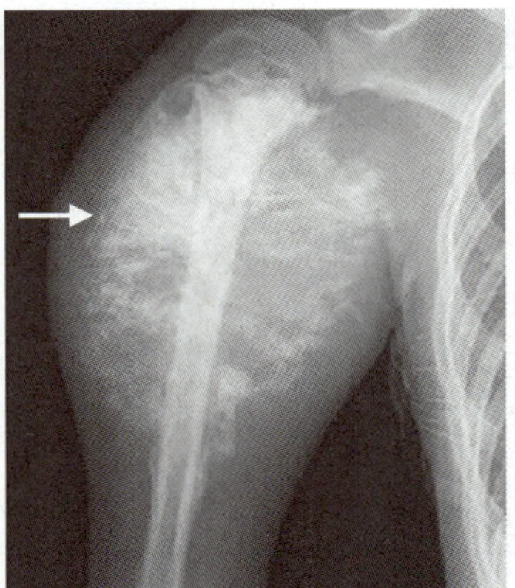

Fig. Sun-ray appearance

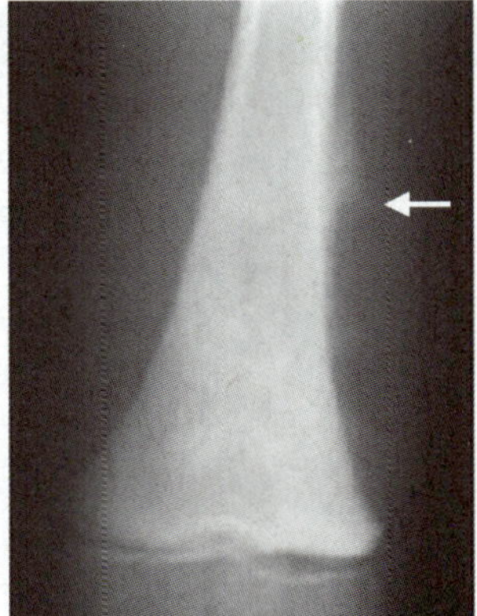

Fig. Codman's triangle

V J. PAGET'S DISEASE

- *'Cotton-wool'* skull [Q]
- Picture-frame vertebrae

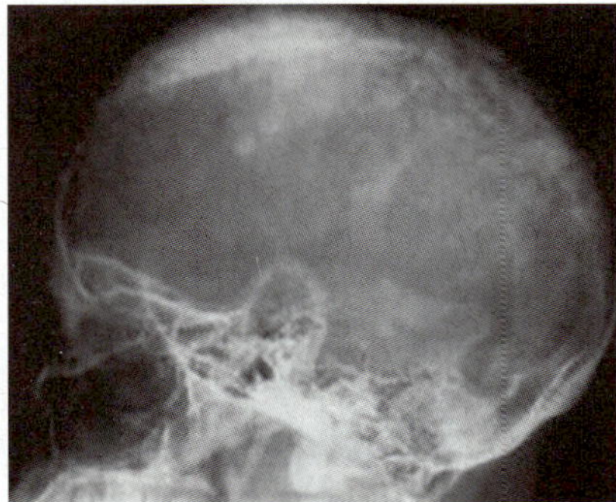

Fig. Cotton-wool skull

V K. RICKETS [MNEMONIC: SACHINCREATED BATTING RECORD IN LAST WORLD CUP] [Q]

- ***S**aucer epiphysis*: Widening of growth plate
- ***C**upping, fraying, splaying* [Q]
- **B**owing of legs [Q]
- **R**ickety rosary
- **L**oss of provisional zone of calcification (Earliest sign) [Q]
- **W**hite line of healing
- **C**raniotabes

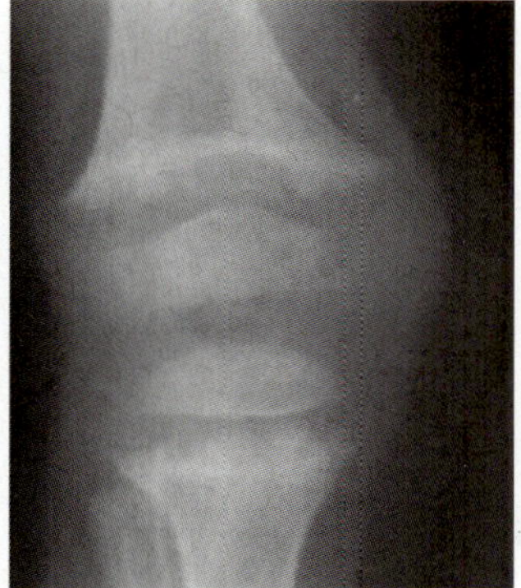
Fig. Cupping, fraying, splaying

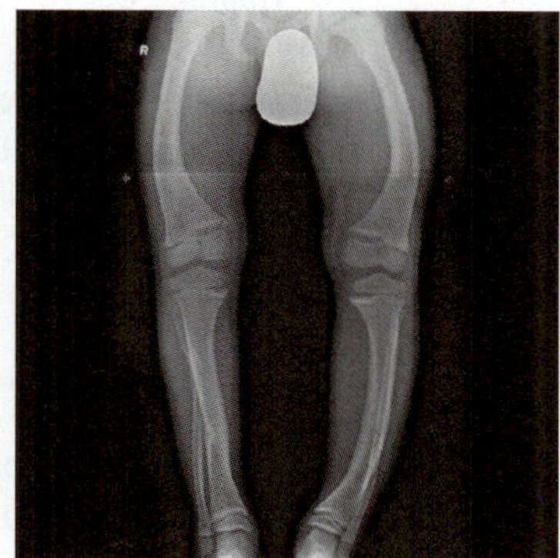
Fig. Bowing of legs

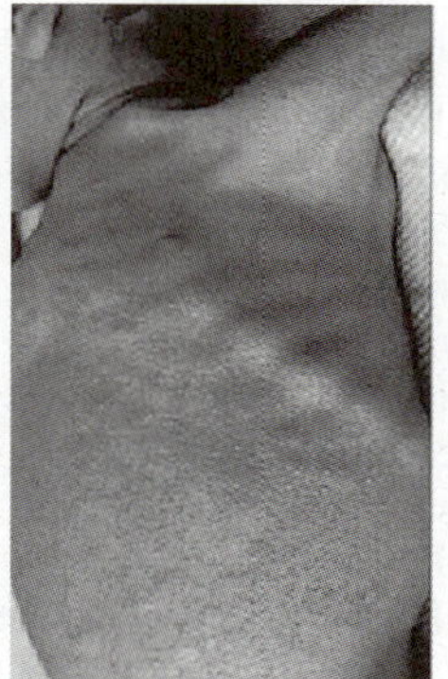
Fig. Rickety rosary

V L. SCURVY (VITAMIN C DEFICIENCY)[MNEMONIC: POST WAR GREAT PLANES FLY] [Q]

- ***P**elkan spur* [Q]
- **O**steoporosis
- **S**ubperiosteal haemorrhages [Q]
- ***T**rummerfeld zone* [Q]
- ***W**imberger's sign*: Sclerotic rim around epiphysis [Q]
- **G**round-glass appearance of bones [Q]
- **P**encil-thin cortex [Q]
- ***F**rankel's (White) line* [Q]

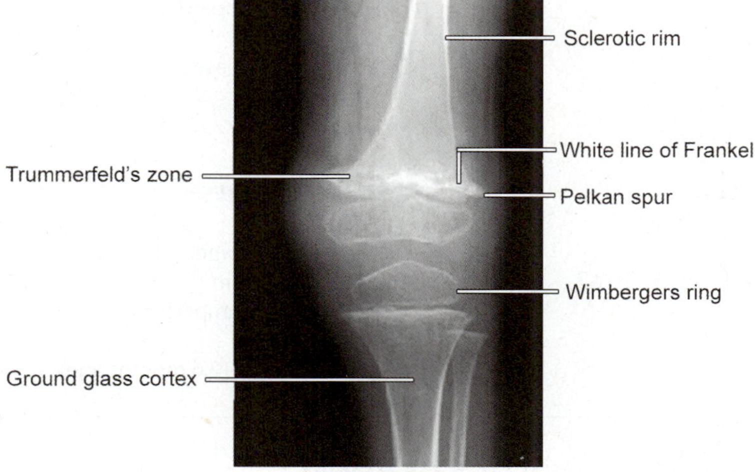

Fig. Scurvy

V M. SECONDARIES

- Hypoechoic (most cancers as primary source), Isoechoic or Hyperechoic (Colon cancer, Ovarian cancer) well-defined, multiple, oval lesions

V N. DIFFERENTIAL DIAGNOSIS IN ORTHOPEDICS

INTERVERTEBRAL DISC CALCIFICATION[Q]	VERTEBRA PLANA[Q]
• Idiopathic • Alkaptonuria • Ankylosing spondylitis • Gout • Pseudogout • Hemochromatosis • Juvenile idiopathic arthritis • Degenerative spondylosis	• **M**etastasis • **M**elanoma • **E**osinophilic granuloma • **L**ymphomas • **T**umours • **T**uberculosis • **T**rauma [Mnemonic: MELT]
POSTERIOR SCALLOPING OF VERTEBRA	**BONE-WITHIN-BONE APPEARANCE[Q]**
• **N**eurofibromatosis • **A**chondroplasia • **S**yringomyelia • **M**arfan's syndrome • **A**cromegaly • **C**ommunicating hydrocephalus • **M**ucopolysaccharidosis • **S**pinal cord tumors **[Mnemonic: NASA C**an **M**onitor **M**eteor **S**hower]	• **H**ypervitaminosis D • **S**arcoidosis/ **S**yphilis (Congenital) • **T**horostat • **O**steopetrosis • **P**aget's disease • **S**ickle cell anaemia • **G**aucher's disease • **H**eavy metal poisoning **[Mnemonic: H**ealing **STOPS G**ut **H**aemorrhage]
LOOSER'S ZONES/MILKMAN FRACTURE[Q]	**WINDSWEPT DEFORMITY**
• Osteomalacia[Q] • Paget's disease • Renal osteodystrophy • Hyperparathyroidism • Osteogenesis imperfecta • Neurofibromatosis • Vitamin D deficiency	• Rheumatoid arthritis • SLE • Rickets[Q] • Osteochondromatosis • Epiphyseal dysplasia • Jaccoud's arthropathy
INCREASED BONE DENSITY (GENERALIZED)	**ACRO-OSTEOLYSIS[Q]**
• Fluorosis[Q] • Renal osteodystrophy[Q] • Myosclerosis[Q] • Caffey's disease[Q] • Hypoparathyroidism[Q] • Hyperparathyroidism[Q] • Osteopetrosis[Q] • Hypercalcemia • Lead poisoning • Gaucher's disease • Hyperphosphatasia	• Hyperparathyroidism[Q] • Scleroderma • Psoriasis • Rheumatoid arthritis • Epidermolysis bullosa • Diabetic neuropathy • Syringomyelia • Raynaud's disease • Trauma • Thermal injury
HAIR-ON-END/CREW-CUT SKULL[Q]	**WORMIAN BONES[Q]**
• Thalassemia major (MCC) [Q] • G6PD deficiency • Severe iron deficiency anemia • Hemangioma • Sickle cell anemia • Hereditary spherocytosis • Cyanotic heart disease	• Idiopathic • Down's syndrome • Hypothyroidism • Osteogenesis imperfecta • Rickets • Normal infant (0-6 months age) • Progeria

V O. FEW IMPORTANT SIGNS IN RADIOLOGY OF BONES

- **Bamboo spine**[Q]: Ankylosing spondylitis
- Beheaded Scottish terrier dog sign[Q]: Spondylolisthesis
- Calvarial thickening[Q]: Hypoparathyroidism
- **Celery-stalk appearance of long bones**[Q]: Congenital syphilis, Congenital rubella (MCC), Congenital cytomegalovirus
- **Champagne glass pelvic inlet** [Q]: Achondroplasia

- Chondrocalcinosis[Q]: Pseudogout
- **Codman's triangle**[Q]: Osteosarcoma
- Cotton-wool appearance[Q]: Paget's disease of bone (Skull)
- **Cupping, Splaying, Fraying of metaphysis**[Q]: Rickets
- Driven snow appearance[Q]: Pindborg tumor
- **Geographic skull**[Q]: Langerhans cell histiocytosis (Eosinophilic granuloma)
- Hinged/ Fallen fragment sign[Q]: Simple (Unicameral) bone cyst
- Inverted Napoleon's Hat sign[Q]: Spondylolisthesis
- Loss of Lamina dura[Q]: Hyperparathyroidism
- Molten wax appearance[Q]: Melorheostosis
- **Onion-peel appearance**[Q]: Ewing's sarcoma of bone
- Patellar squaring, Widened elbow/knee trochlear[Q]: Hemophilic arthropathy
- **Pepper pot skull**[Q]: Hyperparathyroidism
- **Polka dot sign (CT scan)**: Vertebral hemangioma
- **Punched-out osteolytic lesions**[Q]: Multiple myeloma
- **Scottish Terrier dog sign**[Q]: Spondylolysis
- **Sun-ray/Sunburst appearance**[Q]: Osteosarcoma
- **Tram-track appearance**[Q]: Sturge-Weber syndrome (Skull)
- **Trident hand**[Q]: Achondroplasia
- **White line of Frankel**: Scurvy, lead poisoning, phosphorus poisoning
- **Wormian bones**:[Q] Down's syndrome, osteogenesis imperfecta, cretinism, cleidocranial dysplasia
- **White line of Frankel**, Wimberger sign, Pelkan spur[Q]: Scurvy
- **Windswept deformity**[Q]: Rheumatoid arthritis

IMAGE-BASED QUESTIONS

1. **Identify the fracture shown in the X-ray photograph** ***[Recent Question 2016]***

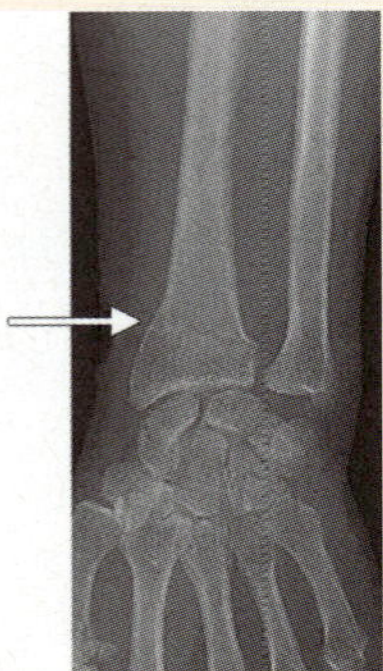

a. Barton's fracture
b. Colles' fracture
c. Smith's fracture
d. Bennett's fracture

2. **Identify the bony disorder as sown in X-ray photograph** ***[Recent Question 2016]***

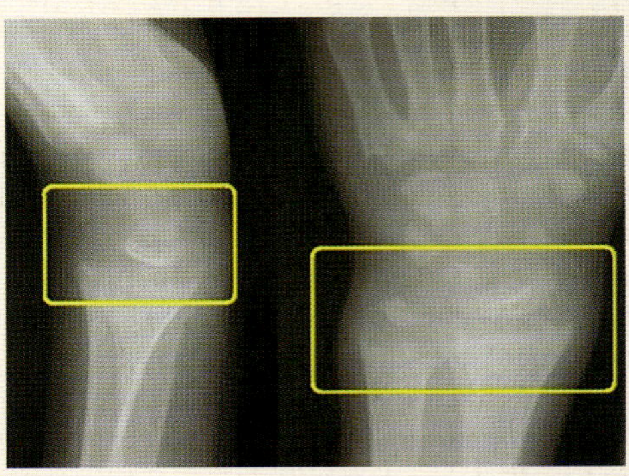

a. Scaphoid fracture
b. Osteoporosis
c. Colles' fracture
d. Rickets

3. **Diagnose the underlying disorder shown in X-ray photograph** ***[Recent Question 2016]***

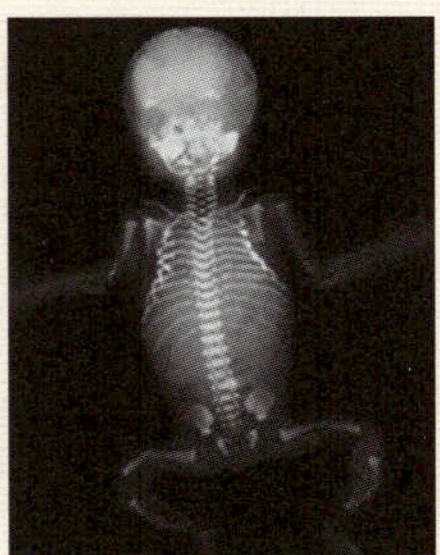

a. Battered baby syndrome
b. Osteogenesis imperfecta
c. Hypoparathyroidism
d. Juvenile osteoporosis

4. **Identify the disorder of vertebra shown in MRI photograph** ***[Recent Question 2016]***

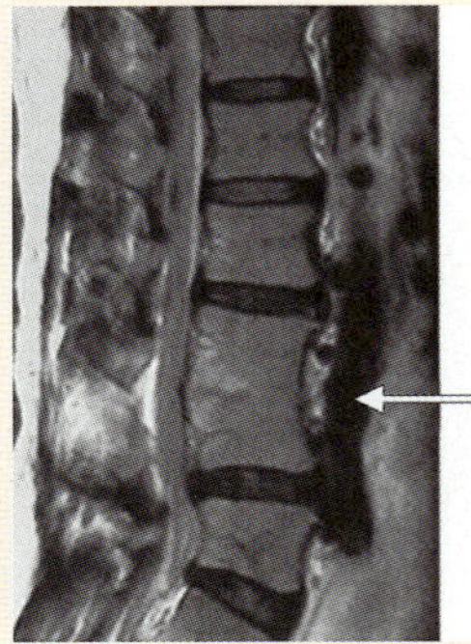

a. Hemi vertebra
b. Block vertebra
c. Butterfly vertebra
d. None of the above

5. **Diagnose underlying bone disorder shown in X-ray photograph** ***[AIIMS November 2016]***

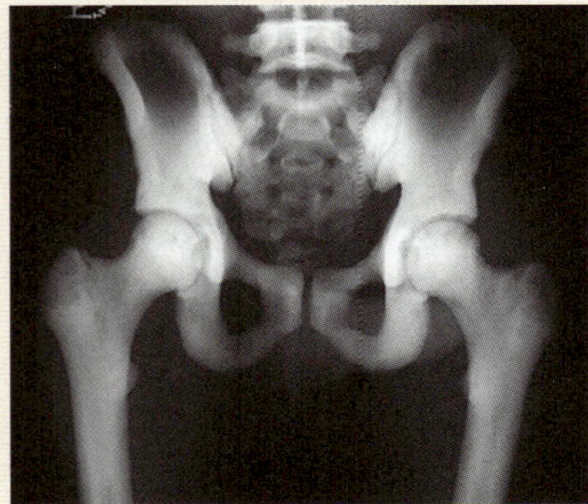

a. Osteoporosis
b. Osteopoikilosis
c. Osteopetrosis
d. Hyperparathyroidism

6. **Choose the FALSE statement regarding the photograph depicted here** ***[Recent Question 2016]***

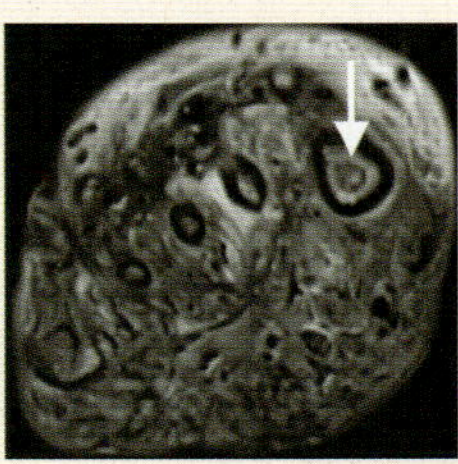

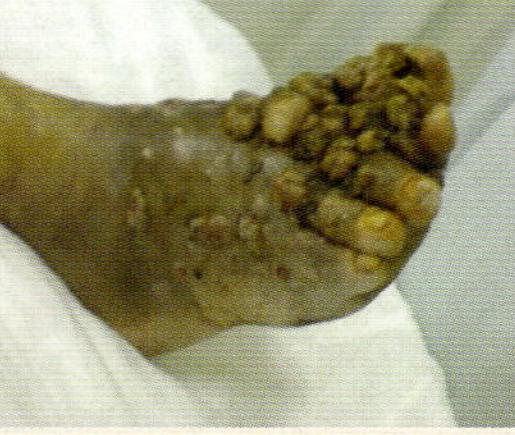

a. MRI shows typical dot-in-circle sign
b. X-ray shows Sun-ray appearance and Codman's triangle
c. Classical triad of symptoms is painful swelling, sinuses and bleeding on touch
d. This is an image of madura foot

7. Diagnose disorder by sign (arrows) shown in photograph ***[Recent Question 2012]***

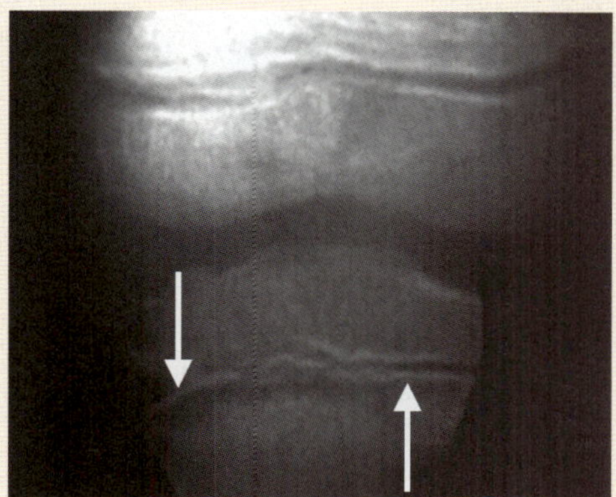

a. Rickets
b. Osteomalacia
c. Scurvy
d. Osteoporosis

8. Condition (arrow) shown in photograph is ***[Recent Question 2012, Recent Question 2013]***

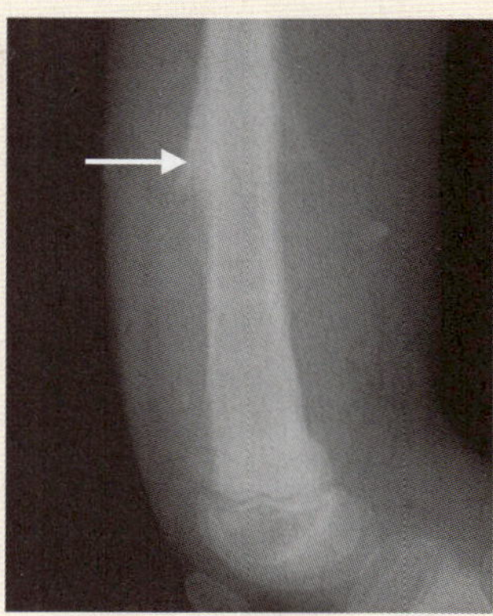

a. Chondroblastoma
b. Chondrosarcoma
c. Osteosarcoma
d. Giant cell tumour

9. Appearance of femur shown in photograph is seen in

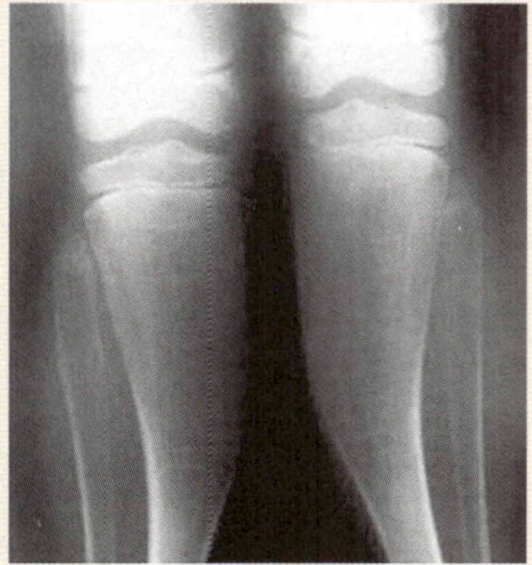

a. Osteomalacia
b. Osteosarcoma
c. Ankylosing spondylitis
d. Osteopetrosis

10. Reaction (arrow) in photograph is characteristic of ***[Recent Question 2014]***

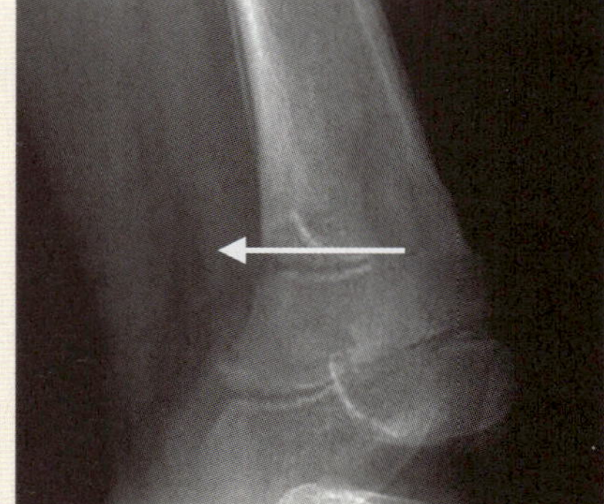

a. Osteosarcoma
b. Ewing's sarcoma
c. Osteoma
d. Osteoclastoma

11. Appearance of vertebrae (photograph) is seen in

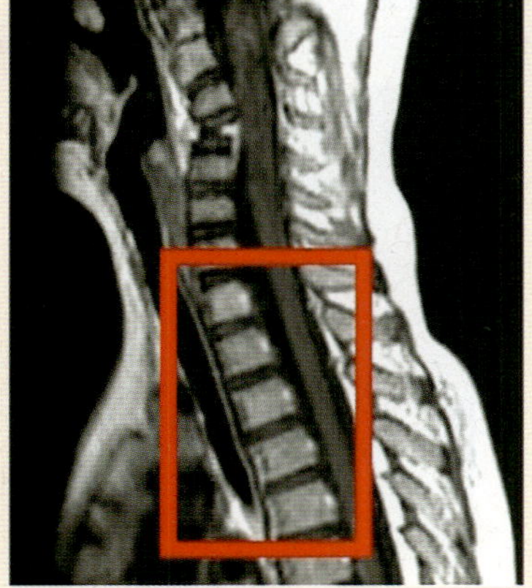

a. Tuberculosis
b. Multiple myeloma
c. Osteogenesis imperfecta
d. All of the above

12. Disorder characterized by zones (arrow) shown in photograph ***[Recent Question 2014]***

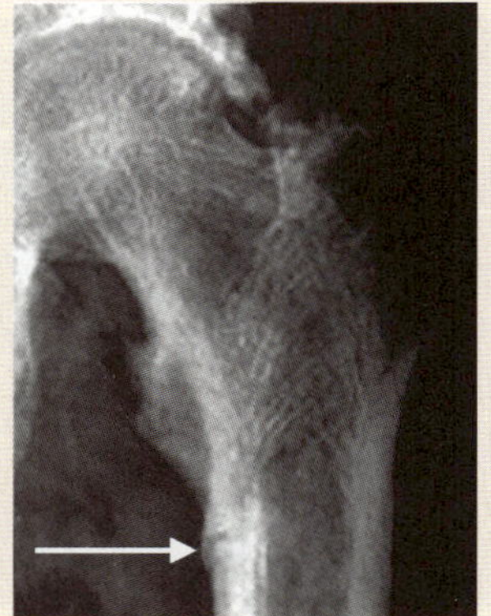

a. Osteoporosis
b. Osteomalacia
c. Osteopetrosis
d. Scurvy

13. Typical spine appearance (arrows) in photograph is characteristic of

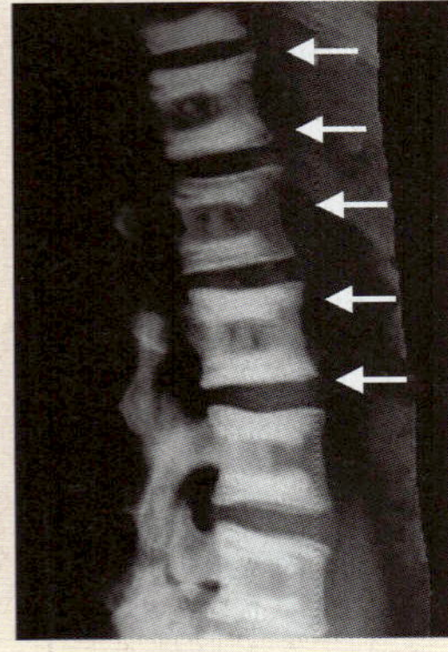

a. Tuberculosis of spine
b. Osteomalacia
c. Rickets
d. Renal osteodystrophy

14. Appearance (arrows) shown in photograph is seen in ***[Recent Question 2014]***

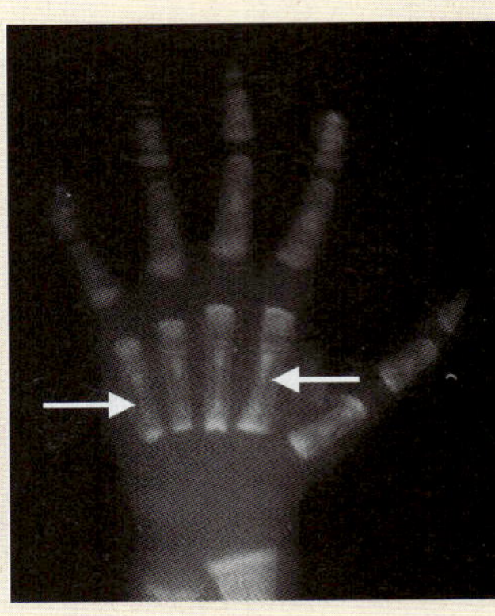

a. Osteoporosis
b. Osteopetrosis
c. CML
d. Bone infarct

15. Typical phalangeal appearance (arrows) in photograph is characteristic of

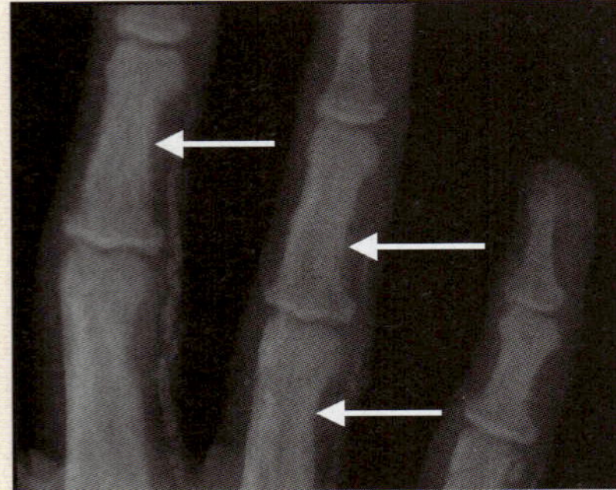

a. Hypothyroidism
b. Hyperthyroidism
c. Hypoparathyroidism
d. Hyperparathyroidism

16. Typical appearance of pelvis (box) shown in photograph indicate

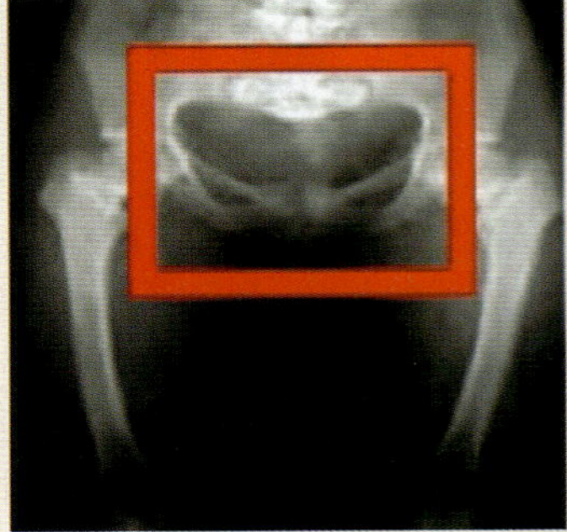

a. Marfan's syndrome
b. Klippel-Feil syndrome
c. Achondroplasia
d. Rickets

17. Appearance (arrows) shown in photograph is mainly characteristic of ***[Recent Question 2012]***

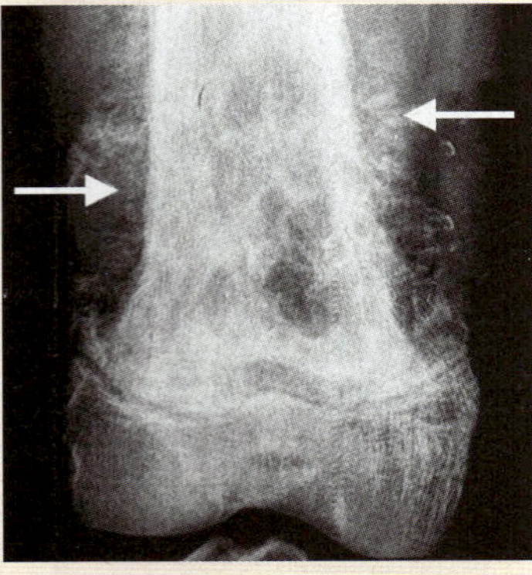

a. Osteogenic sarcoma
b. Ewing's sarcoma
c. Metastasis
d. Chondrosarcoma

18. A patient presented with neck pain and rigidity which gets relieved after bathing in hot water and also after exercises. Cervical X-ray is shown below. What is your diagnosis? ***[AIIMS PG November 2015]***

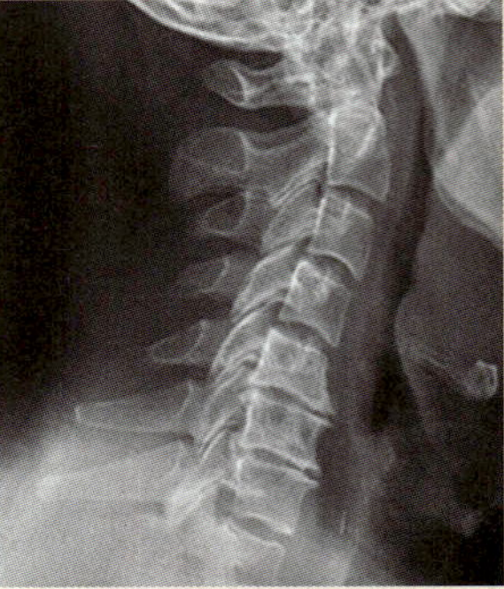

a. Spondylolisthesis
b. Spondylosis
c. Spondyloptosis
d. Spondylitis

19. A 20-year-old male presented with pain on movement and X-ray shows lytic lesion on the upper end of tibia identify the lesion? ***[AIIMS PG November 2015]***

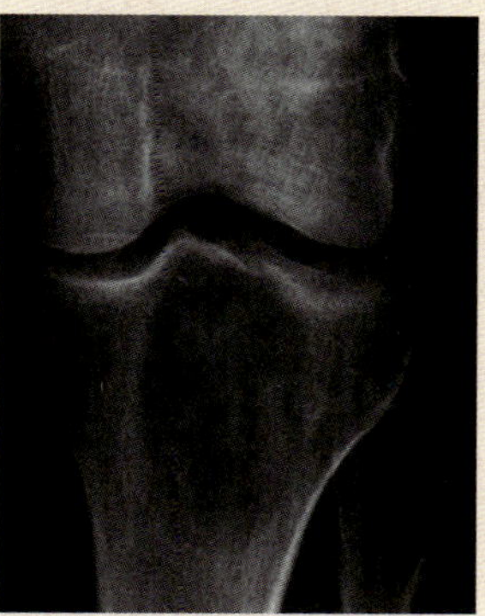

a. GCT
b. Adamantinoma
c. Simple bone cyst
d. Ewing's sarcoma

20. Diagnose the underlying disorder from the X-ray given below ***[Recent Question 2018]***

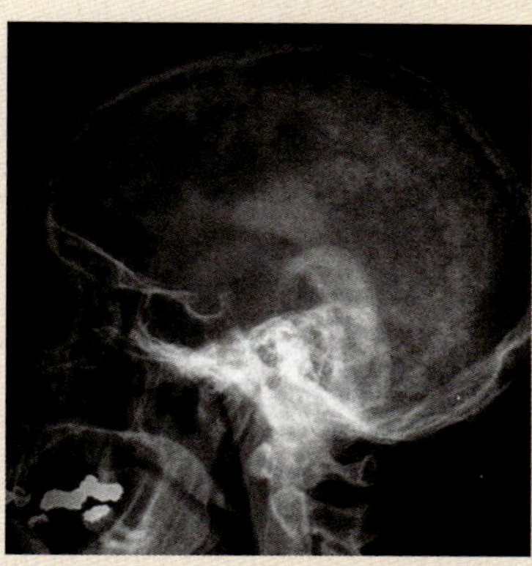

a. Paget's disease
b. Multiple myeloma
c. Osteosarcoma
d. Osteomyelitis

ANSWERS WITH EXPLANATIONS OF IBQs

1. Ans. (b) Colles' fracture *[Ref. Adult Orthopaedic Nursing by Schoen, 1/e p129]*

Fractures Forearm & Hand

- Barton's fracture: Intra-articular fracture of distal radius
- Bennett's fracture: Intra-articular fracture of base of first metacarpal
- Colles' fracture: Distal radius, extra-articular fracture with dorsal tilt of distal fragment **(Photograph)**
- Smiths' fracture: Distal radius fracture, extra-articular with volar tilt of the distal fragment

2. Ans. (d) Rickets *[Ref. Pearls in Practical Pediatrics by Magon, 1/e p187]*

Rickets [Mnemonic: Sachin Created Batting Record in Last World Cup]

- **S**aucer epiphysis: Widening of growth plate
- **C**upping, fraying, splaying **(Boxes in Photograph)**
- **B**owing of legs
- **R**ickety rosary
- **L**oss of provisional zone of calcification (Earliest sign)
- **W**hite line of healing
- **C**raniotabes

3. Ans. (b) Osteogenesis imperfecta *[Ref. Principles of Bone X-ray Diagnosis by Simon, 3/e p4]*

Plain Radiology in Osteogenesis Imperfecta

- Head, neck and spine: Wormian bones, Kyphoscoliosis, Basilar invagination, Vertebral compression fractures, Codfish vertebrae
- Chest: Pectus excavatum/carinatum
- Pelvis: Acetabular protrusion, Coxa vara
- General Skeleton:
  - Severe osteoporosis
  - Cortical thinning
  - Hyperplastic callus formation
  - Popcorn calcification
  - Deformed, over-tubulated bones
  - Zebra stripe sign (Sclerotic growth recovery lines in long bones formation of pseudoarthrosis at sites of healing fractures)

4. Ans. (b) Block vertebra *[Ref. Essentials of Skeletal Radiology by Yochum & Rowe, Volume 1, 3/e p279]*

Block Vertebra

- Type of vertebral anomaly where there is a failure of separation of two or more adjacent vertebral bodies
- In a block vertebra, there is partial or complete fusion of adjacent vertebral bodies

5. Ans. (c) Osteopetrosis *[Ref. Radiology in Medical Practice by Abdullah, 4/e p236]*

Osteopetrosis Radiology
- Generalized osteosclerosis
- Erlenmeyer flask deformity
- Rugger-Jersey spine **(Photograph)**
- Bone-within-bone appearance (Endobone) **(Photograph)**

6. Ans. (c) Classical triad of symptoms is painful swelling, sinuses & bleeding on touch
[Ref. MCQs and EMQs in Surgery - A Bailey & Love Revision Guide, 2/e p58]

Madura Foot
- Chronic infection of skin and underlying tissues caused by both bacteria (Actinomycetomas) and fungi (Eumycetomas)
- Presentation: **(Photograph)**
  - Following initial injury, disease has slow chronic course with painless swelling and intermittent discharge of pus
  - Deep itching sensation
  - Pain may occur due to Secondary bacterial infection or bone invasion
  - After some years, massive swelling of the area occurs, with induration, skin rupture and sinus tract formation
  - As the infection spreads, old sinuses close and new ones open
  - Exudates are typically granular
- X-ray:
  - Multiple large cavities with well-defined margins and periosteal reaction typical of eumycetoma
  - Periosteal reaction with new bone spicules may create a Sun-ray appearance and Codman's triangle
- MRI Dot-in-circle sign **(Photograph)**: Tiny hypodense foci, believed to be grains, within high hyperintensity spherical lesions (Granulomas scattered by fibrosis)

7. Ans. (c) Scurvy` *[Ref. Sumer K Sethi, 5/e p54]*
- *White line of Frankel*: A dense zone of provisional calcification at growing epiphysis
  - Scurvy
  - Lead poisoning
  - Phosphorus poisoning

8. Ans. (c) Osteosarcoma *[Ref. Sumer K Sethi, 5/e p59]*

Codman's Triangle
- Description:
  - A type of periosteal reaction seen with aggressive bone lesions
  - With aggressive lesions, the periosteum does not have time to ossify with shells of new bone, so only the edge of the raised periosteum will ossify
- Seen in:
  - Osteosarcoma
  - Ewing's sarcoma
  - Osteomyelitis
  - Giant cell tumor
  - Aneurysmal bone cyst
  - Metastasis
  - Chondrosarcoma
  - Malignant fibrous histiocytoma

9. Ans. (d) Osteopetrosis *[Ref. Sumer K Sethi, 5/e p56]*

Erlenmeyer Flask Deformity
- Description: A radiographic appearance typically on a femoral radiograph where there is relative constriction of the diaphysis and flaring of the metaphysis
- Seen in:
  - Marrow infiltration/expansion: Thalassemia, Gaucher's disease, Niemann-Pick disease, Sickle cell disease
  - Bone dysplasia: Fibrous dysplasia, Osteopetrosis, Achondroplasia, Ollier's disease, Metaphyseal dysplasia
  - Metabolic bone disease: Rickets, Rheumatoid disease, Hypophosphatasia
  - Heavy metal poisoning, Lead poisoning
  - Down's syndrome

10. Ans. (b) Ewing's sarcoma *[Ref. Sumer K Sethi, 5/e p60]*
- Onion peel appearance is a laminated periosteal reaction seen in Ewing's sarcoma

11. Ans. (d) All of the above *[Ref. Sumer K Sethi, 5/e p52]*

Vertebra Plana or Pancake Vertebra

- Description: Vertebral body has lost almost its entire height anteriorly and posteriorly, representing a very advanced crush fracture
- Seen in:
  - Trauma
  - Osteoporosis
  - Osteomyelitis
  - Multiple myeloma
  - Vertebral hemangioma
  - Spinal tuberculosis
  - Osteogenesis imperfecta
  - Vertebral metastases
  - Lymphoma
  - Leukemia
  - Eosinophilic granuloma

12. Ans. (b) Osteomalacia *[Ref. Sumer K Sethi, 5/e p54]*

Looser Zones/Cortical Infractions/Milkman's Lines

- Description: Pseudofractures and Insufficiency fractures
  - Wide transverse lucencies traversing part way through a bone, usually at right angles to the involved cortex
  - Sclerotic irregular margins, and are often symmetrical.
- Seen in:
  - Osteomalacia
  - Rickets
  - Renal osteodystrophy
  - Fibrous dysplasia
  - Hyperthyroidism
  - Paget's disease of bone
  - Osteogenesis imperfecta
  - X-linked hypophosphatemia

13. Ans. (d) Renal Osteodystrophy *[Ref. Sumer K Sethi, 5/e p54]*

Rugger-Jersey Spine

- Description: Prominent sub-endplate densities at multiple contiguous levels to produce an alternating dense-lucent-dense appearance
- Seen in:
  - Renal osteodystrophy
  - Osteopetrosis
  - Hyperparathyroidism

14. Ans. (b) Osteopetrosis *[Ref. RadDaily.com]*

Bone-Within-Bone Appearance

- Description: Indicative of osteonecrosis
- Seen in: [**Mnemonic:** Healing **STOPS G**ut **H**aemorrhage]
  - **H**ypervitaminosis D
  - **S**arcoidosis/**S**yphilis (Congenital)
  - **T**horostat
  - **O**steopetrosis
  - **P**aget's disease
  - **S**ickle cell anaemia
  - **G**aucher's disease
  - **H**eavy metal poisoning

15. Ans. (d) Hyperparathyroidism *[Ref. Sumer K Sethi, 5/e p53]*

- Subperiosteal bone resorption is the most consistent and specific finding of Hyperparathyroidism and is virtually pathognomonic of the condition
- Terminal tufts of the phalanges are the most commonly involved bones

16. Ans. (c) Achondroplasia *[Ref. Musculoskeletal Imaging by Pope, 2/e p1234]*

Champagne Glass Pelvis

- Description:
  - Iliac blades are flattened, giving rise to a pelvic inlet resembling a champagne glass
  - Acetabular angles are increased
  - Sacrosciatic notch is small
- Seen in: Achondroplasia

17. Ans. (a) Osteogenic sarcoma *[Ref. Sumer K Sethi, 5/e p59]*

Sunburst Appearance

- Description:
  - Type of periosteal reaction giving the appearance of a sunburst secondary to an aggressive periostitis
  - Sunburst appearance occurs when the lesion grows too fast and the periosteum does not have enough time to lay down a new layer and instead the Sharpey's fibres stretch out perpendicular to the bone
- Seen in:
  - Osteosarcoma
  - Ewing's sarcoma
  - Osteoblastic metastases (prostate, lung or breast cancer)

18. Ans. (b) Spondylosis *[Ref. Turek's Orthopedics, 6/e p503]*

Cervical Degenerative Spondylosis

- Grade 0 (normal): No degenerative changes.
- Grade 1 (minimal/early): Minimal anterior osteophyte formation
- Grade 2 (mild): Definite anterior osteophyte formation, Subtle or no reduction in Intervertebral disc height (<25%), Just recognisable sclerosis of the endplates
- Grade 3 (moderate): Definite anterior osteophyte formation, Moderate narrowing of the disc space (25-75%), definite sclerosis of the endplates and osteophyte sclerosis
- Grade 4 (gross): Large and multiple large osteophyte formation (C5, C6, C7 in Photograph), Severe narrowing of the disc space (>75% in Photograph), Sclerosis of the endplates with irregularities (Photograph)

19. Ans. (a) GCT *[Ref. Musculoskeletal Radiology by Griffiths, 1/e p219]*

- Giant cell tumours (GCTs) of bone, also known as osteoclastomas, are relatively common bone tumours, usually benign which are arising from metaphysis and typically extending into the epiphysis of the long bones
- Radiology:
  - Occurs only with a closed growth plate
  - Abuts articular surface
  - Well defined with non-sclerotic margin
  - Eccentric

20. Ans. (a) Paget's disease *[Ref. X-ray Diagnosis of the Skull by Boulay, 2/e p55]*

Paget Disease of the Bone

- Common, chronic bone disorder characterised by excessive abnormal bone remodelling
- Frequently affects the pelvis, spine, skull and proximal long bones
- Early phase features osteolytic (lucent) region which is later followed by coarsened trabeculae and bony enlargement; sclerotic changes occur much later in the disease process.
- Osteoporosis circumscripta: Large, well-defined lytic lesion
- Cotton wool appearance: Mixed lytic and sclerotic lesions of the skull
- Tam o'Shanter sign: Frontal bone enlargement, with the appearance of the skull falling over the facial bones
- Diploic widening

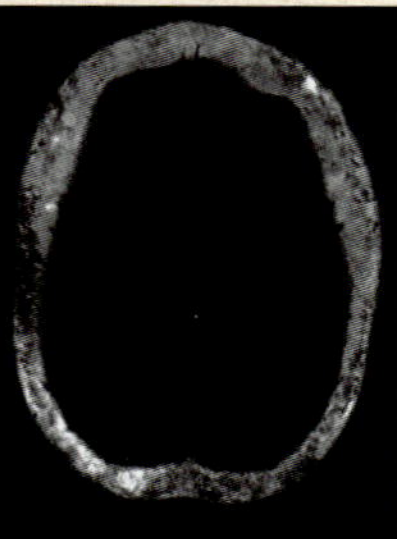

Fig. Paget's disease of skull

Radiodiagnosis and Radiotherapy

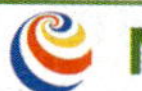 NEET/NBE PATTERN MCQs 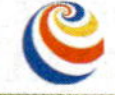

1. X-ray view of choice for pisiform bone fracture *[Recent Question 2016]*
a. Anteroposterior view b. Lateral view
c. Oblique view d. None of the choice

2. Radiological investigation of choice for soft tissue sarcoma is *[Recent Question 2016]*
a. X-ray b. USG
c. CT scan d. MRI

3. 'Looser's zones' are a feature of *[NBE FMGE September 2010]*
a. Osteomalacia b. Cushing's syndrome
c. Paget's disease d. Multiple myeloma

4. Codman's triangle is seen in *[Recent Question 2012]*
a. Chondroblastoma b. Osteosarcoma
c. Chondrosarcoma d. GCT

5. X-rays findings of fibrous dysplasia *[NBE DNB 2009]*
a. Ground glass density b. Calcifications
c. Cortical thickening d. Bony expansion

6. "Sunray appearance" on X-ray is suggestive of *[Recent Question 2012]*
a. Chondrosarcoma
b. Metastatic tumour in the bone
c. Osteogenic sarcoma
d. Ewing's sarcoma

7. Wimberger's sign is found in *[NBE FMGE March 2010]*
a. Lead poisoning b. Rickets
c. Osteomalacia d. Scurvy

8. Bone within bone appearance is seen in *[Recent Question 2012, 2017]*
a. CML b. Osteoporosis
c. Osteopetrosis d. Bone infarct

9. 'Spoke-wheel pattern' of calcification within an osteolytic lesion of bone is characteristic of *[NBE FMGE March 2010]*
a. Hemangioma b. Secondaries
c. Plasmacytosis d. Hydatid disease

PLEASE NOTE: Match the X-ray land marks of foetal development with the period (Questions 10-14) *[NBE DNB 1994, 1995]*
a. 32 weeks b. 36 weeks
c. 24 weeks d. 12 weeks
e. 38 weeks

10. Distal femoral epiphysis

11. Foetal fat line

12. Calcaneous

13. Proximal tibial epiphysis

14. Spine and skull

15. 'Celery stalk' appearance of long bones in infants is seen in all except *[NBE FMGE March 2010]*
a. Congenital syphilis b. Congenital rubella
c. Congenital varicella d. Congenital cytomegalovirus

16. At the end of one year age, the number of carpal bones seen in the skiagram of the hand is? *[NBE DNB 2008, 2009]*
a. Nil b. 1
c. 2 d. 3

17. Calcification of intervertebral disc is seen in *[Recent Question 2012]*
a. Gout b. Rheumatoid
c. Alkaptonuria d. Psoriasis

18. Multiple 'rain-drop' like osteolytic lesions in skull is seen in *[NBE FMGE March 2010]*
a. Lead poisoning b. Letterer-Siwe disease
c. Intracranial tension d. Multiple fractures

19. Earliest sign in Rheumatoid Arthritis is *[NBE DNB 1998, NBE DNB 1999]*
a. Decreased joint space
b. Periarticular osteoporosis
c. Periarticular soft tissue swelling
d. Reduced joint space

20. Frankel's line is seen in *[Recent Question 2012, 2013]*
a. Rickets b. Scurvy
c. Osteomalacia d. None

21. Which of the following is not a radiological feature of Rickets? *[NBE FMGE September 2009]*
a. Bowing of legs b. Cupping
c. Metaphyseal widening d. Frankel's line

22. In normal X-ray of shoulder which is superior most structure *[Recent Question 2012]*
a. Greater tubercle b. Surgical neck of humerus
c. Coracoid process d. Head of humerus

23. Thickness of skull is increased in *[NBE DNB 1998, 2000, 2005]*
a. Rickets b. Osteomalacia
c. Hyperparathyroidism d. Thalassemia

24. Radioactive substance used in a bone scan is *[NBE FMGE September 2009]*
a. Gallium-67 b. Iodine-131
c. Phosphorus-32 d. Technetium-99

25. Pseudofracture or Looser's zone is seen in *[Recent Question 2012, 2015]*
a. Osteoporosis b. Osteopetrosis
c. Osteomalacia d. Scurvy

26. Hair on end appearance is seen in *[Recent Question 2017, NBE DNB 2009]*

a. Thalassemia b. Scurvy
c. Rickets d. Hemochromatosis

27. 'Punched-out' lesions in skull of an elderly patient is diagnostic of *[NBE FMGE September 2008]*
a. Lymphoma b. Metastasis
c. Multiple myeloma
d. Chronic granulomatous infection

28. Radiological feature of osteosarcoma is *[NBE FMGE September 2008]*
a. Onion-peel appearance b. Sun-ray appearance
c. Tram-track appearance d. Cotton-wool appearance

29. "Bone with a Bone" appearance is seen in *[NBE DNB 1993, 2007]*
a. Osteogenesis imperfecta
b. Osteopetrosis
c. Scurvy d. Rickets

30. Osteoblastic metastasis is seen *[Recent Question 2013]*
a. Prostate carcinoma b. Multiple myeloma
c. Thyroid carcinoma d. Renal carcinoma

31. White line of Frankel on radiology of long bones is seen in *[NBE FMGE September 2008]*
a. Scurvy b. Rickets
c. Mercury poisoning d. Stress fractures

32. Radiological changes in Rickets are all except *[NBE FMGE September 2007]*
a. Bowing of bones b. Fractures of bones
c. Smaller epiphysis with pencil-thin cortex
d. Narrowing/absent zone of provisional calcification

33. Onion-peel appearance is seen in *[Recent Question 2012, 2017]*
a. Ewing's sarcoma b. Osteoma
c. Osteosarcoma d. Osteoclastoma

34. Linear striations are typically seen in *[NBE DNB 2009, 2010]*
a. Vertebral myeloma b. Vertebral lymphangiomas
c. Vertebral metastases d. Vertebral haemangiomas

35. 'Bone-within-bone' appearance of X-ray is classic of *[NBE FMGE March 2006]*
a. Osteogenesis imperfecta
b. Osteopetrosis
c. Renal osteodystrophy d. Achondroplasia

36. All of the following are the radiological features of Osteomalacia, except *[NBE DNB 2008, 2009]*
a. Triradiate pelvis b. Milkman's fractures
c. Osteopenia d. Lytic lesions

37. 'Bone-within-bone' appearance is seen in *[NBE FMGE March 2004]*
a. Syphilis b. Congenital syphilis
c. Gaucher's disease d. All of the above

38. X-ray skull showing "crew-cut-hair-on-end" appearance is seen in *[NBE DNB 2011, NBE FMGE September 2012]*
a. Sickle cell anemia
b. Cerebellar hemangioblastoma
c. Thalassemia major
d. Down's syndrome

39. 'Notching of ribs' is seen in *[NBE FMGE September 2006]*
a. ASD b. PDA
c. Coarctation of aorta d. All of the above

40. "Diffuse axonal Injury" is best detected on *[NBE FMGE September 2011]*
a. Non contract CT b. Contrast CT
c. MRI d. Transcranial Doppler

41. Subperiosteal bleeds are seen in radiology of *[NBE FMGE September 2012]*
a. Scurvy b. Rickets
c. Renal osteodystrophy d. Rheumatoid arthritis

42. Pencil-cup appearance on plain X-ray of hand/foot is suggestive of *[NBE FMGE March 2012]*
a. Diabetic foot
b. Leprosy
c. Raynaud's phenomenon
d. Frostbite

43. Inferior rib notching is seen in *[Recent Question 2013, 2014]*
a. Coarctation of aorta b. SLE
c. RA d. Scl erodenna

44. Block vertebrae are seen in *[Recent Question 2013]*
a. Pagets disease b. Leukemia
c. TB d. Klippel-Feil syndrome

45. Punctuated lesions and floating teeth are seen in *[Recent Question 2013]*
a. Metastasis b. Osteitis fibrosa
c. Histiocytosis d. Asbestosis

46. Bamboo spine sign is seen in *[Recent Question 2014]*
a. Rheumatoid arthritis
b. Osteoarthritis
c. Ankylosing spondylitis
d. Juvenile Rheumatoid arthritis

47. All of the following are seen in X-ray in Rickets except *[Recent Question 2014, 2015]*
a. Cupping b. Fraying
c. Splaying d. Bone hyperdensity

48. Scan of choice to detect metastasis to bone *[Recent Question 2014]*
a. Tc99 pyrophosphate b. Th201
c. Tc99 DMSA d. Tc99 sulphur colloid

49. Earliest sign indicative of sacroiliitis on X-ray is? *[Recent Question 2017]*
a. Osteophytes b. Erosion
c. Blurring of SI joint d. Sclerosis

50. Salt pepper skull is seen in? *[Recent Question 2017, 2018]*
a. Multiple myeloma b. Hyperparathyroidism
c. Sickle cell anemia d. Fibrous dysplasia

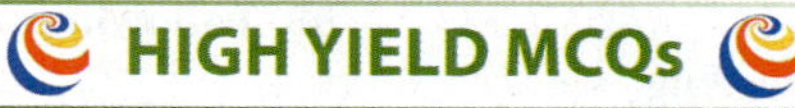

HIGH YIELD MCQs

1. What is the Gold standard method for diagnosing Gout? *[Bihar PG 2016]*
a. CT scan
b. MRI
c. Microscopic exam of synovial fluid
d. All of the above

2. Investigation of choice for bony metastasis *[AIPGMEE 2011, Recent Question 2017]*
a. X-ray b. CT scan
c. MRI d. Bone scan

3. 'Scottish terrier sign' is seen in *[All India 1995]*
a. AP view b. PA view
c. Lateral view d. Oblique view

4. 'Beheaded Scottish terrier' sign is *[AIIMS 1992] [JIPMER 1990, 1999]*
a. Spondylosis b. Spondylolisthesis
c. Lumbar canal stenosis d. Slipped disc

5. Which one of the following tumors shows calcification on CT scan *[All India PGMEE 1995]*
a. Ependymoma b. Medulloblastoma
c. Meningioma d. CNS lymphoma

6. Vertebra plana is seen in *[PGI 2005]*
a. Eosinophilic granuloma b. Trauma
c. Paget's disease d. Malignancy

7. Epiphyseal enlargement is seen in *[AIIMS PGMEE 1997]*
a. Rickets
b. Scurvy
c. Spondylepiphyseal dysgenesis
d. Juvenile rheumatoid arthritis

8. Fraying and cupping of metaphyses of long bones in a child does not occur in *[All India PGMEE 2003]*
a. Rickets
b. Lead poisoning
c. Metaphyseal dysplasia
d. Hypophosphatasia

9. Wind-swept deformity is seen in *[AIIMS PGMEE 1998]*
a. Ankylosing spondylitis b. Scurvy
c. Rheumatoid arthritis d. Rickets

10. 'Trident hand' is seen in *[AIIMS PGMEE 1998]*
a. Achondroplasia b. Mucopolysaccharidosis
c. Diphyseal achlasia d. Cleidocranial dysostosis

11. 'Champagne glass pelvis' is seen in *[JIPMER PGMEE 2002]*
a. CDH b. Down's syndrome
c. Cretinism d. Achondroplasia

12. 'Bone within bone' appearance is seen in *[AIIMS PGMEE 1993, JIPMER PGMEE 2000]*
a. CML b. Osteoporosis
c. Osteopetrosis d. Bone infarct

13. Pseudofracture of Looser's zone is seen in *[AIIMS PGMEE 1997]*
a. Osteoporosis b. Osteopetrosis
c. Osteomalacia d. Scurvy

14. Looser's zones is seen in *[PGI 2002]*
a. Osteoporosis b. Hyperparathyrodism
c. Osteomalacia d. Renal osteodystrophy
e. Paget's disease

15. 'Sunray appearance' on X-rays is suggestive of *[AIIMS PGMEE 2004]*
a. Chondrosarcoma
b. Metastatic tumour in the bone
c. Osteogenic sarcoma
d. Ewing's sarcoma

16. X-ray of which bone (s) would be diagnostic in hyperparathyroidism? *[PGI 2000]*
a. Skull b. Phalanges
c. Long bones d. Scapula
e. Spine

17. Heberden's nodes are found in *[AIIMS PGMEE 2005]*
a. PIP joints in osteoarthritis
b. DIP joints in osteoarthritis
c. PIP joints in rheumatoid arthritis
d. DIP joints in rheumatoid arthritis

18. Tufting of distal phalanx is characteristically seen in *[AIIMS PGMEE 1991]*
a. Gout b. Psoriatic arthropathy
c. Hypoparathyroidism d. Hyperparathyroidism

19. Chondrocalcinosis is seen with *[AIIMS PGMEE 1991]*
a. Gout b. Osteoarthritis
c. Pseudogout d. Septic arthritis

20. Calcification of intervertebral disc is seen in *[AIIMS PGMEE 1990]*
a. TB spine
b. Prolapse of intervertebral disc (PID)
c. Non rheumatic ankylosis
d. Rheumatic ankylosis

21. Calcification of meniscal cartilage is feature of *[All India PGMEE 1991]*
a. Achondroplasia b. Hyperparathyroidism
c. Gaucher's disease d. Pseudogout

22. Calcification around the joint is seen in *[PGI 1999]*
a. Pseudogout b. Hyperparathyroidism
c. Rheumatoid arthritis d. Gout

23. Which one of the following is a recognized X-ray feature of rheumatoid arthritis? *[All India PGMEE 2003]*
a. Juxta-articular osteosclerosis
b. Sacroiliitis
c. Bone erosions
d. Periarticular calcification

24. Radiological feature of osteosarcoma is *[AIIMS PGMEE 1999]*
a. New bone formation b. Sunray appearance
c. Cotton wool appearance d. Osteoid formation

25. Lytic lesion in skull are seen in following except *[PGI 1997]*
a. Multiple myeloma b. Metastasis ca bronchus
c. Thalassemia d. Carcinoma prostate

26. X-ray finding of osteomyelitis within 8 day is *[PGI 1999]*
a. Cystic swelling b. Soft tissue swelling
c. New bone formation d. Sequestrum formation

27. Intracranial calcification with cystic lesion in plain X-ray skull is seen in *[AIIMS PGMEE 1996]*
a. Meningioma b. Glioma
c. Craniopharyngioma d. All of the above

28. Pathognomonic feature of hyperparathyroidism *[AIIMS PGMEE 1992, 1998]*
a. Osteopenia
b. Loss of Lamina dura
c. Brown's tumor
d. Subperiosteal resorption of phalanges

29. "Hair-on end" appearance is seen in *[AIIMS PGMEE 2008]*
a. Thalassemia b. Sickle cell anaemia
c. Hemochromatosis d. Megaloblastic anaemia

30. Looser's zones in seen in *[PGI 2002]*
a. Osteoporosis b. Hyperparathyroidism
c. Osteomalacia d. Multiple myeloma
e. Paget's disease

31. A lady Dimple has a lytic lesion in X-ray of upper end of humerus. The diagnosis is *[AIIMS PGMEE 1999]*
a. Osteosarcoma b. Osteochondroma
c. Unicameral bone cyst d. Osteoclastoma

32. A classical expansive lytic lesion in the transverse process of a vertebra is seen in *[All India PGMEE 2003]*
a. Osteosarcoma b. Aneurysmal bone cyst
c. Osteoblastoma d. Metastasis

33. Wide diploic space of skull with brush border (hair on end) appearance is characteristic of *[All India PGMEE 1991]*
a. Congenital haemolytic anaemia
b. Multiple myeloma
c. Raised intracranial tension
d. Meningioma

34. All are radiological features of sickle cell anaemia except *[PGI 2008]*
a. Vertebra plana b. Floating teeth
c. Bone infarct d. Marrow hyperplasia
e. Secondary osteomyelitis

35. Investigation of choice for temporal bone injury *[AIIMS PGMEE 2010]*
a. CT scan b. MRI
c. Angiography d. Plain X-ray

36. C1 C2 best seen in *[AIIMS PGMEE 2009]*
a. Lateral view
b. Oblique view
c. AP view
d. Odontoid view

37. The gold standard for the diagnosis of osteoporosis is *[AIIMS PGMEE 2004]*
a. Dual energy X-ray absorptiometry
b. Single energy X-ray absorptiometry
c. Ultrasonography
d. Quantitative computed tomography

38. Following can cause rib notching except *[AIIMS PGMEE 2009]*
a. Blalock Taussig shunt
b. Waterston Cooley's shunt
c. Pulmonary atresia with large VSD
d. Aorta disruption

39. Superior rib notching is/are caused by *[PGI 2009]*
a. Hyperparathyroidism b. Poliomyelitis
c. Blalock-Tausig shunt d. Marfan's syndrome
e. Coarctation of aorta

40. All are radiological sign of vitamin C deficiency except *[AIIMS PGMEE 1995]*
a. White line of Frankel b. Wimberger line
c. Osteoporosis of bone d. Widening of epiphysis

41. Radiological features of rickets include *[PGI 2005]*
a. Narrowing of epiphysis b. Cupping of metaphysis
c. Rachitic rosary d. Pelkan's spur

42. Splaying and cupping of the metaphysis is seen in *[PGI 1999]*
a. Rickets b. Scurvy
c. Paget's disease d. Lead poisoning

43. X-ray shows soap bubble appearance of lower end of radius, treatment of choice is *[AIIMS PGMEE 1998]*
a. Local excision b. Excision & bone grafting
c. Amputation d. RT

44. Tracheal bifurcation on X-ray corresponds to *[PGI 2001]*
a. T5T6 b. T1T5
c. Sternal angle d. Thoracic inlet

45. Vertebrae plana is seen in *[AIIMS PGMEE 1998]*
a. Malignancy b. Fracture
c. Tuberculosis d. Eosinophilic granuloma

46. Schober's sign is for *[PGI 1998]*
a. Flexion of lumbar spine
b. Chest expansion
c. Pain with motion of hip
d. Neck pain and stiffness

47. Dense metaphyseal band is seen on *[PGI 2008]*
a. Hypervitaminosis A b. Hypervitaminosis B
c. Scurvy d. Hypervitaminosis D

48. In Spondylolisthesis following radiological features seen *[PGI 2006]*
a. Scotty dog
b. Scotty dog wearing a collar
c. Beheaded Scotty dog terrier sign
d. Napoleon sign

49. Radiographic appearance of Pindborg's tumor is *[All India PGMEE 2002]*
a. Onion-peel appearance
b. Sun burst appearance
c. Cherry-blossom appearance
d. Driven-snow appearance

50. Radiological investigation shows sun ray appearance in *[AIIMS PGMEE 1995, PGI 2005]*
a. Osteosarcoma b. GCT
c. Osteomyelitis d. Ewing's sarcoma

51. Calcification of Intervertebral disc is seen in *[All India PGMEE 2000]*
a. Gout b. Rheumatoid
c. Alkaptonuria d. Psoriasis

52. Radiological features of scleroderma are all except *[All India PGMEE 1993]*
a. Diffuse periosteal reaction
b. Esophageal dysmotility
c. Erosion of tip of phalanx
d. Lung nodules

53. In scurvy all the following radiological signs are seen except *[All India PGMEE 2004]*
a. Pelican spur
b. Soap bubble appearance
c. Zone of demarcation near epiphysis
d. Frankel's line

54. Radiological findings of scurvy are all except *[PGI 1999]*
a. Epiphyseal widening b. Metaphyseal porosis
c. Metaphyseal infarction d. Pelkan spur

55. Earliest evidence of healing in rickets is provided by *[All India PGMEE 1995]*
a. S. Calcium
b. S. Phosphate
c. Radiological examination of growing bone ends
d. Serum alkaline phosphate level

56. Fraying and cupping of metaphyses of long bones in a child does not occur in *[All India PGMEE 2003]*
a. Rickets b. Lead poisoning
c. Metaphyseal dysplasia d. Hypophosphatasia

57. Flaring of anterior ends of the ribs is characteristically seen in *[All India PGMEE 2008]*
a. Neurofibromatosis b. Scurvy
c. Rickets d. Hypothyroidism

58. Which endocrine disorder is associated with epiphyseal dysgenesis? *[All India PGMEE 2003]*
a. Hypothyroidism b. Cushing's syndrome
c. Addison's disease d. Hypoparathyroidism

59. 76 year old man presents with lytic lesion in the vertebrae. X-ray skull showed multiple punched out lesions. The diagnosis is *[AIIMS PGMEE 2000]*
a. Metastasis b. Multiple myeloma
c. Osteomalacia d. Hyperparathyroidism

60. Dense calcification is seen in *[AIIMS PGMEE 1996]*
a. Chondroblastoma b. Chondrosarcoma
c. Osteosarcoma d. Fibrosarcoma

61. Expansible pulsating secondary metastasis is a feature of *[AIIMS PGMEE 1990]*
a. Basal cell carcinoma b. Renal cell carcinoma
c. Osteogenic sarcoma d. Carcinoma prostate

62. An eight year old boy presents with back pain and mild fever. His plain X-ray of the dorsolumbar spine reveals a solitary collapsed dorsal vertebra with preserved disc spaces. There was no associated soft tissue shadow. The most likely diagnosis is *[All India PGMEE 2003]*
a. Ewing's sarcoma b. Tuberculosis
c. Histiocytosis d. Metastasis

63. Which of the following is not true regarding ossified posterior longitudinal ligament [OPLL]? *[All India PGMEE 2009]*
a. Most commonly involves thoracic spine
b. Gradient echo MR sequence may overestimate the canal stenosis
c. MRI is best for diagnosis
d. Low signal intensity on all MR sequences

64. Best radiographic view for fracture of C1, C2 vertebrae is *[AIIMS PGMEE 2004]*
a. AP view b. Odontoid view
c. Lateral view d. Oblique view

65. Best investigation for traumatic paraplegia *[AIIMS PGMEE 1992]*
a. CT scan b. MRI
c. X-ray spine d. Myelography

66. The gold standard for the diagnosis of osteoporosis is *[All India PGMEE 2005]*
a. Dual energy X-ray absorptiometry
b. Single energy X-ray absorptiometry
c. Ultrasound
d. CT scan

67. Shenton's line is seen in *[AIIMS PG May 2015]*
a. Shoulder b. Knee
c. Hip joint d. Pelvis

68. Investigation of choice for stress fracture is *[AIIMS PG May 2015]*
a. MRI b. CT scan
c. Bone scan d. X-ray

69. Radiographic latent period for acute osteomyelitis in extremities and spine respectively is *[PGMCET 2015]*
a. 8 to 10 days and 21 days
b. 21 days and 21 days
c. 10 days and 10 days
d. 21 days and 8-10 days

70. Which is the earliest radiological sign of bone infection? *[PGMCET 2015]*
a. Destructive lytic lesion
b. Presence of periosteal reaction
c. Soft-tissue edema
d. Appearance of sequestra

NEET/NBE PATTERN MCQs ANSWERS WITH EXPLANATIONS 

1. Ans. (c) Oblique view
[Ref. Essentials of Skeletal Radiology by Yochum & Rowe, 3/e Vol-1 p912]

PISIFORM FRACTURE

- Usual mechanism: Direct impacting blow (Fall on an outstretched hand)
- MC type: Vertical fracture
- Radiology: Reverse oblique wrist projection view (Best)

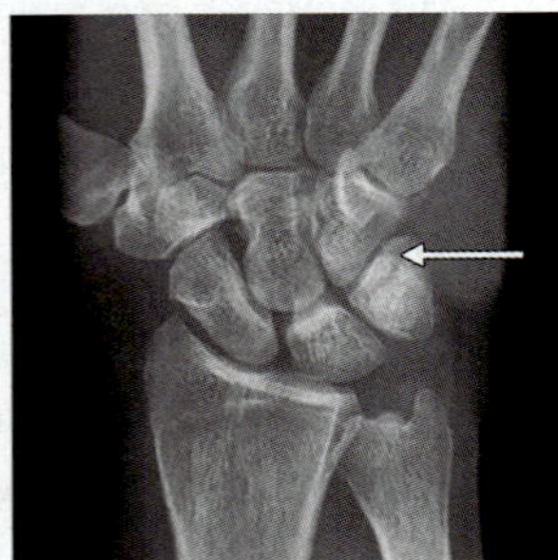

Fig. Pisiform fracture

Also Remember

Useful Radiological Views in Carpal-bones Fractures

- Pisiform fracture: Oblique view with forearm in 20° supination, carpal tunnel views
- Triquetrum fracture: Slightly oblique, pronated lateral view
- Trapezium fracture: Carpal tunnel view, True AP (Robert) view
- Trapezoid fracture: Oblique view

2. Ans. (d) MRI
[Ref. SRB's Surgery for Dental Students, 2/e p233]

Radiology in Soft Tissue Sarcoma

- Incision biopsy is the mainstay of diagnosis
- Excision biopsy is done, if tumor size <3 cm
- CT or MRI can be used to see extent and invasion
- MRI is the radiological investigation of choice: Determines vascularity, relation to vessels and fascial planes

3. Ans. (a) Osteomalacia
[Ref. Sumer K Sethi, 5/e p54]

Radiology in Osteomalacia

- *Looser's zones/Pseudofractures*: Hallmark feature
- *Triradiate pelvis*
- *Cod-fish vertebrae*: Biconcave vertebrae

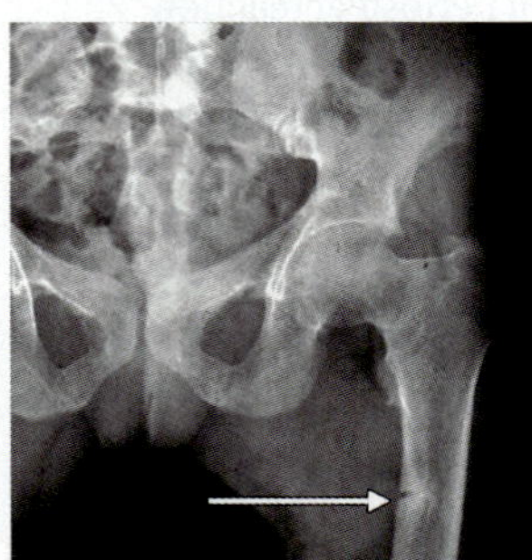

Fig. Looser's zones

Also Remember

- Paget's disease:
  - *'Cotton-wool'* skull
  - Picture-frame vertebrae
- Multiple myeloma:
  - *'Punched-out lesions'* in bones
  - *Pepper-pot skull*: Small punched out lesions in skull (Diagnostic feature)

4. Ans. (b) Osteosarcoma
[Ref. David Sutton, 7/e p1154]

- Buttressing and elevation of periosteal new bone at tumour margins leads to Codman's triangle which is usually indicative of a malignant tumour (Osteosarcoma)

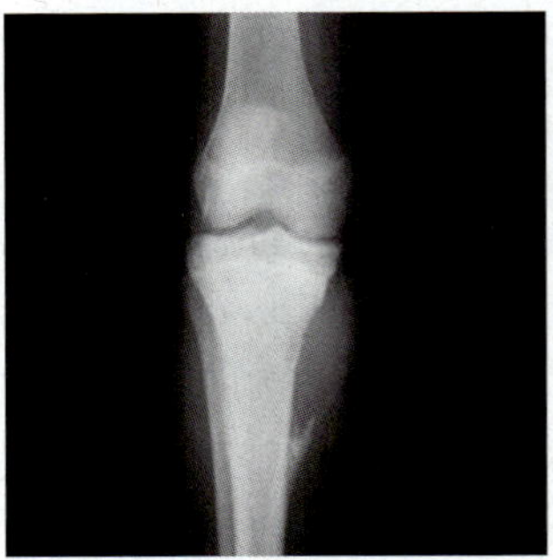

Fig. Codman's triangle

5. Ans. (a) Ground glass deformity
[Ref. Sumer K Sethi, 6/e p108]

Fibrous Dysplasia

- Ground glass appearance on X-ray
- Shepherd crook deformity of femur
- Leonine facies
- McAlbright syndrome (Polyostotic fibrous dysplasia with precocious puberty)
- Increased uptake of radionuclide scanning

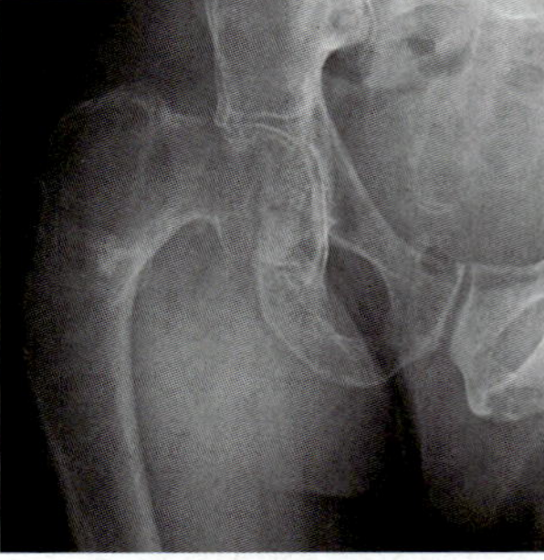

Fig. Ground-glass appearance

6. Ans. (c) Osteogenic Sarcoma
[Ref. Sumer K Sethi, 6/e p106]

- Sunray appearance and Codman's triangle are characteristic of osteosarcoma

7. Ans. (d) Scurvy
[Ref. Sumer K Sethi, 5/e p36]

Radiology in Scurvy (Vitamin C Deficiency) [Mnemonic: POST War Great Planes Fly]

- ***P**elkan spur*
- **O**steoporosis
- **S**ubperiosteal haemorrhages
- ***T**rummerfeld zone*
- ***W**imberger's sign*: Sclerotic rim around epiphysis
- **G**round-glass appearance of bones
- **P**encil-thin cortex
- ***F**rankel's (White) line*

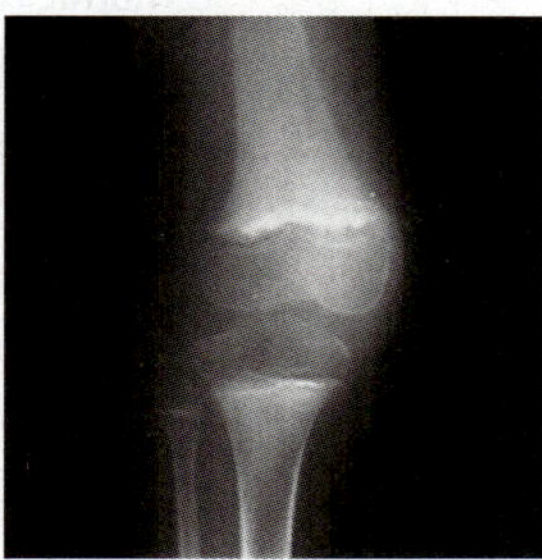

Fig. Scurvy

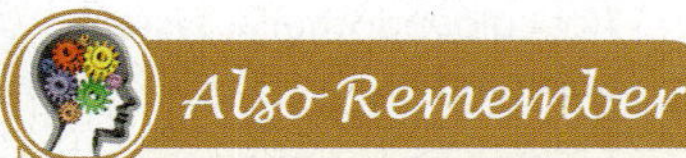

RICKETS **[Mnemonic: S**achin **C**reated **B**atting **R**ecord in **L**ast **W**orld **C**up**]**

- ***S**aucer epiphysis*: Widening of growth plate
- ***C**upping, fraying, splaying*
- **B**owing of legs
- **R**ickety rosary
- **L**oss of provisional zone of calcification (Earliest sign)
- **W**hite line of healing
- **C**raniotabes

8. Ans. (c) Osteopetrosis
[Ref. Sumer K Sethi, 6/e p99]

Osteopetrosis

- Bone within bone appearance
- Increased bone density
- Rugger Jersey/Sandwich appearance

9. Ans. (a) Hemangioma
[Ref. Maheshwari, 4/e p229; Sumer K Sethi, 5/e p62]

Radiology in Hemangioma Bone

- X-rays:
  - *Spoke-wheel pattern/Sun-burst appearance* of calcification
  - *Corduroy cloth appearance*: Vertical striations
- CT scan:
  - *Polka-dot appearance*

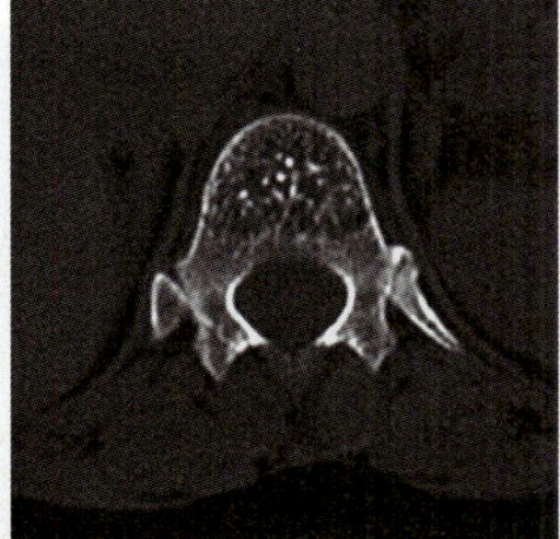

Fig. Polka-dot appearance

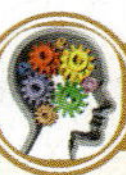

- Secondaries: Hypoechoic (Most cancers as primary source), Isoechoic or Hyperechoic (Colon cancer, Ovarian cancer) well-defined, multiple, oval lesions
- Plasmacytosis: Non-specific findings
- Hydatid disease: CT scan is Investigation of choice
  - *'Floating membrane/ Camalote (Water-lily) sign'* in liver
  - Cysts, Hydatid sand, Cystic membranes, Septae

10. Ans. (a) 32 weeks

11. Ans. (c) 24 weeks

12. Ans. (c) 24 weeks

13. Ans. (e) 38 weeks

14. Ans. (d) 12 weeks

15. Ans. (c) Congenital varicella
[Ref. Medcyclopaedia]

- ***Celery-stalk appearance of long bones***: Longitudinal radiolucent strands in metaphysis
  - Congenital syphilis
  - Congenital rubella (Most common cause)
  - Congenital cytomegalovirus

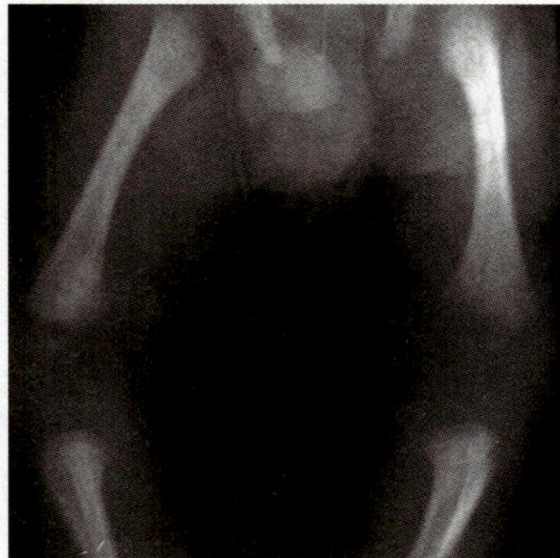

Fig. Celery stalk

16. Ans. (c) 2
[Ref. Textbook of Paediatrics by Desai, 1/e p24]

17. Ans. (a) Gout
[Ref. Bipin Valchandji Daga, 1/e p270]

GOUT

- Acute gouty arthritis: Joint effusion (Earliest sign)
- 'Overhanging' bony edge along the bone counter (Hallmark)
- Chondrocalcinosis
- Elbow: Olecranon bursa "rising sun" sign
- Punched out bony lesion
- Intervertebral disk calcification
- Aural calcification

18. Ans. (b) Letterer-Siwe disease
[Ref. Bone and Joint Disorders by A Francis, 2/e p114]

Langerhans Cells Histiocytosis

- Lesions seen:
  - Lytic lesions in skull
  - 'Floating teeth' appearance of mandible
  - Vertebra plana

- Clinical types:
  - *Eosinophilic granuloma*: *'Hole-in-bone'* (Solitary lytic lesion)
  - *Hand-Schuller-Christian disease*: *'Geographic skull'* (large lytic skull lesions)
  - *Letterer-Siwe disease*: Multiple, lytic, *'rain-drop'* pattern lesions in skull

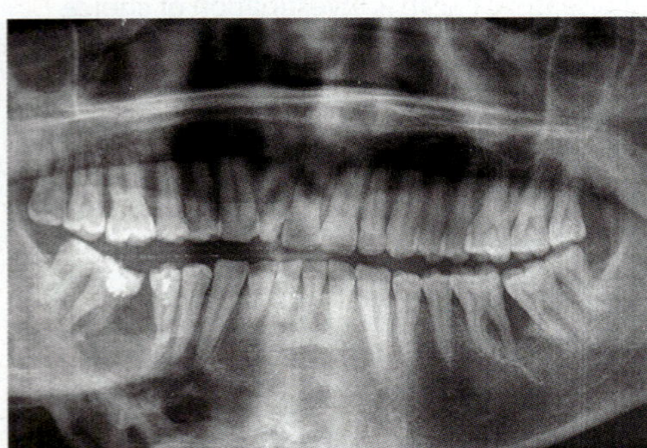

Fig. Floating teeth

19. Ans. (b) Periarticular osteoporosis
[Ref. Grainger & Allison's Diagnostic Radiology Essentials by Lee A Grant, 5/e Table 50.4]

- Periarticular osteoporosis reflects localized hyperaemia and is most pronounced in acute stages of disease

20. Ans. (b) Scurvy
[Ref. Sumer K Sethi, 6/e p97]

- White line of Frankel: Dense zone of provisional calcification at the growing metaphysis

21. Ans. (d) Frankel's line
[Ref. Sumer K Sethi, 5/e p54]

- *White line of Frankel*: A dense zone of provisional calcification at growing epiphysis
  - Scurvy
  - Lead poisoning
  - Phosphorus poisoning

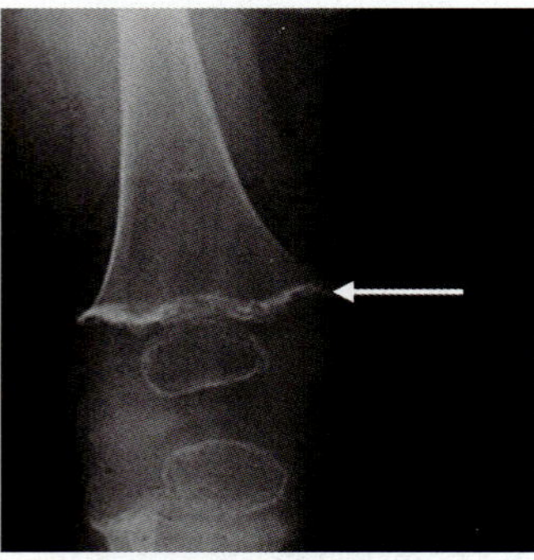

Fig. Frankel's line

22. Ans. (c) Coracoid process
[Ref. X-ray Anatomy by Simon, 1/e p41]

23. Ans. (c) Hyperparathyroidism
[Ref. Principles of X-ray Diagnosis by Trapnell, 1/e p 214]

24. Ans. (d) Technetium-99
[Ref. Sumer K Sethi, 5/e p19]

- *Most common used substance in bone scanning*: Methylene Diphosphonate Technetium-99 (MDP Tc-99)

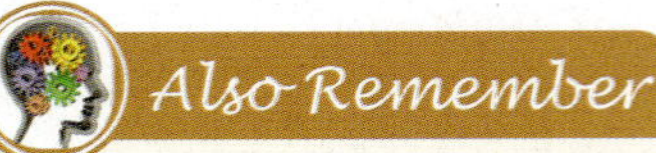

- *Most commonly used radioisotope in imaging*: Tc-99
- *Uses of Tc-99 in radiology*:

Tc-99 based scan	Use
Tc-99 HIDA scan	Investigation of choice for Acute cholecystitis
Tc-99 GTPA	Dynamic renography (GFR)
Tc-99 DMSA	Scars in reflux nephropathy
Tc-99 pyrophosphate scintigraphy	Myocardial infarction
Tc-99 MAA	Perfusion agent in V:P scan (Pulmonary TE)
Tc-99 erythrocyte scan	Minimal GIT bleeding
Tc-99 MDP	Bone scanning
Thallium-Tc99 subtraction scan	Parathyroid imaging
Tc-99 sulphur colloid scan	Reticuloendothelial system scanning
Tc-99 pertechnetate scan	Ectopic gastric mucosa (Meckel's diverticulitis)
SPECT scan with Tc-99	3D image generation

25. Ans. (c) Osteomalacia
[Ref. Sumer K Sethi, 6/e p96]

Osteomalacia

- Hallmark is presence of Looser's zone (Pseudofractures)
- Another feature is Cod-fish vertebra

26. Ans. (a) Thalassemia
[Ref. Sumer K Sethi, 6/e p96]

- Diploic widening (sparing the occiput) with 'Hair on end' or 'crew cut' or 'hair brush' appearance is seen in thalassemia

27. Ans. (c) Multiple myeloma
[Ref. Maheshwari, 4/e p236]

Radiology in Multiple Myeloma

- *'Punched-out lesions'* in bones
- *Pepper-pot skull*: Small punched out lesions in skull (Diagnostic feature)
- *Wedge collapse of vertebrae*
- Rarefaction of bones
- Erosion of ribs-borders

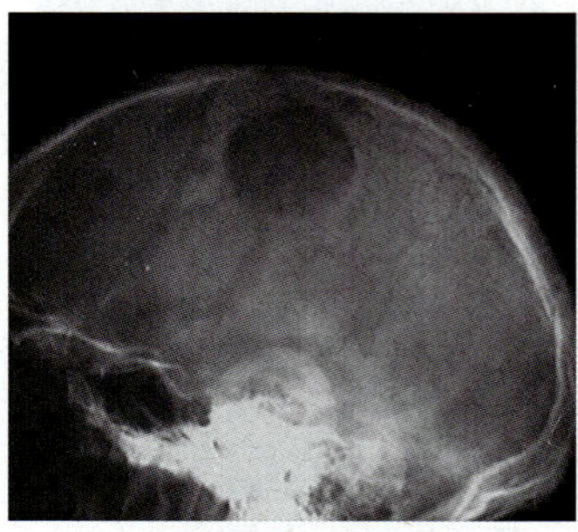

Fig. Punched-out lesions

28. Ans. (b) Sun-ray appearance
[Ref. Sumer K Sethi, 5/e p59]

Radiology in Osteosarcoma

- *Sun-ray appearance*
- *Codman's triangle*
- Periosteal reaction

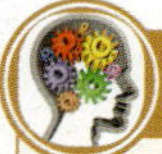

Also Remember

- *Onion-peel appearance is seen in*: Ewing's sarcoma of bone
- *Tram-track appearance is seen in*: Sturge-Weber syndrome (Skull)
- *Cotton-wool appearance is seen in*: Paget's disease of bone (Skull)

29. Ans. (b) Osteopetrosis
[Ref. Sumer K Sethi, 6/e p99]

30. Ans. (a) Prostrate Carcinoma
[Ref. BipinValchandji Daga, 1/e p287]

Osteoblastic Bone Secondaries Arise from

- Prostrate carcinoma
- Breast carcinoma
- Lymphoma
- Medulloblastoma
- Bladder carcinoma
- Pancreas cancer
- Neuroblastoma

31. Ans. (a) Scurvy
[Ref. Sumer K Sethi, 5/e p54]

32. Ans. (c) Smaller epiphysis with pencil-thin cortex
[Ref. Sumer K Sethi, 5/e p54]

33. Ans. (a) Ewing's sarcoma
[Ref. Sumer K Sethi, 6/e p107]

Ewings Sarcoma

- Onion peel appearance
- Soft tissue extension
- Diaphyseal in location

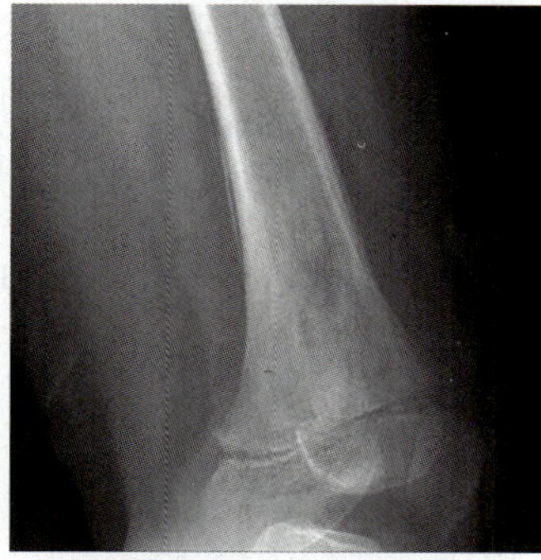

Fig. Onion-peel appearance

34. Ans. (d) Vertebral haemangiomas
[Ref. David Sutton, 7/e p1662]

- **Vertebral haemangiomas**: Usually asymptomatic tumours are diagnosed by observing the characteristic increase of prominence of the secondary bone trabeculae of the vertebral body causing a striate/ honeycomb pattern

35. Ans. (b) Osteopetrosis
[Ref. RadDaily.com]

- *'Bone-within-bone appearance'* is indicative of osteonecrosis **[Mnemonic: H**ealing **STOPS G**ut **H**aemorrhage**]**
  - **H**ypervitaminosis D
  - **S**arcoidosis/**s**yphilis (Congenital)
  - **T**horostat
  - **O**steopetrosis
  - **P**aget's disease
  - **S**ickle cell anaemia
  - **G**aucher's disease
  - **H**eavy metal poisoning

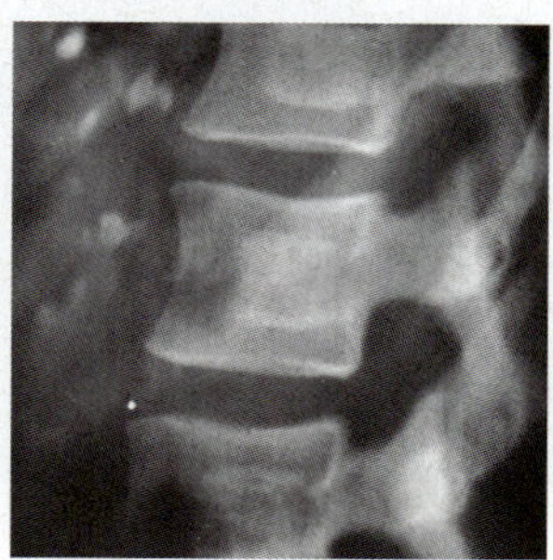

Fig. Bone within bone

36. Ans. (d) Lytic lesion
[Ref. David Sutton, 7/e p1351]

37. Ans. (d) All of the above
[Ref. RadDaily.com]

38. Ans. (c) Thalassemia major
[Ref. Sumer K Sethi, 6/e p96]

39. Ans. (c) Coarctation of aorta
[Ref. Sumer K Sethi, 5/e p44]

Unilateral Inferior notching	Bilateral Inferior notching	Superior notching
• Subclavian artery operation • Blalock-taussig operation	• Coarctation of aorta • Aortic thrombosis • Subclavian obstruction • SVC/IVC obstruction • Pulmonary AV malformation • Hyperpara-thyroidism • Neurogenic	• Rheumatoid arthritis • SLE • Scleroderma • Marfans syndrome • Poliomyelitis • Hyperpara-thyroidism

40. Ans. (c) MRI
[Ref. Lippincott's MRI of the Brain, 2/e p35]

Diffuse Axonal Injury (DAI)

- *Most sensitive diagnostic modality*: Immunocytochemistry
  - Presence of beta-amyloid precursor protein in damaged axons
- *Most sensitive radiological/imaging modality*: MRI
  - Majority of DAI is too small to be detected by CT scanning
- *Newly developed imaging modality*: Diffusion tensor imaging MRI

41. Ans. (a) Scurvy
[Ref. Sumer K Sethi, 6/e p97]

42. Ans. (b) Leprosy
[Ref. Various sources]

- **'Cup and pencil' or 'licked candy stick' appearances**: Thickening and irregularity of the soft tissues, presumably the result of chronic infection in the soft tissues
- *Pencil-in-cup deformity is characteristic of*: Psoriatic arthropathy

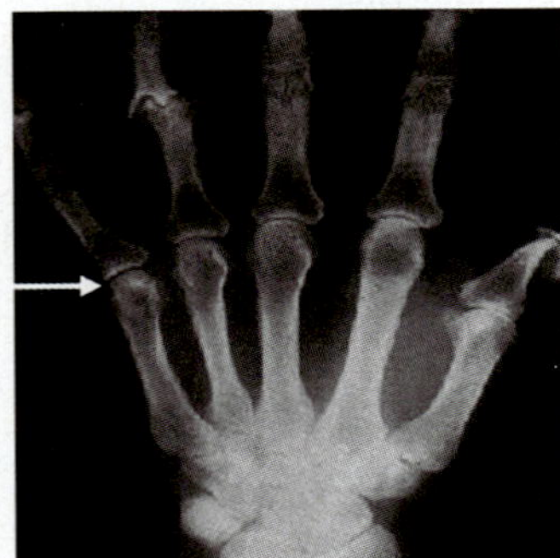

Fig. Pencil-in-cup deformity

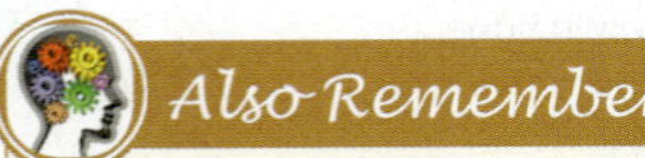

Also Remember

- *Pencil-in-cup deformity is also seen in (although not absolutely correct)*
  - Leprosy
  - Sarcoidosis
  - Rheumatoid arthritis

43. Ans. (a) Coarctation of aorta

44. Ans. (d) Klippel-Feil syndrome
[Ref. Spinal Fusion: Science and Technique edited by Jerome M. Cotler, 1/e p252]

- Klippel-Feil Deformity: Includes all patients with a congenital fusion of cervical vertebrae
- This may be limited to two segments, to an isolated congenital cervical blocked vertebra, or may involve the entire cervical spine
- Block vertebra is failure of fusion of 2 adjacent vertebrae

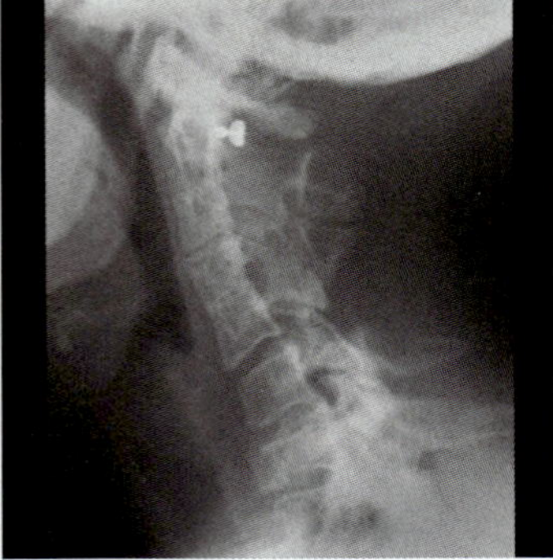

Fig. Block vertebra

45. Ans. (b) Osteitis fibrosa
[Ref. Endodontics by Kishor Gulabivala, 1/e p 379]

- Lack of bone around the teeth, gives the appearance of "teeth floating in space"

46. Ans. (c) Ankylosing spondylitis
[Ref. Radiology 101 by Smith, 3/e p288]

Radiology in Ankylosing Spondylitis: X-ray Lumbar Spine

- Squaring of vertebrae
- Syndesmophytes (Bridging osteophytes)
- 'Bamboo-spine appearance'
- Loss of lumbar lordosis

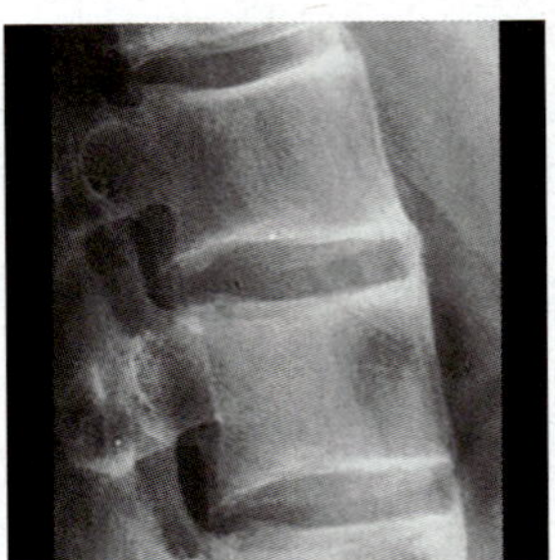

Fig. Syndesmophytes

47. Ans. (d) Bone hyperdensity
[Ref. MCQs in Pediatrics by Nayak, 1/e p101]

Rickets Radiology

- Saucer epiphysis: Widening of growth plate
- Cupping, fraying, splaying
- Bowing of legs
- Rickety rosary
- Loss of provisional zone of calcification **(Earliest sign)**
- White line of healing
- Craniotabes

48. Ans. (a) Tc99 pyrophosphate
[Ref. CRC Manual of Nuclear Medicine Procedures by Keyes, 3/e p7]

49. Ans. (c) Blurring of SI joint
[Ref. Clinical Cases & Pearls in Medicine by Sainani, 1/e p369]

Sacroiliitis in Ankylosing Spondylitis (Radiology)

- Grade 1: Mild blurring of SI joints and periarticular osteopenia
- Grade 2: Erosions with pseudowidening of joint space and subchondral sclerosis
- Grade 3: Partial joint space narrowing (ankylosis)
- Grade 4: Total ankylosis

50. Ans. (b) Hyperparathyroidism
[Ref. Internal Medicine by Al-Tubaikh, 1/e p135]

Salt-and-pepper skull

- Radiograph of the skull in a patient with primary hyperparathyroidism
- A classic salt-and-pepper appearance is indicative of trabecular resorption

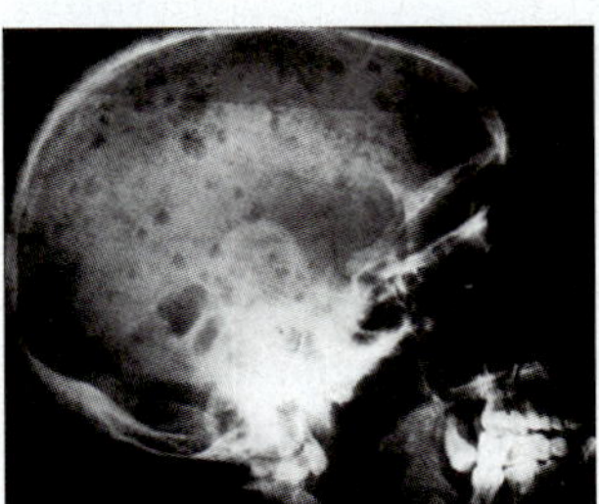

Fig. Salt and pepper skull

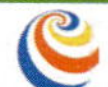 HIGH YIELD MCQs ANSWERS WITH EXPLANATIONS 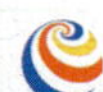

1. **Ans. (c) Microscopic exam of synovial fluid**
   [Ref. Pathobiology of Human Disease by McManus, 1/e p1946]
   - Synovial fluid microscopy is Gold standard investigation for diagnosis of crystal arthritis
   - Examination of synovial fluid under polarized light may reveal either urate or pyrophosphate crystals caused by gout or pseudogout

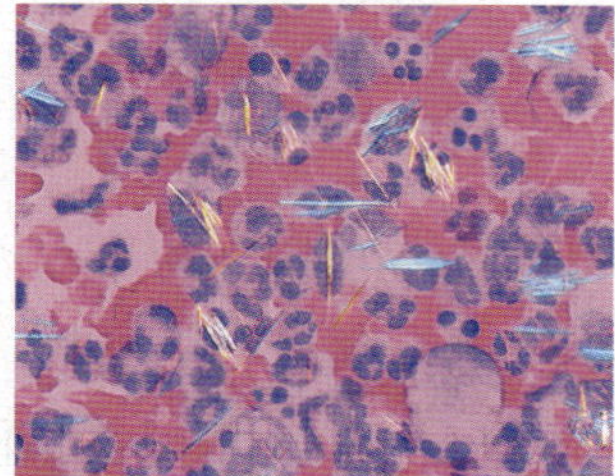

Fig. Synovial fluid (polarised light)

2. **Ans. (d) Bone scan**
   [Ref. David Sutton, 7/e p1248-1249]

3. **Ans. (d) Oblique view**
   [Ref. Turek's Orthopaedics: Principles and their Application, 6/e 503]
   - Oblique view of spine display the lamina and articular processes more clearly than AP view/Lateral view

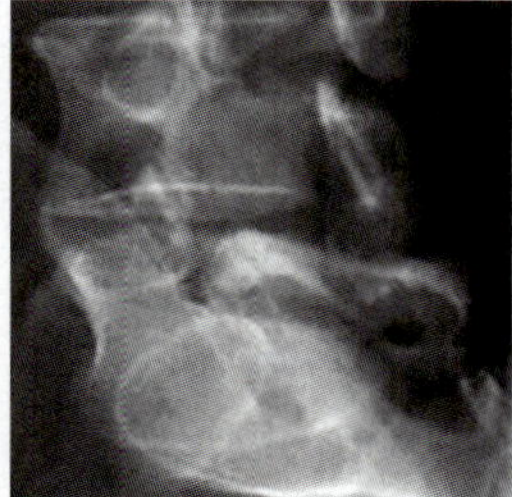

Fig. Scottish Terrier sign

4. **Ans. (b) Spondylolisthesis**
   [Ref. Turek's Orthopaedics: Principles and their Application, 6/e 503]
   - **Spondylolysis**: Shadow of neural arch resembles that of Scottish terrier dog.
   - **Spondylolisthesis**:
     - Beheaded Scottish terrier sign
     - Inverted napoleons hat sign

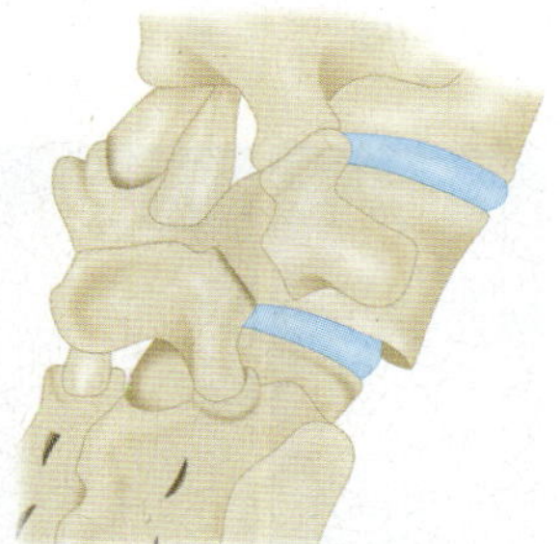

Fig. Beheaded Scottish Terrier sign

5. **Ans. (c) Meningioma**
   [Ref. David Sutton, 7/e p1585]
   - **Meningiomas** are dense fibrous tumours with a high degree of cellularity and little extracellular fluid calcification is common. Plain films may show widening of the optic canal, or hyperostosis of the sphenoid wing. CT generally shows a dense, sharply defined tubular mass.

6. **Ans. (a) Eosinophilic granuloma; (d) Malignancy**
   [Ref. David Sutton, 7/e p1660]
   - Commonest tumors affecting the vertebrae are metastatic
   - Those from the breast and prostate and neuroblastoma frequently induce sclerotic bone reactions, also a feature of Lymphoma and Histiocytosis X
   - Sclerotic vertebra plana in children is characteristically due to the eosinophil granulomatous form of Histiocytosis X

7. **Ans. (d) Juvenile rheumatoid arthritis**
   [Ref. Sumer K Sethi, 6/e p104]
   - Juvenile rheumatoid arthritis is characterized by epiphyseal enlargement, erosions and periosteitis

8. **Ans. (b) Lead poisoning**
   [Ref. Bipin Valchandji Daga, 1/e p266]
   - In lead poisoning normal variant lucent metaphyseal lines are seen

9. **Ans. (c) Rheumatoid arthritis**
   [Ref. Imaging of Arthritis and Metabolic Bone Disease by Barbara N Weissman, 1/e p345]
   - **Wind swept deformity** represents one of a variety of MCP and PIP joint deformities
   - Patients with this deformity have symmetric ulnar subluxations and dislocations of the MCP joint

10. **Ans. (a) Achondroplasia**
    [Ref. Congenital Hand Anomalies and Associated Syndromes by Ghazi M Rayan, 1/e p186]
    - Dwarfism with short extremities, particularly in the proximal (rhizomelic) segments, large head with frontal bossing, hypoplasia of the midface, and trident hands

11. **Ans. (d) Achondroplasia**
    [Ref. David Sutton, 7/e p1140]

    Pelvis in Achondroplasia
    - Pelvis is small and its diameters reduced
    - Iliac blades are particularly small and rather square-the **'tombstone' appearance**
    - Acetabula are set posteriorly and the acetabular roofs are horizontal
    - L5 is deeply set and excessive pelvic tilt causes prominence of the buttocks and an illusion of lordosis
    - Sacrosciatic notch is narrow, with a prominent medially directed spur
    - Pelvic inlet resembles a 'Champagne glass'

12. **Ans. (c) Osteopetrosis**
    [Ref. Sumer K Sethi, 6/e p99]

13. **Ans. (c) Osteomalacia**
    [Ref. Sumer K Sethi, 6/e p96]
    - Osteomalacia: Hallmark is presence of Looser's zone (Pseudofracture)
    - Another feature is cod-fish vertebra

14. Ans. (c) Osteomalacia
[Ref. Sumer K Sethi, 6/e p96]

15. Ans. (c) Osteogenic sarcoma
[Ref. Sumer K Sethi, 6/e p106]

16. Ans. (a) Skull; (b) Phalanges
[Ref. David Sutton, 7/e p1173]

17. Ans. (b) DIP joints in osteoarthritis
[Ref. Sumer K Sethi, 6/e p104]
- Bouchard nodes: PIP
- Heberden nodes: DIP
  (B is proximal to H in alphabet series)

18. Ans. (b) Psoriatic arthropathy
[Ref. Chapman & Nakielny's Aids to Radiological Differential Diagnosis by Stephen G Davie, 1/e p32]
- Resorption of the tuft in Psoriatic arthropathy can precede the skin changes

19. Ans. (c) Pseudogout
[Ref. Gout and Other Crystal Arthropathies by Robert Terkeltaub, 1/e p12]
- Calcium pyrophosphate dihydrate **(CPPD) crystals** can induce low-grade cellular inflammation or incite an episode of acute inflammation, presenting clinically as acute pseudogout

20. Ans. (c) Nonrheumatic ankylosis
[Ref. Rapid Review of Radiology p 219]

21. Ans. (d) Pseudogout
[Ref. Gout and Other Crystal Arthropathies by Terkeltaub, 1/e p12]

22. Ans. (a) Pseudogout
[Ref. Gout and Other Crystal Arthropathies by Terkeltaub, 1/e p12]

23. Ans. (c) Bone erosion
[Ref. Sumer K Sethi, 6/e p104]
- Most important in rheumatoid arthritis is subchondral erosion
- Ball Catchers view is used to detect erosion

24. Ans. (b) Sunray appearance
[Ref. Sumer K Sethi, 6/e p106]

25. Ans. (d) Carcinoma of prostate
[Ref. Bipin Valchandji Daga, 1/e p287]
- Prostrate carcinoma causes osteoblastic lesion

26. Ans. (b) Soft tissue swelling
[Ref. David Sutton, 7/e p1504]

27. Ans. (c) Craniopharyngioma
[Ref. Duke Radiology Case Review by Provenzale, 2/e p318-321]
- **Craniopharyngiomas** can often be suspected on plain skull X-rays on the basis of nodular or curvilinear calcification in the suprasellar region
- On CT scanning cystic components are present with ring or nodular calcification in most children and 80 percent of adults

28. Ans. (d) Subperiosteal resorption of phalanges
[Ref. Sumer K Sethi, 6/e p95]
- **Subperiosteal resorption** which is a hallmark of hyperparathyroidism is best seen on radial aspect of middle phalanx of 2nd and 3rd finger

29. Ans. (a) Thalassemia
[Ref. Sumer K Sethi, 6/e p96]

30. Ans. (c) Osteomalacia
[Ref. Sumer K Sethi, 6/e p96]

31. Ans. (c) Unicameral bone cyst
[Ref. Diagnostic Imaging Trauma, 1/e p140]
- Unicameral bone cyst arises most commonly in proximal humerus.

32. Ans. (b) Aneurysmal bone cyst
[Ref. David Sutton, 7/e p1295-1297]

33. Ans. (a) Congenital haemolytic anemia
[Ref. Sumer K Sethi, 6/e p96]

34. Ans. (b) Floating teeth
[Ref. David Sutton, 7/e p1323-1324]

35. Ans. (a) CT scan
[Ref. Surgery of the Ear and Temporal Bone by Nadol, 1/e p75]
- Diagnostic study of choice for temporal bone injury is CT scan of the temporal bones

36. Ans. (d) Odontoid view
[Ref. Turek's Orthopaedics, 5/e p806]
- Open mouth odontoid view is the best radiographic view to visualize upper cervical C_1 and C_2 vertebra

37. Ans. (a) Dual energy X-ray absorptiometry
[Ref. Harrison's Principles of Internal Medicine, 16/e 227]
- Dual energy X-ray absorptiometry or DEXA is now the gold standard and investigation of choice

38. Ans. (b) Waterston's Cooley's shunt
[Ref. David Sutton, 7/e p48]

39. Ans. (a) Hyperparathyroidism; (b) Poliomyelitis; (d) Marfan's syndrome
[Ref. David Sutton, 7/e p48]

40. Ans. (d) Widening of epiphysis
[Ref. Sumer K Sethi, 6/e p96]

41. Ans. (b) Cupping of metaphysis
[Ref. Sumer K Sethi, 6/e p96]
- Rachitic rosary is a clinical finding and not a radiological feature.

42. Ans. (a) Rickets
[Ref. Sumer K Sethi, 6/e p96]

Rickets
- Saucer epiphysis
- Cupping, fraying, splaying
- Bowing of legs
- Rachitic rosary
- Loss of provisional zone of calcification
- White line of healing
- Craniotabes

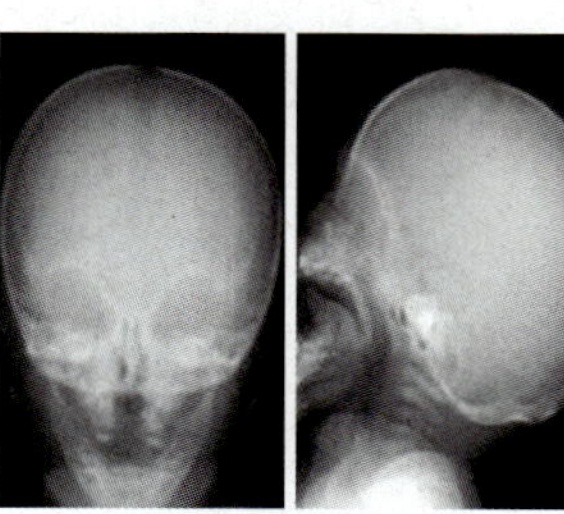

Fig. Craniotabes

43. Ans. (b) **Excision & Bone grafting**

[Ref. Principles, Techniques and Applications in Microsurgery by Ti-Sheng Chang, 1/e p293]

- The initial diagnosis is giant cell tumour
- Usually the management is distal radius resection under epidural anaesthesia with brachial plexus block and the resulting gap to be replaced by a free vascularised bone gap (preferably from ipsilateral fibula)

44. Ans. (b) **T1 T5; (c)** **Sternal angle**

[Ref. Principles and Practice of Anesthesia for Thoracic Surgery edited by Peter Slinger, 1/e p36]

- The tracheal bifurcation is located at the level of the sternal angle anteriorly and the fifth thoracic vertebra posteriorly

45. Ans. **ALL CHOICES**

[Ref. David Sutton, 7/e p1341]

Vertebra Plana [Mnemonic: MELT]

- **M**etastasis
- **M**elanoma
- **E**osinophilic granuloma
- **L**ymphomas
- **T**umours
- **T**uberculosis
- **T**rauma

Fig. Vertebra plana

46. Ans. (a) **Flexion of lumbar spine**

[Ref. Systematic Musculoskeletal Examination by Herbert Frisch, 1/ep84]

Schober's Sign

- With the patient standing, a tape measure is used to measure 10 cm upward from the S1 spinous process
- Then the patient bends the trunk forward, and the increase in the distance between the two reference points is measured
- The normal increase is 4-6 cm
- Smaller increases indicate hypomobility, greater increases mean hypermobility

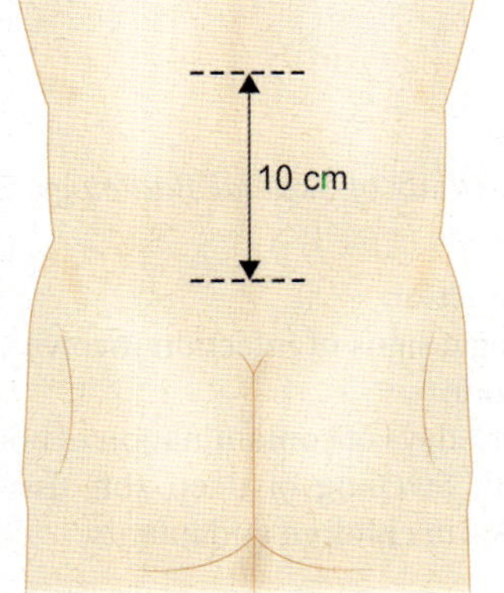

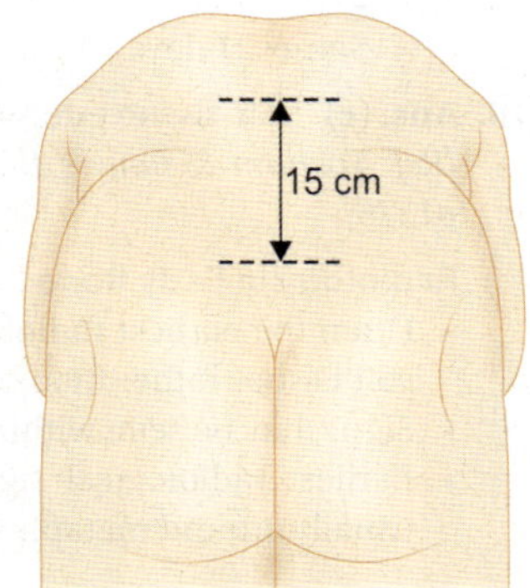

Fig. Schober's sign

47. Ans. (d) **Hypervitaminosis D**

[Ref. Clinical Imaging: An Atlas of Differential Diagnosis by Ronald L Eisenberg, 1/e p10]

- Dense metaphyseal bands are sometimes seen in newborn infants with congenital syphilis
- Hypercalcemia and hypervitaminosis D are less common causes of a single radiodense metaphyseal band

48. Ans. (c) **Beheaded scotty dog terrier sign; (d)** **Inverted napoleons hat sign**

[Ref. Turek's Orthopaedics: Principles and their Application, 6/e 503]

49. Ans. (d) **Driven snow appearance**

[Ref. Essentials of Anatomic Pathology edited by Liang Cheng, 1/e p1097]

- Pindborg tumor appears as a well-demarcated multi-locular radiolucency with calcifications ("Driven snow" appearance)

50. Ans. (a) **Osteosarcoma**

[Ref. Sumer K Sethi, 6/e p106]

51. Ans. (c) **Alkaptonuria**

[Ref. Rapid Review of Radiology p 219]

52. Ans. (a) **Diffuse periosteal reaction**

[Ref. David Sutton, 7/e 197, 538, 565, 1353]

53. Ans. (b) **Soap bubble appearance**

[Ref. Sumer K Sethi, 6/e p96-97]

54. Ans. (a) **Epiphyseal widening**

[Ref. Sumer K Sethi, 6/e p96-97]

55. Ans. (c) **Radiological examination of growing bone ends**

[Ref. Essential Handbook of Practical Orthopaedic Examinations, 1/e p24]

- First (3-6 months) radiological sign of healing is the reappearance of the epiphyseal plate (Caffey) as a faint transverse linear

56. Ans. (b) **Lead poisoning**

[Ref. Bipin Valchandji Daga, 1/e p266]

57. Ans. (c) **Rickets**

[Ref. Sumer K Sethi, 6/e p96-97]

58. Ans. (a) **Hypothyroidism**

[Ref. Pediatric Orthopedics in Practice by Fritz Hefti, 1/e p826]

- Hypothyroidism either occurs as a congenital condition or is acquired as a result of a goiter
- Specifically, the appearance of the epiphyseal ossification centers is delayed (Epiphyseal dysgenesis)
- Abnormal endochondral ossification and epiphyseal dysgenesis are evidenced by the presence of "stippled epiphyses" on X-rays

59. Ans. (b) **Multiple myeloma**

[Ref. Sumer K Sethi, 6/e p110]

- MM shows classical 'rain drop' appearance due to punched out lytic lesion in skull.

60. Ans. (b) **Chondrosarcoma**

[Ref. Sumer K Sethi, 6/e p107]

61. Ans. (b) **Renal cell carcinoma**

[Ref. Sumer K Sethi, 6/e p135]

- Bony metastasis:Lytic expansile lesion

62. Ans. (c) Histiocytosis
[Ref. David Sutton, 7/e p1341]

63. Ans. (a) Most commonly involves thoracic spine
[Ref. David Sutton, 7/e p1663]

- Degeneration in ligaments can lead to fibrocartilaginous metaplasia, calcification, ossification or myxomatous degeneration, all of which can result in diffuse thickening or a focal mass which may compress neural tissue
- Process can involve the posterior longitudinal ligament, the cruciform ligament at the craniocervical junction, the ligamenta flava and the capsular ligaments of the facet joints
- Includes entities, such as ossification of the posterior longitudinal ligament (OPLL), Retro-odontoid pseudo-tumour, Ossification of the ligamentum flavum, Synovial cysts
- Accelerated degenerative changes are seen in such conditions as Ochronosis and Charcot's spine Destructive discovertebral lesions due to non-specific degenerative processes may be seen at one or more levels in ankylosing spondylitis, rheumatoid arthritis, chronic renal failure (dialysis) or as isolated phenomenon
- Process is distinguishable from infection on MRI by absent or non-uniform high signal in the involved disc, and irregularity or fragmentation of the vertebral end-plates rather than destruction

64. Ans. (b) Odontoid view
[Ref. Turek's Orthopaedics: Principles and their Application, 5/e p806]

- Open mouth odontoid view is the best radiographic view to visualize upper cervical C_1 and C_2 vertebra

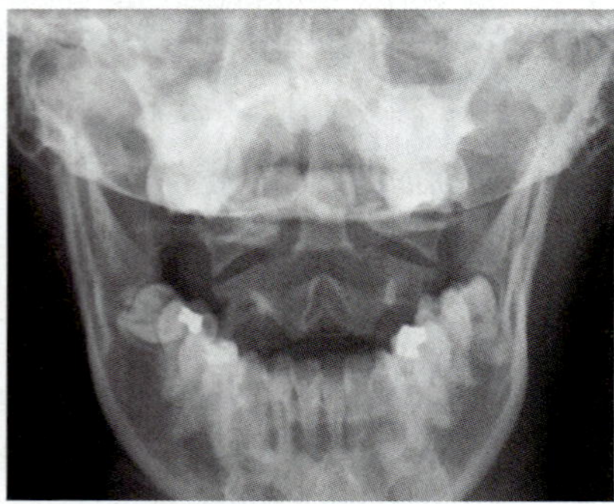

Fig. Open-mouth odontoid view

65. Ans. (b) MRI
[Ref. Bipin Valchandji Daga, 1/e p57]

MRI Spine Indications

- Traumatic paraplegi(a)
- Retroperitoneal tumour with spine extension
- Cauda equina syndrome
- Discitis
- Arachnoiditis
- Radiculopathy
- Syringomyelia

66. Ans. (a) Dual energy X-ray absorptiometry
[Ref. Sumer K Sethi, 6/e p98]

67. Ans. (c) Hip joint
[Ref. Turek's Orthopedics, 6/e p448]

Shenton Line

- An imaginary line drawn along the inferior border of the superior pubic ramus (superior border of the obturator foramen) and along the inferomedial border of the neck of femur
- Normal anatomy: Shenton's line should be continuous and smooth
- Interruption of Shenton's line is seen in:
  - Fracture neck of femur
  - Developmental dysplasia of hip

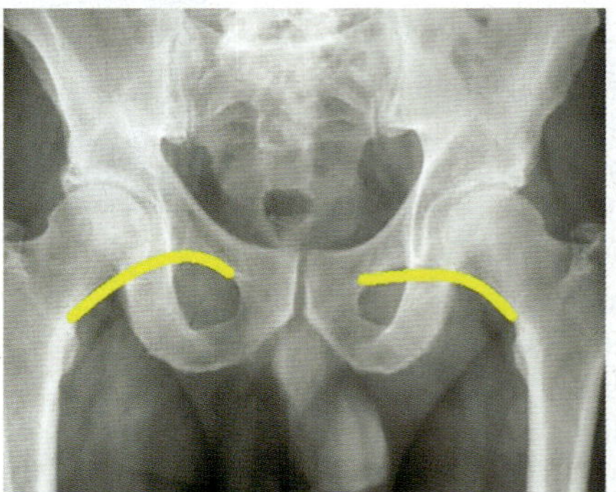

Fig. Shenton's line

68. Ans. (a) MRI
[Ref. Tendon Injuries by Nicola, 1/e p156]

- Stress fractures are often not evident on plain radiographs because of the lack of callous formation
- Therefore, if a stress fracture is suspected, a bone scan or MRI is the investigation of choice

69. Ans. (a) 8 to 10 days and 21 days
[Ref. Yochum & Rowe's Essentials of Skeletal Radiology, 3/e p1378]

- Radiographic Latent period for Acute osteomyelitis
  - Extremities: 10 days
  - Spine: 21 days

70. Ans. (c) Soft-tissue edema
[Ref. Yochum & Rowe's Essentials of Skeletal Radiology, 3/e p1376]

Radiology in Early Bone Infection

- Often the earliest radiologic signs of infection involve the soft tissues rather than bone
- Signs may be seen within 3 days of contamination of bone
- Earliest radiological sign: Swelling of deep soft tissues usually around metaphysis in children and infants

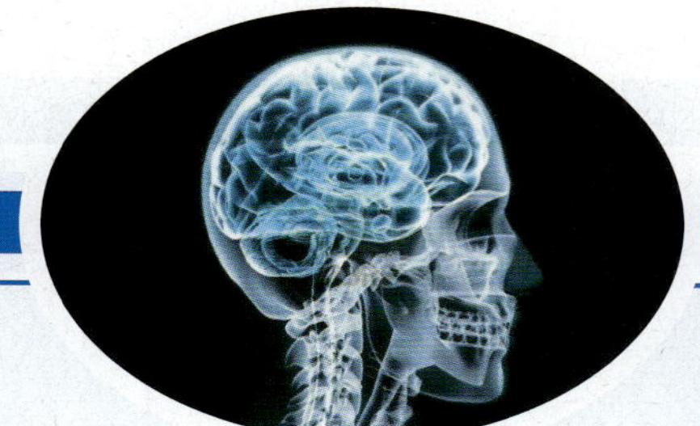

Chapter 6

Central Nervous System and Head & Neck

THEORETICAL CONCEPTS

VI A. SUBARACHNOID HEMORRHAGE

- Investigation of choice for Acute Subarachnoid hemorrhage **(<48 hours)**[Q]: **CT scan**
- Investigation of choice for Chronic Subarachnoid hemorrhage **(>48 hours)** [Q]: **MRI**

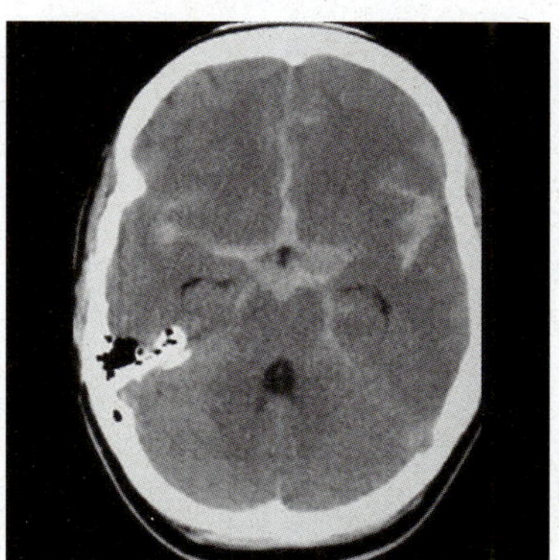

Fig. Sub-arachnoid hemorrhage

VI B. BASAL GANGLIA CALCIFICATION

Common causes	Other causes
Hypoparathyroidism	Birth hypoxia
Hyperparathyroidism	Hallervorden Spatz syndrome
Hypothyroidism	Pseudohypoparathyroidism
Toxoplasmosis	Pseudo-pseudohypoparathyroidism
Wilson disease	Neurocysticercosis
Mitochondrial cytopathies	TORCH
Cockayne syndrome	CNS tuberculosis
Lead poisoning	Methotrexate
Carbon monoxide poisoning	Down's syndrome
Idiopathic (Ageing)	Wilson's disease
Fahr syndrome	Hypothyroidism (Rare cause)
[Mnemonic: High **T**ension **W**ires **M**ay **C**ause **L**eukemic **C**ancer **I**n **F**emales]	

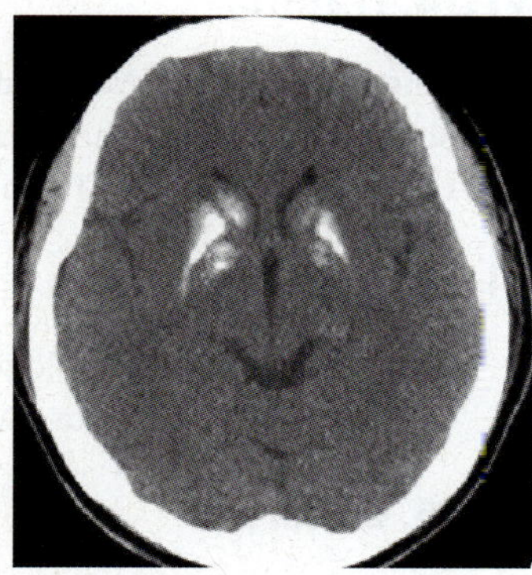

Fig. Basal ganglia calcification

VI C. KEY SIGNS/FEATURES IN CNS RADIOLOGY

- Bracket calcification: Corpus callous lipoma
- **Copper-beaten appearance**: Raised intracranial tension
- Dawson's fingers: Multiple sclerosis
- Dural tail/Flair sign: Meningioma
- Erosion of Dorsum sellae: Raised intracranial tension
- **J-shaped sella**[Q]: Chronic hydrocephalus
- Mother-in-law sign: Meningioma
- **Periventricular calcification**[Q]: Cytomegalovirus
- Radial sunburst, Prolonged bush appearance on angiography: Meningioma
- Suture diastasis[Q]: Raised intracranial tension
- **Tram-track/Rail road calcification**[Q]: Sturge Weber syndrome
- Trouser leg appearance (Myelography) [Q]: Intramedullary block

VI D. PREFERRED INVESTIGATIONS IN CNS, HEAD & NECK CONDITIONS

VI D1. Hemorrhage

- **Acute parenchymal**: CT, MR
- **Subacute/chronic**: MRI
- **Subarachnoid hemorrhage: CT, CTA, lumbar puncture, angiography**
- Aneurysm: Angiography > CTA, MRA

VI D2. Ischemic Infarction

- Hemorrhagic infarction: CT or MRI
- Bland infarction: MRI > CT, CTA, angiography
- Carotid or vertebral dissection: MRI/MRA
- Vertebral basilar insufficiency: CTA, MRI/MRA
- Carotid stenosis: CTA > Doppler ultrasound, MRA

VI D3. Suspected Mass Lesion

- Neoplasm, primary or metastatic: MRI + contrast
- Infection/abscess: MRI + contrast
- Immunosuppressed with focal findings: MRI + contrast
- Vascular malformation: MRI +/– angiography
- White matter disorders: MRI
- Demyelinating disease: MRI +/– contrast
- Dementia: MRI > CT

VI D4. Trauma

- **Acute trauma: CT (Non-contrast)**
- Shear injury/chronic hemorrhage: MRI
- Headache/migraine: CT (Non-contrast)/MRI

VI D5. Seizures

- First time, no focal neurologic deficits: CT as screen +/– contrast
- Partial complex/refractory: MRI with coronal T2W imaging

VI D6. Others

- Cranial neuropathy: MRI with contrast
- Meningeal disease: MRI with contrast

VI D7. Spine

- Low back pain (No neurologic deficits): MRI or CT after 4 weeks
- Low back pain (With focal deficits): MRI > CT
- Spinal stenosis: MRI or CT
- Cervical spondylosis: MRI or CT myelography
- Infection: MRI + contrast, CT
- Myelopathy: MRI + contrast > myelography
- Arteriovenous malformation: MRI, myelography/angiography

IMAGE-BASED QUESTIONS

1. Identify the anatomical structure shown (Arrows) in CT scan of brain in Photograph
[Recent Question 2016]

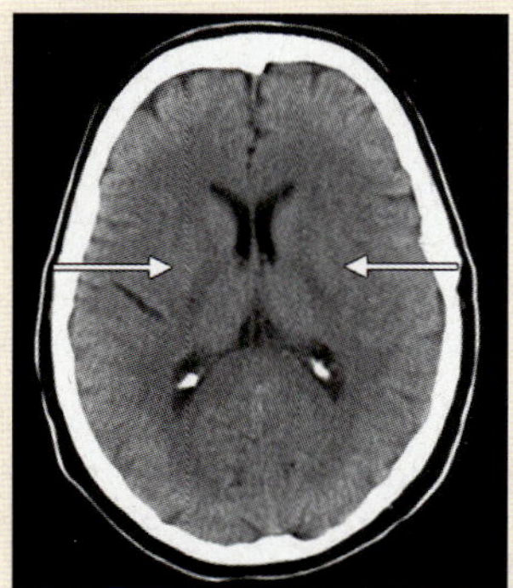

a. Caudate nucleus
b. Lenticular nucleus
c. Thalamus
d. Occipital lobe

2. Diagnose the condition as shown in CT scan head
[Recent Question 2016]

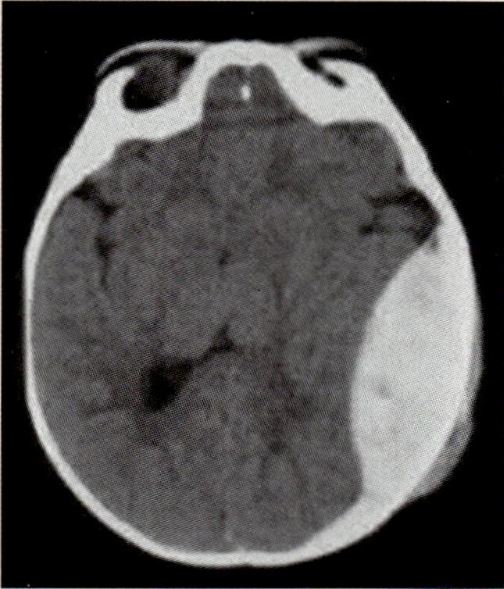

a. Epidural hemorrhage
b. Subdural hemorrhage
c. Subarachnoid hemorrhage
d. Intracerebral hemorrhage

3. Diagnose the condition as shown in CT scan head
[Recent Question 2016]

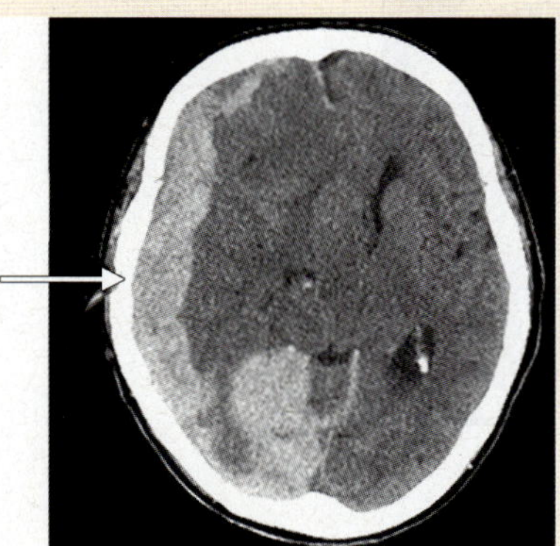

a. Epidural hemorrhage
b. Subdural hemorrhage
c. Subarachnoid hemorrhage
d. Intracerebral hemorrhage

4. Identify the imaging technique shown in Photograph
[Recent Question 2016]

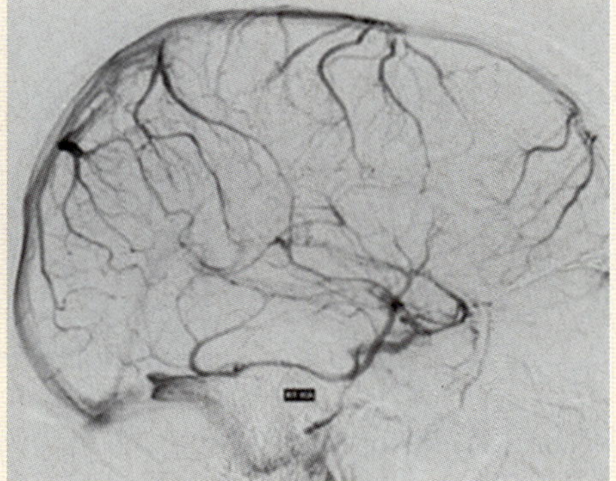

a. Transcranial Doppler Ultrasonography (TDU)
b. Echo-MRI scan
c. DSA (Digital subtraction angiography)
d. MRA (Magnetic resonance angiography)

5. **Plain CT scan of a male who sustained an injury with a baseball bat is given below. Which of the following statements are TRUE regarding this condition?** ***[APPG 2016]***
   P. Middle meningeal artery is the vessel commonly injured
   Q. Usually occurs several weeks after a trivial injury, often forgotten
   R. Lucid interval is classical but seen only in 1/5 to 1/3 patients
   S. May be associated with a Hutchinson pupil

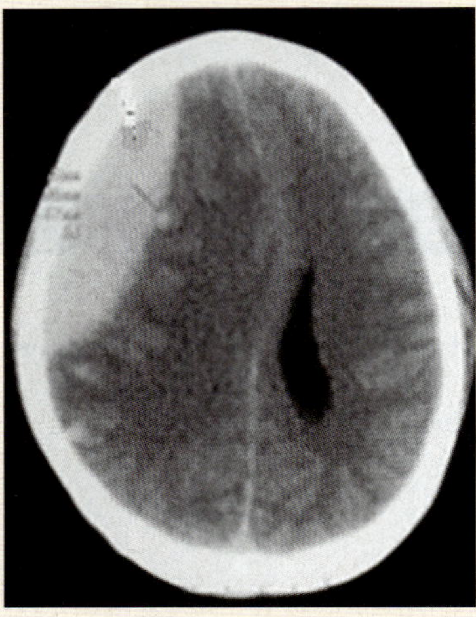

a. Only P, R, S are correct b. Only Q, R, S are correct c. P, Q, R, S all are correct d. Only P, R are correct

6. **These images depict a disease that may present with seizures. Select one True statement.** ***[APPG 2016]***

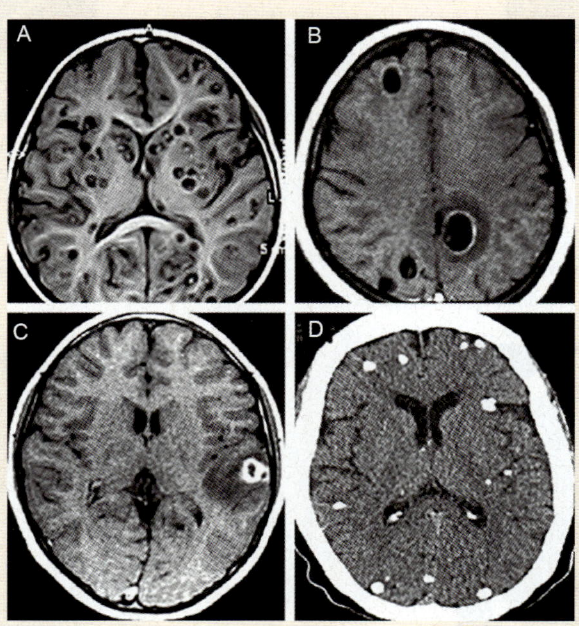

a. IV contrast enhancement of MRI or CT is the preferred imaging mode
b. X-ray of the legs may show multifocal rice grain like calcification
c. Viable cysts appear as thin walled cysts with mural nodule
d. All these statements are true

7. Typical appearance (Arrow) of skull shown in Photograph is found in

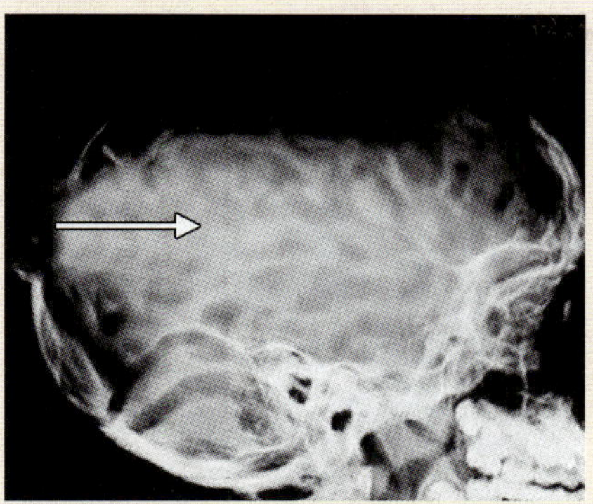

a. Meningioma
b. Craniopharyngioma
c. Raised ICT
d. Tuberous sclerosis

8. X-ray position shown in Photograph is to visualize
[Recent Question 2013]

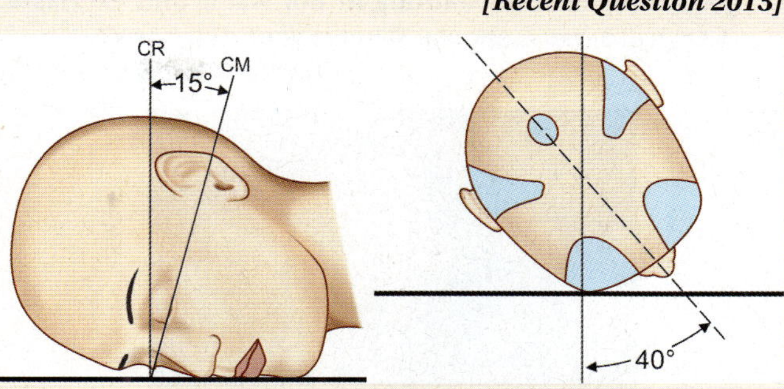

a. Sella turcica
b. Optic foramen
c. Inferior orbital foramen
d. Superior orbital foramen

9. Diagnose Underlying disorder based on Sign (Box) in Photograph

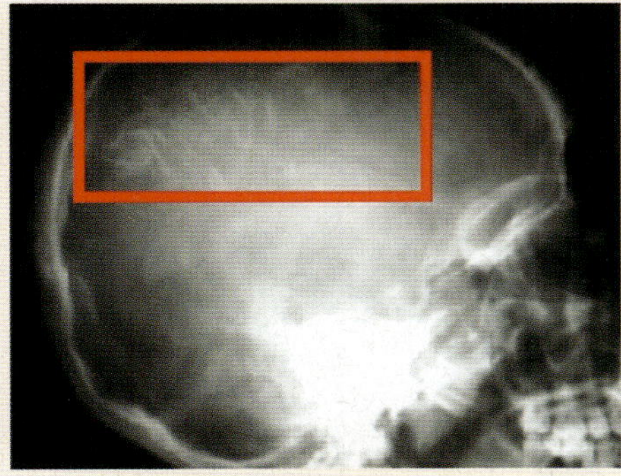

a. Von Hippel-Lindau syndrome
b. Tuberous sclerosis
c. Neurofibromatosis
d. Sturge-Weber syndrome

10. Skull shape shown in the X-ray Photograph is known as

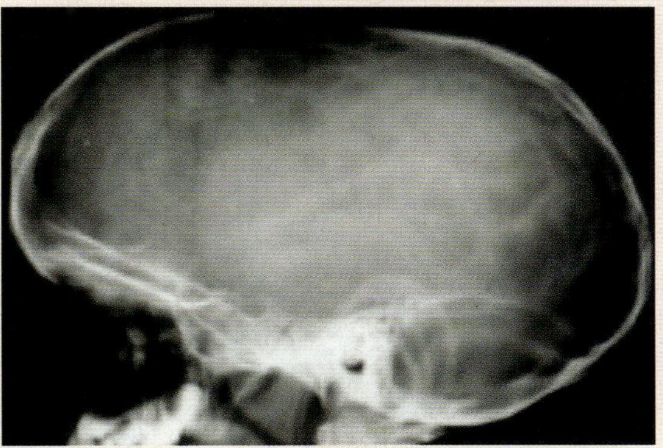

a. Plagiocephaly
b. Macrocephaly
c. Dolichocephaly
d. Platybasia

11. Ego-expansion of Modality shown in Photograph is
[Recent Question 2012]

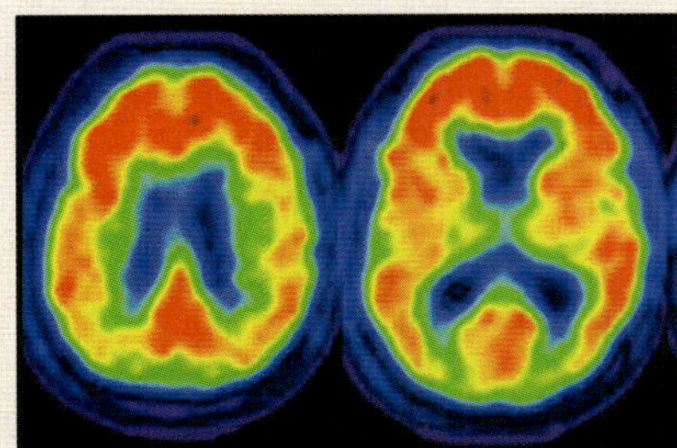

a. Proton Electron Therapy
b. Positive Electron Therapy
c. Photon Emission Tomography
d. Positron Emission Tomography

12. Skull condition (Arrows) in Photograph is characteristic of
[Recent Question 2013]

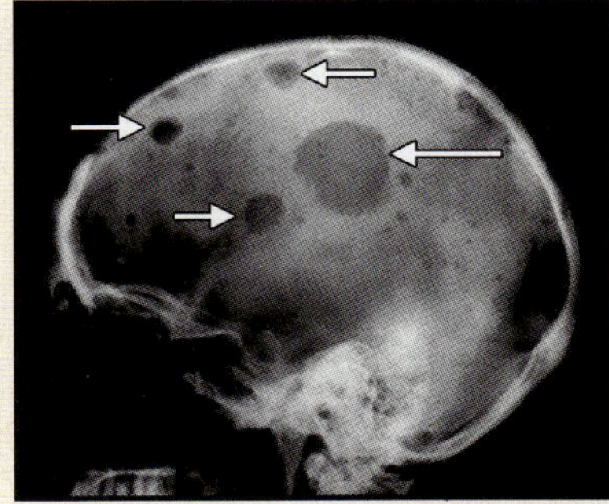

a. Multiple myeloma
b. Pagets disease
c. Tuberculosis
d. Hyperparathyroidism

13. Patient presented with neck pain, rigidity which gets relieved after bathing in hot water and exercises. Cervical X-ray is shown. What is your diagnosis?
[AIIMS PG November 2015]

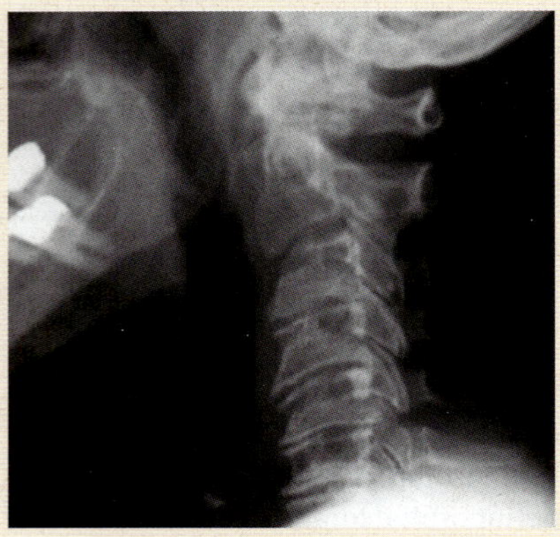

a. Spondylolisthesis
b. Spondylosis
c. Spondyloptosis
d. Spondylitis

14. Identify the salivary gland affected as shown in MRI scan photograph ***[Recent Question 2015]***

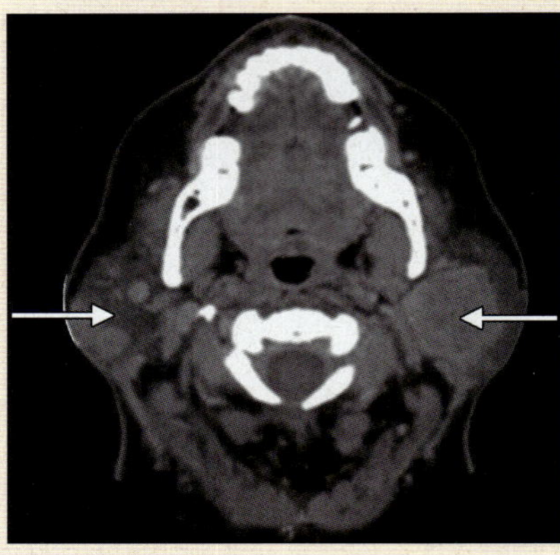

a. Parotid gland
b. Submandibular gland
c. Sublingual gland
d. None of the above

15. MRI of skull is given in the Photograph below. Identify the condition/ structure marked by arrow
[Recent Question 2018]

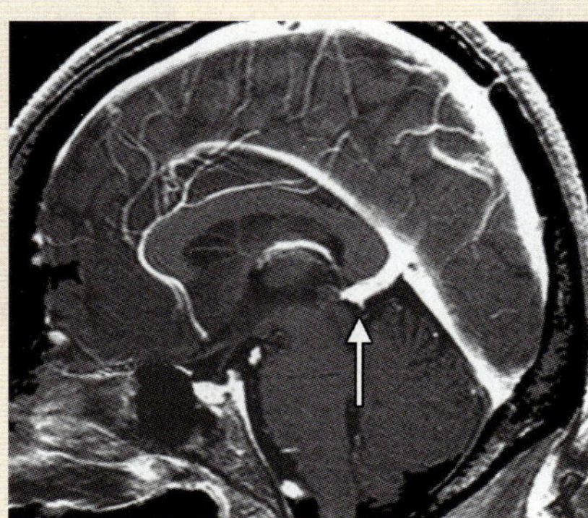

a. Dandy Walker Syndrome
b. Vein of Galen
c. Crouzon syndrome
d. Pneumocephalus

 ANSWERS WITH EXPLANATIONS OF IBQs 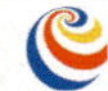

1. Ans. (b) Lenticular nucleus *[Ref. Clinical Radiology by Daffner, 3/e p455]*

CT Scan Brain Anatomical Landmarks

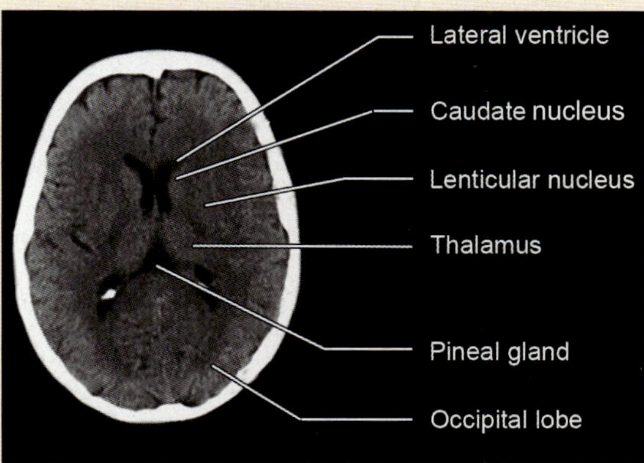

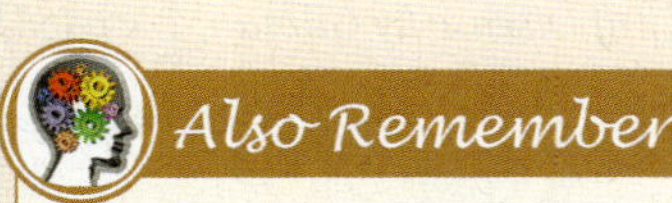

Lentiform nucleus
- Involved in maintaining the muscular tone of the body and assisting in controlling movement, mainly of the limbs of the human body
- In addition is it involved in making find precision movements by reducing any extraneous or unwanted movements

2. Ans. (a) Epidural hemorrhage *[Ref. High-Yield Gross Anatomy by Dudek, 5/e p254]*

Epidural Hematoma
- Location: Lies between skull and outer endosteal layer of Dura mater
- Vessels involved:
  - **Middle meningeal artery (Temporo-parietal locus): Most common**
  - Anterior ethmoidal artery (Frontal locus)
  - Transverse or sigmoid sinus (Occipital locus)
  - Superior sagittal sinus (Vertex locus)
- Presentation:
  - Symptoms develop soon after injury
  - Lucid interval in 20% of cases
- CT appearance: Biconvex lens **(Photograph)**

3. Ans. (b) Subdural hemorrhage *[Ref. High-Yield Gross Anatomy by Dudek, 5/e p254]*

Subdural Hematoma
- Location: Lies between Dura mater and arachnoid mater
- Vessels involved: Bridging veins (Draining into Dura sinus)
- CT appearance: Crescent shape **(Arrow in Photograph)**

4. Ans. (c) DSA (Digital subtraction angiography) *[Ref. Diseases of the Brain, Head & Neck, Spine by Schulthess, 1/e p22]*

Radiological Assessment Methods for Cerebral Vessels
- Cerebral blood flow velocities measurement:
  - Transcranial Doppler Ultrasonography (TCD)
- Structural imaging techniques:
  - Catheter-based Digital Subtraction Angiography (DSA)
  - CT Angiography (CTA)
  - MR Angiography (MRA)
- Physiologic assessment:
  - PET
  - HMPAO SPECT

- 133Xe Clearance
- Xenon-Enhanced CT (Xe/CT)
- Perfusion CT (PCT)
- Diffusion-Weighted/MR Perfusion Imaging

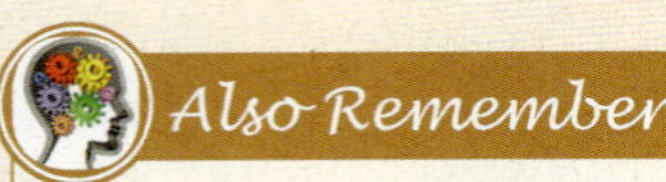

Digital Subtraction Angiography (DSA)

- First introduced (1980) as a direct method of Vessel caliber assessment
- DSA improvised previous angiographic methods: High contrast, high resolution, low artifact images using digital subtraction
- DSA is a fluoroscopic examination:
  - Images acquired through time-controlled X-rays are synchronized to the injection of an iodinated contrast medium into the vasculature via a catheter
  - Images are produced by digitally subtracting extraneous aspects of the image so that the vessels can be visually isolated and evaluated
  - "Digital subtraction" involves recording a precontrast image ("Mask") and subsequently removing the mask from later images

5. Ans. (a) Only P, R, S are correct *[Ref. High-Yield Gross Anatomy by Dudek, 5/e p254]*

- Given CT scan **Photograph** shows a case of epidural hemorrhage

6. Ans. (d) All these statements are true *[Ref. Neurobiology of Disease by Gilman, 1/e p465]*

Neurocysticercosis (Photograph)

- IV contrast enhancement of MRI or CT is the preferred imaging mode
- Viable cysts are thin walled (typically 1-2 cm in diameter) with a mural nodule that represents the invaginated scolex
- "Rice grain calcification" is characteristic of infection with Taenia solium (cysticercosis); when the inflammatory response of the host kills the larval cysts (cysticerci), they undergo granulomatous change and become calcified

7. Ans. (c) Raised ICT *[Ref. Sumer K Sethi, 5/e p85]*

- Copper beaten/Beaten brass skull: Prominence of convolutional markings (gyral impressions on the inner table of the skull) seen throughout the skull vault, a sign of Intracranial tension

8. Ans. (b) Optic foramen *[Ref. Radiological Anatomy by Nagy, 1/e p464]*

- Rhese Method: Parieto-Orbital oblique Position is used to visualize Optic canal/foramen

9. Ans. (d) Sturge Weber syndrome *[Ref. Sumer K Sethi, 5/e p87]*

- 'Tram-track' subcortical calcification is seen in Sturge Weber Syndrome

10. Ans. (c) Dolichocephaly *[Ref. Neuroradiology by Nadgir, 3/e p300]*

Craniostenosis/Craniosynostosis (and Suture Involved)

- Dolicocephaly (Long and thin skull): Sagittal suture
- Brachycephaly (Round and Foreshortened): Coronal suture
- Turricephaly (High riding top): Lambdoid suture
- Plagiocephaly (Asymmetric): Any unilateral suture
- Trigonocephaly (Anteriorly pointed head): Metopic suture

11. Ans. (d) Positron Emission Tomography *[Ref. Sumer K Sethi, 5/e p20]*

Basic Principle of Pet Scan

- Concentration of marker is higher at the critical spots (FDG Fluorodeoxyglucose) because of the increased sugar consumption of the cancerous cells
- When the positron created during the decay of the isotope in the marker meets an electron, they annihilate, resulting in the simultaneous release of two 511 keV gamma photons travelling in nearly opposite directions
- Detection of these pairs can determine the activity concentration using the density of the LORs (line of response) connecting the detection points

12. Ans. (a) Multiple myeloma *[Ref. Skeletal Radiology by Rowe, 3/e p1172]*

Punched-Out/Rain-Drop Skull

- Description:
  - Appearance of multiple, well-defined lytic lesions (punched out lesions) of various size scattered throughout the skull
  - Analogy to rain hitting a surface and splashing, where it leaves a random pattern of dark spots
- Seen in: Multiple myeloma

13. Ans. (b) Spondylosis *[Ref. Lippincott's Anatomy and Embryology, 1/e p103]*

- Spondylitis: Inflammatory spine leading to pain and stiffness in neck
- Spondylosis: Stiffening of spine (ankylosis) due to any degenerative lesion, causing pressure on nerve roots (pain and paraesthesia)
  - Pain is relieved by gentle heat and massage
  - X-ray: Osteophytes, Narrowed joint space, Endplate sclerosis
- Spondylolysis: Defect in Pars interarticularis of affected vertebra
- Spondylolisthesis: Anterior displacement of a vertebra in relation to one below
- Spondyloptosis: Most extreme form of spondylolisthesis where posterior edge of upper vertebra is at Anterior margin of lower vertebra (Just about to 'fall off')

14. Ans. (a) Parotid gland *[Ref. Radiopedia.org]*

- CT and MRI provide useful additional diagnostic imaging if a malignancy is suspected
- Sensitivity of CT/MRI approaches 100% for detecting parotid neoplasms

15. Ans. (b) Vein of Galen *[Ref. Neuroradiology by Castillo, 3/e p118]*

Vein of Galen

- Located under the cerebral hemispheres and drains the anterior and central regions of the brain into the sinuses of the posterior cerebral fossa
- Vein of Galen (Great cerebral vein/Great vein of Galen): Short trunk formed by the union of the two internal cerebral veins and basal veins of Rosenthal (Lying in the quadrigeminal cistern)
- Vein of Galen aneurysmal malformation is a choroidal type of arteriovenous malformation involving the vein of Galen forerunner and is distinct from an arteriovenous malformation with venous drainage into a dilated, but already formed, vein of Galen
- Aneurysmal malformations of the vein of Galen (VGAM) typically result in high-output congestive heart failure or may present with developmental delay, hydrocephalus, and seizures.

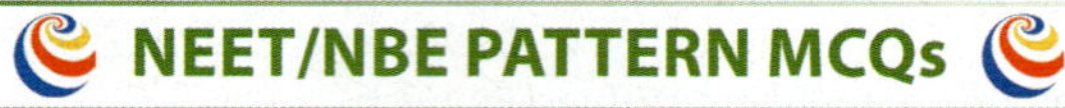

NEET/NBE PATTERN MCQs

1. Investigation of choice in Acute Stroke is *[Recent Question 2016]*
a. X-ray b. USG
c. CT scan d. MRI scan

2. Intracranial calcification can be best diagnosed by *[NBE FMGE September 2010]*
a. Plain X-ray b. CT scan
c. MRI d. PET scan

3. Cerebral calcification is a feature of *[NBE DNB 1996, 1999]*
a. Congenital syphilis
b. Cytomegalic inclusion disease
c. Alzheimer's syndrome
d. Toxoplasmosis
e. Fanconi's syndrome

4. Tiger eye sign on MRI is seen in *[Recent Question 2012]*
a. Hallervorden-Spatz disease
b. CHPS
c. Achalasia Cardia d. Tuberculosis

5. Sun ray calcification in brain is seen in *[NBE DNB 1992]*
a. Hypoparathyroidism b. Tuberous sclerosis
c. CMV infection d. Meningioma

6. Features of increased ICT are following, except *[NBE DNB 1996, 1999]*
a. Suture separation
b. Erosion of post clinoid process
c. Erosion of ant. clinoid process
d. Osteosclerosis

7. A patient is suspected to have vestibular schwannoma. The investigation of choice for its diagnosis is
a. Contrast enhanced CT scan *[Recent Question 2012]*
b. Gadolinium enhanced MRI
c. SPECT
d. PET scan

8. Radiological diagnosis of multiple sclerosis can be done by *[NBE FMGE March 2010]*
a. CT scan b. MRI
c. Carotid angiography d. Pneumoencephalography

9. Earliest radiological sign of raised intracranial tension in a child is *[NBE DNB December 2011]*
a. Sutural widening b. Silver Beaten Skull
c. Erosion of Dorsum sella d. Widening of Optic canal

10. Investigation of choice for intramedullary SOL is *[Recent Question 2012]*
a. MRI b. USG
c. CT d. X-ray

11. Signs of increased intracranial tension in a child in a skull X-ray *[NBE DNB 1996, 2007]*
a. Separation of the sutures
b. Tense anterior fontanelle
c. Silver beaten appearance of the bones
d. All of the above

12. Investigation of choice for acute subarachnoid haemorrhage is *[NBE FMGE March 2006]*
a. Lumbar puncture
b. Computerised tomography
c. MRI
d. Trans-cranial Doppler

13. Investigation of choice for acute subarachnoid hemorrhage is *[NBE DNB 2011]*
a. MRI b. CT scan
c. Plain X-ray skull d. Angiography

14. Commonest calcified brain tumour is *[NBE DNB 1993]*
a. Craniopharyngioma
b. Meningioma
c. Tuberculoma d. Medulloblastoma

15. Basal ganglia calcification is seen in all except *[NBE FMGE September 2007]*
a. Acromegaly b. Hypothyroidism
c. Hypoparathyroidism d. Hyperparathyroidism

16. Intracranial calcifications are preferably diagnosed by *[NBE FMGE September 2012]*
a. X-rays b. Ultrasonography
c. CT scan d. MRI scan

17. Best route for Cerebral angiography
a. Transbrachial route *[NBE FMGE March 2009]*
b. Transradial route
c. Transaxillary route
d. Transfemoral route

18. Investigation of choice in acute subarachnoid hemorrhage is *[NBE FMGE September 2011, September 2012]*
a. Ultrasound
b. Non-contrast CT
c. Contrast-enhanced CT
d. Contrast –enhanced MRI

19. Rhese view is used for *[Recent Question 2013]*
a. Superior orbital foramen
b. Inferior orbital foramen
c. Optic foramen
d. Sella turcica

20. CT scan finding in carotid cavernous sinus fistula is *[Recent Question 2013]*
a. Enlarged superior ophthalmic vein
b. Enlarged inferior ophthalmic vein
c. Enlarged superior ophthalmic artery
d. Enlarged inferior ophthalmic artery

21. Prevertebral space thickness in adult is *[Recent Question 2013, 2015]*
a. 7 mm b. 14 mm
c. 22 mm d. 30 mm

22. X-ray view for supra orbital fissure *[Recent Question 2013]*
a. Towne's b. AP
c. Caldwell d. Basal

23. Epidermoid cyst can be differentiated from arachnoid cyst by *[Recent Question 2013]*

a. MRI b. USG
c. Myelography d. CT scan

24. Punched out lesions in skull are seen in *[Recent Question 2013, 2015]*

a. Multiple myeloma b. Hyperparathyroidism
c. Paget's disease d. None

25. In fracture of nose, which view X-ray taken *[Recent Question 2013, 2015]*

a. Waters view b. Caldwells view
c. Lateral view d. Occlusive anterior view

26. On imaging diffuse axonal injury is characterized by *[Recent Question 2013]*

a. Multiple small petechial hemorrhage
b. Patch ill defined low density lesion mixed with small hyperdense of petechial hemorrhage
c. Crescentic extra-axial hematoma
d. White matter lucencies

27. Investigation of choice for focal neurologic deficit in emergency room is *[Recent Question 2013, 2014]*

a. CT b. MRI
c. Lumbar puncture d. CECT

28. Investigation of choice for retinoblastoma is *[Recent Question 2014, 2015]*

a. X-ray b. USG
c. CECT d. MRI

29. Brain infarct is earliest diagnosed by *[Recent Question 2015]*

a. X-ray b. Diffusion weighted MRI
c. NCCT d. CECT

30. Soap bubble appearance on MRI brain is characteristic of *[Recent Question 2017]*

a. Tubercular meningitis b. Neurocysticercosis
c. Cryptococcal cysts d. Ependymoma

31. "Lemon sign" & "Banana sign" are see in *[Recent Question 2017]*

a. Down syndrome b. Spina bifida
c. Turner syndrome
d. Periventricular leukomalacia

32. Stenver's view is used for *[Recent Question 2017]*

a. Superior orbital foramen
b. Inferior orbital foramen
c. Internal auditory canal
d. Sella turcica

33. In Multiple sclerosis, on MRI lesions are seen in *[Recent Question 2017]*

a. White matter b. Grey matter
c. Thalamus d. Basal ganglia

34. Characteristic CT finding in Acute Subdural hemorrhage *[Recent Question 2017]*

a. Crescent shaped hyperdense lesion
b. Biconvex hyperdense lesion
c. Biconcave hyperdense lesion
d. Crescent shaped hypodense lesion

35. Delta sign on CT is seen in *[Recent Question 2017]*

a. Gradenigo syndrome b. Subdural hematoma
c. Extradural hematoma d. Sagittal sinus thrombosis

36. Hummingbird sign in brain MRI is seen in *[Recent Question 2017]*

a. Multiple sclerosis
b. Progressive supranuclear palsy
c. Parkinson's disease
d. Alzheimer disease

37. Lyre sign is seen in *[Recent Question 2017]*

a. Meningioma b. Acoustic neuroma
c. Sagittal sinus thrombosis
d. Carotid body tumor

38. Pepper pot appearance of skull is seen in *[Recent Question 2017]*

a. Multiple myeloma b. Hyperparathyroidism
c. Sickle cell anemia d. Fibrous dysplasia

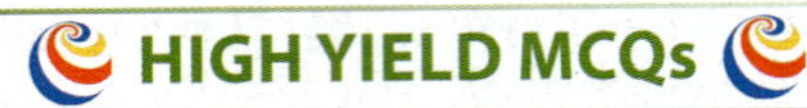

HIGH YIELD MCQs

1. **X-ray view for supra orbital fissure** *[AIIMS PGMEE 1997]*
   a. Towne's b. AP
   c. Caldwell d. Basal

2. **'Tram-track appearance' on CT scan of head is seen in** *[Recent Question 2017, AIIMS PGMEE 2001]*
   a. Sturge Weber syndrome
   b. Von Hipple Lindau syndrome
   c. Tuberous sclerosis
   d. Neurofibroma

3. **Geographic lytic lesions in vault of skull with beveled edges are seen with** *[AIIMS PGMEE 1997]*
   a. Multiple myeloma b. Eosinophilic granuloma
   c. Hyperparathyroidism d. Reticular cell carcinoma

4. **Multiple Punched out lesions on skull X-ray is found in** *[Recent Question 2017, AIIMS PGMEE 1994]*
   a. Down's syndrome b. Hyperparathyroidism
   c. Multiple Myeloma d. All of the above

5. **All are X-ray findings of retinoblastoma except** *[AIIMS PGMEE 1999]*
   a. Widening of optic canal
   b. Intra cerebral calcification
   c. Intraocular calcification
   d. Secondaries in cranial bones

6. **Intracranial calcification with cystic lesion in plain X-ray skull is seen in** *[AIIMS PGMEE 1996]*
   a. Meningioma b. Glioma
   c. Craniopharyngioma d. Medulloblastoma

7. **All are the characteristics of raised ICT on a plain radiology except** *[AIIMS PGMEE 1998]*
   a. Erosion of dorsum sellae
   b. Ballooning of sella
   c. Increased convolutions
   d. Sutural diastasis

8. **Findings in meningioma are all except** *[PGI 1997]*
   a. Vascular markings around falx
   b. Calcification
   c. Erosion d. Osteosclerosis

9. **Meningioma on plain radiography reveals** *[PGI 2009]*
   a. Calcification b. Erosion
   c. Sutural diastasis d. Osteosclerosis
   e. Vascular erosion

10. **Suprasellar calcification with growth retardation is seen in** *[AIIMS PGMEE 1995]*
    a. Pineal body tumour b. Pituitary tumour
    c. Thalamic tumour d. Craniopharyngioma

11. **Commonest calcifying brain tumour in a child is** *[AIIMS PGMEE 1993]*
    a. Medulloblastoma b. Craniopharyngioma
    c. Glioma d. Meningioma

12. **Investigation which should not be done in a patient with brain tumour** *[All India PGMEE 1997]*
    a. CT Scan b. Lumbar Puncture
    c. MRI d. X-ray

13. **Sonographic finding of Spina bifida** *[PGI 2004]*
    a. Ventriculomegaly
    b. Obliteration of cisterna magna
    c. Small BPD
    d. Abnormal curvature of cerebellum
    e. Club foot

14. **On MRI the differential diagnosis of spinal cord edema is** *[AIIMS PGMEE 2006]*
    a. Myelodysplasia b. Myelomalacia
    c. Myeloschisis d. Cord tumors

15. **Basal ganglia calcification is seen in all except** *[All India PGMEE 2007]*
    a. Hypoparathyroidism b. Wilson's disease
    c. Perinatal hypoxia d. Fahr's syndrome

16. **Subdural haematoma most commonly results from** *[AIIMS PGMEE 2001]*
    a. Rupture of intracranial aneurysm
    b. Rupture of cerebral AVM
    c. Injury to cortical bridging veins
    d. Hemophilia

17. **Characteristic of subdural hematoma is** *[AIIMS PGMEE 1998]*
    a. Convex hyperdense
    b. Concavo-convex hyperdense
    c. Biconvex hyperdense
    d. Concavo-convex hypodense

18. **Investigation of choice for acute subarachnoid haemorrhage** *[All India PGMEE 1998]*
    a. Angiography b. CT-Scan
    c. MRI d. Enhanced MRI

19. **Calcification of basal ganglia is seen in all except** *[AIIMS PGMEE 1997]*
    a. Berry's aneurysm b. Cysticercosis
    c. Idiopathic hyperparathyroidism
    d. Wilson's disease

20. **Which of the following is the best choice to evaluate radiologically a posterior fossa tumour?** *[All India PGMEE 2003]*
    a. CT scan b. MRI
    c. Angiography d. Myelography

21. **Basal ganglia calcification is seen in** *[PGI 2003]*
    a. Hyperparathyroidism b. Hyperthyroidism
    c. Hypoparathyroidism d. Hypothyroidism
    e. Acromegaly

22. **Calcification is best detected by** *[PGI 2003]*
    a. X-ray b. USG
    c. CT scan d. MRI
    e. PET scan

23. **Which one of the following is the most preferred route to perform cerebral angiography?** *[All India PGMEE 2005]*
    a. Transfemoral route b. Transaxillary route
    c. Direct carotid puncture d. Transbrachial route

24. Contrast media of choice for myelogram is *[AIIMS PGMEE 1993]*
a. Urografin 7% b. Conray 47
c. Iohexol d. Biligrafin

25. Suprasellar calcification is characteristic of *[All India PGMEE1992]*
a. Toxoplasmosis b. Cysticercosis
c. Craniopharyngioma d. CMV

26. Physiological calcification of Skull in X-ray is seen in *[PGI 2001]*
a. Pineal gland b. Choroid plexus
c. Red nucleus d. Basal ganglion

27. Periventricular calcification is often due to *[PGI 1997]*
a. Toxoplasmosis b. Cytomegalic infection
c. Congenital syphilis d. All of the above

28. Local cerebral lesion with ring on CT scan is caused by *[PGI 2002]*
a. Toxoplasmosis b. Intracranial hemorrhage
c. Cysts d. Hamartoma

29. A new born presents with congestive heart failure resistant to treatment; on examination has bulging anterior fontanelle with a bruit on auscultation. Transfontanellar USG shows a hypoechoic midline mass with dilated lateral ventricles. Most likely diagnosis will be *[AIIMS PGMEE 2010]*
a. Encephalocele
b. Medulloblastoma
c. Arachnoid cyst
d. Vein of Galen malformation

30. Which of the following is not a MRI feature of Mesial temporal sclerosis? *[All India PGMEE 2009]*
a. Atrophy of mammilary body
b. Atrophy of fornix
c. Blurring of Grey white matter junction of ipsilateral temporal lobe
d. Atrophy of hippocampus

31. A 48-year-old woman comes with b/l progressive weakness of both lower limbs, spasticity, urinary hesitancy & mild impairment of respiratory movements. MRI shows an intradural mid-dorsal midline enhancing lesion. What is the likely diagnosis? *[AIIMS PGMEE 2006, 2010, All India PGMEE 2007]*
a. Intradural lipoma b. Meningioma
c. Neuroenteric cyst d. Dermoid cyst

32. Tumor associated with extracranial spread *[AIIMS PGMEE 2010]*
a. Ependymoma b. Medulloblastoma
c. Glioblastoma multiforme
d. Choroid plexus papilloma

33. In 7-year-old posterior fossa mass with cyst formation, hypodense on CT, hyper intense on T2WI and showing post gadolinium nodule enhancement is *[AIIMS PGMEE 2010]*
a. Medulloblastoma b. Ependymoma
c. Astrocytoma d. Cysticercous

34. A male was brought unconscious to the hospital with external injuries. CT shows no midline shift, but basal cisterns were full with multiple small haemorrhage. The most probable diagnosis is *[All India PGMEE 2007, AIIMS PGMEE 2006]*
a. Brain contusion b. Diffuse axonal injury
c. Subdural hemorrhage d. Multiple infarct

35. A middle aged man presents with progressive atrophy weakness of hand & forearms. On examination he is found to have slight spasticity of the leg, generalized hyper-reflexia and increased signal in the corticospinal tracts on T2 weighted MRI. The most likely diagnosis
a. Multiple sclerosis *[AIIMS PGMEE 2004]*
b. Amyotrophic lateral sclerosis
c. Subacute combined degeneration
d. Progressive spinal muscular atrophy

36. Which of the following is the most common cause of a mixed cystic and solid suprasellar mass seen on cranial MR scan of a 1 year old child? *[AIIMS PGMEE 2005]*
a. Pituitary Adenoma. b. Craniopharyngioma
c. Optic chiasma glioma d. Germinoma

37. A 6-year-old boy has been complaining of headache, ignoring to see the objects on the side for 4 months. On Examination, he is not mentally retarded, his grades at school are good & visual acuity is diminished in both the eyes, visual charting showed significant field defect. CT scan of the head showed suprasellar mass with calcification. Which of the following is the most probable diagnosis? *[AIIMS PGMEE 2004]*
a. Astrocytoma b. Craniopharyngioma
c. Pituitary adenoma d. Meningioma

38. A 15-year-old boy had 1-12 partial complex seizures per day in spite of adequate 4 drug antiepileptic regime. He had history of repeated high grade fever in childhood. MRI for epilepsy protocol revealed normal brain scan. What should be the best non-invasive strategy to make a definite diagnosis so that he can be prepared to undergo epilepsy surgery? *[AIIMS PGMEE 2002]*
a. Interictal scalp EEG
b. Video EEG
c. Interictal 18F-FDg PET
d. Video EEG with Ictal 99m Tc-HMP AO Brain SPECT

39. Extensive involvement of deep white matter with bilateral hyperdense thalami on non-contrast CT scan of the brain is virtually diagnostic of *[AIIMS PGMEE 2007]*
a. Alexander's disease
b. Krabbe's disease
c. Canavan's disease
d. Metachromatic leukodystrophy

40. Which of the following is classic CT appearance of an acute Subdural hematoma? *[All India PGMEE 2004]*
a. Lentiform-shaped hyperdense lesion
b. Crescent-shaped hypo dense lesion
c. Crescent-shaped hyperdense lesion
d. Lentiform-shaped hypo dense lesion

41. The first investigation of choice in a patient with suspected subarachnoid haemorrhage should be *[All India PGMEE 2004]*

a. Non-contrast computed tomography
b. CSF examination
c. Magnetic resonance imaging [MRI]
d. Contrast-enhanced computed tomography

42. Best test to determine etiology of SAH *[AIIMS PGMEE 1995]*

a. Enhanced CT b. Unenhanced CT
c. Intra arterial digital Substraction Angiography
d. MRI

43. CT scan of a patient with history of head injury shows a biconvex hyperdense lesion displacing the grey-white matter interface. The most likely diagnosis is *[All India PGMEE 2003]*

a. Subdural hematoma b. Diffuse axonal injury
c. Extradural hematoma d. Hemorrhagic contusion

44. Investigation of choice for Juvenile nasoangiofibroma *[AIIMS PGMEE 1997]*

a. X-ray b. Angiography
c. USG
d. CT Scan - contrast enhanced

45. A patient is suspected to have Vestibular Shwannoma. The investigation of choice for its diagnosis is *[All India PGMEE 2004]*

a. Contrast enhanced CT scan
b. Gadolinium enhanced MRI
c. SPECT
d. PET scan

46. Best view for visualizing Sella turcica on X-ray *[All India PGMEE 1994]*

a. AP View b. Town's view
c. Lateral view d. Open mouth view

47. Parameningeal Rhabdomyosarcoma is best diagnosed by *[AIIMS PGMEE 2001]*

a. MRI b. CT scan
c. SPECT d. PET

48. A 30-year-old man presents with 6 month history of nasal discharge, facial pain and fever. On antibiotic therapy, fever subsided. After 1 month again had symptoms of mucopurulent discharge from the middle meatus and the mucosa of the meatus appeared congested and oedematous. Next best investigation would be *[AIIMS PGMEE 2007]*

a. MID of the sinuses.
b. Non-Contrast CT of the nose and para-nasal sinuses
c. Plain X-ray of the para-nasal sinuses
d. Inferior meatus puncture

49. Which one of the following is the most preferred route to perform cerebral angiography? *[All India PGMEE 2005]*

a. Transfemoral route b. Transaxillary route
c. Direct carotid puncture d. Transbrachial route

50. Investigation of choice in acute head injury is *[AIIMS November 2014]*

a. NCCT b. MRI
c. CECT d. X-ray

51. Radiological investigation of choice for diagnosis of Neurocysticercosis is *[Recent Question 2014]*

a. X-ray plain b. CECT
c. Non contrast CT d. MRI

52. Diagnostic investigation of choice for Orbital fractures is *[Recent Question 2014]*

a. X-ray b. CT scan
c. Thin slice CT scan d. MRI scan

53. Expansion of space on myelography is seen in *[AIIMS PG May 2015]*

a. Intramedullary tumor
b. Intradural tumor
c. Extramedullary intradural tumor
d. Extradural tumor

54. On CT scan, extradural hemorrhage is *[PGMCET 2015]*

a. Biconvex in shape
b. Concavo-convex in shape
c. Shows extension within sulci
d. Cannot cross midline

55. Most accurate diagnostic method for detecting Intracranial haemorrhage is *[PGMCET 2015]*

a. Digital Substraction Angiography (DSA)
b. CT scan
c. MRI d. Trans Cranial Doppler

56. All are the characteristics of raised ICT on a plain radiograph EXCEPT *[PGMCET 2015]*

a. Sellar erosion b. Suture diastasis
c. Ballooning of sella
d. Increased convolutional markings

 NEET/NBE PATTERN MCQs ANSWERS WITH EXPLANATIONS 

1. Ans. (d) MRI scan
[Ref. Oxford Desk Reference: Geriatric Medicine, 1/e p312]

Radiological IOC in Few Neurological Conditions

- Acute stroke: MRI (Diffusion weighted imaging)
- Subarachnoid/Intracerebral hemorrhage: CT scan
- Hydrocephalus: MRI scan
- Bone injury: CT scan
- Brain stem/Cerebellar pathology: CT scan
- Encephalitis: CT scan
- Meningitis/Meningeal pathology: CT scan
- Spinal cord compression: CT scan

2. Ans. (b) CT scan
[Ref. David Sutton, 6/e p215]

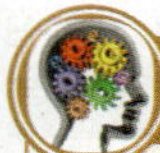

Also Remember

Causes of Intracranial Calcification

- *Age-related and physiologic*: Pineal gland, choroid plexus, falx cerebri, tentorium cerebelli, dura mater, sagittal sinus
- *Congenital*: Sturge-Weber syndrome, tuberous sclerosis, neurofibromatosis, lipoma
- *Infectious*: TORCH diseases, granulomatous infections, chronic viral encephalitis
- *Endocrine and metabolic*: Hypothyroidism, hypoparathyroidism, hyperparathyroidism
- *Vascular*: Primary atherosclerosis, malformation, aneurysms, chronic vasculitis
- *Neoplastic*: Oligodendroglioma, craniopharyngioma, germ cell neoplasms, neurocytoma, ependymoma, meningioma, medulloblastoma, astrocytoma, dermoid, epidermoid, calcified metastases

3. Ans. (b) Cytomegalo inclusion disease; (d) Toxoplasmosis
[Ref. Radiology Review Manual by Dahnert, 6/e p330]

4. Ans. (a) Hallervorden-Spatz disease
[Ref. Radiology Review Manual by Dahnert, 6/e p245]

Tiger Eye on MRI

- Cause: Excess iron accumulation and Central gliosis
- Associated with:
  - Hallervorden-Spatz syndrome (Pentothenate kinase associated neurodegeneration)
  - Other disorders: Dementia, tetraparesis, Neurofibrillary tangles, Retinitis pigmentosa, Acanthocytosis, Pallidal degeneration, X-linked disorders with mental retardation + Dandy-Walker malformation, Disorders with Lewy bodies, Extrapyramidal parkinsonian disorders, Progressive supranuclear palsy

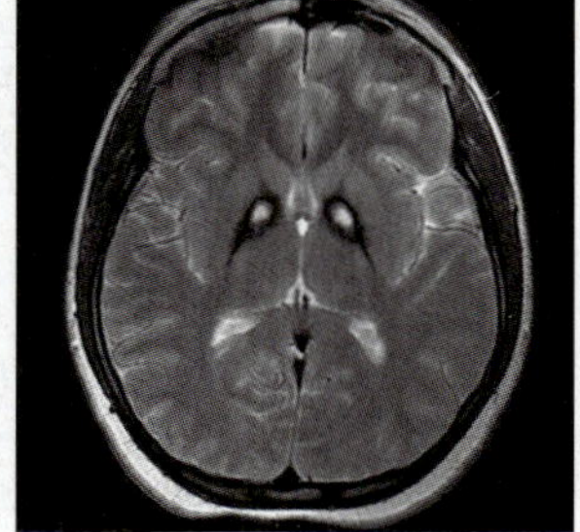

Fig. Tiger eye

5. Ans. (d) Meningioma
[Ref. Radiation Oncology by Jiade, 1/e p475]

- Although plain X-ray is not recommended routinely, "sunray effect," in X-ray helps in diagnosis and evaluation of meningioma

6. Ans. (d) Osteosclerosis
[Ref. Neuropsychological Disorders by Chad, 1/e 374]

7. Ans. (b) Gadolinium enhanced MRI
[Ref. Radiology Review Manual by Dahnert, 6/e p319]

MRI (Most Sensitive Test with GD-DTPA Enhancement)

- Isointense/Slightly hypointense on T1WI relative to brain.
- Intensely enhancing homogeneous mass/Ring-like enhancement (if cystic) after Gd-DTPA
- Hyperintense on T2WI (Differential diagnosis: Meningioma remains hypointense/isointense)

8. Ans. (b) MRI
[Ref. Harrisons, 15/e p2456]

- *MRI has revolutionised diagnosis and management of Multiple sclerosis*:
  - Plaques of demyelination
  - Lesions of anterior corpus callosum
  - Lesions of white matter/ periventricular region

9. Ans. (a) Sutural widening
[Ref. David Sutton, 7/e p1626]

- **Suture diastasis**, the first and most important sign in small children, may be the only sign of raised pressure
- Sellar erosion may occur but is a late sign and implies longstanding chronic pressure
  - In children under 10 years age, Sellar erosion without suture diastasis is likely to be due to a local erosive lesion rather than raised pressure
  - Above this age cellar changes are more likely to be due to raised pressure

Also Remember

- Chronological sequence of Suture widening in rasied ICT: Coronal (First), Sagittal, Lambdoid, Squamosal suture

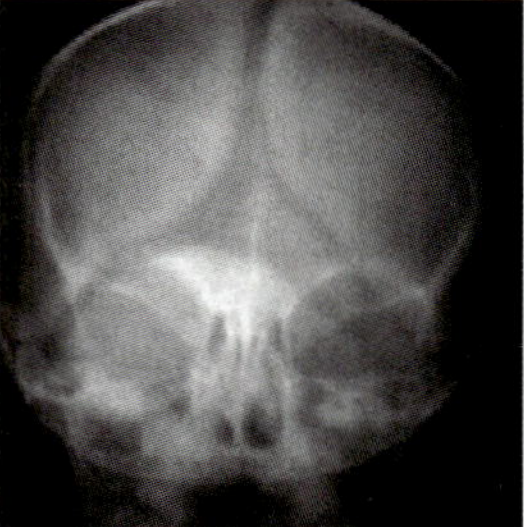

Fig. Sutural diastasis

10. Ans. (a) MRI
[Ref. CT and MRI in Oncology edited by Didier Buthiau, 1/e p92].

11. Ans. (d) All of the above

12. Ans. (b) Computerised tomography
[Ref. Sumer K Sethi, 5/e p89]

- Investigation of choice for Acute Subarachnoid haemorrhage (<48 hours): CT scan (Non-contrast)
- Investigation of choice for Chronic Subarachnoid haemorrhage (>48 hours): MRI

13. Ans. (b) CT scan
[Ref. Sumer K Sethi, 5/e p89]

14. Ans. (a) Craniopharyngioma
[Ref. David Sutton, 7/e p1752]

Craniopharyngioma
- MC Supratentorial tumor in children
- MC cause of Suprasellar calcification
- MC Calcifying brain tumor in a child

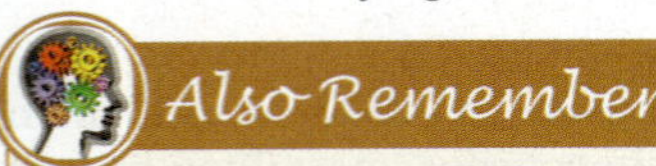

Craniopharyngioma
- Tumours of epithelial origin (3% of primary intracranial tumours)
- Bimodal age distribution (Aged 6-10 years and fifties)
- Half of childhood suprasellar tumours
- Calcification present in over 80% of the childhood cases (Often absent in adults)
- Grow above the sella and adhere tightly to the floor of the third ventricle and infundibulum usually, making surgical extirpation difficult or impossible
- 15% grow into pituitary fossa and produce enlargement and deformity of sella

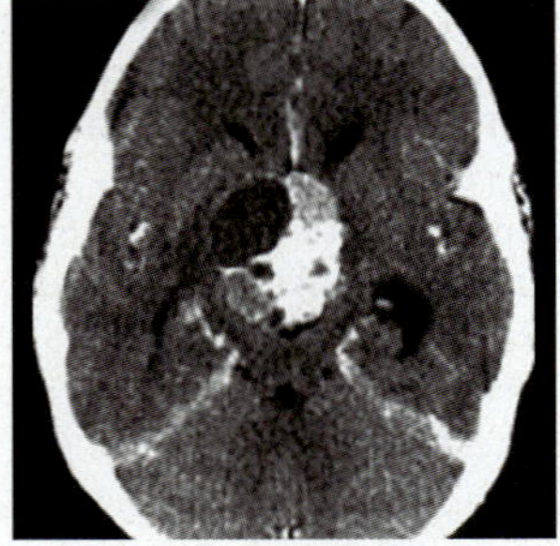

Fig. Craniopharyngioma

15. Ans. (a) Acromegaly
[Ref. Radiology Review Manual by Dahnert, 6/e p244]

Basal Ganglia Calcification

Common causes	Other causes
Hypoparathyroidism Hyperparathyroidism Hypothyroidism Toxoplasmosis Wilson disease Mitochondrial cytopathies Cockayne syndrome Lead poisoning Carbon monoxide poisoning Idiopathic (Ageing) Fahr syndrome **[Mnemonic: H**igh **T**ension **W**ires **M**ay **C**ause **L**eukemic **C**ancer **I**n **F**emales**]**	Birth hypoxia Hallervorden Spaz syndrome Pseudohypoparathyroidism Pseudo-pseudohypoparathyroidism Neurocysticercosis TORCH CNS tuberculosis Methotrexate Down's syndrome Wilson's disease Hypothyroidism (Rare cause)

16. Ans. (c) CT scan
[Ref. David Sutton, 7/e p1621]

17. Ans. (d) Transfemoral route
[Ref. Sumer K Sethi, 5/e p14]

Routes for Invasive Radiological Techniques
- *Cerebral angiography*: Transfemoral route (*Seldinger technique*; Catheter introduced thorough a major vessel, threaded through circulatory system and dye injected into carotid artery)
- *Conventional 4-vessel angiography*: 2 internal carotids and 1 vertebral (fourth vessel fills by reflux)
- *Lymphangiography*: First web space of foot
- *Phlebography*: Dorsal metatarsal vein

18. Ans. (b) Non-contrast CT
[Ref. David Sutton, 6/e p227]

19. Ans. (c) Optic foramen
[Ref. Imaging of the Globe and Orbit by Hosten, 1/e p6]

Structure visualized	Best view
Skull trauma	Lateral view
Internal auditory canal	Stenver's view
Orbital roof/ floor fracture	Water's view
Orbital lesion / supra orbital fissure	Caldwell's view (or Occipitofrontal view)
Optical foramen	Rhese view
Mastoid process	Schuller's view/ Lateral oblique
Paranasal sinuses	Water's view

20. Ans. (a) Enlarged superior ophthalmic vein
[Ref. Imaging in Trauma by King, 1/e p9]

21. Ans. (a) 7 mm

22. Ans. (c) Caldwell
[Ref. Diseases of the Sinuses by Gershwin, 1/e p 64]

23. Ans. (a) MRI
[Ref. Imaging of the Spine by Thomas P. Naidich, 1/e p287]
- MRI has largely replaced myelography in differentiating epidermoid cyst and a non-communicating arachnoid cyst

24. Ans. (a) Multiple myeloma
[Ref. Sumer K Sethi, 6/e p110]
- MM shows classical 'rain drop' appearance due to punched out lytic lesion in skull

25. Ans. (c) Lateral view
[Ref. Diseases of ENT & Head and Neck Surgery by Dhingra, 6/e p434]
- Lateral view of nasal bones (both right & left): Fracture line and depression or elevation of the fractured segment is seen
  - Lower part of nasal bone (best viewed here) is thin and fractured more frequently
  - Best view to evaluate trauma to face, Nasal fracture
- Occlusal view of nasal bone: Both side of nasal pyramid are seen
  - Fracture line and lateral displacement of the nasal pyramid is clearly seen

- Water's view: Gives end on view of nasal arch
  - Fracture of right and left nasal bones and their lateral displacement can be seen

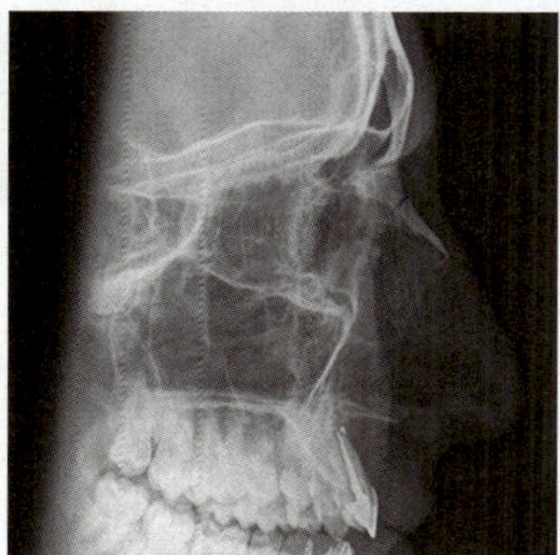

Fig. Lateral view (Fracture nose)

26. Ans. (a) Multiple small petechial hemorrhage
[Ref. Sumer K Sethi, 6/e p144]

27. Ans. (a) CT
[Ref. Harrison's Internal Medicine, 17/e Table 362-1]

- Patient with focal deficit is better judged by MRI than CT
- But in Emergency, CT is always readily available option making it the screening investigation of choice

28. Ans. (c) CECT
[Ref. Radiodiagnosis by Daga, 1/e p39]

- **CECT is investigation of choice for calcified tumors**:
  - Retinoblastoma
  - Craniopharyngioma
  - Oligodendrioglioma
  - Central neurocytoma

29. Ans. (b) Diffusion weighted MRI
[Ref. Brain Edema IX by Ito, p207]

- MR-DWI will contribute to the diagnosis and treatment of early stages of cerebral ischemia

30. Ans. (c) Cryptococcal cysts
[Ref. Epilepsy Board Review by Koubeissi, 1/e p285]

MRI in Cryptococcosis

- Soap bubble appearance with Pseudocysts in mid-brain and parenchyma
- Parenchymal cryptococcomas
- Leptomeningeal involvement
- Spread along perivascular spaces with dilation of perivascular spaces

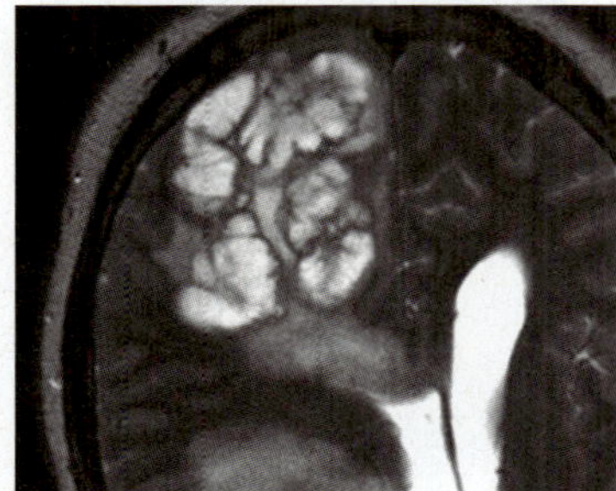

Fig. Soap bubble appearance with pseudocysts

31. Ans. (b) Spina bifida
[Ref. Pediatric Rehabilitation by Murphy, 5/e p377]

Spina bifida on USG

- Lemon sign: Relates to the abnormal shape of the head (In the second trimester, fetuses with open spina bifida tend to have a disproportionately small BPD for the gestational age)
- Banana sign: Related to herniation of the cerebellar vermis through the banana-shaped foramen magnum

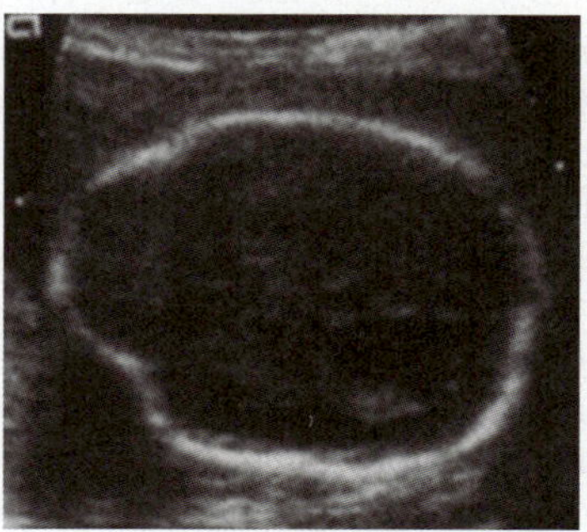

Fig. Lemon sign

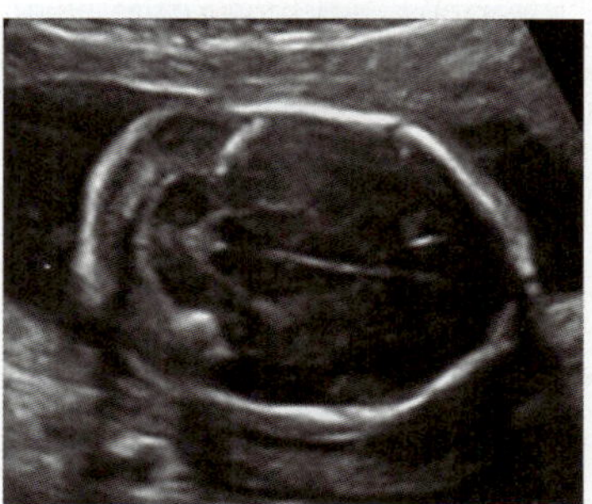

Fig. Banana sign

32. Ans. (c) Internal auditory canal
[Ref. Head and Neck Imaging by Vogl, 1/e p6]

- Stenver's view is a special oblique projection used to demonstrate Petrous ridge, Petrous apex, and Internal auditory canal and its contents (Semi-circular canals, Cochlea)

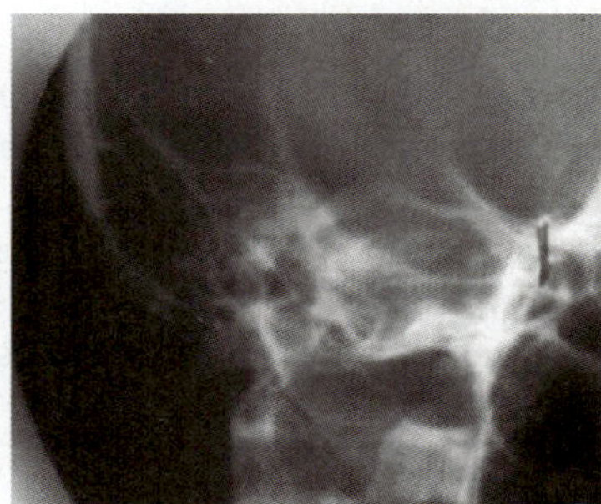

Fig. Stenver's view

33. Ans. (a) White matter
[Ref. Magnetic Resonance in Multiple Sclerosis by Miller, 1/e p31]

- A confident diagnosis of Multiple sclerosis requires the demonstration of clinically disseminated central nervous system (CNS) white matter lesions both in time and space
- MRI aids diagnosis by providing paraclinical evidence for dissemination in space

34. Ans. (a) Crescent shaped hyperdense lesion

[Ref. Diagnostic Imaging: Brain by Osborn, 1/e p1987]

- Acute subdural hematomas appear as hyperdense, crescent-shaped lesions located between the Calvarium and underlying cortex

35. Ans. (d) Sagittal sinus thrombosis

[Ref. Imaging of the Brain by Naidich, 1/e p475]

Empty Delta Sign (CT)

- Major diagnostic finding in Cerebrovenous thrombosis on standard contrast enhanced CT is a filling defect within the dural sinus that is surrounded by intense enhancement in the wall of the dural sinus (empty delta sign)
- Empty delta sign is appreciated most easily on scans perpendicular to the thrombosed dural sinus and is therefore most often seen in the superior sagittal sinus torcular and sigmoid sinus
- It may not be appreciated when there is short segment thrombosis

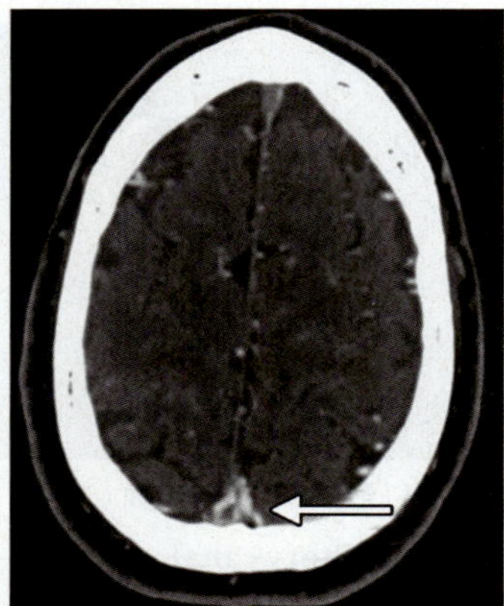

Fig. Delta sign on CT

36. Ans. (b) Progressive supranuclear palsy

[Ref. Brain Imaging with MRI and CT by Rumboldt, 1/e p115]

Penguin/ Hummingbird Sign

- Distinguishing feature of progressive supranuclear palsy
- **Shape of the atrophic midbrain resembles bill of a hummingbird** or a penguin's head
- Most rostral midbrain, the midbrain tegmentum, the pontine base, and the cerebellum appears to correspond to the bill, crown, body, and wing, respectively, of a hummingbird

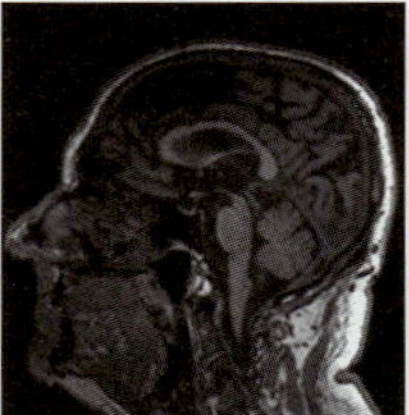

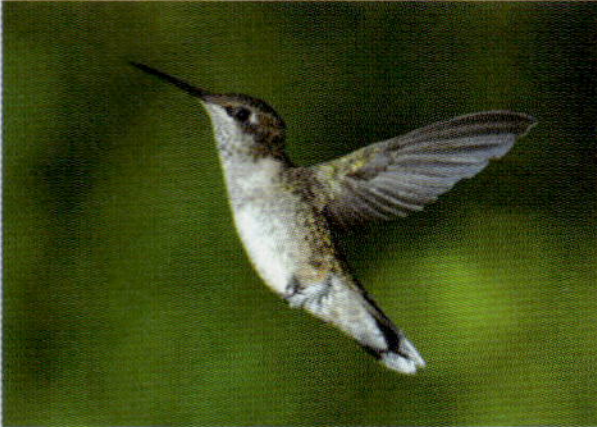

Fig. Hummingbird sign

37. Ans. (d) Carotid body tumor

[Ref. Head & Neck Surgery and Oncology by Thankappan, 1/e p67]

Lyre sign

- Seen in Carotid body tumors
- Tumor completely fills and 'splays the carotid bifurcation'
- Characterized as a bowing and displacing of the internal and external carotid arteries

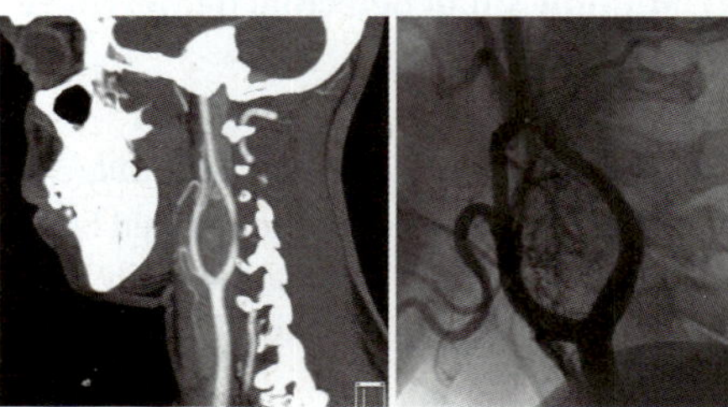

Fig. Lyre's sign

38. Ans. (b) Hyperparathyroidism

[Ref. Endocrinology by Newton, 1/e Vol2 p145]

Pepper-pot skull

- Occasionally used in place of Salt and pepper skull to describe the typical radiographic appearance of multiple small radiolucent lesions of the skull vault
- Classically seen in Hyperparathyroidism
- Sometimes used (inaccurately) to describe the raindrop skull of Multiple myeloma

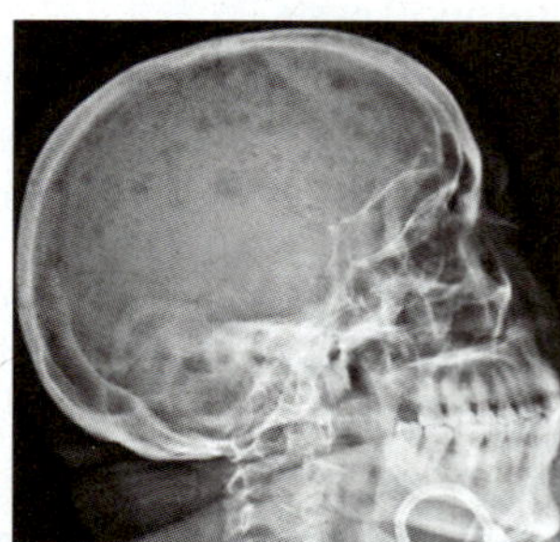

Fig. Pepper-pot skull

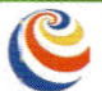 HIGH YIELD MCQs ANSWERS WITH EXPLANATIONS 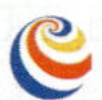

1. **Ans. (c) Caldwell**
   [Ref. Diseases of the Sinuses by Gershwin, 1/e p 64]

2. **Ans. (a) Sturge Weber syndrome**
   [Ref. Sumer K Sethi, 6/e p140]
   - Tram track calcification: Mainly occipital region

3. **Ans. (b) Eosinophilic granuloma**
   [Ref. David Sutton, 7/e p1637]
   - Histiocytosis commonly involves the skull, particularly in Letterer-Siwe and Hand-Schuller-Christian disease where the **typical 'geographic' skull defects** may be seen
   - Eosinophil granuloma may also produce similar lesions in the skull, although it may present as an isolated lesion.

4. **Ans. (c) Multiple myeloma**
   [Ref. Sumer K Sethi, 6/e p110]

5. **Ans. (b) Intra cerebral calcification**
   [Ref. David Sutton, 7/e p1563]

6. **Ans. (c) Craniopharyngioma**
   [Ref. David Sutton, 7/e p1753]

7. **Ans. (b) Ballooning of sella**
   [Ref. David Sutton, 7/e p1626]

Radiological Signs of Raised Intracranial Pressure
- Suture diastasis
- Sellar erosion
- Pineal displacement
- Increased convolutional marking

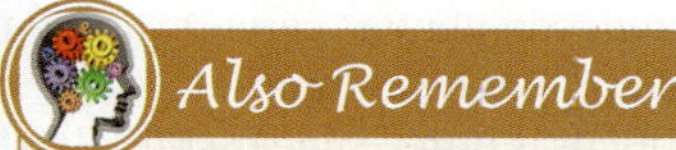

- Signs seen in infants and children are quite different from those seen in adults because once the sutures are united they cannot be affected by raised pressure

8. **Ans. (c) Erosion**
   [Ref. Radiation Oncology by Lu, 1/e p475]

9. **Ans. (a) Calcification**
   [Ref. Radiation Oncology by Lu, 1/e p475]

10. **Ans. (d) Craniopharyngioma**
    [Ref. David Sutton, 7/e p1725]

11. **Ans. (b) Craniopharyngioma**
    [Ref. David Sutton, 7/e p1752]

12. **Ans. (b) Lumbar puncture**
    [Ref. Pediatric Oncology by Chan, 1/e p33]
    - A lumbar puncture is relatively contraindicated in patients with suspected intracranial tumours and possible ICP

13. **Ans. (a) Ventriculomegaly; (b) Obliteration of cistern magna; (d) Abnormal curvature of cerebellum**
    [Ref. Diagnostic Imaging of Fetal Anomalies by Nyberg, 1/e p1002]

14. **Ans. (b) Myelomalacia**
    [Ref. MRI Atlas of the Spine by Cohen, 1/e p90]
    - Presence or absence of Gd-enhancement generally narrows the differential diagnostic possibilities
    - Spinal cord oedema is easily demonstrated with MR as ill defined, diffuse, intramedullary high signal intensity on T2 weighted images

15. **Ans. (b) Wilson's disease**
    [Ref. Sumer K Sethi, 6/e p137]

16. **Ans. (c) Injury to cortical bridging veins**
    [Ref. Traumatic Brain Injury by Mahapatra, 1/e p158]
    - An acute subdural hematoma is a collection of fresh blood under the dura, which may compress the brain
    - Source of acute subdural blood is bridging cortical vein near sagittal sinus, veins from sylvian fissure to sphenoparietal sinus
    - Another source of bleeding that can result in subdural hematoma is laceration or rupture of small cortical arteries and veins

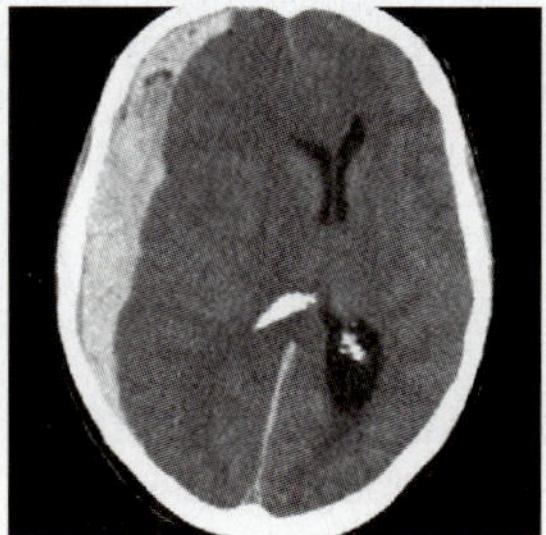

Fig. Subdural hematoma

17. **Ans. (b) Concavo-convex hyperdense**
    [Ref. Understanding X-Rays by Gelderen, 1/e p502]

18. **Ans. (b) CT scan**
    [Ref. Harrison's Internal Medicine, 17/e Table 362-1]

19. **Ans. (a) Berry's aneurysm**
    [Ref. Sumer K Sethi, 6/e p137]

20. **Ans. (b) MRI**
    [Ref. Harrison's Internal Medicine, 17/e Table 362-1]

21. **Ans. (a) Hyperparathyroidism; (c) Hypoparathyroidism; (d) Hypothyroidism**
    [Ref. Sumer K Sethi, 6/e p137]

22. **Ans. (c) CT scan**
    [Ref. Oxford Textbook of Medicine by Warrell, 4/ p936]
    - Radiological hallmark is calcification, best detected on CT scanning
    - Body CT scans without IV contrast are helpful in delineating fine bony detail, calcifications and lung parenchyma

23. **Ans. (a) Transfemoral route**
    [Ref. Vascular and Endovascular Surgery, 7/e p362]
    - Axillary or brachial artery approaches are also used for cerebral angiography when the transfemoral route is not possible. Trans femoral is preferred option.

24. **Ans. (c) Iohexol**
    [Ref. The Adult and Pediatric Spine, Volume 1 by Frymoyer, 3/e p51]

- Iopamidol and iohexol are the agents of choice for myelography
- Iohexol (Omnipaque) is a non-ionic iodinated contrast agent that seems to be quite safe

25. Ans. (c) Craniopharyngioma
[Ref. David Sutton, 7/e p1725]

26. Ans. (a) Pineal gland; (b) Choroid plexus
[Ref. Sumer K Sethi, 6/e p137]

Normal Intracranial Calcification
- Pineal
- Choroid plexus
- Dura
- Ligaments
- Pacchionian bodies
- Basal ganglia and dentate nucleus
- Pituitary
- Lens

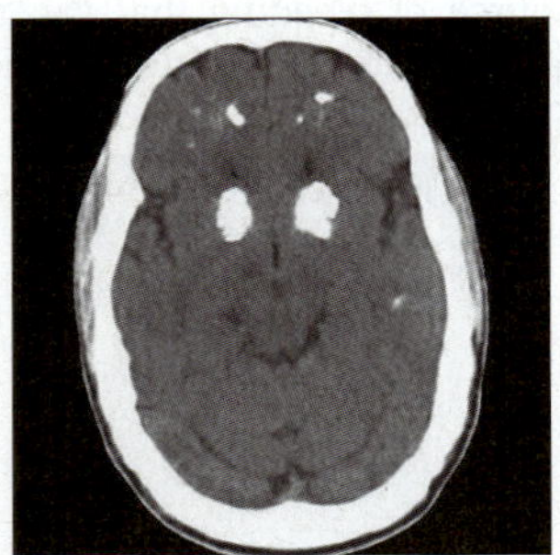

Fig. Intracranial calcification

27. Ans. (b) Cytomegalic infection
[Ref. Neuropathology by Prayson, 2/e p346]
- Periventricular calcification with associated hydrocephalus is typical of cytomegalovirus infection in neonates.

28. Ans. (a) Toxoplasmosis
[Ref. David Sutton, 7/e p1633]

Toxoplasmosis
- Most human infestation with the protozoan is derived from cats
- Healthy adults may be symptomless carriers but unfortunately a pregnant carrier can infect the fetus in utero: Involve the brain, widespread granulomas with calcification, severe brain atrophy with ventricular dilatation, and bilateral choroidoretinitis
- Calcification in congenital toxoplasmosis is characteristic, consisting of multiple scattered flecks in the cortex and linear streaks in the basal ganglia

29. Ans. (d) Vein of Galen malformation
[Ref. David Sutton, 7/e p1715]

30. Ans. (c) Blurring of grey white matter junction of ipsilateral temporal lobe
[Ref. Neuroradiology Companion by Mauricio Castillo,3/e p189]

31. Ans. (b) Meningioma
[Ref. Sumer K Sethi, 6/e p140]

32. Ans. (b) Medulloblastoma
[Ref. Sumer K Sethi, 6/e p138]
- Extracranial spread of tumours: Medulloblastoma > Ependymoma > Choroid plexus papilloma

33. Ans. (c) Astrocytoma
[Ref. David Sutton, 7/e p1739]

34. Ans. (b) Diffuse Axonal injury
[Ref. Sumer K Sethi, 6/e p144]

35. Ans. (b) Amyotrophic lateral sclerosis

36. Ans. (b) Craniopharyngioma
[Ref. David Sutton, 7/e p1725]

37. Ans. (b) Craniopharyngioma
[Ref. David Sutton, 7/e p1725; Nelson's Pediatrics, 18/e p2135]
- Suprasellar calcification along with presence of visual field defect and headache suggest the diagnosis of Craniopharyngioma

38. Ans. (d) Video EEG with Ictal ^{99}m Tc -HMPAO Brain SPECT
[Ref. Grainger & Allison's Diagnostic Radiology Essentials by Lee, 5/e Chapter 50]

SPECT Scan
- Radionuclide imaging of the brain requires radiopharmaceuticals that cross the blood–brain barrier
- SPECT images are formed from detection of gamma rays emitted during radionuclide decay as part of a nuclear medicine examination
- SPECT may be used to produce images of a rCBF using the radiopharmaceuticals 133Xe, 123I isopropyl iodoamphetamine (IMP), ^{99}mTc ethyl cysteinate dimer (ECD) or ^{99}mTc hexamethylpropylene amine oxide (HMPAO)
- Gamma rays or photons are detected by a gamma camera which, if rotated about the patient's head, allows reconstruction of tomographic slices of distribution of activity in that part of the patient
- Clinical applications include dementia, cerebrovascular disease, epilepsy, encephalitis and head injury
- If localization of epileptic focus is unrevealed on MRI, Ictal SPECT with HMPAO is the most practical and best method
  - Addition of video EEG further helps in localizing of epileptic foci.

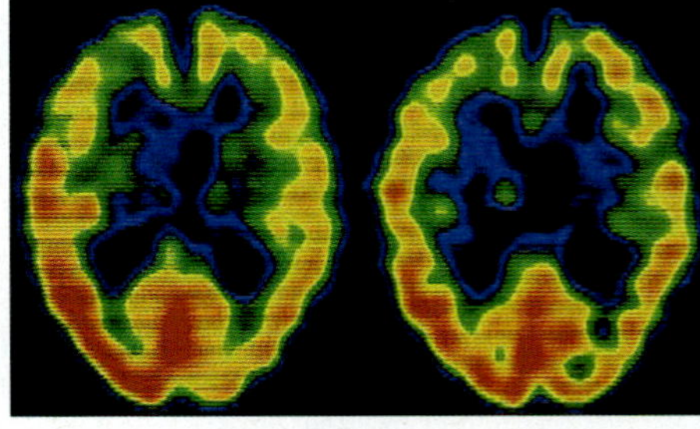

Fig. HMPAO spect

39. Ans. (b) Krabbe's disease
[Ref. David Sutton, 7/e p1801]

40. Ans. (c) Crescent shaped hyperdense lesion
[Ref. David Sutton, 7/e p1779]
- **Subdural haematoma**: The appearances vary considerably depending mainly on age
- Acute subdural haematoma, i.e. within 48 hours of the injury, can sometimes closely resemble the acute extradural lesion, but is more frequently concavo-convex, spreading over the surface of the cerebral hemisphere

- In acute stage, the haematoma is usually of high density, often situated in the frontoparietal regions or middle cranial fossa, and associated with ipsilateral brain swelling
- Subdural collections are generally of higher attenuation than brain for about 2 weeks, and after 3-4 weeks are of lower attenuation, eventually approaching that of CSF

41. Ans. (a) Non contrast CT
[Ref. David Sutton, 7/e p1769]

42. Ans. (c) Intra arterial digital subtraction Angiography
[Ref. David Sutton, 7/e p1677]
- Main indications for direct intra arterial angiography is investigation of definite intracranial subarachnoid hemorrhage

43. Ans. (c) Extradural haematoma
[Ref. Osborn's Brain 1/e p208]
- Biconvex hyperdense lesion on CT after a head injury suggest the diagnosis of extradural haematoma

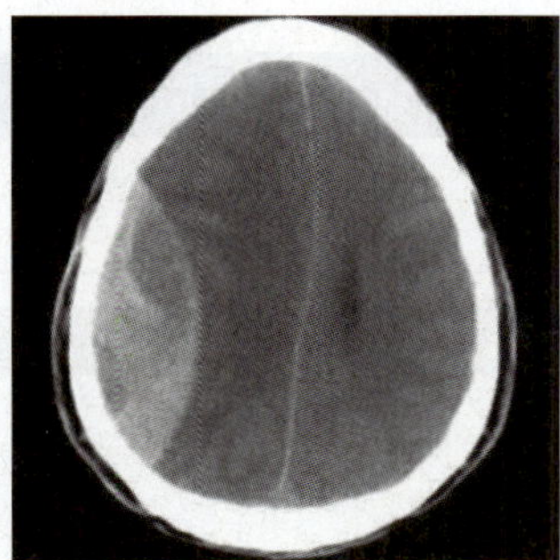

Fig. Extradural hematoma

44. Ans. (d) CT scan contrast enhanced
[Ref. Paediatric Otolaryngology, Volume 6 p7]
- CT scanning is the investigation of choice for Juvenile nasopharyngeal angiofibroma

45. Ans. (b) Gadolinium enhanced MRI
[Ref. Radiology Review Manual by Dahnert, 6/e p319]
- MRI (most sensitive test with Gd-DTPA enhancement) for Vestibular Schwannoma

46. Ans. (c) Lateral view
[Ref. The Pituitary by Melmed, 3/e p 678]
- Sella turcica is best visualized on lateral views of the skull
- Sellar floor can be studied on frontal radiographs angled tangentially to the plane of the floor (Caldwell view)

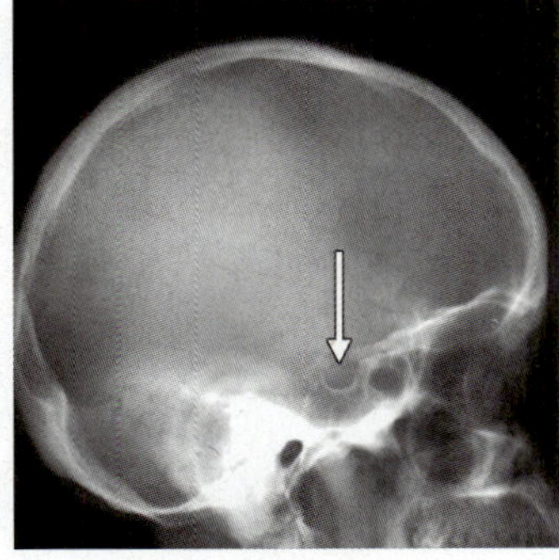

Fig. Sella turcica (lateral view skull)

47. Ans. (a) MRI
[Ref. Radiology Illustrated by Kim, 1/ep327]

48. Ans. (b) Non-contrast CT of the nose and para nasal bone

49. Ans. (a) Transfemoral route
[Ref. Vascular and Endovascular Surgery, 7/e p362]
- Transfemoral is preferred option for Cerebral angiography
- Axillary or brachial artery approaches are also used for cerebral angiography when the transfemoral route is not possible

50. Ans. (a) NCCT
[Ref. Accident and Emegency by Dolan, 3/e p57]

51. Ans. (d) MRI
[Ref. Neurosurgery by Kaye, 3/e p134]
- Diagnostic serological test of choice: Electro-immuno transfer blot assay (EITB)
- Radiological investigation of choice to determine pathological stage of cyst: MRI

52. Ans. (c) Thin slice CT scan
[Ref. Clinical Strabismus Management by Santiago, 1/e p313]
- Investigation of choice for Orbital fractures: Non-enhanced, thin-slice, direct axial and direct coronal CT scans

53. Ans. (c) Extramedullary intradural tumor
[Ref. Practical Small Animal MRI by Bagley]

Intradural-Extramedullary Tumor on Myelographic Spinal Imaging

- "Golf tee appearance": Expansion of Subarachnoid space, and outlining of tumor in negative shadow
- "Dumbbell-shaped appearance": Nerve sheath also expand on either side, where it transverses the dura

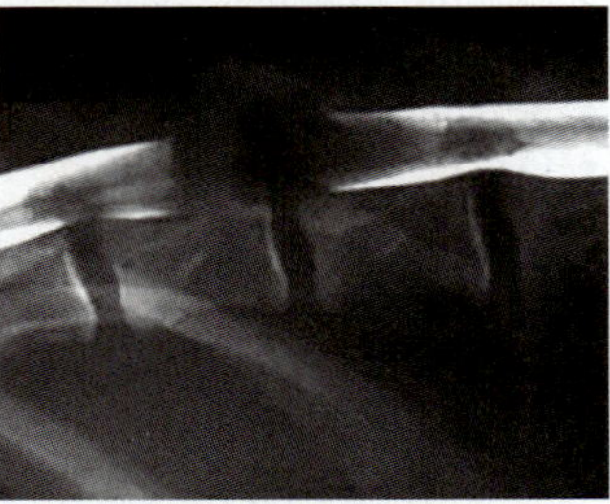

Fig. Golf tee defect

54. Ans. (a) Biconvex in shape
[Ref. Handling Difficult Situations by Wijdicks, 1/e p132]

CT Scanning in Brain Hemorrhages

- Extradural hemorrhage: Biconvex configuration
- Subdural hemorrhage: Crescent-shaped configuration
- Subarachnoid hemorrhage: Located in Cisterns, Fissures, Sulci
- Intracranial hemorrhage: Located in Lobe, Putamen, Caudate, Thalamus

55. Ans. (b) CT scan
[Ref. Acute Ischemic Stroke by Lev, 2/e p43]
- Speed, widespread availability, low cost, and accuracy in detecting subarachnoid and intracranial hemorrhage have led conventional computed tomography (CT) scanning to become the first-line diagnostic test

56. Ans. (c) Ballooning of sella
[Ref. Imaging of Bones and Joints by Gupta, 1/e p287]

Raised Intracranial Pressure

- Sutural distases **(Widening of sutures): First prominent change**, MC in Coronal suture
- Sellar erosion
- Increased convolutional markings

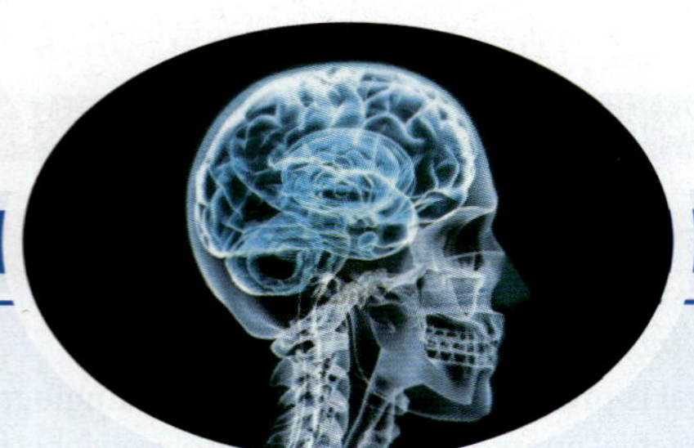

Chapter 7

Genitourinary System

THEORETICAL CONCEPTS

VII A. NEPHROLITHIASIS (RENAL STONES)[Q]

Radio-opaque stones (90%)	Radio-lucent stones (10%)
• Calcium oxalate • Calcium phosphate • Struvite • Cystine • Matrix	• Uric acid • Xanthine

VII B. HYDRONEPHROSIS

- Intravenous urogram/pyelogram (IVU/IVP) in hydronephrosis:
  - *Earliest change*: Dilatation of renal pelvis
  - 'Crescent/foot-pad' sign
  - ***'Rim sign'*** (Severe hydronephrosis)

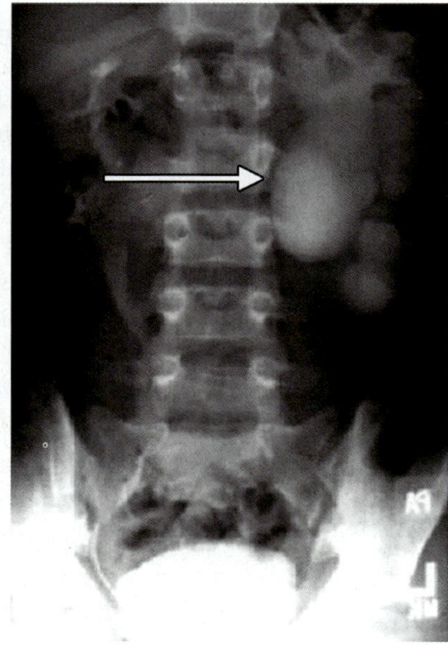

Fig. Hydronephrosis

VII C. KEY SIGNS/FEATURES IN GENITOURINARY RADIOLOGY

- **Bilateral spider leg deformity** Q: Polycystic kidney disease
- **Cobra-head/Adder-head sign** Q: Intravesical (Orthotopic) ureterocoele
- Crescent sign Q: Hydronephrosis
- Drooping-lily/Drooping flower sign Q: Ectopic ureter
- Egg-in-cup appearance: Renal papillary necrosis
- Fir-tree/Pine-tree/**Christmas-tree bladder** Q: Neurogenic bladder
- Flower vase ureter Q: Horse-shoe kidney
- Foetal head calcified bladder Q: Schistosomiasis/Bilharziasis
- Lobster claw/Ball on ate of Renal pyramids: Renal papillary necrosis
- Paint-brush appearance Q: Medullary sponge kidney
- **Putty/Cement kidney** Q: Renal tuberculosis
- **Rim sign** Q: Chronic hydronephrosis, Acute tubular necrosis, Renal vein thrombosis, Renal artery occlusion
- **Saw tooth/Cork-screw ureters**: Tuberculous ureteritis
- Soap-bubble nephrogram: Hydronephrosis
- String of beads/Pile of plates appearance (Angiography): Fibromuscular dysplasia
- Sun-burst nephrogram: Polycystic kidney
- Sun-burst bladder: Extraperitoneal bladder rupture
- Swiss cheese nephrogram: Adult polycystic kidney disease
- Tear-drop bladder Q: Pelvic abscess, Pelvic hematoma, Pelvic lipomatosis, Intraperitoneal bladder rupture
- **Thimble bladder**: Tubercular cystitis

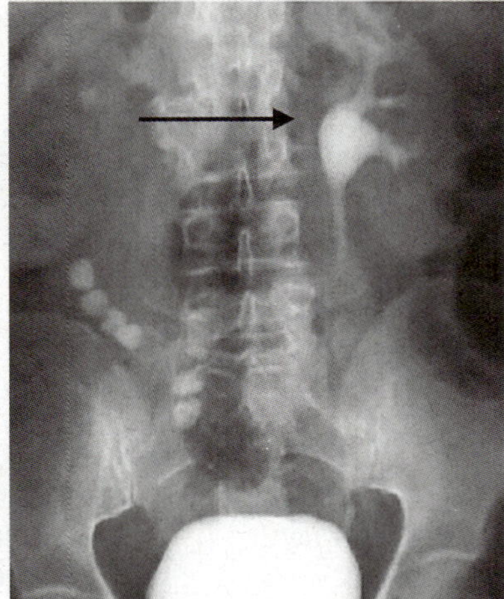
Fig. Spider-leg deformity

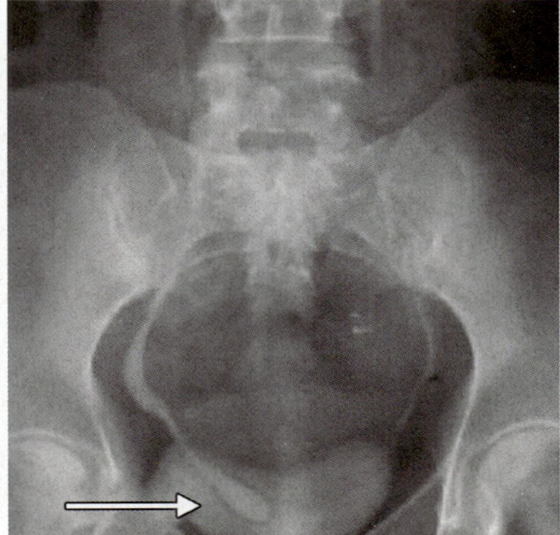
Fig. Cobra/Adder head sign

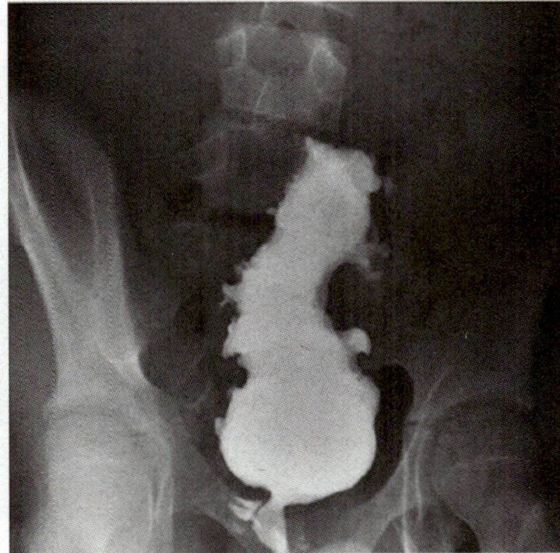
Fig. Christmas-tree bladder

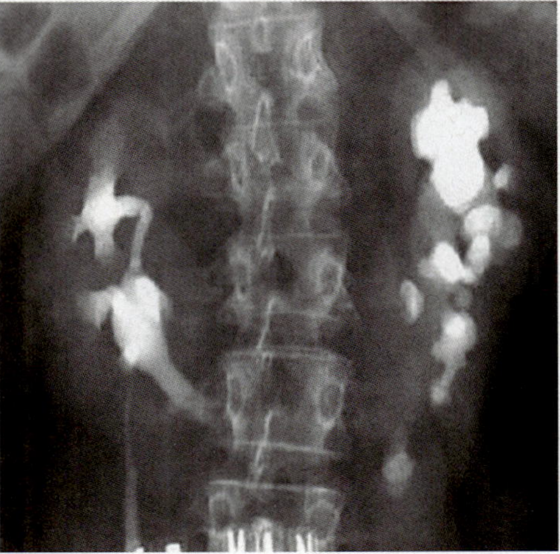
Fig. Flower-vase ureters

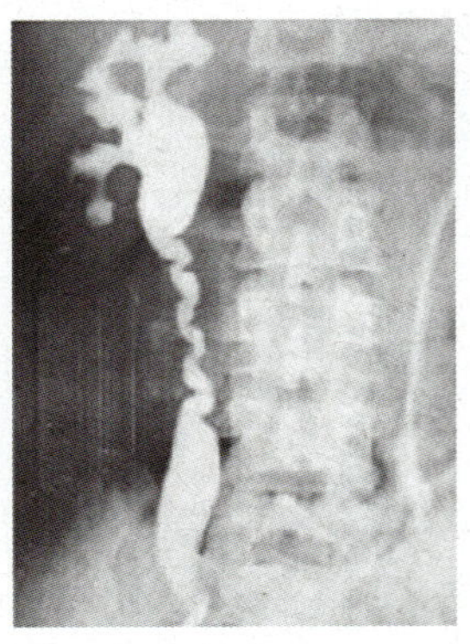

Fig. Cork-screw ureter

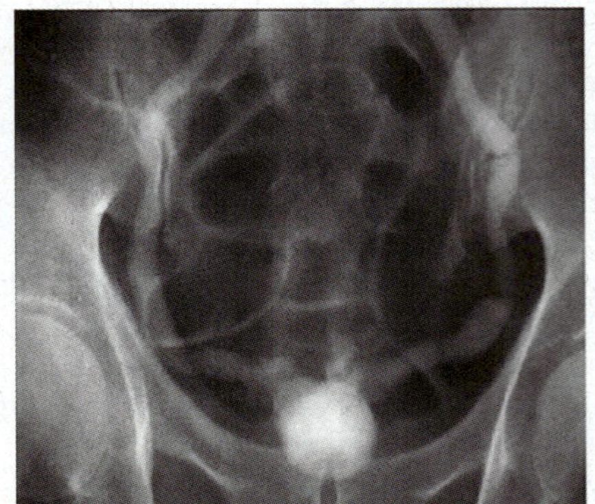

Fig. Thimble bladder

IMAGE-BASED QUESTIONS

1. Identify the anomaly shown (Arrow) in the X-ray Photograph ***[Recent Question 2016]***

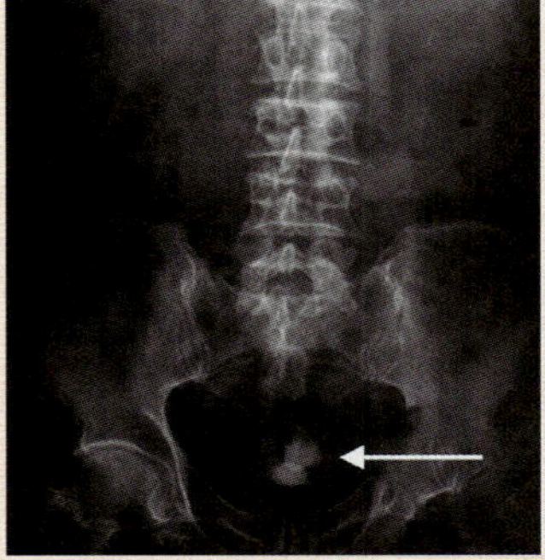

a. Thimble bladder
b. Ureteric calculus
c. Bladder calculus
d. Prostatic carcinoma

2. Most sensitive test for detection of disorder (Arrow in Photograph) ***[Recent Question 2013]***

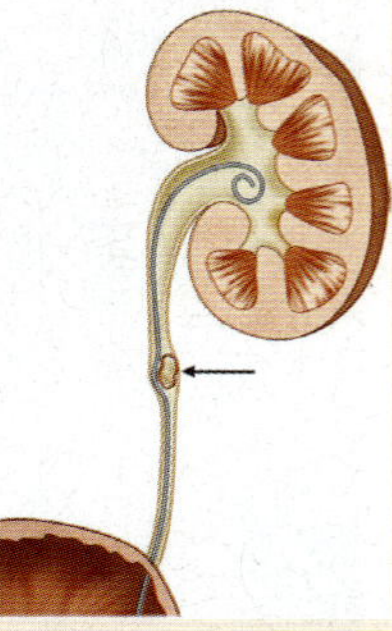

a. KUB X-ray
b. USG
c. NCCT
d. CECT

3. Diagnose the Condition (Arrow) shown in Photograph

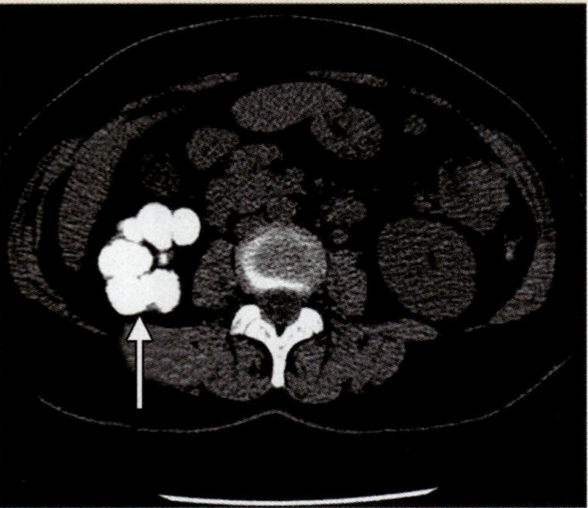

a. Renal carcinoma
b. Nephrolithiasis
c. Renal tuberculosis
d. Adrenal carcinoma

4. Bladder (arrow) appearance is seen in ***[Recent Question 2014]***

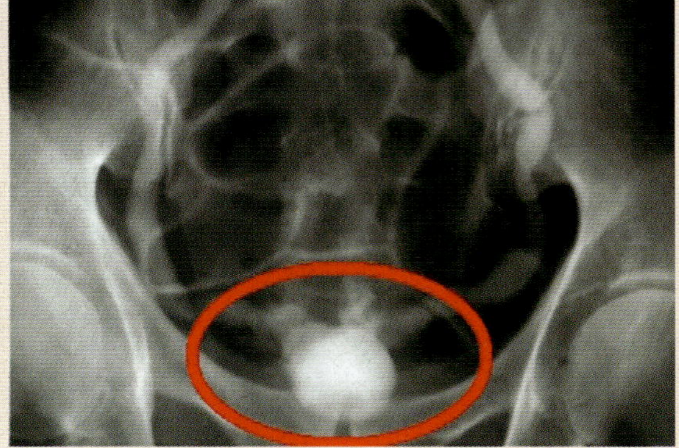

a. Tuberculosis
b. Schistosomiasis
c. Neurogenic bladder
d. Pelvic abscess

5. Bladder (Arrow) appearance is seen in ***[Recent Question 2013]***

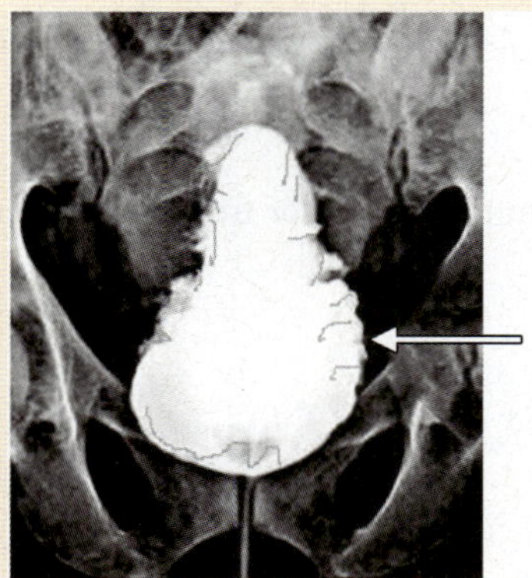

a. Tuberculosis
b. Schistosomiasis
c. Neurogenic bladder
d. Pelvic abscess

6. Ureter (Arrow) appearance shown in Photograph is found in

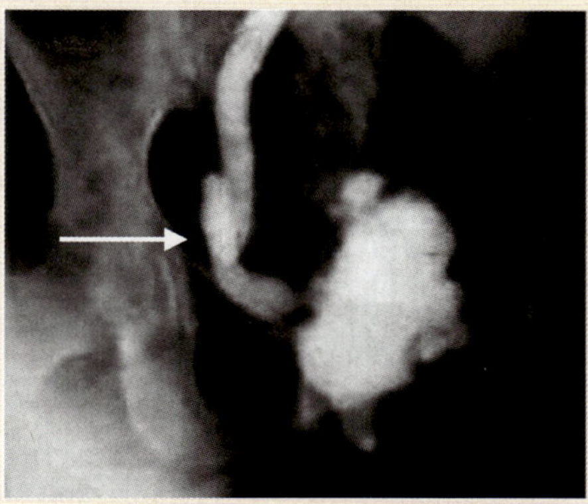

a. Tuberculosis
b. Schistosomiasis
c. Carcinoma
d. Stricture

7. USG of Kidney shown in Photograph is found in

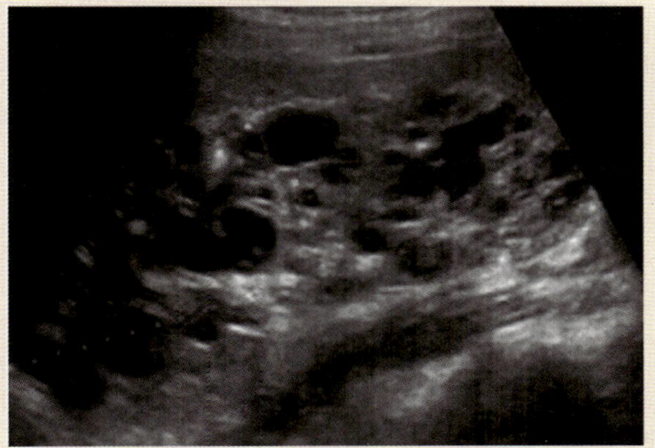

a. Horse shoe kidney
b. Renal agenesis
c. Tuberculosis
d. Polycystic kidney

8. Renal condition shown in Photograph is characterized by all except

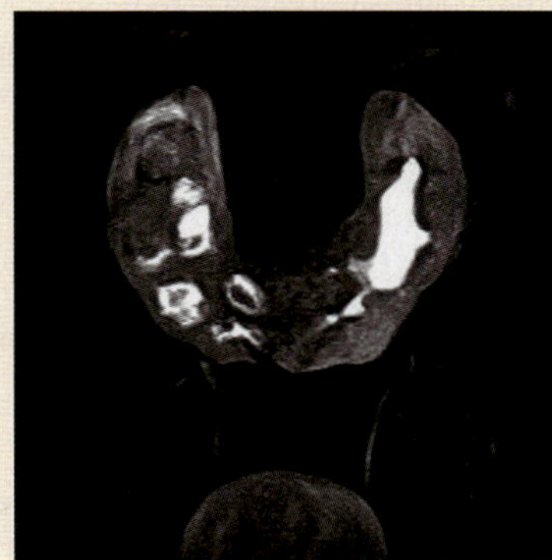

a. Flower vase appearance
b. Shaking hand sign
c. Adder head appearance
d. Prone to obstruction

9. Diagnose the Condition (Box) shown in Photograph

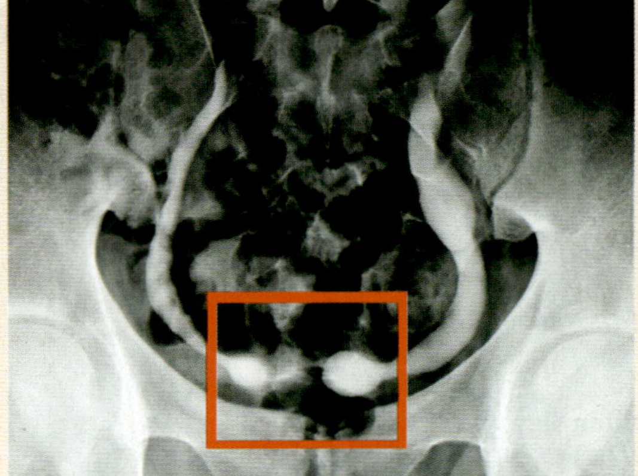

a. TB ureters
b. Carcinoma ureter
c. Ureterocoele
d. Ureteric stone

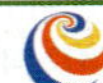 ANSWERS WITH EXPLANATIONS OF IBQs 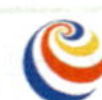

1. Ans. (c) Bladder calculus *[Ref. Clinical Manual of Surgery by Rao, 1/e p672]*

Bladder Calculi

- Development: Occur either from migrated renal calculi or urinary stasis
- Primary bladder calculi: Stones form *de novo* in the bladder
- Secondary bladder stones: Stones are from renal calculi (which migrate down into bladder) or from concretions on foreign material (example: urinary catheters)
- Epidemiology: MCC is urinary stasis
  - Bladder outlet obstruction
  - Cystocoele
  - Neurogenic bladder
  - Foreign body
- Plain radiograph:
  - Usually densely radiopaque
  - Single or multiple (**Arrow in Photograph**) and are often large
  - Frequently lamination internally (Onion-skin)

2. Ans. (c) NCCT *[Ref. Issues in Acoustic and Ultrasound Technology by Action, 2013/e p81]*

- NCCT can reliably characterize the location and size of an offending ureteral calculus, identify complications, and diagnose alternative etiologies of abdominal pain
- Sensitivity: 97%, Specificity: 95%

3. Ans. (c) Renal tuberculosis *[Ref. Sumer K Sethi, 5/e p79]*

- Putty kidney: Pattern of renal calcification associated with renal TB conventionally described on plain radiography
- Calcification characteristically is very homogeneous and ground glass like, representing calcified caseous tissue

4. Ans. (a) Tuberculosis *[Ref. Sumer K Sethi, 5/e p79]*

Renal Tuberculosis

- Putty kidney (Autonephrectomy)
- Thimble bladder (Photograph)
- Pipestem/ Cork-screw ureters
- 'Feathery appearance' of calyces (Earliest sign on IVP)
- 'Golf-hole' ureters (on Sigmoidoscopy)

5. Ans. (c) Neurogenic bladder *[Ref. Nephrology by Nammalwar, 1/e p323]*

Pine Cone/Fir Tree/Christmas Tree Bladder

- Cystogram appearance in which the bladders elongated and pointed with thickened trabeculated wall
- Typically seen in severe Neurogenic bladder with increased sphincter tone (Detrusor sphincter dyssynergia) due to Suprasacral lesions (above S2-S4) or Epiconal lesions (in and around S2-S4)

6. Ans. (a) Tuberculosis *[Ref. Sumer K Sethi, 5/e p79]*

- Cork-screw or Beaded ureters are seen in Tuberculosis

7. Ans. (d) Polycystic kidney *[Ref. Sumer K Sethi, 5/e p80]*

Polycystic Kidney Disease

- Simple renal cysts will appear anechoic with well-defined imperceptible walls, posterior acoustic enhancement (amplification) and lateral shadowing (extinction)
- Cysts with hemorrhage or infection will demonstrate echogenic material within the cyst, without internal blood flow
- Calcification may develop

8. Ans. (c) Adder head appearance *[Ref. Sumer K Sethi, 5/e p80]*

Horse Shoe Kidney

- Flower vase appearance
- Shaking hand sign
- Prone to Obstruction, Trauma, Wilm's tumor

9. Ans. (c) Ureterocoele *[Ref. Sumer K Sethi, 5/e p80]*

Adder-Head/Cobra-Head/Spring Onion Sign

- Description: Dilatation of the distal ureter, surrounded by a thin lucent line
  - Lucent 'hood' of cobra represents the combined thickness of the ureteral wall and prolapsed bladder mucosa, outlined by contrast material within the bladder lumen
  - Lucent line should be thin and well defined
- Seen in: Ureterocoele

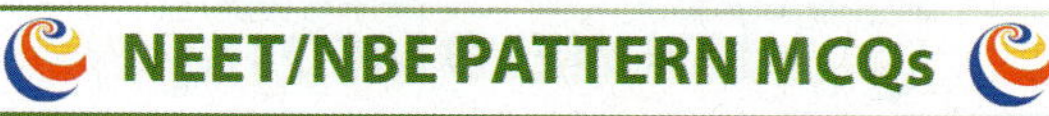

NEET/NBE PATTERN MCQs

1. **All of the following are radio-opaque stones except** *[NBE FMGE September 2009]*
   a. Cystine b. Struvite
   c. Uric acid d. Calcium
2. **Central stellate scar on CT scans are seen in** *[NBE DNB 2008, 2009]*
   a. Renal haemangiomas b. Renal oncocytomas
   c. Wilm's tumors d. Papillomas
3. **'Crescent sign' on IVU is positive in** *[NBE FMGE March 2006]*
   a. Pyelonephritis b. Hydronephrosis
   c. Polycystic kidney d. Renal cell carcinoma
4. **Renal Cortical imaging is done by** *[Recent Question 2012]*
   a. DTPA b. DMSA
   c. MAG3 d. UIH
5. **The 'String of beads' or sausage appearance of the renal artery is due to** *[NBE DNB 1998, 1999, 2005, 2006]*
   a. Fibromuscular hyperplasia
   b. Subadventitial fibroplasia
   c. Medial fibroplasia with aneurysms
   d. Outercoat fibroplasia with aneurysms
   e. None of the above
6. **Spider leg appearance on IVP is suggestive of** *[NBE FMGE September 2012]*
   a. Renal stones
   b. Renal carcinoma
   c. Polycystic kidney disease
   d. Horse shoe kidney
7. **Bead cystogram is used for the diagnosis of** *[NBE DNB 1997, 2004, 2007]*
   a. Ca bladder b. Stress incontinence
   c. Thimble bladder d. Diverticulum
8. **Investigation of choice for hydronephrosis** *[Recent Question 2012]*
   a. Excretory Urography b. USG
   c. MRI d. Cystourethrography
9. **'Thimble' bladder is seen in** *[NBE DNB 2007]*
   a. Cystitis cystica
   b. Chronic tubercular cystitis
   c. Neurogenic bladder
   d. Acute tubercular cystitis
10. **Vesico-urethral reflex is best evaluated by** *[NBE FMGE September 2012]*
    a. Plain X-rays
    b. Micturating cystourethrogram (MCU)
    c. Ultrasound
    d. IVP
11. **Ultrasonography finding of Chronic renal disease is** *[NBE FMGE March 2009]*
    a. Normal kidney b. Shrunken kidney
    c. Enlarged kidney d. Any of the above
12. **Most sensitive imaging modality for diagnosis of ureteric stones in a patient with acute colic is** *[Recent Question 2013]*
    a. X-ray KUB region b. Ultrasonogram
    c. Non contrast CT scan of the abdomen
    d. Contrast enhanced CT scan of the abdomen
13. **All of the following form radiolucent stones except** *[Recent Question 2012, 2013]*
    a. Xanthine b. Cysteine
    c. Uric acid d. Orotic acid
14. **Rim sign in IVP is seen in** *[Recent Question 2012]*
    a. Polycystic kidney b. Hydronephrosis
    c. Chronic pyelonephritis d. Hypernephroma
15. **Sonography in a case of chronic renal disease can show all of following except** *[NBE FMGE March 2012]*
    a. Loss of corticomedullary differentiation
    b. Increased renal size
    c. Smooth renal outline
    d. Increase in renal parenchymal echogenicity
16. **Most sensitive test for ureteric stone is** *[Recent Question 2013, 2014]*
    a. CECT b. KUB
    c. USG d. NCCT
17. **Fir tree appearance of bladder is seen in** *[Recent Question 2013, 2015]*
    a. Schistosomiasis b. Tuberculosis
    c. Neurogenic bladder d. Pelvic abscess
18. **Most sensitive test to detect early Renal TB is** *[Recent Question 2013, 2015]*
    a. Intravenous urography b. CT
    c. MRI d. USG
19. **Keyhole sign on Ultrasound is seen in** *[Recent Question 2017]*
    a. Polycystic kidney b. Hydronephrosis
    c. Chronic pyelonephritis d. Posterior urethral valves
20. **'Drooping lily sign' is seen in** *[Recent Question 2017]*
    a. Polycystic kidney
    b. Duplicated collecting system
    c. Chronic pyelonephritis d. Hypernephroma
21. **Most commonly used investigation for Urinary tract obstruction is** *[Recent Question 2017]*
    a. CECT b. MRI
    c. USG d. Angiography
22. **The best investigation to detect Renal stone is** *[Recent Question 2017]*
    a. X- ray b. CT
    c. MRI d. USG
23. **Which of the following is not a contraindication of Intravenous pyelography?** *[Recent Question 2017]*
    a. Previous hypersensitivity
    b. Recurrent UTI
    c. Multiple myeloma d. Pregnancy

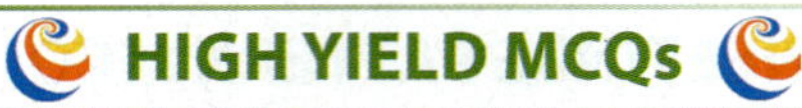

HIGH YIELD MCQs

1. **Which of the following answer choices regarding the diagnosis of ureteroarterial fistulas is TRUE?** *[Bihar PG 2016]*
   a. CT abdomen/pelvis often readily detects Ureteroarterial fistulas
   b. Selective iliac arteriography has a sensitivity approaching 90% for the diagnosis of ureteroarterial fistulas
   c. Provocative maneuvers, including ureteral stent removal over a guidewire, may aid in the diagnosis
   d. Cystoscopy provides no clues towards diagnosis

2. **Renal GFR is best measured by** *[PGI 2005]*
   a. Tc99 DMSA b. Tc99 Pyrophosphate scan
   c. Tc99 DTPA d. Creatinine clearance
   e. Tc99 albumin scan

3. **'Rim sign' in IVP is seen in** *[AIIMS PGMEE 1998]*
   a. Polycystic Kidney b. Hydronephrosis
   c. Chronic pyelonephritis d. Hypernephroma
   e. Cardiomegaly

4. **Bilateral 'spider leg sign' on IVP suggests** *[Delhi PGMEE 2006]*
   a. Renal stone b. Polycystic kidney
   c. Hypernephroma d. Hydronephrosis

5. **GFR is measured with which of the following?** *[All India PGMEE 2008]*
   a. Iodohippurate
   b. Tc99m-DTPA
   c. Tc99m-MAG3
   d. Ic99m-DMSA

6. **Impaired Renal Function is assessed by** *[All India PGMEE 1999]*
   a. MAGS b. IodoHippurate
   c. DMSA Scan d. DTPA

7. **All of the following form radiolucent stones except** *[AIIMS PGMEE 2003]*
   a. Xanthine b. Cysteine
   c. Aliopurinol d. Orotic acid

8. **Papillary necrosis features are all except** *[AIIMS PGMEE 2009]*
   a. Egg in cup b. Hyperdense nephrogram
   c. Calyceal horns d. "Ring shadows"

9. **Renal GFR is estimated by** *[All India PGMEE 1995]*
   a. TC99 DMCA
   b. TC99 DMSA
   c. Tc99 DTPA
   d. Tc90 – Gallium

10. **The posterior urethra is best visualized by** *[AIIMS PGMEE 2005]*
    a. Static cystogram b. Retrograde urethrogram
    c. Voiding cystogram d. CT cystogram

11. **Causes of bladder calcification are** *[PGI 2006]*
    a. Schistosomiasis b. Urethral cell
    c. Tuberculosis d. Carcinoma

12. **The investigations of choice for imaging of urinary tract tuberculosis is** *[AIIMS PGMEE 2004]*
    a. Plain X-ray b. Intravenous urography
    c. Ultrasound d. Computed tomography

13. **Most important investigation for posterior urethral valve is** *[AIIMS PGMEE 1997]*
    a. Urethroscopy
    b. IVP
    c. Retrograde cystogram
    d. Micturating cystourethrogram (MCU)

14. **Investigation of choice to demonstrate vesico-ureteral reflux** *[All India PGMEE 1992]*
    a. Isotope cystogram
    b. Contrast Micturating Cystourethrogram
    c. IVP
    d. Cystoscopy

15. **'Cobra head deformity' is characteristic of** *[AIIMS PGMEE 1997, Recent Question 2014]*
    a. Posterior urethral valve
    b. Ureterocoele
    c. Bladder tumor
    d. Cystitis

16. **IVP of polycystic kidney disease shows** *[PGI 2009]*
    a. Cobra head
    b. Dropping lily
    c. Flower base appearance
    d. Spider leg deformity
    e. Fish hook appearance

17. **Excretory urography should be cautiously performed in** *[All India PGMEE1991]*
    a. Bone 2° b. Multiple myeloma
    c. Neuroblastoma d. Leukemia

18. **Spider leg appearance is found in** *[PGI 1999]*
    a. Polycystic kidney b. Pyelonephritis
    c. Hydronephrosis d. Renal artery stenosis

19. **A dense persistent nephrogram may be seen in all of the following except:** *[AIIMS PGMEE 2002]*
    a. Acute ureteral obstruction
    b. Systemic hypertension
    c. Severe hydronephrosis
    d. Dehydration

20. **A dense renogram is obtained by** *[All India PGMEE 2010]*
    a. Dehydrating the patient
    b. Increasing the dose of contrast media
    c. Rapid [Bolus] injection of dye
    d. Using non ionic media

21. **The most important sign of significance of renal artery stenosis on an angiogram is** *[All India PGMEE 2006]*
    a. A percentage diameter stenosis >7%
    b. Presence of collaterals
    c. A systolic pressure gradient >2 mm Hg across the lesion
    d. Post stenotic dilatation of the renal arte]

22. Non-visualisation of kidney in excretory urogram is seen in *[PGI 2004, PGI 2005]*
a. Duplication b. Renal vein thrombosis
c. Hydronephrosis d. Hypoplasia

23. A patient presented with ARF with complete anuria but a normal ultrasound. Next investigation is *[All India PGMEE 1999]*
a. IVP b. Antegrade Pyelography
c. Retrograde Pyelography
d. Radiorenogram

24. Abdominal Ultrasonography in a 3-year-old boy show a solid circumscribed hypoechoic renal mass. Most likely diagnosis is *[All India PGMEE 2002]*
a. Wilm's tumor b. Renal cell carcinoma
c. Mesoblastic nephroma d. Oncocytoma

25. Which of the following is not an appropriate investigation for anterior urethral stricture? *[AIIMS PGMEE 2003]*
a. Magnetic Resonance Imaging
b. Retrograde urethrogram
c. Micturating cystourethrogram
d. High frequency ultrasound

26. Transrectal ultrasonography in carcinoma prostate is most useful for *[All India PGMEE 2008]*
a. Guided prostatic biopsies
b. Seminal vesicle involvement
c. Measurement of prostatic volume
d. To detect hypoechoic area

27. Hypoechoic lesion within prostate in USG seen in *[PGI 2004]*
a. Adeno CA b. Normal prostate tissue
c. Infertility d. Urethral obstruction
e. BPH

28. A 40-year-old male/female patient on long term steroid therapy presents with recent onset of severe pain in the right hip. Imaging modality of choice for this problem is *[AIIMS PGMEE 2005]*
a. CT scan b. Bone scan
c. MRI d. Plain X-ray

29. Which of the following imaging modality is most sensitive to detect early renal tuberculosis? *[AIIMS PGMEE 2002, 2003, All India PGMEE 2006]*
a. Intravenous urography
b. Ultrasound
c. Computed tomography
d. Magnetic resonance imaging

30. Most sensitive and specific investigation for screening of Renovascular hypertension *[AIIMS PGMEE 2001]*
a. MRI
b. Captopril enhanced radionuclide scan
c. Spiral CT Scan
d. Duplex - Doppler flow study

31. In Renal cell carcinoma investigation of choice to evaluate Inferior vena cava & renal vein for thrombus *[AIIMS PGMEE 1999]*
a. IVP b. Color Doppler
c. USG d. CT scan

32. Renal tuberculosis can be diagnosed earliest by
a. CT scan b. IVP [AIIMS PGMEE 1998]
c. Angiography d. USG

33. Investigation of choice for studying Renal Cortical mass *[AIIMS PGMEE 1993]*
a. 99 Tc DTPA b. 53 Cr Study
c. 99 Tc DMSA d. 99 Tc Pyrophosphate

34. The most sensitive imaging modality for diagnosis of Ureteric stones in a patient with acute colic is
a. X-ray KUB region *[All India PGMEE 2005]*
b. Ultrasonogram
c. Non contrast CT scan of the abdomen
d. Contrast enhanced CT scan of the abdomen

35. Functional analysis of kidney is best done by *[PGI 1997]*
a. Radionuclide scanning b. IVP
c. Ultrasound d. MRI

36. Marker of contrast induced nephropathy is
a. Serum cystatin C[JIPMER PGMEE 2014]
b. Serum creatinine
c. Nephrogram 24 hours later
d. None

37. Invertogram in newborn must be done *[JIPMER PGMEE 2014]*
a. Immediately after birth b. 1-2 hours after birth
c. 2-4 hours after birth d. 12-14 hours after birth

38. Most important investigation in VVF *[ESI IMO 2014]*
a. Three swab test b. IVP
c. Cystoscopy d. Vaginal culture

39. Semen analysis of a young man who presented with primary infertility revealed low volume, fructose negative ejaculate with azoospermia. Which of the following is the most useful imaging modality to evaluate the cause of his infertility? **[ESI IMO 2014]**
a. Colour duplex ultrasonography of the scrotum
b. Transrectal ultrasonography
c. Retrograde urethrography
d. Spermatic venography

40. Scan particularly useful to prove that collecting system dilatation is caused by obstruction in renal system *[PGMCET 2015]*
a. 99m Tc-DTPA scan b. MAG-3 scan
c. DMSA scan d. Hippuran scan

41. Retrograde Cystograph showing an exceedingly Contracted (Thimble) bladder in case of *[PGMCET 2015]*
a. Hunner's ulcer b. Cystitis cystica
c. Tuberculous cystitis d. Encrusting cystitis

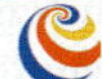

NEET/NBE PATTERN MCQs ANSWERS WITH EXPLANATIONS

1. **Ans. (c) Uric acid**
   [Ref. Sumer K Sethi, 5/e p78]
   - *Types of Nephrolithiasis (Renal stones)*:

Radio-opaque stones (90%)	Radio-lucent stones (10%)
• Calcium oxalate • Calcium phosphate • Struvite • Cystine • Matrix	• Uric acid • Xanthine

2. **Ans. (b) Renal oncocytomas**
   [Ref. Genitourinary Radiology by Zagoria, 2/e p101]
   - **Central stellate scar** is a characteristic imaging finding of oncocytomas on CT or magnetic resonance imaging (MRI)
   - Average size of oncocytomas with central scars is slightly less than that of tumors without scars
   - Oncocytomas are usually isoechoic to the kidney, with well-demarcated margins

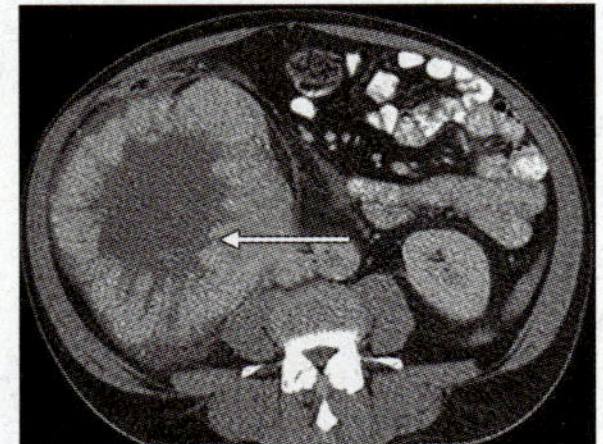

Fig. Central stellate scar

3. **Ans. (b) Hydronephrosis**
   [Ref. Zone Comprehensive Guide to PGMEE, Volume 3, 2009, Pg 861]
   - Intravenous urogram/pyelogram (IVU/IVP) in Hydronephrosis:
     - *Earliest change*: Dilatation of renal pelvis
     - *'Crescent/foot-pad' sign*
     - *'Rim sign'* (Severe Hydronephrosis)
4. **Ans. (b) DMSA**
   [Ref. Comprehensive Clinical Nephrology by Johnson, 5/e p67]
   - Renal cortex imaging is performed with tubular retention agents, usually 99mTc-DMSA.
5. **Ans. (c) Medial fibroplasias with aneurysm**
   [Ref. The Practice of Interventional Radiology by Valji, 1/e p300]
   - Medial fibroplasia, the most common, having the classic aneurysmal **"string of beads" appearance**
   - Angiographically, this typically gives a *string-of-beads* appearance to the *renal artery*
   - Appearance is caused by alternating areas of narrowing *due* to thickened segments

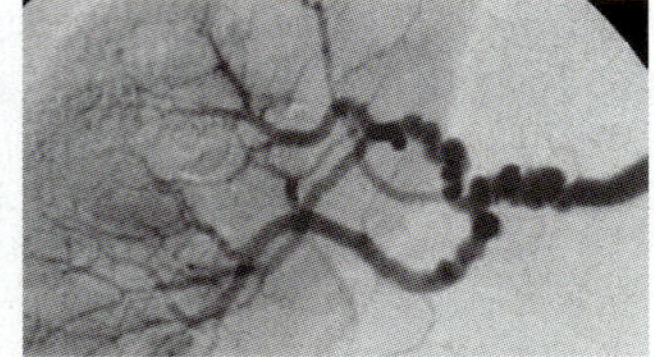

Fig. String of beads

6. **Ans. (c) Polycystic kidney disease**
   [Ref. Sumer K Sethi, 6/e p131]
   - Polycystic kidney (Autosomal dominant or Adult form): Swiss Cheese Nephrogram, also shows spider leg calyces on IVP
7. **Ans. (b) Stress incontinence**
   [Ref. Bipin Valchandji Daga, 1/e p227]
   - Bead cystography measuring the posterior urethra vesical angle is used to evaluate stress incontinence
8. **Ans. (b) USG**
   [Ref. David Sutton, 7/e p923]
   - Two most frequent indications for renal sonography:
     - Evaluation of an antenatal abnormality (hydronephrosis or cystic change)
     - Investigation of a child who has had a urinary tract infection (UTI)
9. **Ans. (b) Chronic tubercular cystitis**
   [Ref. Sumer K Sethi, 6/e p131]
   - Small low capacity thick walled bladder or Thimble Bladder is seen in tuberculosis
10. **Ans. (b) Micturating cystourethrogram (MCU)**
    [Ref. David Sutton, 7/e p924]
    - **Micturating cystourethrography** is used to evaluate siblings of children with vesicoureteric reflex and children with suspected structural abnormalities of the lower urinary tract

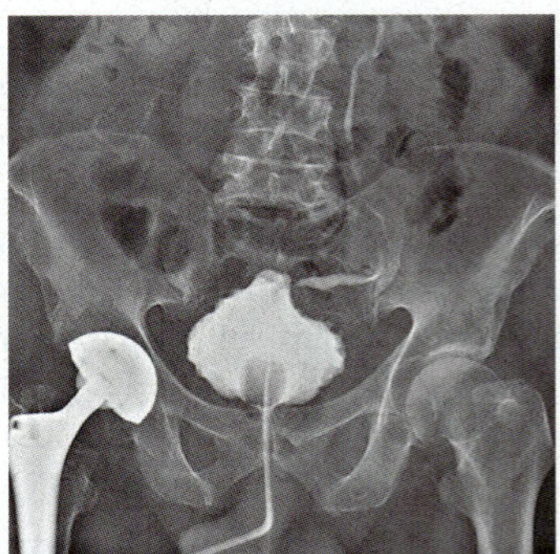

Fig. Micturating cystourethrogram

11. **Ans. (d) Any of the above**
    [Ref. emedicine.net]
    - Generally kidneys are shrunken in Chronic renal disease but may be normal or even enlarged as is seen in Amyloidosis, Adult polycystic kidney disease, Diabetic nephropathy
12. **Ans. (c) Non contrast CT scan of the abdomen**
    [Ref. Campbell's Urology, Volume 1p417]
    - Non-contrast helical CT scan is the most sensitive modality to detect urolithiasis, especially ureteral or small calculi and provides the most anatomic detail of the urinary tract
13. **Ans. (b) Cysteine**
    [Ref. Textbook of Pediatric Emergency Medicine by Fleisher 6/e p1122]
    - Radiopaque stones: calcium, cysteine, struvite
    - Radiolucent stones: uric acid, xanthine, orotic acid

14. Ans. (b) Hydronephrosis

[Ref. Bipin ValchandjiDaga, 1/e p235]

- Hydronephrosis on IVU: Rim sign—'thin band of radio density surrounding calyces' in advance cases

15. Ans. (b) Increased renal size

[Ref. Ultrasound of Urogenital System by Baxter, 1/e p12]

Ultrasonography in Chronic Renal Disease

- Loss of corticomedullary differentiation
- Cortical thinning
- Decreased renal size (<8 cm)
- Smooth renal outline
- Increase in renal parenchymal echogenicity (hyperechoic)

16. Ans. (d) NCCT

[Ref. Campbell's Urology, Volume 1 p417]

- Non-contrast helical CT scan is the **most sensitive modality to detect urolithiasis**, especially ureteral or small calculi and provides the most anatomic detail of the urinary tract

17. Ans. (c) Neurogenic bladder

[Ref. David Sutton, 7/e p999]

- In neurogenic bladder, the detrusor muscle may become hyper-reflexic with frequency urgency and urge incontinence
- Bladder becomes heavily trabeculated and may develop the classical 'fir-tree appearance'
- Alternatively the detrusor muscle may become flaccid, with a smooth over-distended bladder

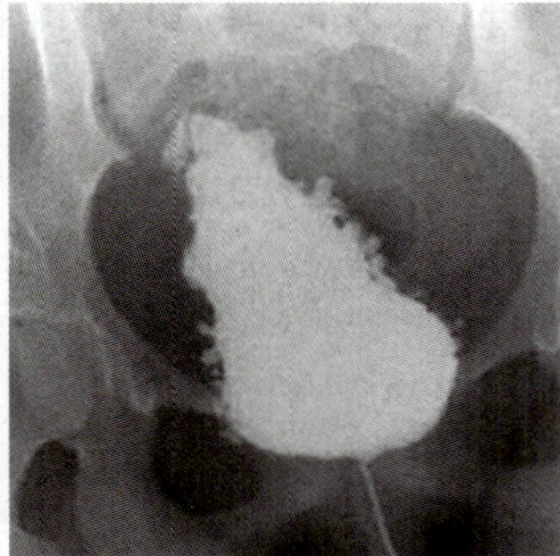

Fig. Fir-tree bladder

18. Ans. (a) Intravenous urography

[Ref. David Sutton, 7/e p980]

Tuberculosis of Kidney & Ureters

- In ureter, it develops as a result of descending infection from renal tuberculosis
- Characteristic features are seen on IVU and include
  - Ulceration in the early stages
  - Multifocal stricturing
  - Calcification with hydroureter and Hydronephrosis
  - Ureter shortened, straightened (Pipestem ureter)

19. Ans. (d) Posterior urethral valves

[Ref. Pediatric Urology by Al-Salem, 1/e p428]

Prenatal USG findings of Posterior Urethral Valves

- Thick walled bladder
- Keyhole sign: Dilated bladder with posterior urethra
- Unilateral/ bilateral hydroureteronephrosis
- Echobright kidneys
- Oligohydramnios

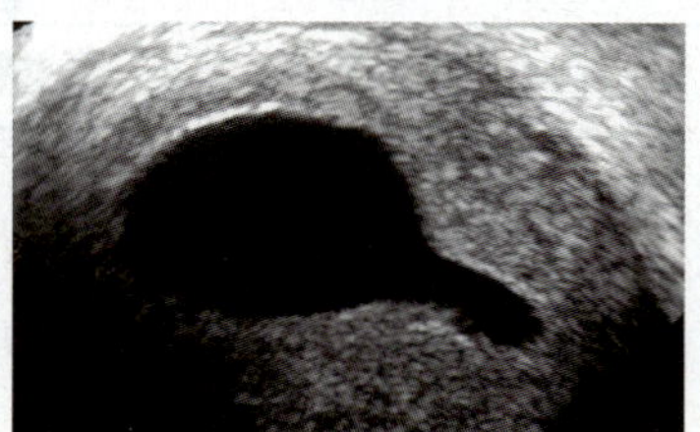

Fig. Keyhole sign

20. Ans. (b) Duplicated collecting system

[Ref. Urologic Imaging by Older, 1/e p3]

Drooping Lily Sign

- Classic sign on IVP of a duplicated collecting system with obstruction
- It results from the obstructed, poorly functioning upper moiety with mass effect on the lower moiety, which is normally functioning
- Excretion into lower moiety's excretory system showing contrast-filled calyces to be bunched together and to resemble drooping petals of a lily

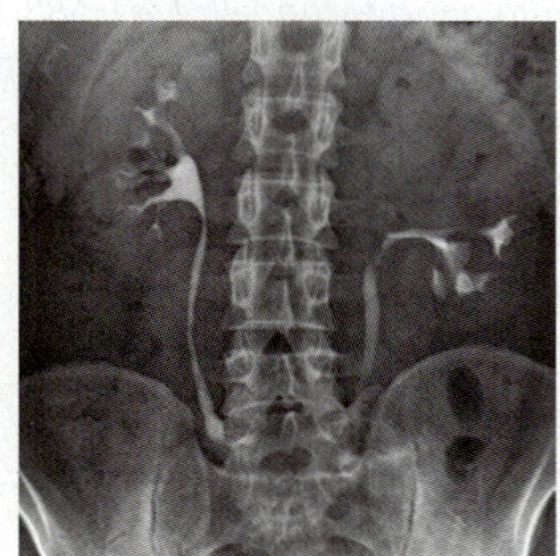

Fig. Drooping lily sign

21. Ans. (c) USG

[Ref. Comprehensive Clinical Nephrology by Johnson, 5/e p710]

- Ultrasound is a useful first-line investigation for any patient with suspected urinary tract obstruction
- Computed tomography (CT) is now the preferred imaging technique when renal calculi are suspected

22. Ans. (b) CT

[Ref. Surgery by Patten, 2/e p179]

Radiology in Renal Stones

- Intravenous urogram and CT scanning (more specifically, CT-KUB) are investigations of diagnostic value for renal stones
- CT scans are able to detect 99% of renal stones and, therefore, are Gold standard diagnostic investigation for renal calculi
- In addition, the CT scan is able to exclude other causes of an acute abdomen and contrast media is not needed unlike IVU which may be nephrotoxic
- X-ray KUB can detect 80% renal calculi so should be the first investigation offered

23. Ans (b) Recurrent UTI

[Ref. Urology Board Review, 3/e p1]

Contraindication to Intravenous pyelography

- Absolute contraindications to IVP: Previous anaphylactic reactions to IV contrast, Positive azotemia (creatinine >2.0)
- Relative contraindications to IVP: Dehydration, Diabetes, Multiple myeloma, Pregnancy

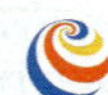

HIGH YIELD MCQs ANSWERS WITH EXPLANATIONS

1. **Ans. (c) Provocative maneuvers, including ureteral stent removal over a guidewire, may aid in the diagnosis**
   [Ref. Urological Emergencies by Wessells, 1/e p191]

Diagnosis of Uretero-arterial fistulas

- Difficult to diagnose radiographically with standard imaging, including CT scan
- Selective iliac arteriography has a sensitivity <50% for diagnosis
- Retrograde pyelogram is non-diagnostic with low sensitivity
- Cystoscopy may reveal lateralizing blood flow that may be pulsatile
- Provocative maneuvers, including Ureteral stent removal over a guidewire, may aid in the diagnosis:
  - 100% sensitivity
  - Additional advantage: Definitive arteriographic embolization can be done if diagnosis is established

2. **Ans. (c) Tc99 DTPA**
   [Ref. Core Radiology by Mandell, 1/e p 582]
   - Tc^{99} DTPA can measure glomerular filtration rate (GFR) and evaluate renal perfusion

3. **Ans. (b) Hydronephrosis**
   [Ref. Bipin Valchandji Daga, 1/e p235]

4. **Ans. (b) Polycystic kidney**
   [Ref. Sumer K Sethi, 6/e p131]

5. **Ans. (b) Tc99 DTPA**
   [Ref. Core Radiology by Mandell, 1/e p582]

6. **Ans. (d) DTPA**
   [Ref. Core Radiology by Mandell, 1/e p582]

7. **Ans. (b) Cysteine**
   [Ref. Textbook of Pediatric Emergency Medicine by Fleisher 6/e p1122]

8. **Ans. (b) Hyperdense nephrogram**
   [Ref. Radiology Review Manual by Dahnert, 6/e p943]

Papillary Necrosis

- Ring shadow
- Egg in cup appearance
- Track & horns from the calyceal fornices
- Decreased nephrogram followed by dense nephrogram

9. **Ans. (c) Tc99 DTPA**
   [Ref. Core Radiology by Mandell, 1/e p582]

10. **Ans. (c) Voiding cystogram**
    [Ref. David Sutton, 7/e p998-999]
    - VCUG is the definitive test for diagnosing posterior urethral valves
    - Anterograde technique: Posterior urethra
    - Retrograde technique: Anterior urethra valves

11. **Ans. (a) Schistosomiasis; (c) Tuberculosis**
    [Ref. Radiology Review Manual by Dahnert, 6/e p899]

Bladder Wall Calcification

- Inflammations:
  - **Schistosomiasis (50%)**
  - Tuberculosis
  - Cystitis:
    1. Bacillary UTI (extremely uncommon)
    2. Encrusted foreign material
    3. Alkaline-encrusted cystitis and pyelitis
- Neoplasms:
  - Primary neoplasm of bladder: TCC, squamous cell carcinoma, leiomyosarcoma, hemangioma, neuroblastoma, osteogenic sarcoma
  - Urachal carcinoma

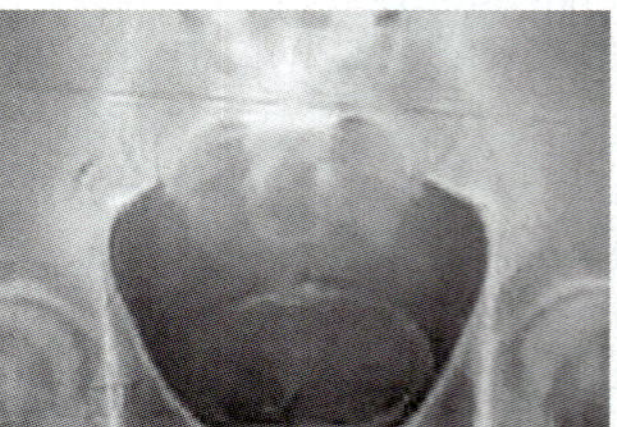

Fig. Bladder wall calcification

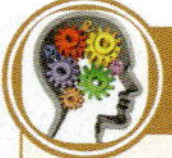

Also Remember

Bladder Calculi

- Stasis calculi (70%): Associated with Gram-negative lower urinary tract infection (Proteus)
- Migrant calculi
- Foreign body nidus calculi (Self-introduced objects, urinary stent, chronic catheterization, bladder wall-penetrating bone fragments, prostatic chips, non-absorbable suture material, fragments of Foley balloon catheter, pubic hair, presence of intestinal mucosa)
- Idiopathic/primary/endemic calculi

12. **Ans. (b) Intravenous urography**
    [Ref. David Sutton, 7/e p980]

13. **Ans. (d) Micturating cystourethrogram (MCU)**
    [Ref. David Sutton, 7/e p998-999]

14. **Ans. (b) Contrast Micturating cystourethrogram**
    [Ref. David Sutton, 7/e p998-999]

15. **Ans. (b) Ureterocoele**
    [Ref. David Sutton, 7/e p935]
    - **Cobra's head appearance**: On IVU the Ureterocele can be seen as a contrast-filled structure with a thin smooth radiolucent wall surrounded by contrast containing urine in the bladder
    - If the Ureterocele is obstructed and the associated kidney non-functioning, it appears as a well-defined radiolucent within the opacified bladder

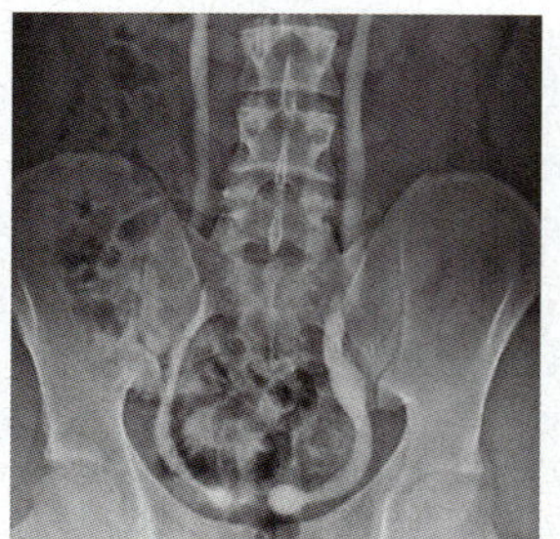

Fig 138. Cobra head appearance

16. Ans. (d) Spider leg deformity
[Ref. Sumer K Sethi, 6/e p131]

17. Ans. (b) Multiple myeloma
[Ref. Blood: Principles and Practice of Hematology, Volume 1 byHandin, 2/e p901]
- Excretory urography is a type of contrast study used to verify and localize upper urinary tract disease.
- Relative contraindications are
  - Multiple myeloma
  - Myeloma kidney
  - Myeloma
  - Allergy
  - Dehydration
  - Obstructive uropathy
  - Jod-Basedow's hyperthyroidism
  - Shock
  - Acute tubular necrosis
  - Acute & chronic Renal failure

18. Ans. (a) Polycystic kidney
[Ref. Sumer K Sethi, 6/e p131]

19. Ans. (b) Systemic hypertension
[Ref. Sumer K Sethi, 6/e p136]
- In acute hypotension (not hypertension) increasingly dense nephrogram is observed

20. Ans. (c) Rapid [Bolus] injection of dye
[Ref. Encyclopedia of Imaging by Albert, 1/e p1927]

21. Ans. (b) Presence of collaterals
[Ref. David Sutton, 7/e p432, 965]
- Hemodynamic significance of renal artery stenosis is determined by
  - Presence of collateral
  - Elevated renin levels in ipsilateral veins ≥1.5:1
  - Greater than 70% stenosis with post stenotic dilatation
  - Decrease in renal size
  - Trans stenotic pressure gradient of + 40 mm Hg

22. Ans. (b) Renal vein thrombosis; (c) Hydronephrosis
[Ref. General Urology, 1/e p322]

23. Ans. (d) Radiorenogram
[Ref. Functional Imaging in Nephro-Urology by Alain Prigent, 1/e p246]
- Renal imaging is useful in case of ARF secondary to obstruction
- Commonly used imaging modalities in this setting are USG and nuclear scan (radiorenogram)

24. Ans. (a) Wilm's tumour
[Ref. Radiology Review Manual by Dahnert, 5/e p927, 933, 950, 984]
- Wilm's tumour occurs in young children
- Renal cell carcinoma and oncocytoma are of adult age group
- Mesoblastic nephroma occur in infants

25. Ans. (a) MRI
[Ref. Sabiston Textbook of Surgery, 16/e p1669]

Radiological Investigation for Urethral Stricture
- Retrograde urethrography
- Micturating cystourethrography
- Endoscopy
- Sonographic urethrogram
- High frequency USG

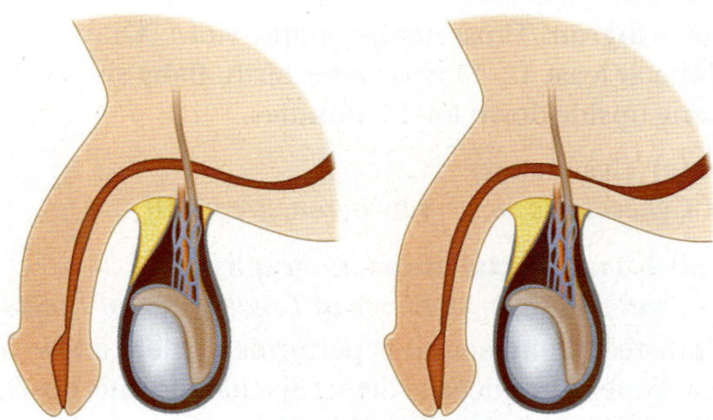

Fig 139. Urethral stricture

26. Ans. (a) Guided prostatic biopsies
[Ref. David Sutton, 7/e p896-897]

27. Ans. (a) Adeno CA; (e) BPH
[Ref. Diagnostic Ultrasound by John P. McGahan, 1/e p255]

28. Ans. (c) MRI
[Ref. Surgery of the Hip Joint, by Tronzo, 2/e p5]
- Systemic steroid administration in virtually every significant series of cases of non-traumatic avascular necrosis of the femoral head
- Investigation of choice is MRI

29. Ans. (a) Intravenous urography
[Ref. David Sutton, 7/e p980]

30. Ans. (c) Spiral CT scan
[Ref. Primary Cardiology by Braunwald, 2/e p291]

31. Ans. (b) Color Doppler
[Ref. Radiology in Surgical Practice by Neuhaus, 1/e 221]
- MRI is investigation of choice
- USG is next best choice

32. Ans. (b) IVP
[Ref. David Sutton, 7/e p980]

33. Ans. (c) 99 Tc DMSA
[Ref. Core Radiology by Mandell, 1/e p 582]

34. Ans. (c) Non contrast CT scan of the abdomen
[Ref. Campbell's Urology, Volume 1 p417]
- Non-contrast helical CT scan is the most sensitive modality to detect urolithiasis, especially ureteral or small calculi and provides the most anatomic detail of the urinary tract

35. Ans. (a) Radionuclide scanning
[Ref. Functional Imaging in Nephro-Urology by Prigent, 1/e p246]

36. Ans. (b) Serum creatinine
[Ref. Contrast Mediaby Thomsen,3/e p75]
- Serum Creatinine value has been used to calculate the risk of contrast-induced nephropathy (CIN) in patients

- Acute contrast-induced renal injury: Rise in Serum Creatinine >25% above baseline or a rise of 0.5 mg/dL within 48 hours of a contrast-based procedure

37. Ans. (d) 12–14 hours after birth

[Ref. Advances in Pediatrics by Sachdeva, 2/ep188]

- Anorectal malformations (Imperforate anus) are a class of congenital birth defect that are represented by a wide spectrum of defects
- **Invertogram**/Cross table-Lateral view: X-ray should be done at least 12–14 hour after birth, Baby should be kept hang upside down for 2-3 minutes.

38. Ans. (c) Cystoscopy

[Ref. Gynecologic Surgery by Byron, 2/e p339]

39. Ans. (b) Transrectal ultrasonography

[Ref. Gender Specific Medicine by Legato, 1/e Vol 1 p543]

- Transrectal ultrasound is performed where a low-volume ejaculate is produced to detect Ejaculatory duct obstruction (Acidic low-volume ejaculate, Absent/ minimal fructose)

40. Ans. (a) 99m Tc-DTPA scan

[Ref. Textbook of Nephrology by Mandal, 2/e p11]

Radiopharmaceuticals in Urinary System

- 99Tc Diethylenetriamine pentaacetic acid (DTPA): Renal perfusion and excretion
- Orthoiodohippurate (OIH): Effective renal plasma flow
- 99mTc Mercaptoacetyl triglycine (MAG3): Effective renal plasma flow (In Renal artery stenosis)
- 99m Tc Dimercaptosuccinic acid (DMSA): Cortical imaging, Space occupying lesions
- 99m Tc Glucoheptonate: Delayed Cortical imaging

41. Ans. (c) Tuberculous cystitis

[Ref. Lower Genitourinary Radiology by Jafri, 1/e p528]

- As with other forms of acute cystitis, Early Tuberculous cystitis shows bullous changes of the bladder mucosa
  - As the disease progresses, the bladder becomes contracted and irregular, and the irregularity may be asymmetric
- In Extensive disease, marked Cicatricial contractions of bladder lead to asymmetric small thick-walled bladder
  - With Irregular bands of fibrosis, Tuberculous bladder may contract to minute proportions, called a "Thimble bladder".

Chapter 8

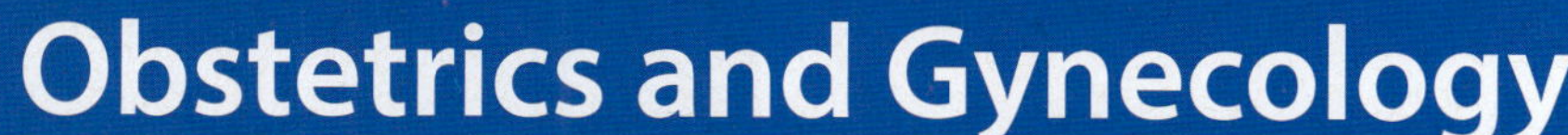

Obstetrics and Gynecology

THEORETICAL CONCEPTS

VIII A. ULTRASONOGRAPHY IN PREGNANCY

- *First investigation of choice in post-term pregnancy*: USG[Q]
  - *USG*: Accurate assessment of gestational age by various parameters
  - *Doppler USG velocitometry*: Assessment of foetal compromise
- *Earliest foetal shadow of vertebral dots can be visualised on USG by*: 16 weeks POG
- ***Best parameters for dating of pregnancy:*** [Q]
  - *First trimester*: Crown-rump length
  - *Second trimester*: Biparietal diameter
  - *Third trimester*: Femur length and head circumference

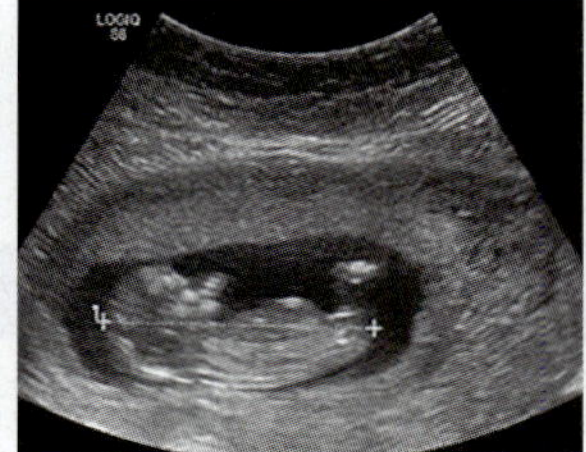

Fig. Crown-rump length

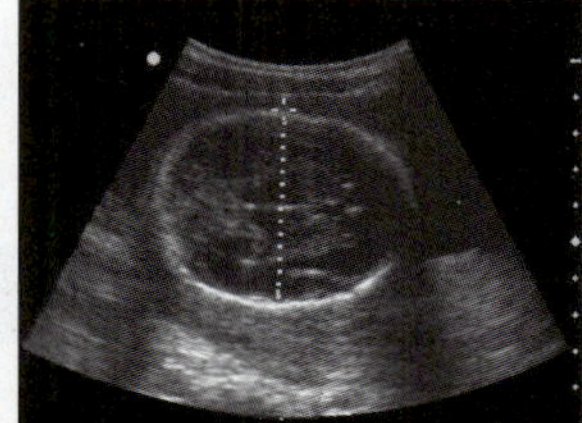

Fig. BPD

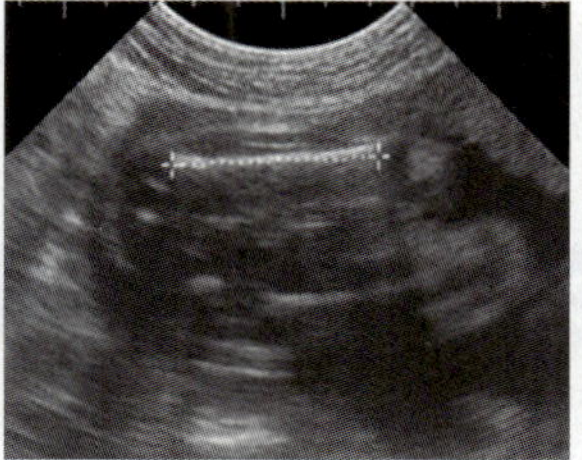

Fig. Femur length

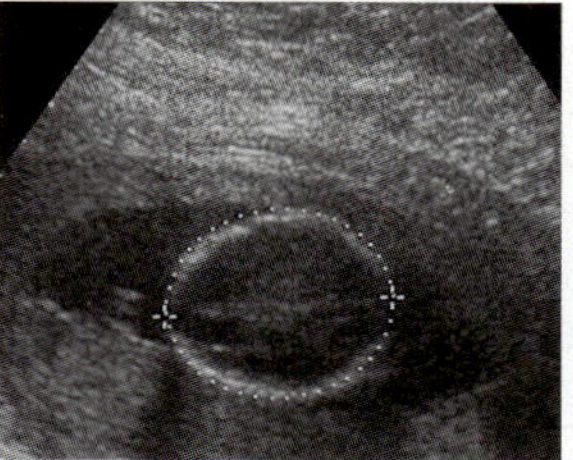

Fig. Fetal head circumference

VIII B. FEW IMPORTANT SIGNS IN RADIOLOGY OBSTETRICS & GYNECOLOGY

- *Robert's sign (Gas in heart/ blood vessels within 12 hours after birth)*: Foetal death[Q]
- ***Spalding's sign*** *(Overlapping of cranial bones)*: Foetal death
- ***Snow-storm appearance on USG:*** Hydatiform mole[Q]

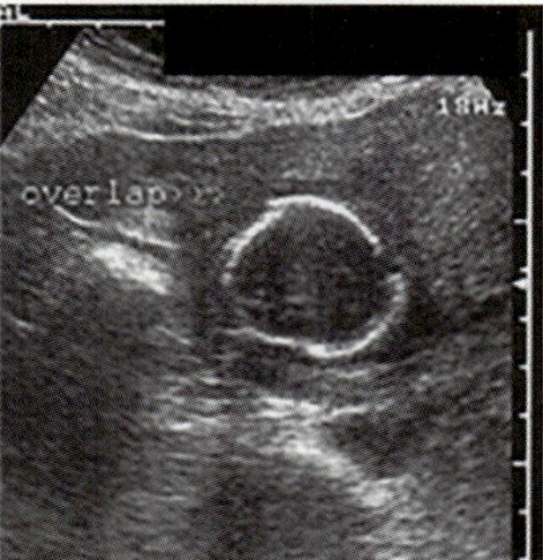

Fig. Spalding sign

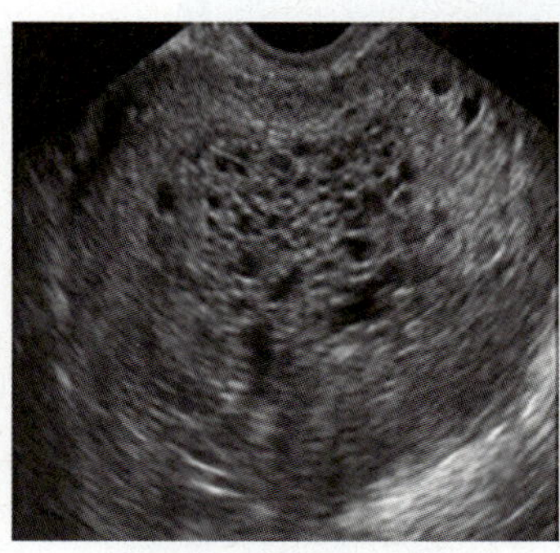

Fig. Snow-storm USG

VIII C. MAMMOGRAPHY IN BREAST CARCINOMA[Q]

- Irregular speculated margins [Q]
- Microcalcifications (**Pathognomonic**[Q])
- Distortions in architecture
- High density lesions

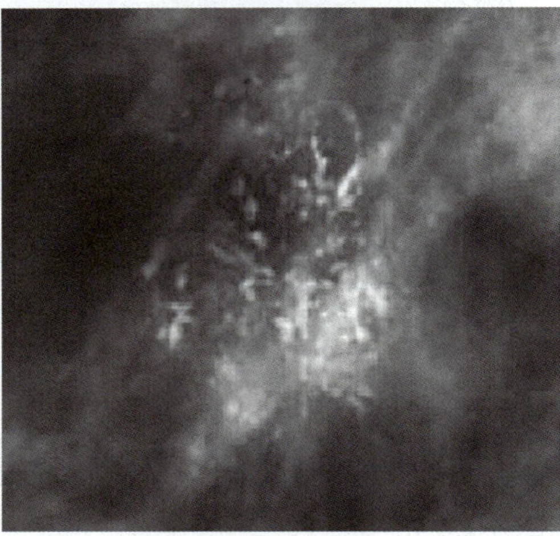

Fig. Microcalcifications

VIII D. BREAST LESIONS CONTAINING FAT[Q]

- Galactocele
- Fat necrosis (Traumatic lipid cyst)
- Hamartoma
- Lipoma
- Oil cyst
- Normal breast fat collections focally

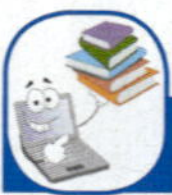

IMAGE-BASED QUESTIONS

1. A 21-year-old G1P0 presents to OPD at 20 weeks of gestation. She was told by her doctor that she has some problem. She comes to you for second opinion. USG image below shows the defect. What is your diagnosis? ***[AIIMS May 2016]***

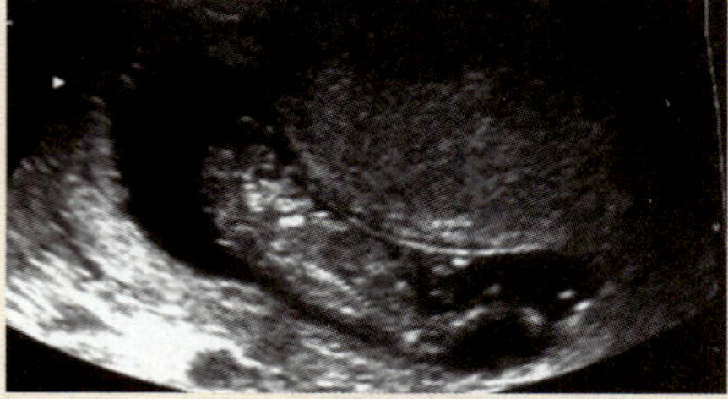

a. Cystic hygroma
b. Anencephaly
c. Omphalocele
d. Encephalocele

2. Sign (Arrow) in imaging of breast is seen in ***[Recent Question 2013]***

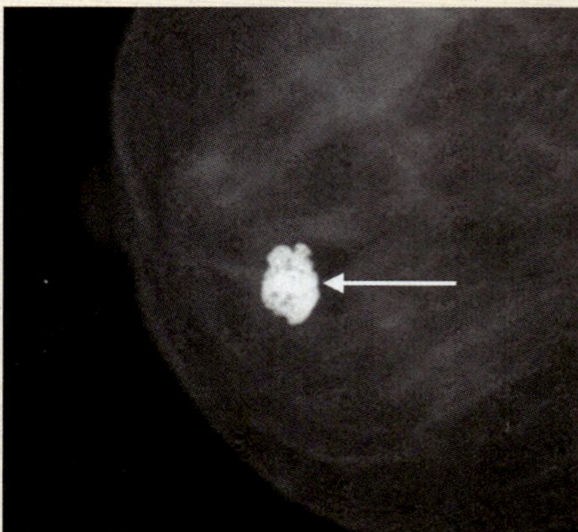

a. Fibroadenoma
b. Fibroadenosis
c. Carcinoma breast
d. Mastitis

3. Identify the measurement used (Arrows) in Antenatal USG *[Recent Question 2013]*

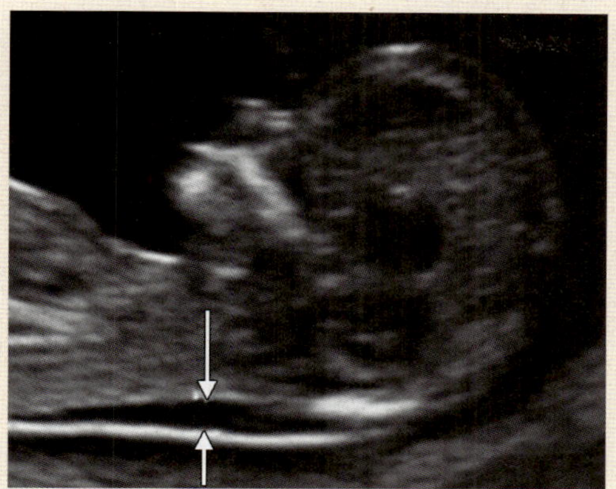

a. Spinal thickness
b. CSF fluid translucency
c. Nuchal translucency
d. None

4. Frequency of waves used in imaging modality (Photograph) *[Recent Question 2014]*

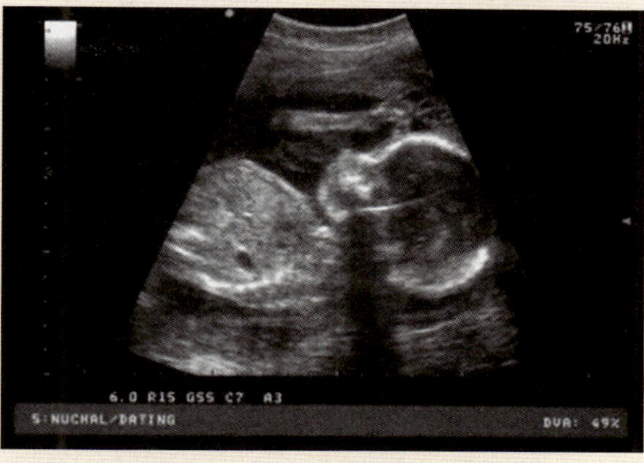

a. 2000 Hz
b. 5000 Hz
c. <2 Mega Hertz
d. >2 Mega Hertz

5. USG appearance in Photograph is characteristic of *[Recent Question 2015]*

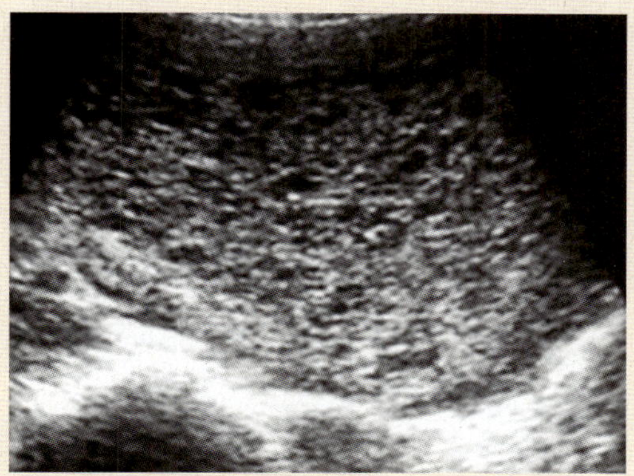

a. Ectopic pregnancy
b. Hydatiform mole
c. Chroriocarcinoma
d. Pelvic malignancy

6. Sign (Arrow) shown in Photograph indicates *[Recent Question 2014]*

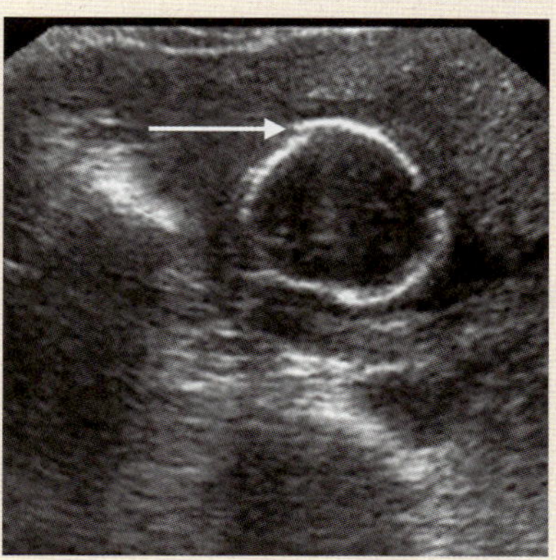

a. Abortion
b. Still birth
c. Intrauterine death
d. Infanticide

7. Diagnose the disorder based on the Image given below *[Recent Question 2018]*

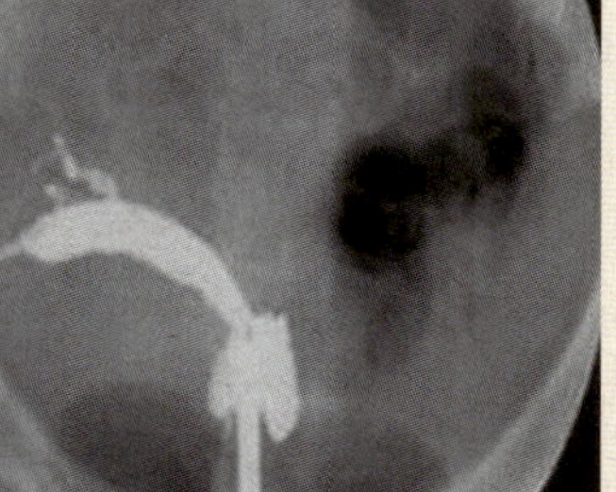

a. Uterus didelphys
b. Septate uterus
c. Unicornuate uterus
d. Bicornuate uterus

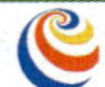 ANSWERS WITH EXPLANATIONS OF IBQs 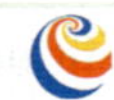

1. Ans. (b) Anencephaly *[Ref. Obstetrics and Gynecology by Arora, 1/e p121]*

USG Photograph: Mid-sagittal section of the fetus

- Head appears abnormally small
- Calcified cranium is absent
- Brain tissue appears dystrophic and distorted and extends beyond the usual location of head
- Thus, it is a case of anencephaly

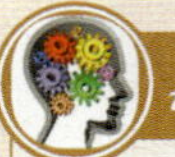

Also Remember

Anencephaly USG Findings

- Absent cranium
- No brain parenchymal tissue above the orbits
- If a small amount of neural tissue is present, it is known as exencephaly
- A "frog eye" or "mickey mouse" appearance may be seen when seen in coronal plane due to absent cranial bone/brain and bulging orbits
- Less than expected value for crown rump length (CRL)
- May show polyhydramnios due to impaired swallowing

2. Ans. (a) Fibroadenoma *[Ref. Common Breast Lesions by Pilnik, 1/e p105]*

Pop-Corn Calcification

- Pulmonary hamartoma
- Fibroadenoma breast
- Uterine fibroid
- Fibrous dysplasia
- Enchondroma
- Chondrosarcoma

3. Ans. (c) Nuchal translucency *[Ref. Medicolegal Radiology by Hare, 1/e p83]*

Nuchal Translucency

- Down's syndrome
- Turner syndrome
- Congenital heart disease
- Omphalocoele
- Skeletal dysplasias
- VACTERL association

4. Ans. (d) >2 Mega Hertz *[Ref. DC Dutta's Obstetrics, 8/e p732]*

- Obstetric USG is generally done at 3–5 MHz
- Commonly used frequency range in obstetrics is 3–5 MHz for abdominal transducers and 5–7 MHz for vaginal tranducers

5. Ans. (b) Hydatiform mole *[Ref. Sumer K Sethi, 5/e p96]*

- Hydatiform mole on USG: Classic sonographic appearance is that of a solid collection of echoes with numerous small anechoic spaces (Snow storm/Granular appearance)

6. Ans. (c) Intrauterine death *[Ref. Sumer K Sethi, 5/e p95]*

- Spalding sign: Overlapping of the fetal skull bones caused by collapse of the fetal brain, usually appearing after a week or more, indicate foetal death.

7. Ans. (c) Unicornuate Uterus 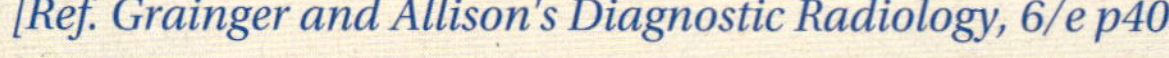 *[Ref. Grainger and Allison's Diagnostic Radiology, 6/e p406]*

Unicornuate Uterus

- Results from failure of normal development of one Müllerian duct, and is associated with increased spontaneous abortion and obstetric complications, and renal abnormalities
- **On Hysterosalpingogram** (See Photograph), endometrial cavity usually assumes a fusiform/banana shape (except for type a where there may a small cavitation filling defect), tapering at the apex and draining into a single fallopian tube (Uterus is generally shifted off the midline).

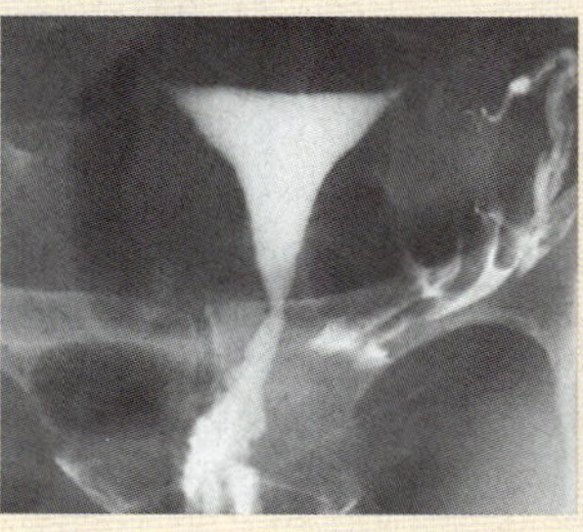

Fig. Normal uterus on HSG

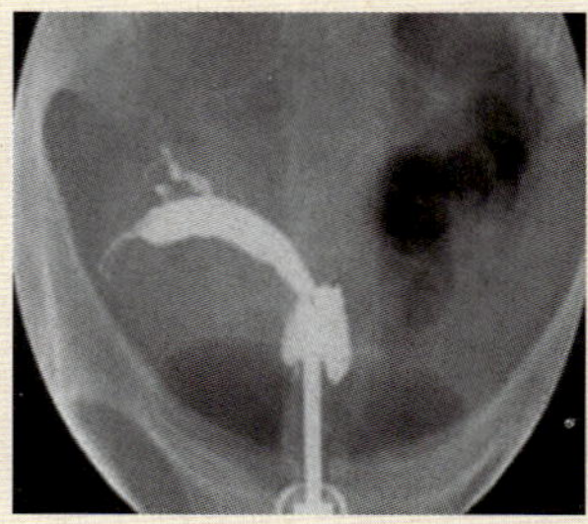

Fig. Unicornuate uterus on HSG

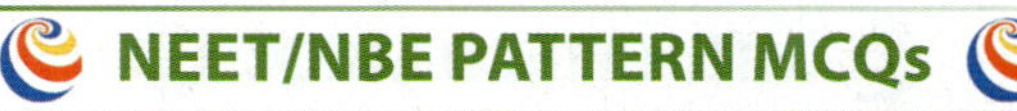

NEET/NBE PATTERN MCQs

1. Most accurate method to diagnose adenomyosis is *[UPSC CMS 2016]*
a. MRI b. PET-CT
c. Transvaginal sonography
d. Hysterosalpingography

2. A female complains of menorrhagia and dysmenorrhea since 10 years on USG the uterus shows salt and pepper pattern. What is your diagnosis? *[Recent Question 2016]*
a. Fibroids b. Carcinoma endometrium
c. Endometriosis d. Adenomyosis

3. Ovarian tumor which can be diagnosed by X-ray is *[Recent Question 2016]*
a. Gonadoblastoma b. Dysgerminoma
c. Choriocarcinoma d. Teratoma

4. First investigation for a woman with post-term pregnancy is *[NBE FMGE March 2007]*
a. X-ray abdomen b. Blood glucose profile
c. Vaginal examination d. Ultrasonography

5. Beaded lumen with fimbrial fluid is seen in *[Recent Question 2012, 2015]*
a. TB of fallopian tube b. TB of endometrium
c. TB of ovary d. None

6. Snow storm appearance on ultrasound of uterus is seen in *[NBE DNB 2007, 2011, Recent Question 2017]*
a. Endometriosis b. Endometrial carcinoma
c. Leiomyoma d. Hydatidiform mole

7. Radiation dose safe in pregnancy is *[Recent Question 2014]*
a. 1 rad b. 5 rads
c. 50 rads d. 500 rads

8. Nuchal translucency is used in *[Recent Question 2012]*
a. Head scan b. MRI neck
c. ANC USG d. Anthropometry

9. Radiographic visualisation of foetus earliest can be done at *[NBE FMGE September 2006]*
a. 8 weeks POG b. 12 weeks POG
c. 16 weeks POG d. 24 weeks POG

10. T sign is seen in *[Recent Question 2013]*
a. Genital TB
b. Membrane in twin pregnancy
c. Molar pregnancy d. Choriocarcinoma

11. Investigation of choice in congenital uterine anomaly *[Recent Question 2013]*
a. MRI c. HSG
b. CT d. Hysteroscopy

12. USG is definitive investigation of *[Recent Question 2013]*
a. Vasa previa b. Abruption placenta
c. Placenta previa d. Imperforate hymen

13. Fetal cardiac activity can be detected earliest by USG at which age of intrauterine life? *[Recent Question 2012]*
a. 1–2 week b. 2–4 weeks
c. 5–6 weeks d. 6–8 weeks

14. Spalding sign is seen in *[Recent Question 2013]*
a. Abortion b. Still birth
c. IUD d. Infanticide

15. Gas shadow in heart and great vessels appears in *[Recent Question 2013, 2015]*
a. IUD b. Abortion
c. Still birth d. None

16. Yolk sac is visible on USG first at *[Recent Question 2014, 2015]*
a. 4th week POG b. Early 5th week POG
c. Late 5th week POG d. 6th week POG

17. Fetal heart activity can be recorded earliest on TVS and TAS USG by .... respectively *[Recent Question 2015]*
a. 1 week and 2 weeks b. 6 weeks and 9 weeks
c. 5 weeks and 6 weeks d. 3 week and 4 weeks

18. Amount of radiation used in Mammography is *[Recent Question 2017]*
a. 0.5 mSv b. 0.7 mSv
c. 0.9 mSv d. 1 mSv

19. Safest radiological investigation in pregnancy is *[Recent Question 2017]*
a. CT b. MRI
c. X-ray d. HRCT

20. Best gestational age to do an anomaly scan is *[Recent Question 2017]*
a. 10–14 weeks b. 14–18 weeks
c. 18–22 weeks d. 22–26 weeks

21. Soft markers on Ultrasonography are helpful in diagnosing *[Recent Question 2017]*
a. Fetal age b. Chromosomal anomalies
c. Fetal size d. Site of pregnancy

22. Ring of fire on USG signifies *[Recent Question 2017]*
a. H. mole b. Ectopic pregnancy
c. PCOD d. Aneuploidy

23. Nuchal translucency is useful in *[Recent Question 2017]*
a. Determination of fetal age
b. Determination of fetal malformations
c. Determination of fetal size
d. Determination of location of placenta

24. Nuchal translucency is best measured at *[Recent Question 2017]*
a. 8–10 weeks b. 11–13 weeks
c. 15–17 weeks d. 18–20 weeks

25. Earliest sign of pregnancy on TVS is *[Recent Question 2017]*
a. Fetal heart sounds b. Fetal pole
c. Yolk sac d. Gestational sac

26. Double decidual sac sign is indicative of *[Recent Question 2017]*
a. Ectopic pregnancy b. Intrauterine pregnancy
c. H. mole d. Twin pregnancy

27. Imaging techniques used in Uterus anomalies EXCEPT *[Recent Question 2018]*
a. HSG b. USG
c. MRI guided HSG d. CT guided HSG

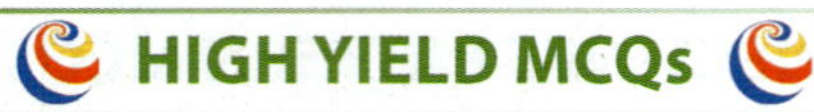

HIGH YIELD MCQs

1. **'Double bleb sign' refers to sonographic presentation of** *[AIIMS May 2016]*
   a. The amnion and chorion
   b. The amnion and yolk sac
   c. Two uterine gestational sacs
   d. Heterotopic pregnancy

2. **Ultrasound frequency used for diagnostic purposes in obstetrics** *[PGI 2001]*
   a. 1–20 MHz b. 20–40 MHz
   c. 40–60 MHz d. 60–80 MHz
   e. 80–100 MHz

3. **All are signs/features of ectopic pregnancy on USG except** *[PGI 2003]*
   a. Pseudo-sac b. Hyperechoic ring
   c. Adnexal mass
   d. Echogenic mass with multicystic spaces within endometrial cavity
   e. Doughnut sign

4. **USG can diagnose all except** *[Kerala PGMEE 2006]*
   a. Anencephaly b. Neural tube defect
   c. Placenta previa d. Down's syndrome

5. **The sensitivity of mammography is low in young females because** *[All India PGMEE 2009]*
   a. Less glandular tissue and more fat
   b. Young females are less cooperative
   c. Young breast have dense tissue
   d. Because of less fat content

6. **USG can defect gestation sac earliest at** *[DPG 2007]*
   a. 5–6 weeks of gestation b. 7–8 weeks of gestation
   c. 10 weeks of gestation d. 12 weeks of gestation

7. **Earliest sign of foetal life is best detected by** *[All India PGMEE 2004]*
   a. X-ray b. Fetoscopy
   c. Real time USG d. Doppler
   e. CT scan

8. **Ultrasonography of umbilical artery is done to know about** *[PGI 1997]*
   a. Heart beat b. Gestational age
   c. Foetal weight d. Foetal maturity

9. **Parameters used to estimate gestational age in last trimester** *[PGI 1997]*
   a. CR length b. Abdominal circumference
   c. BPD d. Femur length

10. **USG done at 18–20 weeks mainly to** *[Rajasthan PGMEE 2005]*
    a. Detect foetal abnormality b. Determine sex
    c. Estimate liquor d. Determine maturity

11. **Anencephaly can be diagnosed by USG at** *[AIIMS PGMEE 1996]*
    a. 10–12 weeks of gestation b. 14–18 weeks of gestation
    c. 20–24 weeks of gestation d. 24–28 weeks of gestation

12. **Best for unruptured ectopic pregnancy is** *[PGI 1997]*
    a. Per abdominal US b. hCG
    c. Transvaginal US d. Amniocentesis

13. **The investigation of choice for an ectopic pregnancy is** *[AIIMS PGMEE 1999, 2008]*
    a. CT scan b. Transvaginal USG
    c. Serum HCG levels d. MRI

14. **Missed IUD (IUCD) is recognized by** *[AIIMS PGMEE 1991]*
    a. X-ray b. USG
    c. Barium meal d. CT Scan

15. **Neural tube defect is best detected by** *[All India PGMEE 1995]*
    a. USG b. Chromosomal analysis
    c. Amniocentesis d. Placentography

16. **Earliest congenital malformation that may be detected on USG is** *[All India PGMEE 1994]*
    a. Down's syndrome b. Hydrocephalous
    c. Anencephaly d. Sacral agenesis

17. **True about antenatal Doppler analysis is all except** *[JIPMER PGMEE 2006, PGI 2006]*
    a. Reduction in end diastolic flow is associated with poor out come
    b. Reduction in EDF is associated with IUGR
    c. In normal gestation placental resistance is high
    d. SID ratio is high in IUGR
    e. Investigation of choice in pregnancy

18. **Which one of the following regarding antenatal assessment of umbilical arteries by color Doppler study is TRUE?** *[All India PGMEE 2008]*
    a. There is decreased SID ratio in smoker and nicotine abusing pregnant females
    b. The reduced diastolic flow at term indicates good prognosis
    c. The flow velocities and the SID ratio are useful to evaluate high risk pregnancies
    d. In otherwise normal pregnancies the increased S/D ratio is normal in smoking females

19. **Which one of the following congenital malformation of the fetus can be diagnosed in first trimester by ultrasound?** *[All India PGMEE 2006]*
    a. Anencephaly b. lnencephaly
    c. Microcephaly d. Holoprosencephaly

20. **Most accurate assessment of gestational age by USG is done by** *[JIPMER PGMEE 2004, Recent Question 2017]*
    a. Femur length
    b. Gestational sac size
    c. Menstrual history
    d. Crown rump length

21. **Ectopic pregnancy, characteristic finding in USG is** *[AIIMS PGMEE 1998]*
    a. Absence of gestational sac in uterus
    b. Complex adnexal mass
    c. Resistance in coloured Doppler
    d. Free fluid in peritoneal cavity

22. On USG finding of cystic hygroma in fetus is suggestive of *[AIIMS PGMEE 1997]*

a. Down's syndrome b. Marphan's syndrome
c. Turner's syndrome d. Klinefelter's syndrome

23. Method to diagnose misplaced intra uterine device is *[AIIMS PGMEE 1991]*

a. Ultrasound
b. X-ray abdomen [Erect view]
c. Uterine sound & hysteroscopy
d. All of the above

24. Radiological investigation of female of reproductive age group is restricted to *[All India PGMEE 1993]*

a. Menstrual period
b. First 10 days of menstrual cycle
c. 10–20 days of menstrual cycle
d. Last 10 days of menstrual cycle

25. Maximum radiopaque shadow in ovary is seen in *[AIIMS PGMEE 1997]*

a. Teratoma b. Dysgerminoma
c. Mucinous cystadenoma d. Granulosa cell tumor

26. Earliest diagnosis of pregnancy can be established by *[AIIMS PG May 2015]*

a. hCG levels b. Maternal Serum AFP
c. Fetal cardiac doppler study
d. USG of fetal cardiac activity

27. Which one of the following is NOT a contraindication for performing the procedure of Hysterosalpingography (HSG)? *[PGMCET 2015]*

a. Abnormal uterine bleeding
b. Pregnancy
c. Sensitivity to contrast medium
d. Pelvic infection including vaginitis and cervicitis

 NEET/NBE PATTERN MCQs ANSWERS WITH EXPLANATIONS 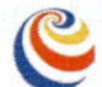

1. **Ans. (a)** **MRI**
[Ref. Chronic Pelvic Pain by Vercellini, 1/e p79]

Radiology in Adenomyosis

- Non-invasive method to assess uterine architecture
- Most accurate method: Magnetic resonance imaging (MRI)
- T2-weighted images: Evaluation of thickness of junctional zone (Inner myometrium >12 mm is diagnosis)

Also Remember

Methods to Diagnose Adenomyosis

- Histology (Definitive diagnosis): Hysteroscopic punch/Excisional biopsies
- USG, MRI
- CA-125 levels
- Hysterosalpingography (HSG)

2. **Ans. (d)** **Adenomyosis**
[Ref. Ultrasound in Subfertility by Jayaprakasan, 1/e p96]

USG for Adenomyosis

- Endometrial tissue proliferating inside myometrium tends to bleed on progesterone withdrawal during menstrual cycle
- Salt and pepper pattern: Uterus develops a typical 'speckled appearance' due to hyperechoic and hypoechoic areas (Rain-in-forest/Swiss cheese pattern)
- Underlying reason: Areas of hemorrhage and clots in myometrium
- Heterogeneous echogenicity has 88% sensitivity for diagnosis

3. **Ans. (d)** **Teratoma**
[Ref. Common Problems in Obstetrics and Gynecology by Goodwin, 5/e p376]

Teratoma of Ovary

- >95% are benign mature cystic teratomas known as 'Dermoid cysts'
- Diagnosis:
  - Clinical examination
  - X-rays: Identification of calcifications, tooth formation, a specific fat-halo sign
  - USG: Characteristic density appearance

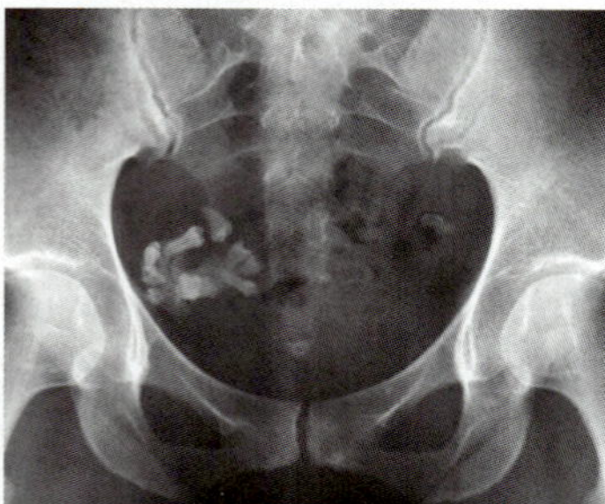

Fig. Ovarian Teratoma

4. **Ans. (d)** **Ultrasonography**
[Ref. Textbook of Obstetrics by DC Dutta, 5/e p116, 339]

- ***First investigation of choice in post-term pregnancy*: USG**
  - *USG*: Accurate assessment of gestational age by various parameters
  - *Doppler USG velocitometry*: Assessment of foetal compromise

5. **Ans. (a)** **TB of fallopian tube**
[Ref. David Sutton, 7/e p1088]

- Genital TB primarily affects the fallopian tubes with tubal disease will have a uterine abnormality
- Tubal tuberculosis leads to a rigid abnormal tube with occlusion in the isthmus
- Ends are frequently clubbed and there are diverticula-like projections from the tubal surface
- Tubal (and very rarely ovarian) calcification can be seen.

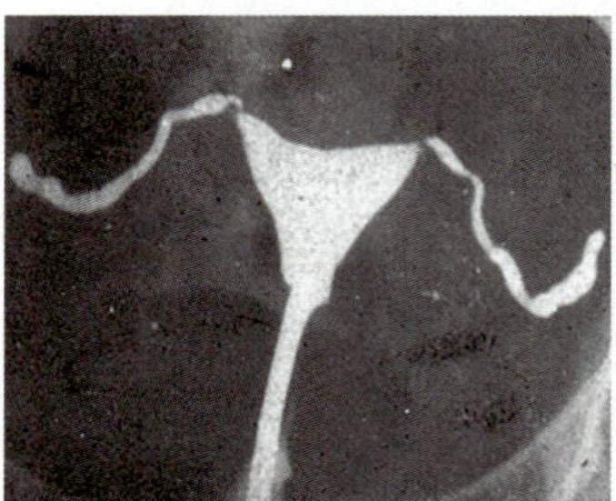

Fig. TB Fallopian tubes

6. **Ans. (d)** **Hydatiform mole**
[Ref. BipinValchandjiDaga, 1/e p406]

7. **Ans. (b)** **5 rads**
[Ref. Handbook of Obstetric and Gynecologic Emergencies by Guy I. Benrubi, 1/e p212]

- Accepted safe cumulative dose of ionizing radiation during pregnancy is 5 rad (0.05 Gy)

8. **Ans. (c)** **ANC USG**
[Ref. David Sutton, 7/e p1048]

- Nuchal translucency may be assessed towards the end of the first trimester
- Increased values may be related to a range of fetal chromosome disorders as well as cardiac abnormalities

9. **Ans. (c)** **16 weeks POG**
[Ref. Textbook of Obstetrics by DC Dutta, 5/e p116, 685]

- *Earliest foetal shadow of vertebral dots can be visualised on USG by*: 16 weeks POG

10. **Ans. (b)** **Membrane in twin pregnancy**
[Ref. Fundamentals in Obstetric Radiology, 2/e p322]

- **T sign** refers to appearance of the inter-twin membrane in a monochronic twin pregnancy

11. **Ans. (d)** **Hysteroscopy**
[Ref. Radiology Review Manual by Dahnert, 6/e p1048]

12. **Ans. (c)** **Placenta previa**
[Ref. David Sutton, 7/e p1064]

- Sonogram is the investigation of choice for placenta previa
- Trans vaginal sonogram (TVS) is reserved when diagnosis becomes doubtful with abdominal USG

13. Ans. (c) 5–6 weeks

[Ref. David Sutton, 7/e p1040]

- Cardiac activity of embryo
- Heart begins to contract at 22 days GA = 36 days MA
- Record the presence or absence or fetal life: This can generally be accomplished by the sixth week (TAS) or fifth week (TVS) counting from the first day of the last menstrual period
- Where there is reasonable doubt as to the viability of an embryo repeat scanning within 7 days should resolve the dilemma

14. Ans. (c) IUD

[Ref. Radiology Review Manual by Dahnert, 6/e p1043]

- **Spanding sign** (overlapping of fetal skull) is a non specific sign not seen before 48 hours after death.

15. Ans. (a) IUD

[Ref. Radiology Review Manual by Dahnert, 6/e p1043]

16. Ans. (b) Early 5th week POG

[Ref. USG in Obstetrics by Kurjak, 1/e p45]

- Yolk sac grows slowly and is visible (earlier than the embryo) on USG:
    - Transabdominal USG: 6th–7th week
    - Transvaginal USG: Early 5th week

17. Ans. (c) 5 weeks and 6 weeks

[Ref. David Sutton, 7/e p1040]

- Recording cardiac activity of embryo: Can generally be accomplished by the sixth week (TAS) or fifth week (TVS) counting from the first day of the last menstrual period
- Where there is reasonable doubt as to the viability of an embryo repeat scanning within 7 days should resolve the dilemma

18. Ans. (b) 0.7 mSv

[Ref. Coronary Heart Disease by Vlodaver, 1/e p90]

Radiation Exposures in Different Procedures

- Standard PA, Lateral chest X-ray: 0.02 mSv
- Invasive coronary angiography: 2-7 mSv
- Stress nuclear scans: 9-11 mSv (Technetium), 18–22 mSv (Thallium) or 26 mSv (Dual-isotope studies)
- Chest and abdominal CT scans: 12 mSv
- Repetitive screening tests (Mammography): 0.7 mSv

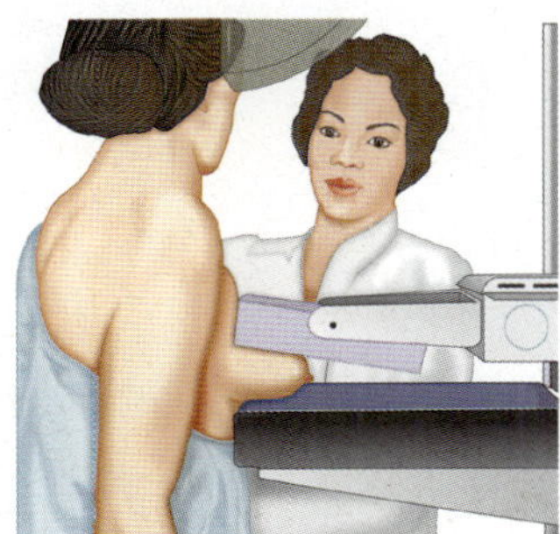

Fig. Mammography

19. Ans. (b) MRI

[Ref. Magnetic Resonance Imaging by Bushong, 4/e p420]

- As with diagnostic ultrasound examination, the stage of pregnancy should not affect the decision to be examined with MRI
- If an ultrasound examination of the abdomen or pelvis of a pregnant patient has been unsuccessful in identifying suspected abnormalities, MRI may be appropriate
- USG is preferable over MRI overall in Pregnancy

20. Ans. (c) 18–22 weeks

[Ref. Ultrasound in Obstetrics & Gynecology by Malhotra, 4/e p378]

- Minimum standard for the 18–20 weeks targeted anomaly scan, gestational age can be established by measurement of BPD, HC, abdominal circumference (AC), and femur length (FL)
- When first trimester scan is missed, the 18–20 weeks targeted anomaly scan provides dating information and diagnosis of multiple pregnancy

21. Ans. (b) Chromosomal anomalies

[Ref. Interpreting Obstetric Ultrasound by Bhide, 1/e p71]

Soft markers on Ultrasonography

- Helpful in diagnosing Chromosomal anomalies
- Include nuchal fold, short humerus, short femur, hydronephrosis, echogenic foci, echogenic bowel, major defect
- Presence of multiple markers increase the risk of chromosomal anomalies
- Value of markers in Pre-screened population is limited

22. Ans. (b) Ectopic pregnancy

[Ref. Gynecologic Ultrasound BY Allison, Vol5 (2) p190]

Ring of fire on USG

- Peripheral blood flow around an ectopic pregnancy
- Concentric enhancement of vessels on color or power Doppler interrogation around the perimeter of a mass
- Not consistently seen, not a reliable sign

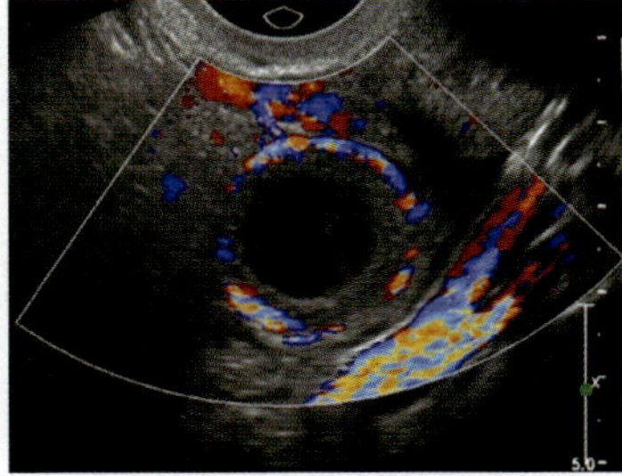

Fig. Ring of fire

23. Ans. (b) Determination of fetal malformations

[Ref. Lashley's Essentials of Clinical Genetics, 2/e p266]

Nuchal Translucency (NT) Screening

- A prenatal screening technique
- Uses ultrasound measurement of fluid in the nape of the fetal neck between 10–14 weeks of gestation to identify possible fetal abnormalities
- Measurement of nuchal translucency (NT) thickness in the first trimester of pregnancy has recently been proposed as the most useful marker in the early screening for fetal chromosomal abnormalities

24. Ans. (b) 11–13 weeks

[Ref. Twining's Textbook of Fetal Abnormalities, 3/e p35]

- Measurement of fetal NT thickness provides effective and early screening for trisomy 21 and other major aneuploidies

- High NT is associated with cardiac defects and a wide range of other fetal malformations and genetic syndromes
- Optimal gestational age for measurement of fetal NT is 11 weeks to 13 weeks and 6 days

25. Ans. (d) Gestational sac

[Ref. Ma and Mateer's Emergency Ultrasound, 3/e p399]

- Transvaginal sonography is now the standard modality for evaluating early pregnancy
- First sonographic sign of early pregnancy: Intradecidual sign (seen at 4-5 weeks)
- Intradecidual sign is a small sac, a useful feature in identifying an early intrauterine pregnancy (IUP) as early as 25 days of gestation (Embryo completely embedded within the endometrial decidua, but that does not displace the endometrial stripe)

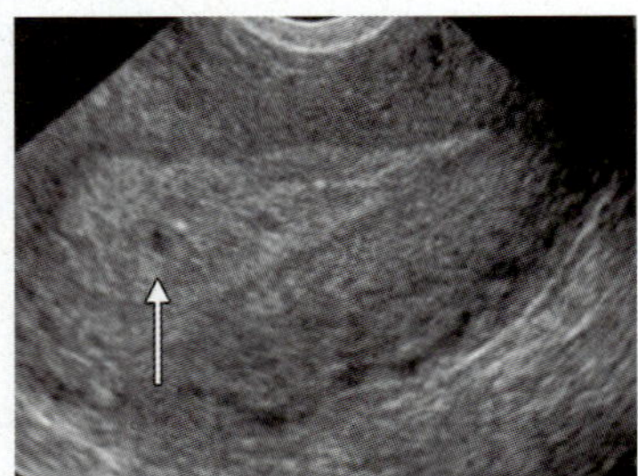

Fig. Intradecidual sign

26. Ans. (b) Intrauterine pregnancy

[Ref. Fundamentals of Diagnostic Radiology by Brant, 3/e p978]

Transvaginal USG findings in Pregnancy

- 3.5–4.0 weeks: Decidual thickening
- > 4.5 weeks: Trophoblastic flow
- > 4.5 weeks: Yolk sac sign
- 4.5–5.5 weeks: Intradecidual sign
- 5.0–5.5 weeks: Visualization of embryo
- 5.5 weeks: Double bleb sign
- > 5.5 weeks: Double decidua sign
- > 5.5 weeks: Cardiac activity

Also Remember

- Double decidual sac sign (DDSS) is a useful feature on early pregnancy ultrasound to confirm an early intrauterine pregnancy (IUP) when the yolk sac or embryo is still not visualised

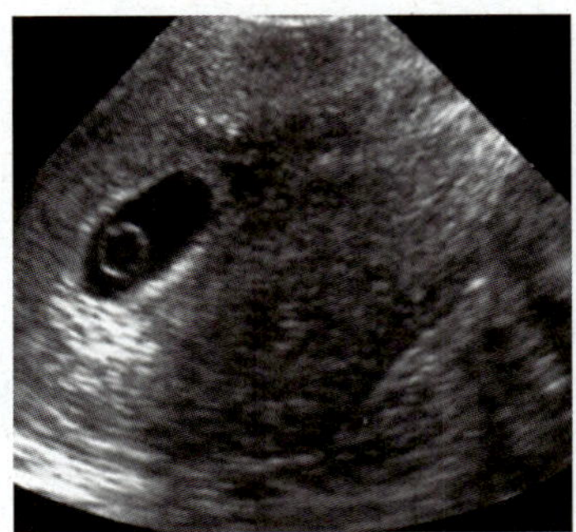

Fig. Double decidua sign

27. Ans. (d) CT guided HSG

[Ref. Hysteroscopy by Tinelli, 1/e p69]

Imaging Techniques for Uterine Anomalies

- Transvaginal USG
- Sonohysterography
- Hysterosalpingography
- MRI

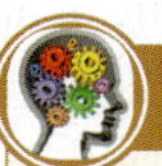

Also Remember

- The role of CT scan in benign gynaecologic conditions has been largely replaced by MRI, though it may be used for investigation of acute pelvic pain where USG has been unhelpful

HIGH YIELD MCQs ANSWERS WITH EXPLANATIONS

1. **Ans. (b) The amnion and yolk sac**
   [Ref. Fundamentals of Diagnostic Radiology by Brant, 3/e p978]

Double Bleb Sign
- Earliest demonstration of embryo on USG
- Produced by amniotic sac and yolk sac with embryonic disc between them

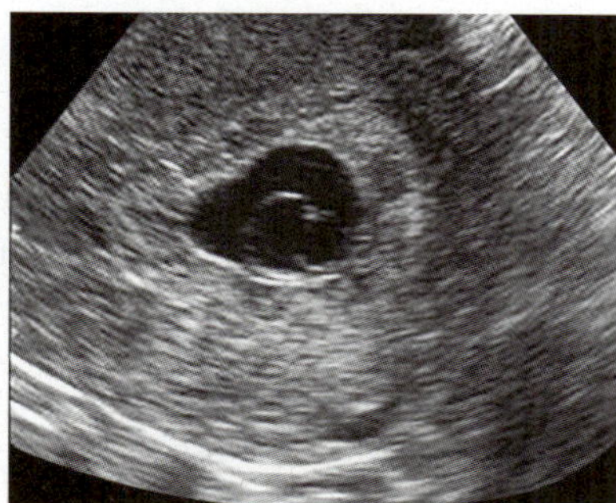

Fig. Double bleb sign

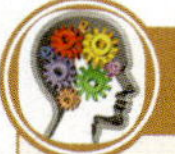

Also Remember

Transvaginal USG findings in Pregnancy
- 3.5–4.0 weeks: Decidual thickening
- >4.5 weeks: Trophoblastic flow
- >4.5 weeks: Yolk sac sign
- 4.5–5.5 weeks: Intradecidual sign
- 5.0–5.5 weeks: Visualization of embryo
- 5.5 weeks: Double bleb sign
- >5.5 weeks: Double decidua sign
- >5.5 weeks: Cardiac activity

2. **Ans. (a) 1–20 MHz**
   [Ref. David Sutton, 7/e p1039]
   - Frequencies for the transducers used in Obstetrics lie between 3 and 5 MHz, the choice being a trade-out between beam penetration and resolution
   - Mechanical sector and phased-array systems are again available, frequencies being in the range 5–7.5 MHz
3. **Ans. (d) Echogenic mass with multicystic spaces within endometrial cavity**
   [Ref. David Sutton, 7/e p1047]
4. **Ans. (d) Down's syndrome**
   [Ref. David Sutton, 7/e p1049]
   - USG can only predict Down syndrome and not for diagnosis
5. **Ans. (c) Young breast have dense tissue**
   [Ref. David Sutton, 7/e p1454]
   - **Mammographic appearance of the breast** depends on the relative amounts of fat and glandular tissue which are present
   - Young woman's breast contains a large proportion of glandular tissue which appears as soft-tissue density on the mammogram and lowers the sensitivity of mammogram

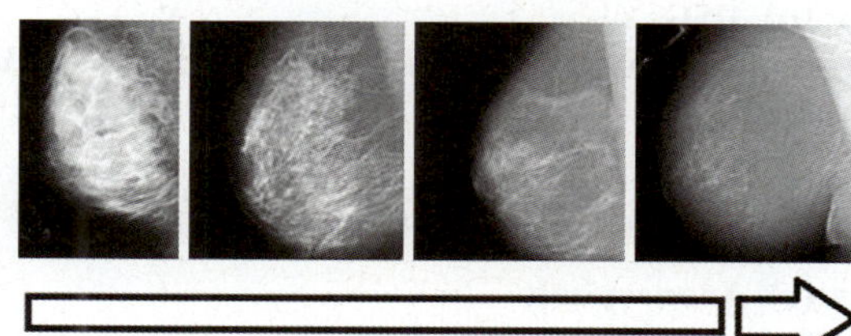

Fig. Mammogram (with increasing age)

6. **Ans. (a) 5–6 weeks of gestation**
   [Ref. David Sutton, 7/e p1041]
   - Gestational sac may be identified by transabdominal scanning at 5 weeks and approximately a week earlier by transvaginal scanning
   - Mean sac diameter (MSD) correlates well with menstrual age during the early first trimester, with similar confidence limits to the crown-rump length during the early first trimester
7. **Ans. (c) Real time USG**
   [Ref. David Sutton, 7/e p1040]
8. **Ans. (c) Foetal weight**
9. **Ans. (b) Abdominal circumference; (c) BPD; (d) Femur length**
   [Ref. Handbook of Anthropometry by Victor R, 1/e p 481]
   - **CRL** is utilized in for estimation of gestational age up to 11th week
   - BPD is best utilized in 2nd trimester. HC, FL, AC are parameters used in 3rd trimester
10. **Ans. (a) Detect foetal abnormality**
    [Ref. Pregnancy at Risk Current Concepts, (FOGSI) p184]
    - Screening for structural malformations is done at **18–20 weeks' gestation**, when fetal abnormalities are large enough to be detected
11. **Ans. (a) 10–12 weeks of gestation**
    [Ref. Sumer K Sethi, 6/e p157]
    - Anencephaly: Symmetric absence of cranial vault and brain structures above large and prominent orbits, diagnosis is suspected by 12-13 weeks and reliable around 15–15 weeks

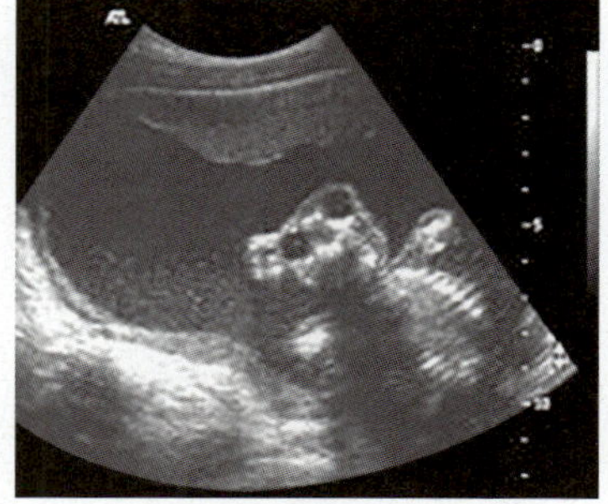

Fig. Anencephaly

12. **Ans. (c) Transvaginal USG**
    [Ref. Sumer K Sethi, 6/e p158]
    - TVS is useful at earliest at 1500–2000 hCG (MIU/mL)

13. Ans. (b) Transvaginal USG
[Ref. Sumer K Sethi, 6/e p158]

14. Ans. (b) USG
[Ref. Clinical Reproductive Medicine and Surgery by Falcone, 1/e p414]

15. Ans. (c) Amniocentesis
[Ref. Danforth's Obstetrics and Gynecology, 10/e p114]

16. Ans. (c) Anencephaly
[Ref. Sumer K Sethi, 6/e p157]

- Anencephaly: Symmetric absence of cranial vault and brain structures above large and prominent orbits, diagnosis is suspected by 12-13 weeks and reliable around 15–15 weeks.

17. Ans. (c) In normal gestation placental resistance is high; (e) Investigation of choice in pregnancy
[Ref. Pregnancy at Risk Current Concepts, (FOGSI), p163]

18. Ans. (c) The flow velocities and the SID ratio are useful to evaluate high risk pregnancies
[Ref. Diagnostic Imaging of Fetal Anomalies by Nyberg, 1/e p 130]

19. Ans. (a) Anencephaly
[Ref. Sumer K Sethi, 6/e p157]

20. Ans. (d) Crown rump length
[Ref. Handbook of Anthropometry by Victor R, 1/e p 481]

- **CRL** is utilized in for estimation of gestational age up to 11th week with an accuracy of more than 95%

21. Ans. (a) Absence of gestational sac in uterus
[Ref. Sumer K Sethi, 6/e p158]

- No intrauterine gestational sac with β-hCG > 1800 mIU/mL suggests a diagnosis of ectopic pregnancy

22. Ans. (c) Turners's syndrome
[Ref. Ultrasound Secrets by Vikram Dogra, p64]

- Approximately 50% of fetuses with large cystic hygroma have Turner syndrome (45XO)

23. Ans. (d) All of the above
[Ref. Operative OBG by Narendra Malhotra, p 638]

24. Ans. (b) First 10 days of menstrual cycle
[Ref. Principles of Imaging Science and Protection by Thompson, 1/e p 429]

25. Ans. (a) Teratoma
[Ref. David Sutton, 7/e p66]

26. Ans. (d) USG of fetal cardiac activity
[Ref. Donald School Textbook of USG in OBG, 2/e p225]

- Paired serum beta-hCG levels though useful, should be used in conjunction with transvaginal ultrasound to establish a diagnosis of pregnancy
- Essential aim of an early pregnancy ultrasound is not only to diagnose a pregnancy, but also to differentiate between normal and abnormal pregnancy
- Serum progesterone has been suggested as a marker for viability and location in early pregnancy

27. Ans. (a) Abnormal uterine bleeding
[Ref. Physicians Desk Reference to Pharmaceutical Specialties and Biologicals, p978]

Contraindications to Hysterosalpingography

- Severe vaginal or cervical infections
- Existing/recent pelvic infection
- Marked cervical erosion or Endocervicitis
- Pregnancy

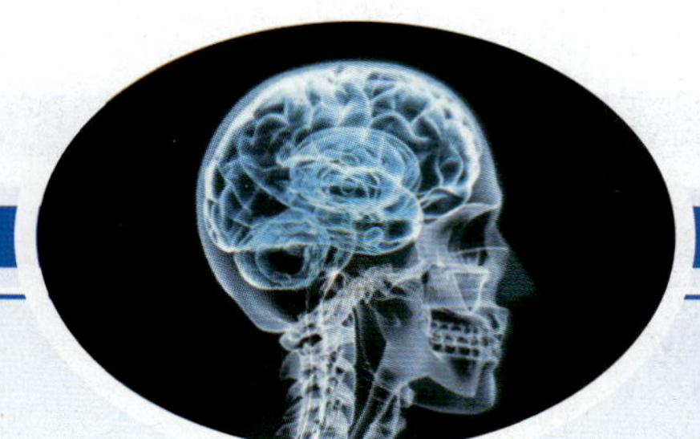

Chapter 9

Principles of Radiotherapy

THEORETICAL CONCEPTS

IX A. TYPES OF RADIATION

Ionizing radiation[Q]	Non-ionizing radiation[Q]
• X-rays • Alpha rays • Gamma rays • Electrons • Positrons • Muons • Neutrons • Protons • Fission fragments • Heavy nuclei • High end ultraviolet rays	• Low end ultraviolet rays • Visible light rays • Infrared rays • Microwave rays • Radiowaves • Extremely low frequency rays • Static field (MRI) rays

Topper's Edge

Types of Radiation

- Radioactivity indicates how many radioactive atoms are disintegrating in a time period and is measured in units of Curies:
  - **One Curie**[Q]: Amount of any radioactive material that will decay at a rate of 37 billion disintegrations per second (based upon the disintegration rate of 1 g of radium-226)
- Rate of nuclear decay is measured in terms of Half-lives:
  - Half-life of any radioactive material is the length of time necessary for one half of the atoms of that material to decay to some other material[Q]
- Radiation emitted by radioactive material can produce ionizations and, therefore, is called ionizing radiation:
  - **Ionization** is the process of stripping, knocking off, or otherwise removing electrons from their orbital paths, creating "free" electrons and leaving charged nuclei[Q]
- **Alpha particle** is an ionizing radiation that consists of two protons and two neutrons[Q]
- **Beta Particle** is a high speed ionizing radiation particle that is usually negatively charged
- **Gamma ray** is an ionizing radiation in the form of electromagnetic energy (no rest mass, no charge) similar in many respects to visible light (but far more energetic)
  - Due to the high energy, no charge, and no rest mass, gamma rays can travel thousands of feet in air and can easily pass through the human body
- **Neutron particle** is an ionizing radiation emitted by nuclear fission and by the decay of some radioactive atoms
  - Neutrons can range from high speed, high energy particles to low speed, low energy particles (called thermal neutrons)
  - Neutrons can travel hundreds of feet in air and can easily penetrate the human body

IX B. RADIOSENSITIVITY OF BODY TISSUES

Extremely radiosensitive[Q]	**Highly radiosensitive**
• **Bone marrow** • Lymphoid tissues • Testes • Ovaries • Intestines	• Skin • Cornea • Oral cavity, oesophagus • Rectum • Bladder, ureters • Vagina, uterine cervix
Moderately radiosensitive • Optic lens • Stomach • Growing cartilage/bone • Fine vasculature	**Low radiosensitive** • Mature cartilage/bones • Salivary glands • Respiratory organs • Kidneys, adrenal, pancreas, liver • Thyroid, pituitary gland
Least radiosensitive[Q] • Muscle • **Brain, spinal cord**	
• *Most radiosensitive tissue of body*: Bone marrow[Q] • *Least radiosensitive tissue of body*: Nervous tissue/brain[Q] • *Most radiosensitive blood cell of body*: Lymphocyte[Q] • *Least radiosensitive blood cell of body*: Platelet[Q] • *Most radiosensitive organ of body*: Gonads[Q]	• *Most radiosensitive mucosa of body*: Intestinal mucosa • *Cells are most radiosensitive in*: G2-M interphase[Q] • *Cells are most radioresistant in*: S phase and Late G2 phase • *Cells are most heat sensitive in*: S phase

Topper's Edge

Radiosensitivity

- Radiosensitivity: Relative susceptibility of cells, tissues, organs or organisms to the harmful effect of ionizing radiation
  - **Law of Bergonié and Tribondeau (1906)**[Q]: X-rays are more effective on cells which have a greater reproductive activity
  - **Sensitivity of cells in cell cycle**[Q]: G2-M phase (Highest) > G2 phase > G1 phase > S phase (least)
  - Most sensitive cells[Q]: Undifferentiated, well nourished, dividing quickly and highly active metabolically
- Cell damage classification:
  - Deterministic effects: Have a threshold of irradiation under which they do not appear and above which they are the necessary consequence of irradiation; the damage they cause depends on the dose
  - Stochastic effects: Do not have a threshold of irradiation, are coincidental, and cannot be avoided; they can be divided into somatic and genetic effects.

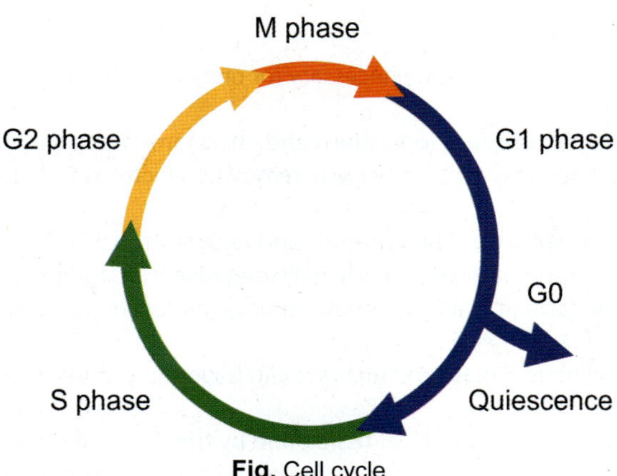

Fig. Cell cycle

IX C. RADIOSENSITIVITY OF TUMOURS

Highly radiosensitive[Q]	**Moderately radiosensitive**
• Lymphoma • Seminoma • Myeloma • Ewing's sarcoma • Wilm's tumour	• Small cell cancer lungs • Breast cancer • Basal cell carcinoma • Medulloblastoma • Teratoma • Ovarian cancer (Most: Dysgerminoma)
Relatively radioresistant	**Extremely radioresistant**[Q]
• Squamous cell carcinoma lung • Hypernephroma • Rectal carcinoma • Bladder carcinoma • Soft tissue sarcoma • Cervical cancer	• Melanoma • Osteosarcoma • Pancreatic carcinoma

IX D. TREATMENT OF CHOICE

- *Radiotherapy is treatment of choice in carcinomas of*: **[Mnemonic: N**one **S**uccessfully **CRAMS H**arrison **B**ook]
  - **N**asal cavity, oropharynx, nasopharynx, hypopharynx, larynx
  - **O**ral cavity, lips, tongue, cheek
  - **S**kin cancer (Except melanoma)[Q]
  - **C**ervical cancer [Q]
  - **R**etinoblastoma
  - **A**strocytoma
  - **M**edulloblastoma
  - **S**eminoma testis [Q]
  - **H**odgkins/Non-Hodgkins lymphoma (early stages only)
  - **B**ladder cancer [Q]

Radiodiagnosis and Radiotherapy

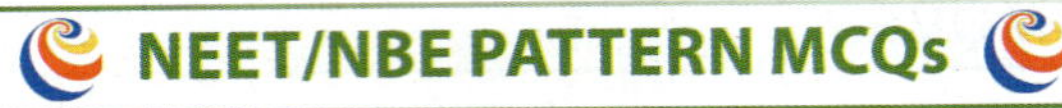

NEET/NBE PATTERN MCQs

1. **Radiosensitive tumor is** *[Recent Question 2016]*
   a. Osteosarcoma b. Melanoma
   c. Lymphoma d. Cervical cancer
2. **Most radiosensitive ovarian tumour is** *[NBE FMGE September 2007]*
   a. Endodermal sinus tumour
   b. Choriocarcinoma c. Dysgerminoma
   d. Serous cystadenocarcinoma
3. **Law of Bergonie and Tribondeau** *[NBE DNB 1992]*
   a. The sensitivity of cells to irradiation is indirect proportion to reproductive activity and inversely to degree of differentiation
   b. Sensitivity of cells indirectly in proportion to degree of differentiation
   c. Sensitivity of cells is inversely proportional to O_2 requirement
   d. Sensitivity of cells is proportional to their size
4. **Most radiosensitive tissue is** *[NBE FMGE March 2007, NBE DNB 1995, 1998, 2003, 2006, 2007, 2008, 2010]*
   a. Liver b. Thyroid
   c. Brain d. Bone marrow
5. **Which of the following is not an ionizing radiation?** *[UPSC 2011]*
   a. Infrared rays b. Gamma rays
   c. X-rays d. Cosmic rays
6. **Cells are most radiosensitive in** *[NBE FMGE September 2006,September 2012] [NBE DNB 2011]*
   a. S-phase b. M-phase
   c. G1-phase d. G0-phase
7. **Which of these tumors is least radiosensitive?** *[NBE DNB 2009]*
   a. Ewing's sarcoma b. Osteosarcoma
   c. Wilm's tumor d. Neuroblastoma
8. **Most radiosensitive cells are** *[NBE DNB 1994, 2000, 2005, 2011, FMGE March 2006]*
   a. Erythrocytes b. Lymphocytes
   c. Neutrophils d. Megakaryocytes
9. **External beam radiotherapy is delivered by** *[NBE DNB 2011]*
   a. CT simulator
   b. Linear accelerator
   c. Positron emission tomography unit
   d. High dose rate brachytherapy unit
10. **Which one of the following is a non-ionizing radiation?** *[NBE DNB 2011]*
    a. Ultraviolet radiation b. X-rays
    c. Gamma rays d. Neutrons
11. **Radiation causing maximum biological effect is** *[NBE FMGE March 2006]*
    a. X-rays b. Gamma rays
    c. Electrons d. Neutrons
12. **In radiotherapy, for the oxygen effect to manifest, oxygen has to be present** *[NBE DNB 2011]*
    a. A short while before irradiation
    b. During or within microseconds after radiation exposure
    c. 5 minutes after irradiation
    d. 10 minutes after irradiation
13. **Which among the following radiations has the highest biologic effect?** *[NBE DNB 2011]*
    a. X-rays b. Gamma rays
    c. Electrons d. Neutrons
14. **Most sensitive structure in a cell for radiotherapy is** *[NBE FMGE September 2011]*
    a. Cell membrane b. Mitochondrial membrane
    c. DNA d. Cell enzymes
15. **Most radiosensitive tumor amongst the following is** *[NBE FMGE March 2012]*
    a. Squamous cell carcinoma
    b. Seminoma
    c. Soft tissue sarcoma
    d. Lympho-epithelioma
16. **Which one of the following has the maximum ionization potential?** *[Recent Question 2013]*
    a. Electron b. Proton
    c. Helium ion d. Gamma photon
17. **Most radiosensitive tumor among following is** *[Recent Question 2013, 2015]*
    a. Bronchogenic carcinoma
    b. Parotid carcinoma
    c. Dysgerminoma
    d. Osteogenic sarcoma
18. **Radioresistant tumor is** *[Recent Question 2014, 2015]*
    a. Ewings sarcoma b. Retinoblastoma
    c. Osteosarcoma d. Neuroblastoma
19. **Most commonly used radiation in Radiotherapy is?** *[Recent Question 2017]*
    a. X-rays b. Beta rays
    c. Alpha rays d. Electron
20. **Gamma knife utilizes** *[Recent Question 2017]*
    a. Strontium 89 b. I-131
    c. Cobalt -60 d. P-32
21. **Non-ionizing radiation among the following is** *[Recent Question 2017]*
    a. MRI b. CT Scan
    c. X-ray
    d. Position emission scintigraphy
22. **All are true about Stereotactic radiosurgery except** *[Recent Question 2017]*
    a. X-rays are used
    b. A form of radiotherapy
    c. Used in AV malformation
    d. Damage to nearby structures is significant

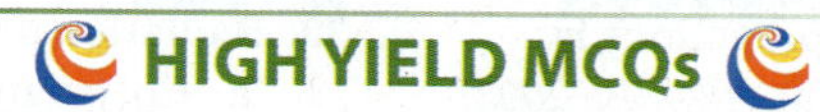

1. **Which one of the following statements is TRUE regarding radiation therapy?** *[APPG 2016]*
   a. Radiotherapy is the treatment of choice in pituitary tumors with visual field defects requiring urgent treatment
   b. Conformal radiotherapy delivers square or rectangular shaped beams which precisely target tumors but increase normal tissue radiation
   c. Radiotherapy is effective in patients with nevoid basal cell carcinoma syndrome
   d. Grenz or Bucky ray therapy helps in treatment of unresponsive scalp psoriasis
2. **All are feature of radiation except** *[All India 1992]*
   a. Biological b. Photographic
   c. Fluorescent d. Non penetrating
3. **Which of the following is the most ionizing radiation?** *[All India PGMEE 2010]*
   a. Alpha b. Beta
   c. X-ray d. Gamma
4. **Which of the following has most penetrating power?** *[All India PGMEE 2002]*
   a. Alpha-particle b. Beta-particle
   c. Gamma-radiation d. Electron beam
5. **Principle used in radiotherapy is** *[All India PGMEE 1997]*
   a. Cytoplasmic coagulation b. Ionization of molecule
   c. DNA damage d. Necrosis of tissue
6. **Which of these tumors is least radiosensitive?** *[AIIMS PGMEE 2007]*
   a. Ewing's sarcoma b. Osteosarcoma
   c. Wilm's tumor d. Neuroblastoma
7. **Which of the following is the most radiosensitive tumour?** *[AIIMS PGMEE 2005]*
   a. Ewing's Tumour
   b. Hodgkin's disease
   c. Carcinoma cervix
   d. Malignant fibrous histiocytoma
8. **Radiosensitive tumors are** *[PGI 2006]*
   a. Seminoma b. Lymphoma
   c. Sarcoma d. Ewing's sarcoma
   e. Leukemia
9. **Most harmful to individual cell** *[PGI 1998]*
   a. X-rays b. Alpha-particles
   c. Beta-particles d. X-rays (gamma rays)
10. **Beams can be used for cancer treatment are** *[PGI 2002]*
   a. Gamma-rays b. Alpha-rays
   c. Neutrons d. Protons
   e. X-rays
11. **Most common used rays for radiotherapy** *[PGI 2006]*
   a. X-rays b. Gamma rays
   c. Alpha rays d. Beta rays
12. **In Teletherapy setup all are used except** *[AIIMS PGMEE 1998]*
   a. Iridium b. Co-60
   c. Simulator d. Computer
13. **Most radiosensitive ovarian tumour is** *[AIIMS PGMEE 1997]*
   a. Serus cystadenoma b. Dysgerminoma
   c. Dermoid cyst d. Teratoma
   d. Craniopharyngioma
14. **Most radiosensitive testicular tumour is** *[AIIMS PGMEE 1993]*
   a. Yolk sack tumour b. Embryonal cell tumour
   c. Teratoma d. Seminoma
15. **Most radiosensitive brain tumour is** *[AIIMS PGMEE 1997]*
   a. Astrocytoma b. Ependymoma
   c. Medulloblastoma d. None of the above
16. **The radiation tolerance of whole liver as** *[All India PGMEE 2004]*
   a. 15 Gy b. 30 Gy
   c. 40 Gy d. 45 Gy
17. **Organs sensitive to radiation are** *[PGI 2003]*
   a. Gonad b. Bone marrow
   c. Liver d. Fat
   e. Nervous tissue
18. **Functional basis of ionising radiation depends on** *[AIIMS PGMEE 1996]*
   a. Pyrimidine base pairing b. Removal of orbital electron
   c. Linear energy transfer d. Adding orbital electron
19. **Which is not a deep heat therapy?** *[All India PGMEE 2007]*
   a. Short wave diathermy b. Infra Red
   c. USG d. Microwave
20. **What is atomic number?** *[PGI 2001]*
   a. Proton b. Electrons + protons
   c. Protons + neutrons d. Protons + protons
21. **Gray equals** *[PGI 2007]*
   a. 100 rad b. 1000 rad
   c. 10000 rad d. 1 rad
   e. 0.1 rad
22. **Curie is unit of** *[PGI 1997, Recent Question 2017]*
   a. Radiation exposure b. Radiation absorption
   c. Radioactivity d. All of the above
23. **Most commonly radiotherapy uses** *[AIIMS PGMEE 1999]*
   a. X-rays b. Gamma-rays
   c. Alpha-rays d. Electron
24. **Radioactive emissions used in radiotherapy are** *[PGI 2001, PGI 2003]*
   a. Alpha-particles b. Beta-particles
   c. gamma-rays d. X-ray
   e. Infrared rays
25. **Maximum dose of radiation per year in a human which is safe** *[All India PGMEE 1992]*
   a. 1 rads b. 5 rads
   c. 10 rads d. 20 rads

26. Maximum permissible radiation dose in pregnancy is *[AIIMS PGMEE 2003]*
a. 0.5 rad b. 1.0 rad
c. 1.5 rad d. 5 rad

27. Most sensitive tissue to radiation is *[AIIMS PGMEE 1995]*
a. Liver b. Gonads
c. Spleen d. Skin

28. Radiation hazard is absent in *[PGI 2006]*
a. MRI b. Doppler USG
c. Digital subtraction angiography
d. Tc 99 scan

29. The cell most sensitive to radiotherapy is *[AIIMS PGMEE 1993]*
a. Neutrophil b. Lymphocyte
c. Basophil d. Platelet

30. Most sensitive structure in cell for radiotherapy is *[PGI 2002]*
a. Cell membrane b. Mitochondrial membrane
c. DNA d. Enzymes
e. ER

31. Most radiosensitive stage *[All India PGMEE 1996, 1997, 1998, PGI 1997, 2005, AIIMS PGMEE 2002]*
a. S-G_1 phase b. G_2 phase
c. M phase d. G_2-M phase

32. Emergency radiotherapy is given in *[PGI 2005]*
a. Superior vena cava syndrome
b. Pericardial tamponade c. Increased ICP
d. Spinal cord compression

33. Which is provided by linear accelerator? *[AIIMS PGMEE 1995]*
a. Electron b. Neutron
c. Proton d. Infrared rays

34. Which of the following best estimates the amount of radiation delivered to an organ in the radiation field? *[All India PGMEE 2010]*
a. Absorbed dose b. Equivalent dose
c. Effective dose d. Exposure dose

35. Which one of the following has the maximum ionization potential? *[All India PGMEE 2006]*
a. Electron b. Proton
c. Helium ion d. Gamma photon

36. Ionization radiation acts on tissue leading to *[All India PGMEE 1998]*
a. Linear acceleration injury
b. Excitation of electron from orbit
c. Formation of pyramidine dimer
d. Thermal injury

37. Principles used in radiotherapy is *[AIIMS PGMEE 1994]*
a. Infrared rays
b. Ionizing molecules
c. Charring of nucleoprotein
d. Ultrasonic effect

38. Radiation produces its effect on tissue by *[AIIMS PGMEE 1993]*
a. Coagulation of cytoplasm
b. Increasing the temperature
c. Charring of nucleoprotein
d. Hydrolysis

39. The technique employed in radiotherapy to counteract the effect of tumour motion due to breathing is known as *[All India PGMEE 2005]*
a. Arc technique b. Modulation
c. Gating d. Shunting

40. Principles of linear accelerators is used in *[PGI 2006]*
a. X-rays b. Gamma-rays
c. Alpha rays d. Infrared rays
e. Alpha particles

41. Most commonly radiotherapy uses *[PGI 2002]*
a. X-rays b. Gamma rays
c. Alpha rays d. Electron

42. Photon transferring some of its energy to electron is *[JIPMER PGMEE 2006]*
a. Photoelectric effect b. Bremsstrahlung effect
c. Compton effect d. Ionization

43. Photoelectric effect is *[All India PGMEE 2008]*
a. Interaction between high energy incident photon and the inner shell electron
b. Interaction between incident photon and the outer shell electron
c. Interaction of the incident photon with the nucleus
d. Interaction between a photon and electric current

44. Ionizing radiation most sensitive in *[PGI 2005]*
a. Hypoxia b. S phage
c. G_2M phage d. Activating cell

45. The phase of cell cycle, most sensitive to radiation is/are *[PGI 2009]*
a. M phase b. G_2 phase
c. S phase d. Early G_1 phase
e. Go phase

46. What is radioresistant? *[AIIMS PGMEE 1997]*
a. Cartilage b. Seminoma
c. Ewings sarcoma d. GI epithelium

47. Most radiosensitive tumor *[AIIMS PGMEE 1995]*
a. Brenner's tumor b. Dysgerminoma
c. Mucinous cystadenoma d. Teratoma

48. All are highly radiosensitive except *[AIIMS PGMEE 1995]*
a. Osteogenic sarcoma b. Lymphoma
c. Ewing's sarcoma d. Seminoma

49. Most radiosensitive tumour among the following is *[All India PGMEE 2006]*
a. Bronchogenic carcinoma b. Carcinoma parotid
c. Dysgerminoma d. Osteogenic sarcoma

50. Most Radiosensitive lung CA is *[AIIMS PGMEE 1993]*
a. Squamous cell b. Small cell
c. Adeno d. Large cell

51. Which of the following malignant tumors is radio resistant? *[All India PGMEE 2006]*
- a. Ewing's sarcoma
- b. Retinoblastoma
- c. Osteosarcoma
- d. Neuroblastoma

52. Most radiosensitive tumor of the following is *[All India PGMEE 2001]*
- a. Ca Kidney
- b. Ca Colon
- c. Ca Pancreas
- d. Ca Cervix

53. Tumor[s] most responding to radiotherapy *[PGI 2003]*
- a. Sarcoma
- b. Seminoma
- c. Lymphoma
- d. Leukaemia

54. Tumor responding best to radiation include following *[PGI 1997]*
- a. Melanoma
- b. Dysgerminoma
- c. Teratoma
- d. Choriocarcinoma

55. Radioactivity is measured by *[PGI November 2014, Recent Question 2017]*
- a. Curie
- b. Bacquerel
- c. Sievert
- d. Gray
- e. Rad

56. As per International Commission of radiation Units and Measurements - Report No. 38, High dose Brachytherapy is *[PGMCET 2015]*
- a. 0.4–2 Gy/hr
- b. 12 Gy/hr.
- c. 2–12 Gy/hr
- d. 0.01–0.3 Gy/hr

 NEET/NBE PATTERN MCQs ANSWERS WITH EXPLANATIONS 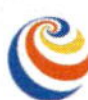

1. Ans. (c) Lymphoma

[Ref. Sumer K Sethi, 5/e p108-109]

Highly radiosensitive tumors	Moderately radiosensitive tumors
Lymphoma	Small cell cancer lungs
Seminoma	Breast cancer
Myeloma	Basal cell carcinoma
Ewing's sarcoma	Medulloblastoma
Wilm's tumour	Teratoma
	Ovarian cancer (Most: Dysgerminoma)

2. Ans. (c) Dysgerminoma

[Ref. Outcome and reproductive function after Chemotherapy for Ovarian Dysgerminoma, Journal of Clinical Oncology, 1999, Pg 2670]

- **Most radiosensitive ovarian tumour: Dysgerminoma**

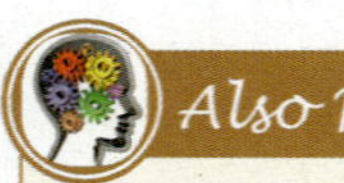

Also Remember

- *Radio-sensitivity of tumours*:

Highly radiosensitive	Moderately radiosensitive
• Lymphoma • Seminoma • Myeloma • Ewing's sarcoma • Wilm's tumour	• Small cell cancer lungs • Breast cancer • Basal cell carcinoma • Medulloblastoma • Teratoma • Ovarian cancer (Most: Dysgerminoma)
Relatively radioresistant	**Extremely radioresistant**
• Squamous cell carcinoma lung • Hypernephroma • Rectal carcinoma • Bladder carcinoma • Soft tissue sarcoma • Cervical cancer	• Melanoma • Osteosarcoma • Pancreatic carcinoma

Radiotherapy is Treatment of Choice

[**Mnemonic: N**one **S**uccessfully **CRAMS H**arrison **B**ook]

- **N**asal cavity, Oropharynx, Nasopharynx, Hypopharynx, larynx
- **O**ral cavity, lips, tongue, cheek
- **S**kin cancer (Except melanoma)
- **C**ervical cancer
- **R**etinoblastoma
- **A**strocytoma
- **M**edulloblastoma
- **S**eminoma testis
- **H**odgkins/ Non-Hodgkins lymphoma (early stages only)
- **B**ladder cancer

3. Ans. (a) The sensitivity of cells to irradiation is indirect proportion to reproductive activity and inversely to degree of differentiation

[Ref. Tumors of Childhood by Dargeon, 1/e p 59]

- In accordance with this law, rapidly proliferating normal tissues such as intestinal mucosa, bone marrow and skin are particularly susceptible to ionizing radiation and readily show evidence of cytotoxicity

4. Ans. (d) Bone marrow

[Ref. Sumer K Sethi, 5/e p110]

Radiosensitivity of Body Tissues

Extremely radiosensitive	Highly radiosensitive
• Bone marrow • Lymphoid tissues • Testes • Ovaries • Intestines	• Skin • Cornea • Oral cavity, oesophagus • Rectum • Bladder, ureters • Vagina, uterine cervix
Moderately radiosensitive • Optic lens • Stomach • Growing cartilage/bone • Fine vasculature	**Low radiosensitive** • Mature cartilage/bones • Salivary glands • Respiratory organs • Kidneys, adrenal, pancreas, liver • Thyroid, pituitary gland
Least radiosensitive • Muscle • Brain, Spinal cord	

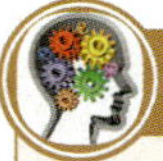

Also Remember

- *Most radiosensitive tissue of body*: Bone marrow
- *Least radiosensitive tissue of body*: Nervous tissue/brain
- *Most radiosensitive blood cell of body*: Lymphocyte
- *Least radiosensitive blood cell of body*: Platelet
- *Most radiosensitive organ of body*: Gonads
- *Most radiosensitive mucosa of body*: Intestinal mucosa
- *Most radiosensitive structure of cell : DNA*

5. Ans. (a) Infrared rays

[Ref. Sumer K Sethi, 6/e p162]

6. Ans. (b) M-phase

[Ref. Sumer K Sethi, 5/e p103]

- ***Cells are most radiosensitive in: G2-M interphase***
- *Cells are most radioresistant in*: S phase and Late G2 phase
- *Cells are most heat sensitive in*: S phase

7. Ans. (b) Osteosarcoma

[Ref. Sumer K Sethi, 6/e p173]

Highly Resistant Tumors

- Melanoma
- Osteosarcoma
- Pancreatic carcinoma

8. Ans. (b) Lymphocytes

[Ref. Sumer K Sethi, 5/e p110]

9. Ans. (b) Linear accelerator

[Ref. The Lymphoid Neoplasms by Magrath, 3/e p895]

- In general, radiation treatment may be delivered through external or internal sources
- Most commonly, for lymphoma, treatment is delivered by external beam radiation therapy using a linear accelerator or cobalt machine

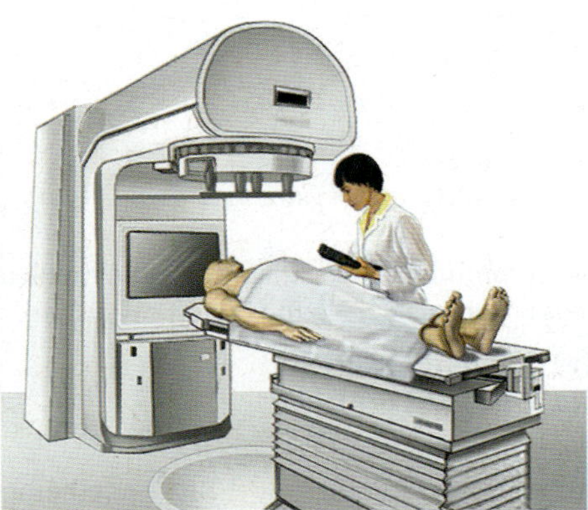

Fig. Linear accelerator (EBR)

10. Ans. (a) Ultraviolet radiation
[Ref. Sumer K Sethi, 6/e p162]

11. Ans. (b) Gamma rays
[Ref. Park, 21/ e p687]

- *Penetration capability of radiation in body tissue*: Gamma rays > X-rays > Beta rays > Alpha rays

12. Ans. (b) During or within microseconds after radiation exposure
[Ref. Sumer K Sethi, 6/e p168]

13. Ans. (d) Neutrons
[Ref. Chemistry by Das, 5/e p126]

- *Biologically* effective dose units: Equal absorbed doses of Alpha rays, *Neutrons*, Beta rays and *Gamma rays* (or X-rays) produce tissue damages in a descending order

14. Ans. (c) DNA
[Ref. Sumer K Sethi, 5/e p103]

15. Ans. (b) Seminoma
[Ref. Sumer K Sethi, 5/e p108]

16. Ans. (c) Helium ion
[Ref. Grainger & Allison's Diagnostic Radiology Essentials by Lee, 4/e p39]

- **Ionization potential**: alpha particle (helium ion) > beta particle > X-ray > gamma ray

17. Ans. (c) Dysgerminoma
[Ref. Sumer K Sethi, 6/e p172]

Highly Radiosensitive Tumors

- Lymphoma
- Germinoma (including dysgerminoma and seminoma)
- Myeloma
- Ewings sarcoma
- Wilms tumor

18. Ans. (c) Osteosarcoma
[Ref. Sumer K Sethi, 6/e p173]

Highly Radio Resistant Tumor

- Melanoma
- Osteosarcoma
- Pancreatic carcinoma

19. Ans. (a) X-rays *[Ref. Radiodiagnosis by Daga, 1/e p468]*

Radiotherapy in Medicine

- MC used Radiation in Radiotherapy: X-rays, Gamma-rays
- Radiation used in treatment of superficial tumours: Beta-rays, Electrons
- Radiation used in research set-up: Heavy ions, Particles, Proton beams, Neutron beams, Pi-masons

20. Ans. (c) Cobalt -60 *[Ref. Sumer K Sethi, 6/e p196-197]*

Gamma Knife

- Gamma Knife is a machine: It delivers a single, finely focused, high dose of radiation to its target, while causing little or no damage to surrounding tissue
- A gamma knife typically contains 201 cobalt-60 sources of approximately 30 curies (1.1TBq), each placed in a circular array in a heavily shielded assembly

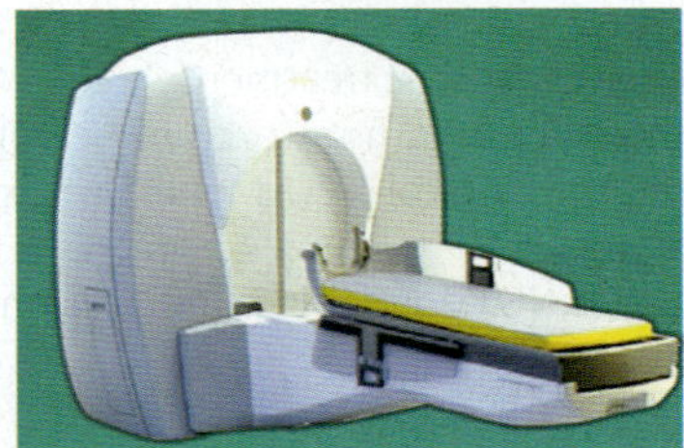

Fig. Gamma knife

21. Ans. (a) MRI
[Ref. Clinical Gynecologic Oncology E-Book by DiSaia, 9/e p389]

- Ionizing radiation include X-rays, Fluoroscopy, Xeroradiography, Mammography, Barium study, Intravenous urography, CT scan, DEXA scan, PET scan
- Non-ionizing radiation include UV rays, Infrared rays (Thermography), Ultrasonography, MRI, Microwaves, Radiofrequency waves

22. Ans. (d) Damage to nearby structures is significant
[Ref. Intracranial Stereotactic Radiosurgery by Pollock, 1/e p543]

Stereotactic radiosurgery (SRS)

- A combination of stereotactic localization techniques invented in neurosurgery and radiation physics used to deliver concentrated energy, in the form of X-rays, gamma rays, and protons, to an image-guided anatomic location
- Deliver a destructive dose of radiation to an intended target while minimizing damage to adjacent structures

HIGH YIELD MCQs ANSWERS WITH EXPLANATIONS 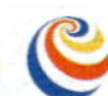

1. Ans. (d) Grenz or Bucky ray therapy helps in treatment of unresponsive scalp psoriasis

[Ref. Davidson's Principles and Practice of Medicine, 22/e p1269]

- Even more superficial ionizing radiation (Grenz or Bucky rays) can be useful for localized dermatoses that are having severe effects on quality of life
- Example: If conventional therapy is ineffective, it may avoid exposure to the risks of systemic therapy for a patient with severe and hitherto unresponsive scalp psoriasis

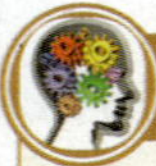

Also Remember

- For pituitary tumors presenting clinically with visual field defects or hypopituitarism, surgery is the treatment of choice, supported as required by radiotherapy
- Conformal radiotherapy:
  - As the radiation beams are very precisely directed, adjacent normal tissues receive less radiation and are able to heal quickly
  - Shaped rather than conventional square or rectangular beams are used
- Nevoid basal cell carcinoma treatment:
  - Effective modalities: Surgical excision, cryotherapy, curettage & diathermy, topical 5-FU, Mohl's microsurgery, CO_2 Laser vapourization
  - Radiotherapy is NOT advisable as new lesions do appear in irradiated field

2. Ans. (d) Non penetrating

[Ref. Sumer K Sethi, 6/e p166]

3. Ans. (a) Alpha

[Ref. Grainger & Allison's Diagnostic Radiology Essentials by Grant,4/e p39]

4. Ans. (c) Gamma radiation

[Ref. Grainger & Allison's Diagnostic Radiology Essentials by Grant,4/e p39]

- Penetrating potential: Gamma rays > X-rays > Beta particle > Alpha article (helium ion)
- Gamma rays penetrate around 50 cm in tissue and 0.3 mm in Lead

5. Ans. (b) Ionization of molecule

[Ref. The Scientific Basis of Urology edited by Anthony R, 3/e p416]

- Radiation used therapeutically is called Ionizing radiation: It causes its effect through the ionization of intracellular molecule
- It is manifested by DNA damage.

6. Ans. (b) Osteosarcoma

[Ref. Sumer K Sethi, 6/e p173]

7. Ans. (a) Ewing's tumor

[Ref. Sumer K Sethi, 6/e p172]

8. Ans. (a) Seminoma; (b) Lymphoma; (d) Ewings sarcoma

[Ref. Sumer K Sethi, 6/e p172]

9. Ans. (b) Alpha particle

[Ref. Grainger & Allison's Diagnostic Radiology Essentials by Lee A Grant,4/e p39]

10. Ans. All choices

[Ref. Sumer K Sethi, 6/e p172]

11. Ans. (a) X-rays

[Ref. Cancer and Cancer Care by Debbie Wyatt, 1/e Chapter 13]

- Most commonly used radiation for the medical purposes: X-rays > Gamma rays in the biological system.

12. Ans. (a) Iridium

[Ref. Sumer K Sethi, 6/e p175]

Teletherapy

- External beam radiotherapy (EBRT)/teletherapy: MC form of radiotherapy
- Co-60 is used for external beam commonly which decays to Nickel-60
- It is also useful to verify a treatment plan

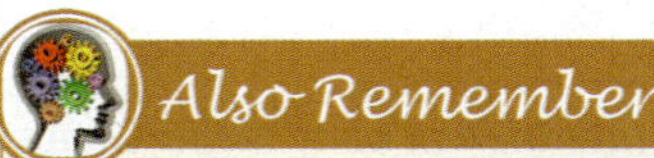

Also Remember

- **Radiotherapy Simulator** helps to diagnose the physical extent of the tumor and its relation to the surrounding tissues for proper selection of the size and orientation of the radiotherapy beams
- Radiotherapy simulator is an essential tool for improving the quality of radiotherapy for the treatment of cancer patients
- Computerized treatment planning systems not only maximize the effectiveness of a medical physics staff through increased productivity, but also improve the quality of patient care through decreased error rates, ability to calculate more complex plans and more detailed calculations of dose distribution

13. Ans. (b) Dysgerminoma

[Ref. Sumer K Sethi, 6/e p172]

14. Ans. (d) Seminoma

[Ref. Sumer K Sethi, 6/e p172]

15. Ans. (c) Medulloblastoma

[Ref. Cancer in Children and Young people by Gibson, 1/e p311]

Most Radiosensitive Brain Tumors

- Germ cell tumor
- Glioma
- Ependymoma
- Medulloblastoma
- Pinealoblastoma
- Primitive neuro ecto dermal tumour (PNET)
- Craniopharyngioma

16. Ans. (c) 40 Gy

[Ref. Normal Tissue Reactions in Radiotherapy and Oncology by Dörr, Vol 3, p65]

- Regeneration capacity of hepatic tissue is high, so higher doses (40-45 Gy) can be administered to small volumes of hepatic tissue.

17. Ans. (a) Gonad; (b) Bone marrow
[Ref. Sumer K Sethi, 6/e p172]

18. Ans. (b) Removal of orbital electron
[Ref. Radiation Oncology Physics by Podgoršak, 1/e p657]

19. Ans. (b) Infra red
[Ref. Therapeutic Modalities by Starkey, 1/e p126]

Application of Therapeutic Heat (Thermotherapy)

- **Superficial agents:** Heat a larger area of tissue, but their limited depth of penetration reduces overall volume of tissue heated
- **Deep heating agents**, Therapeutic ultrasound, Short wave diathermy: Heat tissues located at depths greater than 2 cm.

20. Ans. (a) Proton
[Ref. Practical radiotherapy by Pam Cherry, 2/e p 17]

- **Atomic mass** = total number of neutrons and protons in the nucleus
- **Atomic number** = total number of protons in the nucleus

21. Ans. (a) 100 rad
[Ref. Radiation Physics for Medical Physicists by Podgorsak, 1/e p27]

- **Gray** is the unit of absorbed dose of radiotherapy (100 Rad = 1 Gray)

22. Ans. (c) Radioactivity
[Ref. Radiation Physics for Medical Physicists by Podgorsak, 1/e p27]

- Curie and Becquerel are units of radioactivity

23. Ans. (a) X-rays
[Ref. Medical-Surgical Nursing by Donna D, 8/e p374]

24. Ans. (a) Alpha-particles; (b) Beta-particles; (c) Gamma rays
[Ref. Radiation Physics for Medical Physicists by Podgorsak, 1/e p20-28]

Most Commonly Used Radiations in Radiotherapy

- X-rays
- Gamma rays
- Beta rays
- Electron beam
- Heavy particle beams (neutrons, protons, alpha particles, deuterons, negative pions)

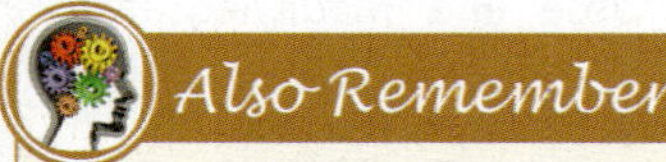

- X-ray is not a radioactive emission, rather produced by linear accelerators

25. Ans. (b) 5 rads
[Ref. Molecular Dosimetry and Human Cancer by Paul L. Skipper, 1/e p98]

- Dose limit for occupational exposure to radiation is 50 mSv, or 5 rad radiation per year

26. Ans. (d) 5 rad
[Ref. Christensen's Physics of Diagnostic Radiology by Curry, 4/e p378]

- Maximum permissible dose in pregnancy is 5 mSv per month

27. Ans. (b) Gonads
[Ref. Radiation Physics for Medical Physicists by Podgorsak, 1/e p178]

Radiosensitivity of Body Tissues

- High radiosensitivity: Gonads, Bone marrow, Lymphoid tissue, GIT epithelium
- Moderate radiosensitivity: Skin, Vascular endothelium, Lung, Kidney, Liver, Lens (eye)
- Low radiosensitivity: CNS, Muscle, Pancreas, Bones, Cartilage, Connective tissue, Vagina, Uterus

28. Ans. (a) MRI; (b) Doppler USG
[Ref. Endocrine imaging by Martin P. Sandler, 1/e p461]

29. Ans. (b) Lymphocyte
[Ref. Harrison's Principles of Internal Medicine 16/e p484-86]

- Blood cells most sensitive to radiation: Lymphocytes
- Blood cells least sensitive to radiation: Platelets

30. Ans. (c) DNA
[Ref. Radiation Physics for Medical Physicists by Podgorsak, 1/e p73]

- Target for radiation induced cell death is DNA

31. Ans. (d) G_2M Phase
[Ref. Principles and Methods of Toxicology by A. Wallace Hayes, 5/e p927]

- Cell cycle **most sensitive** to radiation: G2-M
- Cell cycle **least sensitive** to radiation: Late S phase

32. Ans. All choices
[Ref. Emergencies in Pediatric Oncology by McMaster, 1/e p179]

33. Ans. (b) Neutron
[Ref. Linear Accelerators for Radiation Therapy by Greene,2/e p208]

- The National Bureau of Standards linear accelerator provided a pulsed source of neutrons over the energy range from 0.3 eV to 20 eV

34. Ans. (a) Absorbed dose
[Ref. Frontiers in Neutron Capture Therapy by Hawthorne, Vol1 p572]

- Probability of both deterministic and stochastic effects of radiation in exposed individuals depends on the type and energy of the radiation, the tissue or organ irradiated as well as physical absorbed doses

35. Ans. (c) Helium ion
[Ref. Grainger & Allison's Diagnostic Radiology Essentials by Lee A Grant,4/e p39]

36. Ans. (b) Excitation of electron from orbit
[Ref. Radiation Oncology Physics by Ervin B. Podgoršak 1/e p657]

37. Ans. (b) Ionizing molecules
[Ref. The Scientific Basis of Urology edited by Anthony R, 3/e p416]

38. Ans. (c) Charring of nucleoprotein
[Ref. Sumer K Sethi, 6/e p166]

39. Ans. (c) Gating
[Ref. Sumer K Sethi, 6/e p176]

- Minimizing the planning target volume (PTV) margin and reproducing its position during treatment as well as between treatments are important tasks in external beam radio-therapy
- Patient respiration during radiotherapy can cause significant motion of the tumor volume, which can be mitigated by gating the accelerator beam to patient respiration

40. Ans. (a) X-ray
[Ref. Principles and Practice of Radiation Therapy by Charles M. Washington, 4/e p135]

41. Ans. (a) X-rays; (b) Gamma rays
[Ref. Cancer and Cancer Care by Wyatt, 1/e Chapter 13]

- MC used radiation for the medical purposes: X-ray or Gamma-ray

42. Ans. (c) Compton effect
[Ref. Principles and Practice of Stereotactic Radiosurgery edited by Lawrence S. Chin, 2/e p41]

- It can be seen when a photon collides with a stationary electron, some of the energy and momentum is transferred to the electron (this is known as the Compton effect), but both energy and momentum are conserved in this elastic collision

43. Ans. (b) Interaction between incident photon and the outer shell electron
[Ref. Principles of Radiographic Imaging by Carlton,5/e p202]

44. Ans. (c) G_2M Phase; (d) Activating cells
[Ref. Principles and Methods of Toxicology by Hayes, 5/e p927]

- Cell cycle most sensitive to radiation: G2-M
- Cell cycle least sensitive to radiation: Late S phase
- Cells that are rapidly growing and dividing are radiosen-sitive

45. Ans. (a) M phase; (b) G_2 Phase
[Ref. Principles and Methods of Toxicology by Hayes, 5/e p927]

46. Ans. (a) Cartilage
[Ref. Radiation Physics for Medical Physicists by Podgorsak, 1/e p178]

47. Ans. (b) Dysgerminoma
[Ref. Walter and Miller's Textbook of Radiotherapy by Symonds, 7/e p964]

- **Highly radiosensitive tumours:** Lymphoma, Seminoma, Multiple myeloma, Ewings sarcoma, Wilm's tumour, Dysgerminoma
- **Moderate sensitivity:** Small cell carcinoma of lung, Breast cancer, Basal cell carcinoma, Medulloblastoma, teratoma, Ovarian carcinoma, Nasopharyngeal carcinoma
- **Relatively resistant:** Squamous cell carcinoma, Renal cell carcinoma, Rectal carcinoma, Colonic carcinoma, Bladder carcinoma, Soft tissue sarcoma, Cervical carcinoma
- **Highly resistant:** Osteosarcoma, Melanoma, Pancreatic carcinoma, Hepatic carcinoma

48. Ans. (a) Osteogenic sarcoma
[Ref. Walter and Miller's Textbook of Radiotherapy by Symonds, 7/e p964]

49. Ans. (c) Dysgerminoma
[Ref. Walter and Miller's Textbook of Radiotherapy by Symonds, 7/e p964]

50. Ans. (b) Small cell
[Ref. Walter and Miller's Textbook of Radiotherapy by Symonds, 7/e p964]

51. Ans. (c) Osteosarcoma
[Ref. Walter and Miller's Textbook of Radiotherapy by Symonds, 7/e p964]

52. Ans. (d) Ca Cervix
[Ref. Walter and Miller's Textbook of Radiotherapy by Symonds, 7/e p964]

- Among the options, Renal cell carcinoma, Colonic carcinoma, and Cervical carcinoma are all relatively radioresistant
- In cervical carcinoma, Radiotherapy is treatment of choice beyond stage II B.

53. Ans. (b) Seminoma; (c) Lymphoma
[Ref. Walter and Miller's Textbook of Radiotherapy by Symonds, 7/e p964]

54. Ans. (b) Dysgerminoma
[Ref. Walter and Miller's Textbook of Radiotherapy by Symonds, 7/e p964]

55. Ans. (a) Curie; (b) Bacquerel
[Ref. Radiation by Biddle, p1/e]

- Units of Radioactivity:
  - Curie
  - Bacquerel

Also Remember

Radiation Units

- **Roentgen:** Unit of exposure/radiation absorbed
- **Coulomb per kg:** New unit for exposure/radiation absorbed
- **Rem:** Unit of equivalent dose
- **Sievert (Sv):** New unit of equivalent dose (1 Sv = 100 rem)
- **Rad:** Product of absorbed dose and modifying factors (potential danger to health)
- **Gray (Gy):** Unit of absorbed dose (1 Gray = 100 rad)

56. Ans. (b) 12 Gy/hr
[Ref. Radiation Oncology by Brady, p67]

- According to International Commission on Radiation Units and Measurements (ICRU) - Report No. 38 (5)
  - Low-dose-rate (LDR): 40–200 cGy per hour (0.4-2 Gy per hour)
  - High-dose-rate (HDR) brachytherapy: 0.2 Gy per minute (12 Gy per hour)

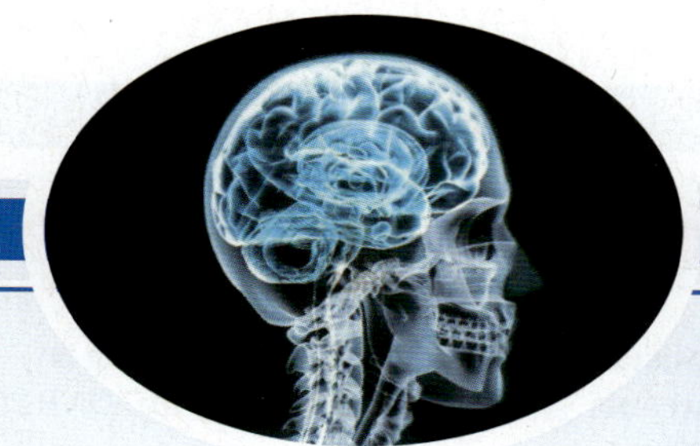

Chapter 10

Principles of Chemotherapy

THEORETICAL CONCEPTS

X A. CHEMOSENSITIVITY OF TUMOURS

Highly chemosensitive[Q]	**Moderately chemosensitive**
• Teratoma testis • Hodgkin's disease • Non-Hodgkin's disease (high grade) • Wilm's tumours • Choriocarcinoma • Acute lymphoblastic leukemia (ALL) • Ewing's sarcoma	• Ovarian cancer • Small cell carcinoma lungs • Non-Hodgkin's disease (low grade) • Breast carcinoma • Myeloma • Acute myeloid leukemia (AML)
Relatively insensitive	**Extremely resistant**[Q]
• Gastric carcinoma • Bladder carcinoma • Squamous cell carcinoma (head, neck) • Soft tissue sarcoma • Cervical carcinoma	• Melanoma • Squamous cell carcinoma lungs • Large bowel carcinoma

Topper's Edge

Chemosensitivity Assay

- Chemosensitivity assay:
  - A laboratory test that measures the number of tumor cells that are killed by chemotherapy
  - The test is done after the tumor cells are removed from the body
  - A chemosensitivity assay may help in choosing the best drug or drugs for the cancer being treated[Q]
- All available chemosensitivity assays are able to report drug 'resistance' information:
  - Resistance implies that when a patient's cancer cells are exposed to a particular chemotherapy agent in the laboratory, the cancer cells will continue to live and grow
- Some chemosensitivity assays also are able to report drug 'sensitivity' information:
  - Sensitivity implies that when a patient's cancer cells are treated with a particular chemotherapy agent in the laboratory, that agent will kill the cancer cells or inhibit their proliferation

NEET/NBE PATTERN MCQs

1. **Which of the following tumours is most Chemosensitive?** *[NBE FMGE September 2008]*
   a. Choriocarcinoma
   b. Gastric cancer
   c. Bladder cancer
   d. Melanoma

2. **Most chemoresistant tumors among the following is** *[NBE DNB 2009]*
   a. Synovial sarcoma
   b. Osteosarcoma
   c. Malignant fibrous histiocytoma
   d. Embryonal rhabdomyosarcoma

HIGH YIELD MCQs

1. **All are chemosensitive except** *[AIIMS PGMEE 1997]*
   a. Small cell carcinoma
   b. Carcinoma cervix
   c. Ewing's tumor
   d. Malignant melanoma

2. **Poor wound healing is seen in** *[AIIMS PGMEE 1993]*
   a. Adriamycin
   b. 5-FU
   c. Methotrexate
   d. Nitrogen mustard

3. **Chemotherapeutic agent of choice in carcinoma pancreas** *[AIIMS PGMEE 1993]*
   a. Mitomycin
   b. 5-FU
   c. Streptozocin
   d. Adriamycin

4. **All are radio sensitizer except** *[AIIMS PGMEE 1997]*
   a. 5-Fu
   b. BUDR
   c. Cyclophosphamide
   d. Hydroxyurea

5. **Radio-protective drug is** *[All India PGMEE 2001]*
   a. Paclitaxel
   b. Vincristine
   c. Amifostine
   d. Etoposide

6. **Tumors that is sensitive to chemotherapy** *[PGI 2003]*
   a. Lymphoma
   b. Germ cell tumour
   c. Leukemia
   d. Choriocarcinoma

 NEET/NBE PATTERN MCQs ANSWERS WITH EXPLANATIONS 

1. **Ans. (a) Choriocarcinoma**
[Ref. Sumer K Sethi, 5/e p109-110]
- *Chemo-sensitivity of tumours*:

Highly chemosensitive	Moderately chemosensitive	Relatively insensitive	Extremely resistant
• Teratoma testis • Hodgkin's disease • Non-Hodgkin's disease (high grade) • Wilm's tumours • Choriocarcinoma • Acute lymphoblastic leukemia (ALL) • Ewing's sarcoma	• Ovarian cancer • Small cell carcinoma lungs • Non-Hodgkin's disease (low grade) • Breast carcinoma • Myeloma • Acute myeloid leukemia (AML)	• Gastric carcinoma • Bladder carcinoma • Squamous cell carcinoma (head, neck) • Soft tissue sarcoma • Cervical carcinoma	• Melanoma • Squamous cell carcinoma lungs • Large bowel carcinoma

2. **Ans. (c) Malignant fibrous histiocytoma**
[Ref. Neuro-Oncology of CNS Tumors by Tonn, 1/e p286]
- Malignant fibrous histiocytoma is both radio-resistant and chemo-resistant
- Recurrence rate is also high.

HIGH YIELD MCQs ANSWERS WITH EXPLANATIONS 

1. **Ans. (d) Malignant melanoma**
[Ref. Walter and Miller's Textbook of Radiotherapy by Symonds, 7/e p964]
- **Highly radiosensitive tumours:** Lymphoma, seminoma, multiple myeloma, Ewings sarcoma, Wilm's tumour, dysgerminoma
- **Moderate sensitivity:** Small cell carcinoma of lung, Breast cancer, basal cell carcinoma, medulloblastoma, teratoma, ovarian carcinoma, nasopharyngeal carcinoma
- **Relatively resistant:** Squamous cell carcinoma, renal cell carcinoma, rectal carcinoma, colonic carcinoma, bladder carcinoma, soft tissue sarcoma, cervical carcinoma
- **Highly resistant:** Osteosarcoma, melanoma, pancreatic carcinoma, hepatic carcinoma

2. **Ans. (d) Nitrogen mustard**
[Ref. The Physiologic Basis of Surgery by O'Leary, 4/e p162]
- Many agents have been examined in experimental models which impair healing are nitrogen mustard, cyclophosphamide, methotrexate, 1,3-bis-(2-chloroethyl)1-nitrosourea (BCNU) (Carmustine), and doxorubicin
- Hypertrophic scars are more likely to be seen in light-skinned individuals, although both occur more frequently in dark-skinned people

3. **Ans. (b) 5FU**
[Ref. Pancreatic Cancer edited by H. Riess, 1/e p80]
- Chemotherapy of Advanced Pancreatic Cancer: 5-FU has been considered the agent of choice with regard to the chemotherapeutic agents.

4. **Ans. (c) Cyclophosphamide**
[Ref. Cancer Nursing by Yarbro, 7/e p256]
- Radiosensitizers are compounds that act to increase radiosensitivity of tumour cells
  - Hypoxic cell radiosensitizers: Nitroimidazoles (Metronidazole, Misonidazole), chemotherapy drugs (Dactinomycin, Bleomycin, Cisplatin, Doxorubicin, 5-FU, Fludarabine, Gemcitabine, Hydroxyurea, Paclitaxel, Mitomycin C, Topotecan, Vinorelbine), Hyperbaric oxygen
  - Non hypoxic radiosensitizers (BUdr, IUdr)

5. **Ans. (c) Amifostine**
[Ref. Cancer Nursing by Yarbro, 7/e p256]
- Radioprotectors protect normal cells (not tumour cells) from radiation effects.
  - Amifostine
  - IL 1, GM CSF, Zinc oxide, pentoxyphylline, extramustine, potassium iodide, melatonin, chlorhexidine, antioxidants (Vitamins CEA)

6. **Ans. (a) Lymphoma; (b) Germ cell tumor; (c) Leukemia**
[Ref. DeVita, Hellman, and Rosenberg's Cancer, Volume 2 8/e p1638]

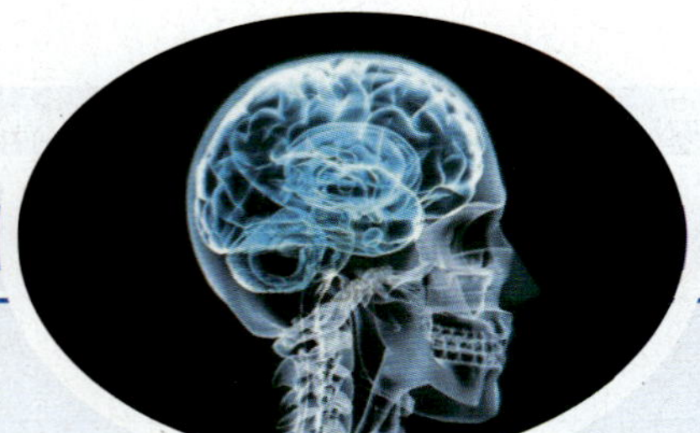

Chapter 11

Prevention and Early Diagnosis of Cancer

THEORETICAL CONCEPTS

XI A. IMPORTANT SCREENING TESTS USED FOR CANCERS

Screening test(s)[Q]	Disease screened
Papanicolaou (Pap) smear test	Cervical cancer
Breast self examination (BSE)	Breast cancer
Mammography	Breast cancer
Bimanual oral examination	Oral cancer
Digital rectal examination (DRE)	Prostate cancer
Prostate specific antigen (PSA)	Prostate cancer
Fecal occult blood test	Colorectal cancer

XI B. SCREENING TESTS FOR BREAST CANCER IN INDIA

- ***Mammography***:
  - **Is *'Most sensitive and specific screening test'*[Q]**
  - **Is NOT indicated for age < 35 years [Q]**
- *Thermography*:
  - Is a less sensitive screening test
  - Does not expose patient to radiation exposure
- ***Breast self examination (BSE)*:**
  - **Is *'Least sensitive and specific screening test'* [Q]**
- *Palpation by physician*:
  - Is unreliable for large breasts

Topper's Edge

Mammography/Mastography

- Process of using low-energy X-rays (usually around 30 kVp) to examine the human breast for diagnosis and screening
- Mammograms use doses of ionizing radiation to create images[Q]:
  - Mo (K-shell X-ray energies of 17.5 and 19.6 keV)
  - Rh (20.2 and 22.7 keV)

- Goal of mammography: Early detection of breast cancer, typically through detection of characteristic masses or microcalcifications
- Central harm of mammographic breast cancer screening: Overdiagnosis (Detection of abnormalities that meet the pathologic definition of cancer but will never progress to cause symptoms or death during a patient's lifetime)
- **BI-RADS score**[Q]:
  - Mammogram results are often expressed in terms of the BI-RADS Assessment Category
  - Categories range from 0 (Incomplete) to 6 (Known biopsy—proven malignancy)

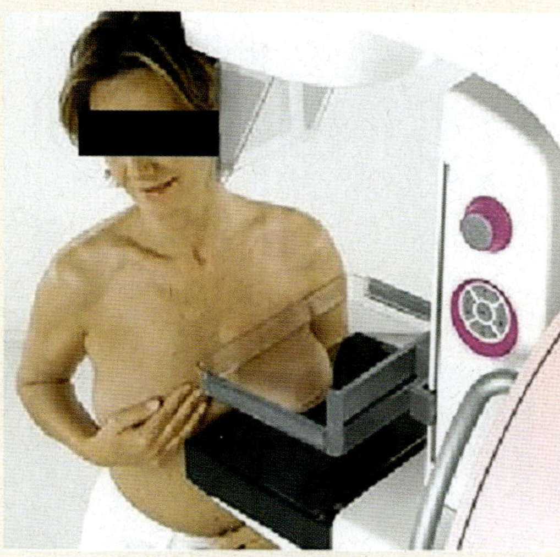

Fig. Mammography

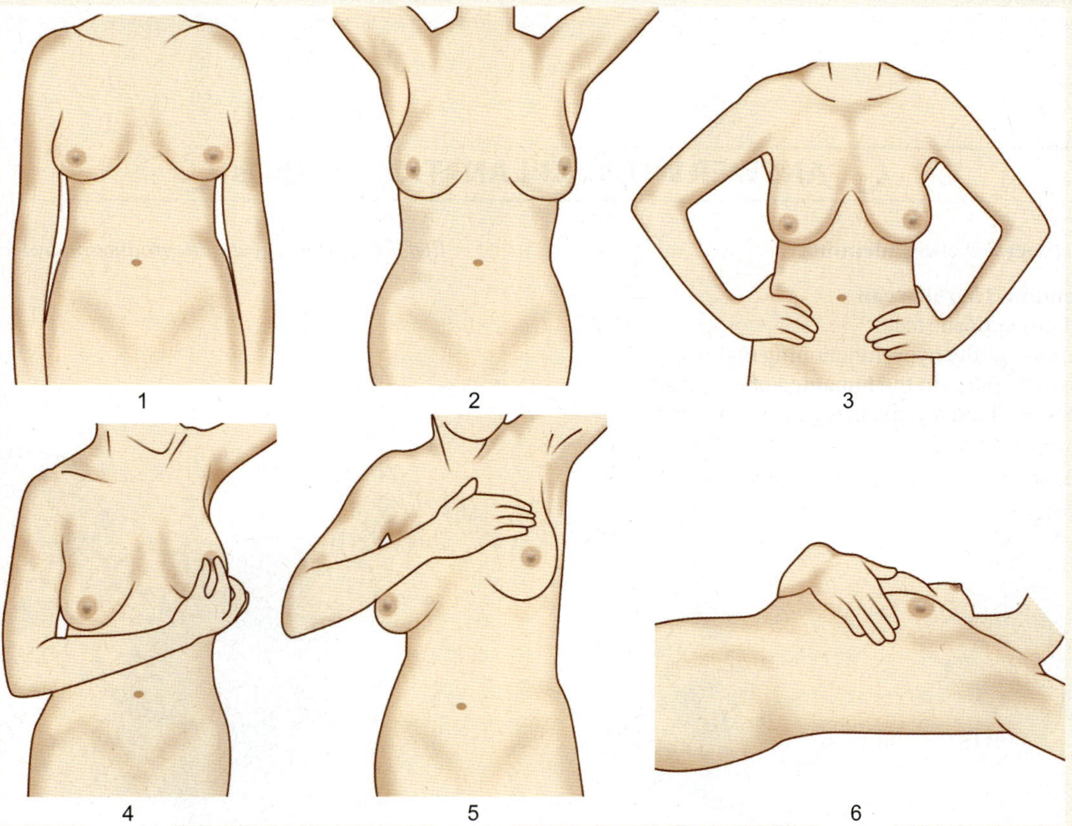

Fig. Breast self examination

IMAGE-BASED QUESTION

1. Radioactive testing scan for thyroid pathology has been carried out on a 32 years old person. Look at the scan image given below. Make a probable diagnosis. *[AIIMS May 2017]*

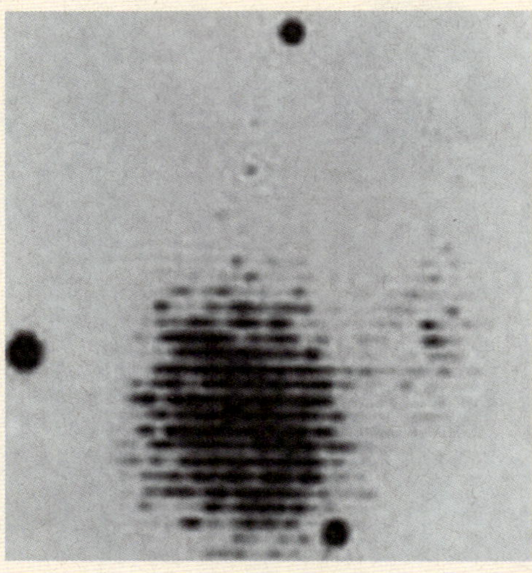

a. Lateral aberrant thyroid
b. Papillary carcinoma thyroid
c. Graves disease
d. Hypersecreting adenoma

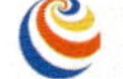 **ANSWER WITH EXPLANATION OF IBQs** 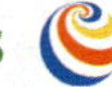

1. Ans. (d) Hypersecreting adenoma *[Ref. Endocrinology and Reproduction by Feldman, 3/e p187]*

Toxic Adenoma Thyroid scan
- Definitive diagnostic test
- Focal uptake in the hyperfunctioning nodules
- Diminished uptake in the remained of the gland
- Suppression of the activity of the normal thyroid

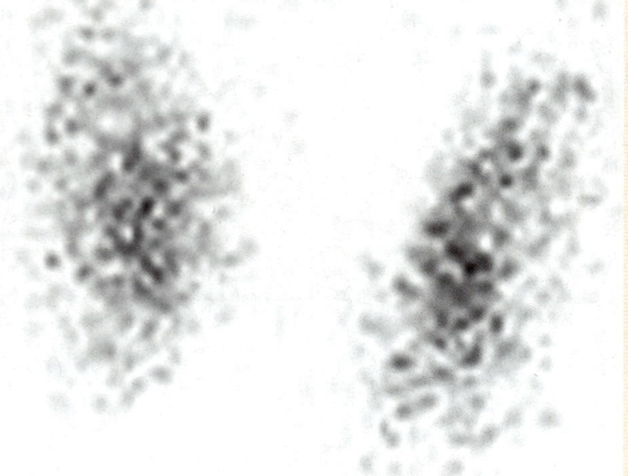

Fig. Normal thyroid scan

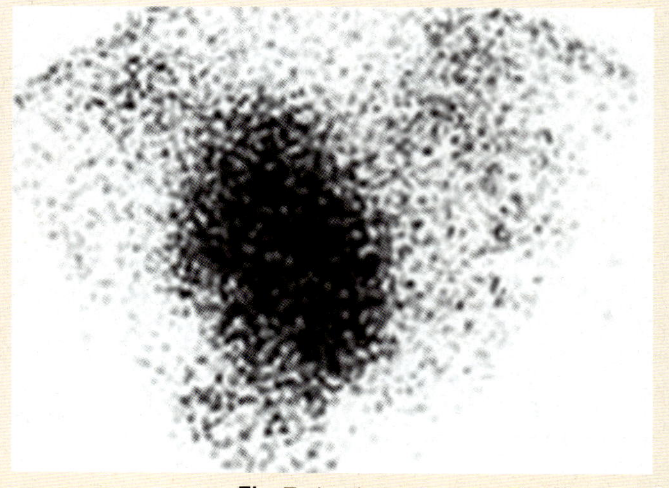

Fig. Toxic adenoma

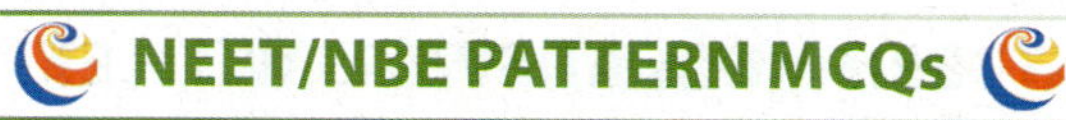

NEET/NBE PATTERN MCQs

1. **Which of the following is not a screening test for breast cancer in India?** *[FMGE, September 2010]*
   a. Mammogram
   b. Breast self examination (BSE)
   c. Thermography
   d. FNAC
2. **'Double-duct' sign is a feature of** *[UPSC 2010]*
   a. Periampullary carcinoma
   b. Gallbladder carcinoma
   c. Klatskin's carcinoma
   d. Hepatocellular carcinoma
3. **Xeroradiography is used in ____ cancer detection** *[NBE DNB 1994, 2000]*
   a. Stomach b. Breast
   c. Colonic d. Pancreatic
4. **In screening mammogram malignancy will be seen as** *[NBE FMGE September 2011]*
   a. Spiculated microcalcifications
   b. Mass lesion
   c. Cavitations d. Crowding of ducts
5. **Popcorn calcification is seen in** *[Recent Question 2013]*
   a. Fibroadenoma b. Fibroadenosis
   c. Carcinoma breast d. None
6. **Best imaging modality in bronchogenic carcinoma** *[Recent Question 2012, 2013]*
   a. CT b. MRI
   c. Bronchoscopy d. None
7. **Thyroid carcinoma USG findings all except** *[NBE DNB 2009]*
   a. Hypoechogenicity b. Hyperechogenicity
   c. Microcalcification d. Irregular margins
8. **Which one of the following statements regarding mammography is false?** *[NBE FMGE March 2012]*
   a. It can detect 85% of early breast cancers
   b. Typically calcification is seen
   c. It can detect non palpable lesions also in at least 50% of patients
   d. Normal mammogram rules out breast cancer

HIGH YIELD MCQs

1. **Least amenable to screening is** *[AIIMS PGMEE 1993]*
   a. Breast CA b. Cervix CA
   c. Lung CA d. Oral cavity CA
2. **Mammographic abnormality seen in carcinoma breast is**
   a. Change in density b. Microcalcification
   c. Change in architecture d. All *[PGI 2005]*
3. **On mammogram all of the following are the features of a malignant tumor except** *[AIIMS PGMEE 2003]*
   a. Spiculation b. Microcalcification
   c. Macrocalcification d. Irregular mass
4. **For which malignancy, intensity modulated radiotherapy (IMRT) is the most suitable** *[AIIMS PGMEE 2005]*
   a. Lung b. Prostate
   c. Leukemias d. Stomach
5. **Prophylactic intracranial irradiations are given in**
   a. Small cell Ca of lung b. Testicular Ca *[PGI 1998]*
   c. Ca breast d. Ca stomach
6. **Triple assessment for carcinoma breast includes** *[All India PGMEE 2009]*
   a. History, clinical examination, biopsy/cytology
   b. Clinical examination, mammography, biopsy/cytology
   c. History, clinical examination, ultrasonography
   d. Observation, ultrasonography, biopsy/cytology
7. **Which of the following features on mammogram would suggest malignancy?** *[AIIMS PGMEE 2006]*
   a. Well defined lesion b. A mass of decreased density
   c. Areas of speculated micro calcifications
   d. Smooth borders
8. **Investigation to diagnose stage-I carcinoma breast**
   a. Bilateral mammogram b. X-ray chest *[PGI 2000]*
   c. Bone scan d. Liver scan
9. **Which of the following does not contain fat on mammography?** *[All India PGMEE 2009]*
   a. Post-traumatic cyst b. Hamartoma
   c. Seborrhic keratosis d. Galactocele
10. **Most sensitive investigation for DCIS (Ductal carcinoma in-situ) of breast?** *[All India PGMEE 2009]*
    a. Mammography b. Ultrasound
    c. MRI d. PET scan
11. **The diagnostic procedure not done in case of pheochromocytoma is** *[AIIMS PGMEE 2007]*
    a. CT scan b. MRI
    c. FNAC d. MIBG scan
12. **Which one of the following imaging modalities is most sensitive for evaluation of extra-adrenal phaeochromocytoma?** *[AIIMS PGMEE 2003]*
    a. Ultrasound b. CT
    c. MRI d. MIBG scan
13. **Which of the following feature of thyroid nodule on ultrasonogram is not suggestive of malignancy?** *[All India PGMEE 2009]*
    a. Hyperechogenicity b. Hypoechogenicity
    c. Nonhomogenous d. Microcalcification
14. **Which of the following is not a CT feature of adrenal adenoma?** *[All India PGMEE 2009]*
    a. Low attenuation
    b. Homogenous density and well-defined borders (regular margins)
    c. Enhances rapidly, contrast stays in it for a relatively longer time and washes out late
    d. Calcification is rare
15. **A 2-year-old boy suffering from leukemia, following are the X-ray finding(s)** *[PGI 2003]*
    a. Osteolytic lesion in flat bones
    b. Metaphyseal osteoporosis
    c. Periosteal new bone formation
    d. Osteosclerosis of long bone
    e. Transverse line of dark band below the growth plate

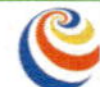 NEET/NBE PATTERN MCQs ANSWERS WITH EXPLANATIONS 

1. Ans. (d) FNAC
[Ref. Park, 21/e p336]

Screening Tests for Breast Cancer in India

- *Mammography*:
  - Is *'Most sensitive and specific screening test'*
  - Is NOT indicated for age < 35 years
- *Thermography*:
  - Is a less sensitive screening test
  - Does not expose patient to radiation exposure
- *Breast self examination (BSE)*:
  - Is *'Least sensitive and specific screening test'*
- *Palpation by physician*:
  - Is unreliable for large breasts

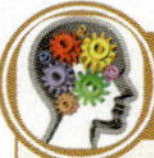 **Also Remember**

- *Examples of important screening tests used for cancers:*

Screening test(s)	Disease screened
Papanicolaou (Pap) smear test	Cervical cancer
Breast self examination (BSE)	Breast cancer
Mammography	Breast cancer
Bimanual oral examination	Oral cancer
Digital rectal examination (DRE)	Prostate cancer
Prostate specific antigen (PSA)	Prostate cancer
Fecal occult blood test	Colorectal cancer

2. Ans. (a) Periampullary carcinoma
[Ref. Pathology of the Gallbladder, Biliary Tract, and Pancreas by Owen, 1/e p342]

Double Duct Sign

- Presence of simultaneous dilatation of the common bile and pancreatic ducts
- Being an anatomical sign it can be seen on all modalities that can visualise the region: MRI, CT, ultrasound, endoscopic retrograde cholangiopancreatography (ERCP)
- **Common causes of the double duct sign**
  - Carcinoma of the head of the pancreas
  - Ampullary tumours (e.g. carcinoma of the ampulla of Vater)
  - Occasionally an impacted gallstone in the distal duct, with associated oedema, can also result in obstruction of the pancreatic duct.

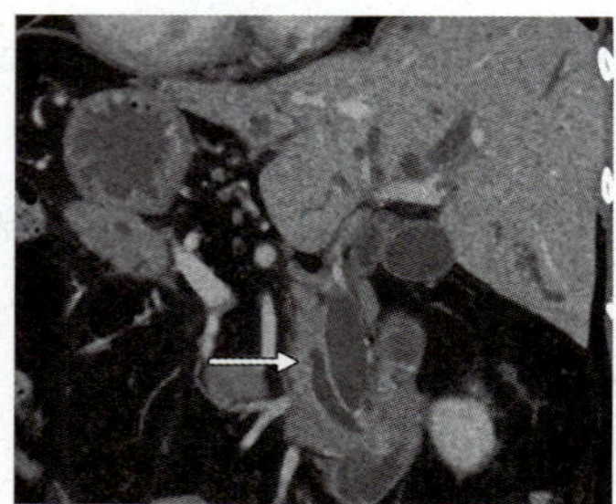

Fig. Double duct sign

3. Ans. (b) Breast
[Ref. Biomedical Image Analysis by Rangayyan, 1/e p1160]

4. Ans. (a) Spiculated micro-calcifications
[Ref. David Sutton, 6/e p240-41]

Radiology of a Typical Carcinoma on Mammography

- High density lesions
- Irregular margins with spiculations
- Fine punctate calcification within lesion
- Overlying skin thickening and dimpling

5. Ans. (a) Fibroadenoma
[Ref. Common Breast Lesions by Pilnik, 1/e p105]

- Coarse dystrophic **(popcorn)** calcifications are frequently seen in involuting fibroadenomas

6. Ans. (a) CT
[Ref. Radiologic Diagnosis of Chest Disease edited by Miriam Sperber, 2/e p 493]

- **CT** is the Imaging modality of choice for the staging of bronchogenic carcinoma
- CT is accepted as the best imaging modality both in pre-intervention assessment and in evaluation of response to treatment

7. Ans. (b) Hyperechogenicity
[Ref. Fundamentals in Oncologic Ultrasound by Catalano, 1/e p129, 143]

Thyroid Malignancy

- Malignant nodules (both carcinoma and lymphoma), typically appear solid and hypoechoic when compared with normal thyroid parenchyma: combination of these two USG features has a sensitivity of 87%
- Marked hypoechogenicity: very suggestive of malignancy

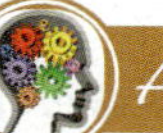 **Also Remember**

- Thyroid calcifications may occur in both benign and malignant disease
  - Thyroid calcifications can be classified as Microcalcification, Coarse calcification, or Peripheral calcification
- Thyroid nodule is ill-defined when > 50% of its border is not clearly demarcated
  - Nodules can be classified according to their contours as smooth and rounded or irregular with jagged edges
  - An ill-defined and irregular margin in a thyroid tumor suggests malignant infiltration of adjacent thyroid parenchyma with no pseudocapsule formation

8. Ans. (d) Normal mammogram rules out breast cancer
[Ref. Bailey and Love, 25/e p828]

Mammography

- *A normal mammography DOES NOT rule out breast carcinoma*:
  - 5-10% breast cancers are missed in mass screening (False-negative rate)
  - 7% false positive rate
  - Tomo-mammography is more sensitive modality
- *Mammography is a safe investigation now-a-days*:

- It uses low energy X-rays
- 0.1cGy dose of radiation only

- *Recommended frequency*: Once every 2-3 years after age 50 years
- *Sensitivity increase with age*: More accurate after 35 years age
- *Advantage*: Is 'Most sensitive and specific screening test'
- *Disadvantage*: Is NOT indicated for age < 35 years.

HIGH YIELD MCQs ANSWERS WITH EXPLANATIONS

1. Ans. (c) Lung Ca

[Ref. Imaging in Oncology by Husband, 2/e p116]

2. Ans. (d) All

[Ref. Sumer K Sethi, 6/e p159]

Breast Density

- Breast density is strictly a mammographic finding
- Density has no relationship to the physical exam: It represents the ratio of glandular tissue (white on a mammogram) to fat (dark on a mammogram)
- Breast density also impacts interpretation of mammograms and the risk of developing breast cancer
- Radiologist evaluates the density and categorizes it into one of 4 categories according to the BIRADS atlas: A, B, C or D
  - Category A represents a breast that is composed almost entirely of fat, and category D represents a breast that is composed almost entirely of glandular tissue
  - Data show that the sensitivity for breast cancer detection is inversely related to density. It is as high as 98% in fatty breasts (category A) and 50-65% in dense breasts (category D).

3. Ans. (c) Macrocalcification

[Ref. Sumer K Sethi, 6/e p159]

- Clustered microcalcification (more than 5 particles in 1 cm^3 of less than 0.5 mm size) is an important sign

4. Ans. (b) Prostate

[Ref. Intensity-Modulated Radiation Therapy by Webb, 1/e p241]

5. Ans. (a) Small cell Ca of Lung

[Ref. Textbook of Therapeutics by Helms, 8/e p2462]

6. Ans. (b) Clinical examination, mammography, biopsy/cytology

[Ref. Oxford Desk Reference: Oncology by Ajithkumar, 1/e p52]

7. Ans. (c) Areas of speculated microcalcification

[Ref. Review of Radiology by Sumer K Sethi, 6/e p159]

8. Ans. (a) Bilateral mammogram

[Ref. Perez & Brady's Principles and Practice of Radiation Oncology by Halperin, 6/e p1060]

9. Ans. (c) Seborrheic keratosis

[Ref. Mosby's Basic Science for Soft Tissue and Movement Therapies, 1/e p464]

10. Ans. (c) MRI

[Ref. Management of Breast Diseases edited by Ismail Jatoi, 1/e p203]

- For diagnostic assessment and screening, MRI found to be more sensitive than mammography in detecting DCIS
- Sensitivity varies 40-100%

11. Ans. (c) FNAC

[Ref. Pediatric Oncology by Gupta, 1/e p25]

- FNAC is contraindicated in pheochromocytoma

12. Ans. (d) MIBG scan

[Ref. Principles and Practice of Endocrinology and Metabolism by Becker 3/e p957]

- Overall sensitivity in the localization of pheochromocytoma was 98% for magnetic resonance imaging (MRI), 89% for CT, and 81% for MIBG scan
- MRI is a useful diagnostic tool because it provides sufficient histologic specificity
- MIBG is most sensitive to identify extra-adrenal pheochromocytoma

13. Ans. (a) Hyperechogenicity

[Ref. Oncologic Ultrasound by Catalano, 1/e p129, 143]

14. Ans. (c) Enhances rapidly, contrast stays in it for a relatively longer time and washes out late

[Ref. Fundamentals of Body CT by Webb, 2/e p285]

15. Ans. (a) Osteolytic lesions in flat bones; (c) Periosteal new bone formation; (d) Osteosclerosis of long bone; (e) Transverse line of dark band below the growth plate

[Ref. Understanding X-rays: A Synopsis of Radiology by Gelderen, 1/e p288]

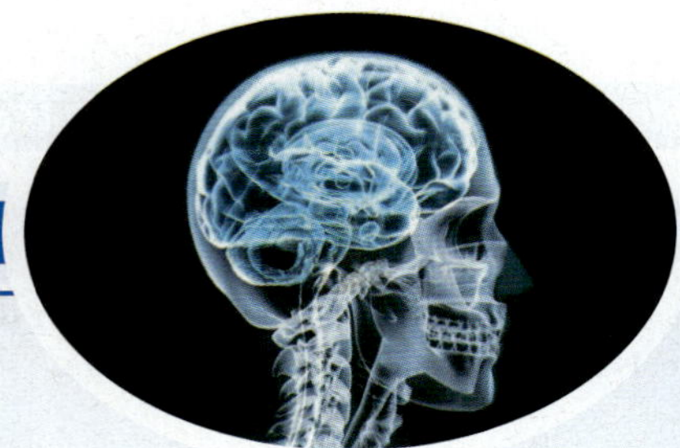

Chapter 12

Principles of Nuclear Medicine and Interventional Radiology

THEORETICAL CONCEPTS

XII A. SCINTIGRAPHY

- *Uses of Gamma/Scintillator/Angel camera*: *Scintigraphy* (Imaging gamma radiation emitting isotopes)
  - Early drug development
  - Nuclear medical imaging
  - Measuring radioactivity in samples (e.g. blood)

Topper's Edge

Common Interventional Radiology Procedures

- **Angiography**: Imaging the blood vessels to look for abnormalities with the use of various contrast media, including iodinated contrast, gadolinium based agents, and CO_2 gas
- **Balloon angioplasty/stent**: Opening of narrow or blocked blood vessels using a balloon; may include placement of metallic stents as well (both self-expanding and balloon expandable)
- **Cholecystostomy**: Placement of a tube into the gallbladder to remove infected bile in patients with cholecystitis, an inflammation of the gallbladder, who are too frail or too sick to undergo surgery
- Drain insertions: Placement of tubes into different parts of the body to drain fluids (e.g. abscess drains to remove pus, pleural drains)
- Endovascular aneurysm repair
- **Embolization**: Blocking abnormal blood (artery) vessels (e.g. for the purpose of stopping bleeding) or organs (to stop the extra function e.g. embolization of the spleen for hypersplenism) including uterine artery embolization for percutaneous treatment of uterine fibroids
  - Various embolic agents are used, including alcohol, glue, metallic coils, polyvinyl alcohol particles, embospheres, encapsulated chemo-microsphere, and gel-foam
  - Chemoembolization: Delivering cancer treatment directly to a tumour through its blood supply, then using clot-inducing substances to block the artery, ensuring that the delivered chemotherapy is not "washed out" by continued blood flow
  - Radioembolization: Embolization of tumors with radioactive microspheres of glass or plastic, to kill tumors while minimizing exposure to healthy cells
- **Thrombolysis**: Treatment aimed at dissolving blood clots (e.g. pulmonary emboli, leg vein thrombi, thrombosed hemodialysis accesses) with both pharmaceutical (TPA) and mechanical means
- Biopsy: Taking of a tissue sample from the area of interest for pathological examination from a percutaneous or transjugular approach
- **Ablation procedures**[Q]:
  - Radiofrequency ablation (RF/RFA): Localized destruction of tissue (e.g. tumours) by heating
  - Cryoablation: Localized destruction of tissue by freezing
  - Microwave ablation: Localized destruction of tissue by heating

- Central venous catheter placement: Vascular access and management of specialized kinds of intravenous devices (IVs) (e.g. PIC lines, Hickman lines, subcutaneous ports including translumbar and transhepatic venous lines)
- IVC filters: Metallic filters placed in the inferior vena cavae to prevent propagation of deep venous thrombus, both temporary and permanent
- **Vertebroplasty**[Q]: Percutaneous injection of biocompatible bone cement inside fractured vertebrae
- Nephrostomy placement: Placing a catheter directly into the kidney to drain urine in situations where normal flow of urine is obstructed
  - NUS catheters are nephroureteral stents which are placed through the ureter and into the bladder
- Radiologically inserted gastrostomy or RIG: Placement of a feeding tube percutaneously into the stomach and/or jejunum
- Dialysis access and related interventions: Placement of tunneled hemodialysis catheters, peritoneal dialysis catheters, and revision/thrombolysis of poorly functioning surgically placed AV fistulas and grafts
- **TIPS**[Q]: Placement of a Transjugular Intrahepatic Porto-systemic Shunt (TIPS) for management of select patients with critical end-stage liver disease and portal hypertension
- Biliary intervention: Placement of catheters in the biliary system to bypass biliary obstructions and decompress the biliary system
- Endovenous laser treatment of varicose veins: Placement of thin laser fiber in varicose veins for non-surgical treatment of venous insufficiency

Nuclear Medicine Imaging

- A medical specialty involving the application of radioactive substances in the diagnosis and treatment of disease.
  - Small amounts of radioactive materials (Radiotracers) are typically injected into bloodstream, inhaled or swallowed
  - Radiotracer travels through the area being examined and gives off energy in the form of gamma rays which are detected by a special camera and a computer to create images of the inside of body
  - Nuclear medicine imaging provides unique information that often cannot be obtained using other imaging procedures and offers the potential to identify disease in its earliest stages
- **Two MC modalities**[Q]:
  - Single Photon Emission Computed Tomography (SPECT)
  - Positron Emission Tomography (PET)

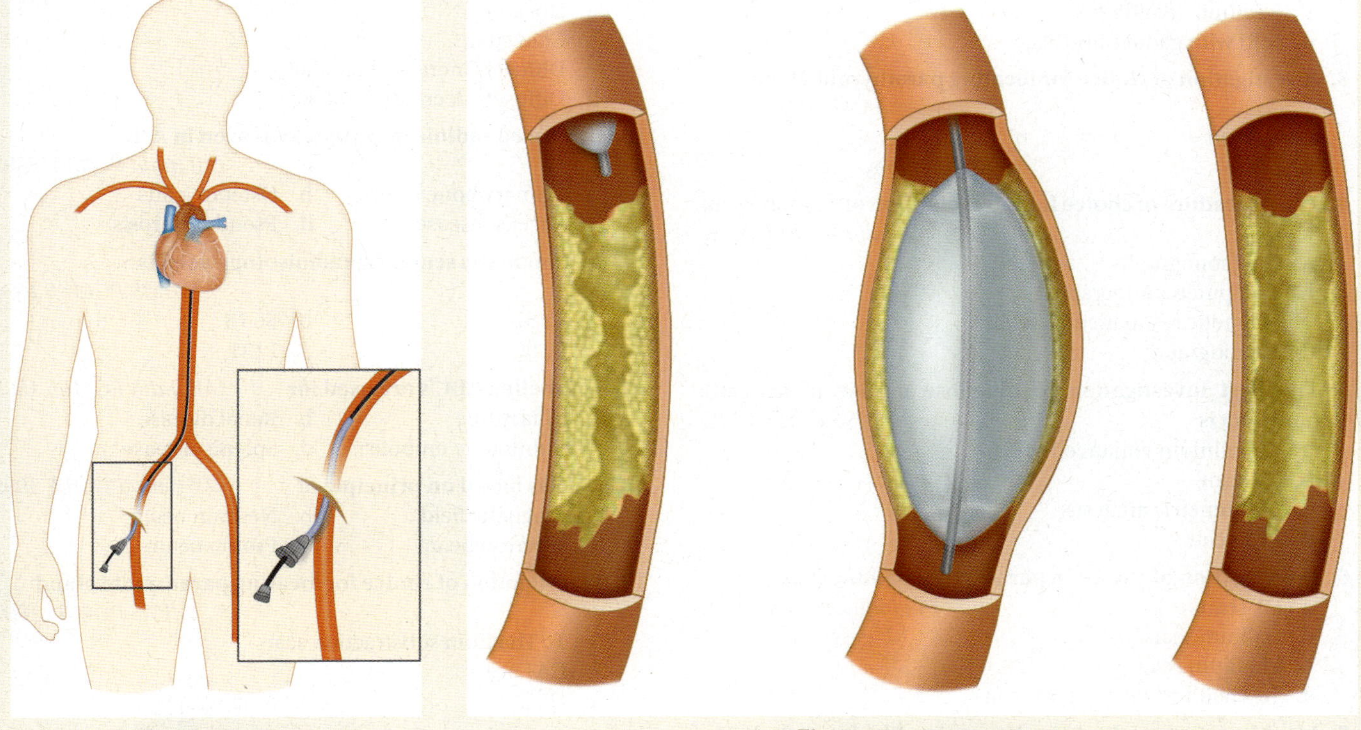

Fig. Angiogram

Fig. Balloon angioplasty

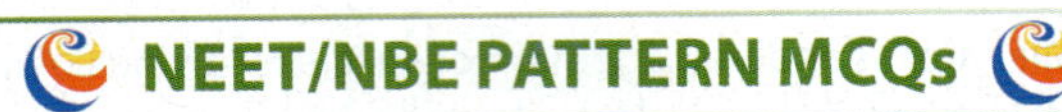

1. Gamma-camera is used for *[NBE FMGE September 2007]*
a. Measuring the radioactivity
b. Radionuclide scans
c. Both
d. None

2. PET imaging of tumour utilizes *[NBE FMGE September 2011]*
a. ^{18}FDG
b. ^{11}C methionine
c. Indium III-DTPA
d. 99 m Tc-DTPA

3. PET scan uses *[Recent Question 2012]*
a. 2-Fluorodeoxyglucose
b. Technetium
c. Chromium
d. Cobalt

4. Alpha particle contains *[NBE FMGE September 2011]*
a. One proton and three neutrons
b. Two protons and two neutrons
c. Three protons and one neutron
d. Four protons only

5. Mode of administration of Radioactive iodine is *[Recent Question 2017]*
a. Intravenous
b. Subcutaneous
c. Oral
d. All of the above

6. Bragg peak effect is most pronounced in *[Recent Question 2018]*
a. X-ray
b. Neutron
c. Electron
d. Proton

HIGH YIELD MCQs

1. NMR based in the principle of *[AIIMS PGMEE 2000]*
a. Electron beam
b. Proton beam
c. Magnetic field
d. Neutron beam

2. Best imaging modality for neuroendocrinal tumors *[AIIMS PGMEE 2001]*
a. PET
b. CECT
c. Radionucleotide scan
d. MRI with gadolinium scan

3. Investigation of choice for locating parathyroid gland *[AP PGMEE 1999]*
a. Tc scan
b. CAT scan
c. USG
d. Angiography

4. The procedure of choice for the evaluation of an aneurysm is *[All India PGMEE 2006]*
a. Ultrasonography
b. Computed tomography
c. Magnetic resonance imaging
d. Arteriography

5. The best investigation to diagnose a case of acoustic neuroma is *[AIIMS PGMEE 2008]*
a. Gadolinium enhanced MRI
b. CT scan
c. Audiometric analysis
d. PET scan

6. Investigation of choice in parathyroid pathology is *[All India PGMEE 1995]*
a. CT scan
b. Gallium scan
c. Thallium scan
d. Tc-Thallium subtraction scan

7. Ideal imaging method for diagnosis of hydrocephalus in infant is *[All India PGMEE 1993]*
a. X-ray
b. CT scan
c. USG
d. MRI

8. Test of choice for reversible myocardial ischemia *[All India PGMEE 2009]*
a. Thallium scan
b. MUGA scan
c. Resting ECHO
d. Coronary angiography

9. Bone scan in multiple myeloma shows *[AIIMS PGMEE 2006]*
a. Hot spot
b. Cold spot
c. Diffusely increased uptake
d. Diffusely decreased uptake

10. Increased radioisotope uptake is seen in A/E *[All India PGMEE 1993]*
a. Primary bone tumor
b. Osteomyelitis
c. Paget's disease
d. Pseudoarthrosis

11. In pancreatic scanning radioisotope used is *[AIIMS PGMEE 1994]*
a. Cr 51
b. Se 75
c. Tc 99
d. I 131

12. Tc labelled RBC's are used for *[All India PGMEE 1995]*
a. Biliary tree
b. Renal disease
c. Pulmonary embolism
d. Splenic disease

13. NMR is based on principle of *[All India PGMEE 1999]*
a. Magnetic field
b. Neutron beam
c. Electron beam
d. Proton beam

14. Investigation of choice for locating parathyroid gland *[AIIMS PGMEE 1991]*
a. Tc Thallium substraction scan
b. CAT scan
c. USG
d. Angiography

15. Gamma camera in nuclear medicine is used for *[All India PGMEE 2005]*
a. Organ imaging
b. Measuring the radioactivity
c. Monitoring the surface contamination
d. RIA

16. Distribution of functional renal tissue is seen by *[JIPMER PGMEE 2005, PGI 2005]*

a. DMSA
b. DTPA
c. MAG3 - Tc 99
d. I-123 iodocholesterol

17. Vesicoureteric reflux is demonstrated by using *[JIPMER PGMEE 2006, TN PGMEE 2004]*

a. DMSA
b. DTPA
c. MAG3-Tc99
d. 1^{123} iodocholesterol

18. A patient presents with acute renal failure and anuria. The USG is normal. Which of the following investigation will give best information regarding renal function? *[All India PGMEE 2010]*

a. Intravenous pyelogram
b. Retrograde pyelography
c. Antegrade pyelography
d. DTPA scan

19. Hot spot in MI is seen in *[AIIMS PGMEE 1996]*

a. Th-20
b. Gallium
c. Pyrophosphate Tc99
d. DMSA

20. Which test is performed to detect reversible myocardial ischemia? *[AIIMS PGMEE 2003]*

a. Coronary angiography
b. MUGA scan.
c. Thallium scan
d. Resting echocardiography

21. Which of the following technique is the best for differentiating recurrence of brain tumour from radiation therapy induced necrosis? *[AIIMS PGMEE 2009, 2005]*

a. MRI
b. Contrast enhanced MRI
c. PET scan
d. CT scan

22. In radionuclide imaging the most useful radio-pharamaceutical for skeletal imaging is: *[All India PGMEE 1994, 1995, 2005, PGI 2004]*

a. Gallium 67 [^{67}Ga]
b. Technetium-sulphur-colloid [^{99m}Tc-Sc]
c. Technetium-99m [^{99m}Tc]
d. Technetium-99m linked to methylene disphosphonate [^{99m}Tc-MDP]

23. Isotope used in ventriculography is *[AIIMS PGMEE 1994]*

a. Gallium
b. Lipoidate
c. Technetium [Tc]
d. Diatrizoate

24. Sestamibi Scan is used in *[PGI 2003]*

a. Ectopic thyroid
b. Ectopic parathyroid
c. Parathyroid adenoma
d. Extra adrenal pheochromocytoma
e. Adrenal pheochromocytoma

25. Isotope for thyroid scanning *[PGI 2003]*

a. 1^{129}
b. 1^{131}
c. Technetium^{99}
d. Selenium

26. Amount of I-131 used for thyroid scan is *[AIIMS PGMEE 1994]*

a. 5 Microcuries
b. 50 Microcuries
c. 50 Millicuries
d. 500 Millicuries

Radiodiagnosis and Radiotherapy

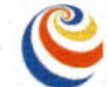 NEET/NBE PATTERN MCQs ANSWERS WITH EXPLANATIONS 

1. Ans. (c) Both

[Ref. Sumer K Sethi, 5/e p16]

- *Uses of Gamma/Scintillator/Angel camera: Scintigraphy* (Imaging gamma radiation emitting isotopes)
  - Early drug development
  - Nuclear medical imaging
  - Measuring radioactivity in samples (e.g. blood)

2. Ans. (a) ^{18}FDG

[Ref. Sumer K Sethi, 5/e p20]

- *Radioisotope substances Used in Radiology:*

Technique	Substance used
PET (Positron Emission Tomography) scan	^{18}FDG (18 Fluorodeoxyglucose)
SPECT (Single Photon Emission CT)	Tc-99 labelled agents
Bone scanning	Tc-99 MDP (Methylene diphosphonate)
Parathyroid TT Subtraction scanning	Tc-99 Thallium
Thyroid functional scanning	I-123
Ventilation-perfusion (VP) scan	V agent: Xe-133, Kr-81, Tc-99 aerosols P agent: Tc-99 MAA (macroaggregates of albumin)
Cardiac perfusion scanning	Thallium-201
Meckel's (diverticulitis) scan	Tc-99 pertechnetate
Cardiac infarct scintigraphy	Tc-99 pyrophosphate
Functional/dynamic renal imaging	Tc-99 DTPA
Anatomical/static renal imaging	Tc-99 DMSA
Inflammatory tissue scanning	Gallium-67

3. Ans. (a) 2-Fluorodeoxyglucose

[Ref. Imaging in Oncological Urology by Rosette, 1/e p308]

4. Ans. (b) Two protons and two neutrons

[Ref. Sumer K Sethi, 5/e p98]

Forms of Radiotherapy

- *X-rays*: Electromagnetic radiation of short wavelength (0.01-200 nm)
  - Produced when high-speed electrons strike solid target (anode)
- *Gamma rays*: Highly penetrating rays not deflected by magnetic or electric field
- *Electrons*: Elementary particle with negative charge
- *Protons*: Stable particle with positive charge (mass 1 amu)
- *Neutrons*: Elementary particle with zero charge and mass equivalent to that of proton
- *Positrons*: Elementary particle with positive charge
- *Alpha particle*: Positively charged particle (+2 charge) that is nucleus of helium atom
  - Consists of 2 protons + 2 neutrons

5. Ans. (d) All of the above

[Ref. Biology of Radioiodine by Bustad, 1/e p137]

- Radioactive iodine can be administered subcutaneously, intravenously, or orally
  - Intravenous administration has been the traditional route
  - When using oral administration, higher doses are required and the risk of radiation spillage is substantial, vomiting might occur with oral administration
  - Subcutaneous injection of radioactive iodine is therefore preferred, over the intravenous route as its easier to administer, effective and safe
- A lower uptake and a longer effective half-life were seen following topical administration

6. Ans. (d) Proton

[Ref. Proton and Charged Particle Radiotherapy by Laney, 1/e p11]

Bragg Peak

- A pronounced peak on the Bragg curve which plots the energy loss of ionizing radiation during its travel through matter
- For protons, α-rays, and other ion rays, the peak occurs immediately before the particles come to rest; this is called Bragg peak, after William Henry Bragg who discovered it in 1903
- Bragg peak is clearly visible for the protons and the carbon ions, as they have high charge
- This effect is also more pronounced for protons in comparison to ions, due to the lower proton mass

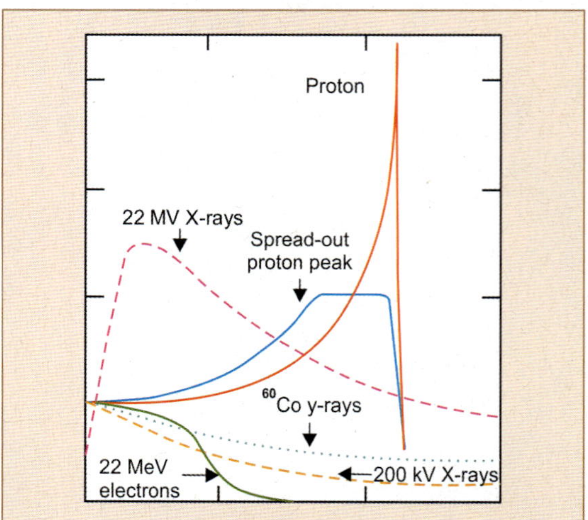

Fig. Bragg peak

HIGH YIELD MCQs ANSWERS WITH EXPLANATIONS 

1. **Ans. (b) Proton beam**
   [Ref. MRI of CNS Diseases by Huk, 1/e Chapter 1]

2. **Ans. (c) Radionucleotide scan**
   [Ref. Tumor Board Review by Todd, 2/e p118]

3. **Ans. (a) Tc scan**
   [Ref. General Surgery Outpatient Decisions by Gaun, 2/e p33]
   - Parathyroid isotope scan Technetium-sestamibi is the investigation of choice in the localisation of parathyroid
   - MRI is a useful technique for locating ectopic parathyroid glands, although angiography and venous sampling are more accurate

4. **Ans. (a) Ultrasonography**
   [Ref. Ultrasonography in Vascular Diagnosis by Schäberle, 2/e p73]
   - Duplex ultrasound is the method of first choice, yielding reliable information on the diameter of the aneurysm

5. **Ans. (d) PET scan**
   [Ref. Psychiatry Test Preparation and Review Manual by Spiegel, 2/e p211]

6. **Ans. (d) Tc-Thallium subtraction scan**

7. **Ans. (c) USG**
   [Ref. Home Care by High Risk Infant by Ahmann, 2.e p270]
   - Investigation of choice for hydrocephalus in infants:
     - Before fontanelle closure: USG
     - After fontanelle closure: CT scan

8. **Ans. (a) Thallium scan**
   [Ref. David Sutton, 7/e p63]
   - Perfusion scan is used to identify areas of reversible ischemia and the most commonly used radioisotope is thallium.

9. **Ans. (b) Cold spot**
   [Ref. Radiology Review Manual by Dahnert, 5/e p1068]
   - Conditions in which there is no osteoblastic activity, do not show radiotracer uptake on bone scan: These areas are seen as cold spots
     - Multiple myeloma
     - Fibrous cortical defect
     - Non ossifying fibroma
     - Pseudoarthrosis
     - Osteopoikilosis

10. **Ans. (d) Pseudoarthrosis**
    [Ref. Radiology Review Manual by Dahnert, 5/e p1081]

    Increased Radiotracer Uptake (Hot Spot on Bone Scan)
    - Osteomyelitis
    - Trauma
    - Paget's disease
    - Avascular necrosis (Perthes disease)
    - Hyperparathyroidism
    - Osteoblastic metastasis
    - Bone tumours (Enchondroma, Exostosis, Fibrous dysplasia, Eosinophilic granuloma)

11. **Ans. (b) Se 75**
    [Ref. Nuclear Medicine, Ultrasonics, and Thermography by Nudelman, Vol 1, 1/e p112]
    - Pancreatic scanning uses radioisotope Selenomethionine Se 75

12. **Ans. (d) Splenic disease**
    [Ref. Radiology Review Manual by Dahnert, 5/e p1088]
    - Tc 99 labelled RBCs provide information regarding RBC pooling, and is used to detect hemangiomas, identify GI bleeders, and for splenic disease workup

13. **Ans. (d) Proton beam**
    [Ref. Magnetic Resonance Imaging of CNS Diseases by Huk, 1/e Chapter 1]

14. **Ans. (a) Tc-Thallium substraction scan**
    [Ref. General Surgery Outpatient Decisions by Gaun, 2/e p33]
    - Parathyroid isotope scan Technetium-sestamibi is the investigation of choice in the localisation of parathyroid
    - Tc 99 sestamibi is scanning procedure of choice for parathyroid: It is very sensitive to detect ectopic parathyroid
    - To prevent thyroid imaging disturbances, dual phase Tc 99 MIBI may be used
    - Previously Tc thallium subtraction scan was used

15. **Ans. (b) Measuring radioactivity**
    [Ref. Nuclear Oncology: Pathophysiology and Clinical Applications by Strauss, 1/e p 93]
    - Gamma camera records distribution of radiopharmaceutical taken up by specific organ or tissue of interest

16. **Ans. (a) DMSA**
    [Ref. Genitourinary Imaging by Zagoria, 3/e p 439]
    - Static renal scintigraphy is used to detect vascular flow and tubular function and delineates functional renal mass
    - DMSA is used for assessment of:
      - Investigation of UTI
      - Assessment of reflux nephropathy (renal scarring
      - Space occupying lesion (cortical mass)
      - Horse shoe kidney, ectopic kidney

17. **Ans. (a) DMSA**
    [Ref. Genitourinary Imaging by Zagoria, 3/e p 439]

    DMSA Scan
    - Investigation of UTI
    - Assessment of reflux nephropathy (renal scarring)
    - Space occupying lesion (cortical mass)
    - Horse shoe kidney, Ectopic kidney

18. **Ans. (d) DTPA scan**
    [Ref. Applied Pharmacokinetics and Pharmacodynamics by Burton, 4/e p188]
    - DTPA scan assesses renal function

19. **Ans. (c) Pyrophosphate Tc99**
    [Ref. Radiology Review Manual by Dahnert, 5/e p1102]
    - Pyrophosphate Tc 99 accumulates in damaged myocardium and the area of infarct appear as "hot spot" due to radiotracer uptake

20. Ans. (c) Thallium scan

[Ref. David Sutton, 7/e p63]

- Perfusion scan is used to identify areas of reversible ischaemia and the most commonly used radioisotope is thallium

21. Ans. (c) PET scan

[Ref. Brain Tumor Imaging edited by Elke Hattingen,1 /e p129]

- PET scanning is of greater use in distinguishing tumor recurrence from radiation necrosis than either MRI or CT because radiation necrosis is hypometabolic. Glucose metabolism is increased in tumour tissue but decreased in radiation necrosis.

22. Ans. (d) Technetium-99m linked to methylene diphosphonate

[Ref. Insights into specialty inorganic chemicals by Thompson, 1/e p52]

- Diphosphonate ligand is used in radiopharmaceuticals for skeletal imaging as it is deposited on sites of actively growing bones

23. Ans. (c) Technetium (Tc)

[Ref. Radiology Review Manual by Dahnert, 5/e p1088]

- Tc 99 labelled RBCs provide information regarding RBC pooling, and is used to detect hemangiomas, identify GI bleeders, cardiac ventriculography and for splenic disease workup

24. Ans. (c) Parathyroid adenoma

25. Ans. (b) I^{131}; (c) Technetium^{99}

[Ref. Surgery of the Thyroid and Parathyroid Glands by Oertli, 2/e p232]

- Isotopes used for thyroid scan is I^{123}, I^{131}, Tc 99

26. Ans. (b) 50 Microcuries

[Ref. Nuclear Medicine, The Requisites by Ziessman, 4/e p428]

- I-131 scan substernal goiter (50 μCi)

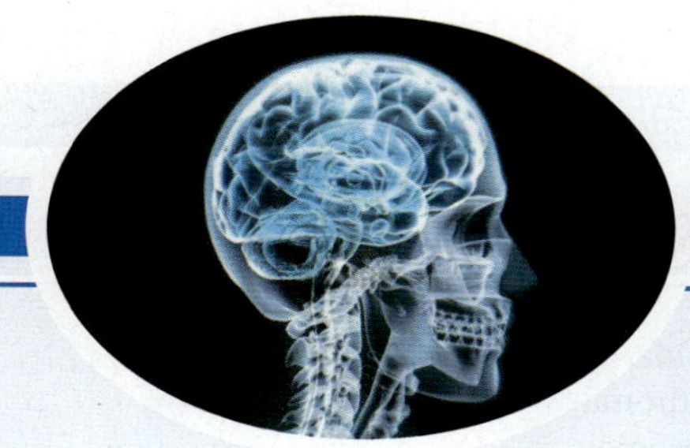

Chapter 13

Radiation Reactions and Management

THEORETICAL CONCEPTS

XIII A. IMAGING PROCEDURES AND RADIATION EXPOSURE

- ***Common imaging procedures causing radiation exposure:***[Q]
  - X-rays
  - Mammography
  - Fluoroscopy
  - Xeroradiography
  - Barium enema/Barium swallow
  - Intravenous pyelogram
  - CT scan
  - Angiographs (Cerebral, cardiac, vascular)
  - DEXA
  - PET scan
  - SPECT scan
- ***Common imaging procedures NOT causing radiation exposure:***[Q]
  - Ultrasonography
  - MRI

XIII B. INTERNATIONAL GUIDELINES

- *Maximum permissible radiation exposure per person per year*: **5 rem**[Q]
- *Latest international recommendations on maximum permissible doses*:

Group	Maximum permissible exposure
Occupational exposure	20 mSv per annum
General public	1 mSv per annum
Pregnancy	2 mSv for entire term

NEET/NBE PATTERN MCQs

1. Most common radiation induced thyroid cancer is *[Recent Question 2016]*
   a. Follicular carcinoma   b. Medullary carcinoma
   c. Anaplastic carcinoma   d. Papillary carcinoma

2. Maximum permissible radiation exposure per person per year is *[Recent Question 2017, NBE FMGE March 2009]*
   a. 2 rem   b. 5 rem
   c. 8 rem   d. 11 rem

3. Most common hormone deficiency seen after intracranial radiation therapy *[NBE DNB 2009]*
   a. Prolactin   b. Gonadotropins
   c. ACTH   d. Growth hormone

4. Most common malignant bone tumour postirradiation is *[NBE FMGE March 2006]*
   a. Ewing's sarcoma   b. Osteosarcoma
   c. Osteochondroma   d. Osteoid osteoma

5. A female child took radiation for some Illness during her childhood. Bone marrow depression was observed in her future life the organ sensitive to radiation was *[NBE DNB 2008]*
   a. Thyroid   b. Lungs
   c. Bone marrow   d. Stomach

6. Most common postradiation malignant bone tumor seen is *[NBE DNB 2011]*
   a. Osteosarcoma
   b. Osteochondroma
   c. Ewing's sarcoma
   d. All of the above

7. Radiation exposure does not occur in *[Recent Question 2015, NBE FMGE September 2005, September 2006]*
   a. X-ray   b. CT scan
   c. MRI   d. Fluoroscopy

8. Radiation induced brain necrosis can be diagnosed by *[NBE DNB 2010]*
   a. PET scan   b. MRI
   c. CT scan   d. Biopsy

9. Largest source of radiation exposure to general population is *[NBE FMGE September 2011]*
   a. Computers   b. Diagnostic radiology
   c. Nuclear weapons   d. Freon industry

10. Minimum radiation dose which may lead to Oligospermia is *[Recent Question 2017]*
   a. <1 Gy   b. 2-3 Gy
   c. 7–10 Gy   d. 15 Gy

11. Threshold radiation dose for Hematological syndrome is *[Recent Question 2017]*
   a. 2 Gy   b. 6 Gy
   c. 15 Gy   d. 50 Gy

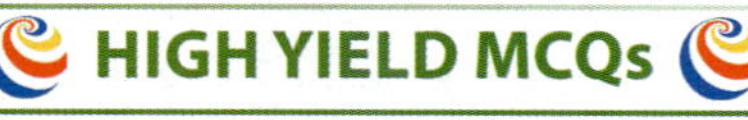

HIGH YIELD MCQs

1. Dose of radiation which leads to hematological syndrome is *[All India PGMEE 2011]*
   a. 2.5–5 cGy   b. 10 cGy
   c. 100 cGy   d. 200 cGy

2. Most common presentation of radiation carditis is *[All India PGMEE 1997]*
   a. Pyogenic pericarditis   b. Pericardial effusion
   c. Myocardial fibrosis   d. Atheromatous plaque

3. Most common hormone deficiency seen after intracranial radiation therapy *[AIIMS PGMEE 2007]*
   a. Prolactin   b. Gonadotropins
   c. ACTH   d. Growth hormone

4. Most common cancer due to Radiation *[PGI 2007]*
   a. Leukemia
   b. Bronchogenic ca
   c. Thyroid ca
   d. Breast cancer
   e. Bone tumour

5. Radiation exposure during infancy has been linked to which one of the following carcinoma? *[All India PGMEE 2003]*
   a. Breast   b. Melanoma
   c. Thyroid   d. Lung

NEET/NBE PATTERN MCQs ANSWERS WITH EXPLANATIONS

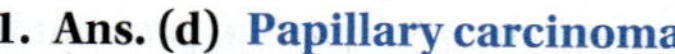

1. Ans. (d) Papillary carcinoma

[Ref. Essential Physics of Medical Imaging by Bushberg, 3/e p818]

- Radiation-induced thyroid cancers do not usually include anaplastic and medullary types
- Papillary adenocarcinomas are by far MC type of radiation-induced thyroid cancer, with lower percentage being follicular form

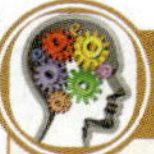

Also Remember

- Papillary carcinoma is the main type of thyroid cancer in populations exposed to radiation after the Chernobyl accident

2. Ans. (b) 5 rem

[Ref. Park, 21/e p686]

- *Maximum permissible radiation exposure per person per year*: 5 rem

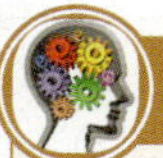

Also Remember

- *Latest international recommendations on maximum permissible doses*:

Group	Maximum permissible exposure
Occupational exposure	20 mSv per annum
General public	1 mSv per annum
Pregnancy	2 mSv for entire term

3. Ans. (d) Growth Hormone

[Ref. Oncology in Primary Care by Michal Rose, 1/e p260]

- Development of hormonal abnormalities correlates strongly with irradiation dosage and the time interval after completion of radiotherapy
- Up to two-thirds of patients ultimately develop hormone insufficiency after a median dose of 50 Gy (5000 rad) directed at the skull base
- Development of hypopituitarism occurs over 5–15 years and usually reflects hypothalamic damage rather than primary destruction of pituitary cells: GH deficiency is most common, followed by gonadotropin and ACTH deficiency
- When deficiency of one or more hormones is documented, the possibility of diminished reserve of other hormones is likely: Anterior pituitary function should be evaluated over the long term in previously irradiated patients, and replacement therapy instituted when appropriate

4. Ans. (b) Osteosarcoma

[Ref. Maheshwari, 4/e p232]

- *Most common malignant bone tumour postirradiation*: Sarcoma
  - Bone (Most common: Osteosarcoma)
  - Blood
  - Vessels

5. Ans. (a) Thyroid

6. Ans. (a) Osteosarcoma

[Ref. Radiology Recall by Gay, 1/e p368]

- Postradiation osteosarcoma develops after 3–50 years of radiation therapy

7. Ans. (c) MRI

[Ref. Sumer K Sethi, 5/e p1-10]

Common Imaging Procedures causing Radiation Exposure

- X-rays
- Mammography
- Fluoroscopy
- Xeroradiography
- Barium enema/Barium swallow
- Intravenous pyelogram
- CT scan
- Angiographs (Cerebral, cardiac, vascular)
- DEXA
- PET scan
- SPECT scan

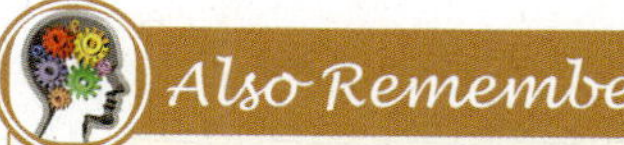

Also Remember

- *Common imaging procedures NOT causing radiation exposure*:
  - Ultrasonography
  - MRI

8. Ans. (d) Biopsy

[Ref. Relative Radiation Sensitivities of Human Organ Systems by Lett, 1/e p264]

- Although a CT scan may suggest radiation-induced changes, if the injury occurs at the tumor site, only biopsy can confirm the diagnosis

9. Ans. (b) Diagnostic radiology

[Ref. Park, 21/e p686]

- *Greatest source of radiation to man*: Extra terrestrial radiation (Cosmic rays - Radon)
- *Greatest man-made source of radiation to man*: X-rays
- *Greatest man-made source of radiation to man WITHIN HOUSE*: TV (Radon)

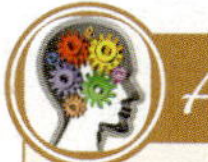

Also Remember

Maximum Permissible Radiation Exposure

- *Workers/radiologists*: 5 rem/person/year
- *General public*: 0.5 rem/person/year

10. Ans. (a) <1 Gy

[Ref. Radiation Oncology by Halperin, 5/e p346]

- Temporary oligospermia can occur after low radiation (<1 Gy) doses
- Permanent azoospermia results from exposure to > 3-4 gray

11. Ans. (a) 2 Gy

[Ref. ALERT by Rubin, 1/e p297]

Doses inducing Radiation Syndrome

Syndrome	Radiation dose
Haematological syndrome	> 2 Gy
Gastrointestinal syndrome	5–10 Gy
Dermatological syndrome	5–6 Gy
Pulmonary syndrome	5–10 Gy
CNS syndrome	> 10 Gy

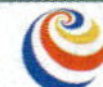 HIGH YIELD MCQs ANSWERS WITH EXPLANATIONS 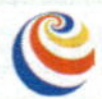

1. **Ans. (c) 100 cGy**

   [Ref. Clinical Radiotherapy Physics by Jayaraman, 2/e p422]

   Acute Radiation syndrome

   - <25 cGy: No detectable acute effect
   - Up to 100 cGy: Nausea, lack of appetite, reduction in RBCs/WBCs/Platelets/Lymphocytes
   - 300–600 cGy: Severe bone marrow damage (Serious haematological symptoms)
   - >600 cGy: Damage to CNS

2. **Ans. (b) Pericardial effusion**

   [Ref. Biological Effects of Radiation by Coggle, 1/e p102]

   - Pericardial involvement is the most common presentation of radiation carditis and includes pericardial effusion and constrictive pericarditis

3. **Ans. (d) Growth hormone**

   [Ref. Oncology in Primary Care by Rose, 1/e p260]

4. **Ans. (a) Leukemia**

   [Ref. Harrison's Principles of Internal Medicine 17/e p517, 2610]

   - Leukemia is most common radiation induced cancer

5. **Ans. (c) Thyroid**

   [Ref. Harrison's Principles of Internal Medicine 17/e p2590]

   - Papillary carcinoma thyroid may develop due to radiation exposure in infancy

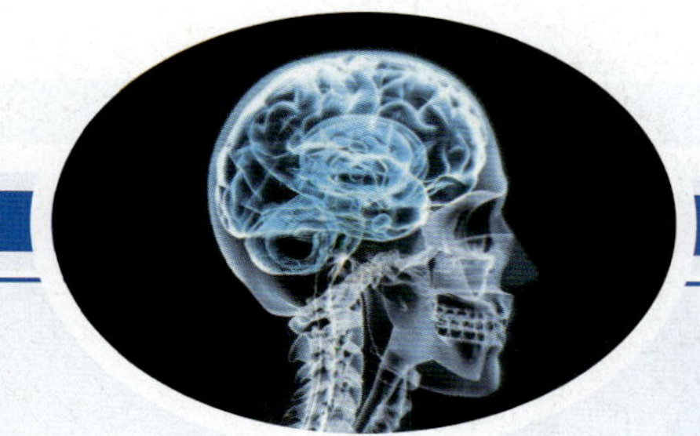

Chapter 14

Radiotherapy and Chemotherapy in Cancers

THEORETICAL CONCEPTS

XIV A. BRACHYTHERAPY

- *Most commonly used radioactive substance for intracavitatory radiotherapy in carcinoma cervix*: Iridium-192[Q]
- *Most commonly used radioactive substance for intracavitatory radiotherapy in early ovarian cancer*: Phosphorus-32

XIV B. ISOTOPES USED IN BRACHYTHERAPY[Q]

- Caesium-137
- Cobalt-60
- Gold-198
- Iridium-192
- Radium-226
- Radon-222
- Strontium-90
- Tantalum-182
- Yttrium-90

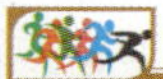

Topper's Edge

Radiotherapy (RT)

- Therapy using ionizing radiation, generally as part of cancer treatment to control or kill malignant cells and normally delivered by a linear accelerator
  - RT may be curative in a number of types of cancer if they are localized to one area of the body
  - RT may also be used as part of adjuvant therapy, to prevent tumor recurrence after surgery to remove a primary malignant tumor
  - RT is synergistic with chemotherapy, and has been used before, during, and after chemotherapy in susceptible cancers
  - Subspecialty of oncology concerned with RT is called radiation oncology
  - **Side effects of RT[Q]**:

Acute side effects	Late side effects	Cumulative side effects
Nausea and vomiting	Fibrosis	Effects on reproduction
Damage to epithelium	Epilation	Effects on pituitary system
Mouth/throat/stomach sores	Dryness	Radiation therapy accidents
Intestinal discomfort	Lymphedema	
Swelling	Secondary malignancies	
Infertility	Heart disease	
	Cognitive decline	
	Radiation enteropathy	

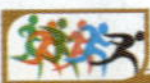

Topper's Edge

TYPES OF RADIOTHERAPY

Teletherapy

- Radioactivity source is away from body
- External beam RT
- **Methods used**[Q]:
  - Cobalt machine: Cobalt-60 produces Nickel-60, Gamma rays and Beta rays
  - LINAC (Linear accelerator): Treatment of cancer is done by X-rays and Electrons

Brachytherapy

- **Types of BT**:
  - Sealed BT: Keep isotope in contact with tumor or in cavity or in substance
  - Unsealed BT: Systemic administration of isotopes
- **Methods of BT**[Q]:
  - Iridium-192: Produces high dose of radiation (>12 Gy/hour)
  - Caesium-137: Produces low dose radiation (0.4-2.0 Gy/hour)

NEET/NBE PATTERN MCQs

1. **Which radioactive substance is used for intracavitatory irradiation for carcinoma cervix?** *[NBE FMGE March 2007]*
   a. Cobalt b. Caesium
   c. Iridium d. Thallium
2. **T1 lesion on lateral border of mobile tongue is best treated by** *[NBE DNB 2011]*
   a. Interstitial brachytherapy
   b. External beam radiotherapy
   c. Combination of interstitial brachytherapy + external beam radiotherapy
   d. Combination of Interstitial brachytherapy + external beam radiotherapy + chemotherapy
3. **Radiotherapy is the treatment of choice for**
   a. Nasopharyngeal carcinoma T3N1 *[NBE DNB 2010]*
   b. Supraglottic CAT3N0
   c. Glottic CA T3N1
   d. Subglottic CA T3N0
4. **Stereotactic radiosurgery uses all, except** *[NBE DNB 2009]*
   a. Proton b. Electron
   c. Linear accelerator d. Gamma knife
5. **Prophylactic cranial irradiation is used in lung cancer when the diagnosis is** *[NBE DNB December 2011]*
   a. Small cell carcinoma b. Squamous cell carcinoma
   c. Adenocarcinoma d. Alveolar carcinoma
6. **Treatment of choice in choriocarcinoma is**
   a. Chemotherapy *[NBE FMGE March 2012]*
   b. External beam radiotherapy
   c. Hysterectomy
   d. Intracavitary brachytherapy
7. **Point A in radiotherapy for carcinoma cervix correspond to** *[Recent Question 2015]*
   a. Lateral pelvic lymph nodes
   b. Urinary bladder
   c. Rectum
   d. Uterine vessels crossing ureter
8. **Radiation used most commonly for pain management due to bone metastasis is** *[Recent Question 2017]*
   a. Co-60 b. Iridium-192
   c. Tritium d. Tin-117
9. **Permanent implant for brachytherapy are all except** *[Recent Question 2017]*
   a. Cesium-131 b. Gold-198
   c. Radon-222 d. Iridium-192
10. **Electron beam therapy is used for which tumor?** *[Recent Question 2017]*
    a. Renal carcinoma b. Kaposi sarcoma
    c. Hepatic carcinoma d. AML

HIGH YIELD MCQs

1. **A patient is receiving external beam radiation for metastatic endometrial carcinoma. Which of the following organs in the field is radiosensitive?** *[AIIMS May 2106]*
   a. Ovary b. Bladder
   c. Vagina d. Rectum
2. **Post-irradiation thyroid tumor is** *[AIIMS PGMEE 1992]*
   a. Follicular Ca b. Papillary Ca
   c. Lymphoma d. Hurthle cell tumour
3. **Radio iodine is used in treatment of** *[All India PGMEE 1992]*
   a. Papillary carcinoma thyroid
   b. Medullary carcinoma thyroid
   c. Follicular carcinoma thyroid
   d. Anaplastic carcinoma thyroid
4. **Intraoperative radiotherapy is given in** *[AIIMS PGMEE 1998]*
   a. Ca Cervix b. Ca Breast
   c. Ca Pancreas d. Ca Thyroid
5. **Point B in treatment of Ca cervix corresponds to** *[AIIMS PGMEE 1993]*
   a. Mackenrodt's ligament b. Obturator lymph node
   c. Ischial tuberosity d. Round ligament
6. **Cardiotoxicity caused by radiotherapy & chemotherapy is best detected by** *[All India PGMEE 1999]*
   a. ECHO
   b. ECG
   c. Radionuclide scan
   d. Endomyocardial biopsy
7. **For teletherapy, isotopes commonly used are** *[PGI 2002]*
   a. I-123 b. Cs-137
   c. Co-60 d. Tc-99
   e. Ir-191
8. **Features of interstitial therapy are all except** *[PGI 2006]*
   a. Only used in head & neck
   b. Used for easily accessible organ
   c. Temporary or permanent
   d. Only iridium used
   e. None
9. **All may be used in interstitial brachytherapy except** *[All India PGMEE 1999]*
   a. Cs 137 b. Au 198
   c. Ir 192 d. Co 60
10. **Which is used in teletherapy and brachytherapy both?** *[AIIMS PGMEE 1998]*
    a. Iridium 127 b. Cobalt 60
    c. Palladium d. Iodine 131
11. **Isotope[s] used in high brachytherapy** *[PGI 2009]*
    a. Ir-192
    b. Co-60
    c. Cs-133
    d. Ra-226
    e. Pd-103

12. Craniospinal irradiation is used in the treatment of
a. Oligodendroglioma *[All India PGMEE 2002]*
b. Pilocytic astrocytoma
c. Mixed oligoastrocytoma
d. Meduloblastoma

13. Advantage of brachytherapy *[PGI 2004]*
a. Non-invasive
b. Less radiation hazard to normal tissue
c. Maximum radiation to diseased tissue
d. Can be given in all malignancies
e. Does not require trained personnel

14. Prophylactic cranial irradiation not indicated in treatment of *[All India PGMEE 2002]*
a. Small cell Ca of lung b. ALL
c. Hodgkin's lymphoma d. NHL

15. Stereotactic Radio-surgery is a form of *[AIIMS PGMEE 2003]*
a. Radiotherapy b. Radioiodine therapy
c. Robotic surgery d. Cryo surgery

16. Gamma knife *[PGI 2006]*
a. Steel knife
b. Used for cutting tumours in difficult location
c. Cobalt is used d. Recovery delayed

17. Radiation therapy to hypoxic tissues may be potentiated by the treatment with *[AIIMS PGMEE 2003]*
a. Mycostatin b. Metronidazole
c. Methotrexate d. Melphalan

18. Which of the following is not an indication of RT in pleomorphic adenoma of parotid?
a. Involvement of deep lobe *[All India PGMEE 2004]*
b. 2nd histologically benign recurrence
c. Microscopically positive margins
d. Malignant transformation

19. For mobile tumor of vocal cord treatment of choice is
a. Surgery b. Chemotherapy
c. Radiotherapy d. None *[AIIMS PGMEE 1992]*

20. What dose of radiation therapy is recommended for pain relief in bone metastases? *[AIIMS PGMEE 2004]*
a. 8 Gy in one fraction b. 20 Gy in 5 fractions
c. 30 Gy in 1 fractions d. Above 70 Gy

21. Radiotherapy is used for which stage-I cancer?
a. Colon b. Larynx *[PGI 2001]*
c. Anterior 2/3 of tongue d. Lung
e. Stomach

22. Radiotherapy is treatment of choice for
a. Nasopharyngeal carcinoma T3N1 *[AIIMS PGMEE 2009]*
b. Supraglottic carcinoma T3NO
c. Glottic carcinoma T3N1
d. Subglottic carcinoma T3NO

23. Which of the following is used in the treatment of differentiated thyroid cancer? *[All India PGMEE 2006]*
a. ^{131}I b. ^{99}Tc
c. ^{32}P d. ^{131}I-MIBG

24. Which one of the following therapeutic mode is commonly employed in intraoperative radiotherapy? *[AIIMS PGMEE 2003]*
a. Electron b. Photon
c. X-ray d. Gamma rays

25. For the treatment of deep seated tumors, the following rays are used *[AIIMS PGMEE 2003]*
a. X-rays and Gamma-rays b. Alpha rays and Beta-rays
c. Electrons and positrons d. High power laser beams

26. In which malignancy postoperative radiotherapy is minimally used? *[All India PGMEE 2004]*
a. Head and neck b. Stomach
c. Colon d. Soft tissue sarcomas

27. The ideal timing of radiotherapy for Wilms Tumour after surgery is *[All India PGMEE 2006]*
a. Within 10 days b. Within 2 weeks
c. Within 3 weeks d. Any time after surgery

28. Intercavitatory radiotherapy is treatment modality for *[AIIMS PGMEE 1999]*
a. Ca cervix b. Ca esophagus
c. Ca stomach d. Renal cell Ca

29. A patient with cancer received extreme degree of radiation toxicity. Further history revealed that the dose adjustment of a particular drug was missed during the course of radiotherapy. Which of the following drugs required a dose adjustment in that patient during radiotherapy in order to prevent radiation toxicity? *[AIIMS PGMEE 2004]*
a. Vincristine b. Dactinomycin
c. Cyclophosphamide d. 6-Mercaptopurine

30. Amifostine, protects all of the following except *[All India PGMEE 2009]*
a. CNS b. Salivary glands
c. Kidneys d. GIT

31. Which of the following statements about 'Stochastic effects' of radiation is true? *[Delhi PGMEE 2009]*
a. Severity of effect is a function of dose
b. Probability of effect is a function of dose
c. It has a threshold
d. Erythema and cataract are common examples

32. Late effects of radiation therapy *[PGI 2002]*
a. Mucositis b. Enteritis
c. Nausea and vomiting d. Pneumonia
e. Somatic mutations

33. Most common skin manifestation seen after 2 days of radiation therapy is *[All India PGMEE 1998]*
a. Erythema b. Atopy
c. Hyperpigmentation d. Dermatitis

34. On 3 phase ^{99}mTc-MDP bone scan, which of the following bone lesions will show least osteoblastic activity? *[AIIMS PGMEE 2003]*
a. Paget's disease b. Osteoid Osteoma
c. Fibrous Dysplasia d. Fibrous cortical defect

35. Which of the following monoclonal antibody can be used with concurrent radiotherapy in advanced head and neck cancer? *[PGMCET 2015]*
a. Trastuzumab b. Bevacizumab
c. Cetuximab d. Rituximab

36. Rhabdomyosarcoma is treated by *[PGMCET 2015]*
a. Chemotherapy b. Radiation
c. Surgery d. All of the above

 NEET/NBE PATTERN MCQs ANSWERS WITH EXPLANATIONS 

1. **Ans. (c) Iridium**
   [Ref. Sure Success in PGMEE by B. Ramgopal, 1/e p130]

Brachytherapy

- *Most commonly used radioactive substance for intra-cavitatory radiotherapy in carcinoma cervix*: Iridium-192[Q]
- *Most commonly used radioactive substance for intra-cavitatory radiotherapy in early ovarian cancer*: Phosphorus-32

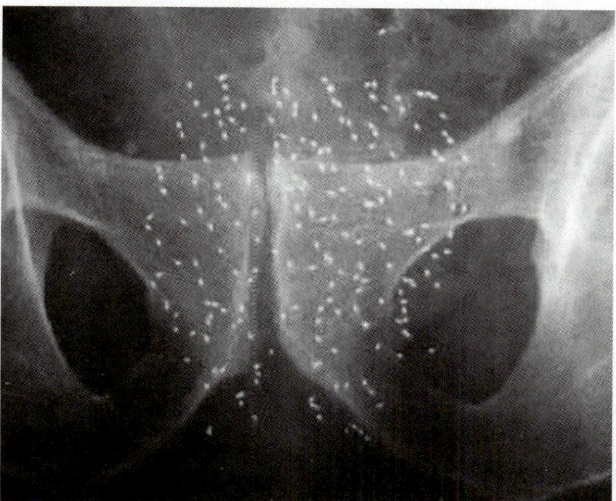

Fig 154. Brachytherapy prostate

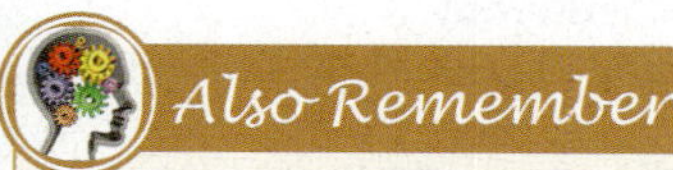

Isotopes Used in Brachytherapy

- Caesium-137
- Cobalt-60
- Gold-198
- Iridium-192
- Radium-226
- Radon-222
- Strontium-90
- Tantalum-182
- Yttrium-90

2. **Ans. (c) Combination of interstitial brachytherapy + external beam radiotherapy**
   [Ref. Principles and Practice of Radiation Therapy by Washington, 4/e p667]

3. **Ans. (a) Nasopharyngeal carcinoma T3N1**
   [Ref. Neurological Surgery of the Ear and the Skull Base by Ugo Fisch, 1/e p 256]

4. **Ans. (b) Electron**
   [Ref. Principles and Practice of Stereotactic Radiosurgery by Lawrence S,2/e p107]

5. **Ans. (a) Small cell carcinoma**
   [Ref. Lung Cancer and Mesothelioma by Gutman, 1/e p304]
   - Prophylactic cranial irradiation is indicated following complete response to induction therapy in small cell lung cancer

6. **Ans. (a) Chemotherapy**
   [Ref. Sumer K Sethi, 5/e p109-110]

7. **Ans. (d) Uterine vessels crossing ureter**
   [Ref. Radiation Therapy by Levitt, 5/e p540]

Radiotherapy for Cervical Cancer

- Point-A: 2 cm superior to vaginal fornix, 2 cm lateral to cervical canal
  - Point-A corresponds to: Uterine vessels crossing urter
- Point-B: 3 cm lateral to Point-A
  - Point-B corresponds to: Lateral pelvic lymph nodes (Obturator LN)

8. **Ans. (d) Tin-117**
   [Ref. Radiation Oncology by Halperin, 5/e p1997]
   - Re-irradiation of sites of metastatic bone pain following initial irradiation is recommended, particularly where this follows an initial period of response
   - Strontium-89, Samarium153 are the agents most commonly utilized in clinical practice
   - Phosphorus-32, Rhenium-186, Tin-117m have also been used

9. **Ans. (d) Iridium-192**
   [Ref. Biomedical Physics in Radiotherapy by Marcu, 1/e p229]
   - Ra-226 and Radon-222 were the first and only radioisotopes used in the early days of brachytherapy
   - Cs-131 is currently used in the form of seeds for permanent prostate implants
   - Today radon has been replaced by Iodine- 125 or Gold-198 seeds, which are put directly in a tumor and permanently left in place

10. **Ans. (b) Kaposi sarcoma**
    [Ref. Principles and Practice of Radiation Therapy by Washington, 4/e p598]
    - Radiation therapy is used in treatment of Kaposi sarcoma for skin lesions and lymph node regions
    - Electrons are used for superficial areas, and photons for deeper seated lymph node tumors

HIGH YIELD MCQs ANSWERS WITH EXPLANATIONS

1. Ans. (a) Ovary

[Ref. Radiation Protection in Medical Radiography by Sherer, 7/e p152]

- Radiation sensitivity: Ovaries > Rectum > Bladder > Vagina

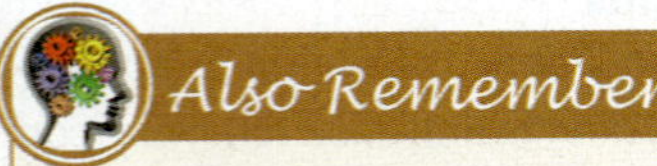

Radiosensitivity of Ovaries

- Damage oocytes, premature menopause (Ovarian failure of estrogen production)
- After menopause: Arteries and veins develop endarteritis obliterans, ovaries partially atrophied
- Oocytes undergo meiosis and are relatively radioresistant; however, proliferating granulosal cells are very radiosensitive and their demise leaves oocytes without support and Graffian follicles cannot be formed
- Therefore, a total dose of 24 Gy (fractionated in 2-Gy single doses) leads to ablation of ovaries due to the loss of granulosa cells

2. Ans. (b) Papillary Ca

[Ref. Molecular Basis of Thyroid Cancer by Farid, 1/e p199]

- Papillary carcinoma is by far the most common type of thyroid tumors associated with radiation via RET/PTC rearrangement

3. Ans. (c) Follicular carcinoma thyroid

[Ref. Thyroid Cancer by Braunstein, 1/e p162]

4. Ans. (c) Ca pancreas

[Ref. Perez and Brady's Principles and Practice of Radiation Oncology by Halperin, 5/e p404]

Intraoperative Radiotherapy

- Pancreatic carcinoma
- Early stage breast cancer after conservative surgery
- Gastric carcinoma
- Colorectal carcinoma
- Head & neck cancer
- Retroperitoneal sarcoma
- Genitourinary cancer
- Brain tumor

5. Ans. (b) Obturator lymph node

[Ref. Shaw's Gynecology by Padubidri, 16/e p534]

- **In the Manchester system, the point B corresponds to location of the obturator nodes**
- **Point B** is defined around the same level as point A (2 cm lateral to the center of the uterine canal and 2 cm superior to the mucosa of the lateral fornix), but 5 cm from the midline
- Unlike **point A** which can change with the geometry of uterus, the location of the point B does not change

6. Ans. (d) Endomyocardial biopsy

[Ref. Cancer and the Heart by Michael S. Ewer, 1/e p247]

- Specimens from endomyocardial biopsy demonstrated a significantly higher incidence of histopathologic changes
- Endomyocardial biopsy represents the most reliable method for evaluation of myocardial damage but it is very limited feasibility in daily clinical practice limits its use in cardiotoxicity monitoring

7. Ans. (b) Cs-137; (c) Co-60

[Ref. Shaw's Gynaecology by Padubidri, 16/e p534]

8. Ans. (a) Only used in head and neck; (b) Used for easily accessible organs; (d) Only iridium used

[Ref. Interstitial Brachytherapy by Anderson, 1/e p5]

9. Ans. (b) Au^{198}

[Ref. Brachytherapy by Devlin, 1/e p52]

Isotopes Used in Brachytherapy

- Radium-226 (First isotope used historically)
- Radon-222
- Iridium-192 (Interstitial temporary; MC used)
- Iodine-125 (Interstitial permanent)
- Cobalt-60
- Caesium-137 (Intracavitary temporary)
- Gold-198
- Palladium-103
- Phosphorus-32 (Intracavitary permanent)
- Yttrium-90
- Strontium-90

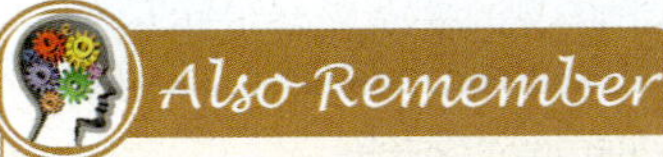

Common Isotopes Used in Brachytherapy

- Interstitial Brachytherapy: Iridium-192, Cobalt-60, Caesium-137, Iodine-125
- Intracavitary Brachytherapy: Phosphorus-32, Yttrium-90
- Low dose rate (LDR) Brachytherapy: Caesium-137, Iridium-192
- High dose rate (HDR) Brachytherapy: Cobalt-60, Iridium-192

10. Ans. (b) Cobalt 60

[Ref. Sumer K Sethi, 6/e p175-177]

Isotopes Used in Teletherapy

- Radon-222
- Iridium-192
- Cobalt-60 (Most widely used)
- Caesium-137

11. Ans. (a) Ir-192; (b) Co-60

[Ref. Sumer K Sethi, 6/e p177]

12. Ans. (d) Medulloblastoma

[Ref. Medical Oncology by Kaye, 3/e p323]

- Craniospinal irradiation is generally given because these tumors spread through the CSF pathways
- Radiation dose for the posterior fossa is well established at 54-55Gy

13. Ans. (b) Less radiation hazard to normal tissue; (c) Maximum radiation to diseased tissue

[Ref. Sumer K Sethi, 6/e p176-177]

14. Ans. (c) Hodgkin's lymphoma

[Ref. Neuropsychology of Cancer and Oncology by Noggle, 1/e p209]

Prophylactic Cranial Irradiation (PCI)/ Radiotherapy (PCRT)

- Technique: Combat the occurrence of metastasis to the brain in highly aggressive cancers that commonly metastasize to brain
- It is used in
  - Small-cell lung cancer
  - ALL
  - NHL
  - Medulloblastoma
  - Seminoma

15. Ans. (a) Radiotherapy

[Ref. Sumer K Sethi, 6/e p196]

- Goal of stereotactic radiosurgery is to deliver enough radiation to destroy or stop the growth of a lesion

16. Ans. (b) Used for cutting tumour in difficult location; (c) Cobalt is used

[Ref. Sumer K Sethi, 6/e p196-197]

Gamma Knife

- Gamma Knife is an advanced radiation treatment for adults and children with small to medium brain tumors, abnormal blood vessel formations called arteriovenous malformations, epilepsy, trigeminal neuralgia, a nerve condition that causes chronic pain, and other neurological conditions
- **Gamma Knife is not knife but is a machine**: It delivers a single, finely focused, high dose of radiation to its target, while causing little or no damage to surrounding tissue
- Abnormalities measuring less than 3 centimeters, or 1 inch in diameter, can be treated with the Gamma Knife
- A gamma knife typically contains **201 cobalt-60 sources** of approximately 30 curies (1.1 TBq), each placed in a circular array in a heavily shielded assembly

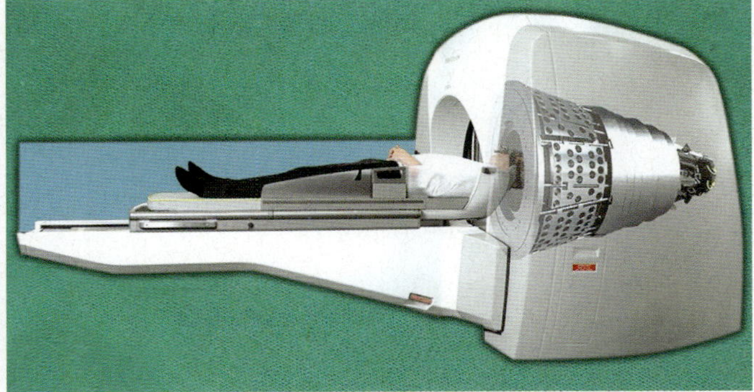

Fig. Gamma Knife

17. Ans. (b) Metronidazole

[Ref. Lung Cancer: Clinical Diagnosis and Treatment by Straus, 1/e p228]

- A newly discovered class of radiosensitizers includes electron-affinic compounds such as metronidazole (Flagyl) and related compounds
- These drugs sensitize hypoxic cells with no effect on well-oxygenated normal tissue

18. Ans. (d) Malignant transformation

[Ref. Salivary Gland Disorders by Myers, 1/e p278]

19. Ans. (c) Radiotherapy

[Ref. Radiotherapy for Head and Neck Cancers by Ang, 3/e p126]

20. Ans. (a) 8 Gy in one fraction

[Ref. Stereotactic Body Radiation Therapy by Lo, 1/e p346]

- Radiation therapy is used for painful bone metastasis. The radiation is given in
  - Single fraction: 8 Gy (Treatment of choice)
  - Multiple fraction: 20 Gy (5 fraction) OR 30 Gy (6 fraction)

21. Ans. (b) Larynx; (c) Anterior 2/3 of tongue

[Ref. Head and Neck Cancer by Ensley, 1/e p477]

22. Ans. (a) Nasopharyngeal carcinoma T3N1

[Ref. Head and Neck Cancer by Ensley, 1/e p477]

23. Ans. (a) ^{131}I

[Ref. Thyroid Cancer edited by Glenn D. Braunstein, 1/e p293]

24. Ans. (a) Electron

[Ref. Intraoperative Radiation Therapy by Ralph R. Dobelbower, 1/e p14]

Intraoperative Radiotherapy

- Methods of IORT: can be delivered using electron beams (electron IORT), Orthovoltage (250-300 kV), X-rays (X-ray IORT), High dose rate brachytherapy (HDR-IORT), or Low energy (50 kV) X-rays (low-energy IORT)
- Electron IORT: Being able to carefully control the depth of radiation penetration while providing a very uniform dose to the tumor bed
  - Applied with energies in the range of 3 MeV to 12 MeV, electron IORT can treat to depths of 4 cm over areas 300 cm^2 in 1–3 minutes only
- X-ray IORT: Poor uniformity of dose as a function of depth of penetration, the radiation does not stop at a pre-defined depth but continues to deposit radiation to underlying structures, and can do damage to boney structures if too high a dose is delivered

25. Ans. (a) X-rays and gamma rays

[Ref. Jatin Shah's Head and Neck Surgery and Oncology, 4/e p773]

- For deep seated tumors, radiation with highest penetrating power will be used (Supervoltage 1.25 MV, Cobalt 60 gamma ray & megavoltage linear accelerator X-ray)
- NB Orthovoltage (250 kV) X-ray is used for superficial lesion.

26. Ans. (b) Stomach

[Ref. Principles of Surgery by Seymour I. Schwartz, 7/e p336]

There is no role of radiotherapy in carcinoma of stomach except palliation of pain.

27. Ans. (a) Within 10 days

[Ref. Pediatric Oncology by Gupta, 1/e p513]

- Postoperative radiotherapy in Wilms tumor is started within 10 days
- Delay in starting RT beyond 10 days leads to tumor cell repopulation and increase in relapse rate

28. Ans. (a) Ca cervix

[Ref. Sumer K Sethi, 6/e p177]

29. Ans. (b) Dactinomycin

[Ref. Cancer Nursing by Yarbro, 7/e p 256]

- Actinomycin D (Dactinomycin) is a well-known radiosensitizer
- It should be reduced during radiotherapy to prevent radiation toxicity

30. Ans. (a) CNS

[Ref. Principles and Methods of Toxicology by Hayes, 5/e p914]

- Amifostine does not protect CNS because of blood-brain barrier

31. Ans. (b) Probability of effect is a function of dose

[Ref. Sumer K Sethi, 6/e p185]

32. Ans. (a) Mucositis; (b) Enteritis; (d) Pneumonia; (e) Somatic mutations

[Ref. Pediatric Hematology by Arceci, 3/e p 471]

33. Ans. (a) Erythema

[Ref. Biological Effects of Radiation by Coggle, 1/e p 78]

- Erythema is the earliest manifestation followed by desquamation

34. Ans. (d) Fibrous cortical defect

[Ref. Radiology Review Manual by Dahnert, 5/e p1068]

Cold Spots

- Conditions in which there is no osteoblastic activity, do not show radiotracer uptake on bone scan
- Multiple myeloma
- Fibrous cortical defect
- Non ossifying fibroma
- Pseudoarthrosis
- Osteopoikilosis

35. Ans. (c) Cetuximab

[Ref. Treatment of Cancer by Price, 6/e p69]

- At present, in the United Kingdom Cetuximab can be used in patients with Advanced Head and neck tumours where concurrent chemotherapy would be contraindicated

36. Ans. (d) All of the above

[Ref. Childhood Cancer Survivorship by Simone, 1/e p46]

- Surgery is a common treatment for rhabdomyosarcoma, sometimes in combination with chemotherapy and radiation.

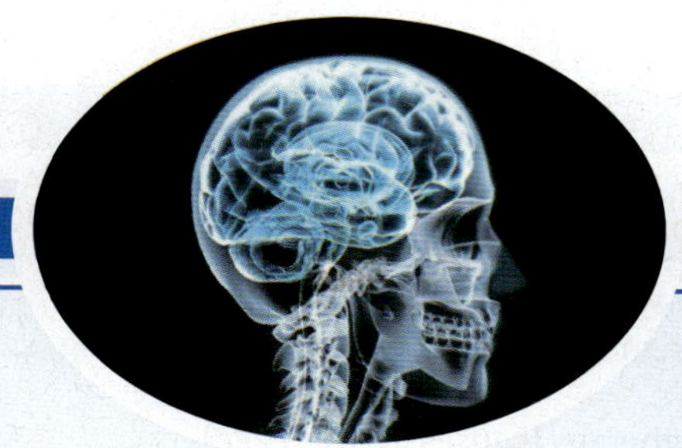

Chapter 15

Radioisotopes in Diagnosis and Therapy

THEORETICAL CONCEPTS

XV A. PARTICLES EMITTED BY COMMON RADIOACTIVE SUBSTANCES

- *Radium can emit all rays*: Alpha, Beta, Gamma
- *Main types of particles emitted by common radioactive substances*:

Alpha emitters	Beta emitters	Gamma emitters[Q]
• Radium • Radon • Thorium • Uranium	• Radium • Strontium-90 • Carbon-14 • Sulphur-35 • Tritium • Phosphorus-32	• Radium-226 • Iodine-131 • Caesium-137 • Cobalt-60 • Technetium-99

XV B. HALF-LIVES OF A FEW IMPORTANT RADIOACTIVE SUBSTANCES

Substance	Half-life
Iodine-132[Q]	**2.3 hours**
Technetium-99	6 hours
Iodine-123	**13 hours**
Gold-198	2.7 days
Gallium-67	3.3 days
Iodine-131[Q]	**8 days**
Phosphorus-32	14.3 days
Iodine-125	59 days
Iridium-192	**74 days**
Cobalt-60[Q]	**5.3 years**
Strontium-90	29.1 years
Caesium-137	**30 years**
Radium-226[Q]	**1600 years**
Uranium-238[Q]	**4.5 billion years**

XV C. IODINE ISOTOPES USED IN RADIOLOGY/RADIOTHERAPY

- ***I-131***: Due to beta radiation causing carcinogenicity in thyroid, it is not used for diagnostic purposes
- ***I-123***: Due to gamma emitting radiation and shorter half-life, it is preferably used in diagnostic testing (esp. thyroid scanning)
- ***I-125***:
  - Due to low energy gamma radiation without beta component, it is useful in brachytherapy (causes less damage)
  - Due to its longer half-life it is used in diagnosis

XV D. RADIOISOTOPES IN THYROID GLAND SCANNING

Isotope	Half-life	Uses
I-131	2–8 days	Localise and treat metastasis after thyroid ablation
I-123	2–13 hours	Thyroid function evaluation

XV E. TECHNETIUM RADIOISOTOPES IN RADIOLOGY

- *Most commonly used radio-isotope in imaging*: Tc-99[Q]
- *Uses of Tc-99 in radiology*:

Tc-99 based scan	Use
Tc-99 HIDA scan[Q]	**Investigation of choice for acute cholecystitis**
Tc-99 GTPA	Dynamic renography (GFR)
Tc-99 DMSA	Scars in reflux nephropathy
Tc-99 pyrophosphate scintigraphy	Myocardial infarction
Tc-99 MAA[Q]	**Perfusion agent in V:P scan (Pulmonary TE)**
Tc-99 erythrocyte scan	Minimal GIT bleeding
Tc-99 MDP	Bone scanning
Thallium-Tc99 subtraction scan	**Parathyroid imaging**
Tc-99 sulphur colloid scan	Reticuloendothelial system scanning
Tc-99 pertechnate scan[Q]	**Ectopic gastric mucosa (Meckel's diverticulitis)**
SPECT scan with Tc-99	3-D image generation

 NEET/NBE PATTERN MCQs 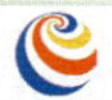

1. Half-life of radioactive Iodine-131 is *[NBE FMGE March 2009]*
a. 8 hours b. 8 days
c. 16 days d. 60 days

2. The half-life of Cobalt-60 is *[Recent Question 2017, NBE DNB 1994, 1999]*
a. 2.6 years b. 5.2 years
c. 8 years d. 200 years
e. 60 years

3. Half-life of Caesium is ____ years *[NBE DNB 1992]*
a. 5.2 b. 11.2
c. 33 d. 1600

4. Substance of choice for thyroid scan is *[NBE FMGE September 2008]*
a. Carbimazole b. Metrimazole
c. I-131 d. PTU

5. Which of the following is a pure B (beta) ray emitter? *[NBE DNB 2011]*
a. Cobalt 60 b. Iodine 131
c. Gold 198 d. Phosphorous 32

6. I-125 is more consistently used in diagnosis than I-131 because it *[NBE FMGE March 2006]*
a. Emits gamma radiations mainly
b. Has lower energy
c. Has comparatively longer half life
d. All of the above

7. Half-life of Technetium-99 is *[NBE FMGE September 2005]*
a. 2 hours b. 4 hours
c. 6 hours d. 8 hours

8. Which of the following has longer half-life? *[NBE FMGE March 2009]*
a. I-123 b. I-131
c. I-132 d. All have equal half lives

9. Half-life of Iodine 131 is *[Recent Question 2013]*
a. 8 hours b. 8 days
c. 8 weeks d. 8 months

10. Radium emits *[NBE FMGE September 2005]*
a. Alpha rays b. Beta rays
c. Gamma rays d. All of the above

11. Substances which have the same atomic number but different mass number are called *[NBE FMGE September 2011]*
a. Isobases b. Isodoses
c. Isotopes d. Isomers

12. The half of Co-60, radio-isotope commonly used in teletherapy is *[NBE FMGE September 2011]*
a. 5.3 years b. 10.6 years
c. 21.2 years d. 1620 years

13. Radio isotope scan used in the diagnosis of Meckel's diverticulum is *[NBE FMGE March 2012]*
a. Tc 99 b. I 131
c. HIDA d. RBC labeled

14. The radioisotope used for ablation of thyroid gland is *[NBE FMGE March 2012]*
a. Iodine 123 b. Iodine 125
c. Iodine 131 d. Technetium 99

15. Phosphorous 32 emits *[Recent Question 2013]*
a. Beta particle
b. Alpha particle
c. Neutron
d. X-rays

16. Radioactive Iodine in thyroid carcinoma is given by *[Recent Question 2015]*
a. Oral route b. IV route
c. Topical route d. Intra-arterial route

17. Half-life of Tritium is *[Recent Question 2017]*
a. 10.2 years b. 12.3 years
c. 15.5 years d. 20.7 years

18. MIBG dose is *[Recent Question 2017]*
a. 40–80 MBq b. 80–100 MBq
c. 100–120 MBq d. 120–150 MBq

19. Acute myocarditis Scintigraphy is done with *[Recent Question 2017]*
a. Thallium b. Technetium
c. Gallium d. None

20. Half-life of Tc-99 is *[Recent Question 2017]*
a. 6 hours b. 8 days
c. 3-2 days d. 4 months

HIGH YIELD MCQs

1. The advantage of using 18 F-fluoride for PET/CT compared with Tc-99m MDP for detecting bone metastases include all the following except *[Bihar PG 2016]*
a. 18 F-fluoride has higher specific bone uptake
b. Proteins bind to 18 F-fluoride less than Tc-99m MDP
c. Lower dosage of 18 F-fluoride is required for imaging
d. 18 F-fluoride is more rapidly cleared from the blood

2. All isotopes are used for thyroid except *[PGI 2002]*
a. I-131 b. I-123
c. I-122 d. I-125
e. I-129

3. Used in radiotherapy *[PGI 2007]*
a. 1-131 b. Co-60
c. Ir 192 d. Id-125

4. Following radioactive isotopes is not used for brachytherapy *[AIIMS PGMEE 2005]*
a. Iodine-125 b. Iodine-131
c. Cobalt-60 d. Iridium-192

5. Artificial radioisotopes *[PGI 2002]*
a. Radium
b. Uranium
c. Plutonium
d. Iridium
e. Cobalt

6. Radioactive isotopes that are used in treatment of cancer are *[PGI 2003]*
a. Cesium
b. Cobalt
c. Carbon
d. Technetium
e. Nitrogen

7. Longest half-life is seen in *[AIIMS PGMEE 1997]*
a. Radon
b. Radium
c. Uranium
d. Cobalt

8. The half-life of Cobalt-60 is *[AIIMS PGMEE 1997]*
a. 3.4 years
b. 5.2 years
c. 1.2 years
d. 2.3 years

9. Half-life of I^{131} is *[All India PGMEE 1994]*
a. 4 hours
b. 12 days
c. 24 days
d. 8 days

10. Half-life of Technetium is *[All India PGMEE 1993]*
a. 6 hours
b. 12 hours
c. 24 hours
d. 26 hours

11. Most suitable radioisotope of Iodine for treating hyperthyroidism is *[All India PGMEE 2003]*
a. I^{123}
b. I^{125}
c. I^{131}
d. I^{132}

12. True about Cobalt 60 *[PGI 2004]*
a. Natural radioactive agent
b. Atomic weight 59
c. Emits beta and gamma-rays
d. Half life is 5.3 yrs
e. Used in both brachy and teletherapy

13. Properties of Helium include *[PGI 2007]*
a. Atomic number 2
b. Viscosity is zero
c. Used in COPD
d. All of the above

14. Which of the following is obsolete in modern day clinical use? *[AIIMS PGMEE 2009]*
a. Ra 226
b. C0 60
c. Ir 192
d. Cs 137

15. Isotope used in RAIU *[All India PGMEE 2007]*
a. I^{131}
b. I^{123}
c. I^{125}
d. I^{127}

16. Isotopes used for radiotherapy *[PGI 2000]*
a. Radon
b. Cobalt-60
c. Iridium
d. Caesium
e. NONE

17. All of the following radioisotopes are used an systemic radionuclide, except *[All India PGMEE 2006]*
a. Phosphorus-32
b. Strontium-89
c. Iridium-192
d. Samarium-153

18. Which one of the following radioisotope is not used as permanent implant? *[All India PGMEE 2005]*
a. lodine-125
b. Palladium-l3
c. Gold-198
d. Caesium-137

19. Radio isotopes are used in the following techniques except *[All India PGMEE 2004]*
a. Mass spectroscopy
b. RIA
c. ELISA
d. Sequencing of nucleic acid

20. Which of the following radioisotopes is commonly used as a source for external beam radiotherapy in the treatment of cancer patients? *[All India PGMEE 2003]*
a. Strontium-89
b. Radium-226
c. Cobalt-59
d. Cobalt-60

21. Radium emits which of the following radiations? *[PGl 2000, PGI 2001]*
a. Alpha rays
b. Beta rays
c. Gamma rays
d. X-rays
e. Neutrons

22. Radiation emitted by Ir-192 *[PGI 2007]*
a. 0.5 Mev
b. 0.6 Mev
c. 0.66 Mev
d. 0.666 Mev
e. 0.47 Mev

23. Phosphorous-32 emits *[All India PGMEE 2006]*
a. Beta particles
b. Alfa particles
c. Neutrons
d. X-rays

24. True about Cobalt 60 *[PGI 2004]*
a. Natural radioactive agent
b. At.wt.59
c. Emits beta and gamma-rays
d. Half life is 5.3 years.
e. Used in both brachy and teletherapy

25. Regarding I-131, true is/are *[PGI November 2014]*
a. Emits alpha
b. Only isotope of Iodine used in treatment
c. Contraindicated in lactation
d. Emits beta
e. Half life 13 hours

26. Half life of Cesium is .... *[PGMCET 2015]*
a. 5.27 years
b. 30.17 years
c. 74.2 days
d. 1602 years

27. In Brachytherapy, Isotope used is *[CGPG 2015]*
a. Polonium
b. Iridium
c. Strontium
d. Cadmium

 NEET/NBE PATTERN MCQs ANSWERS WITH EXPLANATIONS 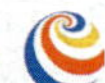

1. **Ans. (b)** **8 days**
[Ref. Sumer K Sethi, 5/e p18 and Integrated Environment Management, Inc.]
- *Half-lives of few important radioactive substances*:

Substance	Half-life
Iodine-132	2.3 hours
Technetium-99	6 hours
Iodine-123	13 hours
Gold-198	2.7 days
Gallium-67	3.3 days
Iodine-131	8 days
Phosphorus-32	14.3 days
Iodine-125	59 days
Iridium-192	74 days
Cobalt-60	5.3 years
Strontium-90	29.1 years
Caesium-137	30 years
Radium-226	1600 years
Uranium-238	4.5 billion years

2. **Ans. (b)** **5.2 years**
[Ref. Sumer K Sethi, 6/e p175]

Cobalt 60
- Half life of 5.27 years
- Decays into Nickel 60

3. **Ans. (c)** **33**
[Ref. Sumer K Sethi, 6/e p177]

4. **Ans. (c)** **I-131**
[Ref. Sumer K Sethi, 5/e p18]
- *Radioisotopes in Thyroid gland scanning*:

Isotope	Half-life	Uses
I-131	2–8 days	Localise and treat metastasis after thyroid ablation
I-123	2–13 hours	Thyroid function evaluation

5. **Ans. (d)** **Phosphorous 32**
[Ref. Sumer K Sethi, 6/e p177]

Phosphorous 32
- Form in which used: Sodium orthophosphate solution
- Half life: 14.3 days
- Radiation emitted: Beta rays
- Method of administration: Intravenous injection

6. **Ans. (d)** **All of the above**
[Ref. Wikipedia]

Iodine Isotopes Used in Radiology/Radiotherapy
- *I-131*: Due to beta radiation causing carcinogenicity in thyroid, it is not used for diagnostic purposes
- *I-123*: Due to gamma emitting radiation and shorter half life, it is preferably used in diagnostic testing (esp. thyroid scanning)
- *I-125*:
  - Due to low energy gamma radiation without beta component, it is useful in brachytherapy (causes less damage)
  - Due to its longer half life it is used in diagnosis

7. **Ans. (c)** **6 hours**
[Ref. Sumer K Sethi, 5/e p15]

8. **Ans. (b)** **I-131**
[Ref. Sumer K Sethi, 5/e p18 and Integrated Environment Management, Inc.]

9. **Ans. (b)** **8 days**
[Ref. Sumer K Sethi, 6/e p177]

Iodine 131
- Form in which used: Sodium iodide solution
- Half life: 8 days
- Radiation emitted: Beta/Gamma rays
- Method of administration: Oral

10. **Ans. (d)** **All of the above**
[Ref. Wikipedia]
- *Radium can emit all rays*: Alpha, Beta, Gamma
- *Main types of particles emitted by common radioactive substances*:

Alpha emitters	Beta emitters	Gamma emitters
• Radium • Radon • Thorium • Uranium	• Radium • Strontium-90 • Carbon-14 • Sulphur-35 • Tritium • Phosphorus-32	• Radium-226 • Iodine-131 • Caesium-137 • Cobalt-60 • Technetium-99

11. **Ans. (c)** **Isotopes**
[Ref. David Sutton, 6/e p10-11]
- *Isotopes*: Substances with same atomic number but different mass number
  - Same chemical and biological behaviour
  - Different energy state

Also Remember
- *Isomers*: Compounds with same molecular formula but different structural formula
  - May not have similar properties
- *Isobases*: A line drawn on map to connect places of similar height
- *Isodoses*: A radiation dose of equal intensity to more than one body area

Radiodiagnosis and Radiotherapy

12. Ans. (a) **5.3 years**
[Ref. Sumer K Sethi, 5/e p114]

13. Ans. (a) **Tc99**
[Ref. Bailey and Love, 25/e p1159]

14. Ans. (c) **Iodine 131**
[Ref. Sumer K Sethi, 5/e p18]

Uses of Iodine Isotopes in Thyroid

- *Uses of Iodine-131*:
  - Thyroid ablation
  - Localize and treat metastasis
- *Uses of Iodine-123*:
  - Thyroid function evaluation
- *Uses of Iodine-125*:
  - Prostate and brain cancer brachytherapy
  - DVT diagnosis

15. Ans. (a) **Beta particle**
[Ref. Sumer K Sethi, 6/e p177]

16. Ans. (a) **Oral route**
[Ref. Medical-Surgical Nursing by Williams, 1/e p1381]

17. Ans. (b) **12.3 years**
[Ref. Radiology by Zabel, Vol 2, 2/e p20]

Radioactive Hydrogen (Tritium)

- One proton, two neutrons, 12.3 year half-life
- Emits a beta particle, no gamma emission
- An ideal tracer for studying ground waters

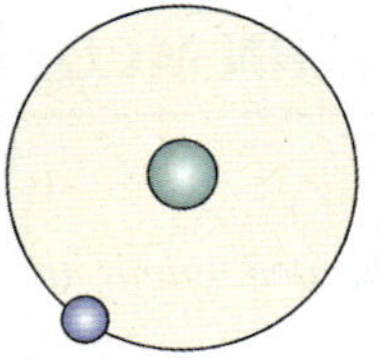
Protium (^1H)

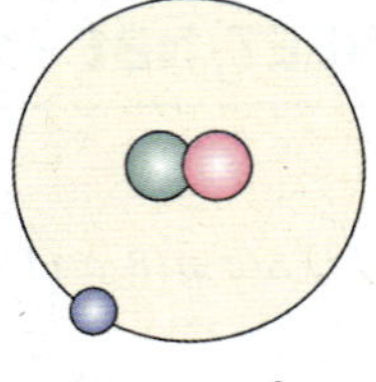
Deuterium (^2H)

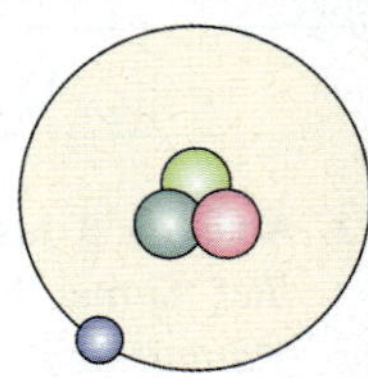
Tritium (^3H)

Fig. Isotopes of hydrogen

18. Ans. (a) **40–80 MBq**
[Ref. Clinical Nuclear Medicine by Biersack, 1/e p457]

Doses for Meta-iodo-guanyl benzidine (MIBG)

- I-131 MIBG (adults): 40-80 MBq
- I-123 MIBG (adults): 400 MBq
- I-131 MIBG (children): 35 MBq
- I-123 MIBG (children): 80 MBq

19. Ans. (c) **Gallium**
[Ref. Cardiovascular Imaging by Zamorano, 2/e p538]

- Gallium-67 citrate injected intravenously binds to transferrin, and it is incorporated into the transferrin receptor of inflammatory cells or malignant tumor cells
- Because of the above-mentioned properties, Gallium-67 scintigraphy is used to detect a focus of active inflammation or malignant lesion
- Gallium-67 scintigraphy is useful for examination of heart disease including cardiac sarcoidosis and acute myocarditis because Gallium-67 does not accumulate physiologically in the heart

20. Ans. (a) **6 hours**
[Ref. Learning Radiology by Herring, 2/e p16]

- Physical Half-Life Technetium 99m is 6 hours

HIGH YIELD MCQs ANSWERS WITH EXPLANATIONS

1. Ans. (c) **Lower dosage of 18 F-fluoride is required for imaging**
[Ref. Dynamic bone imaging with 99mTc-labeled diphosphonates and 18F-NaF: mechanisms and applications. JMJ]

18 F-fluoride for PET/CT vs Tc-99m MDP for detecting Bone Metastases

- 18 F-fluoride has higher specific bone uptake
- Proteins bind to 18 F-fluoride less than Tc-99m MDP
- 18 F–fluoride is more rapidly cleared from the blood: Reduced imaging time
- 18 F-fluoride provide quantitative information
- 18 F-fluoride has higher sensitivity
- 18 F-fluoride provide higher contrast and spatial resolution
- Lower dosage of 18 F-fluoride if required for imaging
- 18 F-fluoride barely binds to serum protein whereas 99mTc-MDP shows significant protein bindings: Lesser imaging time with 18F
- Rapid uptake of 18F-fluoride occurs preferentially at sites of high osteoblastic activity where bone remodeling is greatest

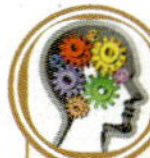

Also Remember

- Mechanism of accumulation of fluoride in 18-F PET/CT: After diffusion through capillaries into bone extracellular fluid, fluoride ion exchanges slowly with hydroxyl groups in hydroxyapatite crystal of bone to form fluoroapatite, and is deposited preferentially at the surfaces of bone, where remodeling and turnover is greatest
- Combining 18F-fluoride PET with other imaging, such as CT, improves the specificity and overall accuracy of skeletal 18F-fluoride PET

2. Ans. (c) **I-122; (e) I-129**
[Ref. Surgery of the Thyroid and Parathyroid Glands by Daniel Oertli, 2/e p232]

- Isotopes used for thyroid scan is I^{123}, I^{124}, I^{125}, I^{131}, Tc^{99}

3. Ans. **All choices**
[Ref. Sumer K Sethi, 6/e p177]

4. Ans. (b) **Iodine-131**
[Ref. Radiotherapy and Brachytherapy by Lemoigne, 1/e p91]

- Permanent implants of interstitial brachytherapy: Cesium-137, Yttrium, Gold-198, I-125, Radon-222, Pallidum-103
- Temporary implants of interstitial brachytherapy: Iridium-192, Cesium-137, Cobalt-60, Californium, Radium-226, Tantalum

5. Ans. (d) Iridium; (e) Cobalt
[Ref. Principles and Practice of Radiation Therapy by Washington, 3/e p143]

Important Artificial Radionuclides
- Tritium-1
- Carbon-14
- Cobalt-60
- Strontium-89
- Strontium-90
- Iodine-131
- Cesium-134
- Cesium-137
- Plutonium-239
- Iridium
- Tc 99

6. Ans. (a) Caesium; (b) Cobalt
[Ref. Radiotherapy and Brachytherapy by Lemoigne, 1/e p91]

7. Ans. (c) Uranium
[Ref. Sumer K Sethi, 6/e p164, 177]
- Half-life
  - Uranium: 4.468 billion years
  - Radium: 1622 years
  - Radon: 3.8 days
  - Cobalt: 5.26 years

8. Ans. (b) 5.2 years
[Ref. Sumer K Sethi, 6/e p177]

9. Ans. (d) 8 days
[Ref. Sumer K Sethi, 6/e p177]

10. Ans. (a) 6 hours
[Ref. Uranium Processing and Properties by Morrell, 1/e p271]
- Technetium-99m is the product of molybdenum-99 decay, has an atomic number of 43, and a half-life of 6 hours

11. Ans. (c) I^{131}
[Ref. Thyroid Cancer by Fagin, 1/e p42]
- I-131 emits short-ranged beta particles that destroy or severely injure thyroid follicular cells (1–2 mm from source) causing them to die over a period of several weeks
- A typical treatment dose for hyperthyroidism is 5-15 mCi

12. Ans. (c) Emits beta and gamma rays; (d) Half life is 5.3 years; (e) Used in both brachy and teletherapy
[Ref. Sumer K Sethi, 6/e p175]

13. Ans. (d) All of the above
[Ref. Helium by Hasan, 1/e p19]

14. Ans. (a) Ra 226
[Ref. Comprehensive Brachytherapy by Venselaar, 1/e p31]

15. Ans. (b) I^{123}
[Ref. Clinical Medicine by Das, 4/e p333]

16. Ans. All choices
[Ref. Radiotherapy and Brachytherapy by Lemoigne, 1/e p91]

17. Ans. (c) Iridium-192
[Ref. Harrison's Principles of Internal Medicine, 16/e p1486]

Systemic Radionucleide
- I-131
- Samarium-153
- Yttrium
- Strontium-89
- P32

18. Ans. (d) Caesium-137
[Ref. Radiotherapy and Brachytherapy by Lemoigne, 1/e p91]

19. Ans. (c) ELISA
[Ref. Radioisotopes in Biology by Slater, 2/e p230]

20. Ans. (d) Cobalt-60
[Ref. Sumer K Sethi, 6/e p175]

21. Ans. (a) Alpha rays; (b) Beta rays; (c) Gamma rays; (e) Neutrons
[Ref. Handbook of Radioactivity Analysis by L'Annunziata, 3/e p77]
- Radium emits alpha, beta, gamma rays
- Radium bromide also produces neutrons when mixed with beryllium

22. Ans. (e) 0.47 MeV
[Ref. Trends in NDE Science and Technology, Vol 1, p31]
- Iridium 192 has a complex gamma ray spectrum with lines from 0.13 MeV to 0.89 MeV with the principal lines at 0.31 and 0.47 MeV

23. Ans. (a) Beta particles
[Ref. Sumer K Sethi, 6/e p177]

24. Ans. ALL CHOICES
[Ref. Sumer K Sethi, 6/e p175]

25. Ans. (b) Only isotope of iodine used in treatment; (c) Contraindicated in lactation; (d) Emits beta
[Ref. Sumer K Sethi, 5/e p252]

Iodine-131
- Half-life: 8 days
- Mode of decay: Beta rays
- Uses of I-131:
  - Imaging: Thyroid, Liver function, Renal blood flow, Urinary obstruction
  - Treatment: Thyrotoxicosis, Thyroid carcinoma, Pheochromocytoma, Neuroblastoma
- Contraindicated in lactation

26. Ans. (b) 30.17 years
[Ref. Radiation Source Use and Replacement, 1/e p27]
- Radionuclide Caesium-137 is produced by fission in a nuclear reactor, has a 30.17 years half-life and decays by beta decay to Barium-137 or Barium-137m

27. Ans. (b) Iridium
[Ref. Brachytherapy by Devlin, 1/e p52]

Radioisotopes Used in Brachytherapy
- Radium-226
- Radon-222
- Iridium-192
- Iodine-125
- Cobalt-60
- Caesium-17
- Gold-198
- Palladium-103

AIIMS PG 2018 MCQs

1. Venous Doppler Flow Image shown in Photograph depicts *[AIIMS May 2018]*

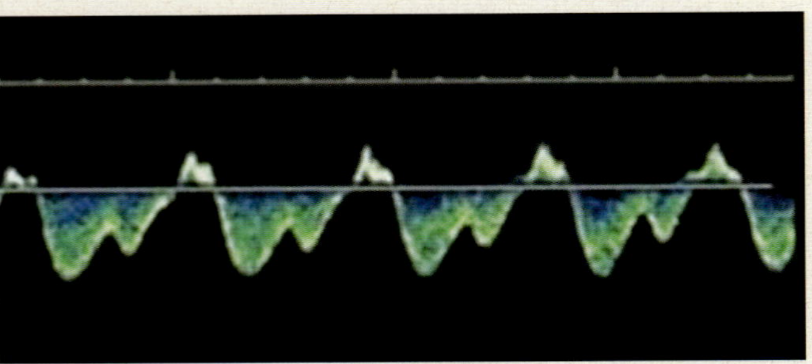

a. Monophasic flow
b. Biphasic flow
c. Triphasic flow
d. None of the above

2. Diagnose the condition shown in the CT Scan image given below *[AIIMS May 2018]*

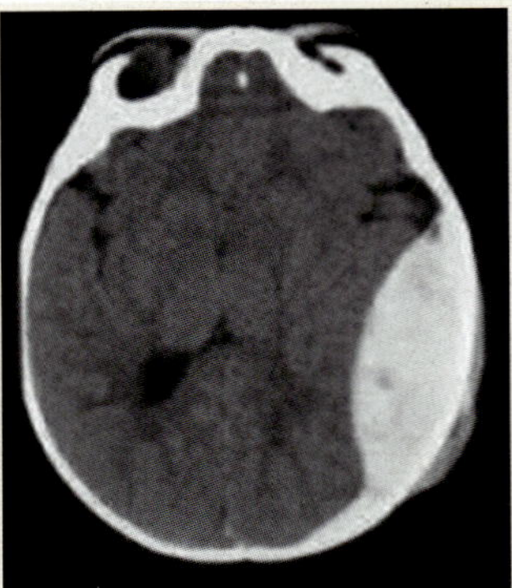

a. Epidural hemorrhage
b. Subdural hemorrhage
c. Subarachnoid hemorrhage
d. ICSOL

EXPLANATORY ANSWERS

1. Ans (c) Triphasic flow

[Ref. Duplex and Color Doppler Imaging of the Venous System by Mostbeck, 1/e p120]

Doppler Waveforms

- Triphasic pattern (two antegrade waves below the baseline and one presystolic retrograde wave above the baseline)
- Biphasic pattern (with absent reversed pre-systolic wave)
- Monophasic pattern (with a flat pattern)

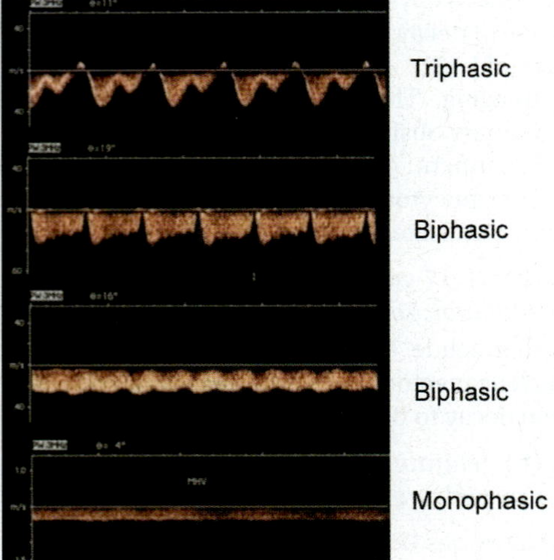

Fig. Doppler Waveforms

2. Ans. (b) Subdural hemorrhage

[Ref. High-Yield Gross Anatomy by Dudek, 5/e p254]

Subdural Hematoma

- Location: Lies between Dura mater and arachnoid mater
- Vessels involved: Bridging veins (Draining into Dura sinus)
- CT appearance: Crescent shape

Radiodiagnosis and Radiotherapy

Psychiatry

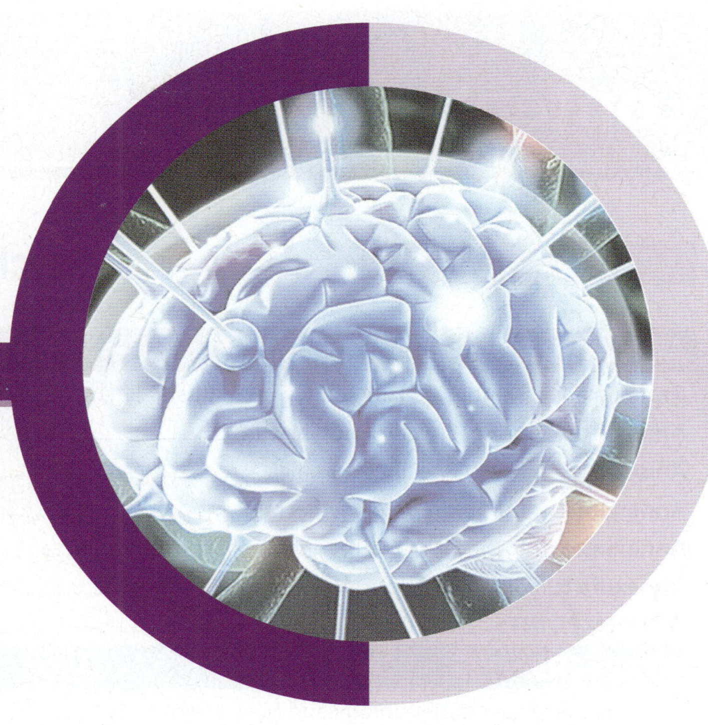

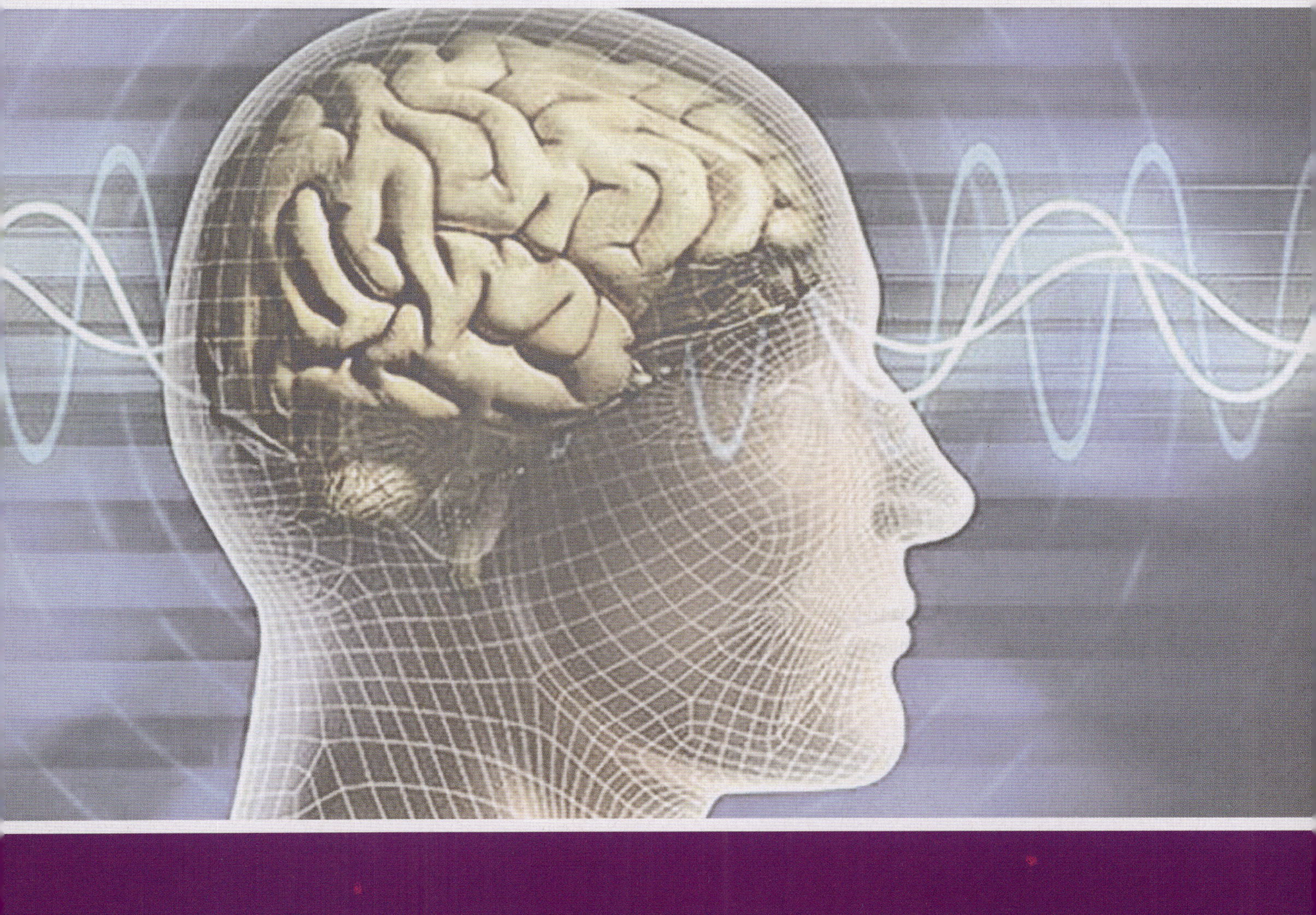

Contents

Psychiatry

ANNEXURES

CHAPTERS

EACH CHAPTER DIVIDED INTO FOLLOWING SECTIONS

Theoretical Concepts (Including Images)
Image-Based Questions
Answers with Explanations of IBQs
NEET/NBE Pattern MCQs
High Yield MCQs
NEET/NBE Pattern MCQs Answers with Explanations
High Yield MCQs Answers with Explanations
AIIMS PG 2018 MCQs with Explanatory Answers

Annexures

ANNEXURE 1. FAMOUS SCIENTISTS AND PSYCHIATRISTS

Scientist/Psychiatrist	Contribution
Aaron T Buck	Father of cognitive therapy
Alfred Binet	Stanford-Binet test of intelligence
Alois alzheimer	Presenile dementia (Alzheimer disease)
Berger	Electroencephalogram (EEG)
BF Skinner	Operant conditioning; Positive reinforcement
Carl Jung	Analytical psychology
Carletti, Bini	Electroconvulsive therapy (ECT)
Cloninger	Two alcoholic species based on environment and genetic factors
Emil Kraepelin	Founder of modern scientific psychiatry
Eugene Bleuler	Renamed Dementia-precox as Schizophrenia; Fundamental symptoms of schizophrenia
Franz Alexander	Father of psychosomatic medicine; 7 classic symptoms of psychosomatic illness
Ganeshan/Kartik Bose	First successful treatment of psychoses with reserpine
Heinroth	Coined term 'Psychosomatic disorders'
Hermann Rorschach	Inkblot (Rorschach) test
Jean Piaget	Cognitive development
Jellinek	Five alcoholic species based on pattern of use
Johann Christian Heinroth	Father of psychiatry
Julius Von Wagner Jauregg	Malaria treatment of general paresis of insane; Pyrotherapy treatment of mental disorders
Kurt Schneider	First/Second rank symptoms of schizophrenia
Manfred Sakel	Insulin shock treatment of schizophrenia
Moniz	Nobel Prize for leucotomy (Psychosurgery)
Phillippe Pinel	Father of modern psychiatry
Ronald David Laing	Anti-psychiatry
Sigmund Freud	Psychoanalysis; Father of psychoanalysis
Carlsson/Greengard/Kandel	Nobel Prize for work on neurotransmitters

Scientist	Terms coined
Braid	Hypnosis
Ernst von Feuchter Sleben	Psychosis
Henneberg	Cataplexy
Ivan Pavlox	Conditioned reflex
Johann Christian Reil	Psychiatry (1808)
Joshua Bierer	Social psychiatry
Kahlbaum	Catatonia
William Cullen	Neurosis
Sigmund Freud	Psychoanalysis

ANNEXURE 2. LIST OF SPECIFIC PHOBIAS

Phobia	Description
Acrophobia	Fear of height
Agoraphobia	Fear of being in places from which escape might be difficult
Agraphobia	Fear of sexual abuse
Algophobia	Fear of pain
Anthophobia	Fear of flowers
Aquaphobia	Fear of water
Arachnophobia	Fear of spiders
Barophobia	Fear of gravity
Cherophobia	Fear of happiness
Cibophobia/Sitophobia	Anorexia nervosa
Claustrophobia	Fear of closed spaces
Enochlophobia	Fear of crowds
Gamophobia	Fear of marriage/commitment
Genophobia/Coitophobia	Fear of sexual intercourse
Glossophobia	Fear of speaking in public
Gynophobia	Fear of women
Heliophobia	Fear of sun/sunlight
Hypnophobia	Fear of sleep
Iatrophobia	Fear of doctors
Icthyophobia	Fear of fish
Necrophobia	Fear of death/dead
Nosocomephobia	Fear of hospitals
Nyctophobia	Fear of darkness
Oneirophobia	Fear of dreams
Pedophobia	Fear of dolls
Pharmacophobia	Fear of medications
Pyrophobia	Fear of fire
Sociophobia	Fear of people
Thanatophobia	Fear of dying
Tokophobia	Fear of pregnancy/child birth
Traumatophobia	Fear of having an injury
Trypanophobia	Fear of medical procedures (needles, etc.)
Xenophobia	Fear of strangers
Zoophobia	Fear of animals

ANNEXURE 3. LIST OF SPECIFIC PARAPHILIA

Paraphilia	Focus of erotic interest
Algolagnia	Pain involving erogenous zone
Anthropophagy	Ingesting human flesh
Autoerotic asphyxiation	Self-induced asphyxiation
Coprophilia/Scatophilia	Faeces
Exhibitionism	Exposing one's genitals to unsuspecting and unconsenting others
Frotteurism	Rubbing against a non-consenting person
Gerontophilia	Elderly persons
Kleptophilia/Kleptolagnia	Stealing
Klismaphilia	Enemas
Masochism	Suffering, being beaten, bound or otherwise humiliated
Morphophilia	Particular body shapes/sizes
Nasophilia	Nose
Necrophilia	Corpses
Pedophilia	Prepubescent children
Podophilia	Feet
Piquerism	Piercing flesh of another person
Pyrophilia	Fire
Sadism	Inflicting pain on others
Sexual fetishism	Non-living objects
Stigmatophilia	Body piercings, tattoos
Transvestism	Wearing clothes of opposite sex
Trichophilia	Hair
Urolagnia	Urination
Vampirism	Blood
Voyeurism	Watching others while naked or having sex
Zoophilia	Animals

ANNEXURE 4. COMMON DEFENCE MECHANISMS

Defence mechanism	Description
PATHOLOGICAL DEFENCE MECHANISMS	
Delusional projection	Persecutory delusions of external reality
Conversion	Intrapsychic conflict, hysteria
Denial	Refusal to accept external reality
Distortion	Gross reshaping of external reality to meet internal needs
Splitting	Compartmentalizing experiences of self and others into all-good or all-bad
Extreme projection	Denial of moral deficiency perceived as deficiency in another
Superiority complex	Feelings of superiority counter or conceal his or her feelings of inferiority
Inferiority complex	Feeling of not measuring up to society's standards
IMMATURE DEFENCE MECHANISMS	
Acting out	Direct expression of an unconscious wish or impulse in action
Fantasy	Retreat into fantasy in order to resolve inner and outer conflicts
Wishful thinking	Making decisions pleasing to imagine instead of by appealing to evidence, rationality
Idealisation	Perceive another individual as having more desirable qualities
Passive aggression	Aggression towards others expressed indirectly or passively
Projection	Perceiving and reacting to unacceptable inner impulses as they were alien
Projective identification	Object of projection invokes in that person precisely the thoughts, feelings or behaviours projected
Somatization	Transformation of uncomfortable feelings towards others into uncomfortable feelings toward oneself
NEUROTIC DEFENCE MECHANSIMS	
Displacement	Shifts sexual or aggressive impulses to a more acceptable or less threatening target
Dissociation	Separation or postponement of a feeling to avoid emotional distress
Hypochondriasis	Excessive preoccupation or worry about having a serious illness
Intellectualization	Avoiding unacceptable emotions by focusing on the intellectual aspects
Isolation	Separation of feelings from ideas and events
Rationalization	Convincing oneself that no wrong has been done through faulty and false reasoning
Reaction formation	Taking the opposite belief because the true belief causes anxiety
Regression	Reversion of ego to an earlier stage of development than handling unacceptable impulses
Repression	Repel desires towards pleasurable instincts
Undoing	'Undo' an unhealthy, destructive threatening thought by acting out reverse of unacceptable
Withdrawal	Removing oneself from events, stimuli under threat of being reminded of painful thoughts
Social comparisons	Means of self-evaluation to perceive one better by comparing to worse-off
MATURE DEFENCE MECHANISMS	
Respect	Willingness to show consideration or appreciation
Moderation	Eliminating or lessening extremes and staying within reasonable limits
Patience	Level of endurance under difficult circumstances one can take before negativity
Courage	Mental ability/willingness to confront conflicts, fear, pain, danger, obstacles
Humility	A person, considering their own defects, has a humble self-opinion
Mindfulness	Particular orientation toward one's experiences, with by curiosity, openness, acceptance
Acceptance	Assent to reality of a situation without attempting to change it, protest, or exit
Gratitude	Thankfulness or appreciation involving appreciation of a wide range of people and events
Altruism	Constructive service to others that brings pleasure and personal satisfaction
Tolerance	Deliberately allowing or permitting a thing of which one disapproves
Mercy	Compassionate behavior on the part of those in power
Forgiveness	Cessation of anger as a result of a perceived offence, disagreement, or mistake

Contd...

Contd...

Defence mechanism	Description
Anticipation	Realistic planning for future discomfort
Humour	Overt expression of ideas and feelings that gives pleasure to others
Identification	Unconscious modelling of one's self upon another person's character and behaviour
Introjection	Identifying with some idea or object so deeply that it becomes a part of that person
Sublimation	Transformation of unhelpful emotions or instincts into healthy actions or emotions
Thought suppression	Conscious process of pushing thoughts into the preconscious
Emotional self-regulation	Respond to ongoing demands of experience with socially tolerable range of emotions
Emotional self-sufficiency	Not being dependent on the validation (approval or disapproval) of others

ANNEXURE 5. SYMPTOMS AND PROGNOSIS OF SCHIZOPHRENIA

Eugen Bleuler's Fundamental Symptoms (4A's of Bleuler)	
• *Ambivalence*	• Inability to decide for or against
• *Autism*	• Withdrawal into self
• *Affect disturbance*	• Inappropriate affect
• *Association disturbance*	• Loosening of association/thoughts

Schneider's First Rank Symptoms of Schizophrenia (SFRS)*	
***S**omatic passivity*	Body sensations imposed by others
***M**ade feelings/affect*	Imposed by others
***M**ade impulses*	Imposed by others
***M**ade volition/acts*	Imposed by others
***D**elusional perception*	Private illogical meaning
***V**oices heard arguing*	Auditory hallucinations
***V**oices commenting on one's action*	Auditory hallucinations
***A**udible thoughts*	Thought echo
***T**hought withdrawal*	Thoughts cease, removed by someone
***T**hought insertion*	Thoughts imposed by someone else
***T**hought diffusion/broadcasting*	Thoughts escaping and experienced by others

*[*Mnemonic: **S**chizophrenic **M**an **D**oes **V**alue **A**udible **T**houghts; **SAM³V²T³D**]*

Factor	Good prognosis	Bad prognosis
Type of onset	Acute	Insidious
Age of onset	More than 35 years	Less than 20 years
Sex of patient	Females	Males
Physique	Fat	Asthenic (thin)
Type of Schizophrenia	Catatonic	Hebephrenic/Simple
Duration	Less than 6 months	More than 2 years
Stressor precipitating	Present	Absent
Depression	Present	Absent
Type of symptoms	Positive	Negative
Social support	Good	Poor
Type of treatment	Out-patient	Institutionalised
CT scan	Normal	Ventricular enlargement

ANNEXURE 6. SIDE EFFECTS OF DRUGS USED IN PSYCHIATRY

Side effect	Maximum with	Minimum with
ANTI-PSYCHOTIC DRUGS		
Autonomic side effects*	Chlorpromazine	Haloperidol
Parkinsonian syndrome	Haloperidol	Clozapine
Akathisia	Haloperidol	Clozapine
Acute dystonia	Haloperidol	Clozapine
Neurolept malignant syndrome	Haloperidol	–
Tardive dyskinesia	–	Clozapine
Seizures	Clozapine	Trifluperazine
Cholestatic jaundice	Chlorpromazine	Haloperidol
Agranulocytosis	Clozapine	Haloperidol
ANTI-DEPRESSANT DRUGS		
Autonomic side effects*	Amitriptyline	Fluoxetine
Impotence	Amitriptyline	Mirtazapine
Seizures	Bupropion	Nomifensine
Tachycardia	Amitriptyline	Trazodone
Arrhythmias	Amitriptyline	Fluoxetine
Hypertension	Venlafaxine	SSRIs
Agranulocytosis	Mianserin	–

(Dry mouth, constipation, cycloplegia, mydriasis, urinary retention)*

Psychiatry

Golden Points

MC organic mental disorder seen in clinical practice	Delirium
Earliest disorientation in delirium	Time disorientation
MC hallucinations type in delirium	Visual
Most severe alcohol withdrawal syndrome	Delirium tremens
MC clinical type of dissociative disorder	Dissociative amnesia
MC type of dissociative amnesia	Circumscribed amnesia
Dissociative identity disorder is	Multiple personality disorder
Most severe form of absence of insight	Anosognosia
MC sub-type of mental retardation	Mild mental retardation
MC phobia encountered in clinical practice	Agoraphobia (60%)
Fear of open spaces is known as	Agoraphobia
Fear of closed spaces is known as	Claustrophobia
Acrophobia is fear of	Heights
Kleptomania is a type of	Impulse disorder
Impulse for setting fire is known as	Pyromania
Delusion of doubles is seen in	Capgras' syndrome
Capgras' syndrome is most commonly seen in disorder	Paranoid schizophrenia
Prosopagnosia is	Inability to recognise faces
False unshakeable belief not according to person's background	Delusion
MC type of delusions seen	Persecutory delusions
Role reversal of sexual sadism is seen in	Sexual masochism
Sexual arousal due to exposure of one's genitalia is	Exhibitionism
Necrophilia is sexual arousal with	Corpses (dead bodies)
Klismaphilia is sexual arousal with	Enemas
MC obsessive compulsive disorder is	Washers
Obsessive compulsive disorders in India is more common in	Unmarried males
MC type of hallucinations in psychosis	Auditory
Antipsychotic drug with least extra pyramidal side effects	Clozapine
Antipsychotic drug with maximum autonomic side effects	Chlorpromazine
Antipsychotic drug with least autonomic side effects	Haloperidol
Antipsychotic drug with maximum extrapyramidal side effects	Haloperidol
Antipsychotic drug with least extrapyramidal side effects	Clozapine
MC ECG change seen with anti-psychotic drugs	QT prolongation
MC cause of dementia is	*Alzheimer's* disease
MC cause of multi-infarct dementia	Hypertension
Vitamins used in treatment of Alzheimer's disease	Vitamin C, vitamin E

Contd...

Contd...

MC cause of organic amnestic syndrome	Wernicke's-Korasoff psychosis
Worst disease affecting mankind	Schizophrenia
Schneider's first rank symptoms are used for	Schizophrenia
4A's of Bleuler are used for	Schizophrenia
Hallucinations characteristic of Schizophrenia	Third person hallucinations
Incidence of schizophrenia	0.5 per 1000 population
Schizophrenia with worst prognosis	Hebephrenic schizophrenia
Schizophrenia with good prognosis	Catatonic schizophrenia
Schizophrenia with marked disturbance of motor behaviour	Catatonic schizophrenia
Most difficult to diagnose schizophrenia	Simple schizophrenia
Schizophrenia with mental retardation	Pfropf schizophrenia
Van Gogh syndrome is characterised by	Self mutilation
First drug used in treatment of schizophrenia	Reserpine
Surgical treatment of choice for schizophrenia	Limbic leucotomy
Potential serious side effect of Clozapine (Antipsychotic)	Agranulocytosis
Inability to experience pleasure is known as	Anhedonia
Drug of choice for an episode of mania	Lithium
Involutional melancholia is a form of	Severe depression
Kleine-Levin syndrome is characterised by excess of	Sleeping and eating
MC side effect of lithium therapy	Tremor
MC cardiovascular side effect of Lithium therapy	T-wave depression
MC cause of death among psychiatric patients	Suicide
Depression increases the risk of suicides by	25 times
MC mode of suicides in India	Ingestion of poisons
MC genetic cause of chorea	Huntington's disease
Disulfiram like reaction occurs due to accumulation in blood of	Acetaldehyde
MC alcohol withdrawal syndrome is	Hangover (next morning)
Most severe alcohol withdrawal syndrome is	Delirium tremens
MC symptom of alcohol withdrawal syndrome is	Tremors
Magnan's symptoms are characteristic of	Chronic cocaine use
Dipsomania is	Compulsive drinking
Species of alcohol dependence having dipsomania is	Epsilon species
CAGE questionnaire is used to identify	Alcoholism
MC type of hallucinations in alcoholism	Auditory
MC side effect of phenytoin therapy	Gum hyperplasia
MC psychiatric emergency	Suicide
First and most important indication for ECT	Severe depression with suicidal risk
Brain damage in ECT	Never occurs
MC non-organic psychiatric disorder	Auditory hallucinations
MC aversion therapy for alcohol dependence	Apomorphine
MC psychiatric disorder in general population	Generalised anxiety
MC psychiatric symptom in clinical practice	Anxiety

Contd...

Contd…

MC disorder of sleep is	Dyssomnias
MC post-partum psychoses	Depressive episode
MC mental retardation type	Mild mental retardation
MC type of attention-deficit disorder association	Hyperactivity
Developmental language/communication disorder is	Dysphasia
High functioning autism is known as	Asperger's syndrome
Disintegrative psychosis is known as	Heller's syndrome
Strauss syndrome/Hyperkinetic disorder is	Attention-deficit disorder
Last symptoms to appear in Tourette's syndrome	Obsessions and compulsions
MC cause of eneuresis	Psychological
Drug of choice for Alzheimer's disease	Donezepil
Drug of choice for prophylaxis in bipolar mood disorders	Lithium
Drug of choice for phobias	Alprazolam
Drug of choice for obsessive compulsive disorders	Fluoxetine
Drug of choice for Gilles de la tourette syndrome	Haloperidol
Drug of choice for nocturnal enuresis	Imipramine
Drug of choice for narcolepsy	Modafinil
Drug of choice for attention deficit disorder in children	Methylphenidate
Drug of choice for attention deficit disorder in adults	Atomoxetine
Drug of choice for status epilepticus	Lorazepam
Drug of choice for generalised anxiety disorder	Benzodiazepines
Drug of choice for panic disorder	Antidepresssants

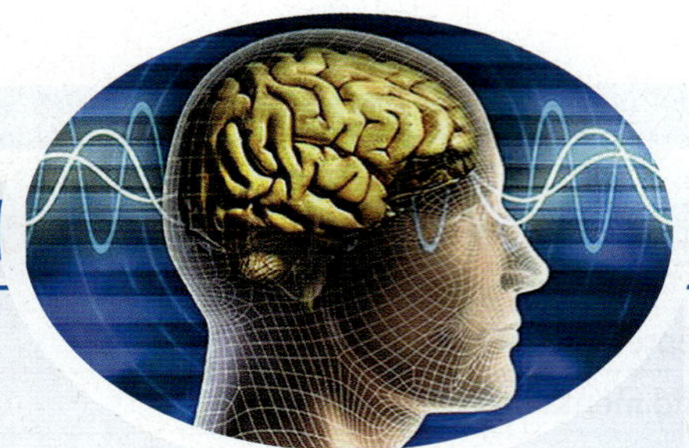

Chapter 1

History Aspects, Physiology and Mental Illness

THEORETICAL CONCEPTS

I A. SCIENTISTS AND THEIR CONTRIBUTION IN PSYCHIATRY

Scientist	Contribution
Sigmund Freud	**Psychoanalysis**[Q]
Jellinek	Five alcoholic species based on pattern of use
Cloninger	Two alcoholic species based on environment and genetic factors
Eugene Bleuler	Renamed Dementia-precox as Schizophrenia **Fundamental symptoms of Schizophrenia**[Q]
Kurt Schneider	**First/Second rank symptoms of Schizophrenia**[Q]
Heinroth	Coined term 'Psychosomatic disorders'
Franz Alexander	Father of Psychosomatic medicine Seven classic symptoms of psychosomatic illness Specificity hypothesis
Julius Von Wagner Jauregg	Nobel prize for Malaria treatment of General paresis of insane Pyrotherapy treatment of mental disorders
Manfred Sakel	Insulin shock treatment of Schizophrenia
Ganeshan/Kartik Bose	First successful treatment of Psychoses with Reserpine
Moniz	Nobel prize for Leucotomy (Psychosurgery)

Fig. Sigmund Freud

Fig. Eugene Bleuer

Topper's Edge

History of Psychiatry

- Term **'Psychiatry'** was coined by[Q]: JC Reil
- Earliest known texts on mental disorders[Q]: Charaka Samhita (Ayurvedic text, India)
- First to classify neurotic disorders: Avicenna
- Lunacy Act 1845 (England): Changed the status of mentally ill people to patients who required treatment[Q]

I B. INSIGHT IN PSYCHIATRIC DISORDERS

I B1. Definition

- **Insight is** ability to recognise one's own mental illness
  - Recognising consequences of one's behaviour
  - Recognising need for treatment

IB 2. Insight present in[Q]	IB 3. Insight absent in[Q]
Neurosis	Schizophrenia
Phobias	Psychoses
Obsessions	Korsakoff's psychosis
Compulsions	Post partum psychosis
Obsessive compulsive disorders	Mood disorders
Paranoid personality disorder	Alzheimer's disease

Topper's Edge

Insight

- Insight: Ability to recognize one's own mental illness[Q]
  - Conscious awareness and understanding of one's own psychodynamics and symptoms of maladaptive behavior
  - Include multiple dimensions, such as recognizing the need for treatment, and recognizing consequences of one's behavior as stemming from an illness
  - Highly important in effecting changes in the personality and behavior of a person
- **Grades of Insight:**
  - Grade 1: Complete denial of illness
  - Grade 2: Slight awareness of being sick and needing help but denying it at the same time
  - Grade 3: Awareness of being sick but blaming it on others, on external events, on medical or unknown organic factors
  - Grade 4 (Intellectual Insight): Admission of illness and recognition that symptoms or failures in social judgment are due to irrational feelings or disturbances; without applying that knowledge to future experiences
  - **Grade 5 (True Emotional Insight[Q]):** Emotional awareness of the motives and feelings within, of the underlying meaning of symptoms; and whether this awareness leads to changes in personality and future behavior, openness to new ideas and concepts about self
- Impaired Insight:
  - Diminished ability to understand the objective reality of a situation
  - Most extreme form of Impaired Insight: Anosognosia (Total absence of insight into one's mental illness)
- Insight Vs Judgment:

Insight[Q]	Judgment[Q]
Denotes **"Looking-in"**	Denotes **"Looking-out"**
Self-appraisal and self esteem	Appraisal of major social relationships
Understanding of current circumstances	Understanding of personal roles, responsibilities
Ability to describe personal, psychological and physical status	

I C. MEMORY DISORDERS

I C1. Agnosia

- *Definition*: Inability to recognise objects, persons, sounds
- *Underlying cause*:
  - Stroke
  - Dementia
  - Injury to temporal/parietal lobes
- *Important types of agnosias*:

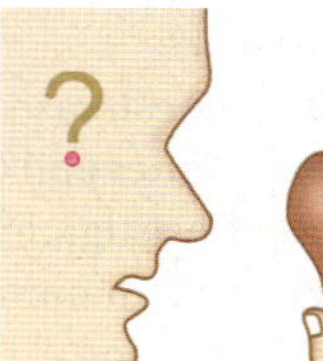

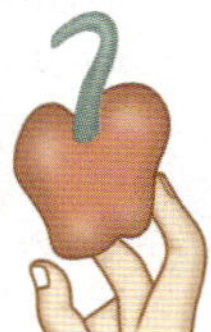

Fig. Agnosia

Agnosia	Description
Alexia[Q]	Inability to recognise text
Alexithymia	Deficiency in understanding, processing emotions
Anosognosia	Unawareness of own's disability
Apraxia[Q]	Disability to map out physical actions

Contd...

Psychiatry

Contd...

Agnosia	Description
Prosopagnosia	Inability to recognise familiar faces
Astereognosis[Q]	Difficulty in recognising object by touch (texture/size/weight)
Tactile agnosia	Difficulty in recognising object by touch alone
Visual agnosia[Q]	Difficulty in recognising object by seeing

Topper's Edge

Agnosia

- **Agnosia:** Loss of ability to recognize objects, people, sounds, shapes, or smells[Q]
  - Inability to attach appropriate meaning to objective sense-data
  - Used when the primary sense organ involved is not impaired
  - Disorder of perceptual recognition that takes place at a higher level than processing of primary sensory information
- Aphasia: Inability to comprehend and formulate language because of damage to specific brain regions[Q]
  - Global aphasia: Most severe form; Patients can produce few recognizable words and understand little or no spoken language, can neither read nor write
  - **Broca's (non-fluent) aphasia[Q]:** Speech output is severely reduced and limited mainly to short utterances of less than four words, Vocabulary access is limited and formation of sounds by persons is laborious and clumsy
  - **Wenicke's (Fluent) aphasia[Q]:** Ability to grasp the meaning of spoken words is chiefly impaired, while the ease of producing connected speech is not much affected
  - Anomic aphasia[Q]: Persistent inability to find the words for the very things they want to talk about—particularly the significant nouns and verbs
  - Primary Progressive Aphasia (PPA): Language capabilities become slowly and progressively impaired, caused by neurodegenerative diseases
- **Apraxia[Q]:** Disorder of the brain and nervous system in which a person is unable to perform tasks or movements when asked, even though:
  - The request or command is understood
  - They are willing to perform the task
  - The muscles needed to perform the task work properly
- The task may have already been learned ts on mental disorders[Q]: Charaka Samhita (Ayurvedic text, India)
- First to classify neurotic disorders: Avicenna
- Lunacy Act 1845 (England): Changed the status of mentally ill people to patients who required treatment[Q]

I C2. Alzheimer's Dementia

- *Definition*: Progressive degenerative fatal brain disease with gradual loss of cell-to-cell connections in brain (leading to dementia)
- *Underlying cause*[Q]:
  - Decreased brain choline acetyltransferase (CAT)
  - Decreased brain acetylcholinesterase (AchE)
- *Treatment*[Q]:
  - Cholinesterase inhibitors
    - **Donezepil**[Q]
    - Rivastigmine
    - Galantamine
  - Memantine
  - Piracetam
  - Vitamin C, Vitamin E

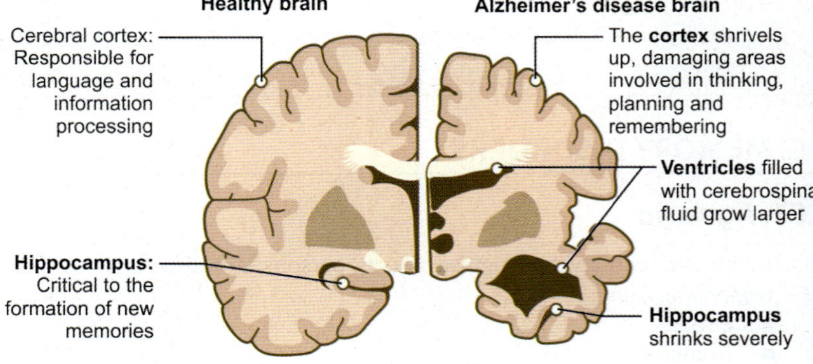

Fig. Alzheimer's disease
Source: Alzheimer's Association

Topper's Edge

Dementias

- Progressive impairment of cognitive functions occurring in clear consciousness (In absence of delirium)
- Essential feature: *'Global impairment of intellect'* – manifested as difficulty in memory, attention, thinking and comprehension

Types of Dementia[Q]
- Alzheimer's dementia: **MC type[Q],** Increases with increasing age (Parieto-temporal lesions)
- Vascular dementia **(Multi-infarct dementia[Q]): 2nd MC type,** Related to Cerebrovascular disease especially Hypertension affecting small and medium sized cerebral vessels
- Binswanger's disease (Subcortical arteriosclerotic encephalopathy[Q]): Multiple small infarctions of white matter sparing cortical regions
- Pick's disease[Q]: Neuronal loss, gliosis, atrophy **(Fronto-temporal lesions[Q])**
- Lewy body disease: Hallucinations, Parkinsonian features, Extrapyramidal signs **(Cerebral cortex affected[Q])**
- Huntington's disease: Subcortical dementia with higher motor anomalies **(Basal ganglia disease[Q])**
- Parkinson's disease: Depression, Bradyphrenia (Basal ganglia disease)
- HIV-related dementia: Encephalopathy (Parenchymal abnormality)
- Dementia pugilistica **(Punch drunk syndrome[Q]):** Head trauma **(Boxers[Q]),** Impulsivity, Emotional lability, Dysarthria
- Substance abuse related dementia: Alcohol, Inhalants, Sedatives, Hypnotics, Anxiolytics

I C3. Amnesia

- *Definition*: Affection of memory and learning disproportionate to other cognitive functions
- *Types of amnesia*:
  - Anterograde amnesia: Inability to recall recent memories BUT long term (remote) memories are intact[Q]
  - Retrograde amnesia: Inability to recall both recent and remote memories[Q]
  - Post traumatic amnesia

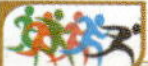

Topper's Edge

Types of Amnesia
- **Anterograde amnesia[Q]:** Inability to form new memories due to inability to consolidate what is perceived or inability to retrieve storage
- **Retrograde amnesia[Q]:** Loss of memory for events that occurred prior to an event/condition
- Post-traumatic amnesia: Memory loss from time of accident till patient can give clear account of recent events
- **Psychogenic amnesia[Q]:** Sudden inability to recall important personal data
- False memory: Confabulation, report of false events which never occurred
- **Transient global amnesia[Q]:** Abrupt onset of disorientation, loss of ability to load recent memories and retrograde amnesia for variable durations (Ischemia of hypothalamus-fornix-hippocampus system)
- Amnestic syndrome: Impaired short term memory (related to Wernicke's Korsakoff syndrome)
- Amnesia involving episodic memory

Differential Diagnosis of Amnesia and Site of Lesion
- Wernicke's Korsakoff psychosis: **Mammillary bodies, Medial dorsal nucleus of thalamus[Q]**
- Neoplasms: Temporal lobe, fornix, hypothalamus, thalamus
- Surgery (Lobectomy): Temporal lobe
- Subarachnoid hemorrhage: Fornix
- Head trauma: Hippocampus
- Stroke (Posterior cerebral artery): Hippocampus
- Anoxia: Hippocampus
- Hypoglycemia: Hippocampus
- Herpes simplex encephalitis: Hippocampus
- Alzheimer's disease: Hippocampus[Q]
- Transient global ischemia: Hippocampus

I C4. Dementia

Definition: **Progressive deterioration of thinking ability and memory due to brain damage**

Types and Causes of Dementia

***Fixed cognitive impairment*:**	***Slowly progressive dementia[Q]*:**
• Traumatic brain injury	• **Alzheimer's dementia**
• Stroke	• Dementia with Lewy bodies
• Seizures	• Vascular dementia
• Hydrocephalus	• Hypothyroidism
• Excessive alcohol use	• Vitamin B12, B3, B9 deficiency

Contd...

Psychiatry

Contd...

Rapidly progressive dementia:	**Associated disorders:**
• Creutzfeldt Jacob disease • Alzheimer's dementia • Dementia with Lewy bodies	• Parkinson's disease • SLE • Sarcoidosis • Behcet's syndrome

I C5. Other Memory Disorders

- Huntington's syndrome
- Parkinson's syndrome
- Wernicke's Korsakoff psychosis

I C6. Memory Disturbances in Psychiatric Disorders

	Memory types		
	Immediate	**Recent**	**Remote**
Delirium[Q]	Impaired	Impaired	Intact
Dementia[Q]	Intact	Impaired	Impaired
Organic amnestic syndrome[Q]	Intact	Impaired	Impaired
Korsakoff psychosis[Q]	Intact	Impaired	Impaired

I D. ORGANIC AMNESTIC SYNDROME

- *Definition*:
  - Impaired memory due to organic cause

Memory	Impairment
Recent/short term memory	Severe impairment
Remote/long term memory	Impairment
Immediate memory	No impairment

  - No severe disturbance of consciousness and attention
  - No global disturbance of intellectual functioning, thinking, personality
- *Underlying causes*:
  - **Thiamine deficiency:** Chronic alcohol dependence/Wernicke's-Korsakoff, psychosis **(Most common cause**[Q]**)**
  - Lesions involving inner limbic system
    - Head trauma
    - Bilateral surgical temporal lobectomy
    - Hypoxia
    - Stroke
    - Herpes simplex encephalitis
    - 3rd ventricle space occupying lesions
- *Treatment*:
  - Treatment of underlying cause
  - Supportive care

IE. CLASSIFICATION OF COMMON MENTAL HEALTH DISORDERS

Group	Disorder(s)
Learning/Memory disorders	Autism, Down's syndrome
Neurosis	Anxiety disorders, OCD, Dissociative/Conversion disorders
Organic mental disorders	Delirium, Dementia, Amnestic disorders
Psychosis	Schizophrenia, Mood disorders (Mania, depression, Bipolar), *Delusional* disorders, Schizoaffective disorders
Personality disorders	Dissociative, Histronic, Narcissistic, Paranoid, Schizoid, Schizotypal

Contd...

Contd…

Group	Disorder(s)
Somatoform disorders	Somatization disorder
Stress disorders	Acute stress reaction, Post-traumatic stress reaction, adjustment disorders
Substance use disorders	Alcohol use disorders, Opiate dependence

IF. WERNICKE-KORSAKOFF SYNDROME

- Underlying cause: **thiamine (B1) deficiency**[Q]
- Underlying precipitating factors[Q]:
  - **Chronic alcoholism (Most common)**
  - Malnutrition due to prolonged starvation
  - Marasmus
  - Hemodialysis for CRF
  - HIV
  - Hyperemesis gravidarum
  - GIT malignancy

Wernicke's Encephalopathy	Korsakoff Syndrome
Pathology[Q] • Petechial hemorrhages in Thalamus, mammillary bodies, Periaqueductal grey matter, Peripheral nerves	**Pathology**[Q] • Atrophy of Mamillary bodies, Medial thalamic nuclei, Hippocampus
Impairments • **Nystagmus (MC ocular abnormality**[Q]**)** • Pupillary abnormalities[Q] • **Global confusion**[Q] • **Ataxic gait**[Q] • Peripheral polyneuropathy • Encephalopathy	**Impairments** • **Severe Anterograde amnesia**[Q] • Less severe Retrograde amnesia[Q] • Impairment of New learning[Q] • **Impaired Recent memory**[Q] • Relatively preserved Remote memory[Q] • Deficit of Explicit/Conscious/Declarative memory[Q] • **Confabulation**[Q]
Classical feature • **Classical triad** of Ataxia, Ophthalmoplegia, Confusion[Q]	**Classical feature** • Preservation of Intelligence, Language, Motor & Perceptual skills[Q]

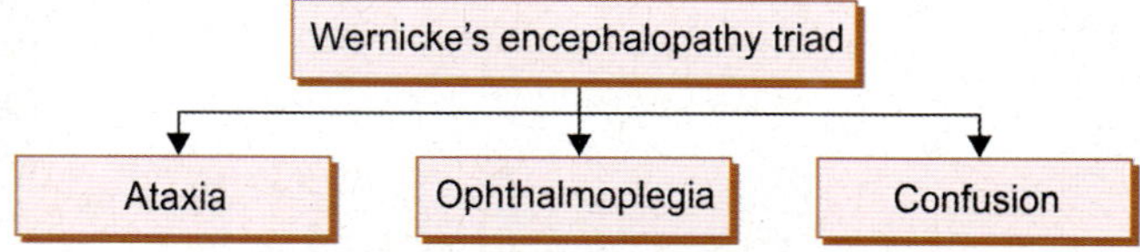

Fig. Wernicke's encephalopathy triad

Topper's Edge

Wernicke-Korsakoff syndrome

- Description:
  - Wernicke-Korsakoff syndrome classically evolves through an acute phase of Wernicke's encephalopathy characterized by ophthalmoplegia, ataxia, and delirium
  - If the responsible thiamine deficiency is not reversed, the patient will progress into Wernicke-Korsakoff syndrome that includes persistent amnesia, nystagmus, and ataxia
- Underlying pathology[Q]:
  - Mammillary bodies are affected in the Wernicke-Korsakoff syndrome and by brain tumors[Q]
  - Medial thalamic nuclei are involved in Wernicke-Korsakoff syndrome, brain tumors, and some strokes[Q]

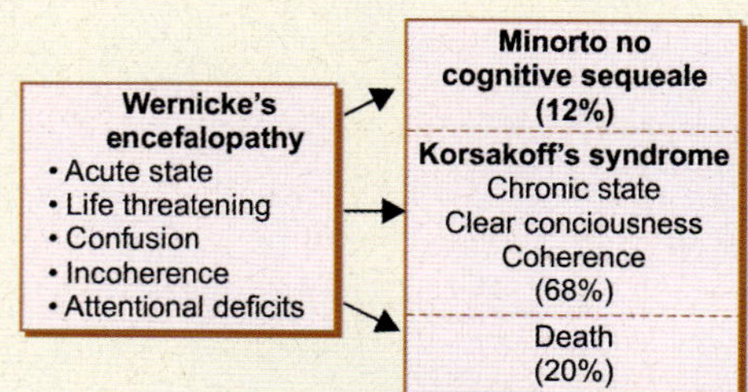

Fig. Wernicke's encephalopathy

IMAGE-BASED QUESTIONS

1. **Identify the Neurologist shown in Photograph** ***[Recent Question 2012]***

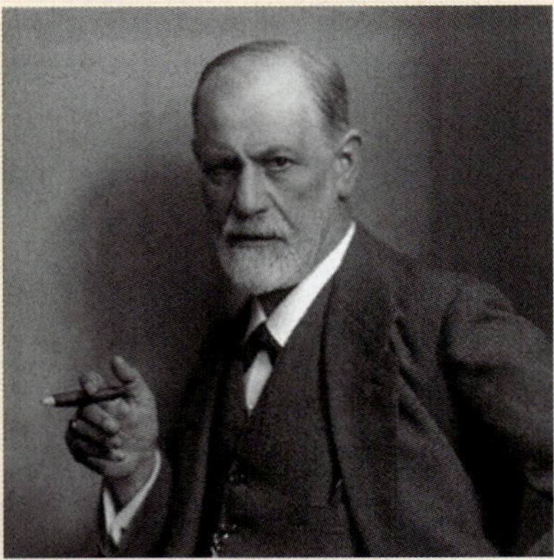

a. Eugene Bleuer
b. Cloninger
c. Sigmund Freud
d. Jellinek

2. **Physician shown in the Photograph is known as Father of ....**

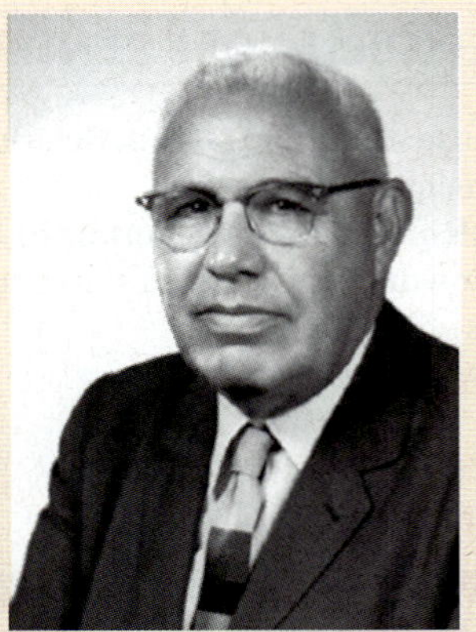

a. Psychiatry
b. Psychosomatic medicine
c. Psychotherapy
d. Mental Health

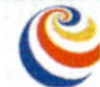 ANSWERS WITH EXPLANATIONS OF IBQs 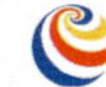

1. Ans. (c) Sigmund Freud *[Ref. Sigmund Freud by Wolheim, 1/e CoverPage]*

- Contributions of Sigmund Freud (1856-1939):
  - Founding Father of Psychoanalysis
  - Theory of Psychosexual development
  - Id, Ego, Superego
  - Dram interpretation
  - Free association

2. Ans. (b) Psychosomatic medicine *[Ref. Psychosomatic Medicine by Franz Alexander, 1/e p1]*

- Franz Alexander (1891-1964):
  - Father of Psychosomatic Medicine
  - Wrote book: Psychosomatic Medicine - Its Principles and Applications

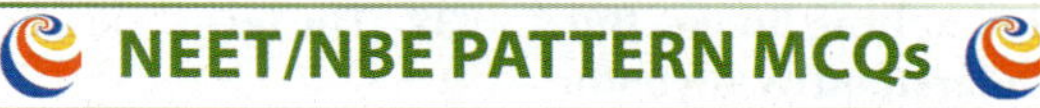

NEET/NBE PATTERN MCQs

1. **Which is not a perceptional disorder?** *[Recent Question 2016]*
   a. Hallucination b. Illusion
   c. Synaesthesia d. Imagery
2. **Wrong statement about Psychoanalysis is** *[Recent Question 2016]*
   a. Parapraxis has meaning
   b. Transference is patient's feeling for therapist
   c. Counter transference is clinician's feelings for patient
   d. Unguided communication has no meaning
3. **Most common mental health disorder is** *[Recent Question 2016]*
   a. Anxiety b. Depression
   c. Phobia d. Schizophrenia
4. **Illusion is a disorder of** *[Recent Question 2016]*
   a. Thought b. Perception
   c. Affect d. Emotion
5. **Highest insight is** *[Recent Question 2016]*
   a. Intellectual b. Emotional
   c. Psychological d. Affective
6. **Emile Durkheim is linked with work on which condition in psychiatry?** *[Recent Question 2016]*
   a. Suicide
   b. Obsessive compulsive disorder
   c. Anxiety disorder
   d. Schizophrenia
7. **All of the following are true about Pseudo-hallucinations except** *[Recent Question 2016]*
   a. Arises in inner subjective self
   b. Patient describes the sensations being perceived by mind eye
   c. Are under voluntary control
   d. Distressing flashback of PTSD is an example
8. **Extracampine hallucinations term was given by** *[Recent Question 2016]*
   a. Eugene Bleuler b. William Harvey
   c. Robert Macinoff d. Eden Speroff
9. **Elderly patient awakens scared at night and he mistakes rope for a snake. What is the diagnosis?** *[Recent Question 2016]*
   a. Illusion b. Hallucination
   c. Delusion d. Pseudo-hallucination
10. **Kleine Levin syndrome which of the following is not true** *[Recent Question 2016]*
    a. Hypersomnia
    b. Hyposexuality
    c. Spontaneous resolution
    d. Also called Sleeping Beauty syndrome
11. **How many Axes in DSM 4?** *[Recent Question 2016]*
    a. 2 b. 3
    c. 4 d. 5
12. **Most common psychiatric illness** *[Recent Question 2016]*
    a. Depression b. Bipolar
    c. Mania d. Cyclothymia
13. **Phantom limb is an example of disorder of** *[Recent Question 2016]*
    a. Thought b. Perception
    c. Cognition d. None of the above
14. **ICD-10 Chapter 1 describes** *[Recent Question 2016]*
    a. Poisoning and consequences
    b. Diseases of the nervous system
    c. Infectious and parasitic diseases
    d. Psychiatric diseases
15. **Hallucination is** *[NBE FMGE September 2005, Recent Question 2017]*
    a. False belief
    b. False interpretation of a stimulus
    c. False sense perception without a stimulus
    d. Irresistible desire
16. **"Hallucination is perception without a stimulus" (false perception) was said by** *[NBE DNB 1993]*
    a. Bleuler b. Janet
    c. Schneider d. Esquirol
17. **Consultation—liaison [C-L] psychiatry involves diagnosing** *[NBE DNB 2006, SGPGI 2004]*
    a. Psychiatric illness in medically ill
    b. Medical illness in psychiatric patients
    c. Suicidal tendency in psychiatric patients
    d. Suicidal tendency in medically ill
18. **Which is not a perceptional disorder?** *[Recent Question 2012, 2015]*
    a. Hallucinations b. Illusion
    c. Delusion d. None
19. **Impaired insight is evident in** *[AIIMS PGMEE 1992, NBE DNB 2009]*
    a. Psychosomatic disorder
    b. Anxiety neurosis
    c. Post Traumatic Stress Disorder
    d. Schizophrenia
20. **All of the following are features of Parkinsonism EXCEPT** *[NBE DNB December 2011]*
    a. Rest-tremors
    b. Mask like face
    c. Rigidity
    d. Preserved postural reflexes
21. **Which of the following is not true about hallucinations?** *[NBE FMGE September 2010]*
    a. It is a disorder of perception
    b. It is always pathological
    c. It is different from imagery
    d. It occurs on objective space
22. **An 8-year-old child after a tonsillectomy sees a bear in her room. She screams in fright. A nurse who rushes in switches on the light, finds a rug wrapped on an armchair. She pacifies the child. What the child experienced was a** *[Kerala PGMEE 1997, NBE DNB 2011]*
    a. Delusion b. Illusion
    c. Hallucination d. None of the above

23. Lallo 40-years-old has recently started writing books. But the matter in this book could not be understood by anybody since it contained words which were never there in any dictionary and the theme was very disjoint. Nowadays he has become very shy and self-absorbed. When he addresses people he speaks about metaphilosophical ideas. What is likely diagnosis?

[AIIMS PGMEE 2000, NBE DNB 2007]

a. Mania　b. Schizophrenia
c. A genius writer　d. Delusional disorder

24. Perception without stumuli is

[All India PGMEE 1998, AIIMS PGMEE 1996, NBE DNB 2010, Recent Question 2015]

a. Delusion　b. Illusion
c. Hallucination　d. Delirium

25. Hallucination are *[All India PGMEE 1999, NBE DNB 2010]*

a. Feeling of familiarity with unfamiliar thing
b. Alteration of perception of ones reality
c. Misinterpretation of stimuli
d. Perception occurring without external stimulation

26. All of the following feature of hallucination EXCEPT

[All India PGMEE 2002, SGPGI 2003, NBE DNB 2010]

a. Depends on will of observer and is under voluntary control
b. Occur in inner subjective space
c. It is vivid as sensory perception
d. It occurs in absence of perceptual stimulus

27. All of the following are features of hallucinations, except

[All India PGMEE 2003, NBE DNB 2011]

a. It is independent of the will of the observer
b. Sensory organs are not involved
c. It is as vivid as that in a true sense perception
d. It occurs in the absence of a perceptual stimulus.

28. Hallucinations are seen in All except

[MP PGMEE 1999, NBE DNB 2003]

a. Schizophrenia
b. Seizure due to Intracerebral space occupying lesions
c. LSD
d. Anxiety

29. A 30-year-old unmarried woman of average socio-economic background believes that her boss is in secretly love with her. She rings him up at odd hours and writes love letter to him despite his serious warning not to do so. She holds this belief despite contradiction from family members & his denial. However she is able to manage her daily activities as before. She is most likely to be suffering from

[AIIMS PGMEE 2004, NBE DNB 2010]

a. Depression　b. Schizophrenia
c. Delusional disorder　d. No psychiatric ailment

30. Visual hallucinations are seen in

[PGI PGMEE 2009, NBE DNB 2010]

a. Hebephrenic schizophrenia
b. Residual schizophrenia　c. Simple schizophrnia
d. Delirium　e. Temporal lobe epilepsy

31. Reflex hallucination is a morbid variety of

[AIIMS PGMEE 2009, NBE DNB 2010]

a. Kinesthesia　b. Parasthesia
c. Hypersthesia　d. Synaesthesia

32. The term "Dementia precox" was coined by

[Recent Question 2012, 2015, PGMCET 2015]

a. Freud　b. Bleuler
c. Kraepelin　d. Schneider

33. Psychogenic amnesia is characterized by

[AIIMS PGMEE 1997, NBE DNB 2000]

a. Antegrade Amnesia　b. Retrograde Amnesia
c. Both with confabulation
d. Patchy impairment of Personal memories

34. The contributions of Sigmund Freud are all except

[NBE DNB 1996]

a. Effects of cocaine
b. Interpretation of dream
c. Psychosexual stages of development
d. Superiority inferiority complex

35. Match the following *[NBE DNB 1993]*

I. Cade (i) Chlorpromazine
II. Cohen (ii) Chlordiazepoxide
III. Hoffman (iii) Lithium
IV. Delay-Deniker (iv) Lysergic acid

a. I (ii), II (iii), III (iv), IV (ii)
b. I (i), II (ii), III (iv), IV (iii)
c. I (iii), II (iv), III (iv), IV (i)
d. I (iii), II (iv), III (ii), IV (i)

36. Hallucination is disorder of *[Recent Question 2012, 2015]*

a. Thought　b. Perception
c. Memory　d. Intelligence

37. Perseveration is *[All India PGMEE 2005, NBE DNB 2007]*

a. Persistent and inappropriate repetition of the same thoughts
b. When a patient feels very distressed about it
c. Characteristic of schizophrenia
d. Characteristic of obsessive compulsive disorder [OCD]

38. Confabulation is a disorder of

[MP PGMEE 2000, NBE DNB 2004]

a. Perception　b. Thought
c. Memory　d. Mood

39. True about confabulation

[Jharkhand PGMEE 2004, NBE DNB 2000]

a. A memory disorder
b. Synonymous with false memory
c. It is congenital　d. It is age related disease

40. Unfamiliarity of familiar things is seen in

[Kerala PGMEE 1999, JIPMER PGMEE 2002, Karnataka PGMEE 1994, NBE DNB 1998]

a. Deja vu　b. Jamais vu
c. Deja entend　d. Deja pence

41. Most common psychiatric illness seen in majority in India is *[NBE DNB 2005, NBE DNB 2008]*

a. Mania　b. Depression
c. Schizophrenia　d. OCD's

42. The term 'id' was coined by

[Recent Question 2012, 2013, 2015]

a. Freud　b. Skinner
c. Wayker　d. Blueler

43. The maximum DALY loss is for the following disease *[Recent Question 2012, 2013, 2015]*
a. Schizophrenia b. Unipolar depression
c. Bipolar depression d. Mania

44. Which year may be regarded as the beginning of biological psychiatry research in India *[NBE DNB 1992]*
a. 1951 b. 1953
c. 1955 d. 1957

45. Narcolepsy is due to abnormality in *[Recent Question 2012, 2015]*
a. Hypothalamus b. Neocortex
c. Cerebellum d. Medulla oblongata

46. Cognitive model of depression was given by *[NBE DNB 2008]*
a. Beck b. Skinner
c. Cerletti d. Freud

47. Kleine-Levin syndrome *[Recent Question 2012, 2015]*
a. Insomnia b. Anxiety
c. Depression d. Hypersomnia

48. A fundamental technique used in psychoanalysis is *[Karnataka PGMEE 1996, NBE DNB 2006]*
a. Concentration b. Hypnosis
c. Empathy d. Free association

49. Life span of Sigmund Freud was *[JIPMER PGMEE 2000, NBE DNB 2007]*
a. 1856-39 and he passed most of his life in Austria
b. 1859-36 and he passed most of his life in Austria
c. 1859-36 and he passed most of his life in Germany
d. 1859-36 and he passed most of his life in France

50. The term 'free association' was coined by *[JIPMER PGMEE 2001, NBE DNB 2007]*
a. Freud b. Adler
c. Erikson d. Juna

51. Following name[s] is/are associated with Psychodynamic theory *[PGI 2009, NBE DNB 2011]*
a. Carl Jung b. Sigmund Freud
c. Emil Kraepelin d. Eugen Bleuler
e. Kurl Schneider's

52. Who introduced cocaine in psychiatry? *[Kerala PGMEE 1998, NBE DNB 2003]*
a. Freud b. Jung
c. Milar d. Stanley

53. The term "Ambivalence" was coined by *[PGI 1999, AIIMS PGMEE 1995, NBE DNB 2004, Recent Question 2017]*
a. Hippocrates b. Eugen Bleuler
c. Kraepelin d. Sigmund Freud

54. Moral treatment of mentally ill patient was first stressed by *[AIIMS PGMEE 1995, Karnataka PGMEE 2001, TN PGMEE 2004, NBE DNB 2005]*
a. Pinel b. Morel
c. Kraepelin d. Sigmund Freud

55. When information memorized afterwards is interfered by the information learnt earlier, it is called *[AIIMS PGMEE 2004, NBE DNB 2005]*
a. Retroactive inhibition b. Proactive inhibition
c. Simple inhibition d. Inhibition

56. The eight stage classification of human life is proposed by *[WB PGMEE 2000, WB PGMEE 2004, UP PGMEE 2005, NBE DNB 2008]*
a. Sigmund Freud b. Pavel
c. Strauss d. Erikson

57. Which of the following scientist propagated 'therapeutic-community concept? *[Karnataka PGMEE 2000, Bihar PGMEE 2003, NBE DNB 2006]*
a. J B Watson b. Maxwell Jones
c. Freud d. Adler

58. Term catatonia was used by *[UP PGMEE 2003, NBE DNB 2006]*
a. Karl Kahlbaum b. Adolf Meyer
c. Leo Kanner d. Karen Homey

59. Ross classified five stages of *[MP PGMEE 2006, NBE DNB 2008, PGMCET 2015]*
a. Schizophrenia b. Delusion
c. Death d. None

60. Most common postoperative psychiatric condition *[NBE DNB 1994, NBE DNB 2003]*
a. Schizophrenia b. Delirium
c. Chronic brain syndrome
d. Depression e. Mania

61. Drug which causes hallucinations is *[NBE FMGE March 2008]*
a. Ketamine b. Gallamine
c. D-tubocurare d. Pancuronium

62. According to recent rounds by DSM what code is given to psychiatric diseases in ICD 10? *[Recent Question 2012, 2015]*
a. E b. F
c. P d. G

63. The term "Dementia precox" was coined by *[All India PGMEE 2008]*
a. Freud b. Bleuler
c. Kraepelin d. Schneider

64. Cognitive model of depression is given by? *[AIIMS PGMEE 2008, NBE DNB 2000]*
a. Ellis b. Beck
c. Godfrey d. Meicheinbanon

65. Preservation is *[NBE DNB 2007]*
a. Persistent and inappropriate repetition of the same thoughts
b. When a patient feels very distressed about it
c. Characteristic of schizophrenia
d. Characteristic of obsessive compulsive disorder (OSD)

66. Perceptual misinterpretation of a real object is *[NBE DNB 2009]*
a. Illusion b. Delusion
c. Hallucination d. Schizophrenia

67. Hallucinations are produced by *[Recent Question 2013, 2015]*
a. Amphetamine b. Morphine
c. Paraxetine d. Chlorpromazine

68. Match the following *[NBE DNB 1996]*

Finding Disease

I. Psychomotor epilepsy (i) Cerebellar illness
II. Apraxia (ii) Brain stem disease
III. Papilloedema (iii) Parietal lobe lesions
IV. Cranial nerve palsy (iv) Temporal lobe epilepsy

a. I (ii), II (i), III (iii), IV (iv)
b. I (i), II (iii), III (ii), IV (iv)
c. I (ii), II (iv), III (i), IV (iii)
d. I (iv), II (iii), III (i), IV (ii)

69. A Patient has been seeking repeated admissions in various hospitals with a variety of symptoms. He had undergone appendicectomy, cholecystectomy, and other exploratory laparotomies on previous admissions. The most likely diagnosis is *[UPSC 1995]*

a. Conversion reaction b. Hypochondriasis
c. Munchausen syndrome d. Ganser's syndrome

70. Insight is present in all except *[NBE FMGE September 2005]*

a. Neurosis
b. Obsessive compulsive disorders
c. Phobias d. Psychosis

71. Gegenhalten is *[Recent Question 2015]*

a. Cogwheel rigidity b. Paratonic rigidity
c. Claspknife rigidity d. Lead pipe rigidity

72. Which is not disorder of perception? *[Recent Question 2015]*

a. Hallucinations b. Imagery
c. Synaesthesia d. Illusion

73. All are true about Dementia except

a. Loss of short term memory *[Recent Question 2014, 2015]*
b. Loss of long term memory
c. Deterioration of personality
d. Impaired learning

74. Axis II of DSM-IV criteria relate to *[Recent Question 2014, 2015]*

a. Disorders diagnosed in childhood and adolescence
b. Personality disorders
c. Endocrinal, nutritional disorders
d. Psychosocial, environmental disorders

75. Anhedonia is *[Recent Question 2017]*

a. Absence of pain on previously painful site
b. Loss of emotions
c. Somatic symptoms of pain
d. Inability to experience pleasure

76. Term 'Psychoanalysis' was coined by *[Recent Question 2017]*

a. Eysenck b. Freud
c. Jung d. Adler

77. Difference between Illusion and Delusion is

a. Illusion is false belief *[Recent Question 2017]*
b. Delusion is altered perception
c. Illusion is a thought disorder
d. Delusion is associated with faulty reasoning

78. Most common psychiatric disorder post-Stroke is *[Recent Question 2017]*

a. Anxiety b. Depression
c. Mania d. Bipolar disorder

HIGH YIELD MCQs

1. In a patient with psychiatric disorder, the Personal history does not include *[AIIMS May 2016]*

a. Occupation history b. Academic history
c. Food preference history d. Marital history

2. In India, Psychiatrists are not posted in *[AIIMS May 2016]*

a. District hospitals b. Military hospitals
c. Primary health centres
d. Hospitals attached to medical colleges

3. Semantic memory includes all of the following except

a. Words b. Events *[AIIMS May 2016]*
c. Rules d. Languages

4. Maslow hierarchy is *[AIIMS November 2016]*

a. Safety, Self-actualization, Belonging, Esteem, Physiological
b. Safety, Physiological, Belonging, Esteem, Self-actualization
c. Self-actualization, Physiological, Safety, Belonging, Esteem
d. Physiological, Safety, Belonging, Esteem, Self-actualization

5. Visual hallucinations is seen in *[TN PGMEE 1998]*

a. Alcoholism b. Mania
c. Depression d. Phobia

6. Auditory hallucinations not seen in *[TN PGMEE 1990]*

a. Schizophrenia b. Mania
c. Hysteria d. Amphetamine toxicity

7. Cognition is *[All India 1997, JHARKHAND PGMEE 2003]*

a. Perception b. Thought
c. Action d. Feeling

8. Emotion is controlled by *[PGI 1997]*

a. Incongruent effect b. Euphoria
c. Labile affect d. Split personality

9. Alexithymia is *[Kerala PGMEE 2000]*

a. A feeling of intense rapture
b. Affective flattening
c. Inability to recognise and describe feelings
d. Inappropriate mood
e. Pathological sadness

10. Hallucination is disorder of *[All India 1999]*

a. Thought b. Perception
c. Memory d. Intelligence

11. A patient saw a rope and fears like a snake. It is called

a. Illusion b. Hallucination *[PGI 2003]*
c. Delusion d. Depersonalization
e. Derealisation

12. Altered perception of real objects is *[AIIMS November 2007]*
a. Illusion b. Delusion
c. Hallucination d. Delirium

13. False sense of perception without any external object or stimulus is known as *[AIIMS May 2003, JHARKHAND PGMEE 05]*
a. Illusion b. Impulse
c. Hallucination d. Phobia

14. Which is not true about hallucination?
a. It is as vivid as normal stimulus *[AIIMS May 2009]*
b. It occurs to inner subjective space
c. It is independent of will of observer
d. It occurs in absence of perceptual stimuli

15. Formed visual hallucinations are seen in lesion of
a. Frontal b. Occipital *[PGI June 2006]*
c. Temporal d. Arcuate fasciculus
e. Dentate nucleus

16. What is hypnopampic phenomenon? *[Bihar PGMEE 2006]*
a. It experienced while falling asleep
b. It experienced while awakening
c. After head trauma
d. After convolution

17. Hallucinations which occur at the 'start' of sleep is
a. Hypnagogic hallucinations *[JIPMER 2002]*
b. Hypnopompic hallucinations
c. Jactationocturna capitis
d. Non-specific hallucinations

18. Preservation is *[Bihar PGMEE 2006]*
a. Persistent repetition of words
b. Found in depression c. After panic attack
d. None

19. Confabulation is defect of *[AIIMS 1998]*
a. Memory b. Intelligence
c. Attention d. Concentration

20. Confabulation is *[Recent Question 2017, SGPGI 2003]*
a. A state of confusion where patient is not able to describe the details
b. Purposefully fabricating stones to project a certain image
c. Filling up to gaps by fabrication to cover lapses in memory
d. Seen in delirium

21. Confabulation means *[All India 1991]*
a. Misinterpretation of stimuli
b. Perception in absence of stimuli
c. Making stories to cheat some one
d. Making stories to fill gaps in memory loss

22. The term 'id' was coined by *[WB PGMEE 2001]*
a. Freud b. Skinner
c. Weyker d. Blueler

23. Concept of super ego was given by *[JIPMER 1991, DPG 1993]*
a. Eric fromm b. Sigmund Freud
c. Eric Erikson d. Carl lung

24. Psychoanalysis was founded by which of the following scientist? *[Karnataka PGMEE 2000]*
a. Eysenck b. Freud
c. Jung d. Adler

25. Oedepius complex has been described by *[UP PGMEE 2006, Bihar PGMEE 2005, All India 1998]*
a. Plato b. Socrates
c. Freud d. Huxley

26. Pavlov's experiment is an example of *[All India 2006]*
a. Operant conditioning b. Classical conditioning
c. Learned helplessness d. Modelling

27. Lack of insight is not a feature of *[All India 2005, SGPGI 2003]*
a. Panic disorder b. Schizophrenia
c. Mania d. Reactive Psychosis

28. Impaired insight is found in *[PGI 1997]*
a. Traumatic psychosis
b. Schizophrenia
c. Anxiety neurosis
d. Obsessive compulsive neurosis

29. Disturbed orientation is seen in *[MP PGMEE 1999]*
a. Schizophrenia b. Neurosis
c. Paranoid personality d. Organic mental disorder

30. Organic Mental Disease is indicated by *[AIIMS 1991]*
a. Incoherence b. Delusion
c. Flight of idea d. Preservation of speech

31. Methods of learning in psychiatry are all except *[AIIMS November 2007]*
a. Modelling b. Catharsis
c. Exposure d. Response prevention

32. Most common psychiatric disorder is *[All India 1992]*
a. Dementia b. Schizophrenia
c. Depression d. Paronia

33. Loss of insight is seen *[AIIMS 1995]*
a. Hysteria b. Anxiety
c. OCN d. Schizophrenia

34. Lack of insight is not a feature of *[AIIMS November 2002]*
a. Panic disorder b. Schizophrenia
c. Mania d. Reactive Psychosis

35. Amnesia is found in *[All India 2000]*
a. Head injury b. Mania
c. Schizophrenia d. Psychiatric state

36. A young female presented with Halo's abdominal pain and amnesia she is likely to be suffering from *[All India 1997]*
a. Conversion disorder
b. Dissociative disorder
c. Depersonalization disorder
d. Mania

37. Term 'Psychiatry' was coined by *[JIPMER PGMEE 2014]*
a. Skinner b. Sigmund Freud
c. Christian Reil d. Eugene Blueur

38. Nobel Prize for experiments on Split brain was given to *[NIMHANS PGMEE 2014]*
a. M. Morgia b. Penfield
c. M. Gazzaniga d. Roger Sperry

39. Emotion is controlled by *[PGMCET 2015]*
a. Limbic system b. Frontal lobe
c. Temporal lobe d. Occipital lobe

40. Co-occurrence of how many psychiatric disorders in a single patient can be termed comorbidity? *[PGMCET 2015]*
   a. 2 b. ≥ 2
   c. ≥3 d. 3

41. Delusion association include all except *[CGPG 2015]*
   a. Personality disorder
   b. Organic brain disease
   c. Dissociative disorder
   d. Obsessive compulsive disorder

42. Perceptional diseases include *[PGI November 2014]*
   a. Illusion b. Delusion
   c. Depersonalization d. Obsession
   e. Hallucination

43. First neurological disorder found due to neurotransmitter deficiency *[AIIMS November 2014]*
   a. Alzheimer's disease b. Parkinson's disease
   c. Huntington's chorea d. Schizophrenia

44. Immediate memory is tested by *[AIIMS November 2017]*
   a. Subtraction test 20–1
   b. Subtraction test 100–7
   c. Digit span forward and backward
   d. Recall for remote personal history

 NEET/NBE PATTERN MCQs ANSWERS WITH EXPLANATIONS 

1. **Ans. (d) Imagery**
[Ref. Oxford Textbook of Psychiatry by Cowen, 6/e p6]
Perception
- Process of becoming aware what is presented through sense organs
- Sense of reality present
- Can be attended to or ignored
- Cannot be terminated by effort or at will

Imagery
- Awareness of percept generated within the mind
- Can be called up or terminated at will
- Lack sense of reality
- Terminated on start of perception

2. **Ans. (d) Unguided communication has no meaning**
[Ref. Kaplan and Sadock's, 10/e p192]
Psychoanalysis
- Parapraxes have been shown by psychoanalytic investigation to be meaningful psychic formations: Concept of parapraxis—in Italian, the term for this notion (for example, a slip of the tongue) is lapsus, which has the primary meaning "fall" or "tumble" - returns in the framework of Classical psychoanalysis
- Transference: Tendency to "transfer" feelings to a therapist similar to those patient had
  - Positive transference: When the feelings attached to the therapist are those of love or admiration
  - Negative transference: When the feelings attached to the therapist are those of hostility or envy
- Counter transference: Clinician's feelings for patient
- In Classical psychoanalysis, Unguided free associations are considered mandatory in order to circumvent conventional resistances to unconscious content

3. **Ans. (a) Anxiety**
[Ref. Niraj Ahuja, 7/e p89]

4. **Ans. (b) Perception**
[Ref. Behavioural Science by Fadem, 3/e p104]
- **Disorders of Perception:** Hallucination, Illusion
- **Disorder of Thought content:** Delusion, Idea of reference
- **Disorders of Form of thought:** Loose associations, Tangentiality

5. **Ans. (b) Emotional**
[Ref. Exposure Treatments for Anxiety Disorders by Rosqvist, 1/e p157]
- True emotional insight is representative of the highest level of insight possible: Patients' awareness and understanding of thoughts, feelings and motives can be used to change behavior

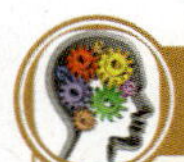 Also Remember

Four Types of Insight
- True emotional insight
- Intellectual insight
- Partially internally based and externally based insight
- Denial of illness

6. **Ans. (a) Suicide**
[Ref. Comprehensive Textbook of Suicidology by Berman, 1/e p51]
David Émile Durkheim [1858-1917]
- Institutionalization of Sociology
- Introduction of Sacred Profane Dichotomy (Central characteristic of Religion)
- Social and cultural influences on Suicide

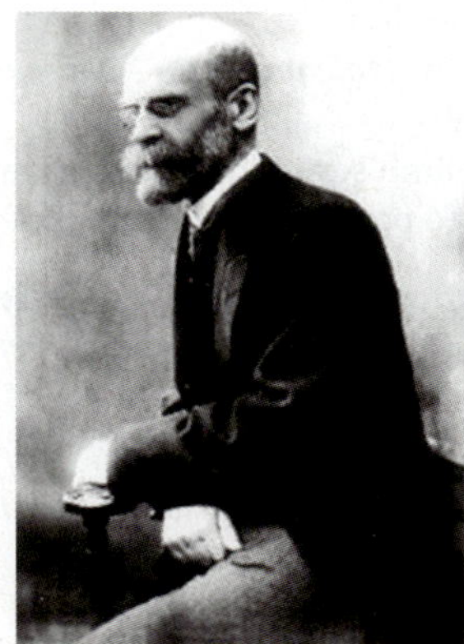

Fig. David E Durkheim

7. **Ans. (c) Are under voluntary control**
[Ref. Life, Knowledge and Confidence by Esomba, 1/e p61]
Pseudo-hallucinations
- False perceptions occurring in internal subjective space ("inside the head")
- Patient describes the sensations being perceived by mind eye
- Lively perceptual conceptions/images
- Are NOT under voluntary control
- Example: Distressing flashback of PTSD

8. **Ans. (a) Eugene Bleuler**
[Ref. Hallucinations by Blom, 1/e p161]
- Extracampine hallucinations: Hallucinations occurring outside the regular field of perception (Bleuler, 1903)

9. **Ans. (a) Illusion**
[Ref. Psychiatry by Namboodri, 3/e p107]

10. **Ans. (b) Hyposexuality**
[Ref. Niraj Ahuja, 7/e p139]
Kleine-Levin syndrome (KLS)
- **Sleeping Beauty syndrome**
- Rare sleep disorder with persistent episodic hypersomnia and cognitive or mood changes
- Many patients also experience hyperphagia, hypersexuality and other symptoms
- Patients commonly have about 20 episodes over about a decade

11. **Ans. (d) 5**
[Ref. DSM-IV-TR in Action by Dziegielewski, 1/e p56]

DSM-IV Multiaxial Assessment

- Axis I: Clinical disorders, Pervasive developmental disorders, Learning motor skills, Communication disorders
- Axis II: Personality disorders, Mental retardation
- Axis III: General mental conditions
- Axis IV: Psychosocial & Environmental problems
- Axis V: Global assessment of functioning (GAF)

12. Ans. (a) Depression

[Ref. Scully's Medical Problems in Dentistry, 7/e p311]

- Anxiety and Depression are the most common Psychiatric disorders

13. Ans. (b) Perception

[Ref. Individual Differences in Conscious Experience by Wallace, 1/e p91]

- A phantom limb sensation is a non-painful perception of the continued presence of an amputated limb

14. Ans. (c) Infectious and parasitic diseases

[Ref. ICD-10-CM Diagnostic Coding System by Dalgleish, 1/e p156]

ICD-10 Chapters

- *Chapter I (A00–B99): Certain infectious and parasitic diseases*
- Chapter II (C00–D48): Neoplasms
- Chapter III (D50–D89): Diseases of the blood and blood-forming organs and certain disorders involving the immune mechanism
- Chapter IV (E00–E90): Endocrine, nutritional and metabolic diseases

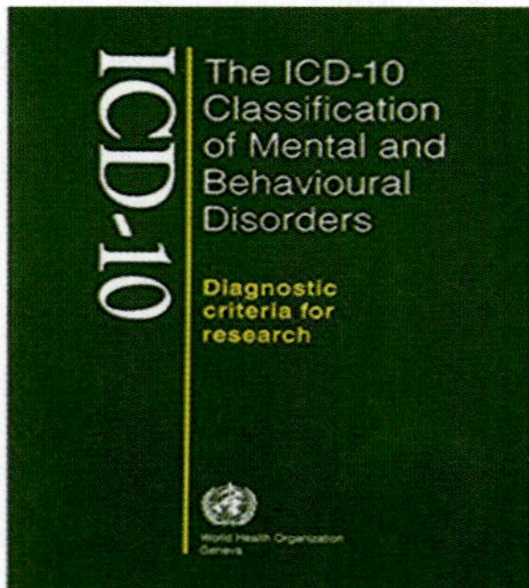

Fig. ICD-10

- ***Chapter V (F00–F99): Mental and behavioural disorders***
- Chapter VI (G00–G99): Diseases of the nervous system
- Chapter VII (H00–H59): Diseases of the eye and adnexa
- Chapter VIII (H60–H95): Diseases of the ear and mastoid process
- Chapter IX (I00–I99): Diseases of the circulatory system
- Chapter X (J00–J99): Diseases of the respiratory system
- Chapter XI (K00–K93): Diseases of the digestive system
- Chapter XII (L00–L99): Diseases of the skin and subcutaneous tissue
- Chapter XIII (M00–M99): Diseases of the musculoskeletal system and connective tissue
- Chapter XIV (N00–N99): Diseases of the genitourinary system
- Chapter XV (O00–O99): Pregnancy, childbirth and the puerperium
- Chapter XVI (P00–P96): Certain conditions originating in the perinatal period
- Chapter XVII (Q00–Q99): Congenital malformations, deformations and chromosomal abnormalities
- Chapter XVIII (R00–R99): Symptoms, signs and abnormal clinical and laboratory findings, not elsewhere classified
- Chapter XIX (S00–T98): Injury, poisoning and certain other consequences of external causes
- Chapter XX (V01–Y98): External causes of morbidity and mortality
- Chapter XXI (Z00–Z99): Factors influencing health status and contact with health services
- *Chapter XXII (U00–U99): Codes for special purposes*

15. Ans. (c) False sense perception without a stimulus

[Ref. Niraj Ahuja, 7/e p13, 28]

Hallucinations

- *Definition*: Hallucination is a disorder of perception experienced in the 'absence of stimulus'
  - Organic cause
  - Non-organic cause
- *Types of hallucinations*:
  - Auditory (Paracusia – Most common in non-organic disorders)
    1. Schizophrenia
    2. Temporal lobe epilepsy
    3. Endocrinal disorders
  - Visual
  - Tactile
    1. Cocaine, amphetamine
    2. Alcohol, benzodiazepine withdrawal
  - Olfactory (Phantosmia)
    1. Viral infection, tumour, trauma, surgery, drugs
    2. Olfactory cortex epilepsy
  - Gustatory
    1. Temporal lobe epilepsy
  - Command hallucinations
    1. Schizophrenia
- *Features of hallucinations*:
  - Experienced like a true perception
  - Seems to come from an external objective space
- *Organic hallucinosis*: **[Mnemonic: Brazil TEAM IS Deadly]**
  - **B**rain-stem lesions
  - **T**emporal arteritis
  - **E**pilepsy
  - **A**lcohol (Auditory hallucinations – Most common)
  - **M**igraine
  - **I**CSOL
  - **S**ensory pathway disease (Release hallucinations)
  - **D**rugs (LSD, Cocaine, Cannabis)

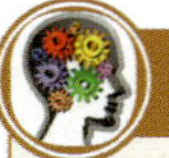

Also Remember

- *Pseudohallucinations*: Feeling does not appear to be a true perception and come from subjective inner space
- *Normal hallucinations*:
  - Hypnagogic hallucinations: Occur as one is falling sleep
  - Hypnapompic hallucinations: Occur as one is waking up
- *Hallucination and other disorders*:

Psychiatry

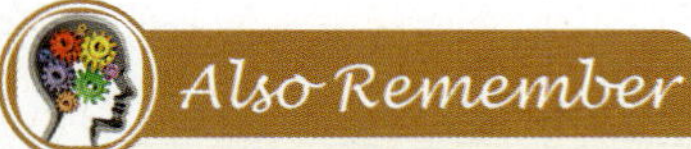

Disorder	Key differentiating point
Hallucination	Perception in absence of stimulus
Dreaming	Does not involve wakefulness
Illusion	Involves distorted and misinterpreted real perception
Imagery	Does not mimic real perception and is under voluntary control
Pseudohallucination	Does not mimic real perception and is not under voluntary control
Delusion	Correctly sensed, interpreted stimulus is given additional significance

16. Ans. (d) Esquirol

[Ref. A Historical Dictionary of Psychiatry by Edward Shorter 2005]

Esquirol Definitions

- *Hallucinations*: Perceptions without a real external stimulus
- *Illusions*: Sensory disorders with distortion or misinterpretation of a real perception

17. Ans. (a) Psychiatric illness in medically ill

[Ref. Kaplan & Sadock's Concise Textbook of Clinical Psychiatry, 3/e p400]

Consultant Liaison Psychiatry

- CL Psychiatry: Study, practice and teaching of relation between medical and psychiatric disorders
- Psychiatrists serve as,
  - Bridge between Psychiatry and other specialties
  - Consultants to Medical colleagues (Non-psychiatrist physicians) and other Mental health professionals (Psychologist, Nurse, Social worker)

18. Ans. (c) Delusion

[Ref. Behavioural Science by Fadem, 3/e p104]

- *Disorders of Perception*:
  - Hallucination
  - Illusion
  - Image disturbance
  - Derealization
  - Depersonalization
- *Disorder of Thought content*:
  - Delusion
  - Idea of reference
- *Disorders of Form of thought*:
  - Loose associations
  - Tangentiality

19. Ans. (d) Schizophrenia

[Ref. Niraj Ahuja, 7/e p57]

Presence of insight	Absence of insight
• Neurosis • Phobias • Obsessions • Compulsions • Obsessive Compulsive disorders • Paranoid personality disorder	• Alzheimer's disease • Schizophrenia • Psychosis • Korsakoff's psychosis • Post partum psychosis • Mood disorders

20. Ans. (d) Preserved postural reflexes

[Ref. Internal Medicine: An Illustrated Radiological Guide by Tubaiikh, 1/e p91]

- *Features of Parkinsonism*:
  - Rigidity
  - Resting tremor
  - Mask-like facies
  - Bradykinesia

21. Ans. (b) It is always pathological

[Ref. Concise Medical Dictionary by E. Martin, 9/e p338]

- *Hallucinations are not always pathological*: For example, Hypnagogic hallucinations at beginning and end of sleep

22. Ans. (b) Illusion

[Ref. A Historical Dictionary of Psychiatry by Edward Shorter 2005]

- Illusions: Sensory disorders with distortion or misinterpretation of a real perception

23. Ans. (b) Schizophrenia

[Ref. Niraj Ahuja, 7/e p56]

Clinical Presentation of Schizophrenia

Thought and speech disorders	
Autistic thinking	Private illogical rules
Loosening of associations	Incoherent disjointed speech
Thought blocking and withdrawal	Sudden interruption without recall
Neologisms	Newly formed phrases/words
Paraphasias	Word approximations
Poverty of speech, ideation	Decreased, non-informative speech
Echolalia	Repetition of other's words
Mutism	No speech production
Perseveration	Persistent repetition of words
Verbigeration	Senseless repetition of same words
Autochthonous/Primary delusions Secondary delusions	Non-explainable on basis of other perceptions Explainable on basis of other perceptions

Contd...

Contd...

Thought and speech disorders	
Perception disorders	
Hallucinations	
Affect disorders	
Apathy, Emotional blunting	
Anhedonia	Inability to experience pleasure
Motor behaviour disorders	
Increased/decreased motor activity	Mannerisms, grimacing, stereotypes
Catatonic features	Catatonic schizophrenia
Negative symptoms	
Attention impairment	
Affective flattening	
Social withdrawal	
Alogia	Lack of speech output
Other symptoms	
Loss of ego boundaries	
Absence of insight	
Normal consciousness, orientation	
Normal memory, intelligence	
Suicidal behaviour	

24. Ans. (c) Hallucination

[Ref. Niraj Ahuja, 7/e p56]

- *Hallucination*: Perception without a real external stimulus
- *Illusion*: Sensory disorder with distortion or misinterpretation of a real perception
- *Delusion*: False unshakeable belief not keeping in with patients' socio-cultural/educational background
- *Delirium*: A transient, usually reversible, cause of cerebral dysfunction and manifests clinically with a wide range of neuropsychiatric abnormalities

25. Ans. (d) Perception occurring without external stimulation

[Ref. Niraj Ahuja, 7/e p56]

26. Ans. (a) Depends on will of observer and is under voluntary control

[Ref. Neuroscience of Visual Hallucinations, 1/e p62]

- Hallucinations are vivid, clear with full-force and impact of normal perception NOT under voluntary control
- Hallucinations, depending on sensory organs involved, may be auditory, visual, tactile, gustatory or olfactory

27. Ans. (b) Sensory organs are not involved

[Ref. Niraj Ahuja, 7/e p56]

28. Ans. (d) Anxiety

[Ref. Niraj Ahuja, 7/e p28]

29. Ans. (c) Delusional disorder

[Ref. Niraj Ahuja, 7/e p83]

Erotomanic Delusions

- **Delusion of being loved by another**
- Generally seen in women who believe that perceived suitor, mostly more socially prominent than herself, is in love with her
- Denials are seen as affirmations of love

30. Ans. (a) Hebephrenic schizophrenia; (d) Delirium; (e) Temporal lobe epilepsy

[Ref. API Textbook of Medicine, 9/e p1653]

- *Conditions with Visual hallucinations*:
  - Schizophrenia (Hebrephrenic, Paranoid)
  - Lewy body disease
  - Alzheimer's dementia
  - Focal brain lesions (Stroke, tumours)
  - Epilepsy
  - Narcolepsy
  - Delirium

31. Ans. (d) Synaesthesia

[Ref. Psychiatry by Neel Burton, 2n Ed., Pg 25]

- *Reflex hallucination*: Stimulus in one modality produce hallucination in another modality
  - Example: Visual hallucination triggered by a running tap
- *Synaesthesia*: Sensory stimulus in one modality produce stimulus in another sensory modality
  - Example: Piece of music is perceived as a Concert of colours

32. Ans. (c) Kraepelin

[Ref. Niraj Ahuja, 7/e p61]

- *Terms coined by Kraepelin*:
  - Manic depressive insanity
  - Dementia praecox
  - Delirious mania
  - Alzheimer's disease

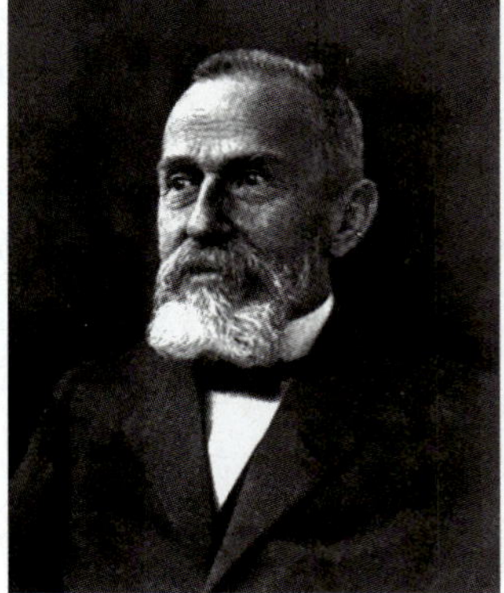

Fig. Emil Kraepelin

33. Ans. (d) Patchy impairment of Personal memories

[Ref. ICD-9-CM for Physicians, Pg 7]

- Dissociative psychogenic amnesia: Sudden patchy impairment of amnesia following a traumatic/stressful event

34. Ans. (d) Superiority inferiority complex

[Ref. A Short Textbook of Psychiatry by Niraj Ahuja, 7/e p205]

Contributions of Sigmund Freud

Theories and major contributions	Major works
• The Conscious and unconscious mind • The Id, Ego, and Superego • Life and death instincts • Psychosexual development • Defence mechanisms	• The Interpretation of dreams • The Psychopathology of everyday life • Totem and Taboo • Civilization and Its discontents • Psychoanalysis

35. Ans. (c) I (iii), II (iv), III (iv), IV (i)

36. Ans. (b) Perception

[Ref. Niraj Ahuja, 7/e p56]

37. Ans. (a) Persistent and inappropriate repetition of the same thoughts

[Ref. A Short Textbook of Psychiatry by Niraj Ahuja, 7/e p56]

38. Ans. (c) Memory

[Ref. Clinical Process in Psychiatry by Nurcombe. 1/e p157]

- *Confabulation*:
  - A false memory that patient believes is true
  - Inconsistent and fanciful
  - Commonly fills memory gaps in Amnestic syndrome

39. Ans. (a) A memory disorder; (b) Synonymous with false memory

[Ref. The Confabulating mind by Schnider, 1/e p45]

- *Types of Confabulations*:
  - *Amnestic confabulations*: False products from memory
  - *Non-amnestic confabulations*: Emanating from false perceptions of bodily states, outer world and other failures

40. Ans. (b) Jamais vu

[Ref. A Dictionary of Neurological Signs by Larner, Pg 199]

- ***Jamais vu:*** "Never seen", is sensation of strangeness or unfamiliarity about visual stimuli that have been experienced previously
- ***Déjà vu:*** "Already seen", is the phenomenon of having the strong sensation that an event or experience currently being experienced, has already been experienced in the past, whether it has actually happened or not
- ***Deja entendu:*** A new voice that sounds familiar
- ***Deja pensee:*** A new idea that seems familiar

41. Ans. (b) Depression

[Ref. WHO Mental Illness in General Health Care, Pg 79]

- *Most common Mental health disorder in India*: Depressive neurosis

42. Ans. (a) Freud

[Ref. Niraj Ahuja, 7/e p205]

43. Ans. (b) Unipolar depression

[Ref. WHO Global Burden of Disease Report 2004, Pg 43]

Leading causes of Daly's Lost in World

Cause	DALY's lost (millions)
Lower respiratory infections	94
Diarrhoeal diseases	73
Unipolar depression	65
Ischemic heart disease	63
HIV	58

44. Ans. (c) 1955

[Ref. Indian Journal of Psychiatry, Volume 44, Pg 5]

- *Watershed year of Biological Psychiatry research in India*: 1955

45. Ans. (a) Hypothalamus

Narcolepsy

- *Description*: Excessive day-time sleepiness, disturbed night-time sleep, disturbances in REM-sleep
- *Hallmark feature*: Decreased REM latency
- *Classical tetrad of symptoms*:
  - Sleep attacks (Most common)
  - Cataplexy
  - Hypnagogic hallucinations
  - Sleep paralysis (Least common)

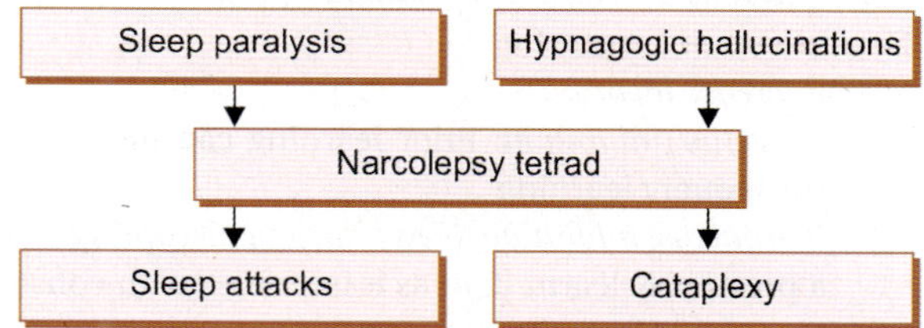

Fig. Narcolepsy tetrad

46. Ans. (a) Beck

[Ref. Cognitive Therapy of Depression by AT Beck, Pg 10]

- ***Beck's Cognitive Model of Depression:***
  - Cognitive triad: Negative views of himself, experiences and future
  - Schemas: Maintenance of self-defeating attitudes despite positive factors in life
  - Cognitive errors

47. Ans. (d) Hypersomnia

[Ref. Niraj Ahuja, 7/e p139]

Kleine-Levin Syndrome

- Hypersomnia (always present)
- Hyperphagia (usually present)
- Hypersexuality (always present)

48. Ans. (d) Free association

[Ref. Comprehensive Dictionary of Psychoanalysis by S. Akhtar, Pg 115]

Fundamental rule of Psychoanalysis: Sigmund Freud gave up the Concept of Hypnosis for Free association (speak without censoring thoughts)

49. Ans. (a) 1856-39 and he passed most of his life in Austria

[Ref. Sigmund Freud's Christin Unconsciousness, Pg 199]

50. Ans. (a) Freud

[Ref. Comprehensive Dictionary of Psychoanalysis by S. Akhtar, Pg 115]

51. Ans. (b) Sigmund Freud

[Ref. Psychology: Concepts and Applications by Nevid, 4/e p480]

- *Sigmund Freud developed the First Psychodynamic theory of personality*: Personality is shaped by underlying conflicts between opposing forces within the mind

52. Ans. (a) Freud

[Ref. Psychiatry Update by Hales & Frances, Annual Review, Volume 5, Pg 161]

- *Sigmund Freud first used Cocaine in Psychiatry*: To treat Morphine addiction (consequent upon treating nerve pain) in his friend

53. Ans. (b) Eugen Bleuler

[Ref. Symptoms of Schizophrenia by Costello, 1/e p202]

54. Ans. (a) Pinel

[Ref. Psychiatry and Religion, Pg 95]

- *Moral treatment of Insanity (Pinel)*: Occupational therapy, exercise, entertainment, good food, attractive surroundings, meetings with hospital attendants

55. Ans. (b) Proactive inhibition

[Ref. Examination Notes in Psychiatry by Malhi, 2/ e p9]

Hypothesis of Forgetting

- *Interference theory*:
  - *Proactive inhibition*: Prior learning can interfere with subsequent learning
  - *Retroactive inhibition*: New learning disrupting recall of a previously learnt item as it interferes with consolidation of that item
- *Decay theory*: Fading of memories with time
- *Repression*: Deliberate (motivated) forgetting
- *Displacement*: If Short-term memory is full, new information displaces old information

56. Ans. (d) Erikson

[Ref. Healing the Eight Stages of Life by Linn, Mathew, Pg 23]

Erikson Eight Stages of Psychosocial Development

Age	Virtues	Psychosocial crisis	Significant relationship
0–2 y	Hope	Basic trust vs Mistrust	Mother
2–4 y	Will	Autonomy vs Shame/ Doubt	Parents
4–5 y	Purpose	Initiative vs Guilt	Family
5–12 y	Competence	Industry vs Inferiority	Neighbours, School
13–19 y	Fidelity	Identity vs Role confusion	Peers, Role model
20–39 y	Love	Intimacy vs Isolation	Friends, Partners
40–64 y	Care	Generativity vs Stagnation	Household, Workmates
65+ y	Wisdom	Ego integrity vs Despair	Mankind, Mykind

57. Ans. (b) Maxwell Jones

[Ref. The Therapeutic Community Movement by Manning, Pg 184]

- *Therapeutic Community (Maxwell Jones)*: Group-based approach to mental illness, personality disorders and drug-addiction
  - Includes Milieu therapy, Group psychotherapy, Practical activities

58. Ans. (a) Karl Kahlbaum

[Ref. Catatonia: A Clinician's Guide to Diagnosis & Treatment by Fink & Taylor, 1/e p3]

- *Catatonia (Karl Ludwig Kahlbaum)*: Brain disease with cyclical alternating course, in which mental symptoms are, consecutively, melancholy, mania, stupor, confusion, and eventually dementia

59. Ans. (c) Death

[Ref. A Physician's Guide to Coping with Death and Dying by Swanson & Cooper, 1/e p14]

- *Five Stages of Death (Elisabeth Kubler Ross)*:
  - Denial
  - Anger
  - Bargaining
  - Depression
  - Acceptance

60. Ans. (b) Delirium

[Ref. Handbook of Consultant Liaison Psychiatry by Leigh, 2/e p410]

- *Delirium* is the *most common disorder* during the early *postoperative* period
- *Other conditions*: Major depressive disorder, Persistent depressive disorder, Adjustment disorder

61. Ans. (a) Ketamine

[Ref. Niraj Ahuja, 7/e p49]

Hallucinogenic Drugs

- *Psychedelics (Classical hallucinogens)*: Makes a person manifest a hidden but real aspect of mind
  - LSD
  - Mescaline
  - Psilocybe
- *Dissociative drugs*: Produce analgesia, amnesia and catalepsy at anaesthetic doses
  - Ketamine
  - Dextromethorphan
  - Nitrous oxide
  - Amanita
- *Deliriants (True hallucinogens)*: Anticholinergic agents which cause acute confusional state
  - Datura
  - Tobacco (large amounts)
  - Diphenhydramine
  - Hydroxyzine

62. Ans. (b) F

[Ref. Niraj Ahuja, 7/e p2]

ICD-10 Chapter F

- *Classification*: Psychiatric Disorders as Mental & Behavioural Disorders (MBDs)
- *Coding*: Alpha-numeric system F00-F99

63. Ans. (c) Kraepelin
[Ref. Niraj Ahuja, 7/e p61]

64. Ans. (b) Beck
[Ref. Niraj Ahuja, 7/e p10]

65. Ans. (a) Persistent and inappropriate repetition of the same thoughts
[Ref. Niraj Ahuja, 7/e p56]

66. Ans. (a) Illusion
[Ref. A Historical Dictionary of Psychiatry by Edward Shorter 2005]

67. Ans. (a) Amphetamine
[Ref. Human Drug metabolism by Coleman, 1/e p236]

- *Amphetamine like drugs*: Elevated amine levels, especially dopamine, can cause Hallucinations

68. Ans. (d) I (iv), II (iii), III (i), IV (ii)
[Ref. Multiple Sources]

69. Ans. (c) Munchausen syndrome
[Ref. Niraj Ahuja, 7/e p119]

Munchausen's Syndrome (Factitious Disorder)

- *Synonyms*: Hospital addiction, Hospital hoboes, Professional patients
- *Description*: Patients who repeatedly simulate or fake diseases for the sole purpose of obtaining medical attention
  - Patients present with Physical/psychological signs/ symptoms
  - Pseudologia fantastica: Patients distort clinical histories, laboratory tests reports
- *Prognosis*: Poor

70. Ans. (d) Psychosis
[Ref. Niraj Ahuja, 7/e p83, 89]

Insight

- *Definition*: Insight is ability of one to recognize one's own illness

***Types of insight*: (6-point scale: 1-6)**

- Complete denial of illness
- Slight awareness but denial
- Awareness but sickness attributed to external factors
- Awareness with sickness attributed to something unknown in self
- Intellectual insight: Total awareness but does not apply this knowledge to current/future experiences
- True emotional insight: Total awareness and this knowledge leads to changes in future behaviour and personality

Presence of insight	Absence of insight
• Neurosis • Phobias • Obsessions • Compulsions • Obsessive Compulsive disorders • Paranoid personality disorder	• Alzheimer's disease • Schizophrenia • Psychosis • Korsakoff's psychosis • Post partum psychosis • Mood disorders

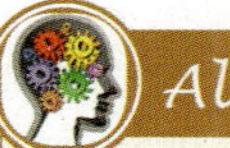

Also Remember

- *Anosognosia*: Total absence of insight into one's own illness (most severe form of insight)

71. Ans. (b) Paratonic rigidity
[Ref. Dictionary of Neurological Signs by Larner, 3/e p158]

- Gegenhalten: Variable resistance to passive movement of a limb when changing its position or posture, seen in Bilateral frontal lobe dysfunction

72. Ans. (c) Synaesthesia
[Ref. Fish's Clinical Psychopathology, 3/e p14]

Disturbances in Perception

- Sensory disturbances:
  - Hypoaesthesia, Hyperaesthesia
  - Dysmegalopsia (Changes in spatial form)
- Sensory deceptions:
  - Illusions
  - Hallucinations
- Body image distortions (Paraschemazia):
  - Hyperchemazia
  - Hyposchemazia

73. Ans. (b) Loss of long term memory
[Ref. Niraj Ahuja, 7/e p22]

Dementia

- Impaired memory (Recent)
- Impaired intellectual functions
- Deterioration of personality
- Consciousness, orientation, attention, sleep-wake cycle: Normal

74. Ans. (b) Personality disorders
[Kaplan & Sadock's Psychiatry, 9/e p33]

DSM-IV-TR Multiaxial System

- Axis-I: Clinical disorders, Other conditions that may be a focus of clinical attention
- Axis-II: Personality disorders, Mental retardation
- Axis-III: Physical/Genetic disorder is present in addition to Psychiatric disorder

75. Ans. (d) Inability to experience pleasure
[Ref. Niraj Ahuja, 7/e p56-57]

Anhedonia

- Anhedonia is the inability to experience pleasure from activities usually found enjoyable, e.g. exercise, hobbies, sexual activities or social interactions (Older model)
- Anhedonia is a negative symptom
- Anhedonia is seen in: Mood disorders (Depression), Schizoaffective disorder, Schizoid personality disorder. Schizophrenia, Post traumatic stressed disorders, Sexual dysfunctions
- Newer models of Anhedonia:
  - Motivational anhedonia: Lack of motivation or desire to engage in an activity
  - Consummatory anhedonia: Lack of level of enjoyment of activity itself

76. Ans. (b) Freud

[Ref. Niraj Ahuja, 7/e p205]

- The credit for 'invention' of Psychoanalysis belongs to Sigmund Freud (1856-1939),

77. Ans. (d) Delusion is associated with faulty reasoning

[Ref. Behavioural Science by Fadem, 3/e p104]

Illusion Vs Delusion

	Illusion	Delusion
Disorder of	Perception	Thought content
Description	Perceptual misinterpretation	False belief
Involves	Distorted, misinterpreted real perception	Correctly sensed, interpreted stimulus given additional significance
Faulty reasoning	Absent	Present
Can be convinced for reality	Yes	No

78. Ans. (b) Depression

[Ref. Shorter Oxford Textbook of Psychiatry, 7/e p377]

- Depression is the most common psychiatric disorder that adversely affects stroke outcome and is often underdiagnosed or inadequately treated
- It may contribute to the apparent intellectual impairment or basis of the syndrome is thought to involve altered dopamine function and aberrant cortico-striatal connectivity

HIGH YIELD MCQs ANSWERS WITH EXPLANATIONS

1. Ans. (c) Food preference history

[Ref. Kaplan & Sadock, 10/e p228]

Personal history in Psychiatry

- Childhood and developmental history
- Occupational history
- Marital/relationship history
- Military history
- Educational history
- Religion history
- Social activity history
- Legal history
- Sexual history

2. Ans. (c) Primary health centres

[Ref. IPHS PHC Standards, MoHFW, GOI]

- Sub-centres, Primary health centres, Community health centres do not have a mental health professional
- All district hospitals are provided with a team consisting of Psychiatrist, Clinical psychologist, Psychiatric social worker, Psychiatric nurse, Statistician
- Medical college staff include all Preclinical, Paraclinical and Clinical specialists and Superspecialists

3. Ans. (b) Events

[Ref. Psychology of Language by Carroll, 5/e p51]

Two major types of memory—Implicit and Explicit

- Implicit memory involves things we need not actively remember
  - Example: Swimming—One need not remember how to swim every time
- Explicit memory has two components: Episodic memory (Events) and Semantic memory (Facts—Words, Rules, and Language)
  - Episodic is the ability to remember personal events over time
  - Semantic memory is abstract, referring to knowledge without context. It includes things that are common knowledge, such as the names of colors, the capitals of countries
  - Example: If you try to remember your first day in a new city, it would be episodic memory as an event will flash in front of one's eyes; If you try to remember MC cancer in males, it would be a semantic memory as one is thinking about a fact

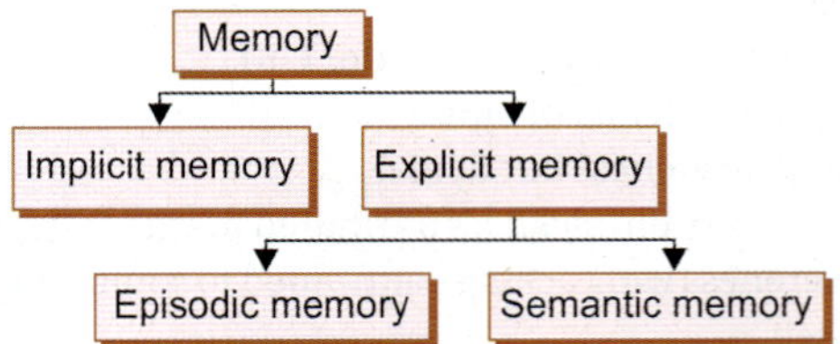

Fig. Types of memory

4. Ans. (d) Physiological, Safety, Belonging, Esteem, Self-actualization

[Ref. Maslow's Hierarchy of Needs Model by Rakowski 1/e p4]

MASLOW'S HIERARCHY OF NEEDS

- A theory in psychology proposed by Abraham Maslow
- Maslow used the terms "physiological", "safety", "belongingness" and "love", "esteem", "self-actualization", and "self-transcendence" to describe the pattern that human motivations generally move through
- Structure of his pyramid starts from the bottom and proceeds upwards
- It represents the priority of human needs which determine human behaviour

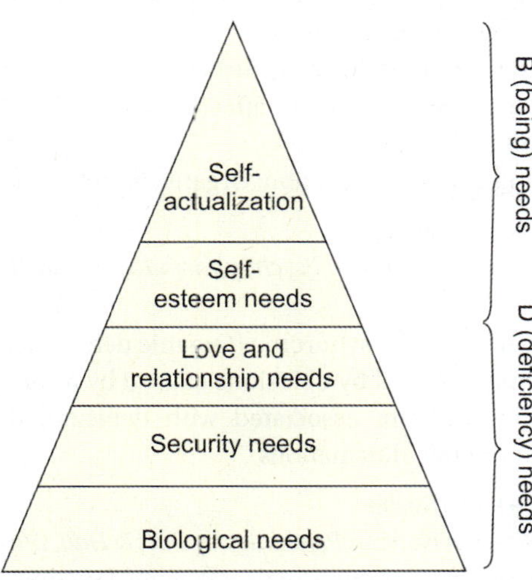

Fig. Maslow's hierarchy of needs

5. Ans. (a) Alcoholism

[Ref. A Dictionary of Hallucinations by Blom, 1/e p536]

Visual Hallucinations in Psychiatry

- Delirium
- Alcoholic hallucinosis
- Alzheimer's dementia
- Other dementias
- Schizophrenia
- Drug related Flash-backs
- PTSD Flash-backs

6. Ans. (c) Hysteria

[Ref. Psychiatry in Medical Practice by Goldberg, Gask & Morriss, 3/e p36]

Auditory Hallucinations in Psychiatry

- Schizophrenia
- Organic brain syndromes
- Mood disorders (manic depressive illness)
- Substance abuse (Cocaine, Amphetamine toxicity)

7. Ans. (b) Thought

[Ref. A Dictionary of Psychology by Colman, 4/e p41]

Cognition

- Description: Ability to acquire, store and use knowledge
- Major cognitive functions: Consciousness, Attention, Perception, Language, Memory, Numeracy, Executive function, Praxia

8. Ans. (b) Euphoria

[Ref. Psychiatry by Neel Burton, 2/e p20]

- *Emotional reactions*: Anxiety, Irritability, Depression, Anhedonia, Euphoria, Ecstasy, Apathy

9. Ans. (c) Inability to recognize and describe feelings

[Ref. Campbell's Psychiatric Dictionary, 9/e p39]

- *Alexithymia*: Difficulty in describing or recognizing one's emotions
  - *Primary alexithymia*: Personality trait
  - *Secondary alexithymia*: State reaction to effects of serious physical illness

10. Ans. (b) Perception

[Ref. Behavioural Science by Fadem, 3/e p104]

11. Ans. (a) Illusion

[Ref. A Historical Dictionary of Psychiatry by Edward Shorter 2005]

- *Illusion*: Sensory disorders with distortion or misinterpretation of a real perception

12. Ans. (a) Illusion

[Ref. A Historical Dictionary of Psychiatry by Edward Shorter 2005]

13. Ans. (c) Hallucination

[Ref. A Historical Dictionary of Psychiatry by Edward Shorter 2005]

- *Hallucinations*: Perceptions without a real external stimulus

14. Ans. (b) It occurs to inner subjective space

[Ref. Neuroscience of Visual Hallucinations, 1/e p62]

- Hallucinations
- Vivid, clear with full-force and impact of normal perception NOT under voluntary control
- Independent of will of observer
- Depending on sensory organs involved, may be auditory, visual, tactile, gustatory or olfactory

15. Ans. (c) Temporal

[Ref. DeJong's Neurologic Examination by Campbell, 7/e p72]

- *Occipital lobe lesions*: Visual hallucinations
- *Temporal lobe lesions*: Auditory hallucinations

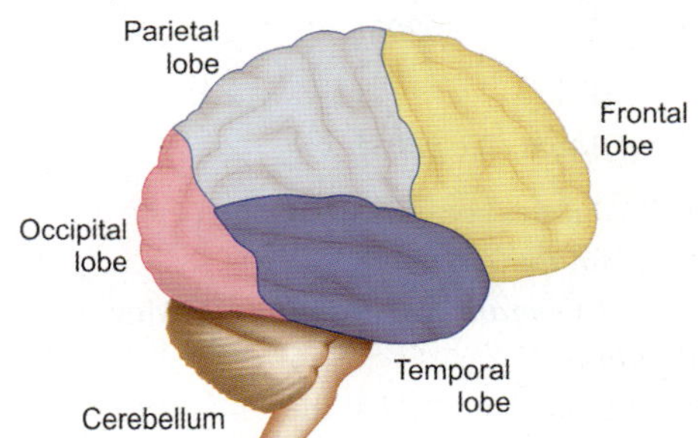

Fig. Lobes of brain

16. Ans. (b) It experienced while awakening

[Ref. Niraj Ahuja, 7/e p138]

- ***Hypnagogic hallucinations*:** Vivid dream-like perceptions, occurring at onset of sleep and associated with fearfulness
- ***Hypnapompic hallucinations*:** Vivid dream-like perceptions, occurring while awake

17. Ans. (a) Hypnagogic hallucinations

[Ref. Niraj Ahuja, 7/e p138]

18. Ans. (a) Persistent repetition of words

[Ref. Niraj Ahuja, 7/e p56]

19. Ans. (a) Memory

[Ref. Clinical Process in Psychiatry by Nurcombe. 1/e p157]

- ***Confabulation*:**
  - A false memory that patient believes is true, Inconsistent and fanciful
  - Commonly fills memory gaps in Amnestic syndrome

20. Ans. (c) Filling up to gaps by fabrication to cover lapses in memory

[Ref. Clinical Process in Psychiatry by Nurcombe. 1/e p157]

- ***Confabulation:***
  - A Confabulation is a type of Paramnesias where there is unintentional filling of gaps of memory with untrue and fanciful material
    - Symptom of generalized brain dysfunction with marked memory impairment
    - The patient uses rationalizations and various cover stories to hide the extent of mental dysfunction from himself and others
    - Bizarre, unrealistic, inaccurate responses to questions
  - Disorders related to Confabulation: Chronic alcoholism, Amnestic syndromes, Korsakoff's syndrome, Syphilis, Senile dementia, Schizophrenic psychosis

21. Ans. (d) Making stories to fill gaps in memory loss

[Ref. Clinical Process in Psychiatry by Nurcombe. 1/e p157]

22. Ans. (a) Freud

[Ref. Niraj Ahuja, 7/e p205]

23. Ans. (b) Sigmund Freud

[Ref. Niraj Ahuja, 7/e p205]

24. Ans. (b) Freud

[Ref. Niraj Ahuja, 7/e p205]

25. Ans. (c) Freud

[Ref. Niraj Ahuja, 7/e p205]

26. Ans. (b) Classical conditioning

[Ref. Niraj Ahuja, 7/e p214]

- *Classical/Operant conditioning*: Pavlov (Dog salivation experiment)
- *Operant conditioning*: Skinner

27. Ans. (a) Panic disorder

[Ref. Panic Disorders and Agoraphobia by Baldwin, 1/e p7]

Presence of insight	Absence of insight
• Neurosis • Phobias • Obsessions • Compulsions • Anxiety • Panic disorder • Obsessive Compulsive disorders • Paranoid personality disorder • Dissociative disorder • Conversion disorder	• Alzheimer's disease • Schizophrenia • Psychosis • Korsakoff's psychosis • Post-partum psychosis • Reactive psychosis • Mood disorders • Delusional disorder • Delirium • Dementia

28. Ans. (b) Schizophrenia

[Ref. Insight & Psychosis by David, Pg 21]

29. Ans. (d) Organic mental disorder

[Ref. Handbook of Emergency Psychiatry by Petit, Pg 71]

Confusion (Disorientation)

- Description: State of disturbed orientation in regard to time, place and person, affecting the clarity & coherence of one's thinking
  - Most often association: Organic brain disease

30. Ans. (b) Delusion

[Ref. Clinical Geriatric Psychopharmacology by Salzman, 4/e p121]

- Organic mental syndrome (Organic delusional syndrome) is characterized by delusions caused by a specific organic factor, and not associated with delirium, dementia or prominent hallucinations

31. Ans. (b) Catharsis

[Ref. Revision Notes in Psychiatry by Puri & Hall, 2/e p415]

- Behavioural methods of Psychological treatment:
  - Modeling
  - Exposure
  - Response prevention

(Catharsis is Intensive affective discharge to provide emotional relief)

32. Ans. (c) Depression

[Ref. WHO Global Burden of Disease Report 2004, Pg 43]

Leading causes of DALY'S Lost in World

Cause	DALY's lost (millions)
Lower respiratory infections	94
Diarrhoeal diseases	73
Unipolar depression	65
Ischemic heart disease	63
HIV	58

33. Ans. (d) Schizophrenia

[Ref. Insight & Psychosis by David, Pg 21]

34. Ans. (a) Panic disorder

[Ref. Panic Disorders and Agoraphobia by Baldwin, 1/e p7]

35. Ans. (a) Head injury

[Kaplan & Sadock's Study Guide and Self-examination Review in Psychiatry, 9/e p188]

Causes of Amnesia

- Epileptic seizure
- Head trauma
- Alcoholic black-outs
- Korsakoff psychosis
- Stroke
- Post-operative amnesia
- Post-infectious amnesia
- Post-ECT
- Surgery
- Infection
- Transient global amnesia
- Cerebrovascular disease
- Metabolic abnormalities

36. Ans. (b) Dissociative disorder
[Ref. Textbook of Cultural Psychiatry by Bhugra, Pg 201]

37. Ans. (c) Christian Reil
[Ref. Approach to Psychiatric Patient by Barnhill, 1/e p29]
- Term Psychiatry was coined by Christian Reil & JCA Heinroth

38. Ans. (d) Roger Sperry
[Ref. Atoms of Mind by Klemm, Pg 187]
- *1981 Nobel Prize in Physiology & Medicine for Split-brain research*: Roger Sperry, Hubel & Weisel

39. Ans. (b) Frontal lobe
[Ref. Human Anatomy by Saladin, 1/e p452]
- Emotional response is controlled by:
  - Hypothalamus
  - Amygdala
  - Prefrontal cortex

40. Ans. (b) ≥2
[Ref. Foundations of Psychiatric Mental Health Nursing by Varcarolis, 7/e p417]

Comorbidity
- Description: Two or more disorders existing together in the same person, with the potential for interaction or exacerbation of symptoms
  - Combination of two or more psychiatric disorders
  - Combination of two or more medical disorders
  - Combination of a psychiatric and medical disorder

41. Ans. (c) Dissociative disorder
[Ref. Encyclopedia of Neurological Scinces by Daroff, 2/e p959]

Delusions in Psychiatric Disorders
- Depression
- Bipolar disorder
- Mania
- Obsessive compulsive disorder
- Schizophrenia
- Schizoaffective disorder
- Delusional disorder
- Capgras syndrome
- Clerambault syndrome
- Parkinson's disease
- Alzheimer's disease
- Organic mental states
- Paranoid personality disorder

42. Ans. (a) Illusion; (c) Depersonalization; (e) Hallucination
[Ref. Behavioural Science by Fadem, 3/e p104]

43. Ans. (b) Parkinson's disease
[Ref. Pharmacology by Thorpe, 1/e p222]
- First neurological disorder found due to neurotransmitter deficiency: Parkinson's disease

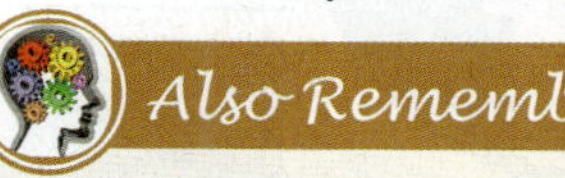

Psychiatric Disorders associated with Neurotransmitters

Disorder	Neurotransmitter(s)
Schizophrenia	Dopamine (Increased), NE (Increased), Serotonin (Increased)
Depression	NE (Decreased), Serotonin (Decreased)
Mania	NE (Increased)
Alzheimer's disease	Acetylcholine (Decreased)
Anxiety	GABA (Decreased), NE (Increased)
Psychotic thinking	Glutamate (Decreased)
Neuronal death (Excitotoxicity)	Glutamate (Increased)
Obsessive Compulsive disorder	Serotonin receptor (Hypersensitivity)
Attention Deficit Hyperactivity Disorder	Dopamine (Decreased), Serotonin (Decreased)
Tourette syndrome	Dopamine (Decrease in Frontal regions/Substantia nigra), Dopamine (Increase in Nucleus accumbens/striatum), Serotonin (Decreased)

(NE: Norepinephrine)

44. Ans. (c) Digit span forward and backward
[Ref. Consultation-Liaison Psychiatry by Leigh, 1/e p24]

Digit Span Test
- Digit span forward is tested by asking the patient to repeat a number of random digits, not including Zero
- Most patients can repeat six digits forward; failure to do so indicate cognitive impairment
- Digit span backward is tested by asking patient to repeat the numbers in reverse order
- Most patients can repeat four digits backward; ability to repeat five digits backward rule out brain dysfunction
- Digit span tests Short term memory and concentration, working memory and language requirement of repetition

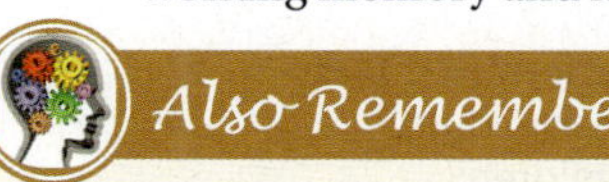

Serial Sevens' test
- Patient is asked to subtract 7 from 100, and then keep subtracting 7 from results
- Is mainly used as test for attention and concentration

Psychiatry

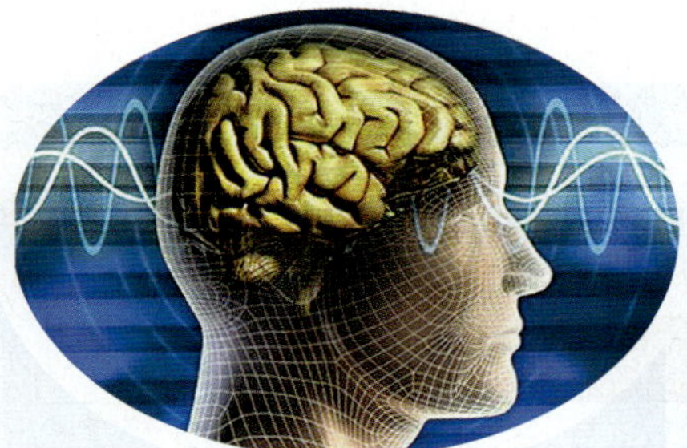

Chapter 2

Mental Status Examination

THEORETICAL CONCEPTS

II A. INTELLIGENCE QUOTIENT

- *Definition(IQ)*: Is a score derived from one of several different standardized tests attempting to measure intelligence
- *First intelligence tests were developed by*: **Binet and Simon (1896)**
- *Stern's IQ* Test: Originally *IQ was calculated for children*[Q]
- *Wechsler Adult Intelligence Scale (WAIS)*: David Wechsler (1939) published the first intelligence test designed for an adult population
    - It was the ***'first IQ test based on Normal/Gaussian distribution'***
- *Levels of Intelligence based on IQ levels*:

Levels of intelligence	IQ range
Idiot	0–24
Imbecile[Q]	25–49
Moron[Q]	50–69
Borderline	70–79
Low normal	80–89
Normal[Q]	90–109
Superior	110–119
Very superior	120–139
Near Genius[Q]	140 and over

Topper's Edge

Commonly used Intelligence Quotient (IQ) Tests
- Wechsler Adult Intelligence Scale for adults[Q]
- Wechsler Intelligence Scale for Children[Q]
- Stanford-Binet Intelligence Scales[Q]: Average score is 90–109
- Woodcock-Johnson Tests of Cognitive Abilities: Detailed analysis of cognitive abilities
- Kaufman Assessment Battery for Children
- Cognitive Assessment System
- Differential Ability Scales: Battery of cognitive and achievement tests

Less Commonly used IQ Tests
- Raven's Progressive Matrices: Measure abstract reasoning, Non-verbal estimate of fluid intelligence
- Cattell Culture Fair III: Measure of cognitive abilities that accurately estimated intelligence devoid of sociocultural and environmental influences
- Reynolds Intellectual Assessment Scales: Includes a co-normed, supplemental measure of memory
- Multidimensional Aptitude Battery II: Group-administered intelligence test to measure Verbal, Performance and Full Scale IQ
- Das-Naglieri cognitive assessment system: Test of cognitive functioning for children and adolescents
- Thurstone's Primary Mental Abilities

- *Categories of mental retardation based on IQ levels*: (Normal IQ is 70 IQ points and over)

Mental retardation	IQ range	Contribution	Features
Mild MR	50–69	90-95% cases	**Educable** up to 6th class; supervised care required under stressful conditions[Q]
Moderate MR	35–49	10%	Drop-out after 2nd class; **trainable** for unskilled/ semi-skilled work[Q]
Severe MR	21–34	2-3%	Poor motor development and poor communication; dependents
Profound MR	20 or below	1-2%	Physical disorders; Require nursing care or life support

Topper's Edge

MENTAL RETARDATION

Causes of Mental Retardation

- Genetic conditions: Down syndrome, Klinefelter syndrome, Fragile X syndrome, Neurofibromatosis, Congenital hypothyroidism, Williams syndrome, Phenylketonuria (PKU), and Prader–Willi syndrome[Q]
- Problems during pregnancy: Alcoholism
- Problems at birth: Hypoxic brain damage
- Exposure to disease or toxins: Whooping cough, Measles, Meningitis, Lead, Mercury exposure
- Iodine deficiency
- Malnutrition
- Absence of the arcuate fasciculus.

Intellectual Developmental Disorders (IDDs)[Q]

- **ICD-11 working group proposes replacing mental retardation with IDDs[Q]**
- IDD: A group of developmental conditions characterized by significant impairment of cognitive functions, which are associated with limitations of learning, adaptive behavior and skills
- New term proposed for DSM-5 is Intellectual disability (ID)/IDD
- Critical components of intelligence proposed in both DSM-5 and the ICD-11:
  - Verbal comprehension
  - Working memory
  - Perceptual reasoning
  - Cognitive efficacy

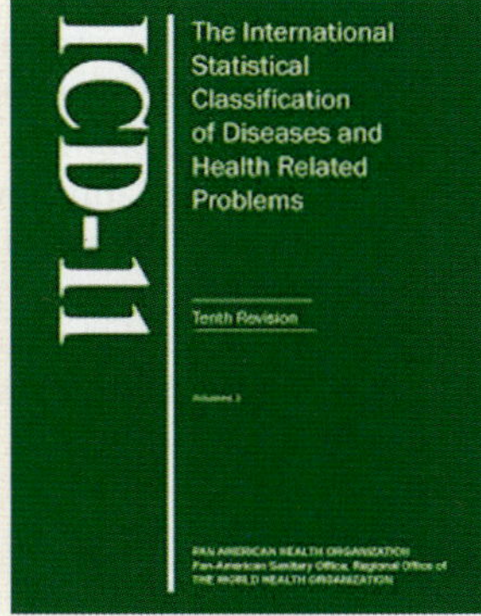

Fig. ICD-11

II B. FIVE PSYCHOSEXUAL STAGES OF DEVELOPMENT (SIGMOND FREUD[Q])

- **PHASE I. ORAL PHASE**
  - *Age range*: Birth–1½ years
  - *Major site of gratification*: Oral region
  - *Normal development*:
    - Oral erotic phase (Sucking)
    - Oral sadistic phase (Biting)
  - *Disorders resulting due to fixation/regression to this phase*:
    - Alcohol dependence
    - Drug dependence
    - Schizophrenia
    - Mood disorders
    - Dependent personality disorder
- **PHASE II. ANAL PHASE**
  - *Age range*: 1–3 years
  - *Major site of gratification*: Anal/peri-anal region
  - *Normal development*:
    - Anal erotic phase (Excretion)
    - Anal sadistic phase (Holding/Letting go)
  - *Disorders resulting due to fixation/regression to this phase*:
    - Obsessive compulsive disorders

- **PHASE III. PHALLIC/OEDIPAL PHASE**
  - *Age range*: 3–5 years[Q]
  - *Major site of gratification*: Genital area
  - *Normal development*:
    - Males: Castration anxiety (replace father in mother's affections), Oedipus complex (aggressive impulses towards father)[Q], Oedipus rex (killing father, marrying mother)
    - Females: Penis envy (fantasy of loss of penis leading to female genitalia), Electra complex (identification with mother)[Q]
  - *Disorders resulting due to fixation/regression to this phase*:
    - Sexual dysfunctions
    - Sexual deviations
    - Neurotic disorders
- **PHASE IV. LATENCY PHASE**
  - *Age range*: 5–12 years
  - *Major feature*: Relative sexual quiescence
  - *Normal development*:
    - Oedipus/Electra complex resolution
    - Super-ego formation
    - Socially appropriate goals formation
  - *Disorders resulting due to fixation/regression to this phase*:
    - Neurotic disorders
- **PHASE V. GENITAL PHASE**
  - *Age range*: 12 years onwards
  - *Major feature*: True self-identity development
  - *Normal development*:
    - Adult sexuality development
    - Gradual release of parental control
    - More influence of peer groups
  - *Disorders resulting due to fixation/regression to this phase*:
    - Neurotic disorders

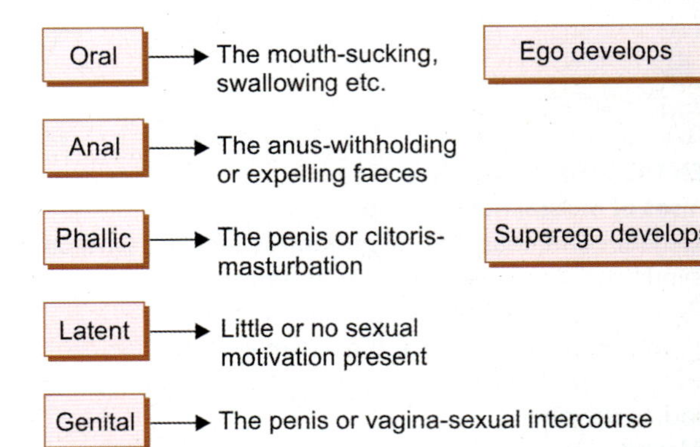

Fig. Stages of psychosexual development (Freud)

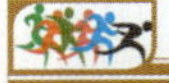

Topper's Edge

Freud's Structural Model of Personality Development

- Human personality consisted of three interworking parts - Id, Ego and Superego
- All parts become unified as a child works through the five stages of psychosexual development
  - **The Id[Q]:** Largest part of the mind, is related to desires and impulses and is the main source of basic biological needs
  - **The Ego[Q]:** Related to reasoning and is the conscious, rational part of the personality; it monitors behavior in order to satisfy basic desires without suffering negative consequences
  - **The Superego[Q]** (Conscience): Develops through interactions with others (mainly parents) who want the child to conform to the norms of society
- The Superego restricts the desires of Id by applying morals and values from society
- Freud believed that a struggle existed between these levels of consciousness, influencing personality development and psychopathology

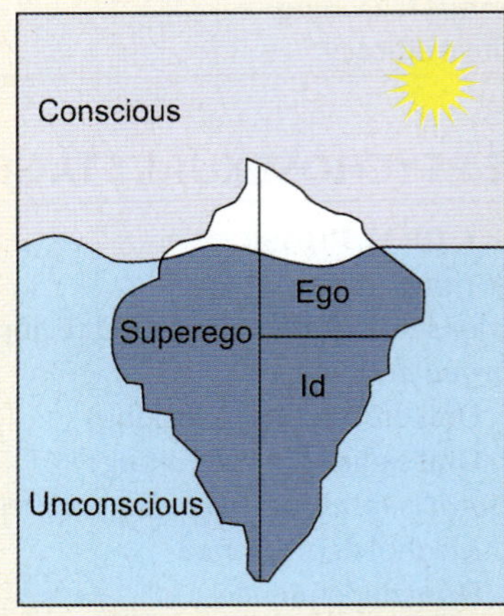

Fig. Freud's structural model of personality

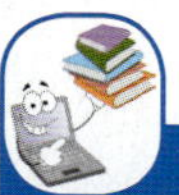

IMAGE-BASED QUESTIONS

1. Maximum score of test shown in Photograph is

[Recent Question 2013, 2015]

MMSE
Mini-Mental® State Examination

a. 13
b. 30
c. 47
d. 55

2. Identify the Chart used in Psychiatry as given in the Photograph

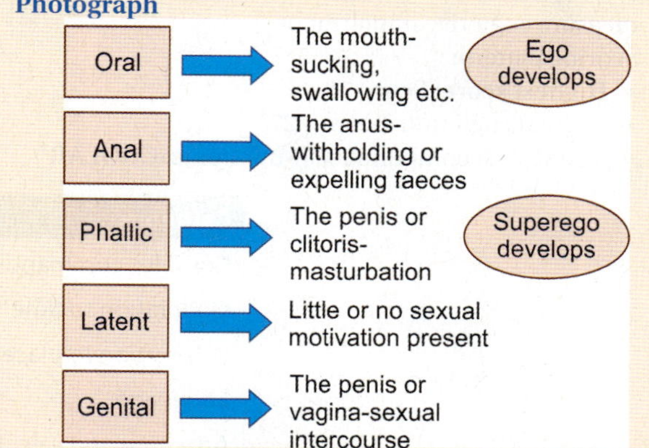

a. First ranks symptoms of Schizophrenia
b. Wechsler classes of IQ level
c. Stages of Psychosexual development
d. MMSE

3. Identify the contribution of Psychologist shown in Photograph

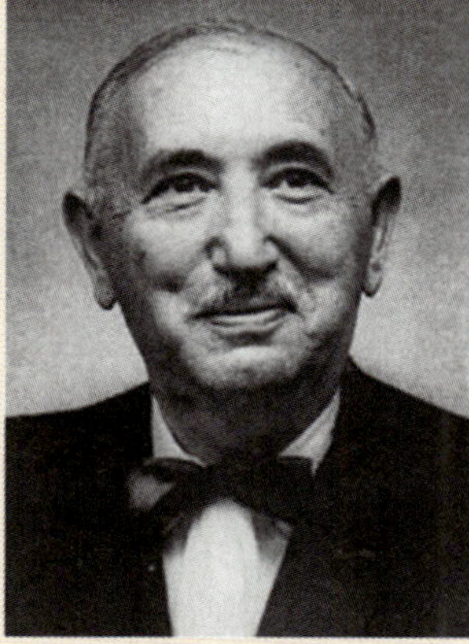

a. First rank symptoms of Schizophrenia
b. Psycho-somatic medicine
c. Psychoanalysis
d. Intelligence scales

ANSWERS WITH EXPLANATIONS OF IBQs

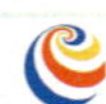

1. Ans. (b) 30 *[Ref. Neuropsychology by Goldstein, 1/e Pg 191]*

Mini-Mental Status Examination

- Description: A sensitive, valid and reliable 30-point questionnaire that is used extensively in clinical and research settings to measure cognitive impairment
- Scoring pattern:
  - **Highest score: Score 30**
  - Normal cognition: Score $\geq$ 27
  - MMSE Test components: [Mnemonic: COOLAR[3]]

Category	Possible points
Complex commands	6
Orientation to time	5
Orientation to place	5
Language	2
Attention and calculation	5
Recall	3
Registration	3
Repetition	1

2. Ans. (c) Stages of Psychosexual development *[Ref. Niraj Ahuja, 7/e p211-12]*

Five psychosexual stages of development (Sigmund Freud)

- Phase I. Oral Phase (Birth-1½ years)
- Phase II. Anal Phase (1-3 years)
- Phase III. Phallic/Oedipal Phase (3-5 years)
- Phase IV. Latency Phase (5-12 years)
- Phase V. Genital Phase (12 years - later)

3. Ans. (d) Intelligence scales *[Ref. Encyclopedia for World's Psychologists, p1568]*

David Wechsler (1896-1981)

- Developed Wechsler Adult Intelligence Scale (WAIS)
- Developed Wechsler Intelligence Scale for Children (WISC)

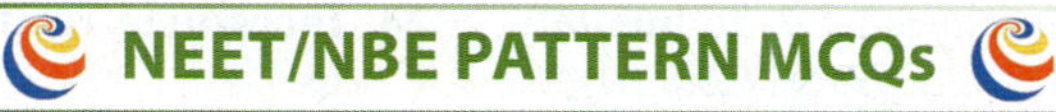

NEET/NBE PATTERN MCQs

1. A patient with IQ 30 is called *[Recent Question 2016]*
a. Mild mental retardation
b. Moderate mental retardation
c. Severe mental retardation
d. Profound mental retardation

2. Serial 7 subtraction is used to test *[Recent Question 2016]*
a. Working memory
b. Long term memory
c. Mathematical ability
d. Recall power

3. Which of the following are Sections of Mental state examination? *[Recent Question 2016]*
a. Mood and affect
b. Speech and language
c. Cognition
d. All the above

4. Bedside test for mental status *[Recent Question 2016]*
a. MMSE
b. GCS
c. MMPI
d. WAIS

5. Which is not used for Narcoanalysis?
a. Scopolamine
b. Hyoscine
c. Thiopentone
d. Ketamine

6. IQ is *[Recent Question 2016]*
a. Mental age/chronological age × 100
b. Chronological age/mental age × 100
c. Mental age + chronological age × 100
d. Mental age – chronological age × 100

7. IQ level of 45 is called *[NBE FMGE September 2005]*
a. Mild mental retardation
b. Moderate mental retardation
c. Severe mental retardation
d. Profound mental retardation

8. Mental retardation is diagnosed if IQ (Intelligence quotient) is less than *[NBE DNB 1998, 2005]*
a. 90
b. 80
c. 70
d. 60

9. Total score in Mini Mental Status Examination (MMSE) is *[Recent Question 2012]*
a. 25
b. 30
c. 32
d. 35

10. Mini mental status is *[JIPMER 2002, NBE DNB 2007]*
a. Method to investigate common psychiatric problem
b. 30-point programme to evaluate cognitive function
c. To evaluate schizophrenia
d. Instrument to measure delirium

11. Capacity to make a will is called *[NBE DNB 1992, 2003]*
a. Civic responsibility
b. Criminal responsibility
c. Testamentary capacity
d. Recreption order

12. Patient with IQ of 65 has *[AIIMS PGMEE 1995, NBE DNB 2004]*
a. Mild Mental Retardation
b. Moderate M.R.
c. Severe M.R.
d. Profound M.R.

13. Patients suffering from which of the following disease as per ICD/DSM criteria are eligible for disability benefit as per National Trust Act? *[All India PGMEE 2009, NBE DNB 2011]*
a. Schizophrenia
b. Bipolar disorder
c. Dementia
d. Mental retardation

14. Oedipal stage of mental development occurs at age of *[NBE FMGE September 2003]*
a. 2 years
b. 4-5 years
c. 5-6 years
d. 6-8 years

15. That part of mind which is working on reality principle is *[Recent Question 2017, Karnataka PGMEE 2001, NBE DNB 2004]*
a. ID
b. Ego
c. Super ego
d. Ego-ideal

16. Interpretation of dreams by Freud *[UP PGMEE 2001, Karnataka PGMEE 2002, NBE DNB 2003]*
a. 1990
b. 1900
c. 1956
d. 1919

17. True regarding mind theory is all except *[PGI 2008, NBE DNB 2011]*
a. Id is reservoir of instincts & drives
b. Ego is executive organ of id
c. Superego predominantly consciously offers approval & disapproval
d. Conscious is common component of id, ego & super ego

18. Fixation of Hysteria is *[WB PGMEE 2002, J & K PGMEE 2004, PGI 2005, NBE DNB 2003]*
a. Genital
b. Anal
c. Oral
d. Phallic

19. Severe mental retardation is *[Recent Question 2012, 2015]*
a. 50-70
b. 35-50
c. 20-35
d. <20

20. Stage of Psychosocial development Vs Conflict *[NBE DNB 1993]*
I. Oral (i) Autonomy versus shame
II. Anal (ii) Initiative versus guilt
III. Genital (iii) Industry versus inferiority
IV. Latent (iv) Trust versus mistrust

a. I (i), II (ii), III (iv), IV (iii)
b. I (ii), II (ii), III (iii), IV (iii)
c. I (iv), II (i), III (ii), IV (iii)
d. I (iv), II (iii), III (ii), IV (i)

21. What cut-off score of Mini-Mental State Examination (MMSE) is used to detect dementia? *[NBE FMGE September 2011]*
a. Less than 20
b. Less than 24
c. Less than 27
d. Less than 29

Psychiatry

22. Which of the following Genetic disorders leads to mental retardation? *[UPSC CMS 2015]*
a. Haemophilia
b. Phenylketonuria
c. Cystic fibrosis
d. Sickle cell anaemia

23. Most appropriate test for child psychologist to evaluate the intellectual ability of a 3-year-old is *[Recent Question 2017]*
a. Stanford Binet scale
b. Denver development scale
c. Alexander's pass along test
d. Rorschach inkblot test

24. Incestuous relationship between mother and son is called as *[Recent Question 2017]*
a. Oedipus complex
b. Electra complex
c. Family incest
d. None

25. Oedipus complex develops in which phase? *[Recent Question 2017]*
a. Oral
b. Anal
c. Genital
d. Phallic

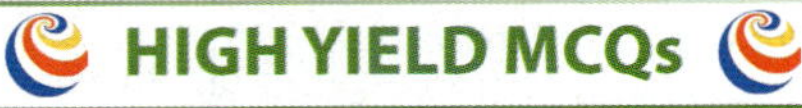

HIGH YIELD MCQs

1. MMSE examination is used for evaluation of *[AIIMS May 2016]*
a. Thought process
b. Mood and effect
c. Cognition
d. Insight

2. Oedipus complex (given by Sigmund Freud) is seen in *[PGI 1998, DPG 1998, Assam PGMEE 2004]*
a. Boys of 1-3 years of age
b. Girls of 1-3 years of age
c. Boys of 3-5 years of age
d. Girls of 3-5 years of age

3. In psychoanalytic terms, obsessive compulsive disorder is fixed at *[DPG 1998, TN PGMEE 2002, Maharashtra PGMEE 2003]*
a. Oedipal stage
b. Genital stage
c. Oral stage
d. Anal stage

4. According to Disabilities Act, 1995, seventh disability is usually referred to as? *[AIIMS November 2008]*
a. Neurological abnormality
b. Mental illness
c. Substance abuse
d. Disability due to road traffic accident

5. A 16-year-old male is found to have a mental age of 9 years on IQ testing. He has *[AIIMS May 2005]*
a. Mild Mental Retardation
b. Moderate Mental Retardation
c. Severe Mental Retardation
d. Profound Mental Retardation

6. X-linked disease leading to mental retardation is *[PGI 2000]*
a. Myotonic dystrophy
b. Fragile-X syndrome
c. Tuberous sclerosis
d. Phenylketonuria

7. In a child of IQ 50, which of the following is true? *[PGI 2001]*
a. Can look after himself independently
b. Can study up to eighth standard
c. Can follow simple verbal commands
d. Can handle money
e. Recognize family members

8. IQ - 40 level of mental retardation *[Recent Question 2012]*
a. Mild
b. Moderate
c. Severe
d. Profound

9. Following are major components of Mental Status Examination EXCEPT *[PGMCET 2015]*
a. Abstract Thinking
b. Test Judgment
c. Logical reasoning
d. Perceptual Disturbances

10. Mini-Mental State Examination (MMSE) is a screening instrument/test for *[PGMCET 2015]*
a. Depression
b. Dementia
c. Schizophrenia
d. Mania

11. New name of 'Mental retardation' according to American Association of Mental Retardation *[Recent Question 2018]*
a. Feeble Mindedness
b. Intellectual disability
c. Mentally unstable
d. Madness

Psychiatry

 NEET/NBE PATTERN MCQs ANSWERS WITH EXPLANATIONS 

1. **Ans. (c) Severe mental retardation**
   [Ref. Niraj Ahuja, 7/e p156]

2. **Ans. (a) Working memory**
   [Ref. Traumatic Brain Injury by Granacher, 3/e p138]

Uses of Serial 7 Subtraction Test

- Divided attention and concentration
- Working memory
- Poor auditory attention

3. **Ans. (d) All the above**
   [Ref. Psychiatric Mental Status Examination by Trzepacz, 1/e p11]

Sections of Mental State Examination

- Appearance, attitude, activity
- Mood and affect
- Speech and language
- Thought process, thought content, perception
- Cognition
- Insight, Judgment

4. **Ans. (a) MMSE**
   [Ref. Neurology in Clinical Practice by Bradley, 4/e p72]
   - Several versions of bedside mental status testing have been published with most widely used being Folstein's Mini-Mental State Examination (MMSE)

5. **Ans. (d) Ketamine**
   [Ref. Healthy Marriage by Swaroop, 1/e p91]

Narcoanalysis

- Truth-Serum test
- Principle:
  - Drugs used suppress reasoning power without affecting memory or speech
  - Subject's imagination is neutralized, reasoning faculty is affected making him semi-conscious
  - Person can respond to simple questions based on facts
  - Lying becomes difficult
- Drugs recommended: Seconal, Hyoscine (Scopolamine), Sodium pentothal, Sodium amytal, Phenobarbital

6. **Ans. (a) Mental age/chronological age × 100**
   [Ref. Niraj Ahuja, 7/e p156]

7. **Ans. (b) Moderate mental retardation**
   [Ref. Niraj Ahuja, 7/e p156]
   - *Categories of mental retardation based on IQ levels*:

Mental status	IQ range
Normal IQ	70 and over
Mild mental retardation	50 – 69
Moderate mental retardation	35 – 49
Severe mental retardation	21 – 34
Profound mental retardation	20 or below

Also Remember

- ***Sentience Quotient (SQ):*** Is a measure of the efficiency of an individual brain, not its relative intelligence
- ***Emotional Intelligence Quotient (EQ):*** Describes an ability, capacity, or skill to perceive, assess, and manage the emotions of one's self, of others, and of groups
- ***Social intelligence:*** Is the ability to understand and manage men and women, boys and girls, to act wisely in human relations

8. **Ans. (c) 70**
   [Ref. Niraj Ahuja, 7/e p156]

9. **Ans. (b) 30**
   [Ref. Neuropsychology by Goldstein, Pg 191]

Mini-Mental Status Examination

- Description: A sensitive, valid and reliable 30-point questionnaire that is used extensively in clinical and research settings to measure cognitive impairment
- Scoring pattern:
  - Highest score: Score 30
  - Normal cognition: Score ≥ 27
  - MMSE Test components: **[Mnemonic: COOLAR]**

Category	Possible points
Complex commands	6
Orientation to time	5
Orientation to place	5
Language	2
Attention and calculation	5
Recall	3
Registration	3
Repetition	1

10. **Ans. (b) 30-point programme to evaluate cognitive function**
    [Ref. Neuropsychology by Goldstein, Pg 191]

11. **Ans. (c) Testamentary capacity**
    [Ref. Niraj Ahuja, 7/e p230-31]
    - *Testamentary capacity*: To make a valid will, a person must have mental capacity to understand the meaning of material in the will

12. **Ans. (a) Mild Mental Retardation**
    [Ref. Niraj Ahuja, 7/e p156]

13. **Ans. (d) Mental retardation**
    [Ref. National Trust Website]
    - National trust works for People with,
      - Autism

- Cerebral Palsy
- Mental Retardation
- Multiple Disabilities

- Concerned legislation: The National Trust for the Welfare of Persons with Autism, Cerebral Palsy, Mental Retardation and Multiple Disabilities Act, 1999

14. Ans. (b) 4-5 years

[Ref. Niraj Ahuja, 7/e p211]

Phase III. Phallic/ Oedipal Phase (Stage III of Psychosexual Development)

- *Age range*: 3-5 years[Q]
- *Major site of gratification*: Genital area
- *Normal development*:
  - Males: Castration anxiety (replace father in mother's affections), Oedipus complex (aggressive impulses towards father)[Q], Oedipus rex (killing father, marrying mother)
  - Females: Penis envy (fantasy of loss of penis leading to female genitelia), Electra complex (identification with mother)[Q]
- *Disorders resulting due to fixation/regression to this phase*:
  - Sexual dysfunctions
  - Sexual deviations
  - Neurotic disorders

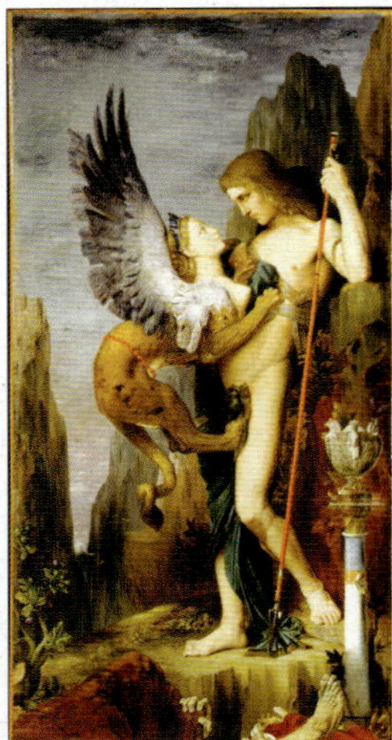

Fig. Phallic - Oedipal Phase

15. Ans. (b) Ego

[Ref. Niraj Ahuja, 7/e p206]

Structural Theory of Mind (FREUD)

- *The Id*: Original state of human mental status with which a newborn is born
  - Primary process: Unconscious containing basic drives and instincts concerned with survival, sexual drive and aggression
  - Pleasure principle
  - Lack link with reality
- *The Ego*: Conscious, intellectual, self-preservative and defensive functions of mental apparatus
  - Balance between the Id and the Super-Ego on one hand with reality on other
  - Guided by: The Reality principle
- *The Super Igo*: Unconscious division of mental apparatus developing from Ego
  - *The Ego-Ideal*: Approvals and rejections, involved in setting of goals and aspirations

16. Ans. (b) 1900

[Ref. Interpretation of Dreams Sigmund Freud (1900) by Sigmund Freud]

17. Ans. (c) Superego predominantly consciously offers approval & disapproval; (d) Conscious is common component of id, ego & super ego

[Ref. Niraj Ahuja, 7/e p206]

18. Ans. (d) Phallic

[Ref. Basic Psychoanalytic Concepts by Nagera, Pg 117]

Freud's Fixation Points in Neuroses

Condition	Fixation point
Hysteria	Phallic oedipal phase
Obsessional neurosis	Anal-sadistic phase
Psychoses	Phase of Auto-erotism & Narcissism
Paranoia	Stage of Narcissism
Schizophrenia	Beginning of course of Auto-erotism to love
Melancholia	Oral sadistic phase

19. Ans. (c) 20-35

[Ref. Niraj Ahuja, 7/e p156]

20. Ans. (c) I (iv), II (i), III (ii), IV (iii)

Comparison of Freud's & Erikson's Stage Theories

Age	Freud's stages	Erikson's stages
Infancy	Oral	Trust vs Mistrust
1.5-3 years	Anal	Autonomy vs Shame/Doubt
3-5.5 years	Phallic	Initiative vs Guilt
5.5-12 years	Latency	Industry vs Inferiority
12-18 years	Genital	Identity vs Role confusion
18-35 years		Intimacy vs Isolation
35 years-Retirement		Generativity vs Stagnation
Post-retirement		Ego identity vs Despair

21. Ans. (b) Less than 24

[Ref. Niraj Ahuja, 7/e p13]

Mini-Mental State Examination (MMSE)

- *Definition*: MMSE/Folstein test is a brief 30-point questionnaire test that is used to screen for cognitive impairment
- *Based on testing of*: Arithmetic, memory and orientation
- *Application*: Used for screening of dementia
- *Test features*: **[Mnemonic: COOLAR[3]]**

Category	Possible points
Complex commands	6
Orientation to time	5
Orientation to place	5
Language	2
Attention and calculation	5
Recall	3
Registration	3
Repetition	1

- *Scoring of MMSE*:

Score	Interpretation
30	Maximum total score
25-30	Normal

Contd...

Contd...

Score	Interpretation
21-24	Mild dementia
10-20	Moderate dementia
≤ 9	Severe dementia

22. Ans. (b) Phenylketonuria

[Ref. Mental Retardation by Olley, 3/e p135]

Common Genetic Disorders associate with Mental Retardation

- Phenylketonuria
- Galactosemia
- Homocystinuria
- Argininemia
- Lesch Nyhan disease
- Maple syrup urine disease
- Tyrosinemia
- Tuberous sclerosis
- Neurofibromatosis
- Rett syndrome
- Sturge Weber syndrome

23. Ans. (a) Stanford Binet scale

[Ref. Braddom's Physical Medicine and Rehabilitation, 5/e p49]

Tests for Intellectual Ability in Children

- Stanford-Binet Intelligence scale: 2 years to adulthood; Provides detailed diagnostic assessment including mental age and IQ, provides guidelines for motor/ visual/hearing handicaps
- Wechsler Preschool and Primary Scale of Intelligence Revised (WPPSI-R): 3-6.5 years age
- Wechsler Intelligence Scale for Children Revised (WISC-R): 6-16 years age
- Kaufmann Assessment Battery for Children: 2.5-12 years age

24. Ans. (a) Oedipus complex

[Ref. Niraj Ahuja, 7/e p211]

- Oedipus complex is the subconscious desire of a son for incestuous relations with his mother

25. Ans. (d) Phallic

[Ref. Niraj Ahuja, 7/e p211]

Phase III. Phallic/ Oedipal Phase (Stage III of Psychosexual Development)

- Age range is 3-5 years, with major site of gratification being genital area
- Normal development:
  - Males: Castration anxiety (replace father in mother's affections), Oedipus complex (aggressive impulses towards father), Oedipus rex (killing father, marrying mother)
  - Females: Penis envy (fantasy of loss of penis leading to female genitalia), Electra complex (identification with mother)

HIGH YIELD MCQs ANSWERS WITH EXPLANATIONS 

1. Ans. (c) Cognition

[Ref. Niraj Ahuja, 7/e p13]

- Most widely used cognitive outcome measure in dementia trials: **Mini-Mental State Examination (MMSE)**
- MMSE takes approximately 10 minutes to administer, can be administered by trained staff, and is relatively easy to interpret
- Do not to over-interpret MMSE scores, because low levels of education and speech impairment will reduce its validity

Also Remember

- MMSE tool can be used to systematically and thoroughly assess mental status
- It's a 11-question measure that tests 5 areas of cognitive function: Orientation, Registration, Attention and calculation, Recall, and Language
- **Maximum score is 30**
- Score of 23 or lower is indicative of cognitive impairment
- Score below 20 indicates definite cognitive impairment of dementia

2. Ans. (c) Boys of 3-5 years of age

[Ref. Niraj Ahuja, 7/e p211-12]

Five Psychosexual Stages of Development (Sigmund FREUD)

Phase	Age group	Normal development	Disorders
Phase I. Oral Phase	Birth-1½ years	• Oral erotic phase • Oral sadistic phase	• Alcohol dependence • Drug dependence • Schizophrenia • Mood disorders • Dependent personality disorder
Phase II. Anal Phase	1-3 years	• Anal erotic phase • Anal sadistic phase	• Obsessive compulsive disorders
Phase III. Phallic Phase (Oedipal Phase)	3-5 years	• Castration anxiety (males) • Oedipus complex (males) • Oedipus rex (males) • Penis envy (females) • Electra complex (females)	• Sexual dysfunctions • Sexual deviations • Neurotic disorders

Contd...

Contd...

Phase	Age group	Normal development	Disorders
Phase IV. Latency Phase	5-12 years	• Oedipus complex resolution • Electra complex resolution • Super-ego formation • Social goals formation	• Neurotic disorders
Phase V. Genital Phase	12 years - later	• Adult sexuality development • Release of parental control • Influence of peer groups	• Neurotic disorders

3. **Ans. (d) Anal stage**
   [Ref. Niraj Ahuja, 7/e p211-12]

4. **Ans. (b) Mental illness**
   [Ref. PRS Website, GOI]
   - *The Persons with Disabilities (Equal Opportunities, Protection of Rights and Full Participation) Act, 1995*:
     - *Seven disabilities*:
       1. Blindness
       2. Low vision
       3. Leprosy cured
       4. Hearing impairment
       5. Locomotor disability
       6. Mental retardation
       7. Mental illness
   - *The Rights of Persons with Disability Bill 2014*: Now replaces The Disability Act 1995
     - Covers 19 conditions

5. **Ans. (a) Mild Mental Retardation**
   [Ref. Niraj Ahuja, 7/e p156]

Mental retardation	IQ range
Mild MR	50 – 69
Moderate MR	35 – 49
Severe MR	21 – 34
Profound MR	20 or below

In the given question,
IQ = Mental age/Chronological age × 100;
so IQ = 9/16 × 100 = 56 IQ points
Thus, girl is having Mild Mental retardation

6. **Ans. (b) Fragile-X syndrome**
   [Ref. Niraj Ahuja, 7/e p157]
   - *Chromosomal causes of Mental retardation*:
     - Down's syndrome
     - Fragile X syndrome
     - Turner's syndrome
     - Klinefelter's syndrome

7. **Ans. (a) Can look after himself independently; (c) Can follow simple verbal commands; (d) Can handle money; (e) Recognize family members**
   [Ref. Niraj Ahuja, 7/e p156]

Type of MR	Referred as	Features
Mild MR	Educable	• Progress up to 6th class • Achieve vocational/ social sufficiency with support
Moderate MR	Trainable	• Reach up to 2nd class • Trained to support themselves • Work best in supervised occupational settings
Severe MR	Dependent	• Poor motor development • Markedly delayed speech • Can be taught to talk
Profound MR	–	• Associated physical disorders • Markedly delayed developmental milestones • Need nursing care or life support in structured environment

8. **Ans. (b) Moderate**
   [Ref. Niraj Ahuja, 7/e p156]

9. **Ans. (c) Logical reasoning**
   [Ref. Psychiatry by Young, p147]
   - *Major components of Mental Status Examination*: General appearance, Orientation, Speech, Motor activity, Affect and mood, Thought production, Thought content, Perceptual disturbance, Suicidal/homicidal ideation, Attention/Concentration/Memory, Abstract thinking, Insight/Judgement

10. **Ans. (b) Dementia**
    [Ref. Niraj Ahuja, 7/e p13]

Mini-Mental State Examination (MMSE)
- Definition: MMSE/Folstein test is a brief 30-point questionnaire test that is used to screen for cognitive impairment
- Based on testing of: Arithmetic, memory and orientation
- Application: Used for screening of dementia

11. **Ans. (b) Intellectual disability**
    [Ref. Psychiatry by Tasman, 4/e]
    - **"Mental retardation" (MR)** is a cluster of syndromes and disorders characterized by low intelligence and associated limitations in adaptive behaviour
    - WHO is in the process of revising the ICD-10 into ICD-11 (2018): Replacement of conceptualization of MR with the concept of Intellectual developmental disorders (IDD) in ICD-11
    - Also referred to as Intellectual and Developmental Disabilities

Psychiatry

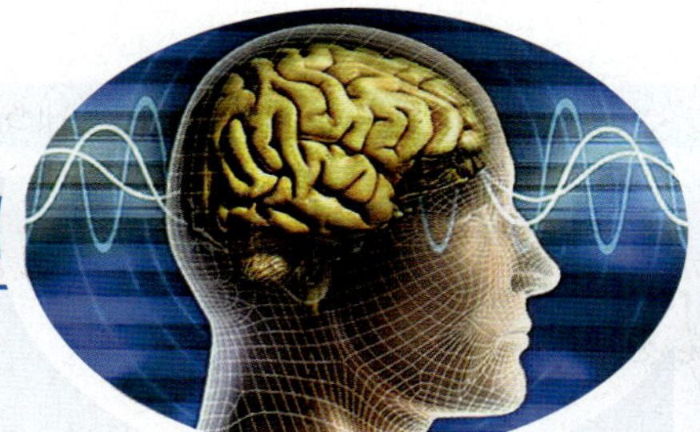

Chapter 3

Behavioral Sciences

THEORETICAL CONCEPTS

III A. PHOBIAS

- *Definition*: An irrational/morbid fear of a specific object/situation/activity which often lead to its persistent avoidance
  - Is a type of anxiety disorder[Q]
- *Underlying cause*:
  - Displacement: Psychodynamic theory (anxiety is transferred form a dangerous to a neutral object)
  - Conditioned reflex: Behavioral theory
  - Hormone release by amygdala: Neuro-biological theory
- *Types of phobias*:
  - Agoraphobia
  - Social phobia
  - Simple/Specific phobia
- *Treatment*:
  - Psychotherapy[Q]
  - Behavior therapy
  - Drug therapy
    - Benzodiazepines (Alprazolam- Drug of choice)[Q]
    - Anti-depressants (SSRIs Paroxetine- Drug of choice)[Q]

III A1. Agoraphobia

- *Characteristic feature*: **Irrational fear of being away from familiar setting of home**[Q]
  - Open spaces
  - Public places
  - Crowded places
- *MC group affected*: 20-40 years old females
- *Clinical presentation*: Classical symptoms of panic
  - Agoraphobia without panic disorder: Dizziness, tachycardia
  - Agoraphobia with panic disorder: Full blown panic attack
  - Severe dependence on Phobic companions (close relatives/ friends whom patient only leaves home with)
- *Associated disorders*:
  - Panic disorder
  - Obsessive compulsive disorder (OCD)
  - Post traumatic stress disorder (PTSD)
  - Separation anxiety disorder
  - Necrophobia (fear of death)

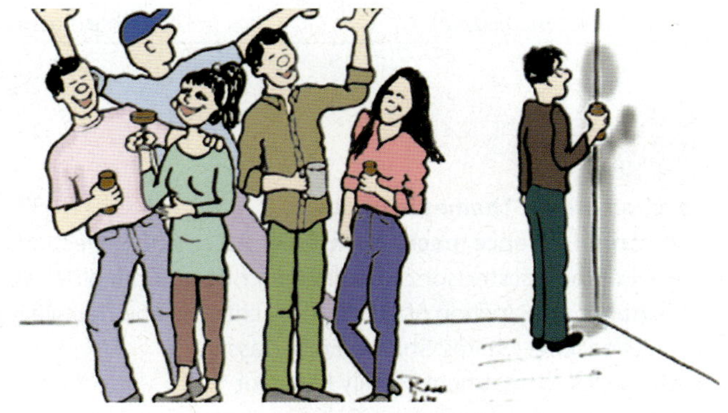

Fig. Agoraphobia

III A2. Social Phobia

- *Characteristic feature*: **Irrational fear of activities or social interactions in front of others**
- *MC group affected*: 20–40 years old females
- *Clinical presentation*: Classical symptoms of panic
  - Erythrophobia: Fear of blushing
  - Glossophobia: Fear of Public speaking
  - Stage fright: Fear of public performance
  - Shy bladder: Fear of urinating in public places[Q]
- *Associated disorders*:
  - Unipolar depression (Most common)[Q]
  - Panic disorder
  - Anxiety disorder
  - Post traumatic stress disorder (PTSD)
  - Substance use disorder
  - Suicide

III A3. Simple/Specific Phobia

- *Characteristic feature*: Irrational fear of objects or situations
  - Stimulus is well circumscribed
- *MC group affected*: Female children/adolescents
- *Clinical presentation*:
  - Avoidance due to anticipatory anxiety
  - Panic attack due to confrontation

III A4. List of Few Specific Phobias

Description	Phobia	
Fear of height	**Acrophobia**[Q]	
Fear of darkness	Nyctophobia	
Fear of animals	Zoophobia	
Fear of strangers	**Xenophobia**[Q]	
Fear of pain	Algophobia	
Fear of closed spaces	**Claustrophobia**[Q]	
Fear of medical procedures (needles, etc)	Trypanophobia	**Fig.** Acrophobia
Fear of sexual abuse	Agoraphobia	
Fear of spiders	**Arachnophobia**[Q]	
Fear of death	Necrophobia	
Fear of water	Aquaphobia	
Fear of doctors	Iatrophobia	
Fear of taking medication	Pharmacophobia	**Fig.** Claustrophobia

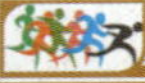

Topper's Edge

Psychodynamic Themes in Phobias

- **Principal defence mechanisms[Q]:** Displacement, Projection, Avoidance
- Environmental stressors: Humiliation/criticism from older sibling, Parental fights, Loss/separation from parents
- Features: Anticipation of humiliation, criticism and ridicule is projected onto individuals in environment
- Principal affect states: Shame, Embarrassment
- Obstacles to treatment: Family behavior
- Basic principle of treatment: Self-exposure to feared situation

III B. IMPULSE DISORDERS

- *Definition*: Impulsive behavior which patient cannot resist or control
- *Characteristic features*[Q]:
  - **Feeling of release of tension by act**
  - **Feeling of guilt after the act is over**

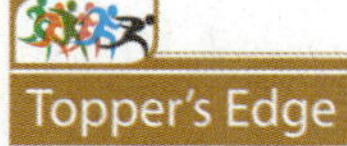

Topper's Edge

IMPULSE CONTROL DISORDERS

DSM-IV Impulse Control Disorders (ICDs) Classification

- ICDs not elsewhere specified: Intermittent explosive disorder, Kleptomania, Pyromania, Pathological gambling, Trichotillomania
- ICDs not otherwise specified: Impulsive-compulsive sexual disorder, Impulsive-compulsive self-injurious disorder, Impulsive-compulsive internet-usage disorder, Impulsive-compulsive buying disorder
- Other disorders with impulsivity: Childhood conduct disorders, Binge eating disorders, Bulimia nervosa, Paraphilias, Bipolar disorder, Attention deficit hyperactivity disorder, Substance use disorders, Cluster-B personality disorder, Neurological disorder with disinhibition

Core Features of Impulse Control Disorders (ICDs)

- **Essential features:** Failure to resist an impulse, drive, or temptation to perform an act that is harmful to the person or others
- **Before the act:** Person feels an increasing sense of tension or arousal
- **At the time of committing an act:** Individual experiences pleasure, gratification or relief
- **After the act:** Individual experiences sense of relief from urge; Individual may or may not regret, self-approach or guilt

III B1. Pathological Gambling

- *Definition*: **2 or more episodes of gambling per year** without any profitable outcome, continued despite personal distress and interference with daily functioning
- *Underlying cause*: Low levels of nor-epinephrine
- *Features*:
  - Intense urge to gamble
  - Preoccupation with thoughts and mental image of gambling
- *Association with other disorders*:
  - Substance use disorders
  - Anxiety and mood disorders
  - Personality disorders
  - Suicidal ideation
- *Treatment*:
  - Cognitive therapy
  - Exclusion therapy

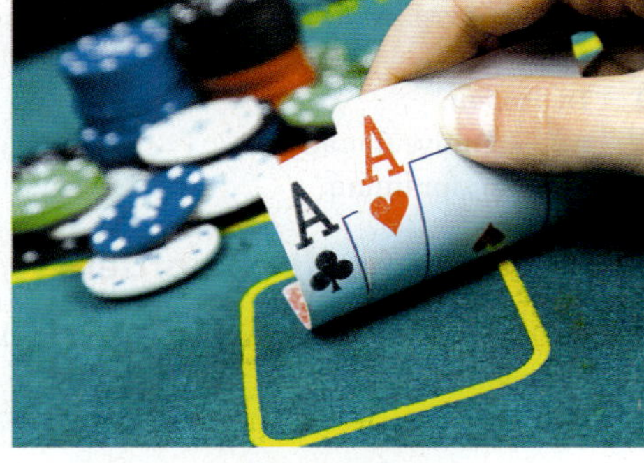

Fig. Gambling

III B2. Pyromania

- *Definition*: **2 or more episodes of fire-setting without a motive**[Q]
- *Underlying cause*:
  - Juvenile delinquency
  - Childhood sexual abuse
  - Parental neglect
- *Age group affected*: Male children and adolescents
- *Features*:
  - Intense urge to set fire[Q]
  - Feeling of tension before and sense of relief after the act[Q]
  - Preoccupation with thoughts and mental image of fire-setting[Q]
- *Treatment*:
  - Cognitive therapy
  - Psychotherapy

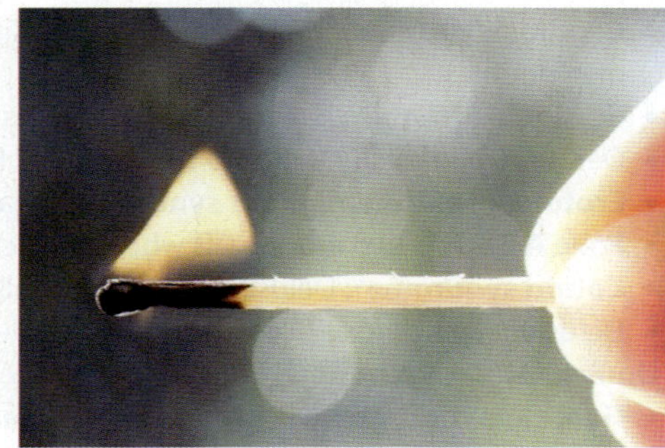

Fig. Pyromania

III B3. Kleptomania

- *Definition*: **2 or more episodes of theft of trivial items without a motive or personal gain**[Q]
- *Underlying cause*: Coexistence with Obsessive compulsive disorders[Q]
- *Age group affected*: Females with bulimia
- *Features*:
  - Intense urge to steal
  - Feeling of tension before and sense of relief after the act
- *Association with other disorders*:
  - Personality disorders (Schizoid, borderline, paranoid)
  - Carbon-monoxide poisoning
  - Traumatic brain injury
- *Treatment*:
  - Cognitive therapy
  - Rational emotive therapy

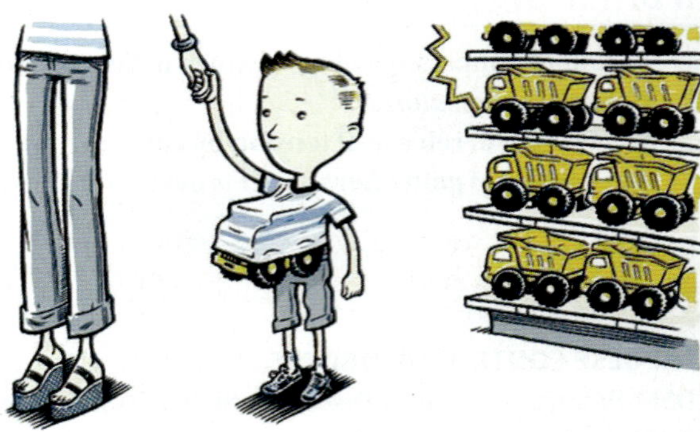

Fig. Kleptomania

III B4. Trichotillomania

- *Definition*: **Recurrent persistent impulse to pull out hair**
- *Underlying cause*: Coexistence with Obsessive compulsive disorders
- *Age group affected*: Early adolescent females
- *Features*:
  - Intense urge to pull out hair
  - Feeling of tension before and sense of relief after the act
  - Stress
  - Carpal tunnel syndrome
- *Association with other disorders*:
  - Anxiety
  - Depression
  - OCD
- *Treatment*:
  - Cognitive therapy
  - Clomipramine

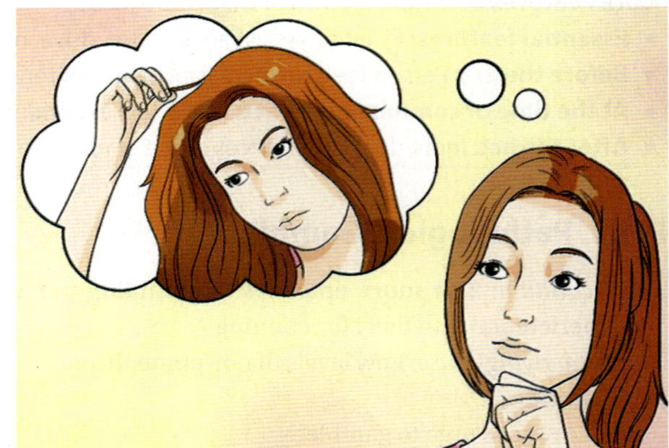

Fig. Trichotillomania

III B5. Other Impulse Disorders

- *Intermittent explosive disorder*: Extreme expressions of anger leading to rage
- *Onychophagia*: Compulsive nail biting
- *Dermatillomania*: Pathological impulse of picking skin

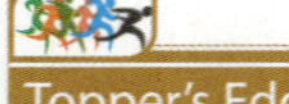

Topper's Edge

UNUSUAL PSYCHOTIC & NON-PSYCHOTIC SYNDROMES

Unusual Psychotic Syndromes

- **Capgras' syndrome[Q]:** Syndrome with delusional conviction that other persons in the environment are not their real selves but are their own doubles
- **Illusion de fregoli[Q]:** Patient falsely identifies strangers as familiar persons
- Delusion of infidelity **(Othello syndrome[Q]):** False belief that spouse/lover is having an affair without proof
- **Erotomania (Clerambault's syndrome[Q]):** False belief that another person is in love with him/her
- **Folie A Deux[Q]:** Two individuals who have a close relationship and shared delusions as seen in Paranoid disorder
- **Cotard syndrome[Q]:** Delusional belief that all body parts are rotten, decomposing or missing, or even dead
- Delusional parasitosis (Ekbom syndrome): Delusion of infestation

Unusual Non-psychotic Syndromes

- **Ganser's syndrome**[Q] (Hysteria pseudodementia[Q]): Approximate answers **(Vorbeireden**[Q]**)**—wrong answers but person understands the nature of question
- Couvade syndrome: Pregnancy symptoms in expectant fathers
- **Munchausen syndrome**[Q] **(Factitious disorder**[Q]**):** Intentionally produced physical symptoms[Q] with a purpose to obtain medical attention

III C. CAPGRAS' SYNDROME (DELUSION OF DOUBLES)[Q]

- *Definition*: Syndrome with delusional conviction that other persons in the environment are not their real selves but are their own doubles[Q]
- Capgras' syndrome is more common in females
- *Types of Capgras' syndrome*:
  - ***Illusion des sosies*** *(Typical Capgras' syndrome)*: Patient sees a familiar person as a complete stranger who is imposing on him as a familiar person
  - ***Illusion de fregoli*:** Patient falsely identifies strangers as familiar persons
  - ***Syndrome of subjective doubles*:** Patient's own self is perceived to be replaced by a double
  - ***Intermetamorphosis*:** Patient misidentifies completely (external appearance + personality)

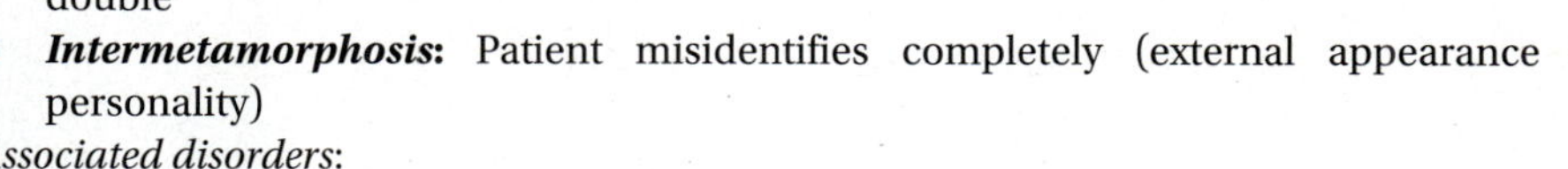

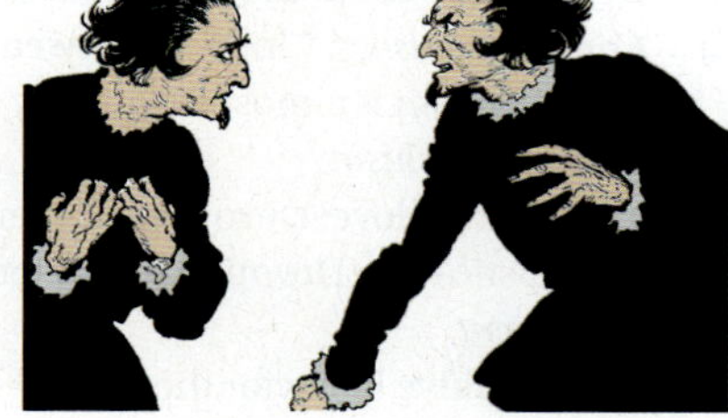

Fig. Capgras' syndrome

- *Associated disorders*:
  - Paranoid schizophrenia **(Most common)**[Q]
  - Brain injury
  - Dementia
  - Delusional disorders
  - Organic delusional disorders

III D. DELUSIONS

- *Definition*: Delusion is a false unshakeable belief/conviction despite presence of superior evidence[Q]
  - Certainty (absolute conviction)
  - Incorrigibility (not changeable even with proof)
  - Impossibility (not plausible)
- *Associated disorders*:
  - Schizophrenia
  - Paraphrenia
  - Bipolar disorder (during manic episodes)
  - Psychotic depression
- *Types of delusions*:
  - *Bizarre delusion*: Strange implausible delusion
  - *Non-bizarre delusion*: False but possible delusion
  - *Mood-congruent delusion*: Delusion with content consistent with depressive or manic mood
  - *Mood-neutral delusion*: Delusion not relating to emotional state
- *Themes of delusions*:
  - ***Delusion of control (passivity)*:** False belief that another person or external force controls one's general thoughts, feelings, impulses, or behavior[Q]
  - ***Nihilistic delusion*:** False belief that one does not exist or has become deceased[Q]
  - ***Delusion of infidelity (Othello syndrome)*:** False belief that spouse/lover is having an affair without proof[Q]
  - *Delusion of guilt*: False feeling of remorse or guilt of delusional intensity
  - ***Delusion of reference*:** Falsely belief that insignificant remarks, events, or objects in one's environment have personal meaning or significance
  - ***Erotomania (Clerambault's syndrome)*:** False belief that another person is in love with him/her
  - *Religious delusion*: Any delusion with a religious or spiritual content
  - *Somatic delusion*: A delusion whose content pertains to bodily functioning, bodily sensations, or physical appearance
  - *Delusional parasitosis*: A delusion where one feels infested with insects, lice, spiders, bacteria
  - *Delusion of poverty*: Strong belief that one is financially incapacitated
  - ***Delusion of persecution*:** Person believes that he/she is going to get harmed[Q]
  - ***Delusion of doubles (Capgras' syndrome)*:** Conviction that other persons in the environment are not their real selves but are their own doubles
  - *Autochthonous (primary) delusions*: Delusions arise de novo and cannot be explained on basis of other experiences
  - ***Hypochondriacal delusions*:** False belief that one is physically ill, in extreme form feeling of organs getting rotten/destroyed[Q]
  - ***Delusions of grandeur*:** False belief of one's own importance, power, or knowledge or that one is, or has a special relationship with, a deity or a famous person[Q]
- *Treatment*:
  - Psychotherapy
  - Anti-psychotics

III E. PARAPHILIAS – DISORDERS OF SEXUAL PREFERENCE

III E1. Fetishism

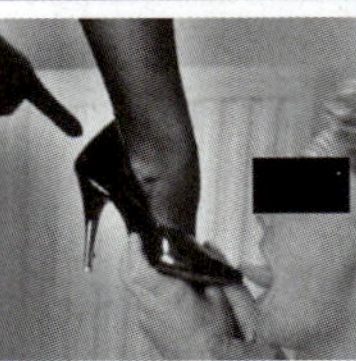
Fig. Fetishism

- *Definition*: **Sexual arousal occurs due to an inanimate object closely associated with human body**[Q]
- *Common fetishes*: Clothes, **footwear,** body parts, leather items
    - Fetishism is almost exclusively seen in males
- *Types of fetishism*:
    - Spiritual love: Devotion for mental phenomena
    - Plastic love: Devotion for material objects
- *Treatment*:
    - Cognitive behavior therapy
    - Psychoanalysis

III E2. Fetishistic Transvestism

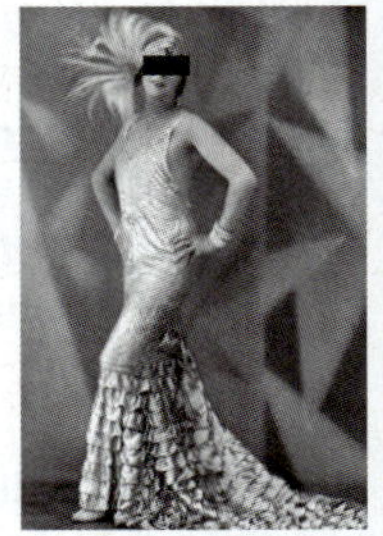
Fig. Transvestism

- *Definition*: **Sexual arousal occurs due to cross-dressing**
- Fetishistic transvestism is associated with fantasy of other males approaching a person who is in female dress
- It is not cross-dressing for entertainment of others

III E3. Sexual Sadism

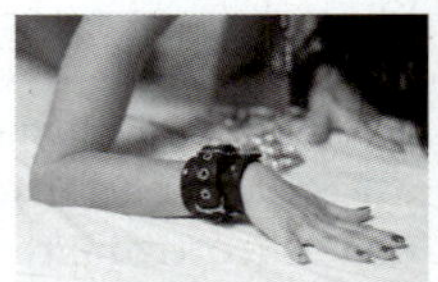
Fig. Sadism

- *Definition*: **Sexual arousal occurs due to physical and/or psychological humiliation of sexual partner** (victim) by a person (sadist)[Q]
    - Usually sadist is a male
- *Methods used*: Tying, beating, burning, cutting, stabbing, rape, killing

III E4. Sexual Masochism

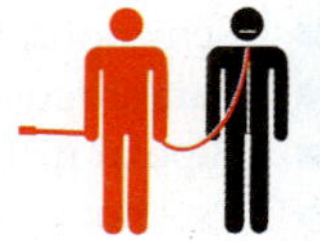
Fig. Sadomasochism

- *Definition*: **Sexual arousal occurs due to receiving of physical and/or psychological humiliation on self** by another person (sadist)[Q]

III E5. Exhibitionism

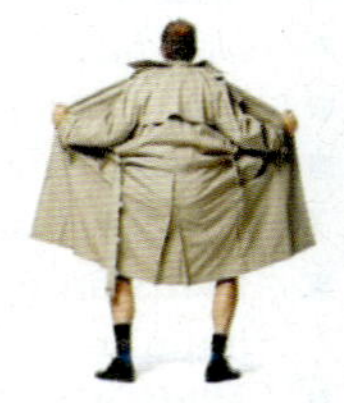
Fig. Exhibitionism

- *Definition*: **Sexual arousal occurs due to exposure of one's genitalia to an unsuspecting stranger**
    - Usually exhibitionist is a male
- *Types of exhibitionism*:
    - Flashing: Exposing breasts to strangers
    - Streaking: Running nude in a public place
    - Mooning: Exposure of buttock to strangers

III E6. Voyeurism

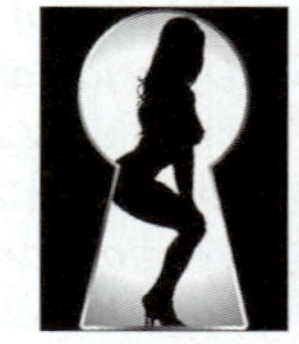
Fig. Voyeurism

- *Definition*: **Sexual arousal occurs due to observing other unsuspecting person disrobing, naked or engaged in sexual activity**[Q]
- Is spying on a person's intimate behaviors
- Usually voyeurist is a male

III E7. Frotteurism

Fig. Frotteurism

- *Definition*: **Sexual arousal occurs due to touching or rubbing against an unsuspecting non-consenting person**[Q]
- Is usually seen in crowded places
- Usually frotteurist is an adolescent male

III E8. Pedophilia

Fig. Pedophilia

- *Definition*: **Sexual attraction in a adult (>16 years age) to pre-pubescent children leading to sexual acts with them**[Q]
- Is a punishable offence in many countries

III E9. Bestiality (Zoophilia)

- *Definition*: **Sexual involvement with animals**[Q]
- May be associated with transmission of zoonoses

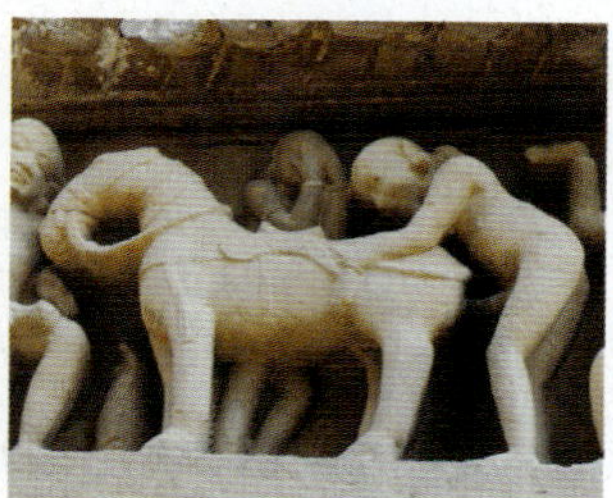

Fig. Bestiality

III E10. Other Paraphilias

Paraphilia	Feature
Urophilia[Q]	Sexual arousal with urine
Coprophilia[Q]	Sexual arousal with faeces
Necrophilia[Q]	Sexual arousal with corpses
Klismaphilia[Q]	Sexual arousal with enemas
Kleptophilia	Sexual arousal with stealing
Podphilia	Sexual arousal with feet

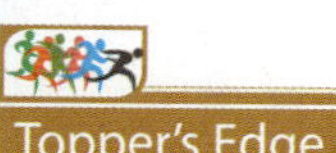

Topper's Edge

Treatment of Paraphilias
- External control
- Reduction of sexual drives
- Treatment of co-morbid conditions (Anxiety, Depression)
- Cognitive behavior therapy
- Dynamic psychotherapy

III F. OBSESSIVE COMPULSIVE DISORDERS (OCDS)

III F1. Definitions

- *Obsession*:
  - Idea/impulse/image repeatedly intrudes into conscious awareness
  - Recognised as one's own BUT perceived as ego-alien
  - Irrational and absurd
  - Patient tries to resist but fails to do so
  - Failure to resist leads to stress
- *Compulsion*:
  - Form of behavior following an obsession
  - Irrational, excessive nature of behavior
  - Used to prevent/neutralise stress
  - **'Insight is present'**[Q]
  - Subjective compulsion to perform

III F2. Underlying cause

- *Psychodynamic theory*:
  - Incomplete isolation of affect: Neutral ideas become anxiety provoking
  - Undoing: Leads to compulsions to prevent/allay feared consequences
  - Reaction formation: Lead to obsessive compulsive personality
  - Displacement: Lead to phobic symptoms
- *Behavioral theory*:
  - Obsessions are conditioned stimuli to anxiety
  - Compulsions are Learned behaviors to reduce anxiety
- *Biological theory*:
  - Hereditary
  - 5-HT system involvement
  - Lesion in cingulum/gyrus/temporal lobes

- Associated disorders
  - **Gilles de la Tourette syndrome**
  - Basal ganglia lesions
  - Von economo's encephalitis
  - Hypothalamic lesions
  - Third ventricle lesions

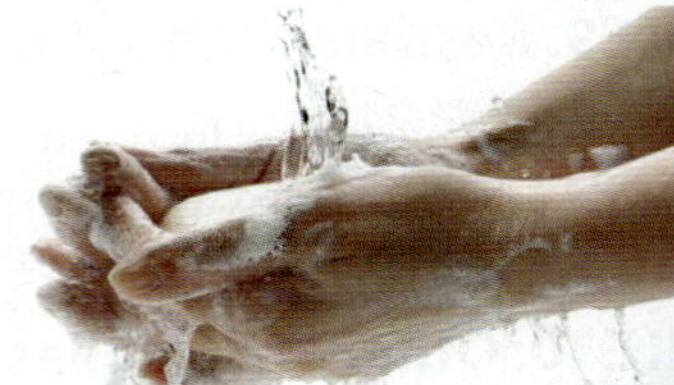

Fig. Washers

III F3. Clinical Syndromes of OCDs

- ***Washers*:**
  - *Occurrence*: **Most common type of OCDs**[Q]
  - *Obsession*: Contamination with dirt/germs
  - *Compulsion*: Repeated washing of hands/body/clothes/room/personal articles
- ***Checkers*:**
  - *Obsession*: Multiple doubts e.g. door has not been locked, kitchen gas left open, counting of money is wrong
  - *Compulsion*: Checking repeatedly to remove doubt
- ***Pure obsessions*:** Repeated intrusive thoughts/images/impulses WITHOUT compulsive acts
  - Content usually sexual or aggressive
  - Obsessions dealt by counter-thoughts
  - *Obsessive rumination*: Person constantly thinks about pros and cons of act
- ***Primary obsessive slowness*:** Severe obsessive ideas in absence of manifested anxiety

III F4. Scale used for OCDs

- **Y-BOCS** (Yale-Brown Obsessive Compulsive scale) Scale: Used for eliciting symptomatology and rating severity

III F5. Treatment

- Cognitive behavior therapy
- Drug therapy
  - **Benzodiazepines**[Q]
  - Antidepressants – **SSRIs:** Clomipramine, Fluoxetine[Q]
  - Antipsychotics
  - Buspirone
- Electroconvulsive therapy: Indicated if risk of suicide
- Psychosurgery

IMAGE-BASED QUESTIONS

1. **Identify the Behavioral syndrome as shown in Photograph** ***[Recent Question 2013]***

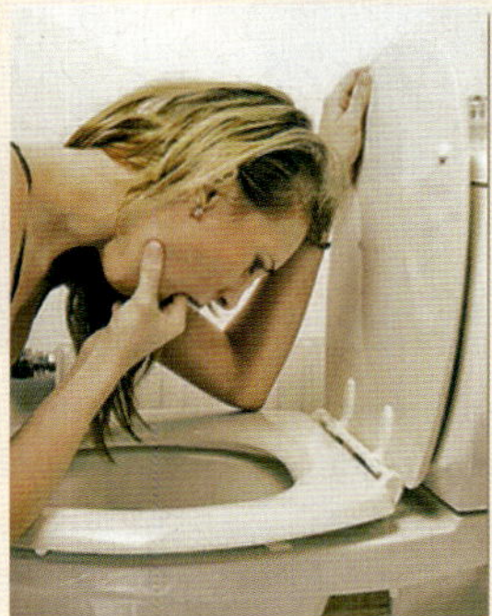

a. Anorexia nervosa
b. Bulimia nervosa
c. Obesity
d. Binge-eating disorder

2. **Fear of Situation shown in the Photograph is known as** ***[Recent Question 2012]***

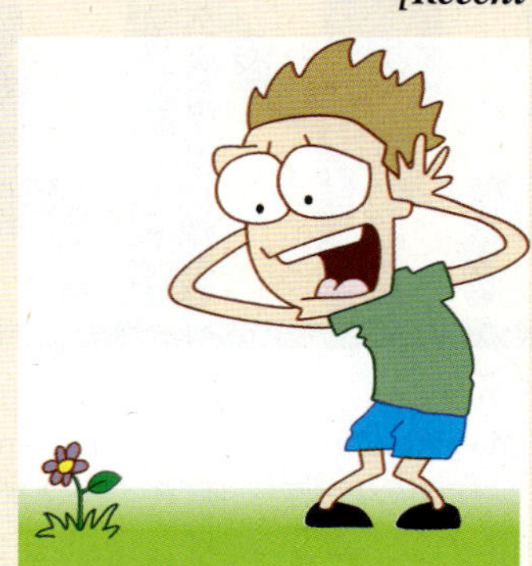

a. Xenophobia
b. Algophobia
c. Anthophobia
d. Claustrophobia

3. **Identify the Behavioral syndrome as shown in Photograph** ***[Recent Question 2013]***

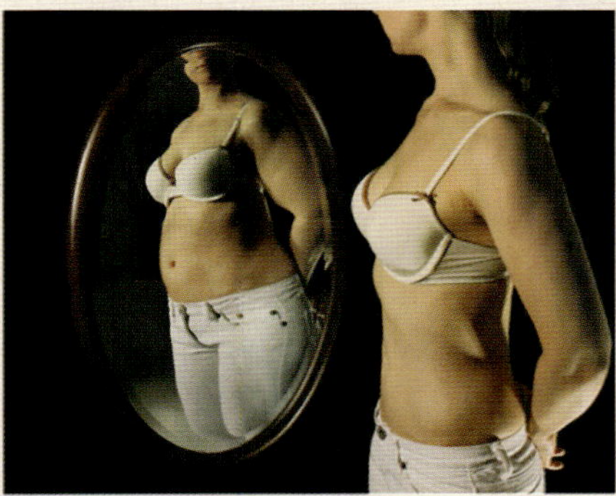

a. Anorexia nervosa
b. Bulimia nervosa
c. Obesity
d. Binge-eating disorder

4. **Diagnose the Underlying Skin disorder shown in the Photograph** ***[Recent Question 2012]***

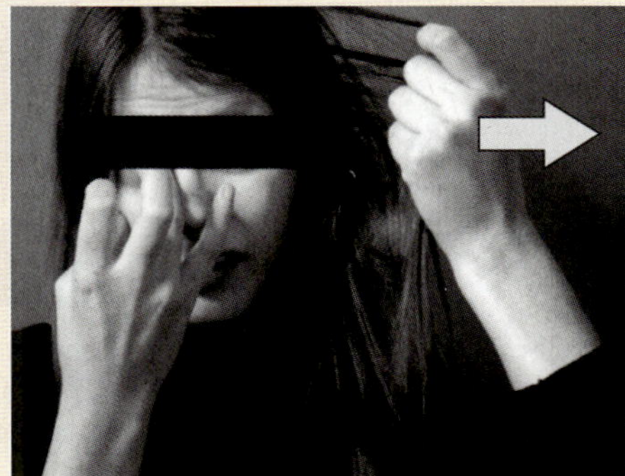

a. Traction alopecia
b. Trichotillomania
c. Telogen effluvium
d. Hirsutism

5. **Delusion of Doubles (Photograph) is characteristic of** ***[Recent Question 2013]***

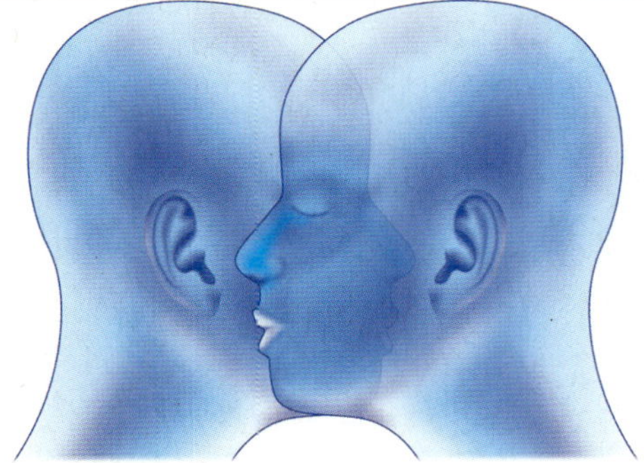

a. Xenophobia
b. Cotard syndrome
c. Capgras syndrome
d. Othello syndrome

6. **Identify Obsession seen in a Patient shown in Photograph**

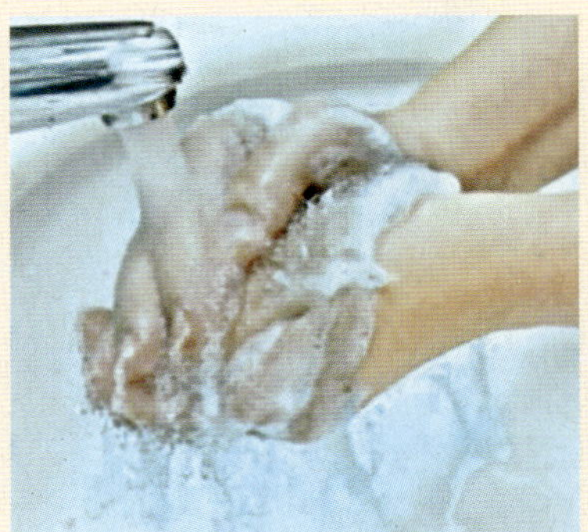

a. Checkers
b. Washers
c. Cleaners
d. None

Psychiatry

7. Identify Paraphilia shown in Photograph

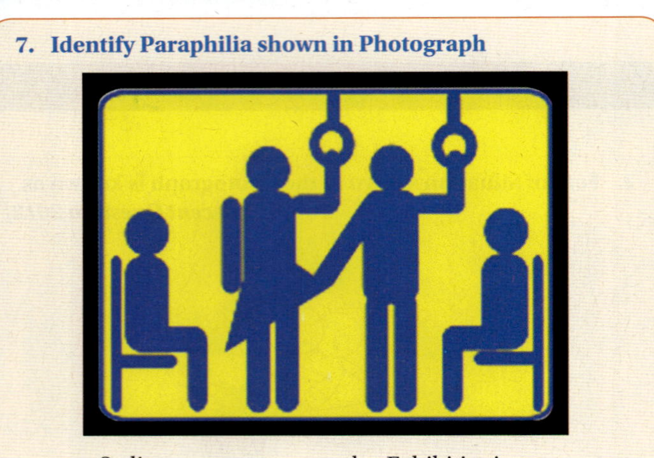

a. Sadism
b. Exhibitionism
c. Sexual masochism
d. Frotteurism

8. Identify Syndrome as shown in Photograph
[Recent Question 2013]

a. Fregoli Syndrome
b. Cotard syndrome
c. Capgras syndrome
d. Clerambaults' syndrome

9. Identify Syndrome as shown in Photograph

a. Xenophobia
b. Cotard syndrome
c. Capgras syndrome
d. Clerambaults' syndrome

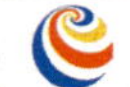

ANSWERS WITH EXPLANATIONS OF IBQs

1. Ans. (b) Bulimia nervosa *[Ref. Niraj Ahuja, 7/e p144]*

- Bulimia Nervosa: Early onset in teens/adolescence, Intense fear of becoming obese, Body-image disturbance, Persistent pre-occupation with eating, Irresistible craving with food, Attempts to counteract effects of over-eating, Self-induced Vomiting, Purgative/laxative abuse, Starvation

2. Ans. (c) Anthophobia *[Ref. Psychiatry by Namboodri, 3/e p210]*

- Xenophobia: Fear of strangers
- Algophobia: Fear of pain
- Anthophobia: Fear of flowers
- Claustrophobia: Fear of closed spaces

3. Ans. (a) Anorexia nervosa *[Ref. Niraj Ahuja, 7/e p142]*

- Anorexia Nervosa (Sitophobia): Onset in females adolescents, Intense fear of becoming obese, Body-image disturbance, Significant weight loss (>25%), Final weight <85% of original, Amenorrhoea (Primary/Secondary), Mood disorders (Depression, OCD), Hypothermia, Self-imposed dietary restrictions, Preoccupation with food, Self-induced vomiting, Hypokalemia, Bulimic episodes

4. Ans. (b) Trichotillomania *[Ref. Niraj Ahuja, 7/e p119]*

- Trichotillomania: Recurrent persistent impulse to pull out hair, generally seen in early adolescent females
- Features: Intense urge to pull out hair, Feeling of tension before and sense of relief after the act, Stress, Carpal tunnel syndrome

5. Ans. (c) Capgras syndrome *[Ref. Niraj Ahuja, 7/e p87]*

- Xenophobia: Fear of strangers
- Cotard syndrome: Walking Corpse Syndrome, a rare neuropsychiatric disorder in which people hold a delusional belief that they are dead, do not exist, are putrefying, or have lost their blood or internal organs
- Capgras syndrome: Delusion of doubles, that someone close has been replaced by an impostor
- Othello syndrome: Delusion of infidelity, a false belief that spouse/lover is having an affair without proof

6. Ans. (b) Washers *[Ref. Niraj Ahuja, 7/e p95-96]*

Washers

- MC type of Obsessive compulsive disorder
- Obsession: Contamination with dirt, germs, body excretions, etc.
- Compulsion: Washing of hands/body repeatedly many times a day

7. Ans. (d) Frotteurism *[Ref. Niraj Ahuja, 7/e p125]*

- Frotteurism: Sexual arousal occurs due to touching or rubbing against an unsuspecting non-consenting person
  - Is usually seen in crowded places
  - Usually frotteurist is an adolescent male

8. Ans. (a) Fregoli Syndrome *[Ref. Niraj Ahuja, 7/e p87]*

- *Fregoli delusion:* Delusion of doubles, is a rare disorder in which a person holds a delusional belief that different people are in fact a single person who changes appearance or is in disguise

9. Ans. (d) Clerambaults' syndrome *[Ref. Niraj Ahuja, 7/e p84]*

- Xenophobia: Fear of strangers
- Cotard syndrome: Walking Corpse Syndrome, a rare neuropsychiatric disorder in which people hold a delusional belief that they are dead, do not exist, are putrefying, or have lost their blood or internal organs
- *Capgras syndrome*: Delusional conviction that other persons in environment are not their real selves but their own doubles (impostors)
- *De Clerambault's syndrome*: Erotomanic delusions of a person that other person is in love with him.

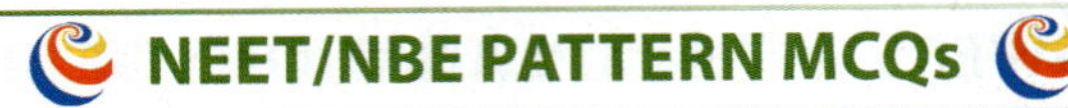

NEET/NBE PATTERN MCQs

1. Skinnerian conditioning is *[Recent Question 2016]*
a. Pavlov method b. Classical conditioning
c. Operant conditioning d. Stimulus response

2. All of the following are true about obsession except *[AIIMS May 2016]*
a. Continues to persist despite resistance
b. Can be present in schizophrenia
c. Comes under thought content in MMSE
d. Ego dystonic

3. 25-year-old gentleman has repeated thoughts that he has not locked his car door properly, frequently checks it while driving, he repeatedly checks locks in his house. Diagnosis *[Recent Question 2016]*
a. OCD b. OPCD
c. Phobia d. Personality disorder

4. Spouse jealousy is a feature of *[Recent Question 2016]*
a. Othello syndrome b. Chronic alcoholism
c. Stockholm syndrome d. Clerambault's syndrome

5. Which is the most common type of persistent delusional disorder? *[Recent Question 2016, 2017]*
a. Delusion of persecution b. Somatic delusion
c. Delusion of jealousy d. Delusion of grandeur

6. Which of the following is a Paraphilia? *[Recent Question 2016]*
a. Fetishism b. Sadism
c. Masochism d. All the above

7. Obsessive attention by an individual towards another person is called *[Recent Question 2016]*
a. Stalking b. Perceiving
c. Following d. Pressurizing

8. Following are the major symptoms of obsessive compulsive disorders *[Recent Question 2016]*
a. Contamination b. Pathological doubts
c. Intrusive thoughts d. All of the above

9. Woman firmly and persistently feels her husband is cheating on her and she disapproves to accept any proof given in the husbands support. The other family members do not support her belief. This is an example of *[Recent Question 2016]*
a. Illusion b. Delusion
c. Hallucination d. Perversion

10. Which of the following is/are a Thought disorder? *[Recent Question 2016]*
a. Circumstantiality b. Tangentiality
c. Prolixity d. All of the above

11. If a person is asked, "What will he do if he sees a house on fire"? Then what is being tested in that person *[Recent Question 2016]*
a. Social judgement b. Test judgement
c. Response judgement d. None of the above

12. Typical change in problem behavior shows how many stages? *[Recent Question 2016]*
a. 2 b. 3
c. 4 d. 5

13. More common in Binge eating compared to Bulimia nervosa is *[Recent Question 2016]*
a. Obesity b. Self-induced vomiting
c. Menstrual disorder d. Short duration

14. Psychosurgery is indicated in *[Recent Question 2016]*
a. Schizophrenia
b. Conduct disorder
c. Generalized anxiety disorder
d. OCD

15. Fear of strangers *[Recent Question 2016]*
a. Algophobia b. Xenophobia
c. Mysophobia d. Thanatophobia

16. Most common major symptom in obsessive compulsive disorder is *[Recent Question 2016]*
a. Compulsive washing of hand
b. Compulsive thinking about same
c. Compulsive checking
d. Obsessive precision

17. Obsessive personality disorder is also called *[Recent Question 2016]*
a. Anankastic b. Dissocial
c. Eccentric d. Histrionic

18. Following are true about Bulimia nervosa except *[Recent Question 2016]*
a. Uncontrolled eating
b. Overweight individuals
c. Depressive symptoms present
d. Sexually active patients

19. A person wanders in public places by removing his clothes it is called *[Recent Question 2016]*
a. Voyeurism b. Frotteurism
c. Exhibitionism d. Undinism

20. Abnormal fear of a particular situation is *[Recent Question 2016]*
a. Social phobia b. Simple phobia
c. Aerophobia d. Agoraphobia

21. Agoraphobia is fear of *[NBE FMGE March 2007, NBE FMGE September 2003, ESI IMO 2014, Recent Question 2017]*
a. Agar b. Strangers
c. Open spaces d. Closed spaces

22. Which of the following has been found to be useful in the treatment of tics, hair pulling, nail biting and skin pulling? *[NBE DNB December 2011]*
a. Social Skill Training b. Habit Reversal Training
c. Mindfulness d. CBT

23. Fear of closed spaces is called as *[NBE FMGE September 2006]*
a. Agoraphobia b. Xenophobia
c. Claustrophobia d. Acrophobia

24. Infidelity & jealousy involving spouse is the thought content of which of the following disorder? *[NBE DNB December 2011]*
a. Othello syndrome
b. Capgras syndrome
c. Hypochondriacal paranoia
d. De Clerambault's syndrome

25. Pyromania is a type of *[NBE FMGE September 2005, NBE FMGE March 2003]*
a. Phobia b. Impulse
c. Delusion d. Obsession

26. A 22-years-old medical student has a parotid gland abscess and an excessive number of dental caries. She is of normal weight for her height, but seems distressed when the doctor questions her about her eating habits. This young woman is most likely to be suffering from
a. Bulimia nervosa *[NBE DNB December 2011]*
b. Anorexia nervosa
c. Conversion disorder
d. Avoidant personality disorder

27. Capgras syndrome is *[NBE FMGE September 2005, Recent Question 2017]*
a. Delusion of love
b. Delusion of infidelity
c. Delusion of pregnancy
d. Delusion of doubles

28. The following symptoms are common in anorexia nervosa, except *[NBE DNB 1998, NBE DNB 2000]*
a. Weight loss b. Dehydration
c. Mood changes d. Menorrhagia

29. Panic attack is characterised by all except *[UPSC 2001]*
a. Fear of dying b. Visual hallucinations
c. Choking sensation d. Fear of losing control

30. Sexual stimulation obtained through some inanimate object is known as *[NBE FMGE September 2003]*
a. Transvestitism b. Fetishism
c. Voyeurism d. Zoophilia

31. All of the following may be seen in Anorexia Nervosa, except *[NBE DNB 2003]*
a. Repeated vomiting after meals
b. Increased commitment to work
c. Distortion of body image
d. Body weight < 85% of the predicted

32. Drug most useful in treatment of obsessive compulsive disorder is *[NBE DNB 1997, 2000, 2001, 2003, 2005, 2006, 2007]*
a. Amoxapine b. Fluoxetine
c. Doxepin d. Dothiepin

33. Learned behavior which is permanent but can be changed is *[NBE DNB 2010]*
a. Attitude b. Culture belief
c. Knowledge d. Practice

34. Commonest type of phobia seen in clinical practice *[NBE DNB 1992, 2004]*
a. Social phobia b. Simple phobia
c. Agoraphobia d. Claustrophobia

35. Which condition doctor is passive?
a. Classical psychoanalysis *[Recent Question 2012, 2015]*
b. Psychoanalytic psycoanalysis
c. Both
d. None

36. Phobia is defined as *[Recent Question 2012, 2015]*
a. Palpitation on thinking about a definite entity
b. Excessive unreasonable fear about a specific situation
c. Perception without stimulation
d. Altered perception

37. Oniomania is a disorder of compulsive *[Recent Question 2017, NBE DNB 2008, 2010]*
a. Stealing b. Gambling
c. Buying d. Hair pulling

38. Paranoid delusions are incompatible with diagnosis of *[NBE FMGE September 2003]*
a. Organic brain syndrome b. Involutional melancholia
c. Acute mania d. None of the above

39. Desensitization is a type of *[Recent Question 2012, 2013 , 2015]*
a. Psychotherapy b. Psychoanalysis
c. Behavioral therapy d. None

40. According to Freudian theory agoraphobia is due to *[NBE DNB 1992]*
a. Fear of father b. Fear of being promiscuous
c. Fear of strangers d. Fear of animals

41. Anorexia nervosa is characterized by all except *[UPSC 1996]*
a. Amenorrhoea b. Weight loss
c. Hypothermia d. Alopecia

42. Repetitive times work doing for premonition of *[Recent Question 2012]*
a. Obsession b. Compulsion
c. Anxiety d. None

43. Obsession is appearance of persistent and irresistible *[NBE FMGE March 2003]*
a. Thought b. Emotion
c. Impulse d. All of the above

44. Excessive eating followed by purging using Laxatives in a 20 years old females *[NBE DNB 2009]*
a. Bulimia nervosa b. Anorexia nervosa
c. Binge eating disorder d. Schizoprenia

45. Kleptomania means *[Recent Question 2013, 2015, 2017]*
a. Irresistible desire to set fire
b. Irresistible desire to steal things
c. Compulsive hair pulling
d. Pathological gambling

46. Agoraphobia is a disorder characterized by all, except
a. Visual hallucinations *[NBE DNB 2008]*
b. Avoidance of situations in which it occurs
c. Presence of panic symptoms
d. Avoidance of being outside alone

47. *"If I'm so persecuted then I must be someone of the great importance"* is *[NBE DNB 1992]*
a. Delusion of grandiosity b. Paranoid delusion
c. Nihilistic delusion d. Delusion of reference

48. Adverse effects of televised violence on the viewers are not mediated by *[NBE FMGE September 2011]*
a. Observational learning b. Operant conditioning
c. Disinhibition d. Desensitization

49. Pseudologia fantastica is typically seen in *[NBE DNB 1994, 1999, 2003]*
a. Alzheimer's disease b. Cotard's syndrome
c. Ekbom's syndrome d. Manchausen's syndrome

50. Delusion is a disturbance of *[NBE FMGE September 2011, Recent Question 2015]*
a. Form of thought b. Content of thought
c. Possession of thought d. Perception

51. Which of following statement differentiates the obsessional idea from delusions? *[NBE DNB 2009, Recent Question 2015]*
a. The idea is not a conventional belief
b. The idea is held in spite of contrary evidence
c. The idea is regarded as senseless by patient
d. The idea is held on inadequate ground

52. Delusion is a disorder of *[NBE DNB 2009]*
a. Thought b. Perception
c. Insight d. Cognition

53. A person who laughs one minute and cries the next without any clear stimulus is said to have *[NBE DNB 2009]*
a. Incongruent affect b. Euphoria
c. Labile affect d. Split personality

54. Which of the following is not a stage of reaction to impending death as described by Kubler-Ross? *[NBE FMGE March 2012]*
a. Denial b. Distortion
c. Depression d. Anger

55. Following is an Eating disorder *[Recent Question 2015]*
a. Enuresis b. Bulimia nervosa
c. Encopresis d. Tourette disorder

56. A 25-years-old male thought that he had accident and has injured someone. Now he is very fearful to drive car and he is repeatedly goes to that place where he thought that he had accident to check if no one is injured. Diagnosis is *[Recent Question 2015]*
a. OCD b. OCPD
c. A specific phobia d. Personality disorder

57. Excessive sexual desire in females is called *[Recent Question 2017]*
a. Nymphomania b. Satyriasis
c. Frigidity d. Impotency

58. Nihilistic delusion is *[Recent Question 2017]*
a. False feeling of remorse of guilt
b. False belief about severe medical illness
c. False belief that world is about to end
d. False belief that one is infested with small but visible organisms

59. A 25-years-old male is not happy with its gender and is always in distress due to this. He wants to change sex and have vagina. It comes under *[Recent Question 2017]*
a. Transsexualism b. Dual role transvestism
c. Gender dysphoria d. Sexual maturation disorder

60. Agoraphobia is most commonly associated with *[Recent Question 2017]*
a. Depression
b. Mania
c. Panic
d. Generalized anxiety disorder

61. Trichotillomania is a symptom of *[Recent Question 2017]*
a. Delusion
b. Obsession
c. Impulse
d. Compulsion

62. Flooding is method of treatment in *[Recent Question 2017]*
a. Phobia
b. Depression
c. Schizophrenia
d. Organic brain syndrome

63. Scatologia is *[Recent Question 2017]*
a. Eating disorder b. Sleep disorder
c. Paraphilia d. Defense mechanism

64. Sexual perversion in which one has the desire to see other person/wife having sex with others is *[Recent Question 2017]*
a. Sadism
b. Exhibitionism
c. Voyeurism
d. Fetishism

65. Phobia in elevator is an example of *[Recent Question 2017]*
a. Acrophobia
b. Social phobia
c. Claustrophobia
d. Algophobia

66. Arachnophobia is fear of *[Recent Question 2017]*
a. Dogs b. Spiders
c. Death d. Eating

67. Which of the following is Cotard syndrome? *[Recent Question 2017]*
a. Persecutory delusions
b. Religious delusions
c. Nihilistic delusions
d. Hypochondriacal delusions

68. Masturbation is also known as *[Recent Question 2017]*
a. Onanism b. Satyriasis
c. Autierection d. All of the above

69. Treatment modality used for Phobia is *[Recent Question 2017]*
a. Psychotherapy
b. Behavior therapy
c. SSRI
d. All of the above

70. Delusion of persecution is *[Recent Question 2017]*
a. Delusion of jealousy
b. Delusion of being cheated
c. Delusion of defective body part
d. Delusion of love

71. Pathological jealousy is *[Recent Question 2017]*
a. Delusion of infidelity b. Delusion of love
c. Delusion of double d. Delusion of grandiose

72. In OCD, if patient tries to resist obsession, then patient develops *[Recent Question 2017]*
a. Depression b. Mania
c. Anxiety d. Delusion

73. A 32-year-old female starts developing suspicion on her husband of having an affair with his secretory for 2 weeks. Diagnosis is *[Recent Question 2017]*
a. Illusion b. Delusion
c. Hallucination d. Delirium

74. Recurrent thoughts of doing something are known as *[Recent Question 2017]*
a. Obsession b. Compulsion
c. Preoccupation d. Confabulations

75. Aversion therapy is used in treatment of *[Recent Question 2017]*
a. Paraphilias b. Tribaldism
c. Cunnilingus d. Nymphomania

76. When a person I asked about his blood sugar level, he answers like "Diabetics have sweet urine... urine and feces are excreta"... Before finally telling his blood sugar. It is an example of? *[Recent Question 2017]*
a. Tangentiality b. Circumstantiality
c. Flight of ideas d. Loosening of association

77. A depressed patient thinks her intestines are rotten. It is an example of *[Recent Question 2017]*
a. Hallucination b. Illusion
c. Ekbom syndrome d. Nihilistic delusion

78. A girt falls in love with a film star & believes that he also loves her. It is best exemplified by *[Recent Question 2017]*
a. Persecutory delusion b. Grandiose delusion
c. Erotomania d. Nymphomania

79. A person thinks that others are implanting a machine on his head. It is an example of *[Recent Question 2017]*
a. Bizarre delusions b. Non-bizarre delusions
c. Hallucinations d. Illusion

80. A 40-years-old male always doubts his neighbor and fights with him without any reason. Rest behavior is normal. This can be due to *[Recent Question 2017]*
a. Delusion of grandiose
b. Nihilistic delusion
c. Delusion of persecution
d. Delusion of infidelity

HIGH YIELD MCQs

1. Which of the following statements is true for a diagnosed case of OCD? *[AIIMS November 2016]*
1. Repression and reaction formation are defence mechanisms
2. DOC is SSRIs
3. Risperidone can be used as an augmentation agent
4. Systemic desensitization is the psychotherapy of choice

a. 1 and 3 b. 1, 2, 3
c. 1, 4 d. 1, 2, 3, 4

2. Delusion is a disorder of *[Recent Question 2015, AIIMS PGMEE 2006, All India PGMEE 2007]*
a. Thought b. Perception
c. Insight d. Cognition

3. The primary delusion is disorder of *[All India PGMEE 1999]*
a. Thought
b. Perception
c. Loosening of association
d. Memory

4. Persistent belief in something which is not a fact is *[USPC 1995, WB PGMEE 2001]*
a. Illusion b. Hallucination
c. Delusion d. Delirium

5. Three years back a woman suffered during an earthquake and she was successfully saved. Meter recovery she has nightmares about the episode and she also gets up in the night and feels terrified. The most probable diagnosis is *[AIIMS PGMEE 2002]*
a. Major depression
b. Post-traumatic stress disorder
c. Mania
d. Schizophrenia

6. True for PTSD are all except *[PGI 2001]*
a. Past h/o psychiatric illness
b. Women are more predisposed
c. Occur in intelectuals
d. Numbness
e. Detachment

7. A lady while driving a car meet with an accident. She was admitted in an ICU for 6 months. After being discharged, she often gets up in night and feels terrified and has fear to sit in car again. The diagnosis is *[AIIMS PGMEE 1999, All India PGMEE 2000]*
a. Panic Attack
b. Phobia
c. Conversion Disorder
d. Post Traumatic stress Disorder

8. A false belief unexplained by reality, shared by a number of people is *[JIPMER PGMEE 1998, AIIMS PGMEE 2003, AIIMS PGMEE 2004]*
a. Superstition
b. Illusion
c. Delusion
d. Obsession

9. A person of 35 years is having firm belief about infidelity involving the spouse. And he never allows her to go out of home alone. He often locks his house, while going office. Inspite of this entire, he is persistently suspicious about her character. The probable diagnosis is

a. Schizophrenia [AIIMS PGMEE 1999]
b. Delusional parasitosis
c. Clerambault's syndrome
d. Othello syndrome

10. Delusion that someone from high socioeconomic status is loving you is in *[PGI 1998]*
a. Othello syndrome
b. Capgras syndrome
c. De Clerambault syndrome
d. Franklin syndrome

11. Infidelity & jealousy involving spouse is the thought content of which disorder? *[PGI 1999, All India PGMEE 1998, Recent Question 2014, 2017]*
a. Capgras syndrome
b. Othello syndrome
c. Hypochondrial paranomia
d. Declerambault's syndrome

12. Which of the following is not a cognitive error/dysfunction? *[All India PGMEE 2010]*
a. Catastrophic thinking b. Arbitrary inference
c. Overgeneralization d. Thought block

13. Psychodynamic theory of mental illness is based on *[Recent Question 2015, AIIMS PGMEE 2007]*
a. Unconscious internal conflict
b. Maladjusted reinforcement
c. Organic neurological problem
d. Focus on teaching patient to restrain absurd thoughts

14. A man hits his neighbour next day he feels that police is behind him and his brain is being controlled by radio waves by his neighbour. The probable diagnosis is *[All India PGMEE 2000]*
a. Personality disorder b. Passivity feeling
c. Delusion of persecution d. Organic brain syndrome

15. Basanti 27 years old female thinks her nose is ugly. Her idea is fixed and not shared by anyone else. Whenever she goes out of home she hides her face. She visits a surgeon for plastic surgery. Next step would be *[All India PGMEE 2001]*
a. Investigate & then operate
b. Reassure the patient
c. Immediate operation
d. Refer to psychiatrist

16. A 41 year old woman working as an Executive Director is convinced that the management has denied her promotion by preparing false reports about her competence and have forged her signature on sensitive documents so as to convict her. She files a complaint in the police station and requests for security. Despite all this she attends to her work and manages the household. She is suffering from *[All India PGMEE 2004]*
a. Paranoid Schizophrenia
b. Late onset Psychosis
c. Persistent Delusional Disorder
d. Obsessive Compulsive Disorder

17. Patient of contamination phobia was asked by therapist to follow behind and touch everything he touches in patient's house. Therapist kept talking quietly & calmly all the time. And the patient was asked to repeat the procedure twice daily. The procedure is *[AIIMS PGMEE 2010]*
a. Flooding b. Modelling
c. Positive reinforcement d. Aversion therapy

18. Behavior therapy to change maladaptive behavior using response as reinforcer uses the principles of *[All India PGMEE 2003]*
a. Classical conditioning b. Modeling
c. Social learning d. Operant conditioning

19. Operant condition where paradigm pain stimulus are given to a child for decreasing a certain undesired behavior can be classified as *[All India PGMEE 1997]*
a. Positive Reinforcement b. Negative reinforcement
c. Punishment d. Negotiation

20. Delusion of infidelity of part of the sexual partner is known as *[JIPMER PGMEE 1990, NIMHANS PGMEE 1994]*
a. De Clerambault's syndrome
b. Couvade syndrome
c. Othello syndrome
d. Ekbom's syndrome

21. Delusion of persecution occur in *[PGI 2009]*
a. Schizophrenia b. Paranoid psychosis
c. Manic episode d. Melancholia
e. Megalomania

22. Delusions are seen in all the following except
a. Obsessive compulsive disorder *[SGPGI 2002]*
b. Depression
c. Mania
d. Schizophrenia

23. Loosening of association is an example of *[All India PGMEE 2006]*
a. Formal thought disorder
b. Schneider's first symptoms
c. Perseveration
d. Concrete thinking

24. Many of our bad habits of day to day life can be removed by *[AIIMS PGMEE 2004]*
a. Positive conditioning b. Negative conditioning
c. Bio feed back d. Generalization

25. Delusions are characteristically seen in *[All India PGMEE 1993]*
a. Schizophrenia b. Delirium
c. Dementia d. Depression

26. Delusion of doubles is found in *[AIIMS PGMEE 1999]*
a. Schizo-affective Disorder
b. Capgras' syndrome
c. Reactive psychosis
d. Paranoid schizophrenia

27. The content of thought in delusional paranoia is
a. Erotic b. Infidelity *[PGI 1997]*
c. Love d. Foul odour

28. The features of OCD are A/E *[All India 1993, Recent Question 2015]*
a. Irrational thought b. Egosyntonic
c. Resisting the idea d. Persistence of idea

29. Abnormal thought possession is found in
a. Organic Brain syndrome *[All India PGMEE 1994]*
b. Hysteria
c. Obsessive compulsive disorder
d. Neuroasthenia

30. Defence mechanism in OCD *[PGI 2007]*
a. Repression b. Undoing
c. Rationalization d. Sublimate
e. Displacement

31. Most appropriate treatment of panic disorder is *[AIIMS PGMEE 2009, Recent Question 2017]*
a. Buspirone + Benzodiazepine
b. Benzodiazepine + Supportive therapy
c. Short term benzodiazepine + SSRI + CBT
d. Long term BDZ + Venalafexine

32. Drugs used in generalized anxiety disorder are
a. Alprazolum b. Paroxetine *[PGI 2007]*
c. Venlafaxine d. Buspirone
e. Carbamazepine

33. Thanatophobia is fear of *[UP PGMEE 1998]*
a. Closed spaces b. Flights
c. High places d. Death

34. Claustrophobia means *[JIPMER PGMEE 1995]*
a. Fear of heights b. Fear of lizards
c. Fear of closed spaces d. Fear of open spaces

35. Acrophobia is *[SGPGI 2003]*
a. Getting caught in places from where escape would be difficult
b. Fear of heights
c. Fear of animals
d. Fear of closed spaces

36. Definitive treatment of all types of phobias *[PGI 2008]*
a. Behavior therapy b. Social therapy
c. Avoidance d. Drug therapy

37. Differential diagnosis of panic disorder *[PGI 2004]*
a. Pheochromocytoma b. Myocardial infarction
c. Mitral valve prolapse d. Depression
e. Carcinoid syndrome

38. Treatment of Choice in Phobic disorder *[AIIMS PGMEE 1994, Assam PGMEE 1999]*
a. Psychotherapy b. Benzodiazepines
c. Behavior therapy d. 5-HT reuptake inhibitor

39. Agoraphobia treated with *[PGI 2007]*
a. Systemic desensitization b. Psychodynamic therapy
c. Exposure therapy d. Relaxation therapy
e. Behavior therapy

40. Features of obsessive-compulsive neurosis are
a. Repetitiveness b. Irresistibility *[PGI 2002]*
c. Unpleasantness d. Poor personal care

41. True about obsessive compulsive disorder is/are
a. Irresistible desire to do a thing repeatedly *[PGI 2001]*
b. Is a dissociative disorder
c. Denial is the defence mechanism against OCD
d. Patient is conscious about the disorder
e. Can cause severe distress

42. Transmitters mainly involved in OCN is
a. GABA b. NE *[AIIMS PGMEE 1995]*
c. Dopamine d. Serotonin

43. An obsessive compulsive neurosis patient is likely to develop *[AIIMS PGMEE 1993]*
a. Hallucination b. Depression
c. Delusion d. Schizophrenia

44. Obsessive Compulsive Neurosis patient is likely to progress into *[AIIMS PGMEE 1990]*
a. Paranoia b. Endogenous Depression
c. Secondary Depression d. Dissociation

45. Treatment of choice for OCD *[MP PGMEE 2006]*
a. Behavior therapy
b. Drug therapy
c. Psychosurgery
d. Combination of behavior and drug therapy

46. In obsessive compulsive disorder, which is not given? *[JHARKHAND PGMEE 2006]*
a. Clormipramine b. Haloperidol
c. Sertaline d. Carbamazepine

47. In OCD treatment is based on *[Bihar PGMEE 2005]*
a. Serotonergic receptor b. Dopaminergic receptor
c. NA receptor d. Glutamate receptor

48. For severe intractable obsessional neurosis the psycho-surgery of choice is *[PGI 1990]*
a. Rifrontal tractotomy b. Cingulotomy
c. Amygdalotomy d. Temporal lobe lesion

49. Drug of choice for Obsessive Compulsive Disorder *[AIIMS PGMEE 2010]*
a. Imipramine b. Fluoxetine
c. Nortryptiline d. Clomipramine

50. Drug of choice for Obsessive Compulsive Neurosis is *[All India PGMEE 1993, 1994, 1996, 1998, JHARKHAND PGMEE 2005, JIPMER 1995]*
a. Imipramine b. Chlorpromazine
c. Carbamazepine d. Clomipramine

51. Drug of choice for Panic Disorder *[AIIMS PGMEE 1994]*
a. Fluoxetine b. Lithium
c. Diazepam d. Chlorpromazine

52. Phobia is *[All India PGMEE 1998, JHARKHAND PGMEE 2005, Assam PGMEE 1997]*
a. Psychosis b. Anxiety
c. Fear of animal d. Neurosis

53. Agoraphobia is *[SGPGI 2003]*
a. Getting caught in places from where escape would be difficult
b. Fear of heights
c. Fear of animals
d. Fear of closed spaces

54. All drugs are used for treatment of OCD except *[PGI 1999, JIPMER PGMEE 2002]*
a. Carbamazepine b. Lithium
c. Fluoxetine d. Diazepam

55. All are treatment modalities of OCD except *[All India PGMEE 1996]*
- a. Exposure & response prevention
- b. Psychoanalytic psychotherapy
- c. Clomipramine
- d. MAO inhibitors

56. Excessive sexual desire in males is known as *[Recent Question 2017, AIIMS PGMEE 2008]*
- a. Nymphomania
- b. Satyriasis
- c. Tribadism
- d. Sadism

57. Squeeze Technique is used for *[All India PGMEE 2000, Recent Question 2017]*
- a. Impotence
- b. Premature ejaculation
- c. Infertility
- d. Priaprism

58. Most accurate treatment of erectile dysfunction *[PGI 2002]*
- a. Sildenafil
- b. Master and Johnson technique
- c. B-blockers
- d. Papaverine

59. Kleptomania is *[PGI 2007]*
- a. Delusion
- b. Obsession
- c. Impulse
- d. Compulsion
- e. Hallucination

60. Kleptomania means *[All India PGMEE 1999]*
- a. Irresistible desire to set fire
- b. Irresistible desire to steal things
- c. Compulsive hair pulling
- d. Pathological gambling

61. All of the following are impulse control disorders except *[All India PGMEE 2003]*
- a. Pyromania
- b. Trichotillomania
- c. Kleptomania
- d. Capgras' syndrome

62. Oniomania is a disorder of compulsive *[JIPMER PGMEE 2000]*
- a. Buying
- b. Cellular phone use
- c. Internet use
- d. Self mutation

63. Which of the following is not a common feature of Anorexia Nervosa? *[All India PGMEE 2006]*
- a. Binge eating
- b. Amenorrhoea
- c. Self perception of being fat
- d. Under weight

64. With regard to anorexia nervosa the following is true except *[Recent Question 2015, Kerala PGMEE 2000]*
- a. Phobic avoidance of normal weight
- b. Over-perception of body image
- c. Self induced vomiting
- d. Menorrhagia
- e. Excessive exercise

65. False regarding Anorexia Nervosa *[Kerala PGMEE 1997, Recent Question 2015]*
- a. Evident psychosis
- b. Vigour exceeding physical ill being
- c. Weight loss
- d. Decreased appetite

66. A young lady is present with H/O repeated episode of over eating (binge) followed by purging using laxatives she probably suffering from *[AIIMS PGMEE 2010, All India PGMEE 2007, UP PGMEE 2004, J&K PGMEE 2001]*
- a. Bulimia nervosa
- b. Schizophrenia
- c. Anorexia pervosa
- d. Benign eating disorders

67. Drug of choice for OCD is *[PGI 2005]* *[Recent Question 2017]*
- a. Fluoxetine
- b. Imipramine
- c. Diazepam
- d. Haloperidol

68. Delusion is *[TN PGMEE 1998, Karnataka PGMEE 2003]*
- a. Comprehensible
- b. Reasonable
- c. Both
- d. None

69. The following is suggestive of an organic cause of the behavioral symptoms *[All India PGMEE 2002]*
- a. Formal thought disorder
- b. Auditory hallucinations
- c. Delusion of fruit
- d. Prominent visual hallucination

70. A person who laughs one minute and cries the next without any clear stimulus is said to have *[AIIMS PGMEE 2005]*
- a. Incongruent effect
- b. Euphoria
- c. Labile affect
- d. Split personality

71. Kallu a 24 year old occasional alcoholic had got a change in behavior. He has become suspicious that people are trying to conspire against him, though his father states that there is no reason for his fears. He is getting hallucinations of voices commenting on his actions. What is most probable diagnosis? *[AIIMS PGMEE 2000]*
- a. Delirium tremens
- b. Alcohol induced psychosis
- c. Schizophrenia
- d. Delusional disorder

72. Delusion is disorder of *[AIIMS PGMEE 1997, Jharkhand PGMEE 2004]*
- a. Perception
- b. Memory
- c. Thinking
- d. Intelligence

73. A 25-year-old university student had a fight with the neighboring boy. On the next day while out, he started feeling that two men in police uniform were observing this movements. When he reached home in the evening he was frightened. He expressed that police was after him and would arrest him. His symptoms represent *[AIIMS PGMEE 2003]*
- a. Delusion of persecution
- b. Ideas of reference
- c. Passivity
- d. Thought insertion

74. A patient complains that people living upstairs are always talking about him and conspires against him. His son complains about his weird behavior like keeping shoes in Fridge and wearing vest over shirt. The likely diagnosis is *[AIIMS PGMEE 1999]*
- a. Depression
- b. Delusional disorder
- c. Dementia
- d. Schizophrenia

75. A man hits his neighbour. Next day he feels that police is behind him and his brain is being controlled by radio waves by his neighbour. The probable diagnosis is *[AIIMS PGMEE 1999]*
- a. Thought insertion
- b. Passivity feeling
- c. Delusion of persecution
- d. Obsessive Compulsive Disorder

76. Delusion is not present in *[All India PGMEE 2002]*
a. Delirium b. Mania
c. Depression d. Compulsive disorder

77. Delusion is not seen in *[Recent Question 2017, JIPMER PGMEE 1990, JIPMER PGMEE 1995]*
a. Depression b. Anxiety
c. Schizophrenia d. Mania

78. Which of the following is a stage of intuitive thoughts appearance in Jean-Piaget scheme? *[PGI 1999]*
a. Sensorimotor b. Concrete
c. Preoperational stage d. Formal operations stage

79. A 30-year-old unmarried woman from a low socio-economic status family believes that a rich boy staying in her neighbourhood is in deep love with her. The boy clearly denies his love towards this lady. Still the lady insists that his denial is a secret affirmation of his love towards her. She makes desperate attempts to meet the boy despite resistance from her family. She also develops sadness at times when her effort to meet the boy does not materialize. She is able to maintain her daily routine. She however, remains preoccupied with the thoughts of this boy. She is likely to be suffering from *[All India PGMEE 2004]*
a. Delusional disorder b. Depression
c. Mania d. Schizophrenia

80. A 25-year-old housewife came to the Psychiatry out patient department [OPD] complaining that her nose was longer than usual. She felt that her husband did not like her because of the deformity and had developed relationship with the neighbouring girl Further she complained that people made fun of her. It was not possible to convince her that there was no deformity. Her symptoms include *[All India PGMEE 2004]*
a. Delusion b. Depersonalization
c. Depression d. Hallucination

81. A 25-year-old female presents with 2 year history of repetitive, irresistible thoughts of contamination with dirt associated with repetitive hand washing. She reports these thoughts to be her own and distressing; but is notable to overcome them with medications. She is most likely to benefit from which of the following therapies given? *[All India PGMEE 2005, AIIMS May 2015]*
a. Exposure and response prevention
b. Systematic desensitization
c. Assertiveness training
d. Sensate focusing

82. All of the following are done in behavior therapy to increase a behavior except *[All India PGMEE 2010]*
a. Punishment b. Operant conditioning
c. Negative reinforcement d. Reward

83. True about social phobia is *[UP PGMEE 2001]*
a. Fear of closed spaces
b. Irrational fear of situation
c. Irrational fear of activities
d. Irrational fear of specified objects

84. Agoraphobia is *[PGI 1997]*
a. Fear of open spaces b. Fear of closed spaces
c. Fear of heights d. Fear of crowded places

85. All of the following are parts of cognitive behavior change technique except *[All India PGMEE 2010]*
a. Pre-contemplation b. Consolidation
c. Action d. Contemplation

86. A lady while driving a car meets with an accident. She was admitted in an ICU for 6 months. After being discharged she often gets up in night and feels terrified. She is afraid to sit in a car again. The diagnosis is *[All India PGMEE 2001]*
a. Anxiety disorder b. Phobia
c. Conversion disorder
d. Post Traumatic Stress Disorder

87. A man taking 2 cigarettes per day, started coughing, his family suggested quitting cigarettes. He is ready to quit but think that quitting will make him irritable, the best health planning model followed is *[AIIMS PGMEE 2009]*
a. Cost and survival
b. Persuasion
c. Precontemplation and preparation
d. Belief

88. Which of the following statements differentiates the obsessional idea from delusions? *[AIIMS PGMEE 2005]*
a. The idea is not a conventional belief
b. The idea is held in spite of contrary evidence
c. The idea is regarded as senseless by patient
d. The idea is held on inadequate ground

89. A person going to temple gets irresistible sense of idea to abuse God which can't be resisted. Likely diagnosis is *[AIIMS PGMEE 1999]*
a. Mania
b. Obsessive Compulsive Disorder
c. Schizophrenia d. Delusion

90. True about obsession-compulsive disorder are all except *[All India PGMEE 1995]*
a. Ego-alien b. Patient tries to resist against
c. Ego syntonic d. Insight is present

91. Treatment of obsessive-compulsive disorder includes *[PGI 2008]*
a. Exposure & response prevention
b. Flooding
c. Psychoanalytic therapy
d. Supportive psychotherapy involving family members
e. Systemic desensitization

92. A middle aged person reported to Psychiatric OPD with the complaints of fear of leaving home, fear of traveling alone and fear of being in a crowd. He develops marked anxiety with palpitations and swelling if he is in these situations. He often avoids public transport to go his place of work. The most likely diagnosis is *[AIIMS PGMEE 2006]*
a. Generalized anxiety disorder
b. Schizophrenia
c. Personality disorder
d. Agoraphobia

93. A fifty year old male feels uncomfortable in using lift, being in crowded places and traveling. The most appropriate line of treatment is *[AIIMS PGMEE 2005]*
a. Counselling
b. Relaxation therapy
c. Exposure and response prevention
d. Covert sensitization

94. Behavior therapy is useful in *[PGI 2008]*
a. Psychosis b. OCD
c. Personality disorder d. Panic attack
e. Anxiety

95. Treatment of choice for phobic disorder is *[All India PGMEE 1997, Jharkhand PGMEE 2005]*
a. Psychotherapy b. Behavior Therapy
c. SSRI d. Benzodiazepine

96. A 35-year-old man with an obsessive compulsive personality disorder is likely to exhibit all of the following features, except *[AIIMS PGMEE 2004]*
a. Perfectionism interfering with performance
b. Compulsive checking behavior
c. Preoccupation with rule
d. Indecisiveness

97. A 15-year-old boy feels that the dirt has hung onto him whenever he passes through the dirty street. This repetitive thought causes much distress and anxiety. He knows that there is actually no such thing after he has cleaned, but he is not satisfied and is compelled to think so. This has led to social withdrawal. He spends much of his time thinking about the dirt and contamination. This has affected his studies also. The most likely diagnosis is
a. Obsessive compulsive disorder *[All India PGMEE 2003]*
b. Conduct disorder c. Agoraphobia
d. Adjustment disorder

98. True statements about obsession *[PGI 2003]*
a. It is the repetitive thoughts or images
b. The patient thought that the images or thoughts are imposed by others
c. Content about sex or God
d. The patient gets disturbed when unable to remove the ideas or thoughts
e. None of the above is correct

99. Which of the following behavioral problems would suggest an organic brain lesion? *[SGPGI 2005]*
a. Formal thought disorder
b. Auditory hallucinations
c. Visual hallucinations d. Depression

100. The drug of choice for obsessive compulsive disorder *[All India PGMEE 2007, AIIMS PGMEE 2007, UP PGMEE 2003]*
a. Imipramine b. Fluoxetine
c. Chlopromazine d. Benzodiazepine

101. A patient presented with short lasting episodic behavioral changes which includes agitation & dream like state with thrashing movements of his limbs. He does not recall of these episodes & no precipitating factor is likely. The most likely diagnosis is *[All India PGMEE 2002]*
a. Schizophrenia b. Temporal lobe epilepsy
c. Panic episodes d. Dissociative disorder

102. True about Obsessive compulsive disorders is/are *[PGI May 2014]*
a. Compulsion b. Recurrent intrusions
c. MC type washers d. Absence of insight
e. Anxiety

103. Least useful in treatment of Obsessive compulsive disorders is *[NIMHANS PGMEE 2014]*
a. SSRIs
b. Clomipramine
c. Systemic desensitization
d. CBT

104. Anorexia nervosa true is *[CGPG 2015]*
a. Self-induced vomiting b. Lethargic
c. Menorrhagia d. More common in males

105. Which of the following is not a Behavior Therapy technique? *[ESI IMO 2014]*
a. Flooding b. Counter-transference
c. Counter-conditioning d. Systematic desensitization

106. Behavioral therapy does not include *[PGI November 2014]*
a. Operant conditioning b. Positive reinforcement
c. Assignments d. Social conditioning
e. Contingency contract

107. Post-traumatic stress disorder, treatment of choice is *[AIIMS November 2014]*
a. Cognitive behavior therapy
b. Hypnotise
c. Rational emotive therapy
d. Eye movement desensitization and reprocessing

108. A 35-years-old male patient presented to Psychiatrist OPD. He believes himself to be richest person of the world. He feels his family members and neighbours are plotting against him and planning to harm him but family members disagree with him. Problem in the content of thought is *[AIIMS November 2017]*
a. Delusions of grandeur
b. Delusions of grandeur and persecution
c. Delusions of grandeur, persecution and reference
d. Delusions of persecution

109. Seman's Squeeze technique is used for
a. Erectile dysfunction *[Recent Question 2018]*
b. Premature ejaculation
c. Retrograde ejaculation
d. Antegrade ejaculation

 NEET/NBE PATTERN MCQs ANSWERS WITH EXPLANATIONS 

1. Ans. (c) **Operant conditioning**

[Ref. Psychology by Weiten, 10/e p46]

Operant Conditioning

- Concept given by Skinner
- Form of learning in which voluntary responses come to be controlled by their consequences
- Governs a larger share of human behavior as compared to Classical conditioning (Pavlov conditioning)

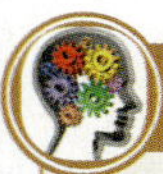

Also Remember

	Classical conditioning	Operant conditioning
Concept by	Pavlov	Skinner
Stimuli	Precede the response	Follow the response
Human response	Reflexive	Voluntary
Types of response	Elicited	Emitted
Example	Salivation on thought of food	Studying for exams

2. Ans. (c) **Comes under thought content in MMSE**

[Ref. Niraj Ahuja, 7/e p13]

Mental Status Examination (MSE)

- An important part of the clinical assessment process in psychiatric practice
- Structured way of observing and describing a patient's psychological functioning at a given point in time
- Domains: Appearance, attitude, behavior, mood and affect, speech, thought process, thought content, perception, cognition, insight and judgment

Mini–Mental State Examination (MMSE)/Folstein test

- A 30-point questionnaire that is used extensively in clinical and research settings to measure cognitive impairment
- Commonly used in medicine and allied health to screen for Dementia
- Domains: Orientation to time, orientation to place, registration, attention and calculation, recall, language, repetition, complex commands

3. Ans. (a) **OCD**

[Ref. Niraj Ahuja, 7/e p96]

Washers Type OCD

- Person has multiple doubts (Door has not been locked, kitchen gas left open)
- Compulsion: Checking repeatedly to remove the doubt
- Any attempt to stop the checking leads to mounting anxiety

Also Remember

Obsessive-Compulsive Personality Disorder (OCPD)

- Overly rigid personality style that does not change much over lifetime
- Not associated with the obsessions and compulsions
- Carry out repetitive behaviors to increase their efficiency or productivity
- See nothing wrong with their behavior and to feel that "other people" are the problem
- Seek treatment because of conflict between themselves and family and friends related to their need to have others conform to their way of doing things
- Rigid views on "right versus wrong"
- More ruled by perfectionism and have a higher need for order and control in both their personal and professional lives
- Overly devoted to work

4. Ans. (a) **Othello syndrome**

[Ref. Niraj Ahuja, 7/e p84]

Few Key syndromes in psychiatry

- **Capgras syndrome (Delusion of doubles):** Patient sees familiar person as stranger
- **Clerambault's syndrome:** Erotomania in which female is convinced that a person with higher status is in love with her
- **Cotard's syndrome:** Delusion that person has lost everything
- **Gilles de la Tourette syndrome:** Multiple motor tics
- **Holiday heart syndrome:** Atrial/ventricular arrhythmia after alcohol-binge
- **Klein Levin syndrome:** Hypersomnia, hyperphagia, hypersexuality
- **Othello syndrome:** Psychosis with jealousy involving spouse
- Pickwickian syndrome: Sleep apnoea in obese
- **Stockholm syndrome:** Psychological condition that causes hostages to develop sympathetic sentiments towards their captors, often sharing their opinions and acquiring romantic feelings for them as a survival strategy during captivity
- **Van Gogh syndrome:** Self-mutilation in schizophrenia

5. Ans. (a) **Delusion of persecution**

[Ref. Psychology by Coon, 14/e p462]

- Most common delusional disorder: Paranoid psychosis (centers on delusions of persecution)
- Paranoid people feel they are being cheated, spied on, followed, poisoned harassed or plotted against
- Hence Paranoid people frequently lead lonely, isolated, and humorless lives dominated by constant suspicion and hostility

6. Ans. (d) All the above
[Ref. Niraj Ahuja, 7/e p124]

Paraphilias – Disorders of Sexual Preference

- **Fetishism:** Sexual arousal occurs due to an inanimate object closely associated with human body (Clothes, footwear, body parts, leather items)
- **Fetishistic Transvestism:** Sexual arousal occurs due to cross-dressing
- **Sexual Sadism:** Sexual arousal occurs due to physical and/or psychological humiliation of sexual partner (victim) by a person (sadist)
- **Sexual Masochism:** Sexual arousal occurs due to receiving of physical and/or psychological humiliation on self by another person (sadist)
- **Exhibitionism:** Sexual arousal occurs due to exposure of one's genitalia to an unsuspecting stranger
- **Voyeurism:** Sexual arousal occurs due to observing other unsuspecting person disrobing, naked or engaged in sexual activity
- **Frotteurism:** Sexual arousal occurs due to touching or rubbing against an unsuspecting non-consenting person
- **Paedophilia:** Sexual attraction in a adult (>16 years age) to pre-pubescent children leading to sexual acts with them
- **Bestiality (Zoophilia):** Sexual involvement with animals

7. Ans. (a) Stalking
[Ref. The Stalker by D'Sylva, 1/e p1]

- **Stalking** is unwanted or obsessive attention by an individual or group toward another person
- Stalking behaviors are related to harassment and intimidation and may include following the victim in person or monitoring them

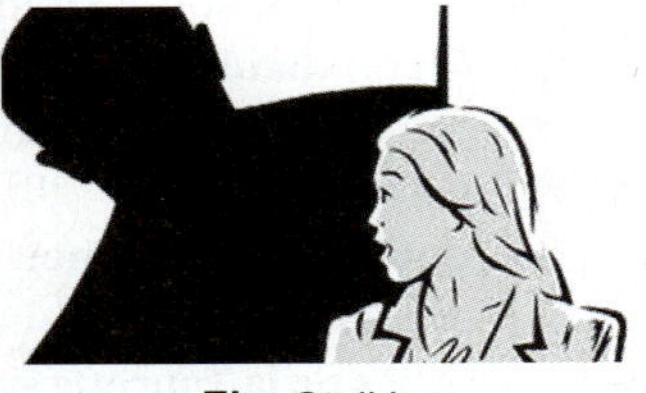
Fig. Stalking

8. Ans. (d) All of the above
[Ref. Residency Handbook of Psychiatry by Rosenquist, 1/e p81]

Symptom-Clusters of OCD

- Contamination: Fear of infection/germs following infection OR avoidance of source of contamination
- Pathological doubts: Obsession of doubt followed by compulsion of checking to avoid guilt/fear
- Intrusive thoughts: Without compulsion usually involving sex/violence
- Symmetry: Need of precision, compulsion for ordering/arranging
- Scrupulosity: Excessive praying or religious concerns
- Hoarding: Collecting objects excessively

9. Ans. (b) Delusion
[Ref. Philosophical Delusion and Its Therapy by Fischer, 1/e p185]

- Jealous delusions involve false beliefs of betrayal or infidelity by a spouse or lover

10. Ans. (d) All of the above
[Ref. Examination Notes in Psychiatry by Malhi, 2/e p73]

Thought and Thought-Disorders

- Flow
- Form:
  - Flight of ideas (Prolixity): Two thoughts are joined by superficial association (Mania)
  - Loosening of association
  - Word salad: Only words
  - Neologism: Coining new words or using old words in unique way—Schizophrenia (Most characteristic sign)
  - Circumstantiality: Unnecessary boring details
  - Tangentiality: Patient gives unnecessary details but substance of idea is not communicated.
- Content: Delusion (Grandiose, Persecution, Reference)

11. Ans. (b) Test judgement
[Ref. Niraj Ahuja, 7/e p15]

Judgement

- Ability to assess a situation correctly and act appropriately
  - Social judgement: Evaluation of Personal judgment during Hospital stay or Interview session
  - Test judgement: Asking person what would he do in certain situations (House on fire/Man lying on road)
- Rating of Judgement: Good/Intact/Normal OR Poor/Impaired/Abnormal

12. Ans. (d) 5
[Ref. Women and Psychiatric Treatment by Henderson, 1/e p178]

Trans-theoretical Model of Change

- Stage 1 (Precontemplation): Neither interested, nor considering change
- Stage 2 (Contemplation): Considering change
- Stage 3 (Preparation): Being ready to change
- Stage 4 (Action): Engaging in change
- Stage 5 (Maintenance): Sustaining the change

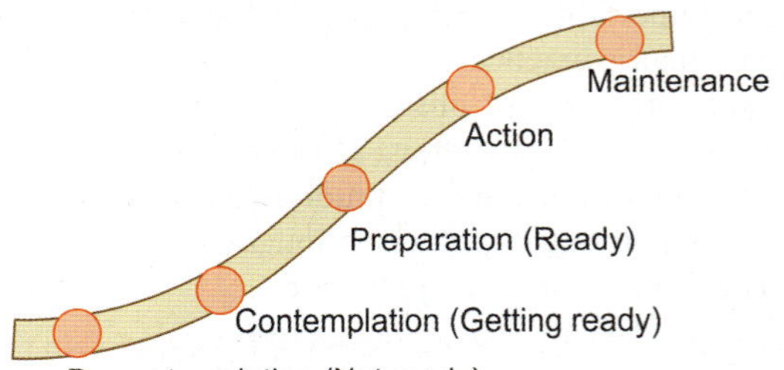

Fig. TT model of change

13. Ans. (a) Obesity
[Ref. The Management of Eating Disorders and Obesity by Goldstein, 2/e p145]

Binge Eating versus Bulimia Nervosa

	Binge eating	Bulimia nervosa
Association with Obesity	Higher chances	Lesser chances
Comorbid psychiatric illness	More prevalence	Less prevalence
Gender	More in males	More in females
Age of onset (Median)	17.2 years	15.7 years
Compensatory behaviors*	Less commonly used	Very commonly used

(* Induced vomiting, Laxatives)

Psychiatry

14. Ans. (d) OCD

[Ref. Niraj Ahuja, 7/e p204]

Psychosurgery

- Surgical intervention to severe fibres connecting one brain part to another, remove/destroy/stimulate brain tissue as a treatment for underlying organic pathology
- Indications:
  - Chronic severe incapacitating depression
  - Chronic severe incapacitating OCD
  - Chronic severe incapacitating anxiety disorder
  - Schizophrenia with chronic depression component
  - Severe pathological uncontrolled aggressive behavior
- Techniques (Indications)
  - Stereotactic subcaudate tractotomy (Severe anxiety, Severe depression, Severe OCD, Schizo-affective disorder)
  - Stereotactic Limbic Leucotomy (Intractable OCD and Schizophrenia)
  - Amygdalotomy (Severe uncontrolled aggression)

15. Ans. (b) Xenophobia

[Ref. Niraj Ahuja, 7/e p93]

16. Ans. (a) Compulsive washing of hand

[Ref. OCD Research by Ling, 1/e p256]

- MC theme of obsession in OCDs reported in different studies include contamination
- Cleaning rituals may take the form of repetitive washing of hands, feet, whole body, doorknobs, chairs, walls

17. Ans. (a) Anankastic

[Ref. General Adult Psychiatry by Stein, 1/e p366]

- Obsessive-compulsive personality disorder (OCPD), as defined by the current versions of the DSM-IV and DSM-5, and termed Anankastic personality disorder in the ICD-10,1 is a disorder characterized by preoccupation with orderliness, perfectionism, and mental and interpersonal control, at the expense of flexibility, openness, and efficiency

18. Ans. (b) Overweight individuals

[Ref. Niraj Ahuja, 7/e p144]

19. Ans. (c) Exhibitionism

[Ref. Niraj Ahuja, 7/e p125]

Exhibitionism

- Definition: Sexual arousal occurs due to exposure of one's genitalia to an unsuspecting stranger
- Usually exhibitionist is a male
- Types of exhibitionism:
  - **Flashing:** Exposing breasts to strangers
  - **Streaking:** Running nude in a public place
  - **Mooning:** Exposure of buttock to strangers

20. Ans. (d) Agoraphobia

[Ref. Abnormal Psychology by Carson, 13/e p195]

- In agoraphobia the most commonly feared and avoided situations include streets and crowded places

21. Ans. (c) Open spaces

[Ref. Niraj Ahuja, 7/e p93]

Agoraphobia

- *Characteristic feature*: Irrational fear of being away from familiar setting of home, i.e. in open spaces, public places or crowded places
- *MC group affected*: 20-40 years old females
- *Clinical presentation*: **Classical symptoms of panic**
  - Agoraphobia without panic disorder: Dizziness, tachycardia
  - Agoraphobia with panic disorder: Full blown panic attack
  - Severe dependence on Phobic companions (close relatives/friends whom patient only leaves home with)
- *Associated disorders*:
  - Panic disorder
  - Obsessive compulsive disorder (OCD)
  - Post traumatic stress disorder (PTSD)
  - Separation anxiety disorder
  - Necrophobia (fear of death)

22. Ans. (d) CBT

[Ref. Niraj Ahuja, 7/e p215-16]

Cognitive Behavior Therapy

- *Description*: Type of Psychotherapy which aims at correcting maladaptive patterns of thinking, thus providing relief from consequent symptoms
- *Hot-Cross Bun Model of CBT*: Cognitive, emotional, behavioral and physiological elements that contribute to individual case formulations, thus helping individual to picture their his problem, reflect on it and generalize it
- *Important techniques in CBT*:
  - Cognitive techniques
  - Behavioral techniques
  - Teaching problem-solving skills
  - Mindfulness
- *Medical uses of CBT*:

In adults	In children/adolescents
• Anxiety disorders • Depression • Eating disorders • Personality disorders • Substance use disorders • Schizophrenia • Psychosis	• Anxiety disorders • Body dysmorphic disorders • Eating disorders & Obesity • Depression, Suicidality • OCD • PTSD • Tics, Trichotillomania, Repetitive disorders

- Obsessive compulsive disorders (OC-disorders) include excoriation disorder (skin picking), trichotillomania (hair pulling), other body-focused repetitive behavior disorders (e.g., nail biting, lip biting, thumb sucking), body dysmorphic disorder (BDD), and hoarding disorder
- Tics are not considered OC-disorders in DSM-V, though their treatment is same.

23. Ans. (c) Claustrophobia

[Ref. Niraj Ahuja, 7/e p93]

Claustrophobia

- *Definition*: Fear of being in a closed space with no escape

- *Situations*: Small rooms, Closed rooms, Caves, Tunnels, Elevators, Aeroplanes
- *Underlying cause*:
  - Smaller right amygdale
  - Classical conditioning (traumatic childhood experience)
- *Treatment*:
  - Cognitive therapy
  - In-vivo exposure (exposures moving from lesser to complete types)

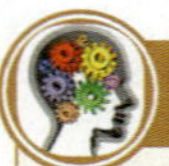

Also Remember

- *List of few specific phobias*:

Description	Phobia
Fear of height	Acrophobia
Fear of darkness	Nyctophobia
Fear of animals	Zoophobia
Fear of strangers	Xenophobia
Fear of pain	Algophobia
Fear of closed spaces	Claustrophobia
Fear of medical procedures (needles, etc.)	Trypanophobia
Fear of sexual abuse	Agaraphobia
Fear of spiders	Arachnophobia
Fear of death	Necrophobia
Fear of water	Aquaphobia
Fear of doctors	Iatrophobia
Fear of taking medication	Pharmacophobia

24. Ans. (a) Othello syndrome

[Ref. Niraj Ahuja, 7/e p84]

- ***Othello Syndrome (Conjugal Paranoia)***: Delusional disorder of jealousy (infidelity) involving the spouse
- ***Capgras syndrome***: Delusional conviction that other persons in environment are not their real selves but their own doubles (impostors)
- ***Hypochondriacal paranoia***: Disorder of Hypochondriacal delusions (Fear of having one or more serious disorders)
- ***De Clerambault's syndrome***: Erotomanic delusions of a person that other person is in love with him

25. Ans. (b) Impulse

[Ref. Niraj Ahuja, 7/e p119]

Pyromania

- *Definition*: Impulsive disorder characterized by 2 or more episodes of fire-setting without a motive
- *Underlying cause*:
  - Juvenile delinquency
  - Childhood sexual abuse
  - Parental neglect
- *Age group affected*: Male children and adolescents
- *Features*:
  - Intense urge to set fire
  - Feeling of tension before and sense of relief after the act
  - Preoccupation with thoughts and mental image of fire-setting
- *Treatment*:
  - Cognitive therapy
  - Psychotherapy

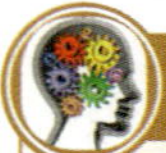

Also Remember

- *List of few impulsive disorders*:

Description	Disorder
Impulse for gambling	Pathological gambling
Impulse for fire-setting	Pyromania
Impulse for stealing	Kleptomania
Impulse for pulling hair	Trichotillomania
Impulse for picking skin	Dermatillomania
Impulse for nail biting	Onychophagia
Impulse for extreme anger leading to rage	Intermittent explosive disorder

26. Ans. (a) Bulimia nervosa

[Ref. Niraj Ahuja, 7/e p144]

Bulimia Nervosa

Features	Treatment
• Early onset in teens/ adolescence • Intense fear of becoming obese • Body-image disturbance • Persistent pre-occupation with eating • Irresistible craving with food • Attempts to counteract effects of over-eating • Vomiting, Purgative/laxative abuse, Starvation	• Behavior therapy • Individual psychotherapy • Antidepressants (SSRI Fluoxetine) • Group therapy • Family therapy

27. Ans. (d) Delusion of doubles

[Ref. Niraj Ahuja, 7/e p87]

Capgras' Syndrome (Delusion of doubles)

- *Definition*: Syndrome with delusional conviction that other persons in the environment are not their real selves but are their own doubles
- *Types of Capgras' syndrome*:
  - Illusion des sosies (Typical Capgras' syndrome): Patient sees a familiar person as a complete stranger who is imposing on him as a familiar person
  - Illusion de fregoli: Patient falsely identifies strangers as familar persons
  - Syndrome of subjective doubles: Patient's own self is perceived to be replaced by a double

- Intermetamorphosis: Patient misidentifies completely (external appearance + personality)
- *Most common associated disorders*: Paranoid schizophrenia

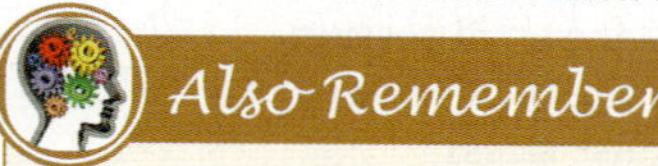

Also Remember

- *Prosopagnosia*: Inability to recognise faces though ability to recognise other objects remain intact

28. Ans. (d) Menorrhagia

[Ref. Niraj Ahuja, 7/e p142]

Anorexia Nervosa

Features	Treatment
• Onset in females adolescents • Intense fear of becoming obese • Body-image disturbance • Significant weight loss (>25%) • Final weight <85% of original	• Behavior therapy • Individual psychotherapy • Hospitalization • Antipsychotics, Antidepressants, Cyproheptadine • Group therapy • Family therapy
• Amenorrhoea (Primary/ Secondary) • Mood disorders (Depression, OCD) • Hypothermia • Self-imposed dietary restrictions • Preoccupation with food • Self-induced vomiting, Hypokalemia • Bulimic episodes	

29. Ans. (b) Visual hallucinations

[Ref. Harrison's Internal Medicine, 18/e p3529]

- *Diagnostic Criteria for Panic Disorder*: Discrete period of intense fear/discomfort during which four or more symptoms develop abruptly and reach peak in 10 minutes
  - Palpitations
  - Sweating
  - Trembling
  - Shortness of breath
  - Feeling of choking
  - Chest pain/discomfort
  - Feeling of uneasiness
  - Nausea/abdominal distress
  - Dizziness/light-headedness, fainting
  - Derealization
  - Fear of losing control
  - Fear of dying
  - Paresthesia
  - Chills/Hot flushes

30. Ans. (b) Fetishism

[Ref. Niraj Ahuja, 7/e p125]

Fetishism

- *Definition*: Sexual arousal occurs due to an inanimate object closely associated with human body
- *Common fetishes*: Clothes, footwear, body parts, leather items
  - Fetishism is almost exclusively seen in males
- *Types of fetishism*:
  - Spiritual love: Devotion for mental phenomena
  - Plastic love: Devotion for material objects
- *Treatment*:
  - Cognitive behavior therapy
  - Psychoanalysis

Also Remember

- *Partialism*: Fetishism towards a particular body part (just like genitalia)

31. Ans. (a) Repeated vomiting after meals

[Ref. Niraj Ahuja, 7/e p142]

32. Ans. (b) Fluoxetine

[Ref. Niraj Ahuja, 7/e p98]

Treatment of OCD

- *Benzodiazepines*: Limited role of Alprazolam, Clonazepam)
- *Antidepressants*:
  - Clomipramine: First drug used for OCD
  - Fluoxetine: Preferred drug due to its better side-effect profile
- *Antipsychotics*: Occasionally used in low doses
- *Buspirone*

33. Ans. (a) Attitude

[Ref. K. Park, 23/e p676]

- ***Emotions***: Strong feelings of whole organism, which motivate human behavior
- ***Value***: The ideals, customs, institutions of a society toward which the people of the group have an affective regard
- ***Opinions***: Views held by people on a point of dispute
  - Are 'temporary, provisional'
  - Is 'subjective in nature'
- ***Belief***: Views derived from parents, grandparents and other people we respect
  - Are 'permanent, unstable, almost unchanging'
  - Is 'subjective in nature'
- ***Attitude***: Relatively enduring organization of beliefs around an object or subject which predisposes one to respond in a preferential manner
  - Acquired characteristics of an individual
  - Is more or less 'permanent ways of behaving'
  - Is 'caught, not taught'
  - Is 'objective in nature'
- ***Habits***: An accustomed way of doing things
  - Habits are acquired through repetitions, are automatic and can be performed only under similar circumstances

34. Ans. (c) Agoraphobia

[Ref. Niraj Ahuja, 7/e p92]

- *Most common Phobia seen in Clinical practice*: Agoraphobia
  - More common seen in women

35. Ans. (a) Classical psychoanalysis

[Ref. Sociolinguistics by U Ammon, 2/e p2533]

- *Classical psychoanalysis*:
  - Non-professional partner is Passive patient
  - Doctor's active interventions cure

36. Ans. (b) Excessive unreasonable fear about a specific situation

[Ref. Niraj Ahuja, 7/e p93]

- *Phobia*: Irrational fear of a specific object/situation/activity, often leading to persistent avoidance of that object/situation/activity

37. Ans. (c) Buying

[Ref. Kaplan and Sadocks Synopsis of Psychiatry, 3/e p370]

- *Oniomania (Kraepelin)*: Compulsive desire to shop

38. Ans. (d) None of the above

[Ref. Niraj Ahuja, 7/e p29, 70, 80]

Paranoid Delusions

- *Definition*: False belief of a conspiracy concerning a perceived threat towards one self (persecutory delusions)
- *Associated conditions*:
  - Organic brain syndrome (Schizophrenia)
  - Involutional melancholia
  - Acute mania
  - Paranoid personality disorders

39. Ans. (c) Behavioral therapy

[Ref. Contemporary Behavior Therapy by Michael D. Spiegler]

- *Systematic desensitization*: Type of behavior therapy used for effectively overcoming phobias and anxiety disorders

40. Ans. (b) Fear of being promiscuous

[Ref. Misogyny, Misandry, and Misanthropy by Ferguson, 1/e p154]

- *Freudian Theory of Agoraphobia*: Agoraphobia in women signify an unresolved Oedipus complex
  - Anxiety of repressed libido manifest as promiscuity on street

41. Ans. (d) Alopecia

[Ref. Niraj Ahuja, 7/e p142]

42. Ans. (b) Compulsion

[Ref. Niraj Ahuja, 7/e p95]

- *Obsession*: Idea/impulse/image intruding into conscious awareness repeatedly
  - Recognized as one's own idea but perceived as 'Ego-alien'
  - Failure to resist lead to distress
  - Insight present (Thought recognized to be irrational, absurd)
- *Compulsion*: Subjective compulsive behavior usually following obsessions
  - Aimed at preventing/neutralizing distress/fear arising out of obsession
  - Irrational/excessive un-realistic behavior of repetitive work/actions
  - Insight present

43. Ans. (d) All of the above

[Ref. Niraj Ahuja, 7/e p95]

- ***Obsession:*** A recurrent, persistent thought, image, or impulse that is unwanted and distressing (ego-dystonic) and comes involuntarily to mind despite attempts to ignore or suppress it
  - Idea/impulse/image repeatedly intrudes into conscious awareness
  - Recognised as one's own BUT perceived as ego-alien
  - Irrational and absurd
  - Patient tries to resist but fails to do so
  - Failure to resist leads to stress
- ***Compulsion:***
  - Form of behavior following an obsession
  - Irrational, excessive nature of behavior
  - Used to prevent/neutralise stress
  - *'Insight is present'*
  - Subjective compulsion to perform

44. Ans. (a) Bulimia nervosa

[Ref. Niraj Ahuja, 7/e p144]

45. Ans. (b) Irresistible desire to steal things

[Ref. Niraj Ahuja, 7/e p119]

Habit & Impulse Disorders

- *Pathological gambling*: Two or more episodes of gambling per year
- *Kleptomania*: Pathological stealing
- *Pyromania*: Pathological fire-setting
- *Trichotillomania*: Compulsive hair-pulling

46. Ans. (a) Visual hallucinations

[Ref. Niraj Ahuja, 7/e p93]

47. Ans. (b) Paranoid delusion

[Ref. Textbook of Clinical Neuropsychiatry and Behavioral Neuroscience by Moore & Puri, 3/e p191]

Few Common Delusions

Delusion	Feeling example
Delusion of Persecution	*'CBI has bugged my room and intends to kill me'*
Delusion of Grandeur	*'I am Lord Krishna'*
Delusion of Reference	*'Some want to send message to me through Newspaper article'*
Delusion of Control/ Influence	*'My dental filling is controlling my thoughts and actions'*
Somatic delusion	*'Doctor say I'm not pregnant. But I am.'*
Nihilistic delusion	*'The World no longer exists'*
Paranoia	*'I won't eat this food. I know it has been poisoned.'*

48. Ans. (b) Operant conditioning

[Ref. A literature review on the portrayal of television violence in the U.S. programs and its impact on viewers, Pg 4]

Adverse Effects of Televised Violence on the Viewers are mediated by

- *Imitation*: Viewers learn behaviors performed by television characters and copy them themselves
- *Observational learning*: Children imitate behaviors of models they observe
- *Disinhibition*: Legitimizing the use of violence by the viewer in real life by undermining social sanctions against behaving violently
- *Desensitization*: Repeated viewing leads to reduced emotional responsiveness to violence on the screen and also to an increased acceptance of violence in real life
- *Arousal*: Immediate emotional reaction of fear

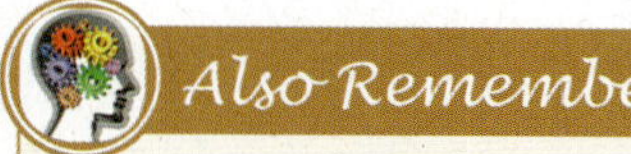

- ***Operant conditioning*:** Individual's behavior is modified by its consequences, i.e. punishment, reward and extinction
  - Operant conditioning plays an important role in aggressive behaviors associated with using interactive video-games

49. Ans. (d) Manchausen's syndrome
[Ref. Niraj Ahuja, 7/e p119]

Munchausen's Syndrome (Factitious Disordr)

- *Synonyms*: Hospital addiction, Hospital hoboes, Professional patients
- *Description*: Patients who repeatedly simulate or fake diseases for the sole purpose of obtaining medical attention
  - Patients present with Physical/psychological signs/symptoms
  - Pseudologia fantastica: Patients distort clinical histories, laboratory tests reports
- *Prognosis*: Poor

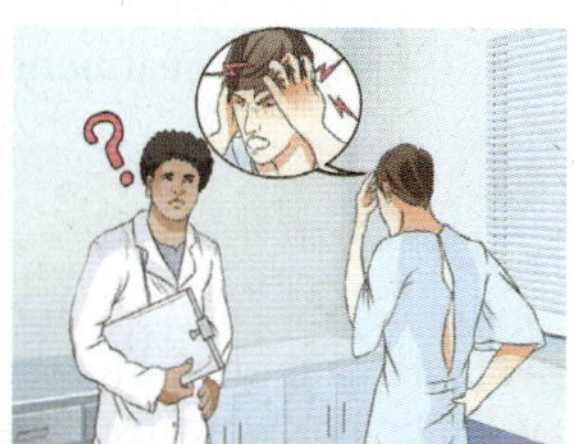

Fig. Manchausen's syndrome

50. Ans. (b) Content of thought
[Ref. Niraj Ahuja, 7/e p56 and A Companion to Fish's Clinical Psychopathology, 1/e p18-36]

- *Disorders of thought form*: Formal thought disorders
  - Schizophrenia
  - Coarse brain disease
- *Disorders of thought content*: Delusions (False, unshakeable belief which is out of keeping with the patients' socio-cultural background)
  - *True delusions*: Schizophrenia, Organic states (Epileptic psychoses)
  - *Delusion-like idea*: (Psychoses, Psychogenic reactions)
- *Disorders of thought possession*:
  - Obsessions and compulsions
  - Thought alienation

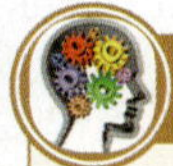

Also Remember

Disorders of Perceptions

- *Sensory distortions*:
  - *Changes in intensity*: Hyperaesthesia and hypoaesthesia
  - *Changes in quality*: Xanthopsia (colouring of yellow), Chloropsia (colouring of green), Erythropsia (colouring of red)
  - *Changes in spatial form (dysmegalopsia)*: Delusions, Atropine poisoning, Temporal lobe lesions
- *Sensory deceptions*:
  - *Illusions*: Delirium, Severe depression with guilt
  - *Hallucinations*: Intense emotions, Sensory deprivation, CNS disorders, Suggestion
- *Disorders of experience of time*: Mania and depression, Acute schizophrenia, Temporal lobe lesions

51. Ans. (c) The idea is regarded as senseless by patient
[Ref. Niraj Ahuja, 7/e p95]

- ***Obsession*:** Idea/impulse/image intruding into conscious awareness repeatedly
  - Recognized as one's own idea but perceived as 'Ego-alien'
  - Failure to resist lead to distress
  - Insight present
- ***Delusion*:** Recognized as one's own idea
  - Not recognized as Ego-alien
  - Not thought to be irrational, so never resisted
- ***Thought insertion*:** Not thought of one's own idea
  - Belief that someone else idea being forcibly inserted into one's mind

52. Ans. (a) Thought
[Ref. Behavioral Science by Fadem, 3/e p104]

- *Disorders of Perception*:
  - Hallucination
  - Illusion
- *Disorder of Thought content*:
  - Delusion
  - Idea of reference
- *Disorders of Form of thought*:
  - Loose associations
  - Tangentiality

53. Ans. (c) Labile affect
[Ref. Niraj Ahuja, 7/e p22]

- *Emotional lability*: Marked variation in emotional expression changing from one extreme to another quickly

54. Ans. (b) Distortion
[Ref. Introduction to Psychology: Minds and Behavior by Coon & Miterer, 1/e p111]

Reactions to Death (Kubler-Ross)

- Denial and Isolation
- Anger
- Bargaining
- Depression
- Acceptance

55. Ans. (b) Bulimia nervosa
[Ref. Niraj Ahuja, 7/e p142]

Eating Disorders

- Anorexia nervosa
- Bulimia nervosa
- Obesity associated with psychosocial disturbances
- Binge eating disorder
- Psychogenic vomiting

56. Ans. (a) OCD
[Ref. The OCD Workbook by Hyman, 2/e p304]

Hit and Run OCD

- Fear of accidentally hitting a pedestrian while driving
- Fears focus on unintentionally killing, injuring, or maiming a victim
- Worry about causing car accidents or causing other vehicles to swerve and hit pedestrians
- Driving back along the same route in order to scan for victims

57. Ans. (a) Nymphomania
[Ref. Niraj Ahuja, 7/e p127]

Nymphomania
- A type of sex addiction characterised by woman's excessive or pathological desire for sex associated with one or more sexual disorders (often include Female organic disorder)
- Intense fear of losing love, tries to satisfy her dependence needs (rather than gratify her sexual impulses)
- Defence mechanism: Compensation

58. Ans. (c) False belief that world is about to end
[Ref. Niraj Ahuja, 7/e p71]

Nihilistic delusions
- False belief that oneself, others or the world is non-existent or about to end
- In severe cases, patient claims nothing, including themselves, exist (Extreme of negation)
- It is belief-centred or focused on theme of no-existence of body parts

59. Ans. (c) Gender dysphoria
[Ref. Psychiatry by Shaffer, 1/e p142]

Gender Dysphoria (Transsexuality)
Syn. **Gender Identity reversal**
- Feeling in a biologically normal person of being a member of the opposite sex
- Etiology: Unknown.
  - It may be a biologic variation secondary to altered physiologic processes at conception and\or during intrauterine development
- Treatment:
  - Surgical correction of external appearance to be consistent with internal feelings
  - No long-term psychotherapeutic process

60. Ans. (c) Panic
[Ref. Niraj Ahuja, 7/e p90]
- Agoraphobia is most commonly associated with panic disorder
- New evidence:
  - Agoraphobia also occurs in many people without any history of panic
  - Agoraphobia also predicts the development of panic disorder

61. Ans. (c) Impulse
[Ref. Niraj Ahuja, 7/e p119]

Trichotillomania
- Recurrent persistent impulse to pull out hair, generally seen in early adolescent females
- Features: Intense urge to pull out hair, Feeling of tension before and sense of relief after the act, Stress, Carpal tunnel syndrome

Also Remember

Impulse control disorder
- A set of psychiatric disorders including intermittent explosive disorder (hot-headedness), kleptomania (stealing), pathological gambling, pyromania (fire starting), and three body-focused repetitive or compulsive behaviors of trichotillomania (a compulsion to pull one's hair out), onychophagia (compulsive nail biting) and dermatillomania (compulsive skin-picking)

62. Ans. (a) Phobia
[Ref. Niraj Ahuja, 7/e p94]

Flooding (Implosion)
- Patients confront the feared object or situation (e.g., a spider) at full intensity for prolonged periods until it is no longer frightening
- Similar to graded exposure in that it involves exposing the patient to the feared object in vivo; however, there is no hierarchy
- Principle: Escaping from an anxiety-provoking experience reinforces the anxiety through conditioning; by using Flooding, clinicians can extinguish the anxiety and prevent the conditioned avoidance behaviour by not allowing patients to escape the situation
- Useful in treatment of Phobias, OCDs

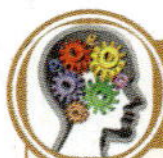

Also Remember

Impulse control disorder
- Systematic desensitization: Based on principle of Counterconditioning, whereby a person overcomes maladaptive anxiety elicited by a situation/object by approaching the feared situation gradually, in a psychophysiological state that inhibits anxiety

63. Ans. (c) Paraphilia
[Ref. Medical Basis of Psychiatry by Fatemi, 3/e p277]

Paraphilias (DSM-IV-TR)
- Sexual disorders characterized by recurrent, intense, sexually arousing fantasies, urges, or behaviors that involve nonhuman objects, children, other non-consenting individuals, or the suffering or humiliation of the individual or partner
- **Eight specific paraphilias:** Fetishism, Transvestic fetishism, Sexual Sadism, Sexual Masochism, Exhibitionism, Voyeurism, Frotteurism, Pedophilia
- **Category of paraphilias not otherwise specified:** Telephone scatologia (obscene phone calls), Klismaphilia (enemas), Necrophilia (corpses), Coprophilia (faeces), Urophilia (urine), Zoophilia (animals), Partialism (focus on body part)

64. Ans. (c) Voyeurism
[Ref. Niraj Ahuja, 7/e p125]

Voyeurism
- Sexual arousal occurs due to observing other unsuspecting person disrobing, naked or engaged in sexual activity
- Is spying on a person's intimate behaviours
- Usually voyeurist is a male

65. Ans. (c) Claustrophobia
[Ref. Niraj Ahuja, 7/e p93]
- Claustrophobia is Fear of being in a closed space with no escape in situations like Small rooms, Closed rooms, Caves, Tunnels, Elevators, Aeroplanes

66. Ans. (b) Spiders
[Ref. Psychiatry Specialty Review and Study Guide by Marks, q412]
- Arachnophobia is the fear of spiders
- Arachnophobia best treated with exposure therapy

67. Ans. (c) Nihilistic delusions
[Ref. Kaplan & Sadock's, 3/e p187]

Cotard syndrome
- Several patients suffer from a syndrome called délire de negation (sometimes referred to as Nihilistic delusional disorder)
- Patients complain of having lost their possessions, status and strength and also their heart, blood and intestines
- Feeling of world coming to nothingness
- May be a precursor to Schizophrenia or Depression episode

68. Ans. (a) Onanism
[Ref. Niraj Ahuja, 7/e p244]
- Tissot, Simon Andre (1728-1797) coined the term 'Onanism', first medical description of masturbation

69. Ans. (d) All of the above
[Ref. Niraj Ahuja, 7/e p94]

Treatment of Phobias
- Psychotherapy
- Behaviour therapy
- Drug therapy
  - Benzodiazepines (Alprazolam- Drug of choice)
  - Anti-depressants (SSRIs Paroxetine- Drug of choice)

70. Ans. (b) Delusion of being cheated
[Ref. Clinical Neuropsychiatry and Behavioral Neuroscience by Moore & Puri, 3/e p191]
- Delusion of persecution: Patient feels being spied against and followed; a conspiracy has been set up; CBI, Police and mafia are involved; Neighbors, family members, coworkers have turned against them and have poisoned their food

71. Ans. (a) Delusion of infidelity
[Ref. General Adult Psychiatry by Stein, 2/e p198]

Delusion of infidelity (Othello syndrome)
- Morbid/pathological jealousy
- False belief that spouse/lover is having an affair without proof

72. Ans. (c) Anxiety
[Ref. Niraj Ahuja, 7/e p95]

Obsession
- An idea, impulse or image which intrudes into the conscious awareness repeatedly, recognised as one's own idea, impulse or image but perceived as ego-alien
- Insight is present: Recognised as irrational and absurd
- Patient tries to resist against it but is unable to; failure to resist, leads to marked distress

73. Ans. (b) Delusion
[Ref. Niraj Ahuja, 7/e p84]
- Delusion of infidelity (Othello syndrome): False belief that spouse/lover is having an affair without proof

74. Ans. (a) Obsession
[Ref. Niraj Ahuja, 7/e p95]
- Examples of obsessions are recurrent thoughts of dirt or germ contamination, a fear of losing things, a need to know or remember something, a need to count or check something, blasphemous thoughts, or concerns about something happening to the self or others

75. Ans. (a) Paraphilias
[Ref. Niraj Ahuja, 7/e p126]

Treatment of Paraphilias
- Psychoanalysis and psychoanalytic psychotherapy
- Behaviour therapy: Aversion therapy is the treatment of choice in severe, distressing paraphilia
- Drug therapy: Antipsychotics, Antiandrogens (Cyproterone acetate or medroxy-progesterone acetate)

76. Ans. (b) Circumstantiality
[Ref. Niraj Ahuja, 7/e p247]
- Circumstantiality: Digression into unnecessary details that distract from the central theme **(Patients talks of urine and faeces in the given question)**; however, the patient returns back to the original theme after digression **(Patient finally tells his blood sugar in the given question).**

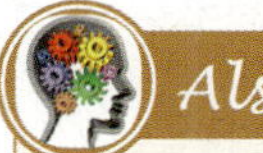

Also Remember
- Tangentiality: Sudden and oblique digression into unnecessary details that completely distract from the central theme; however, the patient never returns back to the original theme after digression

77. Ans. (d) Nihilistic delusion
[Ref. Kaplan & Sadock's, 3/e p187]
- Nihilistic delusional disorder patients complain of having lost their possessions, status and strength and also their heart, blood and intestines

78. Ans. (c) Erotomania
[Ref. Niraj Ahuja, 7/e p84]
- Erotomania is a type of delusional disorder in which an affected person believes that another person, usually a stranger or a famous person, is in love with him or her
- Seen in Psychiatric disorders: Schizophrenia, Bipolar mania

79. Ans. (a) Bizarre delusions
[Ref. Primary Health Care Psychiatry by Baumann, 1/e p718]

Types of delusions:
- Bizarre delusion: Strange implausible delusion
- Non-bizarre delusion: False but possible delusion
- Mood-congruent delusion: Delusion with content consistent with depressive or manic mood
- Mood-neutral delusion: Delusion not relating to emotional state

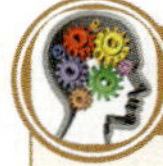

Also Remember
- Bizarre delusions are characteristic of Schizophrenia
- Non-bizarre delusions are more characteristic of Delusional disorders

80. Ans. (c) Delusion of persecution
[Ref. Clinical Neuropsychiatry by Moore, 3/e p191]
- Delusion of persecution: Patient feels being spied against and followed; a conspiracy has been set up; CBI, Police and mafia are involved; Neighbors, family members, coworkers have turned against them and have poisoned their food **(patient doubts neighbour without reason in the given question)**

 HIGH YIELD MCQs ANSWERS WITH EXPLANATIONS 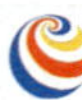

1. Ans. (b) 1, 2, 3
[Ref. Functional Psychiatric Disorders by Chiu, 1/e p67]

Obsessive Compulsive Disorders

- Defence mechanisms associated with OCD: Defective repression, displacement, reaction formation, isolation, undoing, rigidity
- Medications that potently inhibit reuptake of serotonin (SSRIs, Clomipramine) are DOC
- SSRIs have become the first-line medication for the treatment of OCD in children
- Antipsychotic augmentation: Haloperidol, Risperidone, Quetiapine, Olazapine, and Aripiprazole have all been shown in RCTs to augment SSRI response

2. Ans. (a) Thought
[Ref. Behavioural Science by Fadem, 3/e p104]

- *Disorder of Thought content*: Delusion, Idea of reference

3. Ans. (a) Thought
[Ref. Behavioural Science by Fadem, 3/e p104]

4. Ans. (c) Delusion
[Ref. Behavioural Science by Fadem, 3/e p104]

- *Allusion*: Indirect reference
- *Illusion*: Something appearing to be true/real, but actually not existing or different from what it seems
- *Delusion*: Persistent belief contrary to fact/reality

5. Ans. (b) Post-traumatic stress disorder
[Ref. Niraj Ahuja, 7/e p112]

Post-traumatic Stress Disorder

- *Description*: Delayed/protracted response to an exceptionally stressful/catastrophic life event/situation
- *Occurrence*:
  - More common in Individuals with past history of psychiatric illness
  - After a period of latency, within 6 months generally
- *Features of PTSD*:
  - Flash-backs or dreams: Recurrent, intrusive collections of stressful event
  - Marked avoidance of event/situations that may arouse recollection
  - Anxiety, increased arousal
  - Partial amnesia, numbness, anhedonia, detachment
- *Treatment of PTSD*: Prevention, Disaster management, CBT, Antidepressants/Benzodiazepines

6. Ans. (c) Occur in intellectuals
[Ref. Niraj Ahuja, 7/e p112]

7. Ans. (d) Post Traumatic stress Disorder
[Ref. Niraj Ahuja, 7/e p112]

8. Ans. (a) Superstition
[Ref. Annual Progress in Child Psychiatry and Child Development 1998, Pg 69]

- ***Superstition:*** Circumscribed belief in mystical, fantastical external determinants of individual's fate
  - Culturally transmitted or learned through reinforcement
  - Resorted to under conditions of uncertainty
  - Shared belief among groups

9. Ans. (d) Othello syndrome
[Ref. Niraj Ahuja, 7/e p84]

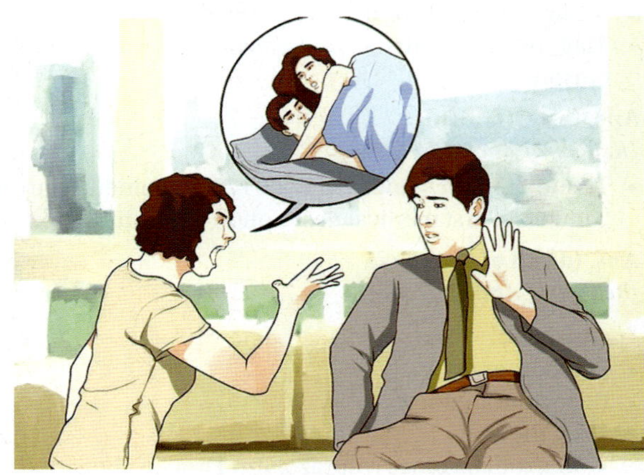

Fig. Othello syndrome

- *Othello Syndrome (Conjugal Paranoia)*: Delusional disorder of jealousy (infidelity) involving the spouse
- *Capgras syndrome*: Delusional conviction that other persons in environment are not their real selves but their own doubles (impostors)
- *Hypochondriacal paranoia*: Disorder of Hypochondriacal delusions (Fear of having one or more serious disorders)
- *De Clerambault's syndrome*: Erotomanic delusions of a person that other person is in love with him

10. Ans. (c) De Clerambault syndrome
[Ref. Niraj Ahuja, 7/e p84]

11. Ans. (b) Othello syndrome
[Ref. Niraj Ahuja, 7/e p84]

12. Ans. (d) Thought block
[Ref. Understanding Anger Disorders by Raymond & Raymond, 2007]

- *Cognitive Distortions (AT Beck)*:
  - Arbitrary interference
  - Selective abstraction
  - All-or-none thinking
  - Overgeneralization
  - Magnification & minimization
  - Catastrophic and probabilistic thinking
  - Personalization
  - Underestimation of social skills

13. Ans. (a) Unconscious internal conflict
[Ref. Understanding Abnormal Behavior by Sue & Sue, 11/e p51]

- *Psychodynamic models view Mental disorders as a result of:*
  - Childhood trauma
  - Anxieties
  - Unconscious conflicts

14. Ans. (c) Delusion of persecution

[Ref. Textbook of Clinical Neuropsychiatry and Behavioral Neuroscience by Moore & Puri, 3/e p191]

- *Delusion of persecution*: Patient feels being spied against and followed; a conspiracy has been set up; CBI, Police and mafia are involved; Neighbors, family members, co-workers have turned against them and have poisoned their food

15. Ans. (d) Refer to psychiatrist

[Ref. Niraj Ahuja, 7/e p84]

- *Delusional Dysmorphophobia*: Delusion of body (or its parts) being ugly or misshapen
  - Refer the patient to Psychiatrist

16. Ans. (c) Persistent Delusional Disorder

[Ref. Niraj Ahuja, 7/e p83]

Persistent Delusional (Paranoid) Disorder

- *Description*: Persistent delusions present for at least 3 months, and can include Delusions of persecution, grandeur, jealousy, somatic, erotomanic or non-bizarre type
- *Etiology*: Multifactorial
- *Features*:
  - Relative stable, chronic course
  - Well systematized delusions of non-bizarre type
  - Individuals are able to carry out near social and occupational life

17. Ans. (b) Modelling

[Ref. Revision Notes in Psychiatry by Puri & Hall, 3/e p26; A Short Textbook of Psychiatry by Niraj Ahuja, 7/e p215]

- ***Observational/Vicarious learning (Modelling):*** Learning of behaviors and skills that can occur by observation, without positive reinforcement
- ***Flooding:*** Patients confront the feared object or situation (e.g., a spider) at full intensity for prolonged periods until it is no longer frightening
- ***Positive reinforcement:*** Involves giving a reward when a desired behavior occurs (e.g., giving a child ice cream after he/she has eaten all of their vegetables)
- ***Aversion therapy:*** An attempt by a clinician to suppress undesirable behavior by punishing it with unpleasant (aversive) stimulation

18. Ans. (d) Operant conditioning

[A Short Textbook of Psychiatry by Niraj Ahuja, 7/e p215]

Operant Conditioning

- *Description*: Learning theory of behavior therapy which assumes that behavior that is followed by a reward is more likely to occur again
- *Operant Conditioning procedures for increasing behavior*:
  - **Positive reinforcement:** Desirable behavior is reinforced by a reward
  - **Negative reinforcement:** Punishment is avoided on desired behavior
  - **Modelling:** Person exposed to model behavior an induced to copy it
- *Operant Conditioning procedures for decreasing behavior*:
  - **Time-out:** Reinforcement withdrawn for some time, when undesired response occurs
  - **Punishment:** Punishment given whenever undesired response occurs
  - **Satiation:** Positive reinforcement of undesired response so that tiring occurs

19. Ans. (c) Punishment

[A Short Textbook of Psychiatry by Niraj Ahuja, 7/e p215]

20. Ans. (c) Othello syndrome

[Ref. Niraj Ahuja, 7/e p84]

21. Ans. (a) Schizophrenia; (b) Paranoid psychosis; (c) Manic episode; (d) Melancholia

[Ref. Niraj Ahuja, 7/e p61, 70, 83]

22. Ans. (a) Obsessive compulsive disorder

[Ref. Niraj Ahuja, 7/e p61, 70, 83]

23. Ans. (a) Formal thought disorder

[Ref. Niraj Ahuja, 7/e p55-56]

- **Thought and speech disorders:**
  - Autistic thinking
  - Loosening of associations
  - Thought blocking
  - Neologisms
  - Delusions

24. Ans. (b) Negative conditioning

[A Short Textbook of Psychiatry by Niraj Ahuja, 7/e p215]

25. Ans. (a) Schizophrenia

[Ref. Niraj Ahuja, 7/e p56]

26. Ans. (b) Capgras' syndrome

[Ref. Niraj Ahuja, 7/e p84]

- *Capgras syndrome*: Delusional conviction that other persons in environment are not their real selves but their own doubles (impostors)

27. Ans. (d) Foul odour

[Ref. Niraj Ahuja, 7/e p84]

- Common Hypochondriacal paranoia:
  - *Delusional halitosis*: Infestation of body by worms/ foreign-body emanating a foul odor
  - *Delusional dysmorphophobia*: Body (or its parts) being ugly or misshapen

28. Ans. (b) Egosyntonic

[Ref. Niraj Ahuja, 7/e p95]

- *Ego-syntonic*: Not distressing patient (Obsessive compulsive personality disorder)
- *Ego-dystonic*: Distressing the patient (Obsessive compulsive disorder)

29. Ans. (c) Obsessive compulsive disorder

[Ref. Niraj Ahuja, 7/e p95]

30. Ans. (a) Repression; (b) Undoing; (e) Displacement

[Ref. Niraj Ahuja, 7/e p207-209]

- ***Major Defence mechanisms in OCD:***
  - Isolation

- Reaction formation
- Undoing
- *Other Defence mechanisms in OCD*:
  - Inhibition
  - Displacement
  - Defective repression
  - Rigidity
  - Denial

31. Ans. (c) Short term benzodiazepine + SSRI + CBT
[Ref. Niraj Ahuja, 7/e p91-92]

32. Ans. (a) Alprazolam; (b) Paroxetine; (c) Venlafaxine; (d) Buspirone
[Ref. Niraj Ahuja, 7/e p91-92]

33. Ans. (d) Death
[Ref. Phobias: Psychology of Irrational fears by Irena & Randi, 1/e p371]

- *Thanatophobia*: Persistent and excessive fear of one's own death

34. Ans. (c) Fear of closed spaces
[Ref. Niraj Ahuja, 7/e p93]

Few Common Phobias

- *Claustrophobia*: Fear of closed spaces
- *Acrophobia*: Fear of high places
- *Zoophobia*: Fear of animals
- *Xenophobia*: Fear of strangers
- *Algophobia*: Fear of pain
- *Agoraphobia*: Irrational fear of situations

35. Ans. (b) Fear of heights
[Ref. Niraj Ahuja, 7/e p93]

36. Ans. (a) Behavior therapy
[Ref. Niraj Ahuja, 7/e p94]

Treatment of Phobias

- *Avoidance*
- *Behavior therapy*: Successful mode if planned properly
  - Flooding
  - Systematic desensitization
  - Exposure & response prevention
  - Relaxation techniques
- *Drugs*:
  - Benzodiazepines
  - SSRIs: Paroxetine
- *Psychotherapy*:
  - Psychodynamic psychotherapy: Usually in personality disorders
  - Supportive psychotherapy: Useful supportive therapy
  - Cognitive behavior therapy

37. Ans. (a) Pheochromocytoma; (b) Myocardial infarction; (c) Mitral valve prolapse; (e) Carcinoid syndrome

[Ref. Textbook of Postgraduate Psychiatry by Vyas & Ahuja, 2/e p256]

Differential Diagnosis of Panic Disorder

Cardiovascular disorders	Neurological disorders	Endocrine disorders
• Angina • Hypertension • Myocardial infarction • Mitral valve prolapse • Alpha-adrenergic state Paradoxical atrial tachycardia	• Cerebrovascular disease • Epilepsy • Huntington's disease • Migraine • Meniere's disease • Wilson's disease • Temporal arteritis • Multiple sclerosis	• Addison's disease • Cushing's disease • Diabetes • Carcinoid syndrome • Hyperthyroidism • Hypoparathyroidism • Pheochromocytoma • Menopausal disorders
Drug intoxication	**Drug withdrawal**	**Other conditions**
• Amphetamines • Amyl nitrite • Anticholinergics • Hallucinogens • Nicotine • Cocaine • Theophylline	• Alcohol • Opioids • Anti-hypertensives • Sedative-hypnotics	• Anemia • Pulmonary conditions • Asthma • B12 deficiency • Heavy metal poisoning • SLE • Uraemia

38. Ans. (c) Behavior therapy
[Ref. Niraj Ahuja, 7/e p94]

39. Ans. ALL CHOICES
[Ref. Niraj Ahuja, 7/e p94]

40. Ans. (a) Repetitiveness; (b) Irresistibility; (c) Unpleasantness
[Ref. Niraj Ahuja, 7/e p95]

41. Ans. (a) Irresistible desire to do a thing repeatedly; (c) Denial is the defence mechanism against OCD; (d) Patient is conscious about the disorder; (e) Can cause severe distress
[Ref. Niraj Ahuja, 7/e p95, 207-209]

42. Ans. (d) Serotonin
[Ref. Niraj Ahuja, 7/e p97]

Causal Theories of OCD

- *Psychodynamic theory*: Defensive regression to Anal-sadistic phase of development, with symptoms produced by
  - Isolation
  - Undoing
  - Displacement
- *Behavioral (Learning) theory*:
  - Obsessions: Conditioned stimuli to anxiety
  - Compulsions: Learned behavior which decreases anxiety associated with obsessions
- *Biological theories*:
  - Serotonin (5-HT) involvement
  - Secondary to many illness

43. Ans. (b) Depression
[Ref. Niraj Ahuja, 7/e p95]

- At least 50% of patients of OCD are associated with Depression

44. Ans. (c) Secondary Depression
[Ref. Obsessive-Compulsive Disorder Spectrum, 1/e p132]
- *Most important depression type seen in OCD*: Secondary depression

45. Ans. (d) Combination of behavior and drug therapy
[Ref. Psychopathology and Psychodynamics of Neurosis by Elzer & Gerlach, 1/e p209]
- SSRIs in combination with Cognitive behavior therapy is quite effective in OCD

46. Ans. (d) Carbamazepine
[Ref. Niraj Ahuja, 7/e p98]
- *Treatments NOT useful in OCD*: Clozapine, Carbamazepine, Lithium, Clonidine, ECT, Stimulants, Sleep-deprivation, Bright light therapy

47. Ans. (a) Serotonergic receptor
[Ref. Niraj Ahuja, 7/e p97-98]

48. Ans. (b) Cingulotomy
[Ref. Niraj Ahuja, 7/e p98]
- *Surgical procedures for Intractable OCD*:
  - Stereotactic limbic leucotomy
  - Stereotactic subcaudate tractotomy
  - Cingulotomy

49. Ans. (b) Fluoxetine
[Ref. Niraj Ahuja, 7/e p98]

Therapy of OCD
- Psychotherapy:
  - Psychoanalytic psychotherapy
  - Supportive psychotherapy
- Behavior therapy & CBT:
  - Thought stopping
  - Exposure & Response prevention (Principal therapy)
  - Systematic desensitization
  - Modelling
  - Flooding
- Drug therapy:
  - **Clomipramine: First drug used** effectively in treatment of OCD
  - **Fluoxetine: Preferred for** its better side-effect profile
  - Other drugs: Fluvoxamine, Paroxetine, Sertraline
  - Antipsychotics (Haloperidol, Risperidone, Planzapine, Pimozide): For severe disability anxiety
  - Buspirone
  - Other drugs: Lithium, Carbamzepine

50. Ans. (d) Clomipramine
[Ref. Niraj Ahuja, 7/e p98]

51. Ans. (a) Fluoxetine
[Ref. Niraj Ahuja, 7/e p92]

52. Ans. (d) Neurosis
[Ref. Niraj Ahuja, 7/e p89]

Neurotic Disorders
- Anxiety states: Panic attack
- Hysteria
- Phobias
- OCD
- Neurotic depression
- Neurasthenia
- Depersonalization syndrome
- Hypochondriasis
- Occupational neurosis

53. Ans. (a) Getting caught in places from where escape would be difficult
[Ref. Niraj Ahuja, 7/e p92]

54. Ans. (d) Diazepam
[Ref. Niraj Ahuja, 7/e p98]

55. Ans. (d) MAO inhibitors
[Ref. Niraj Ahuja, 7/e p98]

56. Ans. (b) Satyriasis
[Ref. Niraj Ahuja, 7/e p127]
- *Excessive sexual drive disorders*:
  - Satyriasis: Men
  - Nymphomania: Women

57. Ans. (b) Premature ejaculation
[Ref. Niraj Ahuja, 7/e p131]
- ***Squeeze technique (Seman's technique)*:**
  - Used in treatment of Premature-ejaculation
  - Female partner manually stimulates penis causing erection
  - Female partner squeezes penis on coronal ridge when male partner experiences ejaculation-inevitability

58. Ans. (a) Sildenafil
[Ref. Niraj Ahuja, 7/e p132]
- *Treatment of choice for erectile dysfunction*: Sildenafil citrate
  - *Mechanism of action*: Competitive, selective inhibition of c-GMP specific PDE-5 (Phosphodiesterase type 5)

59. Ans. (c) Impulse
[Ref. Niraj Ahuja, 7/e p119]

60. Ans. (b) Irresistible desire to steal things
[Ref. Niraj Ahuja, 7/e p119]

61. Ans. (d) Capgras' syndrome
[Ref. Niraj Ahuja, 7/e p119]

62. Ans. (a) Buying
[Ref. Kaplan and Sadocks Synopsis of Psychiatry, 3rd Ed., Pg 370]

63. Ans. (a) Binge eating
[Ref. Niraj Ahuja, 7/e p142]

64. Ans. (d) Menorrhagia
Ref. Niraj Ahuja, 7/e p142]

65. Ans. (d) Decreased appetite
[Ref. Niraj Ahuja, 7/e p142]

66. Ans. (a) Bulimia nervosa
[Ref. Niraj Ahuja, 7/e p144]

67. Ans. (a) Fluoxetine
[Ref. Niraj Ahuja, 7/e p144]

68. Ans. (d) None
[Ref. Niraj Ahuja, 7/e p58, 60]

69. Ans. (d) Prominent visual hallucination
[Ref. Oxford textbook of Old Age Psychiatry by Dening & Thomas, 2/e p154]
- Visual hallucinations predominantly suggest Organic cause
- Prominent in Dementia with Lewy bodies, Acute confusional states

70. Ans. (c) Labile affect
[Ref. Responding to Individuals with Mental Illnesses by Compton, Pg 60]
- Labile affect: A person who has rapidly changing affect, crying one moment and laughing the next moment
- Labile affect is usually present in: Manic episode of Bipolar disorder

71. Ans. (c) Schizophrenia
[Ref. Niraj Ahuja, 7/e p55]

Schneider's First Rank Symptoms of Schizophrenia (SFRS)*	
• Somatic passivity	• Body sensations imposed by others
• Made feelings/affect	• Imposed by others
• Made impulses	• Imposed by others
• Made volition/acts	• Imposed by others
• Delusional perception	• Private illogical meaning
• Voices heard arguing	• Auditory hallucinations
• Voices commenting on one's action	• Auditory hallucinations
• Audible thoughts	• Thought echo
• Thought withdrawal	• Thoughts cease, removed by someone
• Thought insertion	• Thoughts imposed by someone else
• Thought diffusion/ broadcasting	• Thoughts escaping and experienced by others

[*Mnemonic: S*chizophrenic **M***an* **D***oes* **V***alue* **A***udible* **T***houghts*; **SAM^{3}V^{2}T^{3}D]**

72. Ans. (c) Thinking
[Ref. Behavioural Science by Fadem, 3/e p104]

73. Ans. (a) Delusion of persecution
[Ref. Textbook of Clinical Neuropsychiatry and Behavioral Neuroscience by Moore & Puri, 3/e p191]

74. Ans. (d) Schizophrenia
[Ref. Niraj Ahuja, 7/e p55]

75. Ans. (c) Delusion of persecution
[Ref. Textbook of Clinical Neuropsychiatry and Behavioral Neuroscience by Moore & Puri, 3/e p191]

76. Ans. (d) Compulsive disorder
[Ref. Niraj Ahuja, 7/e p95]

77. Ans. (b) Anxiety
[Ref. Niraj Ahuja, 7/e p90-91]

78. Ans. (c) Preoperational stage
[Ref. Niraj Ahuja, 7/e p153-55]

Jean Piaget Theory of Cognitive Development

Period	Age range	Characteristics
Sensori-motor operations	Birth - 2 years	• Actions related to sucking, orality, assimilation of objects • One thought at a time • Out-of-sight means Cease-to-exist
Pre-operations	2–7 years	• Ego-centric intuitive thought • Inability to generalize
Concrete operations	7–11 years	• Reversible, flexible thought process • Ability of abstraction
Formal operations	11–16 years	• Thought comprehensiveness • Ability to develop abstract hypothesis and to test them

79. Ans. (a) Delusional disorder
[Ref. Niraj Ahuja, 7/e p84]
- *De Clerambault's syndrome*: Erotomanic delusions of a person that other person is in love with him

80. Ans. (a) Delusion
[Ref. Niraj Ahuja, 7/e p84]

81. Ans. (a) Exposure and response prevention
[Ref. Niraj Ahuja, 7/e p98]
- Behavior therapy & CBT in OCD:
  - Thought stopping
  - Exposure & Response prevention (Principal therapy)
  - Systematic desensitization
  - Modelling

82. Ans. (a) Punishment
[A Short Textbook of Psychiatry by Niraj Ahuja, 7/e p215]

83. Ans. (c) Irrational fear of activities
[A Short Textbook of Psychiatry by Niraj Ahuja, 7/e p93]

Social Phobia
- Description: Irrational fear of activities or social interaction
- Examples:
  - Erythrophobia (Fear of blushing)
  - Shy bladder (Fear of urinating in public lavaoratory)

84. Ans. (a) Fear of open spaces; (d) Fear of crowded places
[A Short Textbook of Psychiatry by Niraj Ahuja, 7/e p93]

85. Ans. (b) Consolidation
[Ref. CBT for Problem Drinking by Spada, 1/e p30-31]

Cognitive Behavior Change Stages
- **Pre-contemplation stage:** Client unaware of problem or not thinking about it
  - Resistant, Unmotivated, In-denial
- **Contemplative stage:** Client acknowledge problem and tries to think what went wrong
  - Open to information
- **Preparation/Determination stage:** Clear discrepancy between current and desired stage
  - Decision/commitment to change

- **Action stage:** Serious commitment to action
  - Willpower requiring time and energy
- **Maintenance stage:** Active try to implement actions proposed for change, practicing new skills
  - Prevent relapse and consolidate gains

86. Ans. (d) Post Traumatic Stress Disorder
[Ref. Niraj Ahuja, 7/e p112]

87. Ans. (c) Precontemplation and preparation
[Ref. CBT for Problem Drinking by Spada, 1/e p30-31]

88. Ans. (c) The idea is regarded as senseless by patient
[Ref. Niraj Ahuja, 7/e p95]

89. Ans. (b) Obsessive Compulsive Disorder
[Ref. Niraj Ahuja, 7/e p95]

90. Ans. (c) Ego syntonic
[Ref. Niraj Ahuja, 7/e p95]

91. Ans. ALL CHOICES
[Ref. Niraj Ahuja, 7/e p98]

92. Ans. (d) Agoraphobia
[Ref. Niraj Ahuja, 7/e p92]

93. Ans. (c) Exposure and response prevention
[Ref. Niraj Ahuja, 7/e p94]

94. Ans. (b) OCD; (c) Personality disorder; (d) Panic attack; (e) Anxiety
[Ref. Niraj Ahuja, 7/e p91, 92, 98, 115]

95. Ans. (b) Behavior Therapy
[Ref. Niraj Ahuja, 7/e p94]

96. Ans. (d) Indecisiveness
[Ref. Niraj Ahuja, 7/e p95]

97. Ans. (a) Obsessive compulsive disorder
[Ref. Niraj Ahuja, 7/e p95]

Common Clinical OCD Syndromes

- **Washers:**
  - Most common type
  - Obsession: Contamination with dirt, germs, body excretions
  - Compulsion: Washing hands/body repeatedly multiple times a day
- **Checkers:**
  - Obsession: Multiple doubts (door not locked, kitchen gas left open)
  - Compulsion: Repeated checking to remove doubt
- **Pure obsessions:**
  - Obsession: Repetitive intrusive images/thoughts/impulses NOT associated with compulsive actions
  - Associated with Counter-thoughts
- **Primary obsessive slowness:** Marked slowness in daily activities

98. Ans. (a) It is the repetitive thoughts or images; (d) The patient gets disturbed when unable to remove the ideas or thoughts
[Ref. Niraj Ahuja, 7/e p95]

- Insight is present in OCD

99. Ans. (c) Visual hallucinations

[Ref. Oxford textbook of Old Age Psychiatry by Dening & Thomas, 2/e p154]

100. Ans. (b) Fluoxetine

[Ref. Niraj Ahuja, 7/e p98]

- Fluoxetine is the referred drug due to its better side-effect profile in OCD

101. Ans. (b) Temporal lobe epilepsy
[Ref. Niraj Ahuja, 7/e p31]

102. Ans. (a) Compulsion; (b) Recurrent intrusions; (c) MC type washers; (e) Anxiety
[Ref. Niraj Ahuja, 7/e p95]

- Insight is present in OCD

103. Ans. (c) Systemic desensitization
[Ref. Family Medicine: Principles and Practice by Taylor, 5/e p280]

- *Techniques useful for OCD*:
  - Flooding therapy
  - Exposure and Response prevention
  - Modelling
- *Techniques NOT useful for OCD*:
  - Insight therapy
  - Dynamic psychotherapy
  - Systemic desensitization

104. Ans. (a) Self-induced vomiting
[Ref. Niraj Ahuja, 7/e p143]

105. Ans. (b) Counter-transference
[Ref. Complete Psychology by Field, 2/e p515]

Behavior Therapies

- Therapies based on Principles of Classical Conditioning:
  - **Exposure therapies (Extinction principles):**
    1. Flooding: Therapist-led prolonged exposure to provoking stimulus/agent
    2. Counter-conditioning: Therapist tends to attach response to anxiety-provoking events and situations inconsistent with anxiety
    3. Systematic desensitization: Client learns to relax in graded (increasing) anxiety/fear situations; Most effective/widely used/successful behavior therapy technique
  - **Aversion Therapy:** Condition an aversion to a stimulus/event to which a patient is inappropriately attracted
- Therapies based on Principles of Operant Conditioning:
  - **Functional analysis:** Therapist attempts to identify consistencies between problematic behaviors and their consequences
  - **Systematic group therapy:**
    1. Token economy schemes: Participants receive tokens (Positive Reinforcers) for engaging in behaviors defined by the program
- Cognitive behavior therapies:
  - **Beck's cognitive behavior therapy:** Deconstruction of negative themes in patients and replacing them with rational schemes

106. Ans. (d) Social conditioning

[Ref. Complete Psychology by Field, 2/e p515; Gate Encyclopedia of Alternative Medicine, p182]

107. Ans. (a) Cognitive behavior therapy

[Ref. Corsini's Encyclopedia of Psychology and Behavioural Science, 3/e p586]

- *Treatment of choice for PTSD*: Exposure therapy alone or in combination with Cognitive behavior therapy

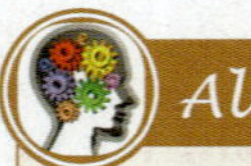

Also Remember

- *New techniques for treatment of PTSD*:
  - Traumatic Incident Reduction (TIR)
  - Eye Movement Desensitization and Reprocessing (EMDR)
  - Thought Field Therapy (TFT)
  - Time Limited Trauma Therapy (T-LTT)
  - Visual Kinesthetic Dissociation (VKD)

108. Ans. (c) Delusions of grandeur, persecution and reference

[Ref. Niraj Ahuja, 7/e p56]

- Delusions of grandeur (*'I am greatest'*): False belief of one's own importance, power, or knowledge or that one is, or has a special relationship with, a deity or a famous person **(Patient feels he is the richest person in the world in the given question)**
- Delusion of reference (*'People are thinking about me'*): Falsely belief that insignificant remarks, events, or objects in one's environment have personal meaning or significance **(Patient feels family members and neighbours are plotting against him in the given question)**
- Delusion of persecution (*'People are against me'*): Person believes that he/she is going to get harmed **(Patient feels family members and neighbours are going to harm him in the given question)**

109. Ans. (b) Premature ejaculation

[Ref. Niraj Ahuja, 7/e p131]

Squeeze technique (Seman's technique)

- Used in treatment of Premature-ejaculation
- Female partner manually stimulates penis causing erection
- Female partner squeezes penis on coronal ridge when male partner experiences ejaculation-inevitability

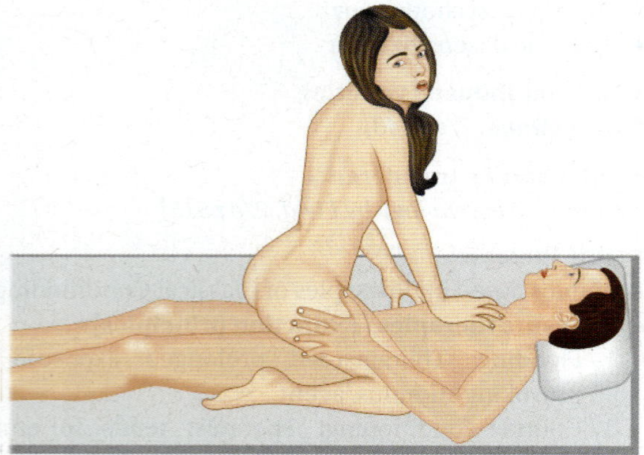

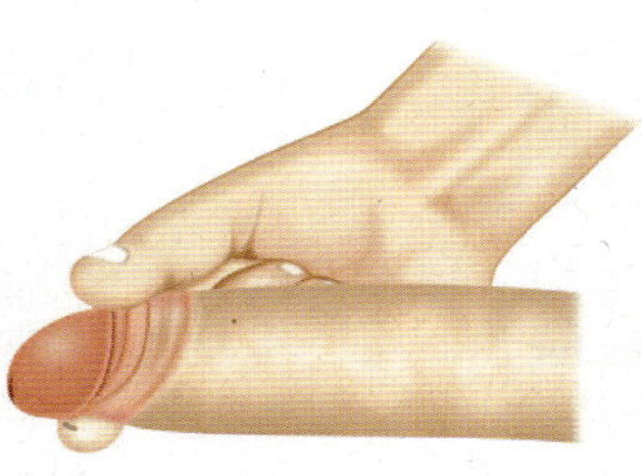

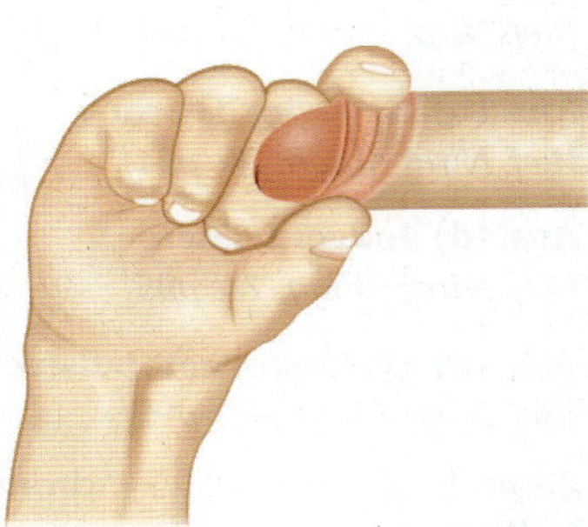

Fig. Squeeze technique

Psychiatry

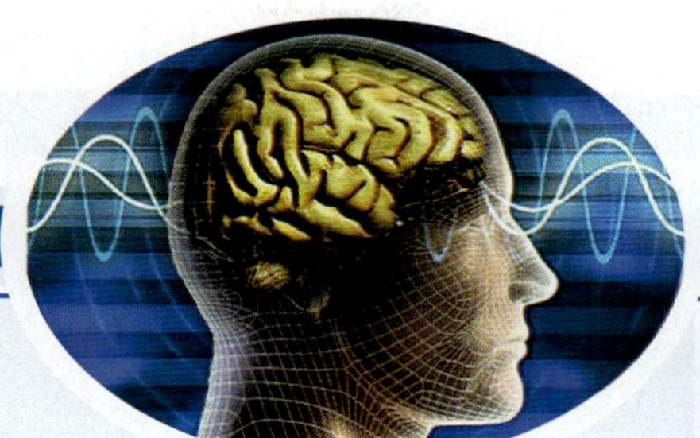

Chapter 4

Psychoses

THEORETICAL CONCEPTS

IV A. PSYCHOSES

IV A1. Definition

- A psychiatric disorder which is characterized by loss of touch with reality
  - Gross impairment in reality testing
  - Marked disturbance in personality
  - Impaired judgement
  - ***Absence of insight***[Q]
  - Characteristic symptoms: Delusions, hallucinations

IV A2. Clinical Presentation

- *Hallucinations*: Sensory perceptions in absence of stimuli
  - **Most common type: Auditory**[Q]
- *Delusions*: A false unshakeable belief/conviction despite presence of superior evidence
  - Primary delusions: Sudden, non-comprehensible in terms of mental processes
  - Secondary delusions: Influenced by the person's background or current situations
- *Thought disorders*: An underlying disturbance to conscious thought and is classified largely by its effects on speech and writing

IV A3. Underlying Causes of Psychosis

Psychiatric disorders		**Medical disorders**	
• Schizophrenia • Depression • Mania in severe depression (Bipolar) • Delusional disorder • Chronic hallucinatory psychosis **Stress** • Sleep deprivation • Sensory deprivation		• Alzheimer's disease • Parkinson's disease • Stroke • Multiple sclerosis • HIV, Malaria, Syphilis, Mumps • Hypo/Hyper- thyroidism/parathyroidism • Hypo-calcemia/glycemia/kalemia/natremia/phosphatemia • Vitamin B_{12} deficiency	
Recreational drugs • Alcohol • Amphetamine • Cannabis • Cocaine • Caffeine	• Heroin • Ketamine • LSD • Phencyclidine	**Medications***[Q] • **A**mphetamine • **P**henytoin • **C**imetidine • **D**igoxin • **I**soniazid	• **A**nxiolytics • **V**igabatrin • **C**orticosteroids • **K**etamine

[***Mnemonic:** ***A**cute **P**sychosis **C**ausing **D**rugs **I**nclude **A** **V**ery **C**ool **K**etamine*][Q]

IV A4. Diagnosis

- 18-item Brief Psychiatric Rating Scale

IV A5. Treatment

- Anti-psychotics
- Cognitive behaviour therapy
- Electro-convulsive therapy (ECT)

IV B. HALLUCINATIONS

Auditory hallucinations[Q] • Schizophrenia • Alcoholic hallucinosis • Manic-depressive illness • Organic brain syndrome • Pontine/Temporal lobe lesions	**Visual hallucinations**[Q] • Organic brain disorders: Delirium, Dementia, Epilepsy • Intoxication: LSD, Amphetamines, Alcohol, Mescaline • Alcohol withdrawal • Occipital/Temporal/Thalamus/Brainstem lesions, Ocular diseases • Schizophrenia
Olfactory hallucinations • Depression • Schizophrenia	**Olfactory and Gustatory hallucinations** • Temporal lobe diseases/Complex partial seizures • Schizophrenia
Gustatory hallucinations • Schizophrenia • Lithium/Disulfiram use	**Tactile hallucinations** • Schizophrenia • Formication[Q] (Cocaine/Methamphetamine use, Alcohol withdrawal)

IV C. THOUGHT DISORDERS

Disorders of Form (Structure)[Q] • Loosening of association • Omission, Substitution • Neologisms • Poverty of content of speech • Tangentiality, Derailment	**Disorders of Stream (Flow)** • Flight of ideas • Perseveration • Thought block • Thought retardation • Circumstantiality
Disorders of Possession (Control) • Obsessions and Compulsions • Thought insertion • Thought withdrawal • Thought broadcast	**Disorders of Content (Themes)** • Delusions of persecution/reference • Delusions of grandiosity • Nihilism • Worthlessness, Helplessness

IV D. SIDE EFFECTS OF ANTI-PSYCHOTIC DRUGS

Side effect	Cause	Maximum with	Minimum risk
Autonomic side effects			
Dry mouth	Cholinergic block	**Chlorpromazine**[Q]	**Haloperidol**[Q], Risperidone
Constipation			
Cyclopegia			
Delirium			
Urinary retention			
Mydriasis		Thioridazine	
Orthostatic hypotension	Adrenergic block	Chlorpromazine	Haloperidol
Impotence			
Impaired ejaculation		Thioridazine	

Contd…

Contd...

Side effect	Cause	Maximum with	Minimum risk
Extra-pyramidal side-effects (EPSE)			
Parkinsonian syndrome[Q]	Dopaminergic block (D2 receptor)	**Haloperidol**[Q]	**Clozapine**[Q]
Akathisia[Q]			
Acute dystonia[Q]			
Rabbit syndrome			
Neuroleptic malignant syndrome[Q]	-		-
Tardive dyskinesia[Q]	D2 hypersensitivity	-	Clozapine
Other CNS effects			
Sedation	Histamine block	Clozapine	Haloperidol
Seizures	Decreased threshold		Trifluperazine
Depression	Decreased catecholamine	-	Ziprasidone
Metabolic and endocrine effects			
Weight gain	Histamine block	Clozapine	Apiprazole
Diabetes	-		
Galactorrhoea	Increased prolactin	Haloperidol	
Allergic effects			
Cholestatic jaundice	Hypersensitivity	Chlorpromazine	Haloperidol
Agranulocytosis[Q]		**Clozapine**	
Cardiac side effects			
QT prolongation	Anticholinergic effect	Thioridazine	Aripiprazole
Sudden death	Ventricular fibrillation	–	–
Ocular side effects			
Corneal deposits	–	Chlorpromazine	Haloperidol
Pigmentary retinopathy	–	Thioridazine	All antipsychotics
Dermatological side effects[Q]			
Contact dermatitis	Allergic	Chlorpromazine	All antipsychotics
Photosensitivity	–		
Blue-gray discolouration	–		

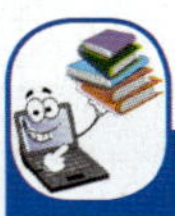

IMAGE-BASED QUESTIONS

1. Identify psychiatrist shown in Photograph *[Recent Question 2014]*

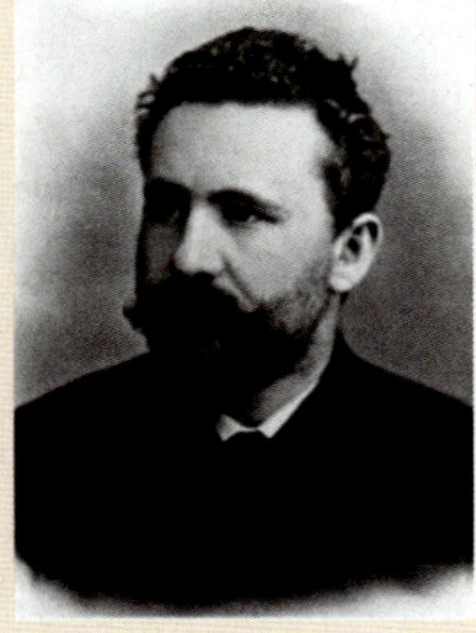

a. Eugene Bleuer b. Emil Kraepelin
c. Freud d. Cloninger

2. Prolongation of Segment shown in ECG Photograph occur due to

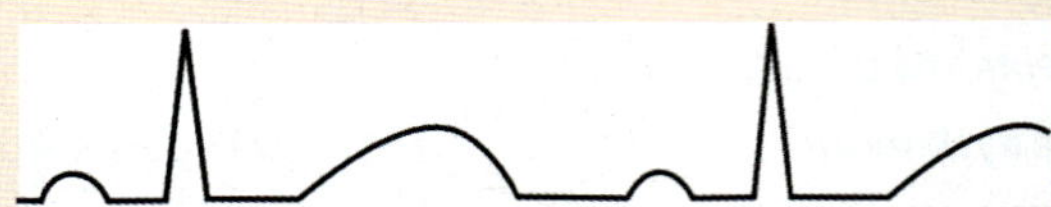

a. Thioridazine
b. Haloperidol
c. Chlorpromazine
d. Clozapine

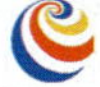 ANSWERS WITH EXPLANATIONS OF IBQs 

1. Ans. (b) Emil Kraepelin *[Ref. Dementia Praecox and Paraphrenia by Kraepelin, 1/e p1]*

Emil Kraepelin (1856-1926)
- Founder of Modern Scientific Psychiatry
- Classification system for Mental illnesses
- Differentiated between Mani-depressive psychosis and Dementia praecox (Schizophrenia)

2. Ans. (a) Thioridazine *[Ref. Niraj Ahuja, 7/e p180]*
- ECG shows: QTc segment prolongation which occur due to Thioridazine, Pimozide, Aripiprazole

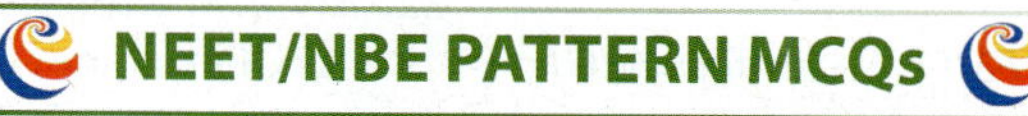

NEET/NBE PATTERN MCQs

1. **Site of lesion in Korsakoff psychosis is** *[Recent Question 2016]*
   a. Frontal lobe b. Corpus striatum
   c. Mammillary body d. Cingulated gyrus
2. **Psychotic patient on antipsychotic drugs develops torticollis within 4 days of therapy. What is the treatment?** *[Recent Question 2016]*
   a. Central anticholinergic b. Peripheral anticholinergic
   c. Beta blocker d. Dantrolene
3. **Not affected in Wernicke's disease** *[Recent Question 2016]*
   a. Hypothalamus b. Thalamus
   c. Hippocampus d. Mammillary bodies
4. **Korsakoff syndrome true is/are** *[Recent Question 2016]*
   a. Can be seen in chronic alcoholics
   b. Absence of intellectual decline
   c. Chronic amnestic syndrome
   d. All of the above
5. **Which is not neurotic defence mechanism?** *[Recent Question 2016]*
   a. Isolation b. Repression
   c. Reaction formation d. Undoing
6. **Antipsychotic drug causing retinal pigment disorder is** *[Recent Question 2016]*
   a. Thioridazine b. Clozapine
   c. Chlorpromazine d. None of the above
7. **Antipsychotic drug with least extrapyramidal symptoms** *[Recent Question 2016]*
   a. Pimozide b. Thioridazone
   c. Clozapine d. Flupromazine
8. **Defence mechanism in phobia is** *[Recent Question 2016]*
   a. Inhibition b. Dissociation
   c. Distortion d. Conversion
9. **What is produced by the supersensitivity of dopamine receptors?** *[Recent Question 2016]*
   a. Dyskinesia b. Hyperphagia
   c. Hyperpathia d. Hypomania
10. **Drug of choice for treatment of Neuroleptic malignant syndrome is** *[Recent Question 2016]*
    a. Dantrolene b. Beta blocker
    c. Central anticholinergic d. None of the above
11. **Effects of long term Levodopa therapy are** *[Recent Question 2016]*
    a. Facial tics b. Nightmares
    c. End of dose effect d. All of the above
12. **Which of the following is a Psychosis?** *[Recent Question 2016]*
    a. OCD b. Phobia
    c. Anxiety d. Mania
13. **Which is Neurotic defence mechanism?** *[Recent Question 2016]*
    a. Repression b. Anticipation
    c. Projection d. Undoing
14. **Which is included in Classical triad of Wernicke's encephalopathy?** *[Recent Question 2016]*
    a. Peripheral neuropathy
    b. Autonomic dysfunction
    c. Ataxia
    d. Abdominal pain
15. **Symptom of Neuroleptic malignant syndrome** *[Recent Question 2016]*
    a. Hypotension
    b. Hypothermia
    c. Increased Magnesium level in blood
    d. Catatonia and stupor
16. **Psychosis can be caused by** *[NBE FMGE September 2009]*
    a. INH b. Ketamine
    c. Steroids d. All of the above
17. **Which drug is the most useful in treating an episode of anti-psychotic-induced acute dystonia?** *[NBE DNB June 2011]*
    a. Lorazepam b. Haloperidol
    c. Promethazine d. Phenobarbitone
18. **A 25-year-old male is taking Haloperidol (Antipsychotic) since last 3 years. He presented to emergency department with protruded tongue, breathing difficulty along with spasm of neck and jaw muscles. Most likely diagnosis is** *[NBE FMGE September 2008, Recent Question 2015]*
    a. Acute dystonia
    b. Drug hypersensitivity reaction
    c. Tardive dyskinesia
    d. Neuroleptic malignant syndrome
19. **Which of the following is not a Schneider's first rank symptom?** *[NBE DNB 1997, 1999, 2001, 2005, 2006, Recent Question 2015]*
    a. Passivity phenomenon
    b. Auditory hallucinations
    c. Delusion of self-reference
    d. Delusional perception
20. **A 20-year-old male manic patient was prescribed haloperidol one week back. For the last two days, he has become restless and kept pacing in the room. On examination, he was found to have tremors of hand. He is most likely suffering from** *[NBE DNB December 2011]*
    a. Anhedonia b. Restless legs syndrome
    c. Dystonia d. Akathisia
21. **Which of the following have a major role to play in pathogenesis of Parkinsonism?** *[NBE FMGE September 2012]*
    a. Acetylcholine b. GABA
    c. Epinephrine d. Dopamine
22. **Antipsychotic drugs mainly work by their action on receptors of** *[NBE FMGE September 2012]*
    a. Dopamine b. Acetylcholine
    c. Epinephrine d. GABA

23. In Korsakoff psychosis, there is *[NBE FMGE September 2005]*
a. Loss of short term memory
b. Loss of long term memory
c. Both short term and long term memory
d. None

24. Parkinson's disease is characterized by all of the following clinical features except *[NBE FMGE September 2012]*
a. Hyperactivity b. Tremor
c. Bradykinesia d. Rigidity

25. Olfactory and gustatory hallucinations are seen in *[NBE DNB 2002]*
a. Depression
b. Paranoia
c. Temporal lobe epilepsy
d. Alzheimer's disease

26. Most common hallucinations seen in functional psychosis is *[NBE DNB 1992]*
a. Visual b. Olfactory
c. Auditory d. Gustatory

27. Patients with depressive psychosis *[NBE DNB 1992]*
a. Feel better in morning
b. Feel better in the evening than in the morning
c. Feel better in morning and evening
d. Don't feel better

28. Gustatory hallucinations are most commonly associated with *[NBE DNB 2008, 2009, 2010]*
a. Temporal lobe epilepsy b. Grand mal epilepsy
c. Anxiety disorders d. Tobacco dependence

29. Which anti-tubercular drug can cause Psychosis? *[NBE FMGE September 2004]*
a. Ofloxacin b. Cycloserine
c. Capreomycin d. Rifampicin

30. Gum hypertrophy is a complication of *[UPSC 1999]*
a. Sodium valproate b. Phenytoin sodium
c. Phenobarbitone d. Clonazepam

31. Most common psychotic feature seen in majority of psychotic problems *[NBE DNB 2008]*
a. Dementia b. Delusions
c. Illusions d. Phobia

32. Atypical antipsychotics are all, except *[NBE DNB 2009]*
a. Olanzapine b. Clozapine
c. Risperidone d. Thioridazine

33. Korsakoff's psychosis is associated with pathological lesions at *[UPSC 1999]*
a. Cerebellum b. Thalamus
c. Mammillary bodies d. Middle cerebral artery

34. Antipsychotic induced "akathisia" is characterized by *[NBE DNB 2008, 2009]*
a. Rigidity
b. Tremor
c. Spasm of muscle/muscle group
d. Restlessness

35. Korsakoff psychosis is due to deficiency of *[NBE FMGE September 2003]*
a. Vitamin B1 b. Vitamin B2
c. Vitamin B3 d. Vitamin B12

36. The commonest form of puerperal psychosis *[NBE DNB 1993, 2003]*
a. Organic b. Schizophreniform
c. Affective d. Anxiety neurosis

37. Antipsychotic induced "akathisia" is characterized by *[NBE DNB 2010]*
a. Rigidity b. Tremor
c. Spasm of muscle/muscle group
d. Restlessness

38. All of the following are maladaptive coping strategies in stress disorder except *[NBE FMGE September 2011]*
a. Use of alcohol
b. Confrontation
c. Aggressive behavior
d. Avoiding offer of help from others

39. Which of the following is NOT a mature defence mechanism? *[NBE FMGE September 2011]*
a. Altruism b. Acting out
c. Sublimation d. Suppression

40. Treatment of choice for Akathisia is? *[Recent Question 2017]*
a. Phenytoin b. Propranolol
c. Dantrolene d. Lithium

HIGH YIELD MCQs

1. All are the features of Wernicke's encephalopathy except *[Bihar PG 2016]*
a. Cogwheel rigidity b. Alteration in mental function
c. Ophthalmoplegia d. Ataxia

2. Most specific of psychosis is *[AIIMS PGMEE 1995]*
a. Neologism b. Incoherence
c. Pressure of speech d. Perseveration

3. Difference between neurosis and psychosis is *[All India PGMEE 1995]*
a. Severity b. Insight
c. Clinical features d. Duration

4. The characteristic symptom of organic psychosis is *[AIIMS PGMEE 1993]*
a. Hallucination b. Depression
c. Transient delusion d. Anxiety

5. Folie a deux is seen in *[PGI 1999]*
a. Hysteria b. Paranoid
c. OCD d. Neurasthenia

6. **Which of the following features is not included in psychosis?** *[PGI 2004]*
   a. Panic attack b. Delusion
   c. Hallucination d. Hypochondriasis

7. **The Psychological disorder most commonly associated with myxoedema** *[All India PGMEE 1992]*
   a. Mania b. Depression
   c. Phobia d. Paronia

8. **Most common type of post puerperal psychosis is**
   a. Depression b. Anxiety *[PGI 1999]*
   c. Mania d. Suicide

9. **A man coming from mountain whose wife died 6 months prior says that his wire appeared to him and asked him to join her. The diagnosis is** *[AIIMS PGMEE 2000]*
   a. Normal grief b. Grief psychosis
   c. Bereavement reaction d. Supernatural phenomenon

10. **The following is not an atypical antipsychotic** *[AIIMS PGMEE 2008]*
   a. Thioridazine b. Clozapine
   c. Olanzapine d. Risperidone

11. **Least Extrapyramidal side-effects are seen in** *[AIIMS PGMEE 1998]*
   a. Haloperidol b. Thioridazine
   c. Clozapine d. Chlorpromazine

12. **Antipsychotic drug with prolonged action** *[All India PGMEE 1993]*
   a. Trifluperazine b. Thioridazine
   c. Penfluridol d. Fluphenazine

13. **A patient of schizophrenia on chlorpromazine develops auditory hallucination again. The next drug to be given is** *[All India PGMEE 2000]*
   a. Haloperidol b. Clozapine
   c. Sulphride d. Tianeptine

14. **Adverse effect of clozapine** *[PGI 1998]*
   a. Hypertension b. Sialorrhea
   c. Extrapyramidal side effects
   d. Neuroleptic malignant syndrome

15. **Tardive dyskinesia is produced by following except**
   a. Fluphenazine b. Haloperidol *[PGI 1998]*
   c. Chlorpromazine d. Clozapine

16. **Irresistible urge to move about with inner restlessness is called** *[All India PGMEE 1999]*
   a. Akinesia b. Hyperkinesia
   c. Dyskinesia d. Akathisia

17. **Malignant neurolept hyperthermia (NMS) seen in all except** *[AIIMS PGMEE 2008]*
   a. Haloperidol b. Metoclopramide
   c. Domperidone d. Amantadine

18. **Akathisia is treated by A/E** *[All India PGMEE 1994]*
   a. Trihexyphenidyl b. Diazepam
   c. Haloperidol d. Propranolol

19. **Carbamazepine may be used in all except** *[All India PGMEE 1997]*
   a. Mania b. Alcohol withdrawal
   c. Schizophrenia d. Trigeminal neuralgia

20. **HIAA is a metabolite of** *[AIIMS PGMEE 2006]*
   a. Serotonin b. Dopamine
   c. Epinephrine d. Histamine

21. **Side effect of SSRI** *[PGI 2007]*
   a. Nausea b. Diarrhoea
   c. Weight gain d. Rash
   e. Sexual dysfunction

22. **Side effects of Fluoxetine are all except** *[AP PGMEE 1994]*
   a. Weigh gain b. Sweating
   c. Urinary retention d. Diarrhoea

23. **Tianeptine acts by** *[AIIMS PGMEE 1998]*
   a. MAO inhibitor b. Serotonin uptake inhibitor
   c. Serotonin uptake enhancer
   d. 5-HT agonist

24. **Mode of action of fluoxetine is** *[AIIMS PGMEE 1996]*
   a. GABA inhibition
   b. Adrenergic neuron blocking action
   c. Inhibition of axonal uptake of 5HT
   d. Adrenergic stimulation

25. **Differentiating features between neurosis and psychosis**
   a. Insight is preserved *[MP PGMEE 2001]*
   b. Lack of insight
   c. Personality and behavior preserved
   d. None

26. **All are seen in organic psychosis except** *[Kerala PGMEE 1996]*
   a. Disorientation in place, time & person
   b. Clouding of consciousness
   c. Hallucination
   d. Normal common knowledge
   e. Intellectual impairment

27. **Characteristic Symptom in induced psychotic disorder is**
   a. Insomnia *[AIIMS PGMEE 1992]*
   b. Profound mood disturbance
   c. Accepting delusions of other person
   d. Suicidal Ideation

28. **All the following statement about clozapine are true except** *[All India PGMEE 1997]*
   a. It is used in schizophrenia
   b. May precipitate seizure
   c. May cause agranulocytosis
   d. Extrapyramidal side effects are seen

29. **A patient presents with one month history of abnormal hallucination and delusion. The patient lacks insight to his changed behaviour. Likely diagnosis is** *[All India PGMEE 1997]*
   a. Paronia b. Depression
   c. Psychosis d. Schizophrenia

30. **Antipsychotic drug with least extrapyramidal effects is** *[PGI 2002]*
   a. Clozapine
   b. Risperidone
   c. Thioridazine
   d. Chlorpromazine
   e. Haloperidol

31. A 25-year-old man with a psychotic illness, was treated with haloperidol 3 mw day. On the third day he developed pacing, and inability to sit still at one place. The medication likely to be helpful is *[Recent Question 2015, AIIMS PGMEE 2002]*

a. Phenytoin b. Propranolol
c. Methylphenidate d. Trihexyphenidyl

32. A patient on treatment for psychiatric disorder takes overdose of a drug, develops bradycardia, hypotension, increased sweating and salivation. The likely drug is *[AIIMS PGMEE 1999]*

a. Amitriptyline b. Lithium
c. Selegiline d. Amphetamine

33. Mode of action of fluoxetine *[All India PGMEE 1999, AIIMS PGMEE 1997]*

a. GABA agonist b. GABA antagonist
c. Inhibit uptake of 5-HT d. Increase uptake of 5-HT

34. The common side effect with fluoxetine therapy is *[All India PGMEE 2006]*

a. Seizure b. Anxiety
c. Hypotension d. Loose stools

35. Vasanti 45 years, was brought to casualty with abnormal movements which induced persistent deviation of neck to right side. One day before she was prescribed Haloperidol 5 mg three times daily from the psychiatry OPD. She also had an alternation with her husband recently. Which of the following is the most likely cause for her symptoms? *[AIIMS PGMEE 2000]*

a. Conversion reaction b. Acute psychosis
c. Acute drug dystonia d. CVA

36. A 60-year-old male comes to causality with acute retention of urine since 12 hours. On examination there was distended bladder. His son gives a history of taking some drug by the patient. Since 2 days as he is suffering from depression. The most likely drug is *[AIIMS PGMEE 2001]*

a. CPZ b. Amitriptyline
c. Haloperidol d. Pimozide

37. A patient on antipsychotic for past 4 weeks is brought to the emergency with complaint of acute onset of fever, excessive sweating confusion, rigidity of limbs & decreased communication. Examination reveals Temperature of 104°F; P/R -12/min BP-15/1 with disorientation. What is the most probable diagnosis? *[PGI 2005]*

a. Lithium toxicity
b. Aggravation of psychosis
c. Dystonia
d. Neuroleptic malignant syndrome
e. Akathisia

38. A patient with acute psychosis, who is on haloperidol 2 mg/day for last 2 days, has an episode characterized by tongue protrusion- oculogyric crisis, stiffness and abnormal posture of limbs and trunk without loss of consciousness for last 2 minutes before presenting to casualty. This improved within a few minutes after administration of diphenhydramine HCl. The most likely diagnosis is *[AIIMS PGMEE 2006]*

a. Acute dystonia
b. Akathisia
c. Tardive dyskinesia
d. Neuroleptic malignant syndrome

39. An elderly woman suffering from schizophrenia is on antipsychotic medication. She developed purposeless involuntary facial and limb movements, constant chewing and puffing of cheeks. Which of the following drugs is least likely to be involved in this side effect? *[AIIMS PGMEE 2003]*

a. Haloperidol b. Clozapine
c. Fluphenazine d. Loxapine

40. True about Neuroleptic malignant syndrome *[PGI 2008]*

a. General antipsychotics are more associated
b. Symptoms include rigidity, fever and palpitation
c. Dantrolene improves symptoms
d. Bromocriptine can be used

41. A 30-year-old man who was recently started on haloperidol 3 mg/day developed hyperpyrexia, muscle rigidity, akinesia, mutism, sweating, tachycardia and increased blood pressure. The investigations showed increased WBC count, increased creatinine phosphokinase. There is no history of any other drug intake or any signs of infection. The most likely diagnosis is *[AIIMS PGMEE 2006]*

a. Drug overdose
b. Neuroleptic malignant syndrome
c. Drug induced Parkinsonism
d. Tardive dyskinesia

42. A patient was on treatment with Trifluperazine for some time. He presents with complaint of hyperthermia, lethargy and sweating. Needed investigations are *[AIIMS PGMEE 2000]*

a. CT Scan brain & hemogram
b. Hemogram, Electrolyte level and creatinine
c. ECG, Chest X-ray and Hemogram
d. Hemogram, CPK and Renal Function Test

43. A 31-year-old male, with mood disorder, on 3 mg of haloperidol and 1 mg of lithium, is brought to the hospital emergency room with history of acute onset of fever, excessive sweating, confusion, rigidity of limbs and decreased communication for a day. Examination reveals tachycardia and labile blood pressure and investigations reveal increased CPK enzyme levels and leucocytosis. He is likely to have developed *[AIIMS PGMEE 2004, Recent Question 2015]*

a. Lithium toxicity b. Tardive dyskinesia
c. Neuroleptic malignant syndrome
d. Hypertensive encephalopathy

44. A 34-years-old patient 'Ram' is suffering from a known case of psychotic disorder. He is currently on treatment with Antipsychotics and Anti-hypertensives. He suddenly developed tachycardia and chest tightness. On medical evaluation Ram was found to have metabolic acidosis. ECG indicated widened QRS complex and prolonged QT interval. Following drug may be responsible for the ECG changes *[AIIMS May 2017]*

a. Chlorthalidone b. Amlodipine
c. Enlapril d. Amytriptyline

 NEET/NBE PATTERN MCQs ANSWERS WITH EXPLANATIONS

1. Ans. (c) Mammillary body
[Ref. Niraj Ahuja, 7/e p39-40]
- Neuropathological lesion in Korsakoff's psychosis is usually widespread
- Most consistent changes: Bilateral dorso-medical nuclei of thalamus and Mammillary bodies
- Other changes: Periventricular & Periaqueductal gray matter, Cerebellum, Parts of brain stem

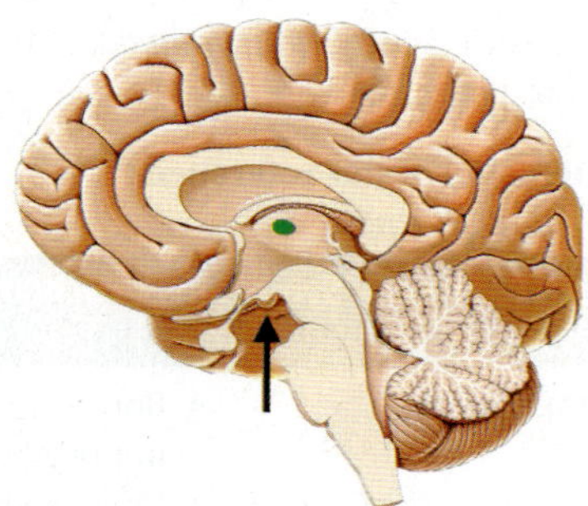

Fig. Mammillary body

2. Ans. (a) Central anticholinergic
[Ref. Geriatric Anesthesia by Kumra, 1/e p383]
- Antipsychotics are used to treat psychosis due to any cause
- Main side effects are Parkinsonism, Muscular dystonias (bizarre muscular spasm mostly involving linguofacial muscle-grimacing, torticollis, locked jaw)
- Central anticholinergics (e.g. Phenothiazines) are DOC

3. Ans. (c) Hippocampus
[Ref. Niraj Ahuja, 7/e p39-40]

4. Ans. (d) All of the above
[Ref. Niraj Ahuja, 7/e p39-40]

5. Ans. (b) Repression
[Ref. Niraj Ahuja, 7/e p210]

Ego-Defence Mechanisms
- **Immature/Neurotic:** Conversion, Dissociation, Displacement, Isolation, Reaction formation, Undoing, Rationalization, Intellectualization, Acting out, Retroflexion, Introjection, Hypochondriasis, Inhibition, Schizoid fantasy
- **Primary:** Repression
- **Psychotic/Narcissistic:** Regression, Denial, Projection, Distortion
- **Mature:** Sublimation, Suppression, Anticipation, Humour, Altruism

6. Ans. (a) Thioridazine
[Ref. Brochert's Crush Step 3 by Movalia, 4/e p146]
- Thioridazine causes retinal pigment deposits
- Clozapine causes agranulocytosis
- Chlorpromazine cause jaundice and photosensitivity

7. Ans. (c) Clozapine
[Ref. Psychiatry by Cutler, 3/e p118]
- Clozapine binds to both dopamine and serotonin receptors, and it has a much lower incidence of extrapyramidal side effects
- Other first generation antipsychotics block only dopamine

8. Ans. (a) Inhibition
[Ref. Kaplan & Sadock, 10/e p599]
- In phobia, the defence mechanisms are Repression, Regression, Displacement, and Projection
- In Social phobia, defence mechanism in children: Inhibition (behavioral)

9. Ans. (a) Dyskinesia
[Ref. Schizophrenic Disorders by Cancro, 1/e p207]

Tardive dyskinesia
- Super-sensitivity of Dopamine receptors which "fight back" after having been blocked for a prolonged period
- Excessive abnormal movements of tardive dyskinesia are representative of side effects of high doses of L-Dopa

10. Ans. (a) Dantrolene
[Ref. The 5-minute Neurology Consult by Lynn, 1/e p301]
- Dantrolene is **DOC** for Malignant hyperthermia, Neuroleptic malignant syndrome

11. Ans. (d) All of the above
[Ref. Competitive Examinations In Pharmacy by Shah, 1/e p2.32]
- Prolonged therapy effect: Facial tics, choreoathetoid movement, nighmares, mania, hallucination and "end of dose" and "on–off" effect

12. Ans. (d) Mania
[Ref. Niraj Ahuja, 7/e p83]
- Psychosis includes Schizophrenia, Schizophreniform disorder, Bipolar illness, Schizoaffective disorder, Depression with psychotic features, Drug-induced psychosis, Organic psychosis, Brief psychotic disorder, Delusional disorder

13. Ans. (a) Repression
[Ref. Psychoanalytic Psychotherapy by Elzer, 1/e p72]

Neurotic Defence Mechanisms
- **Displacement:** Shifts sexual or aggressive impulses to a more acceptable or less threatening target
- **Dissociation:** Separation or postponement of a feeling to avoid emotional distress
- **Hypochondriasis:** Excessive preoccupation or worry about having a serious illness
- **Intellectualization:** Avoiding unacceptable emotions by focusing on the intellectual aspects
- **Isolation:** Separation of feelings from ideas and events
- **Rationalization:** Convincing oneself that no wrong has been done through faulty and false reasoning
- **Reaction formation:** Taking the opposite belief because the true belief causes anxiety
- **Regression:** Reversion of ego to an earlier stage of development than handling unacceptable impulses
- **Repression:** Repel desires towards pleasurable instincts
- **Undoing:** 'Undo' an unhealthy, destructive threatening thought by acting out reverse of unacceptable
- **Withdrawal:** Removing oneself from events, stimuli under threat of being reminded of painful thoughts

- **Social comparisons:** Means of self-evaluation to perceive one better by comparing to worse-off

14. Ans. (c) Ataxia

[Ref. Revision Notes for MCEM, Part 2 by Stacey, 1/e p44]

- **Classical triad of Wernicke's encephalopathy:** Ataxia, Ophthalmoplegia, Confusion

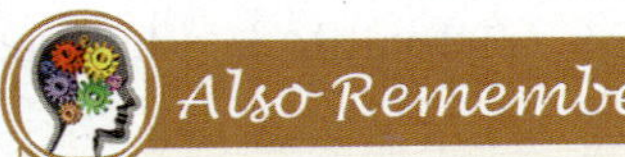

- Beck's Cognitive triad of Depression: Negative views of Self, World, Future

15. Ans. (d) Catatonia and stupor

[Ref. Sims' Symptoms in the Mind, 4/e p382]

- Neuroleptic malignant syndrome show features of Catatonia
- Clinical features of NMS: Rigidity (Lead-pipe rigidity), Hyperthermia, Diaphoresis, Pallor, Dysphagia, Dyspnea, Tremor, Incontinence, Tachycardia, Shuffling gait, Psychomotor agitation, Delirium progressing to lethargy, stupor, coma (Lethal/Malignant catatonia)

16. Ans. (d) All of the above

[Ref. Diagnosis of Psychosis by Cardinal and Bullmore]

- Medications causing Psychosis **[Mnemonic: Acute Psychosis Causing Drugs Include A Very Cool Ketamine]**
  - **A**mphetamine
  - **P**henytoin
  - **C**imetidine
  - **D**igoxin
  - **I**soniazid
  - **A**nxiolytics
  - **V**igabatrin
  - **C**orticosteroids
  - **K**etamine

17. Ans. (c) Promethazine

[Ref. Kaplan & Sadock's Concise Textbook of Clinical Psychiatry, 3/e p483]

- *Drugs used for treatment of Anti-psychotic induced acute dystonia*:
  - Diphenhydramine
  - Promethazine

18. Ans. (c) Tardive dyskinesia

[Ref. Niraj Ahuja, 7/e p179]

Tardive Dyskinesia

- *Definition*: Difficult form of dyskinesia (repetitive body movements) that are tardive (late onset) in nature
  - Is a type of extrapyramidal side-effect of anti-psychotic drugs
  - Is a Late onset oro-facial dyskinesia
- *Clinical presentation*: Repetitive purposeless movements
  - Grimacing
  - Puckering of lips
  - Tongue protrusion
  - Lip-smacking
  - Eye blinking
- ***Underlying cause*: Dopaminergic D2 receptor hypersensitivity**
  - Anti-psychotic drugs
  - Metoclopramide
  - Promethazine
  - Antidepressants
  - Antiepileptics
- *Treatment*: Tetrabenazine

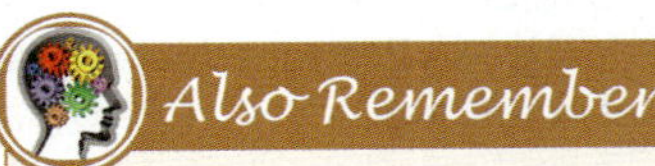

- *Anti-psychotic with least Extra-pyramidal side effects/Tardive dyskinesia:* Clozapine

19. Ans. (c) Delusion of self-reference

[Ref. Niraj Ahuja, 7/e p55]

Schneider's First Rank Symptoms of Schizophrenia (SFRS)*	
• **S**omatic passivity	• Body sensations imposed by others
• **M**ade feelings/affect	• Imposed by others
• **M**ade impulses	• Imposed by others
• **M**ade volition/acts	• Imposed by others
• **D**elusional perception	• Private illogical meaning
• **V**oices heard arguing	• Auditory hallucinations
• **V**oices commenting on one's action	• Auditory hallucinations
• **A**udible thoughts	• Thought echo
• **T**hought withdrawal	• Thoughts cease, removed by someone
• **T**hought insertion	• Thoughts imposed by someone else
• **T**hought diffusion/ broadcasting	• Thoughts escaping and experienced by others

[***Mnemonic:** ***S****chizophrenic* ***M****an* ***D****oes* ***V****alue* ***A****udible* ***T****houghts*; ***SAM³V²T³D***]

20. Ans. (d) Akathisia

[Ref. Psychiatric Side-effects of Prescription and Over the Counter Medications by Brown, 1/e p1650]

Akathisia

- *Description*: Movement disorder characterized by inner restlessness, and compelling need to be in constant motion
- *Causes of Akathisia*:
  - Pontine disorders
  - Drugs induced:
    1. Antipsychotics: Haloperidol
    2. Anti-depressants: Venlafaxine
    3. SSRI: Fluoxetine

21. Ans. (d) Dopamine

[Ref. Textbook of Postgraduate Psychiatry by Vyas & Ahuja, 2/e p479]

- *Principal neurotransmitter affected in Parkinsonism*: Dopamine

22. Ans. (a) Dopamine

[Ref. Niraj Ahuja, 7/e p175]

- *Mechanism of action of Anti-psychotics*:
  - Anti-dopaminergic activity
  - Block D2 receptors
    1. Mesolimbic-mesocortical system: Major site of action
    2. Nigro-striatal system: Extra-pyramidal side-effects
    3. Tubero-infundibular system: Hyperprolactinemia

23. Ans. (c) Both short term and long term memory
[Ref. Niraj Ahuja, 7/e p27]

Wernicke's Korsakoff's Psychosis

- *Wernicke's encephalopathy*: Acute reaction to severe deficiency of thiamine – Vitamin B_1 (Beri-beri)
  - ***Most common cause*: Chronic alcoholism**
  - *Clinical presentation*:
    1. Ocular signs: Nystagmus, Ophthalmoplegia, Retinal hemorrhages, Papilloedema, Impaired vision
    2. Higher mental functions disturbance: Disorientation, memory disturbance, confusion
    3. Peripheral neuropathy
    4. Malnutrition
- *Korsakoff's psychosis*:
  - *Clinical presentation*:
  - Organic amnestic syndrome with impaired memory due to organic cause

Memory	Impairment
Recent/short term memory	Severe impairment
Remote/long term memory	Impairment
Immediate memory	No impairment

  - Confabulation
  - Loss of insight

24. Ans. (a) Hyperactivity
[Ref. Principles and Practice of Geriatric Psychiatry by Agronin & Maletta, 1/e p619]

Features of Parkinson's Disease

Cardinal features	Secondary features	
• Resting tremor • Bradykinesia • Rigidity • Postural instability	• Dystonia • Dysphagia • Dysarthria • Hypomimia • Micrographia • Festination, Freezing, Retropulsion	• Stooping posture, Kyphosis, Scoliosis • Erectile dysfunction • Seborrheic dermatitis • Drooling • Constipation • Over-active bladder

25. Ans. (c) Temporal lobe epilepsy
[Ref. Child and Adolescent Neurology for Psychiatrists by Walker & Kaufman, 1/e p395]

- *Hallucinations in Brain Disorders*:

Region of lesion	Type of hallucinations
Occipital lobe epilepsy	Visual hallucinations
Temporal lobe seizures (Uncus)	Olfactory, Gustatory hallucinations
Occipitoparietal/Occipitotemporal junctions	Complex visual hallucinations
Neocortical temporal cortex	Auditory hallucinations
Frontal/Orbitofrontal seizures	Auditory, Complex visual hallucinations

26. Ans. (c) Auditory
[Ref. Mental and Behavioral Dysfunction in Movement Disorders, 1/e p273]

- *Most common hallucinations seen in Functional Psychosis*: Auditory hallucinations
  - Schizophrenia
  - Bipolar disorder

27. Ans. (b) Feel better in the evening than in the morning
[Ref. Manic Depressive Illness by Clayton & Reich, 1/e p65]

- *Worsening of depression in morning*: Endogenous & Psychotic depression

28. Ans. (a) Temporal lobe epilepsy
[Ref. Child and Adolescent Neurology for Psychiatrists by Walker & Kaufman, 1/e p395]

29. Ans. (b) Cycloserine
[Ref. Diagnosis of Psychosis by Cardinal and Bullmore]

- *Anti-tubercular drugs causing psychosis*:

Commonly leading to psychosis	Uncommon cause of psychosis
• Isoniazid • Ethambutol • Trifluoperazine • Cycloserine • Ciprofloxacin	• Rifampicin • Streptomycin

30. Ans. (b) Phenytoin sodium
[Ref. Adult Emergency Medicine by O' Brien, 1/e p108]

- *Causes of Gum hypertrophy*:
- Drugs: Phenytoin, Cyclosporine, Nifedipine
- Poisonings: Lead, Arsenic
- Other causes: Pregnancy, Scurvy, Leukemias, Poor oral hygiene

31. Ans. (a) Dementia
[Ref. Corsini Encyclopedia of Psychology, Volume 2, 4/e p911]

- *Most common Psychosis*:
  - **Dementia (Most common)**
  - Major depressive disorder with psychosis
  - Delusional disorder

32. Ans. (d) Thioridazine
[Ref. Niraj Ahuja, 7/e p66]

Anti-Psychotic Drugs

First generation/Typical/Traditional	Second generation/Atypical
• Chlorpromazine • Haloperidol • Loxapine	• Clozapine • Olanzapine • Quetiapine

Contd...

Psychiatry

Contd...

First generation/Typical/ Traditional	Second generation/ Atypical
• Pimozide • Prochlorperazine • Thioridazine • Trifluperazine	• Risperidone • Amisulpride • Arpiprazole • Zotepine

33. Ans. (c) Mammillary bodies

[Ref. Niraj Ahuja, 7/e p39-40]

Korsakoff Psychosis

- Description: Organic amnestic syndrome
  - Gross memory disturbance, confabulation
  - Insight is impaired
- Underlying cause: Untreated Thiamine deficiency secondary to Chronic alcohol abuse
- Neuropathological lesions:
  - Major: Dorsomedial nuclei of thalamus, Mammillary bodies
  - Minor: Periventricular/Periaqueductal grey matter, Cerebellum, Brainstem

34. Ans. (d) Restlessness

[Ref. Psychiatric Side-effects of Prescription and Over the Counter Medications by Brown, 1/e p1650]

35. Ans. (a) Vitamin B1

[Ref. Niraj Ahuja, 7/e p38-40]

36. Ans. (c) Affective

[Ref. Kaplan and Sadock's Study Guide and Self Examination Review in Psychiatry, 9/e p139]

- *Most severe form of Post-partum psychiatric illness*: Puerperal psychosis
- *Development of symptoms*: 2-4 weeks after delivery
- *Presentation*: Rapidly evolving affective psychosis with restlessness, irritability, insomnia
  - Agitation
  - Depression
  - Thoughts of infanticide

37. Ans. (d) Restlessness

[Ref. Psychiatric Side-effects of Prescription and Over the Counter Medications by Brown, 1/e p1650]

38. Ans. (b) Confrontation

[Ref. The Maintenance of Anxiety Disorders: maladaptive Coping Strategies by MD Jacofsky and MT Santos]

Coping Strategies in Stress Disorder

Maladaptive/Negative coping strategies	Positive coping strategies
• Dissociation • Aggressive behaviours • Anxious avoidance • Escape (including self-medication) • Substance use • Alcohol/drugs indulgence • Self-blame	• Anticipation • Confrontation • Social support seeking • Good nutrition, exercise and sleep • Humour • Religious coping (Most common) • Meditation

39. Ans. (b) Acting out

[Ref. Niraj Ahuja, 7/e p210]

EGO-Defence Mechanisms

Immature/Neurotic	Primary
• Conversion • Dissociation • Displacement • Isolation • Reaction formation • Undoing • Rationalisation • Intellectualisation • Acting out • Retroflexion • Introjection • Hypochondriasis • Inhibition • Schizoid fantasy	• Repression **Psychotic/Narcissistic** • Regression • Denial • Projection • Distortion **Mature** • Sublimation • Suppression • Anticipation • Humour • Altruism

40. Ans. (b) Propranolol

[Ref. American Psychiatric Publishing Textbook of Psychiatry, 5/e p1089]

Akathisia

- Movement disorder characterized by inner restlessness, and compelling need to be in constant motion
- It is a common reaction that most often occurs shortly after initiation of treatment with a conventional Antipsychotic medication or Aripiprazole
- Treatment of choice: Shift to Atypical agent or Beta-adrenergic blocking drug (Propranolol)

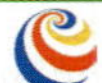 HIGH YIELD MCQs ANSWERS WITH EXPLANATIONS 

1. Ans. (a) Cogwheel rigidity
[Ref. Niraj Ahuja, 7/e p38]

Wernicke's Encephalopathy
- Acute reaction to severe thiamine (Vitamin B1) deficiency
  - Ocular signs: Nystagmus, ophthalmoplegia, retinal hemorrhages, pappilloedema
  - Higher mental function disturbances: Disorientation, confusion, recent memory disturbance, poor attention span
  - Ataxia
  - Peripheral neuropathy
  - Severe malnutrition

2. Ans. (a) Neologism
[Ref. The Psychiatric Mental Status Examination by Baker, 1/e p90]

Neologisms
- *Description*: Idiosyncratic words which are meaningless to others but of significance to psychotic
- *Characteristic disorder*: Psychosis

3. Ans. (b) Insight
[Ref. Evolutionary Psychiatry by Stevens & Price, 2/e p122]

Neurosis vs Psychosis

	Neurosis	Psychosis
Insight	Present	Absent
Personality	Partly involved	Wholly involved
Social adaptation	Fair	Very poor
Contact with reality	Present	Absent
Severity	Mild	Severe
Delusions	Absent	Present
Hallucinations	Absent	Present

4. Ans. (c) Transient delusion
[Ref. Niraj Ahuja, 7/e p56]

5. Ans. (b) Paranoid
[Ref. Basic Concepts of Psychiatric Mental Health Nursing by Shives, 7/e p520]

Folie A Deux
- *Description*: Two individuals who have a close relationship and shared delusions as seen in Paranoid disorder
- *Types of Folie à deux*:
  - Folie imposee: Delusions of a Psychotic person is transferred to a person with sound mind
  - Folie simultanee: Simultaneous appearance of an identical psychosis in two individuals who are intimately associated and morbidly predisposed
  - Folie communique: Recipient develops symptoms after a long period of resistance and maintains the symptoms even after separation
  - Folie induite: New delusions are adopted by a Psychotic individual who is under influence of another individual with psychosis

6. Ans. (a) Panic attack
[Ref. MCAT Psychology and Sociology Review by Princeton, 2015]

Symptoms of Psychosis

Positive symptoms	Negative symptoms
• Delusions • Hallucinations • Disorganized speech • Disorganized/catatonic behavior	• Flat/Blunted affect • Reduced quantity/fluency of speech • Avolition • Hypochondriasis

7. Ans. (b) Depression
[Ref. Hormones, Brain and Behavior, 1/e p239]
- *Most common Psychological disorders associated with Hypothyroidism/Myxedema*:
  - **Depression (Most common)**
  - Cognitive dysfunction
  - Psychotic and delusional symptoms

8. Ans. (a) Depression
[Ref. Kaplan and Sadock's Study Guide and Self Examination Review in Psychiatry, 9thEd., Pg 139]

9. Ans. (b) Grief psychosis
[Ref. Zone Comprehensive Guide to PGMEE Volume 3, 2009, Pg 818]

Grief Reaction
- ***Normal Grief reaction***: Transient self-limiting phenomena
  - Stags of normal grief reaction: Protest, Searching behavior, Despair, Detachment form a loved one, Reorganization to new life
- ***Morbid grief reaction***:
  - Pathological grief reaction: Exaggeration of one or more symptoms of normal grief, or the duration becomes prolonged greater than 6 months without spontaneous recovery
  - Complicated grief reaction: Grief complicated by specific neurotic/psychotic illness, in addition to grief reaction symptoms

10. Ans. (a) Thioridazine
[Ref. Niraj Ahuja, 7/e p66]

11. Ans. (c) Clozapine
[Ref. Niraj Ahuja, 7/e p176-77]

Extrapyramidal Side-Effects in Antipsychotic Use

Maximum EPSE	Least EPSE
• Fluphenazine • Prochlorperazine • Trifluoperazine • Haloperidol • Trifluperidol	• Clozapine • Ziprasidone • Quetiapine • Aripiprazole • Bifeprunox • Asenapine

12. Ans. (d) Fluphenazine

[Ref. Wyatt's Practical Psychiatric Practice, 3/e p143]

- *Long acting Antipsychotics*:
  - Fluphenazine, Haloperidol decanoate
  - Exert action over several weeks
  - Disadvantage: Difficult reversal of side effects

13. Ans. (b) Clozapine

[Ref. Niraj Ahuja, 7/e p66; Treating Mental Illness and Behavior Disorders in Children and Adults with Mental Retardation by Dosen and Day, 1/e p189]

- Clozapine is used for treatment of patients of Schizophrenia who are resistant to treatment with other drugs

14. Ans. (b) Sialorrhea

[Ref. Bipolar Psychopharmacotherapy by Akiskal and Tohel, 2/e, 8.3.3]

- *Side-effects of Clozapine*:
  - Agranulocytosis
  - Seizure disorder
  - Metabolic syndrome
  - Myocarditis
  - Sialorrhoea

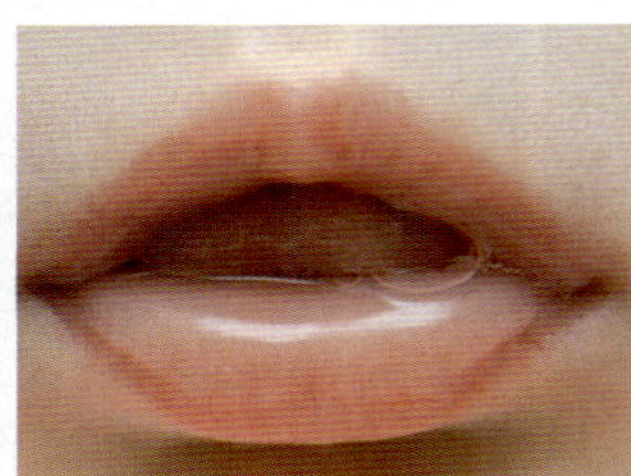

Fig. Sialorrhoea

15. Ans. (d) Clozapine

[Ref. Meyler's Side Effects of Psychiatric Drugs by Aronson, 1/e p267]

- *Tardive dyskinesia*: Involuntary movements of the tongue, lips, face, trunk, and extremities that occur in patients treated with long-term dopaminergic antagonist medications
  - Typical Antipsychotics have a high risk of Tardive dyskinesia
  - Clozapine and Quetiapine carries lowest risk of Tardive dyskinesia

16. Ans. (d) Akathisia

[Ref. Psychiatric Side-effects of Prescription and Over the Counter Medications by Brown, 1/e p1650]

17. Ans. (d) Amantadine

[Ref. The 5-Minute ICU Consult by Yunen & Frendl, 2012, Pg 234]

- *Neurolept Malignant Syndrome (NMS)*: Idiosyncratic reaction to Neuroleptic drugs and Anti-emetics
  - Haloperidol
  - Chlorpromazine
  - Domperidone
  - Metachlopramide

18. Ans. (c) Haloperidol

[Ref. Movement Disorders in Neurologic and Systemic Disease, 1/e p206]

- *Treatment of Akathisia*:
  - Beta-adrenergic blockers (Propranolol – Drug of choice)
  - Anticholinergic agents (Biperiden, Benztropine, Trihexyphenidyl)
  - Benzodiazepines (Lorazepam, Clonazepam, Diazepam)
  - 5-HT antagonists (Mirtazapine, Mianserin, Cyproheptadine)

19. Ans. (c) Schizophrenia

[Ref. Clinical Handbook pf Schizophrenia by Mueser & Jeste, 1/e p188]

- Carbamazepine monotherapy has not shown to be effective in treatment of Schizophrenia

20. Ans. (a) Serotonin

[Ref. Obsessive Compulsive Disorder: Current Science and Clinical Practice by Zohar, 1/e p222]

- 5-Hydroxyindoleacetic acid (5-HIAA) is a major metabolite of Serotonin
  - Urinary 5-HIAA levels are used to estimate Serotonin levels in body

21. Ans. (a) Nausea; (b) Diarrhoea; (c) Weight gain; (e) Sexual dysfunction

[Textbook of Psychiatry by Hales, 5/e p1062]

- *Common side-effects of SSRIs*:
  - Nausea, Vomiting
  - Anxiety
  - Headache
  - Loose bowel movements
  - Increased sweating
  - Insomnia
  - Weight gain
  - SIADH
  - Sexual dysfunction (delayed side-effect)

22. Ans. (c) Urinary retention

[Ref. Textbook of Psychiatry by Hales, 5/e p1062]

23. Ans. (c) Serotonin uptake enhancer

[Ref. Depressive Disorders by Herrman& Sartorius, 3/e p52]

- *Mechanism of action of Tianeptine*: Acts by increasing reuptake of Serotonin, thereby increasing its availability at synaptic level

24. Ans. (c) Inhibition of axonal uptake of 5HT

[Ref. Medical Pharmacology & Therapeutics by Waller & Sampson, 4/e]

- *Mechanism of action of Fluoxetine*: Reduction of neuronal uptake of Serotonin by its Pre-synaptic transporter protein (SERT)

25. Ans. (b) Lack of insight

[Ref. Evolutionary Psychiatry by Stevens & Price, 2/e p122]

26. Ans. (d) Normal common knowledge

[Ref. Chamberlain's Symptoms and Signs in Clinical Medicine, 13/e p224]

Organic Psychosis

- Disorientation, anxiety
- Clouding of consciousness
- Perceptual abnormalities (Illusions, hallucinations)
- Paranoid ideas/delusions
- Fluctuating course with lucid intervals
- Reversible causes

27. Ans. (c) Accepting delusions of other person

[Ref. Assessment and Treatment of Patients with Coexisting Mental Illness and Alcohol and Other Drug Abuse, 1/e p79]

Induced Psychotic Disorder: Dominant partner has delusional psychosis believed and accepted by a passive partner

28. Ans. (d) Extrapyramidal side effects are seen
[Ref. Niraj Ahuja, 7/e p176-77]

29. Ans. (c) Psychosis
[Ref. Evolutionary Psychiatry by Stevens & Price, 2/e p122]

30. Ans. (a) Clozapine
[Ref. Niraj Ahuja, 7/e p176-77]

31. Ans. (b) Propranolol
[Ref. Movement Disorders in Neurologic and Systemic Disease, 1/e p206]

32. Ans. (a) Amitriptyline
[Ref. Multiples sources]

33. Ans. (c) Inhibit uptake of 5-HT
[Ref. Medical Pharmacology & Therapeutics by Waller & Sampson, 4/e]

34. Ans. (b) Anxiety
[Ref. Depression and Anxiety by Swartz, 2007, Pg 29]

- *Most common side effect of Fluoxetine*: Agitation and Anxiety

35. Ans. (c) Acute drug dystonia
[Ref. Handbook of Psychiatric Drug Therapy by Rosenbaum, 5/e p40]

- *Neurolept induced Acute dystonia*: Haloperidol, Fluphenazine

36. Ans. (b) Amitriptyline
[Ref. Physical Rehabilitation by Sullivan, 6/e p1200]

- *Side-effects of Amitriptyline*: Dry mouth, Urinary retention, Constipation, Hypotension, Dizziness, Tachycardia, Hypotension, Blurred vision, Weight gain, Memory impairment

37. Ans. (d) Neurolept malignant syndrome
[Ref. The 5-Minute ICU Consult by Yunen and Frendl, 2012, Pg 234]

- ***Neuroleptic malignant syndrome (NMS):*** A rare, but life-threatening, idiosyncratic reaction to neuroleptic medications that is characterized by fever, muscular rigidity, altered mental status, and autonomic dysfunction
- NMS often occurs shortly after the initiation of neuroleptic treatment, or after dose increases

38. Ans. (a) Acute dystonia
[Ref. Parkinson's Disease by Ebadi, 2/e p677]

- Neurolept induced dystonia is treated with Diphenhydramine hydrochloride as it possess both anti-cholinergic and anti-histaminic properties

39. Ans. (b) Clozapine
[Ref. Niraj Ahuja, 7/e p176-77]

40. Ans. ALL CHOICES
[Ref. The 5-Minute ICU Consult by Yunen & Frendl, 2012, Pg 234]

41. Ans. (b) Neuroleptic malignant syndrome
[Ref. The 5-Minute ICU Consult by Yunen & Frendl, 2012, Pg 234]

42. Ans. (d) Hemogram, CPK and Renal Function Test
[Ref. Drug Intelligence and Clinical Pharmacy, Pg 545]

43. Ans. (c) Neuroleptic malignant syndrome
[Ref. The 5-Minute ICU Consult by Yunen & Frendl, 2012, Pg 234]

44. Ans. (d) Amytriptyline
[Ref. Stahl's Essential Psychopharmacology, 5/e p28]

Torsades de pointes

- Specific form of polymorphic ventricular tachycardia in patients with a long QT interval
  - Rapid, irregular QRS complexes, which appear to be twisting around the ECG baseline
  - This arrhythmia may cease spontaneously or degenerate into ventricular fibrillation
- Drugs which may cause Torsades de pointes **(Based on drugs administered to the patient in the given question)**
  - Antipsychotics: Pimozide, Sertindole, Droperidol, Haloperidol, Thioridazine (Olanzapine, Quetiapine, Risperidone, Ziprasidone do not lead to Torsade de pointes)
  - Anti-depressants: Amitriptyline, Nortriptyline, Imipramine, Desipramine, Mianserin, Doxepin, Citalopram, Escitalopram, Venlafaxine, Bupropion
  - Anit-hypertensives: Quinidine, Amiodarone, Procainamide, Disopyramide, Sotalol

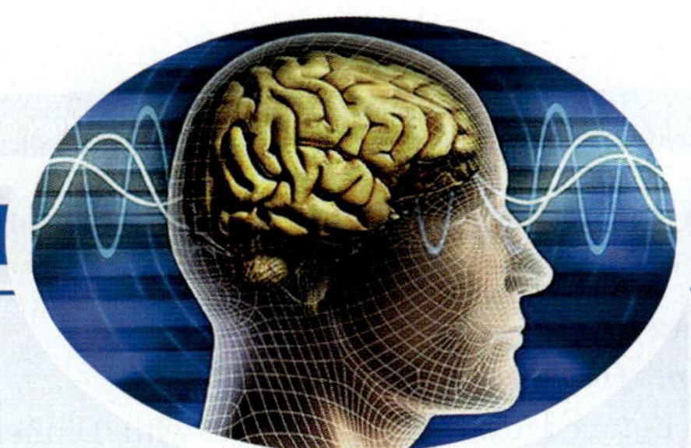

Chapter 5

Schizophrenia

THEORETICAL CONCEPTS

V A. SCHIZOPHRENIA DEFINITION

- Mental disorder characterized by disintegration of thought processes and of emotional responsiveness

Eugen Bleuler's Fundamental symptoms (4A's of Bleuler)[Q]	
• ***A**mbivalence*	• Inability to decide for or against
• ***A**utism*	• Withdrawal into self
• ***A**ffect disturbance*	• Inappropriate affect
• ***A**ssociation disturbance*	• Loosening of association/ thoughts

Schneider's First Rank Symptoms of Schizophrenia (SFRS)*[Q]	
• ***S**omatic passivity*	• Body sensations imposed by others
• ***M**ade feelings/ affect*	• Imposed by others
• ***M**ade impulses*	• Imposed by others
• ***M**ade volition/ acts*	• Imposed by others
• ***D**elusional perception*	• Private illogical meaning
• ***V**oices heard arguing*	• Auditory hallucinations
• ***V**oices commenting on one's action*	• Auditory hallucinations
• ***A**udible thoughts*	• Thought echo
• ***T**hought withdrawal*	• Thoughts cease, removed by someone
• ***T**hought insertion*	• Thoughts imposed by someone else
• ***T**hought diffusion/ broadcasting*	• Thoughts escaping and experienced by others

[***Mnemonic:** ***S**chizophrenic **M**an **D**oes **V**alue **A**udible **T**houghts; **SAM³V²T³D***][Q]

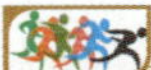

Topper's Edge

DSM-IV-TR Diagnostic Criteria for Schizophrenia

- Criterion A. Characteristic symptoms[Q]: Two or more of following present for significant time during one-month period
  - Delusions
  - Hallucinations
  - Disorganized speech
  - Grossly disorganized or catatonic behavior
  - Negative symptoms (Affective flattening, Alogia, Avolition)
- Criterion B. Social/occupational dysfunction
- Criterion C. Duration: Disturbance >6 months
- Criterion D. Schizoaffective and mood disorder exclusion
- Criterion E. Substance use/general medical condition exclusion
- Criterion F. Relationship to a pervasive developmental disorder

V B. UNDERLYING CAUSES

- *Biological theories*:
  - Hereditary
  - Increased dopamine at post-synaptic receptor
  - Enlarged brain ventricles, cortical atrophy
- *Psychological theories*:
  - Stressful life events
  - Schizophrenic mother, not-real mother, dependency on mother
  - Regression to pre-oral stage of psychosexual development
- *Sociocultural theories*:
  - Lower socioeconomic class
  - Migrants

V C. CLINICAL PRESENTATION

Thought and speech disorders	
Autistic thinking	Private illogical rules
Loosening of associations	Incoherent disjointed speech
Thought blocking and withdrawal	Sudden interruption without recall
Neologisms[Q]	Newly formed phrases/ words
Paraphasias[Q]	Word approximations
Poverty of speech, ideation	Decreased, non-informative speech
Echolalia[Q]	Repetition of other's words
Mutism	No speech production
Perseveration	Persistent repetition of words
Verbigeration	Senseless repetition of same words
Autochthonous/ primary delusions	Non-explainable on basis of other perceptions
Secondary delusions	Explainable on basis of other perceptions
Delusions of persecution	*'People are against me'*
Delusions of reference	*'People are thinking about me'*
Delusions of grandeur	*'I am greatest'*
Delusions of control	*'My friend is controlling me'*
Hypochondriacal delusions	*'Bugs are crawling in my clothes'*
Perception disorders	
Hallucinations	
Auditory hallucinations	Hearing sounds
Thought echo	Audible thoughts
Third person hallucinations	Voices heard arguing about patient
Voices commenting	On patient's actions
Affect disorders	
Apathy	
Emotional blunting	
Emotional shallowness	
Anhedonia[Q]	Inability to experience pleasure
Inappropriate emotional response	
Motor behaviour disorders	
Increased/ decreased motor activity	Mannerisms, grimacing, stereotypes
Catatonic features	Catatonic schizophrenia
Negative symptoms	
Attention impairment	
Affective flattening	
Anhedonia	
Social withdrawal	
Alogia	Lack of speech output

Contd…

Contd…

Other symptoms
Loss of ego boundaries
Absence of insight
Normal consciousness, orientation
Normal memory, intelligence
Suicidal behaviour

V D1. CLINICAL TYPES OF SCHIZOPHRENIA

- ***Paranoid Schizophrenia:***
  - Insidious late onset
  - Well-systemised delusions: Persecution, reference, grandeur, control, infidelity
  - Hallucinations: Persecutory, **grandiose**[Q]
  - Lesser personal deterioration
- ***Hebephrenic (Disorganised) Schizophrenia:***
  - Thought disorder, incoherence, loosening of associations
  - Emotional disturbances
  - **Worst prognosis**[Q]
- ***Catatonic Schizophrenia:*** Marked disturbance of motor behaviour[Q]
  - Excited catatonia: Increased psychomotor activity, increased speech production
  - Stuporous/retarded catatonia: Extreme retardation of psychomotor function
  - Alternating excited-stuporous catatonia
- ***Residual and Latent Schizophrenia:***
  - Prominent negative symptoms
- ***Undifferentiated Schizophrenia:***
  - Features of more than one type seen
- ***Simple Schizophrenia:***
  - **Most difficult to diagnose, poor prognosis**[Q]
  - Negative symptoms
  - Hypochondriacal features
- ***Post-schizophrenic depression:***
  - Depressive features within 12 months of acute episode
  - **Suicidal tendency**[Q]
- ***Other types:***
  - *Pseudoneurotic Schizophrenia*: Neurotic symptoms
  - *Schizophreniform disorder*: Less than 6 months duration of symptoms
  - ***Oneiroid Schizophrenia:*** Dream like states
  - ***Van Gogh syndrome:*** Dramatic self mutilation[Q]
  - *Late Paraphrenia*: Bizarre delusions of persecution
  - *Pfropf Schizophrenia*: Mental retardation
  - *Type I Schizophrenia*: Acute presentation with positive symptoms
  - *Type II Schizophrenia*: Chronic presentation with negative symptoms

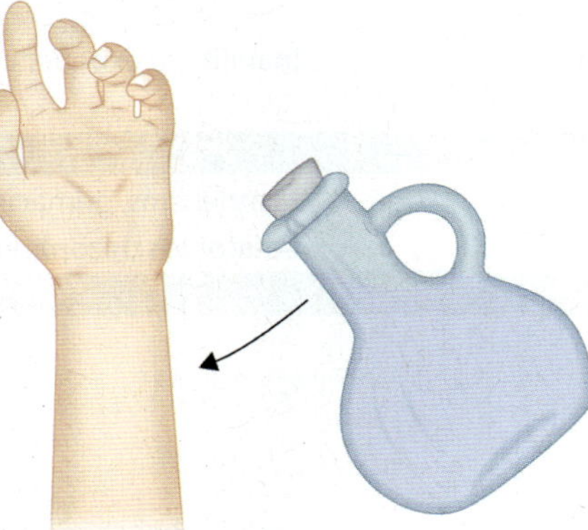

Fig. Deliberate self-harm

V D2. TYPES OF SCHIZOPHRENIC PSYCHOSIS SYNDROMES

	Type I Schizophrenia	Type II Schizophrenia
Predominant profile	Positive symptoms	Negative symptoms
Onset	Acute onset	Chronic course
Prognosis	Good	Poor
Response to Antipsychotics	Favourable	Inadequate
Features	Dopaminergic dysfunction	Intellectual impairment, enlarged ventricular size, cortical atrophy

V E. PROGNOSTIC FACTORS IN SCHIZOPHRENIA

Factor	Good prognosis[Q]	Bad prognosis[Q]
Type of onset	**Acute**	Insidious
Age of onset	**More than 35 years**	Less than 20 years
Sex of patient	**Females**	Males
Physique	**Fat**	Asthenic (thin)
Type of Schizophrenia	**Catatonic**	Hebephrenic/ Simple
Duration	**Less than 6 months**	More than 2 years
Stressor precipitating	Present	Absent
Depression	**Present**	Absent
Type of symptoms	Positive	Negative
Social support	Good	Poor
Type of treatment	Out-patient	Institutionalised
CT scan	Normal	Ventricular enlargement

V F. TREATMENT OF SCHIZOPHRENIA

- *Pharmacotherapy*[Q]:
  - *Typical/ First generation antipsychotics*: Chlorpromazine, Haloperidol, Thioridazine, Trifluperazine, Fluphenazine
  - *Atypical/ Second generation antipsychotics*: Clozapine, Olanzapine,[Q] uetiapine, Riseperidone
- ***Electroconvulsive therapy (ECT)*[Q]:**
  - If there is catatonia
  - If there is acute exacerbation
  - If there are severe side effects of drugs
- *Other treatments*:
  - Limbic leucotomy (Surgical treatment of choice)
- *Psychosocial therapy*:
  - Psychotherapy
  - Psycho education
  - Cognitive behaviour therapy
  - Rehabilitation

IMAGE-BASED QUESTIONS

1. Identify Bleuler's symptom of Schizophrenia shown in Photograph

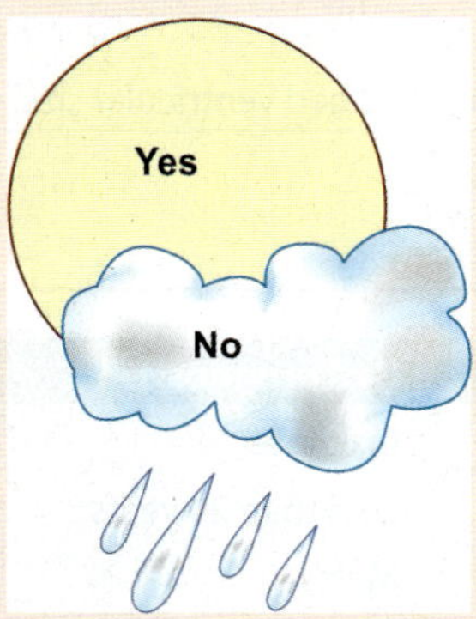

a. Autism
b. Affect disturbance
c. Association disorder
d. Ambivalence

2. Identify type of Schizophrenia shown in Photograph *[Recent Question 2013]*

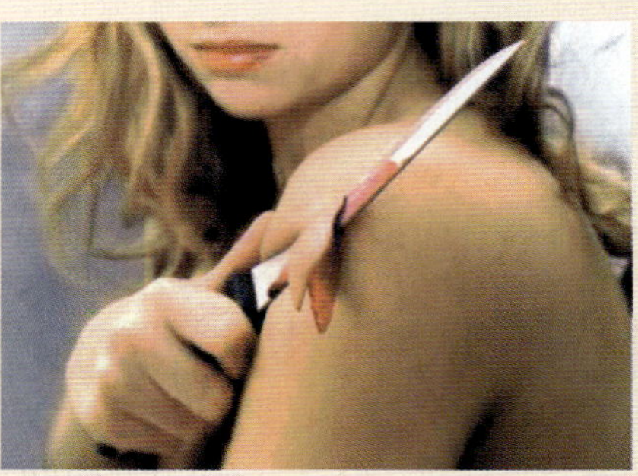

a. Oneiroid schizophrenia
b. Van Gogh syndrome
c. Paranoid schizophrenia
d. Hebrephrenic schizophrenia

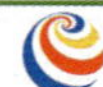 ANSWERS WITH EXPLANATIONS OF IBQs 

1. Ans. (d) Ambivalence *[Ref. Niraj Ahuja, 7/e p55-56]*

- Ambivalence: Co-existence of two opposite impulses towards same thing in same person at same time
- Associated Psychiatric disorders: Schizophrenia (Most characteristic), Obsessive compulsive disorders, Borderline states

2. Ans. (b) Van Gogh syndrome *[Ref. Niraj Ahuja, 7/e p60-61]*

- Van Gogh Syndrome: Subtype of Schizophrenia characterized by dramatic self mutilation

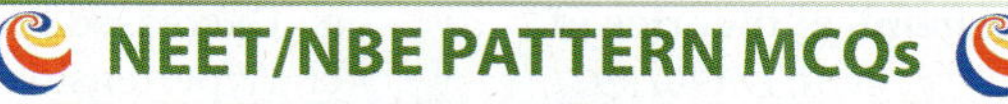

NEET/NBE PATTERN MCQs

1. **Verbigeration is seen in** *[Recent Question 2016]*
   a. Delusional disorders b. Schizophrenia
   c. Mania d. Depression
2. **True about schizophrenia** *[PGI June 2016]*
   a. Q-EEG finding is one of diagnostic criteria for schizophrenia
   b. Psychosurgery can be done for some resistant cases
   c. Family history of schizophrenia is poor prognosis
   d. Depression may be found
   e. Onset only after 40 year of age
3. **Good prognostic factor in schizophrenia is** *[Recent Question 2016]*
   a. Early age of appearance
   b. Male sex
   c. Presence of negative symptoms
   d. None of the above
4. **Erotomania is seen in** *[Recent Question 2016]*
   a. Schizophrenia
   b. Unipolar mania
   c. Neurosis
   d. OCD
5. **Four A's of Eugen Blueler includes which of the following?** *[Recent Question 2016]*
   a. Apathy b. Anhedonia
   c. Avolution d. Ambivalence
6. **Which category of ICD is associated with schizophrenia?** *[Recent Question 2016]*
   a. F0 b. F1
   c. F2 d. F3
7. **Best prognosis is of which type of schizophrenia?** *[Recent Question 2016]*
   a. Hebrephrenic b. Catatonic
   c. Residual d. Undifferentiated
8. **Drug used in Schizophrenia is** *[NBE FMGE September 2006]*
   a. Lithium b. Imipramine
   c. Fluphenazine d. Doxepin
9. **Neurotransmitter which is found in increased quantities in Schizophrenia is** *[NBE DNB 1994, 2004, 2006]*
   a. Noradrenaline b. Serotonin
   c. Dopamine d. All of the above
10. **All of the following are seen in Schizophrenia except** *[NBE FMGE September 2012]*
    a. Thought disorder b. Auditory hallucination
    c. Visual hallucination d. Insight present
11. **In Schizophrenia, all are considered negative symptoms except** *[UPSC 2011]*
    a. Anhedonia
    b. Decreased emotional expression
    c. Impaired concentration d. Hallucinations
12. **Schizophrenia is treated by** *[NBE DNB 2011]*
    a. Anti-depressants b. Anti-psychotics
    c. Anti-epileptics d. Mood stabilizers
13. **Type II schizophrenia is characterized by all, except** *[NBE DNB 2009]*
    a. Negative symptoms
    b. Poor response to treatment
    c. Disorganized behaviour
    d. CT scan abnormal
14. **Wax-molding posture is seen in** *[UPSC 2001]*
    a. Schizoaffective disorder
    b. Manic depressive psychosis
    c. Bipolar-II disorder
    d. Catatonic schizophrenia
15. **Term schizophrenia was coined by** *[Recent Question 2012, 2015]*
    a. Erich muir b. Sigmund Frued
    c. Bleular d. None
16. **Schizophrenia is considered to the due to over-activity of which of the following dopaminergic systems** *[NBE DNB 2007]*
    a. Nigrostriatal b. Tubercule infundibular
    c. Mesocortical d. None of the above
17. **Which one of the following is not considered as first rank symptom of schizophrenia?** *[Recent Question 2012, 2015]*
    a. Auditory hallucinations
    b. Insertion of thoughts
    c. Delusional perceptions
    d. Compulsive acts that relieve the tension
18. **Prognosis in Schizophrenia is less favourable if** *[NBE FMGE September 2003]*
    a. Occurs in women
    b. Anxiety is prominent
    c. Emotional blunting occurs
    d. Rapid onset of psychosis occurs
19. **Following are features of catatonic schizophrenia, except** *[Recent Question 2016, NBE DNB 1997]*
    a. Negativism b. Automatic obedience
    c. Catalepsy d. Cataplexy
20. **First rank symptoms of schizophrenia are all except** *[Recent Question 2012]*
    a. Ambivalence b. Running commentary
    c. Primary delusion d. Somatic passivity
21. **First rank symptoms of schizophrenia are all except** *[Recent Question 2012]*
    a. Depersonalization b. Running commentary
    c. Primary delusion d. Somatic passivity
22. **Good prognosis in schizophrenia is indicated by** *[Recent Question 2012, 2013, 2015]*
    a. Soft neurological signs b. Affective symptoms
    c. Emotional blunting d. Insidious onset
23. **Poor prognostic factor in schizophrenia is** *[NBE DNB 1997, 1999, 2001, 2004, 2006, 2007]*
    a. Acute onset
    b. Middle age
    c. Family history of affective disorder
    d. Gradual onset

24. Match the following Authors and Biochemical theories of Schizophrenia *[NBE DNB 1993]*
I. Stein (i) Serotonin deficiency
II. Murphy and Wyatt (ii) Dopamine activity
III. Randrup and Mukyad (iii) Norepinephrine depletion
IV. Gaddum Wolly and Shaw (iv) Monoamine oxidase inhibitor
a. I (i), II (ii), III (iv), IV (iii)
b. I (ii), II (iii), III (i), IV (iii)
c. I (iv), II (iii), III (ii), IV (iii)
d. I (iii), II (iv), III (ii), IV (i)

25. What is the mean prevalence of schizophrenia? *[NBE DNB December 2011]*
a. 0.5% b. 1.0%
c. 1.5% d. 2.0%

26. The most frequent period for onset of schizophrenia is *[NBE DNB 1994]*
a. Childhood b. Adolescence
c. Middle adulthood d. Old age
e. After trauma

27. Type of schizophrenia with mental retardation *[Recent Question 2013, 2015]*
a. Yon-Gogh syndrome b. Paranoid schizophrenia
c. Catatonic schizophrenia d. Pfropf schizophrenia

28. Which of the following is the treatment of choice for patients with schizophrenia, who refuse to take treatment? *[NBE FMGE March 2012]*
a. Clozapine b. Risperidone
c. Olanzapine d. Fluphenazine

29. Consider the following statements regarding schizophrenia
1. Patient feels that other persons put thoughts into his mind
2. Patient feels that he is being punished for his wrong doings
3. He may be in a state of catatonia

Which of the statements given above is/are correct? *[UPSC CMS 2015]*
a. 1 only b. 2 and 3 only
c. 1 and 3 only d. 1, 2 and 3

30. Schizophrenia drugs mainly act on *[Recent Question 2014, 2015]*
a. D1 Dopamine receptors b. D2 Dopamine receptors
c. D3 Dopamine receptors d. Ach receptors

31. A Schizophrenic patient on Antipscyhotic drugs may develop following side effect *[Recent Question 2014, 2015]*
a. Decreased Prolactin b. Increased Prolactin
c. Hypertension d. Wakefulness

32. Meaning of term 'Schizophrenia' is *[Recent Question 2014, 2015]*
a. Free mind b. Euphoric mind
c. Split mind d. Confused mind

33. Poor prognosis of Schizophrenia is seen in? *[Recent Question 2017]*
a. Female sex
b. Presence of depression
c. Acute onset
d. Predominance of negative symptoms

34. All of the following are associated with good prognosis in Schizophrenia except *[Recent Question 2017]*
a. First episode b. Absence of stressor
c. Late onset d. Presence of depression

35. A 39-year-old male patient present with waxy flexibility, negativism and rigidity. Most probable diagnosis is? *[Recent Question 2017]*
a. Excitatory catatonia b. Stuporos catatonia
c. Paranoid schizophrenia d. None

36. Self-mutilation is a feature of? *[Recent Question 2017]*
a. Von-Gogh syndrome b. Catatonic schizophrenia
c. Paranoid schizophrenia d. Pfropf schizophrenia

37. Most important receptors involved with Schizophrenia are? *[Recent Question 2017]*
a. $GABA_A$ b. $GABA_A$
c. D_2 d. $5\text{-}HT_1$

38. According to ICD-10, how many months should someone be having symptoms to diagnose schizophrenia *[Recent Question 2017]*
a. 1 month b. 2 months
c. 3 months d. 6 months

39. Which is true about age and sex distribution of Schizophrenia? *[Recent Question 2017]*
a. Most common age is >50 years
b. Early onset is a good prognostic factor
c. Male sex is a poor prognostic factor
d. Males are prone for the disease

40. Cataplexy characterized by? *[Recent Question 2017]*
a. Hypnopompic hallucinations
b. Nocturnal penile tumescence
c. Decreased muscle tone
d. Somnambulism

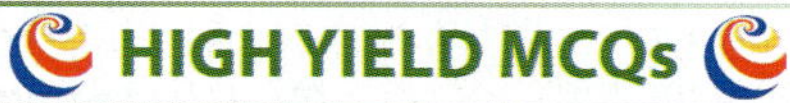

1. Cause of premature deaths in Schizophrenia is *[All India PGMEE 2011]*
a. Hospital acquired infections
b. Homicide
c. Suicide
d. Toxicity of anti-psychotic drugs

2. In schizophrenia, characteristic feature is *[PGI 1997]*
a. Formal thought disorder b. Delusion
c. Hallucination d. Apathy

3. Schizophrenia and depression both have all except *[PGI 2002]*
a. Formal thought disorder b. Social withdrawal
c. Poor personal care d. Decreased interest in sex
e. Suicidal tendency

4. Schizophrenia is a disorder of *[TN PGMEE 2003]*
a. Thought b. Belief
c. Memory d. Perception

5. A patient of Schizophrenia was started on Haloperidol 2 days back. Now he comes back with complaints of torticollis and orofaciolingual movements. This could be due to *[Recent Question 2015, All India PGMEE 2011]*
a. Akathisia b. Acute dystonia
c. Tardive dyskinesia d. Parkinsonism

6. Incidence of schizophrenia in India *[TN PGMEE 1999]*
a. 1–5 per 1000 b. 0.15–0.5 per 1000
c. 5–10 per 1000 d. 10–15 per 1000

7. The following is a Schneider's first rank symptom *[AIIMS PGMEE 2003]*
a. Persecutory delusion
b. Voices commenting on actions
c. Delusion of guilt
d. Incoherence

8. First rank symptoms of Schizophrenia are all except *[All India PGMEE 1998]*
a. Depersonalization b. Running commentary
c. Primary Delusion d. Somatic Passivity

9. Schneider's first rank symptoms in schizophrenia include *[PGI 2001]*
a. Audible thoughts b. Somatic passivity
c. Derealisation d. Depersonalization
e. Hallucinations

10. Schizophrenia is characterized by all except *[AIIMS PGMEE 1998, AIIMS PGMEE 2000]*
a. Delusion b. Auditory Hallucination
c. Elation d. Catatonia

11. Characteristic clinical manifestation of Schizophrenia is *[PGI 1998]*
a. Confusion b. Anxiety
c. Auditory hallucinations d. Visual hallucinations

12. Most common hallucination in Schizophrenia is *[JIPMER PGMEE 1995, CMC PGMEE 1999]*
a. Auditory b. Visual
c. Olfactory d. Tactile

13. Characteristic symptoms of catatonic Schizophrenia is *[AIIMS PGMEE 1993]*
a. Stupor b. Rigidity
c. Negativism d. All of the above

14. Schizophrenia with late onset and good prognosis *[All India PGMEE 1994, All India PGMEE 1991]*
a. Simple Schizophrenia
b. Hebephrenic
c. Catatonic Schizophrenia
d. Paranoid Schizophrenia

15. Most common types of schizophrenia *[AIIMS PGMEE 1995, PGI 2004]*
a. Simple b. Hebephrenic
c. Catatonic d. Paranoid

16. Drug of therapeutic benefit in Schizophrenia is *[All India PGMEE 1993]*
a. Lithium b. Doxepin
c. Imipramine d. Fluphenazine

17. Biochemical abnormalities in schizophrenia *[PGI 2002]*
a. Increased Dopamine
b. Increased dopamine and increased serotonin
c. Decreased Dopamine
d. Increased Dopamine and Decreased serotonin

18. Neurotransmitter related to schizophrenia pathology is/are *[PGI 1997]*
a. Ach b. Dopamine
c. Serotonin d. NA

19. Waxy flexibility is characteristic of *[Orissa PGMEE 2004, JHARKHAND PGMEE 2006]*
a. Excitatory catatonia b. Stuporous catatonia
c. OCD d. All

20. True about schizophrenia *[PGI 2003]*
a. Thought broadcasting b. Third person hallucination
c. Makes violence d. Elated mood
e. Takes good sell care

21. Drug treatment of schizophrenic is/are *[PGI 2003]*
a. Chlordiazepoxide b. Trifluperazine
c. Clozapine d. Rivastigmine
e. Haloperidol

22. Drugs used in schizophrenia include *[PGI 2002]*
a. Chlorpromazine b. Haloperidol
c. Olanzapine d. Imipramine
e. Risperidone

23. Bad Prognostic factor for Schizophrenia is *[AIIMS PGMEE 1997]*
a. Late onset of disease b. Catatonia
c. Presence of depression d. Absence of family history

24. Good prognosis in schizophrenia is indicated by *[PGI 1998]*
a. Soft neurological Signs b. Affective symptoms
c. Emotional blunting d. Insidious onset

25. Schizophrenia mostly occurs in *[AIIMS PGMEE 1999]*
a. Adolescents b. Children
c. Middle age d. Old age

26. The following symptoms of schizophrenia respond quickly to treatment with medication *[AIIMS PGMEE 1992]*
a. Apathy
b. Auditory Hallucinations
c. Poverty of thought content
d. Anhedonia

27. All are examples of form of thought disorder except *[Delhi PGMEE 2002]*
a. Obsessive compulsive Neurosis
b. Delusion
c. Schizophrenia
d. Loosening of association

28. True about thought is all except *[PGI 2007]*
a. Perseveration is out of context repetition
b. Circumstantiality is over inclusion of irrelevant details eventually getting back to original point
c. Verbigeration is senseless repetition
d. Vorbiereden is skirting around end point but never reaching it
e. Loosening of association is logically connected loss of goal directedness

29. Maximum heitability is seen in *[JIPMER PGMEE 2004, SGPGI 2005]*
a. Depression b. Mania
c. Schizophrenia d. Panic Disorder

30. Percentage of monozygotic twins with Schizophrenisa is *[MP PGMEE 2004, WB PGMEE 2003, UP PGMEE 2001]*
a. 0.1% b. 111%
c. 1% d. 50%

31. Bleuler's Criteria for Schizophrenia includes all except *[All India PGMEE 1991]*
a. Ambivalence b. Loosening of association
c. Automatism d. Inappropriate Affect

32. Catatonic features are seen in schizophrenia they are also seen in *[PGI 2008]*
a. Severe depression b. Conversion disorder
c. Personality disorder d. Somatisation disorder

33. Bleur's symptoms of schizophrenia include *[PGI 2005]*
a. Autism b. Automatism
c. Affect disturbance d. Loosening of association
e. Ambivalence

34. Which is not classical 4 A's of Schizophrenia? *[Recent Question 2015, AIIMS PGMEE 1994]*
a. Ambivalence b. Autism
c. Affect d. Automatism

35. Schneider's 1st rank symptoms seen in *[PGI 2004]*
a. Delusion b. Hallucination
c. Schizoid personality d. Schizophrenia

36. Feature(s) suggestive of Schizophrenia rather than organic psychosis is/ are *[PGI 2009]*
a. Third person hallucination
b. Split personality c. Visual hallucination
d. Altered sensorium e. Systemized delusion

37. Ambivalence is most commonly associated with *[MP PGMEE 2002]*
a. Depression
b. Generalized anxiety disorder
c. Schizophrenia
d. OCD

38. The primary disturbance in schizophrenia is *[AIIMS PGMEE 1994]*
a. Hallucination
b. Illusion
c. Psychomotor Retardation
d. Formal Thought Disorder

39. All the following are characteristic of schizophrenia except *[AIIMS PGMEE 2007]*
a. Third person hallucination
b. Inappropriate emotions
c. Intermittent mood changes
d. Formal thought disorder

40. Schizophrenia is characterized by all except *[All India PGMEE 1993]*
a. Delusion of reference b. Delusion of control
c. Waxy flexibility d. Altered sensorium

41. Bad prognostic indicator of Schizophrenia is *[AIIMS PGMEE 1997]*
a. Late onset
b. Family history of Schizophrenia
c. Positive precipitating factors
d. Prominent affective symptoms

42. Which is more appropriate in a case of schizophrenia? *[PGI 2000]*
a. Low socioeconomic group
b. Seen in adolescents
c. Common in primitive societies
d. Affluent society influences the incidence

43. Which symptom of schizophrenia respond earliest to treatment? *[AIIMS PGMEE 1993]*
a. Negativism b. Paranoid delusions
c. Auditory hallucinations d. Apathy

44. Schizophrenia with early onset and poor prognosis is *[All India PGMEE 1991, 1996]*
a. Catatonic b. Hebephrenic
c. Paranoid d. Schizoaffective

45. In catatonic schizophrenia, all are seen except *[JIPMER PGMEE 1991, AIIMS PGMEE 1988]*
a. Mannerism b. Negativism
c. Echolalia d. Flight of ideas

46. A 23-year-old engineering student is brought by his family to he hospital with history of gradual onset of suspiciousness, muttering and smiling without clear reason, decreased socialization, violent outbursts, and lack of interest in studies for 8 months. Mental status examination revealed a blunt affect, thought broadcast, a relatively preserved cognition, impaired judgment and insight. He is most likely to be suffering from *[AIIMS PGMEE 2004]*
a. Delusional disorder b. Depression
c. Schizophrenia d. Anxiety disorder

47. A patient is brought with 6 month history of odd behaviour. There is history of a family member having disappeared some years back. He seems to be talking to himself and sometimes muttering to himself loudly. The likely diagnosis is *[AIIMS PGMEE 2002]*
a. Schizophrenia b. Conversion disorder
c. Major depression d. Delusion

48. A 60 year old male suffering from auditory hallucination says that people staying upwards are talking about him and conspiring against him. He dropped a police compliant against them but the allegations were proved to be wrong. The diagnosis is *[AIIMS PGMEE 2001]*
a. Depression b. Dementia
c. Delusional disorder d. Schizophrenia

49. Schizopherenia is characterized by *[Bihar PGMEE 2003]*
a. Formal through disorder b. Hallucination
c. Delusion d. All

50. 18 years old male hears voices discussing him in 3rd person have *[AIIMS PGMEE 1995]*
a. Obsession b. Depression
c. Mania d. Schizophrenia

51. Defect of conation is typically seen in *[PGI 1997, AIIMS PGMEE 1996, UP PGMEE 2006]*
a. Simple schizophrenia
b. Hebephrenia schizophrenia
c. Catatonic schizophrenia
d. Paranoid schizophrenia

52. A 16 year old boy does not attend school because of the fear of being harmed by schoolmates. He thinks that his classmates laugh at and talk about him. He is even scared of going out to the market. He is most likely suffering from
a. Anxiety neurosis *[AIIMS PGMEE 2000]*
b. Manic Depressive Psychosis
c. Adjustment reaction d. Schizophrenia

53. A 70 year old male, Babulal was brought to the hospital with the history of auditory hallucinations with third person hallucinations. He has no history of similar problems previously. The diagnosis is most likely to be *[AIIMS PGMEE 2001]*
a. Dementia b. Delusional disorders
c. Schizophrenia d. Acute psychosis

54. A 60 year old man is brought to a psychiatrist with a 1 year history that he suspects his neighbours and he feels that whenever he passes by they sneeze and plan against behind his back. He feels that his wife has been replaced by a double and calls police for help. He is quite well groomed alert, occasionally consumes alcohol, likely diagnosis is *[AIIMS PGMEE 2002]*
a. Paranoid personality b. Paranoid schizophrenia
c. Alcohol withdrawal d. Conversion disorder

55. A patient of Schizophrenia on neurolepts, his psychotic symptoms gets relieved but developed sadness, talks less to others, remain on bed, all of following are likely causes except *[AIIMS PGMEE 2000]*
a. Parkinsonism
b. Major depression
c. Negative symptoms are still persisting
d. He is reacting to external stimuli

56. Which subtypes of Schizophrenia carries the best prognosis *[MP PGMEE 2004]*
a. Undifferentiated b. Catatonic
c. Paranoid d. Hebephrenic

57. A 19 year old boy suffering from chronic schizophrenia is put on haloperidol in the dose of 2 mg/day. A week after the initiation of medication the patient shows be restlessness, fidgety, irritability and cannot sit still at one place. The most appropriate treatment strategy is *[AIIMS PGMEE 2004]*
a. Increase in the dose of haloperidol
b. Addition of anticholinergic drug
c. Addition of beta blocker
d. Adding another antipsychotic drug

58. Grossly disorganized, severe personality deterioration and worst prognosis is seen is *[Orissa PGMEE 2007]*
a. Hebephrenic b. Catatonic
c. Simple d. Paranoid

59. A patient of Schizophrenia treated for 5 years developed perioral movements. Likely diagnosis is *[All India PGMEE 1997]*
a. Tardive dyskinesia
b. Muscular dystonia
c. Akathasia
d. Malignant neurolept syndrome

60. First Symptom to go with treatment of schizophrenia *[AIIMS PGMEE 1990, AIIMS PGMEE 1992, AIIMS PGMEE 1993]*
a. Apathy b. Anhedonia
c. Auditory hallucination d. Paucity of thoughts

61. Which of the following hallucinations is pathognomonic of schizophrenia? *[AIIMS PGMEE 2000, Delhi PGMEE 2003]*
a. Auditory hallucinations commanding the patient
b. Auditory hallucinations giving running commentry
c. Auditory hallucinations criticizing the patient
d. Auditory hallucinations talking to patient

62. All of the following are true about paranoid schizophrenia except *[MP PGMEE 1997]*
a. Most common type of schizophrenia
b. Onset in 3rd / 4th decade
c. Delusions of grandeur
d. Rapid deterioration of personality

63. Which of the following is associated with bad prognosis? *[UP PGMEE 2006, WB PGMEE 2007]*
a. Catatonic schizophrenia b. Hebephrenic schizophrenia
c. Paranoid schizophrenia d. Undifferentiated

64. Type two schizophrenia is characterized by all except *[AIIMS PGMEE 2008]*
a. Negative symptoms b. Poor response to TT
c. Disorganised behaviour d. CT scan abnormal

65. Patient presents with waxy flexibility, negativism & rigidity diagnosis is *[All India PGMEE 2001]*
a. Paranoid schizophrenia b. Catatonic schizophrenia
c. Hebephrenic Schizophrenia
d. Simple Schizophrenia

66. Grimacing and Mannerism is *[AIIMS PGMEE 1992]*
a. Simple Schizophrenia
b. Catatonic Schizophrenia
c. Hebephrenic Schizophrenia
d. Phobia

67. Following are feature of catatonic schizophrenia, except *[MP PGMEE2000]*
a. Mutism
b. Echolalia
c. Waxy flexibility
d. Deep tendon reflexes are increased

68. Features like increased psychomotor activity, waxyflexibility at time are seen classically in *[TN PGMEE 1997]*
a. Simple schizophrenia
b. Hebephrenic schizophrenia
c. Catatonic schizophrenia
d. None of the above

69. In which type of Schizophrenia is grimacing a feature of *[Karnataka PGMEE 1998]*
a. Juvenile b. Hebephrenic
c. Paranoid d. Catatonic

70. All are features of catatonia except *[JIPMER PGMEE 1992, Bihar PGMEE 1993]*
a. Automatic obedience b. Cataplexy
c. Catalepsy d. Negativism

71. Delusions of control, persecution and self-reference are seen in *[PGI 1997]*

a. Paranoia
b. Paranoid schizophrenia
c. Mania
d. OCD

72. All of the following are associated with better prognosis in schizophrenia except *[All India PGMEE 2006]*

a. Late onset
b. Married
c. Negative symptoms
d. Acute onset

73. Schizophrenia is associated personalities *[AIIMS PGMEE 1997]*

a. Atheletic
b. Psthesis
c. Asthenic
d. All

74. Which of the following is NOT a part of Catatonia? *[AIIMS PG May 2015]*

a. Ambivalence
b. Akinesia
c. Ambitendency
d. Akathisia

75. An exam-going 21 year old boy having schizophrenia well maintaining on Risperidone 3 mg since last 2 month. For how long medication should be continued for this case? *[AIIMS PG November 2015]*

a. Up to 12 months
b. 2 years
c. 6 months
d. 5 years

76. First rank symptoms for diagnosis of Schizophrenia include *[PGI November 2014]*

a. Visual hallucinations
b. Thought withdrawal
c. Delusions of reference
d. Thought broadcasting
e. Delusional perceptions

77. A 35-years-old Schizophrenic patient has been admitted in Psychiatry ward of a hospital. On seeing the nurse, patient starts beating his wife and claims that she's not rather the nurse is his actual wife. He also accuses nurse of giving wrong medication to him. Most probable diagnosis is *[AIIMS November 2017]*

a. Syndrome of Subjective doubles
b. Cotard syndrome
c. Capgras syndrome
d. Othello syndrome

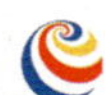

NEET/NBE PATTERN MCQs ANSWERS WITH EXPLANATIONS

1. **Ans. (b) Schizophrenia**
[Ref. Niraj Ahuja, 7/e p59]

Verbigeration/Cataphasia
- Meaningless and stereotyped repetition of words or phrases
- Is a special type of verbal stereotypy
- Does not follow external stimulus
- Seen in schizophrenia, retarded catatonia

2. **Ans. (b) Psychosurgery can be done for some resistant cases; (c) Family history of schizophrenia is poor prognosis; (d) Depression may be found**
[Ref. Niraj Ahuja, 7/e p55, 57, 62]

Schizophrenia
- Though more common in later aged women, it can affect children and adolescents too
- Youngest case recorded in literature is 3 years old
- **Diagnosis (ICD-10):** Minimum 1 clear-cut symptom (or 2 if unclear symptoms) present for atleast 1 month (6 months is DSM-IV criteria used)
- Poor prognostic factors: Insidious onset, Early onset (Less than 20 years age), Males, Thin physique, Family/ past history of schizophrenia, Disorganised/Simple/Undifferentiated/Chronic catatonic subtypes, Absence of depression, Predominant negative symptoms, No proper treatment, Long term hospitalisation, Enlarged ventricles on CT

3. **Ans. (d) None of the above**
[Ref. Niraj Ahuja, 7/e p62]
- **Good prognostic factors in schizophrenia:** Acute onset, Age of onset more than 35 years, Females, Fat physique, Catatonic type, Duration less than 6 months, Stressor precipitating present, Depression, Positive symptoms, Good social support, Out-patient treatment, Normal CT scan

4. **Ans. (a) Schizophrenia**
[Ref. e-Study Guide for Companion to Psychiatric Studies, 1/e Erotomania]

5. **Ans. (d) Ambivalence**
[Ref. Niraj Ahuja, 7/e p55]

6. **Ans. (c) F2**
[Ref. Essentials of Postgraduate Psychiatry by Murray, 3/e p61]

7. **Ans. (b) Catatonic**
[Ref. Niraj Ahuja, 7/e p62]

Prognosis in Schizophrenia Types
- Good prognosis: Catatonic
- Intermediate prognosis: Paranoid
- Poor prognosis: Disorganized, Simple, Undifferentiated, Chronic catatonic

8. **Ans. (c) Fluphenazine**
[Ref. Niraj Ahuja, 7/e p66]
- *Pharmacotherapy for Schizophrenia*:
  - Typical/ First generation antipsychotics: Chlorpromazine, Haloperidol, Thioridazine, Trifluperazine, Fluphenazine
  - Atypical/Second generation antipsychotics: Clozapine, Olanzapine, Quetiapine, Riseperidone

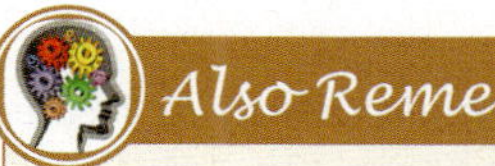

- Clozapine is very effective in Schizophrenia but has a major side effect of Agranulocytosis

9. **Ans. (c) Dopamine**
[Ref. Niraj Ahuja, 7/e p63-64]
- *Biochemical Theory of Schizophrenia*:
  - **Major theory: Functional increase of Dopamine at post-synaptic receptor**
  - Other theories: Involvement of Serotonin, GABA, Acetylcholine

10. **Ans. (d) Insight present**
[Ref. Niraj Ahuja, 7/e p57]

Insight in Psychiatric Disorders

Insight present in	Insight absent in
• Neurosis • Phobias • Obsessions • Compulsions • Obsessive Compulsive disorders • Paranoid personality disorder	• Schizophrenia • Psychoses • Korsakoff's psychosis • Postpartum psychosis • Mood disorders • Alzheimer's disease

11. **Ans. (d) Hallucinations**
[Ref. Niraj Ahuja, 7/e p62]

Symptoms Cluster in Schizophrenia

Positive symptoms	Negative symptoms	Disorganized symptoms
• Delusions • Hallucinations	• Affective flattening • Alogia (Poverty of speech) • Anhedonia-Associality • Avolition-Apathy • Attentional impairment	• Inappropriate affect • Disorganized behavior • Thought disorder • Loosening of associations

12. **Ans. (b) Anti-psychotics**
[Ref. Niraj Ahuja, 7/e p66]

Treatment of Schizophrenia

Pharmacotherapy with Antipsychotics	Psychosocial therapy
• *Typical/ First generation*: Chlorpromazine, Haloperidol, Thioridazine, Trifluperazine, Fluphenazine • *Atypical/ Second generation*: Clozapine, Olanzapine, Quetiapine, Riseperidone	• Psychotherapy • Psycho education • Cognitive behaviour therapy • Rehabilitation

Contd...

Contd...

Electroconvulsive therapy (ECT)	Other treatments
• If there is catatonia • If there is acute exacerbation • If there are severe side effects of drugs	• Limbic leucotomy (Surgical TOC)

13. Ans. (c) Disorganised behavior

[Ref. Handbook of Psychology, Clinical Psychology by Weiner, 1/e p79]

Type I vs Type II Schizophrenia

	Type I Schizophrenia	Type II Schizophrenia
Onset	Acute	Insidious
Course	Episodic	Chronic
Intellectual functioning	Normal	Abnormal
Premorbid adjustment	Good	Poor
Symptoms	Positive	Negative
Characteristics	Hallucinations, Delusions	Poverty of speech, retardation
Underlying cause	Neurochemical disturbance	Structural brain changes
Attributable cause	Dopamine	Enlarged cerebral ventricles
Response to Anti-psychotics	Good	Poor
CT Scan	Normal	Abnormal

14. Ans. (d) Catatonic schizophrenia

[Ref. Clinical Diagnosis to Diagnosis and Treatment of Mental Disorders by First & Tasman, 2/e p247; Niraj Ahuja, 7/e p59]

Catatonic Schizophrenia

- Motoric immobility: Cataplexy (Waxy flexibility) -Stupor
- Extensive purposeless motor activity
- Extreme negativism or mutism
- Peculiar voluntary movements: Rigidity, Posturing (Catalepsy), stereotype movements, prominent mannerisms/grimacing
- Echolalia or echopraxia
- Defect in Conation
- Ambitendency
- Automatic obedience

15. Ans. (c) Bleular

[Ref. Symptoms of Schizophrenia by Costello, 1/e p201]

- *Eugene Bleuler coined terms*: Schizophrenia, Ambivalence

16. Ans. (c) Mesocortical

[Ref. A Clinical Guide for the Treatment of Schizophrenia by Bellack, 1/e p28]

Dopaminergic Systems Involvement in Schizophrenia

- *Mesolimbic-Mesocortical system*: Integrally related to pathogenesis of Schizophrenia
- *Nigrostriatal-Tuberofundibular system*: Related to side-effects

17. Ans. (d) Compulsive acts that relieve the tension

[Ref. Niraj Ahuja, 7/e p55]

Schneider's First Rank Symptoms of Schizophrenia (SFRS)*	
• ***S**omatic passivity* • ***M**ade feelings/ affect* • ***M**ade impulses* • ***M**ade volition/ acts* • ***D**elusional perception* • ***V**oices heard arguing* • ***V**oices commenting on one's action*	• Body sensations imposed by others • Imposed by others • Imposed by others • Imposed by others • Private illogical meaning • Auditory hallucinations • Auditory hallucinations
• ***A**udible thoughts* • ***T**hought withdrawal*	• Thought echo • Thoughts cease, removed by someone
• ***T**hought insertion*	• Thoughts imposed by someone else
• ***T**hought diffusion/ broadcasting*	• Thoughts escaping and experienced by others

[***Mnemonic:** **S**chizophrenic **M**an **D**oes **V**alue **A**udible **T**houghts; **$SAM^3V^2T^3D$**]

18. Ans. (c) Emotional blunting occurs

[Ref. Niraj Ahuja, 7/e p62]

- *Prognostic factors in Schizophrenia*:

Factor	Good prognosis	Bad prognosis
Type of onset	Acute	Insidious
Age of onset	More than 35 years	Less than 20 years
Sex of patient	Females	Males
Physique	Fat	Asthenic (thin)
Type of Schizophrenia	Catatonic	Hebephrenic/ Simple
Duration	Less than 6 months	More than 2 years
Stressor precipitating	Present	Absent
Depression	Present	Absent
Type of symptoms	Positive	Negative
Social support	Good	Poor
Type of treatment	Out-patient	Institutionalised
CT scan	Normal	Ventricular enlargement

- Due to negative symptoms like emotional blunting, Simple and Hebephrenic Schizophrenia have a worse prognosis

19. Ans. (d) Cataplexy

[Ref. Clinical Diagnosis to Diagnosis and Treatment of Mental Disorders by First & Tasman, 2/e p247; Niraj Ahuja, 7/e p59]

20. Ans. (a) Ambivalence

[Ref. Niraj Ahuja, 7/e p55]

21. Ans. (a) Depersonalization

[Ref. Niraj Ahuja, 7/e p55]

22. Ans. (b) Affective symptoms
[Ref. Niraj Ahuja, 7/e p62]

23. Ans. (d) Gradual onset
[Ref. Niraj Ahuja, 7/e p55]

24. Ans. (d) I (iii), II (iv), III (ii), IV (i)
[Ref. Multiple Sources]

25. Ans. (b) 1.0%
[Ref. Best of 5 MCQs for MRCPsych Paper 1, Pg 85]

- *Schizophrenia is a global illness*: Equivalent global prevalence of 1%

26. Ans. (b) Adolescence
[Ref. Adolescent Medicine: Requisites by Slap, 1/e p292]

- *Peak age of Onset of Schizophrenia*: 15-30 years

27. Ans. (d) Pfropf schizophrenia
[Ref. Niraj Ahuja, 7/e p61]

Associations in Few Types of Schizophrenia

Schizophrenia	Association
Pfropf Schizophrenia	Mental retardation
Van Gogh syndrome	Self-mutilation
Pseudoneurotic Schizophrenia	Pan-anxiety, Pan-neurosis, Pan-sexuality
Oneiroid Schizophrenia	Dream like states

28. Ans. (b) Risperidone
[Ref. Niraj Ahuja, 7/e p181]

Treatment of Choices in Schizophrenia

- *First episode*: Olanzapine, Risperidone, Quetiapine, Ziprasidone, Arpiprazole
- ***Suicidal behaviour***: Clozapine
- *Aggressive behaviour*: Clozapine
- ***Tardive dyskinesia***: Clozapine, Olanzapine, Risperidone, Quetiapine, Ziprasidone, Arpiprazole
- ***Extrapyramidal side effects***: Olanzapine, Quetiapine, Ziprasidone, Arpiprazole
- *Prolactin elevation*: Olanzapine, Quetiapine, Ziprasidone, Arpiprazole
- *Weight gain, hyperglycemia, hyperlipidemia*: Ziprasidone, Arpiprazole
- *Refusal to take treatment*: Risperidone (DOC due to least side-effects), Olanzapine, Fluphenazine

29. Ans. (c) 1 and 3 only
[Ref. Niraj Ahuja, 7/e p55]

Schneider's First Rank Symptoms of Schizophrenia (SFRS)

- Audible thoughts: Thought echo
- Thought withdrawal: Perceived removal of thoughts by external force
- Thought insertion: Thoughts experienced as imposed by external force on mind
- Thought broadcasting/diffusion: Thoughts perceived as being experienced by others around
- Made feelings: Imposed by external forces
- Made impulses: Imposed by external forces
- Made volition/acts: Imposed by external forces
- Voices heard arguing: Two or more hallucinatory voices discussing subject in third person
- Voices commenting on one's actions
- Somatic passivity: Bodily sensations perceived as imposed by external force
- Delusional perception: Illogical meaning to a normal perception

30. Ans. (b) D2 Dopamine receptors
[Ref. Physiological Psychology by Wagner, 1/e p239]

31. Ans. (b) Increased Prolactin

Effects on Antipsychotics in Schizophrenia Treatment

- Increased prolactin (Galactorrhea)
- Suppressed LH levels
- Suppressed FSH levels
- Suppressed Testosterone levels

32. Ans. (c) Split mind
[Ref. Schizophrenia by Silber, 1/e p2]

- Word Schizophrenia: Schizo means 'Split', Phrene means 'Mind'
- Schizophrenia term coined by: Eugene Bleuer

33. Ans. (d) Predominance of negative symptoms
[Ref. Niraj Ahuja, 7/e p62]

- **Poor prognostic factors in Schizophrenia:** Insidious onset, Early onset (Less than 20 years age), Males, Thin physique, Family/past history of schizophrenia, Disorganised/Simple/Undifferentiated/Chronic catatonic subtypes, Absence of depression, Predominant negative symptoms, No proper treatment, Long term hospitalisation, Enlarged ventricles on CT
- Symptomatology in Schizophrenia:
  - Positive symptoms include: Delusions, Hallucinations
  - Negative symptoms include: **A**ffective flattening, **A**logia (poverty of speech), **A**nhedonia (asociality), **A**volition (apathy), **A**ttentional impairment **[Mnemonic: 5A's]**
  - Disorganised symptoms include: Disorganised behaviour, Thought disorder, Loosening of associations, Inappropriate affect
- **Negative syndrome Schizophrenia** (Type II Schizophrenia) has been associated with a chronic deteriorating course and poor long-term outcome; Depressive syndrome in schizophrenia has been associated with good prognosis and a remitting course

34. Ans. (b) Absence of stressor
[Ref. Niraj Ahuja, 7/e p62]

- Good prognostic factors in Schizophrenia include acute onset, > 35 years age of onset, female sex, fat physique, Catatonic schizophrenia, duration less than 6 months, presence of precipitating stressor, presence of depression, positive symptoms, good social support, out-patient treatment, normal CT scan
- Availability of family support is associated with better long-term clinical and functional outcomes in first-episode patients

35. Ans. (b) Stuporous catatonia
[Ref. Niraj Ahuja, 7/e p59]

Clinical Features of Stuporous Catatonia

- Mutism, Rigidity, Negativism, Posturing, Stupor, Echolalia, Echopraxia, Waxy flexibility, Ambitendency, Other signs

such as mannerisms, stereotypies, automatic obedience, and verbigeration
- Extreme retardation of psychomotor function
- Delusions and hallucinations

36. Ans. (a) Von-Gogh syndrome
[Ref. Niraj Ahuja, 7/e p60]

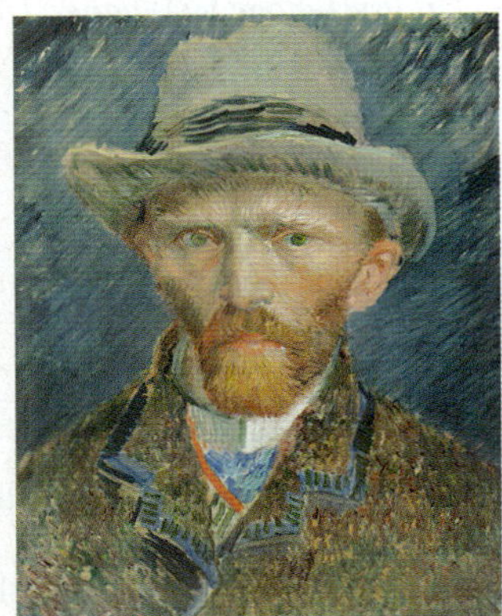

Fig. Vincent Van Gogh

- Subtype of Schizophrenia characterized by dramatic self-mutilation
- Most dramatic example of self-injurious behavior, in patients with schizophrenia include descriptions of unilateral and bilateral eye enucleation, self-laceration, self-amputation of various parts of the body, including the hand, breast, ear, penis, testicles

37. Ans. (c) D_2
[Ref. Medical Biochemistry E-Book by Baynes, 4/e p560]
- There are five known Dopamine receptors, falling into two main groups that differ in their signalling pathways
  - D1like: D1 and D5
  - D2like: D2, D3, and D4
- D1 receptors increase the production of cAMP, whereas D2 receptors inhibit
- Antipsychotic drugs such as phenothiazines and haloperidol tend to inhibit D2 like receptors, suggesting that excessive dopamine activity may be important in causing the symptoms of Schizophrenia

38. Ans. (a) 1 month
[Ref. Niraj Ahuja, 7/e p57]
- According to ICD-10, for the diagnosis of schizophrenia, symptom(s) should have been clearly present for most of the time during a period of 1 month or more
  - If the duration of illness is less than 1 month, then a diagnosis of Acute schizophrenia-like psychotic disorder should be made
- According to DSM-IV-TR, for the diagnosis of schizophrenia, symptom(s) should have been clearly present for most of the time during a period of 6 months or more

39. Ans. (c) Male sex is a poor prognostic factor
[Ref. General Adult Psychiatry by Stein, 1/e p204]

Age and Sex Distribution in Schizophrenia
- Schizophrenia may start at any age, but majority of cases occur in 15-54 years age
- Neither the childhood-onset nor late-onset cases present with any features that are qualitatively different from those characterising Schizophrenia.
- There is a less prominent peak in 20-24 years age group in women, followed by a gradual increase in inception rates for those over 35; with increasing age, with around over 60 years, female onset is more common
- Good prognostic factors include acute onset, late onset (>35 years age), female sex, fat physique

40. Ans. (c) Decreased muscle tone
[Ref. Neurology by Weisberg, 2/e p66]

Narcolepsy (Daytime sleep episodes)
- Cataplexy (Loss of muscle tone in response to intense emotions, e.g., laughing, crying)
- Hypnagogic hallucinations (Hallucinations which occur in drowsy period)
- Sleep paralysis, loss of muscle tone (Occurs upon awakening in the morning)

HIGH YIELD MCQs ANSWERS WITH EXPLANATIONS

1. Ans. (c) Suicide
[Ref. Suicide in Schizophrenia by Tatarelli and Girardi, 1/e p85]
- *Single most important cause of premature death in Schizophrenia*: Suicide
- *Life-time risk of suicide in Schizophrenia*: 4%

2. Ans. (a) Formal thought disorder
[Ref. Essentials of Schizophrenia by Perkins, 1/e p40]
- *Most characteristic of Schizophrenia*:
  - Formal thought disorder
  - Affect disorder

3. Ans. (a) Formal thought disorder
[Ref. Manic Depressive Illness by Goodwin, 2/e p44]
- *Formal thought disorder is more specific for*:
  - Schizophrenia
  - Mania

4. Ans. (a) Thought
[Ref. Essentials of Schizophrenia by Perkins, 1/e p40]

5. Ans. (b) Acute dystonia
[Ref. Handbook of Psychiatric Drug Therapy by Rosenbaum, 5/e p40]
- *Neurolept induced Acute dystonia*: Haloperidol, Fluphenazine

6. Ans. (b) 0.15-0.5 per 1000
[Ref. Delhi psychiatry Journal, 18(1), Pg 95]

Epidemiology of Schizophrenia

Parameter	Rate
Incidence of Schizophrenia in World	1-1.5 per 1000
Prevalence of Schizophrenia in World	2-4 per 1000
Lifetime risk of Schizophrenia	1%
Incidence of Schizophrenia in India	0.4 per 1000
Prevalence of Schizophrenia in India	2-3 per 1000

7. Ans. (b) Voices commenting on actions
[Ref. Niraj Ahuja, 7/e p55]

8. Ans. (a) Depersonalization
[Ref. Niraj Ahuja, 7/e p55]

9. Ans. (a) Audible thoughts; (b) Somatic passivity; (e) Hallucinations
[Ref. Niraj Ahuja, 7/e p55]

10. Ans. (c) Elation
[Ref. Niraj Ahuja, 7/e p55, 59]

11. Ans. (c) Auditory hallucinations
[Ref. Essentials of Schizophrenia by Perkins, 1/e p40]

12. Ans. (a) Auditory
[Ref. Niraj Ahuja, 7/e p56]

13. Ans. (d) All of the above
[Ref. Clinical Diagnosis to Diagnosis and Treatment of Mental Disorders by First & Tasman, 2/e p247; Niraj Ahuja, 7/e p59]

14. Ans. (c) Catatonic Schizophrenia
[Ref. Niraj Ahuja, 7/e p58-60]

Onset & Recovery in Schizophrenia

Type	Onset	Course	Prognosis
Paranoid	Insidious, Later life (3-4th decade)	Progressive	Incomplete recovery
Hebephrenic	Insidious, Early life (Early 2nd decade	Progressive	Worst prognosis
Simple	Early life (Early 2nd decade	Progressive	Poor prognosis
Catatonic	3rd decade	Episodic	Complete recovery

15. Ans. (d) Paranoid
[Ref. Psychology: A Journey by Coon & Mitterer, 4/e p482]

- ***Most common type of Schizophrenia seen*:** Paranoid schizophrenia
  - Onset in Late 3rd or Early 4th decade
  - Well-systematized delusions
  - Persecutory/Grandiose hallucinations
  - Delusions of Persecution/reference/grandeur/control/infidelity
  - No prominent disturbances of speech/volition/affect/behavior
  - Lesser deterioration of personality

16. Ans. (d) Fluphenazine
[Ref. Niraj Ahuja, 7/e p66]

17. Ans. (a) Increased Dopamine; (b) Increased dopamine and increased serotonin
[Ref. High Yield Behavioral Science by B Fadem, 4/e p39]

Neurotransmitters in Major Psychiatry Disorders

Disorder	Neurotransmitter involvement
Schizophrenia	Dopamine (Increased), Serotonin (Increased), Glutamate (Increased/Decreased), Norepinephrine (Increased/Decreased)
Mania	Dopamine (Increased), GABA (Decreased)
Depression	Norepinephrine (Decreased), Serotonin (Decreased), Dopamine (Decreased)
Anxiety	GABA (Decreased), Serotonin (Decreased), Norepinephrine (Increased)
Alzheimer disease	Acetylcholine (Decreased), Glutamate (Increased)

18. Ans. (b) Dopamine; (c) Serotonin; (d) NA
[Ref. High Yield Behavioral Science by B Fadem, 4/e p39]

19. Ans. (b) Stuporous catatonia
[Ref. Clinical Diagnosis to Diagnosis and Treatment of Mental Disorders by First & Tasman, 2/e p247; Niraj Ahuja, 7/e p59]

20. Ans. (a) Thought broadcasting; (b) Third person hallucination; (c) Makes violence
[Ref. Niraj Ahuja, 7/e p55]

21. Ans. (b) Trifluperazine; (c) Clozapine; (e) Haloperidol
[Ref. Niraj Ahuja, 7/e p66]

22. Ans. (a) Chlorpromazine; (b)Haloperidol; (c)Olanzapine; (e) Risperidone
[Ref. Niraj Ahuja, 7/e p66]

23. Ans. (a) Late onset of disease
[Ref. Niraj Ahuja, 7/e p62]

24. Ans. (b) Affective symptoms
[Ref. Niraj Ahuja, 7/e p62]

25. Ans. (a) Adolescents
[Ref. Adolescent Medicine: Requisites by Slap, 1/e p292]

26. Ans. (b) Auditory Hallucinations
[Ref. CMDT 1988, Pg 625]

- *First symptoms of Schizophrenia to respond to treatment*:
  - Auditory hallucinations
  - Psychomotor agitation
  - Racing thoughts

27. Ans. (a) Obsessive Compulsive Neurosis
[Ref. Niraj Ahuja, 7/e p95]

28. Ans. (e) Loosening of association is logically connected loss of goal directedness
[Ref. Multiple Sources]

29. Ans. (c) Schizophrenia
[Ref. Internet]

30. Ans. (d) 50%
[Ref. Advanced Subsidiary Psychology: Approaches and Methods by Brain, 1/e p188]

- *Concordance for Schizophrenia in Twins*:
  - Monozygotic twins: 50%
  - Dizygotic twins: 15%

31. Ans. (c) Automatism
[Ref. Niraj Ahuja, 7/e p55]

Eugen Bleuler's Fundamental symptoms (4A's of Bleuler)	
• *Ambivalence*	• Inability to decide for or against
• *Autism*	• Withdrawal into self
• *Affect disturbance*	• Inappropriate affect
• *Association disturbance*	• Loosening of association/ thoughts

32. Ans. (a) Severe depression; (b) Conversion disorder
[Ref. Niraj Ahuja, 7/e p225]

Psychiatric Disorders with Catatonic Stupor

- Catatonic Schizophrenia
- Depressive stupor
- Mania stupor
- Periodic catatonia
- Conversion and Dissociative disorder
- Reactive psychosis
- Hypnosis

33. Ans. (a) Autism; (c) Affect disturbance; (d) Loosening of association; (e) Ambivalence
[Ref. Niraj Ahuja, 7/e p55]

34. Ans. (d) Automatism
[Ref. Niraj Ahuja, 7/e p55]

35. Ans. (d) Schizophrenia
[Ref. Niraj Ahuja, 7/e p55]

36. Ans. (a) Third person hallucination; (b) Split personality; (e) Systemized delusion
[Ref. Niraj Ahuja, 7/e p55-56]

37. Ans. (c) Schizophrenia
[Ref. Niraj Ahuja, 7/e p55-56]

Ambivalence

- *Description*: Co-existence of two opposite impulses towards same thing in same person at same time
- *Associated Psychiatric disorders*:
  - Schizophrenia **(Most characteristic)**
  - Obsessive compulsive disorders
  - Borderline states

Fig. Ambivalence

38. Ans. (d) Formal Thought Disorder
[Ref. Essentials of Schizophrenia by Perkins, 1/e p40]

39. Ans. (c) Intermittent mood changes
[Ref. Niraj Ahuja, 7/e p55]

40. Ans. (d) Altered sensorium
[Ref. Niraj Ahuja, 7/e p55]

41. Ans. (b) Family history of Schizophrenia
[Ref. Niraj Ahuja, 7/e p62]

42. Ans. (a) Low socioeconomic group; (b) Seen in adolescents
[Ref. Adolescent Medicine: Requisites by Slap, 1/e p292]

43. Ans. (c) Auditory hallucinations
[Ref. CMDT 1988, Pg 625]

44. Ans. (b) Hebephrenic
[Ref. Niraj Ahuja, 7/e p58-60]

45. Ans. (d) Flight of ideas
[Ref. Clinical Diagnosis to Diagnosis and Treatment of Mental Disorders by First & Tasman, 2/e p247; Niraj Ahuja, 7/e p59]

46. Ans. (c) Schizophrenia
[Ref. Niraj Ahuja, 7/e p55]

47. Ans. (a) Schizophrenia
[Ref. Niraj Ahuja, 7/e p55]

48. Ans. (d) Schizophrenia
[Ref. Niraj Ahuja, 7/e p55]

49. Ans. (d) All
[Ref. Niraj Ahuja, 7/e p55]

50. Ans. (d) Schizophrenia
[Ref. Niraj Ahuja, 7/e p55]

- *Third person auditory hallucinations in Schizophrenia*: Patients hearing voices discussing them in third person, sometimes commenting on their actions

51. Ans. (c) Catatonic schizophrenia
[Ref. Platinum Notes USMLE Step 2 - Compete Preparatory Guide by Hassan, Pg 471]

52. Ans. (d) Schizophrenia
[Ref. Niraj Ahuja, 7/e p55]

53. Ans. (c) Schizophrenia
[Ref. Niraj Ahuja, 7/e p55]

54. Ans. (b) Paranoid schizophrenia
[Ref. Psychology: A Journey by Coon and Mitterer, 4/e p482]

55. Ans. (d) He is reacting to external stimuli
[Ref. Niraj Ahuja, 7/e p168-174]

56. Ans. (b) Catatonic; (c) Paranoid
[Ref. Niraj Ahuja, 7/e p55]

- *Prognosis in Schizophrenia types*:
  - ***Best prognosis*:** Paranoid schizophrenia
  - *Good prognosis*: Catatonic schizophrenia
  - *Intermediate prognosis*: Undifferentiated schizophrenia
  - ***Poor prognosis*:** Disorganized (Hebephrenic) schizophrenia, Simple schizophrenia

57. Ans. (c) Addition of beta blocker
[Ref. Zone Comprehensive Guide to PGMEE Volume 3, 2009, Pg 806]

Akathisia

- *Description*: Acute onset, Extrapyramidal side-effects of Antipsychotic therapy (maximum with Haloperidol)
- *Occurrence*: Within 4 weeks of therapy
- *Treatment*: Beta-blocker (TOC), Anticholinergics, Benzodiazepines

58. Ans. (a) Hebephrenic
[Ref. Niraj Ahuja, 7/e p59]

Disorganised/ Hebephrenic Schizophrenia

- Marked thought disorder, incoherence, loosening of associations
- Emotional disturbances, mannerisms, mirror-gazing, disinhibited behavior, poor self are/ hygiene
- Insidious onset, usually in early 2nd decade
- Progressive course, with poor prognosis

59. Ans. (a) Tardive dyskinesia
[Ref. Meyler's Side Effects of Psychiatric Drugs by Aronson, 1/e p267]

- ***Tardive dyskinesia*:** Involuntary movements of the tongue, lips, face, trunk, and extremities that occur in patients treated with long-term dopaminergic antagonist medications
  - Typical Antipsychotics have a high risk of Tardive dyskinesia
  - Clozapine and Quetiapine carries lowest risk of Tardive dyskinesia

60. Ans. (c) Auditory hallucination
[Ref. Brain Evolution, Language and Psychopathology in Schizophrenia by Marini, 1/e p162]

- With Antipsychotic treatment there is marked reduction in Auditory hallucinations within first four weeks

61. Ans. (b) Auditory hallucinations giving running commentary
[The American Psychiatric Publishing Textbook of Schizophrenia by Lieberman & Perkins, 1/e p188]

- *Schneider's First Rank Symptoms*: Focus on pathognomonic symptoms of Schizophrenia
- *Three special forms of auditory hallucinations seen*:
  - Hearing one's thoughts spoken aloud
  - Hearing voices referring to himself/ herself, made in third person
  - Running commentary on one's activity

62. Ans. (d) Rapid deterioration of personality
[Ref. Niraj Ahuja, 7/e p58]

63. Ans. (b) Hebephrenic schizophrenia
[Ref. Niraj Ahuja, 7/e p58]

64. Ans. (c) Disorganized behavior
[Ref. Handbook of Psychology, Clinical Psychology by Weiner, 1/e p79]

65. Ans. (b) Catatonic schizophrenia
[Ref. Clinical Diagnosis to Diagnosis and Treatment of Mental Disorders by First & Tasman, 2/e p247; A Short Textbook of Psychiatry by Niraj Ahuja, 7/e p59]

66. Ans. (b) Catatonic Schizophrenia
[Ref. Niraj Ahuja, 7/e p59]

67. Ans. (a) Mutism
[Ref. Niraj Ahuja, 7/e p59]

68. Ans. (c) Catatonic schizophrenia
[Ref. Niraj Ahuja, 7/e p59]

69. Ans. (d) Catatonic
[Ref. Niraj Ahuja, 7/e p59]

70. Ans. (b) Cataplexy
[Ref. Niraj Ahuja, 7/e p59]

71. Ans. (b) Paranoid schizophrenia
[Ref. Psychology: A Journey by Coon and Mitterer, 4/e p482]

72. Ans. (c) Negative symptoms
[Ref. Niraj Ahuja, 7/e p62]

- *Prognostic factors in Schizophrenia*:

Factor	Good prognosis	Bad prognosis
Type of onset	Acute	Insidious
Age of onset	More than 35 years	Less than 20 years
Sex of patient	Females	Males
Physique	Fat	Asthenic (thin)
Type of Schizophrenia	Catatonic	Hebephrenic/ Simple
Duration	Less than 6 months	More than 2 years
Stressor precipitating	Present	Absent
Depression	Present	Absent
Type of symptoms	Positive	Negative
Social support	Good	Poor
Type of treatment	Out-patient	Institutionalized
CT scan	Normal	Ventricular enlargement

73. Ans. (c) Asthenic
[Ref. Disorders of Personality by Millon, 3/e p13]

- Krestchmer believed that Body types are associated with Personality traits and psychopathologies:
  - ***Asthenic*** *(Thin, small, weak)*: Introversion, Timidity, Schizophrenia
  - ***Pyknic*** *(Stocky, round, fat)*: Friendly, Interpersonally dependent, Gregarious, Manic-depressive illness
  - ***Athletic*** *(Muscular, large boned)*: Later combined into Asthenic/ Lepotosomic

74. Ans. (d) Akathisia
[Ref. Niraj Ahuja, 7/e p59]

- *Clinical features of Retarded Catatonia*: Mutism, Rigidity, Akinesia, Negativism, Echolalia, Echopraxia, Waxy flexibility, Ambivalence, Ambitendency, Posturing, Mannerisms, Verbigeration

75. Ans. (b) 2 years

[Ref. Schizophrenia by Hirsch, 2/e p477]

- Duration of maintenance treatment in Schizophrenia:
  - After 1 episode: 1-2 years
  - After multiple episodes: Minimum five years (preferably lifelong)

76. Ans. (b) Thought withdrawal; (d) Thought broadcasting; (e) Delusional perceptions

[Ref. Niraj Ahuja, 7/e p55]

77. Ans. (c) Capgras syndrome

[Ref. Niraj Ahuja, 7/e p87]

Capgras' Syndrome (Delusion of Doubles)

- Syndrome with delusional conviction that other persons in the environment are not their real selves but are their own doubles
- Types of Capgras' syndrome:
  - Illusion des sosies (Typical Capgras' syndrome): Person holds a delusion that a friend, spouse, parent, or other close family member (or pet) has been replaced by an identical impostor **(Patient claims actual wife as imposter in the given question)**
  - Illusion de fregoli: Patient falsely identifies strangers as familiar persons
  - Syndrome of subjective doubles: Patient's own self is perceived to be replaced by a double
  - Intermetamorphosis: Patient misidentifies completely (external appearance + personality), persons known to patient seem to have exchanged identities with each other
- Associated disorders include Paranoid schizophrenia (MC), Brain injury, Dementia, Delusional disorders and Organic delusional disorders

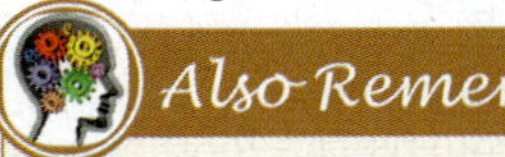

Capgras Vs Fregoli

- Capgras syndrome, causes the patient to think that someone who he or she interacts with on a daily basis has been replaced by an impostor, on the other hand, patients with Fregoli delusion believe that the many people around him or her are actually the same person in many different disguises;
- Capgras is 'hypo-identification', whereas Fregoli is 'hyper-identification'
- Capgras is 'Negative misidentification', whereas Fregoli is 'Positive misidentification'

Chapter 6

Mood Disorders: Mania and Depression

THEORETICAL CONCEPTS

VI A. UNDERLYING CAUSES

- *Biological theories*:
  - Hereditary
  - Biochemical: Abnormality in monoamine system
  - Endocrinal disorders
  - Sleep abnormalities
  - Dilated brain ventricles
- *Psychosocial theories*:
  - Stress
  - Reaction formation (mania) and introjection (depression)

VI B. CLINICAL PRESENTATION

VI B1. Mania

- ***Elevated/expansive/irritable mood***[Q]:
  - Stage I Euphoria: Increased sense of well-being and happiness
  - Stage II Elation: Feeling of confidence and enjoyment with increased psychomotor activity
  - Stage III Exaltation: Intense elation with delusions of grandeur
  - Stage IV Ecstasy: Intense sense of rapture/blissfulness
- *Psychomotor activity*: Increased
- *Speech and thought*:
  - Excessive talking
  - *Flight of ideas*: Rapid speech with abrupt shifts
  - Delusions of grandeur
  - Distractibility
- *Goal directed activity*:
  - Excessive planning
  - Execution of multiple activities
  - High risk activities
- *Other features*:
  - Decreased need for sleep
  - Absence of insight

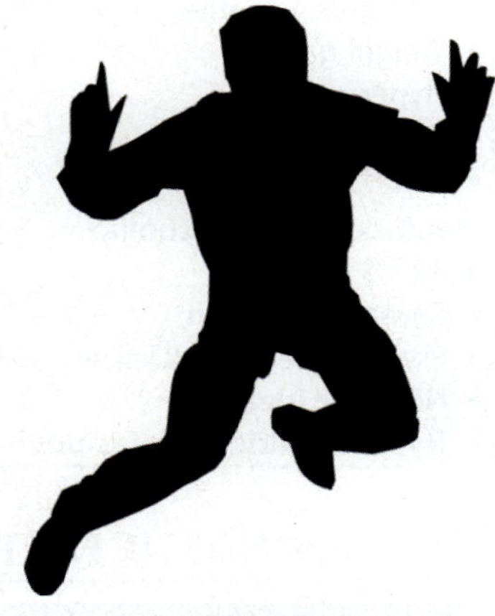

Fig. Mania

VI B2. Depression

- *Depressed mood*:
  - Pervasive and persistent sadness
  - Loss of interest in daily activities
  - **Anhedonia** (inability to experience pleasure)

- *Depressed ideation/cognition*:
  - Hopelessness, helplessness, worthlessness
  - **Suicidal ideas**
  - **Delusions of nihilism**
- *Psychomotor activity*: Anxiety, agitation, restlessness
- *Physical symptoms*:
  - General aches and pains
  - Hypochondriac features
  - Easy fatiguability
- *Biological functions*:
  - **Insomnia**
  - Loss of appetite/weight
- *Psychotic features*:
  - Delusions, hallucinations
  - Inappropriate behaviour
- *Suicidal ideas*
- *Absence of underlying organic cause*

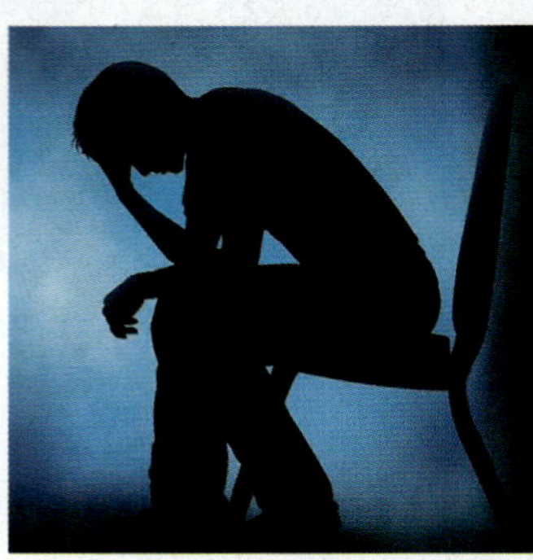

Fig. Depression

VI B3. Diagnostic Criteria for Major Depression

- **Five or more** of the following symptoms must be present **for at least 2 weeks**[Q]:
  - Depressed mood
  - Loss of interest/pleasure in all activities
  - Alteration of appetite
  - Insomnia
  - Psychomotor agitation/retardation
  - Fatigue/weakness/lethargy
  - Feeling of worthlessness/guilt
  - Diminished concentration
  - Recurrent thought of death/suicidal ideation

VI B4. Types of Depression

Major Depression	**Minor Depression**
• 5 or more of above symptoms[Q]	• 2 or more of above symptoms[Q]
Endogenous Depression • Biological features **(Loss of appetite/weight)**[Q] • Psychotic features	**Exogenous/Reactive/Neurotic Depression** • Chronic minor depression **(Dysthymia[Q])** • **Psychotic features absent[Q]**
Atypical Depression • Increased appetite • Weight gain • Hypersomnia • Lethargy • Mood reactivity	**Somatized/Masked Depression** • Chronic pain • Anorexia • Weakness • Insomnia • Depression not evident
Involutional Melancholia[Q] • 40–65 years age • Severe depression • Psychotic features (Delusions, Hallucinations) • **Nihilistic ideas[Q]** • **Hypochondriacal delusions[Q]**	**Agitated Depression** • Severe depression • Marked motor restlessness • Marked agitation • Melancholia

VI C. PROGNOSTIC FACTORS IN MOOD DISORDERS

Good prognosis	Bad prognosis	
• Acute onset • Typical presentation • Severe depression • Well adjusted personality • Good response to treatment	• Co-morbid disorders • Personality disorders • Alcoholism • Double depression	• Ongoing stress • Hypochondriac features • Poor drug compliance

VI D. TREATMENT

VI D1. Antidepressants

- *Tricyclic antidepressants*: Imipramine, Amitriptyline[Q]
- *Selective serotonin reuptake inhibitors (SSRIs)*: Fluoxetine, Sertraline, Citalopram
- *Serotonin norepinephrine reuptake inhibitors (SNRIs)*: Venlafaxine, Duloxetine

VI D2. Electroconvulsive Therapy (ECT)

- ***Indications for ECT***[Q]:
  - **Severe depression with risk of suicide**
  - Severe depression with stupor, retardation, somatic features
  - Severe refractory depression
  - Delusional depression
  - Side effects of therapy

VI D3. Lithium

- *Importance*: **Drug of choice for Manic episode**[Q]
- *Lag period before effect*: 1–2 weeks
- *Lithium has a narrow therapeutic index*

Lithium values in body	
Therapeutic dose range[Q]	**900–1500 mg $LiCO_3$ per day**
Therapeutic level in blood	0.8–1.2 mEq/litre[Q]
Prophylactic level in blood	0.6–1.2 mEq/litre[Q]
Toxicity of lithium	>2.0 mEq/litre
Death	>4.0–4.5 mEq/litre

VI D4. Antipsychotics

- *Indications of Antipsychotics*[Q]:
  - Acute manic episode
    - Along with mood stabilisers
    - If side effects due to mood stabilisers
    - **EMERGENCY TREATMENT of mania**[Q]
  - Delusional depression: Olanzapine, Quetiapine, Risperidone, Ziprasidone
  - Bipolar depression: Quetiapine

VI D5. Other Mood Stabilisers

- Sodium valproate
- Carbamazepine, Oxcarbazepine
- Benzodiazepines
- Lamotrigine
- Thyroid hormones

VI D6. Psychosurgery

- Limbic leucotomy
- Subcaudate tractotomy

VI D7. Psychosocial Treatment

- Cognitive behaviour therapy
- Behaviour therapy
- Interpersonal therapy
- Group/family therapy

VI E. SIDE EFFECTS OF ANTI-DEPRESSANT DRUGS

Side effect	Cause	Maximum risk	Minimum risk
***Autonomic side effects*[Q]**			
Dry mouth	Cholinergic block	**Amitriptyline[Q]**	Fluoxetine[Q]
Constipation			
Cycloplegia			
Mydriasis			
Urinary retention			
Orthostatic hypotension	α-1 adrenergic block		
Sexual side effects			
Impotence	α-1 adrenergic block	Amitriptyline	Mirtazapine Bupropion
Impaired ejaculation			
CNS effects			
Sedation	α-adrenergic block	Amitriptyline	Protriptyline
Tremor & EPSE	Serotonergic	Amoxapine	-
Jitteriness	Adrenergic, Serotonergic	Imipramine[Q]	MAO inhibitors
Seizures	Decreased threshold	Bupropion	Nomifensine
***Cardiac side effects*[Q]**			
Tachycardia	Anticholinergic	Amitriptyline[Q]	Trazodone
ECG changes	Cardiotoxic		Fluoxetine
Arrhythmias			
Hypertension	Noradrenergic	Venlafaxine[Q]	SSRIs
Miscellaneous side effects			
Agranulocytosis	Hypersensitivity	Mianserin	-
Weight gain	-	Mirtazapine	Bupropion

VI F. LITHIUM

- *Indications*:
  - Treatment
    - **Acute mania[Q]**
    - Acute depression
    - Chronic alcoholism and psychoactive substance use disorders
    - Schizo-affective disorder
    - **Cyclothymia** (mild form of bipolar disorder)[Q]
    - Impulsive aggression
    - **Kleine-Levin syndrome** (excessive sleeping and eating)
  - Prophylaxis
    - Bipolar mood disorder
    - Unipolar mood disorder
- *Market preparations*:
  - Lithium carbonate
  - Lithium citrate
- *Lithium has a narrow therapeutic index[Q]*
- *Side effects*

Neurological	**Renal**
• Tremor **(MC side effect overall)**[Q] • Muscular weakness • Seizures • Cog-wheel rigidity • Neurotoxicity	• **Nephrotic syndrome**[Q] • Nephrogenic diabetes insipidus • Polyuria • Polydipsia
Cardiovascular • T-wave depression	**Gastrointestinal** • Nausea, vomiting, diarrhoea, metallic taste
Endocrinal • Goitre, Hypothyroidism • Weight gain	**Dermatological** • Acneiform/papular eruptions • Exacerbation of psoriasis • Alopecia
During pregnancy and lactation • **Ebstein anomaly**[Q]	

- *Contraindications*
  - Pregnancy and lactation
  - Renal, cardiac, thyroid, neurological dysfunction
  - Blood dyscrasia
  - Co-administration of thiazide diuretics, tetracyclines, anesthetics

IMAGE-BASED QUESTIONS

1. Identify the Mental health disorder shown in the Photograph

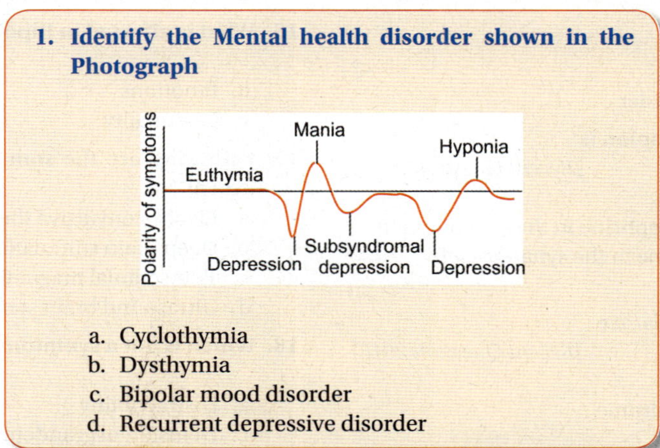

a. Cyclothymia
b. Dysthymia
c. Bipolar mood disorder
d. Recurrent depressive disorder

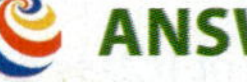 ANSWERS WITH EXPLANATIONS OF IBQs 

1. Ans. (c) Bipolar mood disorder *[Ref. Niraj Ahuja, 7/e p73]*

Bipolar Disorder (Manic Depressive Psychosis)

- Recurrent episodes of Mania and Depression in same patient at different times
- Episodes can occur in any sequence
- Bipolar Type I: Episodes of Severe mania and Severe depression
- Bipolar Type II: Episodes of Hypomania and Severe depression

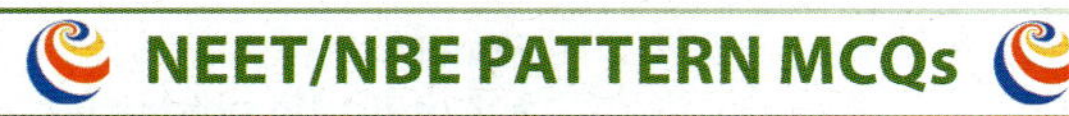

NEET/NBE PATTERN MCQs

1. Dysthymia is seen in *[Recent Question 2016]*
a. Bipolar mood disorder
b. Major depressive disorder
c. Minor depressive disorder
d. Persistent depressive disorder

2. Which of the following is/are not Side-effects of Lithium? *[PGI June 2016]*
a. Seizure
b. Hyporeflexia
c. Nephrogenic diabetes insipidus
d. Alopecia
e. Tremor

3. Phototherapy is used to treat which Psychiatric condition? *[Recent Question 2016]*
a. Depression
b. MR
c. Schizophrenia
d. Obsessive compulsive disorder

4. Which of the following is seen in Catatonia? *[Recent Question 2016]*
a. Cataplexy b. Echolalia
c. Positivism d. Disobedience

5. Catatonia is most commonly seen with *[Recent Question 2016]*
a. Schizophrenia
b. Depression
c. Anxiety disorder
d. Obsessive compulsive disorder

6. Mechanism of action of Bupropion is *[Recent Question 2016]*
a. Increased levels GABA
b. Increased levels of norepinephrine in the synaptic cleft
c. Increased levels of dopamine in the synaptic cleft
d. Both b and c

7. Absolute indications for ECT is/are
a. Suicidal depression *[Recent Question 2016]*
b. Intractable stupor
c. Neuroleptic malignant syndrome
d. All the above

8. Dysthymia is *[Recent Question 2016]*
a. Chronic mild depression
b. Chronic severe depression
c. Bipolar disorder
d. Personality disorder

9. ECT is contraindicated in *[Recent Question 2016]*
a. Raised ICT b. Brain tumor
c. Head injury d. All of the above

10. Which of the following drugs is/are used in treatment of acute mania? *[Recent Question 2016]*
a. Lithium
b. Oxcarbazepine
c. Risperidone
d. All of the above

11. Best use of Lithium is in *[Recent Question 2016]*
a. Treatment of schizophrenia
b. Treatment of recurrent depression
c. Treatment of first depressive episode
d. Prevent recurrence of bipolar mood disorder

12. Mania is characterized by all, except *[Recent Question 2016]*
a. Hypersomnia b. Pressure of speech
c. High self-esteem d. Delusion of grandeur

13. Clinical effects of antidepressant drugs is mainly based on *[Recent Question 2016]*
a. Change in neurotransmitter receptor sensitivity
b. Decreased level of neurotransmitters
c. Change in efficacy of neurotransmitters
d. None of the above

14. SSRIs should be carefully used in the young for the management of depression due to increase in *[Recent Question 2016]*
a. Nihilism ideation b. Guilt ideation
c. Suicidal ideation d. Envious ideation

15. Features of Serotonin syndrome associated with SSRIs, and MOAIs are all, except *[Recent Question 2016]*
a. Tremors b. Agitation
c. Cardiovascular collapse d. Hypothermia

16. What is affected in Bipolar disorders? *[Recent Question 2016]*
a. Emotions b. Perception
c. Personality d. Thought

17. Following are the somatic therapies used in depression, except *[Recent Question 2016]*
a. Electroconvulsive therapy
b. Deep brain stimulation
c. Transcranial magnetic stimulation
d. Ultrasound brain stem stimulation

18. Which is not a symptom of Mania? *[Recent Question 2016]*
a. Distractibility b. Elated mood
c. Delusion of grandeur d. Increased sleep

19. All the following are indications for ECT, except *[Recent Question 2016]*
a. Intractable seizures
b. Depressive stupor
c. Neuroleptic malignant syndrome
d. Acute anxiety

20. Which category of ICD is associated with Mood disorder? *[Recent Question 2016]*
a. F0 b. F1
c. F2 d. F3

21. Persistent feeling of Guilt is seen in *[Recent Question 2016]*
a. OCD b. Depression
c. Mania d. Schizophrenia

22. Post-partum blues is a type of *[Recent Question 2016]*
a. Mood disturbance b. Depression
c. Psychosis d. Dysthymia

23. Catatonic symptoms include *[Recent Question 2016]*
a. Negativism b. Grimacing
c. Mutism d. All of the above

24. A case of Depression is Refractory to Anti-depressant medications. All of the following interventions can be done, EXCEPT *[Recent Question 2016]*
a. Double the dose of Anti-depressant medications
b. Switch the Anti-depressant
c. Augment with Lithium
d. Augment with T3/T4

25. Drugs used to treat mania in an ICU are all, except *[NBE FMGE September 2009]*
a. Lithium b. Haloperidol
c. Benzodiazepine d. Olanzapine

26. Therapeutic level of lithium in serum is *[NBE DNB 1995, 1998, 1999]*
a. 0.1 meq/L b. 0.4 meq/L
c. 1.0 meq/L d. 1.8 meq/L

27. A 50-year-old male presents with a 3 years history of irritability, low mood, lack of interest in surrounding and general dissatisfaction with everything. There is no signification. He is most likely to be suffering from *[NBE DNB December 2011]*
a. Major depression b. No psychiatric disorder
c. Dysthymia d. Chronic fatigue syndrome

28. Following drugs cause CNS depression, except *[NBE DNB 1998]*
a. Amphetamine b. Alcohol
c. Barbiturates d. Diazepam

29. All of the following are used in treatment of Bipolar disorders, except *[NBE FMGE September 2012]*
a. Lithium b. Antipsychotics
c. Phenytoin d. Sodium valproate

30. Lithium toxicity affects all of the following organs, except *[NBE FMGE September 2006]*
a. Liver b. Brain
c. Heart d. Kidney

31. The amino-acid derived neurotransmitter used for treating depression is *[Recent Question 2012, 2015]*
a. Serotonin b. Histamine
c. Acetylcholine d. None

32. True about manic-depressive psychosis is *[NBE DNB 1997, 2000, 2005]*
a. Personality deterioration is common
b. Patient keeps on suffering from mania by depression
c. Unipolar depression is uncommon
d. Patient often remits completely in between attack

33. Early morning insomnia is characteristically seen in *[NBE DNB 1996]*
a. Reactive depression b. Secondary depression
c. Exogenous depression d. Endogenous depression

34. Treatment of choice of bipolar mood disorder *[Recent Question 2012, 2015]*
a. Fluoxetine b. Imipramine
c. Lithium d. Chlorpromazine

35. Not a good prognostic factor in bipolar disorders is
a. Gradual onset *[NBE FMGE September 2012]*
b. Good response to treatment
c. Severe depression
d. Typical features

36. The only definite contraindication to ECT is *[NBE DNB 1995, 2000, 2001, AIIMS PG 1995]*
a. Brain tumour
b. Glaucoma
c. Aortic aneurysm
d. Myocardial disease

37. ECT is contraindicated in *[NBE DNB 1998, 2000, 2004]*
a. Intracranial S.O.L. b. Pregnancy
c. Cardiac disease d. Psychosis

38. All are used in Status epilepticus, except *[NBE FMGE September 2006]*
a. Diazepam b. Phenytoin
c. Phenobarbitone d. Carbamazepine

39. The term "Depressive Equivalent" can be used interchangeably with *[NBE DNB 1992]*
a. Hysteria b. Masked depression
c. OCD d. Opiate dependence

40. All are true of mania, except *[NBE FMGE September 2012]*
a. Impaired judgement b. Heightened concentration
c. Delusions of grandeur d. Restlessness

41. Erotomania is seen in *[Recent Question 2012, 2015]*
a. Bipolar mania b. Unipolar mania
c. Neurosis d. OCD

42. Maximum benefit of electroconvulsive therapy is in
a. Hysteria *[Recent Question 2012, 2015]*
b. Depression with suicidal tendency
c. Chronic schizophrenia
d. Mania

43. Treatment of choice in acute mania is *[Recent Question 2015, NBE FMGE March 2007, September 2004]*
a. Lithium b. Haloperidol
c. Diazepam d. Lithium + Haloperidol

44. Lithium is the drug of choice for *[UPSC 2011, Recent Question 2014, 2015]*
a. Bipolar disorder b. Dysthymia
c. Anxiety neurosis d. Schizophrenia

45. Most common cardiac abnormality associated with use of Lithium in 1st trimester of pregnancy is *[NBE DNB 1992]*
a. Down's syndrome
b. Ebstein's anomaly of tricuspid valve
c. PDA
d. Coarctation of aorta

46. Tricyclic anti-depressant with least cardiotoxicity is *[NBE FMGE March 2004]*
a. Amitriptyline b. Desipramine
c. Doxepin d. Protriptyline

47. First agent shown to be effective in maniac phase of BPD *[Recent Question 2012, 2013, 2015]*
a. Li b. Lamotrigine
c. Valproate d. Carbamazepine

48. All of the following are recognised side effects of lithium carbonate therapy, except *[UPSC 1995]*
a. Hypothyroidism b. Leucocytosis
c. Polyuria d. Hypercalcaemia

49. Long-term use of lithium is associated with the following endocrine abnormality *[NBE DNB 2004, 2008]*
a. Hypothyroidism b. Diabetes mellitus
c. Hyperthyroidism d. Cushing's syndrome

50. DSM IV criterion for depression is *[Recent Question 2012, 2013, 2015]*
a. 1 week b. 2 weeks
c. 3 weeks d. 4 weeks

51. Drug of choice in MDP is *[NBE DNB 1998, 1999, 2004, 2006]*
a. Lithium b. Amphetamine
c. Diazepam d. Alprazolam

52. Absolute contraindication to Lithium therapy *[NBE FMGE March 2004]*
a. Renal failure b. Angina
c. Glaucoma d. Epilepsy

53. The treatment of Acute Manic Episode is *[NBE DNB 2003, 2004]*
a. ECT b. Lithium
c. Diazepam d. Sodium valproate

54. Mania is characterized by following, except *[NBE DNB 1997]*
a. Pressure of speech b. Elation
c. Insomnia d. Lethargy

55. In depressions, there is deficiency of *[Recent Question 2012, 2015]*
a. 5-HT b. Acetylcholine
c. Dopamine d. GABA

56. Cognitive model of depression was given by *[Recent Question 2017, NBE DNB 2010]*
a. Beck b. Skinner
c. Cerletti d. Freud

57. True about voltage and time used in electroconvulsive therapy *[NBE DNB 1993]*
a. 40–60 volts, 2 minutes b. 80–90 volts, 0.01 second
c. 90–120 volts, 0.3 second d. 120–150 volts, 3 minutes

58. A particularly low grade chronic long-lasting depression is known as *[UPSC 2012]*
a. Unipolar depression b. Bipolar depression
c. Dysthymia d. Major depressive disorder

59. All cause depression, except *[NBE DNB 2007]*
a. LSD b. Corticosteroids
c. L-Dopa d. Clonazepam

60. What is the primary disturbance in mania? *[NBE FMGE September 2011]*
a. Heightened affect b. Overactivity
c. Grandiosity d. Decreased need for sleep

61. Indications of ECT are *[NBE DNB 1994]*
a. Endogenous depression
b. Catatonic schizophrenia
c. OCD
d. Phobia

62. A 41-year-old man on treatment for bipolar disorder presents with ataxia, coarse tremors of his upper limbs and diarrhea. He reports that he has been sweating a lot and has not been drinking much water. He is on lithium, fluoxetine and olanzapine and denies having used any other medication or other substances. What is the most likely diagnosis? *[NBE FMGE March 2012]*
a. Olanzapine toxicity b. Fluoxetine toxicity
c. Lithium toxicity d. Serotonin syndrome

63. Neurotransmitter which is found in increased quantities in mania is *[NBE DNB 1997, NBE DNB 2000]*
a. Noradrenaline b. Serotonin
c. Acetylcholine d. GABA

64. All of the following are features of masked depression, except *[NBE FMGE March 2012]*
a. Body aches and pains
b. Gastrointestinal symptoms
c. Functional impairment
d. Depressed mood

65. Lithium carbonate is employed in the following conditions except *[UPSC CMS 2015]*
a. To treat acute episodes of mania
b. To prevent recurrence of mania
c. To prevent depression in bipolar disorders
d. To prevent depression in unipolar disorders

66. Drug of choice in bipolar disorder is *[Recent Question 2017]*
a. Carbamazepine b. Lithium carbonate
c. Imipramine d. Buspirone

67. Treatment of choice for Acute depression is *[Recent Question 2017]*
a. SSRIs
b. Alprazolam
c. ECT
d. Psychotherapy

68. Which of the following is not a side effect of Quetiapine? *[Recent Question 2017]*
a. Dry mouth b. Hair loss
c. Sudden cardiac death d. Dyspepsia

69. Definition of Clinical depression includes *[Recent Question 2017]*
a. Depressed mood
b. Slowed thinking
c. Psychomotor retardation
d. All of the above

70. All are true regarding Depression, except *[Recent Question 2017]*
a. More common in women
b. Most common psychiatric disorder overall
c. Most common age group is middle age
d. Is genetic in origin

71. Duration of the disease for the diagnosis of Dysthymia is *[Recent Question 2017]*

a. 2 years b. 4 years
c. 6 years d. 8 years

72. Endocrine defects involved in depression are all, except *[Recent Question 2017]*

a. Cushing's disease b. Hyperprolactinemia
c. Pheochromocytoma d. Hyperparathyroidism

73. Type II bipolar disorder is characterized by *[Recent Question 2017]*

a. Mania and subclinical depression
b. Hypomania and major depression
c. Hypomania and subclinical depression with normal mood in between
d. Mania and dysthymia

74. A primigravida female feeling depressed and showing emotional liability soon after delivery. Most Likely cause is? *[Recent Question 2017]*

a. Post-partum blues
b. Post-partum psychosis
c. Post-partum depression
d. Post-partum pinks

HIGH YIELD MCQs

1. A 22-year-old lady came to OPD complaining of feeling low and depressed, with insomnia, reduced appetite and lack of interest in surroundings, since past 3 weeks. These symptoms began after losses in a business deal one month ago. Which one of the following statements is TRUE regarding her management? *[APPG 2016]*

a. Counsel her and give supportive therapy
b. Assure her that no treatment is needed as it is triggered by a stressful event
c. Start antidepressant drug therapy
d. Start on a mood stabilizer drug

2. A 40 years old lady presents to psychiatry OPD with the complaints of depressed mood, loss of appetite and loss of interest in surroundings for past 1 year. Associated insomnia is also present. The symptoms have been present since last 1 year after a loss in business. Which of the following is true regarding management? *[Recent Question 2015, All India PGMEE 2011]*

a. SSRIs are most efficacious among available drugs
b. Give combination therapy of two antidepressant drugs
c. Give antidepressant therapy based on the side-effect profile of drugs
d. No treatment is required as symptoms are due to loss in business

3. Nihilistic ideas are seen in *[PGI 2008]*

a. Simple schizophrenia b. Paranoid schizophrenia
c. Cotard's syndrome d. Depression
e. Body Dysmorphic Disorder

4. Stimulation of which of the nerve leads to elevated mood *[AIIMS PGMEE 2009]*

a. Optic b. Olfactory
c. Trochlear d. Vagus

5. Drug of choice in depression in old person is *[All India PGMEE 1996]*

a. Fluoxetine b. Buspirone
c. Amitriptyline d. Imipramine

6. Drugs used for recurrent depressive episode *[PGI 2009]*

a. Imipramine b. Carbamazepine
c. Fluoxetine d. Sodium valproate

7. Treatment of choice in depression with suicidal tendencies *[All India PGMEE 1994]*

a. TCA
b. MAO-Inhibitor
c. Fluoxetine + TCA + MAO inhibitor
d. Electroconvulsive therapy

8. The clinical features of mania include *[PGI 2002, 2006]*

a. Anhedonia b. Elated mood
c. Avolition d. Delusion of grandiosity
e. Distractibility

9. Most common age for depression is *[All India PGMEE 1996, 1998]*

a. Middle age men b. Middle age female
c. Young girl d. Children

10. Not a feature of mania *[AIIMS PGMEE 1991]*

a. Elation b. Disorientation
c. Pressure of speech d. Delusion of grandeur

11. Flight of ideas is seen in *[PGI 2003]*

a. Mania b. Schizophrenia
c. Depression d. Delirium

12. "Nihilistic delusions" are seen in *[PGI 2000]*

a. Endogenous depression
b. Double depression
c. Depression in involutional stage
d. Cyclothymia
e. Dysthymia

13. True about psychotic feature in depression *[PGI 2004]*

a. Found in severe depression
b. Found in moderate depression
c. Mood incongruent psychotic feature
d. Cyclothymia
e. Dysthymia

14. Suicide risk is common with which type of depression *[PGI 2000]*

a. Reactive depression b. Endogenous depression
c. Childhood depression d. Depression in involution

15. Bipolar II disorder includes *[PGI 2002, JIPMER PGMEE 2003, Recent Question 2015]*

a. Cyclothymic disorder
b. Dysthymia
c. Single manic episode
d. Major depression & hypomania

16. **The period of normalcy is seen between two psychoses. The diagnosis is** *[All India PGMEE 1999]*
    a. Schizophrenia
    b. Manic Depressive Psychosis
    c. Alcoholism
    d. Depression

17. **True about bipolar disorder type II is** *[PGI 2005]*
    a. Recurrent depression
    b. Recurrent mania
    c. Repetitive depression & mania
    d. Repetitive mania & hypomania
    e. Repetitive depression & hypomania

18. **Normal Lithium therapeutic level is** *[PGI 2006, 2009]*
    a. 0.5–0.7 mEq/L b. 0.7–1.1 mEq/L
    c. 0.1–0.3 mEq/L d. 1.5–2 mEq/L
    e. 2.5–3 mEq/L

19. **True about Lithium treatment in mania** *[PGI 2009]*
    a. Commonest side effect is tremor
    b. Toxic level is <1.5 mg/dL serum level
    c. Amiloride is DOC for Li induced diabetes insipidus
    d. Lithium is 90% protein bound
    e. Tremor is treated with propranolol

20. **Drugs used for prophylaxis in bipolar disorder** *[PGI 2002]*
    a. Chlorpromazine b. Lithium
    c. Carbamazepine d. Zolpidem
    e. Sodium valproate

21. **Drug not used in prophylaxis of MDP** *[AIIMS PGMEE 1995]*
    a. Haloperidol b. Lithium
    c. Carbamazepine d. Valproate

22. **Lithium is used in prophylaxis of** *[AIIMS PGMEE 1997]*
    a. Recurrent Phobia
    b. Alcohol dependence
    c. Paranoid Schizophrenia
    d. Recurrent manic depressive attacks

23. **Drug(s) used in bipolar disorder is/are** *[PGI 2009]*
    a. $LiCO_3$ b. Sodium valproate
    c. Phenytoin d. Lamotrigine
    e. Carbamazepine

24. **Mania is characterized by** *[PGI 1999]*
    a. Paranoid delusion b. Loss of orientation
    c. High self esteem d. Loss of insight

25. **Lithium is not used in treatment of which of the following?** *[All India PGMEE 2009]*
    a. Major depression
    b. Vascular headache
    c. Neutropenia
    d. Generalized Anxiety disorder

26. **Drug of choice for prophylaxis of Mania is** *[AIIMS PGMEE 1994]*
    a. Diazepam b. Lithium
    c. Haloperidol d. Fluoxetine

27. **All of the following are included in diagnosis of Bipolar disorder, except** *[All India PGMEE 2007]*
    a. Mania alone b. Depression alone
    c. Mania and depression d. Mania and anxiety

28. **Drug not used in prophylaxis for MDP** *[All India PGMEE 1995]*
    a. Carbamazepine b. Valproate
    c. Lithium d. Chlorpromazine

29. **For maintenance of Mania Depressive Psychosis (MDP) following drug is given** *[AIIMS PGMEE 1992]*
    a. Haloperidol b. Ketamine
    c. Carbamazepine d. Chlorpromazine

30. **True about major depressive disorder** *[PGI 2003]*
    a. Commonly seen in females
    b. Recovery is complete after treatment
    c. Associated with hypothyroidism
    d. Family history of major depression

31. **Best marker for electro-convulsive therapy** *[AIIMS PGMEE 2008]*
    a. CSF 5 HIAA
    b. CSF serotonin
    c. Brain derived growth factor
    d. CSF dopamine

32. **Indications for ECT are** *[PGI 2000]*
    a. Paranoid schizophrenia
    b. Depression with suicidal tendency
    c. Catatonic schizophrenia
    d. Neurotic depression
    e. Depression in involutional stage

33. **ECT is not useful in treatment of** *[All India PGMEE 1993]*
    a. Chronic Schizophrenia b. Catatonic Schizophrenia
    c. Endogenous depression d. Acute psychosis

34. **A patient on antidepressant therapy developed sudden hypertension on consuming cheese. The antidepressant is possibly** *[PGI 1999]*
    a. Amitriptyline b. Tranylcypromine
    c. Fluoxetine d. Sertraline

35. **Lithium is best used in** *[AIIMS PGMEE 1991, 1992]*
    a. MDP-Bipolar b. MDP-Unipolar
    c. MDP-rapid cycles d. Depression

36. **Congenital Anomaly produced by lithium therapy is** *[All India PGMEE 1993]*
    a. Limb shortening b. Anencephaly
    c. Heart Block d. Renal Agenesis

37. **Prophylactic maintenance serum level of lithium is** *[All India PGMEE 1994]*
    a. 02–08 mEq/L b. 0.7–1.2 mEq/L
    c. 1.2–2.0 mEq/L d. 2.0–2.5 mEq/L

38. **ECT is most useful in** *[PGI 1997]*
    a. Mania b. Depression
    c. OCD d. Schizophrenia

39. **Maximum benefit of Electro Convulsive Therapy is in** *[AIIMS PGMEE 1993]*
    a. Hysteria
    b. Mania
    c. Depression with Suicidal Tendency
    d. Chronic Schizophrenia

40. **Most common complication of ECT is** *[Recent Question 2015, 2017, AIIMS PG 1991,1996, AIPGME 1992]*
    a. Antegrade Amnesia b. Retrograde Amnesia
    c. Physociasis d. Depression

41. Tricyclic antidepressants have all of the following actions, except *[PGI 1997]*
a. Anti-cholinergic action
b. Anti-MAOI action
c. Blocks 5 HT or NE reuptake
d. Causes sedation

42. Tricyclic Anti-depressant are contraindicated in *[All India PGMEE 1991]*
a. Glaucoma b. Brain Tumor
c. Bronchial Asthma d. Hypertension

43. Non-sedating Antidepressant is *[AIIMS PGMEE 1993]*
a. Fluoxetine b. Mianserine
c. Amoxaprine d. Imipramine

44. The newest Antidepressant is *[AIIMS PGMEE 1993]*
a. Buspirone b. Fluoxetine
c. Penfluridol d. Clozapine

45. A 25-year-old woman complains of intense depressed mood for 6 months with inability to enjoy previously pleasurable activities. This symptom is known as *[AIIMS PGMEE 2005]*
a. Anhedonia b. Avolition
c. Apathy d. Amotivation

46. Bright light treatment has been found to be most effective in treatment of *[All India PGMEE 2006, Recent Question 2015]*
a. Anorexia Nervosa b. Seasonal Affective Disorder
c. Schizophrenia
d. Obsessive Compulsive Disorder

47. Chromosome associated with bipolar disease *[PGI 2005]*
a. Chromosome 16 b. Chromosome 13
c. Chromosome 18 d. Chromosome 11
e. Chromosome 23

48. Neurotransmitters involved in depression are *[Recent Question 2017, All India PGMEE 1995]*
a. GABA and Dopamine
b. Serotonin and Norepinephrine
c. Serotonin and Dopamine
d. Norepinephrine and GABA

49. Otto Veraguth sign is found in *[PGI 2003, Recent Question 2015]*
a. Mania b. Anxiety
c. OCD d. Depression

50. Delusion of Nihilism and Early morning insomnia are characteristic features of *[All India PGMEE 1997, 1998]*
a. Mania b. Major depression
c. Personality disorder d. Schizophrenia
e. Dysthymia

51. Endogenous Depression is characterized by all, except *[All India PGMEE 1992]*
a. Loss of self-esteem
b. Guilt psychosis
c. Third person hallucination
d. None

52. Suicidal tendencies are most common in *[PGI 2000]*
a. Involutional depression b. Reactive depression
c. Psychotic depression d. Childhood depression

53. A 41-year-old woman presented with a history of aches and pains all over the body and generalized weakness for four years. She cannot sleep because of the illness and has lost her appetite as well. She has lack of interest in work and doesn't like to meet friends and relatives. She denies feelings of sadness. Her most likely diagnosis is *[AIIMS PGMEE 2002]*
a. Somatoform pain disorder
b. Major depression
c. Somatization disorder
d. Dissociative

54. A 34-year-old housewife reports a three month history of feeling low, lack of interest in activities, lethargy, multiple body-aches, ideas of worthlessness, decreased appetite and disturbed sleep with early morning awakening. She is likely to benefit from *[AIIMS PGMEE 2004]*
a. Anti-psychotics b. Anti-depressants
c. Anxiolytics d. Hypno-sedatives

55. An 18-year-old student complains of lack of interest in studies for last 6 months. He has frequent quarrels with his parents and has frequent headaches. The most appropriate clinical approach would be *[All India PGMEE 2005]*
a. Leave him as normal adolescent problem
b. Rule out depression
c. Rule out migraine
d. Rule out an oppositional defiant disorder

56. Intense nihilism, somatization and agitation in old age are the hallmark symptoms of *[All India PGMEE 2006]*
a. Involutional melancholia
b. Atypical depression
c. Somatized depression
d. Depressive stupor

57. A 50-year-old man has presented with pain in back, lack of interest in recreational activities, low mood, lethargy, decreased sleep and appetite for two months. There was no history suggestive of delusions or hallucinations. He did not suffer from any chronic medical illness. There was no family history of psychiatric illness. Routine investigations including haemogram, renal function tests, liver function tests, electrocardiogram did not reveal any abnormality. This patient should be treated with *[All India PGMEE 2003, AIIMS PGMEE 2003]*
a. Haloperidol b. Sertraline
c. Alprazolam d. Olanzapine

58. A 60-year-old male is brought by his wife. He thinks that he had committed sins all through his life. He is very much depressed and has considered committing suicide but has not through hot do go about it. He had also attached sessions with a spiritual guru. He is not convinced by his wife that he has lead a pious life. He does not want to hear anything on the contrary. How will you treat him? *[All India PGMEE 2010]*
a. Antipsychotic + Anti-depressant
b. Antidepressant with cognitive behavioural therapy
c. Guidance & recounselling with guru + Anti-depressant
d. Anti-depressant alone

59. Rathi, 26-years-old female diagnosed to be suffering from depression. Now for the past 2 days she had suicidal tendency, thoughts and ideas. The best treatment is *[AIIMS PGMEE 2001]*

a. Amitriptyline b. Selegiline
c. Haloperidol + CPZ d. ECT

60. A 50-year-old male presents with a 3-year history of irritability, low mood, lack of interest in surroundings and general dissatisfaction with everything. There is no significant disruption in his sleep or appetite. He is likely to be suffering from *[AIIMS PGMEE 2005]*

a. Major depression b. No psychiatric disorder
c. Dysthymia d. Chronic fatigue syndrome

61. Which of the following is not seen in mania *[All India PGMEE 1991]*

a. Hypersexuality b. Hyperactivity
c. Decreased sleep d. Clouding of mania

62. Kallu a 22 years old male suffers from decreased sleep, increased sexual activity, excitement and spending excessive money for last 8 days. The diagnosis is *[AIIMS PGMEE 2001]*

a. Confusion b. Disorientation
c. Hyperactivity d. Loss of memory

63. A 20-year-old man has presented with increased alcohol consumption and sexual indulgence, irritability, lack of sleep, and not feeling fatigued even on prolonged periods of activity. All these changes have been present for 3 weeks. The most likely diagnosis is *[All India PGMEE 2003]*

a. Alcohol dependence b. Schizophrenia
c. Mania d. Impulsive control disorder

64. A 67-year-old lady is brought in by her 6 children saying that she has gone senile. Six months after her husband's death she has become more religious, spiritual and gives lot of money in donation. She is occupied in too many activities and sleeps less. She now believes that she has a goal to change the society. She does not like being brought to the hospital and is argumentative on being questioned on her doings. The diagnosis is *[AIIMS PGMEE 2002]*

a. Acute manic excitement b. Delusion
c. Schizophrenia d. Depression

65. In Prophylaxic of Manic Depressive Psychosis drug used is *[All India PGMEE 1996]*

a. Lithium carbonate b. Carbamazepine
c. Valproate d. Haloperidol

66. A 42-year-old male with a past history of a manic episode presents with an illness of 1 month duration characterized by depressed mood, anhedonia and profound psychomotor retardation. The most appropriate management strategy is prescribing a combination of *[AIIMS PGMEE 2004]*

a. Antipsychotics and antidepressants
b. Antidepressants and mood stabilizers
c. Antipsychotics and mood stabilizers
d. Antidepressants and benzodiazepines

67. Drug of choice for rapid cycling MDP is *[All India PGMEE 1999]*

a. Lithium b. Carbamazepine
c. Sodium valproate d. Haloperidol

68. An elderly housewife lost her husband, who died suddenly of Myocardial infarction, couple of years ago. They had been staying alone for almost a decade with infrequent visits from her son and grandchildren. About a week after the death she heard his voice clearly talking to her as he would in a routine manner from the next room. She went to check but saw nothing. Subsequently she often heard his voice conversing with her and she would also discuss her daily matters with him. This however, provoked anxiety and sadness of mood when she was preoccupied with his thought. She should be treated with *[AIIMS PGMEE 2003]*

a. Clomipramine
b. Alprazolam
c. Electroconvulsive therapy
d. Haloperidol

69. A patient of depression is getting chlorpromazine, but his auditory hallucination are not controlled. The next drug is *[AIIMS PGMEE 1999]*

a. Haloperidol b. Clozapine
c. Sulpiride d. Tianeptine

70. A 30-year-old manic patient was prescribed Haloperidol one week back. For the last two days he has become restless and kept pacing in the room for a day. On examination he was found to have tremors of hand. He is most likely suffering from *[AIIMS PGMEE 2003]*

a. Anhedonia b. Dystonia
c. Restless leg syndrome d. Akathesia

71. ECT causes *[AIIMS PGMEE 1998]*

a. Antegrade amnesia b. Retrograde amnesia
c. Both d. None

72. Memory disturbance of ECT recovers in *[AIIMS PGMEE 1996]*

a. Few days to few weeks
b. Few weeks to few months
c. Few months to few year
d. Permanent

73. In Direct ECT, the intraocular tension is *[All India PGMEE 1991]*

a. Increased b. Decreased
c. No change d. Variable

74. ECT is absolutely contraindicated in *[All India PGMEE 1992]*

a. Pregnancy
b. Very ill patient
c. Raised Intracranial Tension
d. Severe heart disease

75. A patient was treated with Amitriptyline for depression, developed urinary retention, constipation & blurring of vision. Most likely cause is *[AIIMS PGMEE 2000]*

a. Symptoms of depression persisting
b. Anti-cholinergic side effects
c. Depression medicamentosa
d. Any of above

76. All are Anti-depressants, except *[All India PGMEE 1997]*

a. Trazodone b. Amitriptyline
c. Fluoxitine d. Pimozide

77. Select the true statements *[PGI 2002]*
a. Imipramine is used in treatment of endogenous depression
b. Fluoxetine causes weight gain
c. Thioridazine cause less anticholinergic effects
d. BZD's have same abuse potential as barbiturates
e. Codeine is an effective antitussive

78. A patient is brought to the casualty in the state of altered sensorium. He was on Lithium treatment for affective disorder and has suffered through an attack of epileptic fits. On examination, he has tremors, increased DTR's and incontinence of urine. He has also undergone an episode of severe gastroenteritis 2 days ago. The serum Lithium was found to be 1.95 mEq/Lit. The probable cause for his present state is *[AIIMS PGMEE 2001]*
a. Lithium toxicity
b. Dehydration
c. Manic Episode
d. None

79. ECT is indicated in *[AIIMS PGMEE 1997]*
a. Neurotic Depression
b. Auditory hallucination
c. Schizophrenia
d. Delusional Depression

80. ECT is useful in *[AIIMS PGMEE 1997]*
a. Mania (Acute)
b. Chronic Schizophrenia
c. Acute Depression
d. Panic Disorder

81. ECT in depressive phase of MDP is useful because it *[PGI PGMEE 1999]*
a. Produces recurrence
b. Reduces recurrence
c. Shortens duration
d. Increases drug effects

82. Mania is characterised by *[PGI May 2014]*
a. Elevated mood
b. Increased need for sleep
c. Grandiosity
d. Pressured speech
e. Slow thoughts

83. Minimum duration length of symptoms in dysthymia is *[JIPMER PGMEE 2014]*
a. 2 days
b. 2 weeks
c. 2 months
d. 2 years

84. Serum Lithium level should be checked earliest after how many days of constant dosing? *[PGMCET 2015]*
a. 3
b. 5
c. 14
d. 20

85. Following is the vegetative disturbance in depression *[PGMCET 2015]*
a. Loss of interest
b. Pseudodementia
c. Hopelessness
d. Insomnia

86. A 32-year-old female presented with mania of 2 weeks duration. Her urine pregnancy test is positive. What is drug of choice? *[AIIMS PG November 2015]*
a. Clonazepam
b. Haloperidol
c. Lithium
d. Promethazine

87. A male patient of bipolar disorder with history of 5 episodes of mania and 1 episode of depression in last 8 years, under control by mood stabilizer, and manic symptoms appears as he tapered down the drugs. Which of following intervention should be carried out to improve drug compliance? *[AIIMS PG November 2015]*
a. Psycho education
b. Insight-oriented psychotherapy
c. Cognitive behavior therapy
d. Supportive psychotherapy

88. A lady presented to emergency with altered sensorium and hypotension. She is taking antidepressant medications. ECG shows wide QRS complex and right axis deviation. What should be given for management of this patient? *[AIIMS PG November 2015]*
a. IV sodium bicarbonate
b. Physostigmine
c. Wait and watch
d. Antiarrhythmics

89. Cognitive triad of depression includes all except? *[AIIMS PG November 2015]*
a. Idea of guilt
b. Hopelessness
c. Helplessness
d. Worthlessness

90. Fatal dose of Lithium is *[AIIMS November 2014]*
a. 2 g
b. 4 g
c. 6 g
d. 8 g

91. Mr Ram presented to Psychiatry OPD with irritability, guilt of not performing well in the office. He has had been having reduced interest in recreational activities since he left college 3 years back. Most likely diagnosis is *[AIIMS November 2017]*
a. Cyclothymia
b. Dysthymia
c. Adjustment disorder
d. Major depressive episode

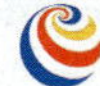 NEET/NBE PATTERN MCQs ANSWERS WITH EXPLANATIONS 

1. Ans. (d) Persistent depressive disorder
[Ref. Essentials of Psychiatric Mental Health Nursing by Varcarolis, 3/e p202]

Persistent depressive disorder (PDD)
- Commonly known as Dysthymia/Chronic depression
- Less notably severe depression characterised by depressive symptoms present for atleast 2 years
- Daytime fatigue, tiredness
- Chronic low depression/irritable mood
- Low self-esteem
- Negative thinking
- Difficulty in sleeping, Hypersomnia
- Eating too much or too little

2. Ans. (b) Hyporeflexia
[Ref. Niraj Ahuja, 7/e p190]

Side-effects of Lithium Therapy
- Neurological: Tremor, Muscular weakness, Seizures, Cog-wheel rigidity, Neurotoxicity
- Renal: Nephrotic syndrome, Nephrogenic diabetes insipidus, Polyuria, Polydipsia
- Cardiovascular: T-wave depression
- Gastrointestinal: Nausea, vomiting, diarrhoea, metallic taste
- Endocrinal: Goitre, Hypothyroidism, Weight gain
- Dermatological: Acneiform/papular eruptions, Exacerbation of psoriasis, Alopecia
- During pregnancy and lactation: Ebstein anomaly

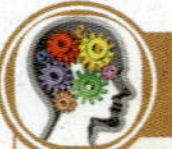
Also Remember
- **MC side-effect of Lithium therapy overall**: Tremor (Symmetric involvement of upper extremities)

3. Ans. (a) Depression
[Ref. Handbook of Depression by Friedman, 2/e p77]
- Phototherapy, the use of light treatment, was developed to treat, and has become the first-line treatment for, individuals with Seasonal affective disorder
  - Treatment of Seasonal and Non-seasonal depression
  - Improvement in Depression, Fatigue, Sleepiness, Health-related Quality of Life
  - Treatment of Pre-menstrual and Ante-partum depression

4. Ans. (b) Echolalia
[Ref. Niraj Ahuja, 7/e p59]

Clinical features of Catatonia
- Mutism (Complete absence of speech)
- Rigidity in posture, Akinesia
- Negativism
- Echolalia (Repetition of phrases/words)
- Echopraxia (Repetition of actions)
- Waxy flexibility (Body-parts maintained in positions of long time)
- Ambivalence, Ambitendency
- Mannerisms
- Verbigeration

5. Ans. (b) Depression
[Ref. Movement Disorders by Fernandez, 1/e p51]

Catatonia
- Common misconception is that catatonia is seen in schizophrenia: A subcategory of Schizophrenia is called catatonic schizophrenia
- Catatonia is a syndrome that is more common in affective disorders, such as bipolar disease
  - More often associated with mania, melancholia, and psychotic depression than with schizophrenia
  - Also seen in autism and in association with general medical conditions (such as metabolic disorders), drug intoxications, neurological disorders

6. Ans. (d) Both b and c
[Ref. Applied Pharmacology by Bardal, 1/e p378]
- **Bupropion** inhibits the presynaptic reuptake of both dopamine (DA) and noradrenaline (NA), leading to increased levels of both of these neurotransmitters in the synaptic cleft

7. Ans. (d) All of the above
[Ref. Niraj Ahuja, 7/e p199-200]
- **Absolute contraindication of ECT**: Raised intraocular tension
- **Relative contraindications of ECT**: Recent MI, Severe hypertension, Cerebrovascular accident, Severe pulmonary disease, Retinal detachment, Pheochromocytoma

8. Ans. (a) Chronic mild depression
[Ref. Niraj Ahuja, 7/e p82]

Dysthymia
- Chronic depressed mood that occurs for most of the day and for most days for over at least 2 years
- Poor appetite/excessive eating, Insomnia/excessive sleepiness, fatigue, poor self-esteem, poor decision making, hopelessness
- More prevalent in women

9. Ans. (d) All of the above
[Ref. Niraj Ahuja, 7/e p201]

10. Ans. (d) All of the above
[Ref. Practical Management of Bipolar Disorder by Young, 1/e p36]

Treatment of Acute Mania
- **First line**: Lithium/Olanzapine/Risperidone/ Quetiapine/ Aripiprazole/Ziprasidone/Divalproex
- Second line: Carbamazepine/Oxcarbazepine/ECT/ Asenapine/Lithium+Divalproex/Peliperidone monotherapy
- Third line: Haloperidol/Chlorpromazine/Lithium+ Haloperidol/ Clozapine/ Tamoxifen

11. Ans. (d) Prevent recurrence of bipolar mood disorder
[Ref. Use and Misuse of Psychiatric Drugs by Paris, 1/e Chap 5]
- Acute manic episodes in bipolar disorder can be controlled with antipsychotics, but lithium has a more specific effect and has been shown to prevent recurrences
- Lithium is the drug with the best evidence for maintenance

12. Ans. (a) Hypersomnia

[Ref. Clinical Neuropsychiatry and Behavioral Neuroscience by Moore, 3/e p694]

Stages of Mania

- Stage I mania: Cardinal manic symptoms of heightened mood, increased energy and decreased need for sleep, pressure of speech, flight of ideas, pressure of activity
- Stage II mania: Delusions appear; Delusions are typically either of grandeur or of persecution, according to the mood of the patient
- Stage III mania: Startling metamorphosis, fragmented speech and behavior, loosening of association, confusion, bizarre delusions

13. Ans. (a) Change in neurotransmitter receptor sensitivity

[Ref. Psychiatric and Neurological Disorders by Bockstaele, 1/e p106]

- Clinical effects of antidepressants are obviously caused by their ability to induce adaptive changes in neurotransmission, mainly serotonergic and noradrenergic

14. Ans. (c) Suicidal ideation

[Ref. Behavioral Aspects of Epilepsy by Holmes, 1/e p354]

- An increase in suicidal ideation and self-injurious behaviors has been reported in children and adolescents treated with SSRIs for Depression
- Although suicidal thoughts are reduced within groups of older adults taking SSRIs, older white men have the highest rates of completed suicides among other age and ethnic groups

15. Ans. (d) Hypothermia

[Ref. Textbook of Therapeutics by Helms, 8/e p1421]

Serotonin syndrome (SS)

- A group of symptoms that may occur following use of certain serotonergic medications
- Triad of mental, autonomic, and neurological disorders
- Degree of symptoms can range from mild to severe
- Symptoms include high body temperature, agitation, increased reflexes, tremor, sweating, dilated pupils, and diarrhea
- Cardiovascular collapse, coma, and death are rare but possible

16. Ans. (a) Emotions

[Ref. Niraj Ahuja, 7/e p70-71]

- Emotional Symptoms of Bipolar Disorder help you recognize if a person is suffering from the condition; they can also help you understand what part of a cycle an individual is in

Manic phase	Depressive phase
• Euphoria • Agitation • Feelings of invincibility • Ongoing happiness	• Feelings of emptiness • Worry • Disinterest • Irritability • Sorrow

17. Ans. (d) Ultrasound brain-stem stimulation

[Ref. Depression by Schwartz, 2/e p166]

New Somatic therapies of Neuro-stimulation for Depression

- Electroconvulsive Therapy
- Transcranial Magnetic Stimulation
- Vagus Nerve Stimulation
- Deep Brain Stimulation

18. Ans. (d) Increased sleep

[Ref. Niraj Ahuja, 7/e p71]

Mania

- Elevated/expansive/irritable mood:
  - **Stage I Euphoria**: Increased sense of well-being and happiness
  - **Stage II Elation**: Feeling of confidence and enjoyment with increased psychomotor activity
  - **Stage III Exaltation**: Intense elation with delusions of grandeur
  - **Stage IV Ecstasy**: Intense sense of rapture/blissfulness
- Psychomotor activity: Increased
- Speech and thought: Excessive talking, Flight of ideas, Delusions of grandeur, Distractibility
- Goal directed activity: Excessive planning, Multiple activities, High risk activities
- Other features: Decreased need for sleep, Absence of insight

19. Ans. (d) Acute anxiety

[Ref. Psychiatry by Deb, 1/e p281]

Indications pf ECT

- Depressive disorder: **MC Indication**
  - Acutely suicidal/homicidal
  - Stupor-Catatonia
  - Severe psychotic symptoms
  - Failed medication trial
  - Non-tolerance to medications (Pregnant women, Geriatric)
- Catatonia
- Manic episode
- Schizophrenia
- Post-partum psychosis
- Other indications: Neuroleptic malignant syndrome, Parkinson's disease, Intractable seizure disorder

20. Ans. (d) F3

[Ref. Essentials of Postgraduate Psychiatry by Murray, 3/e p61]

ICD-10 Chapter V

- F0: Organic, including symptomatic, mental disorders
- F1: Mental and behavioral disorders due to use of psychoactive substances
- F2: Schizophrenia, schizotypal and delusional disorders
- F3: Mood (affective) disorders
- F4: Neurotic, stress-related and somatoform disorders
- F5: Behavioural syndromes associated with physiological disturbances and physical factors
- F6: Disorders of personality and behavior in adult persons
- F7: Mental retardation
- F8: Disorders of psychological development
- F9: Behavioural and emotional disorders with onset usually occurring in childhood and adolescence
- In addition, a group of "unspecified mental disorders"

21. Ans. (b) Depression
[Ref. Depression by Roose, 1/e p108]

Guilt in Depression
- Feelings of pervasive, irrational guilt
- Despite feeling it is irrational, feeling of guilt persist
- Feeling of guilt is ruminative in nature

22. Ans. (a) Mood disturbance
[Ref. Psychiatric and Mental Health Nursing by Elder, 2/e p275]

- **Post-partum blues**: Transient disturbance in mood as normal response to stresses of child birth
  - Features: Labile mood, sadness, dysphoria, subjective confusion
  - Treatment: Self-resolving within days to weeks, Education of mother
- Post-partum depression: Occur within 12 weeks of delivery
  - Features: Depressed mood, excessive anxiety, insomnia, weight-change (may last months-years)
  - Treatment: Regular counselling, Education
- Post-partum psychosis: Rare psychotic disorder
  - Features: Mother's depression, delusions and thoughts of harming herself or child
  - Treatment: Hospitalization, Antipsychotics

23. Ans. (d) All of the above
[Ref. Massachusetts General Hospital Comprehensive Clinical Psychiatry, 2/e p610]

Modified Bush-Francis Catatonia Rating Scale
- 1 out of 14 signs for Diagnosis of Catatonia
- **14 signs**: Excitement, Immobility/ Stupor, Mutism, Staring, Cataplexy/ Posturing, Grimacing, Echopraxia/ Echolalia, Stereotypy, Mannerisms, Verbigeration, Rigidity, Negativism, Waxy flexibility, Withdrawal, Impulsivity, Automatic disobedience, Mitgehen, Gegenhalten, Ambitendency, Grasp reflex, Perseveration, Combativeness, Autonomic abnormality

24. Ans. (a) Double the dose of Anti-depressant medications
[Ref. Niraj Ahuja, 7/e p77]

Alternatives for Patients Refractory to Anti-depressant Medications
- Change of Anti-depressant Medication (Switch)
- Combination of two types of Anti-depressants
- Augmentation with Lithium
- Augmentation with T3 or T4
- Augmentation with Anti-psychotics
- Electroconvulsive therapy
- Use of Newer and Experimental techniques

25. Ans. (a) Lithium
[Ref. Niraj Ahuja, 7/e p78]

Treatment of Mania
- ***Lithium (Drug of choice for Mania)*** *has a lag period of 1-2 weeks before effect*: So it should not be used alone to manage emergency situations
- *Antipsychotics useful in ICUs and emergency situations*:
  - Olanzapine
  - Quetiapine
  - Risperidone
- *Other drugs useful in ICUs and emergency situations*:
  - Sodium valproate
  - Carbamazepine, Oxcarbazepine

26. Ans. (c) 1.0 mEq/L
[Ref. Niraj Ahuja, 7/e p78]

Blood Lithium Levels

Blood level	Significance
0.8–1.2 mEq/L	Therapeutic level
0.6–1.2 mEq/L	Prophylactic level
> 2.0 mEq/L	Toxic dose
> 4.0–4.5 mEq/L	Lethal dose

27. Ans. (a) Major depression
[Ref. Niraj Ahuja, 7/e p71]

Depressed Mood
- Sadness of mood
  - *Pervasive sadness*: Loss of interest/pleasure in all activities
  - *Persistent sadness*: Present throughout the day
- Non responsive to environmental stimuli
- Social withdrawal
- Nihilism
- Early morning insomnia
- Complete anhedonia (inability to experience pleasure) in severe depression

28. Ans. (a) Amphetamine
[Ref. Niraj Ahuja, 7/e p48]

- Amphetamine is a powerful CNS stimulant with peripheral sympathomimetic effects

29. Ans. (c) Phenytoin
[Ref. Niraj Ahuja, 7/e p78-79]

- *Drugs used in Bipolar disorders*:
  - **Lithium (Drug of choice)**
  - Antipsychotics
  - Sodium valproate
  - Carbamazepine, Oxcarbazepine
  - Benzodiazepines (Lorazepam, Clonazepam)
  - Lamotrigine
  - T3, T4

30. Ans. (a) Liver
[Ref. Niraj Ahuja, 7/e p190]

- *Side effects of Lithium therapy*:

Neurological	Renal
• Tremor **(MC side effect overall)** • Muscular weakness • Seizures • Cogwheel rigidity • Neurotoxicity	• Nephrotic syndrome • Nephrogenic diabetes insipidus • Polyuria • Polydipsia
Cardiovascular	**Gastrointestinal**
• T-wave depression	• Nausea, vomiting, diarrhoea, metallic taste

Contd...

Psychiatry

Contd...

Endocrinal	Dermatological
• Goitre, Hypothyroidism • Weight gain	• Acneiform/papular eruptions • Exacerbation of psoriasis
During pregnancy and lactation • Ebstein's anomaly	

Also Remember

- *Toxicity of Lithium is generally seen at level: > 2.0 mEq per litre*

31. Ans. (a) Serotonin
[Ref. Niraj Ahuja, 7/e p77]

32. Ans. (d) Patient often remits completely in between attack
[Ref. Kaplan & Sadock's Concise Textbook of Clinical Psychiatry, 3rd Ed., Pg 214]

33. Ans. (d) Endogenous depression
[Ref. Kaplan & Sadock's Concise Textbook of Clinical Psychiatry, 3rd Ed., Pg 214]

- *Endogenous depression*:
  - Biological basis with an identifiable underlying stress
  - Diurnal variation
  - Delusions
  - Psychomotor retardation
  - Loss of self-esteem
  - Early-morning awakening
  - Feeling of guilt

34. Ans. (c) Lithium
[Ref. Niraj Ahuja, 7/e p78]

35. Ans. (a) Gradual onset
[Ref. Niraj Ahuja, 7/e p74]

Prognostic Factors in Mood Disorders

Good prognostic factors	Poor prognostic factors
• Acute/abrupt onset • Typical clinical features • Severe depression • Well-adjusted premorbid personality • Good response to treatment	• Co-morbid medical/ personality disorder • Double depression • Stress • Marked hypochondriac features • Poor drug compliance

36. Ans. (a) Brain tumour
[Ref. Niraj Ahuja, 7/e p201]

Contraindications for ECT

- ***Absolute contraindications***:
  - **Raised intracranial tension**
- *Relative contraindications*:
  - Myocardial infarction
  - Severe hypertension
  - Cerebrovascular accident (CVA)
  - Severe pulmonary disease
  - Retinal detachment
  - Pheochromocytoma

37. Ans. (a) Intracranial S.O.L.
[Ref. Niraj Ahuja, 7/e p201]

38. Ans. (d) Carbamazepine
[Ref. Emedicine, Wikipedia]

Drugs Used in Status Epilepticus

- Benzodiazepines: Lorazepam **(Drug of choice)**, Diazepam
- Phenytoin/Fosphenytoin
- Sodium valproate
- Propofol (General anesthetic)
- Lidocaine
- Ketamine

39. Ans. (b) Masked depression
[Ref. Depression: Clinical, Experimental and Theoretical Aspects by AT Beck, 1st Ed., Pg 72]

Depressive Equivalents

- *Description*: Patients with somatic complaint but do not show apparent mood depression
- *Synonyms*: Incomplete depression, Latent depression, Atypical depression, Masked depression

40. Ans. (b) Heightened concentration
[Ref. Niraj Ahuja, 7/e p70]

Features of Mania

Elevated/expansive/ irritable mood	Speech and thought
• Stage I Euphoria: Increased sense of well-being, happiness • Stage II Elation: Feeling of confidence, enjoyment • Stage III Exaltation: Intense elation, Delusions of grandeur • Stage IV Ectasy: Intense sense of rapture/ blissfulness	• Excessive talking • Flight of ideas • Delusions of grandeur • Distractibility
Goal directed activity • Excessive planning • Execution of multiple activities • High risk activities	**Other features** • Decreased need for sleep • Absence of insight • Increased psychomotor activity

41. Ans. (a) Bipolar mania
[Ref. e-Study Guide for Companion to Psychiatric Studies, 1st Ed., Erotomania]

Erotomania

- *Description*: A type of delusional disorder in which an affected person believes that another person, usually a stranger or a famous person, is in love with him or her
- *Seen in Psychiatric disorders*: Schizophrenia, Bipolar mania

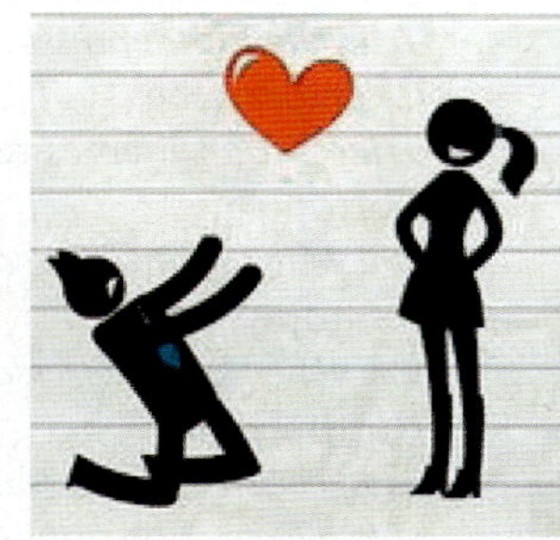

Fig. Erotomania

Psychiatry

42. Ans. (b) Depression with suicidal tendency
[Ref. Niraj Ahuja, 7/e p199]

Indications for ECT

- Severe depression with risk of suicide **(First and most important indication)**
- Severe depression with stupor, retardation, somatic features
- Severe refractory depression
- Delusional depression
- Side effects of therapy
- Severe catatonia
- Severe psychosis

43. Ans. (d) Lithium + Haloperidol
[Ref. Niraj Ahuja, 7/e p78]

- ***Lithium (Drug of choice for Mania)** has a lag period of 1–2 weeks before effect*: So it should not be used alone to manage emergency situations
  - Antipsychotics are used long with Lithium to cover first few weeks

44. Ans. (a) Bipolar disorder
[Ref. Niraj Ahuja, 7/e p78]

45. Ans. (b) Ebstein anomaly of tricuspid valve
[Ref. Niraj Ahuja, 7/e p190]

Side Effects of Lithium Therapy

Neurological	Renal	Endocrine
• Tremor (MC side effect) • Cog wheel rigidity • Seizures • Neurotoxicity • Muscular weakness	• Polyuria • Polydipsia • Nephrotic syndrome • Nephrogenic diabetes insipidus • Tubular changes	• Goitre • Hypothyroidism • Weight gain • Pedal edema • Abnormal thyroid function
Pregnancy/ Lactation	**Gastrointestinal**	**Other**
• Teratogenic • Ebstein's anomaly • Infant toxicity	• Metallic taste • Abdominal pain • Diarrhoea	• CVS: T-wave depression, Leukocytosis, AV block • Skin: Papular eruptions

46. Ans. (c) Doxepin
[Ref. Niraj Ahuja, 7/e p186-188 and KDT, 6/e p442]

Important Facts about Tricyclic Antidepressants

- *Tricyclic antidepressant with highest seizure precipitation*: Clomipramine
- *Tricyclic antidepressant with least seizure precipitation*: Nortriptyline
- *Tricyclic antidepressant with maximum hypotension*: Amitriptyline
- *Tricyclic antidepressant with minimum hypotension*: Nortriptyline
- *Tricyclic antidepressant with maximum antimuscarinic side effects*: Amitriptyline
- *Tricyclic antidepressant with minimum antimuscarinic side effects*: Amoxapine
- *Tricyclic antidepressant with maximum cardiotoxicity*: **Amitriptyline**
- *Tricyclic antidepressant with minimum cardiotoxicity*: **Doxepin**

47. Ans. (a) Li
[Ref. Niraj Ahuja, 7/e p188]

48. Ans. (d) Hypercalcaemia
[Ref. Niraj Ahuja, 7/e p190]

49. Ans. (a) Hypothyroidism
[Ref. Niraj Ahuja, 7/e p190]

50. Ans. (b) 2 weeks
[Ref. Manic Depressive Illness by Goodwin, 2/e p97]

DSM IV Definition of a Major Depressive Episode

- Criterion A1: At least 2 weeks period
- Criterion A2: Loss of interest or pleasure
- Criterion A3: Severe appetite changes
- Criterion A4: Insomnia is most common Sleep disturbance
- Criterion A5: Psychomotor changes including agitation or retardation

51. Ans. (a) Lithium
[Ref. Niraj Ahuja, 7/e p188]

52. Ans. (a) Renal failure
[Ref. Niraj Ahuja, 7/e p191]

Contraindications to Lithium Therapy

- Pregnancy (first trimester)
- Lactation
- Severe renal impairment
- Severe cardiac disease (Sick sinus syndrome, Cardiac failure)
- Sodium imbalance/hyponatremia (Addison's disease)
- Severe hypothyroidism

53. Ans. (d) Sodium valproate
[Ref. Key Topics in Psychiatry by Jones & Roberts, 1/e p67]

- *Treatment of Acute Manic Episode*:
  - Oral Antipsychotic drug or Valproate semi-sodium
  - Lithium can be used if immediate control, or overactive/dangerous behavior is not needed or otherwise be used in combination with an Antipsychotic

54. Ans. (d) Lethargy
[Ref. Niraj Ahuja, 7/e p69-71]

55. Ans. (a) 5-HT
[Ref. Niraj Ahuja, 7/e p74]

- *Biochemical theory in Mania*: Increased Norepinephrine, Increased 5-HT
- *Biochemical theory in Depression*: Decreased Norepinephrine, Decreased 5-HT function

56. Ans. (a) Beck
[Ref. Cognitive Therapy of Depression by AT Beck, Pg 10]

- *Beck's Cognitive Model of Depression*:
  - Cognitive triad: Negative views of himself, experiences and future
  - Schemas: Maintenance of self-defeating attitudes despite positive factors in life
  - Cognitive errors

57. Ans. (c) 90–120 volts, 0.3 second
[Ref. Niraj Ahuja, 7/e p202]

Dose in ECT Session
- Voltage: 90–150 volts (Average 110 volts)
- Duration: 0.1–1.0 seconds
- Current: 200–1600 mA

58. Ans. (c) Dysthymia
[Ref. Niraj Ahuja, 7/e p73, 82]

Dysthymia
- Description: Any mild depression which is not severe enough to be called as Depressive episode, lasting 2 years or more
- Occurrence:
  - More common in females
  - Average age of onset in Late 3rd decade
- Features:
  - Does not require stress as precipitating factor
  - No emphasis on presence of other neurotic symptoms

59. Ans. NONE (All are associated with Depression)
[Ref. Multiple Sources]

60. Ans. (a) Heightened affect
[Ref. Niraj Ahuja, 7/e p13, 28]

Mania
- *Definition of Mania*: Heightened sense of well-being, offset with extreme energy and optimism
- *Severity of manic episode*:

Stage	Type	Mood elevation	Characteristic feature
I	**Euphoria**	Mild	Increased sense of well-being
II	**Elation**	Moderate	Confidence, increased psychomotor activity
III	**Exaltation**	Severe	Delusions of grandeur
IV	**Ecstasy**	Very severe	Sense of rapture, blissfulness

Also Remember

- Depression and Mania are not affect disorders (which are short-lived emotional responses) BUT better called as mood disorders (sustained pervasive emotional responses)

61. Ans. (a) Endogenous depression; (b) Catatonic schizophrenia
[Ref. Niraj Ahuja, 7/e p199]

62. Ans. (c) Lithium toxicity
[Ref. Niraj Ahuja, 7/e p190 and KDT, 6/e 435]

63. Ans. (a) Noradrenaline; (b) Serotonin
[Ref. Niraj Ahuja, 7/e p74]

64. Ans. (d) Depressed mood
[Ref. Niraj Ahuja, 7/e p80]

Masked Depression
- Usually seen in adolescents
- *Clinical features*:
  - Depressive mood is NOT seen (hidden behind somatic symptoms)
  - Chronic body ache and pain
  - Insomnia
  - Atypical facial pain
  - Paraesthesias
  - GIT symptoms
  - Substance abuse
  - Multiple accidents
  - Eating disorders
- *Treatment*: Similar to depressive episode

65. Ans. (c) To prevent depression in bipolar disorders
[Ref. Niraj Ahuja, 7/e p188-189]
- Lithium is less useful in preventing depression Bipolar disorders
- Patients on Lithium often require Tricyclic antidepressant to prevent depressive relapses

66. Ans. (b) Lithium carbonate
[Ref. Niraj Ahuja, 7/e p78]
- Drug of choice for treatment and management of Bipolar disorders has been Lithium carbonate for many decades
- In recent years, good results have been achieved with Anti-convulsant drugs with a mood-stabilising effect with/without Lithium

67. Ans. (a) SSRIs
[Ref. Niraj Ahuja, 7/e p77]
- Because of their fewer side effects, SSRIs (along with SNRIs Selective Norepinephrine reuptake inhibitors) are often the treatment of choice for older adults and for individuals with moderate levels of depression.
- SSRIs also have a relatively lesser risk of high overdose
- SSRIs have become the drug of choice for childhood psychiatric conditions including major depressive disorder (MDD), obsessive compulsive disorder (OCD), and other anxiety disorders
- Venlafaxine and Duloxetine are associated with Hypertension; use them carefully in cardiac disease

68. Ans. (b) Hair loss
[Ref. 2009 Edition Delmar's Nurse's Drug Handbook, p1358]
- Side effects of Quetiapine include fever, weight gain, constipation, dry mouth, dyspepsia, hypotension, tachycardia, sudden cardiac death, Torsades de pointes, rhinitis, pharyngitis, sweating

69. Ans. (d) All of the above
[Ref. Ferri's Clinical Advisor 2001, p203]
- Depressed patient presents with psychomotor retardation with slowed thinking, slowed responses, slowed physical movements, depressed affect and mood, sleep disturbance, appetite disturbance

70. Ans. (b) Most common psychiatric disorder overall
[Ref. Niraj Ahuja, 7/e p89]
- Anxiety disorders overall are the most common type of psychiatric disorder in adults, with a 12-month prevalence of 13–19% and a lifetime prevalence of > 25%

71. Ans. (a) 2 years
[Ref. Niraj Ahuja, 7/e p73]
- Dysthymia is any mild depression which is not severe enough to be called as Depressive episode, lasting 2 years or more
- If symptoms consist of persistent instability of mood between mild depression and mild elation, the disorder is called as Cyclothymia

72. Ans. (c) Pheochromocytoma
[Ref. Developmental Disorders of the Brain by Rinehart, 2/e Table 10.2]

Endocrinal Abnormalities associated with Depression
- Hypothyroidism
- Hyperthyroidism
- Hyperparathyroidism
- Addison's disease
- Cushing's disease
- Hyperprolactinemia
- Porphyrias

73. Ans. (b) Hypomania and major depression
[Ref. Clinical Psychiatry by Castle, 2/e p135]
- Type I Bipolar disorder: Episodes of both Mania and Severe depression occur
- Type II Bipolar disorder: Episodes of Hypomania interspersed by separate and often severe episodes pf Depression

74. Ans. (a) Post-partum blues
[Ref. Psychiatric and Mental Health Nursing by Elder, 2/e p275]
- Post-partum blues is transient disturbance in mood as normal response to stresses of child birth; patient has labile mood, sadness, dysphoria, subjective confusion
- Post-partum depression usually occur within 12 weeks of delivery with depressed mood, excessive anxiety, insomnia, weight-change (may last months-years)
- Post-partum psychosis is a rare psychotic disorder with mother's depression, delusions and thoughts of harming herself or child

HIGH YIELD MCQs ANSWERS WITH EXPLANATIONS 

1. Ans. (c) Start antidepressant drug therapy
[Ref. Niraj Ahuja, 7/e p71]

2. Ans. (a) SSRIs are most efficacious among available drugs
[Ref. Niraj Ahuja, 7/e p77]

3. Ans. (c) Cotard's syndrome; (d) Depression
[Ref. Bipolar Depression: An Evidence-based Guide to Manic Depression by Fountoulakis, 1/e p67]

Cotard Syndrome
- Related to depressive mood
- Delusional belief that all bodyparts are rotten, decomposing or missing, or even dead
- World or everything related to it cease to exist

4. Ans. (d) Vagus
[Ref. The Therapist's Guide to Psychopharmacology by Edwards, Revised 1/e p272]
- *Nerve stimulation causing Mood elevation*: Vagus nerve

5. Ans. (a) Fluoxetine
[Ref. The Frith Prescribing Guidelines for People with Intellectual Disability, 1/e p176]

Drug of Choice in Depression

Patient group with Depression	Drug of choice
Reproductive age women	SSRI (Fluoxetine)
Pregnant women	Imipramine, Amitriptyline, SSRI (Fluoxetine)
Lactating women	Sertraline, Paroxetine, Nortriptyline, Imipramine
Older persons	SSRI (Fluoxetine, Paroxetine, Citalopram, Sertraline)
Down's syndrome	SSRI
Epilepsy	SSRI
Cardiovascular problems	SSRI
Renal impairment	Sertraline, Citalopram
Hepatic impairment	Imipramine, Paroxetine, Citalopram

6. Ans. (a) Imipramine; (c) Fluoxetine
[Ref. Value of Psychiatric Treatment, Volume 24, Number 4, Pg 465]

7. Ans. (d) Electroconvulsive therapy
[Ref. Niraj Ahuja, 7/e p199]

8. Ans. (b) Elated mood; (d) Delusion of grandiosity; (e) Distractibility
[Ref. Niraj Ahuja, 7/e p69-71]

9. Ans. (b) Middle age female
[Ref. Niraj Ahuja, 7/e p71]

10. Ans. (b) Disorientation
[Ref. Niraj Ahuja, 7/e p69-71]

11. Ans. (a) Mania
[Ref. Niraj Ahuja, 7/e p70]

12. Ans. (a) Endogenous depression; (b) Double depression
[Ref. Bipolar Depression: An Evidence-based Guide to Manic Depression by Fountoulakis, 1/e p67]

13. Ans. (a) Found in severe depression; (c) Mood incongruent psychotic feature

[Ref. Niraj Ahuja, 7/e p72]

- *Psychotic features in Depression*:
  - Found in 15–20% patients
  - Psychotic features: Delusions, hallucinations, stupor, grossly inappropriate behavior
  - Types of features:
    1. Mood congruent type: Nihilistic/guilt/poverty delusions
    2. Mood incongruent type: Delusions of control

14. Ans. (b) Endogenous depression; (d) Depression in involution

[Ref. Niraj Ahuja, 7/e p223]

Psychiatric Causes of Suicide

- Depression:
  - Major depression
  - Endogenous depression
  - Involution depression
  - Depression secondary to serious physical illness
  - Reactive depression secondary to life stressors
- Alcoholism and Drug dependence
- Schizophrenia

15. Ans. (d) Major depression and hypomania

[Ref. Niraj Ahuja, 7/e p73]

Subtypes of Bipolar Disorder

- Bipolar Disorder I: Episodes of Severe mania and Severe depression
- Bipolar Disorder II: Episodes of Hypomania and Severe Depression

16. Ans. (b) Manic Depressive Psychosis

[Ref. Niraj Ahuja, 7/e p73]

17. Ans. (e) Repetitive depression and hypomania

[Ref. Niraj Ahuja, 7/e p73]

18. Ans. (b) 0.7–1.1 mEq/L

[Ref. Niraj Ahuja, 7/e p78]

19. Ans. (a) Commonest side effect is tremor; (c) Amiloride is DOC for Li induced diabetes insipidus; (e) Tremor is treated with propranolol

[Ref. Niraj Ahuja, 7/e p190-191]

20. Ans. (b) Lithium; (c) Carbamazepine; (e) Sodium valproate

[Ref. Clinical Pharmacology and Rational Therapeutics by Rataboli, 2/e p149]

- *Drugs used for Prophylaxis of Bipolar disorder*: Lithium, Carbamazepine, Sodium valproate, Lamotrigine

21. Ans. (a) Haloperidol

[Ref. Clinical Pharmacology and Rational Therapeutics by Rataboli, 2/e p149]

22. Ans. (d) Recurrent manic depressive attacks

[Ref. Clinical Pharmacology and Rational Therapeutics by Rataboli, 2/e p149]

23. Ans. ALL CHOICES

[Ref. Clinical Pharmacology and Rational Therapeutics by Rataboli, 2/e p149]

24. Ans. (c) High self-esteem; (d) Loss of insight

[Ref. Niraj Ahuja, 7/e p70]

25. Ans. (d) Generalized Anxiety disorder

[Ref. Manual of Psychiatric Nursing Care Planning by Varcoralis, 4/e p619]

Uses of Lithium

Treatment	Prophylaxis
• Acute mania • Schizoaffective disorder • Cyclothymia • Acute depression • Chronic alcoholism • Impulsive aggression • Kleine Levin syndrome • Neutropenia • Premenstrual syndrome • Bulimia	• Bipolar mood disorder • Unipolar mood disorder • Vascular headache

26. Ans. (b) Lithium

[Ref. Niraj Ahuja, 7/e p78]

27. Ans. (b) Depression alone

[Ref. Niraj Ahuja, 7/e p73]

28. Ans. (d) Chlorpromazine

[Ref. Clinical Pharmacology and Rational Therapeutics by Rataboli, 2/e p149]

29. Ans. (c) Carbamazepine

[Ref. Clinical Pharmacology and Rational Therapeutics by Rataboli, 2/e p149]

30. Ans. (a) Commonly seen in females; (c) Associated with hypothyroidism; (d) Family history of major depression

[Ref. Clinical Pharmacology and Rational Therapeutics by Rataboli, 2/e p149]

31. Ans. (c) Brain derived growth factor

[Ref. Brain Stimulation in Psychiatry by Kellner, 1/e p8]

32. Ans. (b) Depression with suicidal tendency; (c) Catatonic schizophrenia

[Ref. Niraj Ahuja, 7/e p199-200]

33. Ans. (a) Chronic Schizophrenia

[Ref. Niraj Ahuja, 7/e p73]

34. Ans. (b) Tranylcypromine

[Ref. The Complete Guide to Psychiatric Treatment by Drummond, 1/e p271]

Hypertensive Crises following Tranylcypromine

- Drug intake: Antiasthmatics, Antidepressants, Antihypertensives, Antiparkinsonian drugs, Barbiturates, Buspirone, Carbamazepine, Disulfiram, Decongestants
- Food intake: Fermented foods, Cheese, Liver, Dried fruits

35. Ans. (a) MDP-Bipolar

[Ref. Niraj Ahuja, 7/e p78]

36. Ans. (c) Heart Block

[Ref. Niraj Ahuja, 7/e p190]

37. Ans. (b) 0.7–1.2 mEq/L
[Ref. Niraj Ahuja, 7/e p78]

38. Ans. (b) Depression
[Ref. Niraj Ahuja, 7/e p199]

39. Ans. (c) Depression with Suicidal Tendency
[Ref. Niraj Ahuja, 7/e p199]

40. Ans. (b) Retrograde Amnesia
[Ref. Gabbard's Treatment of Psychiatric Disorders, 4/e p453]

Complications of ECT

- Retrograde amnesia (Most common)
- Anterograde amnesia
- Delirium
- Acute confusional state
- Cognitive deficits
- Myalgia
- Headache
- CVS complications
- Cerebrovascular complications
- Regurgitation and aspiration
- Death (Rare)

41. Ans. (b) Anti MAOI action
[Ref. Pharmacology by Bhattacharya, 2/e p292]

42. Ans. (a) Glaucoma
[Ref. Pharmacology for Dentistry by Nayak, 2/e p6]

- *Tricyclic antidepressants are contraindicated in*: Glaucoma, Epilepsy, Ischaemic heart disease, Enlarged prostate

43. Ans. (a) Fluoxetine
[Ref. The Practicing Physician's Approach to Headache by Diamond & Dellesio, 6/e p66]

- *Non-sedative antidepressants*: Fluoxetine, Zolpidem, Sertraline, Venlafaxine, Bupropion

44. Ans. (b) Fluoxetine
[Ref. The Practicing Physician's Approach to Headache by Diamond & Dellesio, 6/e p66]

45. Ans. (a) Anhedonia
[Ref. Niraj Ahuja, 7/e p71]

46. Ans. (b) Seasonal Affective Disorder
[Ref. Seasonal Affective Disorder and Beyond by Lam, 1/e p167]

Uses of Bright Light Therapy

- Seasonal affective disorder
- Delayed sleep phase disorder
- Advanced sleep phase disorder
- Non-24-hour sleep wake rhythm
- Jet lag
- Shift work

47. Ans. (b) Chromosome 13; (c) Chromosome 18
[Ref. Neuroscience for Mental Health Physician by Pliskza, 1/e p203]

- *Chromosomes linked to Bipolar disorders*: 4, 12, 13, 18, 21, 22, X-chromosome

48. Ans. (b) Serotonin and Norepinephrine
[Ref. Niraj Ahuja, 7/e p74]

Neurotransmitters in Mood Disorders

- Mania: Dopamine (Increased), GABA (Decreased)
- Depression Norepinephrine (Decreased), Serotonin (Decreased), Dopamine (Decreased)

49. Ans. (d) Depression
[Ref. Kaplan & Sadock's Concise Textbook of Clinical Psychiatry, 10/e p548]

OTTO Veraguth Sign

- *Description*: Triangle-shaped skin fold running obliquely from lower outside to upper inside on upper eyelid
- *Seen in*: Depression

50. Ans. (b) Major depression
[Ref. Niraj Ahuja, 7/e p71]

51. Ans. (c) Third person hallucination
[Ref. Kaplan & Sadock's Concise Textbook of Clinical Psychiatry, 3/e p214]

52. Ans. (d) Childhood depression
[Ref. Depression and Suicide by Vedrinne, 1/e p249]

- Among child and adolescent psychiatric outpatients with a diagnosis of major depressive disorder, more than 70% reported suicidal ideation or attempts

53. Ans. (b) Major depression
[Ref. Niraj Ahuja, 7/e p71]

54. Ans. (b) Anti-depressants
[Ref. Niraj Ahuja, 7/e p71]

55. Ans. (b) Rule out depression
[Ref. Niraj Ahuja, 7/e p71]

56. Ans. (a) Involutional melancholia
[Ref. Niraj Ahuja, 7/e p80]

Involutional Melancholia

- Severe depression in Involutional period of life (40–65 years age)
- Marked agitation
- Psychotic features (Persecutory delusions, Auditory/tactile hallucinations)
- Somatic symptoms (Hypochondriacal delusions)

57. Ans. (b) Sertraline
[Ref. Niraj Ahuja, 7/e p77]

58. Ans. (a) Antipsychotic + Anti-depressant
[Ref. Niraj Ahuja, 7/e p77]

59. Ans. (d) ECT
[Ref. Niraj Ahuja, 7/e p199]

60. Ans. (c) Dysthymia
[Ref. Niraj Ahuja, 7/e p73, 82]

61. Ans. (d) Clouding of mania
[Ref. Niraj Ahuja, 7/e p70]

62. Ans. (c) Hyperactivity
[Ref. Niraj Ahuja, 7/e p70]

63. Ans. (c) Mania
[Ref. Niraj Ahuja, 7/e p70]

64. Ans. (a) Acute manic excitement
[Ref. Niraj Ahuja, 7/e p70]

65. Ans. (a) Lithium carbonate
[Ref. Niraj Ahuja, 7/e p78]

66. Ans. (b) Antidepressants and mood stabilizers
[Ref. Niraj Ahuja, 7/e p77]

67. Ans. (c) Sodium valproate
[Ref. Niraj Ahuja, 7/e p192]

68. Ans. (d) Haloperidol
[Ref. Niraj Ahuja, 7/e p78]

69. Ans. (b) Clozapine
[Ref. Surviving Manic Depression by Torrey, 1/e p180]
- *Uses of Clozapine*: Acute mania, Mixed states, Rapid cyclers, Depressed phase of MDP

70. Ans. (d) Akathisia
[Ref. Psychiatric Side-effects of Prescription and Over the Counter Medications by Brown, 1/e p1650]

Akathisia
- *Description*: Movement disorder characterized by inner restlessness, and compelling need to be in constant motion
- *Causes of Akathisia*:
  - Pontine disorders
  - Drugs induced:
    1. Antipsychotics: Haloperidol
    2. Anti-depressants: Venlafaxine
    3. SSRI: Fluoxetine

71. Ans. (c) Both
[Ref. Gabbard's Treatment of Psychiatric Disorders, 4/e p453]

72. Ans. (b) Few weeks to few months
[Ref. Niraj Ahuja, 7/e p203]

73. Ans. (b) Decreased
[Ref. Zone's Comprehensive Guide to PGMEE Volume 3, Pg 778]

74. Ans. (c) Raised Intracranial Tension
[Ref. Niraj Ahuja, 7/e p201]

75. Ans. (b) Anti cholinergic side effects
[Ref. Physical Rehabilitation by Sullivan, 6/e p1200]
- *Side effects of Amitriptyline*: Urinary retention, Constipation, Hypotension, Dry mouth, Dizziness, Tachycardia, Blurred vision, Impaired memory, Weight gain

76. Ans. (d) Pimozide
[Ref. Niraj Ahuja, 7/e p66]
- *Uses of Pimozide*: Schizophrenia, Delusional disorder, Motor tics, Tourette syndrome

77. Ans. (a) Imipramine is used in treatment of endogenous depression; (e) Codeine is an effective antitussive
[Ref. Niraj Ahuja, 7/e p77]

78. Ans. (a) Lithium toxicity
[Ref. Niraj Ahuja, 7/e p190]

79. Ans. (d) Delusional Depression
[Ref. Niraj Ahuja, 7/e p199]

80. Ans. (c) Acute Depression
[Ref. Niraj Ahuja, 7/e p199]

81. Ans. (c) Shortens duration
[Ref. Bipolar Disorder by Yatham, 2/e p414]

82. Ans. (a) Elevated mood; (c) Grandiosity; (d) Pressured speech
[Ref. Niraj Ahuja, 7/e p70]

83. Ans. (d) 2 years
[Ref. Niraj Ahuja, 7/e p73, 82]

84. Ans. (b) 5
[Ref. Niraj Ahuja, 7/e p190]

Lithium Levels Stabilization
- Steady state levels of Lithium are achieved: After 7 days of starting treatment
- If any change is made in Lithium dosage, next blood levels is estimated: After atleast 5–7 days of last change

85. Ans. (d) Insomnia
[Ref. Gerontological Nursing by Charlotte, 8/e p430]
- *Vegetative symptoms in Depression*: Insomnia, Fatigue, Anorexia, Weight loss, Constipation, Decreased interest in sex

86. Ans. (b) Haloperidol
[Ref. Management of Mood Disorders by McGrath, 1/e p214]

Treatment of Mania in 1st Trimester of Pregnancy
- Lithium is contraindicated: Can lead to Ebstein's anomaly
- Other drugs contraindicated: Sodium valproate, Lamotrigine, Carbamazepine
- Antipsychotics (especially Atypical antipsychotics) used as Drug of choice: Haloperidol, Trifluoperazine
- Other drugs recommended: Olanzapine, Quetiapine, Risperidone, Clozapine

87. Ans. (a) Psycho education
[Ref. Niraj Ahuja, 7/e p79-80]

Psychosocial Treatment in Mood Disorders
- *Cognitive behavior therapy*: Correction of depressive negative cognitions/ ideations
  - Useful in Mood disorders: Moderate Non-bipolar depression
- *Interpersonal therapy*: Attempts to recognize stressors/ precipitants for depression
  - Useful for Mood disorders: Mild-moderate Unipolar depression
- *Psychoanalytic psychotherapy*: Correction of personality itself
  - Useful in Mood disorders: Dysthymia, Depression with personality disorders, Depression with history of child loss/abuse
- *Behavior therapy*: Provide useful short-term modalities and adaptive techniques
  - Useful in Mood disorders: Mild-moderate depression
- *Group psychotherapy*: Method of Psychoeducation
  - Useful in Mood disorders: Recurrent depression, Bipolar depression

- *Family and Marital therapy*: Decrease intrafamilial/ interpersonal difficulties
  - Useful inMood disorders: Ensure continuity of treatment

88. Ans. (a) IV sodium bicarbonate

[Ref. Hospital Medical Clinics, Volume 3, Issue 1]

- **In the given question**, Altered sensorium and hypotension, ECG shows wide QRS complex and right axis deviation in a woman taking antidepressant medications indicate Tricyclic antidepressants toxicity
- Treatment: Serum alkalization therapy (IV Sodium bicarbonate)
- Dose: 1–2 mEq/ kg
- Target pH: 7.50–7.55
- Outcome monitoring indictors: Narrowing of QRS complex, Increase in Blood pressure

89. Ans. (a) Idea of guilt

[Ref. Depression in Children and Adolescents by Shafi, 1/e p200]

BECK's Cognitive Triad of Depression

- Negative views of self: Worthlessness
- Negative views of world: Helplessness
- Negative views of future: Hopelessness

90. Ans. (b) 4 gm

[Ref. Mental Health Nursing by Fletcher, 3/e p252]

- LITHIUM FATALITY:
  - Dose: 10–60 g
  - Blood level: 4–5 mEq/L

91. Ans. (b) Dysthymia

[Ref. Psychiatric Mental Health Nursing by Varcarolis, 3/e p202]

- Persistent depressive disorder (PDD)/ Dysthymia/Chronic depression is a less notably severe depression characterised by depressive symptoms present for atleast 2 years. It includes daytime fatigue/tiredness, chronic low depression/irritable mood, low self-esteem, negative thinking, difficulty in sleeping, hypersomnia, eating too much or too little **(Patient shows irritability, low self-esteem of not performing well in office since 3 years in the given question)**

Also Remember

- If the symptoms consist of persistent mild depression, the disorder is called as Dysthymia; and if symptoms consist of persistent instability of mood between mild depression and mild elation, the disorder is called as Cyclothymia
- Adjustment disorders: Often precipitated by one or more stressors, it usually represents a maladaptive response to the stressful life event(s). It is characterised by those disorders which occur within 1 month of a significant life change (stressor) with duration usually < 6 months.

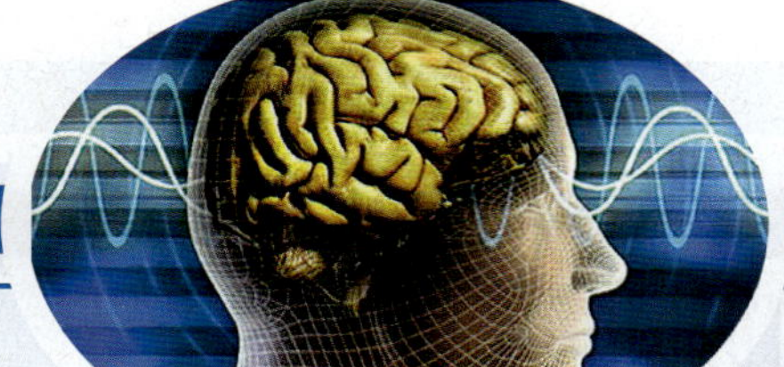

Chapter 7

Anxiety, Hysteria and Somatoform Disorders

THEORETICAL CONCEPTS

VII A. DISSOCIATIVE DISORDERS

- *Definition*: Are conditions that involve disruptions or breakdowns of memory, awareness, identity and/or perception.
- *Features of dissociative disorders*:
  - Disturbed consciousness, identity, memory
  - Sudden onset, abrupt recovery
  - Precipitating factor: Stress

VII A1. Depersonalisation Disorders

- *Definition*: **Alteration in self-perception with temporary loss of one's own reality**
- *Clinical presentation*:
  - Episodes of depersonalisation
  - Marked distress and anxiety
  - Insight present
  - Clear sensorium
  - Feeling of loss over action and speech
  - Sudden onset/termination of episodes
- *Treatment*:
  - Psychotherapy
  - Antidepressants

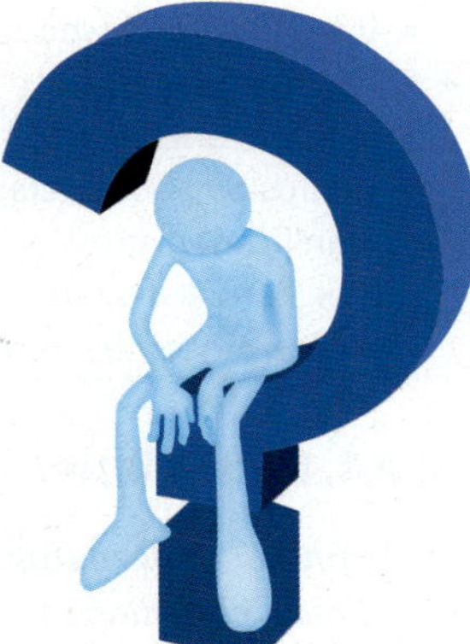

Fig. Depersonalisation

Topper's Edge

DSM-IV Diagnostic Criteria for Depersonalization Disorder

- Persistent/recurrent experiences of felling detached from one's mental process or body
- Reality testing remains intact during depersonalization experience
- Depersonalization causes clinical significant distress or impairment in social/occupational/other areas of functioning
- Depersonalization experience does not occur exclusively during course of another mental disorder, and is not due to direct physiological effects of a substance or a general medical condition

VII A2. Dissociative Amnesia

- *Definition*: **Extreme memory loss due to extensive psychological stress** (No neurobiological cause or damage found)
- *Clinical presentation*:
  - Sudden inability to recall important personal information
  - Usually follows traumatic/ stressful life situation
- *Types of dissociative amnesia*:

Type	Features of amnesia (inability to recall)
Circumscribed amnesia[Q]	All personal events during a circumscribed period of time
Selective amnesia	Few selective personal events during a period of time
Continuous amnesia	All personal events after stressful event till present time
Generalised amnesia	All personal of whole life

VII A3. Dissociative Fugue

- *Definition*: **Physical desertion of familiar surroundings with impaired recall**[Q]
- *Clinical presentation*:
  - Episodes of wandering away from home[Q]
  - Reversible amnesia for personal identity, memories during episode
  - May have establishment of new identity
  - Significant distress
  - Fugue duration varies (hours-months), rapid recovery

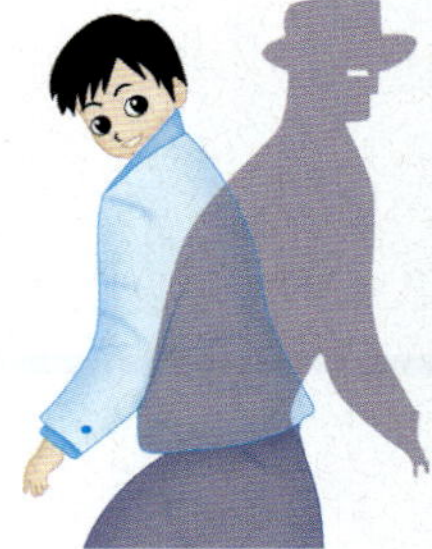

Fig. Dissociative fugue

Topper's Edge

Dissociative Fugue

- **Fugue state, Psychogenic fugue**[Q]:
  - A dissociative disorder
  - A rare psychiatric disorder characterized by reversible amnesia for personal identity, including the memories, personality, and other identifying characteristics of individuality
  - State is usually short-lived (ranging from hours to days), but can last months or longer
  - Dissociative fugue usually involves unplanned travel or wandering, and is sometimes accompanied by the establishment of a new identity
  - It is a facet of dissociative amnesia, according to DSM-5
- DSM-IV definition:
  - Sudden, unexpected travel away from home or one's customary place of work, with inability to recall one's past
  - Confusion about personal identity, or the assumption of a new identity
  - Significant distress or impairment
- Merck Manual definition: One or more episodes of amnesia in which the inability to recall some or all of one's past and either the loss of one's identity or the formation of a new identity occur with sudden, unexpected, purposeful travel away from home

VII A4. Dissociative Identity Disorder

- *Definition*: **Alternation of two or more personality states with impaired recall (due to stress, trauma, child-abuse)**[Q]
- *Clinical presentation*:
  - One personality manifests at one time
  - Amnestic barriers between personalities
  - Depression, memory loss, phobias
  - Multiple dissimilar mannerisms
  - Sudden onset and termination
- *Treatment*:
  - Psychotherapy
  - Behaviour therapy

VII A5. Other Dissociative Disorders

- *Trance and Possession disorders* ***(Possession hysteria)***: Control of person's personality by a spirit during episodes
  - Awareness of existence of possessor is present
- ***Ganser's syndrome*** *(Hysteria pseudodementia)*: Approximate answers ***(Vorbeireden)*** – wrong answers but person understands the nature of question[Q]
  - Commonly seen in prison inmates

VII B. PSYCHOTIC ILLNESSES WITH SOMATIC SYMPTOMS

- **Hypochondriasis**:
  - **Preoccupation with severe/incurable disease**[Q]
  - Misinterpretation of symptoms[Q]
  - Single symptom/illness
  - Doctor shopping
  - Unintentionally produced symptoms[Q]
- **Somatization Disorder**:
  - Multiple somatic symptoms (Pain, GIT manifestations, Sexual)[Q]
  - Unintentionally produced symptoms[Q]
- **Somatoform Pain Disorder**:
  - Pain at one/more sites is ONLY symptom
  - Unintentionally produced symptoms[Q]
- **Hysteria (Conversion disorder)**[Q]:
  - Functional loss (Anesthesia, Seizures, Motor paralysis, Blindness)[Q]
  - Unintentionally produced symptoms[Q]
- **Malingering**:
  - Intentional false/exaggerated physical symptoms[Q]
  - Recognizable motive[Q]
- **Munchausen syndrome/ Factitious disorder**:
  - Intentionally produced physical symptoms[Q]
  - Purpose to obtain medical attention[Q]
  - Multiple scars from earlier treatment[Q]
  - Request for multiple requested investigations[Q]
  - Doctor shopping[Q]

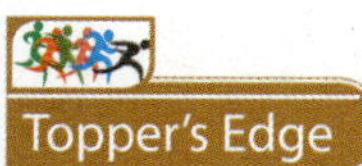

Topper's Edge

Hypochondriasis DSM-IV Diagnostic Criteria

- A. Preoccupation with fears of having, or the idea that one has, a serious disease based on misinterpretation of bodily symptoms
- B. Preoccupation persists despite medical evaluation and reassurance
- C. Belief in A is not delusional intensity (as in somatic delusional disorder), and not restricted to circumscribed appearance (as in body dysmorphic disorder)
- D. Preoccupation cause significant distress or impairment in social/occupation/other functioning
- E. Duration for disturbance is at least 6 months
- F. Preoccupation not accounted for by other psychiatry disorders

Hysteria in Psychiatry

- Hysterical neurosis: Described in ICD-10 under dissociative (conversion) disorder
- Hysterical symptoms: May be seen in depression, anxiety or may complicate organic disease
- Epidemic/Communicable/**Mass hysteria**[Q]: Widespread outbreak of particular hysterical or other symptoms—fainting, hyperventilation, emotional distress, abdominal pain usually seen in young girls in schools starting from a more influential person and spreading to others
- Hysterical/Histrionic personality disorder[Q]: Self-dramatization, exaggerated expression of emotions, easily affected by others, attention seeking attitude, seductiveness, over-concerned with physical attractiveness, egocentric & self-indulgence
- **St Louis Hysteria**[Q] **(Briquet's syndrome)**: Somatization disorder where patient has recurrent, unexplained medical symptoms commencing before age 30 years and are of chronic duration
- Hysterical psychosis/pseudopsychosis: Pseudo-delusions and pseudo-hallucinations seen suddenly after severe emotional stress, ending abruptly in few days
- **Anxiety hysteria: Phobic anxiety**[Q]

Topper's Edge

Malingering

- **Fabricating of symptoms of mental or physical disorders for a variety of "secondary gain" motives**, which may include financial compensation (often tied to fraud); avoiding school, work or military service; obtaining drugs; getting lighter criminal sentences; or simply to attract attention or sympathy
- Not considered a mental illness by many
- MC goals to attain:
  - Drugs
  - Shelter
  - Financial compensation
- Suspicious history:
  - Medicolegal issues
  - Discrepancy between claimed distress and objective findings
  - Antisocial personality disorder
- According to the DSM-V, malingering may be suspected[Q]:
  - When a patient is referred for examination by an attorney
  - When the onset of illness coincides with a large financial incentive, such as a new disability policy
  - When objective medical tests do not confirm the patient's complaints
  - When the patient does not cooperate with the diagnostic work-up or prescribed treatment
  - When the patient has antisocial attitudes and behaviours (antisocial personality)
  - When a patient who claims to be schizophrenic informs the physician about being confused and is eager to discuss the delusions
- Differential diagnosis:
  - Factitious disorder
  - Somatoform disorder
  - Dissociative disorders
  - True medical/psychiatric conditions

MUNCHAUSEN SYNDROME

Munchausen Syndrome

- **Hospital addiction syndrome[Q]**
- Refer to those fabricating an illness in order to receive medical attention **without secondary gain**
- A psychiatric factitious disorder wherein those affected feign disease, illness, or psychological trauma to draw attention, sympathy, or reassurance to themselves
- Fits within the subclass of factitious disorder with predominantly physical signs and symptoms, but patients also have a history of recurrent hospitalization, travelling, and dramatic, extremely improbable tales of their past experiences
- Common signs and symptoms: Recurrent life-threatening events, seizures, bleeding, poisoning, hypoglycemia or hyperglycemia, apnea, CNS depression, repeated infections, diarrhea and vomiting, rashes, fevers

Munchausen Syndrome by Proxy[Q]

- **Physical symptoms are intentionally produced in others, example by a mother in her child**
- Perpetrator has nursing experience
- MC methods used: Poisoning, suffocation
- Father is emotionally, if not physically, absent

IMAGE-BASED QUESTIONS

1. Instrument shown in Photograph is used for diagnosis of

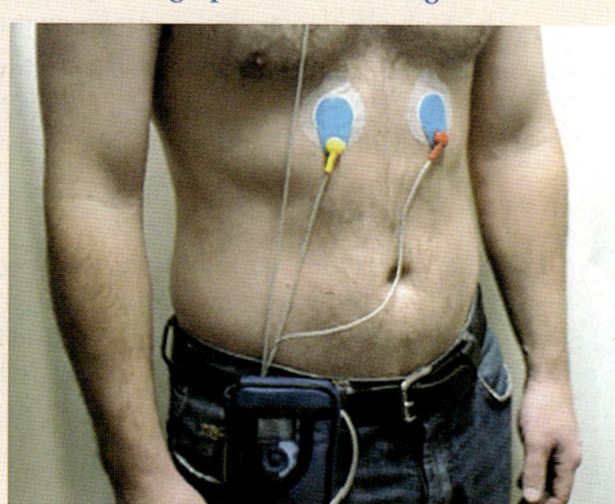

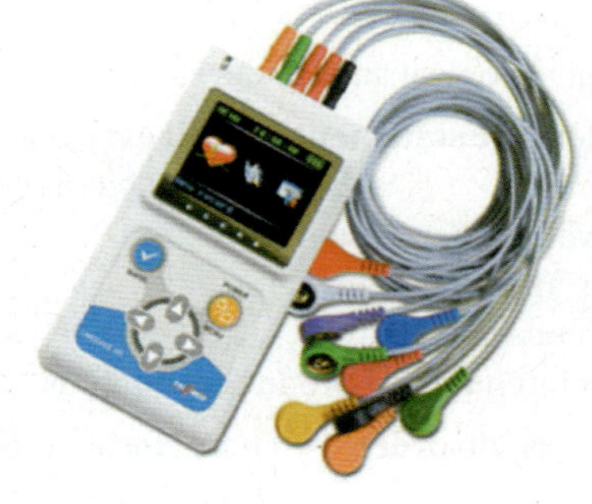

a. Seizures b. Panic disorder c. Sleep disorders d. Dementia

2. Identify syndrome as shown in Photograph

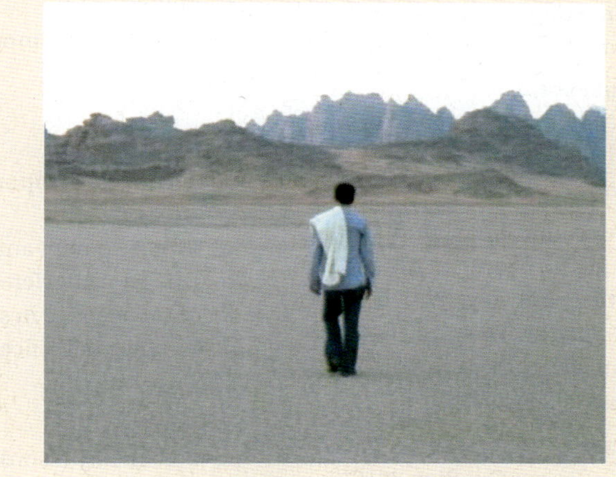

a. Ganser's Syndrome b. Cotard syndrome
c. Dissociative fugue d. Possession hysteria

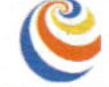

ANSWERS WITH EXPLANATIONS OF IBQs

1. Ans. (b) Panic disorder *[Ref. Anxiety Disease Research by Velotis, 1/e p86]*

Holter ECG

- Description: Portable device for continuously monitoring various electrical activity of the cardiovascular system for at least 24 hours
- Holter ECG use in Psychiatry: Used in Panic attacks to differentiate them for arrhythmias

2. Ans. (c) Dissociative fugue *[Ref. Niraj Ahuja, 7/e p101]*

- Dissociative Fugue: Physical desertion of familiar surroundings with impaired recall
- Clinical presentation: Episodes of wandering away from home, Reversible amnesia for personal identity, memories during episode, May have establishment of new identity, Significant distress, Fugue duration varies (hours-months), rapid recovery

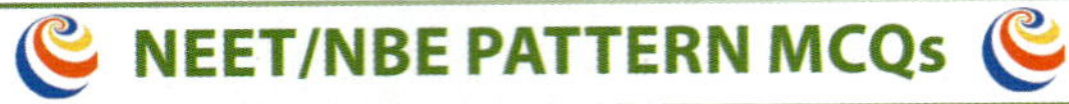

NEET/NBE PATTERN MCQs

1. **All are true regarding Post-traumatic stress disorder except** *[Recent Question 2016]*
   a. Symptoms develop immediately after the event
   b. Symptoms include insomnia, poor concentration
   c. Response to an exceptionally stressful or catastrophic stimuli.
   d. Anxiolytics are given only if anxiety develops.
2. **Conversion disorder true statements are all except** *[Recent Question 2016]*
   a. Autonomic nervous system involved
   b. There is primary and secondary gain
   c. La bella indifference is a feature
   d. Patient does not intentionally produce symptoms
3. **Post-traumatic stress disorder is characterized by all except** *[Recent Question 2016]*
   a. Flash back and night mare
   b. Severe traumatic injury
   c. Re-experiencing stressful events
   d. It does not develop after 6 months of stress
4. **Ganser syndrome is a** *[Recent Question 2016]*
   a. Dementia b. Malingering
   c. Dissociative disorder d. Personality disorder
5. **In Conversion disorder all are found except** *[Recent Question 2016]*
   a. Jealousy b. Paralysis
   c. Anaesthesia d. Abnormal gait
6. **A man with intermittent hiccups feels that he is about to die because he is suffering from gastric cancer. All his radiological investigations prove the contrary. Which is the most probable diagnosis?** *[Recent Question 2016]*
   a. Somatization disorder b. Hypochondriasis
   c. Conversion disorder d. Delusional disorder
7. **La belle indifference seen in all except** *[Recent Question 2016]*
   a. Conversion disorder b. Multiple sclerosis
   c. Parietal lobe lesion d. None of the above
8. **Drug of choice for Generalized anxiety disorder** *[Recent Questions 2016, 2017]*
   a. Alprazolam b. Buspirone
   c. Venlafaxine d. Beta-blockers
9. **Which of the following is not an anxiety reduction technique?** *[NBE FMGE September 2010]*
   a. Using anxiolytics
   b. Biofeedback techniques
   c. Implosion of flooding techniques
   d. Jacobson progressive relaxation
10. **Features of anxiety neurosis are following except** *[NBE DNB 1998, 2007]*
    a. Excessive sweating b. Palpitations
    c. Loss of consciousness d. Tremors
11. **Most common form of dissociation hysteria is** *[NBE DNB 1998]*
    a. Fugue b. Amnesia
    c. Multiple personality d. Somnambulism
12. **Anxiety neurosis is manifested by following, except** *[NBE DNB 1995, 2003, 2004]*
    a. Difficulty in breathing b. Tachycardia
    c. Hyperkinetic movements
    d. Warm hands
13. **A lady feels that her nose is very enlarged but nobody else is able to see that. She is not getting convinced by other people. She is most probably suffering from** *[NBE FMGE September 2012]*
    a. Anxiety disorder
    b. Obsessive compulsive disorder
    c. Body dysmorphic disorder
    d. Hypochondriacal disorder
14. **Derealization and Depersonalization seen in which type of disorder** *[Recent Question 2012, 2015]*
    a. Dissociative disorder b. Personality disorder
    c. Mania d. None
15. **Thyrotoxicosis is most commonly associated with** *[NBE DNB 1993]*
    a. Anxiety b. Paranoid states
    c. Mania d. Delirium
16. **Buspirone as compared to Benzodiazepines** *[NBE FMGE September 2008]*
    a. Is more potent anticonvulsant
    b. Does not interfere with GABAergic transmission
    c. More effective in severe anxiety with panic attacks
    d. Produces significantly more sedation
17. **Anxiety is** *[Recent Question 2012, 2015]*
    a. Neurosis b. Psychosis
    c. Personality disorder d. None
18. **Differentiation of hysterical fits from epileptic fit** *[NBE DNB 1995, 1999, 2001, 2004, 2006]*
    a. Occurs in sleep b. Injuries to person
    c. Incontinence
    d. Occurs when people are watching
19. **Which of the following is FALSE about SOMATIZATION Syndrome?** *[Recent Questions 2012, 2015]*
    a. Involves 2 sexual disturbance symptoms
    b. Two GI symptoms
    c. Four pain symptoms
    d. Multiple recurrent symptoms
20. **Dissociative fugue is characterised by** *[Recent Question 2015, NBE FMGE September 2012]*
    a. Wandering away from home
    b. Irreversible amnesia
    c. Gradual recovery
    d. Normal recall

21. A 44-years-old female disappeared from her residence without informing others. Before this she had no illness but had some unpleasant events in her personal life. Most probable diagnosis is *[NBE FMGE September 2008]*

a. Dementia
b. Dissociative dementia
c. Dissociative fugue
d. Adjustment problem

22. Hysteria is related mainly to body organ *[Recent Question 2015]*

a. Mind
b. Face
c. Eyes
d. Uterus

23. A 35 years old man gets up from sleep with sudden onset breathlessness, anxiety, palpitation, shaking hand, profuse sweating, discomfort in chest and fear of dying. There is history of similar episodes in past. Physical examination is normal. Probable diagnosis is *[Recent Question 2017]*

a. Panic attack
b. Anxiety disorder
c. Conversion disorder
d. Acute psychosis

24. Which of the following is not a Specific somatoform disorder? *[Recent Question 2017]*

a. Somatization disorder
b. Hypochondriasis
c. Conversion disorder
d. Irritable bowel syndrome

25. A group of 4 teenagers while going for a trip met a car accident. Out of four, 3 people died on the spot. Surviving girl was admitted in an ICU for 3 months. After being discharged she often gets up in night and feels terrified. She says that she sees same events in her dreams. She is now afraid of the cars. The diagnosis is? *[Recent Questions 2017, 2018]*

a. Anxiety disorder
b. Phobia
c. Conversion disorder
d. Post-traumatic stress disorder

26. A 25-year-old male c/o recurrent abdominal pain but biochemical assays and ultrasound abdomen is normal. He also complains of constant headache. He suddenly complains of loss of vision of bilateral eyes. Ophthalmologist finds nothing on examination. Symptoms are most probably due to *[Recent Question 2017]*

a. Bilateral optic neuritis
b. Posterior inferior cerebellar artery infarct
c. Malingering
d. Factitious disorder

27. Meena, a 42 years old divorced lady, lives with her mother. She has no significant past medical history, but she frequently makes appointments with her GP problems experienced by her. She complains of feeling 'stressed' all the time and constantly worries about 'anything and everything'. This is also affecting her performance at her work. She describes herself as always having been a 'worrier' but her anxiety has become much worse in the past 12 months since her mother became unwell, and she no longer feels that she can control these thoughts. When worried, she feels tension in her shoulders, stomach and legs, her heart races and sometimes she finds it difficult to breathe. Her sleep is poor with difficulty getting off to sleep due to worrying and frequent wakening. She feels tired and irritable. She does not drink any alcohol. Most likely diagnosis is? *[Recent Question 2017]*

a. Panic disorder
b. Generalized anxiety disorder
c. Depression
d. Conversion disorder

28. Generalized anxiety disorder is diagnosed when anxiety and worry continues for at least? *[Recent Question 2017]*

a. 2 months
b. 4 months
c. 6 months
d. 8 months

29. Hypochondriasis is? *[Recent Question 2017]*

a. Preoccupation with fear of a serious illness
b. Preoccupation with multiple symptoms
c. Maintaining sick role
d. Intentional production of false or exaggerated physical symptoms

30. A 40-year-old male presents with sudden onset breathlessness, anxiety, palpitation, hot flushes, dizziness and chest pain. He is afraid of dying. Physical examination is normal. ECG and X-ray are also normal. What is the diagnosis? *[Recent Question 2017]*

a. Panic attack
b. Anxiety disorder
c. Malingering
d. Acute psychosis

31. Functional somatoform disorder is? *[Recent Question 2017]*

a. Somatization disorder
b. Chronic fatigue syndrome
c. Hypochondriasis
d. Body dysmorphic disorder

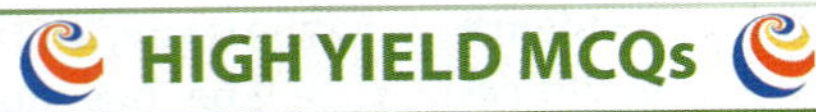

HIGH YIELD MCQs

1. **A 41-year-old presented to emergency with intense gharbharaat, palpitation, tremor, sweating and impending doom. All of the following can be done in emergency to rule out organic cause of anxiety except** *[AIIMS May 2016]*
   a. Haemoglobin b. Blood sugar levels
   c. T3, T4, TSH d. ECG
2. **An old lady survived a place hit by earthquake but lost her belongings and house. She now complains anxiety and constant fear but improved when provided help. Which of the following is correct?** *[AIIMS November 2016]*
   A: Condition is acute stress reaction
   B: She does not need to consult a Psychiatrist
   C: Fluoxetine is treatment of choice
   D: Projection is defence mechanism used
   a. A & C b. A, B & C
   c. A & D d. A, B, C & D
3. **Allodynia is** *[AIIMS PGMEE 1998]*
   a. Feeling pain without stimulus
   b. Feeling pain to a normal non painful stimulus
   c. Both
   d. None
4. **Hypochondriasis is** *[All India PGMEE 1994]*
   a. Normal pre-occupation with abnormal body function
   b. Abnormal pre-occupation with abnormal body function
   c. Normal pre-occupation with normal body function
   d. Abnormal pre-occupation with normal body function
5. **Hypochondriasis is** *[AIIMS PGMEE 1994]*
   a. Fear of fatal disease
   b. Too much concern of own health & misinterpretation of normal body function
   c. Marked mental and Physical fatigue
   d. Repeated hospitalization
6. **All are features of somatisation disorder except** *[JIPMER PGMEE 2003]*
   a. Frequently changing pain site
   b. Sexual symptoms
   c. Paresthesia
   d. Professional patients
7. **Male with symptoms mimicking heart disease with normal ECG & X-ray, the diagnosis is** *[All India PGMEE 2008]*
   a. Angina pectoris b. Panic attack
   c. ANS instability d. Vasovagal attack
8. **Post-traumatic stress syndrome is due to** *[All India PGMEE 1998, Recent Question 2017]*
   a. Head Injury
   b. CVD
   c. Minor Stress
   d. Major life threatening events
9. **Which of the following is NOT a clinical feature of post-traumatic stress disorder (PTSD)?** *[All India PGMEE 2008]*
   a. Flashbacks b. Hyperarousal
   c. Hallucinations d. Emotional numbing
10. **Post-traumatic stress disorder is associated with all except** *[PGI 2000]*
    a. Flash back
    b. Severe traumatic injury
    c. Re-experiencing stressful events
    d. Anhedonia
    e. It doesn't develop after 6 months of stress
11. **All are true for PTSD except** *[PGI 2002]*
    a. Hippocampus & amygdala
    b. Anhedonia
    c. Depression and guilt
    d. Insomnia & poor concentration
    e. Anxiolytic is treatment of choice
12. **True about post-traumatic stress disorder** *[PGI 2000]*
    a. Recall of traumatic events
    b. Associated with major trauma like pelvic fracture
    c. Treatment is ECT
    d. Disturbed sleep
13. **Two months after knowing that his son was suffering from leukemia, a 45-year-old father presents with sleep deprivation, lethargy, headache, and low mood. He interacts reasonably well with others, but has absented himself from work. The most probable diagnosis is** *[All India PGMEE 2008]*
    a. Depression b. Psychogenic headache
    c. Adjustment disorder d. Somatization disorder
14. **Psychosomatic illness can be differentiated from hysteria by** *[All India PGMEE 1994]*
    a. Altered sensorium b. Autonomic disturbance
    c. Involuntary movements d. Skeletal muscles atrophy
15. **All are Dissociative Disorders except** *[AIIMS PGMEE 1992, AIIMS PGMEE 1996]*
    a. Multiple personality b. Fugue
    c. Amnesia d. Deafness (Psychogenic)
16. **Following are included in Dissociative disorder** *[PGI 2000, PGI 2007]*
    a. Multiple personality disorder
    b. Fugue c. Hypochondriasis
    d. Somatisation disorder e. Obsession
17. **Regarding Ganser's syndrome true is** *[AIIMS PGMEE 1998]*
    a. Repeated lying b. Approximate answers
    c. Unconscious episodes d. Malingering
18. **A 45 years old Chandu is always preoccupied with feeling of illness. The diagnosis is** *[All India PGMEE 2000]*
    a. Somatoform disorder b. Hypochondriasis
    c. Munchausen syndrome d. Dissociative disorder
19. **A young 20 years old girl presents with complaints of pain in legs, intermittent vomiting, and headache since 2 months. Her physical examination was normal. What is the most possible diagnosis?** *[AIIMS PGMEE 2009]*
    a. Generalized anxiety disorder
    b. Conversion disorder
    c. Somatoform pain disorder
    d. Somatization disorder

20. La belle indifference is seen in *[AIIMS PGMEE 1998, Recent Question 2015]*
a. Conversion reaction
b. Schizophrenia
c. Mania
d. Depression

21. Hysteria is characterized by *[AIIMS PGMEE 1991]*
a. Flight of ideas
b. Pressure on speech
c. Indifference to suffering
d. Autistic thinking

22. Beta-blockers are indicated in *[AIIMS PGMEE 1995]*
a. Phobia
b. Schizophrenia
c. Anxiety
d. Mania

23. All are anxiolytic Except *[AIIMS PGMEE 1993]*
a. Buspirone
b. Fluoxetine
c. Diazepam
d. Nitrazepam

24. Maintaining sick role by any means is a characteristic feature of *[JIPMER PGMEE 2002, Maharashtra PGMEE 2004, Rohtak PGMEE 2002]*
a. Hypochondriasis
b. Somatization disorder
c. Conversion disorder
d. Factitious disorder

25. A patient says that he feels as if the people he meets are lifeless two dimensional card bord figure. He feels detached, emotionless, but highly unpleasant morbid experiences. Diagnosis is *[AIIMS PGMEE 2008]*
a. Delusional ideas
b. Hallucination
c. Depersonalization
d. Synthesia

26. A 28-year-old male admitted in the hospital with a history of vague pains. His examination revealed many scars of previous surgeries. He was very curious about knowing his diagnosis and was persistently asking for various diagnostic procedures and biopsy. He gave the past history of gall stone & appendicitis pain diagnosed by previous doctors, but the history regarding this was inappropriate and seemed to be manipulative. There were no previous records suggesting this diagnosis. The probable diagnosis is *[JIPMER PGMEE 2000, J & K PGMEE 2002, MAHE PGMEE 2003]*
a. Hypochondriasis
b. Somatization disorder
c. Conversion disorder
d. Factitious disorder

27. The difference between malingering and hysteria is *[All India PGMEE 1994]*
a. Hypnosis
b. Malingering has poor prognosis
c. Hysteria is more common in females
d. Conscious motive in malingering

28. A 41-year-old married female presented with headache for the last 6 months. She had several consultations. All her investigations were found to be within normal limits. She still insists that there is something wrong in her head and seeks another consultation. The most likely diagnosis is *[All India PGMEE 2003]*
a. Phobia
b. Psychogenic headache
c. Hypochondriasis
d. Depression

29. Person preoccupied by worries about ill health is *[Recent Question 2015, PGI 1998]*
a. Hypochondriac
b. Maniac
c. Depressed
d. Delirium

30. A 60-year-old man had undergone cardiac bypass surgery 2 days back. Now he started forgetting things and was not able to recall names and phone numbers of his relatives. What is the probable diagnosis? *[All India PGMEE 2010]*
a. Depression
b. Post-traumatic psychosis
c. Cognitive dysfunction
d. Alzheimer's disease

31. All are true except *[PGI 2008]*
a. Probabilistic learning is from past experiences
b. Implicit learning is procedural skill acquirement
c. Amnestic syndromes lose semantic memory
d. Implicit memory is declarative
e. Anterograde amnesia affects long term memory more

32. One of the following usually differentiates hysterical symptoms from Hypochondriacal symptoms *[All India PGMEE 2005]*
a. Symptoms do not normally reflect understandable physiological or pathological mechanism
b. Physical symptoms are prominent which are not explained by organic factors
c. Personality traits are significant
d. Symptoms run a chronic course

33. A 45-year-old male presents with history of headache, and vague body pains, off & on diarrhoea& constipation, Impotence and tingling and paresthesia in glove stocking pattern. The probable diagnosis is *[All India PGMEE 2000, JIPMER PGMEE 2002]*
a. Hypochondriasis
b. Somatization disorder
c. Conversion disorder
d. Factitious disorder

34. A 35-year-old male, with pre-morbid anxious traits & heavy smoker, believes that he has been suffering from 'lung carcinoma' for a year, No significant clinical finding is detected on examination and relevant investigation. He continues to stick to his belief despite evidence to the contrary. In the process, he has spent a huge amount of money, time and energy in getting himself unduly investigated. He is most likely suffering from *[AIIMS PGMEE 2004]*
a. Carcinoma lung
b. Hypochondriacal disorder
c. Delusional disorder
d. Malingering

35. All are true regarding somatization disorders except *[PGI 2000, JIPMER PGMEE 2004, TN PGMEE 2000]*
a. Maintain sick role
b. Pain symptoms
c. Sexual symptom
d. Pseudo neurological symptom

36. Not a diagnostic/ defining criteria for amnestic disorder *[PGI 2009]*
a. Visual hallucination
b. Transient delusion
c. Impaired concentration/attention
d. Good recall of recent events
e. Ability to form new memories

37. A 40-year-old male is admitted with complaints of abdominal pain and headache. General physical examination revealed six scars on the abdomen from previous surgeries. He seems to maintain a sick role and seeks attention from the nurses. He demands multiple diagnostic tests including a liver biopsy. The treating team failed to diagnose any major physical illness in the patient. His mental status examination did not reveal any major psychopathology.

One of the treating staff recognized him to have appeared in several other hospital with abdominal pain and some other vague complaints. He is most likely suffering from *[AIIMS PGMEE 2003]*

a. Schizophrenia b. Malingering
c. Somatisation disorder d. Factitious disorder

38. A female presented with history of episodes of altered sensorium, involuntary movements, memory deficits and headache since the last 6 months. 4 episodes occurred during the day and 2 during sleep. She has been married since 1 year. Most likely diagnosis is *[AIIMS PGMEE 2008]*

a. Epilepsy b. Somatization disorder
c. Somatoform disorder d. Hypochondriasis
e. Borderline personality

39. A 25-year-old lady presented with sadness, palpitation, loss of appetite and insomnia. There is no complaint of hopelessness, suicidal thoughts and there is no past history of any precipitating event. She is remarkably well in other areas of life. She is doing her office job normally and her social life is also normal. What is the probable diagnosis in this case? *[All India PGMEE 2010]*

a. GAD b. Mixed anxiety depression
c. Adjustment disorder d. Mild depressive episode

40. Baby 20-year-old female complains of sudden onset palpitation and apprehension. She is sweating for last 10 minutes and fears of impending death. Diagnosis is

a. Hysteria *[All India PGMEE 2001]*
b. Generalized anxiety disorder
c. Cystic fibrosis
d. Panic attack

41. A patient presented in casualty with a history of sudden palpitation, sensation of impending doom and constriction in his chest. This lasted for about 10-15 minutes after which he became all right. The diagnosis is likely to be *[AIIMS PGMEE 2001]*

a. Phobia
b. Personality disorder
c. Generalized anxiety disorder
d. Panic attack

42. A person missing from home is found wandering purposefully. He is well groomed and denies of having any amnesia. Most likely diagnosis is *[All India PGMEE 2001]*

a. Dementia b. Dissociative amnesia
c. Dissociative fugue d. Schizophrenia

43. MS. B, a 27-year-old nurse had extracurricular interest in trekking and painting. She broke up relationship with her boyfriend. Two months later she lost interest in her hobbies and was convinced that she would not be able to work again. She thought life was not worth living and has consumed 6 tablets of phenobarbitone to end her life. She is most likely suffering from *[All India PGMEE 2004]*

a. Adjustment disorder
b. Acute stress disorder
c. Depressive disorder
d. Post-traumatic stress disorder [PTSD]

44. All are true for conversion reaction except

a. Secondary gain *[AIIMS PGMEE 1998]*
b. Onset in late age
c. Patient does not consciously produce symptoms
d. Relation with stress

45. Lalu Prasad 45 years old male presents to OPD with complaining the continuous non-progressive headache from last 7 days. He believes that he has brain tumor for that there he is consulting many neurologists in past even all of investigation have been within normal limits. Patient requested for other investigation to reveal that he has brain tumor. Psychiatric evaluation shows the disease on the background of normal investigation. The most probable diagnosis is *[All India PGMEE 2002]*

a. Hypochondriasis
b. Somatization disorder
c. Somatoform pain disorder
d. Conversion disorder

46. An 18-year-old boy came to the Psychiatry OPD with a complaint of feeling changed from inside. He described himself as feeling strange as if he is different from his normal self. He was very tense and anxious yet could not point out the precise change in him. This phenomena is best called as *[All India PGMEE 2005]*

a. Delusional mood b. Depersonalization
c. Autochthonous delusion d. Over valued idea

47. All are true about Ganser's syndrome except *[PGI 1999, JIPMER PGMEE 2000, UP PGMEE 2000]*

a. Approximate answer
b. Apparent clouding of consciousness
c. Only found in prisoners
d. Hallucinations

48. A 20 years old girl Nelu enjoys wearing male clothes. Wearing male clothes gives her feeling of more confidence and after these episodes she is an absolutely normal girl. The likely diagnosis is *[AIIMS PGMEE 1997]*

a. Transsexualism b. Fetishism
c. Dual role transvestism d. Fetishistic transvestism

49. Uncertainty and excessive sense of responsibility is seen in *[AIIMS PG May 2015]*

a. OCD b. Depression
c. Personality disorder d. Generalized anxiety disorder

50. Expression and consequent release of previously repressed emotion is called as *[Recent Question 2018]*

a. Abreaction b. Hypnosis
c. Free association d. Dissociation

 NEET/NBE PATTERN MCQs ANSWERS WITH EXPLANATIONS

1. **Ans. (a) Symptoms develop immediately after the event**
   [Ref. Niraj Ahuja, 7/e p112]
   - **Post-Traumatic Stress Disorder (PTSD)** is a delayed/protracted response to an exceptionally stressful/catastrophic life event/situation
   - Occurs after a period of latency, within 6 months generally
   - More common in individuals with past history of psychiatric illness

2. **Ans. (a) Autonomic nervous system involved**
   [Ref. Niraj Ahuja, 7/e p99]
   - There are usually two types of disturbances in Conversion disorder: Voluntary motor and sensory
   - Autonomic nervous system is typically not involved, except when voluntary musculature is involved, e.g. vomiting, globus hystericus

3. **Ans. (d) It does not develop after 6 months of stress**
   [Ref. Niraj Ahuja, 7/e p112]

4. **Ans. (c) Dissociative disorder**
   [Ref. Kaplan & Sadock's, 10/e p681]

   Ganser syndrome (GS)
   - GS and Multiplex personality disorder are classified under Other dissociative disorders
   - Hysteria pseudodementia
   - Approximate answers (Vorbeireden): Wrong answers but person understands the nature of question
   - Psychogenic physical symptoms, Hallucinations, Apparent clouding of consciousness
   - Commonly seen in prison inmates

5. **Ans. (a) Jealousy**
   [Ref. Kaplan & Sadock's, 10/e p642]

   Conversion disorder
   - Anesthesia and paresthesia are common, especially of the extremities
   - All sensory modalities may be involved
   - Motor symptoms: Abnormal movements, gait disturbance, weakness, and paralysis
   - MC symptoms: Paralysis, Blindness, Mutism

6. **Ans. (b) Hypochondriasis**
   [Ref. Niraj Ahuja, 7/e p105-106]

   Hypochondriasis
   - Preoccupation with severe/incurable disease
   - Misinterpretation of symptoms
   - Single symptom/ illness
   - Doctor shopping
   - Unintentionally produced symptoms

7. **Ans. (d) None of the above**
   [Ref. Principles of Clinical Psychiatry by Ludwig, 1/e p86]

   La bella indifference
   - A condition in which the person is unconcerned with symptoms caused by a conversion disorder
   - Inappropriate lack of emotion or concern for the perceptions by others of one's disability
   - Seen in disorders:
     - Conversion disorder
     - Multiple sclerosis
     - Parietal lobe lesion

8. **Ans. (a) Alprazolam**
   [Ref. Kaplan & Sadock, 3/e p267]
   - Benzodiazepines have been the drugs of choice for generalized anxiety disorder

9. **Ans. (c) Implosion of flooding techniques**
   [Ref. Niraj Ahuja, 7/e p91-92]

   Treatment of Anxiety Disorders
   - Psychotherapy
   - Relaxation techniques
     - Jacobson's progressive relaxation technique
     - Yoga
     - Pranayama
     - Self-hypnosis
     - Meditation
   - Other behaviour therapies
     - Biofeedback
     - Hyperventilation control
   - Drug treatment
     - **Benzodiazepines** (**Drug of choice** for generalised anxiety)
     - Antidepressants (Drug of choice for panic disorder)
     - Propanolol, Atenolol (for anticipatory anxiety)
     - Buspirone

10. **Ans. (c) Loss of consciousness**
    [Ref. Niraj Ahuja, 7/e p90]

    Symptoms of Anxiety

    Physical symptoms
    - *Motor*: Tremors, Restlessness, Muscle twitch, Hyperkinetic movements
    - *Autonomic & Visceral*: Palpitations, Sweating, Tachycardia, Flushes, Dyspnoea, Hyperventilation, Diarrhoea, Mydriasis

    Psychological symptoms
    - *Cognitive*: Distractibility, Poor concentration, Hyperarousal
    - *Perceptual*: Derealization, Depersonalization
    - *Affective*: Apprehension, Fearfulness, Irritability, Feeling of impending doom
    - *Others*: Insomnia, Startle response

11. **Ans. (b) Amnesia**
    [Ref. Modern Synopsis of Comprehensive Book of Psychiatry by Kaplan, 1e p373 and Ref. Niraj Ahuja, 7/e p100]
    - *MC type of Dissociative disorder*: Dissociative amnesia
    - *MC subtype of Dissociative amnesia*: Circumscribed amnesia

12. **Ans. (d) Warm hands**
    [Ref. Niraj Ahuja, 7/e p90]

13. Ans. (c) Body dysmorphic disorder

Body Dysmorphic Disorder

- *Description*: Preoccupation with an imagined defect in appearance that causes significant impairment/ distress in important areas of functioning
  - *MC locations of imagined defect*: Hair (Most common), Nose, Skin, Eyes, Head, Face
  - *Common age of onset*: Adolescence

14. Ans. (a) Dissociative disorder

[Ref. Niraj Ahuja, 7/e p90]

15. Ans. (a) Anxiety

[Neuropsychiatry and Behavioural Neurosciences by Hales, 5/e p813]

16. Ans. (b) Does not interfere with GABAergic transmission

[Ref. Niraj Ahuja, 7/e p197]

Buspirone

- *Type of drug*: Non-benzodiazepine, anti-anxiety drug
- *Mechanism of action*:
  - 5-HT_1 partial agonist
  - Selective DA autoreceptor antagonist
- *Properties*:
  - Non-sedative
  - No anticonvulsant action
  - No muscle relaxant action
  - No addiction/ dependence/ tolerance
- *Dose*: 15-30 mg per day
- *Uses*: Generalised anxiety disorders
- *Side effects*: Dizziness, lightheadedness, headache, diarrhoea
- *Contraindications*:
  - MAO inhibitors use
  - Asthma
  - Diabetes
  - Epilepsy
  - Myocardial infarction
  - Myasthenia gravis

17. Ans. (a) Neurosis

[Ref. Handbook of Childhood and Adolescent OPD Treatment and Community Psychiatry by Ghuman, 1/e p153]

Types of Neurosis

- Anxiety neurosis
- Hysterical neurosis
- Phobic neurosis
- Obsessive compulsive neurosis
- Depressive neurosis
- Neurasthenic neurosis
- Depersonalization neurosis
- Hypochondriacal neurosis

18. Ans. (d) Occurs when people are watching

[Ref. Seminars in General Adult Psychiatry by Stein & Wilkinson, 2/e p385 and Ref. Niraj Ahuja, 7/e p101]

Hysterical Fits vs Epileptic Fits

	Hysterical fits	Epileptic fits
Color	Normal, flushed or pale	Cyanosis or Pallor
Occurrence in sleep	Never	May occur
Occurrence when alone	Never	May occur
Movements	Thrashing type with trunk	Tonic-clonic
Injury and tongue biting	Rare	May occur
Corneal reflex	Retained	Absent
Urinary incontinence	Rare	Common
Amnesia	Partial	Complete
Neurological signs	Absent	Present
Post-ictal confusion	Absent	Present
Duration	Prolonged (20–800 seconds)	Short (30–70 seconds)
Occur when people watching	Common	Rare
Place of occurrence	Indoors at safe places	Anywhere

19. Ans. (a) Involves 2 sexual disturbance Symptoms

[Ref. Clinical Guide to Diagnosis and Treatment of Mental Disorders by Tasman, 2/e p385]

DSM-IV Criteria of Somatization Syndrome

- History of physical symptoms beginning before age of 30 years
- Each of the following criteria:
  - Four pain symptoms
  - Two GIT symptoms
  - One sexual symptom
  - One pseudo-neurological symptom
- Either of the following:
  - B cannot be explained by Medical condition or Substance abuse
  - Physical complaints in excess of related general condition
- Symptoms not intentionally produced or feigned

20. Ans. (a) Wandering away from home

[Ref. Niraj Ahuja, 7/e p101]

- *Dissociative fugue*: Wandering away from home

21. Ans. (c) Dissociative fugue

[Ref. Niraj Ahuja, 7/e p101]

Dissociative Fugue

- *Definition*: Physical desertion of familiar surroundings with impaired recall
- *Clinical presentation*:
  - Episodes of wandering away from home

- Reversible amnesia for personal identity, memories during episode
- May have establishment of new identity
- Significant distress
- Fugue duration varies (hours-months), rapid recovery

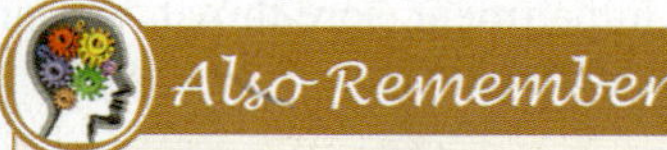

- *Dementia*: Chronic mental disorder with impaired memory, impaired intellectual functions and deterioration of personality
  - Consciousness, orientation, attention, sleep-wake cycle are normal
- *Dissociative dementia*: Dementia due to emotional trauma/ fugue/ cerebral injury
  - Unconsciousness, unconcerned to situations
- *Adjustment disorder*: Maladaptive response to stressful life events within one month
  - Depressive or mixed depressive-anxiety with disturbed emotions and conduct

22. Ans. (a) Mind

[Ref. Medical Bases of Psychiatry by Claytori, 3/e p188]

- *Hysteria is defined as*: Unmanageable emotional excesses
- *Modern concept of Hysteria*: Chronic disorder in which patients have medically-unexplained somatic complaints in all body systems due to 'Psychological disaggregation'
  - Multiple body pains
  - GIT symptoms
  - Sexual/ reproductive symptoms
  - Pseudoneurological problems
- *Neurophysiological basis of Hysteria*: Corticofugal inhibition of afferent stimulation at Reticular activation system (RAS)

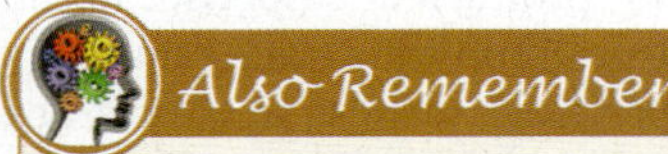

- *Older (now Disproved) concept of Hysteria*: A wandering uterus cause pains in different parts of body

23. Ans. (a) Panic attack

[Ref. Niraj Ahuja, 7/e p90]

Panic Disorder

- Discrete episodes of acute anxiety
- Episode: Sudden in onset, lasts for a few minutes and is characterised by very severe anxiety; symptoms begin unexpectedly ('out-of-the-blue' symptoms)
- Recurrence every few days
- Onset: Early third decade, with a chronic course; 2-3 times more often in females
- No apparent precipitating factor (or sometimes Phobias)
- Life time prevalence of panic disorder: 1.5-2.0 %

24. Ans. (d) Irritable bowel syndrome

[Ref. Shorter Oxford Textbook of Psychiatry, 6/e p394]

- **Somatoform disorders** under DSM-IV include Somatization disorder, Undifferentiated somatoform disorder, Hypochondriasis, Conversion disorder, Pain disorder with psychological factors, Body dysmorphic disorder

25. Ans. (d) Post-traumatic stress disorder

[Ref. Niraj Ahuja, 7/e p112]

- **Post-Traumatic Stress Disorder** is a delayed/ protracted response to an exceptionally stressful/ catastrophic life event/situation, generally occurs after a period of latency, within 6 months generally
- Characterised by recurrent, intrusive collections of stressful event (Flashbacks of same events in dreams, as **in the given question**), marked avoidance of event/ situations that may arouse recollection (victim afraid of cars **in the given question**) anxiety, increased arousal, partial amnesia, numbness, anhedonia, detachment

26. Ans. (d) Factitious disorder

[Ref. Niraj Ahuja, 7/e p119]

- **Factitious Disorder (Munchausen Syndrome)** patients repeatedly simulate or fake diseases with a sole purpose of obtaining medical attention and no other recognizable motive
- Predominant physical signs and symptoms (recurrent abdominal pain **in the given question**), Pseudologica fantastica (distort clinical histories, laboratory test reports), Grid-iron abdomen (evidence of earlier treatment including surgical procedures)
- Treatment is generally unsuccessful and prognosis is poor

27. Ans. (b) Generalized anxiety disorder

[Ref. Niraj Ahuja, 7/e p90]

Characteristics of Generalised Anxiety Disorder (GAD)

- Excessive anxiety/worry over last 6 months (Constant worrying **as in the given question)**
- Associated with (three of more of) restlessness, easy fatigability, difficulty in concentration, irritability, muscle tension, sleep disturbance (Poor sleep **as in the given question**)
- Clinically significant distress in social, occupational functioning (affecting her performance at work **as in the given question**)

28. Ans. (c) 6 months

[Ref. Niraj Ahuja, 7/e p90]

- Generalised Anxiety Disorder has an insidious onset in 3rd decade, stable, usually chronic course with/without episodes of acute anxiety
- Symptoms of anxiety should last for > 6 months for a diagnosis

29. Ans. (a) Preoccupation with fear of a serious illness

[Ref. Niraj Ahuja, 7/e p105]

- Hypochondriasis is characterised by > 6 months of a general and non-delusional preoccupation with fears/idea of having a serious disease based on the person's misinterpretation of bodily symptoms
- Lead to significant distress and impairment in life
- Poor insight

30. Ans. (a) Panic attack

[Ref. Niraj Ahuja, 7/e p247]

Panic Attack

- An acute, intense, overwhelming episode of anxiety which is often associated with feelings of impending doom
- Sudden onset of a discrete, brief period of intense discomfort, anxiety, or fear accompanied by somatic and/ or cognitive symptoms

31. Ans. (b) Chronic fatigue syndrome
[Ref. Treating Somatization by Woolfolk, 1/e p26]

- **Functional somatic syndrome:** Groups of co-occurring symptoms medically unexplained. Polysymptomatic functional somatic syndromes frequently encountered by both mental health and primary care practitioners include
  - Irritable bowel syndrome (IBS)
  - Chronic fatigue syndrome (CFS)
  - Fibromyalgia
- CFS is characterized by unexplained fatigue, lasting at least 6 months, that causes substantial reduction in activities; associated with memory impairment, sore throat, tender lymph nodes, muscle pain, joint pain, etc.

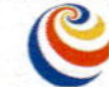 HIGH YIELD MCQs ANSWERS WITH EXPLANATIONS 

1. Ans. (a) Haemoglobin
[Ref. Kaplan & Sadock, 10/e p593]

Organic causes of Anxiety simulating Panic attacks
- Hypo- and hyperthyroid states
- Hyperparathyroidism
- Pheochromocytoma
- Episodic hypoglycaemia with insulinoma
- Arrhythmias
- Asthma

2. Ans. (a) A & C
[Ref. Niraj Ahuja, 7/e p111-112]

Acute Stress Reaction (ASR)
- Immediate and clear temporal relationship between an exceptional stressor (death of a loved one/accident/natural catastrophe) and onset of symptoms
- Disorder is likely to develop in presence of physical exhaustion and extremes of age
- More common in females
- Symptoms resolve rapidly within hours-days
- Treatment:
  - Removal of patients from stressful environment
  - SSRIs are the DOC for ASR as well as PTSD

3. Ans. (b) Feeling pain to a normal non painful stimulus
[Ref. Campbell's Psychiatric Dictionary, 2009, Pg 40]
- ***Allodynia***: Feeling pain to a normally non painful stimulus
- ***Algophobia***: Abnormal fear of pain
- ***Algolagnia***: Psychosexual disorder in which physical/mental pain is an essential part, it may be active (Sadism) or passive (Masochism)

4. Ans. (d) Abnormal preoccupation with normal body function
[Ref. Niraj Ahuja, 7/e p105]
- ***Hypochondriasis***: Persistent preoccupation with fear/belief of having one or more serious disease, based on person's own interpretation of normal body function (or a minor physical abnormality)

5. Ans. (b) Too much concern of own health & misinterpretation of normal body function
[Ref. Niraj Ahuja, 7/e p101]

6. Ans. (d) Professional patients
[Ref. Clinical Guide to Diagnosis and Treatment of Mental Disorders by Tasman, 2/e p385]

7. Ans. (b) Panic attack
[Ref. Psychiatric Nursing: Contemporary Practice by Boyd, 3/e p378]

Panic Attack
- *Description*: Sudden, discrete periods of intense fear or discomfort that are accompanied by significant physical and cognitive symptoms
- *Clinical presentation*:
  - Physical symptoms: Palpitations, chest discomfort, dizziness, discomfort, sweating, trembling, shaking
  - Cognitive symptoms: Disorganized thinking, irrational fears, depersonalization, decreased ability to communicate
  - Fear of death: Mimic heart attack
  - Peak at 10 minutes, Lasts upto 30 minutes

8. Ans. (d) Major Life threatening events
[Ref. Niraj Ahuja, 7/e p112]

Post Traumatic Stress Disorder (PTSD)
- *Description*: Delayed and protracted response to an exceptionally stressful or catastrophic life event/ situation, which is likely to cause pervasive distress in almost any person
- *System involved*: Amygdala-Hippocampus
- *Features of PTSD*:
  - Recurrent and intrusive recollections of stressful event, either in Flash-backs or dreams
  - Associated sense of re-experiencing of stressful event
  - Marked avoidance of events/situations that arouse recollections of stressful event
  - Marked anxiety, Hyperarousal
  - Depression and guilt
  - Partial amnesia, feeling of numbness, anhedonia
- *Treatment*:
  - Prevention: Anticipation of disasters in risk areas
  - Disaster management with good speed of providing practical help
  - Supportive psychotherapy
  - Cognitive behavior therapy
  - Drug therapy: Antidepressants, Anxiolytics (Benzodiazepines)

9. Ans. (c) Hallucinations
[Ref. Niraj Ahuja, 7/e p112]

10. Ans. (e) It doesn't develop after 6 months of stress
[Ref. Niraj Ahuja, 7/e p112]

11. Ans. (e) Anxiolytic is treatment of choice
[Ref. Niraj Ahuja, 7/e p112]

12. Ans. (a) Recall of traumatic events; (b) Associated with major trauma like pelvic fracture; (d) Disturbed sleep
[Ref. Niraj Ahuja, 7/e p112]

13. Ans. (c) Adjustment disorder
[Ref. Niraj Ahuja, 7/e p112]

Adjustment Disorder

- *Description*: A maladaptive response to stressful life event(s)
- *Clinical features*:
  - Usually occur within 1 month of stressor
  - Occur in those vulnerable to poor coping skills or personality factors
  - Duration: Generally less than 6 months
  - Recovery: Within 3 months
- *Treatment*:
  - Supportive psychotherapy (Treatment of choice)
  - Crisis intervention
  - Stress management training, Coping skills training
  - Drug therapy: Antidepressants, Anxiolytics (Benzodiazepines)

14. Ans. (b) Autonomic disturbance
[Ref. Clinical Psychology of Ageing by Seigler, 1/e p190]

Signs of Psychosomatic Illness (vs Hysteria/ Hypochondriasis)

- Involvement of Autonomic nervous system
- Failure of disorder to reduce anxiety
- Evidence of physiologic origin of symptoms
- Definitive somatic threat resulting from structural change

15. Ans. (d) Deafness (Psychogenic)
[Ref. Niraj Ahuja, 7/e p100-102]

Types of Dissociative Disorders

- Dissociative amnesia
- Dissociative fugue
- Multiple personality (Dissociative identity) disorder
- Trance and Possession disorder (Possession hysteria)
- Depersonalization disorder
- Dissociative stupor
- Ganser's syndrome (Hysterical pseudodementia)

16. Ans. (a) Multiple personality disorder; (b) Fugue
[Ref. Niraj Ahuja, 7/e p100-102]

17. Ans. (b) Approximate answers
[Ref. Niraj Ahuja, 7/e p102]

- ***Ganser's syndrome***: Hysterical pseudo-dementia
- Found in prison inmates mostly
- Psychogenic physical symptoms
- Hallucinations
- Apparent clouding of consciousness
- *Vorbeireden*: Approximate answers (Wrong answers though person understands the question)

18. Ans. (b) Hypochondriasis
[Ref. Niraj Ahuja, 7/e p105]

19. Ans. (c) Somatoform pain disorder
[Ref. Somatization Disorder in the Medical Setting by Robert Smith, 1/e p41]

- ***Somatoform pain disorder***: Preoccupation with pain in absence of adequate physical findings that could account for pain or its intensity
- *Central focus*: Pain
  [Somatization disorder has multiple symptoms with predominant chest pain]

20. Ans. (a) Conversion reaction
[Ref. Niraj Ahuja, 7/e p103]

- *La-belle indifference*: Lack of concern towards symptoms, despite apparent severity of disability produced
- *Seen in*:
  - Dissociative (Conversion) disorder
  - Physical illnesses

21. Ans. (c) Indifference to suffering
[Ref. Niraj Ahuja, 7/e p103]

22. Ans. (c) Anxiety
[Ref. Niraj Ahuja, 7/e p92]

Treatment of Anxiety

- Psychotherapy
- Relaxation techniques
- Other behavior therapy techniques:
  - Biofeedback
  - Hyperventilation control
- Drug treatment:
  - Benzodiazepines (Drug of choice): Alprazolam, Clonazepam, Diazepam, Nitrazepam
  - Beta blockers (For anticipatory anxiety): Propranolol, Atenolol
  - Buspirone (No dependence potential)

23. Ans. (b) Fluoxetine
[Ref. Niraj Ahuja, 7/e p92]

24. Ans. (d) Factitious disorder
[Ref. Niraj Ahuja, 7/e p119]

Factitious Disorder/ Munchausen Syndrome

- *Description*: Patients repeatedly simulate or fake diseases
  - Sole purpose of obtaining medical attention
  - No recognizable motive
- *Features*:
  - Predominant physical signs and symptoms
  - *Pseudologica fantastica*: Patients distort clinical histories, laboratory test reports
  - *Grid-iron abdomen*: Evidence of earlier treatment including surgical procedures
- *Treatment*: Unsuccessful
- *Prognosis*: Poor

25. Ans. (c) Depersonalization
[Ref. Niraj Ahuja, 7/e p108]

Depersonalization (Depersonlization-Derealization Syndrome)

- *Description*: Alteration in the perception or experience of self. So that the feeling of one's own reality is temporarily changed or lost

- *Features*:
  - *As if phenomenon*: Person affected in not delusionally convinced about change, but describes it to have occurred, as if
  - *Often accompanied by De-realization*: Alteration in perception/ experience of external world, so that feeling of reality of external world is temporarily lost/ changed

26. Ans. (d) Factitious disorder
[Ref. Niraj Ahuja, 7/e p119]

27. Ans. (d) Conscious motive in malingering
[Ref. Psychiatry in Law by Slovenko, 2/e p364]

- Major difference between Hysteria and Malingering is of 'Degree'
  - *Malingering*: Conscious imitation of illness
    1. Deliberate and persistent planning
    2. Exaggerating physical/mental symptoms
    3. Inconsistent with single disorder
    4. Seen only when person is being observed
  - *Hysteria*: Unconscious simulation of illness
    1. Conscious mind is apartner
    2. Mental/physical symptoms develop subconsciously

28. Ans. (c) Hypochondriasis
[Ref. Niraj Ahuja, 7/e p105]

29. Ans. (a) Hypochondriac
[Ref. Niraj Ahuja, 7/e p105]

30. Ans. (c) Cognitive dysfunction
[Ref. Handbook of Medical Neuropsychology by Morrow, 1/e p86]

- Both short and long term cognitive changes have been observed in patients of CABG

31. Ans. (c) Amnestic syndromes lose semantic memory; (d) Implicit memory is declarative; (e) Anterograde amnesia affects long term memory more
[Ref. Optimizing Cognitive Rehabilitation: Effective Instructional Methods by Turkstra, 1/e p8]

Types of Memory

- *Declarative/Explicit memory*: Information held with conscious awareness
  - *Episodic memory*: Storage of events that are tagged in time and place
  - *Semantic memory*: Storage of facts and concepts
  - *Metamemory*: Awareness of one's own memory functioning
  - *Prospective memory*: Remembering to initiate future intentions
- *Non-declarative/ Implicit memory*: Does not require conscious awareness of learning
  - *Procedural memory*: Acquisition of rules, sequences and perceptual motor skills
  - *Emotional associations*: Association of feelings with people and events
  - *Priming*: Increased probability of producing a response because of having produced it previously

32. Ans. (a) Symptoms do not normally reflect understandable physiological or pathological mechanism
[Ref. Comprehensive Handbook of Psychopathology by Adams & Sutker, 3/e p234]

Hypochondriasis vs Hysteria

- ***Hypochondriasis***:
  - Attention focused and locked onto symptoms
  - Exaggerated concern for symptoms
  - Spend most time looking for relief
- ***Hysteria***:
  - Separation or dissociation of attention from symptoms
  - Lack of concern for symptoms
  - No motivation to seek symptom relief

33. Ans. (b) Somatization disorder
[Ref. Kaplan and Sadock's Synopsis of Psychiatry, 10/e p634]

Somatization Disorder

- *Description*: Illness of multiple somatic complaints in multiple organ systems that occur over a period of several years and result in significant impairment/ treatment seeking
- *Characteristic feature*: Multiplicity of complaints and organs involved
- *Occurrence*: Women of lower socioeconomic status
- *Common associations*: Major depression, Personality disorders, Substance use disorders, Generalized anxiety disorders, Phobias

34. Ans. (b) Hypochondriacal disorder
[Ref. Niraj Ahuja, 7/e p105]

35. Ans. (a) Maintain sick role
[Ref. Clinical Guide to Diagnosis and Treatment of Mental Disorders by Tasman, 2/e p385]

36. Ans. (a) Visual hallucination; (b) Transient delusion; (c) Impaired concentration/attention; (e) Ability to form new memories
[Ref. Addiction Medicine: Science and Practice by Johnson, Volume 1, Pg 106]

ICD-10 Revision Criteria for Amnestic Syndrome

- Memory impairment as shown in impairment of recent memory and learning of new material, disturbance of time sense
- Absence of defect in recent recall, impairment of consciousness or generalized cognitive impairment
- History of objective evidence of chronic use of alcohol/ drugs, includes Korsakoff psychosis/syndrome, induced by alcohol or other psychoactive substance

37. Ans. (d) Factitious disorder
[Ref. Niraj Ahuja, 7/e p119]

38. Ans. (a) Epilepsy
[Ref. Niraj Ahuja, 7/e p28]

39. Ans. (a) GAD
[Ref. Niraj Ahuja, 7/e p90]

Generalised Anxiety Disorder

- MC Psychiatric disorder in population
- One year prevalence 2.5–8%
- Insidious onset in 3rd decade of life
- Chronic course with or without repeated panic attacks
- Symptoms last for 6 months

40. Ans. (d) Panic attack
[Ref. Psychiatric Nursing: Contemporary Practice by Boyd, 3/e p378]

41. Ans. (d) Panic attack
[Ref. Psychiatric Nursing: Contemporary Practice by Boyd, 3/e p378]

42. Ans. (c) Dissociative fugue
[Ref. Niraj Ahuja, 7/e p101]

43. Ans. (a) Adjustment disorder
[Ref. Niraj Ahuja, 7/e p112]

44. Ans. (b) Onset in late age
[Ref. Niraj Ahuja, 7/e p99]

Conversion Disorder

- Sudden onset
- Age affected: Late childhood to early adulthood
- No intention to produce symptoms
- Significant psychosocial stressor(s)
- Symptoms or deficits affecting sensory/motor function, suggesting a medical or neurological disorder
- Secondary gain usually present
- No physical abnormality

45. Ans. (a) Hypochondriasis
[Ref. Niraj Ahuja, 7/e p105]

46. Ans. (b) Depersonalization
[Ref. Niraj Ahuja, 7/e p108]

47. Ans. (c) Only found in prisoners
[Ref. Shorter Oxford Textbook of Psychiatry by Cowen, Harrison & Burns, 6/e p404]

48. Ans. (c) Dual role Transvestism
[Ref. Forensic and Medico-legal Aspects of Sexual Crimes and Unusual Sexual Practices by Aggarwal, 1/e p74]

Transvestism

- *Description*: Unusual sexual behavior where patient derives sexual gratification by wearing clothes usually worn by opposite sex
- *Major types of Transvestism*:

	Fetishistic Transvestism	Dual-role Transvestism
Type of disorder	**Sexual preference disorder**	**Gender identity disorder**
Sexual arousal	High intensity	None or low intensity
Post-orgasm/ decline of arousal	Desire to remove clothing	No such event sequence
Cross-dressing setting	In secret/ closed room	Go out publicly

49. Ans. (d) Generalized anxiety disorder
[Ref. Anxiety by Rachman, 3/e p190]

Unusual Features of Generalized Anxiety Disorder (GAD)

- Maladaptive cognitions
- Unadaptive safety behavior
- Intolerance of uncertainty
- Post-event processing
- Inflated sense of responsibility
- Negative imaging

50. Ans. (a) Abreaction
[Ref. Niraj Ahuja, 7/e p104]

Abreaction

- An emotional release or discharge after recalling a painful experience that has been repressed because it was consciously intolerable
  - Bringing to the conscious awareness, thoughts, affects and memories for the first time.
- A therapeutic effect sometimes occurs through partial discharge or desensitization of the painful emotions and increased insight
  - Once the conflicts have become conscious and their affects (emotions) have been released, the conversion or dissociative symptom disappears
- This may be achieved by hypnosis, free association or Intravenous Thiopentone or Diazepam

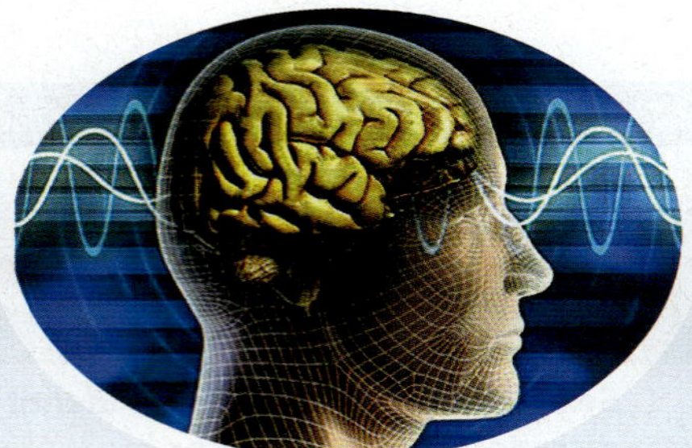

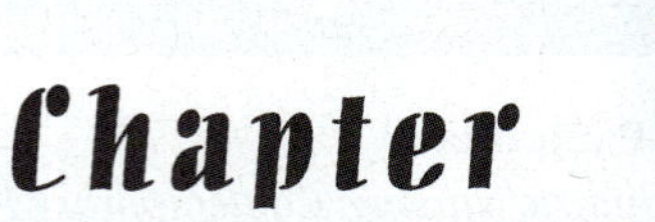

Chapter 8

Delirium and Dementia

THEORETICAL CONCEPTS

VIII A. DELIRIUM

- *Definition*: Delirium (***'acute confusional state'***) is a neuropsychiatric syndrome with core features of acute onset and fluctuating course, attention deficits and generalized severe disorganization of behaviour
- *Causes of delirium*: **[Mnemonic: D**elirium **IS DEMON[Q]]**
  - **D**rugs – Ingestion or withdrawal (Alcohol, Sedatives, Hypnotics, Tricyclic antidepressants, Anticonvulsants, L-dopa, Opiates, Salicylates, Steroids, Penicillin, Insulin, Digitalis, Antihypertensives, Quinidine, Amphetamine, Cocaine, LSD[Q])
    - Poisons: Heavy metals, Mushrooms, Datura, Carbon monoxide, Refrigerants, Solvents)
  - **I**ntracranial causes (Epilepsy, Head injury, Migraine, Stroke, Meningitis, Cerebral malaria)
  - **S**ystemic infections (Endocarditits, Pneumonia)
  - **O**thers (Postoperative state, Sleep deprivation, Heat, Radiation)
  - **M**etabolic (Hypoxia, Hyperglycemia, CO_2 narcosis, Electrolyte imbalance, Anemia, Porphyria)
  - **E**ndocrine (Hypo- and Hyper- pituitarism, thyroidism, parathyroidism, adrenalism)
  - **N**utritional deficiencies (vitamin B1, B3, B6, B9, B12)
- *Clinical presentation*:
  - Acute onset
  - Clouding of consciousness
  - Disorientation (firstly in Time, then place, then finally in person)
  - Hallucinations, illusions, misinterpretations
  - Disturbed sleep-wake cycle
  - **Impaired attention (Hall mark)**
  - Motor symptoms:
    - **Asterixis (flapping tremor[Q])**
    - Carphologia/ flocculation (picking movements at clothes)
    - Myoclonus, reflex abnormalities
  - ***Delirium tremens***: (Shaking frenzy/Spirit fingers[Q])
    - *Definition*: **Most severe alcohol withdrawal syndrome[Q]**
    - *Occurrence*: Within 2-4 days of complete/significant abstinence[Q]
    - *Clinical presentation*: Autonomic disturbances, Hallucinations, Insomnia, Dehydration, Clouding of consciousness, Agitation
    - *Mortality*: 5% (with treatment) – 35% (without treatment)
    - ***Drug of choice*: Benzodiazepines[Q]**
- *Treatment*:
  - Symptomatic (as per the underlying cause)
  - Benzodiazepines (Lorazepam, Diazepam)
  - Anti-psychotics (Haloperidol, Olanzapine)

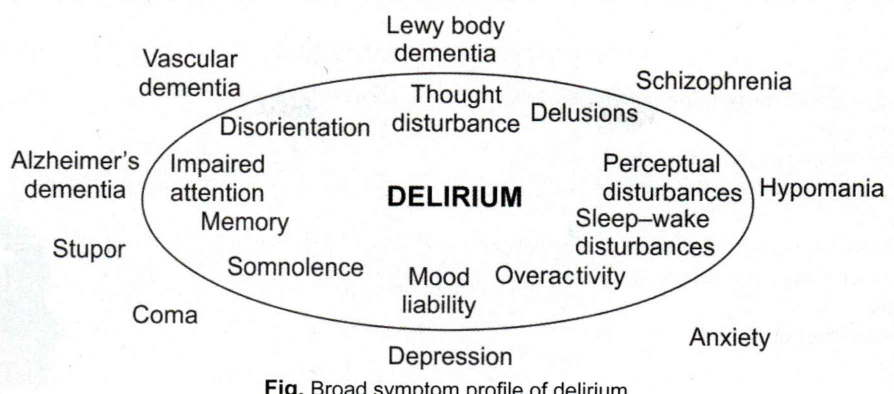

Fig. Broad symptom profile of delirium

VIII B. ALZHEIMER'S DEMENTIA

- Description: Slowly progressive cortical dementia with early memory impairment, alter progressing to disturbances in reasoning, perception, planning and language
- Importance: MC cause of Dementia[Q]
- Epidemiology:

Environmental risk factors	Genetic risk factors
• **Old age** (Most important[Q]) • Lower education rauma • Head rauma • Depression • Diabetes, Hypertension, Stroke	• Family history • Presenilin-1 mutation (Chr 14) • Presenilin-2 mutation[Q] (Chr 1) • Amyloid precursor protein mutation[Q] (Chr 21) • Apo-E gene[Q] (Chr 19) • Ubiquitin-1 gene (Chr 9) • Down's syndrome[Q]
Pathology	**Neurotransmitters involved[Q]**
• **Widening of sulci[Q]** • **Atrophy of gyri[Q]** • Ventricular enlargement • Senile plaques[Q] • **Neurofibrillary tangles[Q]**	• **Decreased Choline acetyltransferase** • **Decreased acetylcholine[Q]** • **Decreased norepinephrine[Q]** • Decreased Somatostatin • Decreased Corticotropin
Protective factors	**Clinical presentation**
• ApoE2 • NSAIDs • Hypolipidemic drugs • Hormone replacement therapy • Physical activity • Cognitive activity	• Presents in 5th-6th decade[Q] • Short term memory impairment (Initially[Q]) • Long term memory impairment (Later[Q]) • **Aphasia[Q], Apraxia[Q], Impaired judgement[Q]** • Visual hallucinations • **Delusions[Q]** (Persecutory, Reference) • **Depression[Q], Anxiety**

- Treatment:
  - Cholinergic activators: Tacrine[Q], Donezepil[Q], Rivastigmine[Q], Galantamine
  - NDMA (Glutamate) antagonist: Memanite
  - Antioxidants: Vitamin E

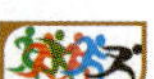

Topper's Edge

ALZHEIMER'S DISEASE

Stages of Alzheimer's Disease

- Effects of ageing on memory but not AD:
  - Forgetting things occasionally
  - Misplacing items sometimes
  - Minor short-term memory loss
  - Not remembering exact details

Contd...

Contd...

- Early stage Alzheimer's:
  - Not remembering episodes of forgetfulness
  - Forgets names of family or friends
  - Changes may only be noticed by close friends or relatives
  - Some confusion in situations outside the familiar
- Middle stage Alzheimer's:
  - Greater difficulty remembering recently learned information
  - Deepening confusion in many circumstances
  - Problems with sleep
  - Trouble knowing where they are
- Late stage Alzheimer's:
  - Poor ability to think
  - Problems speaking
  - Repeats same conversations
  - More abusive, anxious, or paranoid

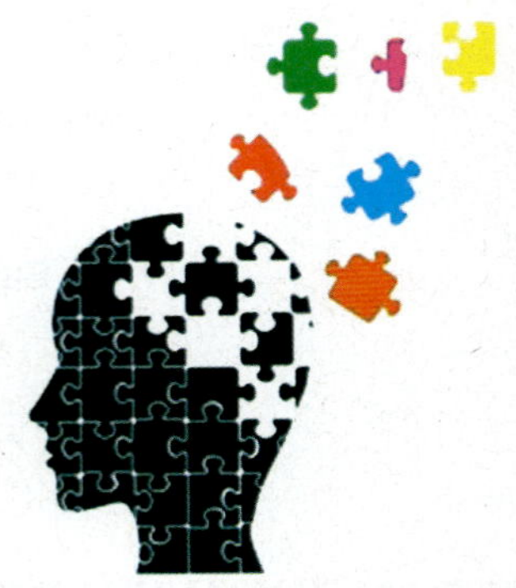

Fig. Alzheimer's dementia

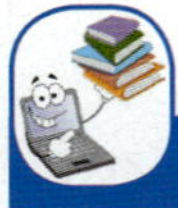

IMAGE-BASED QUESTIONS

1. Psychiatrist shown in Photograph coined the term

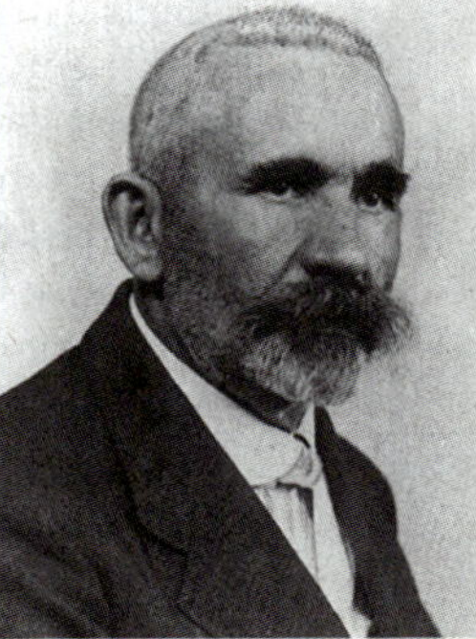

a. Psychiatry
b. Dementia praecox
c. Psychoanalysis
d. Free principle

ANSWERS WITH EXPLANATIONS OF IBQs

1. Ans. (b) Dementia praecox *[Ref. Niraj Ahuja, 7/e p54]*

- Scientist shown in the Photograph: Emil Kraepelin

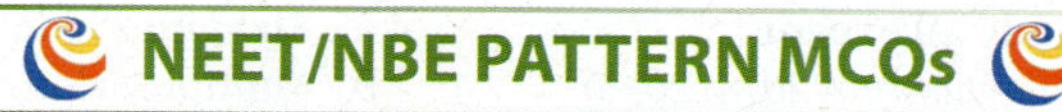

NEET/NBE PATTERN MCQs

1. **Delirium is most commonly seen in** *[Recent Question 2016]*
   a. Alcohol b. Barbiturate
   c. Opium d. Cocaine

2. **Delirium is defined as** *[Recent Question 2016]*
   a. Acute onset of disturbed consciousness
   b. Chronic onset of disturbed consciousness
   c. Progressive generalized impairment of intellectual functions and memory without impairment of consciousness.
   d. Disorientation without clouding of consciousness

3. **Which of the following neurotransmitters are decreased in Alzheimer's disease?** *[Recent Question 2016]*
   a. Acetylcholine b. Norepinephrine
   c. Corticotrophin d. All the above

4. **Pseudodementia is seen in** *[Recent Question 2016]*
   a. Delirium b. Dementia
   c. Depression d. Mental retardation

5. **Alzheimer's disease not associated with**
   a. Short term memory loss *[Recent Question 2016]*
   b. Clouding of consciousness
   c. Loss of judgement d. Acalculia

6. **All of the following regarding Delirium Vs Dementia are true except** *[Recent Question 2016]*
   a. Sleep wake cycle is grossly disturbed in delirium
   b. Orientation is grossly disturbed in dementia
   c. Thoughts are disorganized in delirium
   d. Recent and remote memory are disturbed in dementia

7. **Following is true about Ropinirole** *[Recent Question 2016]*
   a. Selective D2/3 receptor agonist
   b. It is used in restless leg syndrome
   c. Both a and b
   d. None of the above

8. **Most important feature of Delirium**
   a. Impaired attention *[Recent Question 2016]*
   b. Anxiety
   c. Hyperactivity
   d. Clouding of consciousness

9. **Which of the following can cause delirium?** *[NBE FMGE September 2009]*
   a. Cocaine b. Amphetamine
   c. L-Dopa d. All of the above

10. **Which of the following is feature of Alzheimer's disease?**
    a. Early memory loss *[NBE DNB 2007]*
    b. Recent memory loss
    c. Recent and past memory loss
    d. Global memory loss

11. **Delirium is seen in mainly** *[Recent Question 2012]*
    a. Alcohol c. Barbiturate
    b. Opium d. Cocaine

12. **Biochemical etiology of Alzheimer's disease is related to**
    a. Acetylcholine *[NBE DNB 1996]*
    b. GABA
    c. Serotonin
    d. Dopamine

13. **Most common type of Dementia seen is** *[Recent Question 2015, NBE FMGE September 2012]*
    a. Alzheimer's dementia b. Lewy body dementia
    c. AISD dementia complex
    d. Depressive pseudodementia

14. **Dementia is a feature of** *[UPSC 2001]*
    a. Scurvy b. Porphyria
    c. Pellagra d. Thiamine deficiency

15. **Delirium tremens is seen in** *[Recent Question 2012]*
    a. Alcohol withdrawal b. Alcohol overdoses
    c. Morphine poisoning d. Atropine poisoning

16. **Alzheimer's disease is associated with** *[NBE FMGE September 2008]*
    a. Delusion b. Dementia
    c. Delirium d. Depression

17. **Huntington's disease is characterized by all except**
    a. Chorea *[NBE FMGE September 2008]*
    b. Behavioural disturbance
    c. Cog-wheel rigidity
    d. Early onset memory loss

18. **Subcortical dementia is seen in all except** *[AIIMS PG 2009, Recent Question 2011, 2013, 2015]*
    a. Parkinsonism b. Alzheimer's disease
    c. Wilson's disease d. Huntington's chorea

19. **In delirium tremens all are true, except**
    a. Gross tremor *[NBE DNB 2001, 2004, 2005]*
    b. Seen in alcoholic withdrawal
    c. Fits may occur
    d. Orientation clear

20. **True about delirium are all except** *[Recent Question 2012, 2015]*
    a. Preserved attention b. Disturbed sleep
    c. Disorientation d. Hallucination

21. **Most common cause of dementia in India is** *[NBE FMGE March 2005]*
    a. Drug induced dementia b. Vascular dementia
    c. Alzheimer's disease d. Pick's disease

22. **Delirium tremens is characteristically seen in** *[NBE DNB 2007]*
    a. Chronic alcoholism b. B2 deficiency
    c. B12 deficiency d. Niacin deficiency

23. **An organic brain syndrome of old age with abrupt onset of dementia is** *[NBE FMGE September 2003]*
    a. Creutzfeldt-Jacob disease
    b. Vascular dementia
    c. Niemann's-Pick disease
    d. Alzheimer's disease

24. **Drug of choice in Delirium tremens is** *[Recent Question 2014, 2015]*
    a. Acamprosate b. Barbiturates
    c. Benzodiazepines d. Naltrexone

25. Features of Alzheimer's disease include all except
a. More common in females *[Recent Question 2014, 2015]*
b. Recent memory loss
c. MMSE useful for diagnosis
d. Medications offer near 100% cure

26. 'Punch drunk' in boxers is a type of
[Recent Question 2014, 2015]
a. Delirium b. Dementia
c. Depression d. Disability

27. Difference between dementia and delirium is
[Recent Question 2017, 2018]
a. Attention is impaired in delirium
b. Consciousness is impaired in dementia
c. Orientation is normal in dementia
d. All of the above

28. Example of Subcortical dementia is
[Recent Question 2017]
a. Alzheimer's disease
b. Multiple sclerosis
c. Creutzfeldt Jacob disease
d. Pick's disease

29. Amnestic syndrome is characterized by all except
a. No disturbance of consciousness *[Recent Question 2017]*
b. Attention is intact
c. Intact intellect
d. Intact memory

30. True about Delirium is *[Recent Question 2017]*
a. Normal sleep b. Disorientation
c. Attention is intact d. None of the above

31. Most common perceptual disturbance in Delirium is
a. Illusion *[Recent Question 2017]*
b. Decreased perceptions per unit of time
c. Visual Hallucination
d. Auditory hallucination

HIGH YIELD MCQs

1. Subcortical dementia is seen in all except
[JIPMER PGMEE 1998]
a. Parkinsonism b. Alzheimer's disease
c. Wilson's disease d. Huntington's Chorea

2. Dementia is seen in all except
[MP PGMEE 1998, WB PGMEE 2000]
a. Schizophrenia b. Alzheimer's disease
c. Huntington's chorea d. Pick's disease

3. Most common cause dementia in adult
[JHARKHAND PGMEE 2006]
a. Alzheimer's disease b. Multi-infarct dementia
c. Pick disease d. Metabolic cause

4. All are true about Delirium Tremens is
[All India PGMEE 2011]
a. Coarse tremors
b. Visual hallucinations
c. Third nerve palsy
d. Altered consciousness

5. Cognitive disorders are *[PGI PGMEE 2003]*
a. Intellectualization b. Depersonalization
c. Dementia d. Delirium

6. All are features of Delirium except *[AIIMS PGMEE 1996]*
a. Confusion b. Disorientation
c. Hyperactivity d. Loss of memory

7. Illusion with altered sensorium is seen in
[AIIMS PGMEE 1991]
a. Schizophrenia b. Hysteria
c. MDP d. Delirium

8. Features of delirium *[PGI 2008]*
a. Deficit of attention
b. Autonomic instability
c. Altered sleep wake patterns
d. Hallucination
e. Delirium cannot diagnosed clinically

9. Delirium and schizophrenia differ from each other by
[WB PGMEE 2001, Karnataka PGMEE 2004]
a. Change in mood b. Complete consciousness
c. Tangential thinking d. All of the above

10. Delirium tremens is characterized by confusion associated with *[All India PGMEE 2003]*
a. Autonomic hyperactivity and tremors
b. Features of intoxication due to alcohol
c. Sixth nerve palsy
d. Korsakoff psychosis

11. Not a feature of dementia is *[AIIMS PGMEE 1999]*
a. Loss of sensorium b. Wearing of dirty clothes
c. Forget fullness d. Loss of neurons in brain

12. 1 week before incidence recall is called as
[Recent Question 2015, AIIMS PGMEE 2009]
a. Working memory b. Delayed memory
c. Recent memory d. Remote memory

13. True about dementia is all except
[All India PGMEE 1994]
a. Often irreversible
b. Hallucination are not common
c. Clouding of consciousness is common
d. Nootropics have limited role

14. Reversible cause of dementia *[Recent Question 2015, All India PGMEE 1995, AP PGMEE 1996]*
a. Post encephalitis b. Multi infarct
c. Hydrocephalus d. Senile dementia

15. Reversible cause of dementia *[PGI 2004]*
a. Hypothyroidism b. Alzheimer's disease
c. Vitamin B12 deficiency d. Vitamin A deficiency

16. Vascular dementia is characterized by *[PGI 2003]*
a. Disorientation b. Memory deficit
c. Emotional liability d. Visual hallucination
e. Personality deterioration

17. Treatable causes of dementia are *[PGI 2001]*
a. Alzheimer's disease
b. Hypothyroidism
c. Multi-infarct dementia
d. SDH (subdural haemorrhage)
e. Hydrocephalus

18. Protein involved in Alzheimer's disease *[NIMHANS PGMEE 2001]*
a. Apo E gene b. Presel in II
c. Amyloid portion d. All

19. Neurofibrillary tangles with senile plaques are seen in *[PGI 2000]*
a. Parkinson's disease b. Alzheimer's disease
c. Schizophrenia d. Tuberous sclerosis

20. Biochemical etiology of Alzheimer's disease relates it to *[Kerala PGMEE 2005, AIIMS PG 1996]*
a. Acetylcholine b. GABA
c. Serotonin d. Dopamine

21. Following are predispositions to Alzheimer's disease *[All India PGMEE 1999, WB PGMEE 1999]*
a. Down's syndrome b. Head trauma
c. Smoking d. Low education group

22. In case of above 60 years of age psychiatric disorder in India is mostly due to *[WB PGMEE 2000]*
a. Depression b. Dementia
c. Hysteria d. Schizophrenia

23. Donepezil is used in treatment of *[MP PGMEE 2005]*
a. Alzheimer's dementia b. Schizophrenia
c. Anxiety disorder d. Depression

24. Regarding Alzheimer's disease which is/are not true? *[PGI 2008, 2009]*
a. Initial loss of long term memory
b. Delayed loss of short term memory
c. Step ladder pattern
d. Cognitive impairment
e. Judgement impairment

25. Drug of choice in Delirium tremens is *[All India PGMEE 1993, All India PGMEE 1993]*
a. Diazepam b. Phenytoin
c. Chlordiazepoxide d. Morphine

26. True about delirium are all except *[Recent Question 2012, 2013]*
a. Preserved attention b. Disturbed sleep
c. Disorientation d. Hallucination

27. Mutism and akinesis in a person who appears awake and even alert, is best described as *[All India PGMEE 2006]*
a. Twilight state b. Oneroid state
c. Stupor d. Delirium

28. Cognitive disorders are *[PGI 2006, 2007]*
a. Intellectualization b. Deprsonalization
c. Dementia d. Delirium
e. Hallucination

29. Disorientation occurs in *[All India PGMEE 1993]*
a. Schizophrenia b. Organic Brain Syndrome
c. Depression d. Mania

30. The presence of delusion, hallucination and disturbed cognitive functions indicate *[All India PGMEE 1994]*
a. Paranoid Psychosis
b. OCD
c. Organic Brain Syndrome
d. Dissociative disorder

31. Slow waves in EEG activity seen in *[PGI 1998, Recent Question 2015]*
a. Depression
b. Delirium
c. Schizophrenia
d. Mania

32. Patient with altered consciousness, tremors and visual hallucinations, the probable diagnosis is *[AP PGMEE 1993]*
a. Delirium tremens b. Korsakoff psychosis
c. MDP d. Wernicke's encephalopathy

33. A patient semiconscious with altered sensorium with visual hallucination and fragmented delusions is suffering from, which of the following disorder? *[SGPGI 2002]*
a. Delirium b. Delusion
c. Schizophrenia d. Mania

34. A patient with pneumonia for 5 days is admitted to the hospital in altered sensorium. He suddenly ceases to recognize the doctor and staff. He thinks that he is in jail and complains of scorpion attacking him. His probable diagnosis is *[All India PGMEE 2001]*
a. Acute dementia b. Acute delirium
c. Acute schizophrenia d. Acute paronia

35. An alcoholic is brought to the Emergency OPD with the complaint or irrelevant talking. He had stopped using alcohol three days back. On examination, he is found to be disoriented to time, place and person. He also has visual illusions and hallucinations. There is no history of head injury. Most likely diagnosis is *[All India PGMEE 2003]*
a. Dementia praecox b. Delirium tremens
c. Schizophrenia d. Korsakoff psychosis

36. All are true about Delirium tremens except *[AIIMS PGMEE 1998]*
a. Severe depression b. Hallucination
c. Extreme anxiety d. Delusion

37. Biological Amnesia is *[AIIMS PGMEE 1998]*
a. Lack of interest b. Presenile dementia
c. Opioid addiction d. Hypothyroidism

38. Characteristic feature of subcortical dementia is *[AIIMS PGMEE 1999]*
a. Memory loss b. Aphasia
c. Dyslexia d. Tactile agnosia

39. Dementia is seen in all except *[MP PGMEE 1997]*
a. Schizophrenia b. Head injury
c. Huntington's chorea d. Frontal lobe tumour

40. All are examples of cortical dementia except *[JIPMER PGMEE 2003, SGPGI 2001]*
a. Alzheimer's disease
b. Multiple sclerosis
c. Creutzfeldt Jacob disease
d. Pick's disease

41. One of the following is a reversible cause of dementia *[MP PGMEE2003]*
- a. Toxic dementia
- b. Alzheimer's disease
- c. Multi-infarct dementia
- d. Pick disease

42. Reversible cause of dementia is *[All India PGMEE 1995, Recent Question 2015]*
- a. Multi infarct
- b. Senile Dementia
- c. Post Encephalitis
- d. Huntington's chorea

43. The following are the psychiatric sequelae after stroke in elderly *[Recent Question 2017, PGI 2003]*
- a. Depression
- b. Post traumatic stress disorder
- c. Dementia
- d. None

44. A 65-year old male is brought to the outpatient clinic with one year illness characterized by marked forgetfulness, visual hallucinations, suspiciousness, personality decline, poor self-care and progressive deterioration in his condition. His Mini Mental Status Examination [MMSE] Score is 1. His most likely diagnosis is *[AIIMS PGMEE 2002]*
- a. Dementia
- b. Schizophrenia
- c. Mania
- d. Depression

45. Dementia of Alzheimer's type is not associated with one of the following *[AIIMS PGMEE 2005]*
- a. Depressive symptoms
- b. Delusions
- c. Apraxia and aphasia
- d. Cerebral infarcts

46. All the following are featuring Alzheimer's disease except *[WB PGMEE 2002]*
- a. Cerebellar atrophy
- b. Common in 5th and 6th decade
- c. Atrophied gyri widened sulci
- d. Progressive dementia

47. Fronto-temporal dementias include all except *[UP PGMEE 2007]*
- a. Pick's disease
- b. Nonfluent aphasia
- c. Semantic dementia
- d. Alzheimer's disease

48. A 70-year-old man presents with h/o prosopagnosia loss of memory, 3rd person hallucination since 1 month. On examination deep Tendon reflexes are increased, mini mental examination score is 20/30. What is most likely diagnosis? *[AIIMS PGMEE 2001]*
- a. Dissociated Dementia
- b. Schizophrenia
- c. Alzheimer's disease
- d. Psychotic disorder

49. Rivastigmine and Donepezil are drugs used predominantly in the management of *[All India PGMEE2006]*
- a. Depression
- b. Dissociation
- c. Delusion
- d. Dementia

50. Which of the following is not used in delirium? *[PGI 2005]*
- a. Haloperidol
- b. Lithium
- c. Diazepam
- d. Olanzapine
- e. Risperidone

51. A reversible cause of dementia is *[UPSC CMS 2017]*
- a. Alzheimer disease
- b. Huntington chorea
- c. Parkinson disease
- d. Subdural haematoma

52. Mutism and Akinesis are found in a person in awake state. It is a feature of *[AIIMS May 2017]*
- a. Delirium
- b. Twilight state
- c. Oneroid state
- d. Stupor

NEET/NBE PATTERN MCQs ANSWERS WITH EXPLANATIONS

1. Ans. (a) Alcohol
[Ref. Bradley's Neurology in Clinical Practice, 7/e p30]

Delirium
- Frequently seen in people intoxicated with or withdrawing from various substances, most commonly alcohol or BZDs
- Last from less than a week to more than a month
- More protracted in the elderly

2. Ans. (a) Acute onset of disturbed consciousness
[Ref. Neurology in Clinical Practice by Bradley, 4/e p30]

Delirium
- Acute onset of disturbed consciousness
- Attentional deficits
- Disorganized thinking
- Perceptual disturbances
- Disturbed sleep-wake cycle
- Altered psychomotor activity
- Disorientation
- Memory impairment
- Behavioral and emotional abnormalities
- Cognitive deficits

3. Ans. (d) All the above
[Ref. Kaplan & Sadock, 3/e p53]

Neurotransmitters in Alzheimer's disease
- Acetylcholine: Decreased
- Norepinephrine: Decreased
- Somatostatin: Decreased
- Corticotropin: Decreased
- Choline acetyltransferase: Decreased
- Glutamate: Increased

4. Ans. (c) Depression
[Ref. Functional Psychiatric Disorders of the Elderly by Chiu, 1/e p126]

Pseudodementia
- Dementia syndrome developing in context of a psychiatric disorder that subsides when psychiatric symptomatology is ameliorated
- Severity of a functional cognitive disturbance approaches degree of impairment seen in Organic dementing illnesses
- MC associated disorder: Depression
- Other associated disorders: Schizophrenic psychosis, Hysterical personality, PTSD, Malingering, Ganser's syndrome, Mixed mood disorders, Paraphrenias

5. Ans. (b) Clouding of consciousness
[Ref. Case-Based Neurology by Singh, 1/e p277]

Alzheimer's disease: Cortical dementia
- Early symptoms: Depression, insomnia, agitation, anxiety, excitability, mild forgetfulness, impaired judgment
- Middle symptoms: Short-term memory loss, fatigue, decrease in concentration, aphasia, acalculia, getting lost, difficulty following commands
- Late symptoms: Decreased interest, loss of language, confusion

6. Ans. (b) Orientation is grossly disturbed in dementia
[Ref. Clinical Emergency Medicine by Mahadevan, 1/e p180]

Delirium Vs Dementia Vs Acute Psychosis

	Delirium	Dementia	Acute psychosis
Definition	**Acute confusional state**	**Deterioration of higher cortical functions**	**Inability distinguishing reality from imaginary**
Type of disease	Organic	Organic	Functional
Onset	Hours-Days	Months	Hours-Days
Course	Fluctuating	Progressive	Stable
Consciousness	Altered	Normal	Normal
Hallucinations	Visual	None	Auditory
Orientation	Altered	Altered	Normal
Vital signs	Variable fluctuating	Normal	Variable
Miscellaneous	Reversible in 80%	Exacerbations seen	Fixed delusions

7. Ans. (c) Both a and b
[Ref. Pharmacology for Nursing Care by Lehne, 8/e p194]

ROPINIROLE
- Highly selective for D2 D3 receptors
- Used in Parkinson's disease, Restless legs syndrome

8. Ans. (d) Clouding of consciousness
[Ref. Delirium in Critical Care by Page, 2/e p5]
- Greiner suggested that Clouding of consciousness was the main pathogenic feature of Delirium

9. Ans. (d) All of the above
[Ref. Niraj Ahuja, 7/e p19-21]
- *Drugs causing Delirium:*

Medicinal drugs	Psychoactive drugs	Poisons
• Anticholinergics • Antipsychotic • Antihistaminic • Antidepressants • Anticonvulsants • Corticosteroids Sedatives • NSAIDs • Anticancer drugs • Lithium • Cimetidine • Antibiotics • L-dopa	• Ethanol • Marijuana • LSD • Amphetamines • Cocaine • Opiates • Phencyclidine	• Solvents • Carbon monoxide • Refrigerants • Heavy metals • Insecticides • Mushrooms • Datura stramonium • Animal venoms

See Theory also

10. Ans. (b) Recent memory loss
[Ref. Neuroscience in Medicine by Conn, 3/e p378]

Memory Loss in Alzheimer's Disease

- ***Recent memory loss***: Impaired learning (Repetitive questioning, missed appointments, misplaced objects)
  - Insidious onset of memory loss
  - Slowly progressive impairment
  - Neuronal loss in hippocampus
  - Reduction of cholinergic neurons projecting from Basal nucleus of Meynert
- **Relatively intact remote memory**
  - 'Living in the past'

11. Ans. (a) Alcohol
[Ref. Niraj Ahuja, 7/e p21]

Drugs & Poisons Causing Delirium

- Methyl alcohol (mainly),
- Sedatives, Hypnotics (Barbiturates)
- Salicylates, Steroids, Penicillin, Insulin
- Digitalis, Quinidine, Anti-hypertensives
- Tricyclic antidepressants, Antipsychotics, Anticholinergics, Disulfiram
- Anti-convulsants, L-DOPA, Opiates, Cocaine

12. Ans. (a) Acetylcholine
[Ref. Niraj Ahuja, 7/e p25]

Neuro-Chemical Basis of Alzheimer's Disease

- Decreased Acetylcholine levels
- Decreased Choline acetyltransferase
- Decreased Brain acetylcholinesterase

13. Ans. (a) Alzheimer's dementia
[Ref. Niraj Ahuja, 7/e p23]

14. Ans. (c) Pellagra
[Ref. Niraj Ahuja, 7/e p24]

- *Deficiency dementias*:
  - Pernicious anemia
  - Pellagra
  - Folic acid deficiency
  - Thiamine deficiency

15. Ans. (a) Alcohol withdrawal
[Ref. Niraj Ahuja, 7/e p38]

Delirium Tremens

- Most severe alcohol withdrawal syndrome
  - Occurs within 2-4 days of abstinence from heavy alcohol drinking
  - Occur in 5% patients
- Clinical features:
  - Gross coarse tremor
  - Clouded consciousness, Disorientation in time, place
  - Visual/ auditory hallucinations, Delusions
  - Insomnia, Dehydration
  - Poor attention span, Distractibility
  - Autonomic disturbance (Tachycardia, hypertension, sweating)
  - Psychomotor agitation, anxiety, ataxia, seizure
  - Recovery in 3-7 days

16. Ans. (b) Dementia
[Ref. Niraj Ahuja, 7/e p23, 26]

Alzheimer's Dementia

- *Definition*: Progressive degenerative fatal brain disease with gradual loss of cell-to-cell connections in brain (leading to dementia)
- *Underlying cause*:
  - Decreased brain choline acetyltransferase (CAT)
  - Decreased brain acetylcholinesterase (AchE)
- *Changes in brain*:
  - Neurofibrillary tangles
  - Neuritis plaques
  - Senile plaques
- *Treatment*:
  - Cholinesterase inhibitors: Donezepil, Rivastigmine, Galantamine
  - Memantine
  - Piracetam
  - Vitamin C, Vitamin E

17. Ans. (d) Early onset memory loss
[Ref. Niraj Ahuja, 7/e p24]

Huntington's Disease

- *Definition*: Neurodegenerative disorder affecting muscle coordination and leading to cognitive decline and dementia
- *Inheritance*: Autosomal dominant
- *Clinical presentation*:
  - Chorea
  - Saccadic eye movements
  - Sub-cortical dementia
  - Sleep disturbances
  - Seizures
  - Progressive memory loss
  - Cog-wheel rigidity
  - Behavioural disturbance
  - Cognitive impairment
  - Anxiety, depression, addictions, hypersexuality
- *Management*:
  - Tetrabenazine
  - Neuroleptics
  - Benzodiazepines
  - SSRIs
  - Mirtazapine

18. Ans. (b) Alzheimer's disease
[Ref. Primary Care: An Interprofessional Perspective by Singleton, 2/e p714]

Dementias by Site of Involvement

- ***Cortical dementias***:
  - DAT (Dementia of Alzheimer type)
  - Pick's disease
- ***Sub-cortical dementias***:
  - Parkinson's disease
  - Parkinsonian symptoms (Progressive supranuclear palsy)
  - Wilson's disease
  - Huntington's disease
  - Hydrocephalus
  - Multiple sclerosis
  - HIV encephalopathy

- ***Combined Cortical & Sub-cortical dementias***:
  - Vascular dementias (Multi-infarct dementia, Biswanger's disease)
  - Hypoxic dementias
  - Infectious dementias (Creutzfeldt Jakob disease)
  - Miscellaneous dementias (Toxic & metabolic encephalopathy, Neoplasm)

19. Ans. (d) Orientation clear
[Ref. Niraj Ahuja, 7/e p38]

20. Ans. (a) Preserved attention
[Ref. Niraj Ahuja, 7/e p38]

21. Ans. (c) Alzheimer's disease
[Ref. Niraj Ahuja, 7/e p23]

- *MC cause of dementia in India*: Alzheimer's disease

22. Ans. (a) Chronic alcoholism
[Ref. Niraj Ahuja, 7/e p38]

23. Ans. (a) Creutzfeldt-Jakob disease
[Ref. Wikipedia]

Slowly progressive dementia	Rapidly progressive dementia
• **Alzheimer's disease** • Vascular dementia • **Dementia with Lewy bodies** • Hypothyroidism • Normal pressure hydrocephalus • **Huntington's disease** • Homocystinuria • Metachromatic leucodystrophy • Antiphospholipid syndrome • **Niemann-Pick disease** • Wilson's disease • Vitamin deficiency (B12/ folate/niacin) • HIV • Syphilis • SSPE	• Creutzfeldt-Jakob disease • Viral encephalitis • Lymphoma • Glioma • Liver failure • Kidney failure • **Subdural hematoma** • Anti-convulsant drugs toxicity

24. Ans. (c) Benzodiazepines
[Ref. Biology of Alcoholism Volume III, 2/e p242]

- Drug of choice in Delirium tremens: Chlordiazepoxide

25. Ans. (d) Medications offer near 100% cure
[Ref. Niraj Ahuja, 7/e p25]

- At present, Alzheimer's disease is NOT considered a treatable disorder

26. Ans. (b) Dementia
[Ref. Greenfield's Neuropathology, 8/e p786]

Punch Drunk Syndrome

- Synonyms: Chronic progressive traumatic encephalopathy, **Dementia pugilistica**
- Description: Chronic traumatic brain injury (CTBI) as a result of boxing
- Features: Speech difficulties, Unsteady gait, Ataxia, Dementia, Spasticity, Extrapyramidal disturbances
- Histology: Cerebral atrophy, Enlarged ventricles, Large Cavum, Septa pellucida with multiple fenestrations, Degeneration of Substantia nigra, TAU, Neurofibrillary tangles

27. Ans. (a) Attention is impaired in delirium
[Ref. Clinical Emergency Medicine by Mahadevan, 1/e p180]

- In Delirium, alertness, consciousness and orientation are impaired
- In Dementia, alertness and consciousness is normal, orientation only is impaired late in course

28. Ans. (b) Multiple sclerosis
[Ref. Primary Care by Singleton, 2/e p714]

- Sub-cortical dementias are seen in Parkinson's disease, Parkinsonian symptoms (Progressive supranuclear palsy), Wilson's disease, Huntington's disease, Hydrocephalus, Multiple sclerosis, HIV encephalopathy

29. Ans. (d) Intact memory
[Ref. Niraj Ahuja, 7/e p27]

Organic Amnestic Syndrome

- Impairment of memory due to an underlying organic cause
  - Severe impairment of recent/ short-term memory
  - Impaired remote memory or long-term memory
- No severe disturbance of consciousness and attention
- No global disturbance of intellectual function, abstract thinking and personality
- Confabulation (patient uses imaginary events in the early phase of illness)

30. Ans. (b) Disorientation
[Ref. Niraj Ahuja, 7/e p20]

Delirium

- Acute onset, clouding of consciousness, disorientation (firstly in Time, then place, then finally in person), memory impairment, hallucinations, illusions, misinterpretations, disturbed sleep-wake cycle, motor symptoms (Asterixis - flapping tremor, Carphologia/ flocculation - picking movements at clothes, and Myoclonus - reflex abnormalities)
- Impaired attention (Hallmark of Delirium)

31. Ans. (b) Decreased perceptions per unit of time
[Ref. Bradley's Neurology in Clinical Practice E-Book, 7/ p25]

- Clinical Presentation of Delirium include acute onset of mental status change (with fluctuating course), attentional deficits, disorganised thinking, altered conscious, perceptual disturbance, altered sleep-wake cycle, altered psychomotor activity, disorientation and memory impairment, behavioural and emotional problems, other cognitive deficits
- Most common perceptual disturbance is decreased perceptions per unit of time; patients miss things that are going on around them, illusions and misinterpretations occur

HIGH YIELD MCQs ANSWERS WITH EXPLANATIONS 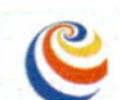

1. **Ans. (b) Alzheimer's disease**
   [Ref. Primary Care: An Interprofessional Perspective by Singleton, 2/e p714]

2. **Ans. (a) Schizophrenia**
   [Ref. Primary Care: An Interprofessional Perspective by Singleton, 2/e p714]

3. **Ans. (a) Alzheimer's disease**
   [Ref. Niraj Ahuja, 7/e p23]

4. **Ans. (c) Third nerve palsy**
   [Ref. Niraj Ahuja, 7/e p38]

5. **Ans. (c) Dementia; (d) Delirium**
   [Ref. Kaplan &Sadock'sConcise Textbook of Clinical Psychiatry, 3/e p47]

Cognitive Disorders

Delirium	Dementia	Amnestic syndromes
• General medical condition • Substance induced • Multiple etiology • Not otherwise specified	• Alzheimer dementia • Vascular dementia • HIV dementia • Parkinson's disease • Huntington's disease • Pick's disease • Creutzfeldt Jakob disease • Head trauma • Substance induced persisting	• General medical condition • Substance induced persisting • Not otherwise specified

6. **Ans. (d) Loss of memory**
   [Ref. Encyclopedia of Neurological Sciences by Daroff, 2/e p954]

Common Presentation of Delirium

Hyperactive delirium	Hypoactive delirium
• Hyperarousal • Vigilance • Hallucination, Illusion • Delusion • Disorientation • Agitation	• Reduced alertness • Lethargy • Sedation • Confusion • Hallucination

7. **Ans. (d) Delirium**
   [Ref. Modern Everyday Psychiatry by Taylor, 1/e p221]

Cardinal Features of Delirium

- Diffuse cognitive impairment
- Altered sensorium
- Fluctuating behavior
- Increased motor activity
- Altered sleep-wake cycle with insomnia & daytime lethargy

8. **Ans. (a) Deficit of attention; (b) Autonomic instability; (c) Altered sleep wake patterns; (d) Hallucination**
   [Ref. Encyclopedia of Neurological Sciences by Daroff, 2/e p954]

9. **Ans. (b) Complete consciousness**
   [Ref. Kaplan &Sadock's Concise Textbook of Clinical Psychiatry, 3/e p51]

Schizophrenia vs Delirium

- More constant and better organized delusions & hallucinations in Schizophrenia
- No change in level of consciousness in Schizophrenia
- No change in orientation in Schizophrenia

10. **Ans. (a) Autonomic hyperactivity and tremors**
    [Ref. Niraj Ahuja, 7/e p38]

11. **Ans. (a) Loss of sensorium**
    [Ref. Synopsis of Psychiatry by Sadock, 10/e p327]
    - Loss of sensorium is a characteristic feature of Delirium not seen in Dementia

12. **Ans. (c) Recent memory**
    [Ref. Memory Rehabilitation by Wilson, 1/e p5]

Types of Memory

- ***Delayed memory***: Events or information that occurred few minutes earlier
- ***Recent memory***: Events or information that occurred in past few day to weeks
- ***Remote memory***: Events or information that occurred years before
- ***Semantic memory***: Memory for general knowledge (facts, meaning of words, appearance of objects)
- ***Episodic memory***: Memory for personal experiences (where did spend your last new year)
- ***Procedural memory***: Memory for skills or routine

13. **Ans. (c) Clouding of consciousness is common**
    [Ref. Alzheimer's and Other Dementias by Hughes, 1/e p26]
    - Clouding of consciousness is a characteristic feature of Delirium not seen in Dementia

14. **Ans. (c) Hydrocephalus**
    [Ref. Psychiatric Nursing by Steele, 7/e p334]
    - *Potentially reversible dementia*:
      - Normal pressure hydrocephalus
      - Vitamin B12 deficiency
      - Toxic dementias
      - Post-encephalitic/ meningiti dementia
      - Myxedema
      - Subdural hematoma

15. **Ans. (a) Hypothyroidism; (c) Vitamin B12 deficiency**
    [Ref. Psychiatric Nursing by Steele, 7/e p334]

16. **Ans. (a) Disorientation; (b) Memory deficit; (c) Emotional liability; (e) Personality deterioration**
    [Ref. Springhouse NCLEXRN, 6/e p156]

Vascular Dementia
- Confusion, Dizziness
- Disorientation
- Depression
- Emotional lability
- Loss of bowel/ bladder control
- Impairment of recent memory
- Slurred speech
- Cognitive deterioration

17. Ans. (b) Hypothyroidism; (d) SDH (Subdural haemorrhage); (e) Hydrocephalus
[Ref. Encyclopedia of Neurological Sciences by Daroff, 2/e p968]

Treatable Causes of Dementia
- Normal pressure hydrocephalus
- Chronic Subdural hematoma
- Metabolic disturbances: Hypothyroidism, Renal failure, Hepatic failure
- Infections: HIV
- Deficiencies: B12 deficiency
- Autoimmune encephalopathy

18. Ans. (a) Apo E gene
[Ref. Memory loss, Alzheimer's Disease & Dementia by Budson, 2/e p56]

19. Ans. (b) Alzheimer's disease
[Ref. Niraj Ahuja, 7/e p38]

Features of Alzheimer's Dementia
- *Macroscopic changes*: Enlarged cerebral ventricles, Widened cerebral sulci, Shrinkage of cerebral cortex
- *Microscopic changes*: Senile plaques, Neurofibrillary tangles, Cortical nerve cell loss, Granulovacuolar degeneration
- *Clinical features*:
  - **4A's: Amnesia, Apraxia, Aphasia, Agnosia**
  - Depression
  - **Hallucinations** (**Visual** > Auditory)
  - Delusions (Persecutory)
  - Progressive dementia
  - Common in 5th - 6th decade

20. Ans. (a) Acetylcholine
[Ref. Niraj Ahuja, 7/e p25]

21. Ans. (c) Smoking
[Ref. Yearbook of Pediatrics 2011 by Stockmann III]

22. Ans. (b) Dementia
[Ref. Niraj Ahuja, 7/e p23]

23. Ans. (a) Alzheimer's dementia
[Ref. Psychopharmacology for Health Professionals by Bullock, 1/e p59]
- ***Acetylcholinesterase inhibitors used in Alzheimer's dementia***:
- Donezepil
- Rivastigmine
- Gallantamine

24. Ans. (a) Initial loss of long term memory; (b) Delayed loss of short term memory; (c) Step ladder pattern
[Ref. Niraj Ahuja, 7/e p23-25]

25. Ans. (c) Chlordiazepoxide
[Ref. Biology of Alcoholism Volume III, 2/e p242]

26. Ans. (a) Preserved attention
[Ref. Niraj Ahuja, 7/e p38]

27. Ans. (c) Stupor
[Ref. Sim's Symptoms in Mind by Oyebode, 5/e p42]

Stupor
- Absence of relational functions: Absence of initiation of Action & Speech
- Mutism
- Akinesis
- Awake, Alert

28. Ans. (c) Dementia; (d) Delirium
[Ref. Kaplan & Sadock's Concise Textbook of Clinical Psychiatry, 3/e p47]

29. Ans. (b) Organic Brain Syndrome
[Ref. Insanity: A Study of Major Psychiatric Disorders by Steinert, 1/e p69]

Features of Chronic Organic Brain Syndrome
- Impaired intellectual function: Persecutory delusions, Visual hallucinations
- Memory impairment
- Diminution of awareness
- Disorientation in time, place, person

30. Ans. (c) Organic Brain Syndrome
[Ref. Insanity: A Study of Major Psychiatric Disorders by Steinert, 1/e p69]

31. Ans. (b) Delirium
[Ref. Essentials of Neuroimaging for Clinical Practice by Dougherty, 1/e p120]
- *EEG in Delirium*: Slow wave rhythm EXCEPT Delirium tremens where it shows fast rhythms

32. Ans. (a) Delirium tremens
[Ref. Niraj Ahuja, 7/e p38]

33. Ans. (a) Delirium
[Ref. Modern Everyday Psychiatry by Taylor, 1/e p221]

34. Ans. (b) Acute delirium
[Ref. Modern Everyday Psychiatry by Taylor, 1/e p221]

35. Ans. (b) Delirium tremens
[Ref. Modern Everyday Psychiatry by Taylor, 1/e p221]

36. Ans. (a) Severe depression
[Ref. Niraj Ahuja, 7/e p38]

37. Ans. (b) Presenile dementia
[Ref. Physiological Psychology by Mahmud, 1/e p205]

38. Ans. (a) Memory loss
[Ref. Lexicon of Psychiatry, Neurology and Neurosciences by Ayd, 2/e p298]
- *Cardinal features of Subcortical dementias*:
  - Cognitive slowing
  - Memory impairment
  - Executive function deficits
  - Mood and personality changes

39. Ans. (a) Schizophrenia
[Ref. Primary Care: An Interprofessional Perspective by Singleton, 2/e p714]

40. Ans. (b) Multiple sclerosis
[Ref. Primary Care: An Interprofessional Perspective by Singleton, 2/e p714]

41. Ans. (a) Toxic dementia
[Ref. Psychiatric Nursing by Steele, 7/e p334]

42. Ans. (c) Post Encephalitis
[Ref. Psychiatric Nursing by Steele, 7/e p334]

43. Ans. (a) Depression; (c) Dementia
[Ref. Principles and Practice of Geriatric Psychiatry by Maletta, 1/e p305]

44. Ans. (a) Dementia
[Ref. Core Clinical Cases Book 1 by Sewan, 2/e p209]

- *MMSE Score suggestive of Dementia*:
  - 28–30: No dementia
  - 25–27: Borderline
  - < 25: Dementia (in absence of acute confusion and depression)

45. Ans. (d) Cerebral infarcts
[Ref. Niraj Ahuja, 7/e p38]

46. Ans. (a) Cerebellar atrophy
[Ref. Niraj Ahuja, 7/e p38]

47. Ans. (d) Alzheimer's disease
[Ref. Communication Disability in the Dementias by Bryan & Maxim, 1/e p95]

48. Ans. (c) Alzheimer's disease
[Ref. Niraj Ahuja, 7/e p38]

49. Ans. (d) Dementia
[Ref. Psychopharmacology for Health Professionals by Bullock, 1/e p59]

50. Ans. (b) Lithium; (c) Diazepam; (d) Olanzapine; (e) Resperidone
[Ref. Meyler's Side Effects of Psychiatric Drugs by Aronson, 1/e p298]

- Haloperidol with Lorazepam is used for treatment of agitated Delirium.

51. Ans. (d) Subdural haematoma
[Ref. Psychiatry E-Book by Bernstein, 4/e p119]

Causes of Dementia

Reversible causes of Dementia	Irreversible causes of Dementia
Normal pressure hydrocephalus Sub-dural hematoma Vasculitis Pernicious anaemia Bromide intoxication Nutritional deficiencies CNS infections (HIV, TB, Fungal, Neurosyphilis, Fungal)	Alzheimer's dementia Multi-infarct dementia Huntington's chorea Multiple sclerosis Pick's disease Parkinson's disease Creutzfeldt-Jakob disease Lewy body dementia Cerebellar degeneration

52. Ans. (d) Stupor
[Ref. Sim's Symptoms in Mind by Oyebode, 5/e p42]

- Stupor is characterised by absence of relational functions (absence of initiation of action & speech), mutism, akinesis, awake, alert

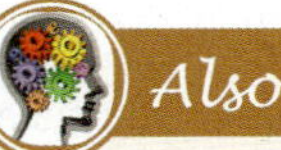

Also Remember

- Delirium is transient acute global impairment of consciousness and cognition, attention, reverse sleep wake cycle with altered psychomotor activity
- Twilight state is abrupt onset of abnormal violent behaviour for variable period, an organic condition seen in epilepsy, alcoholism, brain trauma
- Oneroid state is a dream-like state with impaired consciousness, marked emotional changes, confusion

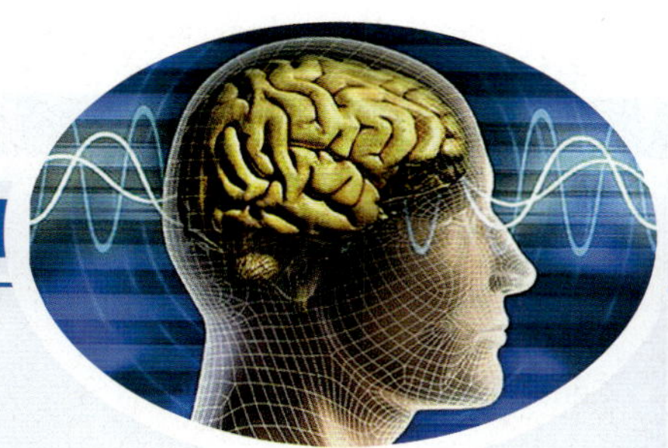

Chapter 9

Alcoholism

THEORETICAL CONCEPTS

IX A. ALCOHOL USE DISORDERS

IX A1. Species of Alcohol Dependence (Jellinek—on the pattern of use)

- ***Alpha species***[Q]:
  - Excessive, inappropriate drinking
  - No loss of control
  - Ability to abstain present
- ***Beta species***:
  - Excessive, inappropriate drinking
  - Physical complications
  - No dependence
- ***Gamma species***:
  - Progressive course
  - Physical dependence, tolerance, withdrawal symptoms
  - Psychological dependence
- ***Delta species***:
  - Tolerance, withdrawal symptoms
  - Inability to sustain
- ***Epsilon species***[Q]:
  - Dipsomania (Compulsive drinking)
  - Spree-drinking

Topper's Edge

Jellinek

- Jellinek coined the expression '**The disease concept of alcoholism**'[Q]: Problem drinking is sometimes caused by a disease of the brain, characterized by altered brain structure and function.
- **Jellinek's Achilles' Heel**: While Jellinek's classification draws a clear (if arbitrary) line between the garden-variety alcoholic and the truly diseased alcoholic, it does not draw such a clear boundary between alcoholism in general and normal drinking

IX A2. Classification of Alcoholism (Cloninger)

	Type I alcoholism	Type II alcoholism
Also known as	Milieu-limited	Male limited
Age	>25 years	<25 years

Contd...

Contd...

	Type I alcoholism	Type II alcoholism
Sex	Both sexes	Males
Underlying cause	Genetic factors + Strong environmental factors	Genetic factors
Family history	May be present	Always present
Clinical presentation	• Psychological dependence • Guilt • Loss of control	• Aggressive behaviour • Spontaneous seeking • No loss of control

Topper's Edge

ALCOHOLISM IN DSM-IV VS DSM-5

DSM-IV Alcoholism

- DSM-IV described two distinct disorders, Alcohol abuse and Alcohol dependence, with specific criteria for each
- Under DSM-IV, the diagnostic criteria for abuse and dependence were distinct: anyone meeting one or more of the "abuse" criteria (Items 1 through 4) within a 12-month period would receive the "abuse" diagnosis
- Anyone with three or more of the "dependence" criteria (see items 5 through 11) during the same 12-month period would receive a "dependence" diagnosis

DSM-5 Alcoholism

- DSM-5 integrates the two DSM-IV disorders, Alcohol abuse and Alcohol dependence, into a single disorder called "Alcohol use disorder (AUD)" with mild, moderate, and severe sub-classifications
- Under DSM-5, anyone meeting any two of the 11 criteria during the same 12-month period would receive a diagnosis of AUD
- Severity of an AUD - Mild, moderate, or severe, is based on the number of criteria met
- DSM-5 eliminates legal problems as a criterion.
- DSM-5 adds craving as a criterion for an AUD diagnosis

DSM-IV CRITERIA FOR ALCOHOL ABUSE & DEPENDENCE

DSM-IV Criteria for Alcohol Abuse[Q]

- A maladaptive pattern of alcohol abuse leading to clinically significant impairment or distress, as manifested by one or more of the following, occurring **within a 12-month period:**
  - Recurrent alcohol use resulting in failure to fulfil major role obligations at work, school, or home
  - Recurrent alcohol use in situations in which it is physically hazardous
  - Recurrent alcohol-related legal problems
  - Continued alcohol use despite persistent or recurrent social or interpersonal problems caused or exacerbated by the effects of the alcohol
- These symptoms must never have met the criteria for alcohol dependence

DSM-IV Criteria for Alcohol Dependence[Q]

A maladaptive pattern of alcohol use, leading to clinically significant impairment or distress, as manifested by three or more of the following seven criteria, occurring at any time in the same 12-month period:

- **Tolerance**, as defined by either of the following:
  - A need for markedly increased amounts of alcohol to achieve intoxication or desired effect
  - Markedly diminished effect with continued use of the same amount of alcohol
- **Withdrawal**, as defined by either of the following:
  - Characteristic withdrawal syndrome for alcohol
  - Alcohol is taken to relieve or avoid withdrawal symptoms
- Alcohol is often taken in larger amounts or over a longer period than was intended
- There is a persistent desire or there are unsuccessful efforts to cut down or control alcohol use
- A great deal of time is spent in activities necessary to obtain alcohol, use alcohol or recover from its effects
- Important social, occupational, or recreational activities are given up or reduced because of alcohol use
- Alcohol use is continued despite knowledge of having a persistent or recurrent physical or psychological problem that is likely to have been caused or exacerbated by the alcohol

IX A3. Laboratory and Other Markers for Alcoholism

- Gamma-glutamyl transferase (GGT) > 40 IU/litre[Q]
- Mean corpuscular volume (MCV) > 92 fl

- Other lab markers (Alkaline phosphatase, Uric acid, Serum triglycerides, Creatinine kinase, ALT, AST)
- Blood alcohol concentration
- Breath analyser
- Michigan alcoholism screening test (**MAST**[Q])
- **CAGE questionnaire** (Score ≥ 2 identifies problem drinkers[Q])
  - Have you ever had to **C**ut down on alcohol amount?
  - Have you been ever **A**nnoyed by people's criticism of alcoholism?
  - Have you ever felt **G**uilty about drinking?
  - Have you ever needed an **E**ye opener drink?

IX A4. Clinical Presentation

IX A4 (i). Acute Intoxication

Blood level of alcohol	Signs of intoxication
150–200 mg%	• CNS depression (after brief excitation) • Increased reaction time, slow thinking, poor motor control • Dysarthria, ataxia, poor motor control • Uninhibited behaviour • Amnesia/ black-outs
300–450 mg%	• Drowsiness • Respiratory depression • Coma
400–800 mg%	• Death

IX A4 (ii). Chronic Alcohol use

- ***Wernicke's encephalopathy***: Acute reaction to severe thiamine (Vitamin B1) deficiency
  - Ocular signs: Nystagmus, ophthalmoplegia, retinal hemorrhages, papilloedema
  - Higher mental function disturbances: Disorientation, confusion, recent memory disturbance, poor attention span
  - Peripheral neuropathy
  - Severe malnutrition
- ***Korsakoff's psychosis***[Q]**:**
  - Organic amnestic syndrome: Gross memory disturbances, confabulation, impaired insight
- ***Marchiafava-Bignami disease***[Q]**:**
  - Epilepsy, ataxia, dysarthria, hallucinations, paralysis
  - Alcohol dementia
  - Peripheral neuropathy
  - Cerebellar degeneration

IX A5. Treatment

IX A5 (i). Detoxification (Treatment of Alcohol Withdrawal Symptoms)

- Benzodiazepines
  - **Chlordiazepoxide**[Q]
  - Diazepam
- Vitamin B1 administration
- Hydration

IX A5 (ii). Alcohol Dependence Treatment

- Behaviour therapy
- Psychotherapy
- Group therapy
- **Deterrent agents**[Q]
  - Disulfiram
  - Metronidazole

- Calcium citrate carbide
- Animal charcoal
- Coprinus atramentarius
- Sulfonylureas
- Cephalosporins
- Griseofulvin

- **Anticraving agents**[Q]
  - Acamprosate
  - Naltrexone
  - SSRIs (Fluoxetine)
- Psychosocial rehabilitation

IX A6. Alcohol Withdrawal

- *Definition*: A set of symptoms when an individual reduces or stops alcohol consumption after prolonged periods of excessive alcohol intake
- *Clinical presentation*:
  - *Hangover next morning*: **Most common withdrawal syndrome**[Q]
  - Mild tremors **(Most common symptom: 34% patients**[Q]**)**
  - Nausea, vomiting
  - Weakness, insomnia, anxiety
  - *Delirium tremens*: **Most severe withdrawal syndrome**[Q]
  - *Alcoholic seizures* ***(Rum fits***[Q]***)***
  - *Alcoholic hallucinosis*
- *Diagnostic criteria (American Psychiatry Association)*:
  - A. Cessation/ reduction in alcohol use that was heavy and prolonged
  - B. ≥ 2 of the following (within hours to a few days after criterion A)
    - Autonomic hyperactivity (e.g, sweating or pulse rate >100)
    - Increased hand tremor
    - Insomnia
    - Nausea or vomiting
    - Transient visual, tactile, or auditory hallucinations
    - Psychomotor agitation
    - Anxiety
    - Grand mal seizures
  - C. The symptoms in criterion B cause clinically significant distress or impairment in social, occupational, or other important areas of functioning
  - D. The symptoms are not due to a general medical condition and are not better accounted for by another mental disorder
- *Appearance of Alcohol withdrawal symptoms*:

Time	Symptoms
6–12 hours	Minor withdrawal symptoms: insomnia, tremulousness, anxiety, GIT upset, headache, diaphoresis, palpitations, anorexia
12–24 hours	Alcoholic hallucinosis: visual, auditory, or tactile hallucinations
24–48 hours	Withdrawal seizures: generalized tonic-clonic seizures
48–72 hours	Delirium tremens: visual hallucinations, disorientation, tachycardia, hypertension, low-grade fever, agitation, diaphoresis[Q]

- *Treatment*:
  - Chlordiazepoxide
  - Diazepam
  - Lorazepam
  - Clonidine
  - Haloperidol

IX B. DISULFIRAM

- Disulfiram is '**tetraethylthiuram disulfide**', a deterrent agent used for alcohol
- Dose:

- First week: 250-500 mg per day
- Maintenance treatment: 250 mg per day

- *Mechanism of action*: When a person on Disulfiram ingests alcohol, alcohol-derived acetaldehyde cannot be oxidised to acetate; this leads to accumulation of acetaldehyde in blood
  - It leads to '**Disulfiram-ethanol reaction (DER)**: Flushing, tachycardia, hypotension, tachypnoea, palpitations, headache, sweating, nausea, vomiting, giddiness
  - DER onset occurs in 30 minutes: Full blown in 1 hour and subsides in 2 hours)
  - DER can be life threatening: Shock, convulsions, coma, myocardial infarction, hypoxia
- *Contraindications*[Q]:
  - Pregnancy (first trimester[Q])
  - Coronary heart disease
  - Live failure
  - Chronic renal failure
  - Peripheral neuropathy
- *Other alcohol-deterrent agents*[Q]:
  - Metronidazole
  - Calcium citrate carbide
  - Animal charcoal
  - Coprinus atramentarius
  - Sulfonylureas
  - Cephalosporins
  - Griseofulvin

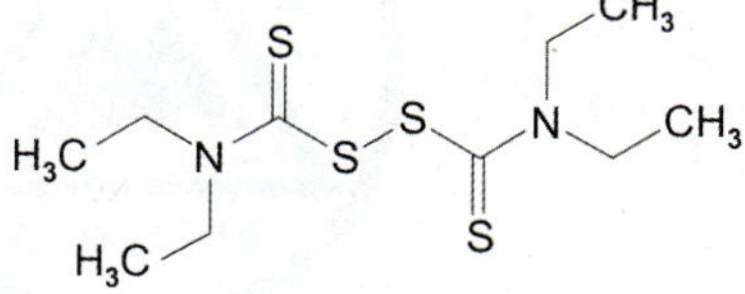

Fig. Disulfiram

Topper's Edge

Disulfiram Effect

- Disulfiram effect[Q] refers to an adverse effect of a particular medication in causing an unpleasant hypersensitivity to alcohol, similar to the effect caused by disulfiram administration
  - **Disulfiram**[Q]
  - Antibiotics (Nitroimidazoles): **Metronidazole**[Q]
  - First-generation Sulfonylureas: Tolbutamide, Chlorpropamide
  - Cephalosporin drugs: Cefoperazone, Cefamandole, Cefotetan
  - **Griseofulvin**[Q] (Oral antifungal drug)
  - Procarbazine
  - Temposil (Citrated calcium carbimide)
  - Mushrooms: Coprine (Tippler's bane), Clitocybe clavipes, Suillellus luridus

IMAGE-BASED QUESTIONS

1. **Anonymous group represented by symbol (photograph) is for** ***[Recent Question 2014]***

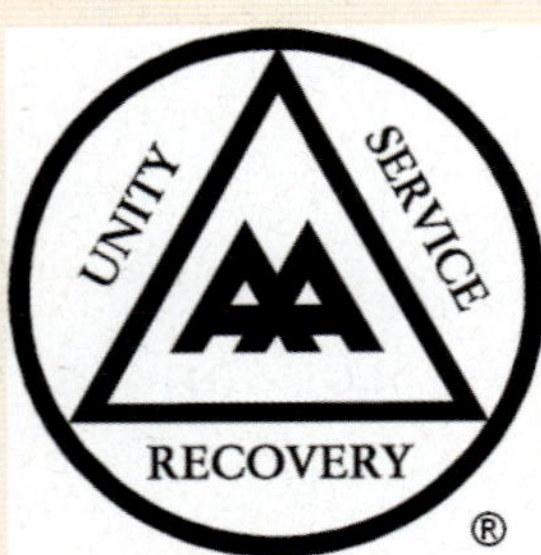

a. Tobacco b. Alcohol
c. Cannabis d. Cocaine

2. **Most severe withdrawal syndrome of dependence shown in photograph is**

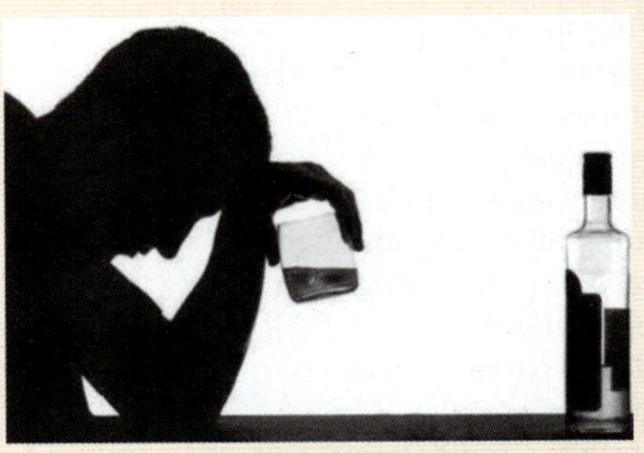

a. Delirium tremens b. Alcoholic seizures
c. Alcoholic hallucinosis d. Vomiting

3. **Deterrent agents used for substance shown in photograph include all except**

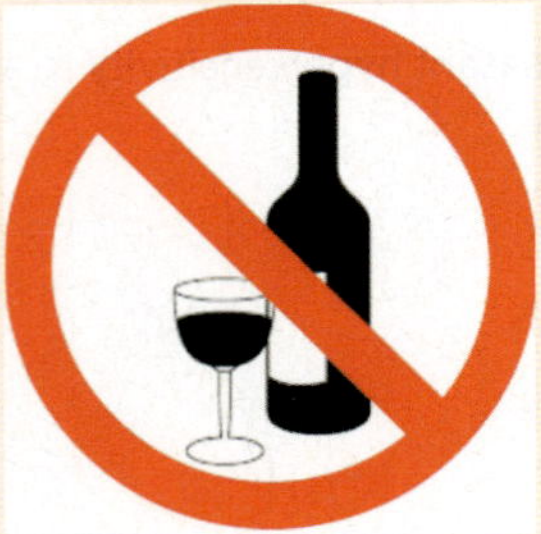

a. Disulfiram
b. Citrate calcium carbide
c. Acamprosate
d. Metronidazole

4. **Body fluid level of substance use at which coma occur .....** ***[Recent Question 2013]***

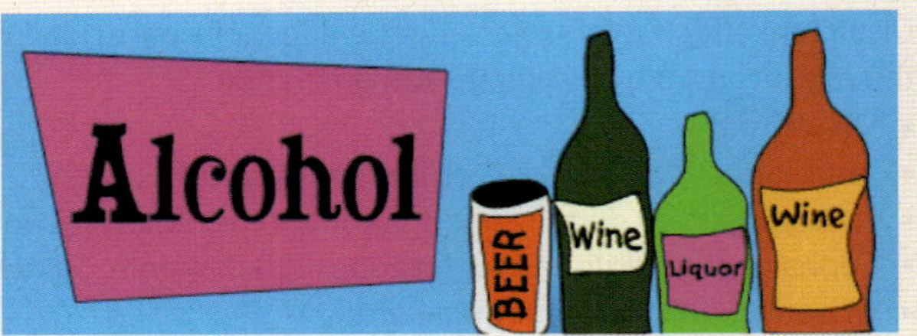

a. 50–100 mg%
b. 100–200 mg%
c. 200–300 mg%
d. >350 mg%

Psychiatry

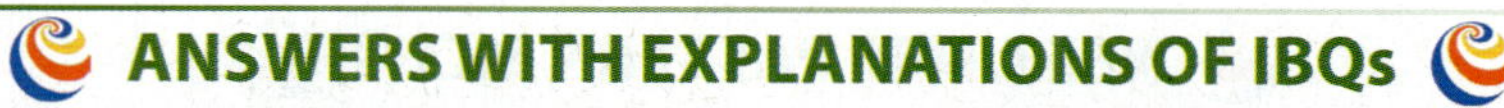

ANSWERS WITH EXPLANATIONS OF IBQs

1. Ans. (b) Alcohol *[Ref. Alcoholics Anonymous]*

- Alcoholics anonymous: An international mutual aid fellowship founded in 1935 by Bill Wilson and Dr. Bob Smith in Akron, Ohio
- AA states that its primary purpose is to help alcoholics "to stay sober and help other alcoholics achieve sobriety

2. Ans. (a) Delirium tremens *[Ref. Niraj Ahuja, 7/e p38,41]*

- Alcohol withdrawal: A set of symptoms when an individual reduces or stops alcohol consumption after prolonged periods of excessive alcohol intake
- Clinical presentation: Hangover next morning (MC withdrawal syndrome), Mild tremors (MC symptom), Nausea/vomiting, Weakness/insomnia/anxiety, Delirium tremens (Most severe withdrawal syndrome), Alcoholic seizures (Rum fits), Alcoholic hallucinosis

3. Ans. (c) Acamprosate *[Ref. Niraj Ahuja, 7/e p42]*

Treatment of Alcohol Dependence

- Detoxification agents: Benzodiazepines, Chlordiazepoxide, Diazepam, Vitamin B1 administration
- Anticraving agents: Acamprosate, Naltrexone, SSRIs (Fluoxetine)
- Deterrent agents: Disulfiram, Metronidazole, Calcium citrate carbide, Animal charcoal, Coprinus atramentarius, Sulfonylureas, Cephalosporins, Griseofulvin

4. Ans. (d) >350 mg% *[Ref. Niraj Ahuja, 7/e p39]*

- Alcohol intoxication with blood level of alcohol:
  - 150-200 mg%: CNS depression (after brief excitation), Increased reaction time/Slow thinking/Poor motor control, Dysarthria/Ataxia/Poor motor control, Uninhibited behaviour, Amnesia/black-outs
  - 300-450 mg%: Drowsiness, Respiratory depression, Coma
  - 400-800 mg%: Death

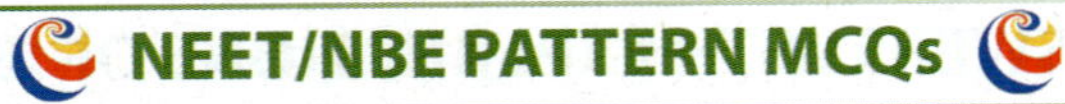

NEET/NBE PATTERN MCQs

1. **Alcohol withdrawal is treated with** *[Recent Question 2016]*
   a. Naltrexone b. Disulfiram
   c. Chlordiazepoxide d. Acamprosate
2. **All of the following drugs are used to prevent release and maintain abstinence in cases of alcohol withdrawal except** *[Recent Question 2016]*
   a. Disulfiram b. Acamprosate
   c. Naltrexone d. Propranolol
3. **Following is true about Alcoholic dependence syndrome except** *[Recent Question 2016]*
   a. No tolerance b. Withdrawal symptoms
   c. CAGE questionnaire d. Physical dependence
4. **Drugs used for treatment of Delirium tremens is/are** *[Recent Question 2016, 2017]*
   a. Diazepam b. Quetiapine
   c. Chlordiazepoxide d. Both a and c
5. **Drug of choice for Alcohol withdrawal** *[Recent Question 2016]*
   a. Metronidazole b. Chlordiazepoxide
   c. Disulfiram d. Naltrexone
6. **Alcoholic patient feels like insects running over him, it is known as** *[Recent Question 2016]*
   a. Formication b. Delusion
   c. Dementia d. Delirium
7. **Cage test in used for diagnosis of** *[Recent Question 2016]*
   a. Opioid abuse b. Schizophrenia
   c. Alcoholism d. Paranoid psychosis
8. **Disulfiram like reaction is not seen with** *[NBE FMGE September 2008]*
   a. Disulfiram b. Amoxycillin
   c. Metronidazole d. Cefoperazone
9. **A 40-year-old man presents with a 20-year history of alcohol intake with a 10-year history of a dependence pattern. He presents with a 2 day history of altered behavior, restlessness, tremors, sleep disturbance, irritability and difficulty in walking. On examination he has gaze palsy and is disoriented. What is the most likely diagnosis?** *[Recent Question 2017, NBE DNB June 2011]*
   a. Delirium tremens
   b. Wernicke's encephalopathy
   c. Korsakoff's psychosis
   d. Alcohol induced psychosis
10. **Wernicke's encephalopathy features are all except** *[Recent Question 2012]*
    a. Confusion b. Ataxia
    c. Aphasia d. Nystagmus
11. **The Disulfiram-alcohol reaction occurs due to the inhibition of which enzyme?** *[NBE DNB June 2011]*
    a. Alcohol reductase
    b. Alcohol dehydrogenase
    c. Aldehyde reductase
    d. Aldehyde dehydrogenase
12. **Most common symptom of Alcohol withdrawal is** *[NBE FMGE September 2006, AIIMS May 2015, Recent Question 2015]*
    a. Body ache
    b. Tremor
    c. Diarrhoea
    d. Nasal stuffiness
13. **Least severe type of alcoholism is** *[NBE DNB 1992]*
    a. Alpha b. Beta
    c. Gamma d. Epsilon type
14. **Wernicke's encephalopathy is due to deficiency of** *[NBE FMGE September 2012]*
    a. Vitamin A b. Vitamin B1
    c. Vitamin B6 d. Vitamin B12
15. **Magnan's phenomenon is seen in addiction of** *[NBE FMGE September 2006]*
    a. LSD b. Cocaine
    c. Amphetamine d. Alcohol
16. **Wernicke's encephalopathy is characterised by** *[UPSC 2010]*
    a. Mental impairment, ophthalmoplegia, cerebellar ataxia
    b. Delirium, facial palsy, cerebellar ataxia
    c. Ophthalmoplegia, hearing loss, cerebellar ataxia
    d. Ophthalmoplegia, facial palsy, cerebellar ataxia
17. **Combination of alcohol and Disulfiram results in nausea and hypertension as a result of accumulation of** *[NBE FMGE March 2007]*
    a. NADH b. Methanol
    c. Acetate d. Acetaldehyde
18. **Heavy users of alcohol are from** *[NBE DNB 1992]*
    a. Upper social class
    b. Middle class
    c. Lower class
    d. None of social class predominance
19. **Delirium and amnestic reaction are seen with** *[NBE FMGE September 2005]*
    a. Alcohol b. Opiates
    c. Cannabis d. Amphetamines
20. **Direct evidence of alcohol addiction is** *[NBE DNB 1995]*
    a. Memory disturbance b. Confabulation
    c. Cirrhosis d. Withdrawal symptoms
21. **Alcohol hallucinations occur within** *[NBE FMGE September 2005]*
    a. 24 hours b. 36 hours
    c. 72 hours d. 96 hours
22. **Following are withdrawal symptoms of alcohol, except** *[NBE DNB 1996]*
    a. Tremors b. Hallucinations
    c. Seizures d. Drowsiness
23. **Most severe Alcohol withdrawal syndrome** *[NBE FMGE September 2005]*
    a. Tremors
    b. Delirium tremens
    c. Hangover
    d. Nausea and vomiting

24. Hangover following alcohol consumption can be treated with *[Recent Question 2012, 2015]*
a. Pyridoxine b. Thiamine
c. Riboflavin d. Niacin

25. Recommended treatment for extremely agitated behaviour by a person who is grossly intoxicated with alcohol is *[NBE FMGE March 2003]*
a. Diazepam b. Phenobarbital
c. Chlorpromazine d. Haloperidol

26. The FAST questionnaire is used for identification of *[NBE FMGE September 2011]*
a. Smoking problems b. Alcohol problems
c. Sleep problems d. Memory problems

27. Match the following blood alcohol concentration and characteristics *[NBE DNB 1993]*
I. 0.015-0.055 (i) Slurred speech
II. 0.100 (ii) Emotional instability
III. 0.150-0.200 (iii) Legally intoxicated
IV. 0.200-0.300 (iv) Blurred vision
a. I (i), II (iii), III (ii), IV (iv)
b. I (iii), II (ii), III (iv), IV (i)
c. I (iv), II (ii), III (iii), IV (i)
d. I (i), II (ii), III (iii), IV (iv)

28. All are associated with Wernicke's encephalopathy except *[Recent Question 2012][AIIMSPG 2005]*
a. Cog wheel rigidity
b. Alteration in mental function
c. VIth nerve palsy
d. Ataxia

29. After cessation of drinking in a person dependent on alcohol, when does the risk of alcoholic seizures peak? *[NBE FMGE March 2012]*
a. 1-12 hrs after cessation of alcohol
b. 12-24 hrs after cessation of alcohol
c. 24-48 hrs after cessation of alcohol
d. 48-72 hrs after cessation of alcohol

30. Alcohol ingestion may give Disulfiram-like-reaction with *[UPSC 1998]*
a. Hydroxyquinolone b. Furazolidone
c. Sulphonamide d. Metronidazole

31. All of the following may be used for detoxification therapy of chronic alcoholism except *[NBE FMGE March 2012]*
a. Naltrexone b. Disulfiram
c. Flumazenil d. Acamprosate

32. Alcohol withdrawal is not associated with? *[Recent Question 2017]*
a. Seizure
b. Amnesia
c. Tremors
d. Delirium

33. Irresistible urge to drink alcohol is called? *[Recent Question 2017]*
a. Kleptomania
b. Pyromania
c. Dipsomania
d. Trichotillomania

34. Loading dose of diazepam for alcohol withdrawal is? *[Recent Question 2017]*
a. 80 mg
b. 50 mg
c. 40 mg
d. 20 mg

35. Tolerance is seen in? *[Recent Question 2017]*
a. Alcohol dependence syndrome
b. Schizophrenia
c. OCD
d. All of the above

36. Most common hallucination seen in Alcoholics is? *[Recent Question 2017]*
a. Visual
b. Auditory
c. Tactile
d. Olfactory

37. Alcohol dependence is seen which of the following phase *[Recent Question 2017]*
a. Oral b. Phallic
c. Anal d. Latency

38. Chronic alcoholism with thiamine deficiency leads to which enzyme defect? *[Recent Question 2017]*
a. Transaldolase
b. Glucose deaminase
c. Glycogen dehydrogenase
d. Pyruvate dehydrogenase

39. Morbid jealousy is associated with which addiction? *[Recent Question 2017]*
a. Alcohol b. Heroin
c. LSD d. Charas

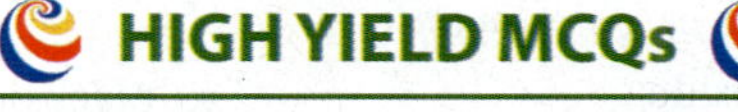

1. Which of the following drugs approved for alcoholism acts as an antagonist to NMDA (N-methyl-D-aspartate) receptor? *[APPG 2016]*
a. Acamprosate b. Naltrexone
c. Oxazepam d. Disulfiram

2. Which one of the following is TRUE regarding alcoholism? *[APPG 2016]*
a. Haloperidol is the drug of choice in rehabilitation of alcoholics
b. DSM-5 requires at least 7 of 11 criteria to be fulfilled to label as Alcohol use disorder
c. Elevated blood levels of GGT, CDT and uric acid
d. Alcohol reduces GABA & dopamine in the brain

3. Which drug is NOT used to treat Alcohol-dependence? *[All India PGMEE 2011]*
a. Naltrexone b. Flumazenil
c. Disulfiram d. Acamprosate

4. Wernicke's encephalopathy can be prevented by *[PGI 2001, AIIMS PGMEE 1998, Recent Question 2015]*
   a. IV saline
   b. Large amounts of glucose
   c. Thiamine supplement
   d. Imipramine

5. Korsakoff's psychosis is diagnosed by *[All India PGMEE 2000]*
   a. Peripheral neuropathy
   b. Visual hallucination
   c. Impairment of long term memory
   d. Seizures

6. Korsakoff's syndrome true is *[PGI 2000, UP PGMEE 2003, JIPMER PGMEE 2001]*
   a. Cerebral cortex is mostly affected
   b. Learning is relatively normal
   c. Retrograde memory is not affected
   d. Cannot be caused by malnutrition
   e. Confabulation may be present

7. Not a feature of Wernicke's Korsakoff syndrome *[AIIMS PGMEE 1994]*
   a. Ataxia
   b. Confusion
   c. Normal pupillary response
   d. Ophthalmoplegia

8. Site of lesion in Korsakoff's psychosis is *[AIIMS PGMEE 1996]*
   a. Frontal lobe b. Corpus striatum
   c. Mammillary Body d. Cingulate gyrus

9. True about alcoholic dependence syndrome *[PGI 2009]*
   a. Tolerance b. Withdrawal
   c. CAGE questionnaire d. Physical dependence
   e. No psychological dependence

10. Psychiatric complications of alcohol dependence *[PGI 2001]*
   a. Anxiety b. Suicide
   c. Depression d. Schizophrenia
   e. Mania

11. Wernicke's encephalopathy involves which part of CNS *[PGI 2000]*
   a. Mammillary body b. Thalamus
   c. Frontal lobe d. Arcuate fasciculus

12. Most common symptom of alcohol withdrawal is *[Recent Question 2015, All India PGMEE 2007]*
   a. Body ache b. Tremor
   c. Diarrhoea d. Rhinorrhea

13. Characteristic of alcohol withdrawal *[AIIMS PGMEE 1991]*
   a. Hallucination b. Illusion
   c. Delusion d. Drowsiness

14. In alcohol withdrawal drug of choice is *[AIIMS PGMEE 1990]*
   a. Benzodiazepine b. Chlordiazepoxide
   c. Lithium d. Haloperidol

15. Alcoholic paranoia is associated with *[All India PGMEE 2010]*
   a. Fixed delusions b. Hallucinations
   c. Drowsiness d. Impulse agitation

16. Which ones are used for long term alcohol withdrawal? *[PGI 2009]*
   a. Acamprosate b. Disulfiram
   c. Naloxone d. Naltrexone
   e. Monosulfiram

17. Disulfiram acts by *[All India PGMEE 1999]*
   a. Inhibiting alcohol dehydrogenase
   b. Inhibiting aldehyde dehydrogenase
   c. Both d. None

18. 35-year-old male comes with history of 1 year of alcoholism and past history of ataxia with bilateral lateral rectus palsy. He was admitted and treated what changes expected to see *[PGI 2008]*
   a. Progression to Korsakoff's psychosis
   b. Residual ataxia in 5% of patients
   c. Extraocular palsy disappear in hour
   d. Immediate relief from symptoms

19. All are the features of Korsakoff's syndrome except *[JIPMER PGMEE 1998, UP PGMEE2002]*
   a. Confabulation b. Retrograde amnesia
   c. Antegrade amnesia d. Defective motor skill

20. All are relatively normal in Korsakoff's psychosis except *[MAHE PGMEE 2003, Karnataka PGMEE 2003, J & K PGMEE 2000]*
   a. Implicit memory b. Intelligence
   c. Language d. Learning

21. True statement about Korsakoff's psychosis is *[Rohtak PGMEE 2000, JIPMER PGMEE 1999, UP PGMEE 1999, PGI 1997]*
   a. Severe anterograde + Mild retrograde memory defect
   b. Mild anterograde + severe retrograde memory defect
   c. Only anterograde memory defect
   d. Only retrograde memory defect

22. Confabulation is typically seen in *[MP PGMEE 1997, Recent Question 2015]*
   a. Mania b. Depression
   c. Alcoholism d. Delirium

23. In Korsakoff psychosis all are seen except *[JIPMER PGMEE 1998]*
   a. Loss of remote memory
   b. Loss of intellectual function but preservation of memory
   c. Lack of insight, unable to understand the disability
   d. Reversible state

24. Korsakoff's psychosis is seen in *[Rajasthan PGMEE 2002]*
   a. CRF b. Alcoholism
   c. Marasmus d. Cirrhosis

25. Not a feature of Korsakoff psychosis is *[AIIMS PGMEE 1994]*
   a. Normal sensorium
   b. Loss of recent memory
   c. Loss of long term memory
   d. Confabulation

26. By which alcohol dependence is best indicated *[AIIMS PGMEE 1995]*
   a. Black outs b. Early morning drinking
   c. Withdrawal symptoms d. Physical dependence

27. Features of alcohol withdrawal are all except *[All India PGMEE 1998]*
   a. Epileptic seizure b. Restlessness
   c. Hypersomnolence d. Hallucination

28. A 30-year-old male with history of alcohol abuse for 15 years is brought to the hospital emergency with complaints of fearfulness, misrecognition, talking to self, aggressive behavior, tremulousness and seeing snakes and

reptiles that are not visible to others around him. There is history of drinking alcohol two days prior to the onset of the present complaints. He is most likely suffering from *[AIIMS PGMEE 2003]*

a. Delirium tremens b. Alcoholic hallucinosis
c. Schizophrenia d. Seizure disorder

29. An alcohol addicted presents in emergency with irrelevant talking & disoriented to time, place and person there is H/O not taking alcohol from last 3 days & no head injury. He also have visual hallucination. The diagnosis is *[All India PGMEE 2002]*

a. Dementia praecox b. Delirium tremens
c. Schizophrenia d. Korsakoff's psychosis

30. A 45-year-old male with a history of alcohol dependence presents with confusion, nystagmus and ataxia. Examination reveals 6th cranial nerve weakness. He is most likely to be suffering from *[All India PGMEE 2005]*

a. Korsakoff's psychosis b. Wernicke encephalopathy
c. De clerambault syndrome
d. Delirium tremens

31. True about delirium tremens *[PGI 2005]*

a. Clouding of consciousness
b. Coarse tremors
c. Chronic delirious behaviour
d. Hallucination
e. Autonomic dysfunction

32. A 40-year-old male, with history of daily alcohol consumption for the last 7 years, is brought to the hospital emergency room with acute onset of seeing snakes all around him in the room, not recognizing family members,violent behavior and tremulousness for few hours. There is history of his having missed the alcohol drink since 2 days. Examination reveals increased blood pressure, tremors, increased psychomotor activity, fearful affect, hallucinatory behaviour, disorientation, impaired judgment and insight. He is most likely to be suffering from *[All India PGMEE 2005]*

a. Alcoholic hallucinosis
b. Delirium tremens
c. Wernicke encephalopathy
d. Korsakoff's psychosis

33. A 40-year-old man presents to casualty with history of regular and heavy use of alcohol for ten years and morning drinking for one year. The last alcohol intake was three days back. There is no history of head injury or seizures. On examination, there is no icterus, sign of hepatic encephalopathy or focal neurological sign. The patient had coarse tremors, visual hallucinations and had disorientation to time. Which of the following is the best medicine to be prescribed for such a patient? *[All India PGMEE 2004]*

a. Diazepam b. Haloperidol
c. Imipramine d. Naltrexone

34. In an uncomplicated case of alcohol withdrawal, the drug which can be given safely is *[AIIMS PGMEE 2008]*

a. Benzodiazepines b. Clonidine
c. Morphine d. Disulfiram

35. Treatment of Alcohol withdrawal *[PGI 2007]*

a. Beta-blocker b. BZD
c. Amitriptyline d. SSRIs

36. Treatment of Delirium tremens is *[AIIMS PGMEE 1991]*

a. Promethazine b. Chlordiazepoxide
c. Diazepam d. Haloperidol

37. All are anticraving agent for alcohol except *[AIIMS PGMEE 2009, NIMSET 2015]*

a. Lorazepam b. Naltrexone
c. Topiramate d. Acamprosate

38. Infants born to mothers who are heavy drinkers are at increased risk of which of the following problems? *[ESI IMO 2014]*

a. Mental retardation b. Chronic liver disease
c. Excessive birth weight d. Chorioretinitis

39. Alcohol intake during pregnancy causes, all except *[ESI IMO 2014]*

a. Brachycephaly b. Microcephaly
c. Hyperkinetic movements d. Congenital anomalies

40. False about Korsakoff syndrome is/are *[PGI November 2014]*

a. Insight present b. Retrograde amnesia
c. Thiamine deficiency d. Chronic alcohol abuse
e. Severe malnutrition

41. A patient taking 120 mL alcohol daily since last 12 years is brought to a hospital by wife. He is diagnosed as Alcohol dependency syndrome. Drug not to be given is *[AIIMS November 2014]*

a. Disulfiram b. Acamprosate
c. Naltrexone d. Phenytoin

42. A 55 years aged chronic alcoholic male, presented with irrelevant talks, tremor and sweating. He had his last drink 3 days back. What will the probable diagnosis? *[Recent Question 2018]*

a. Delirium tremens
b. Korsakoff psychosis
c. Post-acute withdrawal syndrome
d. Discontinuation syndrome

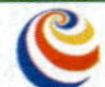 **NEET/NBE PATTERN MCQs ANSWERS WITH EXPLANATIONS** 

1. Ans. (c) Chlordiazepoxide

[Ref. Adult Clinical Psychology by Carr, 2/e p209]

- Benzodiazepines (e.g. chlordiazepoxide) represent the current treatment of choice for acute withdrawal of alcohol

2. Ans. (d) Propranolol

[Ref. Niraj Ahuja, 7/e p41-42]

Detoxification (Treatment of Alcohol Withdrawal Symptoms)

- Benzodiazepines: Chlordiazepoxide, Diazepam
- Vitamin B1 administration
- Hydration

Alcohol Dependence Treatment

- Behaviour therapy
- Psychotherapy
- Group therapy
- Deterrent agents: Disulfiram, Metronidazole, Calcium citrate carbide, Animal charcoal, Coprinus atramentarius, Sulfonylureas, Cephalosporins, Griseofulvin
- Anticraving agents: Acamprosate, Naltrexone, SSRIs (Fluoxetine)
- Psychosocial rehabilitation

3. Ans. (a) No tolerance

[Ref. Niraj Ahuja, 7/e p35]

- Alcohol use is associated with Physical dependence, Psychological dependence and Tolerance

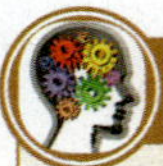

Also Remember

- Cocaine is NOT associated with Tolerance
- LSD is NOT associated with Physical dependence

4. Ans. (d) Both a and c

[Ref. MRCP 1 by Waring, 3/e p108]

- Long-acting agents (Diazepam, Chlordiazepoxide) are used for the prevention and treatment of delirium tremens in the setting of acute alcohol withdrawal

5. Ans. (b) Chlordiazepoxide

[Ref. Niraj Ahuja, 7/e p40]

Treatment of Alcohol Withdrawal

- Long- acting benzodiazepines are required for the
- Drug of choice is Chlordiazepoxide
- Diazepam may be used, especially if an intravenous agent is required
- Lorazepam is the DOC in chronic liver disease

6. Ans. (a) Formication

[Ref. Primary Health Care Psychiatry by Baumann, 1/e p79]

Formication

- Tactile hallucinations with sensation of insects crawling under one's skin
- Seen in:
  - Cocaine use
  - Methamphetamine use
  - Alcohol withdrawal

7. Ans. (c) Alcoholism

[Ref. Clinical Topics in Addiction by Day, 1/e p114-15]

- **CAGE questionnaire** is a four-item alcohol screening instrument with demonstrated relevance for primary care in clinical, educational, and research settings
- Family CAGE is intended to screen for alcohol problems in families, not to diagnose family alcoholism

8. Ans. (b) Amoxycillin

[Ref. Niraj Ahuja, 7/e p42]

Alcohol Deterrent/ Sensitizing Agents

[**Mnemonic:** **A**gents **C**ausing **D**isulfiram-like-reaction **M**ainly **C**ause **C**oarse **T**remors]

- **A**nimal charcoal
- **C**alcium citrate carbide
- **D**isulfiram
- **M**etronidazole
- **C**oprinus atramentarius
- **C**ephalosporins—first generation: Cefoperazone, Cefotetan
- **T**olbutamide

9. Ans. (b) Wernicke's encephalopathy

[Ref. Niraj Ahuja, 7/e p38]

Wernicke's Encephalopathy

- *Description*: Acute reaction to severe thiamine (Vitamin B1) deficiency in chronic alcohol use
- *Features*:
  - Ocular signs: Nystagmus, Ophthalmoplegia, Retinal hemorrhages, Papilledema
  - Higher mental function disturbances: Disorientation, Confusion, Recent memory disturbance, Poor attention span, Ataxia
  - Peripheral neuropathy, VI nerve palsy
  - Severe malnutrition

10. Ans. (c) Aphasia

[Ref. Niraj Ahuja, 7/e p38]

11. Ans. (d) Aldehyde dehydrogenase

[Ref. Niraj Ahuja, 7/e p42]

Disulfiram Ethanol Reaction (Mechanism of Action)

- Disulfiram inhibits liver enzyme aldehyde dehydrogenase
- Alcohol derived acetaldehyde cannot be oxidized to acetate
- Accumulation of acetaldehyde in blood

12. Ans. (b) Tremor

[Ref. Niraj Ahuja, 7/e p38]

Clinical Presentation of Alcohol Withdrawal

- *Hangover next morning*: Most common withdrawal syndrome
- Mild tremors (Most common symptom: 34% patients)
- Nausea, vomiting
- Weakness, insomnia, anxiety
- *Delirium tremens*: Most severe withdrawal syndrome
- *Alcoholic seizures (Rum fits)*
- *Alcoholic hallucinosis*

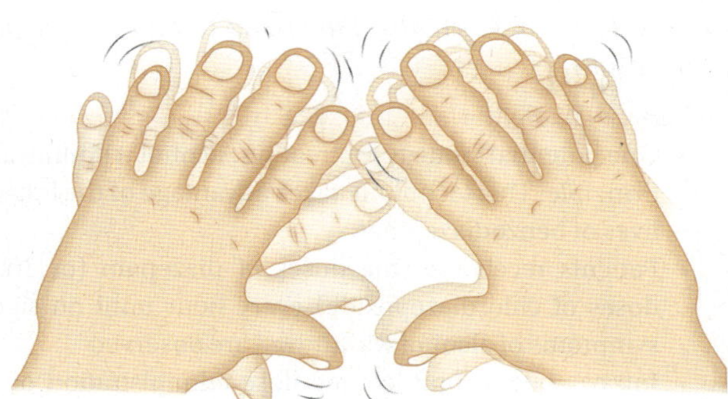

Fig. Fine tremor

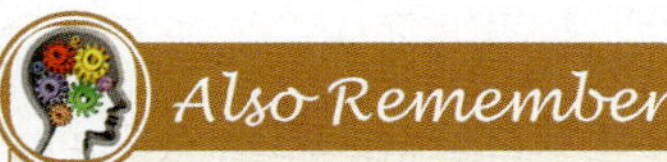

- *Kindling*: Repeated withdrawal from benzodiazepines or alcohol leads to increasingly severe withdrawal symptoms, including an increased risk of seizures

13. Ans. (d) Epsilon type
[Ref. Niraj Ahuja, 7/e p36]

14. Ans. (b) Vitamin B1
[Ref. Niraj Ahuja, 7/e p38]

15. Ans. (b) Cocaine
[Ref. Niraj Ahuja, 7/e p46-48]

- ***Acute intoxication of Cocaine*:**
  - Tachycardia, hypertension, sweating, nausea, vomiting
  - Hypomania with increased psychomotor activity
  - Impaired judgement and occupational functioning
- ***Chronic use of Cocaine*:**
  - *Magnan's symptoms (Cocaine bugs)*: Tactile hallucinations of insects crawling beneath skin surface
  - Acute anxiety, psychotic episodes, delirium, delusional episodes
  - Respiratory depression, myocardial infarction

16. Ans. (a) Mental impairment, ophthalmoplegia, cerebellar ataxia
[Ref. Niraj Ahuja, 7/e p38]

17. Ans. (d) Acetaldehyde
[Ref. Niraj Ahuja, 7/e p41]

- *Mechanism of action of Disulfiram*: When a person on Disulfiram ingests alcohol, alcohol-derived acetaldehyde cannot be oxidised to acetate; this leads to accumulation of acetaldehyde in blood
  - ***Main mechanism of action*: Inhibition of acetaldehyde dehydrogenase**
  - *It leads to 'Disulfiram-ethanol reaction (DER)*

18. Ans. (d) None of social class predominance
[Ref. Niraj Ahuja, 7/e p36]

19. Ans. (a) Alcohol
[Ref. Niraj Ahuja, 7/e p27, 38]

- *Clinical presentation of alcoholism*:

Acute intoxication	• CNS depression (after brief excitation), Increased reaction time, slow thinking, poor motor control, Dysarthria, ataxia, poor motor control, Uninhibited behaviour • Amnesia/ black-outs • Drowsiness, Respiratory depression • Coma, Death
Chronic alcohol use	• Wernicke's encephalopathy • Korsakoff's psychosis • Marchiafava-Bignami disease • Alcohol dementia • Peripheral neuropathy • Cerebellar degeneration
Alcohol withdrawal	• Hangover next morning • Mild tremors • Nausea, vomiting • Weakness, insomnia, anxiety • Delirium tremens • Alcoholic seizures (Rum fits) • Alcoholic hallucinosis

20. Ans. (d) Withdrawal symptoms
[Ref. Niraj Ahuja, 7/e p38]

21. Ans. (a) 24 hours
[Ref. Niraj Ahuja, 7/e p38]

Alcohol Withdrawal Syndrome

- *Delirium tremens*: Within 2-4 days of alcohol withdrawal
- *Alcoholic seizures (rum fits)*: Within 12-48 hours of alcohol withdrawal
- *Alcoholic hallucinosis*: Within 12-24 hours of alcohol withdrawal

22. Ans. (d) Drowsiness
[Ref. Niraj Ahuja, 7/e p38]

23. Ans. (b) Delirium tremens
[Ref. Niraj Ahuja, 7/e p38]

24. Ans. (b) Thiamine
[Ref. Basic Pharmacology for Nurses by Clayton, 16/e p837]

25. Ans. (a) Diazepam
[Ref. Niraj Ahuja, 7/e p40]

- *Treatment of alcohol withdrawal symptoms (Detoxification)*:
  - Benzodiazepines
    1. Chlordiazepoxide
    2. Diazepam
  - Vitamin B1 administration
  - Hydration

26. Ans. (b) Alcohol problems
[Ref. Clinical Topics in Addiction by Ed Day, 1/e p114-15]

Alcohol use Screening Questionnaires

- **CAGE Questionnaire**: Cut down, Annoyed, Guilt, Eye opener
  - Disadvantage: Does not assess risky levels of consumption
- **AUDIT Questionnaire**: Alcohol use disorder identification test
  - Disadvantage: Lengthier questionnaire

- **FAST Questionnaire**:
  - Advantage: Quicker to administer and score
  - Scoring: Minimum 0; Maximum 16; Hazardous drinking ≥ 3

27. Ans. (c) I (iv), II (ii), III (iii), IV (i)
[Ref. Niraj Ahuja, 7/e p39]

28. Ans. (a) Cog wheel rigidity
[Ref. Niraj Ahuja, 7/e p38]

29. Ans. (c) 24-48 hrs after cessation of alcohol
[Ref. Oxford's Alcohol, Science, Policy and Public Health, 1/e p 291]

Alcohol Withdrawal Seizures (RUM FITS)
- Occurrence: 7-38 hours after cessation of alcohol drinking
- Peak: 24-48 hours after cessation of alcohol drinking

30. Ans. (d) Metronidazole
[Ref. Clinically Oriented Psychopharmacology by Buch, 1/e p226]

Drugs causing Disulfiram like Reaction
- Metronidazole
- Chloramphenicol
- Furazolidone
- Cefamandole
- Cefoperazone
- Chlorpropamide
- Ritonavir

31. Ans. (c) Flumazenil
[Ref. Niraj Ahuja, 7/e p40-42]

Treatment of Alcohol Dependence

Detoxification agents	Deterrent agents
• Benzodiazepines • Chlordiazepoxide • Diazepam • Vitamin B1 administration	• Disulfiram • Metronidazole • Calcium citrate carbide • Animal charcoal
Anti-craving agents • Acamprosate • Naltrexone • SSRIs (Fluoxetine)	• Coprinus atramentarius • Sulfonylureas • Cephalosporins • Griseofulvin

32. Ans. (b) Amnesia
[Ref. Niraj Ahuja, 7/e p37-38]
- Alcohol withdrawal may lead to hangover next morning (MC withdrawal syndrome), Mild tremors (MC symptom), Nausea/ vomiting, Weakness/ insomnia/ anxiety, Delirium tremens (Most severe withdrawal syndrome), Alcoholic seizures (Rum fits), Alcoholic hallucinosis

33. Ans. (c) Dipsomania
[Ref. Niraj Ahuja, 7/e p34, 36]

Dipsomania
- Episodic or periodic excessive alcohol abuse between periods of relative abstention
- It corresponds to Jellinek's 'epsilon alcoholism'
- Though rare, dipsomania is likely to be associated with quite severe personality disorders

Also Remember
- Dipsomania must be distinguished from 'Mania a potu': In Mania a potu, acute psychotic excitement follows ingestion of relatively small amounts of alcohol

34. Ans. (d) 20 mg
[Ref. American Psychiatric Publishing Textbook of Psychiatry, 5/e p1084]

Benzodiazepine loading-dose technique (Sellers et al. 1983)
- One potential strategy for treating Alcohol withdrawal
- Principle: This technique takes advantage of the long half-lives of benzodiazepines
- Patients receive 20 mg doses of diazepam (or 100 mg doses of chlordiazepoxide) every hour until no signs or symptoms of alcohol withdrawal are observed
- Intravenous or oral loading dose administration of diazepam is a simple, rapid, and effective treatment for alcohol withdrawal

35. Ans. (a) Alcohol dependence syndrome
[Ref. Niraj Ahuja, 7/e p35]
- Based on Jellinek's species of Alcohol dependence, Gamma (γ) subtype (Malignant alcoholism) is characterised by Progressive course, Physical dependence with tolerance and withdrawal symptoms, Psychological dependence, with inability to control drinking

36. Ans. (b) Auditory
[Ref. Niraj Ahuja, 7/e p38]
- Alcoholic hallucinosis differs from hallucinogen-induced hallucinosis in that the hallucinations are primarily auditory rather than visual
- Alcoholic hallucinosis is a condition in which hallucinations occur in the context of cessation or decrease in alcohol use in an alcohol-dependent patient, later visual hallucinations may follow

37. Ans. (a) Oral
[Ref. Sexuality Now by Carroll, 6/e p29]
- In Freud's theories, alcoholics have never passed beyond the oral phase of development in which the mouth maintains contact with the world
- The oral stage, lasts through the first 18 months of life
- According to Freud's theory, problems during this stage could result in an oral fixation, leading to behaviors such as cigarette smoking, overeating, fingernail chewing, or alcohol abuse

38. Ans. (d) Pyruvate dehydrogenase
[Ref. 100 Cases in Psychiatry by Dave, 1/e p70]
- **Thiamine (Vitamin B1),** critical for glucose metabolism, is a cofactor of alpha-ketoglutarate dehydrogenase and Pyruvate dehydrogenase enzymes (TCA cycle) and Transketolase enzyme (Pentose phosphate pathway)
- Chronic alcoholism may lead to severe B1 deficiency, usually associated with Wernicke's encephalopathy

39. Ans. (a) Alcohol
[Ref. Addiction Behaviour by Belle Glass, 1/e]

Pathological/morbid Jealousy
- Feelings of jealousy become so extreme that they can impinge destructively on the lives of those involved
- Association with alcoholism is well recognized, and it may be symptomatic of other psychiatric illnesses like Paranoid schizophrenia and depressive illness

 HIGH YIELD MCQs ANSWERS WITH EXPLANATIONS 

1. **Ans. (a) Acamprosate**
   [Ref. Drugs for Relapse Prevention of Alcoholism by Spanagel, 1/e p92]
   - Anticraving compound Acamprosate acts as a weak NMDA-receptor antagonist
   - Also modulates NMDA-receptor subunit expression

2. **Ans. (c) Elevated blood levels of GGT, CDT and uric acid**
   [Ref. Niraj Ahuja, 7/e p37]

Laboratory and Other Markers for Alcoholism
- Gamma-glutamyl transferase (GGT) > 40 IU/litre
- Mean corpuscular volume (MCV) > 92 fl
- Other lab markers (Alkaline phosphatase, Uric acid, Serum triglycerides, Creatine kinase, ALT, AST)
- Blood alcohol concentration
- Breath analyser
- Michigan alcoholism screening test (MAST)
- CAGE questionnaire (Score > 2 identifies problem drinkers)

Also Remember
- DSM-5 requires at least 2 of 11 criteria to be fulfilled to label as Alcohol use disorder
  - 2-3 criteria; Mild
  - 4-5 criteria: Moderate
  - 6 or more: Severe

3. **Ans. (b) Flumazenil**
   [Ref. Niraj Ahuja, 7/e p41-42]

Drugs for Treatment of Alcohol Dependence

Deterrent agents	Anticraving agents	Other agents
• Disulfiram • Citrated calcium carbide • Metronidazole • Animal charcoal	• Acamprosate • Naltrexone • SSRIs (Fluoxetine) • Topiramate	• Benzodiazepines • Antidepressants • Antipsychotics • Lithium, Carbamazepine

4. **Ans. (c) Thiamine supplement**
   [Ref. Basic Pharmacology for Nurses by Clayton, 16/e p837]

5. **Ans. NONE**
   [Ref. Niraj Ahuja, 7/e p39]

6. **Ans. (e) Confabulation may be present**
   [Ref. Niraj Ahuja, 7/e p39-40]

Korsakoff Psychosis
- **Damage to Dorsomedial nuclei of thalamus, Mammillary bodies**
- Confusion, Ataxia, Nystagmus
- Compensatory confabulation
- Impaired insight
- Ophthalmoplegia
- Memory loss (Usually recent memory impaired; Long term remote memory beyond retrograde amnesia usually spared)
  - Severe anterograde amnesia
  - Mild retrograde amnesia
- Defects in learning
- Death

7. **Ans. (c) Normal pupillary response**
   [Ref. Niraj Ahuja, 7/e p39-40]

8. **Ans. (c) Mammillary body**
   [Ref. Niraj Ahuja, 7/e p39-40]

9. **Ans. (a) Tolerance; (b) Withdrawal; (c) CAGE questionnaire; (d) Physical dependence**
   [Ref. Niraj Ahuja, 7/e p39]

10. **Ans. (a) Anxiety; (b) Suicide; (c) Depression**
    [Ref. Psychiatry at a Glance by Robertson, 5/e p43]

Complications of Alcohol Dependence

Neuropsychiatric complications	Psychiatric complications
• Wernicke's encephalopathy • Peripheral neuropathy • Erectile/ejaculatory impotence • Cerebellar degeneration • Dementia	• Depression • Suicidal ideas/ attempts • Severe anxiety • Insomnia

11. **Ans. (a) Mammillary body**
    [Ref. Niraj Ahuja, 7/e p39-40]

12. **Ans. (b) Tremor**
    [Ref. Clinical Neurology of Older Adult by Malamut, 2/e p517]

Alcohol Withdrawal Syndrome
- Tremor—Rest, postural, action (MC manifestation)
- Nausea/vomiting
- Hallucination/Illusion
- Delirium
- Agitation, restlessness
- Autonomic dysfunction
- Confabulation
- Generalized tonic-clonic seizures

13. **Ans. (a) Hallucination**
    [Ref. Clinical Neurology of Older Adult by Malamut, 2/e p517]

14. **Ans. (b) Chlordiazepoxide**
    [Ref. Niraj Ahuja, 7/e p40]

Drugs for Treatment of Alcohol Withdrawal
- Chlordiazepoxide **(DOC)**, Diazepam, Lorazepam
- Thiamine, Folic acid, Multivitamin
- Magnesium sulphate
- Phenytoin

15. Ans. (a) Fixed delusions
[Ref. Alcoholism: A Treatment Guide for Practitioners by Hewitt, 1/e p54]

- *Alcohol paranoia*: As alcoholism progresses, these usually become more pronounced and can very easily end up as fixed delusions

16. Ans. (a) Acamprosate; (b) Disulfiram; (d) Naltrexone
[Ref. Niraj Ahuja, 7/e p41-42]

17. Ans. (b) Inhibiting aldehyde dehydrogenase
[Ref. Niraj Ahuja, 7/e p42]

18. Ans. (b) Residual ataxia in 5% of patients; (c) Extraocular palsy disappear in hour
[Ref. Niraj Ahuja, 7/e p38]

19. Ans. (d) Defective motor skill
[Ref. Niraj Ahuja, 7/e p39-40]

20. Ans. (d) Learning
[Ref. Niraj Ahuja, 7/e p39-40]

21. Ans. (a) Severe anterograde + Mild retrograde memory defect
[Ref. Niraj Ahuja, 7/e p39-40]

22. Ans. (c) Alcoholism
[Ref. Clinical Neurology of Older Adult by Malamut, 2/e p517]

23. Ans. (a) Loss of remote memory
[Ref. Niraj Ahuja, 7/e p39-40]

24. Ans. (b) Alcoholism
[Ref. Niraj Ahuja, 7/e p39-40]

25. Ans. (a) Normal sensorium
[Ref. Niraj Ahuja, 7/e p39-40]

26. Ans. (c) Withdrawal symptoms
[Ref. Niraj Ahuja, 7/e p37]

27. Ans. (c) Hypersomnolence
[Ref. Clinical Neurology of Older Adult by Malamut, 2/e p517]

28. Ans. (a) Delirium tremens
[Ref. Niraj Ahuja, 7/e p38]

29. Ans. (b) Delirium tremens
[Ref. Niraj Ahuja, 7/e p38]

30. Ans. (b) Wernicke encephalopathy
[Ref. Niraj Ahuja, 7/e p38]

31. Ans. ALL CHOICES
[Ref. Niraj Ahuja, 7/e p38]

32. Ans. (b) Delirium tremens
[Ref. Niraj Ahuja, 7/e p38]

33. Ans. (a) Diazepam
[Ref. Niraj Ahuja, 7/e p40]

34. Ans. (a) Benzodiazepines
[Ref. Niraj Ahuja, 7/e p40]

35. Ans. (b) BZD
[Ref. Niraj Ahuja, 7/e p40]

36. Ans. (b) Chlordiazepoxide
[Ref. Niraj Ahuja, 7/e p40]

37. Ans. (a) Lorazepam
[Ref. Niraj Ahuja, 7/e p41-42]

38. Ans. (a) Mental retardation
[Ref. Pediatric Nutrition by Ekvall, 2/e p119]

Fetal Alcohol Syndrome

- Mental retardation (Mild to moderate)
- Microcephaly
- Hypotonia, Poor coordination
- Irritability (Infancy)
- Hyperactivity (Childhood)
- Less than 2 SD for height and weight
- Adipose tissue reduction
- Short palpebral fissures in eyes
- Short upturned nose
- Hypoplastic philtrum
- Hypoplastic maxilla
- Retrognathia, thin upper vermillion
- Micrognathia, relative prognathia (Adolescence)

39. Ans. (a) Brachycephaly
[Ref. Pediatric Nutrition by Ekvall, 2/e p119]

40. Ans. (a) Insight present
[Ref. Niraj Ahuja, 7/e p39]

41. Ans. (a) Disulfiram
[Ref. Niraj Ahuja, 7/e p40]

42. Ans. (a) Delirium tremens
[Ref. Niraj Ahuja, 7/e p38]

Delirium tremens (Shaking frenzy/ Spirit fingers)

- Most severe alcohol withdrawal syndrome
- Occurrence: Within 2-4 days of complete/significant abstinence
- Clinical presentation:
  - Autonomic disturbances (Tachycardia, fever, hypertension, sweating and pupillary dilatation)
  - Hallucinations, Insomnia, Dehydration, Clouding of consciousness, Agitation, Insomnia
  - Poor attention span and distractibility.
  - Vivid frightening visual (and also auditory) hallucinations and illusions,
  - Tactile hallucinations of insects crawling over the body
- Mortality: 5% (with treatment)—35% (without treatment)
- Drug of choice: Benzodiazepines

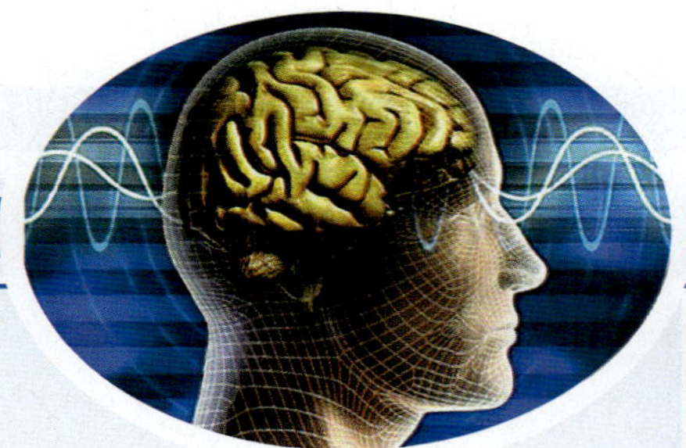

Chapter 10

Substance/Drug Abuse

THEORETICAL CONCEPTS

X A. DEFINITIONS AND CONCEPTS

- ***Drug***: Any substance that, when taken into living organism, may modify one or more of its functions
- ***Drug abuse***: Persistent or sporadic excessive drug use inconsistent with or unrelated to acceptable medical practice[Q]
  - Includes both drug addiction and habituation
- ***Drug addiction***: A state of periodic or chronic intoxication detrimental to an individual and society, produced by the repeated consumption of a drug (natural/synthetic[Q])
  - An overpowering desire or need to continue taking the drug and to obtain it by any means
  - A tendency to increase the dose
  - A psychic and something physical dependence on the effects of drug
- ***Drug dependence***: A state, psychic and sometimes also physical, resulting from the interaction between a living organism and a drug, characterized by behavioral and other responses that always include a compulsion to take the drug on a continuous or periodic basis in order to experience its psychic effects, and sometimes to avoid the discomfort of its absence
  - Tolerance may or may not be present
  - A person may be dependent on more than one drug
- ***Withdrawal syndrome***: After the repeated administration of certain dependence producing drugs, e.g. opioids, barbiturates and alcohol, abstinence can increase the intensity of drug seeking behavior because of the need to avoid or relieve withdrawal discomfort and/or physiological changes of sufficient severity to require medical treatment

X B. COCAINE USE DISORDER

- *Cocaine*: An alkaloid derived from Erythroxylum coca[Q]
- *Most common form used*: Cocaine HCl
- ***Mode of administration***: Oral, intranasal (***snorting***), smoking (*free basing*), parenterally[Q]
- *Mechanism of action*: Inhibits reuptake of dopamine, norepinephrine, serotonin
- *Mechanism of use*:
  - Cocaine runs: Binges
  - Cocaine crashes: Interruptions of use
  - **Speed balls**: Used in combination with opiates (heroin[Q])
- *Acute intoxication*:
  - Tachycardia, hypertension, sweating, nausea, vomiting
  - Hypomania with increased psychomotor activity
  - Impaired judgement and occupational functioning

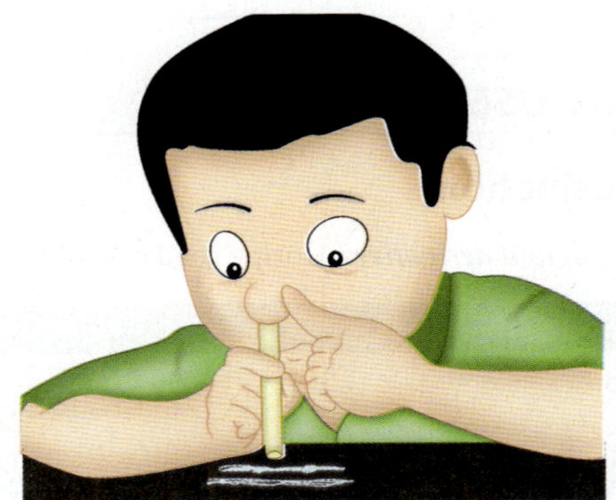

Fig. Snorting

- *Chronic use:*
  - **Magnan's symptoms (Cocaine bugs)**: Tactile hallucinations of insects crawling beneath skin surface[Q]
  - Acute anxiety, psychotic episodes, delirium, delusional episodes
  - Respiratory depression, myocardial infarction
- *Triphasic withdrawal syndrome*:

Phase	Substage	Duration	Clinical features
I (Crash phase)	i ii iii	9 hrs - 4 days	• Agitation, depression, craving, anorexia • Fatigue, depression, sleepiness • Exhaustion, hypersomnia, hyperphagia
II	i ii	4–7 days	• Normal sleep, improved mood • Anxiety, anhedonia, craving
III (Extinction phase)	i	7–10 days	• No symptoms but tendency to relapse

- *Treatment*:
  - *Treatment of overdose*:
    - Oxygenation, muscle relaxants
    - IV thiopentone
    - IV diazepam
    - IV propanolol
    - Haloperidol
  - *Treatment of chronic use*:
    - Bromocriptine
    - Amantadine
    - Desipramine, imipramine, trazodone
    - Supportive psychotherapy
    - Behaviour therapy

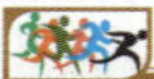

Topper's Edge

"CRACK" AND COCAINE

Cocaine

- Powder form (Cocaine hydrochloride)
- Usually "snorted" intranasally, producing a "high" of less intensity
- A high temperature (195°C) is required to vaporize cocaine hydrochloride powder for smoking
- Powder has a slower onset of action to produce the euphoric effects compared with Crack

Crack

- Crack is cocaine (cocaine base), but not in the powder form[Q]
- A solid formed by mixing cocaine powder with water and baking soda
- Transformation makes Crack a drug that is easier and more economical to market and, consequently, much less expensive
- Crack is in a form that allows it to be vaporized at a much lower temperature (98°C), without burning and destroying excess cocaine
- Getting cocaine into a vapor form or smoke is important to Cocaine users:
  - When smoked, the drug is delivered through the lungs to the brain almost immediately: Causes release of brain chemicals in the pleasure centers of the brain, resulting in the desired stimulating, euphoric effect
  - Crack form does not waste Cocaine by burning it up

X C. OPIOID USE DISORDERS

X C1. Introduction

- *Source of opioid derivatives*: Unripe seed capsules of Papaver somniferum[Q]

Natural opioid derivatives[Q]	Synthetic opioid derivatives[Q]	
• Morphine • Codeine • Thebaine • Noscapine • Papaverine	• Heroin • Nalorphine • Methadone • Dextropropoxyphene • Mepridine/ Pethidine	• Cyclazocine • Levallorphan • Diphenoxylate • Hydromorphone

- *Mechanism of action*: Bind to opioid receptors
  - **Mu receptors**: Heroin, morphine[Q]
  - **Kappa receptors**: Pentazocine, Butorphanol, Dynorphin[Q]
  - **Delta receptors**: Enkephalin, beta-endorphin[Q]
  - Sigma receptors: Phencyclidine
  - Epsilon receptors
  - Lambda receptors

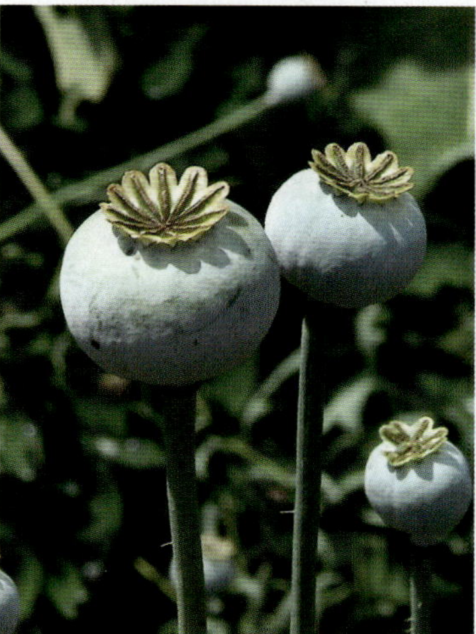

Fig. Opium (Papaver somniferum)

X C2. Clinical Presentation

- ***Acute intoxication***[Q]**:**
  - Apathy
  - Bradycardia
  - Hypotension
  - Respiratory depression
  - Sub-normal body core temperature
  - Pin-point pupils (Dilated pupils in severe intoxication due to hypoxia)
- ***Withdrawal syndrome***[Q]**:**
  - Lacrimation, Rhinorrhoea
  - Pupillary dilation
  - Sweating, Diarrhoea
  - Tachycardia, Hypertension
  - Insomnia
  - Body ache, muscle cramps
  - Nausea, vomiting, anorexia
- *Complications*:
  - Due to illicit drug use: Parkinsonism, transverse myelitis, peripheral neuropathy, ambylopia
  - Due to intravenous use: Pulmonary embolism, thrombophlebitis, hepatitis, tetanus, endocarditis
  - Social complications
- *Laboratory testing*:
  - Naloxone challenge test[Q]
  - Urinary opioid testing

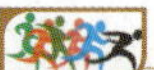

Topper's Edge

Opioid Use Disorder Diagnostic Criteria (DSM-5)

A problematic pattern of opioid use leading to clinically significant impairment or distress, as manifested by at least two of the following, occurring within a 12-month period:

- Often taken in larger amounts or over a longer period than was intended
- Persistent desire or unsuccessful efforts to cut down or control use
- A great deal of time is spent to obtain, use or recover from its effects
- Craving, or a strong desire or urge to use opioids
- Recurrent opioid use resulting in a failure to fulfill major role obligations
- Continued opioid use despite having persistent social or interpersonal problems
- Important social, occupational, or recreational activities are given up or reduced
- Recurrent opioid use in situations in which it is physically hazardous
- Continued use despite knowledge of having a persistent physical/psychological problem
- Tolerance
  - A need for markedly increased amounts of opioids to achieve desired effect
  - A markedly diminished effect with continued use of same amount of an opioid
- Withdrawal
  - Characteristic opioid withdrawal syndrome
  - Opioids are taken to relieve or avoid withdrawal symptoms

X C3. Treatment

- *Opioid overdose treatment*: **Narcotic antagonists**[Q]
  - Naloxone[Q]
  - Naltrexone[Q]

- *Detoxification*: Abrupt taking-off opioids
  - Substitution drugs: **Methadone**[Q]
  - Clonidine
  - Naltrexone with clonidine
  - Other drugs:
    - LAAM
    - Propoxyphene
    - Buprenorphine
- *Maintenance therapy*:
  - **Agonist substitution/Methadone maintenance**[Q]
  - Opioid antagonists:
    - Naltrexone
    - Naltrexone with clonidine
  - Psychotherapy
  - Behaviour therapy
  - Psychosocial rehabilitation

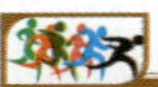

Topper's Edge

Opioid Replacement Therapy (ORT)

Opioid substitution therapy (Opioid maintenance therapy) involves replacing an opioid, such as Heroin, with a longer acting but less euphoric opioid

- Commonly used substitution agents[Q]:
  - **Methadone**
  - **Buprenorphine**
- Less commonly used substitution agents:
  - Diamorphine
  - Dihydrocodeine
  - Heroin-assisted treatment
  - Morphine
  - Naltrexone

X D. DRUG DEPENDENCE AND WITHDRAWAL

Dependence/Withdrawal	Substances/Drugs
Only Psychological dependence[Q]	Cannabis, Cocaine
Physical and Psychological dependence[Q]	Opioids (Highest), Alcohol, Barbiturates, Nicotine, Amphetamines, Benzodiazepines (Least)
Minimal Physical dependence[Q]	LSD (Absent), Cannabis, Cocaine, Phencyclidine, Solvents
Significant withdrawal symptoms[Q]	Alcohol, Opioids, Nicotine, Amphetamines, Cocaine, Benzodiazepines, Barbiturates
Lesser Withdrawal symptoms[Q]	LSD, Cannabis

X E. KEY FEATURES OF COMMON SUBSTANCE USE DISORDERS

Morphine/ Heroin Intoxication	**Alcohol Intoxication**
• **Pin-point pupil**[Q] • **Cyanosis**[Q] • **Hypotension**[Q] • Shallow breathing • Hypothermia	• **Nystagmus**[Q] • **Slurred speech**[Q] • Hypotension • Hypoglycemia[Q] • Hypothermia

Contd...

Contd…

Morphine/Heroin Withdrawal • **Lacrimation**[Q] • **Sweating**[Q] • **Yawning**[Q] • **Rhinorrhea**[Q] • **Goose flesh (Piloerection)**[Q] • Mydriasis[Q] • Insomnia • Diarrhoea • Raised BP	**Alcohol Withdrawal** • **Hangover (Most common)**[Q] • **Mild tremor**[Q] • Nausea, Vomiting • Insomnia • Restlessness • Anxiety • Delirium tremens (Most severe)[Q] • Alcoholic seizures (Rum fits)[Q] • Alcoholic hallucinosis[Q]
Cocaine Abuse • Psychotic episodes • Persecutory delusions[Q] • **Formication (Tactile hallucinations[Q])** • **Cocaine bugs[Q] (Magnan symptoms[Q])** • **Black tongue/teeth**[Q]	**Amphetamine Abuse** • Paranoid hallucinations[Q] • Delusion of persecution • Auditory/visual hallucination[Q] • Clear consciousness[Q] • **Formication (Tactile hallucinations)**[Q]
Cannabis Toxicity • **Flash backs**[Q] • **A motivational syndrome**[Q] • **Run amok**[Q] • Red eye[Q] • Increased appetite[Q] • Synesthesia[Q] • Dry mouth • Mild tachycardia	**LSD Intoxication** • **Synesthesia**[Q] • **Bad trip**[Q]/Acute panic • Increased tendon reflexes • Depression • Confusion • Tachycardia • Tremors • Mydriasis

IMAGE-BASED QUESTIONS

1. **Countries shown in Photograph constitute** ***[Recent Question 2013]***

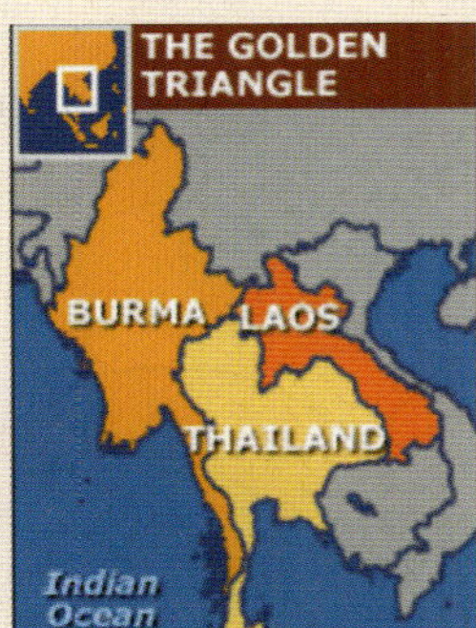

a. Golden crescent
b. Golden triangle
c. Golden trap
d. Bermuda triangle

2. **Opioid shown in Photograph act mainly via ……… receptors** ***[Recent Question 2013]***

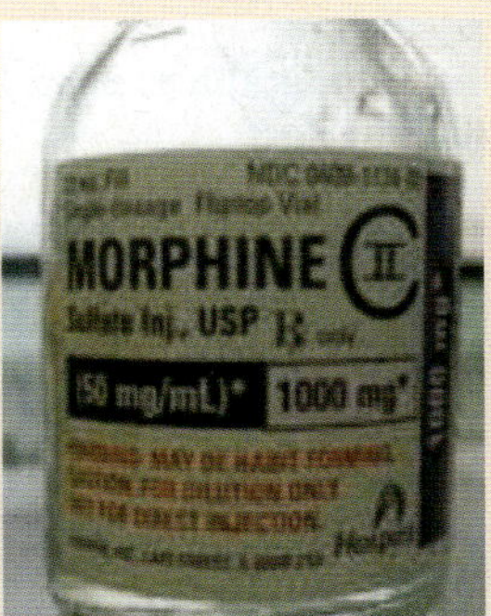

a. mu
b. kappa
c. delta
d. sigma

Psychiatry

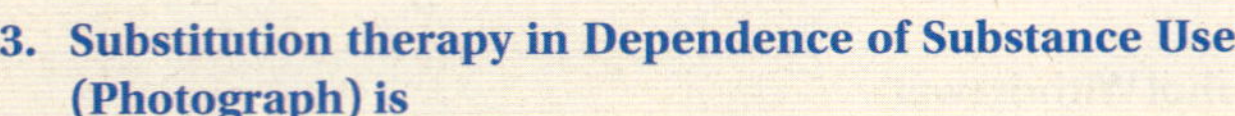

3. Substitution therapy in Dependence of Substance Use (Photograph) is

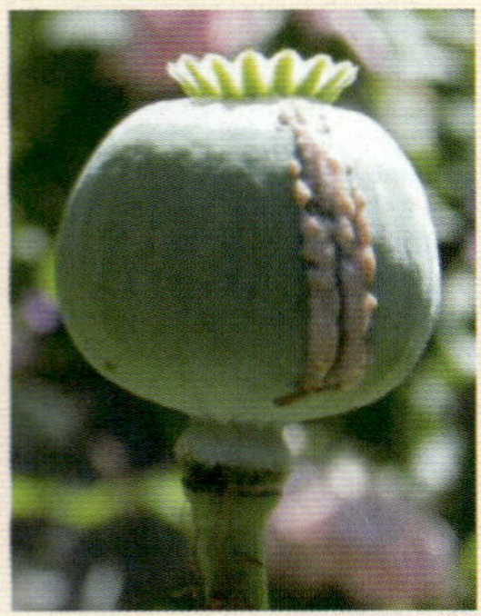

a. LAAM
b. Naltrexone
c. Methadone
d. Clonidine

4. Dried leaves, flowering shoots and cut tops of the Plant (Photograph) provide ***[Recent Question 2013]***

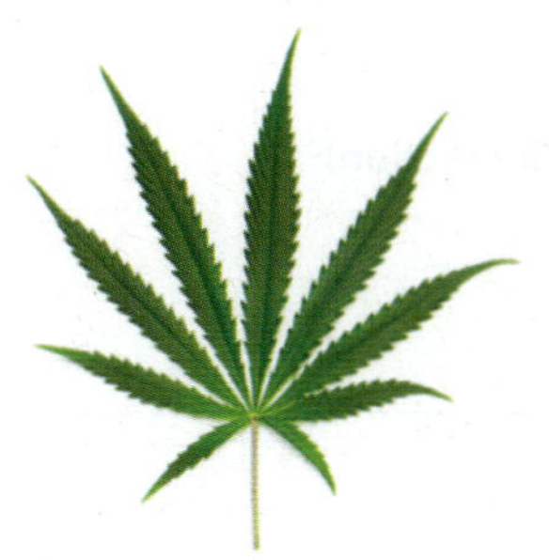

a. Charas
b. Bhang
c. Ganja
d. Hash oil

5. Method of Substance use shown in Figure is mainly used for

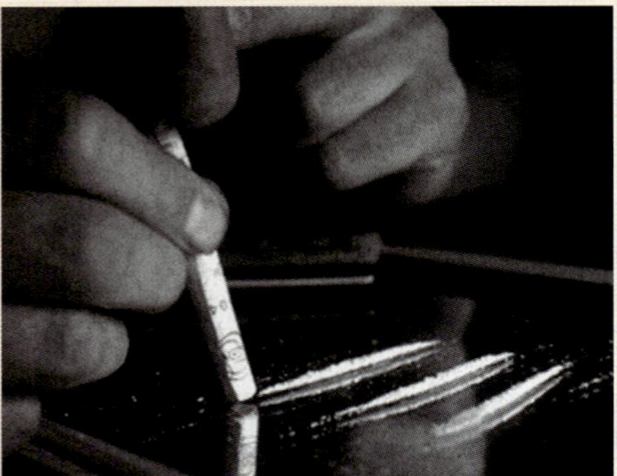

a. Ganja
b. Bhang
c. Charas
d. Cocaine

6. Countries shown in Photograph constitute zone known as ***[Recent Question 2014]***

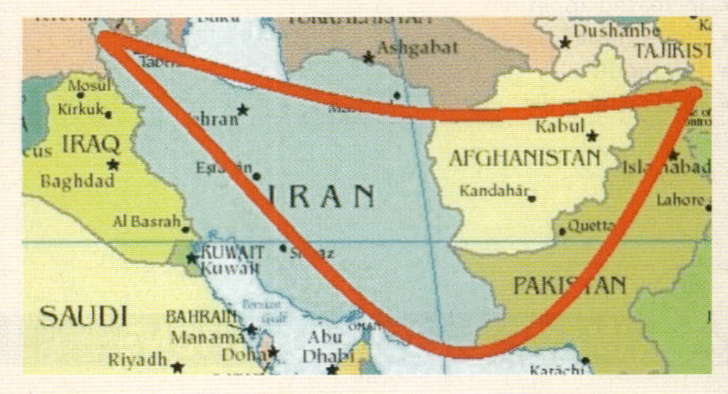

a. Golden crescent
b. Golden triangle
c. Golden trap
d. Bermuda triangle

7. Plant shown in Photograph is used for production of which recreational drug?

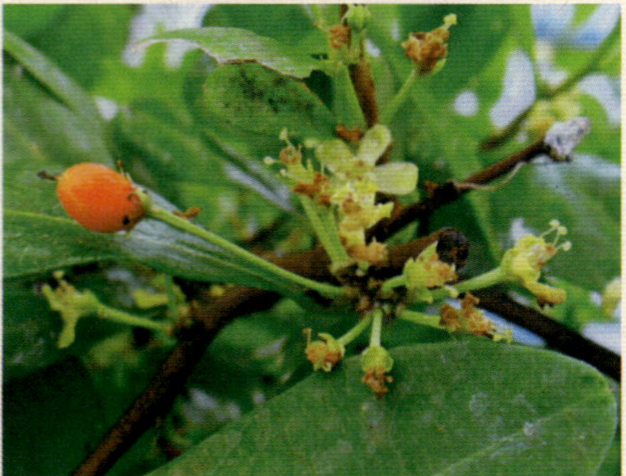

a. Cocaine
b. Cannabis
c. LSD
d. Heroin

8. 'Flash-backs' as shown in Photograph are seen in

a. LSD
b. Cocaine
c. Opiate
d. Amphetamine

ANSWERS WITH EXPLANATIONS OF IBQS

1. Ans. (b) Golden triangle *[Ref. Drug Trafficking by Sherman, 1/e p40]*
- World's Opium supply comes from 2 major areas:
  - Golden triangle: Myanmar (Burma), Thailand, Laos
  - Golden crescent: Afghanistan, Iran, Pakistan

2. Ans. (a) mu *[Ref. Niraj Ahuja, 7/e p43]*
- Mechanism of action of Opioids: Bind to opioid receptors
  - Mu receptors: Heroin, morphine
  - Kappa receptors: Pentazocine, Butorphanol, Dynorphin
  - Delta receptors: Enkephalin, beta-endorphin
  - Sigma receptors: Phencyclidine
  - Epsilon receptors
  - Lambda receptors

3. Ans. (c) Methadone *[Ref. Kaplan's & Sadocks's Psychiatry, 3/e p526]*
- Photograph shows Opium Poppy plant (Papaver sominiferum)
- Substitution therapy in opioid withdrawal: Methadone, Levomethadyl, Buprenorphine

4. Ans. (b) Bhang *[Ref. Niraj Ahuja, 7/e p45]*
- Plant shown is Cannabis sativa
- Cannabis preparations:
  - Hashish/Charas: Resinous exudate from flowering tops of cultivated plants
  - Ganja: Small leaves and inflorescence of highly cultivated plants
  - Bhang: Dried leaves, flowering shoots, cut tops of uncultivated plants
  - Hash oil: Lipid soluble plant extract

5. Ans. (d) Cocaine *[Ref. Cocaine by Weiss, 1/e p15]*
- Method shown: Snorting (intranasal absorption)

6. Ans. (a) Golden crescent *[Ref. Drug Trafficking by Sherman, 1/e p40]*
- World's Opium supply comes from 2 major areas:
  - Golden triangle: Myanmar (Burma), Thailand, Laos
  - Golden crescent: Afghanistan, Iran, Pakistan

7. Ans. (a) Cocaine *[Ref. Niraj Ahuja, 7/e p45]*
- Plant shown: Erythroxylon coca

8. Ans. (a) LSD *[Ref. Niraj Ahuja, 7/e p50]*
- Flashbacks: Spontaneous recurrence of LSD use experience in a drug-free state
- Usually occur weeks-months after last experience
- Induced by Stress, Fatigue, Alcohol, Severe physical illness, Marihuana intoxication

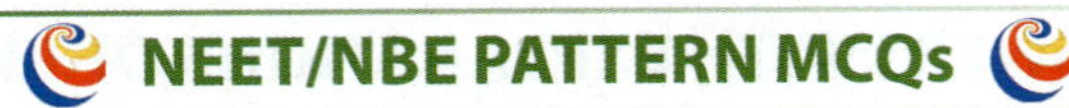

NEET/NBE PATTERN MCQs

1. Date rape drug among the following is *[Recent Question 2016]*
a. Diazepam b. Lorazepam
c. Temazepam d. Flunitrazepam

2. Grass/Weed/Pot slang is used for *[Recent Question 2015, 2016]*
a. Cocaine b. Cannabis
c. LSD d. Opioid

3. Trip word in LSD is defined as *[Recent Question 2016]*
a. Occasional use with long abstinence
b. Frequent use with short abstinence
c. Single use for lifetime
d. Occasional use with short abstinence

4. Withdrawal of which of the following causes Piloerection? *[Recent Question 2016]*
a. Morphine b. Cannabis
c. Smoking d. Alcohol

5. Drugs which cause both physical and psychological dependence are *[Recent Question 2016]*
a. Opioids b. Alcohol
c. Nicotine d. All the above

6. Bad trip is seen with *[Recent Question 2016]*
a. Cocaine b. Cannabis
c. LSD d. Heroin

7. Opioid dependence produces *[Recent Question 2016]*
a. Physical dependence
b. Psychological dependence
c. Both a and b
d. None of the above

8. A motivational syndrome caused by *[Recent Question 2015, 2016]*
a. Cannabis abuse b. Opioid abuse
c. Alcohol abuse d. Heroin abuse

9. Most common substance of abuse in India is *[Recent Question 2016]*
a. Tobacco b. Alcohol
c. Cannabis d. Opium

10. Morning blues seen with *[Recent Question 2016]*
a. Nitrates
b. Opioids
c. Amlodipine
d. Clozapine

11. Methadone is used in Opioid deaddiction as *[Recent Question 2016]*
a. It is not addictive
b. Less analgesic than morphine
c. Longer t½ therefore less withdrawal
d. Reduces adrenergic side effects

12. Opiate withdrawal causes *[Recent Question 2016]*
a. Mydriasis
b. Dry skin and mouth
c. Tremors
d. Constipation

13. Drug dependence is a term which *[NBE FMGE March 2010]*
a. Includes drug addiction but excludes drug habituation
b. Includes both drug addiction and habituation
c. Includes drug habituation but excludes drug abuse
d. None of the above

14. Physical withdrawal symptoms are absent in patients abusing *[Recent Question 2017, NBE DNB 1994, 2000]*
a. Pethidine b. Cannabis
c. Opium d. Alcohol

15. All of the following are associated with caffeine withdrawal symptoms EXCEPT *[NBE DNB December 2011]*
a. Headache b. Nervousness
c. Hallucinations d. Depression

16. Following are features of morphine withdrawal, except *[NBE DNB 2002]*
a. Piloerection b. Insomnia
c. Discharge from nose d. Constipation

17. MC used body fluid in screening for drugs of abuse *[NBE FMGE September 2006]*
a. Blood b. Serum
c. Saliva d. Urine

18. Not related to development of dependence is *[NBE DNB 2010, AIIMS PG 2009]*
a. Family history b. Personality
c. Peer pressure d. Intelligence

19. LSD is also known as *[NBE DNB 1992]*
a. Brown sugar b. Mind blocker
c. Mind expander d. Glue

20. Etheromanias refer to *[Recent Question 2012]*
a. Acute psychosis post ether anaesthesia
b. Ether addiction
c. Excessive ether use drug anaesthesia
d. None of the Above

21. Which of the following is least narcotic? *[NBE DNB 2010]*
a. Codeine b. Morphine
c. Papaverine d. Pethidine

22. Most commonly abused opioid *[Recent Question 2012]*
a. Morphine b. Diacetylmorphine
c. Oxycodine d. Bupremorphine

23. Features of Opioid intake include all except *[NBE FMGE September 2006]*
a. Relaxation b. Analgesia
c. Euphoria d. Dilated pupils

24. Following is/are withdrawal symptoms of opiate *[NBE DNB 1996]*
a. Miosis b. Rhinorrhoea
c. Constipation d. Dry and warm skin

25. Formication and delusion of persecution occurs together in *[NBE DNB 2009]*
a. Cocaine b. Amphetamine
c. Cannabits d. LSD

26. Hallucinations, psychosis, hypertension and tachycardia are adverse effects typically associated with which of the following narcotics *[NBE FMGE September 2011]*

a. Morphine b. Meperidine
c. Pentazocine d. Buprenorphine

27. Drug which is used for long term maintenance in opioid addiction *[Recent Question 2017, NBE DNB 2009]*

a. Naloxone b. Nalophine
c. Butaphenol d. Methadone

28. Cocaine overdose presents with all of the following except *[NBE FMGE September 2011]*

a. Diaphoresis
b. Hypertension
c. Constricted pupils
d. Agitation

29. Methadone is used for opioid withdrawal because *[Recent Question 2015]*

a. It is antagonist at opioid receptor
b. It is partial antagonist at opioid receptor
c. It is agonist at opioid receptor
d. It is partial agonist at opioid receptor

30. Buprenorphine drug is a type of *[Recent Question 2014, 2015]*

a. 'Mu' agonist
b. 'Mu' partial agonist
c. 'Mu' antagonist
d. 'Mu' partial antagonist

31. Narcotic Drugs and Psychotropic Substance Act was passed in which year? *[Recent Question 2017]*

a. 1983 b. 1985
c. 1990 d. 1993

32. Which of the following antidepressant is also used in cessation of smoking? *[Recent Question 2017]*

a. Sertraline
b. Bupropion
c. Venlafaxine
d. Amitriptyline

33. Tolerance means? *[Recent Question 2017]*

a. Increase effect of drug on same dose
b. Decrease effect of drug on same dose
c. Same effect on lesser doses
d. None

HIGH YIELD MCQs

1. Treatment is not required in withdrawal of *[All India PGMEE 1996, PGMCET 2015]*

a. Cannabis b. Alcohol
c. Amphetamine d. LSD

2. Following are opioid withdrawal symptoms except *[AIIMS PGMEE 1992]*

a. Insomnia b. Piloerection
c. Rhinorrhea d. Constipation

3. Tactile Hallucination are seen in *[All India PGMEE 1992]*

a. Alcohol b. Heroin
c. Cocaine d. Phenergan

4. Feeling of creeping insects is seen in *[AIIMS PGMEE 1994]*

a. Alcohol withdrawal b. Lead Poisoning
c. Schizophrenia d. Cocaine abuse

5. Formication and delusion of persecution, both are together seen in *[AIIMS PGMEE 2009]*

a. LSD psychosis
b. Amphetamine psychosis
c. Cocaine psychosis
d. Cannabis psychosis

6. Most common substance abuse in India is *[AIIMS PGMEE 2007, 2010, All India 2007]*

a. Tobacco b. Cannabis
c. Alcohol d. Opium

7. Naltrexone is used in opioid dependence to *[AIIMS PGMEE 2010, All India PGMEE 2007]*

a. Prevent respiratory depression
b. Treat withdrawal symptoms
c. Prevent relapse
d. Detoxification of opioid over dose

8. Drug which is used for long-term maintenance in opioid addiction *[AIIMS PGMEE 2006]*

a. Naloxone b. Nalorphine
c. Butorphanol d. Methadone

9. Which of the following is an alternative to methadone for maintenance treatment of opiate dependence? *[AIIMS PGMEE 2005]*

a. Diazepam
b. Chlordiazepoxide
c. Buprenorphine
d. Dextropropoxyphene

10. Opiate withdrawal is treated with *[AIIMS PGMEE 1995]*

a. CPZ b. Nalorphine
c. Pethidine d. Methadone

11. Which is not used in treatment of heroin dependence? *[AIIMS PGMEE 2010]*

a. Disulfiram b. Buprenorphine
c. Clonidine d. Lofexidine

12. Which of the following drugs is not used in opioid dependence? *[AIIMS PGMEE 2009]*

a. Disulfiram b. Clonidine
c. Lorazepam d. Naltrexone

13. In patients of substance-abuse, drugs used are *[PGI 2002]*

a. Naltrexone b. Naloxine
c. Clonidine d. Lithium
e. Disulfiram

14. All are adulterants of Heroin except *[AIIMS PGMEE 2005]*

a. Chalk powder b. Quinine
c. Charcoal d. Fructose

15. **Drugs used in Heroin withdrawal are all except** *[AIIMS PGMEE 1998]*
   a. Buprenorphine b. Clonidine
   c. Dextropropoxyphene d. Haloperidol
16. **Active substance in Hashish is** *[All India PGMEE 1991]*
   a. Morphine b. LSD
   c. Mescaline d. Tetrahydrocannabinol
17. **Which of the following is not an opioid peptide?** *[AIIMS PGMEE 2005]*
   a. Beta-Endorphin b. Epinephrine
   c. Leu5-enkephalin d. Met-enkephalin
18. **Yawning is a common feature of** *[AIIMS PGMEE 2003]*
   a. Alcohol withdrawal b. Cocaine withdrawal
   c. Cannabis withdrawal d. Opioid withdrawal
19. **Physical withdrawal symptoms are absent in patient abusing** *[All India PGMEE 1991]*
   a. Alcohol
   b. Cannabis
   c. Opium
   d. Pethidine
20. **Physical dependence is not seen with** *[AIIMS PGMEE 1995]*
   a. Alcohol b. Raw opium
   c. Cannabis d. Benzodiazepines
21. **Flash-back are seen with** *[AIIMS PGMEE 1990]*
   a. LSD b. Cocaine
   c. Opiate d. Amphetamine
22. **Symptomatic treatment is not required in withdrawal of** *[All India PGMEE 1998]*
   a. Cannabis b. Morphine
   c. Alcohol d. Cocaine
23. **After use of some drug, a person develops episodes of age in which he runs about and indiscriminately injures a person who is encountered in way. He is probably addict of** *[AIIMS PGMEE 1997]*
   a. Alcohol b. Cannabis
   c. Opium d. Cocaine
24. **Drugs abuse with symptoms similar like paranoid schizophrenia are seen in** *[AIIMS PGMEE 1990, 1997, MPPG 1998]*
   a. LSD b. Cannabis
   c. Heroin/Cocaine d. Amphetamine
25. **Features of opioid withdrawal are all except** *[All India PGMEE 1993]*
   a. Diarrhoea
   b. Lacrimation
   c. Miosis
   d. Rhinorrhoea
26. **Acute opioid withdrawal is characterized by** *[PGI 2004]*
   a. Rhinorrhoea
   b. Piloerection
   c. Miosis
   d. Insomnia
27. **Naltrexone is used in opioids addiction because** *[AIIMS PGMEE 2006, AIIMS PGMEE 2007]*
   a. To treat withdrawal symptoms
   b. To treat overdose of opioids
   c. Prevent relapse
   d. Has addiction potential
28. **'Angel dust' is term used for** *[NIMHANS PGMEE 2014]*
   a. LSD b. PCP
   c. Heroin d. Cocaine
29. **Heroin withdrawal symptom(s) include the following** *[PGI November 2014]*
   a. Restlessness
   b. High blood pressure
   c. Insomnia
   d. Depressed heart rate
   e. Loss of appetite

 NEET/NBE PATTERN MCQs ANSWERS WITH EXPLANATIONS 

1. Ans. (d) Flunitrazepam

[Ref. Date Rape Drugs by Kehner, 1/e p13]

Date-rape Drugs

- Also known as **Predator drug**, is any drug that is an incapacitating agent which, when administered to another person, incapacitates the person and renders them vulnerable to a drug facilitated sexual assault (DFSA), including rape
- Older Date-rape drugs: Alcohol, Marijuana, Benzodiazepines, Chloral hydrate, Barbiturates, Heroin, Morphine, Methaqualone, LSD
- Newer Date-rape drugs: **Rohypnol** (Flunitrazepam), Gamma-hydroxy butyrate, Ketamine
- Abusers often consider Rohypnol the Date-rape drug of choice

2. Ans. (b) Cannabis

[Ref. Niraj Ahuja, 7/e p45]

Slang names of Cannabis

- Common names: Grass, Weed, Pot, Mary jane, Marijuana, Reefer
- Less common names: Herb, Smoke, Dope, Shit, Bush, Tea, Texas tea, Locoweed, Hay, Griefo, Hemp, Jive, Rope, Boo, Wacky-backy, Black

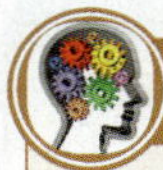

Also Remember

Common Slang Names of Other Drugs of Abuse

- Heroin: Smack, Junk, Brown sugar
- Cocaine: Coke, Snow, Stardust, Rock, Crack, Snuff, Snort
- Morphine: God's medicine
- Amphetamines: Speed, Crystal
- Phencyclidine: PCP, Angel dust, Peace pill
- Ketamine: Green, Purple, Mauve, Jet

3. Ans. (a) Occasional use with long abstinence

[Ref. Niraj Ahuja, 7/e p49]

- LSD Trip: Occasional use of LSD followed by long periods of abstinence
- Characterised by perception of one's minds' unknown aspects and creative exuberance

4. Ans. (a) Morphine

[Ref. Kaplan & Sadock, 3/e p139]

Morphine/Heroin Withdrawal: Lacrimation, Sweating, Yawning, Rhinorrhea, Goose flesh (Piloerection), Mydriasis, Insomnia, Diarrhoea, Raised BP

5. Ans. (d) All the above

[Ref. Niraj Ahuja, 7/e p35]

Psychoactive Substance Use Dependence

- Agents causing both Physical and Psychological dependence: Alcohol, Amphetamines, Barbiturates, Opioids, Nicotine, Caffeine, Benzodiazepines
- Agents causing mainly Psychological dependence: cannabis, cocaine, PCP, volatile solvents
- Agents causing only Psychological dependence: LSD

Also Remember

- Psychoactive substance use **NOT** associated with Tolerance: Cocaine

6. Ans. (c) LSD

[Ref. Drug Use and Abuse by Abadinsky, 8/e p100]

- A bad trip is actually an acute anxiety or panic reaction following the ingestion of LSD
- On a bad trip, painful or frightening feelings are intensified

7. Ans. (c) Both a and b

[Ref. Niraj Ahuja, 7/e p35]

Opioid use is associated with high levels of physical dependence, psychological dependence and tolerance

8. Ans. (a) Cannabis abuse

[Ref. Handbook of Psychiatry by Lader, 1/e p234]

Amotivational syndrome

- Long-term effects of cannabis include amotivational syndrome and brain damage
- Phrase coined to describe a condition of chronic apathy
- A social, non-direction behavior with no goals in life

9. Ans. (a) Tobacco

[Ref. Genomics and Health in the Developing World by Kumar, 1/e p1136]

According to National Health Survey 2004 India, excluding tobacco, alcohol is the most common substance of abuse in India

10. Ans. (a) Nitrates

[Ref. www.valuemd.com]

Monday morning blues

- Tolerance to nitrates develops with uninterrupted usage
- Persons exposed to nitrates throughout their work do not feel the side effects, but when they return on Monday, they feel adverse drug reactions and thus feel "blue"

Also Remember

Monday disease

- Toxicity that happens to those who are exposed to Nitroglycerin or isosorbide dinitrate industrially, like who work in construction or demolition industries, mix concrete, do plaster
- During the week, Monday to Friday, they are exposed to the vasodilating action, so they build up a tolerance
- If they are off on Saturday and Sunday the tolerance is lost. So when they go back to work on Monday the tachycardia, hypotension, flusing and headache return, but a tolerance is built up again by the next day

11. Ans. (a) It is not addictive

[Ref. Pharmacology by Seth, 3/e pIII.142]

Methadone as Substitution Therapy

- Methadone is absorbed from GIT and 90% is bound to plasma proteins
- On repeated administration, there is gradual accumulation in tissues

- On discontinuation of drug, low concentrations are maintained in plasma by slow release from extravascular tissues
- There is occurrence of relatively mild protracted withdrawal syndrome

12. Ans. (a) Mydriasis

[Ref. Niraj Ahuja, 7/e p43]

Morphine/Heroin Withdrawal: Lacrimation, Sweating, Yawning, Rhinorrhea, Goose flesh (Piloerection), Mydriasis, Insomnia, Diarrhoea, Raised BP, Raised body temperature, Anxiety

13. Ans. (b) Includes both drug addiction and habituation

[Ref. WHO Technical Report Series, 1969]

- ***Drug dependence***: A state, psychic and sometimes also physical, resulting from the interaction between a living organism and a drug, characterized by behavioral and other responses that always include a compulsion to take the drug on a continuous or periodic basis in order to experience its psychic effects, and sometimes to avoid the discomfort of its absence
  - Tolerance may or may not be present
  - A person may be dependent on more than one drug

14. Ans. (b) Cannabis

[Ref. Niraj Ahuja, 7/e p46]

Physical dependence withdrawal symptoms are mild in Cannabis: Due to long half-life of THC

15. Ans. (c) Hallucinations

[Ref. Clinical Guide to the Diagnosis and Treatment of Mental Disorders by Tasman, 2/e p176]

Caffeine Withdrawal

- Headache
- Tiredness, fatigue
- Drowsiness
- Depression
- Dysphoria
- Irritability, Anxiety
- Muscle aches/stiffness

16. Ans. (d) Constipation

[Ref. Niraj Ahuja, 7/e p43]

Opiate Withdrawal

- Lacrimation, Rhinorrhea, Sweating, Diarrhoea, Yawning
- Pupillary dilation
- Tachycardia, Hypertension
- Insomnia, Anorexia
- Raised body temperature, Muscle cramps, Bodyache
- Anxiety, Piloerection

17. Ans. (d) Urine

[Ref. www.labtestblog.com]

- Urine is the **biological fluid of choice** for screening for drugs of abuse
- Specimen collection is non-invasive
- Large quantities are available for analysis

18. Ans. (d) Intelligence

[Ref. Clinical Consult for Psychiatric Mental Health Care by Rhoads, 1/e p56]

Risk Factors for Dependence

- History: Family history, Mental illness, Emotional/physical/sexual abuse
- Peer pressure
- Educational level: Low
- Economic status: Low
- Untreated physical pain
- Unemployment
- Poor social coping skills
- Chaotic home environment

19. Ans. (c) Mind expander

[Ref. From Healing to Hell by Wall, 1/e p185]

Lysergic acid diethylamide (LSD): Mind-expander, Acid, Acid-trip

20. Ans. (b) Ether addiction

[Ref. An Excess of Manias & Phobias by Robertson, 1/e p82]

Etheromania: A morbid addiction to consumption of ether or other inhalants as a stimulant/ intoxicant

21. Ans. (a) Codeine

[Ref. A-Level Chemistry by Ramsden, 4/e p713]

Codeine

- Last potent opiate
- One-sixth as effective as Morphine
- Less additive than other narcotics

22. Ans. (b) Diacetylmorphine

[Ref. In a Page: Emergency Medicine by Kahan, 1/e p171]

MC abused Opioid: Heroin (Diacetyl morphine)

23. Ans. (d) Dilated pupils

[Ref. Niraj Ahuja, 7/e p43]

Clinical Presentation of Opioid Use

Acute intoxication	Withdrawal syndrome
• Apathy • Bradycardia • Hypotension • Respiratory depression • Subnormal body core temperature • Pin-point pupils	• Lacrimation, Rhinorrhoea • Pupillary dilation • Sweating, Diarrhoea • Tachycardia, Hypertension • Insomnia • Bodyache, muscle cramps • Nausea, vomiting, anorexia

24. Ans. (b) Rhinorrhoea

[Ref. Niraj Ahuja, 7/e p43]

25. Ans. (a) Cocaine

[Ref. drug Injury by Donnell & Ahuja, 2/e p617]

Cocaine Disorer

- Bull-horrors (Paranoid psychotic state)
- Delusions of persecution
- Formication (Cocaine bugs): Tactile hallucinations, Feeling of creeping insects under skin

26. Ans. (c) Pentazocine

[Ref. Essentials of Medical Pharmacology by KD Tripathi, 6/e p464-65]

Side Effects of Opioids

Morphine (natural opioid)	*Meperidine/Pethidine (synthetic opioid)*
• Bradycardia • Hypotension • Blurring of vision • Urinary retention • Psychological dependence • Physical dependence	• Lesser analgesic potency • Tachycardia • Hypotension • Safer in asthmatics • Does not suppress cough • Lesser urinary retention

Contd...

Psychiatry

Contd...

Pentazocine (Agonist-antagonist)	*Buprenorphine (Partial agonist, Antagonist)*
• Hallucinations • Psychosis • Hypertension • Tachycardia	• Bradycardia • Hypotension • Lower tolerance • Lower dependence

27. Ans. (d) Methadone

[Ref. Niraj Ahuja, 7/e p44]

Treatment/ Maintenance Agents for Opioid Addiction

- Methadone (Major maintenance agent)
- Buprenorphine (Major maintenance agent, alternative to Methadone)
- LAAM (Levo-o-acetylmethadol)
- Naltrexone (prevent relapse)
- Clonidine
- Lofexidine
- Lorazepam
- Dextropropoxyphene
- Diphenoxylate

28. Ans. (c) Constricted pupils

[Ref. Niraj Ahuja, 7/e p48]

Acute Cocaine Overdose

- Pupillary dilation
- Tachycardia
- Hypertension
- Sweating
- Diaphoresis
- Nausea, vomiting
- Hypomania (Increased psychomotor activity, grandiosity, mood-elation, agitation)
- Impaired judgement

Also Remember

- *Treatment of Cocaine overdose*:
  - **IV Propanolol (specific antagonist)**
  - IV Thiopentone
  - IV Diazepam
  - Oxygenation
  - Craving reducers: Bromocriptine, Amantadine, Despriamine, Imipramine

29. Ans. (c) It is agonist at opioid receptor.

[Ref. Kaplan's and Sadocks's Psychiatry, 3/e p526]

Substitution Therapy in Opioid Withdrawal

- Methadone:
  - Pure agonist at opioid mu-receptors
  - Negligible agonist or Antagonist activity at opioid delta/kappa receptors
- Levomethadyl:
  - Pure agonist at opioid mu-receptors
  - Negligible agonist or Antagonist activity at opioid delta/kappa receptors
- Buprenorphine:
  - Partial agonist at opioid mu-receptors
  - Potent Antagonist activity at opioid kappa receptors
  - Neither Agonist or Antagonist activity at opioid delta receptors

30. Ans. (b) 'Mu' partial agonist

[Ref. Substance Abuse by Kaye, 1/e p312]

- Buprenorphine:
  - Partial agonist at Mu-receptor
  - Antagonist at Kappa-receptor

31. Ans. (b) 1985

[Ref. Niraj Ahuja, 7/e p233]

Legislations for Substance Use in India

- The Opium Act of 1857 (The first Act for drug abuse and dependence in India)
  - The Opium Act, 1878
  - The Opium and Revenue Laws Act, 1950
- The Dangerous Drug Act of 1930,
- The Narcotic Drugs and Psychotropic Substances Act, 1985 (NDPS Act)
  - Prohibits a person to produce/manufacture/cultivate, possess, sell, purchase, transport, store, and/or consume any narcotic drug or psychotropic substance
  - Repealed all above-mentioned Acts of India
  - Act includes narcotic drugs (cannabis, cocaine, coca leaf, opium, poppy straw and all manufactured 'drugs') and psychotropic substances (76 drugs and their derivatives are listed in the schedule, e.g. diazepam, pentazocine, phenobarbital)
  - Punishment includes rigorous imprisonment < 1 year or with a fine < ₹10,000 (small quantity involvement), rigorous imprisonment < 10 year or with a fine < ₹100,000 (more than small quantity but lesser than commercial quantity involvement) and rigorous imprisonment < 20 year or with a fine < ₹100,000–200,000 (commercial quantity involvement)

32. Ans. (b) Bupropion

[Ref. Kaplan & Sadock's, 3/e p492]

Bupropion

- Although increasingly used as first-line monotherapy or as add-on therapy to other antidepressants (SSRIs)
- Marketed as Zyban for use in smoking cessation regimens.

33. Ans. (b) Decrease effect of drug on same dose

[Ref. Niraj Ahuja, 7/e p172]

Tolerance (Is defined by either of the following)

- A need for markedly increased amounts of drug/substance to achieve intoxication or desired effect
- Markedly diminished effect with continued use of the same amount of drug/substance

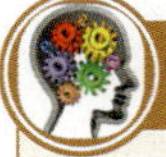

Also Remember

- Tolerance: After repeated administration, a given dose of drug produces a decreased effect or increasingly larger doses must be administered to obtain the effect observed with the original dose.
- Behavioural tolerance: Ability of the person to perform tasks despite the effects of the drug.
- Cross-tolerance: Ability of one drug to be substituted for another, each usually producing the same physiological and psychological effect.

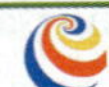 HIGH YIELD MCQs ANSWERS WITH EXPLANATIONS 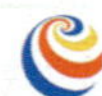

1. **Ans. (d) LSD**
   [Ref. Niraj Ahuja, 7/e p50]
   - No withdrawal syndrome has been described with LSD use
   - ***Bad-trip***: Spontaneous recurrence of LSD use experience in a drug-free state
     - Seen weeks-months after last experience
     - Episode induced by fatigue, stress, alcohol, physical illness, marihuana intoxication

2. **Ans. (d) Constipation**
   [Ref. Niraj Ahuja, 7/e p43]

3. **Ans. (c) Cocaine**
   [Ref. drug Injury by Donnell & Ahuja, 2/e p617]

4. **Ans. (d) Cocaine abuse**
   [Ref. drug Injury by Donnell & Ahuja, 2/e p617]

5. **Ans. (c) Cocaine psychosis**
   [Ref. drug Injury by Donnell & Ahuja, 2/e p617]

6. **Ans. (a) Tobacco**
   [Ref. Research on Tobacco in India by C. Ray, p18]

7. **Ans. (c) Prevent relapse**
   [Ref. Niraj Ahuja, 7/e p44]

8. **Ans. (d) Methadone**
   [Ref. Niraj Ahuja, 7/e p44]

9. **Ans. (c) Buprenorphine**
   [Ref. Niraj Ahuja, 7/e p44]

10. **Ans. (d) Methadone**
    [Ref. Niraj Ahuja, 7/e p44]

11. **Ans. (a) Disulfiram**
    [Ref. Niraj Ahuja, 7/e p44]

12. **Ans. (a) Disulfiram**
    [Ref. Niraj Ahuja, 7/e p44]

13. **Ans. (a) Naltrexone; (b) Naloxone; (c) Clonidine; (e) Disulfiram**
    [Ref. Niraj Ahuja, 7/e p41, 44]

14. **Ans. (c) Charcoal**
    [Ref. Smart Study Series Psychiatry by Deb, 1/e p51]

    Adulterants of Heroin
    - Noscapine, Scopalamine, Paracetamol, Quinine
    - Fructose, Sucrose
    - Flour
    - Powdered milk
    - Chalk, Caffeine

15. **Ans. (d) Haloperidol**
    [Ref. Niraj Ahuja, 7/e p44]

16. **Ans. (d) Tetrahydrocannabinol**
    [Ref. Niraj Ahuja, 7/e p45]

    Cannabis Chemicals
    - *Identifiable chemicals produced*: 400
    - *Total cannabinoids*: 40
    - *Most active component*: Delta-9 tetrahydrocannabinol (Δ9 THC)

17. **Ans. (b) Epinephrine**
    [Ref. Sensory Systems II: Senses Other than Vision by Adelman, 1/e p9]

    Opioid Peptides

Opioid peptide	Amino acids	Receptor preference
Enkephalins	5–8	Delta
Dynorphins	10–17	Kappa
Beta-endorphin	31	Mu, Delta

18. **Ans. (d) Opioid withdrawal**
    [Ref. Niraj Ahuja, 7/e p43]

19. **Ans. (b) Cannabis**
    [Ref. Niraj Ahuja, 7/e p46]
    Withdrawal symptoms are usually mild in Cannabis use disorder

20. **Ans. (c) Cannabis**
    [Ref. Niraj Ahuja, 7/e p46]

21. **Ans. (a) LSD**
    [Ref. Niraj Ahuja, 7/e p50]

22. **Ans. (a) Cannabis**
    [Ref. Niraj Ahuja, 7/e p46]

23. **Ans. (b) Cannabis**
    [Ref. Textbook of Forensic Medicine and Toxicology by Vij, 5/e p515]
    Run amok: Acute psychotic reaction with homicidal frenzy

24. **Ans. (d) Amphetamine**
    [Ref. Manual of Drug and Alcohol Abuse by Westermeyer, 1/e p143]

25. **Ans. (c) Miosis**
    [Ref. Niraj Ahuja, 7/e p43]

26. **Ans. (a) Rhinorrhoea; (b) Piloerection; (d) Insomnia**
    [Ref. Niraj Ahuja, 7/e p43]

27. **Ans. (c) Prevent relapse**
    [Ref. Niraj Ahuja, 7/e p44]

28. **Ans. (b) PCP**
    [Ref. Niraj Ahuja, 7/e p52]

    Phencyclidine (PCP)
    - Dissociative anesthetic agent
    - Atypical hallucinogen
    - *'Angel dust'*
    - *'Peace pill'*
    - Antagonize NDMA
    - No clearcut withdrawal syndrome

29. **Ans. (a) Restlessness; (c) Insomnia; (e) Loss of appetite**
    [Ref. Niraj Ahuja, 7/e p43]
    Heroin withdrawal symptoms: Lacrimation, Rhinorrhoea, Sweating, Diarrhoea, Pupillary dilation, Yawning. Tachycardia, Insomnia, Mild hypertension, Raised body temperature, Muscle cramps, Bodyache, Anxiety, Piloerection, Nausea, Vomiting, Anorexia

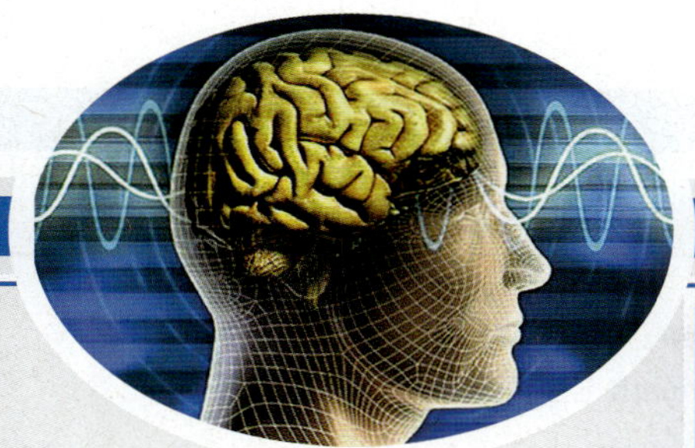

Chapter 11

Psychiatric Emergencies

THEORETICAL CONCEPTS

XI A. COMMON PSYCHIATRIC EMERGENCIES

- **Suicides (Most common[Q])**
- Stupor and catatonic syndrome
- Excited behaviour and violence
- Severe depression
- Hyperventilation syndrome
- Side effects of psychotropic drugs
- Pseudo-seizures (Conversion/dissociation hysteria)
- Anorexia nervosa
- Battered child syndrome
- Grief
- Drug/alcohol use disorders
- Panic disorders
- Acute psychosis

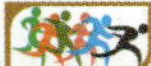

Topper's Edge

Psychiatric Emergencies

- **Major emergencies[Q]:**
  - Suicidal patients
  - Agitated and violent patients
- **Minor emergencies:**
  - Disaster
  - Grief reaction
  - Panic attack
  - Rape
- **Medical emergencies in psychiatry:**
  - Deliriums due to life-threatening conditions
  - Neuroleptic malignant syndrome
  - Serotonin syndrome
  - Over-dosages of common psychiatric medications
  - Over-dosages and withdrawal from addicting substances

Psychiatric Disorders Associated with Violent Behaviour

- Schizophrenia (especially Paranoid)
- Mania
- Paranoid psychosis
- Personality disorder especially antisocial type
- Alcohol intoxication or withdrawal
- Substance intoxication with cocaine, amphetamines, anabolic steroids, phencyclidine
- Substance withdrawal
- Post-traumatic stress disorder
- Dementia
- Learning disorder

XI B. SUICIDES

XI B1. Definition

- *Suicide*: Deliberate self-harm which is intentional and associated with self-inflicted death
- *Attempted suicide*: Unsuccessful suicidal act with a non-fatal outcome
- *Suicidal gesture*: Attempted suicide where intention is never to die by the act

XI B2. Epidemiology (Most Recent Data 2018)

- ***Suicide rate in India*: 10.6 per 100,000 population per year (M : F = 2 : 1)**
- *Highest number of suicides in India*: Maharashtra (12% of total in India)
- *Highest suicide rate in India*: Pondicherry (40.4 per 100,000 population per year)

XI B3. Underlying Cause

***Risk factors*: [Mnemonic: Having Suicidal Thoughts In A Major Illness Is Psychiatric Disorder[Q]]**

- **H**istory of suicidal attempts
- **S**taying Single
- **T**rauma (Recent major stressful life event)
- **I**mpulsivity
- **A**ge > 40 years
- **M**ale sex
- **I**llnesses
- **I**solation
- **A**lcohol/drug dependence
- **Pr**e-occupation with suicidal plans and thoughts
- **D**epression

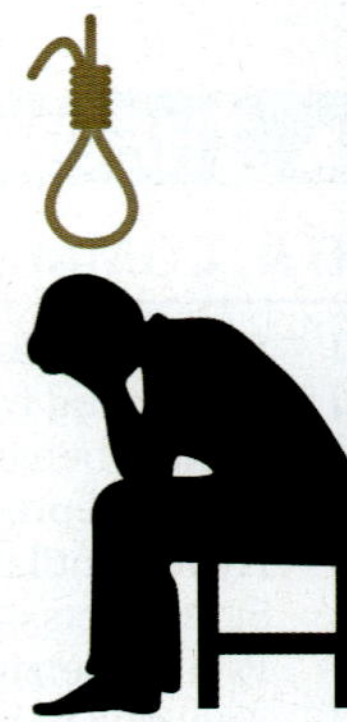

Fig. Suicide

***Underlying causes*:**

- Psychiatric disorders
  - Depression
  - Depression secondary to illness
  - Alcohol/drug dependence
  - Schizophrenia
  - Borderline personality
- Physical disorders (incurable/painful)
  - Cancer
  - AIDS
- Psychosocial factors
  - Failure in examinations
  - Failure in love
  - Marital difficulties
  - Family problems

XI B4. Modes Used

- Hanging (**MC in India**[Q])
- Ingestion of poisons
- Burning
- Drowning

XI B5. Medico-legal Aspects

- *Section 309, IPC*: Attempt to suicide/commission of such is an offence[Q] *[Passive euthanasia permitted by Supreme Court in March 2018]*

XI B6. Management

- Seeking help of Psychiatrist
- Psychiatric emergency interview
- Counselling and guidance
- Treatment of psychiatric disorders

IMAGE-BASED QUESTIONS

1. Not a Risk factor for Psychiatric emergency shown in Photograph is

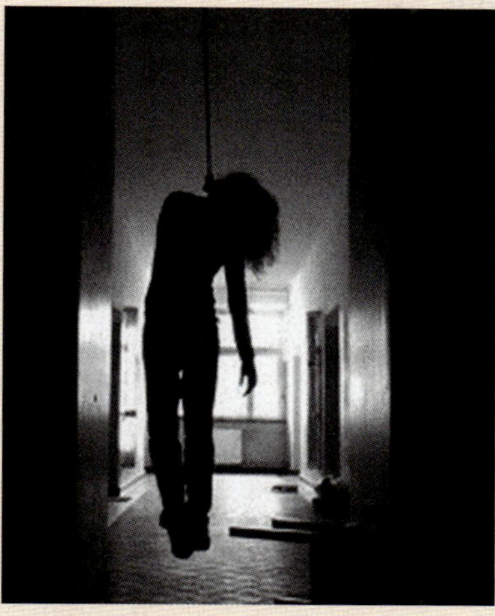

a. Prior history of similar attempt
b. Alcohol dependence
c. Married life
d. Depression

ANSWERS WITH EXPLANATIONS OF IBQs

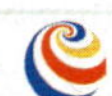

1. Ans. (c) Married life *[Ref. Niraj Ahuja, 7/e p72]*

- Risk factors of Suicide: History of suicidal attempts, Staying Single, Trauma (Recent major stressful life event), Impulsivity, Age > 40 years, Male sex, Illnesses, Isolation, Alcohol/drug dependence, Pre-occupation with suicidal plans and thoughts, Depression

NEET/NBE PATTERN MCQs 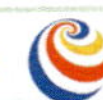

1. **Risk factor for suicide** *[Recent Question 2016]*
   a. Female sex b. Unmarried
   c. Age 30 years d. Married
2. **Increased suicidal tendency is associated with** *[Recent Question 2016]*
   a. Increased Noradrenaline
   b. Decreased Serotonin
   c. Decreased Dopamine
   d. Increased GABA
3. **Recurrent suicidal tendencies are seen in** *[NBE FMGE September 2009]*
   a. Schizophrenia
   b. Severe depression
   c. Borderline personality disorders
   d. All of the above
4. **Risk factors for contemplated suicide include** *[NBE DNB 1998]*
   a. Being married
   b. Age under 20 years
   c. Alcoholism
   d. A history of having discussed suicide with a friend
5. **Suicidal tendencies are least common with** *[Recent Question 2013, 2015]*
   a. Alone
   b. Depression
   c. Male
   d. Married person
6. **Suicidal tendencies are most commonly seen in** *[NBE FMGE March 2003]*
   a. Mania
   b. Hypomania
   c. Involutional melancholia
   d. Anxiety neurosis
7. **All are side-effects of prolonged Phenytoin therapy except** *[NBE FMGE September 2008]*
   a. Osteomalacia b. Gum hyperplasia
   c. Gynaecomastia d. Megaloblastic anaemia
8. **Which of the following anti-epileptic drugs act by affecting levels of GABA?** *[NBE FMGE September 2008]*
   a. Phenytoin sodium
   b. Ethosuximide
   c. Sodium valproate
   d. Carbamazepine
9. **Most common psychiatric emergency** *[NBE FMGE March 2005]*
   a. Rape b. Violence
   c. Panic attack d. Suicide
10. **Anorexia nervosa is an eating disorder characterized by all except** *[NBE FMGE March 2012]*
    a. Menorrhagia
    b. Salivary gland enlargement
    c. Acrocyanosis
    d. Bradycardia
11. **Which of the following is a Psychiatric emergency?** *[Recent Question 2014, 2015]*
    a. Capgras syndrome
    b. Suicide
    c. Acute Schizophrenia
    d. Cocaine use
12. **Psychiatric emergencies include all except** *[Recent Question 2014]*
    a. Suicide b. Panic disorder
    c. Drug use disorder d. Insomnia
13. **Risk factor for Suicide is?** *[Recent Question 2017]*
    a. Increased serotonin b. Drug abuse
    c. Female sex d. Married person

HIGH YIELD MCQs

1. **Incidence of suicide in India is** *[Recent Question 2017, PGI 2005]*
   a. 8-10/100 population
   b. 8-10/10000 population
   c. 8-10/1 lac population
   d. 8-10/10 lac population
   e. 8-10/1 billion population
2. **The neurotransmitter that is associated with suicidal tendencies is** *[AIIMS PGMEE 2008]*
   a. Serotonin
   b. GABA
   c. Nor-epinephrine
   d. Acetylcholine
3. **Suicidal tendency seen in** *[PGI 2002]*
   a. Schizophrenia b. PTSD
   c. Depression d. OCD
   e. Anxiety disorder
4. **Most common mental disorder as a cause of suicide** *[JIPMER PGMEE 2002, SGPGI PGMEE 2003]*
   a. Mania b. Depression
   c. Alcohol dependence d. Schizophrenia
5. **Suicidal tendencies seen in** *[PGI PGMEE 2006]*
   a. Depression
   b. Posttraumatic stress disorder
   c. Schizophrenia
   d. Substance abuse
   e. Anxiety
6. **A patient presents to the emergency department with self-harm and indicates suicidal intent. Which of the following conditions does not warrant an immediate specialist assessment?** *[All India PGMEE 2010]*
   a. Formal thought disorder
   b. Acute Alcohol intoxication
   c. Chronic Severe physical illness
   d. Social isolation

7. Anorexia nervosa can be differentiated from bulimia by

[AIIMS PGMEE 2008]

a. Intense fear of weight gain
b. Disturbance of body image
c. Adolescent age
d. Peculiars patterns of food handing

8. Which of the following conditions characterized by episodes of excessive and uncontrolled eating

[UP PGMEE 2006, Jharkhand PGMEE 2007, TN PGMEE 2005]

a. Anorexia nervosa
b. Bulimia nervosa
c. Body dysmorphobia
d. All of the above
e. None of the above

9. In Bulimia all are seen except

[JIPMER PGMEE 1998, Recent Question 2015]

a. Parotitis
b. Menorrhagia
c. Oligomenorrhea
d. Caries Teeth

10. What is most common cause of suicide in India according to National Crime Records Bureau 2014?

[AIIMS PG November 2015]

a. Hanging
b. Drowning
c. Poisoning
d. Fall from height

11. Mood stabiliser having an Anti-suicidal role is

[AIIMS May 2017]

a. Lamotrigine
b. Carbamazepine
c. Valproate
d. Lithium

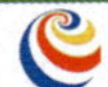 NEET/NBE PATTERN MCQs ANSWERS WITH EXPLANATIONS 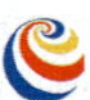

1. Ans. (b) Unmarried

[Ref. Niraj Ahuja, 7/e p72]

- **Risk factors for Suicide**: History of suicidal attempts, Staying Single, Trauma (Recent major stressful life event), Impulsivity, Age > 40 years, Male sex, Illnesses, Isolation, Alcohol/drug dependence, Pre-occupation with suicidal plans and thoughts, depression

2. Ans. (b) Decreased Serotonin

[Ref. Understanding Abnormal Behavior by Sue, 11/e p280]

- Reduced availability of serotonin and Low serotonin levels are associated with Suicide
- These abnormalities are also seen in depression

3. Ans. (d) All of the above

[Ref. Niraj Ahuja, 7/e p222-224]

Underlying Causes of Suicidal Behaviour

- Psychiatric disorders
  - Depression
  - Depression secondary to illness
  - Alcohol/drug dependence
  - Schizophrenia
  - Borderline personality
- Physical disorders (incurable/painful)
  - Cancer
  - AIDS
- Psychosocial factors
  - Failure in examinations
  - Failure in love
  - Marital difficulties
  - Family problems

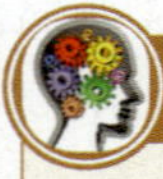

Also Remember

- **Recurrent suicidal behaviour is seen in**
  - Borderline personality disorder
  - Depression (secondary to severe illness)
  - Alcohol/drug dependence
  - Schizophrenia

4. Ans. (c) Alcoholism; (d) A history of having discussed suicide with a friend

[Ref. Niraj Ahuja, 7/e p72]

5. Ans. (d) Married person

[Ref. Niraj Ahuja, 7/e p72, 222]

6. Ans. (c) Involutional melancholia

[Ref. Niraj Ahuja, 7/e p191]

7. Ans. (c) Gynaecomastia

[Ref. Essentials of KDT, 6/e p405]

- *Side effects of Phenytoin therapy:*

At therapeutic levels	At higher plasma levels
Gum hyperplasia **(Most common)** Hirsutism Hypersensitivity reactions Megaloblastic anemia Osteomalacia Hyperglycaemia Foetal hydantoin syndrome	Cerebellar/ vestibular manifestations Drowsiness, confusion, hallucinations Epigastric pain, nausea, vomiting Local vascular injury (on IV injection) Hypotension (on IV injection) Cardiac arrhythmias (on IV injection)

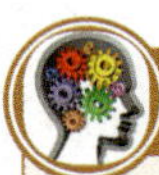

Also Remember

Drugs causing Gynaecomastia

[**Mnemonic: DESI G**ossypol **R M**ost **C**ommon Causeo**FG**ynaecomastia in **K**ommon **P**eople]*

- **D**igitalis
- **E**thionamide, Estrogen
- **S**pirinolactone
- **I**NH
- **G**ossypol, **G**riseofulvin
- **R**eserpine
- **M**ethyldopa
- **C**yproterone acetate, **C**imetidine
- **C**lomiphene, **C**alcium antagonist
- **F**lutamide
- **G**oserelin
- **K**etoconazole
- **P**henytoin (rare cause)

(***M**nemonic has been taken from http://bestmedicalmnemonics.blogspot.com)

8. Ans. (c) Sodium valproate

[Ref. Essentials of Medical Pharmacology by KD Tripathi, 6/e p404]

- *Mechanism of action of anti-epileptic drugs:*

Prolongation of sodium channel inactivation	Facilitator of GABA-mediated Cl^- channel opening	Inhibitor of T-type Ca^{++} current
• Phenytoin • Carbamazepine • Valproate • Lamotrigine • Topiramate • Zonisamide	• Barbiturate • Benzodiazepine • Vigabatrin • Valproate • Gabapentin • Tiagabine	• Ethosuximide • Trimethadione • Valproate

9. Ans. (d) Suicide

[Ref. Niraj Ahuja, 7/e p222]

Common Psychiatric Emergencies
- Suicides **(Most common)**
- Stupor and catatonic syndrome
- Excited behaviour and violence
- Severe depression
- Hyperventilation syndrome
- Side effects of psychotropic drugs
- Pseudo-seizures (Conversion/dissociation hysteria)
- Anorexia nervosa
- Battered child syndrome
- Grief
- Drug/alcohol use disorders
- Panic disorders
- Acute psychosis

10. Ans. (a) Menorrhagia
[Ref. Niraj Ahuja, 7/e p142-43]

Clinical Features of Anorexia Nervosa
- General: Hypothermia
- CVS: Bradycardia, Hypotension
- Dermatological: Alopecia, Acrocyanosis, Oedema
- GIT: Salivary (Parotid) gland enlargement, Constipation
- Hematological: Normocytic-normochromic anaemia, Leucopenia
- Electrolyte: Hypokalemia, Hyponatremia
- Endocrine: Low LH/ FSH, Amenorrhoea

11. Ans. (b) Suicide
[Ref. Niraj Ahuja, 7/e p222]

12. Ans. (d) Insomnia
[Ref. Niraj Ahuja, 7/e p221]

13. Ans. (b) Drug abuse
[Ref. Niraj Ahuja, 7/e p72]
- Risk factors for Suicide: History of suicidal attempts, Staying Single, Trauma (Recent major stressful life event), Impulsivity, Age > 40 years, Male sex, Illnesses, Isolation, Alcohol/drug dependence, Pre-occupation with suicidal plans and thoughts, depression
- Suicide is associated with decreased levels of Serotonin

HIGH YIELD MCQs ANSWERS WITH EXPLANATIONS 

1. Ans. NONE
[Ref. Developments in Psychiatry in India by Malhotra & Chakrabarti, 1/e p203]
- *Suicide rate in India*: 10.6 per 100,000 population

2. Ans. (a) Serotonin
[Ref. Pathology: Implications for Physical Therapist by Good man & Fuller, 4/e p116]
- *Proposed role of Serotonin in Suicide*: Fewer Serotonin transporter sites with local reduction of Serotonin binding

3. Ans. (a) Schizophrenia; (c) Depression
[Ref. Niraj Ahuja, 7/e p223]

Psychiatric Disorders with Suicide
- Depression
  - Major depression
  - Reactive depression
  - Depression secondary to serious physical illness
- Alcoholism and Drug dependence
- Schizophrenia
- Bipolar disorder
- Cluster B Personality disorder

4. Ans. (b) Depression
[Ref. Niraj Ahuja, 7/e p223]
- *MC mental illness associated with Suicide*: Depression

5. Ans. (a) Depression; (c) Schizophrenia; (d) Substance abuse
[Ref. Niraj Ahuja, 7/e p223]

6. Ans. (b) Acute Alcohol intoxication
[Ref. Niraj Ahuja, 7/e p223]

7. Ans. (d) Peculiar patterns of food handing
[Ref. Niraj Ahuja, 7/e p142-145]

8. Ans. (b) Bulimia nervosa
[Ref. Niraj Ahuja, 7/e p144]

9. Ans. (b) Menorrhagia
[Ref. Niraj Ahuja, 7/e p144]

10. Ans. (a) Hanging
[Ref. Accidental Deaths and Suicides in India 2014, NCRB p208]

Prominent Means of Committing Suicides in India
- Hanging (41.8%)
- Consuming Poison (26.0%)
- Self-Immolation (6.9%)
- Drowning (5.6%)

11. Ans. (d) Lithium
[Ref. Suicide in Psychiatric Disorders by Tatarelli, 1/e p110]

Lithium: Anti-suicidal Agent
- Recent evidence show for patients with bipolar or recurrent unipolar depressive disorders, Lithium may have specific anti-suicidal properties over and above its mood-stabilizing properties
- Relative reduction of risks of suicides and attempts
- Reduction of lethality (increased attempts: suicide ratio)

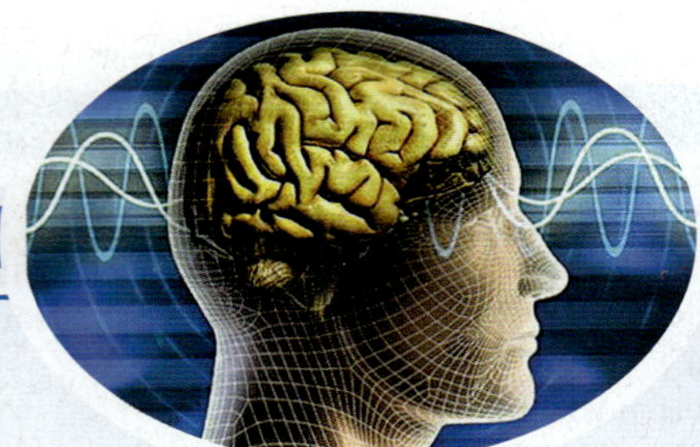

Chapter 12

Disorders of Childhood and Adolescence

THEORETICAL CONCEPTS

XII A. SPECIFIC DEVELOPMENT DISORDERS

- ***Dyslexia***: Developmental reading disorder[Q]
  - Serious delay in learning to read
  - Omissions, distortion, substitution of words
  - Impaired spelling and writing
- ***Dyscalculia***: Developmental arithmetic/ mathematical disorder[Q]
  - Difficulty in recognising mathematical signs
  - Difficulty in calculations
  - Difficulty in learning mathematical tables
- ***Dysphasia***: Developmental language/ communication disorder[Q]
  - *Dyslalia*: Below par accuracy in use of speech sounds
  - Expressive language disorder
  - Receptive language disorder
- ***Motor dyspraxia***: Clumsy child syndrome
  - Poor coordination in daily activities

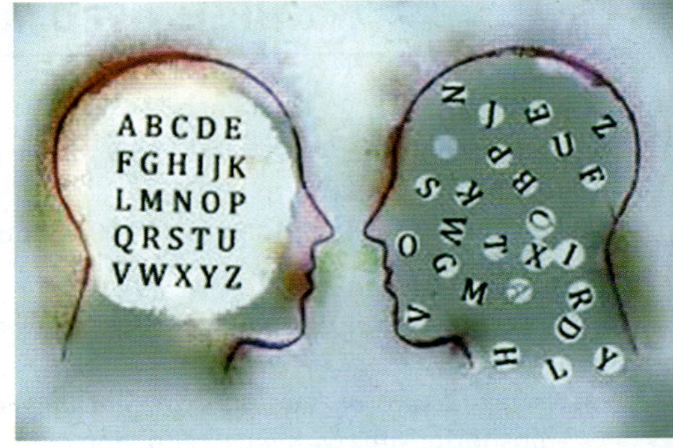

Fig. Dyslexia

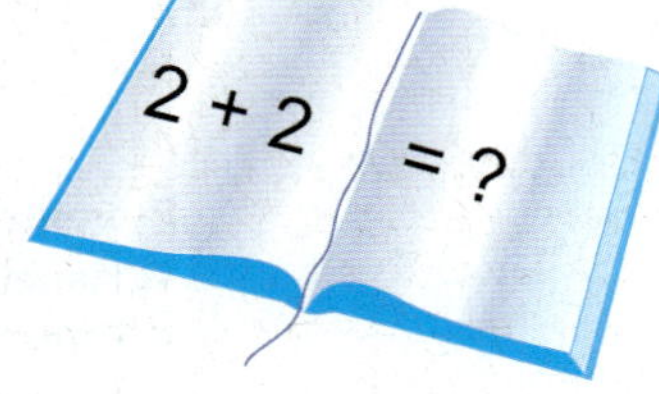

Fig. Dyscalculia

Topper's Edge

Dyslexia
- Reading disorder:
  - A learning difficulty that primarily affects the skills involved in accurate and fluent word reading and spelling and is characterized by difficulties in phonological awareness, verbal memory and verbal processing speed
  - Characterized by trouble with reading despite normal intelligence
- Causes of Dyslexia:
  - Two types of cause: Related to language processing and Related to visual processing
  - Acquired dyslexia or alexia may be caused by brain damage due to stroke or atrophy
- Associated Learning Disabilities[Q]:
  - Dysgraphia: Difficulties with writing or typing
  - Attention deficit hyperactivity disorder (ADHD)
  - Auditory processing disorder: Listening disability affecting ability to process auditory information
  - Developmental coordination disorder

XII B. CHILDHOOD AUTISM

- *Prevalence*: 0.5 per 1000 population
- *Clinical presentation*:
  - Marked impairment in social and interpersonal interaction[Q]
    - Absent social smile
    - Treats people as furniture
    - Lack of attachment to parents/ Absent separation anxiety
    - Absence of fear when in danger
    - Marked impairment in making friends
  - Marked impairment in language and non-verbal communication
    - Absent/delayed speech
    - Abnormal speech patterns
  - Abnormal behavioural characteristics
  - Mental retardation
- *Treatment*:
  - Behaviour therapy
  - Psychotherapy
  - Pharmacotherapy
    - Haloperidol
    - Risperidone

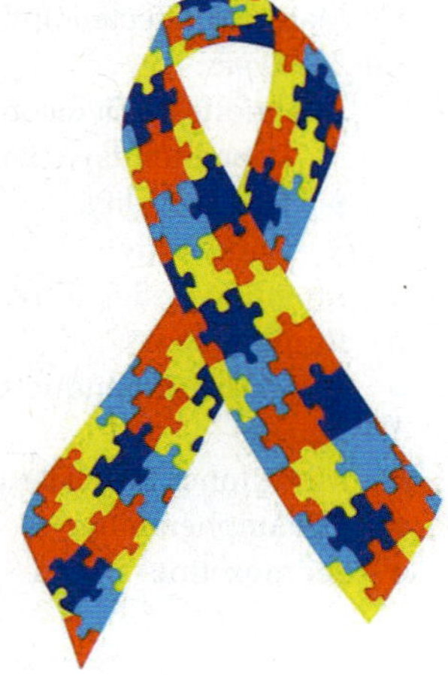

Fig. Autism logo

Topper's Edge

Autism

- A neurodevelopmental disorder characterized by **impaired social interaction, verbal and non-verbal communication, and restricted and repetitive behavior**
- Parents usually notice signs in the **first two years of their child's life**

Clinical Presentation of Autism

- Social development[Q]:
  - **Social impairments**, lack the intuition about others that many people take for granted
  - Less attention to social stimuli, smile and look at others less often, and respond less to their own name, Less eye contact
  - Inability to use simple movements to express themselves, to exhibit social understanding, to approach others spontaneously, to imitate and respond to emotions, to communicate nonverbally
  - Making and maintaining friendships often proves to be difficult
- Communication:
  - **Do not develop enough natural speech to meet their daily communication needs**
  - Delayed onset of babbling, unusual gestures, diminished responsiveness, and vocal patterns
  - Less likely to make requests or share experiences
  - Difficulty with imaginative play and with developing symbols into language
- Repetitive behavior:
  - **Stereotyped behaviors**: Repetitive movements (Hand flapping, head rolling, or body rocking)
  - **Compulsive behaviors**: Placing objects in a specific order, checking things, or hand washing
  - Sameness: Resistance to change
  - Ritualistic behavior: Unvarying pattern of daily activities, such as an unchanging menu or a dressing ritual
  - Restricted interests: Preoccupation with a single television program, toy, or game
  - Self-injury: Eye-poking, skin-picking, hand-biting and head-banging
- Other symptoms:
  - **Unusual abilities**, ranging from splinter skills such as the memorization of trivia to the extraordinarily rare talents of prodigious autistic savants
  - Superior skills in perception and attention, relative to the general population
  - Sensory abnormalities are found in over 90% of those with autism
  - Unusual eating behavior: Selectivity

Pathophysiology

- Autism affects the amygdala, cerebellum, and many other parts of the brain[Q]

Diagnosis

- Based on behavior, not cause or mechanism
- Under the DSM-5, autism is characterized by persistent deficits in social communication and interaction across multiple contexts, as well as restricted, repetitive patterns of behavior, interests, or activities
- These deficits are present in early childhood, typically before age three, and lead to clinically significant functional impairment
- Sample symptoms include lack of social or emotional reciprocity, stereotyped and repetitive use of language or idiosyncratic language, and persistent preoccupation with unusual objects
- The disturbance must not be better accounted for by Rett's syndrome, intellectual disability or global developmental delay
- ICD-10 uses essentially the same definition

XII C. ATTENTION-DEFICIT DISORDER (HYPERKINETIC DISORDER[Q])

- *Age on onset*: 4–7 years[Q]
  - Males are affected upto 6-8 times more than females[Q]
- *Clinical types*:
  - Attention-deficit disorder with hyperactivity (Hyperkinetic disorder)
    - Poor attention span with distractibility
    - Hyperactivity
    - Impulsivity
  - Attention-deficit disorder without hyperactivity
  - Residual type
  - Hyperkinetic conduct disorder
- *Treatment*:
  - Methylphenidate **(Drug of choice[Q])**
  - Dexamphetamine
  - Atomoxetine

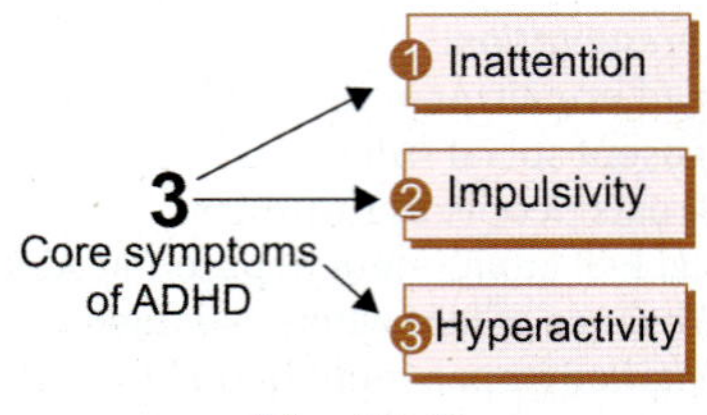

Fig. ADHD

Topper's Edge

ATTENTION DEFICIT HYPERACTIVITY DISORDER (ADHD)

- A brain disorder marked by an ongoing pattern of inattention and/or hyperactivity-impulsivity that interferes with functioning or development
- A mental disorder of the neurodevelopmental type characterized by problems paying attention, excessive activity, or difficulty controlling behavior which is not appropriate for a person's age
  - **Inattention**: Person wanders off task, lacks persistence, has difficulty sustaining focus, and is disorganized; and these problems are not due to defiance or lack of comprehension
  - **Hyperactivity**: Person seems to move about constantly, including in situations in which it is not appropriate; or excessively fidgets, taps, or talks. In adults, it may be extreme restlessness or wearing others out with constant activity
  - **Impulsivity**: Person makes hasty actions that occur in the moment without first thinking about them and that may have high potential for harm; or a desire for immediate rewards or inability to delay gratification

Types of ADHD[Q]

- ADHD predominantly inattentive type (ADHD-PI): Being easily distracted, forgetful, daydreaming, disorganization, poor concentration, and difficulty completing tasks
- ADHD predominantly hyperactive-impulsive type: Excessive fidgetiness and restlessness, hyperactivity, difficulty waiting and remaining seated, immature behavior; destructive behaviors
- ADHD combined type: Combination of the first two subtypes

Associated Disorders of ADHD[Q]

- **Learning disabilities**
- **Tourette syndrome**
- Oppositional defiant disorder (ODD) and conduct disorder (CD)
- Primary disorder of vigilance
- Sluggish cognitive tempo (SCT)
- Mood disorders
- Anxiety disorders
- Obsessive-compulsive disorder (OCD)
- Substance use disorders
- Restless legs syndrome
- Sleep disorders
- Persistent bed wetting
- Obesity, asthma and sleep disorders, celiac disease and migraine
- Pathophysiology of ADHD
- Associated with functional impairments in brain's neurotransmitter systems, particularly involving dopamine and norepinephrine

Contd...

Contd...

Management of ADHD

- Behavioral therapies:
  - Psychoeducational input, behavior therapy, cognitive behavioral therapy (CBT), interpersonal psychotherapy, family therapy, school-based interventions, social skills training, behavioral peer intervention, organization training, parent management training, and neurofeedback
  - Parent training and education
  - Training in social skills, behavioral modification and medication
  - Regular physical exercise
- Medication:
  - Stimulant medications - **Pharmaceutical treatment of choice: Methylphenidate**
  - Non-stimulant medications: Atomoxetine, Bupropion, Guanfacine, Clonidine
- Diet:
  - Free fatty acid supplementation
  - Decreased eating of artificial food coloring
  - Iron, magnesium and iodine supplementation
  - Zinc supplementation

XII D. TOURETTE'S SYNDROME[Q]

- Multiple motor tics
- Multiple vocal tics
- Obsessions and compulsions
- Duration more than 1 year

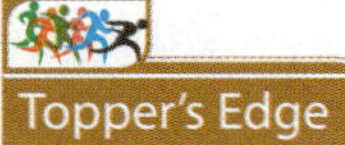

Topper's Edge

Tourette's Syndrome

- Tourette's Syndrome:
  - Common neuropsychiatric disorder with onset in childhood[Q]
  - **Characterized by multiple motor tics and at least one vocal (phonic) tic**[Q]
  - Tics characteristically wax and wane, can be suppressed temporarily, and are typically preceded by an unwanted urge or sensation in the affected muscles
  - Common tics: Eye blinking, coughing, throat clearing, sniffing, facial movement
- Diagnosis of TD (DSM-IV): Multiple motor tics, and at least one phonic tic, are present for more than a year
- Pathophysiology: Dysfunction in cortical and subcortical regions, the thalamus, basal ganglia and frontal cortex[Q]
- Treatment
  - Medication with most proven efficacy: **Typical and Atypical neuroleptics** (Risperidone, Ziprasidone, Haloperidol, Pimozide, Fluphenazine)
  - Cognitive behavior therapy
  - Relaxation techniques

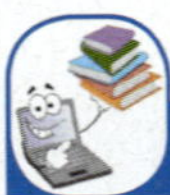

IMAGE-BASED QUESTIONS

1. Symbol shown in Photograph is related to .... disorder

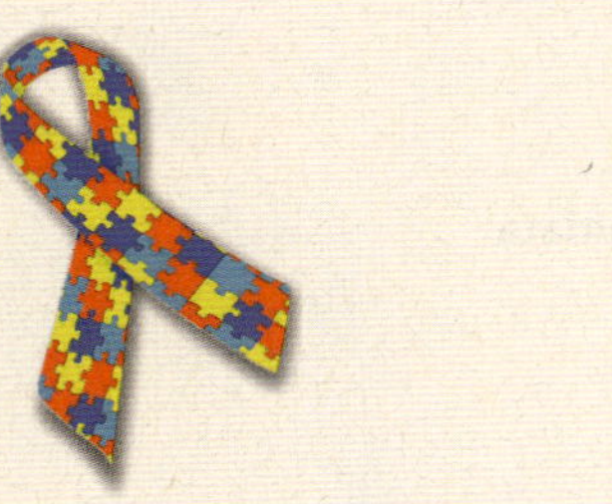

a. Alcoholism b. Depression
c. Substance use disorders d. Autism

2. Identify the Child Psychiatric disorder as shown in Photograph

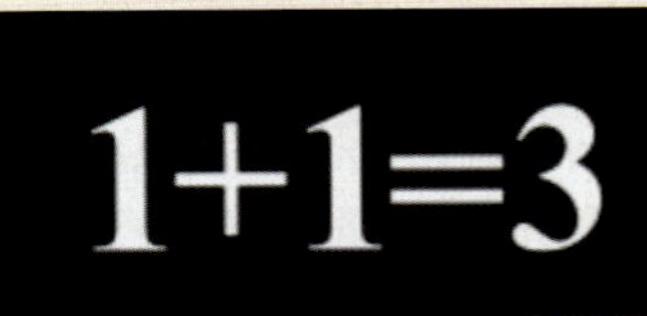

a. Dyscalculia b. Dysphasia
c. Dyspraxia d. Echolalia

3. Identify the Child Psychiatric disorder as shown in Photograph

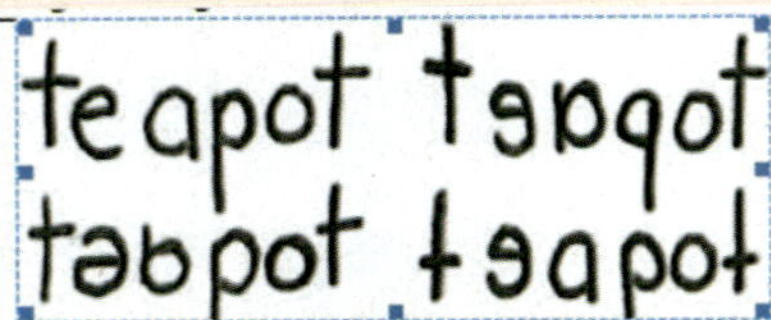

a. Dyscalculia
b. Dysphasia
c. Dyslexia
d. Echolalia

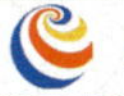 ANSWERS WITH EXPLANATIONS OF IBQs 

1. Ans. (d) Autism *[Ref. Autism Society]*

Autism Awareness Ribbon

- Puzzle pattern reflects: Complexity of the autism spectrum
- Different colors and shapes represent: Diversity of the people and families living with the condition
- Brightness of the ribbon signals: Hope that through increased awareness of autism, and through early intervention and access to appropriate services/supports, people with autism will lead full lives able to interact with the world on the own terms

2. Ans. (a) Dyscalculia *[Ref. Child Psychology and Psychiatry by Skuse, 1/e p69]*

- Dyscalculia: Severe difficulty in making arithmetic calculations
- Dysphasia: Language disorder marked by deficiency in the generation of speech, and sometimes also in its comprehension
- Dyspraxia: Motor learning disability leading to problems with coordination and movements
- Echolalia: Meaningless repetition of another person's spoken words

3. Ans. (c) Dyslexia *[Ref. Neuroscience of Clinical Psychiatry by George, 1/e p208]*

- Dyslexia: An unexpected difficulty in reading in a person with otherwise normal intelligence and motivation
- It represents developmental reading disorder, Impaired writing and spelling.

NEET/NBE PATTERN MCQs

1. Rett's syndrome is characterized by all except *[Recent Question 2016]*
 a. Regression of acquired skills
 b. Breath holding spells
 c. Autistic behavior
 d. Macrocephaly

2. Following drugs are used in treatment of ADHD *[Recent Question 2016]*
 a. Amphetamine b. Modafinil
 c. Methylphenidate d. All of the above

3. Which personality disorder/s can be a part of Autistic spectrum of disorders? *[Recent Question 2016]*
 a. Schizoid b. Schizotypal
 c. Borderline d. All the above

4. A neurodevelopmental disorder characterized by impaired social interaction, verbal and non-verbal communication, and restricted and repetitive behavior is description for *[Recent Question 2016]*
 a. Autism b. Anxiety disorder
 c. Antisocial personality d. Paranoid schizophrenia

5. Appetite for Non-nutritive substance is called *[Recent Question 2016]*
 a. Pica b. Appepritant
 c. Bulimia d. Bolean

6. Autism is characterized by all except *[Recent Question 2016]*
 a. Lack of social play in child
 b. Language problems
 c. Stereotyped behavior
 d. Depression

7. Drug of choice in Tourette syndrome is *[Recent Question 2016, 2017]*
 a. Valproate b. Carbamazepine
 c. Haloperidol d. Methadone

8. Characteristic disorder appears in Late childhood and continues in Adulthood *[Recent Question 2016]*
 a. Somatoform disorder b. Personality disorder
 c. Anxiety disorder d. Mood disorder

9. 10-year-old child presents with impaired social interaction, communication and stereotyped behavior. He has normal IQ and language skills. What is the most probable diagnosis? *[Recent Question 2016]*
 a. Asperger syndrome b. Rett syndrome
 c. Autism d. Childhood depression

10. Adverse effect due to Sodium valproate seen only in children is *[NBE FMGE March 2007]*
 a. Tremor b. Hepatitis
 c. Anorexia d. Loss of hair

11. The treatment of choice in attention deficit hyperactivity disorder is *[Recent Question 2012, 2013, AIIMS PG 2003]*
 a. Haloperidol b. Imipramine
 c. Methylphenidate d. Alprazolam

12. Stimulant drug is given to child for *[Recent Question 2012]*
 a. Conduct disorder
 b. Speech developmental disorder
 c. Pervasive disorder
 d. ADHD

13. Bruxism is *[Recent Question 2012]*
 a. Walking during sleep
 b. Nocturnal enuresis
 c. Grinding of teeth during sleep
 d. Sleep apnoea

14. Fluoxetine is used in which of the following childhood condition *[NBE DNB 2002]*
 a. Depression b. Autism
 c. Enuresis d. None of these

15. A 14 years old boy presents with history of frequent fighting at school disciplinary problems, stealing money, truancy and vandalism. What is the most appropriate diagnosis? *[NBE FMGE March 2012]*
 a. Attention deficit hyperactivity disorder
 b. Autistic disorder
 c. Narcissistic personality disorder
 d. Conduct disorder

16. A 10-year-old child "blanks out" in class (e.g. stops talking midsentence and then continues as if nothing had happened). During spells there is slight quivering of lips. What is the most probable diagnosis? *[UPSC CMS 2015]*
 a. Mutism b. Autism
 c. Adjustment disorder d. Absence seizure

17. Tourette is a disorder of *[Recent Question 2015]*
 a. Attention deficit
 b. Tics
 c. Autism
 d. Mental retardation

18. Autistic spectrum disorder? *[Recent Question 2017]*
 a. Defective communication
 b. Absent separation anxiety
 c. Impaired concentration
 d. More common in girls

19. All are true about Tourette syndrome, except? *[Recent Question 2017]*
 a. Motor tics
 b. More common in females
 c. Associated with OCD
 d. Neuroleptics are useful in the treatment

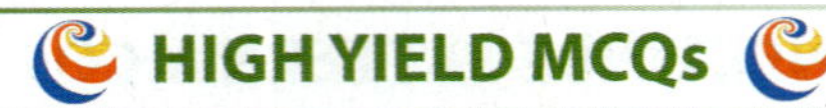

HIGH YIELD MCQs

1. A 6-years-old child presents with bed wetting at night. There is no history of any day time symptoms. The urine microscopy is normal, the specific gravity of urine is 1.020 and other investigations are normal. What should be advised? *[AIIMS May 2016]*
a. Reassurance and revisit after 6 months
b. CT pelvis
c. USG kidney and bladder
d. Refer to child psychiatrist

2. Coprolalia is seen in *[Recent Question 2015, JIPMER PGMEE 1990, AIIMS PGMEE 1995]*
a. Delirium
b. Alcoholic intoxication
c. Mania
d. Tourette's syndrome

3. True about treatment of nocturnal enuresis *[PGI 2005]*
a. Imipramine
b. CPZ
c. Alprazolam
d. Haloperidol

4. Most useful drug in Enuresis is *[AIIMS PGMEE 1996]*
a. Haloperidol
b. Diazepam
c. Trimipramine
d. Chlorpromazine

5. DOC of night terrors *[PGI 1998]*
a. Meprobamate
b. Tricyclic antidepressant
c. Clonazepam
d. Diazepam

6. A 9-year-old child disturbs other people, is destructive, and interferes when two people are talking, does not follow instructions and cannot wait for his turn while playing a game. He is likely to be suffering from *[AIIMS PGMEE 2005]*
a. Emotional disorders
b. Behavioural problems
c. No disorder
d. Attention deficit hyperactivity disorder

7. Which of the following is not seen in hyperkinetic child? *[All India PGMEE 1991]*
a. Aggressive outburst
b. Decreased attention span
c. Left to right disorientation
d. Soft neurological signs

8. Drug(s) used in treatment of Attention-Deficit Hyperactivity Disorder *[PGI 2008]*
a. Atomoxetine
b. Methylphenidate
c. Dexmethylphenidate
d. Quetiapine
e. Dextroamphetamine

9. Treatment of hyperkinetic syndrome include *[PGI 2001, 2006]*
a. Imipramine
b. Methylphenidate
c. Haloperidol
d. Clozapine
e. Amphetamine

10. Infantile autism is characterized by *[PGI 2004]*
a. Impaired vision
b. Impaired neurobehavioral development
c. Impaired folate level
d. A socioeconomic hazard
e. Parenting

11. Autism is *[PGI 2000]*
a. Neuro-developmental disorder
b. Social and language communication problem
c. Metabolic disease
d. Mainly due to hypothalamus damage

12. Autism is *[PGI 2001]*
a. Biological causation
b. Pervasive social and language communication problem
c. Metabolic disease
d. Mainly due to hypothalamus damage
e. Onset after 23 years usually

13. Lack of development of speech in a child can be due to *[PGI 2006]*
a. Tongue tie
b. Deafness
c. Mental subnormality
d. Laryngomalacia
e. Psychosocial

14. A 14-year-old boy has difficulty in expressing himself in writing and makes frequent spelling mistakes. He passes his examination with poor marks. However his mathematical ability & social adjustment are appropriate for his age. Which of the following is the most likely diagnosis? *[AIIMS PGMEE 2004]*
a. Mental Retardation
b. Specific learning disability
c. Lack of interest in studies
d. Examination anxiety

15. Conduct disorder in a child manifests with *[PGI 2001]*
a. Disregard for right of others
b. Doesn't care for authority
c. Backward in studies
d. Decreased head circumference
e. Steals things

16. An eleven months old boy is all the time so restless that the rest of the class is unable to concentrate. He is hardly ever in his seat but roams around the hall. He has difficulty playing quietly. The most likely diagnosis is *[Recent Question 2017, All India PGMEE 2002]*
a. Attention-deficit hyperactivity disorder
b. Conduct disorder
c. Depressive disorder
d. Schizophrenia

17. ADHD in childhood can lead to what in future? *[PGI 2000]*
a. Schizophrenia
b. Alcoholism
c. Intellectual changes
d. Antisocial behaviour
e. Academic underachievement

18. A 9 years old child is restless. He is hyperactive and his teacher complains that he does not listen to the teachings. Disturbs other students he also shows less interest in playing. The likely diagnosis is *[AIIMS PGMEE 2002]*
a. Cerebral palsy
b. Attention deficit hyperkinetic child
c. Delirium
d. Mania

19. A child 10-years-old present with hyperactivity, in attention. Parents are extremely worried, what would you say to the parents? *[AIIMS PGMEE 2008]*
a. Normal behaviour
b. Behavioural problem and behavior therapy
c. Serious problem and medical therapy
d. Change in environment

20. A 6-year-old child has history of birth asphyxia does not communicate well has slow mental and physical growth, does not mix with people, has limited interests gets widely agitated if disturbed. Diagnosis is *[AIIMS PGMEE 2001]*
a. Hyperkinetic child
b. Autistic Disorder
c. Attention deficit Disorder
d. Mixed Receptive-Expressive Language Disorder

21. A two years old girl child is brought to the outpatient with features of hand wringing stereotype movements, impaired language and communication development, breath-holding spells, poor social skills and deceleration of head growth after six months of age. The most likely diagnosis is *[AIIMS PGMEE 2003, Recent Question 2015]*
a. Asperger syndrome
b. Rett's syndrome
c. Fragile X syndrome
d. Cotard syndrome

22. A 3-year-old child presents with delayed speech and poor concentration. He has difficulty in communication and also difficulty in making friends. The likely diagnosis is *[AIIMS PGMEE 2006, 2010]*
a. Autism
b. ADHD
c. Specific learning disability
d. Mental retardation

23. Autistic disorder is characterized by all of the following, except *[All India PGMEE 2010]*
a. Visual impairment
b. Lack of social interaction
c. Delayed development of speech
d. Stereotypic movements

24. A young patient with 10 years history of eye blinking and grunting which has now increased so much so that it disturbs his routine activity. He will be benefitted by *[AIIMS PG May 2015]*
a. Carbamazepine
b. Risperidone
c. Methylphenidate
d. Imipramine

25. 'Idiot Savants', who have prodigious rote memories or calculating abilities, are found in *[PGMCET 2015]*
a. School Refusal
b. Oppositional defiant disorder
c. Severe mental retardation
d. Autistic disorder

26. Which of the following is not true about the Autistic specific disorders? *[ESI IMO 2014]*
a. Impaired communication
b. Impaired imagination
c. Language development is delayed
d. Vision problems

27. Asperger's syndrome, true is/ are *[PGI November 2014]*
a. Autism disorder
b. Linguistic and cognitive development preserved
c. Poor auditory perception
d. Viral disease in origin
e. Poor visual perception

28. All are habit disorder except *[Recent Question 2018]*
a. Nail biting
b. Temper tantrum
c. Tics
d. Thumb sucking

29. Minimal brain dysfunction syndrome seen in *[Recent Question 2018]*
a. Dyslexia
b. ADHD
c. Mental subnormality
d. Down's syndrome

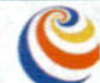 NEET/NBE PATTERN MCQs ANSWERS WITH EXPLANATIONS 

1. Ans. (d) Macrocephaly
[Ref. Concise Neurology by Espay, 1/e p165]

Rett's Syndrome
- X-linked dominant disorder, Lethal in males
- Developmental regression and autistic behavior in girls
- Acquired microcephaly
- Hand stereotype movements
- Gait apraxia, ataxia
- Hyperventilation and Breath holding spells

2. Ans. (d) All of the above
[Ref. Niraj Ahuja, 7/e p167]
- **Drugs used in treatment of ADHD**: Amphetamine, Dextroamphetamine, Modafinil, Methylphenidate, Methamphetamine, Lisdexamfetamine, Atomoxetine

3. Ans. (d) All the above
[Ref. Essential Psychopathology Casebook by Kilgus, 1/e p141]

4. Ans. (a) Autism
[Ref. Zitelli and Davis' Atlas of Pediatric Physical Diagnosis, 6/e p102]

Autism Spectrum Disorder
- Neurodevelopmental disabilities of varying severity
- Deficits in social interaction
- Deficits in verbal/non-verbal communication used for social interaction
- Limited social reciprocity
- Difficulty in maintaining peer relationships
- Restricted interests
- Repetitive behaviors
- Limited eye-to-eye gaze
- Unusual facial expressions

5. Ans. (a) Pica
[Ref. Clinical Child Psychology by Shyam, 1/e p313]
- Pica is a medical disorder characterized by a persistent appetite for largely non-nutritive substances (e.g., coal, soil, faeces, chalk, paper, soap) for at least one month
- Seen in all ages especially children, pregnant women

6. Ans. (d) Depression
[Ref. Child Psychotherapy and Counseling by Brems, 3/e p216]

Autistic Disorder
- Impairment in social interaction, verbal and nonverbal communication
- Repetitive or stereotyped patterns of behaviors and activities
- Lack of empathy for others feelings
- Inability to form relationships
- Lack of social play
- Delay or lack of spoken language

7. Ans. (c) Haloperidol
[Ref. How to Live with Your Children by Fontenelle, 1/e p445]
- Since the 1960s, haloperidol has been the drug of choice for treating Tourette syndrome
- Haloperidol is most effective at low doses

8. Ans. (b) Personality disorder
[Ref. Learning Disabilities and Mental Health by Raghavan, 1/e p75]
- According to ICD-10, Personality disorder tends to appear in late childhood or adolescence and continues to be manifest into adulthood
- They are NOT secondary to any other brain disease or mental disorder BUT they may precede or coexist with other disorders

9. Ans. (a) Asperger syndrome
[Ref. Niraj Ahuja, 7/e p165]

10. Ans. (b) Hepatitis
[Ref. KD Tripathi, 6/e p407]

Side Effects of Sodium Valproate
- Anorexia
- Drowsiness
- Ataxia
- Tremor
- Alopecia
- Thrombocytopenia
- Fulminant hepatitis (only in children <3 years age)
- Pancreatitis (only in children)
- PCOD (only in girl children)
- Menstrual irregularities (only in girl children)
- Teratogenic: Spina bifida, neural tube defects

11. Ans. (c) Methylphenidate
[Ref. Niraj Ahuja, 7/e p167]

Pharmacotherapy for ADD
- Stimulant medication:
  - Methylphenidate: Drug of choice
  - Dextroamphetamine, Dexamphetamine
- Other medication: Clonidine, Imipramine, Bupropion, Venlafaxine, Chlorpromazine, Thioridazine, Lithium carbonate, Atomoxetine

12. Ans. (d) ADHD
[Ref. Niraj Ahuja, 7/e p167]

13. Ans. (c) Grinding of teeth during sleep
[Ref. Niraj Ahuja, 7/e p140]

Parasomnias
- Somnabulism: Sleep walking
- Pavor nocturnus: Sleep/ night terrors
- Bedwetting: Sleep related enuresis
- Bruxism: Teeth grinding
- Somniloquy: Sleep talking

14. Ans. (a) Depression
[Ref. Pharmacotherapy of Child and Adolescent Psychiatric Disorders by Rosenberg, 3/e p135]

15. Ans. (d) Conduct disorder
[Ref. Niraj Ahuja, 7/e p167]

Conduct Disorders
- *Definition*: Persistent and significant pattern of conduct where basic rights of others are violated or rules of society are not followed

- *Occurrence*: Less than 18 years age, More in males
- *Types of conduct disorders*:
  - Socialized conduct disorder (Most common)
  - Unsocialized conduct disorder
  - Oppositional defiant disorder
  - Conduct disorder confined to family context
- *Characteristic features of conduct disorders*:
  - Frequent lying
  - Stealing, robbery
  - Running away from home, school
  - Physical violence (rape, fire-setting, assault, break-in, weapon-use)
  - Cruelty towards other people/animals

16. Ans. (d) Absence seizure

[Ref. AAOS Emergency, 10/e p587]

- **Absence seizure**:
  - *Blank* stare and subject typically does not respond to voice command
  - Brief lapse of consciousness without generalized body twitching
  - Lip smacking
  - Eye blinking

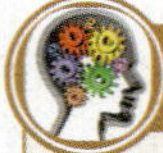

Also Remember

- **Mutism**: Marked, emotionally determined, selective speaking despite presence of language competence in school or in front of strangers
- **Autism**: Marked impairment in reciprocal/ interpersonal interaction, Marked impairment in language/ non-verbal communication, Abnormal behavior characteristics, Mental retardation
- **Adjustment disorder**: Maladaptive response to stressful life event(s) usually seen in adults

17. Ans. (b) Tics

[Ref. Niraj Ahuja, 7/e p168]

Tourette's Syndrome

- Multiple motor tics
- Multiple vocal tics
- Obsessions and compulsions
- Duration more than 1 year

18. Ans. (a) Defective communication

[Ref. Niraj Ahuja, 7/e p164]

- Autism spectrum disorders (ASDs) are a heterogeneous group of neurodevelopmental disorders characterized by social communication deficits and stereotyped behaviors with restricted interests (American Psychiatry Association [APA], 2013)
  - Autism (marked impairment in reciprocal social and interpersonal interaction)
  - Marked impairment in language and non-verbal communication
  - Abnormal behavioural characteristics (Mannerisms, stereotyped behaviours, hyperkinesis)
  - Mental retardation
  - Other features: Enjoy music, prodigious rote memory or calculating ability, and musical abilities, epilepsy

19. Ans. (b) More common in females

[Ref. Niraj Ahuja, 7/e p168]

Gilles de la Tourette's syndrome (Tourette's disorder)

- Multiple motor tics, multiple vocal tics, duration > 1 year, and onset usually < 11 years of age (almost always < 21 years of age)
- 3 times more common in males
- Prevalence rate 0.5 per 1000 people

HIGH YIELD MCQs ANSWERS WITH EXPLANATIONS

1. Ans. (d) Refer to child psychiatrist

[Ref. Niraj Ahuja, 7/e p169]

ENURESIS

- Repetitive voiding of urine, either at day or night, at inappropriate places
- Diagnosis only done after 5 years age (or 4 years mental age)
- Cause: Biopsychological
- Types of enuresis:
  - Organic enuresis: Mostly diurnal in adolescents
  - Primary enuresis: Bladder control never achieved
  - Secondary enuresis: Enuresis after one year of bladder control
- Treatment:
  - Restriction of fluid intake after 8 pm
  - Positive reinforcement for bladder holding in daytime
  - Interruption of sleep before expected time of bed-wetting
  - Conditioning devices
  - Supportive psychotherapy of child, parents, family
  - Pharmacotherapy: Not a preferred option

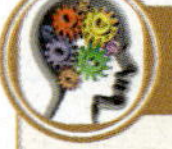

Also Remember

- Pharmacotherapy for Enuresis: Imipramine (DOC), Intranasal desmopressin

2. Ans. (d) Tourette's syndrome

[Ref. Niraj Ahuja, 7/e p168]

Vocal Tics in Tourette Disorder

- Simple vocal tics: Coughing, barking, throat clearing, sniffing, clicking
- Complex vocal tics:
  - Echolalia: Repetition of heard phrases
  - Palilalia: Repetition of heard words
  - Coprolalia: Use of obscene words
  - Mental coprolalia: Thinking of obscene words

3. Ans. (a) Imipramine
[Ref. Niraj Ahuja, 7/e p169]

Pharmacotherapy for Nocturnal Enuresis
- Tricyclic antidepressant
  - Imipramine (Drug of choice)
  - Trimipramine
- Intranasal desmopressin
- Other drugs: Dexamphetamine, Propantheline, Oxybutynin, Terodiline

4. Ans. (c) Trimipramine
[Ref. Niraj Ahuja, 7/e p169]

5. Ans. (d) Diazepam
[Ref. Handbook of Child Behavior Therapy by Gresham, 1/e p213]

Pharmacotherapy for Night Terrors
- Diazepam (Drug of choice)
- Other drugs: Alprazolam, Diphenhydramine, Imipramine, Trimeprazine, Melatonin

6. Ans. (d) Attention deficit hyperactivity disorder
[Ref. Niraj Ahuja, 7/e p166]

Attention Deficit Hyperkinetic Disorder
- Poor attention span with distractibility (Fails to finish task, shift from one task to another, no listening, loses things)
- Hyperactivity (Difficulty in sitting at one place, moving about, excessive talking, fidgety, interfering, outburst)
- Impulsivity (Acts before thinking, difficulty in waiting for turn)
- Soft neurological signs

7. Ans. (c) Left to right disorientation
[Ref. Niraj Ahuja, 7/e p166]

8. Ans. (a) Atomoxetine; (b) Methylphenidate; (c) Dexmethylphenidate; (e) Dextroamphetamine
[Ref. Niraj Ahuja, 7/e p167]

9. Ans. (b) Methylphenidate; (e) Amphetamine
[Ref. Niraj Ahuja, 7/e p167]

10. Ans. (b) Impaired neurobehavioral development; (d) A socioeconomic hazard
[Ref. Niraj Ahuja, 7/e p164]

Infantile Autism
- Autistic disorder, Pervasive developmental disorder, Pseudodefective psychosis
- Biological causation: Perinatal CNS insult, EEG abnormalities, Increased 5-HT
- Autism: Marked impairment in reciprocal social and interpersonal interaction
- Marked impairment in language and non-verbal communication
- Abnormal behavioural characteristics
- Mental retardation
- Other features: Epilepsy, Enjoy music, Idiot savant syndrome (Certain islets of splinter functions remain)

11. Ans. (b) Social and language communication problem
[Ref. Niraj Ahuja, 7/e p164]

12. Ans. (a) Biological causation; (b) Pervasive social and language communication problem
[Ref. Niraj Ahuja, 7/e p164]

13. Ans. (b) Deafness; (c) Mental subnormality
[Ref. Human Exceptionality: School, Community & Family by Hardman, Drew & Egan, 11/e p254]

Causes of Delayed Speech
- Deafness
- Mental sub-normality (Most common cause)
- Cerebral palsy
- Emotional disturbance
- Prolonged negativism

14. Ans. (b) Specific learning disability
[Ref. Learning & Learning Difficulties: A Handbook for Teachers by Westwood, 1/e p71]
- *Specific learning disability*: Students with least average intelligence, free from sensory impairments, absent physical health problems/emotional disturbance BUT fail to gain normal proficiency in basic skills of reading/writing despite appropriate teaching

15. Ans. (a) Disregard for right of others; (b) Doesn't care for authority; (c) Backward in studies; (e) Steals things
[Ref. Niraj Ahuja, 7/e p167]

16. Ans. (a) Attention-deficit hyperactivity disorder
[Ref. Niraj Ahuja, 7/e p166]

17. Ans. (b) Alcoholism; (d) Antisocial behaviour; (e) Academic underachievement
[Ref. Managing ADHD in K-8 Classroom: A Guide for Teachers by Flick, 1/e p25]

Long Term Outcomes for AHD
- Alcoholism
- Antisocial behavior
- Academic underachievement, Poor academic performance
- Hysteria
- Social and marital problems
- Suicides, Accidental injuries

18. Ans. (b) Attention deficit hyperkinetic child
[Ref. Niraj Ahuja, 7/e p166]

19. Ans. (c) Serious problem and medical therapy
[Ref. Niraj Ahuja, 7/e p166]

20. Ans. (b) Autistic Disorder
[Ref. Niraj Ahuja, 7/e p164]

21. Ans. (b) Rett's syndrome
[Ref. Niraj Ahuja, 7/e p165]

Rett's Syndrome
- Autistic disorder among girls
- Normal early development, Normal head circumference at birth
- Deceleration of head growth in 5-30 months age
- Loss of purposive hand movements and acquired fine motor manipulative skills

- Stereotyped movements of hands
- Severe mental handicap

22. Ans. (a) Autism
[Ref. Niraj Ahuja, 7/e p164]

23. Ans. (a) Visual impairment
[Ref. Niraj Ahuja, 7/e p164]

24. Ans. (b) Risperidone
[Ref. Niraj Ahuja, 7/e p168-169]
- 10 years history of eye-blinking and grunting indicate Motor-Tic disorder
- Treatment of Tic disorders: Haloperidol, Riseperidone, Olanzapine, Aripiprazole, Ziprasidone, quetiapine, Sulphuride

25. Ans. (d) Autistic disorder
[Ref. Schizophrenia and Other Psychotic Disorders by Noll, 3/e p42]

Autistic Savants/ Idiot Savants
- Term coined by: J. Landon Down
- Description: Children who, being feeble-minded, exhibit special faculties capable of being cultivated to a great extent
  - More commonly seen in Males
  - 10% autistic children have this syndrome
- Clinical subtypes:
  - *Savant I (**Talented Savant**)*: Have skills that are remarkable simple in contrast to handicap
  - *Savant II (**Prodigious Savant**)*: Ability or brilliance is remarkable not only in contrast to handicap but would also be spectacular if viewed in a normal person

26. Ans. (d) Vision problems
[Ref. Niraj Ahuja, 7/e p164]

Clinical Presentation of Autism
- Marked impairment in social and interpersonal interaction
  - Absent social smile
  - Treats people as furniture
  - Lack of attachment to parents/Absent separation anxiety
  - Absence of fear when in danger
  - Marked impairment in making friends
- Marked impairment in language and non-verbal communication
  - Absent/delayed speech
  - Abnormal speech patterns
- Abnormal behavioural characteristics
  - Mannerisms
  - Stereotype d behaviours (head-banging)
  - Hyperkinesis
- Mental retardation
  - Moderate to profound Mental retardation

27. Ans. (a) Autism disorder; (b) Linguistic and cognitive development preserved
[Ref. Niraj Ahuja, 7/e p165]

Asperger's Syndrome
- Description: Pervasive developmental disorder with Autistic features
- Features:
  - More common in boys
  - High functioning autism (Mild case of autism)
  - No significant delay in language/ cognitive development, intelligence
- Diagnostic **(Schatzmari Criteria)**:
  - Social isolation (No friends, Loner)
  - Impaired social interaction (One sided response to peers, Indifference to others' feelings)
  - Impaired non-verbal communication (Limited facial expression, Avoid looking at others)
  - Speech and language peculiarities (Over-talkative, Repetitions, Non-communicative)

28. Ans. (c) Tics
[Ref. The Encyclopedia of Human Behavior by Goldenson, 1/e p1335]

Adjustment Reaction of Childhood
- Habit disturbances: Nail biting, thumb-sucking, enuresis, masturbation, temper tantrums, feeding problems
- Conduct disturbances: Truancy, stealing, destructiveness, sexual offenses, fire-setting, vandalism, cruelty, use of alcohol, and running away from home
- Neurotic traits: Tics, somnambulism, stuttering, over activity, phobias

29. Ans. (b) ADHD
[Ref. Niraj Ahuja, 7/e p166]

Attention-deficit hyperactivity disorder (ADHD)
- Outdated term 'Minimal cerebral dysfunction' has been replaced by the now widely used term Attention-deficit hyperactivity disorder (ADHD) (American Psychiatric Association, 1994)
- Synonyms: Minimal brain dysfunction (MBD), Hyperkinetic syndrome, Strauss syndrome, Organic drivenness and Minimal brain damage
- 3% of school age children, males are 6-8 times more often affected, onset occurs < 7 years age
- Four clinical types: With hyperactivity, Without hyperactivity, Residual type, and With conduct disorder

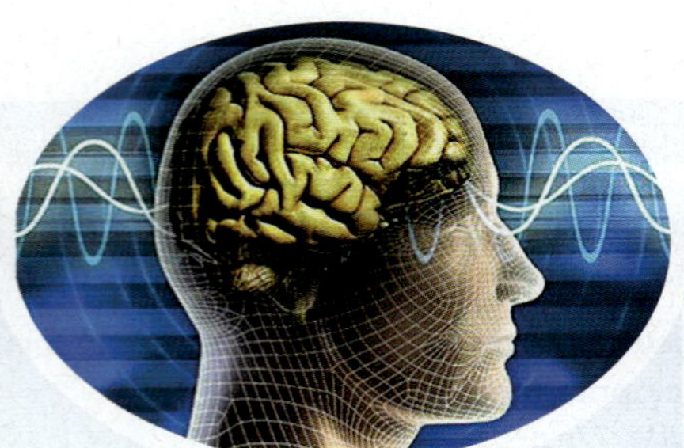

Chapter 13

Personality Disorders

THEORETICAL CONCEPTS

XIII A. CLASSIFICATION

Type-A personality disorders: Odd-eccentric; 'Schizophrenic-continuum'	
Paranoid	Irrational suspicions and mistrust of others
Schizoid	Lack of interest in social relationships, does not share time
Schizotypal	Odd behavior or thinking
Type-B personality disorders: Dramatic-emotional-erratic; 'Psychopathic continuum'	
Antisocial (Dissocial)	disregard for the law and the rights of others
Histrionic	Attention-seeking behaviour
Narcissistic	Grandiosity, need for admiration
Borderline	Extreme 'black-and-white' thinking
Type-C personality disorders: Anxious-fearful; Introvert	
Anxious (Avoidant)	Social inhibition
Dependent	Psychological dependence on others
Obsessive-compulsive (Anankastic)	Rigid conformity to rules, moral codes

Topper's Edge

GENERAL PERSONALITY DISORDER (DSM-5 & DSM-IV CRITERIA)

Importance

- These criteria should be met by all personality disorder cases before a more specific diagnosis can be made[Q]

ICD-10 General Guideline Criteria

- Markedly disharmonious attitudes & behavior (Several areas of functioning): Affectivity, arousal, impulse control, ways of perceiving/thinking, style of relating to others
- Abnormal behavior pattern is enduring, long standing, not limited to episodes of mental illness
- Abnormal behavior pattern is pervasive and clearly maladaptive to a broad range of personal and social situations
- Above manifestations always appear during childhood or adolescence and continue into adulthood
- Considerable personal distress but this may only become apparent late in its course
- Usually, but not invariably, associated with significant problems in occupational and social performance

Contd...

Contd...

DSM-5 Criteria

- An enduring pattern of inner experience and behavior that deviates markedly from the expectations of the individual's culture, pattern manifested in $\geq$ 2 of the following areas:
  - Cognition (ways of perceiving and interpreting self, other people, and events)
  - Affectivity (range, intensity, lability, and appropriateness of emotional response)
  - Interpersonal functioning
  - Impulse control
- Enduring pattern is inflexible and pervasive across a broad range of personal-social situations
- Enduring pattern leads to clinically significant distress or impairment in social, occupational, or other important areas of functioning
- Pattern is stable and of long duration, and onset traceable to adolescence or early adulthood
- Enduring pattern is not better explained as a manifestation or consequence of another mental disorder
- Enduring pattern is not attributable to the physiological effects of a substance or another medical condition

Dimensional System of Classifying Personality Disorders

Level of Severity	Description	Definition by Categorical System
0	No personality disorder	Does not meet actual or subthreshold criteria for any personality disorder
1	Personality difficulty	Meets subthreshold criteria for one or several personality disorders
2	Simple personality disorder	Meets actual criteria for one or more personality disorders within the same cluster
3	Complex personality disorder*	Meets actual criteria for one or more personality disorders within more than one cluster
4	Severe personality disorder	Meets criteria for creation of severe disruption to both individual and to many in society

(* Diffuse personality disorder)

XIII B. PARANOID PERSONALITY DISORDER

- *Features*:
  - Excessive sensitiveness
  - Tendency to bear grudges
  - Significant suspiciousness
  - Sense of personal right
  - Suspicions of partner infidelity
  - Excessive self-importance
  - Preoccupation with conspiratorial explanation of events
- *Underlying defense mechanism*: **Projection**[Q]
- *Seen in*: Paranoid schizophrenia

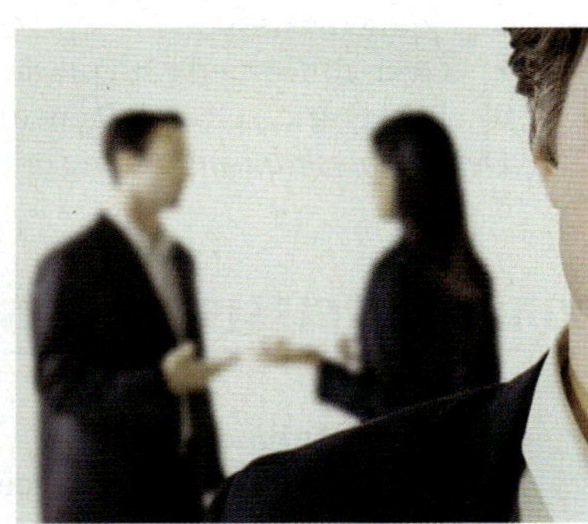

Fig. Paranoid personality

XIII C. SCHIZOID PERSONALITY DISORDER

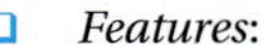

- *Features*:
  - **Emotional coldness**[Q]
  - **Lack of pleasure from activities**[Q]
  - **Inability to express feelings**[Q]
  - Indifference to praise/criticism
  - Little interest in sexual experiences
  - Likes solitary activities
  - Fantasy loving
  - Lack of close friends
  - Insensitivity to social norms
- *Seen in*: Cold and aloof parenting in a child with introverted temperament

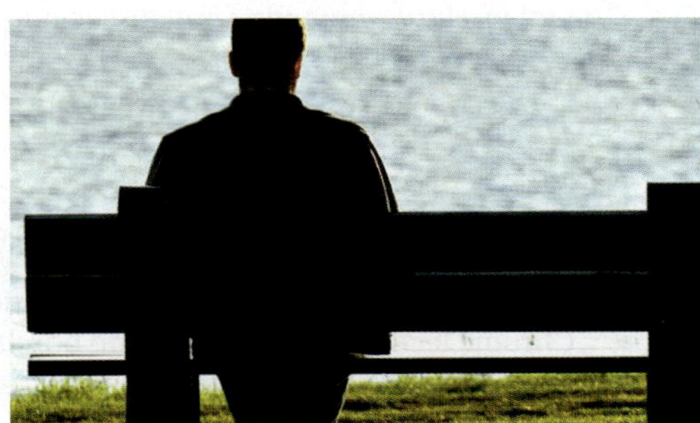

Fig. Schizoid personality

Psychiatry

XIII D. SCHIZOTYPAL PERSONALITY DISORDER

- *Features*:
  - Eccentric behaviour
  - Anomalies of thinking and affect
  - Poor rapport with others
  - Social withdrawal
  - Odd beliefs or magical thinking
  - Suspicious/paranoid ideas
  - Obsessive ruminations
  - Unusual perceptual experiences
  - Stereotyped thinking
  - Transient psychotic episodes
- *Lies between*: Schizoid personality and Schizophrenia

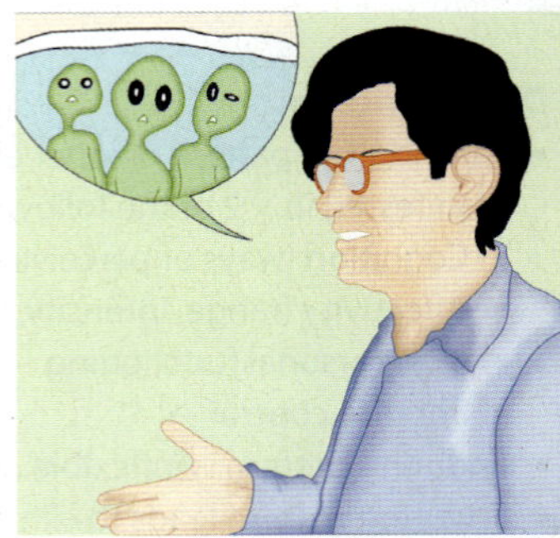

Fig. Schizotypal personality

XIII E. ANTISOCIAL (DISSOCIAL) PERSONALITY DISORDER

- *Features*: ***'Psychopaths'***
  - No concern for others' feelings[Q]
  - Irresponsible attitude[Q]
  - **Disregard for social norms**[Q]
  - Inability to maintain relationships
  - Inability to experience guilt
  - Low threshold for aggression
  - Proneness to blame others
- *Seen in*: History of conduct disorder in childhood and adolescence

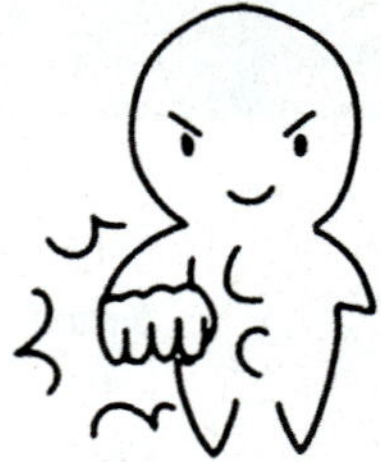

Fig. Antisocial personality

XIII F. HISTRIONIC PERSONALITY DISORDER

- *Features*:
  - **Self-dramatization**[Q]
  - **Exaggerated expression of emotions**[Q]
  - Easily affected by others
  - Attention seeking attitude
  - Seductiveness
  - Over-concerned with physical attractiveness
  - Egocentric, self-indulgence
- *Defence mechanisms*: Acting out, dissociation

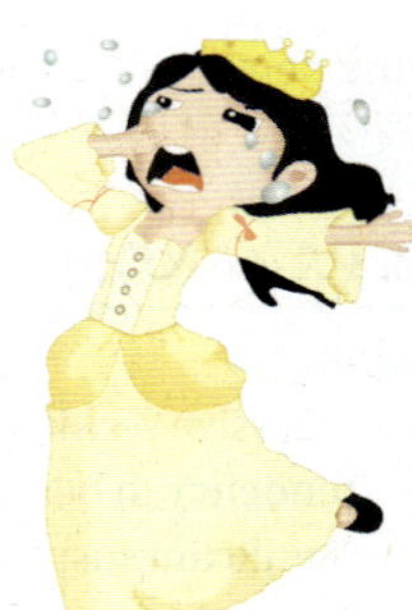

Fig. Histrionic personality

XIII G. NARCISSISTIC PERSONALITY DISORDER

- *Features*:
  - **Ideas of grandiosity**[Q]
  - Fantasies of unlimited success
  - **Attention seeking, dramatic behaviour**[Q]
  - Exploitative behaviour
  - **Shaky self-esteem with sense of inferiority**[Q]
- *Defence mechanisms*: Acting out, dissociation

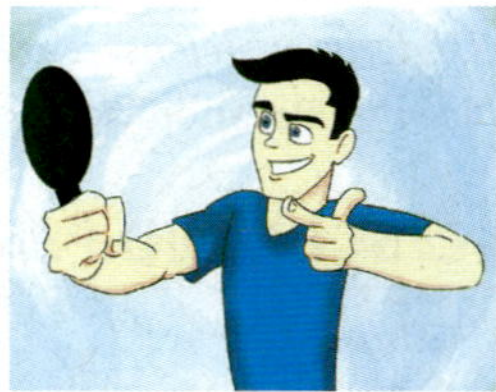

Fig. Narcissistic personality

XIII H. BORDERLINE PERSONALITY DISORDER

- *Features*:
  - **Emotional instability**[Q]
  - **Unclear self-image**[Q]
  - Unstable interpersonal relationship patterns[Q]
  - Chronic feelings of emptiness and boredom
  - Deliberate self-harm: Self-mutilation, suicidal, accident-prone[Q]
- *Defence mechanisms*: Splitting

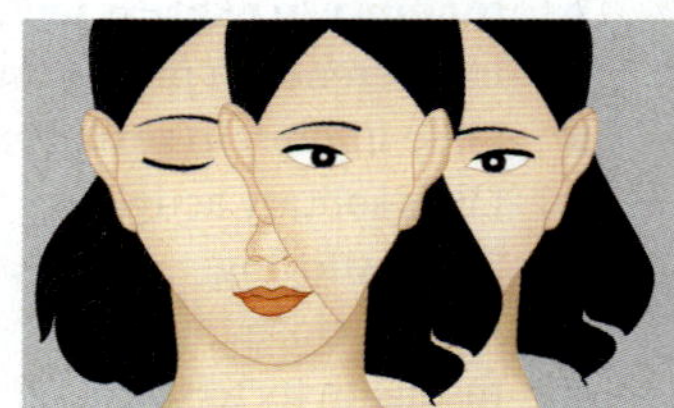

Fig. Borderline personality

XIII I. ANXIOUS (AVOIDANT) PERSONALITY DISORDER

- *Features*: ***'Inferiority complex'***[Q]
  - Persistent feelings of tension and apprehension
  - Feeling of self-inferiority
  - Feeling of being rejected
  - Avoidance of social and occupational activities

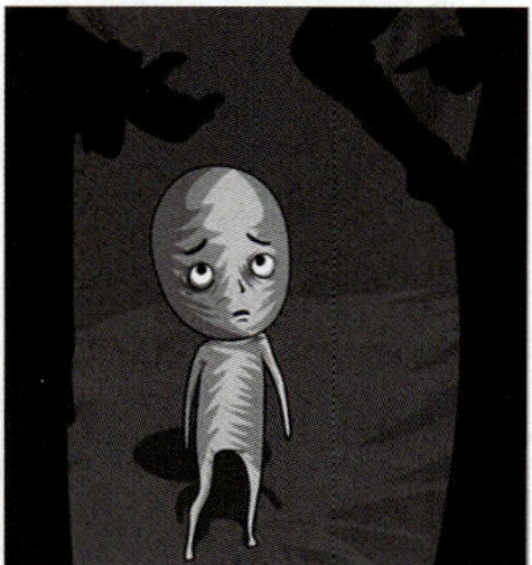

Fig. Avoidant personality

XIII J. DEPENDENT PERSONALITY DISORDER

- *Features*:
  - Allowing others to make decisions for them
  - Unwillingness to make demands
  - Fear of being abandoned by loved ones
  - Inability to make everyday decisions
  - Feeling of helplessness
  - Masochism (sometimes)

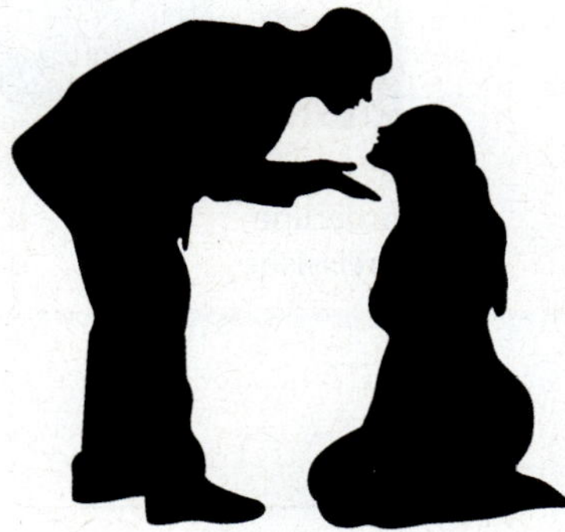

Fig. Dependent personality

XIII K. OBSESSIVE-COMPULSIVE (ANANKASTIC) PERSONALITY DISORDER

- *Features*:
  - Feelings of excessive doubt
  - Perfectionism interfering with task completion
  - Rigidity and stubbornness
  - Depressive episodes
- *Defence mechanisms*: Reaction formation

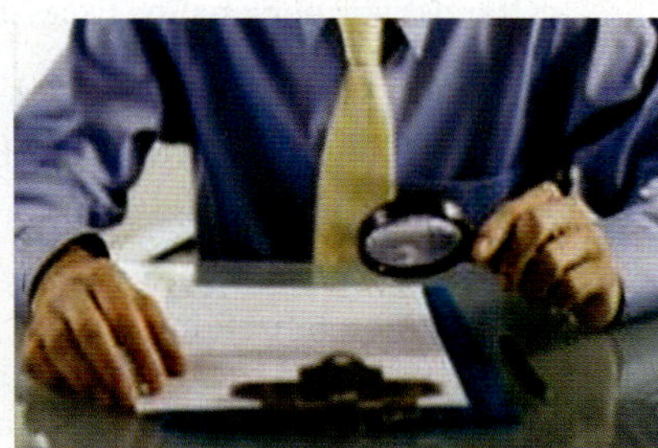

Fig. Anankastic personality

Topper's Edge

Sex Differences in Frequency of Personality Disorders

- **Male Predominance**[Q]**:**
  - Paranoid personality disorder
  - Schizoid personality disorder
  - Schizotypal personality disorder
  - Antisocial personality disorder
  - Narcissistic personality disorder
  - Obsessive-compulsive personality disorder
- **Female Predominance**[Q]**:**
  - Borderline personality disorder
  - Histrionic personality disorder
  - Dependent personality disorder
- **Equal dominance**[Q]**:**
  - Avoidant personality disorder

IMAGE-BASED QUESTIONS

1. Identify personality disorder shown in photograph

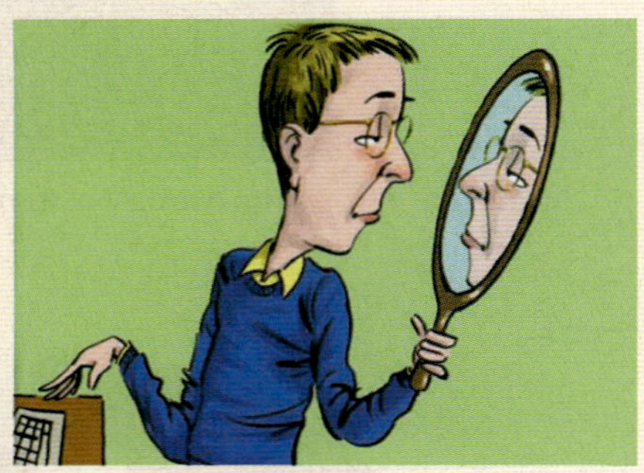

a. Borderline
b. Anxious
c. Narcissistic
d. Dependent

2. Personality disorder shown in photograph

a. Histrionic
b. Anxious
c. Narcissistic
d. Avoidant

 **ANSWERS WITH EXPLANATIONS OF IBQs** 

1. Ans. (c) Narcissistic *[Ref. Niraj Ahuja, 7/e p116]*

- Narcissistic personality: Excessive excessively preoccupied with personal adequacy, power, prestige and beauty
  - Ideas of grandiosity
  - Inflated sense of importance
  - Attention seeking, dramatic behaviour

2. Ans. (a) Histrionic *[Ref. Niraj Ahuja, 7/e p116]*

- Histrionic personality: Exaggerated expression of emotions
  - Self-dramatization
  - Continual attention seeking attitude
  - Over-concern with physical attractiveness

NEET/NBE PATTERN MCQs

1. A girl has disturbance of self-identity and shows impulsive and suicidal behavior. She is a case of *[Recent Question 2016]*

a. Antisocial personality
b. Anxious personality
c. Histrionic personality
d. Borderline personality

2. Cardinal feature of antisocial personality *[Recent Question 2016]*

a. Violation of rules of society
b. Attention-seeking behavior
c. Unstable interpersonal relationship
d. Grandiose behavior

3. Patients who are grandiose and require admiration from others has which type of personality? *[Recent Question 2016]*

a. Narcissistic
b. Histrionic
c. Borderline
d. Antisocial

4. Schizotypal personality belongs to which cluster of personality disorders? *[Recent Question 2016]*

a. A
b. B
c. C
d. D

5. All of the following are cluster-A personality disorders except *[NBE FMGE September 2005]*

a. Paranoid
b. Schizoid
c. Schizotypal
d. Histrionic

6. Impulsivity, deliberate self harm, identity disturbance, chronic feeling of emptiness and micropsychotic episodes is often found in *[NBE DNB December 2011]*

a. Antisocial personality disorder
b. Dependent personality disorder
c. Borderline personality disorder
d. Avoidant personality disorder

7. Most effective treatment in borderline personality disorders *[Recent Question 2012, 2017]*

a. Pharmacotherapy
b. Behavior therapy
c. Combination of both pharmacotherapy and behavioral therapy
d. None

8. Schizoid personality disorder all are seen except *[Recent Question 2013]*

a. Aloof and detached
b. Prone to fantasy
c. Suspicious
d. Introspective

9. Impulsivity, deliberate self harm, identity disturbance, chronic feeling of emptiness and micropsychotic episodes is often found in *[NBE DNB December 2011]*

a. Antisocial personality disorder
b. Dependent personality disorder
c. Borderline personality disorder
d. Avoidant personality disorder

10. Life long theatricality of behaviour is seen in *[NBE DNB 1992]*

a. Obsessive personality
b. Schizoid personality
c. Hysterical personalities
d. Avoidant personalities

11. Type C personality disorder *[Recent Question 2012, 2013, 2015]*

a. Avoidant personality disorder
b. Histrionic personality disorder
c. Paranoid personality disorder
d. Narcissistic personality disorder

12. Classical combination of personality change and intellectual deterioration is seen in *[NBE DNB 1992]*

a. Temporal lobe tumour
b. Occipital lobe tumour
c. Frontal lobe cerebral tumour
d. Parietal lobe tumour

13. Antisocial personality disorder is characterized by *[Recent Question 2014, 2015]*

a. Excessive sensitivity and suspiciousness
b. Emotional coldness, lack of pleasure
c. Unconcern for feeling of others, disregard for social norms
d. Self dramatization, exaggerated expression of emotions

14. Borderline personality is characterized by? *[Recent Question 2017]*

a. Unstable and intense interpersonal relationship
b. Violation of the rules
c. Grandiose
d. Attention seeking behavior

15. A 40-year-old married male thinks that he is multitalented and is always overconfident. He never listens to his family or friends. Infact whenever anyone gives him any advice, he thinks that they have some motive against him. He is always suspicious of his wife. All these are feature of? *[Recent Question 2017]*

a. Borderline personality disorder
b. Schizoid personality disorder
c. Paranoid personality disorder
d. Histrionic personality disorder

16. Cluster C personality disorder is? *[Recent Question 2017]*

a. Obsessive compulsive
b. Paranoid
c. Schizoid
d. Borderline

17. False about borderline personality disorder? *[Recent Question 2017]*

a. Self-image issues
b. Disturbed relationships
c. Self-mutilation behavior
d. Attention seeking behavior

18. Cluster B personality is seen in? *[Recent Question 2017]*
a. Psychopath
b. Shy and socially inhibited
c. Markedly detached
d. Emotionally cold

19. Characteristic of Histrionic personality disorder is? *[Recent Question 2017]*
a. Violation of rules of society
b. Attention seeking behavior
c. Unstable interpersonal relationship
d. Grandiose behavior

20. A 24-year-girl named Heena is often flamboyantly dressed and goes out on dates frequently. Although she changed boyfriend almost monthly but she used to plan her marriage and future with each of them with equal enthusiasm and optimism. She would often make stories to seek attention. She would feel uncomfortable at big parties leave them midway. Heena made promises to other people that were impossible to keep but seemed to be aimed at winning their approval; when she broke the promise, she usually made up a story designed to elicit sympathy and compassion. Diagnosis is *[Recent Question 2017]*
a. Borderline personality disorder
b. Histrionic personality disorder
c. Dependent personality disorder
d. Antisocial personality disorder

21. Narcissistic is which type of personality disorder? *[Recent Question 2017]*
a. Cluster A
b. Cluster B
c. Cluster C
d. Cluster D

22. True about Borderline personality disorder is? *[Recent Question 2017]*
a. Delusion of persecution
b. Antisocial behavior
c. Self mutilation behavior
d. Attention seeking behavior

23. OCD is associated with which personality disorder? *[Recent Question 2017]*
a. Anankastic
b. Borderline
c. Narcissistic
d. Histrionic

24. A person is very impatient, competitive and works like a perfectionist. He/she can be best described as *[Recent Question 2017]*
a. Type A personality
b. Type B personality
c. Type C personality
d. Type D personality

HIGH YIELD MCQs

1. A person has different multiple personality is suffering from *[PGI 1997]*
a. Mania
b. Personality disorder
c. Paranoid schizophrenia
d. Dissociative disorder

2. Not a personality trait *[AIIMS PGMEE 2009]*
a. Sensation seeking b. Neuroticism
c. Open to experience d. Problem solving

3. True about personality disorder *[PGI 2003]*
a. Typically onset at early childhood & adolescent
b. Matured around age 30-40 years
c. Egodystonic
d. Dramatic and maladaptive behaviour

4. All are cluster B disorders of personality except *[Recent Question 2017, PGI 1999]*
a. Antisocial b. Narcissistic
c. Avoidant d. Borderline

5. A person having the habit of repeated self inflicted injuries, what is the type of personality *[PGI 2004]*
a. Borderline personality disorder
b. Schizoid personality disorder
c. Histrionic personality disorder
d. Narcissistic personality disorder
e. Depressive disorder

6. Markedly inappropriate sensitivity, self importance and suspiciousness are clinical features of *[Recent Question 2015, AMU PGMEE 2002, TN PGMEE 1999]*
a. Antisocial b. Historic
c. Schizoid d. Paranoid

7. Characteristic feature of Schizoid personality is *[AIIMS PGMEE 1999]*
a. Conversion reaction
b. Not concerned with disease
c. Checks details of all things
d. Emotional coldness

8. Antisocial personality is seen with *[PGI 1999]*
a. Drug abuse b. Paranoid schizophrenia
c. OCN d. None

9. A female presents with the history of slashed wrists and attempted suicide, now presents with similar history. The diagnosis is *[AIIMS PGMEE 2001]*
a. Borderline personality b. OCD
c. Conversion reaction d. Histrionic personality

10. False regarding type A personality *[AIIMS November 2007]*
a. Hostile
b. Time pressure
c. Competitiveness
d. Mood fluctuations

Psychiatry

11. True about personality disorder *[PGI 2007]*
a. Onset in early childhood and adolescent
b. Matures around adulthood
c. Not associated to social norms
d. Direct result of disease or damage

12. A person has poor performance in front of his seniors in public place, has tachycardia when he has to deliver a lecture, avoids going to parties. The diagnosis is *[AIIMS PGMEE 1999]*
a. Panic disorder
b. Schizophrenia
c. Social phobia
d. Avoidant personality

13. Oddities of speech, mannerism and clothing with magical thinking is seen in which type of personality disorder *[JIPMER PGMEE 2000]*
a. Schizoid
b. Paranoid
c. Schizotype
d. Border line

14. Which personality disorder of DSM-IV is not classified as PD & is placed with schizophrenia in ICD 1 *[WB PGMEE 1998]*
a. Schizoid
b. Paranoid
c. Narcissistic
d. Schizotype

15. True about personality disorder *[PGI 2008]*
a. It arises during childhood
b. It matures during adulthood
c. Suspiciousness is seen in paranoid personality disorder
d. Excessive preoccupation with fantasy seen in schizoid

16. A 16-year-old girl was brought to the psychiatric emergency after she slashed her wrist in an attempt to commit suicide. On enquiry her father revealed that she had made several such attempts of wrist slashing in the past, mostly in response to trivial fights in her house. Further she had marked fluctuations in her mood with a pervasive pattern of unable interpersonal relationship. The most probable diagnosis is *[AIIMS PGMEE 2002]*
a. Borderline personality disorder
b. Major depression
c. Histrionic personality disorder
d. Adjustment disorder

17. A young lady was admitted after taking overdose of diazepam after broken affair. She has history of slitting her wrist previously. Most likely diagnosis is *[AIIMS PGMEE 2000]*
a. Narcissistic personality disorder
b. Dependent personality disorder
c. Borderline personality disorder
d. Histrionic personality disorder

18. Eccentric behaviour, magical thinking and social withdrawal is characteristic of .... personality *[Recent Question 2017, NIMHANS PGMEE 2014]*
a. Narcissistic personality disorder
b. Schizotypal personality disorder
c. Borderline personality disorder
d. Histrionic personality disorder

19. Histrionic, shy, avoidant symptoms come under which cluster? *[Recent Question 2015, AIIMS PG May 2015]*
a. A
b. B
c. C
d. D

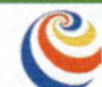 NEET/NBE PATTERN MCQs ANSWERS WITH EXPLANATIONS 

1. Ans. (d) Borderline personality
[Ref. Niraj Ahuja, 7/e p117]

- ***Borderline personality disorder***: Emotional instability, Unclear self-image, Unstable interpersonal relationship patterns, Chronic feelings of emptiness and boredom, Deliberate self-harm (Self-mutilation, suicidal, accident-prone)

Also Remember

- ***Antisocial personality (Psychopaths)***: No concern for others' feelings, Irresponsible attitude, Disregard for social norms, Inability to maintain relationships, Inability to experience guilt, Low threshold for aggression, Proneness to blame others, History of conduct disorder in childhood and adolescence
- ***Anxious personality (Inferiority complex)***: Persistent feelings of tension and apprehension, Feeling of self-inferiority, Feeling of being rejected, Avoidance of social and occupational activities
- ***Histrionic personality***: Self-dramatization, Exaggerated expression of emotions, Easily affected by others, Attention seeking attitude, Seductiveness, Over-concerned with physical attractiveness, Egocentric, self-indulgence

2. Ans. (a) Violation of rules of society
[Ref. Forensic Neuropsychology by Young, 1/e p8]

- Antisocial behavior is a cardinal feature of conduct disorder and antisocial personality disorder
- Antisocial behavior may also be seen in acquired brain injury, learning disability, dementia, aggression and violence

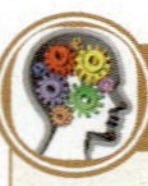

Also Remember

- Features of antisocial personality **(Psychopaths)**: No concern for others feelings, Irresponsible attitude, Disregard for social norms, Inability to maintain relationships, Inability to experience guilt/remorse, Low threshold for aggression, Proneness to blame others

3. Ans. (a) Narcissistic
[Ref. Niraj Ahuja, 7/e p116]

Narcissistic personality disorder

- Ideas of grandiosity
- Fantasies of unlimited success
- Attention seeking, dramatic behavior
- Exploitative behavior
- Shaky self-esteem with sense of inferiority

4. Ans. (a) A
[Ref. Psychiatry by Hales, 5/e p823]

Clusters of Personality Disorders

- **Cluster A (the "odd, eccentric" cluster)**: Paranoid, Schizoid, and Schizotypal personality disorders
  - Common features: Social awkwardness and social withdrawal
  - Dominated by distorted thinking
- **Cluster B (the "dramatic, emotional, erratic" cluster)**: Borderline, Narcissistic, Histrionic, Antisocial personality disorders
  - Problems with Impulse control and emotional regulation
- **Cluster C (the "anxious, fearful" cluster)**: Avoidant, Dependent, and Obsessive-compulsive personality disorders
  - High level of anxiety

5. Ans. (d) Histrionic
[Ref. Niraj Ahuja, 7/e p113]

Type-A personality disorders: Odd-eccentric; 'Schizophrenic-continuum'	
Paranoid	Irrational suspicions and mistrust of others
Schizoid	Lack of interest in social relationships, does not share time
Schizotypal	Odd behavior or thinking
Type-B personality disorders: Dramatic-emotional-erratic; 'Psychopathic continuum'	
Antisocial (Dissocial)	disregard for the law and the rights of others
Histrionic	Attention-seeking behaviour
Narcissistic	Grandiosity, need for admiration
Borderline	Extreme 'black-and-white' thinking
Type-C personality disorders: Anxious-fearful; Introvert	
Anxious (Avoidant)	Social inhibition
Dependent	Psychological dependence on others
Obsessive-compulsive (Anankastic)	Rigid conformity to rules, moral codes

6. Ans. (c) Borderline personality disorder
[Ref. Niraj Ahuja, 7/e p117]

- *Borderline personality disorder*: Emotional instability, Unclear self-image, Unstable interpersonal relationship patterns, Chronic feelings of emptiness and boredom, Deliberate self-harm (Self-mutilation, suicidal, accident-prone)

7. Ans. (b) Behavior therapy
[Ref. Niraj Ahuja, 7/e p117]

Treatment of Borderline Personality Disorder

- Cognitive behavior therapy (Best approach)
- Psychoanalysis
- Supportive psychotherapy
- Drug therapy: Antidepressants, Antipsychotics, Lithium, Valproate, Carbamazepine

8. Ans. (c) Suspicious
[Ref. Niraj Ahuja, 7/e p114]

- ***Schizoid personality disorder***: Emotional coldness, Lack of pleasure from activities, Inability to express feelings, Indifference to praise/criticism, Little interest in sexual experiences, Likes solitary activities, Fantasy loving, Lack of close friends, Insensitivity to social norms

9. Ans. (c) Borderline personality disorder
[Ref. Niraj Ahuja, 7/e p117]

10. Ans. (c) Hysterical personalities
[Ref. Dimensions of Personality by Eysenck, 1/e p53]

Hysterical Personality

- Life-long theatricality of behavior
- Desire to impress and gain sympathy
- Contrast in shallowness and expression of feelings
- Contrast of external shyness and intense erotic interest
- Lack of persistence of emotion and effort
- Compensatory day-dreaming

11. Ans. (a) Avoidant personality disorder
[Ref. Niraj Ahuja, 7/e p113]

12. Ans. (c) Frontal lobe cerebral tumour
[Ref. Textbook of Psychological Medicine: An Irish Perspective by Brian O'Shea, 1/e p344]

- *Frontal lobe tumors*: Intellectual deterioration, impaired consciousness, unexplained personality changes

13. Ans. (c) Unconcern for feeling of others, disregard for social norms
[Ref. Niraj Ahuja, 7/e p115]

Antisocial (Dissocial) Personality Disorder (Psychopaths)

- No concern for others' feelings
- Irresponsible attitude
- Disregard for social norms
- Inability to maintain relationships
- Inability to experience guilt
- Low threshold for aggression
- Proneness to blame others

14. Ans. (a) Unstable and intense interpersonal relationship
[Ref. Niraj Ahuja, 7/e p117]

Borderline personality disorder

- Emotional instability, Unstable interpersonal relationship patterns
- Chronic feelings of emptiness and boredom, Unclear self-image/identity, Deliberate self-harm (Self-mutilation, suicidal, accident-prone)
- Extreme 'black-and-white' thinking
- Impulsivity
- Defence mechanisms: Splitting

15. Ans. (c) Paranoid personality disorder
[Ref. Niraj Ahuja, 7/e p114]

Paranoid Personality Disorder

- Features: Excessive sensitiveness, tendency to bear grudges, significant suspiciousness, sense of personal right, suspicions of partner infidelity, excessive self-importance, preoccupation with conspiratorial explanation of events
- Underlying defense mechanism: Projection

16. Ans. (a) Obsessive compulsive
[Ref. Niraj Ahuja, 7/e p113]

- Cluster C (the "anxious, fearful" cluster) personality disorders include Avoidant (Anxious), Dependent, and Obsessive-compulsive personality disorders (Anankastic)

17. Ans. (d) Attention seeking behavior
[Ref. Niraj Ahuja, 7/e p117]

- Borderline personality disorder is characterised by Emotional instability, Unclear self-image, Unstable interpersonal relationship patterns, Chronic feelings of emptiness and boredom, Deliberate self-harm (Self-mutilation, suicidal, accident-prone)
- Defence mechanisms: Splitting

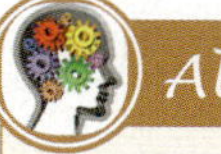

Also Remember

- Attention seeking behaviour is seen in Histrionic and Narcissistic personality types

18. Ans. (a) Psychopath
[Ref. Niraj Ahuja, 7/e p113]

- Type-B personality disorders (Dramatic-emotional erratic; 'Psychopathic continuum') include Antisocial (Dissocial - disregard for the law and the rights of others), Histrionic (Attention-seeking behaviour), Narcissistic (Grandiosity, need for admiration) and Borderline (Extreme 'black-and-white' thinking) personality types

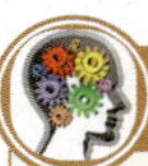

Also Remember

- Type-A personality disorders: Odd-eccentric; 'Schizophrenic-continuum'
- Type-B personality disorders: Dramatic-emotional erratic; 'Psychopathic continuum'
- Type-C personality disorders: Anxious-fearful; Introvert

19. Ans. (b) Attention seeking behavior
[Ref. Niraj Ahuja, 7/e p116]

- Histrionic personality is characterised by Self-dramatization, Exaggerated expression of emotions, Easily affected by others, Attention seeking attitude, Seductiveness, Over-concerned with physical attractiveness, Egocentric, self-indulgence

20. Ans. (b) Histrionic personality disorder
[Ref. Niraj Ahuja, 7/e p116]

- Histrionic personality disorder is characterized by **self-dramatization**, exaggerated expression of emotions, **easily affected by others, attention seeking attitude**, seductiveness, over-concerned with physical attractiveness, egocentric, self-indulgence (features **as given in the question**)
- Defence mechanisms used: Acting out, dissociation

21. Ans. (b) Cluster B
[Ref. Niraj Ahuja, 7/e p112]

- Cluster B (the "dramatic, emotional, erratic" cluster having problems with impulse control and emotional regulation) include Borderline, Narcissistic, Histrionic, Antisocial personality disorders

- Narcissistic personality: Excessive excessively preoccupied with personal adequacy, power, prestige & beauty, Ideas of grandiosity, Inflated sense of importance, Attention seeking, dramatic behaviour

22. Ans. (c) Self mutilation behavior

[Ref. Niraj Ahuja, 7/e p117]

- Borderline personality disorder is characterised by Emotional instability, Unclear self-image, Unstable interpersonal relationship patterns, Chronic feelings of emptiness and boredom, Deliberate self-harm (Self-mutilation, suicidal, accident-prone)

23. Ans. (a) Anankastic

[Ref. Niraj Ahuja, 7/e p113]

Obsessive-Compulsive (Anankastic) Personality Disorder

- Feelings of excessive doubt, Perfectionism interfering with task completion, Rigidity and stubbornness, Depressive episodes
- Defence mechanisms: Reaction formation

24. Ans. (a) Type A personality

[Ref. Fundamentals of Psychology by Eysenck, 1/e p92]

- Type A personality includes three elements, a strong competitive orientation, impatience and time urgency, and anger and hostility. They are ambitious, hard-driving perfectionists who are exceedingly time conscious, routinely trying to do several things at once.
- Type B personality are relaxed, easy-going, able to engage in leisure activities without worrying of work

HIGH YIELD MCQs ANSWERS WITH EXPLANATIONS 

1. Ans. (d) Dissociative disorder

[Ref. Multiple Personality Disorder by Goodwin, 1/e p3]

- *Multiple personality disorder was formally known as*: Dissociative disorder
  - At least two distinct enduring personality types together

2. Ans. (d) Problem solving

[Ref. Media Choice: A Theoretical & Empirical View by Hartmann, 1/e p57]

Five Fundamental Personality Traits

- Extroversion (Sensation seeking)
- Neuroticism
- Openness to experience
- Agreeableness
- Conscientiousness

3. Ans. (a) Typically onset at early childhood & adolescent; (b) Matured around age 30-40 yrs; (d) Dramatic and maladaptive behavior

[Ref. Niraj Ahuja, 7/e p113]

Personality Disorders

- Life-time prevalence in general population: 5-10%
- Recognizable by early adolescence, diagnosed not before early adult life; Less obvious after 40 years age
- Inflexible, maladaptive, dramatic behavior
- Significant social or occupational impairment
- Significant subjective stress
- Ego-syntonic; Do not seek psychiatric help

4. Ans. (c) Avoidant

[Ref. Niraj Ahuja, 7/e p113]

Clusters of Personality Disorders

- Cluster A (the "odd, eccentric" cluster) include Paranoid, Schizoid, and Schizotypal personality disorders. They are characterized by Social awkwardness and Social withdrawal, Distorted thinking
- Cluster B (the "dramatic, emotional, erratic" cluster) include Borderline, Narcissistic, Histrionic, Antisocial personality disorders. They are characterized by impulse control and emotional regulation
- Cluster C (the "anxious, fearful" cluster) include Avoidant, Dependent, and Obsessive-compulsive personality disorders. They are characterized by high level of anxiety

5. Ans. (a) Borderline personality disorder

[Ref. Niraj Ahuja, 7/e p117]

6. Ans. (d) Paranoid

[Ref. Niraj Ahuja, 7/e p114]

- ***Paranoid personality disorder***: Excessive sensitiveness, Tendency to bear grudges, Significant suspiciousness, Sense of personal right, Suspicions of partner infidelity, Excessive self-importance, Preoccupation with conspiratorial explanation of events

7. Ans. (d) Emotional coldness

[Ref. Niraj Ahuja, 7/e p114]

- ***Schizoid personality disorder***: Emotional coldness, Lack of pleasure from activities, Inability to express feelings, Indifference to praise/criticism, Little interest in sexual experiences, Likes solitary activities, Fantasy loving, Lack of close friends, Insensitivity to social norms

8. Ans. (a) Drug abuse

[Ref. Evidence Based Treatments for Alcohol and Drug Abuse by Vedel, 1/e p165]

- *Common psychiatric disorders in substance users*:
  - Antisocial personality disorder
  - Conduct disorder
  - Antisocial adult behavior

9. Ans. (a) Borderline personality

[Ref. Niraj Ahuja, 7/e p117]

10. Ans. (d) Mood fluctuations

[Ref. Fundamentals of Psychology by Eysenck, 1/e p92]

- ***Type A Personality***: Hard-driving, Competitive, Aggressive, Time pressure, Impatience, Hostility
- ***Type B Personality***: Relaxed, easy-going, Able to engage in leisure activities without worrying of work

11. Ans. (a) Onset in early childhood & adolescent; (b) Matures around adulthood; (c) Not associated to social norms

[Ref. Niraj Ahuja, 7/e p113]

12. Ans. (c) Social Phobia

[Ref. Niraj Ahuja, 7/e p93]

- *Social phobia*: Irrational fear of activities or social interaction (during performance of activities in front of others)

13. Ans. (c) Schizotype

[Ref. Niraj Ahuja, 7/e p115]

- ***Schizotypal personality disorder***: Eccentric behavior, Anomalies of thinking and affect, Poor rapport with others, Social withdrawal, Odd beliefs or magical thinking, Suspicious/paranoid ideas, Obsessive ruminations, Unusual perceptual experiences, Stereotyped thinking, Transient psychotic episodes

14. Ans. (d) Schizotype

[Ref. Niraj Ahuja, 7/e p113]

15. Ans. ALL CHOICES

[Ref. Niraj Ahuja, 7/e p113-118]

16. Ans. (a) Borderline personality disorder

[Ref. Niraj Ahuja, 7/e p117]

17. Ans. (c) Borderline personality disorder

[Ref. Niraj Ahuja, 7/e p117]

18. Ans. (b) Schizotypal personality disorder

[Ref. Niraj Ahuja, 7/e p115]

19. Ans. (c) C

[Ref. Companion to Psychiatric Studies by Lawrie, 8/e p516]

Personality Cluster C

- Avoidant personality disorder: Avoidant, Shy, Anxious, Social inhibition
- Dependence personality disorder: Need care from a dominant partner
  - Frequently associated disorders: Borderline, Avoidant, Histrionic
- Obsessive-compulsive personality disorder: Rigid conformity to rules, Perfectionism orderliness

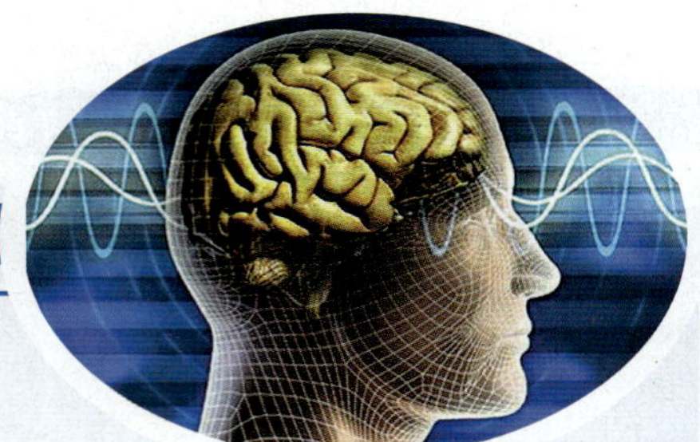

Chapter 14

Other Psychiatric Disorders

THEORETICAL CONCEPTS

XIV A. ELECTRO-CONVULSIVE THERAPY (ECT)

XIV A1. Definition

- Induction of seizures in anesthetized psychiatric patients for therapeutic effect

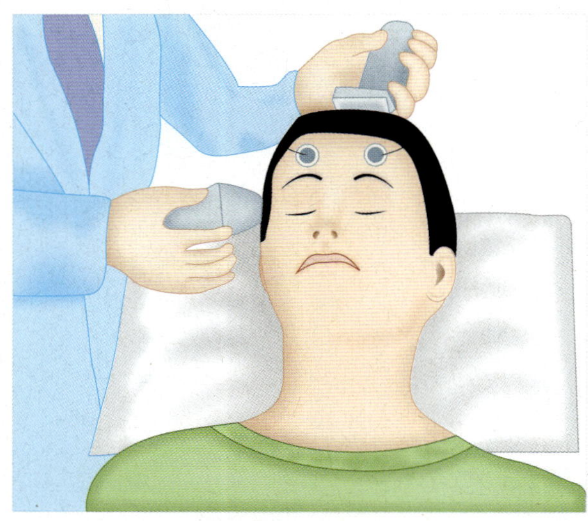

Fig. ECT

XIV A2. Indications

Major severe depression[Q]	Severe catatonia[Q]	Severe psychosis[Q]
• **With suicidal risk (first and most important indication)** [Q] • With stupor • With poor food/ fluids intake • With psychotic features • With partial response to drug therapy • Where drugs are contraindicated • For faster recovery	• With stupor • With poor food/ fluids intake • With partial response to drug therapy • Where drugs are contraindicated • For faster recovery	• With suicidal/ homicidal/assault risk • With partial response to drug therapy • Where drugs are contraindicated • With prominent depressive features

XIV A3. Contraindications

Absolute contraindications[Q]	*Relative contraindications*
• Raised intracranial tension	• Myocardial infarction • Severe hypertension • Cerebrovascular accident (CVA) • Severe pulmonary disease • Retinal detachment • Pheochromocytoma

XIV A4. Technique

- *Direct ECT*: Without muscular relaxation and general anesthesia
- *Modified ECT*: With drug-induced muscular relaxation and general anesthesia
- *Unilateral ECT*
- *Bilateral ECT*
- *Duration of ECT*: ≤ 3 ECTs per week (Total 06–10 treatments)
- *Mechanism of action*:
  - Affects catecholamine pathways between diencephalon and limbic system
  - Increase threshold for further seizures (anti-convulsant action)

XIV A5. Side Effects

- Deaths (mainly due to anaesthesia[Q])
- Memory disturbances
- Confusion
- Headache, apnea, prolonged seizure

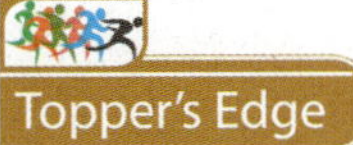

Topper's Edge

Electroconvulsive Therapy (ECT)

Reasons for Unilateral Vs Bilateral Electrode Placement[Q]

- Unilateral Electrode Placement:
  - Speed of response is less important
  - Previous good response to Unilateral ECT
  - Minimizing memory impairment is critical
- Bilateral Electrode Placement:
  - Speed of response is a priority
  - Failure of Unilateral ECT
  - Previous good response to Bilateral ECT without any significant memory problems
  - Where determination of cerebral dominance is difficult

Psychiatric Drugs and ECT

- Drugs that raise seizure threshold[Q]:
  - Benzodiazepines/ Barbiturates
  - Anticonvulsants
- Drugs that lower seizure threshold[Q]:
  - Antipsychotics
  - Antidepressants
  - Lithium

XIV B. COMMON DEFENCE MECHANISMS

Disorder	Defence mechanisms
Anxiety[Q]	**Repression**
Phobias[Q]	**Displacement**
Paranoid personality	Projection

Contd…

Psychiatry

Contd...

Disorder	Defence mechanisms
Histrionic personality	Acting out + Dissociation
Borderline personality[Q]	**Splitting**
Obsessive compulsive personality[Q]	**Reaction formation**
Suicide[Q]	**Retroflexion**
Hysteria	Conversion
Delusions of grandiosity	Distortion
Persecutory delusions	Projection
Nymphomania	Compensation

Topper's Edge

Vaillant's Four-level Classification of Defence Mechanisms[Q]
- Level I: Pathological defences (Psychotic denial, Delusional projection)
- Level II: Immature defences (Fantasy, Projection, Passive aggression, Acting out)
- Level III: Neurotic defences (Intellectualization, Reaction formation, Dissociation, Displacement, Repression)
- Level IV: Mature defences (Humour, Sublimation, Suppression, Altruism, Anticipation)

DEFENCE SEQUENCES IN A NARCISSIST

Narcissistic Defences
- Processes whereby the idealized aspects of the self are preserved, and its limitations denied
- Tend to be rigid and totalistic
- Often driven by feelings of shame and guilt, conscious or unconscious
- Typically runs through a sequence of defences to discharge painful feelings until he or she finds one that works

Sequence of Defences[Q]
- Unconscious repression
- Conscious denial
- Distortion (including exaggeration and minimization) and lies
- Psychological projection (blaming somebody else)
- Enlisting the help of one or more of his or her codependent friends who will support his or her distorted view

XIV C. PSYCHOLOGICAL TESTS

XIV C1. Intelligence Tests

- Wechsler adult intelligence scale (WAIS)
- Stanford-Binet test
- Binet Kamath test
- Bhatia's battery test of intelligence

XIV C2. Personality Tests

Objective personality tests	Projective personality tests
Minnesota multiphasic personality inventory (MIMPI)	Rorschach inkblot test[Q]
Millian clinical multiaxial inventory (MCM1)	Thematic Apperception test (TAT)[Q]
16 Personality Assessment inventory (PM)	Draw a person test
Edwards Personal Preference schedule (EPPS)	Sentence completion test
Adjective checklist (ACL)	Holtzman inkblot technique (HIT)

XIV C3. Neuropsychological Tests: To Identify Cognitive Defect in Organic Mental Disorders[Q]

- Wisconsin card sorting test
- Luria Nebraska test

- Bender Gestalt test[Q]
- Halstead-Reitan battery test
- Wechsler memory scale
- PGI battery of brain dysfunction
- Benton visual retention test
- PGI Memory scale

XIV D. HALSTEAD-REITAN BATTERY TEST

- Use: To determine the location and the effect of specific brain lesions
- Composition: Battery is comprised of 10 tests
  - Category test
  - Speech-sound perception test
  - Time sense test
  - Tactual performance test[Q]
  - Trail-making test
  - Aphasia screening test
  - Rhythm test[Q]
  - Critical flicker frequency
  - Sensory-perceptual test
  - Finger - Oscillation test[Q]

IMAGE-BASED QUESTIONS

1. **Identify Defence mechanism shown in Photograph** ***[Recent Question 2012]***

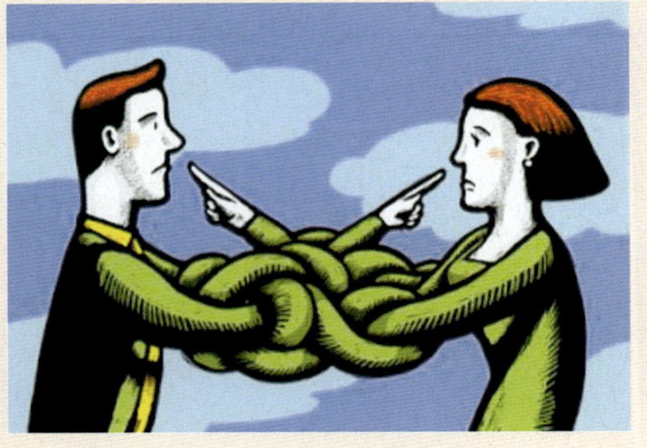

a. Repression b. Projection
c. Denial d. Distortion

2. **Indication for Treatment shown in Photograph**

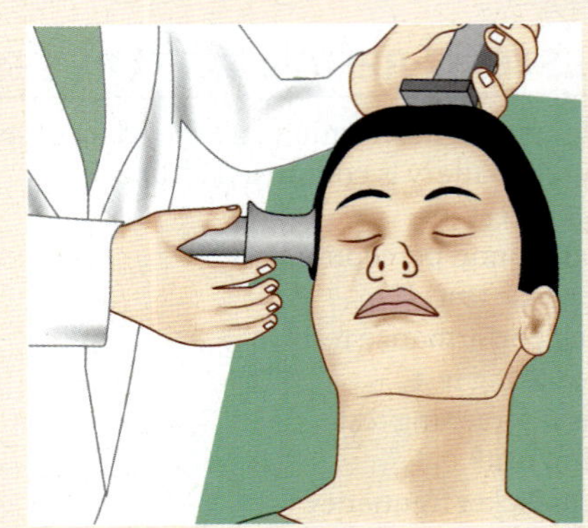

a. Mild depression
b. Severe depression
c. Severe refractory depression with suicidal tendency
d. Depression during Pregnancy

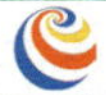 ANSWERS WITH EXPLANATIONS OF IBQs 

1. Ans. (b) Projection *[Ref. Psychology by Nevid, 3/e p386]*

- Projection: Projecting one's own unwanted/ unacceptable feelings/wishes/urges/impulses to another person

2. Ans. (c) Severe refractory depression with suicidal tendency *[Ref. Niraj Ahuja, 7/e p200]*

- Treatment shown: Electroconvulsive therapy
- Indications of ECT:
  - Major severe depression: With suicidal risk, with stupor, with poor food/fluids intake, with psychotic features, with partial response to drug therapy, where drugs are contraindicated, for faster recovery
  - Severe catatonia: With stupor, with poor food/fluids intake, with partial response to drug therapy, where drugs are contraindicated, for faster recovery
  - Severe psychosis: With suicidal/homicidal/assault risk, with partial response to drug therapy, where drugs are contraindicated, with prominent depressive features

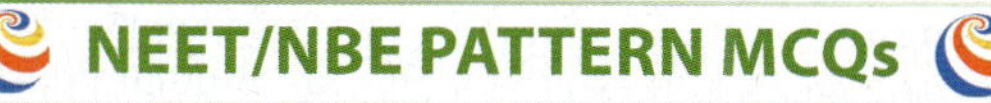

NEET/NBE PATTERN MCQs

1. **Night walking is seen in** *[Recent Question 2016]*
   a. Awake position b. REM sleep
   c. NREM sleep d. Light sleep
2. **True about Sleep are all except** *[Recent Question 2016]*
   a. NREM is followed by REM
   b. NREM constitute for 20% of total sleep
   c. 1 sleep cycle for 90–100 minutes
   d. Total sleep is 4–5 sleep cycles
3. **Maximum duration of time spent is in NREM stage** *[Recent Question 2016]*
   a. I b. II
   c. III d. IV
4. **All is true about Pseudocyesis except** *[Recent Question 2016]*
   a. Abdominal enlargement
   b. Patient is pregnant
   c. Labour pains at EDD
   d. Amenorrhea
5. **What is a feature of Narcolepsy?** *[Recent Question 2016, 2017]*
   a. Insomnia b. Hypersomnia at day time
   c. Bruxism d. Somnambulism
6. **Hypomimia is** *[Recent Question 2016]*
   a. Decreased ability to copy
   b. Decreased execution
   c. Deficit of expression by gesture
   d. Deficit of fluent speech
7. **Patient wants to scratch for itching in his amputated limb is an example of** *[Recent Question 2016]*
   a. Illusion
   b. Pseudohallucination
   c. Phantom limb hallucination
   d. Autoscopy hallucination
8. **Myxedema madness includes** *[Recent Question 2016]*
   a. Auditory hallucinations and paranoia
   b. Visual hallucinations and depression
   c. Auditory hallucinations and depression
   d. Paranoia and depression
9. **Phototherapy is used for** *[Recent Question 2016]*
   a. Sensory deprivation syndrome
   b. Schizophrenia
   c. Sleep disorder
   d. Mania
10. **Which of the following is not seen in Paradoxical sleep?** *[Recent Question 2016]*
    a. Increased muscle tone
    b. Penile erection
    c. Autonomic hyperactivity
    d. Rapid eye movement
11. **Which of the following are false about erectile dysfunction?** *[Recent Question 2016]*
    a. Psychogenic erectile dysfunction is distinguished from organic erectile dysfunction by PIPE therapy
    b. Sildenafil is used for treatment
    c. Nocturnal penile tumescence is maintained in psychological erectile dysfunction
    d. Sensate focus therapy aims at sensitizing non-genital areas
12. **Substance responsible for erection of penis** *[Recent Question 2016]*
    a. Clomipramine b. Papaverine
    c. Buspirone d. Amitriptyline
13. **The balance between REM and NREM sleep is maintained by** *[Recent Question 2016]*
    a. Pituitary gland b. Cerebellum
    c. Suprachiasmatic d. Gracile nucleus
14. **Ponto-geniculo-occipital spike is characteristic of Sleep stage** *[Recent Question 2016]*
    a. Stage 1 NREM b. Stage 2 NREM
    c. Stage 4 NREM d. REM
15. **Which of the following should not be used in a patient who is to receive ECT?** *[NBE FMGE September 2003]*
    a. Diazepam b. Phenytoin
    c. Reserpine d. Barbiturate
16. **In DSM III-R Premenstrual tension syndrome has been designated as** *[NBE DNB 1992]*
    a. Depressive equivalent
    b. Variant of somatoform disorder
    c. Late luteal phase dysphoric disorder
    d. Variant of hypochondriasis
17. **True about REM sleep is** *[Recent Question 2013]*
    a. Night mares b. Night terror
    c. Somniloquy d. None
18. **Match the following** *[NBE DNB 1996, 1999, 2001]*
    I. Hysteria (i) Displacement
    II. Obsessional (ii) Identification
    III. Depression (iii) Isolation
    IV. Phobia (iv) Turning on the self
    a. I (ii), II (iii), III (iv), IV (i)
    b. I (iii), II (iv), III (ii), IV (i)
    c. I (iv), II (iii), III (i), IV (ii)
    d. I (i), II (ii), III (iv), IV (iii)
19. **Reflex hallucination is a morbid variety of** *[NBE DNB 2009]*
    a. Kinesthesia b. Paresthesia
    c. Hyperesthesia d. Synaesthesia
20. **Drug used for reducing sex drive in sexual offenders** *[NBE DNB 1992]*
    a. Penfluridol b. Trifluridol
    c. Benperidol d. Molindone
21. **Max duration of time spent is in NREM stage** *[Recent Question 2012, 2013]*
    a. I b. II
    c. III d. IV

22. "Learned helplessness" is typically seen in *[Recent Question 2015, NBE DNB 1993, NBE DNB 2003, Bihar PG 2016]*
a. Delirium b. Dementia
c. Schizophrenia d. Depression

23. All of the following are NREM (Stage-IV) disorders, except *[NBE DNB 1998, NBE DNB 1999]*
a. Nocturnal enuresis b. Night terror
c. Nightmare d. Somnambulism

24. How to differentiate between psychological and organic erectile dysfunction? *[Recent Question 2012]*
a. Nocturnal penile tumescence
b. PIPE therapy
c. Sildenafil induced erection
d. Squeeze technique

25. In phobic neurosis, main ego defence used by the patient is *[NBE DNB 2007]*
a. Repression b. Avoidance
c. Undoing d. Reaction formation

26. HIAA is a metabolite of *[NBE DNB 2009]*
a. Serotonin b. Dopamine
c. Epinophrine d. Histamine

27. NREM Sleep true is *[Recent Question 2012, 2015]*
a. Teeth grinding b. Narcolepsy
c. Nightmares d. Sleep paralysis

28. Defence mechanism in phobia is *[NBE DNB 1997, 2003]*
a. Sublimation b. Displacement
c. Substitution d. Projection

29. Person included in disability act 1999 *[NBE DNB 2008]*
a. Mental retardation b. Phobia disorder
c. Alcohol dependence d. Personality disorder

30. A dishonest person thinks other persons are also dishonest. Defence mechanism used by him is
a. Projection b. Introjection *[UPSC 1991]*
c. Suppression d. Rationalisation

31. Narcolepsy, not true *[Recent Question 2012]*
a. Cataplexy b. Sleep architecture normal
c. Loss of muscle tone d. Hallucination

32. Which of the following is most common psychiatric diagnosis in HIV infected (AIDS) in individuals? *[NBE DNB 1996]*
a. Dementia b. Delirium
c. Paranoid psychosis d. Adjustment reaction

33. True in Narcolepsy is *[Recent Question 2015]*
a. Normal night time sleep b. Normal REM sleep
c. Hypersomnia d. Increased REM latency

34. EEG of a patient sitting silently with eyes closed shows *[Recent Question 2015]*
a. Beta waves b. Theta waves
c. Alpha waves d. Delta waves

35. Phototherapy is used in which Psychiatric illness? *[Recent Question 2014]*
a. Involutional melancholia
b. Seasonal mood disorder
c. Masked depression
d. Bipolar depression

36. A person believes that his penis is getting small and would soon disappear leading to his death. He is a case of *[Recent Question 2015]*
a. Amok b. Koro
c. Dhat d. Brain fag

37. Parkinsonism differ from Atypical Parkinsonism by absence of *[Recent Question 2015]*
a. Resting tremor
b. Postural instability
c. Vertical gaze palsy
d. Gait abnormality

38. EEG waves with prominence in Occipital lobe is *[Recent Question 2015]*
a. Alpha b. Beta
c. Theta d. Gamma

39. Cardinal element of behaviour therapy is *[Recent Question 2017]*
a. Modeling
b. Learning
c. Conditioning
d. Guidance

40. Narcolepsy is characterized by *[Recent Question 2017]*
a. Increased REM sleep
b. Increased daytime sleep
c. Increased night time sleep
d. Normal sleep architecture

41. A 25-year-old male believes that his penis is decreasing in size every day and one day it will disappear. Diagnosis is *[Recent Question 2017]*
a. Obsession
b. Somatization
c. Hypochondriasis
d. Culture bound syndrome

42. Which of the following is not a Culture bound syndrome? *[Recent Question 2017]*
a. Amok b. Latah
c. Dhat d. Van-Gogh

43. DHAT syndrome is? *[Recent Question 2017]*
a. Passage of blood in urine
b. Passage of semen in urine
c. Passage of pus in urine
d. None

44. Sleep disturbances are diagnosed by *[Recent Question 2017]*
a. Polysomnography b. Oximetry
c. Echocardiography d. Orthography

45. A person wakes up in night frightened with remembering fearful dreams. Diagnosis is *[Recent Question 2017]*
a. Narcolepsy b. Nightmares
c. Night terrors d. Somnambulism

46. Tic douloureux is characterized by *[Recent Question 2017]*
a. Multiple tics b. Neuralgia
c. Hallucinations d. Tremors

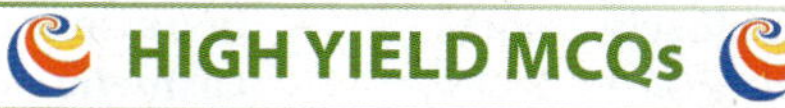

1. **Which of the following is NOT a component of Polysomnography?** *[AIIMS November 2016]*
   a. EEG
   b. EOG
   c. Pulse oximetry
   d. Intra-arterial oxygen assessment
2. **Echolalia is a recognized feature of** *[JIPMER PGMEE 1999, PGI 2001]*
   a. Catatonic schizophrenia
   b. Anorexia nervosa c. Alzheimer's disease
   d. Childhood autism e. Petit mal epilepsy
3. **Following are correctly matched except** *[PGI 1998, Recent Question 2015]*
   a. Schizophrenia-Auditory hallucination
   b. OCD-infidelity
   c. Alcoholism-auditory hallucination
   d. Depression-guilt feeling
4. **Systemic de-sensitization therapy is used for** *[All India PGMEE 2000, AIIMS PGMEE 1997]*
   a. Phobia b. Depression/Mania
   c. Schizophrenia d. Organic brain syndrome
   e. Anxiety
5. **In which behaviour therapy is helpful?** *[AIIMS PGMEE 1995]*
   a. Schizophrenia b. Agoraphobia
   c. Personality disorder d. Neuretic depression
6. **Displacement reaction is characteristically seen in** *[MP PGMEE 1998]*
   a. Mania b. Phobia
   c. Conversion disorder d. Depression
7. **Visual hallucinations without auditory hallucinations is seen in** *[JIPMER PGMEE 1993]*
   a. Organic brain damage
   b. Obsessive compulsive neurosis
   c. Agarophobia
   d. Schizophrenia
8. **Pseudo dementia is seen in** *[PGI 1997, DPG 2003]*
   a. Alcoholism b. Depression
   c. Schizophrenia d. Mania
9. **Deja vu is seen in** *[Kerala PGMEE 1994, Recent Question 2015]*
   a. Temporal lobe epilepsy b. Normal person
   c. Psychosis d. All of the above
10. **Apraxia is a disorder in** *[UP PGMEE 1997]*
    a. Cerebellum b. Sensory system
    c. Motor system
    d. Initiating and planning movement
11. **Rorschach inkblot test is** *[Rohtak PGMEE 2003]*
    a. Projective b. Subjective
    c. Both d. None
12. **Best test for diagnosis of organic mental (Brain) disorders** *[MP PGMEE 2002, AIPG 2000, 2010]*
    a. Bender Gestalt test b. Rorschach test
    c. Thematic apperception d. Sentence completion test
13. **Behaviour therapy is useful in** *[PGI 2008]*
    a. Phobia b. Hysteria
    c. Stuttering d. OCD
14. **Cognitive behaviour therapy deals with** *[PGI 2009]*
    a. Unconscious motive b. Maladaptive assumptions
    c. Psuedo-dynamic conflict
    d. Emotional consciousness of automatic thoughts
15. **'Reinforcement' is used in** *[Recent Question 2015, AIIMS PGMEE 1994, 1999]*
    a. Psychoanalysis b. Hypno-analysis
    c. Abreaction d. Conditioned learning
16. **Most common psychological features of AIDS is** *[AIIMS PGMEE 1994]*
    a. Mania b. Depression
    c. Suicidal Tendency d. Violence
17. **Visual analogue scale (VAS) most widely used in measure** *[Recent Question 2015, AIIMS PGMEE 2003]*
    a. Sleep b. Sedation
    c. Pain intensity d. Depth of Anaesthesia
18. **One of the important defence mechanism is** *[Karnataka PGMEE 2001]*
    a. Allenation b. Confabulation
    c. Repression d. Suppression
19. **Which is not an ego defence mechanism?** *[PGI 1999]*
    a. Rationalization b. Repression
    c. Identification d. Obsession
20. **Most important cause of neurotic reaction is the excessive use of** *[PGI 1998, NIMHANS 2001, Maharashtra PGMEE 2004]*
    a. Projection b. Regression
    c. Suppression d. Sublimation
21. **Widmark Formula is used for** *[AIIMS PGMEE 1993]*
    a. Opium b. Cannabis
    c. Alcohol d. Atrophetamine
22. **Morbid Jealousy is seen with** *[All India PGMEE 1994, Recent Question 2015, 2017]*
    a. Alcohol b. Opium
    c. Cannabis d. Amphetamine
23. **Van Gogh Syndrome is seen in** *[PGI 2003]*
    a. Mania
    b. Depression
    c. Schizophrenia
    d. Obsessive compulsive disorder
24. **Differential diagnosis of premenstrual tension includes all of the following except** *[AIIMS PGMEE 2002]*
    a. Psychiatric depressive disorder
    b. Panic disorder
    c. General anxiety disorder
    d. Chronic fatigue syndrome
25. **Alpha-rhythm is seen in** *[PGI 1997]*
    a. Sleep with eyes closed with mind wandering
    b. Mental activity
    c. Awake with eyes open d. REM sleep

26. Which one of the following phenomenon is closely associated with slow wave sleep? *[AIIMS PGMEE 2004]*
a. Dreaming
b. Sleep walking
c. Atonia
d. Irregular heart rate

27. The Non-REM (NREM) sleep is commonly associated with *[All India PGMEE 2004]*
a. Frequent dreaming
b. Frequent penile erections
c. Increased blood pressure
d. Night terrors

28. True about narcolepsy *[PGI 2006]*
a. Sleep sudden
b. Long duration (>5 hrs) of sleep
c. Cataplexy
d. Presents in IInd decade

29. A homosexual person feels that he is imposed by a female body & persistent discomfort with his sex, diagnosis is *[PGI 2003]*
a. Gender identity disorder
b. Transvestism
c. Voyeurism
d. Paraphilias

30. Not a feature of paradoxical sleep is *[PGI 1999, Recent Question 2015]*
a. Decreased muscle tone
b. Rapid eye movements
c. Brain shows increased metabolism
d. EEG shows decreased activity

31. Ambivalence is most commonly seen in *[AIIMS PGMEE 1996]*
a. Schizophrenia
b. Hysteria
c. Mania
d. OCN

32. A 30-year-old man since 2 months suspects that his wife is having an affair with his boss. He thinks his friend is also involved from abroad and is providing technology support. He thinks people talk ill about him. His friends tried to convince him but he is not convinced at all. Otherwise he is normal, he doesn't have any thought disorder or any other inappropriate behavior. The most likely diagnosis is *[All India PGMEE 2010]*
a. Paranoid Personality disorder
b. Persistent delusion disorder
c. Schizophrenia
d. Acute and Transient psychosis

33. The Halstead Reitan battery involves all except *[PGI 1999]*
a. Finger oscillation
b. Constructional praxis
c. Rhythm
d. Tactual performance

34. Rorschach test measures *[PGI 1999]*
a. Intelligence
b. Creativity
c. Personality
d. Neuriticism

35. Ramu, a 22-year-old single unmarried man is suffering from sudden onset of 3rd person hallucination for the past 2 weeks. He is suspicious of his family members and had decreased sleep and appetite. The diagnosis is *[AIIMS PGMEE 2001]*
a. Schizophrenia
b. Acute Psychosis
c. Acute mania
d. Acute delirium

36. A patient came with complaints of having a deformed, nose and also complained that nobody takes him seriously because of the deformity of his nose. He has visited several cosmetic surgeons but they have sent him back saying that there is nothing wrong with his nose. He is probably suffering from *[AIIMS PGMEE 2001]*
a. Hypochondriasis
b. Somatization
c. Delusional Disorder
d. OCD

37. Modafinil is approved by FDA for treatment of all except *[All India PGMEE 2009]*
a. Obstructive sleep apnea syndrome [OSAS]
b. Shift work syndrome [SWS]
c. Narcolepsy
d. Lethargy in depression

38. Which of the following is a mature defence mechanism? *[JIPMER PGMEE 1991, UP PGMEE 2007]*
a. Projection
b. Reaction formation
c. Anticipation
d. Denial

39. Mature defence mechanism is seen in *[JIPMER PGMEE 1995, WB PGMEE 2005, Assam PGMEE 2006]*
a. Altruism
b. Repression
c. Regression
d. None

40. Ego's defence mechanism "Undoing" is typically seen in *[PGI 2001, AIIMS PGMEE 1993, AIIMS PGMEE 1995]*
a. Depression
b. Schizophrenia
c. Obsessive compulsive neurosis
d. Hysteria

41. All of the following are defence mechanisms of ego except *[Recent Question 2015, All India PGMEE 1991, AIIMSPG 1998]*
a. Projection
b. Conversion
c. Reaction formation
d. Transference

42. Which drug acts through alpha subunit of GABA receptor? *[AIIMS PGMEE 2008]*
a. Benzodiazepine
b. Barbiturate
c. Haloperidol
d. TCA

43. Not a defence mechanism *[PGI 1998]*
a. Derailment
b. Repression
c. Distortion
d. Undoing

44. A reluctant child forced to bring sugar from a shop spills half of it on the way. This is an example of *[JIPMER PGMEE 1997, Delhi PGMEE 2002, Rajasthan PGMEE 2004]*
a. Hysteria
b. Passive aggression
c. Disobedience
d. Active aggression

45. A Chronic alcoholic blames the family environment as a cause of his alcoholism. This is phenomenon of *[AIIMS PGMEE 2000]*
a. Projection
b. Denial
c. Rationalization
d. Sublimation

46. Which of the following excludes painful stimuli from awareness? *[AIIMS PGMEE 1998]*
a. Repression
b. Reaction formation
c. Projection
d. Rationalization

47. Blood of 45 years old male shows Increased HVA. This patient is most likely to show *[AIIMS PGMEE 2008]*
a. PCC b. Schizophrenia
c. Depression d. Parkinson's disease

48. Not true about nocturnal penile tumescence is *[AIIMS PGMEE 1995]*
a. Totals about 1 min / night
b. Normal phenomenon
c. Occurs in NREM sleep
d. Can be used to distinguish between psychological or organic impotence

49. True regarding Narcolepsy is/are *[PGI May 2014, Recent Question 2017]*
a. Cataplexy
b. Sleep paralysis
c. Hypnagogic hallucinations
d. Excessive day time sleepiness
e. Day time wakefulness

50. Feature(s) of Parkinson's disease *[PGI May 2014]*
a. Dystonic tremor b. Resting tremor
c. Rigidity d. Bradykinesia
e. Postural stability

51. Psychiatric disorders are classified in .... blocks of ICD-10 Classification *[JIPMER PGMEE 2014]*
a. A b. F
c. G d. P

52. MC mental health disorder is *[NIMHANS PGMEE 2014]*
a. Anxiety b. Depression
c. Phobia d. Schizophrenia

53. Gilles de la Tourette syndrome is most commonly associated with *[NIMHANS PGMEE 2014]*
a. Parkinsonism b. Depression
c. OCD d. Schizophrenia

54. A smoker is worried about side effects of smoking. But he does not stop smoking thinking that he smokes less as compared to others and takes a good diet. This thinking is called *[AIIMS PG May 2015]*
a. Self protection b. Self exemption
c. Cognitive behavior d. Distortion

55. A patient with psychosis given haloperidol intramuscular, develops irrelevant talks, inability to move his eyes, tremor and rigidity. Which drug should be used for immediate management? *[AIIMS PG May 2015]*
a. Promethazine b. Lorazepam
c. Risperidone d. Diazepam

56. Regarding Parkinsonism, true is/are *[PGI November 2014]*
a. Tremor b. Hyperkinesia
c. Rigidity d. Postural stability
e. Depression

57. A 35-years-old male presents with inability to sleep. He is advised to undergo EE. Following EEG tracing is obtained. This is which stage of Sleep? *[AIIMS November 2017]*

EEG

a. REM sleep b. NREM stage 2
c. NREM stage 3 d. NREM stage 4

58. A 24-year-old female presents to Psychiatry OPD. She has been having thoughts of cutting her own fingers, though she has been planning it and imagining doing it but never actually does it. She's not having remorse for that too but according to her it's distressing for her and she is unable to control them. The thoughts vanish either by ending with a seizure or automatically subsides on its own. Following may be the most likely cause *[AIIMS May 2017]*
a. Crowding of thoughts b. Obsession
c. Thought insertion d. Forced thinking

59. In Freud's theory of Dreams, all of the following are components except *[Recent Question 2018]*
a. Displacement b. Condensation
c. Symbolisation d. Correlation

Psychiatry

NEET/NBE PATTERN MCQs ANSWERS WITH EXPLANATIONS 

1. Ans. (c) NREM sleep
[Ref. Niraj Ahuja, 7/e p140]

Stage 4 Sleep Disorders (Parasomnias)

- Sleep-walking **(Somnabulism)**: Automatic motor activities in sleep, Difficult arousal, Accident-prone
- Sleep-terrors/ Night-terrors **(Pavor nocturnus)**: Wakes up with screaming, Autonomic arousal, Unable to recall later
- Sleep related eneuresis **(Bed-wetting)**: Repetitive voiding of urine during sleep
- Bruxism **(Teeth grinding)**: Involuntary forceful grinding of teeth during sleep
- Sleep talking **(Somniloquy)**: Talks during sleep, Does not remember in morning

2. Ans. (b) NREM constitute for 20% of total sleep
[Ref. Niraj Ahuja, 7/e p133]

Key Characteristics of Sleep

- **Two phases:**
  - Rapid eye movement (REM) sleep: D-sleep/Desynchronized sleep/Dreaming sleep/ Active sleep/Paradoxical sleep
  - Non-REM (NREM) sleep: S-sleep/ Synchronized sleep/ Quiet sleep/ Orthodox sleep
- **NREM sleep has 4 phases:**
  - Stage 1 NREM: First and lightest stage, No alpha waves, Low voltage, Predominant theta activity
  - Stage 2 NREM: Sleep spindles (Waxing and waning amplitude), K-complexes (High voltage spikes)
  - Stage 3 NREM: High voltage, Delta waves
  - Stage 4 NREM: Predominant delta waves
- **Key features of sleep:**
  - Each sleep cycle lasts 90–100 minutes in adults
  - NREM sleep is followed by REM sleep
  - NREM-REM sleep has 3–5 cycles
  - NREM is 80% (6–6.5 hours) while REM is 20% (1.5–2 hours) of total sleep (8 hours)

Also Remember

- Usual sleep duration in a newborn child is 16–18 hours a day
- As age advances, duration of sleep tends to decrease

3. Ans. (b) II
[Ref. Respiratory Care by Hess, 3/e p205]

Sleep Stages in Young Adults

Sleep stage	Time spent
NREM (N) sleep	75–80%
Stage N1	2–5%
Stage N2	45–55%
Stage N3	15–20%
REM (R) sleep	20–25%

Contd…

Contd…

4. Ans. (b) Patient is pregnant
[Ref. Mental Health and Mental Disorders by Sperry, 1/e p879]

Pseudocyesis

- False belief of being pregnant
- False pregnancy, Hysterical pregnancy, Phantom pregnancy
- Symptoms: Weight gain, Abdominal enlargement, Amenorrhea, Mammary gland hyperplasia and lactation, Mucoid vaginal discharge, Restlessness, Nesting, Labor pains on EDD, Mothering of inanimate objects

5. Ans. (b) Hypersomnia at day time
[Ref. Niraj Ahuja, 7/e p138]

- **Narcolepsy** is a chronic, neurological sleep disorder characterized by excessive daytime sleepiness (EDS), cataplexy and abnormal REM sleep
- A person with signs of narcolepsy will experience extreme fatigue and may fall asleep at odd and inappropriate times, such as during work or school

6. Ans. (c) Deficit of expression by gesture
[Ref. A Dictionary of Neurological Signs by Larner, 4/e p168]

Hypomimia/Amimia

- Deficit or absence of expression by gesture or mimicry
- Mask-like facies: Most obvious as a lack of facial expressive mobility
- Seen in: Frontal-subcortical disease (Basal ganglia disease), Frontal lobe lesions

7. Ans. (c) Phantom limb hallucination
[Ref. Individual Differences in Conscious Experience by Wallace, 1/e p91]

- **A phantom limb** is the sensation that an amputated or missing limb is still attached
- Approximately 60–80% of individuals with an amputation experience phantom sensations in their amputated limb, and the majority of the sensations are painful

8. Ans. (a) Auditory hallucinations and paranoia
[Ref. Neurology in Clinical Practice by Bradley, 4/e p109]

Myxedema Madness

- Psychosis with Hypothyroidism
- Typically presents with paranoid delusions and auditory hallucinations
- Fatal if untreated

9. Ans. (c) Sleep disorder
[Ref. Evaluation of Sleep Complaints by Kushida, 1/e p486]

- Phototherapy is another commonly used treatment for Sleep disorders
- Exposure to light at the proper times helps to align the circadian alerting signal

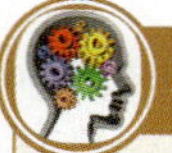

Also Remember

Treatment of Circadian Rhythm Sleep Disorders

- Regular sleep schedule
- Phototherapy
- Cognitive behavior therapy for Insomnia
- Chronotherapy
- Melatonin
- Further treatments: Prescription medications (Sleeping pills, Stimulants), Signals (Timing of social activities, exercise, meals, social activities)

10. Ans. (a) Increased muscle tone

[Ref. Fundamentals of Human Physiology by Sherwood, 4/e p131]

- The behavioral pattern accompanying paradoxical sleep is marked by abrupt inhibition of muscle tone throughout the body

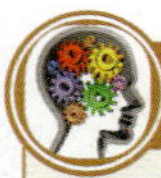

Also Remember

	Slow-wave sleep	Paradoxical sleep
EEG	Slow waves	Similar to alert, awake
Motor activity	Considerable muscle tone	Inhibition of muscle tone
HR, RR, BP	Regular	Irregular
Dreaming	Rare	Common
Arousal	Easy	Difficult
% sleep time	80%	20%
Features	4 stages	REM movements

11. Ans. (a) Psychogenic erectile dysfunction is distinguished from organic erectile dysfunction by PIPE therapy

[Ref. Diabetes in Old Age by Sinclair, 3/e p153]

Erectile Dysfunction (ED)

	Psychogenic ED	Organic ED
Onset	Sudden	Gradual
Initiation	Complete immediate loss	Incremental progression
Morning erection	Present	Absent
Other feature	Varies with partner/ circumstance	Remain same with partners/circumstance

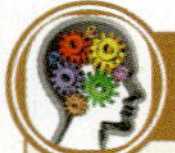

Also Remember

- Technique of Pharmacologically induced penile erection (PIPE) which is now being used both as a diagnostic and a therapeutic tool in ED
- Papaverine HCl, was subsequently utilized for differentiating psychogenic from organic causes of impotence

12. Ans. (b) Papaverine

[Ref. Color Doppler US of the Penis by Bertolotto, 1/e p43]

- Prostaglandins can be responsible for a long standing erection that lasts 3–4 hours associated with pain, which generally disappears spontaneously
- Papaverine is the second most used drug to stimulate erections at a dose ranging from 10–40 mg

13. Ans. (c) Suprachiasmatic

[Ref. Swaiman's Pediatric Neurology, 5/e p926]

- Ultimate command center for the once-a-day (circadian) rhythm of sleep and wakefulness is suprachiasmatic centre of hypothalamus

14. Ans. (d) REM

[Ref. Principles of Physiology by Pramanik, 1/e p469]

PGO spikes (Ponto-geniculo-occipital spikes)

- An important feature of REM sleep is the occurrence of
- Electrical potential changes arising from Pons, passing through lateral geniculate body and ending in occipital cortex

15. Ans. (c) Reserpine

[Ref. MIMS]

Indications of Reserpine	Contraindications of Reserpine
• Hypertension • Dyskinesia in Huntington's disease	• Peptic ulcer disease • Depression • Parkinson's disease • Pheochromocytoma • Electroconvulsive therapy

16. Ans. (c) Late luteal phase dysphoric disorder

[Ref. Menstrual Disorders by Hoffmann, 1/e p125-126]

Premenstrual Syndrome

- DSM-III: Late luteal phase dysphoric disorder
- DSM-IV: Premenstrual dysphoric disorder (PMDD)

17. Ans. (a) Night mares

[Ref. Niraj Ahuja, 7/e p140]

Sleep Disorders

NREM Sleep Disorders	REM Sleep Disorders
• Sleep walking (Somnabulism) • Pavor nocturnus (Sleep/ Night terrors) • Bed-wetting (Sleep enuresis) • Teeth grinding (Bruxism) • Sleep talking (Somniloquy)	• Night mares (Dream anxiety disorders)

18. Ans. (a) I (ii), II (iii), III (iv), IV (i)

[Ref. Niraj Ahuja, 7/e p207-210]

19. Ans. (d) Synaesthesia

[Ref. Hallucinations and Illusions by Parish, 1/e p221]

- *Reflex hallucination:* A special variety of hallucination, in which a stimulus in one modality produces hallucination in another modality

20. Ans. (c) Benperidol

[Ref. Human Sexuality and Its' Problems by Bancroft, 3/e p502]

- *Anti-libido drugs used in Sex offenders*: Benpridol, Depo-Provera, Cyproterone, Medroxyprogesterone acetate

21. Ans. (b) II

[Ref. Sleep Medicine by Smith, 1/e p13]

Time Spent in Sleep

- REM Sleep:15–25% of total sleep
- NREM Sleep: 75–85% of total sleep
  - Phase 1: 5%
  - Phase 2: 50%
  - Phase 3 and 4: 20–25%

22. Ans. (d) Depression

[Ref. Scientific Foundations of Cognitive Theory and Therapy of Depression by Beck, 1/e p41]

- *Most influential theory of Depression*: Learned helplessness theory (Martin Seligman)

23. Ans. (c) Nightmare

[Ref. Niraj Ahuja, 7/e p140]

24. Ans. (a) Nocturnal penile tumescence

[Ref. Niraj Ahuja, 7/e p128]

- *Psychological impotence*: Early morning erections and Erections during REM sleep (Nocturnal penile tumescence) are usually preserved

25. Ans. (b) Avoidance

[Ref. Phobias: The Psychology of Irrational Fear by McCabe, 1/e p323]

- *Commonly observed defences in Phobic neurosis*:
  - Displacement
  - Avoidance

26. Ans. (a) Serotonin

[Ref. Psychiatry Update: The American Psychiatric Association Annual Review by Grinspoon, Volume II, Pg 457]

27. Ans. (a) Teeth grinding

[Ref. Niraj Ahuja, 7/e p140]

28. Ans. (b) Displacement

[Ref. Niraj Ahuja, 7/e p208]

- *Displacement is used as a Defence mechanism in*:
  - Phobia
  - OCD

29. Ans. (a) Mental retardation

[Ref. Income Tax Act 2009, 12/e p540]

- *Disability act 1999 covers*:
  - Autism
  - Cerebral Palsy
  - Mental retardation
  - Multiple disabilities

30. Ans. (a) Projection

[Ref. Niraj Ahuja, 7/e p207]

- *Projection*: Unconscious attribution of one's attitudes and urges to other person(s), because of painful affect aroused by those attitudes and urges

31. Ans. (b) Sleep architecture normal

[Ref. Niraj Ahuja, 7/e p138]

Narcolepsy

- Description: Excessive day time sleepiness, often disturbed night time sleep and disturbances in REM sleep
- Age of onset: 15–25 years age
- Hallmark: Decreased REM latency
- Classical Tetrad of Symptoms:
  - Sleep attacks (Most common): Unable to resist sleep attack anytime of day
  - Cataplexy: Loss of muscle tone in various parts of body
  - Hypnagogic hallucinations
  - Sleep paralysis (Least common)

32. Ans. (d) Adjustment reaction

[Ref. Health and Performance by Smith & Jones, Volume II, Pg 234]

- MC Psychiatric disorder among HIV positives: Adjustment reaction with Depression
- MC Psychiatric symptom among HIV positives: Depression

33. Ans. (c) Hypersomnia

[Ref. Niraj Ahuja, 7/e p138]

34. Ans. (c) Alpha waves

[Ref. Neurological Differential Diagnosis by Patten, 2/e p386]

Waves in Electroencephalogram (EEG)

Wave in EEG	Frequency	Remark
Alpha	8–12 Hz	Subject sitting quietly with eyes closed
Beta	20–22 Hz	• Dream, REM sleep • Sitting quietly with eyes open • Subject sitting quietly with eyes closed but solving problem • Anxious subjects • Sedatives, Tranquilizers
Theta	5–7 Hz	• Light sleep • Visual imagery • Normal children • Over-breathing • Temporal lobe lesions
Delta	1–4 Hz	• Deep restful sleep • Vague dream states • Resting children with over-breathing

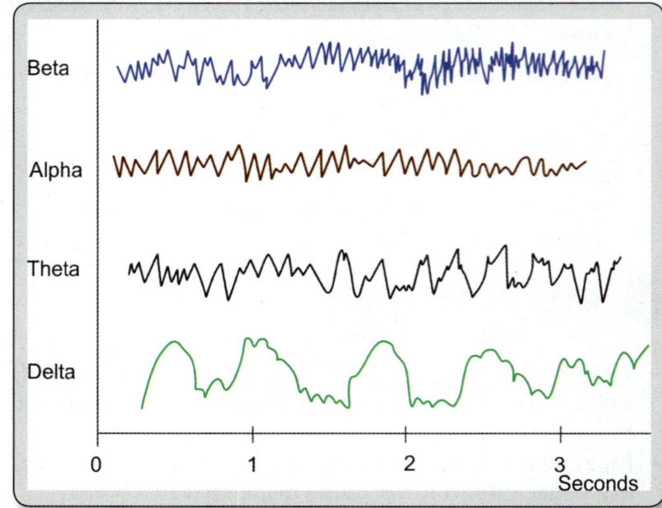

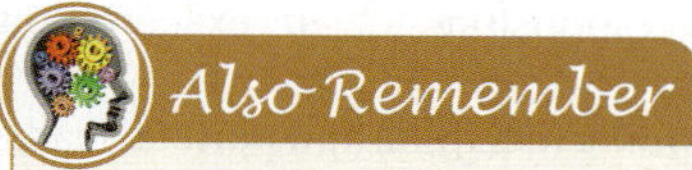

- Father of Electroencephalography: Hans Berger

35. Ans. (b) Seasonal mood disorder
[Ref. Psychiatry by Cowan, 5/e p86]

Phototherapy in Psychiatric Disorders

- Seasonal affective disorder
- Delayed sleep phase syndrome
- Jet lag

36. Ans. (b) Koro
[Ref. Sexual Medicine by Kar, 1/e p445]

Culture Bound Syndromes

- ***Koro***: A man who suffers from Koro has an overpowering belief that his genitals are retracting and will gradually be absorbed by his body
- ***Amok***: A person suffering from Amok suddenly withdraws from family and friends, then bursts into a murderous rage, attacking the people or objects around him with whatever weapon is available
- ***TaijinKyofusho***: Person suffering from TaijinKyofusho are likely to be extremely embarrassed of themselves or displeasing to others when it comes to the functions of their bodies or appearances (Social phobia dealing with social anxiety)
- ***Ghost Sickness***: A person suffering from Ghost Sickness is said to be preoccupied and/or consumed by the red or dying (Sometimes associated with witchcraft and symptoms include weakness, loss of appetite, nightmares and suffocation)
- ***Brain Fag***: A person suffering from Brain Fag is usually a high school or university student with syndromes such as difficulties concentrating, remembering, and thinking, as well as head, neck, and eye pain (Caused by excessive external pressure to be successful among the young)
- ***Ataque de Nervios***: A person suffering from Ataque de Nervios displays syndromes such as uncontrollable screaming or shouting, crying, trembling, sensations of heat rising in the chest and head, and verbal or physical aggression (Usually associated with a stressful event)
- ***Hikikomori***: Phenomenon of reclusive adolescents or young adults who withdraw from social life, often seeking extreme degrees of isolation and confinement in their room, apartment or house for prolonged periods, sometimes measured in years
- ***Dhat***: Person suffering from Dhat is said to report premature ejaculation or impotence, and the belief that they are passing semen in their urine
- ***Falling Out***: Constricted consciousness as a psychological response to anxiety and specific stressors (Sudden collapse and preceded dizziness and spinning sensation)
- ***Evil Eye***: Malevolent look which is believed to be able to cause injury or misfortune for the person at whom it is directed for reasons of envy or dislike
- ***Latah:*** Startle reaction and subsequent imitative behavior with echolalia, echopraxia and coprolalia, altered consciousness and fear. Behavior precipitated by sudden acute stress is seen in Malaysia and Indonesia.

37. Ans. (c) Vertical gaze palsy
[Ref. Movement Disorders by Donaldson, 1/e p429]

- Patients with Atypical Parkinsonism have symptoms similar to Parkinson's' disease, including resting tremors, slowed movement, stiffness, gait difficulty and postural instability
- Parkinsonism plus syndrome (Atypical Parkinsonism) also have additional problems like vertical gaze palsy, early postural instability, procerus sign (worried facial expression)

38. Ans. (a) Alpha
[Ref. Bioelectronic Recording Techniques by Patterson, 1/e p26]

EEG Waves Origins

- Alpha waves: Occipital lobe, Parietal lobe
- Beta waves: Frontal lobe, Precentral parts of brain
- Gamma waves: Frontal lobe, Precentral parts of brain
- Delta waves: Interaction between Thalamus, Cortex and Reticular activation
- Theta waves: Temporal lobe, Frontal lobe
- Kappa waves: Temporal lobes
- Lambda waves: Parieto-occipital lobes
- K-complex: Vertex
- Sleep spindles: Precentral region

39. Ans. (b) Learning
[Ref. Niraj Ahuja, 7/e p214]

Behaviour therapy

- Type of Psychotherapy based on theories of learning
- Aims at modifying maladaptive behaviours and substituting them with adaptive behaviours
- Short duration therapy (6-8 weeks) with cost-effectiveness
- Main Theories of learning:
  - Operant conditioning model (Skinner)
  - Classical conditioning model (Pavlov)
- Main Techniques of Behaviour therapy:
  - Systematic desensitization
  - Operant conditioning to increase behaviour (Positive reinforcement, Negative reinforcement, Modelling) or decrease behaviour (Time-out, Punishment, Satiation)
  - Aversion therapy
  - Flooding
- Other techniques: Token economy, Social skills training, family therapy, marital therapy, cognitive behaviour therapy

40. Ans. (b) Increased day time sleep
[Ref. Niraj Ahuja, 7/e p138]

- Narcolepsy is a chronic, neurological sleep disorder characterized by excessive daytime sleepiness (EDS), cataplexy and abnormal REM sleep
- A person with signs of narcolepsy will experience extreme fatigue and may fall asleep at odd and inappropriate times, such as during work or school
- The first symptom of narcolepsy to emerge is excessive daytime sleepiness, sleep attacks, hypersomnolence, and chronic fatigue in spite of getting an adequate amount of sleep

41. Ans. (d) Culture bound syndrome
[Ref. Sexual Medicine by Kar, 1/e p445]

Culture Bound Syndromes

- Koro: A man who suffers from Koro has an overpowering belief that his genitals are retracting and will gradually be absorbed by his body
- Other Culture bound syndromes include Amok, Taijin-Kyofusho, Ghost Sickness, Brain Fag, Ataque de Nervios, Hikikomori, Dhat, Falling Out, Evil Eye, Latah

42. Ans. (d) Van-Gogh
[Ref. Sexual Medicine by Kar, 1/e p445]

43. Ans. (b) Passage of semen in urine
[Ref. Niraj Ahuja, 7/e p110]

Dhat Syndrome

- Person suffering from Dhat is said to report premature ejaculation or impotence, and the belief that they are passing semen in their urine
- Multiple somatic symptoms, asthenia (physical or mental exhaustion), anxiety or depression, sexual dysfunction

44. Ans. (a) Polysomnography
[Ref. Niraj Ahuja, 7/e p135]

Study of Sleep and Associated Phenomena

- Observation of a sleeping person for externally visible changes
- EEG
- Polysomnography (Preferred method): Polysomnography entails the recording of multiple physiological variables during sleep to ascertain the presence/ absence of sleep disorders. It is an important technique useful to detect if a sleep disorder is responsible for or exacerbating psychiatric symptoms.
  - Continuous EEG recording (occipital and parietal leads)
  - EOG (electrooculography)
  - EMG (electromyography)
  - ECG (cardiac status)
  - Oxymetry, expired CO_2, O_2 saturation (respiratory status)
  - MSLT (Multiple sleep latency test)
  - Penile tumescence, body temperature, GSR (galvanic skin response), and body movements

45. Ans. (b) Nightmares
[Ref. Niraj Ahuja, 7/e p140]

Nightmares/ Dream anxiety disorder

- Occur during the REM-sleep phase
- Characterised by fearful dreams occurring most commonly in the last one-third of night sleep
- Person wakes up very frightened and remembers the dream vividly
- This is in contrast to night terrors which occur early in the night, are a stage 4 NREM disorder, and are characterised by complete amnesia

46. Ans. (b) Neuralgia
[Ref. Kaufman's Clinical Neurology for Psychiatrists, 8/e p187]

Tic douloureux (Trigeminal neuralgia)

- Chronic, recurring disorder consisting of dozens of 20–30 second jabs daily of agonizing, sharp pain extending along one or more of the three divisions of Trigeminal nerve
- Trigeminal neuralgia most commonly affects the V2 division of Trigeminal nerve

HIGH YIELD MCQs ANSWERS WITH EXPLANATIONS 

1. Ans. (d) Intra-arterial oxygen assessment
[Ref. Neurophysiology Board Review by Gupta, 1/e p327]

Components of Polysomnogram

- EEG Scalp
- Electro-oculogram (EOG: Eye movement)
- Respiratory effort (Chest and Abdomen)
- Pulse oximetry (Oxygen saturation)
- EMG Anterior tibialis (Leg movements)
- Body position

2. Ans. (a) Catatonic schizophrenia; (d) Childhood autism
[Ref. Language Development in Exceptional Circumstances by Mogford, 1/e p195]

- **Echolalia** (Repetition of Heard Phrases)
  - Catatonic schizophrenia
  - Tourette syndrome (Vocal tics)
  - Developmental aphasia, transcortical aphasia
  - Congenital blindness
  - Senile dementia
  - Childhood autism

3. Ans. (b) OCD-infidelity
[Ref. Niraj Ahuja, 7/e p76]

4. Ans. (a) Phobia
[Ref. Niraj Ahuja, 7/e p214-215]

Systematic Desensitization

- **Principle of Reciprocal inhibition:** If a response incompatible with anxiety is made to occur at the same time as an anxiety provoking stimulus, then anxiety is likely to reduce
- Steps:
  - Relaxation training
  - Hierarchy reconstruction
  - Systematic desensitization proper
- Treatment of choice in:
  - Phobias
  - Obsessive compulsive disorders

5. Ans. (b) Agoraphobia
[Ref. Niraj Ahuja, 7/e p94]

6. Ans. (b) Phobia
[Ref. Niraj Ahuja, 7/e p208]

7. Ans. (a) Organic brain damage
[Ref. Psychosis: An Integrative Approach by Cullberg, 1st Edition]

8. Ans. (b) Depression
[Ref. Late Life Depression by Roose, 1/e p84]
- *Pseudo-dementia*: Impairment in memory and other cognitive domains resembling dementia but caused by Functional psychiatric disorders such as Depression

9. Ans. (d) All of the above
[Ref. Platinum Notes: USMLE Step 2 by Hassan, Pg 3]
- ***Déjà vu:*** Sense of familiarity
  - Temporal lobe epilepsy
  - Normal person
  - Psychosis

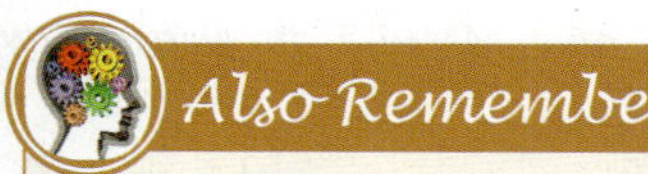

Para-amnesias
- Description: Distorted/falsified recall of events especially in context of details or temporal relationships

Types of Para-amnesias
- **Confabulation:** Unintentional filling of gaps of memory with untrue and fanciful material
  - Related disorders: Chronic alcoholism, Korsakoff's syndrome, Syphilis, Senile dementia, Schizophrenic psychosis
- **Deja vu:** Unfamiliar event/situation feel strangely familiar
  - Related disorders: Normal phenomenon, Schizophrenia, Anxiety, Temporal lobe epilepsy, Dissociative identity disorders, Simple partial seizures
- **Jamais vu:** Feeling of strangeness to familiar situation/ event
  - Related disorders: Amnesia, Epilepsy, Simple partial seizure, Aura of migraine
- **Deja pence:** A thought never entertained before is incorrectly regarded as repetition of a previous thought
- **Deja endendu:** Illusion that what one is hearing one has heard previously
- **Ganser syndrome:** Syndrome of approximate answers, Somatic conversion features, Pseudo-hallucinations and Clouding of consciousness

10. Ans. (d) Initiating and planning movement
[Ref. Padretti's Occupational Therapy, 7/e p640]
- *Apraxia*: Deficit in execution of learned movement which cannot be accounted for by either weakness, incoordination or sensory loss, or by incomprehension of or inattention to commands

11. Ans. (a) Projective
[Ref. The Freud's Encyclopedia: Theory, Therapy and Culture by Erwin, 1/e p428]

Projective Tests
- Most popular test: Rorschach inkblot test
- Other tests: Thematic Apperception test, Holtzman Inkblot test, Children's Apperception test, Blacky pictures, House-Tree-Person test, Lowenfield Mosaic test

12. Ans. (a) Bender Gestalt test
[Ref. Advanced Psychodiagnostic Interpretation of the BGT by Raphael, 1/e p2]

13. Ans. (b) Hysteria
[Ref. Niraj Ahuja, 7/e p103]

14. Ans. (b) Maladaptive assumptions; (d) Emotional consciousness of automatic thoughts
[Ref. Niraj Ahuja, 7/e p216]

Cognitive Behaviour Therapy
- *Cognitive techniques*: Recognizing and correcting negative autonomic thoughts, Teaching reattribution techniques, Increasing objectivity in perspectives, Identifying and testing maladaptive patterns, Decentering
- *Behavioural techniques*: Activity scheduling, Homework assignments, Graded task assignments, Behavioural rehearsal, Role playing, Diversion techniques
- Teaching problem-solving skills
- Mindfulness

15. Ans. (d) Conditioned learning
[Ref. Introduction to Psychology by Mitterer, 1/e p236]

16. Ans. (b) Depression
[Ref. Health and Performance by Smith & Jones, Volume II, Pg 234]

17. Ans. (c) Pain intensity
[Ref. Physical Therapies in Sports and Exercise by Kolt, 1/e p139]

18. Ans. (c) Repression
[Ref. Niraj Ahuja, 7/e p207]
- *COMMON EGO DEFENCE MECHANISMS*
- *Primary defence mechanisms*: Repression
- *Psychotic/Narcissistic defence mechanisms*: Regression, Denial, Projection, Distortion
- *Neurotic/Immature defence mechanisms*: Undoing, Conversion, Dissociation, Displacement, Hypochondriasis, Inhibition, Compensation, Splitting Rationalization, Intellectualization, Acting out, Isolation, Reaction formation, Schizoid fantasy, Retroflexion (Turning against self), Introjection,
- *Mature mechanisms*: Sublimation, Anticipation, Humor, Suppression (Voluntary), Altruism

19. Ans. (d) Obsession
[Ref. Niraj Ahuja, 7/e p207-210]

20. Ans. (b) Regression
[Ref. Niraj Ahuja, 7/e p207]

21. Ans. (c) Alcohol
[Ref. Principles of Clinical Toxicology by Gossel, 3/e p80]

22. Ans. (a) Alcohol
[Ref. Identification and Treatment of Alcohol Dependence by Martin, 1/e p134]

Morbid Jealousy
Syn. Pathological jealousy, Othello syndrome, Delusional jealousy, Jealous husband syndrome
- A psychological disorder in which a person is preoccupied with the thought that their spouse or sexual partner is being unfaithful without having any real proof, along with socially unacceptable or abnormal behaviour related to these thoughts
- MC forms of psychopathology: Delusions and obsessions
- Symptomatology may include accusing partner of looking or giving attention to other people, questioning of the partner's behavior, interrogation of phone calls, not allow-

ing any social media accounts, going through the partner's belongings, controlling the partner's social circle, claiming the partner is having an affair when they withdraw or tries to escape abuse, verbal and/or physical violence towards the partner, the individual who is considered to be the rival, or both, threatening to harm others or themselves, strong association with stalking/ cyber-stalking/ sabotage/ violence
- Associations: Schizophrenia, Delusional disorder (Bipolar disorder), Alcoholism, Sexual dysfunction, After neurological illness

23. Ans. (c) Schizophrenia
[Ref. Niraj Ahuja, 7/e p60-61]

24. Ans. (d) Chronic fatigue syndrome
[Ref. Evidence Based Color Atlas of OBG: Diagnosis & Management by Saxena, 1/e p373]

Differential Diagnosis of Premenstrual Tension
- *Psychiatric disorders*:
  - Anxiety & mood disorders (Depression, Anxiety, Dysthymia, Panic attacks)
  - Personality disorder
  - Anorexia, Bulimia
- *Chronic medical disorders*: Diabetes, Hypothyroidism, Anemia
- *Gynecological conditions*: Dysmenorrhoea, Perimenopause, OCPs, Substance abuse

25. Ans. (d) REM sleep
[Ref. Niraj Ahuja, 7/e p132]

26. Ans. (b) Sleep walking
[Ref. Encyclopedia of Sleep by Kushida, 1/e p203]

27. Ans. (d) Night terrors
[Ref. Niraj Ahuja, 7/e p140]

28. Ans. (a) Sleep sudden; (c) Cataplexy; (d) Presents in IInd decade
[Ref. Niraj Ahuja, 7/e p138]

29. Ans. (a) Gender identity disorder
[Ref. Niraj Ahuja, 7/e p121]
- *Gender identity disorder*: Disturbance in gender identity, i.e. the sense of one's masculinity or feminity is disturbed

30. Ans. (d) EEG shows decreased activity
[Ref. Niraj Ahuja, 7/e p133-134]

31. Ans. (a) Schizophrenia
[Ref. Niraj Ahuja, 7/e p55]

32. Ans. (b) Persistent delusion disorder
[Ref. Niraj Ahuja, 7/e p83]

33. Ans. (b) Constructional praxis
[Ref. Neuropsychology by Sbordone, 3/e p219]

Halstead Reitan Battery
- Importance: Most widely used neuropsychological test battery
- Components:
  - Halstead category test
  - Tactual performance test
  - Sea shore rhythm test
  - Speech sounds perception test
  - Finger oscillation (tapping) test
  - Trail making test
  - Grip strength test
  - Sensory perceptual examination
  - Tactual perceptual examination
  - Modified Aphasia screening test
  - Wechsler Adult Intelligence scale
  - MMPI

34. Ans. (c) Personality
[Ref. Integrating Rorschach and MMPI-2 in Personality Assessment by Genellen, 1/e p2]
- *Widely used Personality tests*:
  - Rorschach test
  - MMPI

35. Ans. (b) Acute Psychosis
[Ref. Niraj Ahuja, 7/e p83, 89]

36. Ans. (c) Delusional Disorder
[Ref. Niraj Ahuja, 7/e p83]

37. Ans. (d) Lethargy in depression
[Ref. Non-motor Symptoms of Parkinson's Disease by Chaudhuri, Pg 250]
- ***FDA Approved uses of Modafinil*:**
  - Narcolepsy
  - Persistent EDS despite treated Obstructive apnea/ hypopnea syndrome
  - Shift work sleep disorder

38. Ans. (c) Anticipation
[Ref. Niraj Ahuja, 7/e p207]

39. Ans. (a) Altruism
[Ref. Niraj Ahuja, 7/e p207]

40. Ans. (c) Obsessive compulsive neurosis
[Ref. Niraj Ahuja, 7/e p208]

Undoing
- Description: Unconscious motivated acts which magically/ symbolically counteract unacceptable thoughts, impulses or acts
- Useful in: Compulsive acts on OCD, Compulsive rituals

41. Ans. (d) Transference
[Ref. Niraj Ahuja, 7/e p207-209]

42. Ans. (a) Benzodiazepine
[Ref. Sleep Medicine Pearls: Expert Consult Online by Wagner, 3rd Ed., Pg 610]
- GABA-A receptor binding:
  - GABA
  - Agonists (Muscimol, Gaboxadol)
  - Antagonists (Bicuculline)
  - Benzodiazepine

43. Ans. (a) Derailment
[Ref. Niraj Ahuja, 7/e p207-209]

44. Ans. (b) Passive aggression

[Ref. Coping with Aggression by Emanuele, 1/e p11]

Aggression

- *Reactive/ impulsive aggression*: Automatic response to an immediate threat marked by strong emotions usually anger
- *Proactive aggression*: Emotionless and cold-blooded
- *Passive aggression*: Passive and Oppositional
- *Inward aggression*: Self destructive behavior, may even lead to suicide

45. Ans. (c) Rationalization

[Ref. Niraj Ahuja, 7/e p209]

- ***Rationalization***: Providing logical explanations for irrational behavior motivated by unacceptable unconscious wishes

46. Ans. (a) Repression

[Ref. The Adapted Mind by Barkow, 1/e p605]

- *Repression decreases anxiety*: By decreasing awareness of painful facts and wishes

47. Ans. (b) Schizophrenia

[Ref. Psychoneuroendocrine Dysfunction by Shah & Donald, 1/e p504]

48. Ans. (c) Occurs in NREM sleep

[Ref. Niraj Ahuja, 7/e p128]

49. Ans. (a) Cataplexy; (b) Sleep paralysis; (c) Hypnagogic hallucinations; (d) Excessive day time sleepiness

[Ref. Niraj Ahuja, 7/e p138]

50. Ans. (b) Resting tremor; (c) Rigidity; (d) Bradykinesia

[Ref. Principles and Practice of Geriatric Psychiatry by Agronin & Maletta, 1/e p619]

Features of Parkinson's Disease

Cardinal features	Secondary features	
• Resting tremor • Bradykinesia • Rigidity • Postural instability	• Dystonia • Dysphagia • Dysarthria • Hypomimia • Micrographia • Festination, Freezing, Retropulsion	• Stooping posture, Kyphosis, Scoliosis • Erectile dysfunction • Seborrheic dermatitis • Drooling • Constipation • Over-active bladder

51. Ans. (b) F

[Ref. Niraj Ahuja, 7/e p2]

52. Ans. (a) Anxiety

[Ref. 21st Century Global Mental health by Sorel, Pg 231]

53. Ans. (c) OCD

[Ref. Kaplan & Sadock's Synopsis of Psychiatry, 10/e p1235]

- OCD co-exist in 1/3–2/3 of children/ adolescents with Tourette syndrome
- OCD co-exist in 1/3 of adults with Tourette syndrome

54. Ans. (b) Self exemption

[Ref. McKenna et al., 2001, Peretti-Watel, Halfen, & Gremy, 2007]

- **Self-Exempting Beliefs:** Smokers are prone to deny their risk of developing smoking-related diseases (McKenna et al., 2001; Weinstein et al., 1998) or rationalize the health consequences of smoking behavior in order to reduce cognitive dissonance (Peretti-Watel, Halfen, & Gremy, 2007)
- An inverse relationship is expected between the self-exempting beliefs and the intention to quit smoking

55. Ans. (a) Promethazine

[Ref. Niraj Ahuja, 7/e p178]

- Rigidity, tremors, irrelevant talks point towards Haloperidol induced Parkinsonism
- Treatment of Haloperidol induced Parkinsonism: Anticholinergics: Promethazine, Procyclidine, Trihexyphenydyl, Orphenadrine, Biperiden

56. Ans. (a) Tremor; (c) Rigidity; (e) Depression

[Ref. Neuroscience by Ekman, p]

Features of Parkinsonism

- Tremor (Pill-rolling)
- Rigidity (Cog-wheel)
- Bradykinesia/Hypokinesia
- Postural instability

57. Ans. (a) REM sleep

[Ref. Biological Psychology by Freberg, 2/e p322]

EEG in Stages of Sleep

- REM stage
- NREM Stage 1: Theta rhythms appaear
- NREM Stage 2: Sleep spindles appear, K-complexes appear
- NREM Stage 3: Delta rhythms appear
- NREM Stage 4: Delta rhythms

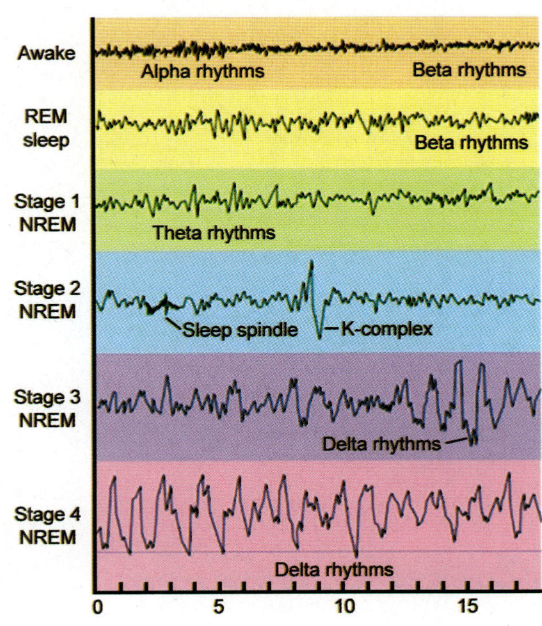

58. Ans. (d) Forced thinking
[Ref. Comprehensive textbook of Ppsychiatry by Kaplan, 1/e p220]

Forced Thinking

- Rare epileptic phenomenon observed in Frontal lobe/ Temporal lobe epilepsy patients
- Recurrent compulsive thought entering the mind to the exclusion of all other thoughts occur in lesions involving Posterior portion Frontal lobe
- Compulsion to think on few restricted topics
- Intrusion of thoughts against the patients will causes distress
- Not under the control of patient
- Disturbance of thought may be a seizure manifestation
- Motor automatism followed by brief seizure activity (< 1 minute) which subside by its own

59. Ans. (d) Correlation
[Ref. Niraj Ahuja, 7/e p212]

Theory of Dreams (Freud)

- Freud analysed dreams as "the royal road to the unconscious"; dreams are conscious expression of unconscious fantasies or impulses which are not accessible to the individual in wakefulness, thereby providing gratification by wish fulfilment.
- Dream work (preservation of sleep along with gratification) comprises of
  - Symbolism
  - Displacement
  - Condensation
  - Projection
  - Secondary elaboration

AIIMS PG 2018 MCQs

1. **A 35 years old woman presents to Psychiatry OPD with emotional coldness. She feels indifferent to praise/criticism, indifference to social relationships and a limited range of emotional expression. She is a case of** *[AIIMS May 2018]*
   a. Obsessive personality b. Schizoid personality
   c. Hysterical personality d. Avoidant personality
2. **A 38 years old woman presents with increased appetite, weight gain, excessive sleep, and weakness. She reports moods that are strongly reactive to environmental circumstances, and feeling extremely sensitive to rejection. Most probable diagnosis is** *[AIIMS May 2018]*
   a. Endogenous depression
   b. Atypical depression
   c. Masked depression
   d. Involutional melancholia
3. **Pathological Doubt is seen in** *[AIIMS May 2018]*
   a. Kleptomania b. Agoraphobia
   c. Suicidal tendencies d. OCD

EXPLANATORY ANSWERS

1. **Ans. (b) Schizoid personality**
   [Ref. Niraj Ahuja, 7/e p114]
   - Schizoid personality disorder is characterised by Emotional coldness, Lack of pleasure from activities, Inability to express feelings, Indifference to praise/criticism, Little interest in sexual experiences, Likes solitary activities, Fantasy loving, Lack of close friends, Insensitivity to social norms
2. **Ans. (b) Atypical depression**
   [Ref. Depressive Disorders by Maj, 2/e p138]
   - Atypical Depression is characterized by increased appetite, weight gain, hypersomnia (excessive sleepiness), lethargy (weakness) and mood reactivity

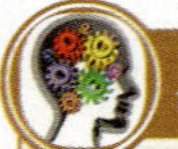

Also Remember

- Endogenous depression is characterized by biological features (Loss of appetite/weight), psychotic features

Contd...

Contd...

- Involutional melancholia is characterized by severe depression, psychotic features (Delusions, Hallucinations), nihilistic ideas and hypochondriacal delusions
- Somatized/Masked Depression is characterized by chronic pain, anorexia, weakness, insomnia, and depression is not evident

3. **Ans. (d) OCD**
   [Ref. Psychiatry by Rosenquist, 1/e p81]

   Pathological Doubts
   - Seen in OCD
   - Obsession of doubt followed by compulsion of checking to avoid guilt/fear
   - It is an irregular worry about having failed to engage in a specific action
   - Pathological doubt can lead to marked avoidance behavior

Note

Orthopedics

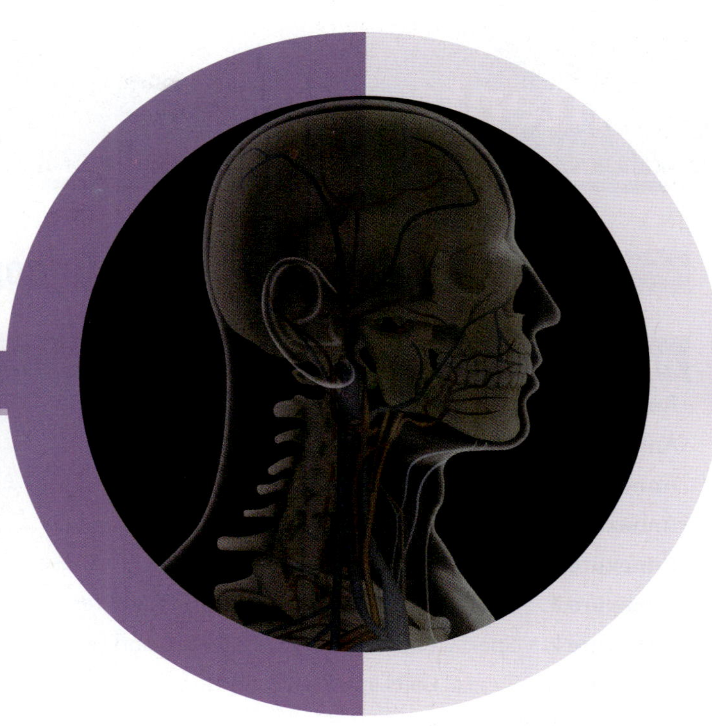

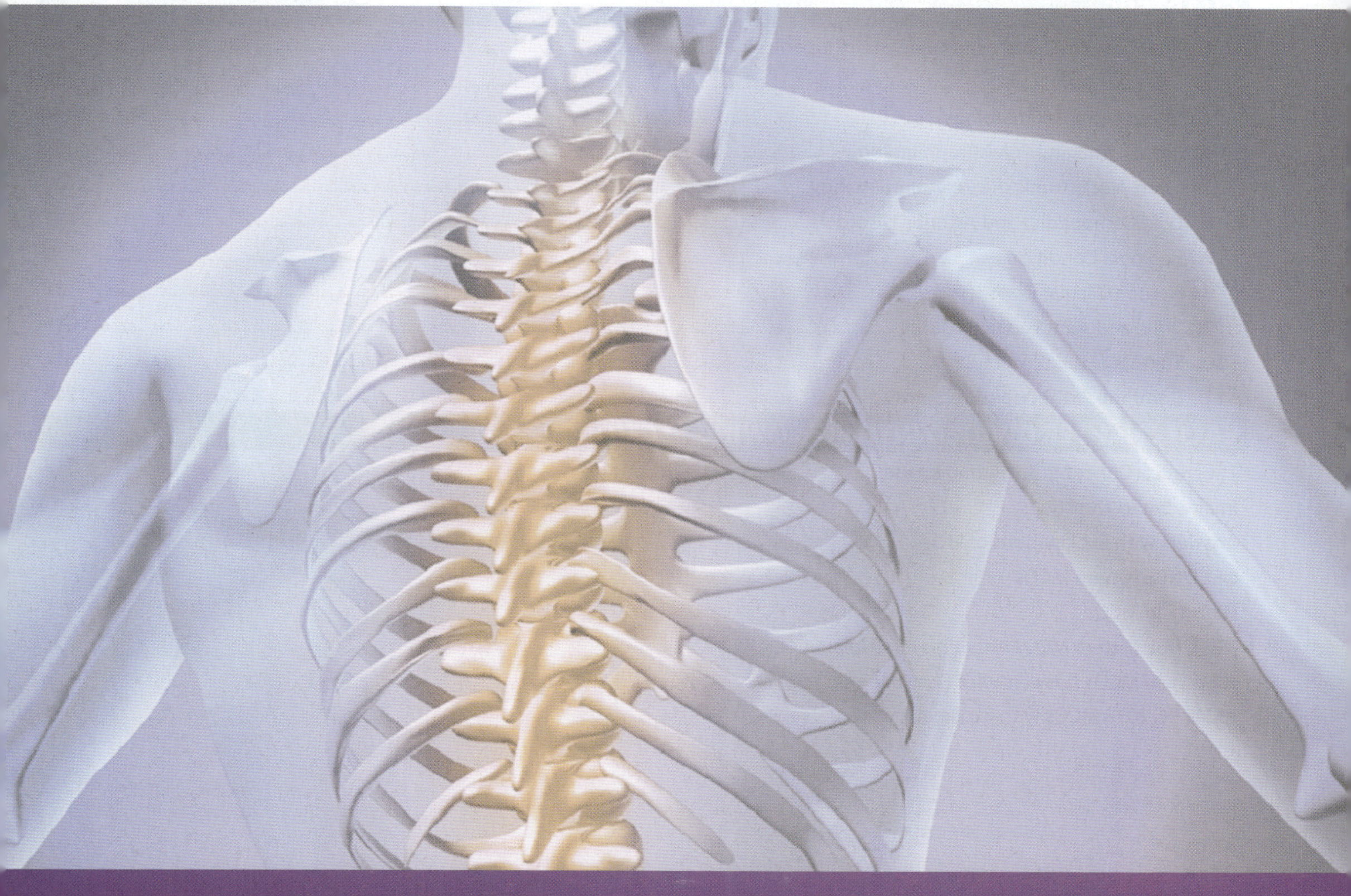

Contents

Orthopedics

ANNEXURES

CHAPTERS

EACH CHAPTER DIVIDED INTO FOLLOWING SECTIONS

Theoretical Concepts (Including Images)

Image-based Questions

Answers with Explanations of IBQs

NEET/NBE Pattern MCQs

High Yield MCQs

NEET/NBE Pattern MCQs Answers with Explanations

High Yield MCQs Answers with Explanations

AIIMS PG 2018 MCQs with Explanatory Answers

Annexures

ANNEXURE 1. IMPORTANT FRACTURES IN ORTHOPEDIC CLINICS

Fracture	Description
Aviators' Fracture	Fracture of neck of talus
Bankart's Fracture	Anterior glenoid fracture with
Barton's Fracture	Intra-articular fracture of distal radius
Bennett's Fracture	Intra-articular fracture of base of first metacarpal
Boxer's Fracture	Fracture of neck of fifth metacarpal
Bumper Fracture	Comminuted fracture of lateral condyle of the tibia
Chance Fracture	Horizontal fracture of vertebral body
Chauffeur's Fracture	Radial styloid fracture
Chopart's Fracture	Foot dislocation through talonavicular and calcaneocuboid joints with fractures
Clay Shovellers' Fracture	Spinous process fracture of C6, C7 or T1
Colle's Fracture	Distal radius, extra-articular fracture with dorsal tilt of distal fragment
Cotton's Fracture	Trimalleolar ankle fracture
Duverney's Fracture	Isolated fracture of Iliac wing
Galleazzi Fracture	Fracture of distal half of radius with dislocation of distal radioulnar joint
Hangman's Fracture	Fracture pedicle—lamina of C-2 vertebra
Hume Fracture	Olecranon fracture with anterior dislocation of radial head
Jones' Fracture	Fracture of the base of the 5th metatarsal
Le Fort Fracture	Serial of facial fractures
LisFranc Fracture	Fracture dislocation of mid-foot
Malgaigne's Fracture	Pelvic ring disruption with both pubic rami and sacroiliac injury on same side
Mallet Fracture	Avulsion of attachment of external tendon from the base of distal phalanx
March Fracture	Stress fracture of shaft of 2nd metatarsal
Monteggia Fracture	Fracture of proximal half of ulna with dislocation of the head of radius
Night stick Fracture	Isolated fracture shaft of the ulna
Potts' Fracture	Bimalleolar ankle fracture
Rolando Fracture	Fracture of base of first metacarpal, intra-articular
Salter Harris Fracture	Fracture involving a growth plate
Shepherds' Fracture	Fracture lateral tubercle of posterior process of talus
Smiths' Fracture	Distal radius fracture, intra-articular with volar tilt of the distal fragment
Tillaux Fracture	Salter Harris III fracture of tibia
Toddlers' Fracture	Undisplaced spiral fracture of tibia among children <8 years age

ANNEXURE 2. KEY TESTS IN ORTHOPEDICS

Test	Use in Orthopaedics
Adson's test	For thoracic outlet syndrome
Allen's test	for testing patency of radial and ulnar arteries
Allis test	For CDH
Anvil test	For testing tenderness of the spine
Anterior drawer test	For ACL injury
Ape thumb	For median nerve injury
Apley's grinding test	For meniscus injury
Apprehension test	For recurrent dislocation of the shoulder
Barlow's test	For CDH
Bryant's test	For anterior dislocation of the shoulder
Callaway's test	For anterior dislocation of the shoulder
Coin test	For dorsolumbar tuberculosis of spine
Clarkes' test	For patellofemoral pain syndrome
Cozen's test	For tennis elbow
Durkan's test	Carpal tunnel syndrome
Finkelstein's test	For de Quervain's tenovaginitis
Gaenslen's test	For inflammation of lumbar vertebrae/sacroiliac joint
Hamilton ruler test	For anterior dislocation of the shoulder
Hawkin-Kennedy test	For Supraspinatous tendon injury
Jobe's test	For anterior shoulder instability
Lasegue's test	For disc prolapse
Lachmann test	For ACL injury
McMurray's test	For meniscus injury
Naffziger test	for disc prolapse
Ober's test	For tight ilio-tibial band (e.g.in polio)
Ortolani's test	For CDH
Patrick's (FABERE) test	For pathology of hip or sacroiliac joint
Pivot shift test	For ACL injury
Posterior drawer test	For PCL injury
Schober's test	For flexion of lower back
Simmonds' test	Rupture of Achilles tendon
Thomas test	For hip flexion deformity
Trendelenburg's test	For unstable hip due to any reason
Watson test	For instability between scaphoid and lunate carpals
Wilsons' test	For osteochndritis dissecans in knee
Yergason's test	For Biceps or glenoid labrum pathology

ANNEXURE 3. KEY SIGNS IN ORTHOPEDICS

Sign	Use in Orthopaedics
Baastrups' sign	Osteophytosis of posterior lumbar spinous process
Blue sclera sign	Osteogenesis imperfecta
Chovstek's sign	For tetany
Claw hand	For ulnar nerve injury
Destot sign	For pelvic fracture
Foot drop	For common peroneal nerve injury
Froment's sign	For ulnar nerve injury
Gaenslen's test	For SI joint involvement
Galleazzi sign	For CDH
Gower's sign	For muscular dystrophy
Kanavel's sign	For infection in ulnar bursa
Kapandji score	For assessment of opposition of thumb
Larry's sign	Scaroilitis
Ludloff's sign	For avulsion of lesser trochanter
Mulder's sign	Morton's neuroma
O'Donoghue triad	Triad of MCL, ACL and medial meniscus injuries occurring together
Phalen's maneuver	Carpal tunnel syndrome
Policeman tip	For Erb's palsy
Runner's knee	For patellar tendinitis
Sulcus sign	For inferior dislocation of the shoulder
Terry Thomas sign	For scapholunate advanced colapse
Tinel's sign	For detecting improving nerve injury
Volkmann's sign	For ischaemic contracture of forearm muscles
Waddell's sign	Chronic back pain
Wrist drop sign	For radial nerve injury

ANNEXURE 4. CLASSIFICATIONS USED IN ORTHOPEDICS

Classification	Use in Orthopedics
Allman classification	For clavicle fractures
Bado classification	For monteggia fractures
Delbert's classification	For proximal femoral fractures
Dennis classification	For sacral fractures
Fraser's classification	For floating knee
Frykman classification	For fracture distal radius
Garden's Classification	For fracture neck of the femur
Gartland classification	For supracondylar fractures (children)
Gustilo Anderson's classification	For open fractures
Hawker's classification	For talar neck fractures
Kellgren-Lawrence Grading	For severity of osteoarthritis of knee
Lauge-Hansen classification	For ankle injuries
Letournel and Judet classification	For acetabular fractures
Mason classification	For fracture radial head
Modified Ellis classification	For tibiofibular shaft fractures
Neer's classification	For upper end of humerus/clavicle fractures
Pauwel's Classification	For fracture neck of the femur
Pipkin classification	For femoral head fractures
Russel Taylor classification	For subtrochanteric fractures
Salter and Harris classification	For epiphyseal injuries
Schatzker classification	For olecranon/proximal tibial fractures
Tile classification	For pelvic ring fractures
Tscherne classification	For closed fractures
Winquist and Hansen classification	For femoral shaft fractures
Young-Burgess classification	For pelvic ring fractures

ANNEXURE 5. NAILS, WIRES, PINS, PLATES, SPLINTS AND PROSTHESES

Nail/ Wire/ Pin/ Plate/ Prosthesis	Use in Orthopedics
Aeroplane splint	Brachial plexus injury
Austin-Moore prosthesis	Fracture neck of the femur
Baksi's prosthesis	Elbow replacement
Bohler Braun splint	Fracture femur
Buttress plate	Condylar fractures of the tibia
Charnley prosthesis	Total hip replacement
Cockup splint	Radial nerve palsy
Condylar blade plate	Condylar fractures of the femur
Dennis Brown splint	CTEV (Club foot)
Dynamic hip screw	Intertrochantric fracture
Ender's nail	Fixing intertrochanteric fracture
GK nail	Femoral or tibial shaft fracture
Gamma nail	Inter or subtrochanteric fracture
Harrington rod	Fixation of the spine
Hartshill rectangle	Fixation of the spine
Herbert screw	Scaphoid fracture
Insall Burstein prosthesis	Total knee replacement
Interlocking nail	Femoral or tibial shaft fracture
Kirschner wire	Small bone fixation
Knuckle bender splint	Ulnar nerve palsy
Kuntscher nail	Fracture shaft of the femur
Luque rod	Fixation of the spine
Milwaukee brace	Scoliosis
Moore's pins	Fracture neck of the femur
Neer's prosthesis	Shoulder replacement
Rush nail	Diaphyseal fractures of the long bones
SP nail with McLaughlin's plate	Intertrochanteric fracture
SP nail	Fracture neck of the femur
Seidel nail	Fracture of the shaft of the humerus
Soutter's prosthesis	Elbow replacement
Steffi plate	Fixation of the spine
Steinmann pin	Skeletal traction
Swanson prosthesis	Finger joint replacement
Talwalkar nails	Fracture of radius and ulna
Thomas splint	Fracture femur
Thompson prosthesis	Fracture neck of the femur
Von Rosen's splint	Congenital dislocation of hip

ANNEXURE 6. IMPORTANT ORTHOPEDIC SURGICAL PROCEDURES

Procedure	Surgical use in Orthopedics
Bankart's procedure	For recurrent dislocation of the shoulder
Bristow's procedure	For recurrent dislocation of the shoulder
Dilwyn Evans operation	For correction of CTEV
Dwyer's osteotomy	For varus of heel in CTEV
Girdlestone arthroplasty	For TB hip
Grice Green operation	For subtalar arthrodesis
Hauser's operation	For recurrent dislocation of patella
Jone's operation	For foot deformity in polio
Keller's operation	For hallux valgus correction
Lambrinudi operation	For correcting equinus deformity of the foot
Meyer's operation	For fracture neck of the femur
Putti-Plat procedure	For recurrent dislocation of the shoulder
Soutter's release	For flexion deformity of the hip in polio
Steindler's release	For cavus deformity of the foot
Tension- band wiring	For fracture patella, olecranon
Turco's procedure	For CTEV
Wilson's release	For flexion deformity of the knee
Yount's release	For flexion deformity of the knee in polio

ANNEXURE 7. SPECIAL RADIOLOGICAL VIEWS, ANGLES AND FEATURES

Special Radiological Views	
Judet view	For acetabular fracture
Mortise view	For ankle injuries
Oblique view of the wrist	For fracture scaphoid
Shenton's line	Hip X-ray in CDH
Sunset view	For patella femoral dysplasia
Von Rosen view	For CDH
Angles	
Bohler's angle	Fracture of the calcaneum
Cobbs' angle	Sagittal plane deformity in thoracolumbar fractures
Carrying angle	Elbow
Kite's angle	Talonavicular angle in CTEV
Neck-shaft angle	Of the femoral neck
Pauwel's angle	Fracture neck of the femur
Classic Features	
Aneurysmal sign	TB spine (anterior type)
Fabella	Sesamoid bone in the lateral head of Gastronemius
Cotton-wool appearance (Skull)	Paget's disease of bone
Driven snow appearance	Pindborg tumour
Hair-on-end (Crew-cut) appearance	Thalassemia
Onion-peel appearance	Ewing's sarcoma
Patchy calcification	Chondrosarcoma
Risser's sign	Epiphysis of iliac bone
Sagging rope sign	Perthe's disease
Salt and pepper appearance (Skull)	Hyperparathyroidism
Shepherd Crook deformity	Fibrous dysplasia
Soap-bubble appearance	Osteoclastoma
Spondylolisthesis	Slip of one vertebra over other
Spondylolysis	Break in posterior elements (at pars interarticularis)
Spondylosis	Degenerative spine disease
Sun-ray appearance	Osteosarcoma
Tonguing of vertebra	Morquio-Brails disease
Trethowan's sign	Slipped capital femoral epiphysis
Wormian bones	Osteogenesis imperfecta

ANNEXURE 8. TYPICAL GAITS AND DISLOCATIONS

Gait	Condition Responsible
Antalgic gait	Painful conditions of lower limb
Charlie Chaplin gait	Tibial torsion, alkaptonuria
Circumduction gait	Hemiplegia
Duck waddling gait	Bilateral CDH, pregnancy, osteomalacia, lumbar lordosis
Festinating gait	Parkinsonism
High stepping gait	Foot drop
Peg-leg gait	Congenital vertical talus
Reeling gait	Alcoholism, cerebellar lesions
Russian march gait	Foot drop (= High stepping gait)
Sailor's gait	Bilateral CDH
Scissoring gait	Cerebral palsy, CVA, Early lathyrism
Stiff hip gait	Ankylosis of the hip
Stamping gait	Tabes dorsalis, alcoholism, B_{12} deficiency, sensory ataxia
Stumbling gait	Bilateral CTEV
Trendelenburg gait	Unstable hip due to CDH, gluteus medius weakness, etc.
Dislocation	**Description**
Chopart's	Dislocation through talonavicular joints
Divergent	Elbow dislocation where ulna and radius dislocate in opposite directions
Lisfranc's	Dislocation through intertarsal joints
Lunate	Wrist injury where lunate bone comes out to lie in front of other carpal bones
Luxatio-erecta	Inferior dislocation of shoulder
Otto pelvis	Gradual shift of the acetabulam into the pelvis
Perilunate	Wrist injury with lunate in place and other carpals dislocate around it dorsally
Spondylolisthesis	Movement of one vertebra over another (MCy L4 over L5)
Sprain	A break in continuity of a ligament
Strain	A break in muscle fibres

Golden Points

Bones in children are break-resistant (only outer cortex breaks)	Greenstick fractures
Rate of axonal recovery/nerve regeneration	1 mm per day
Motor-march phenomenon is absent in	Neuropraxia
Tinel's percussion sign is used for	Nerve regeneration
Nerve grafting is done, if nerve gap is more than	10 cm
Common donor nerve used for nerve grafting	Sural nerve
MCC of deformity of bone	Fractures
Joint most amenable to manipulation	Knee joint
MC donor site for bone grafts	Iliac crest
MC joint in human body to dislocate	Shoulder joint
MC dislocation at shoulder joint	Anterior
MC dislocation at elbow joint	Posterior
Radius head pulled out of annular ligament	Pulled elbow
Best treatment of fracture of forearm bones	Conservative
Fracture head of radius is a type of	Valgus injury
Type of injury causing Monteggia fracture-dislocation	Hyperpronation injury
Most characteristic displacement of Colles' fracture	Dorsal tilt
MC cause of Sudeck's dystrophy in upper limb	Colles' fracture
Glass holding position of cast	Scaphoid cast
Positioning of wrist in Scaphoid cast is reverse of	Colles' cast
Intra-articular fracture at base of 1st metacarpal	Bennet's fracture dislocation
Extra-articular fracture at base of 1st metacarpal	Rolando's fracture
MC pelvic fracture	Ischiopubic rami fracture
Bilateral Ischiopubic rami fracture is known as	Straddle fracture
Unsolved fracture (higher complications)	Fracture neck of femur
Prosthesis used in hemiarthroplasty (fracture neck of femur)	Austin-Moore prosthesis
K-nail is used for fracture of	Shaft of femur
Gallow's traction is used for fracture of	Shaft of femur (infants)
Most frequently injured joint	Knee joint
Comminuted fracture of patella is known as	Stellate fracture
Post fracture neck of talus, Avascular necrosis occurs in	Body of talus
Jefferson's fracture is fracture of	Atlas
Clay Shoveller's fracture is fracture of	Spinous process of D1 vertebra
Cord-hemisection (ipsilateral paralysis, c/l loss of pain)	Brown-Sequard syndrome
MC site of acute osteomyelitis (Hematogenous)	Lower femoral metaphysis
MC complication of acute osteomyelitis	Chronic osteomyelitis
MC cause for chronic osteomyelitis	Delayed/insufficient treatment

Contd...

Contd...

Dense sclerotic bone overlying a sequestrum is	Involucrum
MC clinical presentation of chronic osteomyelitis	Chronic discharging sinus
MC cause of septic arthritis	Staphylococcus aureus
Tom Smith arthritis is	Septic arthritis of infancy (hip)
MC site of gonococcal arthritis	Knee joint
Most common site of bone and joint tuberculosis	Spine (Pott's disease)
Most common site of spinal TB	Dorsolumbar region
Investigation of choice for TB spine	MRI
MC cause of early onset Pott's paraplegia	Abscess
Besides spine, MC site of TB bones	Hip
MC cause of Hip-pain in children in India	TB hip
MC congenital foot deformity	CTEV
Most important muscle related to CTEV	Tibialis posterior
MC cause of cerebral palsy	Birth anoxia
MC type of spina bifida	Spina bifida occulta
Most common primary bone malignancy	Multiple myeloma
Second most common primary bone malignancy	Osteosarcoma
Most common benign tumour of bone	Osteochondroma
Most common 'TRUE' benign tumour of bone	Osteoid osteoma
Most common malignant bone tumour	Secondaries to bone
Most common primary bone malignancy	Multiple myeloma
Second most common primary bone malignancy	Osteosarcoma
Most common benign tumour of bone	Osteochondroma
Most common 'TRUE' benign tumour of bone	Osteoid osteoma
Most common bone tumour in hand	Enchondroma
MC site of vertebral disc proplapse	L4-L5
MC joint affected in rheumatoid arthritis	MP joint (Index finger)
MC joint affected in gout	MP joint (Great toe)
Marie-Strumpell disease is	Ankylosing spondylitis
Squaring of patella is seen in	Hemophilic arthritis
MC site of cervical spondylosis	C5-C6
Dupuytren's contracture is contracture of	Palmar aponeurosis
Medial epicondylitis is	Golfer's elbow
Lateral epicondylitis	Tennis elbow
Pain over radial styloid process is	DeQuervain's tenovaginitis
Constriction of fibrous digital sheath leads to	Trigger finger
Frozen shoulder is common among	Diabetics
Entrapment of lateral cutaneous nerve of thigh in fascia	Meralgia paresthetica
MC metabolic bone disease	Osteoporosis
MC site of fracture in osteoporosis	Dorsolumbar spine
% bone-mass loss in Osteoporosis for seen on X-rays	30%
MC cause of Rickets in children in India	Nutritional deficiency

Contd...

Contd…

Brown's tumour (Expansile bone lesion of osteoclasts) is in	Hyperparathyroidism
In fluorosis of bones, there is excess deposition of	Calcium
Earliest sign of dental fluorosis	Mottling
Best sign to see Mottling of teeth due to fluorosis	Incisors (upper jaw)
Orthopaedic disorders in dwarf circus jokers	Achondroplasia
Diaphyseal achalasia (Multiple exostosis) is due to	Remodeling defect
Trumpet-shaped metaphysic is in	Diaphyseal achalasia
Dense brittle bones/ Marble bones are in	Osteopetrosis
Paget's disease defect (Osteitis deformans)	Osteoclasts
MC osteochondritis	Perthes disease
MC torticollis	Spasmodic
Infantile cortical hyperostosis is	Caffey's disease
Mulitple enchondromatosis is	Ollier's disease
MC cause of congenital torticollis is	Sternocleidomastoid tumor
% population with cervical rib	0.5%
Trethowan's sign is seen in slipping of	Capital femoral epiphysis
MC cause of loose bodies in joints	Osteoarthritis
Blount's disease is a type of	Genu varum
MC cause of hallux valgus	Rheumatoid arthritis

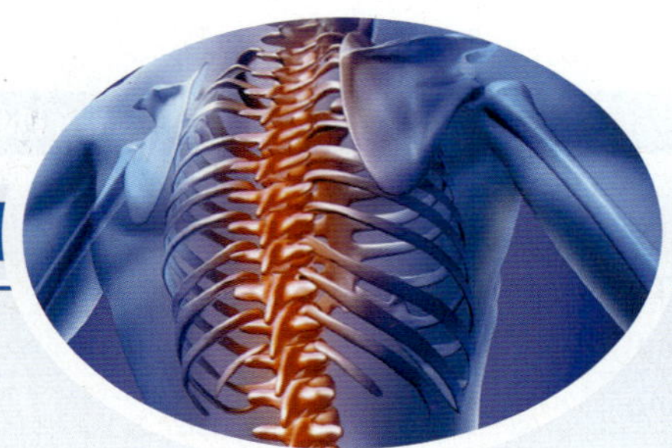

Chapter 1

Anatomy, Physiology and General Orthopedics

THEORETICAL CONCEPTS

I A. ANATOMY OF A TYPICAL LONG BONE

- ***Epiphysis***: Two ends of a long bone.
- ***Diaphysis***: Intermediate portion
- ***Metaphysis***: Part of shaft adjoining epiphysis
- *Epiphyseal plate*: Thin plate of growth cartilage at each end 'separating epiphysis from metaphysis'
- *Corticocancellous junction*: Junction between cortical bone (shaft) and cancellous bone (ends)
- ***Sharpe's fibres***: Strands of fibrous tissue connecting bone to periosteum[q]
- *Osteon*: Basic structural unit of a lamellar bone
  - *Haversion canals*: Central longitudinal canals of concentric lamellae
  - *Volkmann's canals*: Horizontal canals between endosteal and periosteal surfaces

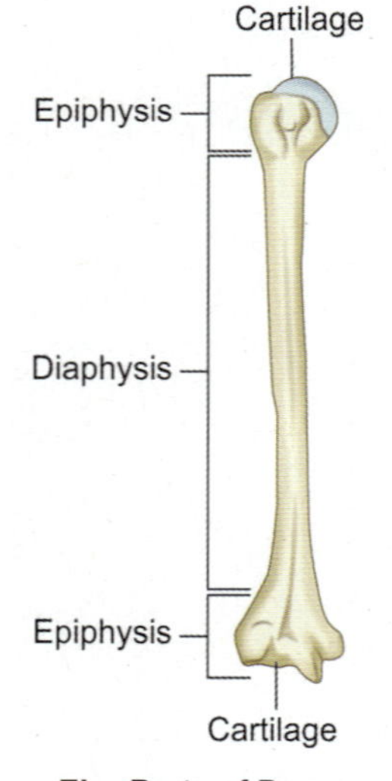

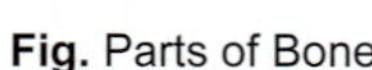

Fig. Parts of Bone

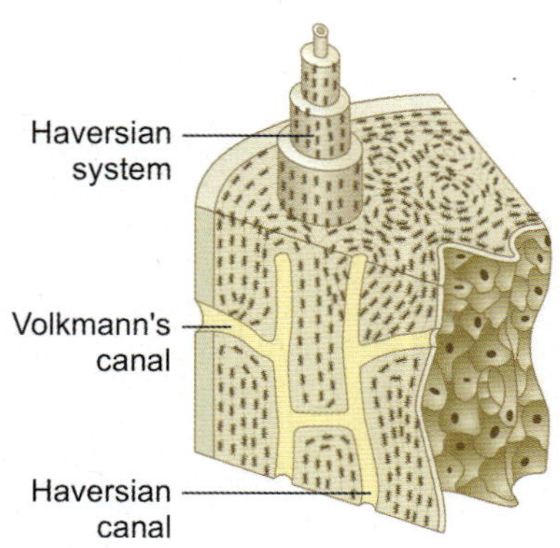

Fig. Osteon

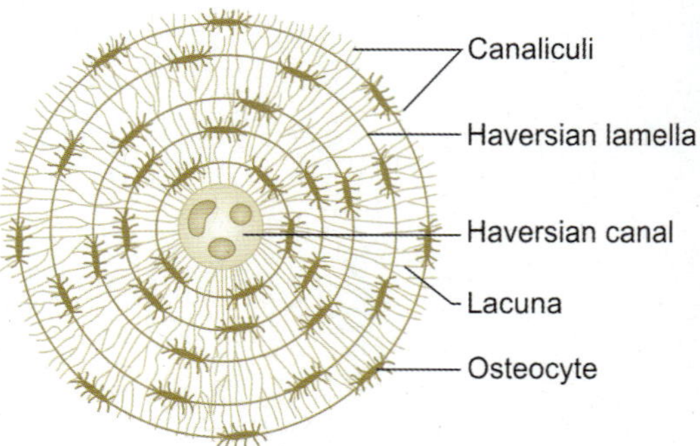

Fig. Haversion System

- *Structural composition*:

Matrix	Composition	% dry weight of bone
Organic matrix	Collagen	30–35%
Inorganic matrix	Calcium phosphorus hydroxyapatite	65–70%[Q]

- *Cellular composition*:

Cell type	Function	Composition
Osteoblasts	Ossification	ALP, glycolytic enzymes, phosphorylases
Osteocytes	Mature bone cells, varying activity	Glycogen, PAS positive granules
Osteoclasts	Mesenchymal cells for bone resorption	Collagenases, acid hydrolases

- *Ossification centres of bones*:
  - *Primary centre*: Middle of shaft; before birth
  - *Secondary centre*: Ends of bones; after birth

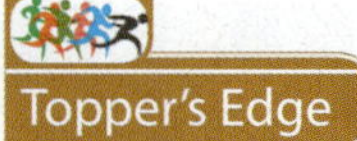

Topper's Edge

BONE ANATOMY AND PHYSIOLOGY

Adult Skeleton

- Bones in adult skeleton[Q]: **206** (80 bones Axial skeleton, 126 bones Appendicular skeleton)
- Bones in adult skeleton: **80% Cortical bones**, 20% Trabecular bones
- Bones in vertebrae: 25% Cortical bones, 75% Trabecular bones

Bone

- Bone formation is higher on periosteal surface, *whereas*, Bone resorption is higher on Endosteal surface of Cortical bones
- **Most metabolically active part of bone[Q]: Endosteum**
- Maximum remodeling in bone occurs at: Endosteal surface
- **Four types of bone cells**:
  - Osteoclasts: Bone forming mononuclear cells
  - Osteoblasts: Bone resorbing multinucleate giant cells
  - Osteocytes: Mature bone involved in maintenance of bone, most abundant cells
  - Osteogenic/Osteoprogenitor cells: Only bone cells that divide

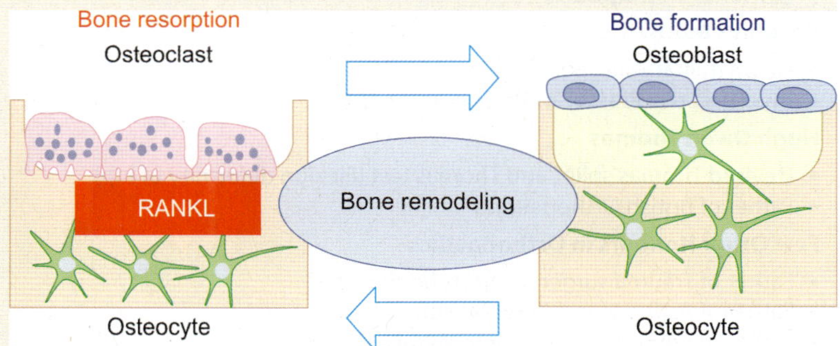

Fig. Bone Cells

Bone Markers

Markers of Bone Formation[Q]	Markers of Bone Resorption[Q]
• Osteocalcin • Bone-specific alkaline phosphatase (BALP) • Total alkaline phosphatase • Procollagen I C-terminal extension peptide • Procollagen I N-terminal extension peptide	**Serum Markers** • Tartrate resistant acid phosphatase (TRACP) • Tartrate resistant acid phosphatase 5b (TRACP 5b) • C-terminal crosslinking telopeptide of Type I collagen (CTX) • N-terminal crosslinking telopeptide of Type I collagen (NTX) • C-terminal crosslinking telopeptide of Type I collagen (ICTX) **Urine Markers** • Deoxypyridinaline (DPD) • Pyridinaline (PYD) • Hydroxyproline (Hyp) • C-terminal crosslinking telopeptide of Type I Collagen (CTX)

I B. STAGES OF FRACTURE HEALING OF CORTICAL BONES (FROST)

Stages	Time	Features
Hematoma formation	< 1 week	Fracture end necrosis + Sensitized precursor cells
Granulation tissue	2-3 weeks	Proliferation of daughter cells—osteoblasts, fibroblasts
Callus formation	**4-12 weeks**[Q]	Mineralisation of granulation tissue
Remodelling	1-2 years	Lamellar bone formation
Modelling	Many years	Modelling of endosteal and periosteal surfaces

- ***Factors promoting faster healing of fractures***[Q]**:**
  - Young age
  - Flat and cancellous bones
  - Spiral and oblique fractures
  - Absence of ischaemia
  - Good apposition
  - Good immobilisation (not for all fractures)
  - Compression

Topper's Edge

HISTORICAL ASPECTS OF ORTHOPEDICS

Nicholas Andry

- **Father of Modern Orthopedic Surgery**[Q]
- **Coined the word 'Orthopaedics'**[Q] [Greek words for "correct/ straight" (*Orthos*) and "child" (*Paidion*)
- Book written: *Orthopaedia* (The Art of Correcting and Preventing Deformities in Children) (1741)

Jean-Andre Venel

- Established the First Orthopedic Institute, Switzerland (1780)
- **Father of Orthopedics**[Q]

Antonius Mathysen

- Dutch military surgeon
- **Invented the Plaster of Paris cast**[Q] **(1851)**

Hugh Owen Thomas

- Devised Thomas splint and Thomas test (Flexion deformity of hip)
- Father of British Orthopaedics

Few Other Honours in Orthopaedics

- Father of Trauma surgery: Lorenz Bohler
- Father of Arthroscopy: Kenji Takagi
- Father of Modern Arthroscopy: Masake Watanabe
- Father of Internal fixation: Albin Lambotte
- Father of Total hip arthroplasty: Sir john Charnley
- Father of Orthopedic Oncology: William F Enneking
- **Father of Sports Medicine**[Q]**: Galen**

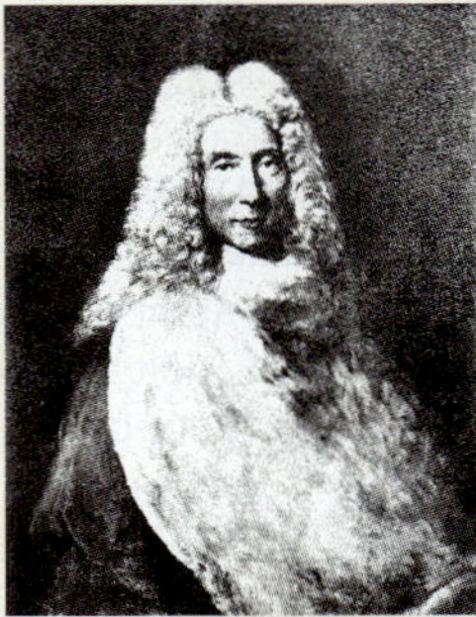

Nicholas Andry

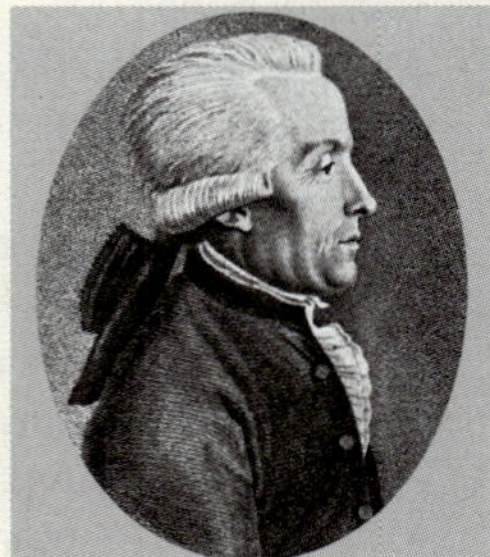

Jean-Andre Venel

IMAGE-BASED QUESTIONS

1. Identify the type of bony fracture shown in Photograph. ***[Recent Question 2012]***

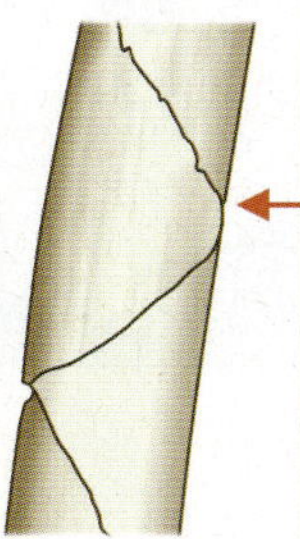

a. Transverse
b. Spiral
c. Oblique
d. Comminuted

2. Identify the deformity shown in the photograph. ***[AIIMS PG November 2016]***

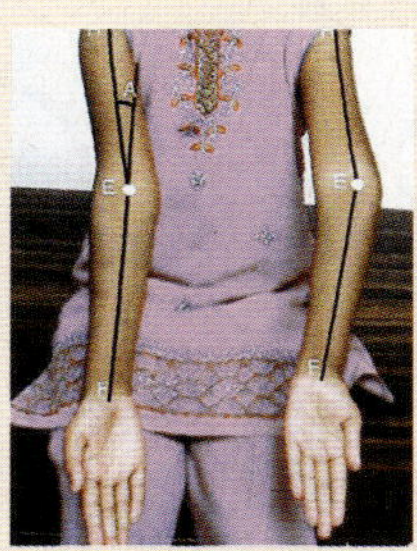

a. Cubitus varus left elbow
b. Cubitus varus right elbow
c. Cubitus valgus left elbow
d. Cubitus valgus right elbow

3. Identify the Orthopedic Prosthesis shown in Photograph.

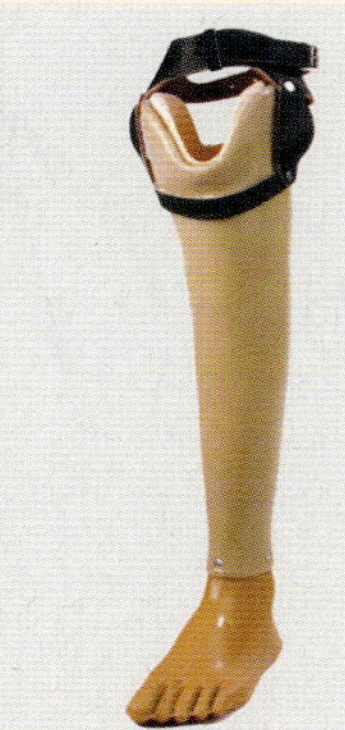

a. CTEV shoes
b. SACH foot
c. Jaipur foot
d. Syme's prosthesis

4. Angle shown in Photograph is used for assessment of .... fracture.

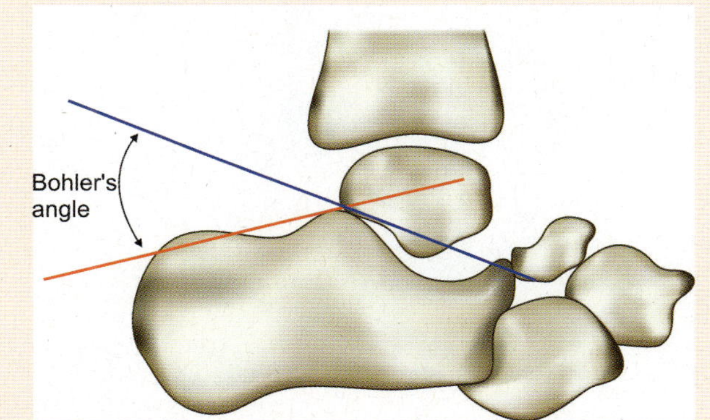

a. Talus
b. Calcaneus
c. Metatarsal
d. Phalangeal

5. Clinical test shown in Photograph is highly sensitive for

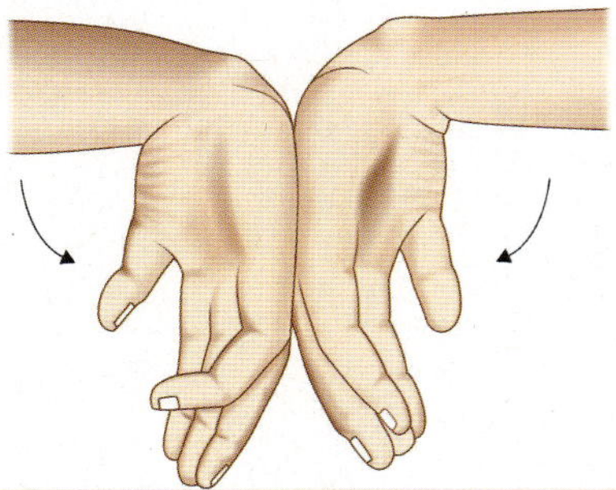

a. Dupuytren's contracture
b. Carpal tunnel syndrome
c. deQuervain's tenosynovitis
d. Student's elbow

6. Clinical test shown in Photograph is characteristic of

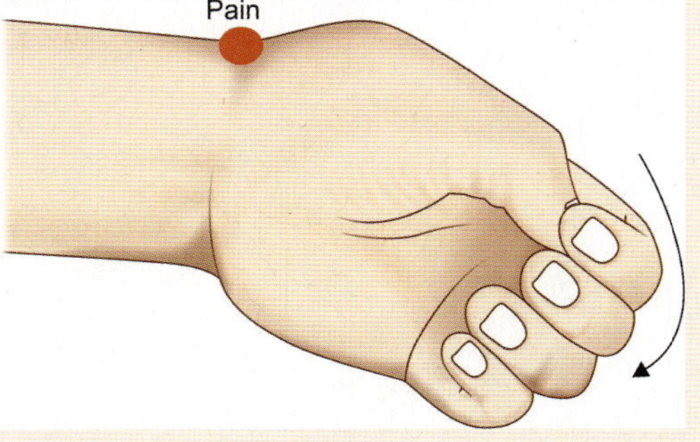

a. Carpal tunnel syndrome
b. Tennis elbow
c. Students' elbow
d. deQuervain's disease

7. Osteochondritis of the bony part (Box) shown in Photograph is known as

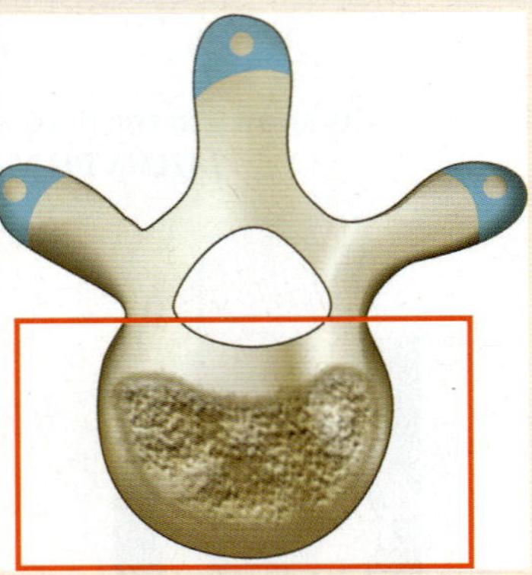

a. Scheuermann's disease
b. Osgood-Schlatter disease
c. Calvé's disease
d. Sever's disease

8. Identify the test being performed in the image below. ***[AIIMS PG November 2015]***

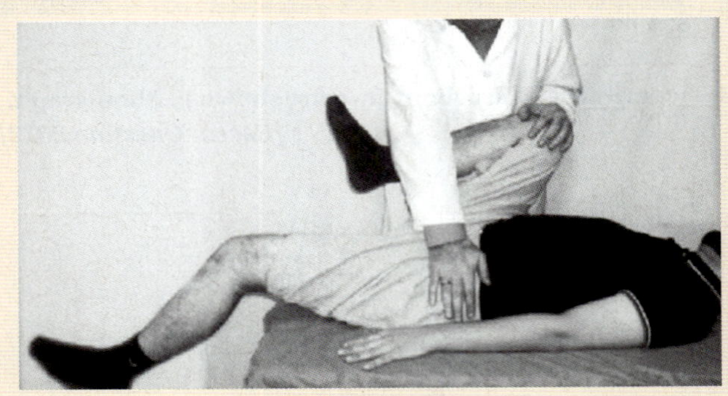

a. Trendelenburg
b. Thomas test
c. Smith
d. Narath

9. Which of the following positions is being tested as shown in the Photograph? ***[AIIMS May 2017]***

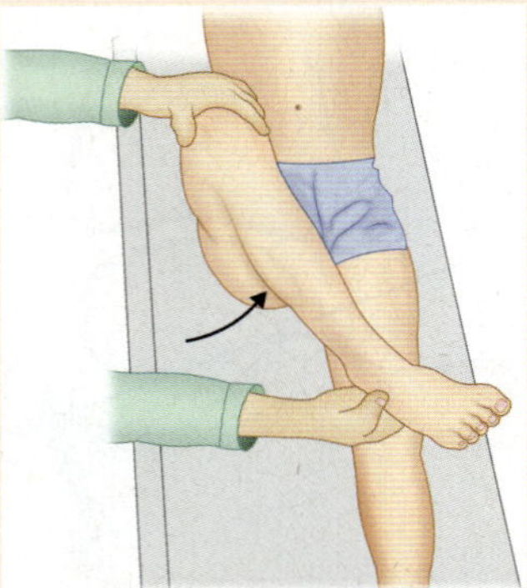

a. Internal rotation
b. External rotation
c. Flexion
d. Extension

10. Bone-holding forceps used in orthopaedic surgeries is ***[AIIMS May 2017]***

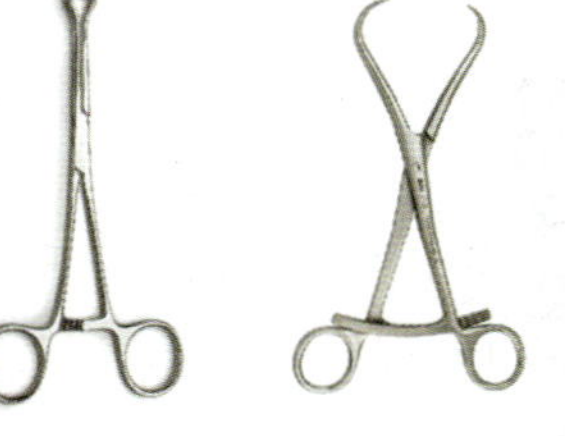

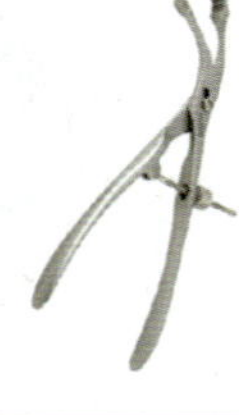

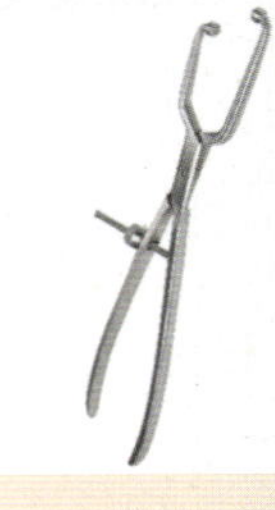

a. b. c. d.

ANSWERS WITH EXPLANATIONS OF IBQs

1. Ans. (b) Spiral *[Ref. Maheshwari, 4/e p275]*

- Transverse fracture: Fracture line is perpendicular to long axis of bone usually caused by bending force
- Spiral fracture: Fracture line runs spirally in more than one plane usually caused by a twisting force
- Oblique force: Fracture line is oblique usually caused by bending force with a component along long axis of bone
- Comminute fracture: Fracture with multiple fragments usually caused by compression/crushing force along long axis of bone

2. Ans. (a) Cubitus varus Left elbow *[Ref. Maheshwari, 4/e p275]*

- Varus deformity: Part of limb is deviated towards the midline of the body
- Cubitus varus of elbow: Common deformity in which the extended forearm is deviated towards midline of the body
- Clinical importance:
  - Cubitus varus is also known as Gunstock deformity
  - MC complication of supracondylar fracture of humerus (Occurs due to Malunion)

3. Ans. (c) Jaipur foot *[Ref. Artificial Parts, Practical Lives by Serlin, 1/e p327]*

- Jaipur Foot (Jaipur Leg): Rubber-based prosthetic leg for people with below-knee amputations
- Discovered by: PK Sethi and RC Sharma

4. Ans. (b) Calcaneus *[Ref. McGlamry's Foot and Ankle Surgery, 3/e p1824]*

Bohler Angle

- Description: Angle between two lines tangent to the calcaneus on the lateral radiograph, with lines drawn tangent to the anterior and posterior aspects of the superior calcaneus
- Normal value for Bohler angle: 20-40 degrees
- Calcaneus fracture: <20 degrees (though not necessary)

5. Ans. (b) Carpal tunnel syndrome *[Ref. Plastic and Reconstructive Surgery by Cugna, 1/e p649]*

Phalen's Test

- **Phalen's test:** Passive flexion of the patients wrists (Pushing dorsal surfaces of both wrists together) for 15-60s
- Positive test: When the patient experiences tingling or numbness in the median nerve distribution in cases of Carpal tunnel syndrome

6. Ans. (d) deQuervain's disease *[Ref. Clinical Signs by Cho, 1/e p20]*

Finkelstein's Test

- Finkelstein's test: Examining physician or therapist grasps the thumb and ulnar deviates the hand sharply
- Positive test: Sharp pain occurs along the distal radius (top of forearm) in cases of De Quervain's tenosynovitis

7. Ans. (a) Scheuermann's disease *[Ref. Maheshwari, 4/e p308]*

Common Osteochondritis

- Perthes disease: Epiphysis of head of femur
- Panner's disease: Capitulum
- Kienbock's disease: Lunate
- Osgood-Schlatter disease: Tibial tuberosity
- Kohler disease: Navicular
- Frieberg's disease: Metatarsal head (2nd > 3rd)
- Scheurmann's disease: Ring epiphysis of vertebrae
- Calve's disease: Central body nucleus of vertebral body

8. Ans. (b) Thomas test *[Ref. Practical Orthopedics by Ebnezar, 1/e p502]*

Thomas Test

- Used to rule out Hip flexion contracture and Psoas syndrome
- Associated with runners, dancers, and gymnasts
- Steps:
  - Step 1: Patient lies supine on the examination table, Clinician passes the palm of his hand beneath the patients spine to identify lumbar lordosis
  - Step 2: Normal hip is flexed till the thigh just touches the abdomen to obliterate the lumbar lordosis
  - Step 3: Measure the angle between the affected thigh and the table to reveal the fixed flexion deformity of the hip

9. Ans. (b) External rotation *[Ref. Systematic Musculoskeletal Examination by Frisch, 1/e p123]*

Testing for internal rotation

- Keeping one hand on the knee and holding the heel with the other hand, lift and guide the leg until both the hip and knee are at 90°
- Then rotate the lower leg outwards so that the thigh rotates inward (internally)

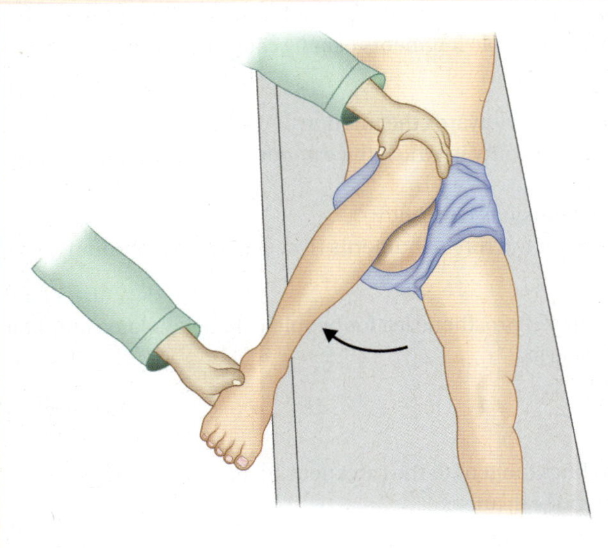

Fig. Testing for Internal Rotation

Testing for external rotation

- Bring the lower leg back to neutral and then rotate it inwards so that the thigh rotates outward (externally)

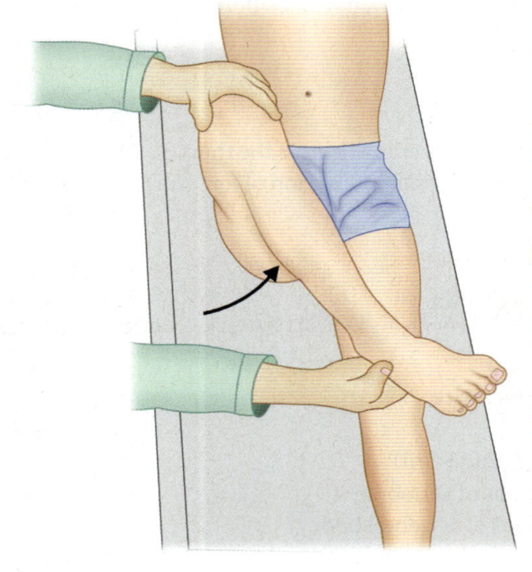

Fig. Testing for External Rotation

10. Ans. (c) *[Ref. Practical Orthopedics by Ebnezar, 1/e p339]*

Instruments given in the Photograph

- a - Babcock forceps
- b - Reduction forceps
- c - Bone-holding forceps
- d - Pelvic reduction forceps

 NEET/NBE PATTERN MCQs 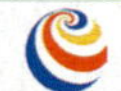

1. **Lift-off test is used for which of the following Muscles?** *[Recent Question 2016]*
   a. Supraspinatus b. Subscapularis
   c. Infraspinatus d. Biceps Brachii
2. **Osteoclasts have all of the following except** *[Recent Question 2016]*
   a. Bone resorption
   b. Receptor for parathormone
   c. Ruffled border
   d. Rank ligand
3. **Most vascular zone of the bone is** *[Recent Question 2016]*
   a. Metaphysis b. Diaphysis
   c. Epiphysis d. Medullary cavity
4. **Extensor carpi radialis longus is** *[Recent Question 2016]*
   a. Extensor and ulnar deviator of wrist
   b. Extensor and radial deviator of wrist
   c. Injured in posterior interosseus nerve injury
   d. Weak extensor of wrist
5. **Thomas test helps to detect** *[Recent Question 2016]*
   a. Adduction deformity of the hip
   b. Integrity of the Abductor mechanism
   c. Fixed flexion deformity of the hip
   d. Apparent shortening at the hip Joint
6. **PTH acts directly on which cells?** *[Recent Question 2016]*
   a. Osteoclasts
   b. Osteocytes
   c. Osteoblasts
   d. Macrophages
7. **Effect of Hypoparathyroidism on bones include** *[Recent Question 2016]*
   a. Brown tumours
   b. Subperiosteal Resorption of Bone
   c. Multiple Cysts in Bone
   d. None of the Above
8. **Bone transport can be used in the management of** *[Recent Question 2016]*
   a. Gap non-union
   b. Deformity Correction
   c. Comminuted shaft femur fracture
   d. Avascular Necrosis of Femoral Head
9. **What structure passes through the Quandrangular space?** *[Recent Question 2016]*
   a. Axillary nerve b. Radial nerve
   c. Median nerve d. Brachial artery
10. **Nutrient and oxygen reach the chondrocytes across perichondrium by** *[Recent Question 2016]*
    a. Capillaries b. Diffusion
    c. Along neurons d. Active transport
11. **Ossification centre of Scaphoid appears at** *[Recent Question 2016]*
    a. 1-6 months b. 1-2 years
    c. 2-4 years d. 4-6 years
12. **Test for DeQuervain's tenovaginitis** *[Recent Question 2016]*
    a. Cozen test b. Finkelstein test
    c. Kanavel's sign d. Phalen test
13. **Wolff's law states that** *[Recent Question 2016]*
    a. If a bone is continuously subjected to a particular stress it will adapt to become stronger to resist that loading
    b. Only diaphysis allows longitudinal growth in childhood
    c. Any infection not showing periosteal reaction within 1 week of symptoms can be ruled out to be osteomyelitis
    d. Angular deformities will progress till the closure of physis
14. **Tensile strength of a bone is due to** *[Recent Question 2016]*
    a. Strands of collagen b. Hydroxyapatite crystals
    c. Periosteum d. Metaphysis
15. **What is the normal orientation of Humeral head?** *[Recent Question 2016]*
    a. Retroversion of 80°
    b. Retroversion of 30°
    c. Anteversion of 15°
    d. Anteversion of 50°
16. **Shenton's line is** *[Recent Question 2016]*
    a. Line joining ASIS and ischial tuberosity
    b. Line joining ASIS and tip of GT
    c. Line joining two ASIS (left and right)
    d. Curve formed by neck of femur and obturator foramen
17. **Z score measures the bone mineral density compared to** *[Recent Question 2016]*
    a. Age, race and sex-matched individuals
    b. Race and sex-matched individuals
    c. Sex-matched individuals
    d. None of the above
18. **Talus bone is supplied by** *[Recent Question]*
    a. Anterior tibial artery b. Posterior tibial artery
    c. Dorsalis pedis artery d. All of the above
19. **Dawbarn sign is seen in** *[Recent Question]*
    a. Infraspinatus tendinitis b. Subacromial bursitis
    c. Achilles tendon injury d. None of the above
20. **Type of collagen found in bone is** *[Recent Question]*
    a. Type 1 b. Type 2
    c. Type 3 d. Type 4
21. **Periosteum is attached to bone by** *[NBE FMGE March 2008]*
    a. Cementum b. Fibroblasts
    c. Sharpe's fibres d. Interstitial lamellae
22. **Talus is supplied by** *[Recent Question 2012]*
    a. Anterior tibial artery b. Posterior tibial artery
    c. Dorsal pedis artery d. All
23. **Osteonecrosis is not seen in** *[Recent Question 2012]*
    a. Ollier's disease b. Kienbock's disease
    c. Kohler's disease d. Perthe's disease
24. **Osteonecrosis is seen in all except** *[Recent Question 2012, 2013]*
    a. Fracture neck femur b. Sickle cell anemia
    c. Perthe's disease d. Paget's disease
25. **Ulnar nerve supplies all except** *[Recent Question 2012]*
    a. FCU b. Interossei
    c. 3rd, 4th lumbricals d. Abductor pollicis brevis
26. **Muscle tested in Froment's sign (Book test) is** *[NBE DNB 1996, 2003, 2007, 2008]*
    a. Adductor pollicis b. Abductor pollicis
    c. Opponens pollicis brevis d. Flexor pollicis brevis

27. **Osteomalacia is due to** *[Recent Question 2012]*
 a. Vitamin C deficiency b. Vitamin D deficiency
 c. Vitamin E deficiency d. None
28. **A Meningomyelocele is most commonly situated in** *[UPSC 2012]*
 a. Cervical spine b. Thoracic spine
 c. Dorsolumbar spine d. Lumbosacral spine
29. **Kanavel's sign is found in** *[NBE DNB 2010]*
 a. Trigger finger b. Tenosynovitis
 c. Carpal tunnel syndrome d. None
30. **Watson-Jones operation is carried out for** *[NBE DNB 2010]*
 a. Club foot b. Valgus deformity
 c. Hip replacement d. Muscle paralysis
31. **Most common bone for which nailing is done** *[Recent Question 2012]*
 a. Radius b. Ulna
 c. Tibia d. Humerus
32. **Sequestrum is best defined as** *[Recent Question 2012]*
 a. A piece of dead bone
 b. A piece of dead bone surrounded by infected tissue
 c. A piece of bone with poor vascularity
 d. None
33. **An adventitious bursa is** *[NBE DNB 1994, 1999, 2004, 2008]*
 a. An infected cyst b. A congenital cyst
 c. Normal bursa type
 d. Abnormality over friction site
34. **Claw hand is seen in** *[NBE DNB 1999]*
 a. Radial nerve injury b. Ulnar nerve injury
 c. Median nerve compression
 d. Axillary nerve dissection
35. **Subperiosteal bone resorption is seen in** *[Recent Question 2012]*
 a. Hypothyroidism b. Hyperthyroidism
 c. Hypoparathyroidism d. Hyperparathyroidism
36. **Anterior drawer test is for** *[Recent Question 2012]*
 a. ACL b. PCL
 c. Medial meniscus d. Lateral meniscus
37. **MC site for Myositis ossificans in body is** *[NBE DNB 1994, 2000, 2003, 2006]*
 a. Shoulder b. Elbow
 c. Hip d. Knee
38. **Fairbank triangle is seen in** *[Recent Question 2012, 2017]*
 a. CDH b. Congenital coxa vara
 c. Perthe's disease d. SCFE
39. **Card test is utilized for** *[NBE DNB 2007]*
 a. Testing function of radial nerves
 b. Testing function of ulnar nerve
 c. Testing function of median nerve
 d. Testing function of axillary nerve
40. **MC muscle-group affected in Polio is** *[NBE DNB 2007]*
 a. Flexors–Hip b. Extensors–Hip
 c. Flexors–Ankle d. Dorsiflexors–Ankle
41. **Plaster of Paris is used for casts for immobilisation of fractures. It consists of** *[UPSC 2003]*
 a. Calcium carbonate b. Calcium sulphate
 c. Calcium oxide d. Calcium hydroxide
42. **Most common site of osteoporosis is** *[Recent Question 2012, 2013]*
 a. Humerus b. Vertebrae
 c. Scapula d. Flat bones
43. **Which of the following is a syndesmosis?** *[Recent Question 2012, 2013]*
 a. Superior tibiofibular joint
 b. Inferior tibiofibular joint
 c. Talocalcaneal joint
 d. Calcaneocuboid joint
44. **Fibrosis is MC in muscle** *[NBE DNB 2007]*
 a. Serratus anterior b. Trapezius
 c. Sternocleidomastoid d. Tendocalcaneous
45. **Hormone exerting maximal influence on bone growth is** *[NBE DNB 1996, 2004]*
 a. Testosterone b. Estrogen
 c. Growth hormone d. Thyroxin
46. **Enzymatic difference between osteoclasts and osteoblasts is** *[NBE DNB 1996]*
 a. Alkaline phosphatase b. Acid phosphatase
 c. Deoxyribonuclease d. None of the above
47. **Periosteal reactions is seen in** *[Recent Question 2012, 2013]*
 a. Osteomyelitis b. Syphilis
 c. Tumor d. All
48. **Who gave the concept of 'Normal bone re-modelling in response to stress'?** *[NBE DNB 2009]*
 a. Kuntscher b. Pauwels
 c. Wolff d. Wheelsberg
49. **Perthe's disease is** *[Recent Question 2012, AIIMS PG 1994]*
 a. Fracture of femoral shaft
 b. Osteochondritis of femoral epiphysis
 c. Infarction of femoral head
 d. Fracture dislocation of femoral neck
50. **MC cause of Kyphosis among males is** *[NBE DNB 1997]*
 a. Tuberculosis b. Trauma
 c. Secondary deposits d. Age related
51. **Trendelenberg test is positive in palsy of** *[Recent Question 2012]*
 a. Gluteus maximus b. Gluteus medius
 c. Rectus femoris d. Vastus medialis
52. **MC cause of pain in anterior knee is** *[NBE DNB 2009]*
 a. Pre-patellar bursitis
 b. Chondromalacia patellae
 c. PLICA syndrome
 d. Congenital discoid menisci
53. **MC type of Spondylolisthesis seen is** *[NBE DNB 2009]*
 a. Traumatic
 b. Degenerative
 c. Congenital dysplastic
 d. Isthmic spondylolytic
54. **Partial anterior dislocation of one segment of the spine over another is** *[Recent Question 2012]*
 a. Spondylosis b. Spondylolisthesis
 c. Kyphosis d. Scoliosis
55. **Von-Rosen splint is used for** *[NBE DNB 1997, 1998]*
 a. Congenital coax vera b. CTEV
 c. Congenital dislocation d. Calve-Perthes disease
56. **Muscles affected in deQuervain's tenosynovitis is/are** *[NBE DNB 2009, NIMS 2000, Recent Question 2018]*
 a. Extensor carpi radialis and Extensor pollicis longus
 b. Extensor pollicis brevis and Abductor pollicis longus
 c. Abductor pollicis longus and Abductor pollicis brevis
 d. Flexor pollicis longus and Flexor pollicis brevis

57. Cloacae are present in *[Recent Question 2012, 2013]*
a. Sequestrum b. Involucrum
c. Normal bone d. Myositis

58. Heterotopic ossification occurs in *[Recent Question 2012]*
a. Bone b. Joint
c. Soft tissue d. None

59. MC site of Venous ulcers in human body is *[Recent Question 2014]*
a. Pubis b. Buttocks
c. Medial malleolus d. Lateral malleolus

60. Loose bodies are most commonly seen in *[Recent Question 2014]*
a. Hip b. Knee
c. Ankle d. Elbow

61. Patella dislocation is prevented by .... muscle *[Recent Question 2014]*
a. Vastus medialis b. Vastus lateralis
c. Vastus intermedius d. None

62. Kite's angle is *[Recent Question 2014]*
a. Calcaneocuboid b. Calcaneonavicular
c. Talocalcaneal d. Talonavicular

63. Most common cause of Amputation in India is *[Recent Question 2014]*
a. Trauma b. Infection
c. Diabetes d. Tumours

64. Gottron's sign is seen in *[Recent Question 2015]*
a. Leprosy b. Dermatomyositis
c. SLE d. Psoriasis

65. Pseudofractures are seen in *[Recent Question 2015]*
a. Osteoarthritis b. Rickets
c. Osteomalacia d. Osteopetrosis

66. Congenital and recurrent abnormality is *[Recent Question 2015]*
a. Rickets
b. Femoral neck fracture
c. Carpal tunnel syndrome
d. Congenital dislocation of hip

67. Pipkin's classification is used for *[Recent Question, 2015]*
a. Acetabular fractures b. Pelvis ring fractures
c. Femoral head fractures d. Femoral shaft fractures

68. Proximal tibial epiphysis fuses at *[Recent Question 2017]*
a. 12–14 years b. 14–16 years
c. 16–18 years d. 18–20 years

69. Anterior gliding of tibia on femur prevented by *[Recent Question 2017]*
a. Anterior cruciate ligament
b. Posterior cruciate ligament
c. Ligament of Humprey
d. Ligament of Wrisberg

70. Which of the following is not an aggressive periosteal reaction? *[Recent Question 2017]*
a. Spiculated b. Laminated
c. Thick and irregular d. Interrupted

71. Continuous fixed traction is provided by *[Recent Question 2017]*
a. Thomas splint b. BB splint
c. Hamilton Russel d. Gallows

72. Primary dynamic stabilizer of Patella against the lateral pull of Vastus lateralis is *[Recent Question 2017]*
a. Vastus medialis longus
b. Vastus medialis obliques
c. Medial patellofemoral ligament
d. Trochlear depth

73. Most mobile segment of vertebral column is *[Recent Question 2017]*
a. Cervical b. Thoracic
c. Lumbar d. Sacral

74. Shenton'ss line is seen in X-ray of *[Recent Question 2017]*
a. Anteroposterior pelvis with both hips
b. Anteroposterior shoulder
c. Lateral cervical spine
d. Lateral lumbosacral spine

75. Most sensitive investigation for Early bone infection is *[Recent Question 2017]*
a. X-ray b. CT scan
c. Bone scan d. USG

76. Autonomous zone of sensory supply by Radial nerve is *[Recent Question 2017]*
a. 1st dorsal webspace b. Tip of index finger
c. Tip of thumb d. Tip of little finger

77. Angle of Gissane is for _____ bone *[Recent Question 2017]*
a. Talus b. Calcaneum
c. Navicular d. Cuboid

78. Denis classification is used to assess *[Recent Question 2017]*
a. Amount of femur head subluxation in dysplastic hips
b. Degree of calcium content
c. Degree of tumor invasion
d. Stability of spine

79. High crural index is seen in *[Recent Question 2017]*
a. Weight-lifters
b. Gymnasts
c. Jumping athletes
d. Long-distance runners

80. "No Man's Land" zone in flexor tendon is *[Recent Question 2017]*
a. Zone I
b. Zone II
c. Zone III
d. Zone IV

81. You are posted as an intern in causality. Which among the following patients with fracture will be your first priority to call orthopedics PG/Senior and inform? *[Recent Question 2018]*
a. 10 cm abrasion
b. Patient can not extend his arm
c. Patient's finger is blackening
d. Intra-articular fracture of elbow joint

82. 8th and 9th rib costal cartilage forms which type of joint? *[Recent Question 2018]*
a. Costochondral joint b. Synovial joint
c. Interchondral joint d. Costovertebral joint

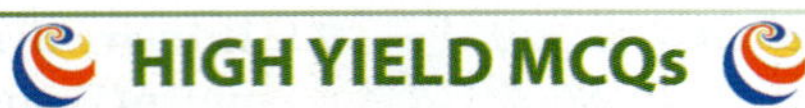

HIGH YIELD MCQs

1. **Type of joint seen in growth plate is:** *[All India PGMEE 2011]*
   a. Primary cartilaginous
   b. Secondary cartilaginous
   c. Fibrous
   d. Plane
2. **Most common site for autologous bone graft is:** *[All India PGMEE 2008]*
   a. Trochanter b. Fibula
   c. Iliac crest d. Tibial tuberosity
3. **Kanaval's sign is positive in** *[AIIMS PGMEE 2007]*
   a. Dupuytren's contracture
   b. Tenosynovitis
   c. Trigger finger
   d. Carpel tunnel syndrome
4. **Bone formation makers is/are** *[PGI 2007]*
   a. Hydroxyapatite b. Procollagen-I
   c. ALP d. Calcitonin
   e. TRAP
5. **Jefferson fracture is** *[AIIMS PGMEE 1995]*
   a. Fracture of atlas
   b. Fracture of axis
   c. Fracture of spinous process of C7
   d. Fracture of any cervical vertebra
6. **Indicators of bone formation are all EXCEPT** *[All India PGMEE 2007]*
   a. Osteocalcin b. Bone scan
   c. Hydroxyproline d. ALP
7. **True about Synovial fluid** *[AIIMS PGMEE 2010]*
   a. Type A synovial cells phagocytic
   b. Exhibit non-sss flow
   c. Contains hyaluronic acid and lubricin
   d. All are true
8. **Bone apposition is best in** *[AIIMS PGMEE 2001]*
   a. Osteoblastic activity at the area of stress
   b. Endochondral ossification
   c. Subperiosteal Cambian layer
   d. Osteoblastic activity in Howship's lacunae
9. **Regarding bone remodeling, all are true EXCEPT** *[AIIMS PGMEE 2001]*
   a. Osteoclastic activity at the compression site
   b. Osteoclastic activity at the tension site
   c. Osteoclastic activity and osteoblastic activity are both needed for bone remodelling in cortical and cancellous bones.
   d. Osteoblasts transforms into osteocytes
10. **Hangman's fracture is** *[Karnataka PGMEE 1998]*
   a. Subluxation of C5 over C6
   b. Fracture dislocation of C2
   c. Fracture dislocation of ankle joint
   d. Fracture of odontoid
11. **Bone resorption markers is/are** *[PGI 2008]*
   a. Serum propeptide of type I procollagen
   b. Osteocalcin
   c. Urine total free deoxypyridinoline
   d. Free glutamic acid crosslinkage
12. **A boy is sitting on the edge of table with knees flexed at 9 degree. When he extends his knee fully, what will happen to the tibial tuberosity in relation to patella**
   a. No change *[AIIMS PGMEE 2010]*
   b. Movement of IT towards medial border of patella
   c. Movement of IT towards lateral border of patella
   d. Movement of IT towards centre of patella
13. **Marker for bone formation is** *[AIIMS PGMEE 1997]*
   a. Tartrate resistant acid phosphate
   b. Osteocalcin
   c. Urinary calcium
   d. Serum nucleotidase
14. **House-maid's knee is bursitis of** *[AIIMS PGMEE 1995]*
   a. Ischial bursa b. Olecranon bursa
   c. Infrapatellar bursa d. Prepatellar bursa
15. **Blount's disease is** *[All India PGMEE 2011, Recent Question 2017]*
   a. Genu valgum b. Genu varum
   c. Genu recurvatum d. Meniscal injury
16. **Most common type of injury to spinal cord is** *[All India PGMEE 2007]*
   a. Flexion b. Extension
   c. Compression d. Flexion-rotation
17. **Major mineral contained in bones is** *[AIIMS PGMEE 2010]*
   a. Calcium carbonate b. Calcium chloride
   c. Calcium oxide d. Hydroxy-apatite
18. **Bankart's lesion is seen in** *[AIIMS PGMEE 2000]*
   a. Anterior surface of glenoid labrum
   b. Posterior surface of glenoid labrum
   c. Anterior part of humeral head
   d. Posterior part of humeral head
19. **Wrist flexion and finger extension test the following nerve root** *[AIIMS PGMEE 2005, JIPMER PGMEE 2003]*
   a. C6 b. C7
   c. C8 d. T3-T4
20. **Hill-Sachs lesion is associated with**
   a. Perthes disease *[JIPMER PGMEE 1992]*
   b. Fracture neck of femur
   c. Recurrent dislocation of shoulder
   d. Recurrent dislocation of hip
21. **Duga's test is used for** *[JIPMER PGMEE 1991]*
   a. Scaphoid fracture
   b. Fracture neck of femur
   c. Anterior dislocation of shoulder
   d. Dislocation of hip
22. **MC site of myositis ossificans** *[UP PGMEE 1996]*
   a. Knee b. Elbow
   c. Wrist d. Hip
23. **Treatment of acute myositis ossificans is** *[AIIMS PGMEE 1991, Recent Question 2017]*
   a. Immobilization b. Active mobilization
   c. Passive mobilization d. Infrared therapy
24. **Myositis ossificans is due to** *[Bihar PGMEE 1990]*
   a. Ossification
   b. New bone formation
   c. Migration of osteoblasts to hematoma
   d. Ossification of subperiosteal hematoma

25. Substance that is used for vertebroplasty is *[AIIMS PGMEE 2008]*
a. Polymethyl methacrylate
b. Polyethyl methacrylate
c. Polymethyl ethacrylate
d. Polyethyl ethacrylate

26. Basic pathology in Myositis ossificans progressive involves *[Bengal PGMEE 1990]*
a. Body collagen b. Serum chemistry
c. Muscle fibres d. Nerve fibres

27. Usual cause of death in a 60-year-old male with myositis ossificans progressive *[AIIMS PGMEE 2000]*
a. Bed sores b. Lung disease
c. Septicaemia d. Nutritional deficiencies

28. Trendelenberg test is positive due to injury of which nerve *[AIIMS PGMEE 2008]*
a. Superior gluteal b. Inferior gluteal
c. Obturator d. Tibial

29. Best diagnostic procedure for Anterior Cruciate ligament injury is *[Delhi PGMEE 1988, JIPMER PGMEE 2002, AIIMS PGMEE 2002, All India PGMEE 2003, 2008]*
a. Lachman's test b. Pivot shift test
c. Anterior drawer test d. Mc Murray's test

30. Trendelenburg test is positive in ALL EXCEPT *[AIIMS PGMEE 1998]*
a. Posterior dislocation of hip
b. Poliomyelitis
c. Fracture neck of femur
d. TB hip joint

31. Telescopic test is used for diagnosing *[ORISSA PGMEE 2008]*
a. Perthes disease
b. Intracapsular fracture neck of femur
c. Malunited Trochanteric fracture
d. Ankylosis of hip joint

32. The pivot test is for *[All India PGMEE 2001]*
a. Anterior cruciate ligament
b. Posterior cruciate ligament
c. Medial meniscus
d. Lateral meniscus

33. A dead piece of bone is known as *[BIHAR PGMEE 1991]*
a. Involucrum b. Sequestrum
c. Cloacae d. All of the above

34. A patient with POP cast for 2 months post-tibial fracture of Left side, now needs mobilization with a single crutch. Crutch will be used on which side? *[AIIMS PGMEE 2000]*
a. Left b. Right
c. Any side d. Both sides

35. Structural integrity of collateral ligaments are tested by *[JIPMER PGMEE 2002, MAHE PGMEE 2004]*
a. Varus/valgus stress test in full flexion
b. Varus/valgus stress test in full extension
c. Varus/valgus stress test in 30° of flexion
d. Varus/valgus stress test in 90° of flexion

36. Physiological locking involves *[Recent Question 2016, All India PGMEE 2008]*
a. Internal rotation of femur over stabilized tibia
b. Internal rotation of tibia over stabilized femur
c. External rotation of tibia over stabilized femur
d. External rotation of femur over stabilized tibia

37. Healing is usually slow below knee joint due to *[JIPMER PGMEE 1991]*
a. Low subcutaneous fat
b. Weight bearing
c. Poor vascularity
d. Increased movements

38. Indicators of bone formation includes all of following except *[All India PGMEE 2007]*
a. Osteocalcin b. Alkaline phosphatase
c. Hydroxyprolin d. Bone scan

39. For growth of bone, which term is most appropriate *[All India PGMEE 1992, AIIMS PGMEE 1991, JIPMER 2014]*
a. Enlargement b. Apposition
c. Hyperplasia d. Hypertrophy

40. Rate of mineralization of newly formed osteoid can be estimated by the following *[All India PGMEE 2009]*
a. Von Kossa staining for calcium
b. Alizarin red stain
c. Labeled tetracycline
d. Immunofluorescence

41. Injury to the medial meniscus is rather impossible when the knee joint does not *[NBE DNB 1989]*
a. Extend b. Flex
c. Rotate d. Abduct adduct

42. Tube-cylinder cast is applied for *[All India PGMEE 2007]*
a. Fracture hip b. Fracture knee
c. Fracture pelvis d. Fracture shoulder

43. Which of the following statements about 'Menisci' is not true? *[Recent Question 2016, All India PGMEE 2010]*
a. Medial meniscus is more mobile than lateral
b. Lateral meniscus covers more tibial articular surface than lateral
c. Medial meniscus is more commonly injured than lateral
d. Menisci are predominantly made up of Type I Collagen

44. Medial meniscus of knee joint is injured more often than the lateral meniscus because the medial meniscus is relatively *[AIIMS PGMEE 2002]*
a. More mobile b. Less mobile
c. Thinner
d. Attached lightly to femur

45. Cock-up splint is used in management of *[AIIMS PGMEE 1995]*
a. Radial nerve b. Ulnar nerve
c. Median nerve d. Axillary nerve

46. Phocomelia is *[AIPGME 1996, 1998]*
a. Absence of short bones
b. Complete absence of extremities
c. Defects of long bones of limbs
d. Partial absence of extremities

47. Site for first order bone grafting *[PGI 2003, 2006]*
a. Pelvis b. Tibial metaphysis
c. Medial malleolus d. Femoral condyle
e. Greater trochanter

48. McMurray's test is positive in injury of *[UPSC 1988]*
a. Anterior cruciate ligament
b. Posterior cruciate ligament
c. Medical meniscus injury
d. Lateral Meniscus injury
e. Popliteal bursitis

49. Surgical excision is done in all except *[AIIMS PGMEE 1995]*
a. Patella
b. Olecranon process
c. Head of radius
d. Lateral condyle humerus

50. Callus induction is hampered in *[PGI 2006]*
a. Hypoxemia
b. Fractured fragments of bone
c. Micromovements
d. Muscle interposition in between fractured fragments
e. Early mobilization

51. Healing of Fracture of bone is affected by *[PGI 2007]*
a. Micromovement
b. Muscle interposition
c. Hypoxia
d. Bone fragments

52. Factors that promotes callus formation *[PGI 2003]*
a. Micromovements between the fracture fragments
b. Appropriate approximation of he fragments
c. Muscle interposed in between the fracture fragment
d. Early initiation of mobilization
e. Ischemia

53. Trethowan's sign is seen in *[AMU PGMEE 1999]*
a. Perthe's disease
b. CDH
c. SCFE
d. Fracture neck femur

54. Ortolani's test is done for *[All India PGMEE 1994, UP PGMEE 1999, Recent Question 2014]*
a. Congenital dislocation of hip
b. Traumatic dislocation of hip
c. Rheumatoid arthritis
d. Tuberculous arthritis

55. Legg-Calve-Perthes disease is *[ORISSA PGMEE 2001]*
a. Mild pyogenic arthritis
b. TB of hip
c. Avascular necrosis of head of femur
d. Slipped femoral epiphysis

56. Metal-on-metal articulation should be avoided in *[All India PGMEE 2010]*
a. Osteonecrosis
b. Young female
c. Inflammatory arthritis
d. Revision surgery

57. Aseptic loosening in cemented total hip replacement, occurs as a result of hypersensitivity response to *[All India PGMEE 2004]*
a. Titanium debris
b. High density polythene debris
c. N. N-dimethyltryptamine (DMT)
d. Free radicals

58. Watson-Jones operation is done for *[AIIMS PGMEE 2008]*
a. Neglected Club foot
b. Muscle paralysis
c. Valgus deformity
d. Hip replacement

59. Watson-Jones operation is done for *[AIIMS PGMEE 2008]*
a. Polio
b. Muscle paralysis
c. Neglected clubfoot
d. Chronic ankle instability

60. Barlow's test is done for testing *[UP PGMEE 1999, Bihar PGMEE 1998]*
a. CDH in child
b. CDH in infancy
c. Femoral neck fracture
d. Slipped femoral epiphysis

61. Ortolani's test and Barlow maneuver is done for *[All India PGMEE 1994, UP PGMEE 1999]*
a. Congenital dislocation of hip
b. Traumatic dislocation of hip
c. Rheumatoid arthritis
d. Tubercular arthritis

62. Most common cause of genu valgum in children is *[AIIMS PGMEE 1993]*
a. Osteoarthritis
b. Rickets
c. Paget's disease
d. Rheumatoid arthritis

63. Sprengel's deformity is *[AIIMS PGMEE 1984]*
a. Absence of clavicle
b. Undescended scapula
c. Undescended neck of scapula
d. Exostosis of scapula

64. Cancellous bone graft taken from *[PGI 2006]*
a. Femoral condyles
b. Pelvis
c. Greater trochanter
d. Tibial metaphysis
e. None

65. Blount's disease is *[PGI 2000]*
a. Genu valgus
b. Tibia vera
c. Flat foot
d. Genu recurvatum

66. Brittle bone disease is *[DPG 1990, NBE DNB 2000]*
a. Osteoporosis
b. Osteomalacia
c. Osteopetrosis
d. Osteogenesis imperfecta

67. Which of the following is true of shoulder joint? *[JIPMER PGMEE 1995, AMU PGMEE 1998]*
a. Composed of only 2 joints
b. Anterior posterior gliding of scapula of never occurs
c. Acromio clavicular joint is more important
d. Allows flexion, rotation and abduction

68. Excision of head of radius in a child should not be done because *[JIPMER PGMEE 2001]*
a. It produces instability of elbow joint
b. It leads to secondary osteoarthritis of elbow
c. It causes subluxation of inferior radioulnar joint
d. It causes myositis ossificans.

69. Most common congenital anomaly among the following is encountered in our country *[TN PGMEE 1994]*
a. Congenital pseudoarthrosis of Tibia
b. Congenital dislocation of hip
c. Congenital talipes equino varus
d. Multiple congenital contractures

70. If head of the radius is removed, it will result in *[PGI 1991]*
a. Lengthening of limb
b. Valgus deformity
c. Varus deformity
d. No deformity

71. The Rotator cuff is composed of four of the following muscles except *[NBE DNB 1990, TN PGMEE 1996]*
a. Teres minor
b. Supraspinatus
c. Infraspinatus
d. Teres major
e. Subscapularis

72. The word "Talipes" refers to *[Bihar PGMEE 1988]*
a. Long feet with spidery toes
b. Flat feet
c. Club feet
d. Hammer toes

73. Weakest portion of shoulder joint capsule is *[All India PGMEE 1992, AIIMS PGMEE 1999, PGI 1993]*
a. Anterior
b. Posterior
c. Inferior
d. Superior

74. Muscle crossing through the shoulder joint is *[PGI 1995, NIMHANS PGMEE 1998]*
a. Biceps short head
b. Biceps long head
c. Triceps long head
d. Coracobrachialis

75. Monteggia fracture is fracture of *[UPSC 1991]*
a. Lower 1/3rd of radius b. Upper 1/3rd of radius
c. Lower 1/3rd of ulna d. Upper 1/3rd of ulna

76. Rotator interval is between *[MAHE PGMEE 2005, AIIMS PGMEE 2006, JIPMER PGMEE 2002]*
a. Supraspinatus and teres minor
b. Teres major and teres minor
c. Supraspinatus and subscapularis
d. Subscapularis and infraspinatus

77. Marble bone disease include *[JIPMER PGMEE 1997]*
a. Osteosarcoma b. Osteopetrosis
c. Osteitis fragilis d. Paget's diseases
e. Osteosclerosis

78. Unaffected in Albers-Schonberg disease is/are *[PGI 2000]*
a. Calcium levels b. Phosphorus levels
c. Parathormone levels d. ALP levels
e. Bone growth

79. Galeazzi fracture is fracture of *[AP PGMEE 1998]*
a. Upper end of ulna b. Lower end of ulna
c. Upper end of radius d. Lower end of radius

80. Increased bone density on X-ray is seen in *[PGI 2008]*
a. Periosteal reaction
b. Osteomyelitis
c. Paget's disease
d. Avascular necrosis
e. Collapse of cancellous bone

81. Triple arthrodesis involves *[All India PGMEE 2001]*
a. Calcaneocuboid, talonavicular and talocalcaneal
b. Tibiotalar, calcaneocuboid and talonavicular
c. Ankle joint, calcaneocuboid and talonavicular
d. None of the above

82. Triple arthrodesis is NOT done before-skeletal maturation because of *[AIIMS PGMEE 1998]*
a. Shortening of foot
b. Recurrence of deformity
c. Inadequate fusion
d. Complete correction not possible

83. Caffey's disease affect *[UP PGMEE 2008]*
a. Infants b. Adolescents
c. Adults d. Old age

84. Rugger-Jersey spine is seen in *[All India PGMEE 2006]*
a. Fluorosis b. Renal osteodystrophy
c. Achondroplasia d. Marfan's syndrome

85. Rocker bottom foot is due to *[AMU PGMEE 1999]*
a. Over corrected club foot
b. Poliomyelitis
c. Vertical talus
d. Deformities of spine

86. Alkaline phosphatase is elevated in all EXCEPT *[AIIMS PGMEE 1997]*
a. Rickets b. Osteomalacia
c. Hypoparathyroidism d. Hypophosphatemia

87. Glass holding cast is also known as *[All India PGMEE 1991]*
a. Coll's cast b. Smith's cast
c. Sarmento cast d. Scaphoid cast

88. Treatment of choice for Paget's disease of bone is *[All India PGMEE 1995]*
a. Vitamin D b. Calcitonin
c. Surgical treatment d. Immobilization of limb

89. Duga's test is helpful in *[JIPMER PGMEE 1991]*
a. Dislocation of hip
b. Scaphoid fracture
c. Fracture neck of femur
d. Anterior dislocation of shoulder

90. Drug treatment of Osteitis deformans (Paget's disease of bone) include all except *[Karnataka PGMEE 2001]*
a. Alendronate b. Etidronate
c. Plicamycin d. Calcitonin

91. Wormian bones are seen in *[Delhi PGMEE 1994]*
a. Osteogenesis imperfecta
b. Scheurmann's disease
c. Paget's disease
d. Osteoclastoma

92. Complications of Paget's disease of bone is *[AIIMS PGMEE 1987]*
a. Deafness b. Heart failure
c. Osteosarcoma d. All of the above

93. Vitamin required for collagen formation *[PGI 1997]*
a. Vitamin A
b. Vitamin B
c. Vitamin C
d. Vitamin D
e. Vitamin E

94. Following are the common sites of avascular necrosis, EXCEPT *[All India PGMEE 1992]*
a. Proximal half of scaphoid
b. The body of talus
c. Patella
d. Head of the femur

95. Albers Schonberg disease is *[PGI 2000, PGI 1998, AP PGMEE 1993]*
a. Osteopetrosis b. Osteoporosis
c. Osteochondritis d. Osteomalacia

96. Bohler's angle is seen in *[All India PGMEE 2007]*
a. Talus b. Navicular
c. Cuboid d. Calcaneum

97. Lift off test is done to assess the function of *[All India PGMEE 2010]*
a. Supraspinatus b. Infraspinatus
c. Teres Minor d. Subscapularis

98. Velpeau bandage and Sling and Swathe splint are used in? *[AIIMS PGMEE 2008]*
a. Shoulder dislocation
b. Fracture scapula
c. Acromioclavicular dislocation
d. Fracture clavicle

99. Disc prolapsed commonly occurs at *[PGI 2001]*
a. C3–C4 b. C4–C5
c. C5–C6 d. L4–L5
e. L5–S1

100. Increased Bone density in X-ray seen in *[PGI 2008]*
a. Increased thickening of trabeculae
b. Fracture and Collapse of cancellous bone
c. Defective mineralization
d. Myositis ossificans
e. Relative disuse atrophy and surrounding bone response

101. Caffey's disease is *[UP PGMEE 2003]*
a. Renal osteodystrophy
b. Infantile cortical hyperostosis
c. Osteomyelitis of jaw in children
d. Chronic osteomyelitis in children

102. Game Keeper's thumb is *[PGI 1992, Karnataka PGMEE 1995, NIMHANS PGMEE 1997]*
a. Ulnar collateral ligament injury of MCP joint
b. Radial collateral ligament injury of MCP joint
c. Radial collateral ligament injury of CMC joint
d. Ulnar collateral ligament injury of CMC joint

103. Mallet finger is *[UPSC 1985, UPSC 1988, Kerala PGMEE 1987]*
a. Avulsion fracture of extensor tendon of distal phalanx
b. Fracture of distal phalanx
c. Fracture of middle phalanx
d. Fracture of proximal phalanx

104. Common vertebral level of spondylolisthesis is *[BIHAR PGMEE 1999]*
a. T12–L1
b. L1–L2
c. L3–L4
d. L4–L5
e. L5–S1

105. Hanging cast is used in *[AIIMS PGMEE 1995]*
a. Fracture femur
b. Fracture radius
c. Fracture tibia
d. Fracture humerus

106. In hand surgery which area is called no man's land? *[AIIMS PGMEE 2000]*
a. Proximal phalanx
b. Distal phalanx
c. Between distal phalanx crease and proximal phalanx
d. Wrist

107. Middle palmar space ends distally *[DNB 1991]*
a. Along the digital sheaths
b. Into the flexor tendon sheaths
c. Into the webspace
d. By mixing with the superficial palmer space

108. Cervical spondylosis is more common at *[UP PGMEE 1999, AIIMS PGMEE 1990]*
a. C1–C2
b. C2–C3
c. C6–C7
d. C4–C5

109. All of the following names are associated with tests/ operations around the hip joint except *[NBE DNB 1990]*
a. Bryant
b. Shenton
c. Mc Murray
d. Salter
e. Nelton

110. Telescopic test is useful to diagnose *[NBE DNB 2008, AMU PGMEE 2009]*
a. Perthe's disease
b. Intracapsular fracture neck of femur
c. Malunited Trochanteric fracture
d. Ankylosis of hip joint

111. Metabolic bone disease is caused by excess intake of which vitamin *[PGI 2001, PGI 2006, PGI 2009]*
a. A
b. B
c. C
d. D
e. E

112. Hallux valgus means *[AP PGMEE 2000]*
a. Outward deviation of fifth toe
b. Inward deviation of fifth toe
c. Outward deviation of great toe
d. Inward deviation of great toe

113. Pauvel's angle is *[Rajasthan PGMEE 1994]*
a. Neck shaft angle of femur
b. The difference between neck shaft angle between two femurs of a patient
c. Formed by joining a line extended from fracture line of femur neck to an arbitrary line depicting the horizontal plane
d. None of the above

114. Garden's classification is applicable to *[UP PGMEE 1994]*
a. Intertrochanteric fracture
b. Fracture neck of femur
c. Epiphyseal separation
d. Posterior dislocation of hip

115. Common injury to baby is *[CMC PGMEE 2002]*
a. Fracture humerus
b. Fracture clavicle
c. Fracture
d. Fracture femur

116. Most common bone fractured during birth *[MP PGMEE 1998]*
a. Clavicle
b. Scapula
c. Radius
d. Humerus

117. Which of the following is ideal site for harvesting bone graft? *[All India PGMEE 2008]*
a. Iliac crest
b. Distal end of humerus
c. Distal end of femur
d. Fibula

118. Sabre tibia is seen in *[AIIMS PGMEE 1991]*
a. Rickets
b. Paget's disease
c. Tuberculous osteomyelitis
d. Syphilitic osteitis

119. Action of Vitamin D is that it *[AMU PGMEE 1991, UPSC 1990]*
a. Stimulates bone marrow
b. Increases calcium loss
c. Stimulates absorption of calcium
d. Stimulates osteoclasts

120. The most common cause of osteomalacia in our country is *[PGI 1990]*
a. Repeated systemic infections
b. Idiopathic steatorrhoea
c. Dietetic deficiency of vitamin D and calcium
d. Poor protein intake
e. Chronic renal disease

121. Fracture shaft of femur in adult unites by *[Bihar PGMEE 1990]*
a. 3 to 4 weeks
b. 3 to 4 weeks
c. 3 to 4 months
d. 4 to 6 months
e. None of these

122. Line joining ant. sup iliac spine to ischial tuberosity and passes a greater trochanter *[AIIMS PGMEE 1999]*
a. Nelaton's line
b. Showmakers line
c. Cniene's line
d. Perkin's line

123. Arthroscopy is contraindicated in *[RAJASTHAN PGMEE 2004]*
a. Hemophilia
b. Chronic joint disease
c. Loose bodies
d. Meniscal tear

124. All of the following are used for giving skeletal traction, except *[AIIMS PGMEE 2006]*
a. Steinmann's pin
b. Kirschner's wire
c. Bohler's stirrup
d. Rushpin

125. Basic pathological defect in rickets is *[UP PGMEE 1997, Rajasthan PGMEE 1998]*
a. Decreased osteoblastic activity
b. Non functional osteoclast
c. Defective osteoclastic resorption of uncalcified osteoid and cartilage
d. Defective proliferation of physis.

126. Bony lesion in Rickets is due to *[AIIMS PGMEE 1991]*
a. Increased parathoromone leading to osteoclastic activity
b. Reduced dietary calcium absorption
c. Increased calcium excretion
d. None

127. Pollicization is *[All India PGMEE 2008]*
a. Amutation of thumb
b. Equalization of fingers
c. Toe to thumb transplantation
d. Reconstruction of thumb

128. "Trendelenburg sign" is positive in damage of the following nerve *[Recent Question 2016, All India PGMEE 1997]*
a. Inferior gluteal nerve b. Pudendal nerve
c. Superior gluteal nerve d. Posterior tibial nerve

129. McMurray's osteotomy is based on the following principle? *[AP PGMEE 1994]*
a. Biological b. Biomechanical
c. Biotechnical d. Mechanical

130. First to appear amongst the ossification centres about the elbow is *[PGI 1996, UP PGMEE 2003, Assam PGMEE 1999]*
a. Radial Head b. Olecranon
c. Lateral epicondyle d. Capitellum

131. The metabolic indicator of Rickets is *[Delhi PGMEE 2001]*
a. Low serum Ca b. Low PO_4
c. Alkaline phosphatase d. Urinary hydroxy proline

132. Brodie's abscess usually involves *[WB PGMEE 1991]*
a. Short bones b. Long bones
c. Flat bones d. Pelvic bones

133. Anterior interosseous nerve is a branch of *[All India PGMEE 1989]*
a. Musculocutaneous b. Radial
c. Median d. Ulnar

134. A diet deficient in calcium will most commonly result in *[All India PGMEE 1990]*
a. Osteomalacia b. Rickets
c. Osteoporosis d. Osteitis fibrosa

135. Most common site of actinomycosis *[All India PGMEE 2003]*
a. Femur b. Tibia
c. Rib d. Mandible

136. Healing below knee joint is slow because of *[JIPMER PGMEE 1991]*
a. Decreased subcutaneous fat
b. Increased movement
c. Weight bearing
d. Poor vascularity

137. Alkaline phosphatase is elevated in all, EXCEPT *[AIIMS PGMEE 1997]*
a. Rickets b. Osteomalacia
c. Hypoparathyroidism d. Hypophosphatemia

138. All of the following statements about synovial fluid are true, Except *[All India PGMEE 2009, AIIMS PGMEE 2010]*
a. Secreted primarily by type A synovial cells
b. Follows non-newtonian fluid kinetics
c. Contains hyaluronic acid
d. Viscosity is variable

139. Which of the following statements about changes in articular cartilage with aging is not true? *[All India PGMEE 2010]*
a. Total proteoglycan content is decreased
b. Synthesis of proteoglycans is decreased
c. Enzymatic degradation of proteoglycans is increased
d. Total water content of cartilage is decrease

140. Most common site of disc prolapse is *[Delhi PGMEE 1988]*
a. C5–C6 b. T8–T9 *[Kerala PGMEE1990]*
c. L4–L5 d. L5–S1

141. The most common site for prolapse of intervertebral disc is *[Orissa PGMEE 1988]*
a. Cervical region b. Lower thoracic region
c. Upper thoracic region d. Lumbar region

142. After L4–S1 the next most common site of intervertebral disc prolapse is *[JIPMER PGMEE 1995]*
a. C6–C7 b. T12–L1
c. L1–L2 d. L2–L3

143. Madura foot is *[All India PGMEE 2005]*
a. Tuberculous infection of the bone
b. Parasitic infection of the bone
c. Water borne disease of the foot
d. Madura mycotic infection of the bone

144. The "Card test" tests the function of *[UPSC 1995]*
a. Median nerve b. Ulnar nerve
c. Axillary nerve d. Radial nerve

145. Finkelstein's test is associated with *[All India PGMEE 1992]*
a. DeQuervains disease
b. Dupuytren's contracture
c. Carpal tunnel syndrome
d. Any of the above

146. Vitamin required for collagen is *[PGI 1997]*
a. Vitamin A b. Vitamin C
c. Vitamin D d. Vitamin E

147. Vitamin C deficiency leads to *[NIMS PGMEE 1998]*
a. Defective mineralisation
b. Defective osteoid formation
c. Normal collagen and Bone matrix
d. X-ray shows normal evidence

148. Froment's sign is present in paralysis of .... nerve *[Recent Question 2016, Delhi PGMEE 1994]*
a. Ulnar b. Radial
c. Median d. Axillary

149. 'Tennis elbow', is characterized by *[All India PGMEE 1997]*
a. Tenderness over the medial epicondyle
b. Tendinits of common extensor origin
c. Tendinitis of common flexor origin
d. Painful flexion and extension

150. Claw hand is seen in *[NBE DNB 1999, All India PGMEE 1993]*
a. Cervical rib carpal tunnel syndrome
b. Multiple sclerosis
c. Radial nerve injury
d. Ulnar nerve injury

151. "Ulnar paradox" is related with the following *[UP PGMEE 1994]*
a. Lumbricals b. Intrinsic muscle
c. Extensor pollicis longus d. Ulnar half of FDP

152. Three point relationship is reversed in all, except *[AIIMS PGMEE 1991, AIIMS PGMEE 2000, Recent Question 2017]*
a. Fracture medial epicondyle
b. Fracture lateral epicondyle
c. Supracondylar fracture
d. Posterior elbow dislocation

153. Three bony point relationship is maintained in *[AIIMS PGMEE 1995]*
a. Supracondylar fracture humerus
b. Dislocation of elbow
c. Fracture lateral condyle
d. Intercondylar fracture

154. Scurvy affects bone by *[AIIMS PGMEE 2010]*
a. Decreasing mineralization of bone
b. Less formation of osteoid matrix
c. Loss of calcium from mineralized matrix
d. Affection of zone of provisional calcification only

155. Brown tumors are seen in *[All India PGMEE 2006]*
a. Hyperparathyroidism
b. Pigmented villonodular synovitis
c. Osteomalacia
d. Neurofibromatosis

156. True about Osteoclast is all except *[PGI 2000]*
a. Derived from monocytes
b. Stimulated by PTH
c. Phagocytosis of foreign bodies
d. Resorption of bone

157. Following structures pass through spiral groove of humerus *[PGI 1990]*
a. Radial nerve
b. Radial artery
c. Anterior circumflex humeral artery
d. Posterior circumflex humeral artery
e. Arteria profunda brachii

158. Major mineral of the bone is *[AIIMS PGMEE 2010]*
a. Calcium chloride b. Hydroxyapatite
c. Calcium oxide d. Calcium carbonate

159. The stability of the ankle joint is maintained by all of the following, except *[AIIMS PGMEE 2003]*
a. Plantar calcaneonavicular (spring) ligament
b. Deltoid ligament
c. Lateral ligament
d. Shape of the superior talar articular surface

160. Which of the following is a primary defect in Paget's disease? *[NBE DNB 2000, Rajasthan PGMEE 2009]*
a. Osteoblast
b. Osteoclast
c. Osteocyte
d. Fibroblast

161. Calcium content of bone is increased in *[MAHE PGMEE 1998]*
a. Prolonged immobilization
b. Glucocorticoid administration
c. Hyperparathyroidism
d. Estrogen supplementation in postmenopausal women

162. Non dynamic splint is *[PGI 1987]*
a. Banjo b. Opponens
c. Cock up d. Brand

163. Which sign is positive in deQuervain's disease? *[Manipal PGMEE 2000]*
a. Phalen's sign b. Froment's sign
c. Cozen's sign d. Finkelstein's sign

164. Posterolateral anconeus triangle is formed by *[JIPMER PGMEE 2000, Karnataka PGMEE 2001]*
a. Head of radius, lateral epicondyle, medial epicondyle
b. Head of radius, lateral epicondyle, olecranon
c. Olecranon, medial epicondyle, neck of radius
d. Neck of radius, head of rafius, lateral epicondyle

165. Which of the following cysts is medially situated? *[NBE DNB 1991, Delhi PGMEE 2006]*
a. Housemaid's knee
b. Clergyman's knee
c. Bursa anserine
d. Semimembranosus bursitis
e. Morrant Baker's cyst

166. Bohler angle measurement gives the reference for *[AII India PGMEE 2007]*
a. Calcaneus b. Talus
c. Navicular d. Cuboid

167. Neutral triangle is seen radiologically in *[NIMS PGMEE 2003]*
a. Neck femur b. Proximal humerus
c. Calcaneus d. Talus

168. Kienboch's disease *[Recent Question 2016, AIIMS PGMEE 2000]*
a. Osteochondritis of lunate
b. Osteochondritis of neck of femur
c. Osteochondritis of navicular
d. Osteochondritis of tibial condyle

169. Common peroneal nerve is related to *[AIIMS PGMEE 2006]*
a. Shaft of tibia b. Neck of fibula
c. Lower tibio-fibular joint d. Shaft of fibula

170. The most common source of bone and joint infection is *[TN PGMEE 1994]*
a. Direct spread b. Percutaneous
c. Lymphatic d. Haematogenous

171. Gunstock deformity is due to *[TN PGMEE 1997, PGI 1993, Recent Question 2017]*
a. Fracture of 1st metacarpal bone
b. Fracture of lower end of radius
c. Supracondylar fracture of humerus
d. Lateral condylar fracture of humerus

172. Commonest cause of spinal cord injuries in our country is *[AMU PGMEE 2002, SGPGI 2003]*
a. Road traffic accident b. Fall from a height
c. Fall into well d. House collapse

173. Phalen's test is positive in *[Delhi PGMEE 2009]*
a. Carpal tunnel syndrome
b. DeQuervain's disease
c. Tennis elbow
d. Ulnar bursitis

174. Test for tight iliotibial band is *[AIIMS PGMEE 2001]*
a. Ober's test b. Osber's test
c. Simmond's test d. Charnley's test

175. Osgood-Schlatter disease *[PGI 2007]*
a. Involve the knee joint
b. Pelvis
c. Wrist joint
d. Cervical spine

176. Stance phase muscle among the following is *[PGI 2001]*
a. Quadriceps
b. Hamstring
c. Gastrocnemius-soleus
d. Tibialis anterior
e. Peroneus longus

177. Perichondrial ring is *[PGI 2008]*
a. Seen around foramen magnum
b. Seen around epiphyseal plate
c. More prominent in adults
d. Shear strength increases with age

178. Iselin's disease is osteochondritis of *[JIPMER PGMEE 1999]*
a. 2nd Metacarpal
b. 5th Metacarpal
c. 2nd Metatarsal
d. 5th Metatarsal

179. Freiberg's osteochondritis is *[All India PGMEE 1990]*
a. 2nd Metatarsal head
b. 5th Metatarsal head
c. 2nd Metatarsal base
d. 5th Metatarsal base

180. Madelung's deformity involves the following *[TN PGMEE 1994]*
a. Knee
b. Wrist
c. Hip
d. Elbow

181. Craniovertebral joint contains all except? *[AIIMS PG November 2015]*
a. Wings of sphenoid
b. Basiocciput
c. Atlas
d. Axis

182. Milkman's Fracture is a type of *[ESI IMO 2014]*
a. Pseudofracture
b. Clavicular fracture
c. Humeral fracture
d. Metacarpal fracture

183. In children, all are true except *[ESI IMO 2014]*
a. Thick Periosteum
b. Soft Bones
c. Dislocations are rare
d. Comminuted fractures are common

184. Craniovertebral joint contains all except? *[AIIMS PG November 2015]*
a. Wings of sphenoid
b. Basiocciput
c. Atlas
d. Axis

185. Ivory vertebra is seen in *[NIMSET 2015]*
a. Osteoporosis
b. Hyperparathyroidism
c. Lymphoma
d. Thalassemia

186. Growth of cartilage following fracture can be increased by *[AIIMS May 2017]*
a. Intramedullary nail
b. K-wire fixation
c. Strict immobilization
d. Repeated tiny movements at the fracture site

187. Talocalcaneonavicular joint is a type of ________ joint *[AIIMS November 2017]*
a. Plane
b. Saddle
c. Ball and socket
d. Ellipsoid

188. First carpal bone to ossify *[AIIMS November 2017]*
a. Trapezoid
b. Capitate
c. Lunate
d. Pisiform

189. Statement not true regarding Posterior cruciate ligament is *[AIIMS November 2017]*
a. Main restraint in Posterior drawer test
b. Extrasynovial structure
c. Main restraint in Internal rotation
d. Originates from Anterolateral aspect of Medial femoral condyle in the area of Intercondylar notch

190. During examination of a patient in supine position, Examiner keeps his hand blow the heel of one foot and asks the patient to flex his other hip against resistance while keeping his leg straight. This sign/ test is called as *[AIIMS November 2017]*
a. Waddell's test
b. O' Donoghue's test
c. McMurray test
d. Hoover's test

NEET/NBE PATTERN MCQs ANSWERS WITH EXPLANATIONS

1. Ans. (b) Subscapularis

[Ref. Orthopedic Physical Assessment by Magee, 5/e p312]

Lift-Off Test

- Given by: Gerber and Krushell (1991)
- Synonym: Gerber's test
- Test procedure:
  - In standing position, patient is asked to place his hand behind back, with dorsum of hand resting in region of Mid-lumbar spine
  - Dorsum of hand is raised off the back by maintaining or increasing internal rotation of humerus and extension at shoulder
  - To perform this test the patient must have full passive internal rotation so that it is physically possible to place the arm in desired position and pain cannot be a limiting factor during the manoeuvre.

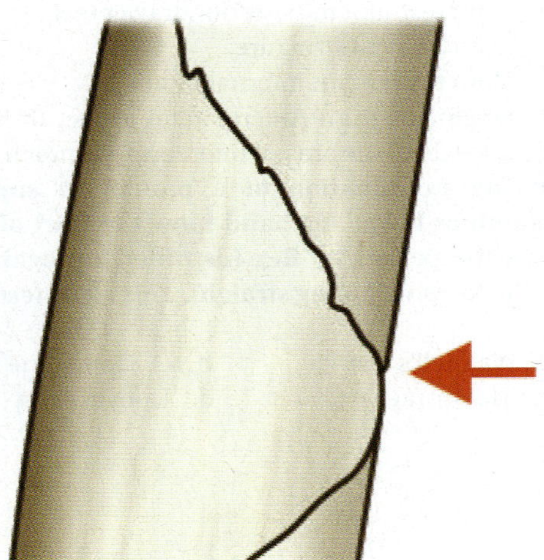

- Results:
  - Ability to actively lift the dorsum of the hand off the back constitutes a NORMAL Lift-off test
  - Inability to move dorsum off the back constitutes an ABNORMAL lift-off test and indicates subscapularis rupture or dysfunction

2. Ans. (b) Receptor for Parathormone

[Ref. Ingle's Endodontics 6, 1/e p504]

Osteoclasts

- When bone cells are activated by PTH or IL-1, they express osteoprogerin-ligand on their surface with two functions:
  1. Binding to surface receptor RANK (Receptor activator of nuclear factor κB) on mononuclear Pro-osteclasts inducing their maturation to multinucleated mature Osteoclasts
  2. Binding to RANK on surface of inactive osteoclasts, activating them to become bone-resorbing cells with Ruffles border

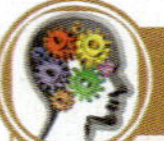

Also Remember

- There are abundant PTH receptors on Osteoblasts but few on Osteoclasts: Bone resorption has to be mediated indirectly by Osteoblasts

3. Ans. (a) Metaphysis

[Ref. Orthopaedics and Trauma Volume 1 by Kulkarni, 2/e p61]

- Metaphyseal arteries freely anastomose with spiral branches of nutrient arteries: Metaphysis is the most vascular area of the long bone
- Hair-pin loops of Nutrient artery loops anastomose with Epiphyseal, Metaphyseal (juxtaepiphyseal) and Periosteal arteries
- In developing bone, newly formed spongy bone from ossification zone of growth cartilage is laid down here

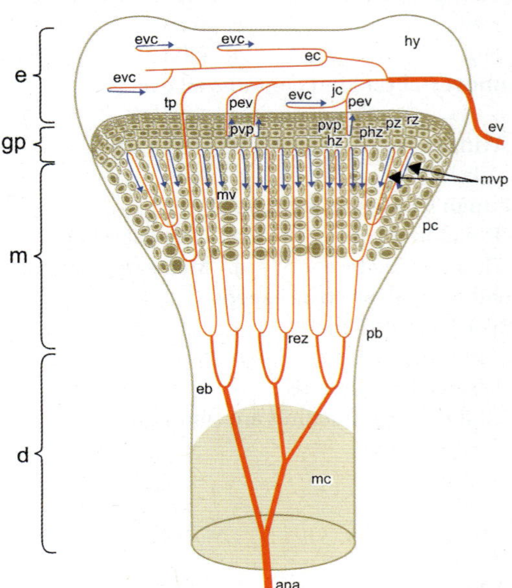

Fig. Hair pin loops in bone

4. Ans. (b) Extensor and radial deviator of wrist

[Ref. Essentials of Kinesiology by Mansfield, 2/e p138]

Deviators of Wrist

Radial deviators	Ulnar deviators
Primary set *(Action on wrist only)* Extensor carpi radialis longus Extensor carpi radialis brevis ***Secondary set*** *(Act on wrist and hand)* Extensor pollicis longus Extensor pollicis brevis Flexor carpi radialis Abductor pollicis longus Flexor pollicis longus	***Primary set*** *(Action on wrist only)* Extensor carpi ulnaris Flexor carpi ulnaris

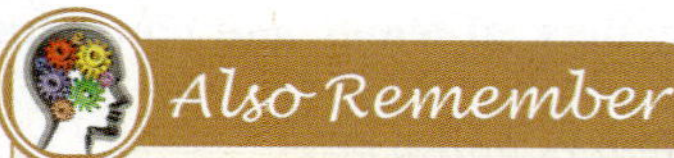

- **Muscles extending the wrist:**
  - Extensor carpi radialis longus
  - Extensor carpi radialis brevis
  - Extensor carpi ulnaris
  - Extensor digitorum
  - Extensor indicis
  - Extensor digit minimi
  - Extensor pollicis longus
  - Extensor pollicis brevis

5. Ans. (c) Fixed flexion deformity of the Hip

[Ref. Practical Orthopedics by Ebnezar, 1/e p502]

Thomas Test

- Used to rule out Hip flexion contracture and Psoas syndrome
- Associated with runners, dancers, and gymnasts
- **Step 1**: Patient lies supine on the examination table, Clinician passes the palm of his hand beneath the patients'spine to identify lumbar lordosis
- **Step 2**: Normal hip is flexed till the thigh just touches the abdomen to obliterate the lumbar lordosis
- **Step 3**: Measure the angle between the affected thigh and the table to reveal the fixed flexion deformity of the hip

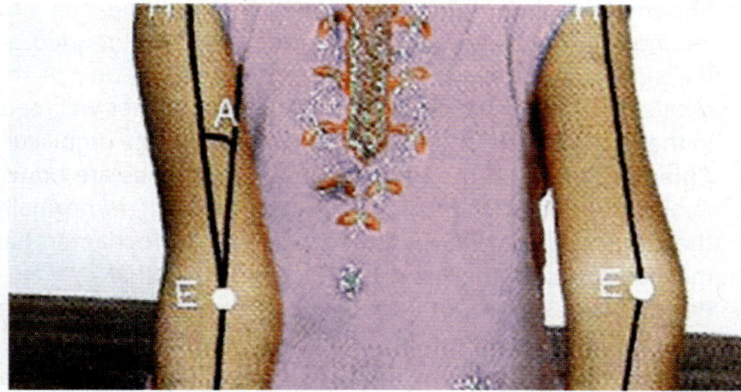

6. Ans. (c) Osteoblasts

[Ref. Krause's Food & the Nutrition Care, 13/e p534]

PTH acts directly on osteoblasts, which increase the production of IL-6 and other cytokines that in-turn stimulate osteoclasts to resorb bone

7. Ans. (d) None of the Above

[Ref. Arthritis and Metabolic Bone Disease by Weissman, 1/e p657]

Hypoparathyroidism of Bones

- Localised/diffuse Osteosclerosis (MC finding)
- Thickening of Facial bones/Cranial vault with widened diploe, sutural diastasis
- Intracranial calcifications, Ligamental calcifications, Subcutaneous calcifications
- Hypoplastic dentition

8. Ans. (a) Gap non-union

[Ref. Plastic Surgery by Stone, 1/e p10]

Management of Bone Gaps

- Non-vascularised bone gaps
- Vascularised bone-gaps
- **Ilizarov techniques**:
  - Limb shortening followed by Distraction osteogenesis
  - Limb held to length followed by Bone transport

9. Ans. (a) Axillary nerve

[Ref. Gray's Basic Anatomy, 2/e p354]

- Axillary nerve and Posterior circumflex humeral artery and vein pass through quadrangular space

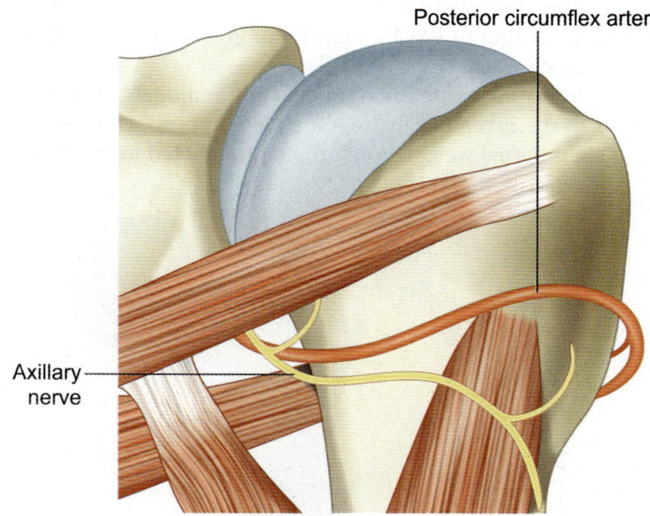

Fig. Quadrangular space

10. Ans. (b) Diffusion

[Ref. Functional Electronic Histology, 1/e p45]

Chondrocytes are supplied with oxygen and nutrients by diffusion of molecules across long distances of semisolid matrix; this fact imposes a limit to the size cartilage can reach before its center begins to die, and it also makes the chondrocytes vulnerable to changes

11. Ans. (d) 4 to 6 years

[Ref. Pediatric Skeletal Trauma by Johnson, 1/e p295]

Ossific nucleus of the scaphoid appears around 4–6 years of age, and ossification is complete at 13-15 years of age

12. Ans. (b) Finkelstein test

[Ref. Clinical Signs by Cho, 1/e p20]

Finkelstein's Test

- Finkelstein's test: Examining physician or therapist grasps the thumb and ulnar deviates the hand sharply
- **Positive test**: Sharp pain occurs along the distal radius (top of forearm) in cases of De Quervain's tenosynovitis

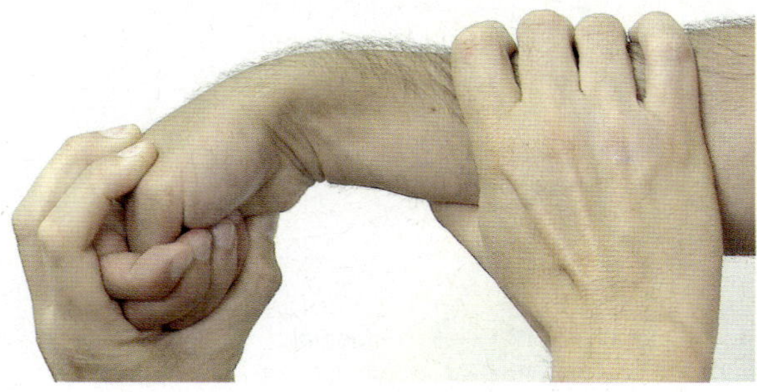

Fig. Finkelstein's test

13. Ans. (a) If a bone is continuously subjected to a particular stress it will adapt to become stronger to resist that loading
[Ref. Bone Histology by Crowder, 1/e p7]

Wolff's Law (Bone Adaptation Theory)

- The form of a bone being given, the bone elements place or displace themselves in the direction of functional forces and increase or decrease their mass to reflect the amount of the functional forces
- According to Wolff's Law, **bone grows in proportion to mechanical stress**
- A healthy living bone models and remodels in response to the mechanical stress it experiences so as to produce a minimal weight structure that is adapted to the stresses acted on it

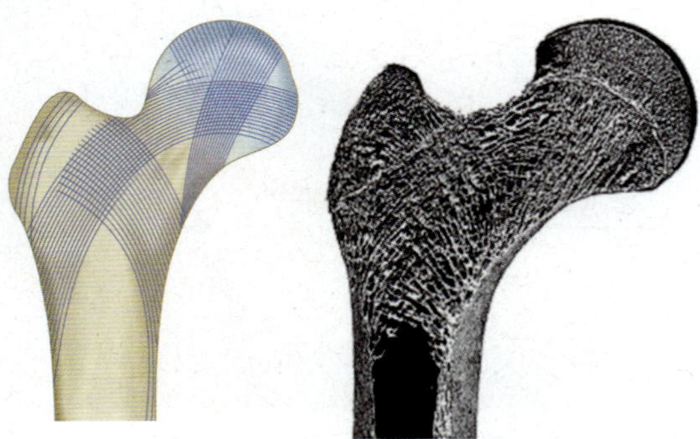

Fig. Wolff's law

14. Ans. (a) Strands of collagen
[Ref. Biophysical Chemistry by Dash, 1/e p59]

- Tensile strength of tissue is due to the presence of collagen and calcium matrix
- Each strand of collagen possesses three chains of tropocollagen appears arranged like a rope
- High tensile strength of collagen is due to its helical structure

15. Ans. (b) Retroversion of 30 degrees
[Ref. The Shoulder, Volume 1 by Rockwood, 4/e p222]

- 30-degree retroversion of articular orientation of Humeral head is complemented by the 30-degree anterior rotation of Scapula on trunk

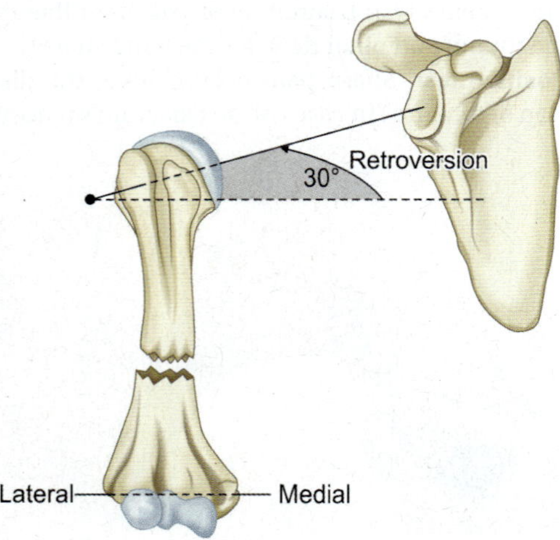

Fig. Retroversion humeral head

16. Ans. (d) Curve formed by neck of femur and obturator foramen
[Ref. Nelson Textbook of Pediatrics, 20/e p3277]

- **Shenton's line**: Smooth curve formed by inferior border of neck of femur with superior margin of obturator foramen

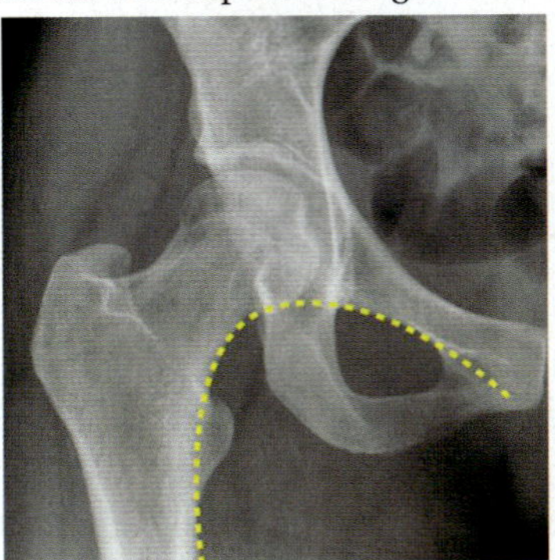

Fig. Shenton's line

Also Remember

- **Nelaton's line**: With the hip 90 degree of flexion, a line joining the ASIS and ischial tuberosity passes through the tip of the greater trochanter on that side; In cases of supratrochanteric shortening the troachanter will be proximal to this line
- **Shoemaker's line**: With the patient lying supine, the line joining ASIS and tip of the greater trochanter is extended on the side of the abdomen on both sides; In case one of the greater trochanter has migrated proximally the lines will meet in the opposite side of the abdomen and below the umbilicus
- **Chiene's line**: With the patient lying supine, lines are brawn joining the two ASIS and the two greater trochanters, normally these make two parallel lines; In case one of the trochanters has moved proximally the line will converge on that side
- **Perkin's line**: A horizontal line is drawn through the triradiate cartilage and a vertical line is drawn down form the outer edge of the acetabulum on both sides, the upper femoral epiphyses normally lies medial to the vertical line and below the horizontal line; But in congenital dislocation of hip the epiphyses will lie on the outer aspect of the vertical line and above the horizontal line
- **Bryant's triangle**: When patient lies supine, the tips of the greater trochanter and ASIS on both sides are marked and a perpendicular is dropped from each ASIS on to the bed; From the tip of the greater trochanter another perpendicular is dropped on to the first one, the tips of the greater trochanter are joined to the ASIS on the respective side. This forms a triangle ABC; Side BC of the triangle measures supratrochanteric shortening of hip.

17. Ans. (a) Age, race and sex-matched individuals
[Ref. Varney's Midwifery, 4/e p353]

"Z" Score

- Relates the measure of bone mineral density figure to the mean value expected for a healthy normal subject matched for age, sex, and race
- This score expresses the difference between a woman's bone mineral density and age-matched mean units for population standard deviation

18. Ans. (d) All of the above

[Ref. Netter's Concise Orthopaedic Anatomy by Thompson, 1/e p373]

Branches of Posterior tibial, Dorsalis pedis, and Peroneal arteries contribute to the Talus; however there are multiple variations

19. Ans. (b) Subacromial bursitis

[Ref. Orthopedic Physical Assessment by Evans, 2/e p192]

Dawbarn's Sign Test

- Shoulder examination used to determine Subacromial bursitis
- Patient seated, examiner palpates anterior to the acromion and observes patient, then examiner passively abducts patient shoulder to 90°
- Positive pain with palpation that disappears after the shoulder is abducted 90° indicates subacromial bursitis.

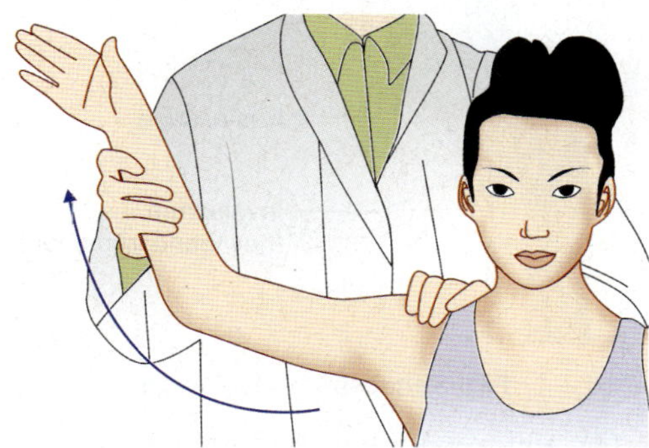

20. Ans. (a) Type 1

[Ref. Musculoskeletal Diseases by Bonakdarpour, 1/e p7]

Components of Bone Matrix

- **Bone proteins**
- **Collagens**:
  - Collagen type 1: Woven, Lamellar bone
  - Collagen type 2: Cartilage
  - Collagen type 3: Certain pathological conditions
- **Non-collagenous proteins**:
  - Calcium binding proteins: Osteonectin, Bone sialo-protein
  - Adhesion proteins: Osteopontin, Fibronectin, Thrombospondin'
  - Mineralisation protein: Osteocalcin
  - Enzymes: Collagenase, ALP, Metalloproteinase
  - Cytokines: PG, IL-1, IL-6
  - Growth factors: IGF-1, TGF-beta, PGDF
  - Hydrated mucopolysaccharide gels

21. Ans. (c) Sharpe's fibres

[Ref. Maheshwari, 4/e p8]

- **Corticocancellous junction**: Junction between cortical bone (shaft) and cancellous bone (ends)
- **Sharpe's fibres**: Strands of fibrous tissue connecting bone to periosteum
- **Osteon**: Basic structural unit of a lamellar bone
  - *Haversion canals*: Central longitudinal canals of concentric lamellae
  - *Volkmann's canals*: Horizontal canals between endosteal and periosteal surfaces

- **Cellular composition**:

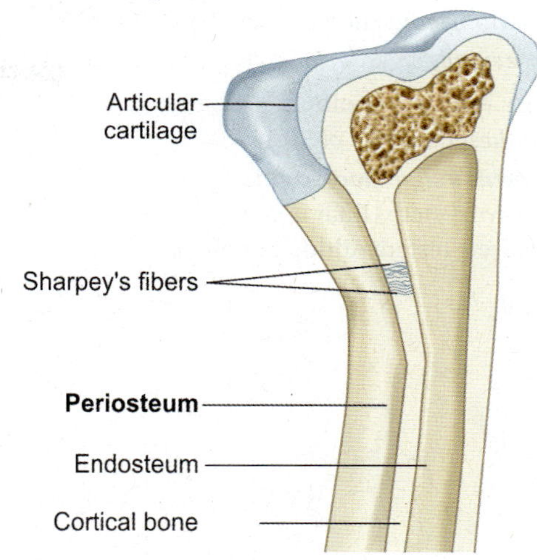

Fig. Periosteum

Cell type	Function	Composition
Osteoblasts	Ossification	ALP, Glycolytic enzymes, Phosphorylases
Osteocytes	Mature bone cells, varying activity	Glycogen, PAS positive granules
Osteoclasts	Mesenchymal cells for bone resorption	Collagenases, Acid hydrolases

22. Ans. (d) All

[Ref. Anatomy of Foot and Ankle by Kelikian, 1/e p344]

- ***Arterial supply of Talus***:
  - Anterior tibial artery/Dorsalis artery
  - Posterior tibial artery
  - Peroneal artery

23. Ans. (a) Ollier's disease

[Ref. Diagnostic Imaging of Musculoskeletal Diseases: A Systematic Approach by Khurana, 1/e p99]

- ***Osteochondrosis with Osteonecrosis***:
  - Legg-Calvé-Perthes disease
  - Kienbock disease
  - Kohler disease
  - Freiberg infraction
  - Osteochondritis dessicans

24. Ans. (d) Paget's disease

[Ref. Radiology Review Manual by Dahnert, 7/e p52]

Causes of Osteonecrosis

[Mnemonic: Infective GPS]

- Idiopathic (Perthes, Kohler)
- Neoplasia
- Fat Alcoholism
- Environmental (Frost bite, Thermal injury)
- Caisson's disease
- Trauma (Femoral neck fracture, hip dislocation)
- Irradiation
- Vasculitis (SLE, PAN, rheumatoid arthritis)
- End stage renal disease, Renal failure, Dialysis
- Sickle cell disease, Steroids
- Polycythemia, Pancreatitis
- Gaucher disease

25. Ans. (d) Abductor pollicis brevis

[Ref. Anatomy and Human Function by Field, 2/e p140]

- *Nerve supply of Abductor pollicis brevis*: Median nerve (T1)

26. Ans. (a) Adductor pollicis

[Ref. Maheshwari, 4/e p65]

- ***Froment's sign/Book sign:***
  - Nerve tested: Ulnar nerve
  - Muscle tested: Adductor pollicis

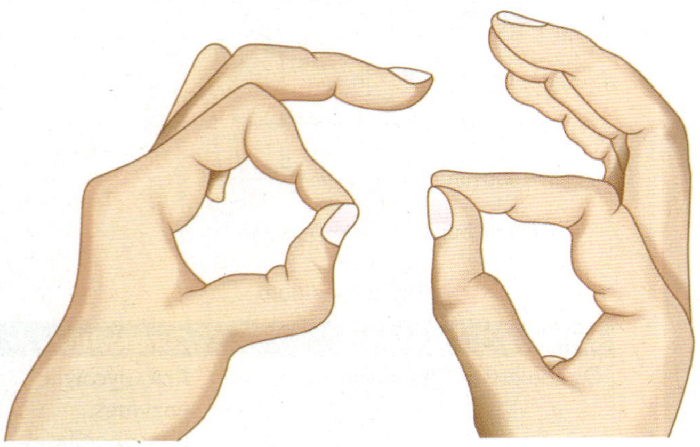

Fig. Froment's sign

27. Ans. (b) Vitamin D deficiency

[Ref. Maheshwari, 4/e p302]

28. Ans. (d) Lumbosacral spine

[Ref. Hankey's Clinical Neurology, 2/e p211]

29. Ans. (b) Teno-synovitis

[Ref. Maheshwari, 4/e p202]

- **Kanavel's sign**: Point of maximum tenderness between transverse palmar creases in case of ulnar bursitis (Acute suppurative tenosynovitis of little finger) or other flexor sheath.

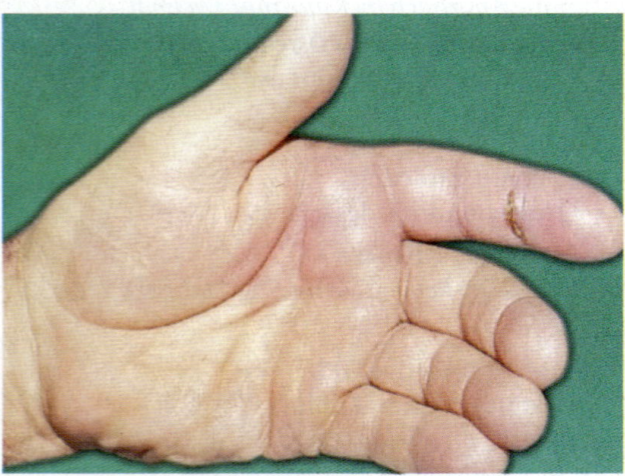

Fig. Kanavel's sign

30. Ans. (c) Hip replacement

[Ref. ICD-9 CM, Pg 1118]

- **Watson-Jones Operation**:
  - Hip arthrodesis
  - Reconstruction of lateral ligaments of ankle
  - Shoulder arthrodesis
  - Tenoplasty

31. Ans. (c) Tibia

[Ref. Orthopedics: Seeking a Balance by Sarmiento, 1/e p248]

32. Ans. (b) A piece of dead bone surrounded by infected tissue

[Ref. Maheshwari, 4/e p166]

- **Sequestrum**: Piece of dead bone surrounded by infected granulation tissue, trying to consume the sequestrum
- **Involucrum**: Dense sclerotic bone overlying a sequestrum, containing some holes (cloacae)

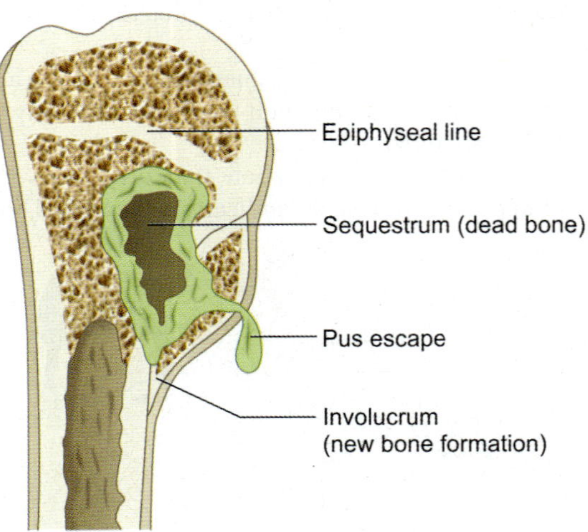

Fig. Sequestrum-Involucrum

33. Ans. (d) Abnormality over friction site

[Ref. Practical Surgery Short Clinical Cases by Goel, 1/e p263]

- **Adventitious bursa**: Abnormal bursa-like structure due to chronic or repeated friction or some mechanical cause that contains fluid-like synovial fluid

34. Ans. (b) Ulnar nerve injury

[Ref. Maheshwari, 4/e p202]

35. Ans. (d) Hyperparathyroidism

[Ref. Maheshwari, 4/e p303]

Radiological Presentation of Hyperparathyroidism

- Sub-periosteal resorption of phalanges **(Diagnostic feature)**
- Salt pepper appearance of skull
- Loss of lamina dura
- Brown's tumour
- Other features: Diffuse rarefaction of bones, central collapse of vertebral body

36. Ans. (a) ACL

[Ref. Maheshwari, 4/e p144]

Test for Injuries of Ligament Injuries

Knee ligament	Test used in injury
Medial collateral	Valgus stress + at 30° knee flexion
Lateral collateral	Varus stress + at 30° knee flexion
Anterior cruciate	Anterior drawer test +, Lachmann test +, Pivot test +
Posterior cruciate	Posterior drawer test +

37. Ans. (b) Elbow

[Ref. Emergency Orthopaedics by Sherman, 6/e p29]

- **MC site of Myositis ossificans**: Brachilais anticus muscle (Anterior to Elbow joint)

38. Ans. (b) Congenital coxa vara

[Ref. Maheshwari, 4/e p313]

- ***Fairbank's triangle***:
  - Description: Separate triangle of bone in inferior portion of metaphysis in femur head
  - Seen in: Congenital coxa vara

39. Ans. (b) Testing function of ulnar nerve

[Ref. Maheshwari, 4/e p64]

40. Ans. (d) Dorsiflexors—Ankle

[Ref. Maheshwari, 4/e p220]

41. Ans. (b) Calcium sulphate

[Ref. Maheshwari, 4/e p17]

Plaster of Paris

- $CaSO_4.½H_2O$ (Dry form)
- $CaSO_4.2H_2O$ (Wet form)

42. Ans. (b) Vertebrae

[Ref. Maheshwari, 4/e p298]

- **MC site of Osteoporosis**: Dorsolumbar spine

43. Ans. (b) Inferiortibio fibular joint

[Ref. Textbook of Therapeutic Exercises by Narayanan, 1/e p142]

44. Ans. (b) Trapezius

45. Ans. (a) Testosterone

46. Ans. (b) Acid phosphatase

[Ref. Basic Orthopaedics Sciences: The Stanmore Guide by Ramachandran, 1/e p117]

- Osteoblasts characterized by: Alkaline phosphatase
- Osteoclasts synthesize: Acid phosphatase

47. Ans. (d) All

[Ref. Pediatric Radiology by Heller & Joshi, 3/e p180]

Causes of Periosteal Reaction

- Infection: Osteomyelitis, Congenital syphilis
- Metabolic: Rickets, Scurvy
- Tumor/tumor-like diseases: Osteosarcoma, Ewing's sarcoma, Histiocytosis
- Idiopathic: Caffey's disease
- Iatrogenic/Toxic: Prostaglandins, Hypervitaminosis A

48. Ans. (c) Wolff

[Ref. The Adult Hip Volume I by Rosenberg, 2/e p207]

Wolff's Law of Bone Remodelling

- Areas of bone under high stress: Respond by increasing bone mass
- Areas of bone under low stress: Respond by lowering bone mass by either getting porous (Internal modelling) or by thinning (External modelling)

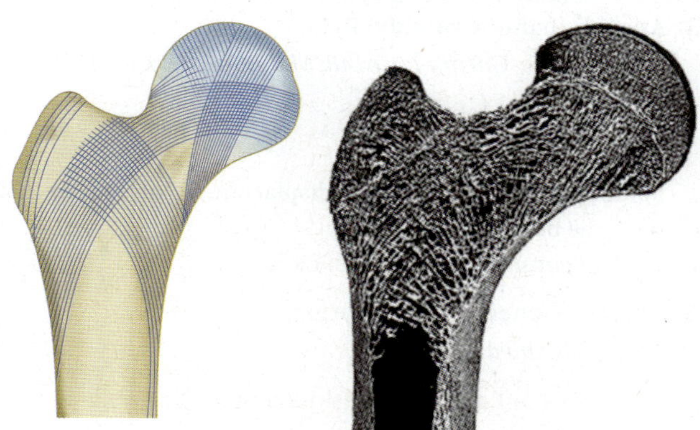

Fig. Wolff's law

49. Ans. (b) Osteochondritis of femoral epiphysis

[Ref. Maheshwari, 4/e p308]

- ***Perthe's disease*** *(Coxa plana/Pseudocoxalgia)*: Osteochon-dritis of Epiphysis of Femoral head

50. Ans. (a) Tuberculosis

51. Ans. (b) Gluteus medius

[Ref. Practical Orthopaedic Examination by Varshney, 2/e p27]

Positive Trendelenburg Test

- Gluteus medius palsy: Polio, Superior gluteal nerve palsy, L5 radiculopathy, Girdle muscular dystrophy, Cerebral palsy
- Lever failure: Fracture neck of femur, trochanteric avulsion, Coxa vara
- Fulcrum failure: Posterior dislocation of hip, Perthe's disease, Osteonecrosis
- Gluteal inhibition: Painful hip due to Arthritis/infection, Sacroilitis

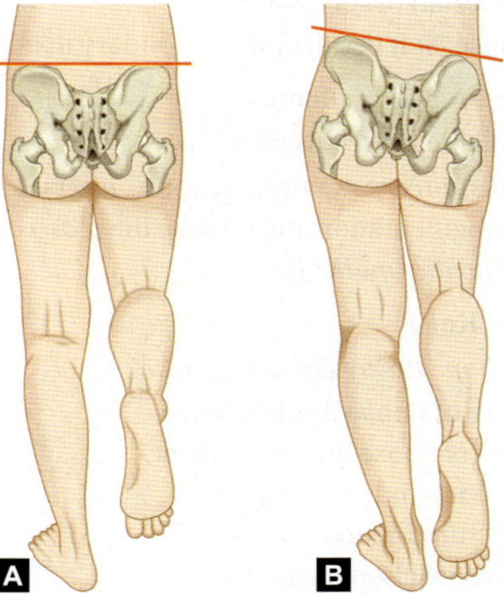

Fig. Trendelenburg test. (A) Normal; (B) Positive trendelenburg (lift side)

52. Ans. (b) Chondromalacia patellae

[Ref. Berman's Pediatric Decision Making by Berman, 5/e p446]

- **MC cause of Anterior knee pain**: Chondromalacia patellae/Patellofemoral pain syndrome

Orthopedics

53. Ans. (d) Isthmic spondylolytic

[Ref. Spine by Garfin, 1/e p148; Maheshwari, 4/e p276]

54. Ans. (b) Spondylolisthesis

[Ref. Maheshwari, 4/e p275]

Spondylolisthesis: Forward displacement of one vertebra over one below it

- Most common occurrence: L5-S1, L4-L5

55. Ans. (c) Congenital dislocation

[Ref. Maheshwari, 4/e p215]

Treatment of Congenital Dislocation of Hip

- Reduction procedures:
  - Closed manipulation
  - Traction followed by closed manipulation
  - Open reduction
- Maintenance of reduction:
  - Plaster cast: Frog-leg/Lorenz cast, Bachelor's cast
  - Von Rosen splint
- Acetabular reconstruction procedures:
  - Salter's osteotomy
  - Chiari's pelvic displacement osteotomy
  - Pemberton's pericapsular osteotomy

56. Ans. (b) Extensor pollicis brevis and Abductor pollicis longus

[Ref. Maheshwari, 4/e p294]

57. Ans. (b) Involucrum

[Ref. Maheshwari, 4/e p275]

58. Ans. (c) Soft tissue

[Ref. Soft Tissue Tumours by Weiss, 6/e p62]

- **Heterotopic ossification**: Localized, self-limiting reparative lesion of soft tissues
  - Cause: Soft tissue injury secondary to obvious trauma

59. Ans. (c) Medial malleolus

[Ref. NMS Medicine Case Book, p88]

- ***Venous ulcers***: Causes painful *ulcers* associated with hyperpigmentation and edema; the *most common location* is the *medial malleolus*

60. Ans. (b) Knee

[Ref. Orthopedics by Ebnezar, 4/e p429]

- **MC site of Loose bodies: Knee**
- Causes of Loose bodies in knee:
  - Osteochondritis dissecans
  - Fractured articular surface
  - Synovial chondromatosis
  - Osteophytes
  - Damaged menisci

61. Ans. (a) Vastus medialis

[Ref. Patellofemoral Disorders by Biedert, 1/e p222]

- ***Patellofemoral ligament*** is dynamized by V*astus medialis* obliquus muscle and the two functions as a complex that acts to *prevent patellar dislocation*

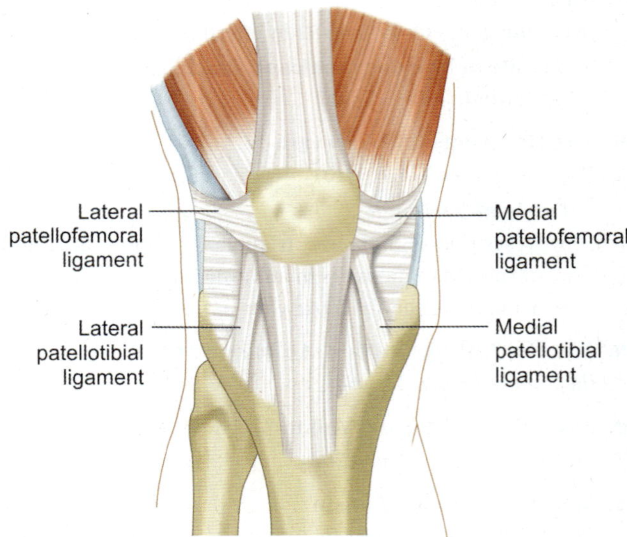

Fig. Ligaments

62. Ans. (c) Talocalcaneal

[Ref. Orthopedic Dictionary by Ziede, 1/e p389]

Kite's Angle: Talocalcaneal Angle

- Normal angle: 20-35 degrees
- Hindfoot valgus: >35 degrees
- Hindfoot varus: <35 degrees

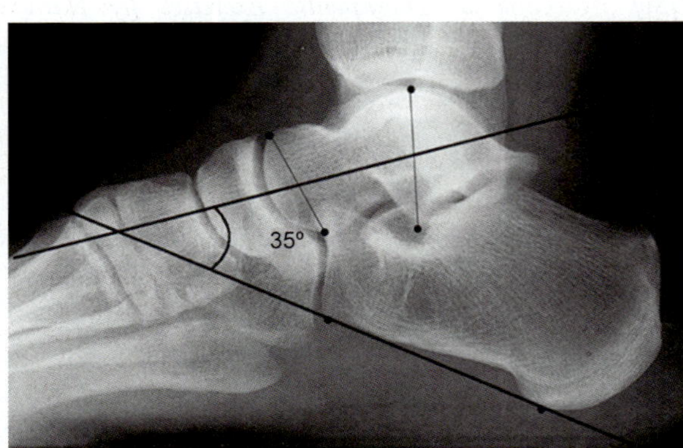

Fig. Kite's Angle

63. Ans. (a) Trauma

[Ref. Foot Ulcers by Acton, 1/e p4]

- **MC cause of Amputation in Developing countries**: Trauma
- MC cause (Non-traumatic) of Amputation in Developing countries: Diabetic foot ulcers

64. Ans. (b) Dermatomyositis

[Ref. Rheumatic Diseases by Klippel, 13/e p364]

- **Gottron's papules** are scaly, erythematous, or violaceous papules and plaques located over bony prominences, particularly over the small joints of the hands, elbows, knees, and ankles
- Seen in: Dermatomyositis

65. Ans. (c) Osteomalacia

[Ref. Rubin's Pathology, 5/e p550]

Pseudofractures of Milkman-Looser Syndrome

- Specific finding in Osteomalacia
- Radiolucent transverse defects
- Seen in: Concave side of long bone, Medial side of femoral neck, Ischial/Pubic rami, Ribs, Scapula

66. Ans. (d) Congenital dislocation of hip

[Ref. Clinical Symposia, Volume 42, p17]

- Recurrence risk for congenital dislocation of the hip is as high as 6%

67. Ans. (c) Femoral head fractures

[Ref. Intraarticular Fractures by Malhotra, 1/e p347]

Pipkin's Classification

- Type I: Fracture distal to the fovea capitis, not involving the weight-bearing surface
- Type II: Fracture proximal to the fovea capitis, involving the weightbearing surface
- Type III: Type I or II fracture with a fracture of the femoral neck
- Type IV: Type I or II fracture with a fracture of the acetabular wall

68. Ans. (c) 16 -18 years

[Ref. Musculoskeletal Emergencies by Browner, 1/e]

Proximal tibial epiphysis and the ossification center of the Tibial tubercle eventually fuse at 13–15 years in girls and 15–19 years in boys

69. Ans. (a) Anterior cruciate ligament

[Ref. Orthopaedic Medicine by Ombregt, 3/e pe266]

- Anterior cruciate ligament (ACL) inserts into the medial side of the lateral femoral condyle, preventing excessive anterior gliding as well as external rotation of Tibia
- During flexion, the femoral condyles tend to roll backwards over the tibia; this is checked by ACL which induces a simultaneous anterior gliding of the femur

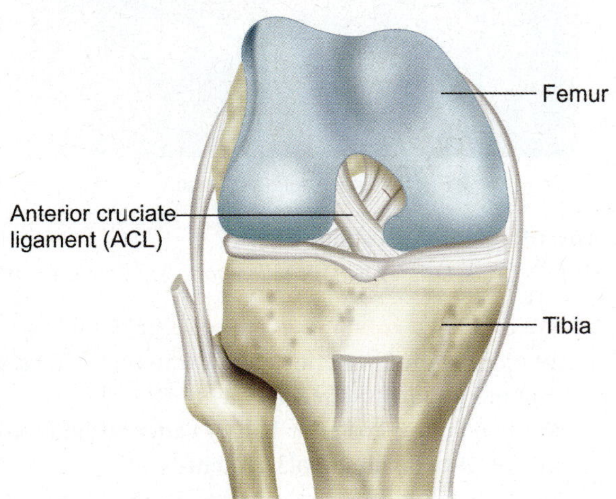

Fig. ACL

70. Ans. (c) Thick and irregular

[Ref. Orthopaedic Medicine by Ombregt, 3/e pe266]

Aggressive PR	Non-aggressive PR
Spiculated (Hair-on-end/ Sunburst)	Thin
Laminated	Solid
Disorganised	Thick and Irregular
Interrupted	Septated
Codman's triangle	

71. Ans. (a) Thomas splint

[Ref. Orthopaedics and Fractures by Duckworth, 4/e p35]

Methods of Holding Reduction (Immobilization)

- Sustained Traction:
  - Traction by gravity
  - Balanced traction (Skin traction, Skeletal traction)
  - Fixed traction (principle is the same as for balanced traction, except that in this case the limb is held in a Thomas's splint and the traction tapes are tied to the distal end of the splint while the proximal padded ring of the splint abuts firmly against the pelvis)
- Cast splintage
- Functional bracing
- Internal fixation
- External fixation

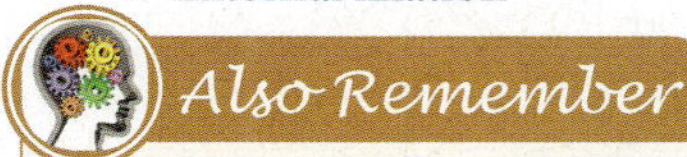

- Fixed Traction
  - Traction is applied against a counter force applied to the patient's body, e.g. a collar and cuff sling utilizes the weight of the arm to apply traction to the upper arm or shoulder
  - Counter force is applied to the part of the sling which passes around the patient's neck

72. Ans. (b) Vastus medialis obliquus

[Ref. The Patellofemoral Joint by Fox, 1/e p356]

- Primary stabilizer to Lateral patellar subluxation is the Vastus medialis obliquus (VMO)
- VMO resists the excessive valgus vector force commonly seen with patellofemoral misalignment

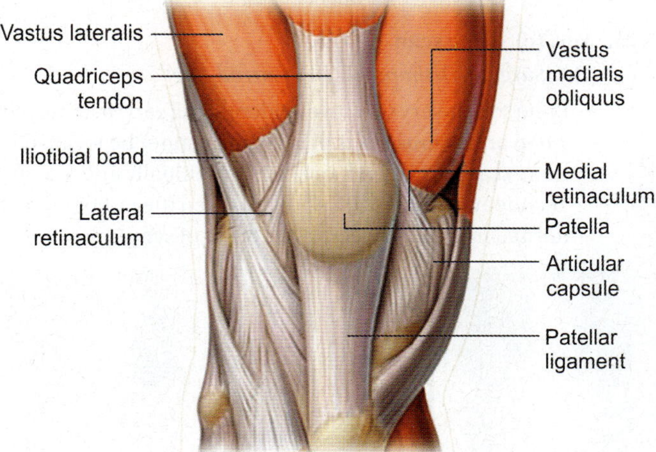

Fig. Vastus medialis obliquus

Orthopedics

73. Ans. (a) Cervical

[Ref. Orthopedic Physical Assessment by Evans, 2/e p63]

- Cervical region is the most mobile of the spinal column with a range of motion of approximately 80-90 of flexion, 70 of extension, 20–45 of lateral flexion, and up to 90 of rotation to both sides

74. Ans. (a) Anteroposterior pelvis with both hips

[Ref. Maheshwari, 4/e p215]

Shenton's Line

- SL is an imaginary line drawn along the inferior border of the superior pubic ramus (superior border of the obturator foramen) and along the inferomedial border of the neck of femur
- SL should be continuous and smooth
- SL is seen on AP view of both hips
- SL is broken in: Fracture neck of femur, developmental dysplasia of hip

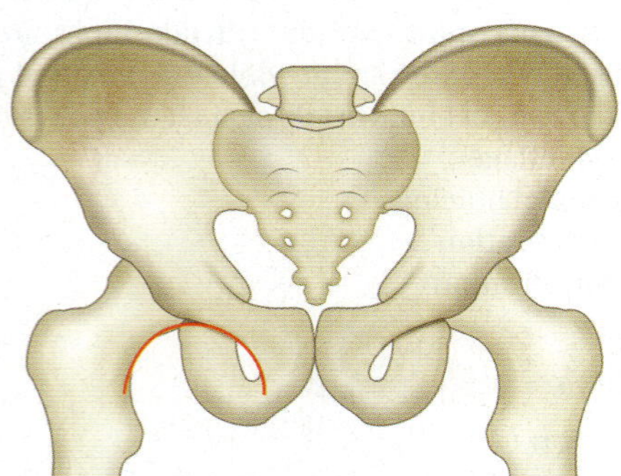

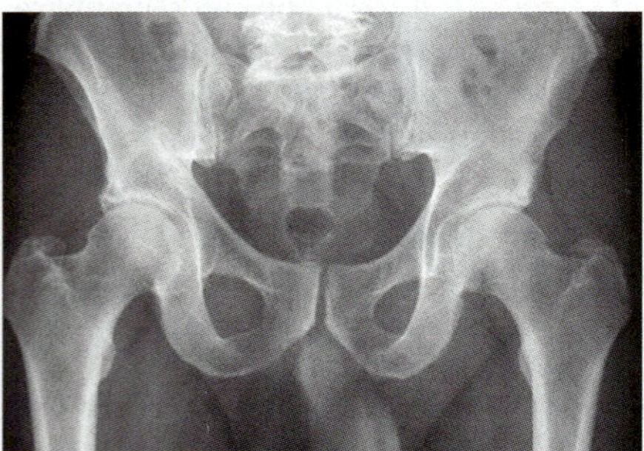

Fig. Shenton's Line

75. Ans. (c) Bone scan

[Ref. Surgery, Orthopaedics by Carroll, 1/e]

- Bone scan is very sensitive in identifying early osteomyelitis when an obvious focus of infection cannot be localized
- Bone scans are often more sensitive initially and a 3-phase Technetium bone scan is helpful when the radiographs are normal in first 2–3 weeks after onset of symptoms

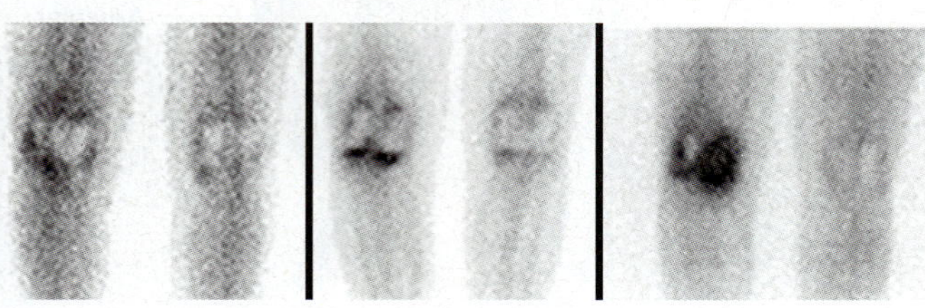

Fig. Bone Scan showing infection

76. Ans. (a) 1st dorsal webspace

[Ref. Rapid Orthopedic Diagnosis by Mostofi, 1/e p122]

Autonomous Zones of Nerves in hand

- Median nerve: Tip of index finger
- Radial nerve: Dorsal 1st webspace
- Ulnar nerve: Tip of little finger

77. Ans. (b) Calcaneum

[Ref. Skeletal Trauma by Browner, 4/e Volume1 p2631]

Gissane Angle (Critical Angle)

- An angular measurement made directly inferior to the Lateral process of the talus
- Formed by the downward and upward slopes of the Calcaneal superior surface
- Better seen on a lateral plain film of the Calcaneus and Hindfoot
- Normal value: 120–145°
- Gissane's angle, together with Böhler's angle, are commonly used to evaluate the severity of a calcaneal fracture, and the goal of a surgical treatment is to restore these angles to normal values

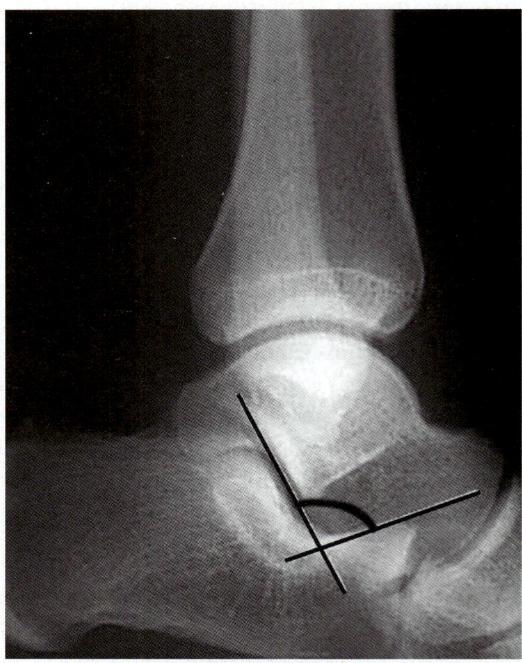

Fig. Critical Angle of Gissane

78. Ans. (d) Stability of spine

[Ref. DeLee & Drez's Orthopaedic Sports Medicine, 1/e p1534]

Denis's model – 3 column system of Spinal Stability

- Anterior column: Anterior half of vertebral bodies, Disks and Anterior longitudinal ligament
- Middle column: Posterior half of vertebral bodies, Disks and Posterior longitudinal ligament
- Posterior column: Neural arches, Posterior ligamentous complex (Supraspinous ligament, Interspinous ligament, Ligamentum flavum, Joint capsules)

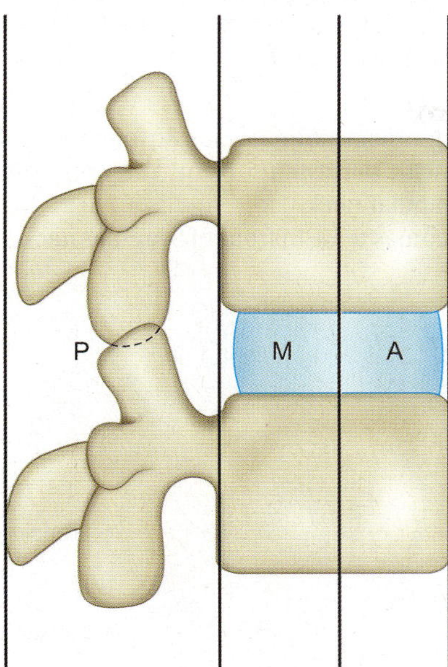

Fig. Denis classification

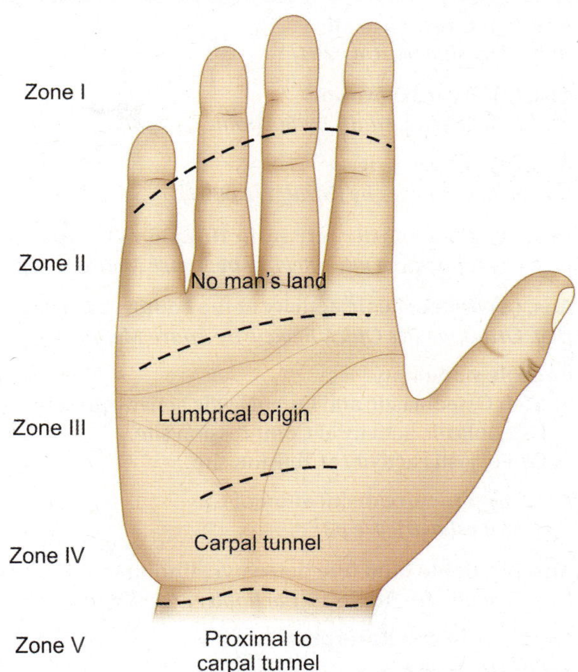

Fig. No Man's Land (Zone II)

79. Ans. (c) Jumping athletes

[Ref. Applied Anatomy and Biomechanics by Ackland, 2/e p259]

- Distance runners have relatively short lower limbs and a low crural index
- Jumpers are among the tallest of elite athletes, with a high relative lower limb length and a high crural index; these proportionality characteristics provide a mechanically advantageous lever system for jumping

80. Ans. (b) Zone II

[Ref. Orthopedic Secrets by Namdari, 4/e p95]

- "No man's land is the area in which both flexor tendons of the fingers pass through the tight fibro-osseous tunnel
- Designated as Zone II, it is the area between the distal palmar crease and the insertion of the FDS at the mid-portion of the middle phalanx
- Repair of tendon lacerations in this region requires meticulous technique and complications are more frequent

81. Ans. (c) Patient's finger is blackening

[Ref. Emergency Triage by ALSG, 3/e p181]

- Blackening of finger after fracture is an indication of cut-off of blood supply
- This vascular compromise may further lead to complication like gangrene
- So this should be the first priority for treatment

82. Ans. (b) Synovial joint

[Ref. Anatomy and Human Movement by Palastanga, 6/e p484]

- Eighth and ninth costal cartilage joints are synovial, while the tenth is more like a Fibrous joint
- Small synovial joints are also formed between the adjacent margins of the fifth to ninth costal cartilages
- All these synovial joints are surrounded by fibrous capsules, strengthened anteriorly and posteriorly by oblique ligaments.

HIGH YIELD MCQs ANSWERS WITH EXPLANATIONS

1. Ans. (a) Primary cartilaginous

[Ref. Medical Sciences by Naish, Student Consult Online]

- **Primary cartilaginous joints (Synchondroses)**: Joint bridged by hyaline cartilage, temporary in nature and associated with growth of bones
  - Example: Epiphyseal growth plates

2. Ans. (c) Iliac crest

[Ref. The Adult and Pediatric Spine Volume 1 by Weisel, 3/e p1191]

- **MC donor site for autologous bone graft: Posterior iliac crest**
- Second MC site for autologous bone graft: Anterior iliac crest

3. Ans. (b) Tenosynovitis

[Ref. Maheshwari, 4/e p202]

4. Ans. (b) Procollagen-I; (c) ALP

[Ref. Fractures in Adults by Buchohlz, 7/e p498]

Markers of Bone Formation

- Osteocalcin
- Bone-specific Alkaline phosphatase (BALP)
- Total Alkaline Phosphatase
- Procollagen I C-terminal extension peptide
- Procollagen I N-terminal extension peptide

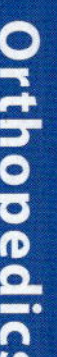

5. Ans. (a) Fracture of atlas
[Ref. Maheshwari, 4/e p264]

6. Ans. (c) Hydroxyproline
[Ref. Fractures in Adults by Buchohlz, 7/e p498]

7. Ans. (d) All are true
[Ref. Sports injuries by Doral, 1/e p694]

8. Ans. (d) Osteoblastic activity in Howship's lacunae
[Ref. Orthopaedics Quick Review by Apurv Mehra, 1/e p11]

9. Ans. (a) Osteoclastic activity at the compression site
[Ref. Orthopaedics Quick Review by Apurv Mehra, 1/e p11]

Bone Remodelling
- Both Osteoblastic and Osteoclastic activity present
- Osteoblastic activity at Compression site
- Osteoclastic activity at Tension site

10. Ans. (b) Fracture dislocation of C2
[Ref. Maheshwari, 4/e p3]

11. Ans. (c) Urine total free deoxypyridinoline
[Ref. Fractures in Adults by Buchohlz, 7/e p498]

Markers of Bone Resorption
- **Serum markers**:
  - Tartrate resistant acid phosphatase (TRACP)
  - Tartrate resistant acid phosphatase 5b (TRACP 5b)
  - C-terminal cross-linking telopeptide of Type I Collagen (CTX)
  - N-terminal cross-linking telopeptide of Type I Collagen (NTX)
  - C-terminal cross-linking telopeptide of Type I Collagen (ICTX)
- **Urine markers**:
  - Deoxypyridinaline (DPD)
  - Pyridinaline (PYD)
  - Hydroxyproline (Hyp)
  - C-terminal cross-linking telopeptide of Type I Collagen (CTX)

12. Ans. (c) Movement of IT towards lateral border of patella; (d) Movement of IT towards centre of patella
[Ref. Basic Biomechanics of Musculoskeletal System by Frankel, 3/e p184]

13. Ans. (b) Osteocalcin
[Ref. Fractures in Adults by Buchohlz, 7/e p498]

14. Ans. (d) Prepatellar bursa
[Ref. Maheshwari, 4/e p292]

15. Ans. (b) Genu varum
[Ref. Maheshwari, 4/e p315]
Blount's disease: Genu varum in which proximal tibial epiphysis (Posteromedial part) fails to grow during first 3 years of life

16. Ans. (a) Flexion
[Ref. Maheshwari, 4/e p259]

17. Ans. (d) Hydroxy-apatite
[Ref. Maheshwari, 4/e p9]

Composition of Bone
- Organic matrix (30–35%): Collagen
- Inorganic matrix (65–70%): Calcium-hydroxyl apatite

18. Ans. (a) Anterior surface of glenoid labrum
[Ref. Maheshwari, 4/e p87]

Bankart's Lesion
- Shoulder dislocation causes Stripping of Glenoid labrum along with periosteum from Anterior surface of glenoid and scapular neck
- Head comes to lie in front of Scapular neck

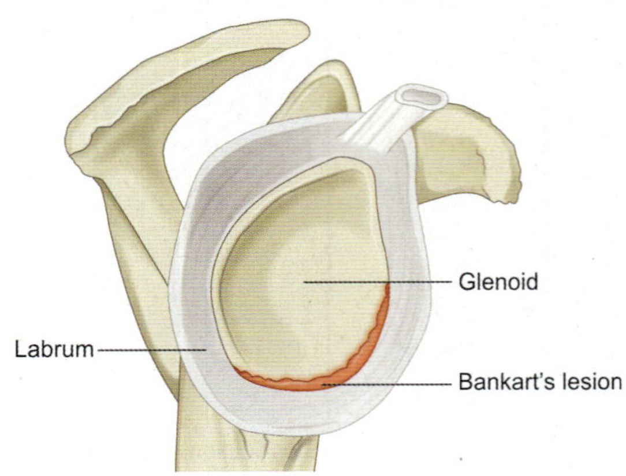

Fig. Bankart's lesion

19. Ans. (b) C7
[Ref. Clinical Examination in Orthopaedics by Iyer, 1/e p37]

Key Movements in Hand
- Wrist extension: C6
- Wrist flexion: C7
- Finger extension: C7
- Finger flexion: C8
- Finger adduction, abduction: T1

20. Ans. (c) Recurrent dislocation of shoulder
[Ref. Maheshwari, 4/e p87]

Hill Sachs Lesion
- Depression on Humeral head in its' Posterolateral quadrant
- Underlying cause: Impingement by Anterior edge of Glenoid on head as it dislocates

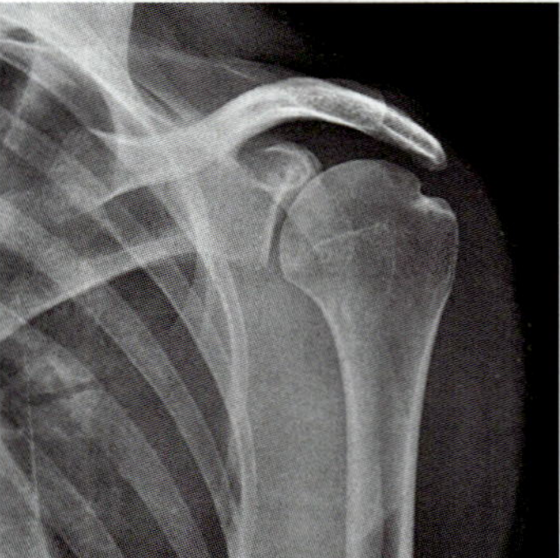

Fig. Hill Sachs lesion

21. Ans. (c) Anterior dislocation of shoulder
[Ref. Maheshwari, 4/e p87]

Tests of Shoulder Dislocation
- Duga's test
- Hamilton's ruler test

22. Ans. (b) Elbow
[Ref. Surgical Anatomy of Hand and Upper Extremity by Doyle, 1/e p405]
- **Myositis ossificans**: Ossification in muscle (Most commonly Brachialis) after trauma especially elbow dislocation

23. Ans. (a) Immobilization
[Ref. Maheshwari, 4/e p51]

Treatment of Myositis Ossificans
- Active stage: Immobilization, Resting of limb
- Late stage: Physiotherapy
- Surgical excision of bone mass
- Massage following injury is Contraindicated

24. Ans. All Choices
[Ref. The New England Journal of Medicine, Volume 185, Pg 49]

25. Ans. (a) Polymethyl methacrylate
[Ref. Reconstructive Surgery by Chiang, 1/e p153]

26. Ans. (c) Muscle fibres
[Ref. Bone and Muscle by Rogers, 1/e p200]

Myositis Ossificans Progressive
- Description: Group after group of muscles become ossified, until individual is completely rigid with difficulty in breathing and swallowing
- **No treatment possible**: Progressive until death occurs, usually due to pulmonary infection secondary to respiratory difficulties (involvement of intercostal muscles)

27. Ans. (b) Lung disease
[Ref. Shafer's Textbook of Oral Pathology, 6/e p860]

28. Ans. (a) Superior gluteal
[Ref. Practical Orthopaedic Examination by Varshney, 2/e p27]

29. Ans. (a) Lachman's test
[Ref. Maheshwari, 4/e p144]

30. Ans. (d) TB hip joint
[Ref. Practical Orthopaedic Examination by Varshney, 2/e p27]

31. Ans. (b) Intracapsular fracture neck of femur
[Ref. Practical Orthopaedics by Ebnezar, 1/e p18]

32. Ans. (a) Anterior cruciate ligament
[Ref. Maheshwari, 4/e p144]

33. Ans. (b) Sequestrum
[Ref. Maheshwari, 4/e p166]

34. Ans. (b) Right
[Ref. Elsevier Comprehensive Guide 2009, p410]

35. Ans. (c) Varus/valgus stress test in 30° of flexion
[Ref. Maheshwari, 4/e p144]

36. Ans. (a) Internal rotation of femur over stabilized tibia
[Ref. Grey's Anatomy, 39th Ed., p1482]

Locking and Unlocking of Knee
- **Locking**: When tibia is stabilized (Foot fixe), Femur rotates medically to lock the knee
  - Locking occurs in last 30 degrees of extension
  - Muscle involved in Knee locking and extension: Quadriceps femoris
- **Unlocking**: Femur moves laterally on Stabilized tibia (Fixed foot)
  - Unlocking is need to intitate flexion at knee
  - Muscle involved: Popliteus

37. Ans. (c) Poor vascularity
[Ref. Sports Medicine by Allman, 2/e p306]

38. Ans. (c) Hydroxyproline
[Ref. Fractures in Adults by Buchohlz, 7/e p498]

39. Ans. (b) Apposition
[Ref. Essential Histology by Cormack, 2/e p185]

40. Ans. (c) Labeled tetracycline
[Ref. Replacement of Renal Function by Dialysis by Maher, 3/e p921]

41. Ans. (c) Rotate
[Ref. Maheshwari, 4/e p146]

42. Ans. (b) Fracture knee
[Ref. Medical Surgical Nursing by Lewis, 9th Ed., p1516]

43. Ans. (a) Medial meniscus is more mobile than lateral
[Ref. Maheshwari, 4/e p146]
- **Medical meniscal injury is more common**: Medial meniscus is less mobile due to its fixation to medial collateral ligament

44. Ans. (b) Less mobile
[Ref. Maheshwari, 4/e p146]

45. Ans. (a) Radial nerve
[Ref. Textbook of Orthopaedics by Ebnezar, 4/e p334]

46. Ans. (c) Defects of long bones of limbs
[Ref. The Netter Collection of Medical Illustrations by Parker, 2/e p161]

Phocomelia
- Intersegmental deficiency with Failure of Proximodistal development
- May be total (Limb/hand directly attached to trunk) or partial (Limb/hand attached to a deficient severely shortened limb)

47. Ans. (a) Pelvis; e. Greater trochanter
[Ref. Frontiers in Fracture Management by Bunker, 1/e p57]

Donor Sites for Bone Graft

Donor sites lower limb	Donor site upper limb
Pelvis (Anterior/Posterior iliac crest) 1st order Greater trochanter 1st order Femoral condyles 2nd order Tibial metaphysis 2nd order Medial malleolus 2nd order	Olecranon 2nd order Radial styloid 2nd order

48. Ans. (c) Medical meniscus injury; (d) Lateral Meniscus injury
[Ref. Physical Medicine and rehabilitation by Delisa, 4/e p58]

49. Ans. (d) Lateral condyle humerus
[Ref. Multiple Sources]

50. Ans. (a) Hypoxemia; (b) Fractured fragments of bone; (d) Muscle interposition in between fractured fragments; e. Early mobilization

[Ref. Classic Papers in Orthopaedics by Kader, 1/e p500]

51. Ans. All Choices

[Ref. Textbook of Oral and Maxillofacial Surgery by Balaji, 1/e p555]

52. Ans. (a) Micromovements between the fracture fragments; (b) Appropriate approximation of the fragments

[Ref. A Textbook of Fractures and Related Injuries by Bonnin, 1/e p140]

53. Ans. (c) SCFE

[Ref. Maheshwari, 4/e p314]

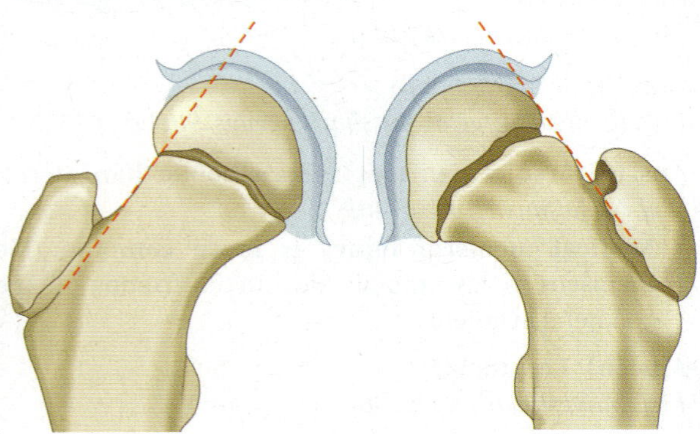

Fig. Normal and Trethowan's sign

Trethowan's Sign

- Description: Line drawn along superior surface of neck remains superior to femoral head
- Seen in: Slipped capital femoral epiphysis

54. Ans. (a) Congenital dislocation of hip

[Ref. Maheshwari, 4/e p214]

Ortolani's Test

- Description: Hips and knees held in flexed position is gradually abducted, a 'click' of entrance felt as femoral head slips into acetabulum
- Seen in: Congenital dislocation of hip

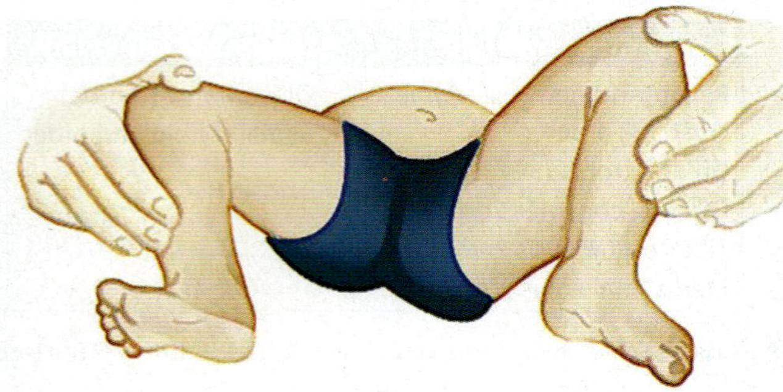

Fig. Ortolani's test

55. Ans. (c) Avascular necrosis of head of femur

[Ref. Orthopaedics for Physical Assistants by Hart, 1/e p9]

56. Ans. (b) Young female

[Ref. Arthritis and Arthroplasty: The Hip by Brown, 1/e p24]

- Metal-on-metal articulation in Hip replacement is problematic in:
  - Young female of child bearing years
  - History of renal or cardiac disease
  - History of metal hypersensitivity

57. Ans. (b) High density polythene debris

[Ref. AIPGME 2004; A Review by Koli, p12]

58. Ans. (d) Hip replacement

[Ref. ICD-9 CM, Pg 1118]

59. Ans. (d) Chronic ankle instability

[Ref. ICD-9 CM, Pg 1118]

60. Ans. (b) CDH in infancy

[Ref. Maheshwari, 4/e p213]

Barlow's Test

- Description:
  - First part: Child knees flexed and hips flexed to right angle then hip is gently adducted
  - Second part: Hips in 90° flexion and fully adducted then thighs are gently abducted
- Seen in: Congenital dislocation of hip

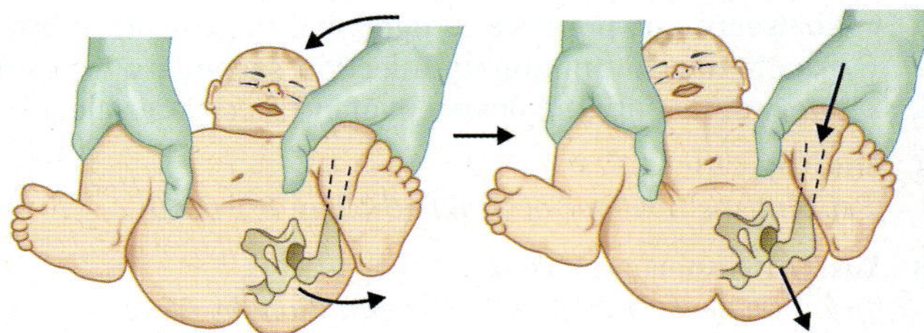

Fig. Barlow's test

61. Ans. (a) Congenital dislocation of hip

[Ref. Maheshwari, 4/e p214]

62. Ans. (b) Rickets

63. Ans. (b) Undescended scapula

[Ref. Maheshwari, 4/e p217]

- **Sprengel's deformity**: Failure of descent of scapula which is developmentally a cervical appendage, i.e. Congenital high scapula

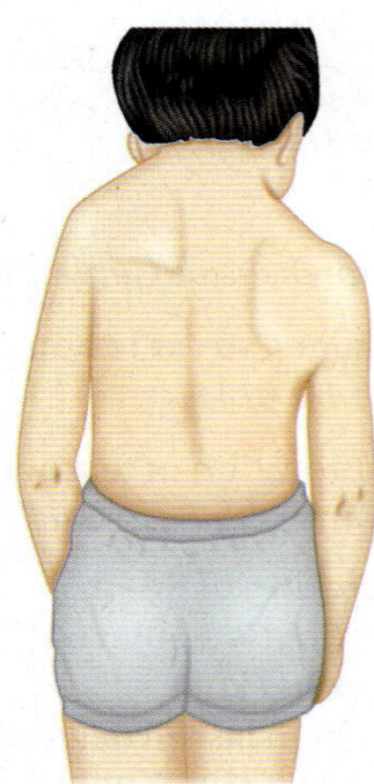

Fig. Sprengel's deformity

64. Ans. (a) Femoral condyles; (b) Pelvis; (c) Greater trochanter; (d) Tibial metaphysis
[Ref. Frontiers in Fracture Management by Bunker, 1/e p57]

65. Ans. (b) Tibia vara
[Ref. Maheshwari, 4/e p315]

66. Ans. (d) Osteogenesis imperfecta
[Ref. Maheshwari, 4/e p307]
Osteogenesis imperfecta: Brittle bone disease, Fragilitas ossium

67. Ans. (d) Allows flexion, rotation and abduction
[Ref. Medical Sciences by Naish & Court, 2/e p425]

68. Ans. (c) It causes subluxation of inferior radioulnar joint
[Ref. Textbook of Orthopaedics and Trauma by Kulkarni, 2/e p2210]

69. Ans. (c) Congenital talipes equino varus
[Ref. Textbook of Orthopedics by Kotwal, 1/e p55]

70. Ans. (b) Valgus deformity; (c)Varus deformity
[Ref. Fundamental Orthopedic Management by Manske, 4/e p430]

71. Ans. (d) Teres major
[Ref. Maheshwari, 4/e p85]

Rotator Cuff Muscles
- Supraspinatus
- Infraspinatus
- Teres major
- Subscapularis

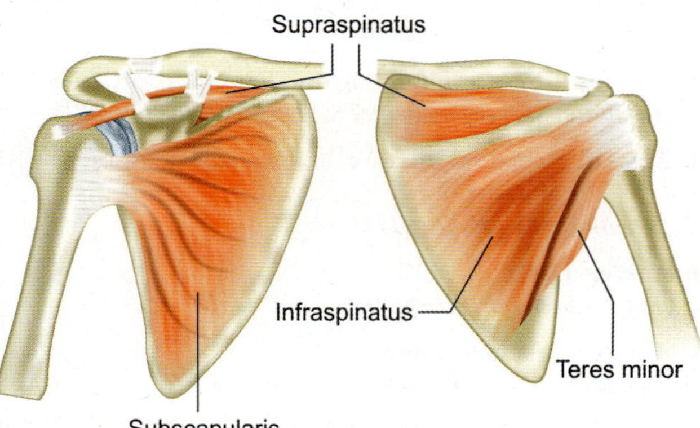

Fig. Rotator Cuff

72. Ans. (c) Club feet
[Ref. professional Guide to Diseases by Williams & Wilkins, 9/e p327]

73. Ans. (c) Inferior
[Ref. Dislocations of Shoulder: Reconstruction by Williams, 3/e p172]

74. Ans. (b) Biceps long head
[Ref. The Scientific and Clinical Application of Elastic Resistance by Page & Ellenbecker, 1/e p48]

75. Ans. (d) Upper 1/3rd of Ulna
[Ref. Maheshwari, 4/e p106]

Monteggia Fracture Dislocation
- Fracture upper 1/3 of ulna
- Dislocation of head of radius

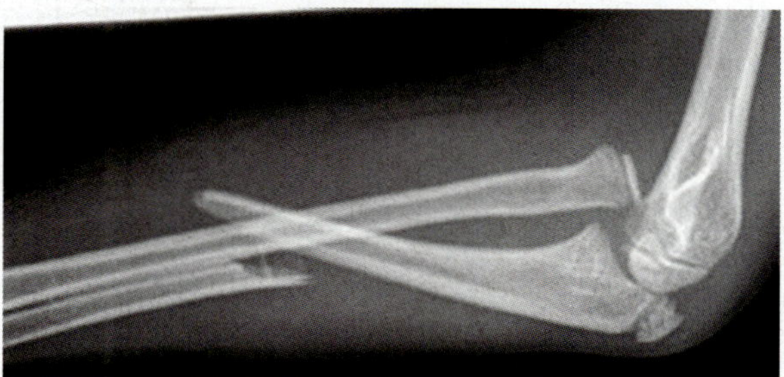

Fig. Monteggia fracture

76. Ans. (c) Supraspinatus and subscapularis
[Ref. Atlas of Orthopaedic Surgery by Zuckerman, 1/e p3]
Rotator interval: Triangular space between supraspinatus and subscapularis tendons

77. Ans. (b) Osteopetrosis; e. Osteosclerosis
[Ref. Encyclopedia of Human Genetics and Disease Volume I, 1/e p618]

78. Ans. (a) Calcium levels; (b) Phosphorus levels; (c) Parathormone levels

79. Ans. (d) Lower end of radius
[Ref. Maheshwari, 4/e p106]

Galeazzi Fracture Dislocation
- Fracture lower 1/3 of radius
- Dislocation/subluxation of distal radioulnar joint

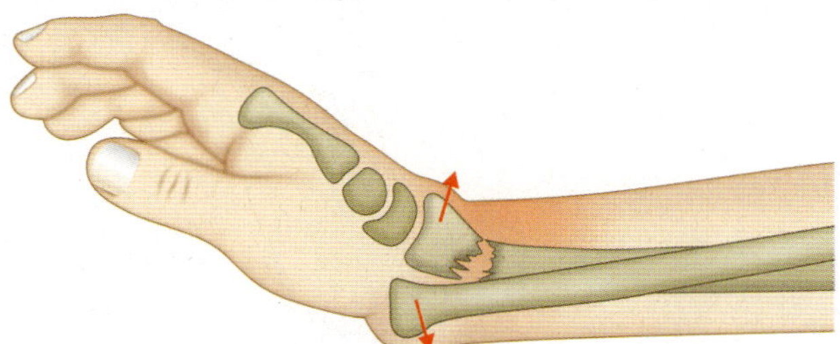

Fig. Galeazzi fracture

80. Ans. All Choices

81. Ans. (a) Calcaneocuboid, talonavicular and talocalcaneal
[Ref. Maheshwari, 4/e p209]

82. Ans. (c) Inadequate fusion
[Ref. Maheshwari, 4/e p209]

83. Ans. (a) Infants
[Ref. Maheshwari, 4/e p310]
Caffey's disease (Infantile cortical hyperostosis): Formation of subperiosteal bone on shafts of long bones and mandible

84. Ans. (b) Renal osteodystrophy
[Ref. Musculoskeletal Imaging by Chew, 3/e p179]

85. Ans. (c) Vertical talus
[Ref. Essentials of Skeletal Radiology by Yochum & Rowe, 3/e p334]

86. Ans. (d) Hypophosphatemia
[Ref. E Study Guide: Bioinorganic Medicinal Chemistry]

87. Ans. (d) Scaphoid cast
[Ref. Maheshwari, 4/e p111]

Scaphoid cast: Glass-holding position (Wrist in slight dorsiflexion and radial deviation)

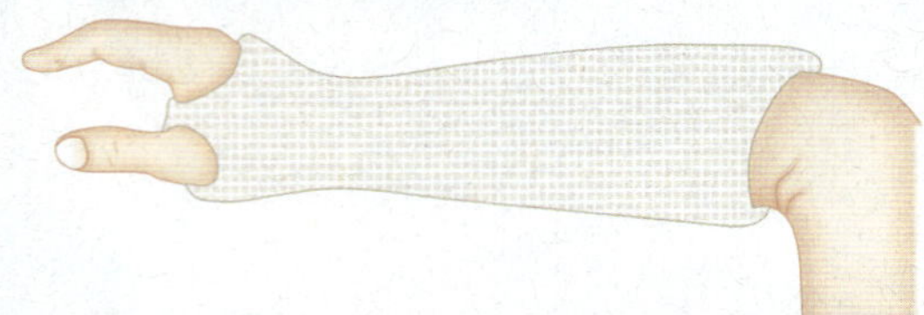

Fig. Scaphoid cast

88. Ans. (b) Calcitonin
[Ref. Maheshwari, 4/e p307]
- Treatment of choice for Paget's disease of bone:
  - Bisphosphonates (Aledronate, Etidronate, Risedronate, Tiludronate, Pamidronate, Zoledronate)
  - Calcitonin

89. Ans. (d) Anterior dislocation of shoulder
[Ref. Maheshwari, 4/e p87]

Duga's Test
- Inability to touch opposite shoulder
- Seen in: Dislocation of shoulder

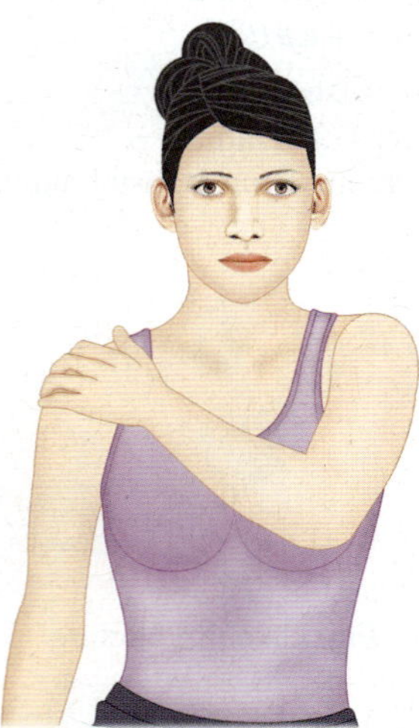

Fig. Duga's test

90. Ans. (c) Plicamycin
[Ref. Maheshwari, 4/e p307]

91. Ans. (a) Osteogenesis imperfecta
[Ref. Human Malformations and Related Anomalies by Hall, 2/e p247]

Conditions with Wormian Bones
- Osteogenesis imperfecta
- Progeria
- Hypothyroidism
- Hypophosphatasia
- Cleidocranial dysostosis
- Mandibular dysplasia

92. Ans. (d) All of the above
[Ref. Current Concepts of Bone Fragility by Hans, 1/e p227]
- **Complications of Paget's disease of bone**:
  - Fractures
  - Spinal/cranial nerve compression
  - Deafness
  - Heart failure
  - Osteosracoma

93. Ans. (c) Vitamin C
[Ref. Essentials of Biochemistry by Naik, 1/e p103]

94. Ans. (c) Patella
[Ref. Essentials of Orthopaedics for Physiotherapists by Ebnezar, 1/e p42]

Common Sites of Avscular Necrosis
- Head of femur (Fracture neck of femur, Dislocation of hip)
- Body of talus (Fracture neck of talus)
- Proximal pole of scaphoid (Fracture through waist of scaphoid)

95. Ans. (a) Osteopetrosis
[Ref. Maheshwari, 4/e p307]

96. Ans. (d) Calcaneus
[Ref. Fractures of Calcaneus by Dhillon, 1/e p16]

97. Ans. (d) Subscapularis
[Ref. Sports Medicine by Busconi, 1/e p189]

98. Ans. (c) Acromioclavicular dislocation
[Ref. Adult Orthopaedic Nursing by Schoen, 1/e p409]

99. Ans. (d) L4–L5
[Ref. International Neurology by Carroll, p580]

100. Ans. (a) Increased thickening of trabeculae; (b) Fracture & Collapse of cancellous bone

101. Ans. (b) Infantile cortical hyperostosis
[Ref. Maheshwari, 4/e p310]

102. Ans. (a) Ulnar collateral ligament injury of MCP Joint
[Ref. hand Surgery by Berger & Weiss, Volume I, p202]

103. Ans. (a) Avulsion fracture of extensor tendon of distal phalanx
[Ref. Maheshwari, 4/e p114]

104. Ans. e. L5-S1
[Ref. Maheshwari, 4/e p275]

105. Ans. (d) Fracture humerus
[Ref. Maheshwari, 4/e p90]
- Hanging cast used for: Lower 1/3 of fractures of Humerus

106. Ans. (c) Between distal phalanx crease and proximal phalanx
[Ref. Hospital for Special Surgery Orthopaedics by Sculco, 1/e p533]

107. Ans. (c) Into the webspace

108. Ans. (c) C6–C7
[Ref. Bonica's Management of Pain by Fishman, 1/e p1031]
- MC site of disc herniation and Cervical spondylosis: C6–C7 > C5–C6

109. Ans. (d) Salter

110. Ans. (b) Intracapsular fracture neck of femur
[Ref. Practical Orthopedics by Ebnezar, 1/e p18]
- **Telescopic test** is significantly positive in: Non-union fracture of Neck of femur

111. Ans. (a) A; (d) D

112. Ans. (c) Outward deviation of great toe
[Ref. Maheshwari, 4/e p90]

Deformities of Toes

- **Hallux Valgus**: Lateral deviation of Great toe at Metatarso-phalangeal joint
- **Hallux rigidus**: Stiff great toe due to osteoarthritis of metatarsophalangeal joint
- **Hammer toe**: Fixed flexion deformity of an Interphalangeal joint of toe, with callosity over prominent proximal joint

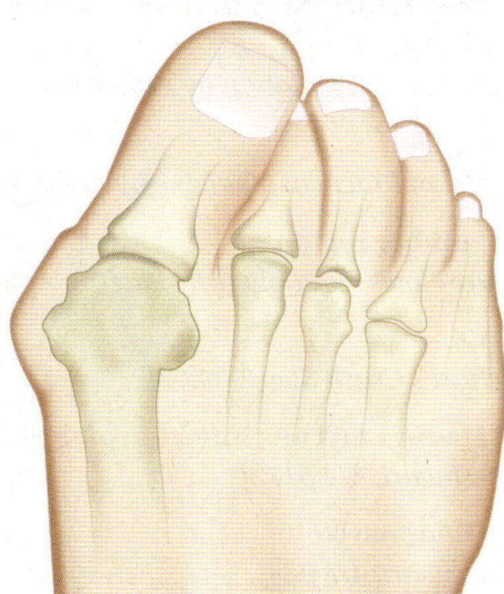

Fig. Hallux valgus

113. Ans. (c) Formed by joining a line extended from fracture line of femur neck to an arbitrary line depicting the horizontal plane
[Ref. Short Textbook of Surgery by Roy, 1/e p372]

114. Ans. (b) Fracture neck of femur
[Ref. Textbook of Orthopedics and Trauma by Kulkarni, Volume 3, 2/e p2029]

Garden's Classification of Femoral Neck Fractures

- Stage I: Incomplete fracture
- Stage II: Complete fracture without displacement
- Stage III: Complete fracture with partial displacement
- Stage IV: Complete fracture with complete displacement

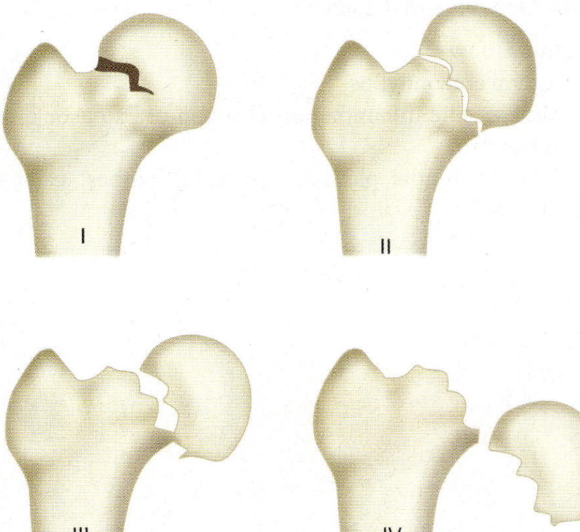

Fig. Garden's classification

115. Ans. (b) Fracture clavicle
[Ref. Textbook of Clinical Pediatrics by Stapleton, 2/e p168]

116. Ans. (a) Clavicle
[Ref. Textbook of Clinical Pediatrics by Stapleton, 2/e p168]

117. Ans. (a) Iliac crest
[Ref. Frontiers in Fracture Management by Bunker, 1/e p57]

118. Ans. (d) Syphilitic osteitis
[Ref. A Short Textbook of Clinical Imaging by Young, 1/e p355]

119. Ans. (c) Stimulates absorption of calcium
[Ref. Robbin's Basic Pathology, 9/e p299]

120. Ans. (c) Dietetic deficiency of vitamin D and calcium
[Ref. Textbook of Orthopedics and Trauma by Kulkarni, Volume 1, 2/e p216]

121. Ans. (c) 3 to 4 months
[Ref. 100 Cases of Orthopaedics and Rheumatology by Singh, 1/e p40]

122. Ans. (a) Nelaton's line
[Ref. Textbook of Orthopedics by Kotwal, 1/e p29]

123. Ans. (a) Hemophilia
[Ref. Oral and Maxillofacoial Surgery by Pogrel, 1st Ed. p1198]

Contraindications of Arthroscopy

Absolute Contraindications	Relative Contraindications
Bony ankyloses Advanced bony resorption Infection in joint areas Malignant tumours	Increased risk of hemorrhage Increased risk of infection Fibrous ankylosis

124. Ans. (d) Rushpin
[Ref. Operative Techniques in Orthopaedic Surgery by Wiesel, 1/e p111]

- **Rushpin** is used for Intermedullary fixation of bones

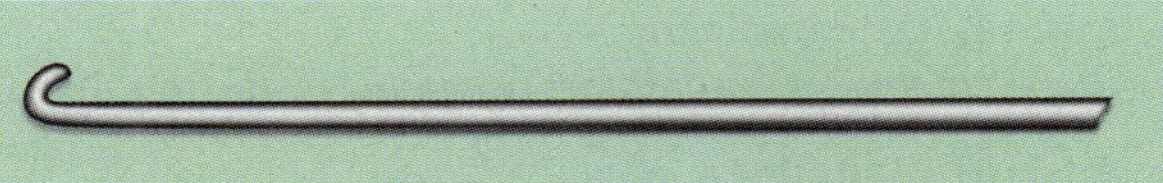

Fig. Rushpin

125. Ans. (c) Defective osteoclastic resorption of uncalcified osteoid and cartilage
[Ref. Metabolic Bone and Stone Disease by Nordin, 1/e p64]

126. Ans. (b) Reduced dietary calcium absorption
[Ref. Nelson's Textbook of Pediatrics, Volume 1, 20th Ed., Pg 338]

127. Ans. (d) Reconstruction of thumb
[Ref. Reconstructive Surgery in Hand Mutilation by Foucher, 1/e p29]

Pollicization

- Transfer of a finger to replace a thumb
- Single stage procedure to uniquely reconstruct the Carpometacarpal joint
- Provides for correct position, stability, strength, length, motion, sensibility and appearance required for thumb reconstruction
- Disadvantage: Sacrifice of a normal functioning of digit to replace the thumb

128. Ans. (c) Superior gluteal nerve
[Ref. Practical Orthopaedic Examination by Varshney, 2/e p27]

129. Ans. (b) Bio-mechanical
[Ref. General Principles of Orthopaedic and Trauma by Iyer, 1/e p5]

McMurray's Osteotomy
- Medial displacement oblique intertrochanteric pelvic support osteotomy
- Used for Fracture neck of femur

130. Ans. (d) Capitellum
[Ref. Rosen's Emergency Medicine by Marx, 8/e p2255]

Sequence of Ossifcation Centres Around Elbow
- Capitellum: 6–12 months age
- Radial head: 4–5 years age
- Medial epicondyle: 5–7 years age
- Trochlea: 8–10 years age
- Olecranon: 8–9 years age
- Lateral epicondyle: 9–13 years age

131. Ans. (c) Alkaline phosphatase
[Ref. Handbook of Nutrition and Food by Heber, 3/e p285]
Rising Alkaline phosphatase in absence of elevated liver enzymes is a strong indicator of Metabolic bone disease

132. Ans. (b) Long bones
[Ref. Pediatric and Adolescent Musculoskeletal MRI by Kleinman, 1/e p715]
Brodie's abscess is usually located in Metaphysis of long bones

133. Ans. (c) Median
[Ref. Surgical Anatomy of Hand and Upper Extremity by Doyle, 1/e p189]
Anterior interosseous nerve: Largest muscular *branch* that originates from Median nerve

134. Ans. (a) Osteomalacia
[Ref. Principle of Ambulatory Medicine by Burton, 7/e p1444]

135. Ans. (d) Mandible
[Ref. MRI Atlas of Head and Neck by Hasso, 1/e p165]

136. Ans. (d) Poor vascularity
[Ref. Surgical Techniques in Sports Medicine by Sekiya, 1/e p313]

137. Ans. (c) Hypoparathyroidism
[Ref. Orthopaedics Nursing Secrets by Zychowicz, 1/e p27]

Levels in Metabolic Bone Disorders

	Calcium	Phosphorus	Alkaline phosphatase
Hyperparathyroidism	Increased	Decreased	Increased
Hypoparathyroidism	Decreased	Increased	Decreased
Osteomalacia	Normal/ Decreased	Normal/ Decreased	Increased
Paget's disease	Normal	Normal	Increased
Rickets	Decreased	Decreased	Increased

138. Ans. (a) Secreted primarily by type A synovial cells
[Ref. Rheumatology Secrets by West, p19]

Synoviocytes
- Type A Synoviocytes: Macrophage like cells, Responsible for Phagocytosis
- Type B Synoviocytes: Fibroblast like cells, Responsible for secretion of Synovial fluid
- Type C Synoviocytes: Transition cells, Unknown function

139. Ans. (c) Enzymatic degradation of proteoglycans is increased
[Ref. Lumbar Disc Herniation by Postacchini, 1/e p63]

140. Ans. (c) L4-L5
[Ref. Manual of Practical Medicine by Alagappan, 5/e p724]

141. Ans. (d) Lumbar region
[Ref. Lecture Notes : Radiology by Patel, 3/e p301]

142. Ans. (a) C6 – C7
[Ref. Brochurt's Crush Step 2, p207]

143. Ans. (d) Madura mycotic infection of the bone
[Ref. Maheshwari, 4/e p172]

144. Ans. (b) Ulnar nerve
[Ref. Maheshwari, 4/e p64]
- Card test is used for Palmar interossei of fingers (Ulnar nerve)

145. Ans. (a) De Quervains disease
[Ref. Hand Secrets by Kasdan, 3/e p75]

146. Ans. (b) Vitamin C
[Ref. User's Guide to Vitamin C by English, p21]

147. Ans. (b) Defective Osteoid formation
[Ref. Partha's Fundamentals of Paediatrics by Parthasarthy, 2/e p79]

148. Ans. (a) Ulnar
[Ref. Maheshwari, 4/e p65]

149. Ans. (b) Tendinitis of common extensor origin
[Ref. Maheshwari, 4/e p293]

Tennis Elbow
- Lateral epicondylitis
- Non-specific inflammation at origin of Extensor muscles of Forearm
- Seen in Tennis players, squeezing clothes, carrying a suitcase

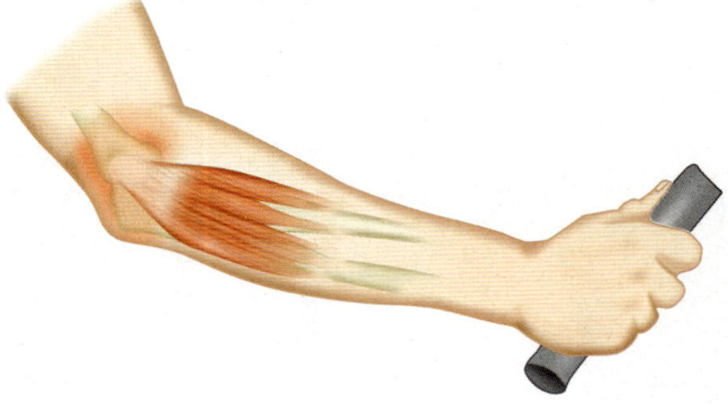

Fig. Tennis elbow

150. Ans. (d) Ulnar nerve injury
[Ref. Maheshwari, 4/e p61]

151. Ans. (b) Intrinsic muscle
[Ref. SRB's Manual of Surgery, 4/e p278]
- **Ulnar paradox**: In Ulnar nerve palsy, higher the injury, lesser the deformity
  - Along with Intrinsic muscles, Extrinsic muscles are also paralyzed

152. Ans. (c) Supracondylar fracture
[Ref. Smart Study Series Orthopedics by Rohilla, p99]

153. Ans. (a) Supracondylar Fracture humerus
[Ref. Smart Study Series Orthopedics by Rohilla, p99]

154. Ans. (b) Less formation of osteoid matrix
[Ref. Mosby's Review for NBDE, Part 1, p263]

Scurvy
- Vitamin C deficiency
- Impaired osteoid formation
- Subperiosteal hemorrhage
- Osteoporosis

155. Ans. (a) Hyperparathyroidism
[Ref. Skeletal Radiology: The Bare Bones by Chew, p282]

Brown Tumours
- Focal areas of bone resorption where the bone has been replaced by fibrous tissue and osteoclasts
- Seen in primary hyperparathyroidism
- Healing occur through ossification

156. Ans. (b) Stimulated by PTH; (c) Phagocytosis of foreign bodies
[Ref. Skeletal Biology and Medicine, Volume 1192, p20]

157. Ans. (a) Radial nerve; (e) Arteria profunda brachii
[Ref. Anatomy by Samar Mitra, p4.37]

158. Ans. (b) Hydroxyapatite
[Ref. General Principles of Orthopedics and Trauma by Iyer, 1/e p1]

159. Ans. (a) Plantar calcaneonavicular (spring) ligament
[Ref. Grey's Basic Anatomy, Internaitonal Ediiton 2012, p320]

160. Ans. (b) Osteoclast
[Ref. Clinical Chemistry by Marshall, Fig 15.4]

Paget's Disease
- Primary defect: Increased osteoclastic activity
- Increased osteoblastic activity
- High serum alkaline phosphatase

161. Ans. (d) Estrogen supplementation in postmenopausal women
[Ref. Primary and Secondary Preventive Nutrition by Bendich, 1/e p319]

162. Ans. (c) Cock up
[Ref. Hand Function in the Child by Pehoski, 2/e p404]

Static Splints
- Finger gutter splint
- Cock-up splint
- Thumb spica
- Resting hand splint

163. Ans. (d) Finkelstein's sign
[Ref. Geriatric Physical Diagnosis by Williams, 1/e p65]

Finkelstein Test
- Method of test: Patient makes a fist over opposed thumb, and then flex and ulnar deviate the fist; Pain over anatomical snuff box or producing a click is a positive test
- Test positive in: DeQuervain disease

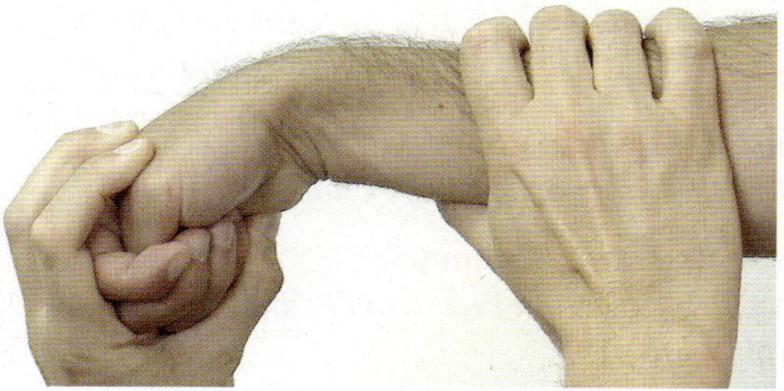

Fig. Finkelstein test

164. Ans. (b) Head of radius, lateral epicondyle, olecranon
[Ref. Orthopedic Physical Assessment by Magee, 6/e p419]

165. Ans. (c) Bursa anserine
[Ref. Oxford American Handbook of Physical Medicine and Rehabilitation by Pober, 1/e p136]

166. Ans. (a) Calcaneus
[Ref. Handbook of Fractures by Koval, 4/e p757]

Calcaneus
- **Bohler Triangle:** Anterior facet of Calcaneus, Posterior face of Calcaneus, Superior border of tuberosity
- **Neutral triangle:** Sparse trabeculae prone to impaction of Posterior facet in Calcaneus fractures

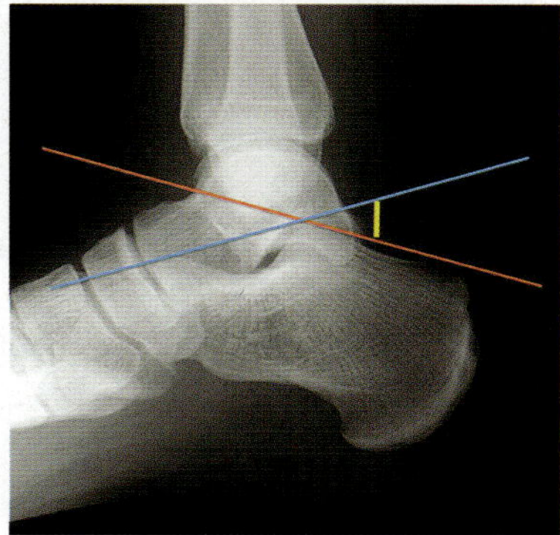

Fig. Bohler angle

167. Ans. (c) Calcaneus
[Ref. Handbook of Fractures by Koval, 4/e p757]

168. Ans. (a) Osteochondritis of lunate
[Ref. Maheshwari, 4/e p308]

Common Osteochondritis

Osteochondritis	Site
Perthes disease	Epiphysis of head of femur
Panner's disease	Capitulum
Kienbock's disease	Lunate

Contd...

Orthopedics

Contd...

Osteochondritis	Site
Osgood-Schlatter disease	Tibial tuberosity
Kohler disease	Navicular
Frieberg's disease	Metatarsal head (2nd > 3rd)
Scheurmann's disease	Ring epiphysis of vertebrae
Calve's disease	Central body nucleus of Verterbral body

169. Ans. (b) Neck of fibula
[Ref. BRS Gross Anatomy by Chung, 7/e p108]

170. Ans. (d) Haematogenous
[Ref. Principles and Practice of Pediatric Infectious Diseases by Prober, 4/e p78]

171. Ans. (c) Supracondylar fracture of humerus
[Ref. Maheshwari, 4/e p98]

- **Gunstock deformity**: Malunion of Supracondylar fracture of humerus leading to Cubitus varus deformity

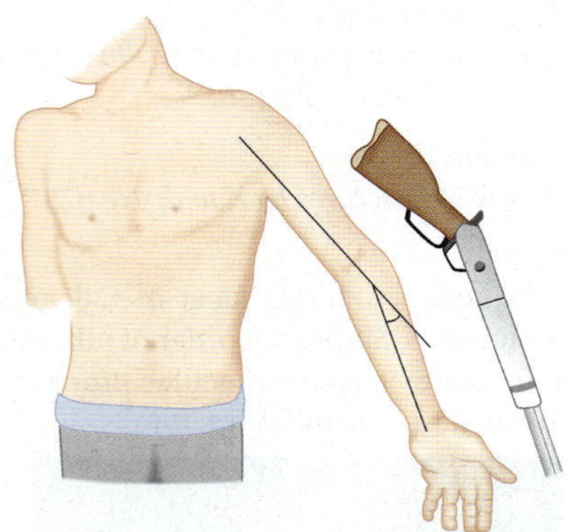

Fig. Gunstock deformity

172. Ans. (b) Fall from a height
[Ref. Neglected Musculoskeletal Injuries by Jain & Kumar, 1/e p161]

- MCC of Spine injuries in developing countries: Fall from height
- MCC of Spine injuries in developed countries: Road-traffic accidents

173. Ans. (a) Carpal tunnel syndrome
[Ref. Textbook of Orthopaedics and Trauma by Kulkarni, 2nd Ed., Volume 3, p2488]

Tests for Carpal Tunnel Syndrome

- **Phalen test**: Patient places elbow on table with forearm vertical and wrist flexed; Numbness and tingling occur in median nerve distribution
- **Reverse Phalen test**: Sustained extension of wrists exacerbate the symptoms
- **Torniquet test**: Inflating cuff on arm over Systolic BP reproduce symptoms over 30-60 seconds
- **Durkan's test**: Direct pressure on Median nerve or Carpal tunnel by thumb/pressure-manometer over 30 seconds produce symptoms

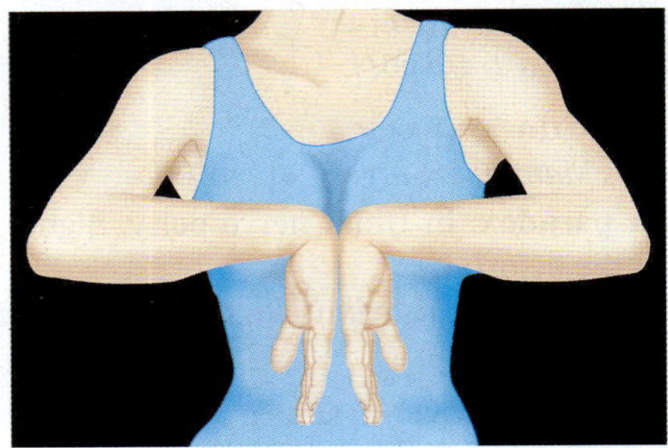

Fig. Phalen's test

174. Ans. (a) Ober's test
[Ref. Length Tension Testing Book 1 by Sanzo, 2/e p47]

175. Ans. (a) Involve the knee joint
[Ref. Maheshwari, 4/e p308]

176. Ans. (a) Quadriceps; (c) Gastrocnemius-soleus
[Ref. Motor Control by Cook, 3/e p307]

177. Ans. (b) Seen around epiphyseal plate
[Ref. Pediatric Orthopedics in Practice by Hefti, 2/e p250]

Perichondrial ring of Fibrous ligaments: Protect Epiphyseal growth plate which is subjected to heavy shearing forces

178. Ans. (d) 5th Metatarsal
[Ref. Pediatric and Adolescent Sports Traumatology by Guzzanti, 1/e p49]

Iselin's disease: Traction apophysitis of Base of 5th Metatarsal at insertion of tendon of Peroneus brevis, with pain aggravated by jumping and running

179. Ans. (a) 2nd Metatarsal head
[Ref. Maheshwari, 4/e p308]

180. Ans. (b) Wrist
[Ref. Nettler's Collections of Medical Illustrations by Parker, 2nd Ed. , Volume 6, p146]

- **Madelung deformity**: Growth disturbance in Volar—Ulnar distal Radial epiphysis at wrist

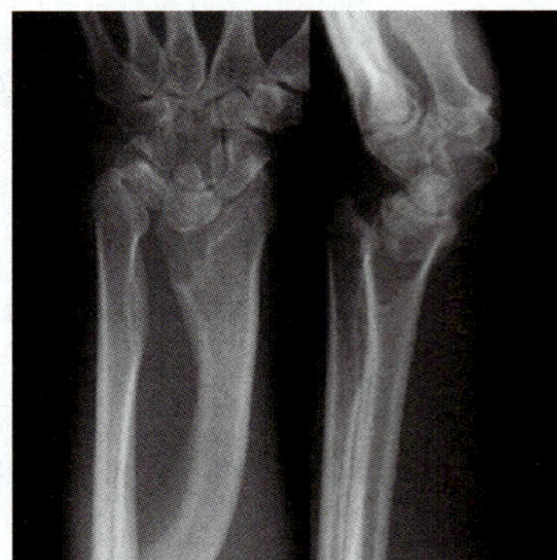

Fig. Madelung deformity

181. Ans. (a) Wings of sphenoid
[Ref. Operative Neurosurgical Techniques by Alfreda, 6/e p2055]

Craniovertebral Joint

- Axis vertebra
- Atlas vertebra
- Basiocciput
- Foramen magnum

182. Ans. (a) Pseudofracture
[Ref. Orthopedics by Joshi, 1/e p194]
Due to decalcification in Osteomalacia, **Milkman's fracture (Pseudofracture)** is commonly observed at the femoral neck, pubis, upper humerus, scapula and ribs

183. Ans. (d) Comminuted fractures are common
[Ref. Wong's Nursing Care of Infants and Children, 10/e p1569]

Bones in Children
- Thicker periosteum, Soft bones
- Higher resilience to stress
- Reduced healing times
- Better remodeling
- Dislocations rare
- Comminuted fractures rare

184. Ans. (a) Wings of sphenoid
[Ref. Gray's, 3/e p843-845]

Craniovertebral Junction
- Basiocciput
- Foramen magnum
- Atlas vertebra
- Axis vertebra

185. (c) Lymphoma
[Ref. The Teaching Files by Som, 1/e p633]

Ivory Vertebra Sign
- *Description*: Diffuse and homogeneous increase in opacity of a vertebral body that otherwise retains its size and contours, and with no change in the opacity and size of adjacent intervertebral disks
- *Causes*:

Children	Adults
Lymphoma	Osteoblastic metastases
Osteosarcoma	Prostate cancer
Osteoblastoma	Breast cancer
Metastatic disease	Lymphoma
Neuroblastoma	Paget's disease of bone
Medulloblastoma	TB spondylitis
Ewing's sarcoma (rare)	Hemangioma

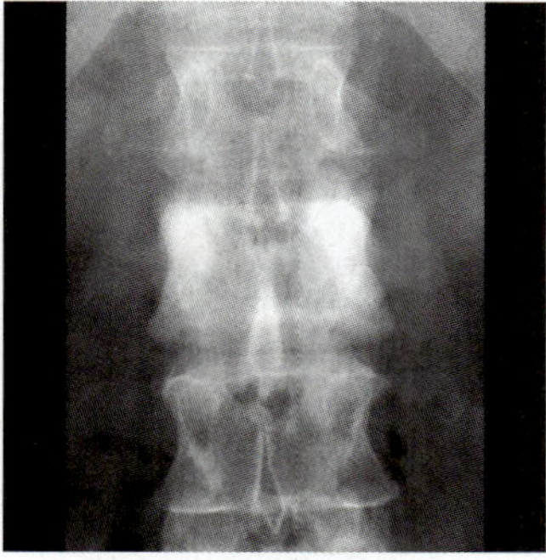
Fig. Ivory vertebra sign

186. Ans. (d) Repeated tiny movements at the fracture site
[Ref. Neglected Musculoskeletal Injuries by Jain, 1/e p33]
- Callus forms more easily than bone and helps to stabilize the fracture site, decrease pain, and lessen the likelihood of a fat embolism
- It also rapidly and efficiently provides a scaffold for further circulation and for cartilage and endosteal bone production
- Amount of movement at the fracture site influences the amount and quality of the callus
- Small amounts of micromovements stimulate the formation of Callus

187. Ans. (c) Ball and socket
[Ref. Anatomy by Mitra, 1/e p3.80]

Talocalcaneonavicular Joint (TCNJ)
- TCNJ is a synovial ball and socket joint, multiaxial with 3° of freedom
- The ball is formed by the anterior and inferior aspects of the head of the Talus
- The rounded head articulates anteriorly with the navicular

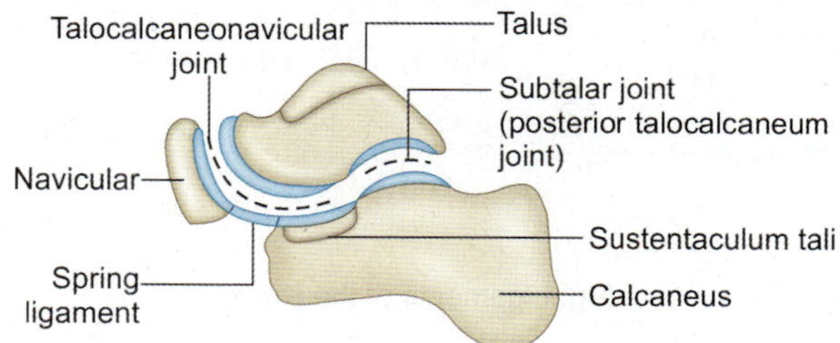

Fig. TCNJ

188. Ans. (b) Capitate
[Ref. Juvenile Skeleton by Scheuer, 1/e p299]
- Each carpal bone ossifies from one center; the Capitate usually is first and the Pisiform usually last, but variability may exist in the order
- Carpal bones ossification:
  - **Capitate: 2.5 months**
  - Hamate: 4-5.5 months
  - Triquetrum: 2 years
  - Lunate: 5 years
  - Trapezium: 6 years
  - Trapezoid: 6 years
  - Scaphoid: 6 years
  - **Pisiform: 12 years**

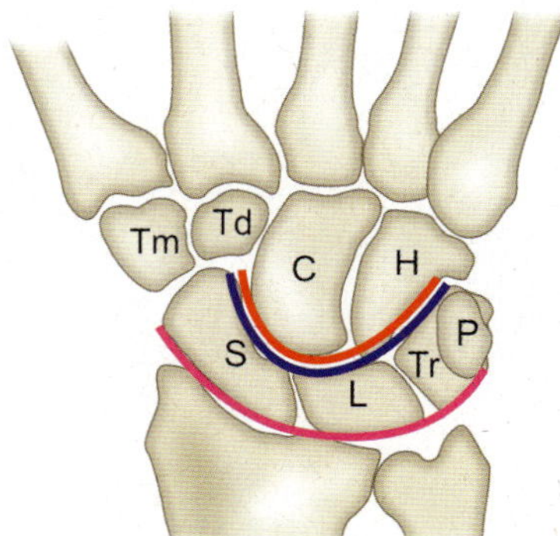

Fig. Carpal Bones

189. Ans. (c) Main restraint in Internal rotation
[Ref. Orthopaedics by Banaszkiewicz, 1/e p141]

Posterior Cruciate Ligament (PCL)
- PCL arises from anterolateral aspect of the medial femoral condyle in the region of the Intercondylar notch; Its origin is anterior to that of the anterior cruciate ligament (ACL)

Orthopedics

- PCL is the primary restraint to posterior translation of the Tibia with respect to the Femur
  - Posterior drawer test is performed with the patient's hip flexed at 45° and the knee flexed at 90°
  - **PCL is primary restraint to posterior drawer up to 5 mm**
- PCL (as well as ACL) within the Intercondylar notch extend from the femur to the proximal tibia as **Intracapsular but Extrasynovial structures**

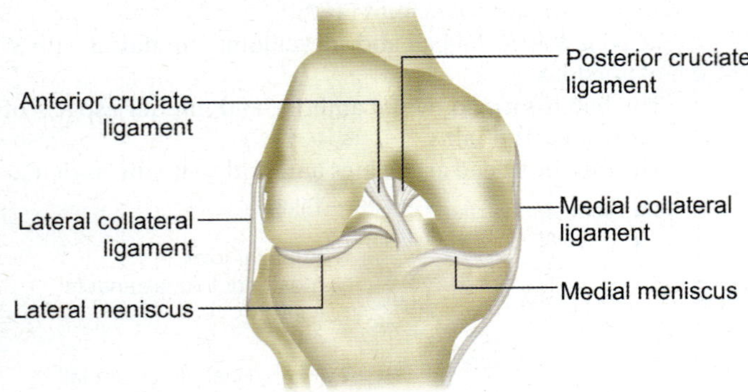

Fig. Ligaments of the Knee

190. Ans. (d) Hoover's test
[Ref. Manual Sports Medicine by Karageanes, 1/e p311]

Hoover's Test

- With the athlete-lying supine, the examiner places a hand under each heel
- Athlete is then asked to raise the affected leg-off the table
- Normal response is to push downward with the contralateral side
- Positive test: Feel a lack of downward force
- Indicates: Lack of effort from Athlete

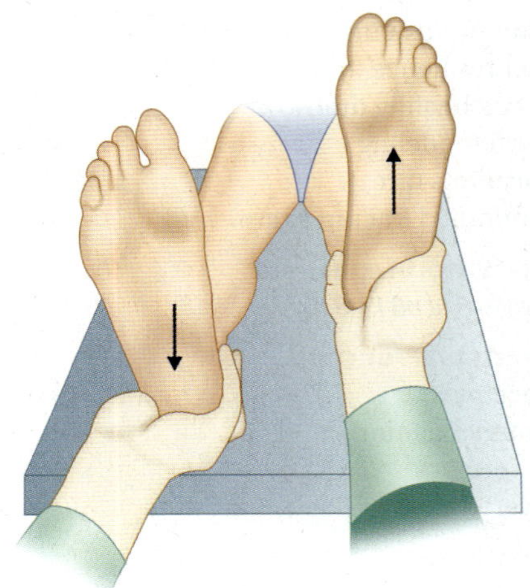

Fig. Hoover's test

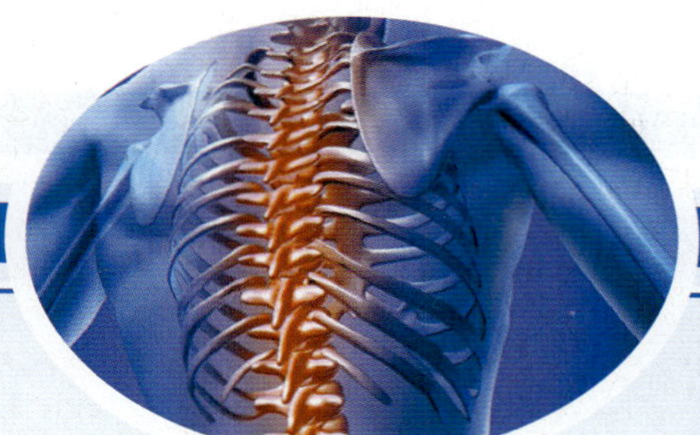

Chapter 2

General Traumatology

THEORETICAL CONCEPTS

Topper's Edge

Classification of Fractures

Based on Fracture Pattern	Based on Etiology	Based on Displacement
Transverse # Oblique # Spiral # Comminuted # Segmental #	Traumatic # Pathological # Stress # Fragility #	Undisplaced # Displaced # Impacted #
Based on Location Intra-articular # Extra-articular #	**Based on Completeness** Complete # Incomplete #	**Based on Radiology** X-ray-based classification CT scan-based classification
Based on Communication with Environment Closed # Open #		

II A. COMPLICATIONS OF FRACTURES

- *Hypovolaemic shock*: **MCC of death after fractures of major bones**[Q]
  - Blood loss in Pelvis fracture: **1500–2000 mL**[Q]
  - Blood loss in Femur fracture: **1000–1500 mL**[Q]
- *Adult respiratory distress syndrome*: Onset 24 hours after injury
- *Fat embolism syndrome*: In severe injuries with multiple fractures
  - **'Snow-storm appearance'** on CxR[Q]
- *DVT and Pulmonary embolism*
- *Crush syndrome*: leads to **Acute renal tubular necrosis**[Q]
- *Injury to major blood vessels*: **MC damaged is Popliteal artery**[Q]
- *Injury to nerves*: **MC damaged is Radial nerve**[Q]
- *Injury to muscles, tendons, joints, viscera*
- *Osteomyelitis infection*
- *Compartment syndrome*
- *Delayed and Non-union (>6 months)*
  - **MC operation for non-union: Bone grafting**[Q]
- *Mal-union*
  - MC operation for non-union: Redoing fracture surgically[Q]
- *Shortening*: Noticeable, if >2 cm
- *Avascular necrosis*: Head of femur, Proximal pole scaphoid, Body talus[Q]

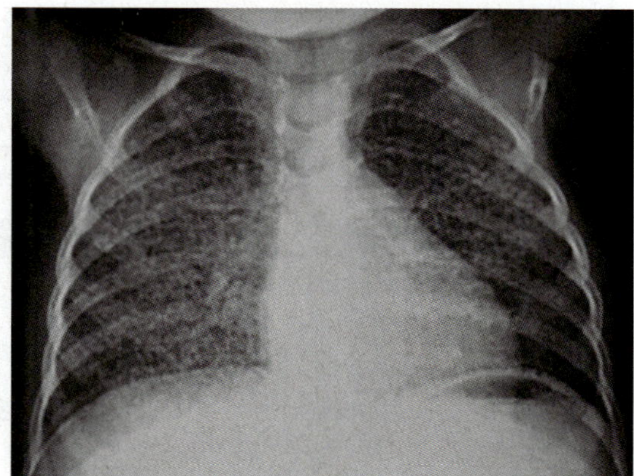

Fig. Snowstorm chest X-ray

- *Stiffness of joints*
- ***Sudeck's dystrophy*: Reflex sympathetic dystrophy**[Q]
  - Sympathetic blocks help in recovery in resistant cases
- ***Myositis ossificans*: Post-traumatic**[Q]
  - Massage after injury is strictly prohibited

Topper's Edge

FRACTURE TRAUMATOLOGY

General Traumatology

- **MC symptom of fracture**[Q]: Pain
- **MC sign of fracture**[Q]: Tenderness
- **Surest sign of fracture**[Q]: Abnormal motility and Loss of transmitted movement

Fractures prone to Malunion[Q]	Fractures prone to Nonunion[Q]
• Supracondylar fracture of humerus • Intertrochanteric fracture femur • Colles' fracture	• Fracture neck of femur • Fracture body of talus • Fracture scaphoid (proximal pole, waist) • Fracture fifth metatarsal (proximal part) • Fracture lateral condyle humerus

Age-wise MC Fractures

- **MC fracture at birth**[Q]: Clavicle
- **MC fracture children**[Q]: Greenstick fractures
- **MC fracture elderly**[Q]: Vertebral fracture

Atypical Fractures

- **Greenstick fractures**[Q]: Occur in children
- Torus fracture[Q]: Buckling of outer cortex in children
- **Stress fracture**[Q]: Common in athletes
- Pathological fracture: Usually in elderly

II B. DISLOCATIONS AND SUBLUXATIONS

- **MCC of dislocations and subluxations**: Injury[Q]
- **Only dislocation where lengthening of limbs occur**: Anterior dislocation of hip[Q]
- Common dislocations in body:

Site	Type
Spine	**Anterior** C5-C6 (cervical spine)[Q]
Hip	**Posterior**[Q]
Shoulder	**Anterior**[Q]
Elbow	Posterior
Wrist	Lunate[Q]

II C. FRACTURES IN CHILDREN

- **Salter-Harris classification of Epiphyseal injuries**[Q]:

Class	Types of Injury	Site
I	Physeal fracture	Radial neck epiphysis
II	Physeal + Metaphyseal fracture	Lower end radius epiphysis
III	Physeal + Epiphyseal fracture	Medial malleolus epiphysis
IV	Physeal + Metaphyseal Epiphyseal fracture	Lateral condyle humerus
V	Physeal crush injury	Lower tibial epiphysis
VI	Perichondrial injury	
Good prognosis: Type I, II		
Thurston-Holland sign[Q]: Type II epiphyseal injury		

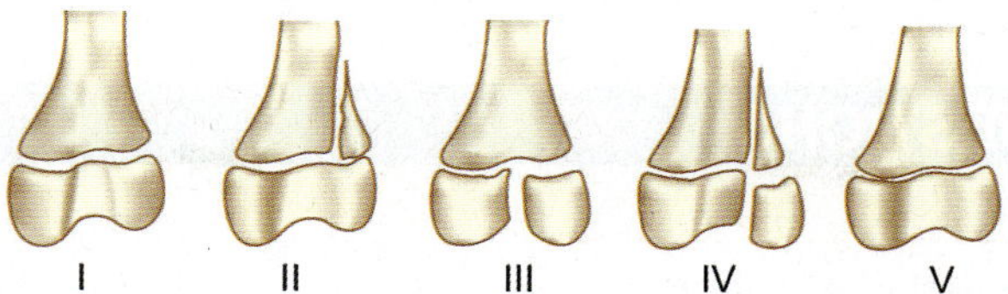

II D. COMMON DEFORMITIES DUE TO FRACTURES

- ***Mallet finger***: Avulsed extensor tendon of base of distal phalanx[Q]
- ***Dinner fork deformity***: Colles' fracture[Q]
- ***Gunstock deformity***: Supracondylar fracture humerus[Q]

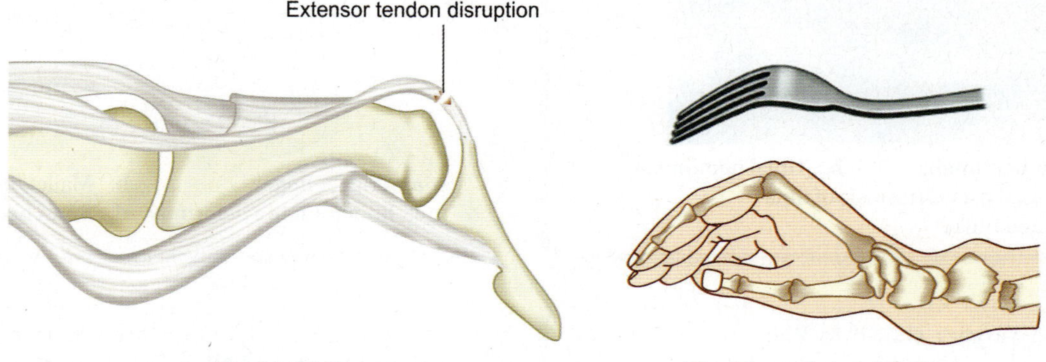

Fig. Mallet finger

Fig. Dinner fork deformity

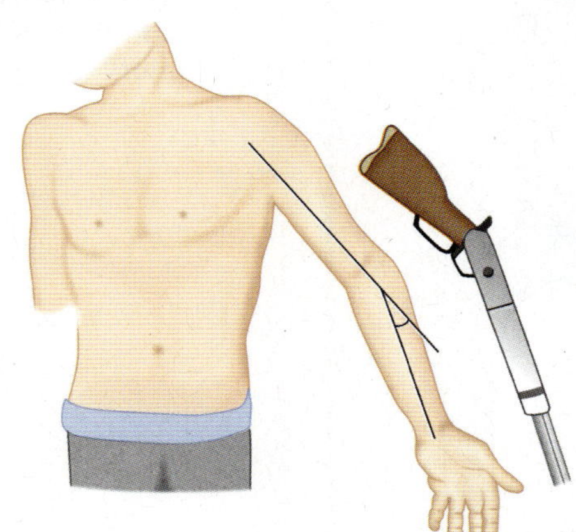

Fig. Gunstock deformity

II E. COMMON OSTEOTOMIES

- ***French osteotomy***: Cubitus varus/Gunstock deformity[Q]
- ***McMurray's osteotomy***: Fracture neck of femur[Q]
- ***Pauwels' osteotomy***: Osteoarthritis hip
- ***Salter's osteotomy***: Congenital dislocation of hip[Q]
- *Chiari Pelvic displacement osteotomy*: Congenital dislocation of hip[Q]
- *Pemberton's pericapsular osteotomy*: Congenital dislocation of hip[Q]

II F. BONE GRAFTING

- ***Autogenous bone grafting***: Graft from same person
  - Cortical grafts for osteogenic reason: Iliac crest
  - Cancellous grafts for stability: Fibula
- ***Allogenous bone grafting***: Graft from another person
- ***Xeno-grafting***: Graft from another species[Q]

IMAGE-BASED QUESTIONS

1. A child presented with deformity as shown in the figure. The most probable diagnosis is ***[AIIMS May 2016]***

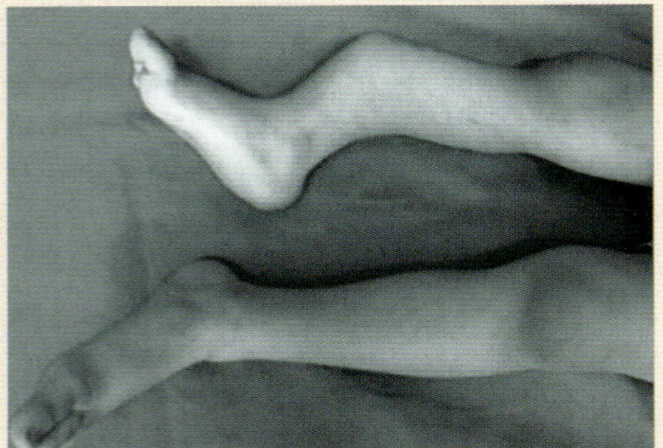

a. Fibular hemimelia
b. Tibial hemimelia
c. Congenital pseudarthrosis of tibia
d. Angulated tibia

2. Identify the Deformity shown in Photograph ***[Recent Question 2012]***

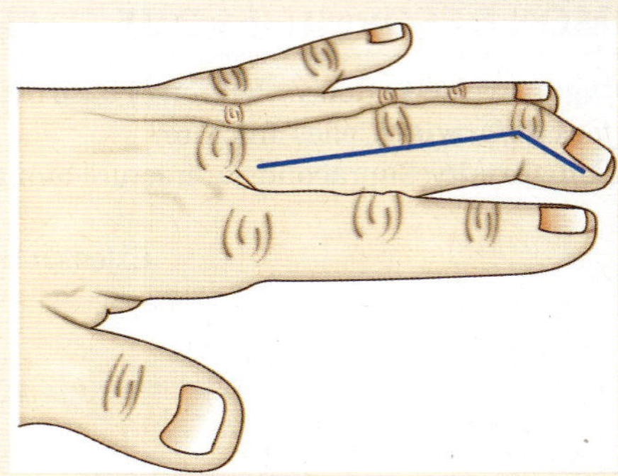

a. Trigger finger
b. Mallet finger
c. Boutanniere's deformity
d. Swan neck deformity

3. Corrective Surgery shown in Photograph used for DDH is

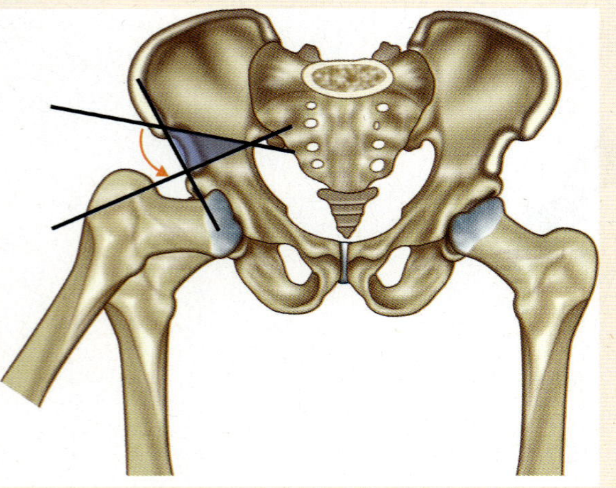

a. Pemberton osteotomy
b. Salter osteotomy
c. Steel's osteotomy
d. Dega osteotomy

4. A 27-year-old patient with complaints of inability to move his 4th and 5th digits. He cannot hold pen and was not able to hold paper between fingers. Site given in Photograph below that could be probable cause of injury to the nerve in question is ***[AIIMS May 2017]***

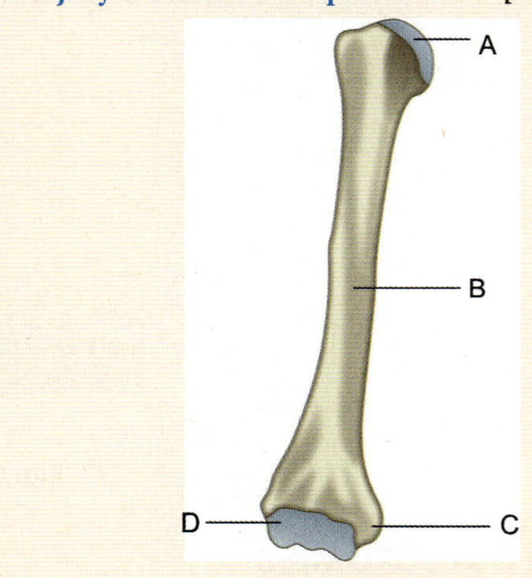

a. A
b. B
c. C
d. D

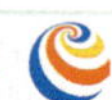 ANSWERS WITH EXPLANATIONS OF IBQs

1. Ans. (c) Congenital pseudarthrosis of tibia *[Ref. Musculoskeletal Imaging by Pope, 1/e p1071]*

Congenital Pseudarthrosis

- CPT refers to nonunion of a tibial fracture that develops spontaneously or after a minor trauma
- A pseudarthrosis is defined as a "false joint" and is a break in the bone that fails to heal on its own
- CPT usually develops within the first two years of life; however, there have been reported cases of CPT development before birth as well as later in life
- Most common bone: Tibia
- Other bones: Fibula, Radius, Ulna, Clavicle, Humerus

2. (b) Mallet finger *[Ref. Maheshwari, 4/e p114]*

- Trigger finger: Constriction of fibrous digital sheath preventing free gliding of contained flexor tendon
- Mallet finger: Avulsion of attachment of extensor tendon from the base of distal phalanx
- Boutanniere's deformity: PIP flexion with DIP hyperextension
- Swan neck deformity: DIP hyperflexion with PIP hyperextension

3. (b) Salter osteotomy

Common Osteotomies

- *French osteotomy*: Cubitus varus/Gunstock deformity
- *McMurray's osteotomy*: Fracture neck of femur
- *Pauwels' osteotomy*: Osteoarthritis hip
- *Salter's osteotomy*: Congenital dislocation of hip (Osteotomy of Iliac bone above Acetabulum)
- *Chiari Pelvic displacement osteotomy*: Congenital dislocation of hip
- *Pemberton's pericapsular osteotomy*: Congenital dislocation of hip

4. (c) C *[Ref. Tachdjian's Pediatric Orthopaedics, 5/e p1308]*

- Inability to move his 4th and 5th digits. He cannot hold pen and was not able to hold paper between fingers indicates **Injury to Ulnar Nerve**
- Bone shown in the Photograph is **Humerus**

Fractures of Humerus & Nerve involvement (part-wise as shown in Photograph):

- Part A: Neck of Humerus—Axillary Nerve
- Part B: Shaft of Humerus—Radial Nerve
- Part C: Medial Epicondyle—Ulnar Nerve
- Part D: Lateral Epicondyle—Causes Tardy ulnar nerve palsy (Due to nonunion)

Orthopedics

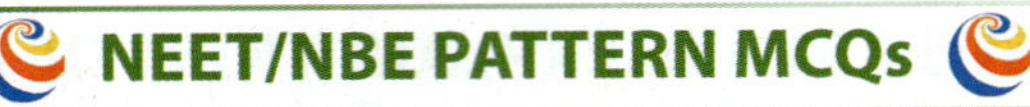

NEET/NBE PATTERN MCQs

1. While performing a Total hip replacement, the surgeon found destruction of the articular cartilage and multiple wedge-shaped subchondral depressions. What is this called? *[Recent Question 2016]*
a. Osteolysis
b. Osteomyelitis
c. Osteonecrosis
d. Osteogenesis

2. AVN of hip may occur following which of the following fractures? *[Recent Question 2016]*
a. Intertrochanteric fracture of the hip
b. Subtrochanteric fracture
c. Transcervical fracture of the neck of femur
d. Fracture of posterior lip of the acetabulum

3. Greenstick/Nightstick fractures are seen in *[Recent Question 2016]*
a. Children
b. Elderly
c. Young adults
d. Common in all age groups

4. VN following transcervical neck femur fractures occurs due to damage to which of the following blood vessels? *[Recent Question 2016]*
a. Lateral retinacular branch of lateral circumflex femoral artery
b. Lateral retinacular branch of medial circumflex femoral artery
c. Medial retinacular branch of lateral circumflex femoral artery
d. Obturator artery

5. Salter-Harris classification is used for *[Recent Question 2016]*
a. Supracondylar humerus fractures in children
b. Estimation of growth of the physes
c. Physeal injuries
d. Severity of degloving injuries to the limb

6. A 4-year-old child suffered from a fall on outstretched hand. X-rays revealed a fracture with the fracture line at the physes with a small metaphyseal fragment. There was no epiphyseal fracture. What type of injury by Salter-Harris Classification is this? *[Recent Question 2016]*
a. I
b. II
c. III
d. IV

7. All of the following are features of Myositis ossificans except *[Recent Question 2016]*
a. Commonly occurs around the elbow
b. It matures from inside out
c. Massaging is a known associated factor
d. Can be post traumatic or occur without trauma also

8. Which of the following injuries can be classified as Gustilo Anderson Grade III injuries? *[Recent Question 2016]*
a. Open fracture with clean wounds less than 1 cm long
b. Open fractures with a laceration more than 1 cm long usually up to 10 cm, with extensive soft tissue damage, flaps or avulsions
c. Open segmental fractures, open fractures with extensive soft tissue damage, traumatic amputation
d. Compartment syndrome with an open fracture

9. Which is the Earliest reliable sign suggestive of Compartment syndrome? *[Recent Question 2016]*
a. Stretch pain
b. Pulselessness
c. Paraesthesia
d. Pallor

10. Which one is not associated with Wound healing? *[Recent Question 2016]*
a. Zinc
b. Copper
c. Vitamin C
d. Vitamin E

11. A patient with fracture of femur shaft develops petechiae, respiratory distress and decreased sPO_2, 5 days after injury. Possible diagnosis is [Recent Question 2016]
a. Hypostatic pneumonia
b. Haemolytic anemia
c. Crush syndrome
d. Fat embolism

12. All are biological factors causing delayed union of fractures, except *[NBE DNB 2009]*
a. Periosteal stripping
b. Insufficient blood supply
c. Severe soft tissue damage
d. Imperfect splint

13. Least commonly affected in traumatic osteonecrosis is *[NBE DNB 2009]*
a. Head of femur
b. Head of radius
c. Proximal part of scaphoid
d. Posterior part of talus

14. Tension band wiring is done in all, except *[Recent Question 2012]*
a. Fracture patella
b. Fracture olecranon
c. Fracture medial malleolus
d. Colles' fracture

15. All are common sites of fracture non-union, except *[NBE FMGE March 2008]*
a. Scaphoid
b. Talus
c. Lateral condyle humerus
d. Distal end of radius (Colles fracture)

16. Avascular necrosis is commonly seen in *[NBE FMGE September 2005]*
a. Capitulum
b. Talus
c. Head of humerus
d. Intracapsular fracture of neck of humerus

17. Most common fracture in elderly *[Recent Question 2013]*
a. TCNF
b. Colles' fracture
c. IT fracture
d. Supracondylar fracture

18. Smith's fracture involves which bone *[Recent Question 2013]*
a. Distal radius
b. Proximal ulna
c. Metatarsal
d. Patella

19. The contraindication to internal fixation *[Recent Question 2013]*
a. Physeal injury
b. Active infection
c. Intra-articular fracture
d. Fracture dislocation

20. Most common organism causing infection after open fracture *[Recent Question 2012]*
a. *Pseudomonas*
b. *Staphylococcus aureus*
c. *Gonococcus*
d. *Klebsiella*

21. Hanging cast is used for *[Recent Question 2012]*
a. Femur fracture b. Radius fracture
c. Humerus fracture d. Tibia fracture

22. Green stick fracture is *[Recent Question 2012]*
a. Fracture in adults b. Complete fracture
c. Incomplete fracture d. Fracture spine

23. Nonunion is common in fracture *[Recent Question 2013]*
a. Scapula b. Talus
c. Neck femur d. None

24. Thurston-Holland sign is seen in *[NBE FMGE March 2004]*
a. Oblique fracture lower 1/3 humerus
b. Reverse oblique fracture of intratrochanteric femur
c. Salter-Harris type-II fracture
d. Coronal fracture of femoral condyles

25. Find incorrect combination of fracture and nails/screws *[NBE DNB 1992]*
a. Neck femur – Smith-Petersen nail
b. Shaft femur – Kutschner nail
c. Shaft tibia – V-shaped nail
d. Shaft ulna – Rush nail
e. Olecranon process – Lag screw

26. True about fracture healing except *[Recent Question 2012, 2013]*
a. Nutrition affects healing
b. Stable fixation promotes healing
c. Compression at fracture site causes nonunion
d. Hormonal status may affect healing

27. A construction worker has sustained a massive crush injury of right lower limb. He soon develops acute renal failure. Which complication has he developed?
a. Necrotizing fasciitis *[NBE FMGE September 2011]*
b. Acute osteomyelitis
c. Compartment syndrome
d. Crush syndrome

28. Non-union is commonly seen in *[NBE DNB 1993]*
a. Coracoid process fracture
b. Ulnar fracture
c. Supracondylar fracture of humerus
d. Lower tibial fracture

29. Avascular necrosis is seen in all except *[UPSC 2012]*
a. Fracture scaphoid
b. Fracture calcaneum
c. Fracture talus
d. Subcapital fracture of femur neck

30. Salter-Harris Classification is based on
a. Metaphyseal fractures *[Recent Question 2014]*
b. Diaphyseal fracture
c. Epiphyseal plate fractures
d. Osteoid matrix

31. Gustilo Anderson Classification is MC classification used for *[Recent Question 2016, 2015]*
a. Open fractures
b. Closed fractures
c. Malunited fractures
d. Non-union of fractures

32. What is the treatment for patient with Hypertrophic nonunion with deformity at fracture site? *[Recent Question 2017]*
a. No treatment required b. Fixation only
c. Bone grafting only d. Fixation with bone grafting

33. Dunlop traction is a type of traction used in management of *[Recent Question 2017]*
a. Fracture humerus b. Fracture radius
c. Fracture femur d. Fracture tibia

34. Greenstick fracture is *[Recent Question 2017]*
a. Incomplete transverse fracture pattern in children
b. Complete transverse fracture pattern in children
c. Incomplete spiral fracture pattern in children
d. Complete spiral fracture pattern in children

35. Which splint is used in management of Fracture shaft femur in age group of 2 -10 years? *[Recent Question 2017]*
a. Split Russell traction b. Gallows traction
c. Bucks traction d. Brandth traction

36. Seat belt injury affects which bone of body *[Recent Question 2017]*
a. Vertebrae b. Pelvis
c. Fracture neck femur d. Clavicle

37. Patient with femur head fracture with associated fracture of acetabulum will fall into Pipkin type *[Recent Question 2017]*
a. I b. II
c. III d. IV

38. Common fractures in childhood are all except *[Recent Question 2017]*
a. Forearm bone fracture
b. Fracture supracondylar humerus
c. Spiral fracture of shaft tibia
d. Fracture of hand bones

39. X-ray appearance of sequestrum is *[Recent Question 2017]*
a. Unnatural radiodense fragments
b. Osteopenic fragment
c. Fragment with honeycomb loculated appearance
d. Radiolucent area with speckled calcification

40. Fracture of necessity is used to describe *[Recent Question 2017]*
a. Cottons fracture b. Galeazzi fracture
c. Monteggia fracture d. Rolando fracture

41. Most common joint to be dislocated in the body is *[Recent Question 2017]*
a. Shoulder b. Hip
c. Elbow d. Knee

42. Locking compression plating for is commonly indicated in the following fracture types *[Recent Question 2017]*
a. Periarticular fractures
b. Transverse or oblique fractures of long bones
c. Intertrochanteric fractures
d. Fracture of long bones

43. Which of the following is false regarding Salter-Harris classification? *[Recent Question 2017]*
a. Classifies epiphyseal injuries
b. Type II is the most common type of epiphvseal injury
c. Type IV classifies injury through epiphysis, physis, metaphysis
d. Type V is the perichondrial ring injury

44. Chauffeur fracture is *[Recent Question 2017]*
a. Extra-articular fracture of styloid process
b. Intra-articular fracture of styloid process
c. Intra-articular fracture of base of 1st metacarpal
d. Extra-articular fracture of base of lst metacarpal

45. Compartment syndrome is commonly seen in *[Recent Question 2017]*
a. Fracture of proximal tibia
b. Fracture shaft humerus
c. Fracture of femur shaft
d. Fracture distal end radius

46. Potts fracture is an eponym used for *[Recent Question 2017]*
a. Bimalleolar ankle fracture
b. Trimalleolar ankle fracture
c. Fracture of distal end radius
d. Pathological fracture in osteomalacia

47. Which structure is usually first repaired in hand injury? *[Recent Question 2017]*
a. Bone
b. Tendon
c. Nerve
d. Artery

HIGH YIELD MCQs

1. Factor which leads to Increased cartilage formation during Fracture healing *[AIIMS November 2016]*
a. Rigid immobility
b. Compression
c. Necrosis of fracture ends
d. Movement at fracture site

2. Direct impact on bone will lead to *[AIIMS PGMEE 2003]*
a. Oblique fracture b. Transverse fracture
c. No fracture seen d. Comminuted fracture

3. Pathological fractures are seen in *[PGI 2000]*
a. Osteogenesis imperfecta b. Osteoporosis
c. Anaemia d. Osteomalacia
e. Radiation

4. In the management of long bone fracture, following can be done *[PGI 2003, 2006]*
a. Intramedullary nailing b. Plating
c. External fixation d. Tension band wiring
e. Screw

5. Last step in healing of fractures is *[Rajasthan PGMEE 1993]*
a. Hematoma b. Callus formation
c. Remodelling d. Consolidation

6. Action of intramedullary 'K' nail is *[Recent Question 2017, All India PGMEE 1996]*
a. Two-point fixation b. Three-point fixation
c. Compression d. Weight concentration

7. Which of the following condition should be given most priority in case of fracture? *[PGI 2008]*
a. Open fracture b. Dislocated fracture
c. Vascular injury d. Malunited fracture
e. Compartment syndrome

8. Which fracture in children requires open reduction? *[AIIMS PGMEE 1991]*
a. Fracture tibial epiphysis
b. Fracture shaft of femur
c. Fracture both bones forearm
d. Fracture femoral condyle

9. Most common cause of non-union of fractures is *[UP PGMEE 1998]*
a. Infection b. Ischaemia
c. Inadequate immobilization
d. Soft tissue interposition

10. Non-union is a complication in fracture of *[AIIMS PGMEE 1998]*
a. Scaphoid b. Colles
c. Inter-trochanteric hip d. Supracondylar humerus

11. Open reduction and internal fixation is done for all of the following fractures, except *[All India PGMEE 1997]*
a. Patella fracture
b. Olecranon fracture
c. Volar Barton's fracture
d. Fracture lateral condyle of humerus

12. Surgical excision is contraindicated in *[AIIMS PGMEE 1995]*
a. Olecranon process b. Patella
c. Head of radius d. Lateral condyle humerus

13. Contraindication for skin traction *[PGI 2006]*
a. Dermatitis
b. Vascularity compromised status of limb
c. Abrasions
d. Hypopigmentation (vitiligo)
e. Bony deformity

14. Skeletal traction is given by *[PGI 2008, PGI 2009]*
a. K-wire b. Pavlik harness
c. Denham Pin d. Steinmann's pin
e. Rush pin

15. Which is the most common fracture in children? *[All India PGMEE 1995, PGI 1996]*
a. Fracture clavicle
b. Supracondylar fracture
c. Green stick fracture of lower end of radius
d. All of the above

16. Which statements pertaining to Green stick fracture is correct? *[All India PGMEE 1993, AIIMS PGMEE 1996]* *[AP PGMEE 1999]*
a. Any fracture in child
b. Is generally incomplete
c. Fracture only in rickety children
d. All of the above

17. One of the features given below is Essential in the diagnosis of a Fracture of a bone *[AP PGMEE 1999]*
a. Deformity b. A crepitus
c. A partial or complete loss of continuity of bone
d. None of the above

18. The one most consistent sign of Fresh fracture is *[PGI 97]*
a. Crepitus b. Bony tenderness
c. Deformity d. Abnormal mobility
e. Shortening of bone

19. Sudeck's atrophy is associated with *[Delhi PGMEE 1999]*
a. Osteoporosis b. Osteophyte formation
c. Osteopenia d. Osteochondritis

20. Sudeck's atrophy is more common in
a. Malunited Colles' fracture *[Karnataka PGMEE 1998]*
b. Malunited fracture femur
c. Pott's fracture
d. Carries spine

21. Stellate ganglion block is useful in *[AIIMS PGMEE 1999]*
a. Sudeck osteodystrophy
b. Compound palmar ganglion
c. Tenosynovitis
d. Osteoarthritis of first CMC joint

22. Regarding Sudeck's osteodystrophy all are true, except
a. Burning pain *[PGI 1993]*
b. Stiffness and swelling
c. Erythematous and cyanotic discolouration
d. Self-limiting and good prognosis

23. In children, all are true, except *[All India PGMEE 2000]*
a. Dislocations are rare
b. Comminuted fractures are conunon
c. Thick periosteum
d. Soft bones

24. In children, best remodelling is seen in fracture with *[AIIMS PGMEE 1997]*
a. Angulation in diaphysis b. Angulation in metaphysis
c. Rotation in diaphysis d. Rotation in metaphysis

25. Pathognomonic sign of Traumatic fracture is *[JIPMER PGMEE 1998]*
a. Redness b. Swelling
c. Crepitus d. Tenderness

26. Direct impact on the bone will produce a *[AIIMS PGMEE 2003]*
a. Transverse fracture b. Oblique fracture
c. Spiral fracture d. Comminuted fracture

27. Type VI Rang's injury includes *[PGI 2008]*
a. Transverse fracture of metaphysic with longitudinal extension into physis
b. Open injury with loss of physis
c. Thurston Holland's sign
d. Perichondrial ring injury
e. Intra-articular fractures

28. Pathologic fracture can occur in all, except *[PGI 2005]*
a. Metabolic bone disease
b. Osteosarcoma
c. Osteochondroma
d. Bone cyst
e. Fluorosis

29. Pathological Fracture is seen in following, except
a. Radiation b. Anaemia *[PGI 2000]*
c. Osteoporosis d. Osteomalacia

30. The most common cause of Pathological fracture in generalized affection is
[JIPMER PGMEE 1997, UP PGMEE 1999]
a. Carcinoma b. Osteoporosis
c. Cyst d. All of the above

31. Compound fracture is defined as *[DPG 1988]*
a. Fracture with artery involvement
b. Fracture with nerve involvement
c. Fracture with muscle involvement
d. Fracture with skin involvement

32. Open fracture is treated by *[UP PGMEE 1998]*
a. Tourniquet b. Debridement
c. Internal fixation d. External fixation

33. Most common bone fracture during birth is *[MP PGMEE 1998]*
a. Radius b. Humerus
c. Scapula d. Clavicle

34. In which of the following condition bilateral symmetrical fractures occur? *[NIMS PGMEE 2000, Delhi PGMEE 1998]*
a. Rickets
b. Osteopetrosis
c. Osteogenesis imperfecta
d. Fluorosis

35. Multiple bone fracture in a new born is seen in *[Delhi PGMEE 1999]*
a. Scurvy b. Syphilis
c. Osteogenesis imperfecta d. Morquio's syndrome

36. Avascular necrosis of bone is most commonly seen in *[JIPMER PGMEE 1991, JIPMER PGMEE 1993]*
a. Calcaneus b. Cervical spine
c. Scaphoid d. Scapula

37. Milkman's fracture is? *[All India PGMEE 2009]*
a. Pseudofracture in adults
b. Fracture of Clavicle in children
c. Fracture humerus
d. Fracture first Metacarpal

38. Oblique view is required to diagnose fracture of *[Assam PGMEE 1995]*
a. Capitate b. Scaphoid
c. Navicular d. Hamate

39. Most common cause of Pathological fracture is *[BIHAR PGMEE 1990]*
a. Delayed union b. Mal union
c. Non union d. Secondary deposits
e. Any of the above

40. Treatment of choice in pathological fractures is *[BIHAR PGMEE 1988]*
a. Internal fixation b. Plaster of Paris casts
c. Skin traction d. External skeletal fixation

41. Mirel's criteria is developed for the evaluation of *[AIIMS PGMEE 1992, JIPMER PGMEE 2000]*
a. Risk of fatigue fracture
b. Severity of osteoporosis
c. Risk of pathological fracture
d. Severity of neurological deficit

42. True about Post traumatic fat embolism syndrome is all, except *[PGI 2009]*

a. Bradycardia occur
b. Systemic hypoxia may occur
c. Fracture mobility is a risk factor
d. Associated diabetes pose a risk
e. More common in closed fracture
f. Liposuction is used for treatment

43. Factors favoring Fat embolism in trauma patient *[PGI 2007]*

a. Diabetes mellitus b. Mobility of joint
c. Respiratory failure d. Hypovolemic shock

44. Internal fixation is probably needed in all of the following, except *[UPSC 1993]*

a. Fracture condyle of humerus
b. Fracture neck of femur
c. Fracture of olecranon
d. Fracture of scaphoid

45. MC cause of Anterior compartment syndrome is *[PGI 1993]*

a. Operative trauma
b. Fractures
c. Post ischaemic swelling
d. Superficial injury to muscles

46. Sudeck's dystrophy is more common in *[Karnataka PGMEE 1998]*

a. Malunited Colles' fracture
b. Malunited fracture of femur
c. Pott's spine
d. Caries spine

47. Garden I fractures are also known as *[Assam PGMEE 1997, UP PGMEE 2003]*

a. Complete fracture without displacement
b. Complete fracture with minimal (partial) displacement
c. Complete fracture with full displacement
d. Valgus impaction fractures

48. Commonest site of fracture leading to fat embolism is *[All India PGMEE 1999]*

a. Tibia fracture b. Femur fracture
c. Humerus fracture d. Ulna fracture

49. Fat embolism syndrome characterized by *[PGI 2004]*

a. Tachycardia b. Hypoxia
c. Fat globules in urine d. Thrombocytosis

50. All of the following factors facilitate non-union, except *[All India PGMEE 1997]*

a. Haematoma formation b. Periosteal injuries
c. Absence of nerve supply d. Chronic infection

51. Initial stage of Clinical union of bone is equivalent to *[Bihar PGMEE 1990]*

a. Callus formation b. Woven bone
c. Haematoma formation d. Calcification only
e. None of the above

52. 5 True about Fat embolism *[PGI 2004, 2007]*

a. Seen one week after injury
b. Petechiae
c. Bradycardia
d. Tachycardia
e. Incidence in multiple fractures

53. Time necessary for healing of fracture depends on the following factors *[WB PGMEE 1989]*

a. Age of the patient
b. Location of the fracture
c. Type of the fracture
d. Degree of damage to soft tissues
e. All of the above

54. Most important factor in fracture healing is *[Rohtak PGMEE 1989]*

a. Good alignment
b. Organization of blood clot
c. Accurate reduction and 100% apposition of fractured fragments
d. Immobilisation
e. Adequate calcium intake

55. Fat embolism may ensue following *[TN PGMEE 1995] [Karnataka PGMEE1997]*

a. Fracture of spine and ribs
b. Fractured fibula
c. Fracture of skull bone
d. Fracture of long bones only

56. Which of the following is true about fat embolism? *[Rohtak PGMEE 1998]*

a. Usually ensues after fracture of the lower limb
b. Uncommon complication of fracture
c. Spontaneously reversible process
d. All of the above

57. Fat embolism is characterized by *[PGI 2004]*

a. Petechial haemorrhages
b. Closed fractures of femur
c. Aggregation of chylomicrons
d. Fall in the haemoglobin
e. Fat globules in sputum & urine

58. Which fracture requires Open reduction in children? *[AIIMS PG 1991, 1992, AIPGME 1991]*

a. Fracture of both bones of forearm
b. Epiphyseal separation of tibia
c. Intercondylar fracture of femur
d. Lateral condyle fracture of humerus

59. Delayed union of fracture of a bone following a surgical treatment may be due to *[NBE DNB 1990, Delhi PGMEE 2004]*

a. Infection
b. Inadequate circulation
c. Inadequate mobilization
d. All of the above

60. True about fat embolism *[PGI PGMEE 2007, 2009]*

a. Bradycardia and systemic hypoxia may occur
b. Is more commonly seen in closed fractures
c. Liposuction is used in treatment
d. Co-existent diabetes mellitus pose a risk
e. Fracture mobility is a risk factor

61. Which of the following fractures would best be treated by Open reduction? *[AMU PGMEE 1989]*

a. Fracture of the femoral shaft of the child
b. Collies' fracture
c. Displaced fracture of the femoral neck
d. Fracture of humeral shaft

62. Non-union is a complication of *[AIIMS PGMEE 1998]*
a. Scaphoid fracture
b. Colles' fracture
c. Inter-trochanteric fracture of hip
d. Supracondylar fracture of the humerus

63. Which of the following is known for Non union in children, if left untreated? *[NBE DNB 1990, AMU PGMEE 1995]*
a. Intercondylar fracture of humerus
b. Fracture shaft of humerus
c. Fracture shaft of femur
d. Fracture distal 1/3rd of tibia
e. Fracture lateral condyle of humerus

64. Glass-holding cast is *[All India PGMEE 1991]*
a. Smith's cast b. Sacremento cast
c. Scaphoid cast d. None

65. Classical example of Muscular violence is *[PGI 1996]*
a. Fracture of fibula b. Fracture of patella
c. Fracture of clavicle d. All of the these

66. Pipkin fracture is defined as *[PGI 2005]*
a. Head of radius fracture
b. Head of femur fracture
c. Fracture dislocation of ankle
d. Fracture neck of femur
e. Fracture of C6 Spine

67. In some old fractures, cartilaginous tissue forms over the fractured bone ends with a cavity in between containing clear fluid. This condition is called as *[All India PGMEE 2004]*
a. Delayed union b. Slow union
c. Non union d. Pseudoarthrosis

68. Pseudoarthrosis may be seen in all of the following conditions, except *[All India PGMEE 1998]*
a. Fracture b. Idiopathic
c. Neurofibromatosis d. Osteomyelitis

69. In an injury with multiple fractures, most important is *[DPG 1988, PGI 1994, AIIMS 1999]*
a. Airway maintenance
b. Blood transfusion
c. Intravenous fluids
d. Open reduction of fractures

70. Tube (Cylinder) cast is applied for the fracture of *[All India PGMEE 2007]*
a. Shoulder b. Hip
c. Pelvis d. Knee

71. Fat embolism ensue after *[TN PGMEE 1995, Karnataka PGMEE 1997]*
a. Fractured spine/ribs
b. Fractured fibula
c. Fractured skull bone
d. Fractured long bones

72. Which of the following causes Acute Compartment syndrome most frequently? *[PGI 1980, AIIMS PGMEE 1986]*
a. Fractures
b. Postischemic swelling
c. Exercise initiated syndrome
d. Soft tissue injury

73. Compartment syndrome is treated by *[UP PGMEE 1999]*
a. Fasciotomy
b. Bicarbonate
c. Chloride rich fluid
d. Early aggressive fluid

74. True regarding fractures *[PGI 2009]*
a. Colles fracture: Distal end of radius fracture with dorsal tilt
b. Bennett's fracture: Oblique intra-articular fracture at base of 1st metacarpal
c. Galeazzi fracture: Distal 1/3 radius fracture with dislocated distal radio-ulnar joint
d. Monteggia fracture: Proximal 1/3 ulna fracture with radial head dislocation
e. Pott's fracture: Trimalleolar ankle fracture

75. Cotton's fracture is *[Recent Question 2017, Bihar PGMEE 1999]*
a. Bimalleolar b. Trimalleolar
c. Avulsion fracture of C7 d. Burst fracture of atlas
e. None

76. Following fractures are known for Non-union, except *[NBE DNB 1990, UP PGMEE 2002]*
a. Fracture of lower half of tibia
b. Fracture of neck of femur
c. Fracture of scaphoid
d. Fracture of patella
e. Supracondylar fracture of humerus

77. Following are principles in the treatment of Compound fractures, except *[JIPMER PGMEE 1993]*
a. Wound debridement
b. Immediate wound closure
c. Tendon repair
d. Aggressive antibiotic therapy

78. True about Eponymous fractures is all, except *[PGI 2009]*
a. Monteggia fracture is fracture of the proximal third of ulna with radial head dislocation
b. Galeazzi fracture is fracture of the distal third of the radius with dislocation of the distal radio-ulnar joint
c. Colles fracture is fracture at cortico-cancellous junction of the distal-end of radius with dorsal tilt
d. Potts fracture Trimalleolar ankle fracture
e. Bennett's fracture is Oblique intra-articular fracture of the base of the 1st metacarpal

79. Vascular injury during childhood is common in fracture of *[AIIMS PGMEE 1994]*
a. Lower end of humerus b. Lower end of radius
c. Upper end of femur d. Upper end of radius

80. Cotton's facture is *[Bihar PGMEE 1989]*
a. Avulsion fracture of C7 b. Trimalleolar
c. Bimalleolar d. Burst fracture of atlas
e. None of these

81. Avascular necrosis is a complication of *[All India PGMEE 1999]*
a. Fracture of talus
b. Fracture of medial condyle of femur
c. Olecranon fracture d. Radial head fracture

82. Internal splints (fixation devices) are used in all except *[Manipal PGMEE 1999]*
a. Compound fractures
b. Multiple fractures
c. Fractures in elderly patients
d. Fracture neck of femur

83. A compound fracture is initially treated by antibiotics, wound toilet and *[Rohtak PGMEE 1998]*
a. Skin cover
b. External splintage
c. Prosthesis
d. Internal fixation

84. In which type of fracture, the tuber-joint angle is reduced to about half *[AMU PGMEE 1990]*
a. Crush fracture of calcaneum
b. Fracture neck of humerus
c. Dislocation of shoulder
d. Spilt fracture of calcaneum

85. Which of the following is the most appropriate hospital treatment of a patient with compound fracture? *[UPSC 1999]*
a. Under anesthesia, thorough scrubbing and cleaning of the area getting the fracture end inside, suturing the wound and applying continuous skeletal traction with adequate antibiotic cover
b. Cleaning and suturing the wound, applying plaster Spica under traction on a Harly's table and administering antibiotics round the clock
c. Scrubbing and cleaning the area, resecting the protruding one inch of the bone, suturing the wound, bringing the fractured ends into alignment and applying plaster Spica with continuous antibiotic cover
d. Thorough cleaning of the area, extending the wound, bringing the fragments into alignment under vision, fixing them with intra-medullary nail and giving antibiotics to the patient.

86. Most common cause of Anterior Compartment syndrome is *[PGI 1993]*
a. Fractures
b. Post ischaemic swelling
c. Superficial injury to muscles
d. Operative trauma

87. Tetanus is noticed usually in *[All India PGMEE 1990]*
a. Burn cases
b. Wounds contaminated with faecal matter
c. Open fractures
d. Gunshot wounds
e. All of the above

88. Which of the following score evaluates chances of Amputation in a traumatized limb? *[JIPMER PGMEE 2002, AMU PGMEE 2001]*
a. Revised trauma score
b. Injury severity score
c. Abbreviated injury score
d. MES score

89. Drawer sign is seen in *[Rajasthan PGMEE 1992]*
a. Scurvy
b. Perthes disease
c. Hyperparathyroidism
d. Cruciate ligament injury

90. What is true about Compartment syndrome? *[PGI 2005]*
a. Loss of pulses is reliable sign
b. Pain on passive stretch is reliable sign
c. Interstitial stretch is reliable sign
d. Fasciotomy is earliest management

91. All are relevant in Compartment syndrome, except *[PGI 2000]*
a. Fasciotomy
b. Splitting of tight pop cast
c. Reexploration
d. Exercise

92. All of the following factors evaluate the chances of amputation in a limb, except *[PGI 1995, MAHE PGMEE 2001]*
a. Age
b. B.P.
c. Velocity of trauma
d. Presence of infection

93. All are correct regarding Compartment syndrome *[PGI 2005]*
a. Pulse is a reliable indicator
b. Pain on passive stretching
c. Interstitial pressure > capillary pressure
d. Hyperesthesia
e. Fasciotomy is the earliest treatment

94. Myositis ossificans is most common around the .... joint *[UP PGMEE 1996]*
a. Knee
b. Elbow
c. Wrist
d. Hip

95. Treatment of Acute Myositis Ossificans is *[AIIMS PGMEE 1991]*
a. Active mobilization
b. Passive mobilization
c. Infra Red Therapy
d. Immobilization

96. In flap method of amputation which structure is kept shorter than the level of amputation? *[NBE DNB 1992, Delhi PGMEE 2010]*
a. Bone
b. Muscles
c. Nerves
d. Skin
e. Vessels

97. MC joint site for Ligament injury *[AP PGMEE 1999]*
a. Shoulder
b. Elbow
c. Knee
d. Ankle

98. Myositis ossificans is due to *[Bihar PGMEE 1990]*
a. Ossification
b. New bone formation
c. Ossification of subperiosteal haematoma
d. Migration osteoblasts to haematoma
e. All of the above

99. Treatment of choice in Acute myositis ossificans is *[TN PGMEE 1991]*
a. Immobilization of elbow
b. Short wave diathermy
c. Passive movements of arm
d. Active exercises

100. Following are recognized F/O Myositis ossificans, except *[Karnataka PGMEE 2002, TN PGMEE 1999]*
a. It is a post traumatic ossification
b. It follows either a posterior dislocation or a supracondylar fracture of elbow joint
c. The complication is less likely in children
d. Diagnosis is made with certainty by skiagraphy

101. Ring sequestrum is seen in *[TN PGMEE 1992]*
a. Typhoid osteomyelitis
b. Chronic osteomyelitis
c. Amputation stump
d. Tuberculosis osteomyelitis

102. Which of the following is true regarding a Phantom limb? *[All India PGMEE 1994]*
a. Occurs in leprosy
b. Follows amputation
c. Follows a psychiatric illness
d. After filariasis

103. Myodesis is employed in amputations for all of the following indications, except *[All India PGMEE 2009]*
a. Trauma
b. Tumor
c. Children
d. Ischemia

104. In Traumatic Myositis ossificans, following are true, except *[PGI 2000]*
a. Hydroxyapatite deposition
b. Common in elbow injury
c. Periosteal hematoma and leakage
d. Injury of tendon over muscle

105. In Myositis ossificans mature bone is seen *[MAHE PGMEE 2004, AMU PGMEE 2003]*
a. At periphery
b. In center
c. Whole muscle mass
d. In the joint capsule

106. Radiological feature differentiating myositis ossificans from bone tumor is *[NIMHANS PGMEE 2003, SGPGI 1999]*
a. Peripheral ossification
b. Central lucency
c. Discontinuity with the bone
d. None

107. Milkman's fracture is *[All India PGMEE 2009]*
a. Fracture humerus
b. Fracture 1st metacarpal
c. Fracture clavicle in children
d. Pseudofracture in adults

108. Traumatic fracture(s) showing Avascular necrosis is/are *[PGI 2007]*
a. Radius lower end
b. Femoral neck
c. Body of talus
d. Cuboid
e. Surgical neck of humerus

109. Which of the following is not true about Myositis ossificans? *[PGI 2000]*
a. Associated with muscle tendon rupture
b. Inflammation around the ruptured muscle (deposition of hydroxyapatite crystals)
c. Common in supracondylar fracture
d. Ossification of musculo-periosteal haematoma

110. False about myositis ossificans progressiva (child with heterotopic ossifications) is *[All India PGMEE 2008]*
a. Pneumonia is common
b. Life longevity is normal
c. Most common site involved is the spine
d. Onset is before 6 year

111. Basic pathology in Myositis Ossificans Progressiva is in *[NBE DNB 1990, Delhi PGMEE 1997]*
a. Muscle fibres
b. Serum chemistry
c. Body collagen
d. None of the above

112. Post-traumatic Avascular necrosis occur in fracture(s) of *[PGI 2000][PGI 2009]*
a. Neck talus
b. Neck femur
c. Surgical neck humerus
d. Neck radius
e. Waist scaphoid

113. A person of 6 years age is suffering from Myositis ossificans progressive. Usual cause of death would be *[AIIMS PGMEE 2000, NIMHANS PGMEE 2001]*
a. Nutritional deficiency
b. Bed sore
c. Lung disease
d. Septicemia

114. All are true regarding myositis ossificans progressive, except *[PGI 2003]*
a. Usually involve children
b. Progressive form of normal myositis
c. Respiratory problems
d. Ankylosis
e. Form normal bone

115. OR is not required in which fracture *[AIIMS PGMEE 1995]*
a. Patella
b. Outer 1/3 of radius
c. Condyle of humerus
d. Olecranon displaced

116. Aseptic necrosis can occur in *[PGI 2008]*
a. Steroid administration
b. Gaucher's disease
c. Slipped capital femoral epiphysis
d. Caisson disease
e. Perthes disease

117. Commonest fracture in childhood is *[All India PGMEE 1989]*
a. Femur
b. Distal humerus
c. Clavicle
d. Radius

118. Ruptured tendon is most commonly seen in *[All India PGMEE 2000]*
a. Stab injury
b. Soft tissue tumour
c. Overuse
d. Congenital defect

119. Compartment syndrome include *[PGI November 2014]*
a. Common in injuries to long bones
b. Decreased pressure
c. Earliest sign stretch test
d. Nerve damage
e. Surgical decompression

120. Earliest way to detect Compartment syndrome in a patient with Cast is *[AIIMS November 2017]*
a. Check radial pulse by displacing the cast
b. Reduced response to analgesia
c. Change in odour of skin
d. Change in colour of fingers

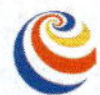 NEET/NBE PATTERN MCQs ANSWERS WITH EXPLANATIONS

1. **Ans. (c) Osteonecrosis**
   [Ref. Mayo Clinic Internal Medicine Board Review, 11/e p816]

   Osteonecrosis
   - Bone death related to loss of blood supply
   - Multiple wedge-shaped subchondral depressions
   - May lead to collapse of articular cartilage surface, i.e. Secondary osteoarthritis
   - **MC site: Femoral head**
   - Common cause: Trauma hampering blood supply

2. **Ans. (c) Transcervical fracture of the neck of femur**
   [Ref. Surgery of the Hip Joint, Volume 2 by Tronzo, 2/e p2]

   Avascular Necrosis of Hip
   - Seen in conjunction with trauma to the region of the hip, usually transcervical fracture or complete dislocation
   - Extracapsular, intertrochanteric, and subtrochanteric fractures are at much less risk for avascular necrosis (AVN) of the femoral head than intracapsular, femoral neck fractures

3. **Ans. (a) Children**
   [Ref. Essentials of Surgical Specialties by Lawrence, 3/e p233]
   - Although most bone fractures are complete, an incomplete buckling of only one cortex is seen in children and is known as a **Greenstick fracture**

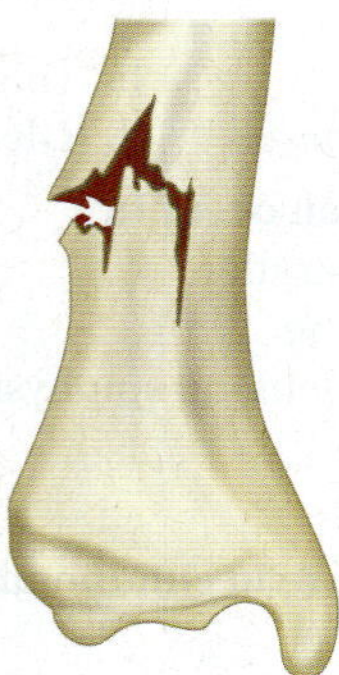

Fig. Greenstick fracture

4. **Ans. (b) Lateral retinacular branch of medial circumflex femoral artery**
   [Ref. Pediatric Femur Fractures by Daniel Hedequist, 1/e p76]
   - Lateral Epiphyseal Vessels supply majority of developing femoral head, and are tributaries of Ascending cervical branches of Medial circumflex femoral artery (MCFA)
   - LFCA nourish Anterior femoral head, but absent by age 2–3 (at which time, its principal supply of Femoral neck metaphysis)
   - Blood supply to the head of the femur is severely compromised by any fracture of the head or neck that involves the Medial circumflex artery, or its posterosuperior and posteroinferior branches

5. **Ans. (c) Physeal injuries**
   [Ref. Rockwood and Wilkins' Fractures in Children, Volume 3, 7/e p98]

   Salter-Harris (SH) Classification of Physeal Fractures
   - Salter and Harris published their commonly used five-part classification of physeal injuries in 1963
   - First four types were adopted from Poland (Types I, II, and III) and Aitken (Aitken type III became SH Type IV)
   - Additional V type was added by SH (Unrecognized compression injury)

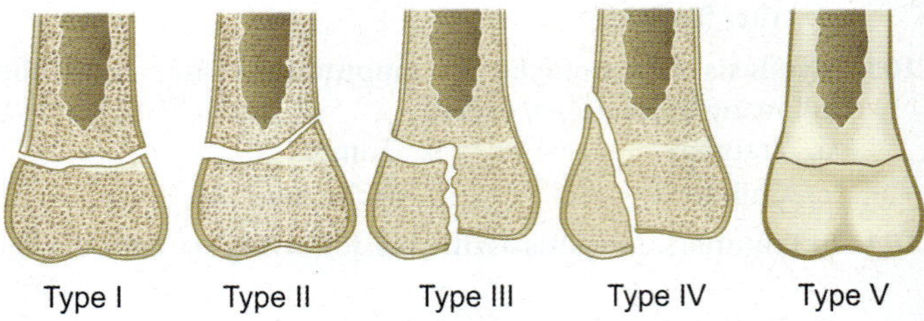

Fig. Salter-Harris classification

6. **Ans. (b) II**
   [Ref. Maheshwari, 4/e p56]

   Salter-Harris Classification of Epiphyseal Injuries
   - I - Physeal fracture (Radial neck epiphysis)
   - II - Physeal + Metaphyseal fracture (Lower end radius epiphysis)
   - III - Physeal + Epiphyseal fracture (Medial malleolus epiphysis)
   - IV - Physeal + Metaphyseal Epiphyseal fracture (Lateral condyle humerus)
   - V - Physeal crush injury (Lower tibial epiphysis)
   - VI - Perichondrial injury

7. **Ans. (b) It matures from inside out**
   [Ref. Comprehensive Board Review in Orthopaedic Surgery by Kamal, Chap7]

   Myositis ossificans
   - Mineralizes from outside inwards with mature bone initially at periphery of lesion; opposite of osteosarcoma, which mineralizes from inside out

8. **Ans. (c) Open segmental fractures, open fractures with extensive soft tissue damage, traumatic amputation**
   [Ref. Oxford Desk Reference - Major Trauma, 1/e p254]

   Gustilo and Anderson Classification of Open Fractures
   - **Type I**: Open fracture with a wound < 1 cm long and clean
   - **Type II**: Open fracture with a laceration > 1 cm long without extensive soft tissue damage, flaps, or avulsions
   - **Type III**: Either an open segmental fracture, an open fracture with extensive soft tissue damage (>10 cm) or a traumatic amputation
     - Type IIIA: Open fractures with adequate soft tissue coverage of a fractured bone despite extensive soft tissue laceration or flaps, or high-energy trauma regardless of the size of the wound
     - Type IIIB: Open fractures with extensive soft tissue injury loss with periosteal stripping and bone exposure, usually associated with massive contamination
     - Type IIIC: Open fractures associated with arterial injury requiring repair

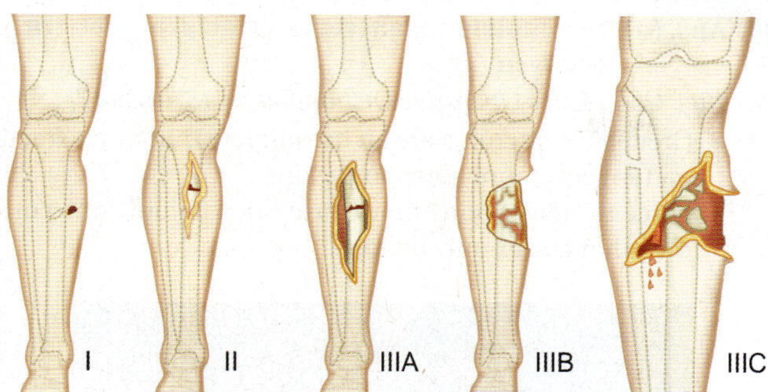

Fig. Gustilo and Anderson classification

9. Ans. (a) Stretch pain

[Ref. Skeletal Trauma by Browner, 1/e p344]

- Pain referred to a compartment on passive stretching of the digits is a **Reliable sign** of an impending Acute compartment syndrome
- **Earliest sign** of an Acute compartment syndrome is a tensely swollen compartment whose palpation reproduces the patient's pain
- **First and most important symptom** of an impending compartment syndrome is pain that is greater than that expected from injury

10. Ans. (d) Vitamin E

[Ref. Wound Care by Sarabahi, VK Tiwari, 1/e p440]

Wound Healing Associations

- **Copper** is associated with increased wound elasticity and resistance
- **Zinc** increase wound elasticity and resistance; Zinc deficiency is associated with deranged fibroblast proliferation and delayed epithelialization resulting in poor wound healing and decreased breaking strength of experimental wounds
- **Vitamin A** increase collagen cross-linkage and wound breaking strength
- **Vitamin D** increase wound breaking strength and improve epithelialization
- **Vitamin C** increase epithelial cell adhesion and tensile strength of tissue

Also Remember

- Vitamin E has a negative impact on Wound healing:
  - Alter Prostaglandin synthesis
  - Reduce collagen production
  - Decrease inflammation

11. Ans. (d) Fat embolism

[Ref. Fractures by Hoppenfeld, 1/e p292]

Fat Embolism Syndrome (FES)

- Multi-organ disorder with potentially serious sequelae that is commonly seen in the orthopaedic patient population after femur fractures
- Major clinical features of FES include hypoxia, pulmonary dysfunction, mental status changes, petechiae, tachycardia, fever, thrombocytopenia, and anemia

12. Ans. (d) Imperfect splint

13. Ans. (b) Head of radius

14. Ans. (d) Colles' fracture

15. Ans. (d) Distal end of radius (Colles fracture)

[Ref. Maheshwari, 4/e p47-49]

Non-Union of Fractures

More common sites	Less common sites
Proximal pole and waist of scaphoid Head and neck of femur Body of talus Fracture healing	Lower 1/3 tibia Lower 1/3 ulna Lateral condyle humerus

Also Remember

- *Common sites for mal-union of fractures*:
  - Supracondylar humerus
  - Intratrochanteric humerus
  - Distal end of radius (Colles fracture)

16. Ans. (b) Talus

[Ref. Maheshwari, 4/e p49]

17. Ans. (b) Colles' fracture

18. Ans. (a) Distal radius

19. Ans. (d) Fracture dislocation

20. Ans. (a) Pseudomonas

21. Ans. (c) Humerus fracture

22. Ans. (c) Incomplete fracture

23. Ans. (c) Neck femur

24. Ans. (c) Salter-Harris type-II fracture

[Ref. Maheshwari, 4/e p56]

- *Salter-Harris classification of Epiphyseal injuries*:

Class	Types of injury	Site
I	Physeal fracture	Radial neck epiphysis
II	Physeal + Metaphyseal fracture	Lower end radius epiphysis
III	Physeal + Epiphyseal fracture	Medial malleolus epiphysis
IV	Physeal + Metaphyseal Epiphyseal fracture	Lateral condyle humerus
V	Physeal crush injury	Lower tibial epiphysis
VI	Perichondrial injury	

- *Good prognosis*: Type I, II
- *Thurston-Holland Sign*:
  - Small separated frogman of bone from growth plate
  - Seen in Type II epiphysial injury
  - Also known as *'Shiny corner sign'*

25. Ans. (d) Shaft ulna - Rush nail

26. Ans. (c) Compression at fracture site causes nonunion

27. Ans. (d) Crush syndrome

[Ref. Ref. Maheshwari, 4/e p43]

Crush Syndrome

- *Causes*:
  - Massive crush injuries
  - Earthquakes, mining accidents, air-raids
  - Application of tourniquet for an excessively long period
- *Pathophysiology*:
  - Crushing of muscles lead to entry of myohemoglobin into circulation

- MyoHb precipitates in renal tubules leading to Acute tubular necrosis
- *Clinical features*:
  - Scanty urine, apathy, restlessness, delirium
- *Treatment*:
  - Application of a tourniquet which is gradually released
  - If oliguria develops: Treat for acute renal failure

28. Ans. (d) Lower tibial fracture

29. Ans. (b) Fracture calcaneum

30. Ans. (c) Epiphyseal plate fractures

[Ref. Maheshwari, 4/e p56]

31. Ans. (a) Open fractures

[Ref. Mercer's Textbook of Orthopedics, 10/e p249]

Gustilo-Anderson Classification of Open Fractures

Type	Wound	Contamina-tion	Soft tissue injury	Bone injury
I	< 1 cm	Clean	Minimal	Minimal comminution
II	> 1 cm	Moderate	Moderate	Moderate comminution
III A	< 10 cm	High	Severe with Crushing	Comminuted
III B	> 10 cm	High	Very severe, Loss of skin	Moderate to severe comminution
III C	> 10 cm	High	Very severe, Loss of skin/ vascularity	Moderate to severe com-minution, Bone coverage poor

32. Ans. (b) Fixation only

[Ref. Orthopedics by Mohindra, 2/e p17]

- Treatment in hypertrophic nonunion, just a stable Internal fixation may promote union
- Treatment of oligotrophic and atrophic non-infected nonunion requires open reduction, debridement followed by Internal fixation with bone grafting

33. Ans. (a) Fracture humerus

[Ref. Pediatric Orthopedics by Staheli, 2/e p66]

Dunlop Traction

- **Used for Supracondylar humeral fractures**
- Advantage: Allows swollen elbow to settle
- Disadvantages:
  - It cannot be applied over skin injuries
  - Elevation of the humeral fracture above the level of the heart is not possible with this method

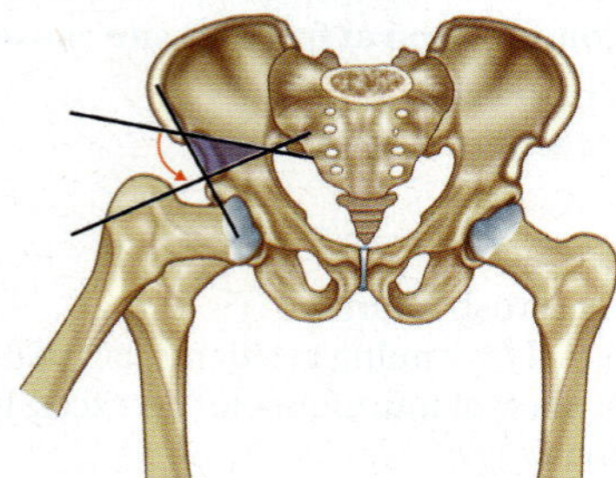

Fig. Dunlop Traction

34. Ans. (a) Incomplete transverse fracture pattern in children

[Ref. Campbell's Operative Orthopaedics, 13/e p1147]

- Greenstick fractures are an incomplete transverse fracture pattern commonly seen in children
- Force to side of bone may cause break in only one cortex; the other cortex only bends

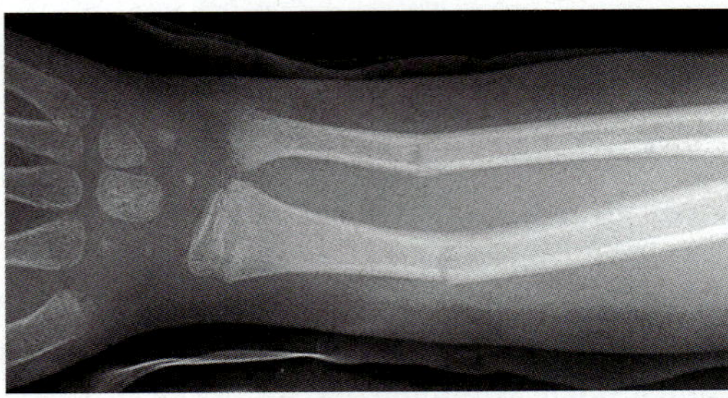

Fig. Green-stick fractures

35. Ans. (a) Split Russell traction

[Ref. The Parkland Trauma Handbook, 1/e p562]

Femur Fractures-Shaft

Infants (0–2 years of age)

- Beware of child abuse
- Almost always is immediately placed in a Spica cast for 4–6 weeks
- Up to 3° angulation and 1 cm shortening are acceptable

Children 2–10 years of Age

- Most can be treated with closed reduction and immediate Spica cast application
- Shortening > 7 cm or multiple injuries are contraindications to immediate spica cast
- Treat with split Russell's or skeletal traction for 2-3 weeks
- Split Russell's traction:
  - Skin traction is applied in the longitudinal axis of the limb
  - A balanced sling with a vertical force is placed under the distal femur or knee and suspended by weights to support the part

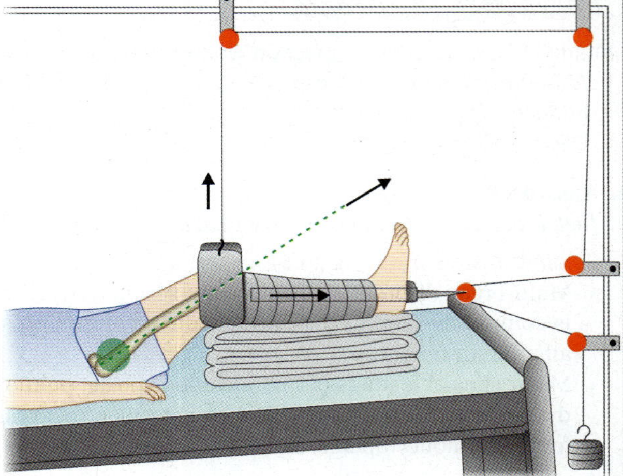

Fig. Split Russell's traction

Orthopedics

36. Ans. (a) Vertebrae

[Ref. Pediatric Orthopedics by Staheli, 2/e p301]

- Seat-belt injuries are due to a **flexion distraction mechanism** causing compression fractures of the lumbar vertebrae thought to be due to the elasticity of the posterior ligamentous structure present in children.

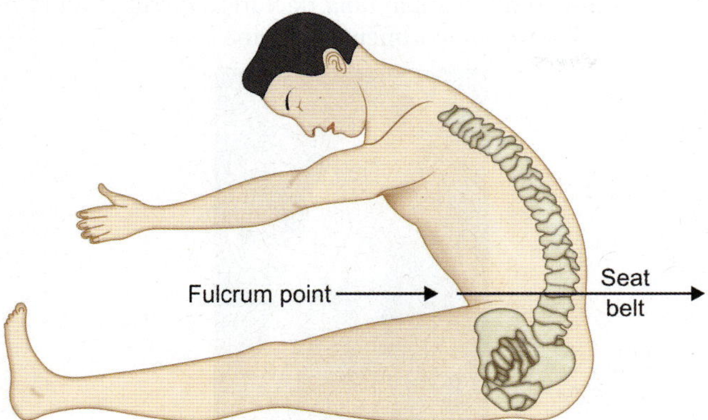

Fig. Seat-belt injury

37. Ans. (d) IV

[Ref. Intra-articular Fractures by Malhotra, 1/e p347]

Pipkin's Classification

- Type I: Fracture distal to the fovea capitis, not involving the weight-bearing surface
- Type II: Fracture proximal to the fovea capitis, involving the weight-bearing surface
- Type III: Type I or II fracture with a fracture of the femoral neck
- Type IV: Type I or II fracture with a fracture of the acetabular wall

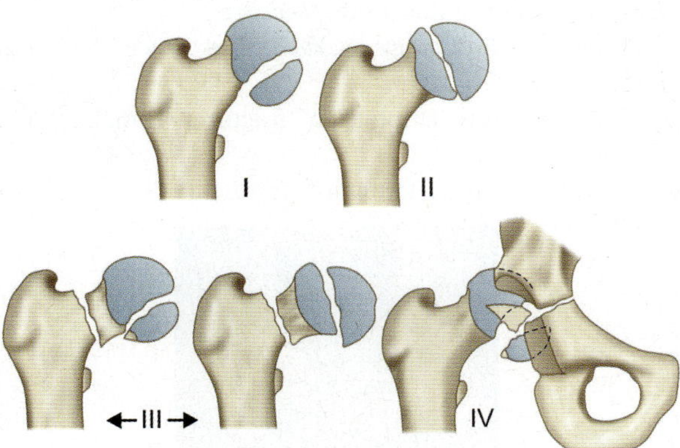

Fig. Pipkin's classification

38. Ans. (d) Fracture of hand bones

[Ref. Musculoskeletal Diseases 2017-2020 by Hodler, 1/e p132]

- Fractures common in children: Forearm bones fractures, Supracondylar fracture of the humerus, Fracture of lateral condyle of the humerus, Epiphyseal injuries, Spiral fracture of Tibial shaft
- Dislocations are uncommon in children
- Fractures of hands and feet are also uncommon in children

39. Ans. (a) Unnatural radiodense fragments

[Ref. Orthopaedic Examination Made Easy by Varshney, 2/e p431]

Sequestra

- Radiodense intraosseous necrotic bone fragments
- In osteomyelitis, Sequestrum maintains it's original bone density, but appears more radiodense due to the tissue density of the Involucrum which is composed of fibrous tissue and vascularized, rarefied living bone

40. Ans. (b) Galeazzi fracture

[Ref. Orthopaedic Dictionary by Hoppenfeld, 1/e p134]

Galeazzi fracture

- Fracture of the distal radius with disruption of the distal radioulnar joint (DRUJ)
- **Fracture of necessity:** Because in adults its management necessitates the surgical treatment with anatomic reduction and stable fixation of both the radial fracture and the DRUJ

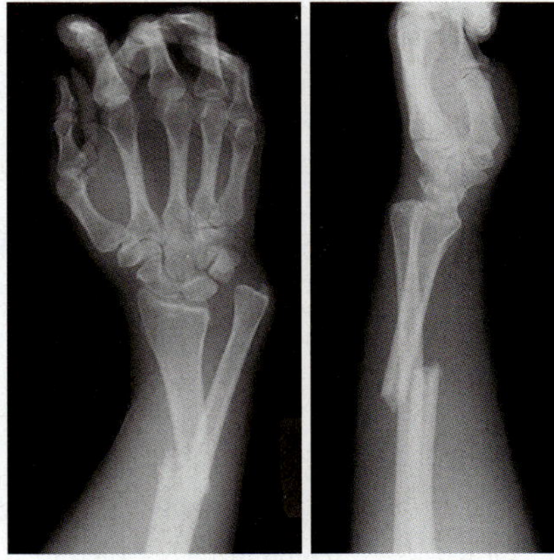

Fig. Galeazzi fracture dislocation

41. Ans. (a) Shoulder

[Ref. Anatomy Upper Limb and Thorax Volume 1 by Vishram Singh, 2/e p82]

Shoulder Joint

- Most freely mobile joint in body
- MC dislocated joint in the body
- MC joint to undergo recurrent dislocation

42. Ans. (a) Periarticular fractures

[Ref. Orthopedics by Mohindra, 1/e p406]

Locking Compression Plate (LCP)

- Especially designed for rigid fixation in cases of periarticular fractures and fractures of osteoporotic bones
- Screws of this plate have threads with high pitch and also have threads in the screw heads that can be locked to the holes in the plates, thereby providing a very rigid fixation

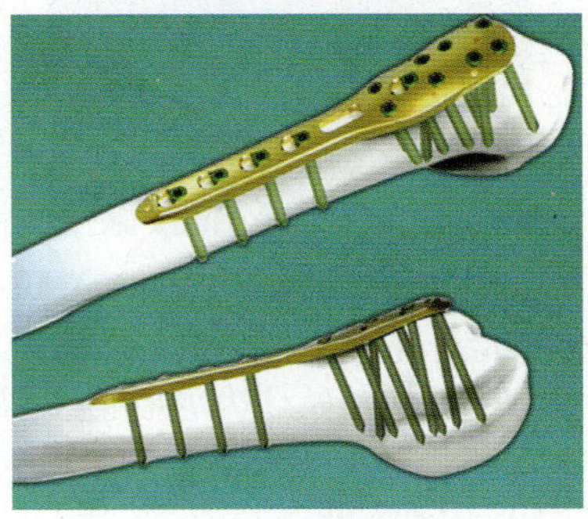

Fig. LCP

Orthopedics

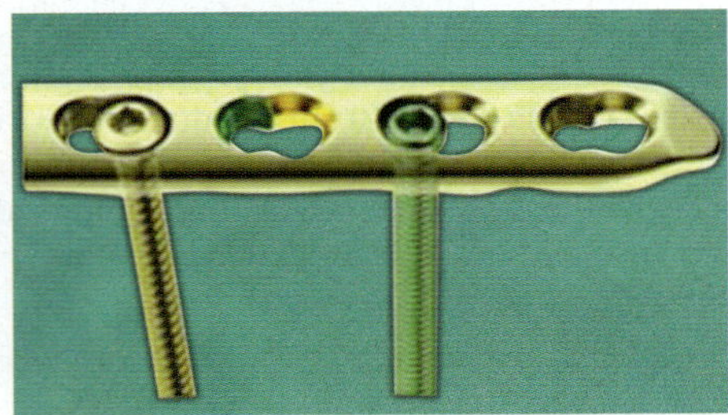

Fig. LCP

43. Ans. (d) **Type V is the perichondrial ring injury**

[Ref. Maheshwari, 4/e p56]

Salter-Harris Classification of Epiphyseal Injuries

- I - Physeal fracture (Radial neck epiphysis)
- II - Physeal + Metaphyseal fracture (Lower end radius epiphysis)
- III - Physeal + Epiphyseal fracture (Medial malleolus epiphysis)
- IV - Physeal + Metaphyseal Epiphyseal fracture (Lateral condyle humerus)
- V - Physeal crush injury (Lower tibial epiphysis)
- VI - Perichondrial injury

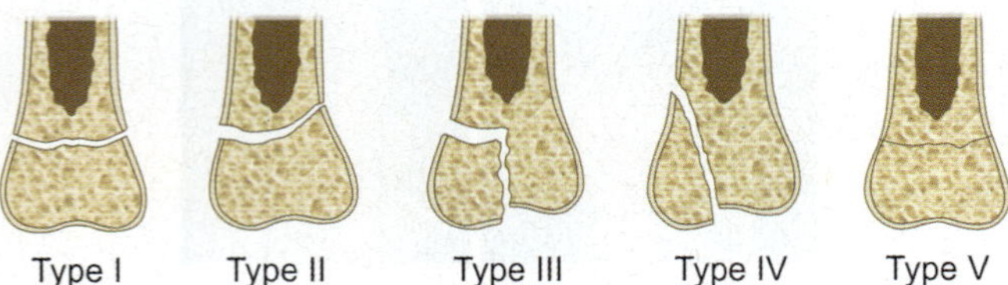

Fig. Salter-Harris classification

44. Ans. (b) **Intra-articular fracture of styloid process**

[Ref. Essential Orthopaedics by Maheshwari, 5/e p3]

Chauffeur Fracture

- Hutchinson's fracture
- An intra-articular, oblique fracture of the styloid process of the radius

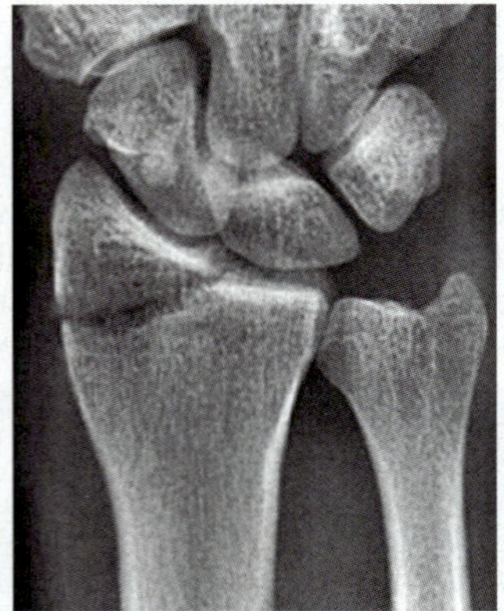

Fig. Chauffer's fracture

45. Ans. **(a) Fracture of proximal tibia**

[Ref. Mercer's Textbook of Orthopaedics and Trauma, 10/e p380]

Compartment Syndrome

- MCC: Fracture
- Syndrome is often caused by higher energy, closed fractures, but can also occur with lower-energy forces and open fractures
- History of direct blunt injury to the limb, such as a tibia struck by the bumper of a ca
- Occur MC with closed tibia fractures, and are particularly common in proximal tibia fractures. Vascular injury can also lead to compartment syndrome

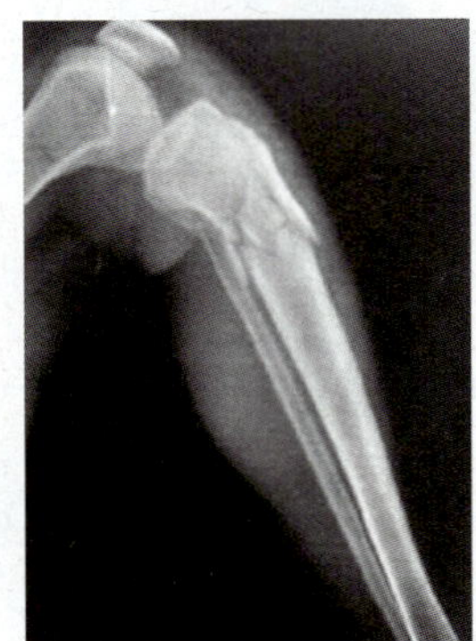

Fig. Fracture proximal tibia

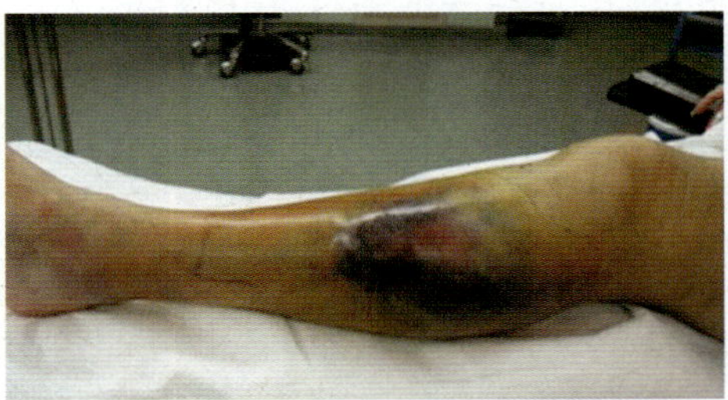

Fig. Compartment syndrome

46. Ans. (a) **Bimalleolar ankle fracture**

[Ref. Skeletal Radiology by Yochum & Rowe, 3/e Volume 1, p877]

- Pott's fracture/Dupuytren fracture: Bimalleolar ankle fractures
- Cotton's fracture: Trimalleolar fracture

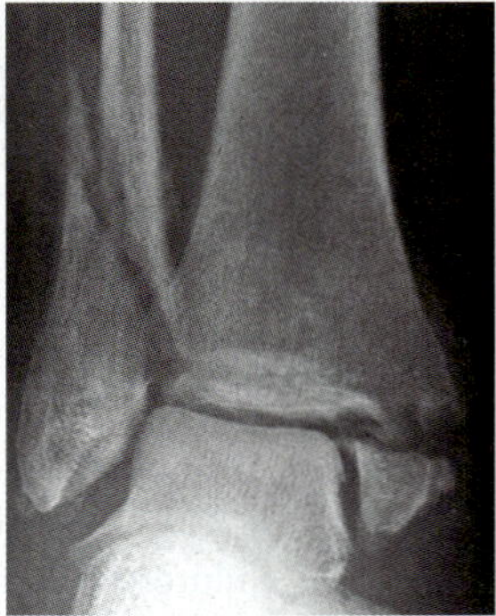

Fig. Pott's fracture

47. Ans. (a) **Bone**

[Ref. Trauma Management by Ilyas, 1/e p20]

- In the part-by-part approach, a surgeon repairs the same anatomic structure of each digit sequentially
- Repair sequence: First bones and then tendons, vessels, nerves, and so forth

HIGH YIELD MCQs ANSWERS WITH EXPLANATIONS 

1. Ans. (b) Compression
[Ref. Maheshwari, 5/e p11]

Factors affecting Fracture Healing
- **Age of patient**: Faster union of fractures in childhood
- **Type of bone**: Flat & Cancellous bones unite faster than Tubular & Cortical bones
- **Pattern of fracture**: Spiral fractures (Fastest union) > Oblique fractures > Transverse fractures > Comminuted fractures (Slowest healing)
- Disturbed pathoanatomy: Soft tissue interposition & Ischaemic fracture ends impair healing
- Type of reduction: Good apposition lead to faster reunion
- Immobilization: Ribs/Scapular fractures heal without immobilization, Fracture neck femur may not heal even after immobilization
- Open fractures: Delayed union & Nonunion
- Compression at fracture site: Enhances rate of union in Cancellous bone (In cortical bones, it increases rigidity of fixation, possibly resulting in Primary bone healing)

2. Ans. (b) Transverse fracture
[Ref. Imaging of Pediatric Bone and Joint Trauma by Martino, 1/e p10]

Transverse Fracture of Bones
- Fracture line perpendicular to major axis of bone
- Seen in Childhood and adolescence
- Result of direct impact or shear forces

3. Ans. (a) Osteogenesis imperfecta; (b) Osteoporosis; (d) Osteomalacia; (e) Radiation
[Ref. Medical Language for Modern Health, 1/e]

Pathological Fractures
- Osteoporosis
- Osteomalacia
- Osteitis
- Osteogenesis imperfecta
- Paget's disease
- Benign bone cyst and tumors
- Primary and secondary malignant bone tumors

4. Ans. (a) Intramedullary nailing; (b) Plating; (c) External fixation
[Ref. Essentials of Terror Medicine by Cole, 1/e p291]

5. Ans. (c) Remodelling
[Ref. Maheshwari, 4/e p10]
- Stages in Fracture healing (Frost): Hematoma, Granulation tissue, Callus, Remodelling, Modelling

6. Ans. (b) Three-point fixation
[Ref. Maheshwari, 4/e p335]

7. Ans. (a) Open fracture; (b) Dislocated fracture; (c) Vascular injury; (e) Compartment syndrome

8. Ans. (a) Fracture tibial epiphysis
[Ref. Campbell's Operative Orthopedics by Beaty, 12/e]

9. Ans. (c) Inadequate immobilization
[Ref. Oral and Maxillofacial Surgery by Pogrel, 1/e p891]
- **Causes of Non-union of fracture**: *Inadequate immobilization (Most common cause), inadequate reduction,* Distraction, Infection, Impaired circulation

10. Ans. (a) Scaphoid
[Ref. Maheshwari, 4/e p112]

11. Ans. (c) Volar Barton's fracture
[Ref. Maheshwari, 4/e p109-110]

12. Ans. (d) Lateral condyle humerus
[Ref. Maheshwari, 4/e p109]

13. Ans. (a) Dermatitis; (b) Vascularity compromised status of limb; (c) Abrasions
- **Contraindications of Skin traction**: Dermatitis, Vascularity compromised status of limb (Impending gangrene/Varicose veins), Abrasions, Lacerations

14. Ans. (a) K-wire; (c) Denham Pin; (d) Steinmann's pin
[Ref. Textbook of Orthopedics by Kotwal, 1/e p8]

15. Ans. (c) Greenstick fracture of lower end of radius
[Ref. The Surgical Examination of Children by Hutson, 2/e p175]

16. Ans. (b) Is generally incomplete
[Ref. Pediatric Physical Therapy by Tecklin, 4/e p459]
- **Incomplete fractures in children**: Greenstick fractures, Torus/ Buckle, Plastic bowing

17. Ans. (c) A partial or complete loss of continuity of bone
[Ref. Maheshwari, 4/e p1]

18. Ans. (b) Bony tenderness
[Ref. Textbook of Orthopedics by Kotwal, 1/e p197]
- **MC symptom of Fracture**: Pain
- **MC sign of Fracture**: Tenderness over bone affected

19. Ans. (c) Osteopenia
[Ref. Imaging of Arthritis and Metabolic Bone Disease by Weissman, 1/6 p607]

Sudeck's Dystrophy
- Reflex sympathetic dystrophy syndrome: Severe localized osteopenia associated with severity of conditions
- **Colles' fracture (MCC in Upper limb)**
- Presentation: Burning pain, stiffness, discoloration
- Treatment: Intensive physiotherapy, Stellate ganglion block/Paravertebral LUMBAR BLOCK (Dramatic reversal)

20. Ans. (a) Malunited Colles' fracture
[Ref. Maheshwari, 4/e p110]

21. Ans. (a) Sudeck osteodystrophy
[Ref. Metabolic Bone Disease by Krane, 1/e p365]

22. Ans. (d) Self-limiting and good prognosis
[Ref. Maheshwari, 4/e p110]

23. Ans. (b) Comminuted fractures are common
[Ref. Rockwood and Wilkins' Fractures in Children by Kasser, 7/e p368]

24. Ans. (b) Angulation in metaphysis
[Ref. musculoskeletal Imaging by Manaster, 4/e p42]

- Remodelling of bones in children is best in presence of: Young age, Metaphyseal involvement, Angulation

25. Ans. (c) Crepitus
[Ref. System of Surgery, Volume 1 p527]

26. Ans. (a) Transverse fracture
[Ref. Differential Diagnosis in Conventional radiology by Francis, 3/e p53]

27. Ans. (d) Perichondrial ring injury
[Ref. The Rehabilitation Specialists' Handbook by Roy, 4/e p162]

Epiphyseal Injuries

- Type I: Complete epiphyseal separation from metaphysis without fracture of bone
- Type II: Line of separation passing through epiphysis and metaphysis to produce triangular fragment
- Type III: Intra-articular fracture extending from joint surface through epiphyseal plate to periphery
- Type IV: Intra-articular fracture extending from joint surface through entire epiphyseal plate thickness, and through portion of metaphysis
- Type V: Severe crushing injury applied through epiphysis to one area of plate
- Type VI: Damage to periosteum or perichondrial ring

28. Ans. (c) Osteochondroma; (e) Fluorosis

29. Ans. (b) Anaemia

30. Ans. (b) Osteoporosis
[Ref. Adam's Outline of Fractures by Adams, 1/e p17]

- **MCC of Pathological fracture due to diffuse/generalized affection**: Osteoporosis
- MCC of Pathological fracture due to **localized/circumscribed lesion**: Metastatic carcinoma

31. Ans. (d) Fracture with skin involvement
[Ref. Delmar's Administrative Medical Assisting by Dahl, 4/e p151]

- **Compound fracture**: Bone protrudes through skin surface creating possibility of an infection

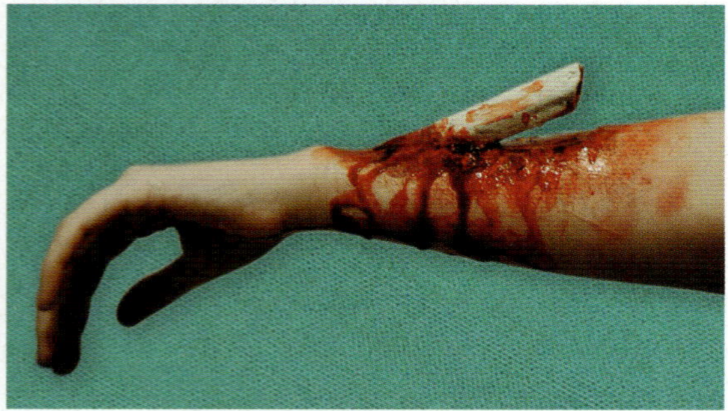

Fig. Compound fracture

32. Ans. (b) Debridement
[Ref. Emergency Procedures and Techniques by Brenner, 4/e p262]

33. Ans. (d) Clavicle
[Ref. The Shoulder by Rockwood, 4/e p394]

34. Ans. (c) Osteogenesis imperfecta

35. Ans. (c) Osteogenesis imperfecta
[Ref. Pediatric Imaging by Donelly, 1/e p168]

- **Causes of Multiple fractures in children**: Osteogenesis imperfecta, Menkes syndrome, Battered baby syndrome (Child abuse)

36. Ans. (c) Scaphoid
[Ref. Maheshwari, 4/e p111]

- MC sites of Avascular necrosis of bones in wrist: **Scaphoid** > Lunate

37. Ans. (a) Pseudofracture in adults
[Ref. Rheumatology Secrets by West, 3/e p397]

- **Pseudo-fractures/Milkman's fractures** in adults: Looser's zones

38. Ans. (b) Scaphoid
[Ref. Rockwood and Wilkinson's Fractures in Children by Kasser, 7/e p272]

39. Ans. (d) Secondary deposits
[Ref. Adam's Outline of Fractures by Adams, 1/e p17]

40. Ans. (a) Internal fixation

41. Ans. (c) Risk of pathological fracture
[Ref. Oncology: An Evidence Based Approach by Strecher, 1/e p1668]

- **Mirel's Objective Scoring System:**

Score	1	2	3
Site of lesion	Upper extremity	Lower extremity	Peri-trochanteric
Pain	Mild	Moderate	Functional
Lesion	Blastic	Mixed	Lytic
Size	< 1/3	1/3–2/3	> 2/3

- **Risk of Pathological Fracture:**

Score	Risk (%)
<6	0
7	4
8	15
9	33
10	72
11	96
12	100

42. Ans. (d) Associated diabetes pose a risk; (f) Liposuction is used for treatment

43. Ans. (b) Mobility of joint; (d) Hypovolemic shock

44. Ans. (d) Fracture of scaphoid
[Ref. Maheshwari, 4/e p111]

- **Treatment of Scaphoid fracture**: Conservative, Scaphoid cast/Glass-holding position cast for 2 weeks

45. Ans. (b) Fractures
[Ref. Compartment Syndromes by Styf, 1/e p49]

46. Ans. (a) Malunited colles' fracture
[Ref. Maheshwari, 4/e p121]

47. Ans. (d) Valgus impaction fractures
[Ref. Hands-on Guide for Surgical Training by Stephenson, 1/e p37]

48. Ans. (b) Femur fracture
[Ref. Diagnostic radiology by Niranjan, 3/e p411]

49. Ans. (a) Tachycardia; (b) Hypoxia; (c) Fat globules in urine
[Ref. Maheshwari, 4/e p42]

50. Ans. (a) Haematoma formation

51. Ans. (b) Woven bone
[Ref. Orthopedics for the Physical Therapist Assistant by Dutton, 1/e p144]

Bone Healing
- Hematoma formation: Inflammation phase
- Soft callus formation phase: Reparative/revascularization phase
- Hard callus **(Modeling phase)**: Clinical union through Woven bone
- Remodeling phase: Conversion of Cancellous to compact bone
- Intercortical bridging: Primary cortical union

52. Ans. (b) Petechiae; (d) Tachycardia; (e) Incidence in multiple fractures
[Ref. Maheshwari, 4/e p42]

53. Ans. (e) All of the above
[Ref. Maheshwari, 4/e p11-12]

Factors Affecting Bone Healing
- Age of patient: Children fractures unite faster than Adults
- Type of bone: Flat/cancellous bones unite faster than Tubular/cortical bones
- Pattern of fracture: Spiral fractures > Oblique fractures > Transverse fractures > Comminuted fractures in terms of union of fracture
- Disturbed pathoanatomy: Soft tissue interposition, Ischemic fracture impair healing
- Type of reduction: Good apposition unite faster
- Open fractures: Go into delayed union and mal-union
- Compression at fracture site: Increase rate of union in cancellous bone

54. Ans. (d) Immobilisation
[Ref. Beasleys' Surgery of Hand, 1/e p139]
- **Most important factors affecting fracture healing**: Blood supply, adequate immobilization

55. Ans. (d) Fracture of long bones only
[Ref. Maheshwari, 4/e p133]

56. Ans. (a) Usually ensues after fracture of the lower limb
[Ref. Maheshwari, 4/e p42]

57. Ans. All Choices
[Ref. Maheshwari, 4/e p42]

58. Ans. (d) Lateral condyle fracture of humerus
[Ref. Maheshwari, 4/e p99]

59. Ans. (d) All of the above
[Ref. Oral and Maxillofacial Surgery by Pogrel, 1/e p891]

60. (a) Bradycardia and systemic hypoxia may occur; (b) Is more commonly seen in closed fractures; (e) Fracture mobility is a risk factor
[Ref. Maheshwari, 4/e p42]

61. Ans. (c) Displaced fracture of the femoral neck
[Ref. Maheshwari, 4/e p131]

62. Ans. (a) Scaphoid fracture
[Ref. Maheshwari, 4/e p112]

63. Ans. (b) Fracture shaft of humerus
[Ref. Maheshwari, 4/e p139]

64. Ans. (c) Scaphoid cast
[Ref. Maheshwari, 4/e p111]

65. Ans. (b) Fracture of patella
[Ref. Complete Encyclopedia of Medicine and Health by Schade, 1/e p511]

66. Ans. (b) Head of femur fracture
[Ref. Handbook of Fractures by Egol, 4/e p374]

Pipkin Classification of Femoral Head Fractures
- Type I: Interfoveal fracture below weight-bearing surface of femoral head
- Type II: Suprafoveal fracture involving weight-bearing surface of femoral head
- Type III: Type I or II PLUS Femoral neck fracture
- Type IV: Type I or II or III PLUS Acetabular fracture

67. Ans. (d) Pseudoarthrosis
[Ref. A Concise Textbook of Oral and Maxillofacial Surgery by Chatterjee, 1/e p257]

68. Ans. (d) Osteomyelitis
[Ref. Quick Review Orthopedics by Mehra, 1/e p69]
- **Causes of Pseudoarthrosis**: Idiopathic, Neurofibromatosis, Congenital, Osteogenesis imperfecta, Fibrous dysplasia, Cleidocranial dysplasia, Ankylosing spondylitis, Post-surgical

69. Ans. (a) Airway maintenance
[Ref. Trauma Manual by Rhodes, 4/e p254]

70. Ans. (d) Knee
[Ref. Maheshwari, 4/e p142]
- Cylinder cast is used for: patter fractures, Other Knee conditions

71. Ans. (d) Fractured long bones
[Ref. Maheshwari, 4/e p42]

72. Ans. (a) Fractures
[Ref. Maheshwari, 4/e p46]

73. Ans. (a) Fasciotomy
[Ref. Maheshwari, 4/e p46]

74. (a) Colles fracture: Distal end of radius fracture with dorsal tilt; (b) Bennett's fracture: Oblique intra-articular fracture at base of 1st metacarpal; (c) Galeazzi fracture: Distal 1/3 radius fracture with dislocated distal radio-ulnar joint; (d) Monteggia fracture: Proximal 1/3 ulna fracture with radial head dislocation

75. Ans. (b) Trimalleolar
[Ref. Maheshwari, 4/e p3]

76. Ans. (e) Supracondylar fracture of humerus
[Ref. Maheshwari, 4/e p47]

Common Fractures Causing Nonunion
- Neck of femur
- Scaphoid fracture
- Lower third of tibia fracture
- Lower third of ulna fracture
- Lateral condyle of Humerus fracture

77. Ans. (b) Immediate wound closure

78. Ans. (d) Potts fracture Trimalleolar ankle fracture
[Ref. Maheshwari, 4/e p3]

79. Ans. (a) Lower end of humerus

80. Ans. (b) Trimalleolar
[Ref. Maheshwari, 4/e p3]

81. Ans. (a) Fracture of talus
[Ref. Maheshwari, 4/e p49]

82. Ans. (a) Compound fractures

83. Ans. (b) External splintage
[Ref. Manual of Fracture Treatment by Cox, 1/e p2]

84. Ans. (a) Crush fracture of calcaneum
[Ref. Insurance Counsel Journal 1961, p286]

85. Ans. (a) Under anesthesia, thorough scrubbing and cleaning of the area getting the fracture end inside, suturing the wound and applying continuous skeletal traction with adequate antibiotic cover

86. Ans. (a) Fractures
[Ref. Compartment Syndromes by Styf, 1/e p49]

87. Ans. (e) All of the above
[Ref. Medical-Surgical Nursing by Lewis, 9/e p1468]

Possible wounds for tetanus: Wounds contaminated with fecal matter, Burn cases, Open fractures, Gunshot wounds, Frostbite cases, Human/animal bites, IV drug use injection sites

88. Ans. (d) MES score
[Ref. Evidence Based Orthopedics by Wright, 1/e p320]

Mangled Extremity Scoring (MES) Systems

Scoring system	Criteria	Score predictive of amputation
MESI	ISS, Skin injury, Nerve injury, Vascular injury, Bone, Age, Pre-existing disease, Shock	>20
PSI	Arterial injury, Bone injury, Muscle injury, Time from surgery to injury	8
MESS	Injury, Ischemia, Shock, Age	7
LSI	Arterial injury, Bone injury, Nerve injury, Skin injury, Muscle injury, Deep vein injury, Warm ischemia time	6
NISSSA	Nerve injury, Ischemia, Skeletal injury, Soft tissue ischemia, Shock, Age	7

89. Ans. (d) Cruciate ligament injury
[Ref. Maheshwari, 4/e p356]

Tests for Ligaments & Menisci
- Medial and Lateral Collateral ligaments: Pain on attempt to open up the joint
- Anterior cruciate ligament: Anterior drawer test, Lachman test
- Posterior cruciate ligament: Posterior drawer test
- Tests for Menisci injury: McMurrays' test, Apley's grinding test

90. Ans. (b) Pain on passive stretch is reliable sign; (d) Fasciotomy is earliest management
[Ref. Maheshwari, 4/e p46]

91. Ans. (d) Exercise
[Ref. Maheshwari, 4/e p98]

92. Ans. (d) Presence of infection
[Ref. Classification and Diagnosis in Orthopedic Trauma by Anwar, 1/e p20]
- **Mangled Extremity Severity Score (MESS)** for predicting limb amputation after Injury:
  - Skeletal soft tissue injury: Velocity of trauma, Type of fracture, Contamination, Dislocations, gunshot injuries
  - Limb ischemia: Pulse, Numbness, Paralysis
  - Shock: Blood pressure
  - Age (years)

93. Ans. (a) Pulse is a reliable indicator
[Ref. Oxford's Handbook of Clinical Skills by Dawson, 1/e p493]

Presence of Peripheral pulse is NOT a reliable indicator of Compartment syndrome: Arteriolar spasm/collapse and subsequent loss of pulse is late and ominous sign

94. Ans. (b) Elbow
[Ref. Essential Handbook of Practical Orthopedic Examination by Banerjee, 3/e p31]
- **MC site of Myositis Ossificans Traumatica**: Elbow joint (Brachialis muscle)

95. Ans. (d) Immobilization
[Ref. Maheshwari, 4/e p51]

96. Ans. (a) Bone

97. Ans. (d) Ankle

98. Ans. (e) All of the above
[Ref. Maheshwari, 4/e p51]

99. Ans. (a) Immobilization of elbow
[Ref. Maheshwari, 4/e p51]

100. Ans. (c) The complication is less likely in children
[Ref. Maheshwari, 4/e p51]

101. Ans. (c) Amputation stump
[Ref. Orthopedics by Biswas, 1/e p103]

Sequestrum
- Description: Piece of dead bone separated from healthy bone
- **Types of Sequestrum:**
  - Ring sequestrum: Bone amputation stump (after it gets infected)

- Feathery sequestrum: Pyogenic infection
- Coarse sandy sequestrum: Tuberculosis
- Dense ivory sequestrum: Syphilis
- Coloured sequestrum: Osteomyelitis of Tibia, Ulna
- Bombay sequestrum: Phalanx and Traumatic amputation
- Coralliform sequestrum: Pyogenic infection
- Button-hole sequestrum: Pin-tract infection

102. Ans. (b) **Follows amputation**
[Ref. The Parkes of Love by Parkes, 1/e p99]

Phantom limb: Sensation that an amputated or missing limb (even an organ, like the appendix) is still attached to the body and is moving appropriately with other body parts.

103. Ans. (d) **Ischemia**
[Ref AIPGMEE 2009: Rapid Review by Koli, 1/e]

104. Ans. (a) **Hydroxyapatite deposition; (d) Injury of tendon over muscle**

105. Ans. (a) **At periphery**
[Ref. Imaging of Soft Tissue Lesions by Kransdorf, 2/e p438]

Myositis ossificans: Progressive degree of cellular maturation from centre to periphery, maturation being lowest in centre and highest (with mature bone formation) at periphery

106. Ans. (c) **Discontinuity with the bone**
[Ref. Pediatric Bone Imaging by Ritter, 1/e p403]

107. Ans. (d) **Pseudofracture in adults**
[Ref. Internal Fixation in Femoral Neck Fractures by Bosch, 1/e p235]

108. Ans. (b) **Femoral neck**
[Ref. Textbook of Orthopedics by Kotwal, 1/e p123]

109. Ans. (a) **Associated with muscle tendon rupture**
[Ref. Imaging of Soft Tissue Lesions by Kransdorf, 2/e p438]

110. Ans. (b) **Life longevity is normal**
[Ref. Orthopedic Dictionary by Zeide, 1/e p268]

In Myositis ossificans progressiva, severe functional disability occurs and is generally fatal due to progressive loss of pulmonary function

111. Ans. (a) **Muscle fibres**
[Ref. Atlas of Skeletal Muscle Pathology by Anderson, 1/e p160]

112. Ans. (a) **Neck talus; (b) Neck femur; (e) Waist scaphoid**
[Ref. Textbook of Orthopedics by Kotwal, 1/e p123]

113. Ans. (c) **Lung disease**
[Ref. Orthopedic Dictionary by Zeide, 1/e p268]

114. Ans. (b) **Progressive form of normal myositis**
[Ref. Orthopedic Dictionary by Zeide, 1/e p268]

115. Ans. (b) **Outer 1/3 of radius**
[Ref. Maheshwari, 4/e p102]

116. Ans. **All Choices**
[Ref. Radiology Review Manual by Dahnert, 7/e p52]

Causes of Aseptic Necrosis

[Mnemonic: PLASTIC GRASP]

- Pancreatitis
- Lupus erythematosus, Legg-Calve-Perthes disease
- Alcoholism, Atherosclerosis
- Steroids
- Trauma (Femoral neck fracture, Hip dislocation)
- Idiopathic, Infection
- Caisson's disease, Collagen disease (SLE)
- Gaucher's disease
- Rheumatoid arthritis, Radiation treatment
- Amyloid
- Sickle cell disease
- Pregnancy

117. Ans. (c) **Clavicle**
[Ref. Textbook of Clinical Pediatrics by Harfi, 2/e p168]

118. Ans. (c) **Overuse**
[Ref. AIPGME 2000 by Koli]

119. Ans. (a) **Common in injuries to long bones; (c) Earliest sign Stretch test; (d) Nerve damage; (e) Surgical decompression**
[Ref. Medical-Surgical Nursing by Bucher, 9/e p1522]

Compartment Syndrome

- **Description:** Increased pressure within a limited space/compartment compromise the function of vessels, nerves and/or tendons passing through
- **Causes of Compartment syndrome:**
  - **Decreased compartment size:** Casts, Splints, Restrictive dressings, Excessive traction
  - **Increased compartment contents:** Edema, Bleeding, Inflammation, IV infiltration
- **Features:**
  - Usually associated with fractures of long bones, trauma, crush injury
  - **Six P's:** Pain (distal to injury and on stretch), Pressure, Paresthesia, Pallor, Paralysis, Pulselessness
- Treatment: Elevate limb, Surgical decompression

120. Ans. (b) **Reduced response to analgesia**
[Ref. NCLEX-RN Q and A by Pearson, 1/e p69]

- Earliest symptom of Compartment syndrome: Unrelenting, progressive pain distal to the injury that is not relieved by analgesics
- Pain characteristic of the syndrome could thus be detected by evaluating the response to analgesics.

Chapter 3

Upper Limb Traumatology

THEORETICAL CONCEPTS

III A. FRACTURE OF CLAVICLE

- ***Most common site***: Junction of Lateral 1/3 and middle 1/3 of bone[Q]
- ***Treatment***: 'Figure of 8' bandage[Q]
- ***Common late complication***: Shoulder stiffness[Q]

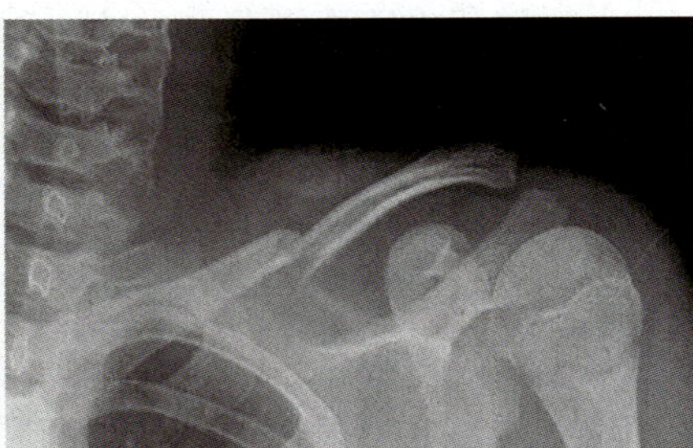

Fig. Fracture clavicle

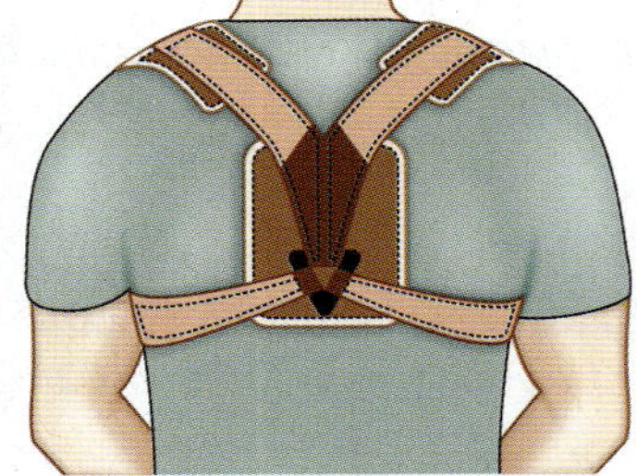

Fig. Figure-of-8 bandage

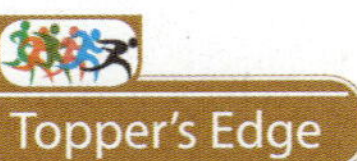

Topper's Edge

Facture Clavicle

- **MC fracture at birth[Q]**
- **MC mode of injury[Q]: Direct mode**
- Nearly all fractures are treated closed
- Open reduction for specific indications
- Malunion is a rule BUT no functional disability[Q]

III B. FRACTURE OF SURGICAL NECK HUMERUS

- *Common among*: Elderly females
- *Treatment*: Triangular sling
- ***Complication*: Axillary nerve palsy[Q]**

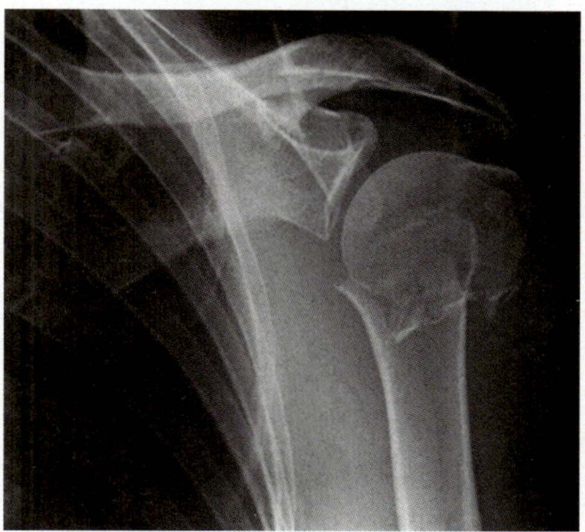

Fig. Fracture surgical neck humerus

III C. FRACTURE OF SHAFT HUMERUS

- *Common among*: All ages
- *Patterns seen*: All types
- ***Treatment*: Hanging cast[Q]**
- ***Complication*: Radial nerve palsy[Q]**

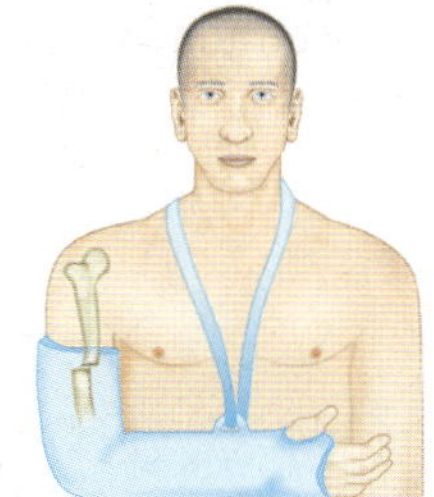

Fig. Hanging cast

III D. SUPRACONDYLAR FRACTURE HUMERUS

- ***Cause*: Fall on out-stretched hand leading to hyperextension of elbow[Q]**
- *Treatment*:
  - Closed reduction
  - Open reduction with K-wire fixation[Q]
- *Complications*[Q]:
  - Brachial artery injury **(most common[Q])**
  - Radial nerve injury **(Median nerve injury—Most common)**
  - Volkman's ischaemia
  - Volkman's Ischaemic Contracture[Q]
  - Mal-union leading to Cubitus varus **(Gun stock deformity[Q])**
  - Myositis ossificans
- *Treatment*:
  - Volkman's splint[Q]
  - Maxpage operation[Q]

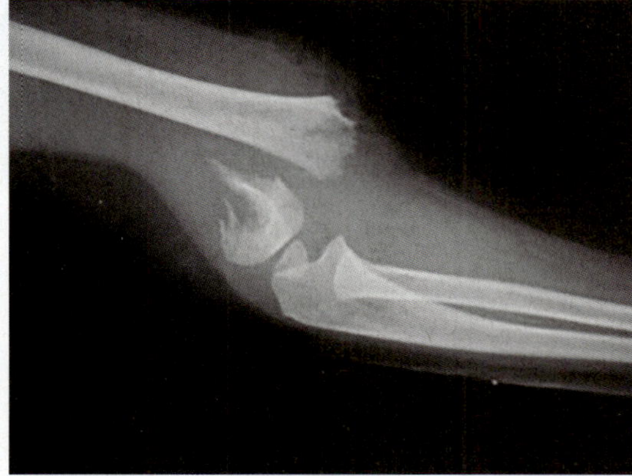

Fig. Supracondylar fracture humerus

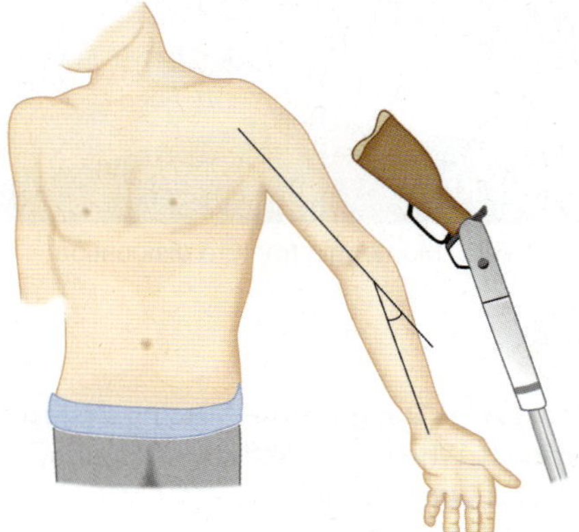

Fig. Gunstock deformity

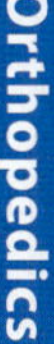

Topper's Edge

Supracondylar fracture Humerus
- 2nd MC fractures (after Forearm fractures) in children
- Characteristic mechanism of injury: Fall on outstretched hand with hyperextension at elbow with abduction/ adduction[Q]
- **MC type: Extension injury type[Q]**
- Closed reduction difficult
- Open reduction in specific indications
- **MC complication[Q]: Cubitus varus**

III E. FRACTURE LATERAL CONDYLE HUMERUS

- *Cause*: Varus injury to elbow in children
- *Treatment*:
  - Non-displaced fracture: Plaster slab
  - Displaced fracture: Open reduction and K-wire fixation[Q]
- *Complications*:
  - **Cubitus valgus** deformity leading to **'Tardy ulnar nerve palsy'**[Q]
  - Non-union

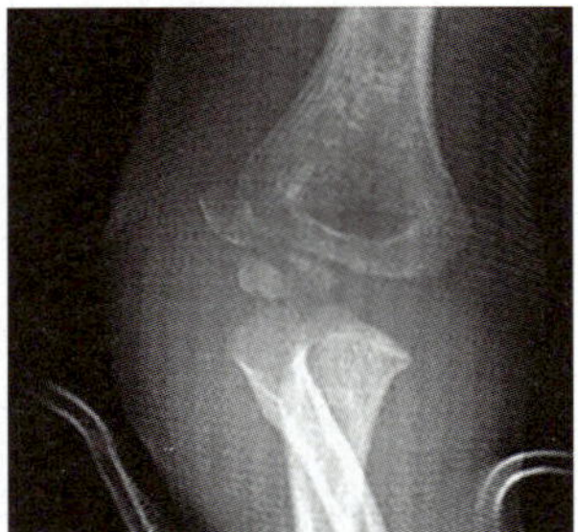

Fig. Fracture lateral condyle humerus

III F. FRACTURE-DISLOCATIONS

- ***Monteggia fracture-dislocation***: Fracture upper 1/3 ulna + dislocation head of radius[Q]
  - Underlying cause: Hyperpronation injury
- ***Galeazzi fracture-dislocation***: Fracture lower 1/3 radius + dislocation/ subluxation of distal radio-ulnar joint[Q]
  - Underlying cause: Fall on an outstretched hand
- ***Bennett's fracture-dislocation***: Intraarticular fracture base 1st metacarpal + dislocation/ subluxation of metacarpal[Q]
  - Underlying cause: Longitudinal force on thumb

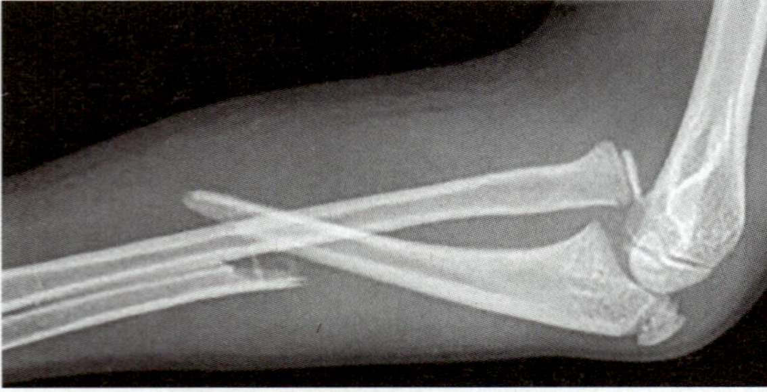

Fig. Monteggia fracture dislocation

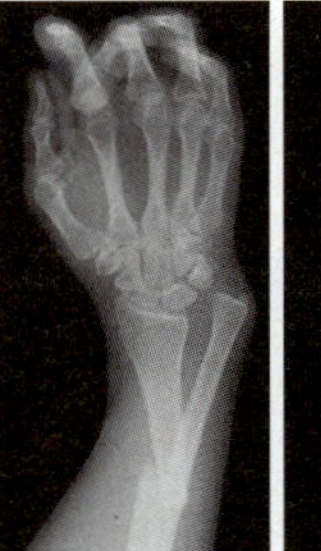

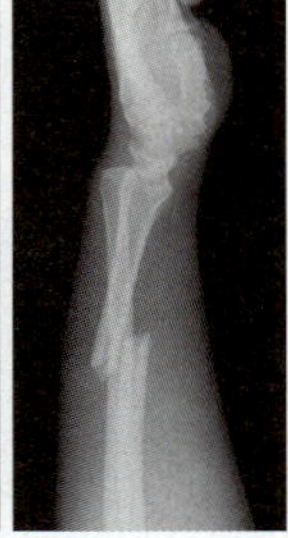

Fig. Galeazzi fracture dislocation

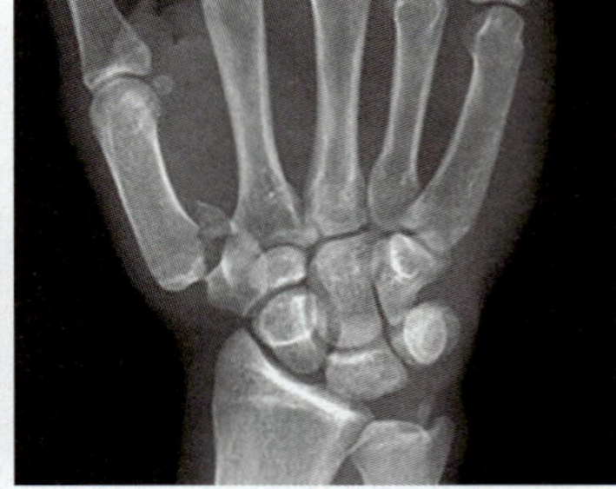

Fig. Bennette fracture

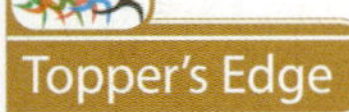

Topper's Edge

Monteggia Fracture is Dangerous—Missing Dislocation of Radius Head
- Missed by patient: When victim reflexly pulls elbow after fall and reduced dislocation unknowingly
- Missed by quack: Due to ignorance
- Missed by physician: He fails to order including elbow in forearm bone fractures
- Missed by radiologist: He fails to utilize McLaughlin's line

III G. COLLES' FRACTURE

- ***Type*: Fracture distal end radius** (Corticocancellous junction[Q])
- *Age group*: Menopausal females above forty years
- *Displacements seen*[Q]:
  - Dorsal displacement
  - Dorsal tilt **(Most characteristic[Q])**
  - Lateral displacement
  - Lateral tilt
  - Supination
- *Clinical presentation*:
  - **Dinner fork deformity[Q]**
- *Treatment*:
  - **Colles' cast** (Wrist in Palmar flexion + Ulnar deviation[Q])
- *Complications of Colles' fracture*:
  - **Finger stiffness (Most common[Q])**
  - Malunion
  - Subluxation of inferior radioulnar joint
  - Carpal tunnel syndrome[Q]
  - Sudeck's osteodystrophy[Q]
  - Rupture extensor pollicis longus tendon[Q]

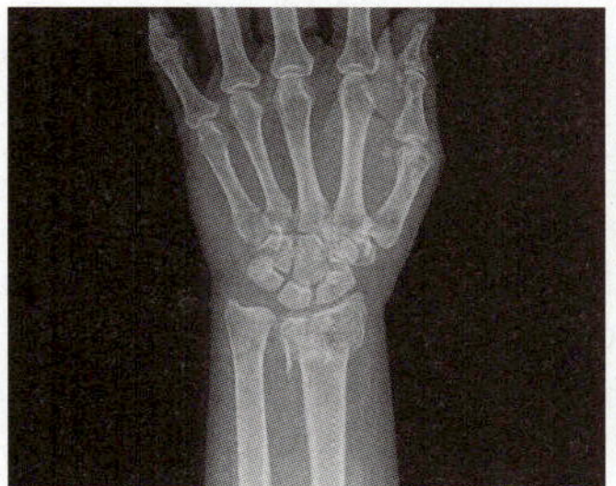
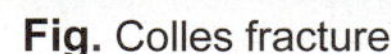

Fig. Colles fracture

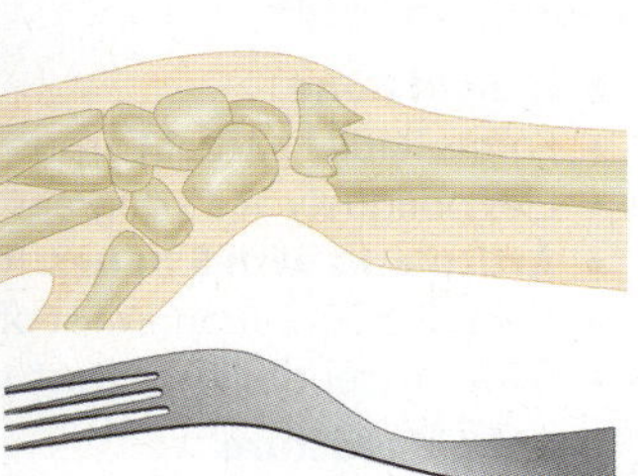

Fig. Dinner fork deformity

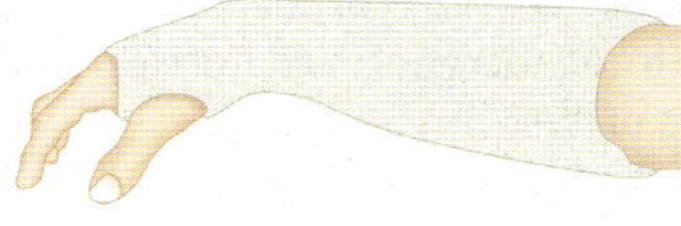
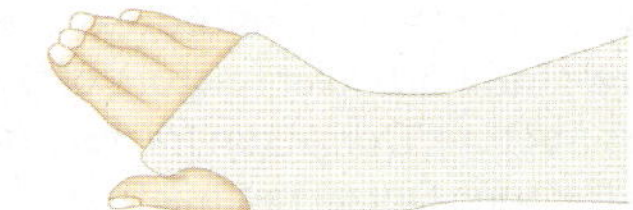

Fig. Colles cast

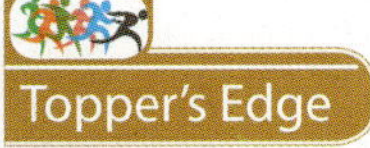

Topper's Edge

Colles' fracture
- Synonym: **'Poutteau fracture'[Q]**
  - MC mode of injury: Fall on outstretched hand with Dorsiflexion 40–90 degrees[Q]
  - Force required: 192 kg (Women) to 282 kg (Men)
- Composition[Q]: Fracture lower end radius PLUS Fracture-dislocation Inferior radioulnar joint
- **Classical deformity [3D's][Q]**: **D**inner fork deformity (Only seen in **D**orsal tilt and **D**orsal displacement)
- Reliable sign[Q]: Styloid process test
- Common complication
  - Finger Stiffness
  - Malunion (MC surgery done: **Darrach's surgery**)

III H. SCAPHOID FRACTURE

- ***MC Type***: Fracture waist of scaphoid[Q]
- *Age group*: Young adults
- ***Clinical presentation***: Tenderness in anatomical snuff box[Q]
- ***X-ray***: Oblique view of wrist[Q]
- ***Treatment***:
  - Scaphoid cast (Wrist in dorsiflexion + Radial deviation: *'Glass holding position'*[Q])
- ***Complications of Colles' fracture***:
  - Avascular necrosis (of proximal pole[Q])
  - Delayed union/ mal-union[Q]

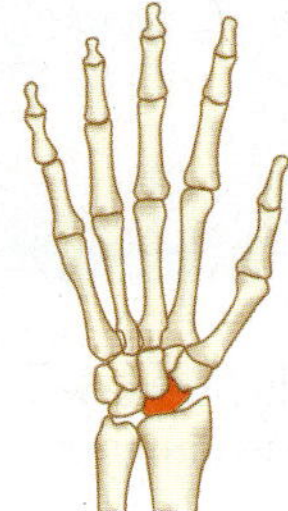

Fig. Scaphoid bone

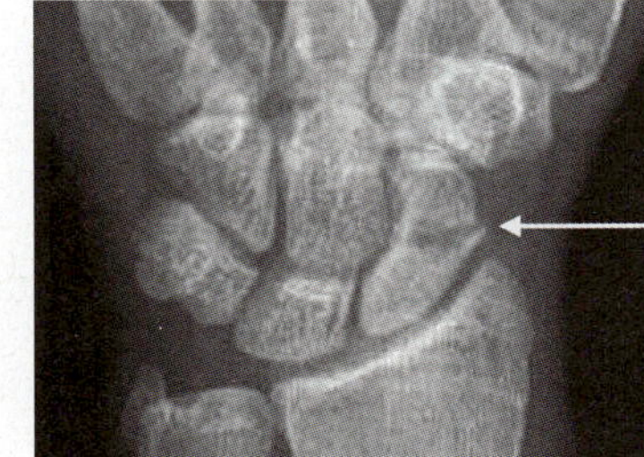

Fig. Scaphoid fracture

Orthopedics

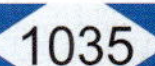

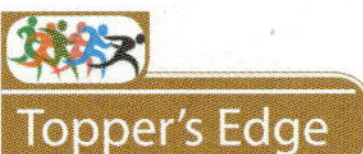

Topper's Edge

Scaphoid Bone

- Forms Radial part of Carpus
- Lies obliquely at 45 degrees to longitudinal axes of 2 rows
- **Articulates with 5 bones**: Radius, Lunate, Triquetral, Trapezium, Capitulum
- Central indentation: Waist of scaphoid
- More susceptibility to fractures[Q]: Since it crosses 2 rows of carpus

Scaphoid Fracture

- 70% of Carpal injuries[Q]
- **Usually results from fall on outstretched hand[Q]**
- Fracture site: Waist (MC[Q]) > Proximal pole > Distal body > Tuberosity
- **Typical finding[Q]**: Tenderness in anatomical snuff box
- High incidence of AVN

Injuries Around the Wrist

- Radial styloid fracture: Chauffer's fracture, Hutchinson's fracture, Backfire fracture
- **Smith's fracture[Q]**: Distal radius fracture, extra-articular with volar tilt of the distal fragment
- **Barton's fracture[Q]**: Intra-articular fracture of Distal radius
  - Dorsal Barton's fracture: Dorsal rim fracture of Distal radius (Variant of Colles' fracture)
  - Volar Barton's fracture: Dorsal rim fracture/ dislocation of Distal radius
- **Colles' fracture[Q]**: Distal radius, extra-articular fracture with dorsal tilt of distal fragment
- Scaphoid fracture
- Lunate fracture

Injuries of the Hand

- **Bennetts'fracture[Q]**: Intra-articular fracture of base of first metacarpal with subluxation/ dislocation of 1st Carpometacarpal joint (MC in Fist-fights)
- **Rolando fracture[Q]**: Fracture of base of first metacarpal, intra-articular nature
- Kaplan's lesion: Hyperextension injury due to buttonholing of metacarpal head through volar capsule into the palm
  - Interposition of Volar plate between Base of proximal phalanx and Head of metacarpal
- **Mallet/ Baseball/Drop finger[Q]**: Avulsion of attachment of extensor tendon from the base of distal phalanx
- **Jersey finger[Q]**: Avulsion of Flexor digitorum profundus tendon from its insertion on Distal phalanx
  - Opposite of Mallet finger
  - Seen in Football, Rugby players

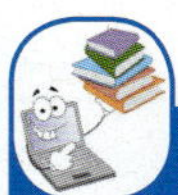

IMAGE-BASED QUESTIONS

1. Eponym for fracture shown in below X-ray is ***[AIIMS May 2016]***

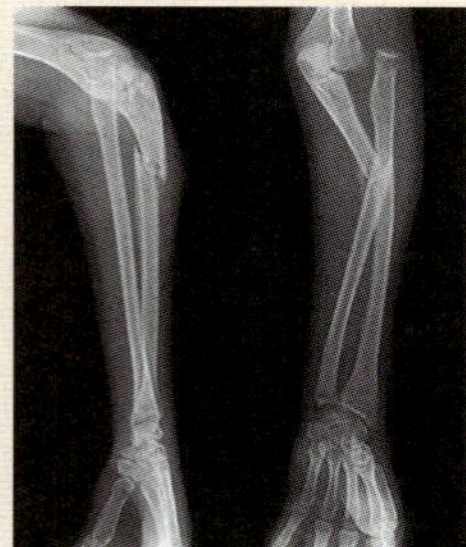

a. Monteggia fracture
b. Colles fracture
c. Galeazzi fracture
d. Smith fracture

2. MC Nerve affected in Condition shown in Photograph is ***[Recent Question 2012]***

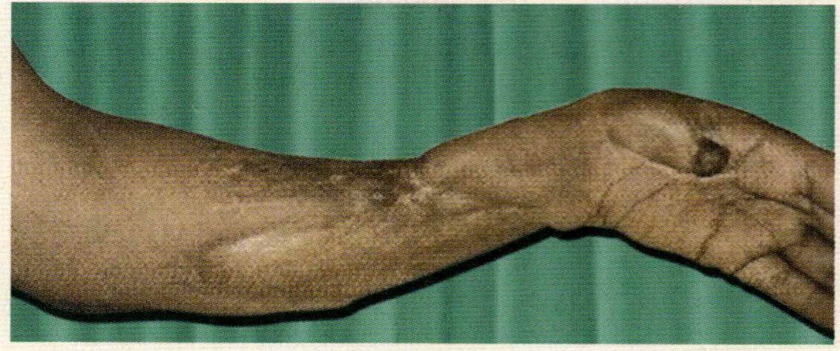

a. Radial nerve
b. Ulnar nerve
c. Median nerve
d. Axillary nerve

3. Identify the Deformity shown in Photograph
[Recent Question 2012]

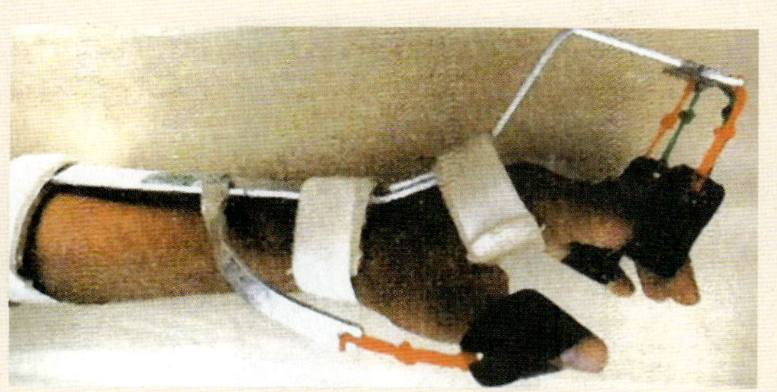

a. Aeroplane splint
b Thomas splint
c. Bohler-Braun splint
d. Cock-up splint

4. Diagnose the Fracture shown in the Photograph

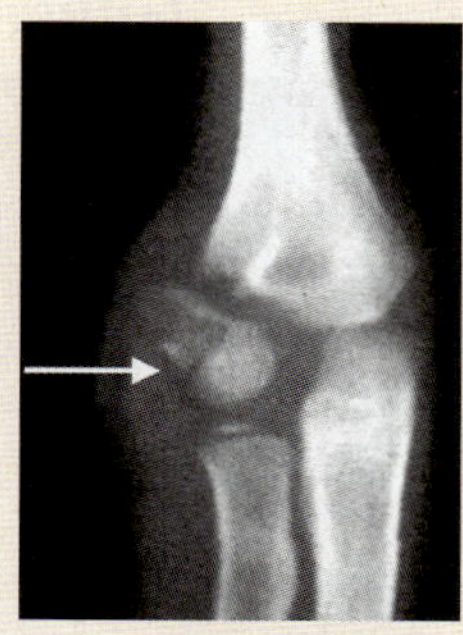

a. Fracture medial epicondyle humerus
b. Fracture lateral epicondyle humerus
c. Intercondylar fracture humerus
d. Fracture fibular neck

5. Bandage shown in Photograph is used in Fracture:
[Recent Question 2012, 2014]

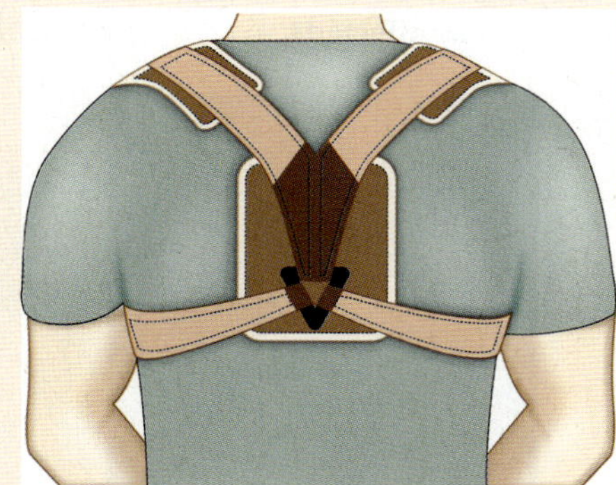

a. Humerus
b. Scapula
c. Clavicle
d. Cervical spine

6. Injury shown in Photograph can lead to Fracture of

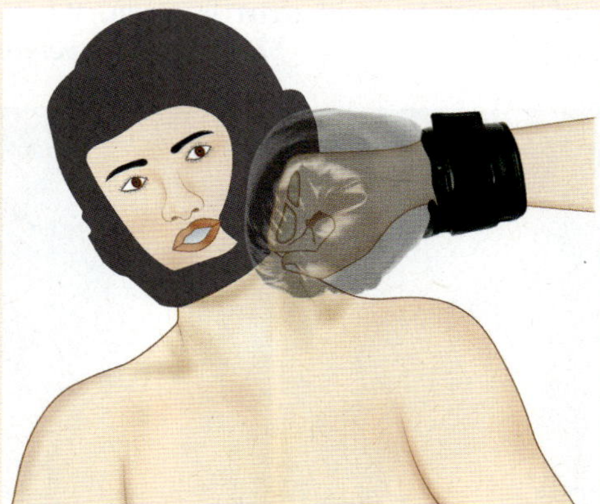

a. Neck of 1st metacarpal
b. Base of 2nd metacarpal
c. Neck of 5th metacarpal
d. Base of 5th metacarpal

7. Fracture shown in the X-ray Photograph is a type of ....
[Recent Question 2012]

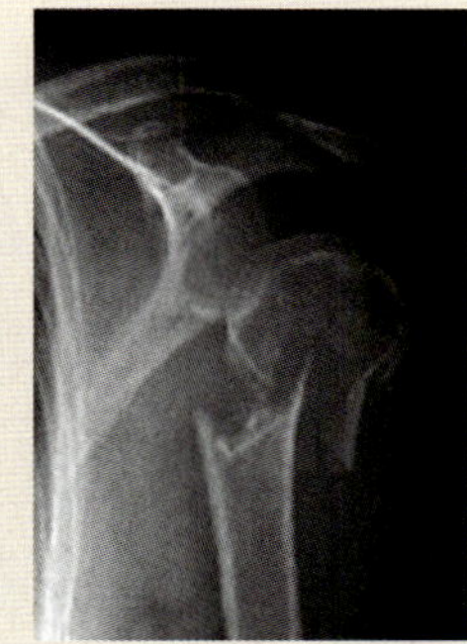

a. Acromioclavicular displacement
b. Sternoclavicular displacement
c. Lateral 1/3 clavicular fracture
d. Proximal humerus fracture

8. Fracture shown in Photograph is
[Recent Question 2013]

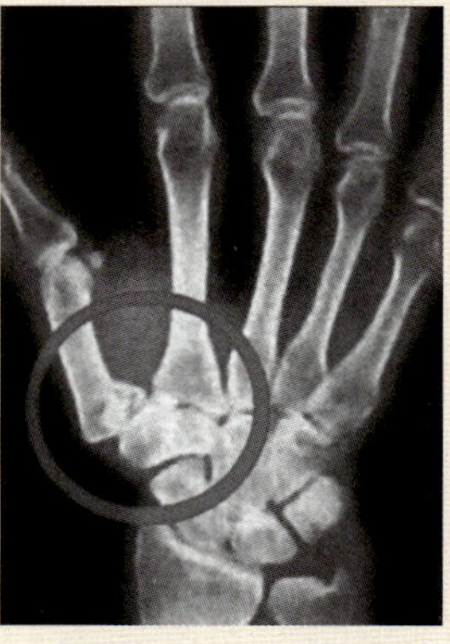

a. Benett's fracture
b. Rolando fracture
c. Kaplan's lesion
d. Mallet finger

9. AP and Lateral View of wrist is given. What is your diagnosis? ***[AIIMS PG November 2015]***

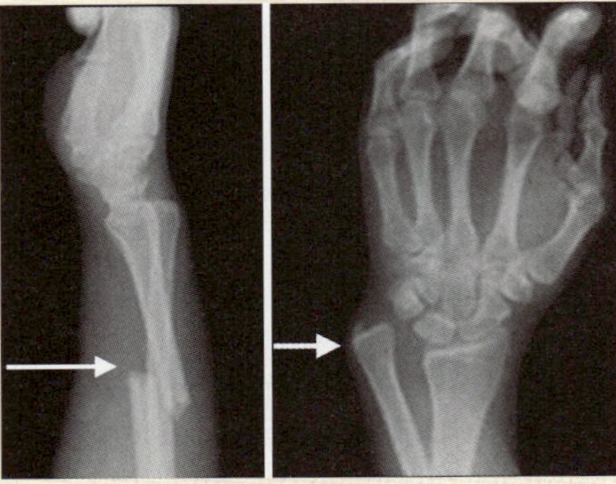

a. Monteggia fracture dislocation
b. Smith fracture dislocation
c. Colles fracture dislocation
d. Galeazzi fracture dislocation

10. Identify the deformity in the image below? ***[AIIMS PG November 2015, AIIMS PG November 2015]***

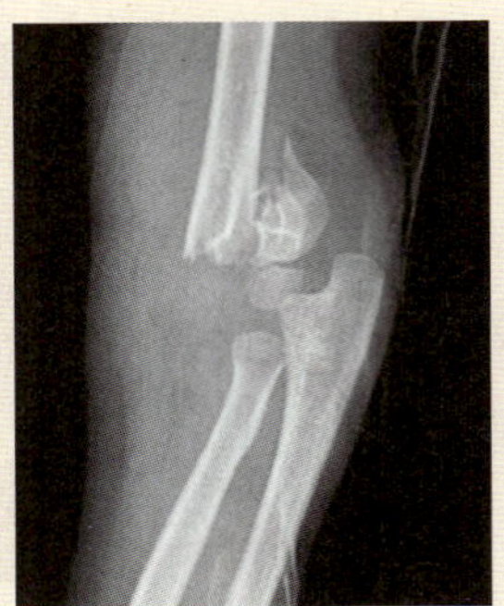

a. Lateral condylar fracture Humerus
b. Supracondylar fracture Humerus
c. Fracture shaft humerus
d. Medial condylar fracture Humerus

11. AP and Lateral View of wrist is given. What is your diagnosis? ***[AIIMS PG November 2015]***

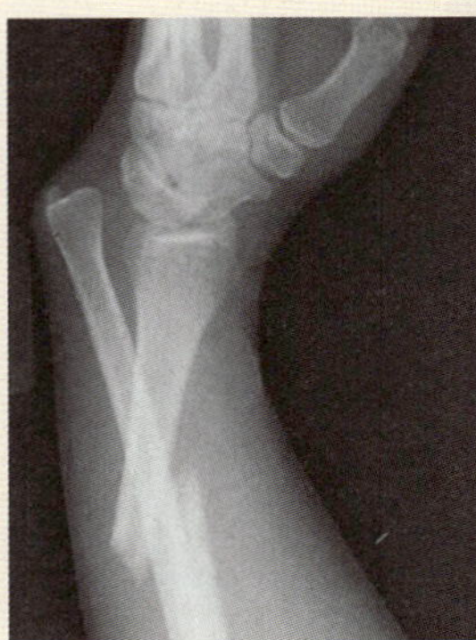

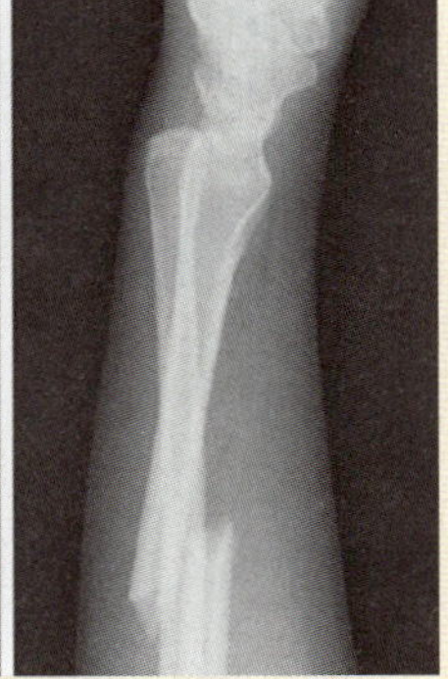

a. Monteggia
b. Smith
c. Colles
d. Galeazzi

12. A four years old boy has a history of fall on outstretched hand. X-ray is given below. Which of the following vessel is most likely to be affected? ***[AIIMS May 2017]***

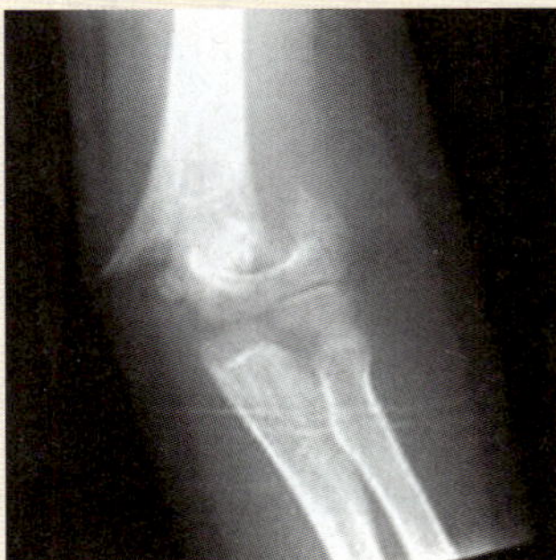

a. Ulnar artery
b. Radial artery
c. Brachial artery
d. Cubital vein

13. Identify the facture classification shown in the X-ray Photograph. ***[AIIMS November 2017]***

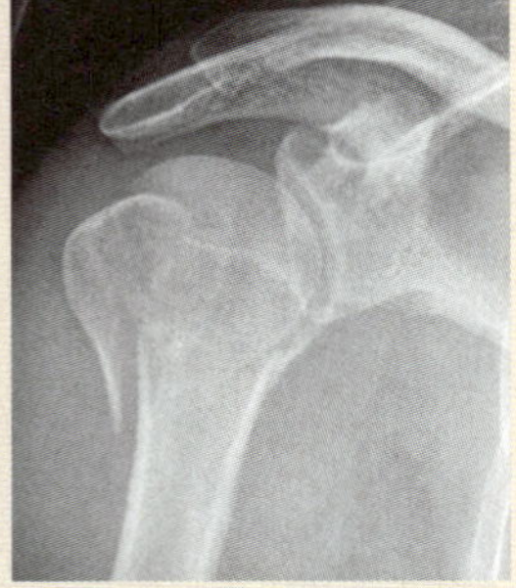

a. Garden classification grade 3
b. Schatzker classification grade 5
c. Ideberg classification grade 4
d. Neer classification grade 4

14. When a person falls on outstretched hand, MC bone injured is. ***[Recent Question 2018]***

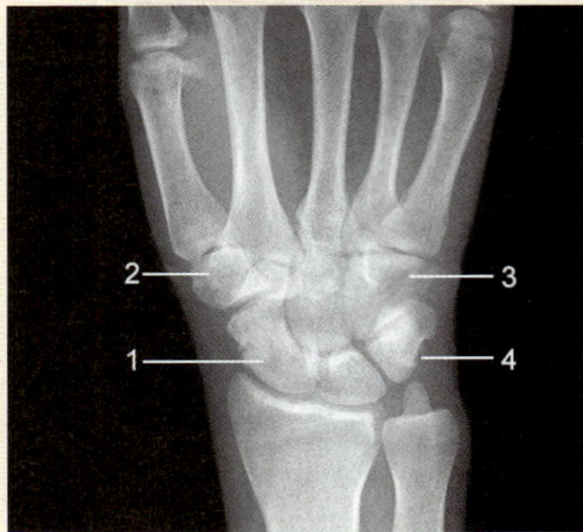

a. 1
b. 2
c. 3
d. 4

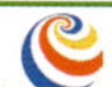 ANSWERS WITH EXPLANATIONS OF IBQs 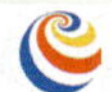

1. Ans. (a) Monteggia fracture *[Ref. Maheshwari, 4/e p106]*

Monteggia Fracture Dislocation (Photograph)
- Fracture upper 1/3 of ulna
- Dislocation of head of radius

2. Ans. (c) Median nerve *[Ref. Neglected Musculoskeletal Injuries by Jain, 1/e p110]*

Volkman's Ischemic Contracture
- Description: Ischemic muscles gradually replaced by fibrous tissue which contracts giving rise to flexion of wrists/ fingers
- Underlying vessel involved: Anterior Interosseous artery (Branch of Brachial artery)
- MC Nerve involved in Volkmann's Ischemic Contracture: Median nerve > Ulnar nerve
- MC affected muscles in Volkmann's ischemia: Flexor digitorum profundus (medial half) > Flexor pollicis longus

3. Ans. (d) Cock-up splint *[Ref. Maheshwari, 4/e p24]*

Uses of Common Splints
- Aeroplane splint: Brachial plexus injury
- Thomas splint: Fracture femur
- Bohler-Braun splint: Fracture of femur
- Cock-up splint: Radial nerve palsy
- Von Rosen splint: Congenital dislocation of hip
- Knuckle bender splint: Ulnar nerve palsy
- Denis Browne splint: CTEV (Clubfoot)

4. Ans. (b) Fracture lateral epicondyle humerus *[Ref. Maheshwari, 4/e p99]*

Fracture Lateral Epicondyle of Humerus
- Occur due to Varus injury to elbow in children
- Fracture line runs upwards and laterally from intercondylar area
- Is type of Salter Harris Type IV injury
- Complications: Non-union, Tardy ulnar nerve palsy, Osteoarthritis
- Treatment:
  - Above-elbow plater cast (Undisplaced fracture)
  - Open reduction and K-wires internal fixation

5. Ans. (c) Clavicle *[Ref. Maheshwari, 4/e p85]*

Figure-of-8 Bandage
- Treatment of Displaced Clavicle fracture in a young adult
- Provides Immobilisation, Pain relief

6. Ans. (c) Neck of 5th metacarpal *[Ref. Maheshwari, 4/e p3]*
- Boxer's fracture: Ventrally displaced fracture occurring through Neck ok 5th metacarpal, usually seen in Boxers

7. Ans. (d) Proximal humerus fracture *[Ref. Maheshwari, 4/e p89]*

Proximal Humerus Fracture
- MC in Elderly women >60 years age
- MC Cause: Domestic fall
- Treatment: Immobilization with a sling, K-wires stabilisation

8. Ans. (a) Bennett's fracture *[Ref. Maheshwari, 4/e p113]*

Bennett's Fracture Dislocation
- Fracture-dislocation of 1st metacarpal base
- Dislocation of 1st CP joint
- Cause: Longitudinal force applied along thumb

9. Ans. (d) Galleazzi fracture dislocation *[Ref. Maheshwari, 4/e p3]*

Galeazzi Fracture-Dislocation

- Description: Fracture lower 1/3 radius PLUS Dislocation/subluxation of distal radio-ulnar joint
- Underlying cause: Fall on an outstretched hand

10. Ans. (b) Supracondylar fracture Humerus *[Ref. Maheshwari, 4/e p94]*

Supracondylar Fracture Humerus

- Mechanism: Fall on outstretched arm forcing elbow into hyperextension
- Types: Extension type (More common), Flexion type
- Examination: Posterior prominence of Olecranon process, Maintained 3-point bony relationship
- Displacements: Posterior shift, Posterior tilt, Proximal shift, Medial/ lateral shift, medial tilt, Internal rotation

11. Ans. (d) Galeazzi *[Ref. Practical Orthopedics by Mercier, 6/e p125-128]*

- Galeazzi fracture: Fracture of the radius with dislocation of the distal radioulnar joint
- Classically involves an isolated fracture of the junction of the distal third and middle third of the radius with associated subluxation or dislocation of distal radioulnar joint

12. Ans. (c) Brachial artery *[Ref. Maheshwari, 4/e p96-98]*

Complications of Supracondylar Fracture Humerus (Given in Photograph)

- Immediate complications: Brachial artery injury, Median nerve injury
- Early complications: Volkmann's ischemia
- Late complications: Mal-union (Gun-stock deformity), Myositis ossificans, Volkmann's ischemic contracture

13. Ans. (d) Neer classification grade 4 *[Ref. Pediatric Orthopedic Imaging by Stein-Wexler, 1/e p148]*

Neer classification of Proximal Humerus Fractures

- **Basis of classification:**
  - Considers 4 major parts of the Proximal humerus, namely, Humeral head with articular surface, Greater tubercle, Lesser tubercle, Diaphysis
  - In the childhood, the four parts are separated by growth plates
  - A fragment is considered separate, when it is displaced by at least 1 cm or angulated by 45 and more degrees
- **Basic division of fractures is based on the number of fragments:** Undisplaced (1-part, 2-part, 3-part, and 4-part) fractures
  - I: Minimal displacement (1-part)
  - II: Anatomical neck (2-part)
  - III: Surgical neck (2-part)
  - IV: Greater tuberosity (2, 3, or 4-part)
  - V: Lesser tuberosity (2, 3, or 4-part)
  - VI: Fracture dislocation (Anterior: 2, 3, 4-part, or articular surface involvement; Posterior: 2, 3, 4-part, or articular surface involvement)

14. Ans. (a) 1 *[Ref. Medical Sciences by Naish, 1/e p427]*

In the given Photograph,

- 1 – Scaphoid (MC Bone injured in fall on outstretched hand)
- 2 – Trapezium
- 3 – Hamate
- 4 – Triquetrum

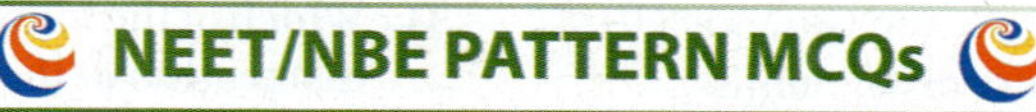

NEET/NBE PATTERN MCQs

1. **4 year old child presented to the clinic with a history of fall on out-stretched hand. Radiographs revealed a broken anterior cortex with an intact posterior cortex of Radius with an exaggerated bowing. Fracture sustained is known as** *[Recent Question 2016]*
   a. Torus Fracture
   b. Greenstick fracture
   c. Galeazzi Fracture
   d. Monteggia Fracture Dislocation
2. **What is Luxatio erecta?** *[Recent Question 2016, 2017]*
   a. Anterior Dislocation of the shoulder joint
   b. Inferior Dislocation of the shoulder joint
   c. Anterior Dislocation of the hip joint
   d. Posterior Dislocation of hip joint
3. **Aeroplane splint is used in -** *[Recent Question 2016]*
   a. Conservative management of proximal humerus fractures
   b. CTEV
   c. Axillary nerve palsy
   d. Brachial plexus injury
4. **Which of the following casts/splints is used for Fracture shaft humerus?** *[Recent Question 2016]*
   a. Hanging casts b. Knuckle bender splint
   c. Aeroplane Splint d. Above elbow cast
5. **Functional bracing is now the Gold standard in Non-operative management of which fractures?** *[Recent Question 2016]*
   a. Fracture shaft humerus
   b. Fractures of both bones of the forearm
   c. Fracture shaft tibia
   d. Fracture shaft femur
6. **Which of the following is true about Colles' Fracture?** *[Recent Question 2016]*
   a. Volar angulation with Radial deviation occurs
   b. It is an intra-articular fracture
   c. It may lead to gunstock deformity due to malunion
   d. It is associated with dorsal angulation
7. **True regarding Mallet finger is which of the following** *[Recent Question 2016, 2017]*
   a. Avulsion of tendon at the base of the middle phalanx
   b. Avulsion of extensor tendon at the base of the distal phalanx
   c. Fracture of distal phalanx
   d. Fracture of the proximal phalanx
8. **Cubitus valgus is seen in** *[Recent Question 2016]*
   a. # Lateral condyle of humerus
   b. # Intercondylar of humerus
   c. # of the olecranon
   d. # Head of the radius
9. **Boxer's fracture is** *[Recent Question 2016, 2017]*
   a. Radial styloid fracture b. Reverse colles fracture
   c. 5th metacarpal fracture d. 1st metacarpal fracture
10. **Most common shoulder dislocation is** *[Recent Question 2016]*
   a. Luxatio erecta b. Posterior
   c. Superior d. Anterior
11. **Trauma to neck of humerus, nerve damaged** *[Recent Question 2012]*
   a. Radial b. Ulnar
   c. Median d. Axillary
12. **Which nerve is most likely to be injured in fracture of shaft of humerus?** *[Recent Question 2017, NBE DNB 2011]*
   a. Median nerve b. Musculocutaneous nerve
   c. Radial nerve d. Dinar nerve
13. **One of the common fractures that occur during boxing by hitting with a closed fist is** *[Recent Question 2012]*
   a. Monteggia fracture dislocation
   b. Galeazzi fracture dislocation
   c. Bennett's fracture dislocation
   d. Smith's fracture
14. **Tardy ulnar nerve palsy is usually seen after malunited ....** *[NBE DNB December 2011]*
   a. Supracondylar fractures b. Lateral condyle fractures
   c. Intercondylar fractures d. Dislocation of the elbow
15. **Pulled elbow means** *[Recent Question 2012]*
   a. Fracture of head of radius
   b. Subluxation of head of radius
   c. Fracture dislocation of elbow
   d. Fracture ulna
16. **True about supracondylar fracture of humerus** *[Recent Question 2012]*
   a. Common in adults
   b. Extension type most common
   c. Flexion type is most common
   d. None
17. **Most common complication of Colles fracture is** *[Recent Question 2012, 2013]*
   a. Malunion b. Avascular necrosis
   c. Finger stiffness d. Rupture of EPL tendon
18. **Malunited fracture supracondylar humerus causes** *[Recent Question 2012, 2017]*
   a. Dinner fork deformity b. Cubitus varus
   c. Cubitus valgus d. None
19. **Most common complication of lateral condyle humerus fracture** *[Recent Question 2013]*
   a. Malunion b. Nonunion
   c. VIC d. Median nerve injury
20. **Following are complications seen in Colles' fracture EXCEPT** *[NBE FMGE March 2004]*
   a. Malunion b. Delayed union
   c. Finger stiffness d. Carpal tunnel syndrome

21. Barton's fracture is *[Recent Question 2013]*
a. Fracture proximal radius b. Fracture distal radius
c. Fracture ulna d. Fracture humerus

22. In Colles' fracture, distal segment is *[NBE FMGE March 2004]*
a. Shifted dorsally b. Angulated radially
c. Supinated d. All of the above

23. The commonest carpal bone to be fractured at wrist is *[NBE FMGE September 2011]*
a. Capitate b. Pisiform
c. Scaphoid d. Triquetral

24. Proximal humerus fracture which has maximum chances of avascular necrosis *[Recent Question 2012]*
a. One part b. Two part
c. Three part d. Four part

25. Monteggia fracture dislocation involves *[NBE DNB 1997, 1999, 2003, 2004]*
a. Upper 1/3 radius b. Lower 1/3 radius
c. Upper 1/3 ulna d. Lower 1/3 ulna

26. Nerve injured in medial epicondylar fracture *[NBE DNB 1993]*
a. Radial b. Ulnar
c. Median d. Axillary

27. MC nerve involved in fracture of surgical neck of humerus is *[NBE DNB 1997]*
a. Radial b. Ulnar
c. Median d. Axillary

28. Dinner fork deformity is seen in *[UPSC 2002, Recent Question 2013]*
a. Colle's fracture b. March fracture
c. Lateral condyle fracture d. Supracondylar fracture

29. Hanging cast is used for *[NBE FMGE September 2011]*
a. Forearm fracture b. Colle's fracture
c. Scaphoid fracture d. Humerus fracture

30. Not true about Fracture of scaphoid is *[UPSC 2001]*
a. Is most commonly fractured carpal bone
b. Persistent tenderness in anatomical snuff box is suggestive of it
c. Immediate x-ray of hand may not reveal fracture line
d. Malunion is a frequent complication

31. Cock-up splint is used in *[NBE FMGE September 2011, March 2012]*
a. Median nerve injury
b. Radial nerve injury
c. Ulnar nerve injury
d. Volkmann's ischemic contracture

32. MC complication of Colles' fracture is *[UPSC 2011]*
a. Malunion b. Delayed union
c. Non union d. Sudeck's dystrophy

33. What is the most common injury sustained after falling on an outstretched hand in a 65 years old person? *[UPSC 2010]*
a. Colles' fracture b. Supracondylar fracture
c. Metacarpals fracture d. Shoulder dislocation

34. Which of the following nerve may be injured in the anterior dislocation of the shoulder joint? *[NBE FMGE March 2012]*
a. Radial nerve
b. Circumflex axillary nerve
c. Median nerve
d. Musculocutaneous nerve

35. In fracture of shaft of humerus, which of the following nerve is most likely to be injured? *[NBE FMGE March 2012]*
a. Median nerve
b. Musculocutaneous nerve
c. Radial nerve
d. Dinar nerve

36. In Mallet's finger, seen is *[NBE DNB 1995, 2000, UPSC 1985, 1988]*
a. Avulsion of terminal slip of flexor tendon to distal phalanx
b. Avulsion of terminal slip of extensor tendon to distal phalanx
c. Avulsion of terminal slip of flexor tendon to proximal phalanx
d. Avulsion of terminal slip of extensor tendon to proximal phalanx

37. Which of the following occur as a complication of Colles' fracture? *[NBE DNB 1995, 2000, 2006, 2008]*
a. Radial nerve palsy b. Ulnar nerve palsy
c. Stiff wrist joint d. All of the above

38. Management of Pulled Elbow include *[Recent Question 2014]*
a. Supination + Pressure over Olecranon process
b. Supination + Pressure over Head of radius
c. Pronation + Pressure over Olecranon process
d. Pronation + Pressure over Head of Radius

39. Variants of Monteggia fracture dislocation include all except *[Recent Question 2015]*
a. Isolated dislocation Head of radius
b. Fracture Shaft ulna with fracture Neck radius
c. Fracture Shaft ulna with fracture Shaft radius
d. Fracture shaft ulna

40. Priority in management of Supracondylar fracture of humerus in a child is *[UPSC CMS 2015]*
a. Preservation of Brachial artery entanglement
b. Debridement of wound
c. Antibiotics
d. Immobilization

41. Which of the following is not true about Galeazzi fracture dislocation? *[Recent Question 2017]*
a. Fracture of distal third of radius and dislocation of distal radioulnar joint
b. Results from fall on outstretched hand
c. The distal end of ulna dislocates volarly after disruption of distal radioulnar joint
d. Radius is angulated medially and anteriorly

42. Most common lesion associated with pathological fracture in Hand is *[Recent Question 2017]*
a. Enchondroma
b. Metastases
c. Osteoid osteoma
d. Osteochondroma

43. Which of the following shoulder movements is/are weak in patients of Supraspinatus tear? *[Recent Question 2017]*
a. Abduction
b. Adduction
c. External rotation
d. Internal rotation

44. Which of the following is not true about Monteggia fracture dislocation? *[Recent Question 2017]*
a. Fracture of proximal third of ulna with dislocation of radial head
b. Extention type is a commoner type
c. Ulna angulates posteriorly in the extension type
d. Malunion occurs commonly in conservatively managed patients

45. Bankarts lesion occurs in patients with *[Recent Question 2017]*
a. Anterior shoulder dislocation
b. Posterior shoulder dislocation
c. Posterior elbow dislocation
d. Posterior hip dislocation

46. Knuckle bender splint is used in management of *[Recent Question 2017]*
a. Radial nerve palsy
b. Ulnar nerve palsy
c. Median nerve palsy
d. Peroneal nerve palsy

47. Most common complication of Supracondylar fracture of humerus *[Recent Question 2017]*
a. Malunion
b. Median nerve injury
c. Myositis ossificans
d. Volkmann's ischemic contracture

48. Management of displaced noncomminuted Intercondylar humerus fracture is *[Recent Question 2017]*
a. Open reduction internal fixation
b. Above elbow plaster slab application
c. Olecranon pin traction
d. External fixation

49. Kocher maneuver is used for *[Recent Question 2017]*
a. Shoulder reduction
b. Elbow reduction
c. Ankle dislocation
d. Knee dislocation

50. A patient presents with wrist trauma. On investigations patient is diagnosed to have a sprained wrist, without any evidence of fracture. There is tenderness in anatomical snuffbox. Which ligament is commonly involved? *[Recent Question 2017]*
a. Scapholunate ligament
b. Radial collateral ligament
c. Lunotriquetral ligament
d. Ulnar collateral ligament

51. Treatment of Scaphoid fracture *[Recent Question 2017]*
a. Conservative
b. Compression Screws
c. Compression Plating
d. Traction

52. All of the following are true regarding fracture of Lateral condyle of humerus except *[Recent Question 2017]*
a. Usually seen at 6–10 years of age
b. Results in Gun stock deformity
c. Cubitus valgus occurs
d. Tardy ulnar nerve palsy is seen

53. Which of the following is true about Colle's fracture? *[Recent Question 2017]*
a. Intraarticular fracture of distal radius with palmar displacement
b. Intraarticular fracture of distal radius with dorsal displacement
c. Extraarticular fracture of distal radius with palmar displacement
d. Extraarticular fracture of distal radius with dorsal displacement

54. Hill Sachs lesion is situated on which part of Humeral head? *[Recent Question 2017]*
a. Anteromedial
b. Posterolateral
c. Posteromedial
d. Anterolateral

55. What is meant by Perilunate dislocations? *[Recent Question 2018]*
a. Lower radius, Scaphoid and Lunate and Capitate all in same plane
b. Lower radius, Scaphoid and Capitate in alignment, Lunate alone out of plane
c. Lower radius, Scaphoid and Lunate in alignment, Capitate alone is out of plane
d. Both Lunate and Capitate are out of plane

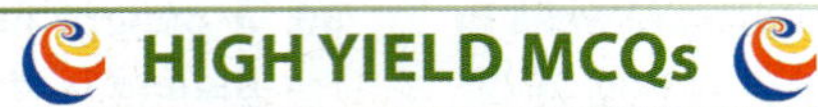

HIGH YIELD MCQs

1. **Keyboard operators and Typists are especially susceptible to injury of** *[UPSC CMS 2016]*
   a. Axillary nerve b. Median nerve
   c. Ulnar nerve d. Radial nerve
2. **Priority in management of Supracondylar fracture of Humerus in a child is** *[UPSC CMS 2016]*
   a. Prevention of Brachial artery entanglement
   b. Debridement of wound
   c. Antibiotics
   d. Immobilization
3. **True Colles fracture** *[PGI November 2016]*
   a. Occur at distal end of radius, about 2 cm from distal articular surface
   b. Fracture also involves radiocarpal joint
   c. Fracture also involves proximal radioulnar joint
   d. Cause ulnar deviation
   e. Common in women
4. **Most common nerve injured in supracondylar fracture of humerus is** *[All India PGMEE 2011, UPSC 1991]*
   a. Median nerve b. Anterior interosseus nerve
   c. Ulnar nerve d. Radial nerve
5. **Mallet finger is due to avulsion of extensor tendon of** *[PGI PGMEE 2001, JIPMER PGMEE 2014]*
   a. Proximal phalanx b. Middle phalanx
   c. Distal Phalanx d. Metacarpals
   e. Any other phalanx
6. **MC complication of Colles fracture is** *[All India PGMEE 1995, 1997, AIIMS PGMEE 1995, 2005]*
   a. Stiffness of fingers b. Sudeck's dystrophy
   c. Nonunion d. Tendon rupture
7. **Commonest complication of Colles fracture among following is** *[Karnataka PGMEE 2000]*
   a. Nonunion b. Malunion
   c. Vascular injury d. Sudeck's osteodystrophy
8. **All of the following can be the complications of a mal-united Colles fracture except** *[All India PGMEE 2004]*
   a. Rupture of flexor pollicis longus tendon
   b. Reflex sympathetic dystrophy (RSD)
   c. Carpal tunnel syndrome
   d. Carpal instability
9. **Rupture of Extensor pollicis longus occurs four weeks after** *[Bihar PGMEE 1999]*
   a. Colles fracture b. Radial styloid fracture
   c. Smith's fracture d. Scaphoid fracture
   e. All of these
10. **Which tendon gets involved in Colles fracture?** *[Rohtak PGMEE 1997, WB PGMEE 1999]*
    a. Abductor pollicis longus b. Extensor pollicis brevis
    c. Extensor pollicis longus d. All the above
11. **Complications of Colles fracture are all except** *[All India PGMEE 1996, All India PGMEE 1998]*
    a. Malunion b. Non union
    c. Sudeck's dystrophy d. Rupture of extensor policis longus
12. **Not a complication of Colles fracture** *[JIPMER PGMEE 2000]*
    a. Stiffness of wrist b. Stiffness of shoulder
    c. Carpal tunnel syndrome d. Wrist drop
13. **Complication of Colles' fracture is** *[NBE DNB 2000, Rajasthan PGMEE 2002]*
    a. Radial nerve palsy b. Stiffness of wrist joint
    c. Ulnar nerve palsy d. None of the above
14. **A patient presented with Claw hand after a Supracondylar fracture was reduced and plaster applied. The diagnosis is** *[All India PGMEE 1992]*
    a. Medial nerve injury
    b. Volkmann's ischaemic contrature
    c. Ulnar nerve injury
    d. Dupuytren's contracture
15. **A lady presents with swelling of hands with shiny skin. She has a history of fracture radius and kept on POP cast for 4 weeks after which she develops this. Give the most likely diagnosis** *[AIIMS PGMEE 2000]*
    a. Myositis ossification
    b. Rupture of external pollicis longus tendon
    c. Reflex sympathetic dystrophy
    d. Malunion
16. **MC complication of Fracture of Clavicle** *[MP PGMEE 1998, Karnataka PG 1999]*
    a. Malunion
    b. Non-union
    c. Injury to brachial plexus
    d. Stiffness of shoulder
17. **MC site of fracture clavicle is** *[DPG 1991, PGI November 2014]*
    a. Junction of Medial 1/3rd and lateral 2/3rd
    b. Junction of medial 2/3rd and lateral 1/3rd
    c. Midpoint of clavicle
    d. Scapular end
18. **A 6-year-old child falls in right-sided forearm region and develops fracture in dorsal surface of mid region of radius. The best treatment is** *[UP PGMEE 1998]*
    a. Antibiotics and sedative
    b. Bone plating and external fixation
    c. Slab with wait for bone remodeling
    d. Break the cortex other side and immobilization by POP
19. **Management of Smith's fracture is** *[All India PGMEE 1994]*
    a. Open reduction and fixation
    b. Plaster cast with forearm in pronation
    c. Closed reduction with below-elbow cast
    d. Above-elbow cast with forearm in supination
20. **Barton's fracture of the wrist** *[TN PGMEE 1992]*
    a. Involves radiocarpal subluxation
    b. Is a severe form of a colles' fracture
    c. Is often treated by open reduction and internal fixation
    d. All of the above

21. All are injuries of Lower end of radius except *[PGI 1995, TN PGMEE 1998]*
a. Smith's fracture b. Colles fracture
c. Night stick fracture d. Barton's fracture

22. Which one of the following statements is NOT correct regarding Fracture of the Scaphoid? *[UPSC 2001]*
a. It is the most commonly fractured carpal bone
b. Persistent tenderness in the anatomical snuffbox is highly suggestive of fracture
c. Immediate X-ray of hand may not reveal fracture line
d. Malunion is a frequent complication

23. Most common site of scaphoid fracture is *[Recent Question 2017, All India PGMEE 1997]*
a. Waist b. Proximal fragment
c. Distal fragment d. Tilting of the lunate

24. Main risk in fracture Scaphoid is *[AMC PGMEE 1989]*
a. Nonunion b. Malunion
c. Delayed union d. Avascular necrosis
e. Carpal tunnel syndrome

25. Complication of fracture Scaphoid is
a. Avascular necrosis of distal part *[Kerala PGMEE 1994]*
b. Injury to radial artery
c. Injury to radial nerve
d. Avascular necrosis of proximal part

26. Best radiological view for fracture scaphoid is *[All India PGMEE 1989]*
a. AP b. PA
c. Lateral d. Oblique

27. Nerve injury commonest fracture of Surgical neck of Humerus is *[PGI 2000]*
a. Radial nerve b. Ulnar nerve
c. Median nerve d. Musculocutaneous nerve
e. Axillary nerve

28. MC injury associated with fracture Medial epicondyle
a. Elbow dislocation *[PGI 1992]*
b. Monteggia fracture dislocation
c. Fracture supracondylar humerus
d. Vacular deficit

29. MC Elbow injury in adolescents is *[UP PGMEE 2001]*
a. Dislocation b. Olecranon fracture
c. Supracondylar fracture d. Physeal injury

30. Carpal bone which fracture commonly *[NIMHANS PGMEE 1987, Kerala PGMEE 1987]*
a. Scaphoid b. Lunate
c. Hammate d. Pisciform

31. A patient reported with a history of fall on an outstretched hand, complains of pain in the anatomical snuffbox and clinically no deformities visible. The diagnosis is *[AIIMS Nov 2017, AIIMS PGMEE 1998, Recent Question 2015, 2017]*
a. Colles' fracture
b. Lunate dislocation
c. Barton s fracture
d. Scaphoid fracture

32. If an adolescent boy falls on an out-stretched hand, the most common bone to be injured is *[AP PGMEE 1999]*
a. Fracture of lower end of radius
b. Fracture of both bones of forearm
c. Scaphoid fracture
d. Supracondylar fracture of humerus

33. In Scaphoid fracture, important views are all except:
a. AP b. Lateral *[PGI 1991]*
c. Oblique d. Cone

34. Gunstock deformity is seen due to *[TN PGMEE 1993]*
a. Fracture 1st metacarpal
b. Fracture lower end radius
c. Fracture lateral condyle humerus
d. Fracture supracondylar humerus

35. Complications after a Fracture Supracondylar humerus is/are *[PGI 2005]*
a. Elbow stiffness b. Malunion
c. Non-union d. Myositis ossificans
e. Gunstock deformity

36. Which of the following Scaphoid fracture is most prone to develop Avascular necrosis? *[Karnataka PGMEE 1992]*
a. Fracture of waist of scaphoid
b. Fracture of tubercle
c. Fracture of distal pole
d. All of the above

37. Fracture scaphoid is usually seen in *[PGI 1995]*
a. Elderly male
b. Elderly postmenopausal female
c. Young active adult
d. Children

38. In children Fracture Scaphoid is through rare but usually involves *[JIPMER PGMEE 1998, AIIMS PGMEE 1992]*
a. Waist b. Proximal pole
c. Neck d. Distal pole

39. Nerve injury in Supracondylar fracture of humerus is *[UP PGMEE 2001]*
a. Radial nerve b. Ulnar nerve
c. Median nerve d. Axillary nerve

40. 19 year old boy had a history of fall on out stretched hand while playing. He developed slight radial side pain and tenderness. On examination pressure along the axis of thumb is painful and X-rays are normal. Most likely diagnosis is *[All India PGMEE 1992, AIIMS PGMEE 1990]*
a. Fracture lower end radius
b. Wrist sprain
c. Scaphoid fracture
d. Perilunate dislocation

41. In Non-union of Scaphoid fracture, Vascularized muscle pedicle graft is taken from *[PGI 1993, AIIMS PGMEE 1990]*
a. Pronator teris b. Brachioradialis
c. Pronator quadratus d. Extensor pollicis longus

42. In Classical Scaphoid cast position of wrist is *[PGI 1994]*
a. Dorsal and ulnar flexion
b. Dorsal and radial flexion
c. Ventral and ulnar flexion
d. Ventral and radial flexion.

43. MC cause of Volkman's Ischaemic Contracture in children is *[AIIMS PGMEE 1999]*
a. Intercondylar fracture of humerus
b. Supracondylar fracture of humerus
c. Lateral condyle fracture of humerus
d. Fracture of radius and ulna simultaneously

44. Which of the following statement(s) is/are true? *[PGI 1992]*
a. Oedema & tenderness over the anatomical snuff box is the pathognomonic features of Fracture of the scaphoid
b. Normally the radial styloid is "12" lower than the ulnar
c. Dinner fork deformity is characteristic of Colle's fracture
d. All of the above

45. First sign of Volkman's Ischaemia is *[PGI 2000]*
a. Paraesthesia b. Swelling of fingers
c. Pain on passive extension of fingers
d. Pain on active extension of fingers

46. MC involvement in Volkmann's Ischaemia seen is that of *[AIIMS PGMEE 1998]*
a. Flexor carpi radialis longus
b. Pronator teres
c. Flexor digitorum superficialis
d. Flexor digitorum profundus

47. Commonly inured carpal bone next to scaphoid is *[NBE DNB 1991, Delhi PGMEE 2010]*
a. Trapeium b. Trapezoid
c. Lunate d. Capitate
e. Hamate

48. Bennett's fracture is fracture dislocation of base of .... metacarpal *[Recent Question 2017, PGI 2000, UP PGMEE 1988, 1999]*
a. 4th b. 3rd
c. 2nd d. 1st

49. Bennett's fracture is used to describe *[Karnataka PGMEE 1989]*
a. Fracture-dislocation of metacarpophalangeal joint of thumb
b. Interphalangeal fracture dislocation of thumb
c. Anterior marginal fracture of distal end of radius
d. Fracture dislocation of trapeziometacarpal joint

50. In Volkman's Ischaemic Contracture, surgery should be done within *[AMU PGMEE 1987, DPG 2006]*
a. 1 hour b. 6 hours
c. 24 hours d. 72 hours

51. Volkman's Ischaemic Contracture is due to *[Karnataka PGMEE 1988]*
a. Arterial injury
b. Venous injury
c. Nerve injury
d. Increased compartment pressure in limb

52. Most common nerve involved in Volkman's Ischaemic Contracture is *[All India PGMEE 1999]*
a. Radial nerve b. Ulnar nerve
c. Median nerve d. Axillary nerve

53. Treatment of Oblique fracture of Olecranon process is *[AIIMS PGMEE 1996]*
a. Excision and re-suturing
b. Tension band wiring
c. Elbow immobilisation in cast
d. Open reduction and external fixation

54. Displacement NOT seen in Colles' fracture is *[AIIMS PGMEE 1997, AIIMS November 2014]*
a. Dorsal tilt b. Ventral tilt
c. Dorsal displacement d. Ventra displacement

55. Position of wrist in Cast of Colles' fracture is *[JIPMER PGMEE 1998]*
a. Dorsal deviation and pronation
b. Dorsal deviation and supination
c. Palmar deviation and pronation
d. Palmar deviation and supination

56. Bennett's fracture is difficult to maintain in a reduced position mainly because of the pull of the *[PGI 1992, Karnataka PGMEE 1999, AIIMS PG 1994]*
a. Flexor pollicis longus b. Flexor pollicis brevis
c. Extensor pollicis brevis d. Abductor pollicis longus

57. Tendon involved in Colles' fracture is *[Rohtak PGMEE 1997, Bengal PGMEE 1999]*
a. APL (abductor pollicis longus)
b. EPL (extensor pollicis longus)
c. EPB (extensor pollicics brevis)
d. None

58. Not a complication of Colles' fracture *[JIPMER PGMEE 2000]*
a. Stiffness of finger b. Stiffness of shoulder
c. Wrist drop d. Carpal tunnel syndrome

59. Avulsion of Extensor tendon gives rise to *[AP PGMEE 1999]*
a. Mallet finger b. Dupuytren's contracture
c. Trigger finger d. Swan neck deformity

60. 'Figure of 8' bandage is used for *[UP PGMEE 2001]*
a. Fracture of scapula b. Fracture clavicle
c. Fracture humerus d. Fracture metacarpals

61. Which of the fractures of scaphoid is most prone to develop Avascular necrosis? *[Karnataka PGMEE 1992]*
a. Tubercle b. Waist
c. Distal pole d. Proximal fragment

62. Most common nerve involved in Lunate dislocation is *[UP PGMEE 1998]*
a. Radial nerve
b. Median nerve
c. Anterior interosseus nerve
d. Posterior interosseus nerve

63. Game keeper's thumb is *[Recent Question 2016, PGI 1992, Karnataka PGMEE 1995]*
a. Ulnar collateral ligament injury of MCP joint
b. Ulnar collateral ligament injury of CMC joint
c. Medial collateral ligament injury of MCP joint
d. Medial collateral ligament injury of CMC joint

64. In Mallet's finger, seen is *[Kerala PGMEE 1987]*
a. Fracture middle phalanx
b. Avulsion of terminal slip of extensor tendon to distal phalanx
c. Fracture proximal phalanx
d. Fracture distal phalanx

65. All true regarding fracture lateral condyle humerus except *[PGI 1993, JIPMER PGMEE 1998]*
a. Salter Harris type IV injury
b. Most common complication of surgically treated cases is cubitus valgus deformity
c. Tardy ulnar nerve palsy occurs
d. Cubitus varus occur more commonly than valgus
e. Open reduction & internal fixation

66. Fracture of Lateral condyle of humerus seen in age group of *[PGI 1990]*
a. 2 - 3 years b. 3 - 5 years
c. 5 - 15 years d. 15 - 25 years
e. 35 - 45 years

67. "Cubitus-valgus" deformity is complication of *[AIIMS PGMEE 1997, AIPGME 2001]*
a. Fracture Lateral condyle of humerus
b. Fracture Intercondylar of humerus
c. Fracture of the olecranon
d. Fracture Head of the radius

68. A 12-year-old child presents with tingling sensation and numbness in the little finger and gives history of fracture in the elbow region 4 years back. The probable fracture is *[Delhi PGMEE 2009, AIIMS PG 1999]*
a. Lateral condyle fracture humerus
b. Injury to ulnar nerve
c. Supracondylar fracture humerus
d. Dislocation of elbow

69. Tardy ulnar nerve palsy occur as a delayed sequel of
a. Supracondylar fracture of humerus *[PGI 1992]*
b. Posterior dislocation of elbow
c. Fracture of lateral condyle of humerus in children
d. Fracture of Olecranon

70. Fracture Scaphoid is more common among *[PGI 1995]*
a. Elderly postmenopausal females
b. Elderly males
c. Young active adults d. Children

71. Fracture Lateral condyle of the humerus is a common injury in children. Which one of the following is the most ideal treatment for a displaced fracture lateral condyle of the humerus in a 7-year-old child? *[Karnataka PGMEE 1989]*
a. Open reduction and plaster immobilization
b. Closed reduction and plaster immobilization
c. Open reduction and internal fixation
d. Excision of the fractured fragment

72. Growth disturbance, nonunion, elbow instability & late ulnar nerve palsy is commonly seen in *[AMU PGMEE 1993, MAHE PGMEE 2002, BHU PGMEE 1996, AIIMS 1991]*
a. Fracture supracondylar humerus
b. Fracture medial condyle
c. Fracture lateral condyle
d. Fracture head radius

73. Medial epicondyle fracture results in injury to .... nerve *[NBE DNB 1993, AMU PGMEE 1995]*
a. Radial b. Median
c. Ulnar d. Axillary

74. Most common associated injury of Fracture Medial epicondyle *[PGI 1992, NIMHANS PGMEE 1995]*
a. Elbow dislocation
b. Monteggia fracture dislocation
c. Fracture supracondylar humerus
d. Vascular defecit

75. Suspected medial Epicondylar fracture of humerus in a 4 year old child requires *[CMC PGMEE 1996, TN PGMEE 1995]*
a. X-ray both arms with elbow for comparison
b. X-ray same limb only
c. Examination under general anaesthesia
d. POP in full flexed position

76. After falling from a height, a child lands on his fully out stretched hands. On examination there is pain and swelling over his right elbow. Give your probable diagnosis *[AP PGMEE 1993, AIIMS PGMEE 2000]*
a. Fracture olecranon
b. Post dislocation of elbow
c. Supra condylar fracture of humerus
d. Fracture both bones forearm

77. Fracture neck of humerus is common in *[TN PGMEE 1997]*
a. Young females b. Elderly males
c. Elderly females d. Infants

78. Most common Elbow injury in Adolescents is *[All India PGMEE 1990, AMU PGMEE 1997, UP PGMEE 2001]*
a. Dislocation b. Physeal injury
c. Supracondylar fracture d. Olecranon fracture

79. Most common Elbow injury in Children is *[Kerala PGMEE 1988]*
a. Extension type of supracondylar fracture of humerus
b. Dislocation of elbow
c. Fracture lateral condyle of humerus
d. Fracture medial epicondyle of humerus

80. In Supracondylar fracture of humerus, the distal segment is often displaced to *[Kerala PGMEE 1988]*
a. Anteriorly b. Laterally
c. Posteriorly d. Medially

81. Most common type of Supracondylar fracture is
a. Neutral b. Flexion *[TN PGMEE 93]*
c. Extension d. Lateral

82. Supracondylar fracture is usually caused by *[MAHE PGMEE 2002, SGPGI 2001]*
a. Hyper flexion injury
b. Axial rotation
c. Extension injury
d. Hyper extension injury

83. In Flexion injuries causing Supracondylar fractures, the distal fragment is often displaced to *[Karnataka PGMEE 1996, TN PGMEE 1999]*
a. Anterior b. Posterior
c. Medial d. Lateral

84. A 10-year-old boy presenting with a Cubitus varus deformity and a history of trauma 3 months back on clinical examination, has the preserved 3 bony point relationship of the elbow. The most probable diagnosis is *[All India PGMEE 1994, AIIMS PGMEE 1994, AIIMS PGMEE 2004]*

a. Old unreduced dislocation of elbow
b. Non-union lateral condylar fracture of humerus
c. Malunited intercondylar fracture of humerus
d. Malunited supracondylar fracture of humerus

85. Malunion of Supracondylar fracture of the humerus most commonly leads to *[AIIMS 1997, 2006, AIPGME 1994, TNPG 1997, PGI 1997, Karnataka 1998]*

a. Flexion deformity
b. Cubitus varus
c. Cubitus valgus
d. Extension deformity

86. Osteotomy done for Malunited Supracondylar fracture is *[J & K PGMEE 2001]*

a. French
b. Shanz's
c. Mc Murry's
d. Mc Alister

87. Following are complications of Supracondylar fracture of humerus in children, except *[AIIMS PGMEE 2006]*

a. Compartment syndrome
b. Myositis ossificans
c. Malunion
d. Nonunion

88. Least common complication of Closed Supracondylar fracture in an 8 year old child is *[TN PGMEE 1996, AMU PGMEE 1998, BHU PGMEE 1999]*

a. Cubitus valgus
b. Cubitus varus
c. Nonunion
d. Vessel injury

89. Which complication may arise after Supra condylar fracture? *[PGI 1995, 2005]*

a. Median nerve injury
b. Damage to brainchild artery
c. Cubitus varus
d. All of the above

90. Tardy Ulnar nerve palsy caused by *[PGI 2002]*

a. Supracondylar fracture
b. Lateral condylar fracture
c. Olecranon fracture
d. Intercondylar fracture
e. Distal radioulnar dislocation

91. All of the following are associated with Supracondylar fracture of humerus, EXCEPT *[All India PGMEE 2002]*

a. It is uncommon after 15 years of age
b. Extension type fracture is more common than the flexion type
c. Cubitus varus deformity commonly results following malunion
d. Ulnar nerve is most commonly involved

92. True statement regarding Supracondylar fracture of the Humerus in children *[Kerala PGMEE 1990]*

a. Admission to hospital is essential following reduction
b. It is due to a fall on the point of the elbow
c. It require open reduction
d. It is usually compound

93. Earliest symptom of Volkmann's Ischaemic is *[JIPMER PGMEE 1993, Orissa PGMEE 1992, TN PGMEE 1991, PGI 2000]*

a. Pain in flexor muscles
b. Absence of pulse
c. Pain on passive extension
d. Cyanosis of limb

94. Most important sign in Volkmann's ischaemic contracture is *[TN PGMEE 1990]*

a. Pain
b. Pallor
c. Numbness
d. Obliteration of radial pulse

95. Volkmann's ischaemic contracture mostly involves *[AIIMS PG 1992, 1998]*

a. Flexor digitorum superficialis
b. Pronator teres
c. Flexor digitorum profundus
d. Flexor carpi radialis longus

96. Earliest ischemic feature after reduction of Supra-condylar fracture is *[AP PGMEE 1989]*

a. Coldness
b. Pain
c. Swelling
d. Tingling

97. One of the following is associated with Volkmann's ischaemic contracture *[PGI 2000]*

a. Supracondylar fracture of humerus
b. Fracture shaft humerus
c. Intercondylar fracture of humerus
d. Dislocation of elbow

98. In Volkmann's ischemia, surgery should be done *[AMU PGMEE 1987]*

a. Immediately
b. After 6 hours
c. 24 hours
d. 72 hours

99. A patient presenting with Volkmann's Ischaemia all of the following are done except *[PGI 2000]*

a. Split open the plaster of Paris cst and bandage
b. Decompression by fasciotomy
c. Exploration
d. Sympathetic ganglion blockade

100. Volkmann's contracture *[UPSC 1998, Bihar 1991]*

a. Is localized thickening of palmar fascia
b. Develops at the ankle in a case of chronic venous ulcer
c. Follows Ischaemia of the forearm
d. Is due to excessive scarring of the skin of the arm following a burn.

101. Volkmann's ischaemic contracture is commonly due to *[Bihar PGMEE 1990]*

a. Tight plaster
b. Tight splint
c. Both
d. None

102. Volkmann's Ischaemic contracture is due to *[Karnataka PGMEE 1988]*

a. Arterial injury
b. Venous injury
c. Nerve injury
d. Increase of compartment pressure in the limb

103. In Below elbow amputation the length of stump should be *[AIIMS PGMEE 1993]*

a. 10-15 cm
b. 15-20 cm
c. 20-25 cm
d. 5-10 cm

104. Distance from Olecranon in amputation should be *[Delhi PGMEE 2007]*

a. 5-10 cm
b. 10-25 cm
c. 15-20 cm
d. 20-30 cm

105. All are TRUE about Clavicle, EXCEPT *[AIIMS PGMEE 1993]*

a. No treatment required for fracture but rest
b. Breaks at mid-point
c. First bone to ossify
d. Ossifies in membrane

106. True statement regarding Fracture of Clavicle is *[All India PGMEE 2000]*

a. Most common Complication is Malunion
b. Occurs at the medial 1/3nd & lateral 2/3nd
c. Usually occurs due to fall on elbow
d. Communited fracture is common

107. Clavicular fracture is usually treated by *[TN PG 1999, APPG 1999, UP PG 2001, JIPMER 1987]*

a. Traction
b. Open Reduction and Internal fixation
c. Figure-of-eight bandage
d. Plate and Screw fixation

108. Fracture of clavicle is commonest at *[Delhi PGMEE 1991]*

a. Junction of medial l/3rd and lateral 2/3rd
b. Junction of medial 2/3rd and lateral 1/3rd
c. Midpoint
d. Scapular end

109. Most common site of Avascular necrosis amongst the following is *[All India PGMEE 1999]*

a. Head of the radius fracture
b. Medical condyle of femur fracture
c. Olecranon fracture
d. Talus fracture

110. Pulled elbow is *[PGI 1994]*

a. A sprain of extensor tendons
b. Dislocation of head of radius
c. Fracture of lateral condyle of humerus
d. Dislocation of elbow

111. A 30 years old male comes to Orthopedics emergency with his 3 years old daughter who is crying. The father gives the history of child being swung by forearm. The most probable diagnosis is *[AIIMS PGMEE 2001, November 2014, TN PGMEE 2002]*

a. Supracondylar humerus fracture
b. Elbow dislocation
c. Stress fracture
d. Pulled elbow

112. A one and a half year old child holding her father's hand slipped and fell but did not let go of her father's hand. After that she continued to cry and hold the forearm in pronated position and refused to move the affected extremity. Which of the following management at this stage is most appropriate? *[AIIMS PGMEE 2004]*

a. Supinate the forearm
b. Examine the child under GA
c. Elevate the limb and observe
d. Investigate for osteomyelitis

113. An oblique Fracture of Olecranon. If displaced proximally. The treatment is *[AIIMS PGMEE 1996]*

a. Excision & resuturing
b. Tension band wiring
c. Elbow is imbolised by cast
d. Open reduction & external fixation

114. In fracture of the Olecronon, excision of the proximal fragment is indicated in all of the following situations except *[All India PGMEE 2004]*

a. Old ununited fractures
b. Non-articular fractures
c. Fracture extending to coronoid process
d. Elderly patient

115. In Monteggia fracture, which is true about Ulnar fracture and Head of radius? *[Recent Question 2016, JIPMER PGMEE 1992, JIPMER PGMEE 2014]*

a. Both ulnar fracture and head of radius is displaced posteriorly
b. Both ulnar fracture and head of radius is displaced anteriorly
c. Ulnar fractures is posteriorly and head of radius is displaced anteriorly
d. Ulnar fracture is anteriorly and head of radius is displaced posteriorly

116. 3-point bony relationship is reversed in all of the following fractures except *[Recent Question 2016, AIIMS PGMEE 1991, AIIMS PG 1993, 2000]*

a. Lateral condyle humerus fracture
b. Supracondylar fracture humerus
c. Dislocation of elbow
d. Intercondylar fracture humerus

117. Galeazzi fracture is *[Karnataka PGMEE 1997]*

a. Supracondylar fracture of the humerus
b. Fracture of the distal radius with inferior radioulnar joint dislocation
c. Fracture radius in the proximal site and dislocation of the elbow
d. Fracture of the radial head

118. Principle in the treatment of fractures of both bones of the forearm is to *[Bihar PGMEE 1991]*

a. Reduce angulation of radius and ulna
b. Restore the normal relationship of radius and ulna
c. Immobilize the elbow only
d. Prevent over riding of fragments
e. All of the above

119. Treatment of choice of fracture of radius and ulna in an adult is *[Delhi PGMEE 1992, Delhi PGMEE 1992]*
a. Plaster for 4 weeks
b. Closed reduction and calipers
c. Only plates
d. Kuntscher nails

120. Cubitus valgus is a deformity seen in *[AIIMS PGMEE 1997, JIPMER PGMEE 2014]*
a. Fracture of Olecranon
b. Fracture of head of radius
c. Fracture humerus (intercondylar)
d. Fracture of humerus (lateral condyle)

121. All are true regarding Clavicular fracture except *[TN PGMEE 1992]*
a. Be caused by a fall on to the outstretched arm
b. Commonly occurs between the insertions of the Coracoclavicular and the Costoclavicular ligaments
c. Jeopardize blood supply to the overlying skin
d. Usually requires careful reduction

122. Fracture neck Humerus is common in *[TN PGMEE 1997]*
a. Elderly woman b. Young lady
c. Elderly man d. All of these

123. In fracture Surgical neck of humerus, the following nerve injury is common *[PGI PGMEE 2000]*
a. Axillary b. Radial
c. Ulnar d. Median
e. Musculocutaneous

124. Fracture of both bone forearm at same level, position of the arm in plaster is *[AIIMS PGMEE 1999]*
a. Full supination b. 10 degree supination
c. Full pronation d. Mid-prone

125. Colles fracture is *[NBE DNB 1990, AMU PGMEE 1992, WB 93]*
a. Common in adolescence
b. A fracture about the ankle joint
c. Common in elderly women
d. A fracture of head of the radius

126. Seen in Colles Fracture all except *[AIIMS PGMEE 1995]*
a. Proximal shift b. Dorsal tilt
c. Lateral tilt d. Pronation

127. Treatment of choice for fracture neck of humerus in a 70 year old male *[PGI PGMEE 1994, MAHE PGMEE 1996]*
a. Analgesic with arm sling
b. U-slab
c. Arthroplasty
d. Open reduction—Internal fixation

128. Medial epicondyle fracture results in injury to *[AMU PGMEE 1995]*
a. Radial b. Ulnar
c. Median d. Axillary

129. Treatment of choice in 65 year old female with impacted Fracture neck of humerus is *[AIIMS PGMEE 1999, UPPG 2000, PGI 2000]*
a. Triangular sling b. Arm chest strapping
c. Arthroplasty d. Observation

130. Which of the following movements will be affected if the Greater tubercle of the humerus is lost? *[AIIMS PGMEE 2002]*
a. Abduction and lateral rotation
b. Adduction and flexion
c. Adduction and medial rotation
d. Flexion and medial rotation

131. In a Fracture shaft humerus, which of the following complication requires immediate surgery? *[AIIMS PGMEE 2000]*
a. Compound fracture
b. Nerve injury
c. Brachial artery occlusion
d. Comminuted fracture

132. Most important cause of Nonunion of Fracture of humeral shaft is *[Orissa PGMEE 1990]*
a. Comminuted fracture
b. Compound (Open) fracture
c. Overriding of fracture ends
d. Distraction at fracture site
e. Operative reduction

133. Increased intercondylar distance is seen in Fracture of all except *[Delhi PGMEE 1993]*
a. Olecranon b. Medial epicondyle
c. Lateral epicondyle d. Lateral condyle

134. About displacement of distal fragment in Colles fracture, true is *[UPSC 1990]*
a. Anteriorly and medially b. Posteriorly and laterally
c. Anteriorly and laterally d. Posteriorly and medially

135. Dinner fork deformity' is present in case of *[Recent Question 2016, PGI 1992, UP PGMEE 1999]*
a. Smith's fracture b. Student's elbow
c. Colles' fracture d. All of these

136. In Colles fracture not seen is *[All India PGMEE 1997]*
a. Proximal impaction b. Lateral rotation
c. Dorsal angulation d. Medial rotation

137. 3 point symmetry is NOT disturbed in which fracture *[AIIMS PGMEE 1993]*
a. Fracture ulna only
b. Fracture radius only
c. Fracture of radius & ulna both bones of forearm
d. Weak posterior capsule

138. True about Monteggia fracture dislocation is/ are *[PGI May 2014]*
a. Fracture lower 1/3 radius
b. Fracture lower 1/3 ulna
c. Fracture upper 1/3 radius
d. Fracture upper 1/3 ulna
e. Radial head dislocation

139. Management of Open fractures include all except *[JIPMER PGMEE 2014]*
a. Internal fixation b. External fixation
c. Torniquet d. Surgical debridement

140. Most common nerve involved in Fracture of Surgical neck of humerus *[ESI IMO 2014]*
a. Ulnar b. Axillary
c. Median d. Radial

141. Complications of Colles fracture include all of the following except *[ESI IMO 2014]*

a. Sudeck's Osteodystrophy
b. Rupture of EPL tendon
c. Malunion
d. Nonunion

142. Most common site of Scaphoid fracture is *[ESI IMO 2014]*

a. Distal fragment
b. Tilting of the lunate
c. Waist
d. Proximal fragment

143. Commonest cause of "Wrist Drop" is *[PGMCET 2015]*

a. Intramuscular injection
b. Fracture Humerus
c. Dislocation of elbow
d. Dislocation of shoulder

144. Most common complication after Supracondylar fracture humerus is *[PGMCET 2015]*

a. Cubitus varus
b. Cubitus valgus
c. Median nerve injury
d. Ulnar nerve injury

145. Chauffeur's fracture involves the *[PGMCET 2015]*

a. Radial head
b. Radial styloid
c. Ulnar styloid
d. Base of 1st Metacarpal

146. Mallet finger is due to rupture of *[PGMCET 2015]*

a. Central extensor slip of finger
b. Distal end of index extensor
c. Distal end of flexor digitorum profundus
d. None of above

147. Following is true regarding Galeazzi fracture dislocation *[AIIMS May 2017]*

a. Interosseous membrane tear with ulnar shaft fracture
b. Radial collateral ligament tear with interosseous membrance tear with radial shaft fracture
c. Interosseous membrane tear with triangular fibrocartilage complex (TFCC) tear and ulnar shaft fracture
d. Interosseous membrane tear with triangular fibrocartilage complex (TFCC) tear and radial shaft fracture

NEET/NBE PATTERN MCQs ANSWERS WITH EXPLANATIONS 

1. Ans. (b) Greenstick fracture

[Ref. Campbell's Operative Orthopaedics, 13/e p1147]

Greenstick Fractures

- An incomplete transverse fracture pattern commonly seen in children
- Force to side of bone may cause break in only one cortex; the other cortex only bends
- An injuring force applied to a bone exceeds the limits of elasticity of that bone; it result in bone's bending to the point of bony disruption and fracture on side opposite to side of applied force
- Characterized by incomplete cortical fracture and angulation and rotation through plastic deformation of the remaining intact cortex
- Often associated with Complete fracture of the other bone of forearm

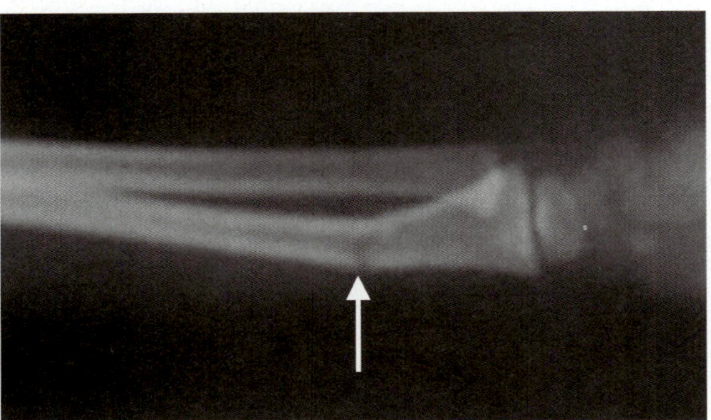

Fig. Greenstick fracture

Also Remember

- Three common incomplete fractures present in children:
  - Greenstick fractures
  - Torus/ buckle fractures
  - Plastic bowing fractures

2. Ans. (b) Inferior Dislocation of the shoulder joint

[Ref. Maheshwari, 4/e p87]

Luxatio Erecta

- Inferior dislocation of Glenohumeral joint/ Shoulder joint
- Least common form of Shoulder dislocation
- Arm appears to be permanently held upward or behind the head, in fixed abduction
- Underlying cause: Hyperabduction of arm that forces humeral head against acromion

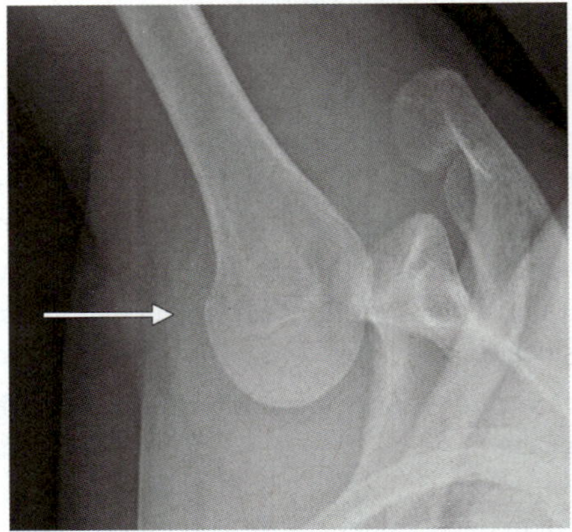

Fig. Luxatio Erecta

3. Ans. (d) Brachial plexus injury

[Ref. Orthopaedics Examination by Banerjee, 1/e p199]

Aeroplane splint

- Shoulder-abduction splint
- Used in Brachial plexus injury

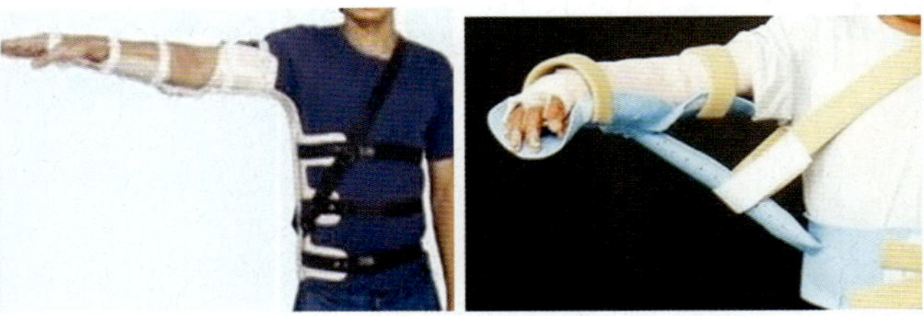

Fig. Aeroplane splint

4. Ans. (a) Hanging casts

[Ref. Manual of Fracture Treatment by Cox, 1/e p23]

Hanging cast

- Most popular method of treating a fracture of Shaft of humerus
- Although use of a hanging cast violates every primary rule of fracture treatment, the system works
- Best used for fractures in Middle 1/3 shaft

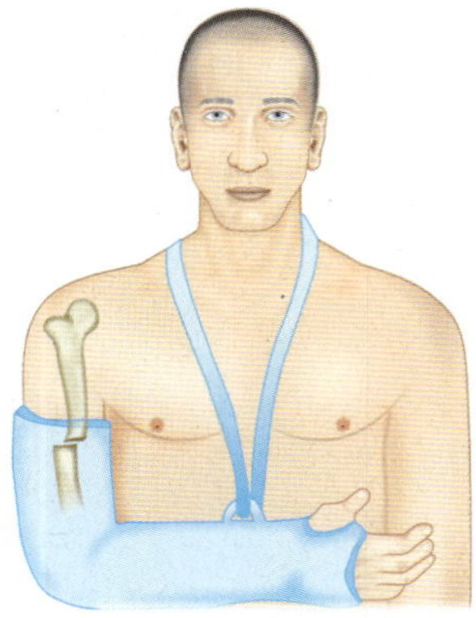

Fig. Hanging cast

5. Ans. (a) Fracture shaft humerus

[Ref. Fractures of the Humerus by Castoldi, 1/e p214]

Functional Bracing

- Orthosis with an anterior and posterior pre-fabricated shell contoured to accommodate arm musculature
- Since its first inception, Functional bracing has become the Gold standard for definitive management of majority of Midshaft humeral fractures

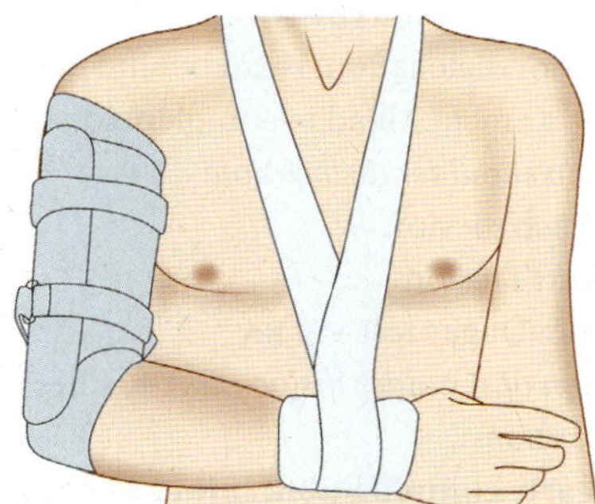

Fig. Functional bracing

6. Ans. (d) It is associated with dorsal angulation

[Ref. Musculoskeletal Radiology by Griffiths, 1/e p10]

- **Colles fracture** is a comminuted, basically horizontal fracture of the distal radius, with dorsal angulation, frequently, but not necessarily, associated with a fracture of the ulnar styloid (only in 60%)
- Dorsal angulation is the most common type of malunion that occurs after Colles fracture

7. Ans. (b) Avulsion of extensor tendon at the base of the distal phalanx

[Ref. Emergency Radiology by Marincek, 1/e p272]

- **Mallet finger**: Intra-articular avulsion fracture of the dorsal base of the distal phalanx or a disruption of the distal terminal extensor tendon without fracture

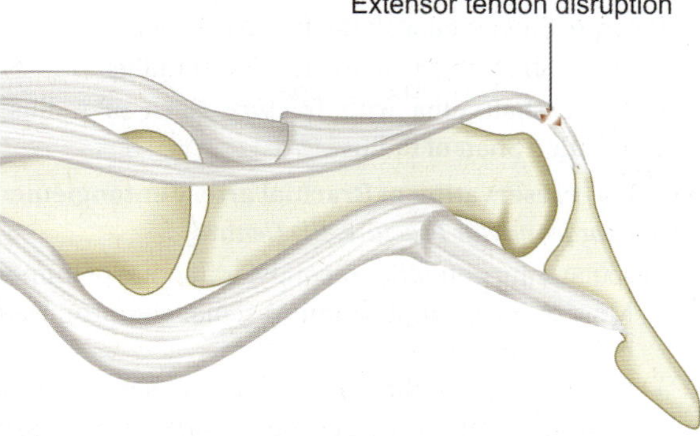

Fig. Mallet finger

8. Ans. (a) Lateral condyle of humerus

[Ref. Orthopaedics & Applied Physiotherapy by Joshi, 1/e p95]

- Non-union of Lateral condylar humerus fracture can cause Cubitus valgus deformity in growing children

9. Ans. (c) 5th metacarpal fracture

[Ref. Maheshwari, 4/e p3]

- **Boxer's fracture**: Ventrally displaced fracture occurring through Neck of 5th metacarpal, usually seen in Boxers

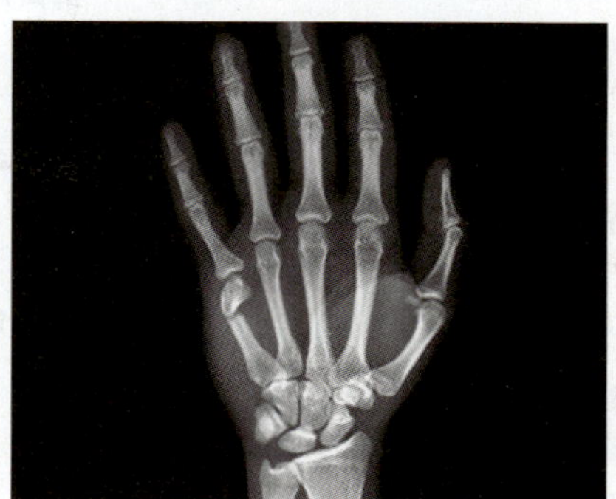

Fig. Boxes's fracture

10. Ans. (d) Anterior

[Ref. Encyclopedia of International Sports Studies by Bartlett, 1/e p92]

- Anterior shoulder dislocation is **MC type of shoulder dislocations** (90–95 per cent)
- This injury is MC in overhead and contact sports

11. Ans. (d) Axillary

12. Ans. (c) Radial nerve

13. Ans. (c) Bennett's fracture dislocation

14. Ans. (b) Lateral condyle fractures

15. Ans. (b) Subluxation of head of radius

16. Ans. (b) Extension type most common

17. Ans. (c) Finger stiffness

18. Ans. (b) Cubitus varus

19. Ans. (b) Nonunion

20. Ans. (b) Delayed union

[Ref. Maheshwari, 4/e p110]

Complications of Colles Fracture

- Finger stiffness **(Most common)**
- Malunion
- Subluxation of inferior radioulnar joint
- Carpal tunnel syndrome
- Sudeck's osteodystrophy
- Rupture extensor pollicis longus tendon

21. Ans. (b) Fracture distal radius

22. Ans. (d) All of the above

[Ref. Maheshwari, 4/e p108]

- ***Colles fracture***: Fracture of distal end of radius
- It is most common fracture in age group: >40 years age
- ***Displacements in Colles fracture*:**
  - Dorsal displacement
  - Dorsal tilt (Most characteristic)
  - Lateral displacement
  - Lateral tilt
  - Supination

23. Ans.(c) Scaphoid

[Ref. Human Anatomy by BD Chaurasia, 5th Ed., Pg 33]

- ***Most common carpal bone to be fractured*: Scaphoid**
- *MC Type*: Fracture waist of scaphoid
- *Age group*: Young adults
- *Clinical presentation*: Tenderness in anatomical snuff box
- *X-ray*: Oblique view of wrist
- *Treatment*: Scaphoid cast (Wrist in dorsiflexion + Radial deviation: ***'Glass holding position'***)

- *Complications of Colles' fracture*:
  - Avascular necrosis (of proximal pole)
  - Delayed union/malunion

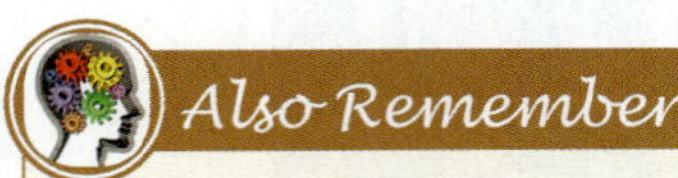

- *Second common carpal bone to be fractured:* Triquetrum

24. Ans. (d) Four part

25. Ans. (c) Upper 1/3 ulna

26. Ans. (b) Ulnar

27. Ans. (d) Axillary

28. Ans. (a) Colles fracture

29. Ans. (d) Humerus fracture
[Ref. Maheshwari, 4/e p90]

Useful Aids/ Procedure in Orthopedics

Orthopedic aid/ procedure	Used in
Austin-Moore prosthesis	**Fracture neck of femur**
Kirschner wire	Small bone fixation
Kuntscher nail	Fracture shaft of femur
Bankart's procedure	Recurrent dislocation of shoulder
Dwyer's osteotomy	CTEV
Meyer's operation	Fracture neck of femur
Thomas splint	**Immobilsation of hip and thigh injuries**
Cock-up splint	**Radial nerve palsy**
Von Rosen's splint	**Congenital dislocation of hip**
Dennis brown splint	**CTEV**
Milwaukee brace	**Scoliosis**
Gallow's traction	**Fracture shaft of femur (Age <2 years)**
Hip spica	Fracture shaft of femur
Russel's traction	Trochanteric fractures
Frog's cast	Congenital dislocation of hip
Batchelor's cast	**Congenital dislocation of hip**
Hanging cast	**Fracture shaft of humerus**
Minerva jacket	**Immobilization of injured cervical spine**

30. Ans. (d) Malunion is a frequent complication

31. Ans. (b) Radial nerve injury
[Ref. Maheshwari, 4/e p24]

32. Ans. (a) Malunion

33. Ans. (a) Colles' fracture

34. Ans. (b) Circumflex axillary nerve
[Ref. Maheshwari, 4/e p88]

Shoulder Dislocation

- *Types of shoulder dislocations*:
  - **Anterior dislocation: Most common**; head of humerus in front of glenoid cavity
  - Posterior dislocation: Head behind glenoid cavity
  - Luxatio erecta: Head in sub-glenoid position
- *Lesions in shoulder dislocation*:
  - Hill-Sach's lesion
  - Bankart's lesion
- *Diagnosis*: Dugas test + X-ray
- *Reduction of shoulder dislocation*: Kocher's manoeuvre
- *Complications*:
  - **MC early complication: Injury to Axillary nerve**
  - MC late complication: Recurrence of dislocation
- *Treatment*: Putti-platt operation, Bankart's operation

35. Ans. (c) Radial nerve
[Ref. Maheshwari, 4/e p90]

- Fracture shaft of humerus may lead to Radial nerve injury causing **'Wrist-drop'**

36. Ans. (b) Avulsion of terminal slip of extensor tendon to distal phalanx

37. Ans. (c) Stiff wrist joint

38. Ans. (b) Supination + Pressure over Head of radius
[Ref. Sports Injuries by Hyde, 2/e p565]

39. Ans. (d) Fracture shaft ulna
[Ref. Orthopedics by Ebnezar, 4/e p174]

Variants of Monteggia Fracture Dislocation

- Isolated dislocation Head of radius
- Fracture Shaft ulna with fracture Neck radius
- Fracture Shaft ulna with fracture Shaft radius
- Fracture shaft ulna with fracture Neck of radius with dislocation Shaft of radius

40. Ans. (a) Preservation of Brachial artery entanglement
[Ref. Supracondylar Fracture, ED Central]

- Vascular injury after Supracondylar fracture of humerus:
  - Most serious complication: Vascular compromise of the brachial artery
  - If not relieved there is a risk of ischaemia of the anterior compartment of the forearm with consequent Volkmann's ischaemic contracture
  - Risk of vascular injury increases with the Grade of Gartland (I < II < III)

41. Ans. (c) The distal end of ulna dislocates volarly after disruption of distal radioulnar joint
[Ref. Maheshwari, 4/e p106]

Galeazzi Fracture Dislocation

- Fracture lower 1/3 of radius ***plus*** Dislocation/ subluxation of Distal radioulnar joint

- Classically involves an isolated fracture of the junction of the distal third and middle third of the radius with associated subluxation or dislocation of distal radioulnar joint
- Underlying cause: Fall on an outstretched hand

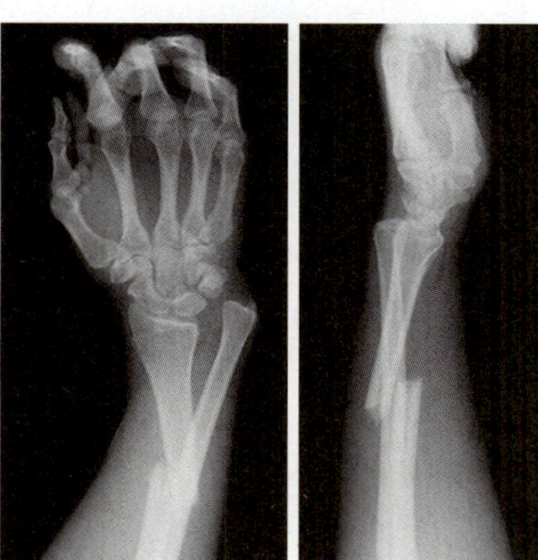

Fig. Galeazzi fracture dislocation

42. Ans. (a) Enchondroma

[Ref. Hand Fractures by Lawton, 1/e]

Pathological Fracture in Hand

- 80% of pathologic fractures of hand are due to Enchondromas
- Solitary enchondroma is the MC bone tumor of the hand, typically afflicting the small tubular bones and more commonly involving the ulnar digits
- More than half of these benign tumors present with pathologic fractures
- Because of this strong association, Pathologic hand fractures literature focuses on the management of fractures associated with Enchondromas

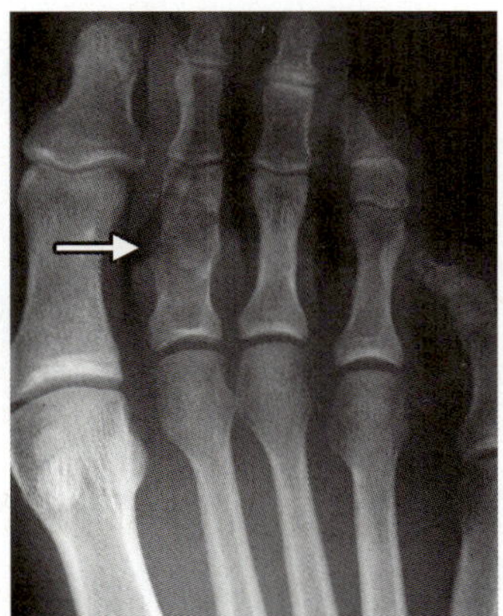

Fig. Pathological fracture (enchondroma)

43. Ans. (a) Abduction

[Ref. MRCEM Part C by Somani, 2/e p230]

- Shoulder abduction is a complex movement involving transition from Glenohumeral to Scapulothoracic movements
- This gradual transition is lost in joint disruption or damage to the tendons that stabilise the joint
- Patient will not be able to initiate the movement in the case of a Supraspinatus tear
- Once initiated, there may be pain on continuing abduction which is a sign of impingement

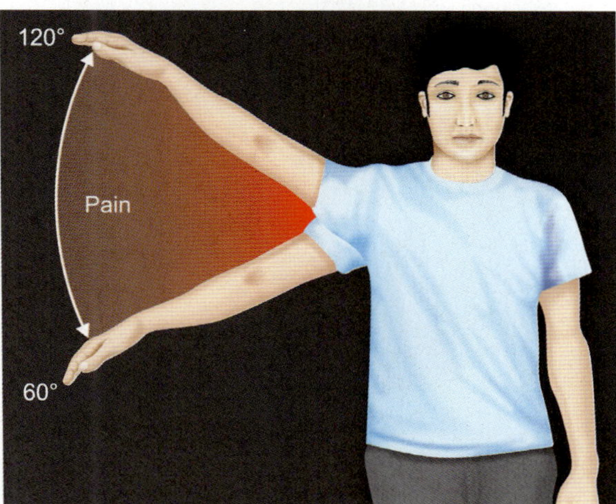

Fig. Abduction restriction (supraspinatus tear)

44. Ans. (c) Ulna angulates posteriorly in the extension type

[Ref. Harris & Harris' Radiology, 5/e p370]

Bado Classification of Monteggia Fracture (Depending upon displacement of Radial head)

- I - Extension type (60%): Ulna shaft angulates anteriorly (extends) and radial head dislocates anteriorly
- II - Flexion type (15%): Ulna shaft angulates posteriorly (flexes) and radial head dislocates posteriorly
- III - Lateral type (20%): Ulna shaft angulates laterally (bent to outside) and radial head dislocates to the side
- IV - Combined type (5%): Ulna shaft and radial shaft are both fractured and radial head is dislocated, typically anteriorly

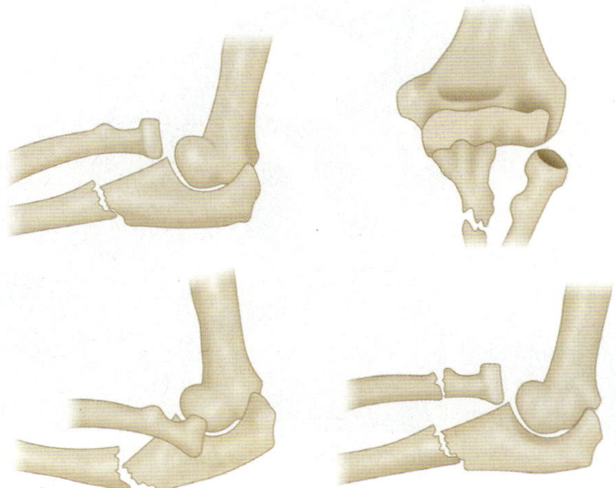

Fig. Bado classification (Monteggia fractures)

45. Ans. (a) Anterior shoulder dislocation

[Ref. Maheshwari, 4/e p87]

Bankart's Lesion

- Shoulder dislocation causes Stripping of Glenoid labrum along with periosteum from Anterior surface of glenoid and scapular neck
- Head comes to lie in front of Scapular neck

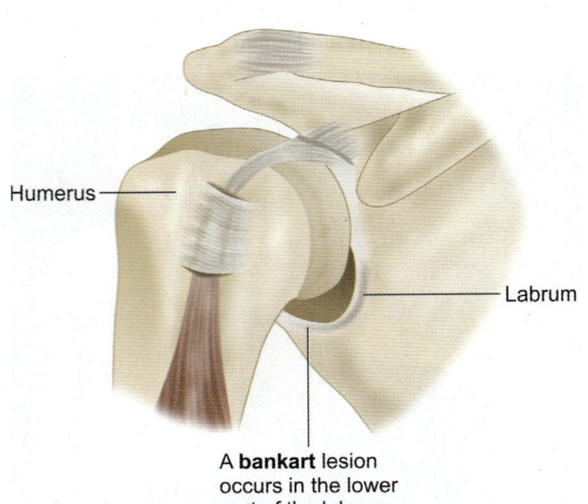

Fig. Bankart lesion

46. Ans. (b) Ulnar nerve palsy

[Ref. Maheshwari, 4/e p294]

Knuckle Bender Splint

- Indications: Ulnar claw hand (Ulnar nerve palsy), Total claw hand (Median nerve + Ulnar nerve palsy)
- Function: Maintain MCP joint in 90 degree flexion and IP joints in extension
  - Immobilization of fingers
  - Stability of wrist in extension
  - Maintenance of transverse palmar arch

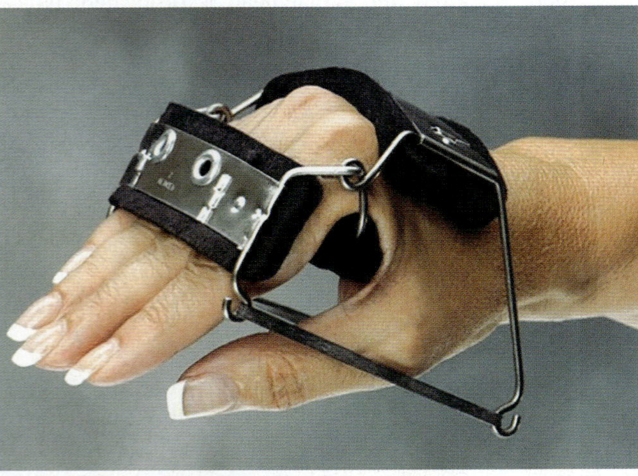

Fig. Knuckle Bender Splint

47. Ans. (a) Malunion

[Ref. Sports Medicine by O'Connor, p361]

Complications of Supracondylar Fracture Humerus

- Cubitus varus, the result of Malunion or medial condyle avascular necrosis, is the most common complication
- Most serious complication of displaced Supracondylar fractures of the Humerus in children is Volkmann's ischemia of nerves and muscles of the forearm

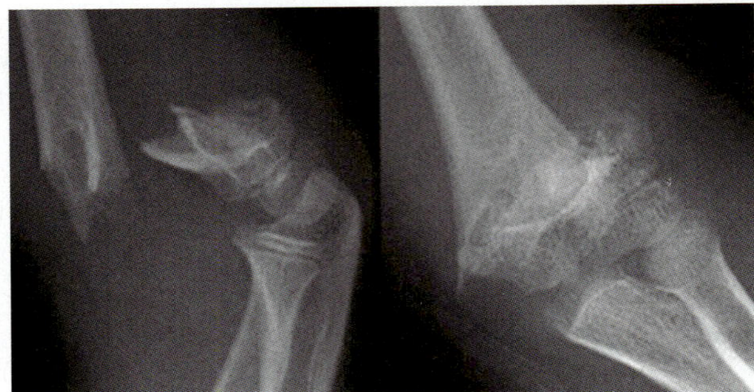

Fig. Supracondylar fracture humerus

48. Ans. (a) Open reduction internal fixation

[Ref. Trauma and Orthopaedic Classifications by Lasanianos, 1/e p62]

Distal Humerus Fractures

- Types of DH Fractures:
  - Type I: No displacement
  - Type II: Slightly displaced with no rotation of condylar fragments
  - Type III: Displacement with rotation of condylar fragments
  - Type IV: Severe comminution of condylar fragments

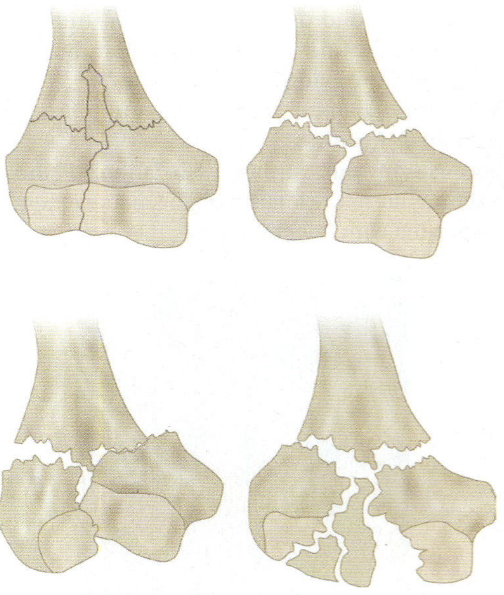

Fig. Types of distal humerus fractures

- Management:
  - Best management: Meticulous open reduction **with** Stable internal fixation
  - Operative management: Plate placement, Total arthroplasty. Hemi-arthroplasty

49. Ans. (a) Shoulder reduction

[Ref. Orthopedics by Biswas, 1/e p490]

- **Kocher's maneuver:** Elbow bent to 90 degrees and held close to body; Slow external rotation to 75 degrees; Point of elbow lifted forward and arm adducted; Arm internally rotated

Orthopedics

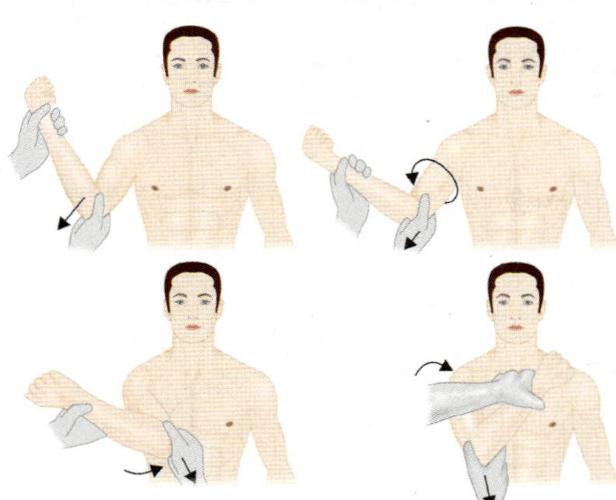

Fig. Kocher's maneuver

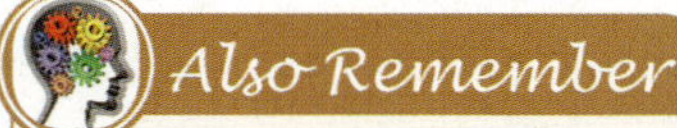

Also Remember

- **Non-operative management of anterior shoulder dislocation**
  - Kocher's manipulation
  - Hippocrates method
  - Stimson technique
  - Milch technique

50. Ans. (a) Scapholunate ligament

[Ref. Soft Tissue Rheumatology by Hazleman, 1/e p398]

- Patient who has pain and swelling in the anatomical snuffbox but negative X-rays, including stress views, may have an occult Scaphoid fracture or rupture of the Interosseous scapholunate ligament

51. Ans. (a) Conservative

[Ref. Scaphoid Fractures by Yao, 1/e p18]

- Treatment of Scaphoid fracture: Scaphoid cast (Wrist in dorsiflexion + Radial deviation: 'Glass holding position')

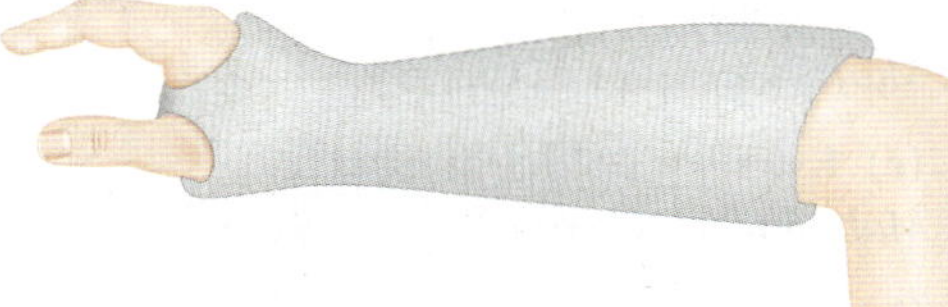

Fig. Scaphoid cast

52. Ans. (b) Results in Gun stock deformity

[Ref. Maheshwari, 4/e p98]

- Mal-union of Supracondylar fracture Humerus lead to Cubitus varus (Gun-stock deformity)

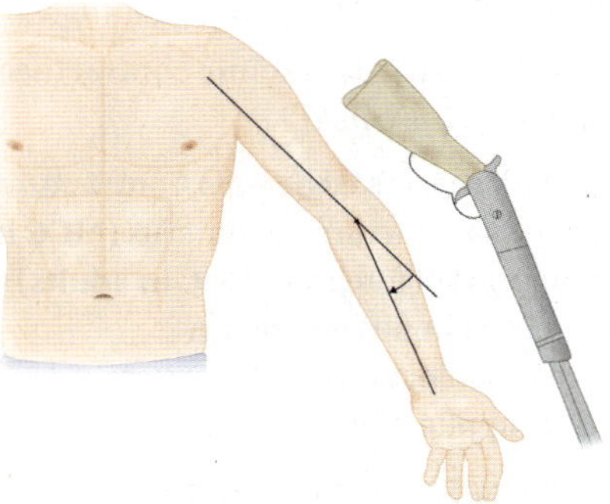

Fig. Gun-stock deformity

53. Ans. (d) Extra-articular fracture of distal radius with dorsal displacement

[Ref. Orthopaedic Trauma by Dawson-Bowling, 1/e p167]

- Colles' fracture is an osteoporotic Extra-articular distal radius fracture with Dorsal displacement
- Smith's fracture is osteoporotic and Extra-articular, but distal fragment is displaced Volarly
- Barton's farcture has Intra-articular involvement of Radiocarpal but Volar/ Dorsal subluxation of carpus

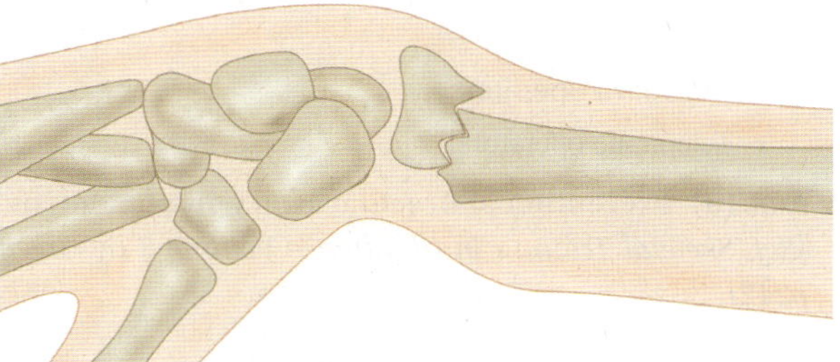

Fig. Colles' fracture

54. Ans. (b) Posterolateral

[Ref. Sports Medicine by Elattrache, 1/e p189

- In 1940, Hill and Sachs, two radiologists, reported that these defects were actually compression fractures produced when the **Posterolateral humeral head** impinged against the Anterior rim of Glenoid

55. Ans. (c) Lower radius, Scaphoid and Lunate in alignment, Capitate alone is out of plane

[Ref. Hand Surgery and Therapy by Trumble, 3/e p85]

Perilunate Dislocation

- Involve traumatic rupture of the Radioscaphocapitate (RSC) ligament, the Scapholunate interosseous ligament, and Lunotriquetral interosseous ligament
- Capitate is initially displaced dorsal to the Lunate

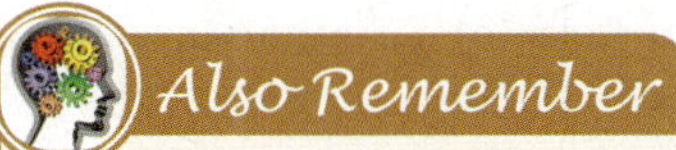

Also Remember

- In the final stage of this injury (Lunate dislocation), the Capitate reduces into the fossa of the radius, displacing the lunate toward the palm

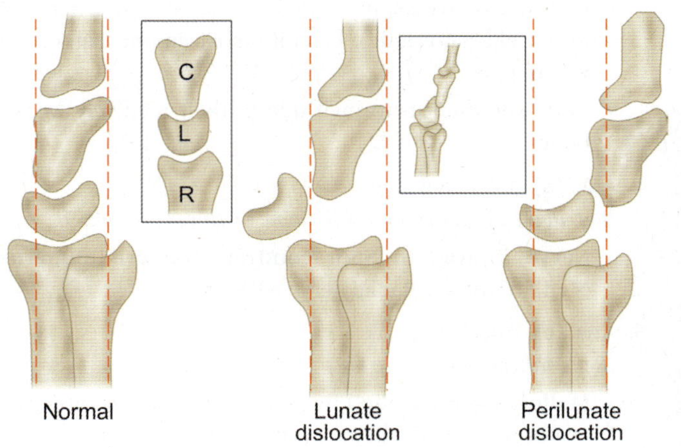

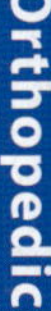

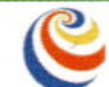 HIGH YIELD MCQs ANSWERS WITH EXPLANATIONS 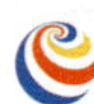

1. **Ans. (b) Median nerve**
[Ref. Natural Medicine by Murray, 3/e p392]
   - Compression of Median nerve **(Carpal tunnel syndrome)** causes weakness; pain in gripping; and burning, tingling, or aching that may radiate to the forearm
   - It is also seen in people who do repetitive lighter work
     - Typists
     - Keyboard operators
     - Telephone operators

2. **Ans. (a) Prevention of Brachial artery entanglement**
[Ref. Skeletal Trauma in Children - Volume 3 by Green, 4/e p212]

Management of Supracondylar Fracture Humerus

- With a Supracondylar fracture, there is a high risk of neurovascular compromise or even a Volkmann ischaemic contracture—a permanent hand contracture
- Most difficult aspect of managing children with Supracondylar fractures, is the question of how to proceed when an apparently satisfactory attempt at closed reduction has failed to re-establish a palpable pulse
- If the lack of radial pulse is associated with poor circulatory status (as shown by pallor, pain, paraesthesia, etc.) then exploration of the brachial artery is indicated
- Use **"Watch and wait" approach** with careful observation and regular assessment of neurovascular status, particularly looking for signs of impending Compartment syndrome

3. **Ans. (a) Occur at distal end of radius, about 2 cm from distal articular surface; (e) Common in women**
[Ref. Essential Orthopaedics by Maheshwari, 5/e p113]

Colles' Fracture

- Fracture of Lower end of Radius within one inch (2.5 cm) of Distal articular surface of Radius
- **Displacements seen**: Dorsal displacement, Dorsal tilt **(Most characteristic)**, Lateral displacement, Lateral tilt, Supination
- More common in women due to their relatively weaker bones

4. **Ans. (a) Median nerve**
[Ref. Pediatric Emergency Medicine by Baren, 1/e p259]
   - **Nerve injured in Supracondylar fracture humerus: Median nerve** > Radial nerve > Ulnar nerve

5. **Ans. (c) Distal Phalanx**
[Ref. Maheshwari, 4/ e p114]
   - **Mallet finger/Baseball finger**: Avulsion of attachment of extensor tendon from the base of distal phalanx

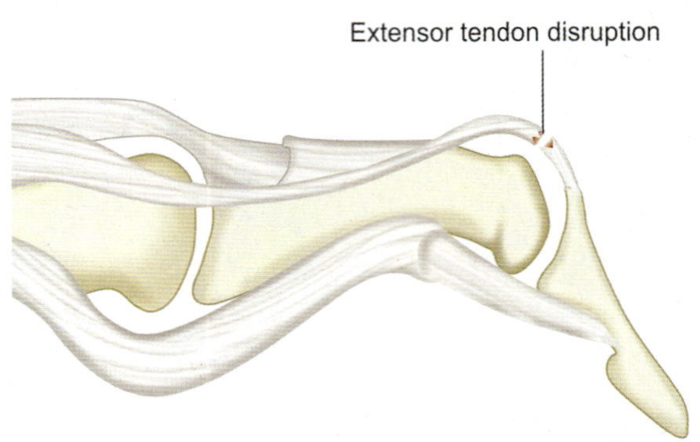

Fig. Mallet finger

6. **Ans. (a) Stiffness of fingers**
[Ref. Maheshwari, 4/e p110]

7. **Ans. (b) Malunion**
[Ref. Maheshwari, 4/e p65]

8. **Ans. (a) Rupture of flexor pollicis longus tendon**
[Ref. Maheshwari, 4/e p110]

Complications of Colles' Fracture

- Finger stiffness (Most common)
- Stiffness of shoulder/wrist/elbow joints
- Malunion
- Subluxation of inferior radioulnar joint
- Carpal tunnel syndrome
- Sudeck's osteodystrophy
- Rupture extensor pollicis longus tendon

9. **Ans. (a) Colles' fracture**
[Ref. Maheshwari, 4/e p110]

10. **Ans. (c) Extensor pollicis longus**
[Ref. Maheshwari, 4/e p110]

11. **Ans. (b) Nonunion**
[Ref. Maheshwari, 4/e p110]

12. **Ans. (d) Wrist drop**
[Ref. Maheshwari, 4/e p110]

13. **Ans. (b) Stiffness of wrist joint**
[Ref. Maheshwari, 4/e p110]

14. **Ans. (b) Volkmann's ischaemic contracture**
[Ref. Maheshwari, 4/e p98]

Causes of Volkmann's Ischaemic Contracture

- Supracondylar fracture of humerus **(MCC in children)**
- Crush injuries of forearm **(MCC in adults)**
- Fracture both bones of forearm
- Intraarterial injections in Drug users
- Improper application of splints

15. **Ans. (c) Reflex sympathetic dystrophy**
[Ref. Maheshwari, 4/e p50]

16. Ans. (a) Malunion

[Ref. Text and Atlas of Complications of Fractures by Ebnezar, 1/e p5]

Complications of Fracture Clavicle

- Malunion **(Most common complication)**
- Shoulder stiffness (Common complication)
- Neuromuscular injury (Subclavian vessels, Median cord of Brachial plexus)
- Non-union (Rare complication)

17. Ans. (b) Junction of medial 2/3rd and lateral 1/3rd

[Ref. Instant Anatomy by Singh, 2/e p34]

- **MC Site of Fracture clavicle**: Junction of Medial 2/3 and Lateral 1/3 (as it is the meeting point of two curvatures)

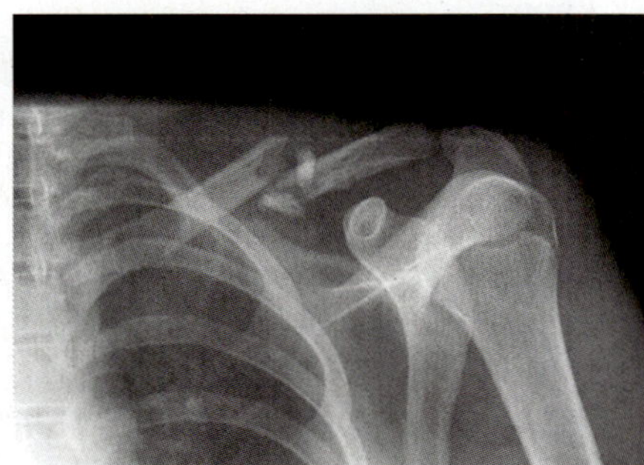

Fig. Clavicle fracture

18. Ans. (d) Break the cortex other side and immobilization by POP

19. Ans. (d) Above-elbow cast with forearm in supination

[Ref. Textbook of Orthopedics and Trauma by Kulkarni, 2/e p2433]

20. Ans. (a) Involves radio carpal subluxation

[Ref. Rosen's Emergency Medicine by Walls, 7/e Volume 1]

21. Ans. (c) Night stick fracture

[Ref. Orthopedics Secrets by Brown, 3/e p169]

- **Nightstick fracture**: An isolated fracture of the ulnar diaphysis, typically in the distal one third of the shaft, occurring due to direct blow to ulna

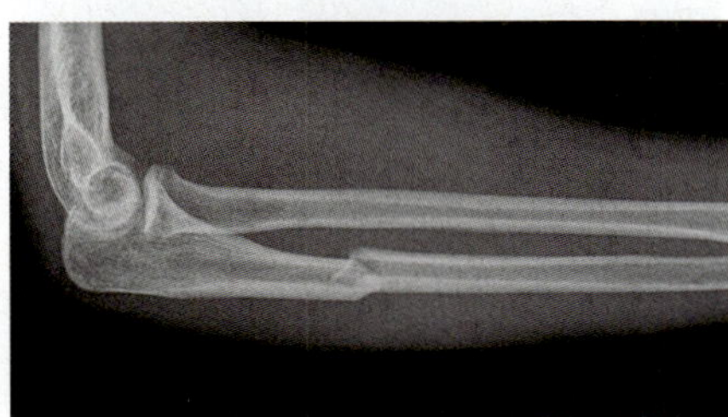

Fig. Ulna fracture rightstick

22. Ans. (d) Malunion is a frequent complication

[Ref. Maheshwari, 4/e p111]

Complications of Scaphoid Fracture

- Avascular necrosis of Proximal part **(Most common)**
- Delayed union, non-union
- Osteoarthritis of wrist

23. Ans. (a) Waist

[Ref. Maheshwari, 4/e p111]

24. Ans. (d) Avascular necrosis

[Ref. Maheshwari, 4/e p111]

25. Ans. (d) Avascular necrosis of proximal part

[Ref. Maheshwari, 4/e p111]

26. Ans. (d) Oblique

[Ref. Rockwood and Wilkinson's Fractures in Children by Kasser, 7/e p272]

27. Ans. (e) Axillary nerve

[Ref. Textbook of Anatomy Upper Limb and Thorax by Singh, 2/e p22]

Few Common Nerve Injuries

- Brachial plexus: Clavicle fracture
- Axillary nerve: Fracture surgical neck of humerus, Shoulder dislocation
- Radial nerve: Fracture shaft of humerus, Supracondylar fracture of humerus
- Ulnar nerve: Fracture medial epicondyle of humerus
- Median nerve: Supracondylar fracture, Lunate dislocation, Volkmann's ischemic contracture
- Sciatic nerve: Posterior dislocation of hip
- Lateral popliteal nerve: Fracture neck of fibula

28. Ans. (a) Elbow dislocation

[Ref. Skeletal Trauma in Children by Green, 4/e p255]

29. Ans. (c) Supracondylar fracture

[Ref. Sports Injuries in Children and Adolescents by Karantanas, 1/e p114]

30. Ans. (a) Scaphoid

[Ref. Current Therapy in Pain by Smith, 1/e p163]

- Carpal bone fractures: Scaphoid > Triquetral > Trapezium > Lunate

31. Ans. (d) Scaphoid fracture

[Ref. Maheshwari, 4/e p111]

32. Ans. (c) Scaphoid fracture

[Ref. Maheshwari, 4/e p111]

33. Ans. (d) Cone

[Ref. The Wrist: Operative and Diagnostic Treatment by Cooney, 2/e p412]

- Views for Scaphoid fracture: AP, PA, Oblique, Lateral, and Scaphoid

34. Ans. (d) Fracture supracondylar humerus

[Ref. Maheshwari, 4/e p98]

- Fracture Supracondylar humerus: Gun-stock deformity (Cubitus varus deformity)

35. Ans. (a) Elbow stiffness; (b) Malunion; (d) Myositis ossificans; (e) Gunstock deformity

[Ref. Maheshwari, 4/e p96-98]

Complications of Supracondylar Fracture Humerus

- Immediate complications: Brachial artery injury, Median nerve injury

- Early complications: Volkmann's ischemia
- Late complications: **Mal-union (Gun-stock deformity)**, Myositis ossificans, Volkmann's ischemic contracture

36. Ans. (a) Fracture of waist of scaphoid
[Ref. Maheshwari, 4/e p111]

37. Ans. (c) Young active adult
[Ref. Maheshwari, 4/e p111]

38. Ans. (d) Distal pole
[Ref. Pediatric Sports Medicine for Primary Care by Birrer, 1/e p377]

- **Fracture scaphoid in children**: Distal pole (75%) > Waist (20%) > Proximal pole (5%)

39. Ans. (c) Median nerve
[Ref. Orthopedic Secrets by Brown, 3/e p169]

40. Ans. (c) Scaphoid fracture
[Ref. Maheshwari, 4/e p111]

41. Ans. (c) Pronator quadratus
[Ref. Hand Surgery by Berger, p573]

42. Ans. (b) Dorsal and radial flexion
[Ref. Maheshwari, 4/e p111]

- **Scaphoid cast**: Wrist maintained in Little dorsiflexion and radial deviation **(Glass-holding position)**

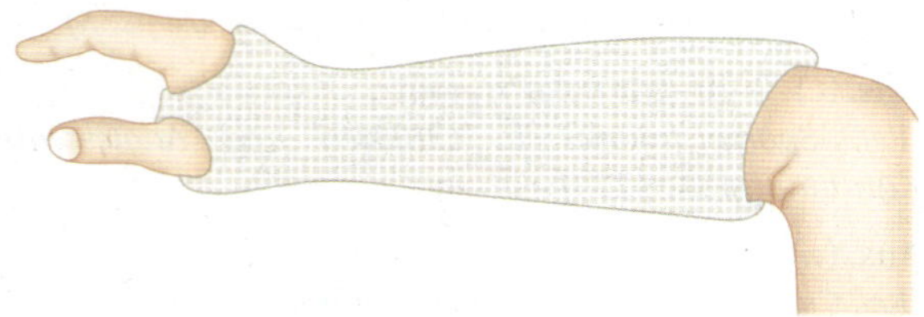

Fig. Scaphoid cast

43. Ans. (b) Supracondylar fracture of humerus
[Ref. Textbook of Orthopedic and Trauma by Kulkarni, 2/e p2348]

44. Ans. (d) All of the above

45. Ans. (c) Pain on passive extension of fingers
[Ref. Skeletal Trauma in Children by Green, 4/e p232]

46. Ans. (d) Flexor digitorum profundus
[Ref. Maheshwari, 4/e p42]

- **MC affected muscles in Volkmann's ischemia:** Flexor digitorum profundus (medial half) > Flexor pollicis longus

47. Ans. (a) Trapezium
[Ref. Current Therapy in Pain by Smith, 1/e p163]

48. Ans. (d) 1st
[Ref. Maheshwari, 4/e p112]

- **Benetts' fracture dislocation**: Oblique intra-articular fracture of base of first metacarpal with subluxation/ dislocation of the metacarpal (Displacement of Trapeziometacarpal joint)

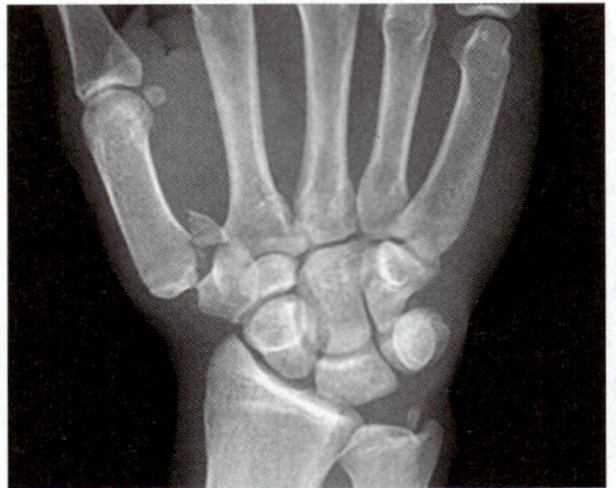

Fig. Bennett fracture

49. Ans. (d) Fracture dislocation of trapeziometacarpal joint
[Ref. Radiography of Upper Extremities by, p103]

50. Ans. (a) 1 hour

51. Ans. (d) Increased compartment pressure in limb
[Ref. Rockwood and Wilkinson's Fractures in Children by Kasser, 7/e p513]

52. Ans. (c) Median nerve
[Ref. Neglected Musculoskeletal Injuries by Jain, 1/e p110]

- **MC Nerve involved in Volkmann's Ischemic Contracture**: Median nerve > Ulnar nerve
- **MC affected muscles** in Volkmann's ischemia: Flexor digitorum profundus (medial half) > Flexor pollicis longus

53. Ans. (b) Tension band wiring
[Ref. Maheshwari, 4/e p102]

Olecranon Fractures

- Type I (Crack without displacement): Above elbow plaster cast in 30 degrees flexion
- Type II (Clean break with separation of fragments): Open reduction and Internal fixation (Tension band wiring)
- Type II (Comminuted fracture):
  - If fragments not separated: Above elbow plaster cast in 30 degrees flexion
  - If fragments separated: Tension band wiring or Excision of fragments

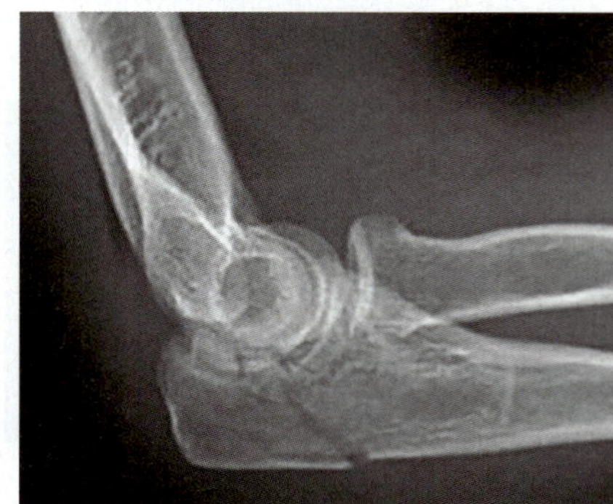

Fig. Olecranon fracture

54. Ans. (b) Ventral tilt
[Ref. Maheshwari, 4/e p108]

- Displacements seen in Colles' fracture: Impaction of fragments, Dorsal displacement, Dorsal tilt, Lateral displacement, Lateral tilt, Supination

55. Ans. (c) Palmar deviation and pronation
[Ref. Maheshwari, 4/e p109]

56. Ans. (d) Abductor pollicis longus
[Ref. Adult Orthopedic Nursing by Schoen, 1/e p395]
- Bennett's fracture is difficult to maintain in position due to: Abductor pollicis brevis and Adductor pollicis muscles

57. Ans. (b) EPL (extensor pollicis longus)
[Ref. Fractures and Injuries of Distal Radius and Carpus by Osterman, 1/e pW4]

58. Ans. (c) Wrist drop
[Ref. Maheshwari, 4/e p110]

59. Ans. (a) Mallet finger
[Ref. Maheshwari, 4/e p114]

60. Ans. (b) Fracture clavicle
[Ref. Maheshwari, 4/e p85]
- Figure-of-8 bandage is used in Clavicular fracture: Gives both immobilization as well as pain relief

61. Ans. (b) Waist
[Ref. Maheshwari, 4/e p111]

62. Ans. (b) Median nerve
[Ref. Carpal Tunnel Syndrome by Amadio, 1/e p4]

63. Ans. (a) Ulnar collateral ligament injury of MCP joint
[Ref. Essentials of Physical Medicine and Rehabilitation by, 3/e p184]

Game Keeper's Thumb

- Synonyms: Skier's thumb, Break-dancer's thumb, Stener's lesion
- Description: Ruptured, displaced ulnar collateral ligament with Interposed adductor aponeurosis

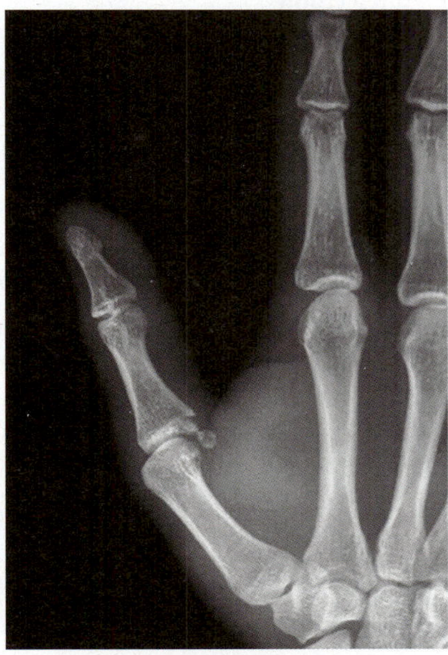

Fig. Game Keeper's thumb

64. Ans. (b) Avulsion of terminal slip of extensor tendon to distal phalanx
[Ref. Maheshwari, 4/ e p114]

65. Ans. (b) Most common complication of surgically treated cases is cubitus valgus deformity
[Ref. Maheshwari, 4/e p100]

66. Ans. (c) 5–15 years
[Ref. Orthopedics Quick review by Mehra, 1/e p14]
- Lateral condyle humerus fracture: 5-15 years
- Supracondylar fracture humerus: 5-8 years

67. Ans. (a) Fracture Lateral condyle of humerus
[Ref. Maheshwari, 4/e p100]
- In Lateral condyle of humerus, Diminished growth at lateral side of distal humerus epiphysis results in **Cubitus valgus deformity**
  - It may result in **Late/Tardy Ulnar nerve palsy** due to friction neuritis of Ulnar nerve as it moves over medial epicondyle when elbow is flexed and extended

68. Ans. (a) Lateral condyle fracture humerus
[Ref. Maheshwari, 4/e p100]

69. Ans. (c) Fracture of lateral condyle of humerus in children
[Ref. Maheshwari, 4/e p100]

70. Ans. (c) Young active adults
[Ref. Maheshwari, 4/e p111]

71. Ans. (c) Open reduction and internal fixation
[Ref. Maheshwari, 4/e p99]

Treatment of Fracture Lateral Condyle Humerus

- Undisplaced fracture: Above-elbow Plaster cast for 2-3 weeks
- Displaced fracture: Open reduction and Internal fixation using 2 K-wires

72. Ans. (c) Fracture lateral condyle
[Ref. Maheshwari, 4/e p99]

73. Ans. (c) Ulnar
[Ref. Maheshwari, 4/e p101]

74. Ans. (a) Elbow dislocation
[Ref. Maheshwari, 4/e p101]
- Fracture Medial epicondyle of humerus is associated with Posterior dislocation of elbow

75. Ans. (a) X-ray both arms with elbow for comparison
[Ref. Maheshwari, 4/e p101]

76. Ans. (c) Supracondylar fracture of humerus
[Ref. Maheshwari, 4/e p93]

77. Ans. (c) Elderly females
[Ref. Maheshwari, 4/e p89]

78. Ans. (c) Supracondylar fracture
[Ref. The Netter Collection of Medical Illustrations by Parker, 2/e p90]

79. Ans. (a) Extension type of supracondylar fracture of humerus
[Ref. The Netter Collection of Medical Illustrations by Parker, 2/e p90]

80. Ans. (c) Posteriorly
[Ref. Maheshwari, 4/e p94]

81. Ans. (c) Extension
[Ref. Maheshwari, 4/e p93]

82. Ans. (d) Hyper extension injury
[Ref. Maheshwari, 4/e p93]

83. Ans. (a) Anterior
[Ref. Maheshwari, 4/e p93]

84. Ans. (d) Malunited supracondylar fracture of humerus
[Ref. Maheshwari, 4/e p93]
- Since Supracondylar fracture of humerus is located above condyles, the three-point bony relationship is maintained as in normal elbow

85. Ans. (b) Cubitus varus
[Ref. Maheshwari, 4/e p98]

86. Ans. (a) French
[Ref. Maheshwari, 4/e p99]

87. Ans. (d) Non Union
[Ref. Maheshwari, 4/e p96-98]

88. Ans. (c) Nonunion
[Ref. Maheshwari, 4/e p96-98]

89. Ans. (d) All of the above
[Ref. Maheshwari, 4/e p96-98]

90. Ans. (a) Supracondylar fracture; (b) Lateral condylar fracture
[Ref. Maheshwari, 4/e p100]

91. Ans. (d) Ulnar nerve is most commonly involved
[Ref. Maheshwari, 4/e p97]

92. Ans. (a) Admission to hospital is essential following reduction
[Ref. Maheshwari, 4/e p94]
- Close monitoring of children (by hospitalization) is required to monitor neurovascular status for serious complication of Volkmann's Ischemic Contracture

93. Ans. (c) Pain on passive extension
[Ref. Essential Accident and Emergency Care by Wilson, 1/e p61]

94. Ans. (a) Pain
[Ref. Skeletal Injury in a Child by Ogden, 3/e p493]

Volkmann's Ischemia
- Five classical signs **(5P's)**: **P**ain, **P**allor (Cyanosis), **P**ulselssness, **P**aresthesia, **P**aralysis
- Most important sign: Pain

95. Ans. (c) Flexor digitorum profundus
[Ref. Orthopedics Illustrated by Gupta, 2/e p42]

96. Ans. (b) Pain
[Ref. Surgery 1000 MCQs by Ram, 6/e p343]

97. Ans. (a) Supracondylar fracture of humerus
[Ref. Maheshwari, 4/e p98]

98. Ans. (a) Immediately

99. Ans. (d) Sympathetic ganglion blockade
[Ref. Maheshwari, 4/e p98-99]

100. Ans. (c) Follows Ischaemia of the forearm
[Ref. Maheshwari, 4/e p98-99]

101. Ans. (c) Both
[Ref. Maheshwari, 4/e p98]

102. Ans. (d) Increase of compartment pressure in the limb
[Ref. Maheshwari, 4/e p98]

103. Ans. (a) 10-15 cm
[Ref. Essentials of Orthopedics and Applied Physiotherapy by Joshi, 1/e p228]

104. Ans. (c) 15-20 cm
[Ref. Essentials of Orthopedics and Applied Physiotherapy by Joshi, 1/e p228]
- Above Elbow amputation: 20 cms long stump measured from the tip of Acromian
- Below elbow amputation: 20 cms long stump measured from tip of Olecranon (minimum length being 7.5 cms)

105. Ans. (b) Breaks at mid-point
[Ref. Maheshwari, 4/e p84]

106. Ans. (a) Most common Complication is Malunion
[Ref. Maheshwari, 4/e p84]

107. Ans. (c) Figure-of-eight bandage
[Ref. Maheshwari, 4/e p84]

108. Ans. (b) Junction of medial 2/3rd and lateral 1/3rd
[Ref. Maheshwari, 4/e p84]

109. Ans. (d) Talus fracture
[Ref. Maheshwari, 4/e p49]

110. Ans. (b) Dislocation of head of radius
[Ref. Maheshwari, 4/e p101]

111. Ans. (d) Pulled elbow
[Ref. Maheshwari, 4/e p101]

112. Ans. (a) Supinate the forearm
[Ref. Maheshwari, 4/e p356]

113. Ans. (b) Tension band wiring
[Ref. Maheshwari, 4/e p101]

114. Ans. (c) Fracture extending to coronoid process
[Ref. Textbook of Orthopedics by Ebnezar, 4/e p164]

Indications of Excision of Proximal Fragment (Olecranon fracture)
- Comminuted fractures
- Delayed or non-union in upper half fractures
- Patient >50 years age

115. Ans. (b) Both ulnar fracture and head of radius is displaced anteriorly
[Ref. Radiology Review Manual by Dahnert, 7/e p90]

116. Ans. (b) Supracondylar fracture humerus
[Ref. Maheshwari, 4/e p94]

117. Ans. (b) Fracture of the distal radius with inferior radio ulnar joint dislocation
[Ref. Maheshwari, 4/e p107]

118. Ans. (a) Reduce angulation of radius and ulna; (b) Restore the normal relationship of radius and ulna
[Ref. Rockwood and Wilkin's Fractures in Children by Kasser, 2/e p369]

119. Ans. (c) Only plates
[Ref. Rockwood and Wilkin's Fractures in Children by Kasser, 2/e p369]

120. Ans. (d) Fracture of humerus (lateral condyle)
[Ref. Maheshwari, 4/e p100]

121. Ans. (d) Usually requires careful reduction
[Ref. Maheshwari, 4/e p84]

122. Ans. (a) Elderly woman
[Ref. Maheshwari, 4/e p89]

123. Ans. (a) Axillary
[Ref. Maheshwari, 4/e p89]

124. Ans. (d) Mid-prone

Positions for Plaster in Fratcure both Bones Forearm

- Proximal third fractures: Supination
- Mid-arm fractures: Mid-prone
- Distal third fractures: Supination

125. Ans. (c) Common in elderly women
[Ref. Maheshwari, 4/e p108]

126. Ans. (d) Pronation
[Ref. Maheshwari, 4/e p108]

127. Ans. (a) Analgesic with arm sling
[Ref. Maheshwari, 4/e p89]

128. Ans. (b) Ulnar
[Ref. Rockwood and Wilkin's Fractures in Children by Kasser, 2/e p515]

129. Ans. (a) Triangular sling
[Ref. Maheshwari, 4/e p89]

130. Ans. (a) Abduction and lateral rotation

131. Ans. (c) Brachial artery occlusion
[Ref. Skeletal Trauma by Browner, 5/e p424]

132. Ans. (d) Distraction at fracture site
[Ref. Disorders of Shoulder by Williams, 2/e p928]

133. Ans. (a) Olecranon
[Ref. Best Orthopedics by Pramod, 1/e p120]

Fractures with Increased Intercondylar Distance

- Fracture medial epicondyle
- Fracture medial condyle
- Fracture lateral epicondyle
- Fracture lateral condyle
- Fracture intercondylar humerus

134. Ans. (b) Posteriorly and laterally
[Ref. illustrated Clinical Anatomy by Craven, 2/e p185]

135. Ans. (c) Colles' fracture
[Ref. Maheshwari, 4/e p108]

136. Ans. (d) Medial rotation
[Ref. Maheshwari, 4/e p108]

137. Ans. (b) Fracture radius only

138. Ans. (d) Fracture upper 1/3 ulna; (e) Radial head dislocation
[Ref. Maheshwari, 4/e p2]

139. Ans. (c) Torniquet
[Ref. Essential of Orthopedics for Physiotherapist by Ebnezar, 1/e p36]

140. Ans. (b) Axillary
[Ref. Radiography of the Upper Extremities by CE4RT, 2015 p231]

Nerve Damage in Humerus Fracture

- Surgical neck fracture: Axillary nerve
- Mid-shaft fracture: Radial nerve
- Supracondylar fracture: Median nerve
- Medial epicondyle fracture: Ulnar nerve

141. Ans. (d) Nonunion
[Ref. Maheshwari, 5/e p114]

- A Colles' fracture always unites, but Malunion occurs in a large proportion of cases

142. Ans. (c) Waist
[Ref. Harris & Harris' The Radiology of Emergency Medicine, 5/e p398]

Scaphoid Fracture

- Most frequently fractured of the carpal bones
- Second only to fractures of the distal radius for all wrist fracture
- MC site of scaphoid fracture: Waist
    - Less common site: Proximal and distal poles
    - Rare site: Distal tubercle fracture

143. Ans. (b) Fracture Humerus
[Ref. Neurologic Differential Diagnosis by Ettinger, 1/e p587]

- In the axilla, fracture of the humerus is one of the most common causes of radial nerve injury and it results in wrist drop

144. Ans. (a) Cubitus varus
[Ref. Sports Medicine by O'Connor, p361]

- Cubitus varus is the most common complication following supracondylar humerus fracture
- Underlying cause: Improper fracture reduction

145. Ans. (b) Radial styloid
[Ref. Orthopedic Secrets by Mehta, 3/e p182]

Chauffeur's/ Back-Fire Fracture

- Type of fracture of the forearm, specifically the Radial styloid process

- Injury is typically caused by compression of the Scaphoid bone of the hand against the styloid process of the distal radius
- It can be caused by fall on outstretched hand

146. Ans. (b) Distal end of index extensor

[Ref. Essentials of Orthopedics for Physiotherapists by Ebnezar, 1/e p29]

147. Ans. (d) Interosseous membrane tear with triangular fibrocartilage complex (TFCC) tear and radial shaft fracture

[Ref. Green's Operative Hand Surgery, 6/e p536]

- Forearm bones articulate proximally at elbow, distally at wrist and rotation-wise (pronation, supination) at both the joints; these components are linked at Proximal radio-ulnar joint by Annular ligament, at Distal radioulnar joint (DRUJ) by Triangular fibrocartilage complex (TFCC), and in the Mid-forearm by the Interosseous membrane
- Galeazzi fracture refers to a fracture at the junction of the middle and distal thirds of the radius with an associated DRUJ (distal radioulnar joint) dislocation
  - Injury involves disruption of the Interosseous membrane
  - TFCC injury is almost inevitably present, although there is a spectrum of DRUJ instability that may be associated

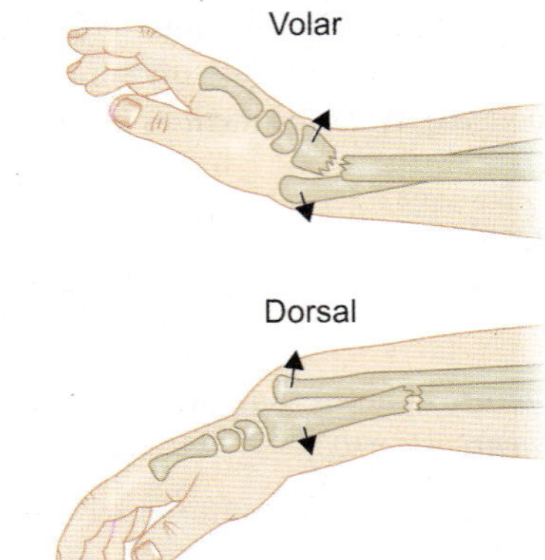

Fig. Galeazzi fracture dislocation

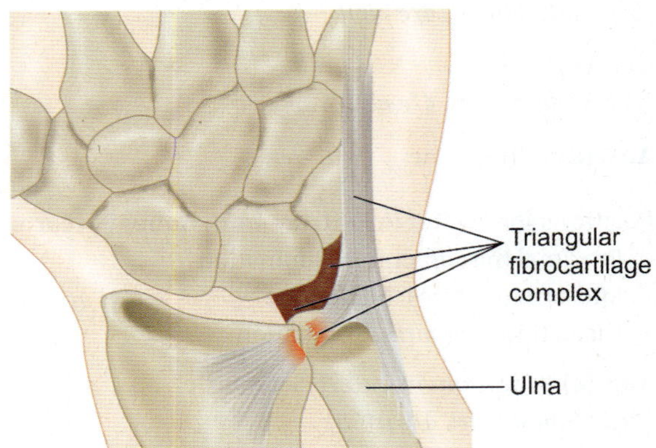

Fig. TFCC injury

Orthopedics

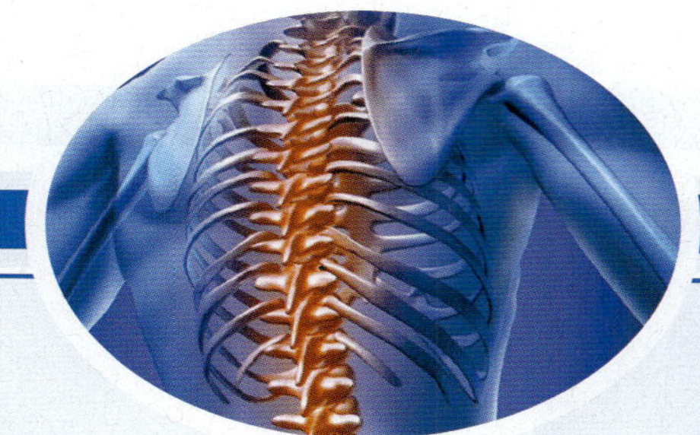

Chapter 4

Lower Limb and Pelvis Traumatology

THEORETICAL CONCEPTS

IV A. FRACTURES NECK OF FEMUR

	Fracture Neck of Femur	Intertrochantric Fracture
Type	**Intracapsular fracture**	**Extracapsular fracture**
Age-sex	Females > 50 years	Males > 60 years
Treatment	Multiple cancellous screws McMurray's osteotomy Hemiarthroplasty Meyer's procedure	Russell's traction Skeletal traction in Thomas splint Smith-Peterson nail
Complications	Nonunion Avascular necrosis of head Osteoarthritis	Malunion Osteoarthritis

Topper's Edge

Fracture Neck of Femur

- Types of Fracture Neck of femur:
  - Extracapsular type
  - Intracapsular type: ***'Orthopedic enigma'*** (No permanent treatment available)
- Common in Elderly women due to senile osteoporosis
- Classifications used[Q]:
  - Broad classification: Intracapsular, Extracapsular
  - Based on character of fracture: Subcapital, Transcervical, Basal, Fracture angle
  - **Pauwels' classification** (Fracture line angle to Horizontal line): I (30 degrees), II (50 degrees), III (70 degrees)
  - Perlington's classification (Fracture line angle to Vertical line): I (70 degrees), II (50 degrees), III (370 degrees)
  - **Garden's classification** (Pattern of fracture line and displacement): Incomplete, Complete-undisplaced, Complete-partial displaced, Complete-total displaced (MC, Most widely used classification)
- Aim of treatment: Early anatomical reduction, Impaction, Rigid internal fixation
- Accepted method of fixation: DHS, Multiple cannulated cancellous screws
- Complications: Non-union, AVN (Leading to Secondary osteoarthritis[Q])

IV B. FRACTURE SHAFT OF FEMUR

- *Site*: Equally common in upper, middle, lower 1/3 shaft
- *Treatment*:
  - **Birth-2 years: Gallow's traction[Q]**
  - 2-16 years: Hip spica, Internal fixation
  - **Adults/ elderly: K-nail** (intramedullary internal fixation[Q])

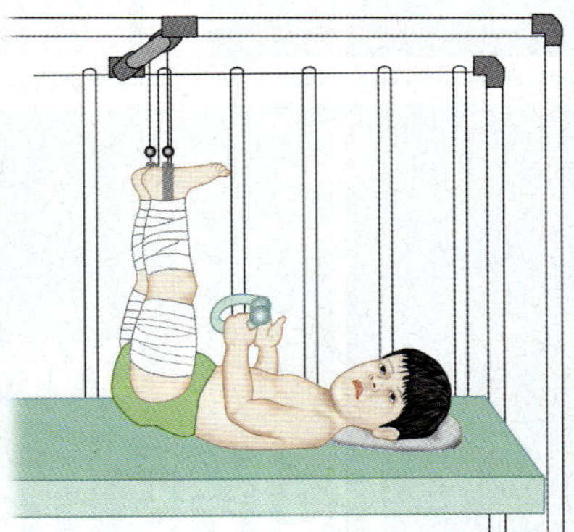

Fig. Gallow's traction

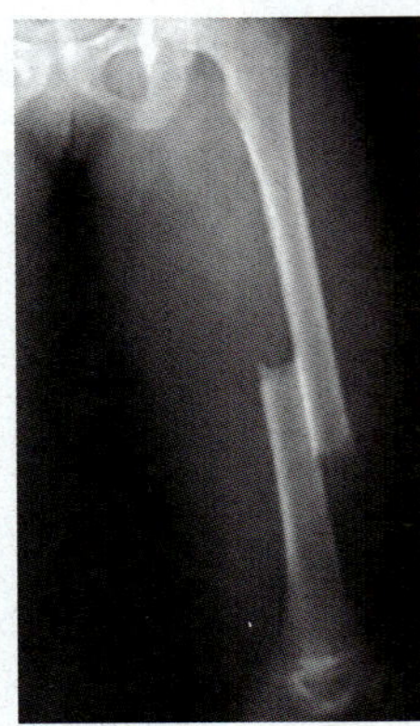

Fig. Shaft of femur

- *Complications*:
  - Shock: 1000–1500 mL blood lost[Q]
  - Fat embolism: after 24–48 hours[Q]
  - Injury to sciatic nerve/femoral artery
  - Non-union, Delayed union
  - Malunion

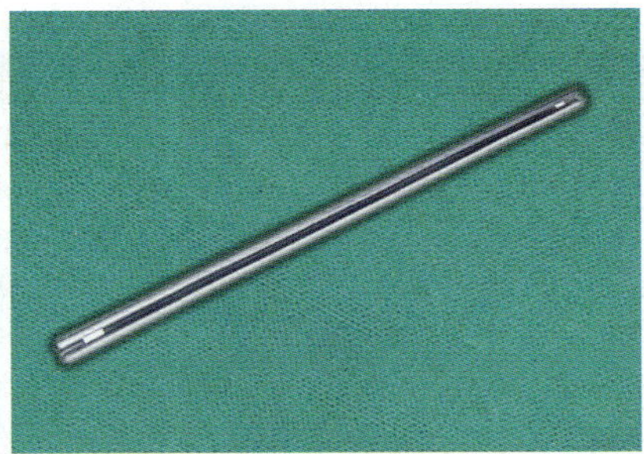

Fig. K-nail

IV C. FRACTURES OF PATELLA

- *Types*:
  - 2-part fracture: Transverse fracture line[Q]
  - Stellate fracture: Comminuted fracture[Q]
- ***X-ray*: Skyline view of patella**[Q]
- ***Treatment*:**
  - Undisplaced fracture: Cylindrical cast
  - 2-part fracture: Tension band wiring[Q]
  - Comminuted fracture: Patellectomy[Q]
- *Complications*:
  - Knee stiffness **(Most common)**[Q]
  - Osteoarthritis

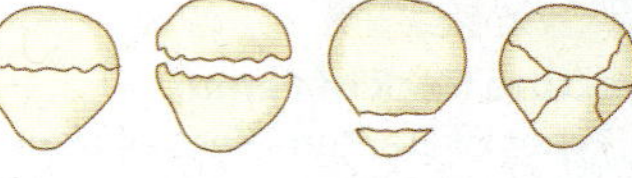

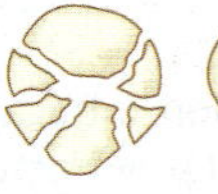

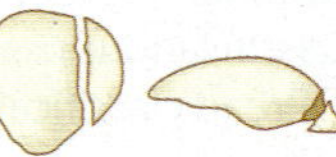

Fig. Fractures of patella

Topper's Edge

Fractures of Patella

- Mechanism of injury:
  - Direct trauma: Dashboard injury/Bumper injury/Direct fall over patella (Stellate fracture is common cause)
  - Indirect trauma: Sudden forceful contraction of Quadriceps (Usually transverse fracture)
- Types of fractures:
  - Undisplaced fracture
  - Displaced fracture: Transverse (MC), Oblique, Vertical, Comminuted
- Bipartite patella and Osteochondral fractures cause confusion in diagnosis

IV D. ANKLE INJURIES

- ***Cotton's fracture*:** Trimalleolar fracture[Q]
- ***Pott's fracture*:** Bimalleolar fracture[Q]
- *Pilon fracture*: Comminuted fracture tibial articular surface + fracture fibula
- *Sprained ankle*: Lateral collateral (anterior tibiofibular) ligament[Q]

Topper's Edge

ANKLE INJURIES

Classifications

- Lauge-Hansen's classification: Based on Position of foot, Direction of injury force mechanism
  - Supination-Adduction
  - Pronation-Abduction
  - Pronation-External rotation
  - Supination-External rotation
- Denis Weber classification: Based on level of Fibular fracture

Common Injuries of Ankle

- **Pott's fracture[Q]:** Bimalleolar ankle fracture
- **Cotton's fracture[Q]:** Trimalleolar ankle fracture
- **Dupuytren's fracture[Q]:** Complete diastosis of Inferior tibiofibular syndesmosis and Comminuted fracture of lower end of fibula
- **Tillaux fracture[Q]:** Avulsion fracture of anterior/posterior tip of inferior fibular facet of tibia
- Lateral ankle ligament sprain:
  - MC musculoskeletal injury among athletes[Q]
  - Due to Inversion of supinated plantar flexed foot
  - MC ligament injured[Q]: Anterior talofibular ligament

IV E. ANKLE SPRAINS

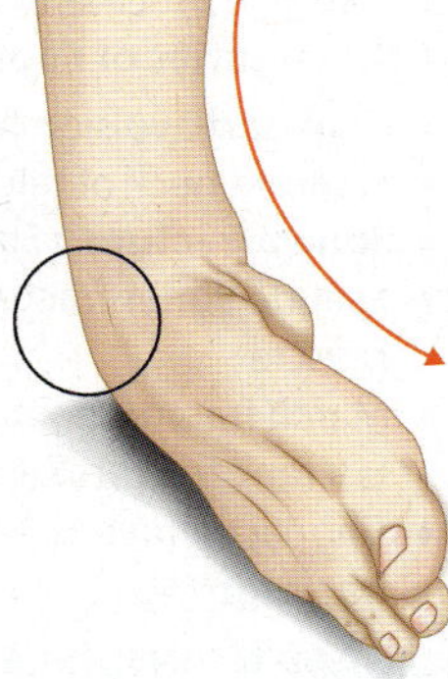

Fig. Ankle sprain

- *Definition*: Ligament injuries of ankle
- ***More commonly involved*: Lateral collateral ligament (inversion injury[Q])**
- *Less commonly involved*: Medial collateral ligament (eversion injury[Q])
- ***Most common ligament part involved*: Anterior talofibular ligament**
- *Injury types and treatment*:
- *General functional treatment*: **PRICE** routine (**P**rotect, **R**est, **I**ce, **C**ompression, **E**levation[Q])
- *Specific treatment according to type***:**

Injury Type	Treatment
Type I sprain	Below knee cast X 2 weeks + Immobilisation
Type II sprain	Below knee cast X 4 weeks + Immobilisation
Type III sprain	Below knee cast X 6 weeks + Immobilisation

IV F. STRESS FRACTURES OF METATARSALS

- *Type of fracture*: Fatigue/stress fracture of metatarsals due to prolonged walking or running (Army recruits)
- *Sites of stress fracture*:
  - 2nd metatarsal **(*March fracture*—most common[Q])**
  - 5th metatarsal **(*Jones fracture/Dancer's fracture*[Q])**

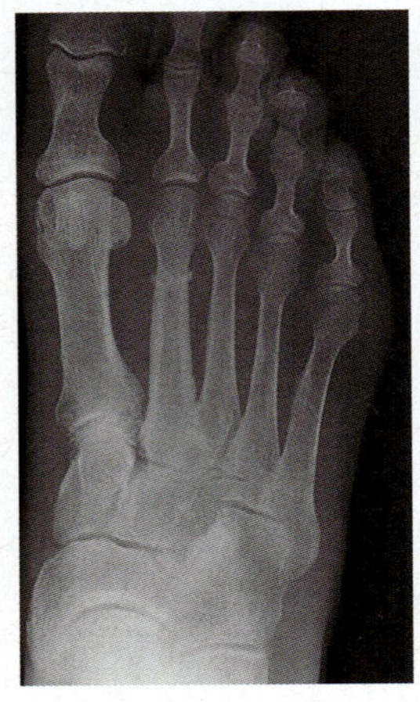

Fig. March fracture

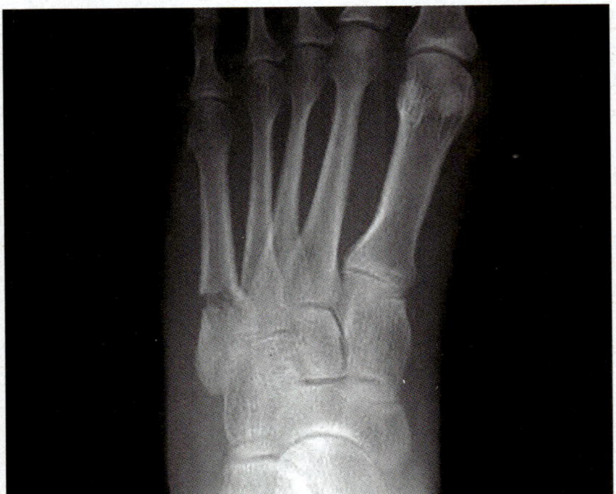

Fig. Jones fracture

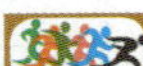

Topper's Edge

INJURIES OF THE FOOT

Calcaneum fractures

- **MC fractures Tarsal bone[Q]: Calcaneum**
- Synonym: Don-Juan fracture, Lover's fracture
- Essex-Lopresti's classification
  - Intra-articular fracture: 75% fractures
  - Extra-articular fracture: Anterior process, Tuberosity, Medial calcaneal process, Sustentaculum tali
- Fracture patterns: Undisplaced, Tongue-shaped, Joint depression, Comminuted
- X-ray view[Q]: Lateral view

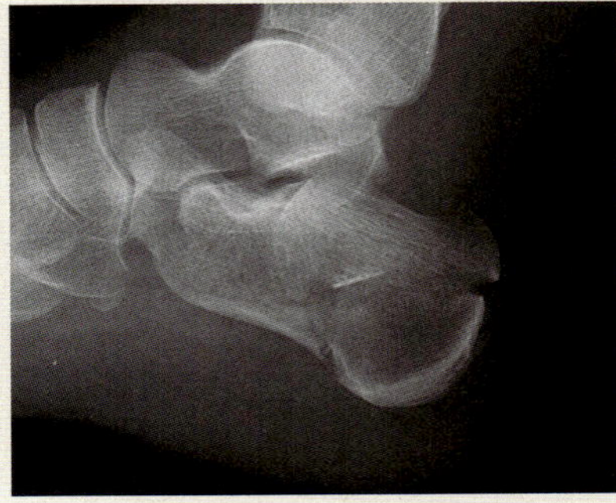

Fig. Calcaneal fracture

Other Injuries of Foot

- Chip-and-avulsion fracture talus: MC Talar fracture[Q]
- Fracture neck of talus: **Aviator's astralgus**[Q]
- **Jones' fracture[Q]:** Fracture of the base of the 5th metatarsal
- Pseudo-Jones fracture **(Tennis fracture[Q])**: Avulsion fracture due to pull of peroneus brevis muscle
- March fracture[Q]: Stress fracture of shaft of 2nd metatarsal
- LisFranc fracture[Q]: Fracture dislocation of mid-foot (Tarso-metatarsal joints)
- Chopart's fracture[Q]: Foot dislocation through talonavicular and calcaneocuboid joints with fractures

LIGAMENT INJURIES AROUND KNEE

Medial Collateral Ligament Injury

- History of valgus and external rotation force in mild sprains (Football, rugby sports)
- **MC tear site[Q]:** MCL insertion at adductor tubercle
- Treatment:
  - I degree sprain: RICE concept (Rest, Ice, Compression with bandage, Elevation of limb), NSAIDs
  - II degree sprain: Long leg cast (4–6 weeks) with knee in 30–40 degrees flexion
  - III degree sprain: Direct surgical repair with non-absorbable sutures

Lateral Collateral Ligament Injury

- Less common injury due to history of Varus force
- MC tear site: LCL insertion at Head of fibula

Anterior Cruciate Ligament Injury

- **MC knee ligament injury**[Q]
- Mechanism:
  - External rotation with abduction of flexed knee or
  - Hyperextension of knee in internal rotation

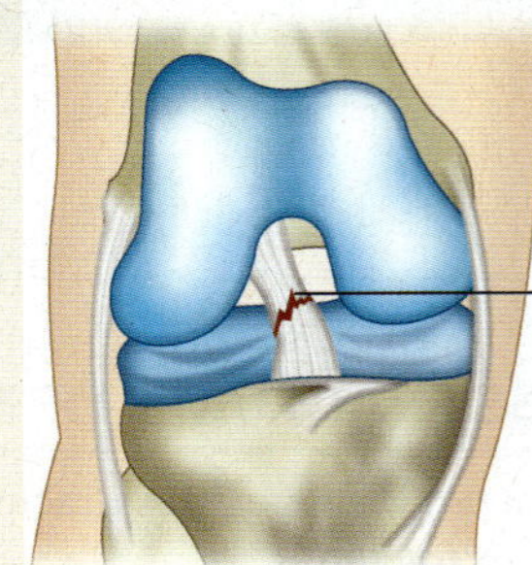

Fig. ACL tear

Orthopedics

- Popping sensation at time of injury; Knee gives-away/buckled at time of injury
- **Tests**[Q]**:** Anterior drawer test, Lachman test
- **Best diagnostic tool**[Q]**:** MRI

Posterior Cruciate Ligament Injury

- Mechanism:
  - Severe rotational injury
  - Dashboard injury
  - Complete dislocation of knee

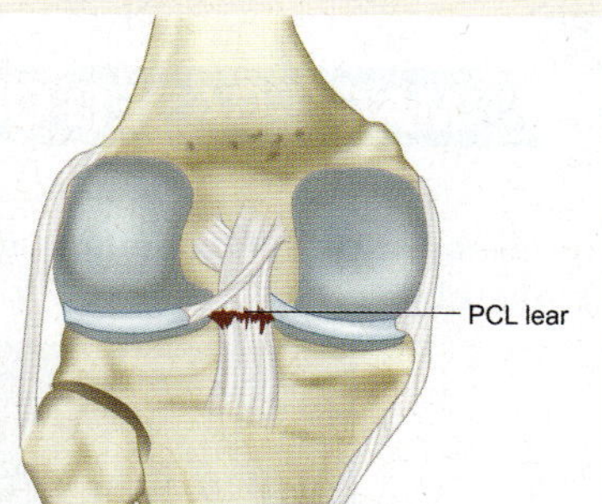

Fig. PCL tear

Medial Meniscus Injury

- **More common (70%) than Lateral meniscus injury**[Q]**:** Lateral meniscus is smaller diameter, thicker periphery, wider, more mobile, attached to both cruciate ligaments, stabilized posteriorly to femoral condyle by popliteus
- Mechanism:
  - Young persons: Weight being taken, knee flexed, twisting strain
  - Older persons: Tear with less force due to fibrosis (reduced mobility) of meniscus
- Types of tear: Horizontal (MC[Q]), Longitudinal, Cystic degeneration, Congenital anomalies, Regenerative lesions
- Tests[Q]: Joint line tenderness, McMurray's test, Apley's test
- Treatment:
  - Conservative: Abstinence from weight bearing, RICE concept, Buck's extension skin traction, Joint aspiration, Quadriceps exercises, Cylindrical cast (If pain persists)
  - Manipulation under anesthesia (If joint locked due to torn menisci)
  - Surgery (If joint unlocked with recurrent symptoms): Closed partial meniscectomy (Better method), Total menisci removal

IMAGE-BASED QUESTIONS

1. **Management of condition shown in Photograph is done by** ***[AIIMS November 2016]***

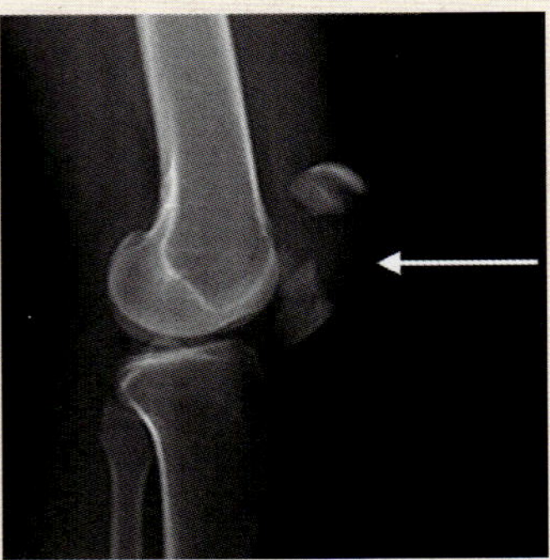

a. K-wire
b. Plating
c. Nails
d. Tension band wiring

2. **Following a road traffic accident, a 28-years-old Male patient came to emergency room. His left lower limb was in a specific position as shown in Photograph. Most likely diagnosis is** ***[AIIMS November 2016]***

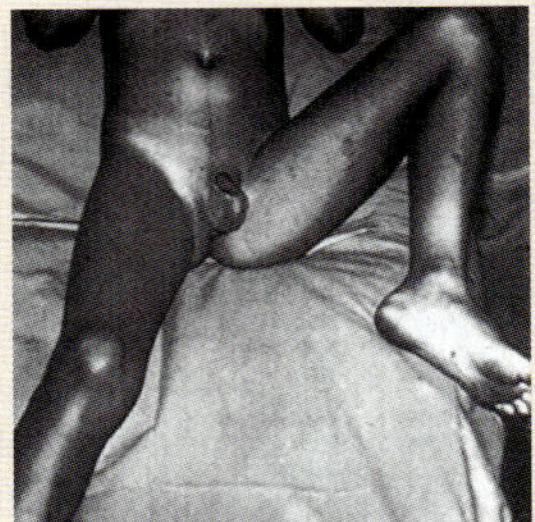

a. Anterior dislocation
b. Central dislocation
c. Posterior dislocation
d. Inferior dislocation

3. **Prosthesis used for Arthroplasty shown in the Photograph is**

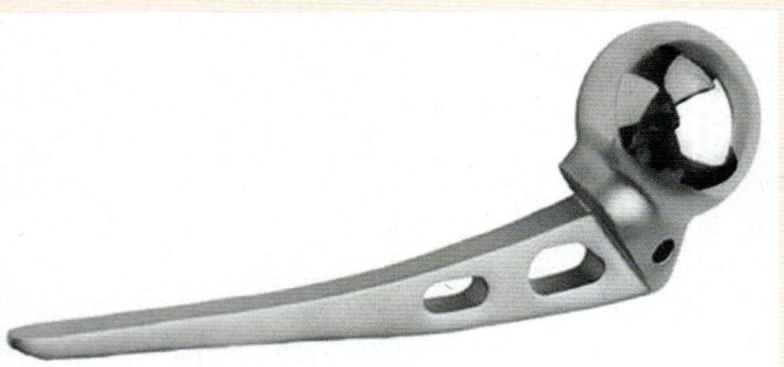

a. Thompson's prosthesis
b. Austin-Moore prosthesis
c. Mueller prosthesis
d. Bipolar prosthesis

4. **Identify Type of traction shown in the Photograph** ***[Recent Question 2013]***

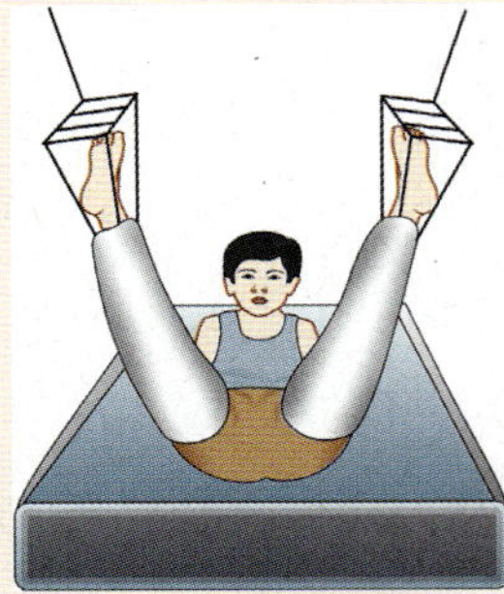

a. Hamilton Russell's traction
b. Gallow's traction
c. Buck's traction
d. Balanced skeletal traction

5. **Type of traction shown in the Photograph** ***[Recent Question 2014]***

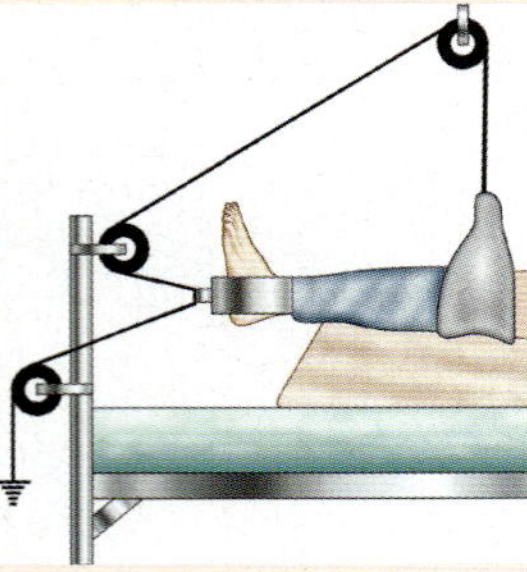

a. Hamilton Russell's traction
b. Gallows traction
c. Buck's traction
d. Balanced skeletal traction

6. **Identify the Clinical test shown in Photograph**

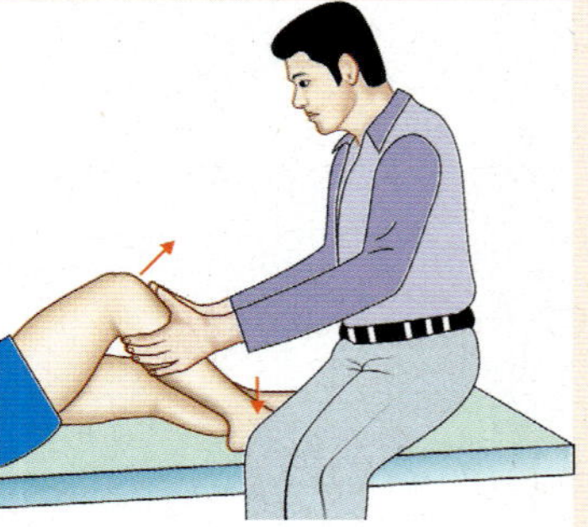

a. Lachmans test
b. Apley's test
c. Anterior drawer test
d. McMurray's test

7. Injury Mechanism (Photograph) lead to
[Recent Question 2013]

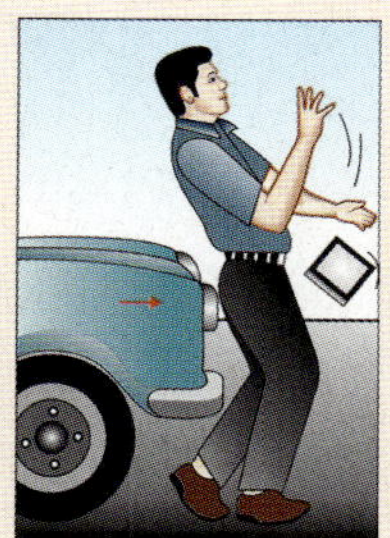

a. Anterior dislocation of hip
b. Posterior dislocation of hip
c. Central dislocation of hip
d. Fracture neck of femur

8. Line (Dashed) shown in Photograph is generally disrupted in

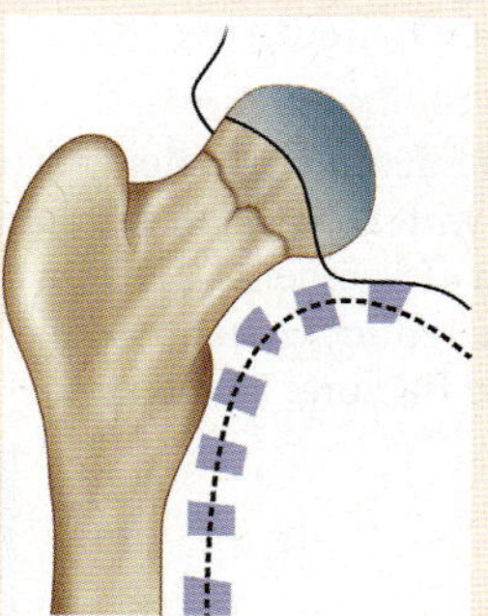

a. Fracture shaft of femur b. Acetabular hip fracture
c. Fracture neck of femur d. Hip dislocation

9. Identify the abnormality shown in Photograph
[AIIMS PG November 2015]

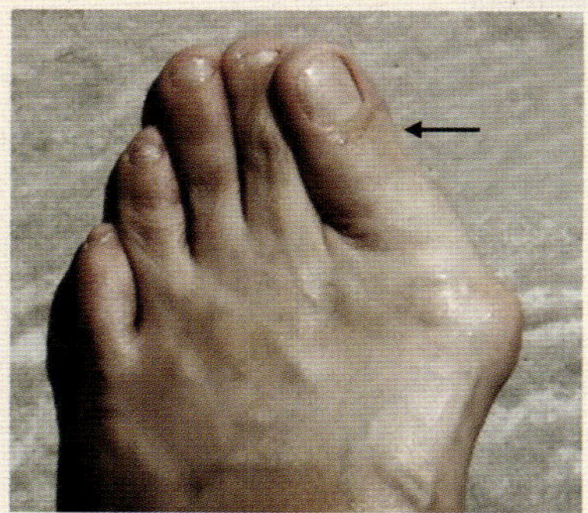

a. Hallux valgus b. Hallux varus
c. Rheumatoid nodule d. Subcutaneous nodule

10. Identify the deformity in the Image below?
[AIIMS PG November 2015]

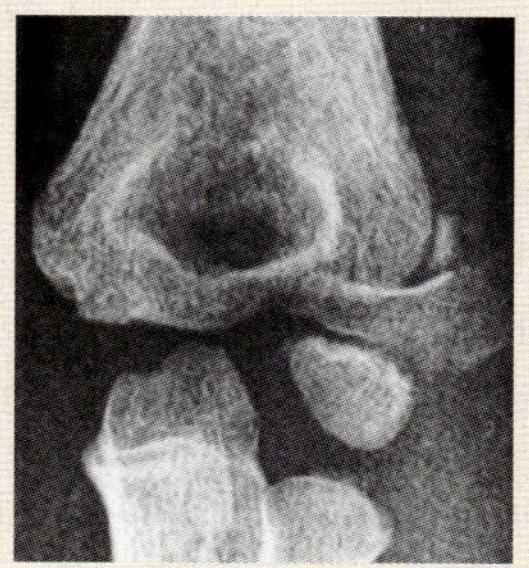

a. Humerus lateral condylar fracture
b. Supracondylar fracture humerus
c. Fracture shaft humerus
d. Medial condyle fracture of humerus

11. A 70-year-old patient slipped in bathroom and sustained injury over his hip. X-ray is shown below. Her attitude of leg will be ***[AIIMS May 2017]***

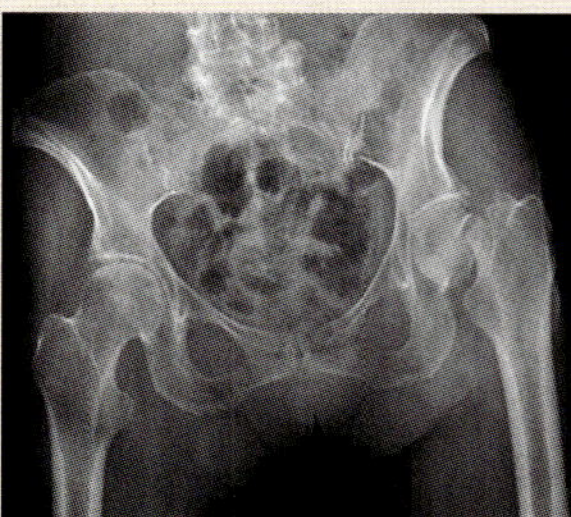

a. Shortened abducted and externally rotated
b. Shortened and abducted
c. Lengthened and internally rotated
d. Flexed and adducted and internally rotated

12. Treatment of fracture shown in the Photograph is
[AIIMS May 2017]

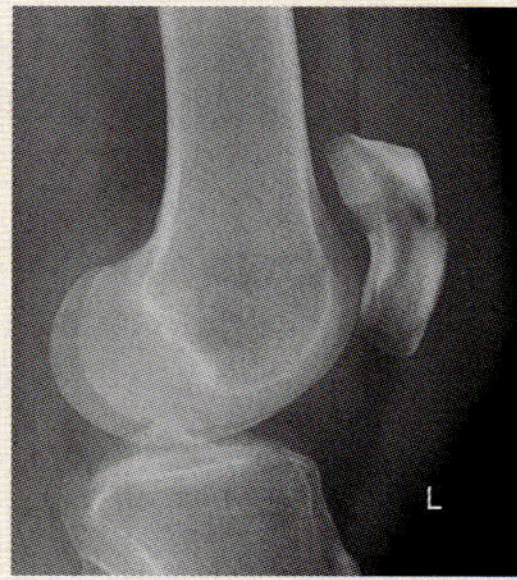

a. Intramedullary nail
b. Tension band wiring
c. Patellectomy
d. Above knee cast

Orthopedics

ANSWERS WITH EXPLANATIONS OF IBQs

1. Ans. (d) Tension band wiring *[Ref. Maheshwari, 4/e p142]*

Treatment of Patellar Fractures

- Undisplaced fracture: Cylinder cast (knee in full extension for 3 weeks), Physiotherapy
- Clean break with Separation of fragments **(Photograph)**:
  - Reduction of fragments, Tension band wiring, Repair of extensor retinaculae
  - If accurate reduction not possible, the Partial or Total patellectomy
- Comminuted fracture: Patellectomy (Excision of patella)

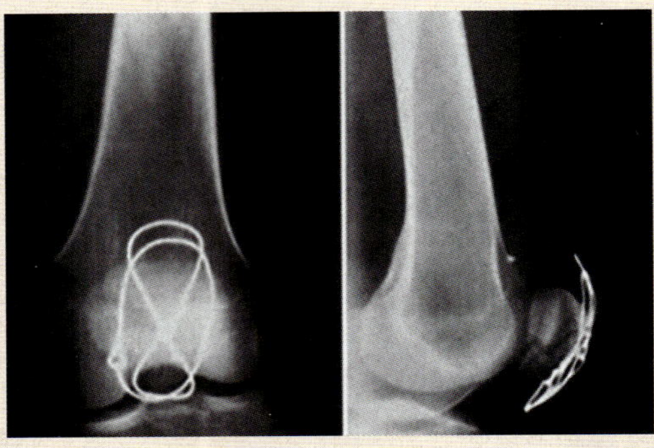

Fig.

2. Ans. (a) Anterior dislocation *[Ref. Maheshwari, 4/e p127]*

Dislocations of Hip Joint

- Anterior dislocation:
  - Cause: Forceful abduction, External rotation of limb
  - Seen in: Fall from a tree, RTA
  - Clinical presentation: Flexion, Abduction, External rotation, True lengthening of limb **(Photograph)**
- Posterior dislocation:
  - Cause: Force along Shaft of femur with Hip in flexed position
  - Seen in: Motor accidents, Dashboard injury
  - Clinical presentation: Flexion, Adduction, Internal rotation, Shortening of limb
- Central dislocation:
  - Cause: Fall from a height or a motor vehicle crash
  - Clinical presentation: Associated with an Acetabular fracture

3. Ans. (b) Austin-Moore prosthesis *[Ref. Maheshwari, 4/e p132]*

Austin-Moore Prosthesis

- *Use:* Hemiarthroplasty *for D*isplaced femoral neck fractures
- Indication: >3 weeks old fracture on Physiologically old (>65 years age) persons where chances of union is very little

4. Ans. (b). Gallow's traction *[Ref. Maheshwari, 4/e p132]*

- Gallow's traction: Used for Fracture shaft of femur (Birth-2 years age group)
- Underlying principle: Hips are kept raised off the bed so that weight of body provides counter-traction, and fracture is reduced
- Maintenance till 3-6 weeks (Till Callus formation is sufficient)

5. Ans. (a) Hamilton Russell's traction *[Ref. Maheshwari, 4/e p135]*

- Hamilton Russel Traction is used for Intertrochanteric fracture
- Method: Pulley system to provide support to femur and apply traction at 30 degrees to horizontal (approximately in line to femur)

6. Ans. (c) Anterior drawer test *[Ref. Maheshwari, 4/e p144]*

Common Clinical Tests in Knee Injuries

- *Anterior cruciate ligament*: Anterior drawer test, Lachman test, Pivot shift test
- *Posterior cruciate ligament*: Posterior drawer test
- *Medial collateral ligament*: Valgus stress test
- *Lateral collateral ligament*: Varus stress test
- *Meniscus injury*: McMurray test, Apley's grinding test

7. Ans. (a) Anterior dislocation of hip *[Ref. Maheshwari, 4/e p127]*

Anterior Dislocation of Hip

- Occur, if legs are forcibly abducted and externally rotated
- Occur, if fall from a tree with stuck foot, Road accident
- Limb attitude: External rotation, True lengthening
- Treatment: Closed/Open reduction

8. Ans. (c) Fracture neck of femur *[Ref. Maheshwari, 4/e p215]*

- *Shenton line:* An imaginary line drawn along the inferior border of the superior pubic ramus (superior border of the obturator foramen) and along the inferomedial border of the neck of femur
  - Shenton line should be continuous and smooth
  - Shenton line is broken in: Fracture neck of femur, Developmental dysplasia of hip

9. Ans. (a) Hallux valgus *[Ref. Maheshwari, 4/e p317]*

Hallux Valgus

- Description: Lateral deviation of Great toe at metatarsophalangeal joint
- Causes: Rheumatoid arthritis, Idiopathic, High heel shoes
- Treatment: Mitchell osteotomy, Mayo's operation, Keller's operation

10. Ans. (a) Humerus lateral condylar fracture *[Ref. Pediatric Orthopedic Deformities by Shapiro, 1/e p562-565]*

11. Ans. (a) Shortened abducted and externally rotated *[Ref. Orthopedic and Trauma by Roth, 1/e p155]*

In Femoral neck fractures (Shown in Photograph), the extremity is held in a slightly shortened, abducted, and externally rotated position, unless the fracture is only a stress fracture or severely impacted.

12. Ans. (b) Tension band wiring *[Ref. Maheshwari, 4/e p142]*

Photograph given shows transverse fracture of patella (Undisplaced)

Treatment of Patellar Fractures

- Undisplaced fracture: Cylinder cast (knee in full extension for 3 weeks), Physiotherapy
- Clean break with Separation of fragments (Transverse fracture):
  - Reduction of fragments, tension band wiring (TBW), repair of extensor retinaculae
  - If accurate reduction not possible, the partial or total patellectomy
- Comminuted fracture: Patellectomy (Excision of patella)

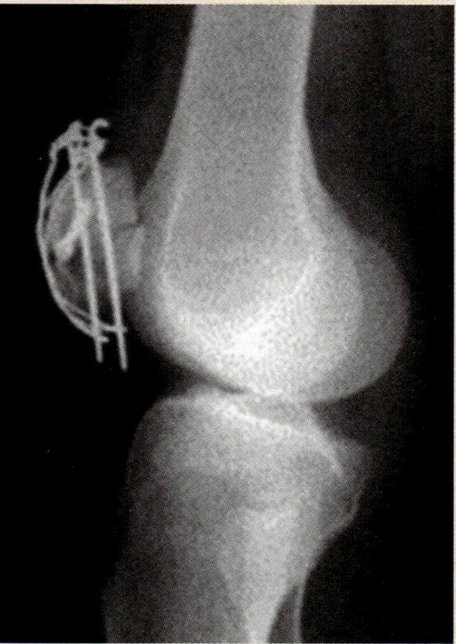

Fig. Tension band wiring

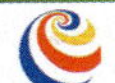 NEET/NBE PATTERN MCQs 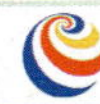

1. **In Uncemented arthroplasty of the hip, the stem remains attached to the bone by** *[Recent Question 2016]*
   a. Bone Ingrowth/ongrowth over the surface of the stem
   b. Mechanical bonding between the stem and bone
   c. Press fitting of the stem in the tight canal
   d. Adhesion between the stem and bone due to adhesive properties of the stem
2. **Which of the following fractures of Neck of femur are associated with maximal compromise in blood supply?** *[Recent Question 2016]*
   a. Intertrochanteric fractures
   b. Basicervical fracture
   c. Transcervical fracture
   d. Subcapital fractures
3. **Sudden dorsiflexion of foot may lead to which of the following injuries?** *[Recent Question 2016]*
   a. Anterior talofibular ligament injury
   b. Tendo-Achilles avulsion injury
   c. Rupture of deltoid ligament
   d. Tarsal tunnel syndrome
4. **Patellar clunk is a known complication of which Surgery?** *[Recent Question 2016]*
   a. Corrective osteotomy for genu valgum
   b. Total Knee Replacement
   c. Medial patellofemoral ligament reconstruction
   d. Bicondylar plating of proximal tibia fracture
5. **Gallow's Traction is used for** *[Recent Question 2016]*
   a. Fracture shaft tibia in children
   b. Fracture shaft femur in children
   c. Fracture shaft tibia in adults
   d. Fracture shaft Femur in adults
6. **Which of the following fractures is associated with high mortality and morbidity?** *[Recent Question 2016]*
   a. Femur Shaft fractures
   b. Pelviacetabular fractures
   c. Subtrochanteric fractures
   d. Shaft tibia fractures
7. **Lisfranc Fracture is** *[Recent Question 2016]*
   a. Fracture dislocation at the tarsometatarsal joint
   b. Intertarsal dislocation
   c. Avulsion of calcaneal tuberosity
   d. Fracture neck of talus
8. **Jones Fracture is** *[Recent Question 2016, 2017]*
   a. Fracture neck of 2nd metatarsal
   b. Fracture base of 5th metatarsal
   c. Fracture dislocation of metatarsophalangeal joints
   d. Fracture neck of talus
9. **Which of the following is a feature of Triple deformity of the knee joint?** *[Recent Question 2016]*
   a. Posterior subluxation of tibia
   b. Internal rotation of tibia
   c. Medial angulation of tibia
   d. Recurvatum
10. **Tripod fracture is** *[Recent Question 2016]*
    a. Displaced fracture of calcaneum
    b. Zygomaticomaxillary fracture
    c. Sphenoid Wing Fracture
    d. Coronal Shear pilon Fracture
11. **What is a Floating knee?** *[Recent Question 2016]*
    a. Damage to both anterior and posterior cruciate ligaments
    b. Condition of knee due to tear in medial and lateral collateral ligaments
    c. Femoral shaft fracture with proximal tibia metaphyseal fracture
    d. Advanced tuberculosis of knee joint
12. **MC complication of Fracture talus is** *[Recent Question 2016]*
    a. Avascular necrosis
    b. Nonunion
    c. Osteoarthritis of ankle joint
    d. Osteoarthritis of subtalar joint
13. **In Complete ACL rupture, the Tibia moves over Femur in which direction?** *[Recent Question 2016]*
    a. Forward b. Backward
    c. lateral d. Medial
14. **Fairbank's triangle is seen in** *[Recent Question 2016]*
    a. CDH b. SCFE
    c. Congenital coxa vara d. Perthes disease
15. **Patella dislocation is prevented by** *[Recent Question 2016]*
    a. Vastus medialis b. Vastus lateralis
    c. Vastus intermedius d. Rectus femoris
16. **Avascular necrosis is common after a fracture of** *[NBE FMGE September 2010, March 2012]*
    a. Cuboid b. Cuneiform
    c. Talus d. Calcaneum
17. **MC complication of fracture of ischiopubic rami of pelvis is:** *[UPSC 2007]*
    a. Rupture of urinary bladder
    b. Rupture of prostatic urethra
    c. Rupture of membranous urethra
    d. Injury to penile urethra
18. **MC medial meniscal tear type is:** *[NBE DNB 2008, 2009]*
    a. Horizontal tear b. Longitudinal tear
    c. Oblique tear d. None of the above
19. **Which of the following fractures reduce Bohler's angle?** *[Recent Question 2017, NBE DNB 2009]*
    a. Talus b. Calcaneum
    c. Cuboid d. Navicular
20. **What is March fracture?** *[Recent Question 2013]*
    a. Fracture of 2nd metatarsal
    b. Fracture of 4th metatarsal
    c. Fracture of cuboids
    d. Fracture of tibia
21. **Injury from lateral side of knee causes damage to** *[Recent Question 2012]*
    a. MCL b. LCL
    c. ACL d. PCL
22. **Bumper fracture involves** *[Recent Question 2014]*
    a. Sternum b. Ribs
    c. Medial tibial condyle d. Lateral tibial condyle
23. **Treatment of choice for fracture neck femur in a 40 years old female** *[Recent Question 2013]*
    a. Multiple screw fixation b. Bipolar hemiarthroplasty
    c. THR d. None

24. Fracture of neck of talus may give rise to *[NBE FMGE September 2005]*
a. Avascular necrosis of head
b. Avascular necrosis of neck
c. Avascular necrosis of body
d. Any of the above

25. Most common ligament injured in ankle sprain is *[NBE FMGE September 2005]*
a. Deltoid
b. Spring
c. Anterior talofibular
d. Posterior talofibular

26. Pott's fracture is *[Recent Question 2012, 2013]*
a. Talus fracture
b. Bimalleolar ankle fracture
c. Trimalleolar ankle fracture
d. None

27. Bone involved in stress fracture is *[Recent Question 2017, NBE FMGE March 2005]*
a. Talus
b. Calcaneum
c. 2nd metatarsal
d. 5th metatarsal

28. Why fracture shaft femur is early stabilized? *[Recent Question 2012]*
a. To prevent blood loss
b. ARDS
c. Nonunion
d. Compartment syndrome

29. All of the following tests are used for anterior cruciate ligament tear EXCEPT *[NBE FMGE March 2005]*
a. Pivot test
b. Lachman test
c. Anterior drawer test
d. Posterior drawer test

30. Gallow's traction for fracture shaft femur is used in which of the following age *[Recent Question 2012, 2014]*
a. < 2 years
b. 3–6 years
c. 7–13 years
d. > 13 years

31. Most common complication of fracture neck of femur *[Recent Question 2012]*
a. Malunion
b. Nonunion
c. AVN
d. Arthritis

32. Nerve injured in fibular neck fracture *[Recent Question 2012]*
a. Common peroneal
b. Tibial
c. Sural
d. Femoral

33. Lachman sign comes positive in which of the following injuries? *[NBE DNB 1993, NBE DNB 2003]*
a. Anterior cruciate ligament injury
b. Posterior cruciate ligament injury
c. Medial meniscus injury
d. Lateral meniscus injury

34. What is March fracture? *[Recent Question 2012]*
a. Fracture of 2nd metatarsal
b. Fracture of 4th metatarsal
c. Fracture of cuboids
d. Fracture of tibia

35. Healing time for fracture of tibia is *[NBE DNB 1994]*
a. 6 weeks
b. 12 weeks
c. 18 weeks
d. 24 weeks

36. McMurray's sign is seen in injury to *[UPSC 1988]*
a. Anterior cruciate ligament
b. Posterior cruciate ligament
c. Medial collateral ligament
d. Medial meniscus

37. Which of the following describes grade 2 fracture neck femur? *[Recent Question 2012]*
a. Incomplete fracture, medial trabeculae intact
b. Complete fracture with undisplaced neck
c. Complete fracture with ischemic head
d. Moderate displacement of neck, vascularity damaged

38. Anterior Drawer sign is positive in *[UPSC 2007]*
a. Anterior cruciate ligament injury
b. Lateral collateral ligament injury
c. Medial meniscal injury
d. Lateral meniscal injury

39. Stress fractures are most common in *[NBE DNB 1995]*
a. Tibial head
b. Femoral head
c. Fibular head
d. Metatarsals

40. Most common complication of Fracture Neck of Talus is *[Recent Question 2014]*
a. Nonunion
b. Malunion
c. Aseptic necrosis
d. Subtalar and ankle arthrosis

41. 'Unhappy triad' involves all except *[Recent Question 2014]*
a. Anterior cruciate ligament
b. Posterior cruciate ligament
c. Medical meniscus
d. Medial collateral ligament

42. Thomas splint is used for *[Recent Question 2014]*
a. Pelvic fracture
b. Femur fracture
c. Tibial fracture
d. Fibular fracture

43. O'Donoghue's triad does not include *[Recent Question 2015]*
a. Anterior cruciate ligament
b. Medial collateral ligament
c. Lateral collateral ligament
d. Meniscus

44. Not true about anterior cruciate ligament *[Recent Question 2017]*
a. It begins just behind the anterior horn of lateral meniscus on tibia
b. It is taut in extension
c. It provides proprioceptive inputs to knee
d. It is intrasynovial

45. Jumpers knee *[Recent Question 2017]*
a. Apophysitis of patellar tendon as it inserts in patella
b. Apophysitis of patellar tendon as it inserts in tibia
c. Apophysitis of quadriceps tendon as it inserts in patella
d. Apophysitis of hamstring tendon as it inserts in tibia

46. CTEV shoe true is *[Recent Question 2017]*
a. It is the same as normal shoe
b. It has straight medial border
c. It has medical shoe raise
d. It has heel with extra length

47. Which of the following is not true about the tests for Hip instability in neonates? *[Recent Question 2017]*
a. Ortolani's test has two parts
b. They are performed at 2–3 days of birth
c. In Ortolani's test examiners fingers rest on the greater trochanter
d. In Barlow's test examiners thumb is placed in the groin

48. Increased Q angle predisposes to *[Recent Question 2017]*
a. Medial patellar subluxation
b. Lateral patellar subluxation
c. Superior patellar subluxation
d. Inferior patellar subluxation

49. Which of the following is not true about Perthes' disease? *[Recent Question 2017]*
a. It is also called Coxa plana
b. Occurs more commonly in females
c. It is caused by interruption in the blood supply of the capital femoral epiphyses
d. Abduction, external rotation and extension of hip are restricted.

50. Which of the following is not true about SCFE? *[Recent Question 2017]*
a. Males are affected more frequently
b. Extension is restricted
c. Commonly occurs during adolescence
d. Varus, adduction and external rotation deformities are present

51. Cobra head plate is used for *[Recent Question 2017]*
a. Hip arthrodesis b. Knee arthrodesis
c. Elbow arthrodesis d. Ankle arthrodesis

52. Which of the following is not true about itracapsular fracture of femur neck? *[Recent Question 2017]*
a. Displacement is less common than extracapsular fractures
b. Malunion is common complication
c. Contour of greater trochanter is normal
d. Tenderness is mainly present over the anterior joint line

53. Popliteal artery injury is commonly seen in which type of Traumatic knee dislocation? *[Recent Question 2017]*
a. Anterior b. Posterior
c. Medial d. Lateral

54. Sudden inversion of foot leads to rupture of *[Recent Question 2017]*
a. Deltoid ligament
b. Anterior talofibular ligament
c. Posterior talofibular ligament
d. Spring ligament

55. Most common complication of Fracture of tibia *[Recent Question 2017]*
a. Infection
b. Compartment syndrome
c. Delayed union
d. Vascular injury

56. All of the following are complications of fracture neck of femur except *[Recent Question 2017]*
a. Nonunion
b. Sciatic nerve injury
c. Avascular necrosis
d. Osteoarthritis

57. Which of the following is not true about ACL injury? *[Recent Question 2017]*
a. It is a component of the O' Donoghue triad
b. ACL is intrasynovial
c. ACL is important for proprioceptive function
d. Anterior drawer test is the most sensitive test

58. Unna boot is used for treatment of *[Recent Question 2017]*
a. Diabetic foot ulcer b. Varicose ulcers
c. Ankle instability d. Calcaneum fracture

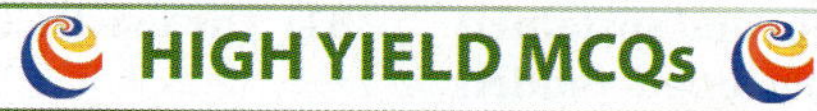

HIGH YIELD MCQs

1. **For assessing the injury of meniscus of knee joint, which of the following test is/are done?** *[PGI November 2016]*
   a. Apley's test b. Lachman test
   c. McMurray's test d. Thessaly test
   e. Hamilton ruler test
2. **Repair is better than removal in which part of meniscal injury?** *[All India PGMEE 2008]*
   a. Inner area
   b. Middle area
   c. Outer area
   d. At junction with cruciate ligaments
3. **Stress fractures affect** *[PGI 2000]*
   a. Second metatarsal b. Fifth metatarsal
   c. Second metacarpal d. Tibia
   e. Calcaneum
4. **Subtrochanteric fractures of femur can be treated by all of the following methods except** *[All India PGMEE 2005]*
   a. Skeletal traction on Thomas' splint
   b. Smith Petersen Nail
   c. Condylar blade plate
   d. Ender's nail
5. **The femur is fractured at birth at** *[Rajasthan PGMEE 1993]*
   a. Upper third of shaft b. Middle third of shaft
   c. Lower third of shaft d. Neck region
6. **In upper one third femoral shaft fracture, the displacement of proximal segment is** *[Rohtak PGMEE 1997]*
   a. Flexion adduction and internal rotation
   b. Flexion, adduction and external rotation
   c. Flexion, abduction and external rotation
   d. Flexion, abduction and internal rotation
7. **Treatment of choice for fracture lower 1/4th of tibia in non-union with multiple scarred wounds and discharging sinuses and about 4 cm shortening of leg?**
   a. Ilizarov fixator b. Plate *[AIIMS PGMEE 2009]*
   c. External fixation d. Intramedullary nail
8. **Maximum shortening of lower limb is seen in:** *[AIIMS PGMEE 1995]*
   a. Fracture shaft femur b. Fracture Neck femur
   c. Fracture intertrochanter d. Transcervical fracture
9. **You have treated the simple and undisplaced fracture of shaft of right tibia in a 9-year-old girl with above knee plaster cast. Parents want to know the prognosis of union of the fractured limb which was affected by poliomyelitis four years ago. What is the best possible advice will you offer to the parents?** *[AIIMS PGMEE 2003]*
   a. Fracture will unite slowly
   b. Fracture will not unite
   c. Fracture will unite normally
   d. Fracture will unite on attaining puberty
10. **An 8-year-old boy with a history of fall from 10 feet height complains of pain in the right ankle. X-ray taken at that time are normal without any fracture line. But after 2 years, he developed a calcaneovalgus deformity. The diagnosis is**
    a. Undiagnosed malunited fracture *[AIIMS PGMEE 2001]*
    b. Avascular nercrosis talus
    c. Tibial epiphyseal injury
    d. Ligamentous injury of ankle joint
11. **Traumatic dislocation of Epiphysial plate of Femur occurs** *[PGI 2002]*
    a. Medially b. Laterally
    c. Posteriorly d. Rotationally
    e. Anteriorly
12. **Fracture shaft of femur in children of less than 2 years old is treated by** *[AP PGMEE 1989]*
    a. Open reduction b. External fixation
    c. Gallow's traction d. Closed reduction
13. **A 3-year-old child presents with fracture of femoral shaft had immobilized on traction constantly for two months. The next step of management is** *[Bihar PGMEE 1999]*
    a. Hip Spica, and if necessary internal fixation
    b. Gallow traction for 2 months
    c. Open reduction and Kuntscher's clover leaf intra-medullary nailing or plating
    d. Traction by Thomas splint
14. **Fracture femur in children is treated by** *[UP PGMEE 1998, WB PGMEE 2000]*
    a. Open reduction b. Gallow's splint
    c. Intramedullary nailing
    d. Closed reduction and splintage
15. **Fracture of femur at the level of Isthmus is best treated by**
    a. Intramedullary nail fixation *[AP PGMEE 1989]*
    b. Plate and screws
    c. Closed method d. External fixation
16. **Intramedullary fixation is ideal in a case of fracture of shaft of femur when there is** *[NBE DNB 1998]*
    a. A transverse fracture
    b. A compound fracture
    c. Soft tissue interposition between the fractured ends
    d. Such a fracture in a child
17. **Treatment of choice for old non-united fracture of Shaft of femur** *[AIIMS PGMEE 1994]*
    a. Compression plating
    b. Bone grafting
    c. Nailing
    d. Compression plating with bone grafting
18. **Treatment of nonunion of Fracture shaft femur** *[AIIMS PGMEE 1996]*
    a. Open reduction with external fixation
    b. Excision of the bone
    c. Bone grafting with internal fixation with K-nail
    d. All of the following
19. **Best treatment of 3 weeks old, fracture shaft femur with nonunion is** *[AIIMS PGMEE 1994]*
    a. Bone graft with internal fixation
    b. External fixation c. Internal fixation only
    d. Prosthesis
20. **An army recruit, Smoker and 6 months into training started complaining of pain at posteromedial aspect of both legs. There was acute point tenderness and the pain was aggravated on physical activity. The most likely diagnosis is** *[All India PGMEE 2004]*
    a. Buerger's disease b. Gout
    c. Lumbar canal stenosis d. Stress fracture

21. A 30-year-old man had road traffic accident and sustained fracture of femur. Two days later, he developed sudden breathlessness. The most probable cause can be *[All India PGMEE 2005]*

a. Pneumonia b. Congestive heart failure
c. Bronchial asthma d. Fat Embolism

22. A 64-year-old hypertensive obese female was undergoing surgery for fracture femur under general anesthesia. Intraoperatively her end-tidal carbon dioxide decreased to 2 from 4 mm of Hg followed by hypotension and oxygen saturation of 85%. What could be the most probable cause? *[All India PGMEE 2003]*

a. Fat embolism b. Hypovolemia
c. Bronchospasm d. Myocardial infarction

23. Commonest site of March fracture is *[PGI 2000, JIPMER PGMEE 2014]*

a. Involves shaft of 2 and 3 metatarsals
b. Avulsion Fracture of 5th metatarsals
c. Calcaneus involved
d. Olecranon involved

24. Stress fracture is treated by *[Delhi PGMEE 1990]*

a. Rest b. Cast immobilization
c. Closed reduction d. Internal fixation

25. What is March fracture? *[PGI 1999]*

a. Fracture of 2nd metatarsal
b. Fracture of 4th metatarsal
c. Fracture of cuboids
d. Fracture of tibia

26. In pelvis fracture, the amount of blood loss is around *[TN PGMEE 1999]*

a. 1-4 units b. 2-4 units
c. 2-6 units d. 4-8 units

27. Ramesh Singh, a 40-years-old man, was admitted with fracture shaft femur following a road traffic accident. On 2nd day, he became disoriented. He was found to be tachypneic, and had conjunctival Petechiae. Most likely diagnosis is *[All India PGMEE 2002]*

a. Pulmonary embolism
b. Sepsis syndrome
c. Fat embolism
d. Hemothorax

28. Management of fat embolism includes all of the following except *[All India PGMEE 2004]*

a. Oxygen b. Heparinization
c. Low Molecular weight dextran
d. Pulmonary Embolectomy

29. If a patient with a suspected fracture of the pelvis has some bleeding from the urethra and is unable to pass urine *[UPSC 1997]*

a. He should be encouraged to pass urine after being given antibiotics and analgesics
b. He should be immediately catheterized in the ward
c. A hot water bottle should be given followed by injection of Carbachol
d. He should be prepared for surgery and catheterization attempted in the O.T.

30. Jumper's fracture is seen in *[PGI 1997]*

a. Calcaneum b. Tibia
c. Pelvis d. Neck femur

31. The usual site of stress fracture includes *[TN PGMEE 1993, Bihar PG 1999]*

a. Tibia
b. First metacarpal bone
c. Second metacarpal bone
d. Second metatarsal bone

32. Stress fracture not involves *[PGI 2000]*

a. Metatarsals b. Metacarpals
c. Tibia d. Calcaneum

33. Open book and bucket handle injuries are seen in *[AMU PGMEE 1999, SGPGI 2002, Rohtak 2002]*

a. Spine b. Pelvis
c. Femur d. Humerus

34. True about Crescent fracture is *[AIIMS PGMEE 2009]*

a. Anteroposterior instability with rotationability
b. Diastasis of pubis with pubic rami fracture
c. Antero-posterior compression is the mechanism of injury
d. Fracture of the iliac bone with sacroiliac disruption

35. Late complication of Acetabular fracture *[PGI 1997]*

a. Avascular necrosis of head of femur
b. Avascular necrosis of lilac crest
c. Fixed deformity of the hip joint
d. Secondary osteoarthritis of hip joint

36. All of the following areas are commonly involved sites in Pelvic fracture except *[All India PGMEE 2005]*

a. Pubic rami
b. Alae of ileum
c. Acetabula
d. Ischial tuberosities

37. Kocher Langenbeck approach for emergency acetabular fixation is done in all except *[AIIMS PGMEE 2009]*

a. Open fracture
b. Progressive sciatic nerve injury
c. Recurrent dislocation inspite of closed reduction and traction
d. Morel-Lavallee lesion

38. Emergency treatment of acetabular Fracture are all except *[AIIMS PGMEE 2009]*

a. Recurrent dislocations despite fixation with traction
b. Open acetabular fracture
c. Progressive aciatic nerve involvement
d. Morel-Lavallee lesion

39. Which is not true about Langenbeck Kocher operation? *[AIIMS PGMEE 2009]*

a. Adequate exposal of posterior segment
b. Anterior segment is not visualized adequately
c. Superior exposure is very adequate
d. Sciatic nerve injury in 1% in the cases

40. An elderly woman was admitted with a fracture of the neck of right femur which failed to unite. On examination, an avascular necrosis of the head of femur was noted. The condition would have resulted most probably from the damage to *[AIIMS PGMEE 2003]*

a. Superior gluteal artery
b. Inferior gluteal artery
c. Acetabular branch of obturator
d. Retinacular branches of circumflex femoral arteries

41. Garden's classification is used for *[UP PGMEE 1994]*
a. Posterior dislocation of hip
b. Epiphyseal injuries
c. Fracture neck of femur
d. Intertrochantric fracture

42. In fracture neck femur, all the trabeculae of pelvis and femur are in alignment in which stage *[AMU PGMEE 1994 [PGI 1992]*
a. State I
b. Stage II
c. Stage III
d. Stage IV

43. Increase in Pauwel's angle indicates *[SGPGI 2000, MAHE PGMEE 2000]*
a. Good prognosis
b. Impaction
c. More chances of displacement
d. Trabecular alignment disrupted

44. A 60-year-old female lands up in emergency with history of fall trauma, the attitude of limb is extension and external rotation, the most probable diagnosis is *[AIIMS PGMEE 1998]*
a. Intracapsular fracture neck of femur
b. Posterior dislocation of hip
c. Intertrochanteric fracture
d. Acetabular fracture

45. A woman aged 60 years suffers a fall. Her lower limb is extended and externally rotated; likely diagnosis is: *[All India PGMEE 2001, PGI 1995]*
a. Neck of femur fracture
b. Intertrochanteric femur fracture
c. Posterior dislocation of hip
d. Anterior dislocation of hip

46. Commonest hip injury in the elderly patients is: *[AMU PGMEE 1999]*
a. Stress Fracture
b. Extracapsular fracture
c. Impacted Fracture neck of femur
d. Subcapital capsular fracture neck of femur

47. Concerning fractures of the neck of the femur which statement is considered now to be incorrect
a. It is common in elderly women *[AMU PGMEE 1996]*
b. It can occur in young adults due to fatigue
c. It can occur in young adults following severe violence applied in the long axis of the femur
d. The bone fractures in an elderly woman because she falls

48. 80-years-old female after fall developed inability to walk with external rotation deformity on examination SLR is not possible and broadening of trochanter is present. The possible diagnosis is *[PGI PGMEE 1993, AMU PGMEE 1996]*
a. Fracture Neck femur
b. Fracture Intertrochanteric femur
c. Fracture Subtrochanteric femur
d. Fracture greater trochanter

49. A 60-year-old man fell in bathroom and was unable to stand on right buttock region ecchymosis with external rotation of the led and lateral border of foot touching the bed. The most probable diagnosis is *[UP PGMEE 1998]*
a. Extracapsular fracture neck of femur
b. Anterior dislocation of hip
c. Intracapsular fracture neck of femur
d. Posterior dislocation of hip

50. Features of fracture neck of femur includes
a. Flexion at hip and lateral rotation *[Manipal PGMEE 1998]*
b. Flexion at hip abduction
c. Shortening and lateral rotation
d. Shortening and flexion

51. Occult fracture of neck femur are best diagnosed by *[SGPGI 2003, AIIMS PGMEE 2006]*
a. Bone Scan
b. MRI
c. X-Ray
d. CT scan

52. Nonunion is a very common complication of intracapsular fractures of the neck of femur. Which of the following is not a very important cause for the same? *[CMC PGMEE 1997, JIPMER PGMEE 1995]*
a. Inadequate immobilization
b. Inadequate blood supply
c. Inhibitory effect of synovial fluid
d. Stress at fracture site due to muscle spasm

53. Most common complication of intertrochanteric fracture femur is *[All India PGMEE 1998]*
a. Malunion
b. Nonunion
c. Osteoarthritis
d. Nerve injury

54. Commonest complication of extracapsular fracture of neck of femur is *[Delhi PGMEE 1997, All India PGMEE 1988, WB PGMEE 1999]*
a. Nonunion
b. Ischemic necrosis
c. Malunion
d. Pulmonary complications

55. A 22-year-old male is admitted with fracture of the left femur. Two days later, he becomes mildly confused, has a respiratory rate of 4/min and scattered petechial rash on his upper torso. Chest X-ray shows patchy alveolar opacities bilaterally. His arterial blood gas analysis is abnormal. The most likely diagnosis is *[TN PGMEE 1994, Kerala PGMEE 1993]*
a. Cerebral edema with early neurogenic pulmonary oedema
b. Pulmonary thrombo-embolism
c. Chest contusion
d. Fat embolism

56. Most common complication of Transcervical fracture of Femur is *[TN PGMEE 1992, WB PGMEE 1992]*
a. Avascular necrosis
b. Malunion
c. Nonunion
d. None

57. In which one of the following femoral fractures is Avascular necrosis common? *[NBE DNB 2000, AIIMS PGMEE 1993]*
a. Pertrochanteric
b. Transcervical
c. Subtrochanteric
d. Shaft of femur

58. Avascular necrosis of head of femur occurs commonly at *[AIPGMEE 1988, AMU PGMEE 1997, NBE DNB 2000, 2003, 2004, 2006, AIIMS PG 1997]*
a. Transcervical region
b. Trochanteric region
c. Subcapital region
d. Subchondral region

59. Most common complication of intracapsular fracture neck of femur is *[JIPMER PGMEE 1990]*
a. Malunion
b. Osteoarthritis
c. Nonunion
d. Shortening

60. AVN is seen in which type of Fracture of femur *[PGI 2008]*
a. Intertrochantric fracture
b. Subcapital fracture
c. Trans cervical fracture
d. Basal fracture

61. After an operation on femur bone, chest X-ray shows widespread mottling throughout the lung field like a snowstorm. It is diagnostic of *[CMC PGMEE 1999]*
a. Fat embolism b. Shock lung
c. Bronchopneumonia d. Atelectasis

62. Most common complication of extracapsular fracture neck of femur is *[All India PGMEE 1988]*
a. Nonunion
b. Malunion
c. Ischaemic necrosis
d. Pulmonary complications

63. Best treatment for fracture neck femur in a 65-year-old lady is *[AIIMS PG 1994, 1998, UPSC 1997, AMU PGMEE 2000, UP 2000]*
a. POP cast
b. Gleotomy
c. Bone grafting and compression
d. Hernireplacement arthroplasty

64. A 50 years male with fracture neck of femur comes after 3 days, treatment of choice is *[AIIMS PGMEE 1999]*
a. Hemiarthroplasty
b. Total hip replacement
c. Hip spika
d. CR & IF

65. True about Fracture shaft femur in infants *[PGI 2006, PGI 2011]*
a. Most common cause is child abuse
b. Sclera must be examined
c. Fat embolism is commonly seen
d. Heals quite rapidly
e. Mostly only traction is required

66. Treatment of choice in fracture neck of femur in a 40-year-old male presenting after 2 days is *[All India PGMEE 1996]*
a. Hemiarthroplasty
b. Closed reduction and Internal fixation by cancellous screws
c. Closed reduction and Internal fixation by Austin-Moore pins
d. Plaster and rest

67. Treatment of choice for one week old fracture neck femur at 65 years age is *[All India PGMEE 1994]*
a. Hemireplacement arthroplasty
b. Closed reduction and internal fixation by cannulated cancellous screws
c. Closed reduction and 'internal fixation by Austin more pins
d. Total hip replacement

68. In 65-year-old male with history of fracture neck of femur 6 weeks old, treatment of choice *[Rajasthan PGMEE 1991, AIIMS PGMEE 1994, AMU 2000, AIPGME 1989]*
a. SP nailing
b. McMurray's osteotomy
c. Hemiarthroplasty
d. None

69. Fracture femur in children is treated by *[UP PGMEE 1998, WB PGMEE 2000]*
a. Open reduction
b. Closed reduction and splintage
c. Intramedullary nail
d. Gallow's splint

70. Management recommended for a three-week old fracture shaft femur with non-union *[AIIMS PGMEE 1994]*
a. Internal fixation
b. External fixation
c. Internal fixation with bone graft
d. Prosthesis

71. Femoral neck fracture of three weeks old in a young adult should be best treated one of the following
a. Total hip replacement *[Bihar PGMEE 1998]*
b. Reduction of fracture and femoral osteotomy with head
c. Prosthetic replacement of femoral head
d. Reduction of fracture and multiple pin or screw fixation
e. Upper femoral displacement osteotomy

72. Prosthetic replacement of femoral head is usually indicated for *[PGI 1990]*
a. Fresh intracapsular fracture head of femur in old patients
b. Fresh intracapsular fracture of femoral neck in a young adult
c. Unreduced posterior dislocation of hip
d. Untreated femoral neck fracture in a patient over 65 years
e. Pathological femoral neck fracture due to secondaries

73. Prosthesis at head of femur applied in *[UP PGMEE 1998]*
a. 40-year-old young male with Fracture head of femur
b. 40-year-old young male with Fracture neck of femur
c. 40-year-old young male with posterior dislocation of hip
d. 65-year-old male with non united fracture neck of femur

74. Fractured neck of femur is associated with all except
a. Causes shortening of the leg *[TN PGMEE 1988]*
b. Causes internal rotation of the leg
c. Be pathological
d. Be treated with hemiarthroplasty

75. Trochanteric fracture of femur is best treated by *[PGI 1993]*
a. Dynamic hip screw
b. Inlay plates
c. Plaster in abduction
d. Plaster in abduction and internal rotation

76. Prosthetic replacement of femoral head is indicated for one of the following sites of fractures *[Bihar PGMEE 1998]*
a. Inter-trochanteric fracture of femoral neck
b. Subcapital fracture neck femur
c. Transtrochanteric fracture femur
d. Basal fracture of femoral neck

77. Meyer's procedure is a method for treatment of *[PGI 1990]*
a. Recurrent shoulder dislocation
b. Habitual dislocation of patella
c. Congenital dislocation of hip
d. Fracture neck of femur

78. A fracture neck femur in a child is best treated by
a. Spica in abduction *[PGI 1993]*
b. Spica in abduction + internal rotation
c. Masterly inactivity
d. Open reduction and internal fixation

79. In a 10-year-old male transcervical fracture, neck femur is best treated by *[MAHE PGMEE 2006, NBE DNB 2005]*
a. Spica b. Austin Moore pins
c. K-Wires d. CC screw

80. In fracture of femur popliteal artery is commonly damaged by *[PGI 1993]*
a. Proximal fragment b. Distal fragment
c. Muscle haematoma d. Tissue swelling

81. Transverse fracture of the patella with separation of fragments is best treated by *[PGI 1992, AIIMS 1987, Kerala PGMEE 1987]*
a. Closed reduction with cylinder cast
b. Open reduction with screw fixation of the fragments
c. Blind fixation of the two fragments with Kirschner wire
d. Open reduction with Kirschner wire fixation of the fragment and tension band wiring

82. In Traumatic injury of the Hip *[PGI 2002]*
a. Anterior dislocation is common
b. Posterior dislocation is common
c. Avascular fracture is common
d. Visceral injury usually associated with fracture femur
e. Open reduction is always necessary

83. Comminuted fracture of the Patella should be treated by
a. Inserting screws and wires *[Bihar PGMEE 1989]*
b. Physiotherapy alone
c. Removal of the entire patella
d. Removal of smallest piece only
e. Plastering and Immobilization

84. Treatment of Displaced transverse fracture of Patella *[PGI 2003, PGI 2006]*
a. POP b. Tension band wiring
c. Screw d. Patellectomy
e. POP cast

85. What is acceptable angulation after reducing the Fracture tibia? *[AIIMS PGMEE 1993]*
a. 5 b. 1
c. 15 d. 20

86. In Fracture neck of fibula, the following nerve is involved *[NIMS PGMEE 2000, APPG 2000, Recent Question 2014]*
a. Common peroneal nerve
b. Anterior tibial nerve
c. Posterior tibial nerve
d. Medial popliteal nerve

87. Patients comes with Fracture femur in an acute accident, the first things to do is *[PGI 1986]*
a. Secure airway and treat the shock
b. Splinting
c. Physical examination
d. X-rays

88. Patellar tendon bearing POP cast is indicated in the following fracture *[All India PGMEE 2002]*
a. Patella b. Tibia
c. Medial malleolus d. Femur

89. Ankle sprain occurs due to rupture of *[All India PGMEE 1999]*
a. Anterior talofibular ligament
b. Posterior talofibular ligament
c. Calcaneofibular ligament
d. Deltoid ligament

90. MC complication of Fracture of Talus is
a. Nonunion *[AIIMS PGMEE 1995]*
b. Avascular necrosis
c. Osteoarthritis ankle joint
d. Osteoarthritis subtalar joint

91. Calcaneum fracture is usually seen along with *[AIIMS PGMEE 1997, DPG 1992]*
a. Fracture of ribs b. Fracture of fibula
c. Fracture of skull d. Fracture of vertebrae

92. Least common chances after fall from a height is fracture of *[AIIMS PGMEE 1994]*
a. Base of skull b. 12th thoracic vertebra
c. Fibula d. Calcaneum

93. Fatigue/stress fractures are most common in *[Bihar PG 1989, 1999]*
a. Tibia b. Fibula
c. Neck of femur d. Metatarsals

94. A patient develops Compartment syndrome (Swelling, pain and numbness) following manipulation and plaster for fracture of both bones of leg. What is the best treatment? *[All India PGMEE 1992, AIIMS PGMEE 1990]*
a. Split the plaster
b. Infusion of low molecular weight dextran
c. Elevate the leg after splitting the plaster
d. Do operative decompression of fascial compartment

95. Characteristic features of the Acute Compartment syndrome in the lower leg include all of the following except *[WB PGMEE 1994, AMU PGMEE 1996]*
a. Acute pain on employing the stretch test
b. Normal pulses
c. Normal sensation distally
d. Venous occlusion

96. In Posterior compartment syndrome which passive movement causes pain? *[AIIMS PGMEE 2008]*
a. Dorsiflexion of foot
b. Foot inversion
c. Toe dorsiflexion
d. Toe planter flexion

97. A patient has 2 months POP cast for Tibial fracture of left leg. Now he needs mobilization with a single crutch. You will use this crutch on which side *[AIIMS PGMEE 2000]*
a. Left side b. Right side
c. Any side d. Both side

98. Most commonly affected component of the lateral collateral ligament complex in an "ankle sprain" is the *[AIIMS PGMEE 2003]*
a. Middle component b. Anterior component
c. Posterior component d. Deeper component

99. Ankle sprain is due to *[All India PGMEE 1998]*
a. Rupture of anterior talofibular ligament
b. Rupture of posterior talofibular ligament
c. Rupture of deltoid ligament
d. Rupture of Calcaneofibular ligament

100. A patient presents with compound fracture of Tibia with 1 cm opening in skin. Which grade it belongs? *[JIPMER PGMEE 2000]*
a. Grade I b. Grade II
c. Grade IIIA d. Grade IIIB

101. Tibial Fracture with > 1 cm wound, slight comminution and moderate crushing is *[JIPMER PGMEE 2003, AMU PGMEE 2003]*
a. Grade I
b. Grade II
c. Grade III A
d. Grade III B

102. Inversion injury at the Ankle can cause all of the following except *[All India PGMEE 2002]*
a. Fracture tip of lateral malleolus
b. Fracture base of the 5th metatarsal
c. Sprain of Extensor digitorum brevis
d. Fracture of sustentaculum tali

103. The mechanism of injury of Transverse fracture of Medial malleolus results due to *[AP PGMEE 1999]*
a. Abduction injury
b. Adduction injury
c. Rotation injury
d. Direct injury

104. Immediate treatment of Compound fracture of tibia is *[Delhi PGMEE 1997]*
a. Intravenous antibiotics
b. Thorough debridement
c. Internal fixation of fracture
d. Amputation of limb

105. Fracture involving both the Malleoli is *[NIMS PGMEE 1992]*
a. Cotton's fracture
b. Potts's fracture
c. Pirogoff fracture
d. Dupuytren's fracture

106. Pott's fracture is fracture of *[PGI 1991]*
a. Lower end of tibia
b. Lower end of tibia + fibula
c. Lower end of tibia + Calcaneum
d. Calcaneum + Talus

107. One of the following fractures require Plaster of paris cast with equines position *[NBE DNB 1996]*
a. Distal fracture both bones leg
b. Distal fracture fibula
c. Bimalleolar
d. Fracture talus

108. MC component of fracture talus is *[AIIMS PGMEE 1995]*
a. Avascular necrosis
b. Nonunion
c. Osteoarthritis of ankle joint
d. Osteoarthritis of subtalar joint

109. Fracture of talus without displacement in X-ray would lead to *[PGI 2002]*
a. Osteoarthritis of ankle
b. Osteonecrosis of head of talus
c. A vascular necrosis of body of talus
d. Avascular necrosis of neck of talus
e. Nonunion

110. Gissane's angle in intra-articular fracture of calcaneum *[AMU PGMEE 2002, MAHE PGMEE 2004]*
a. Reduced
b. Increased
c. Not changed
d. Variable

111. Bohler's angle is decreased in fracture of
a. Calcaneum
b. Talus *[AIIMS PGMEE 2007]*
c. Navicular
d. Cuboid

112. Fracture of Calcaneus management depend upon
a. Type of fracture *[PGI 2008]*
b. Subtalar joint dislocation
c. Duration of presentation
d. Degree of displacement
e. None

113. Positive Pivot shift test in Knee is due to injury to *[AIIMS PGMEE 2000]*
a. Anterior cruciate ligament
b. Posterior cruciate ligament
c. Medial collateral ligament
d. Posterior elbow ligament

114. MC mode of meniscal injury *[AP PGMEE 1999]*
a. Flexion of knee
b. Extension of knee
c. Flexion and rotation movement
d. Extension and rotation movement

115. Bucket handle tear at Knee joint is due to injury to
a. Medial collateral ligament *[ORISSA PGMEE 1991]*
b. Lateral collateral ligament
c. Menisci
d. Ligamentum patellae

116. Tarsometatarsal amputation is also known as *[Recent Question 2016, Karnataka PGMEE 1999, UP PGMEE 1997, AIIMS PGMEE 2006]*
a. Chopart's amputation
b. Lisfranc amputation
c. Pirogoff amputation
d. Symes amputation

117. Amputation is often not required in *[AIIMS PGMEE 1995]*
a. Gas gangrene
b. Buerger's
c. Chronic osteomyelitis
d. Diabetic gangrene

118. In injury to Knee cartilage, investigation of choice is *[AIIMS PGMEE 1994, APPG 2000]*
a. X-ray
b. Aspiration
c. Arthroscopy
d. Arthrography

119. MC Ligament injured around Ankle joint is *[All India PGMEE 1998]*
a. Anterior talofibular
b. Posterior talofibular
c. Deltoid
d. Spring

120. Position for transport of a patient with Fracture lumbar spine in a patient *[Delhi PGMEE 1994]*
a. Neutral
b. Hyperflexion
c. Alternating
d. Hyperextension

121. Bulbocavernosus reflex is elicited by all except *[PGI 1993]*
a. Glans penis
b. Clitoris
c. Tug of foley catheter
d. Perianal stimulation

122. In Anterior cruciate ligament tear, which of these tests are positive *[PGI 2002]*
a. Lachman test
b. McMurry's test
c. Anterior drawer test
d. Posterior drawer test
e. Apley's test

123. Drawer sign seen in *[Rajasthan PGMEE 1992]*
a. Cruciate ligament injury
b. Scurvy
c. Perthes' disease
d. Hyperparathyroidism

124. Avascular necrosis of Head of femur can occur in *[PGI 2009]*
a. Caisson's disease
b. Sickle cell anaemia
c. Diabetes
d. Trochanteric fracture
e. Intra-capsular fracture neck

125. Which activity will be difficult to perform for a patient with an anterior cruciate deficient knee joint? *[AIIMS PGMEE 2002]*
a. Walk downhill
b. Walk uphill
c. Sit cross leg
d. Getting up from sitting

126. Posterior cruciate ligament, true statement is *[AIIMS PGMEE 2006, All India PGMEE 2007]*
a. Attached to the lateral femoral condyle
b. Intrasynovial
c. Prevents posterior dislocation of tibia
d. Relaxed in full flexion

127. A twisting injury of knee in flexed position would result in injury to all except *[AIIMS PGMEE 2002]*
a. Meniscal tear
b. Capsular tear
c. Anterior cruciate ligament
d. Fibular collateral ligament

128. Torsion of knee results in injury most commonly to *[AIIMS PGMEE 2002]*
a. Anterior cruciate ligament
b. Medial meniscus
c. Fibular collateral ligament
d. Tibial collateral ligament

129. Which type of injury causes more damage to the semi-lunar cartilage in the Knee? *[All India PGMEE 1996]*
a. Flexion and extension at the ankle
b. Rotation on a flexed knee
c. Rotation on an extended knee
d. Squatting position

130. Most common type of mode of Meniscal injury is *[AP PGMEE 1999]*
a. Extension of knee
b. Flexion of knee
c. Flexion and rotation movement
d. Extension and rotation of movement

131. Locking of knee joint can be caused by *[PGI 2005]*
a. Osgood shalter
b. Loose body in knee joint
c. Tuberculosis of knee
d. Medial meniscal partial tear

132. A patient gives a history of twisting strain and locking of the knee joint, the most likely diagnosis is *[PGI 1997, All India PGMEE 1993]*
a. Avulsion of tibial tubercle
b. Meniscal tear
c. Tearing of lateral collateral ligament
d. Tear of anterior cruciate ligament

133. Which of the following is correct in Medical meniscus tear? *[JIPMER PGMEE 1987, Kerala PGMEE 1987]*
a. Rotation of femur on tibia
b. Menisci do not heal
c. Locking and unlocking episodes
d. Menisci should be excised
e. All of the above are correct

134. It is wise to keep and repair the meniscus rather than removing it when the injury is to which of the following? *[All India PGMEE 2008]*
a. Medial part of meniscus
b. Mid part of meniscus
c. Lateral part of meniscus
d. Associated with collateral ligament injury

135. All of the following features in the knee are recognized to be consistent with a torn medial meniscus, except *[Manipal PGMEE 1994]*
a. Excessive forward glide b. Giving way
c. Locking d. McMurray's sign

136. A 18 years old boy was playing football, when he suddenly twisted his knee on the ankle and he fell down. He got up after 1 minutes and again started playing but next day his knee was swollen and he could not move it. The most probable cause is *[AIIMS PGMEE 2001]*
a. Medial meniscus tear
b. Anterior cruciate ligament tear
c. Medical collateral ligament injury
d. Posterior cruciate ligament injury

137. Which is the Investigation of choice for a Sport injury of the knee? *[AP PGMEE 1993, TN PGMEE 1997]*
a. Ultrasonography
b. Plain radiography
c. Arthrography
d. Arthroscopy

138. Commonest dangerous complication of Posterior dislocation of knee is: *[AIIMS PGMEE 1999]*
a. Popliteal artery injury
b. Sciatic nerve injury
c. Ischaemia of lower leg compartment
d. Femoral artery injury

139. Management of hemarthrosis is/are: *[PGI 2004]*
a. Compression bandage
b. Needle aspiration
c. POP cast
d. Rest to the joint
e. Synovectomy in recurrent cases

140. Injury around the ankle joint occur at *[Bihar PGMEE 1999]*
a. Inversion of foot
b. Eversion of foot
c. Internal rotation of foot
d. External rotation of foot

141. Most common cause of Insertional tendonitis of tendo-Achilles is *[AIIMS PGMEE 2008]*
a. Overuse b. Improper shoe wear
c. Runners and jumpers d. Steroid injections

142. Operative procedure known as "Microfracture" is done for *[AIIMS PGMEE 2003]*
a. Delayed union of femur
b. Nonunion of tibia
c. Loose bodies of ankle joint
d. Osteochondral defect of femur

143. Indications of Arthoplasty *[PGI 2004]*
a. Osteoarthritis b. Rheumatoid arthritis
c. Ankylosing spondylosis d. Gout
e. Fracture neck femur

144. Major indication(s) for Arthroplasty *[PGI 2000]*
a. Osteoarthritis of hip
b. Ankylosis of elbow
c. Ununited tibial fracture
d. Ununited femoral neck fracture
e. TB spine

145. Most common cause of death after Total Hip Replacement is *[ESI IMO 2014]*
a. Infection b. Pneumonia
c. Anemia d. Thromboembolism

146. Traction NOT used for Lower limb is *[AIIMS PG May 2015]*
a. Perkin b. Gallow's
c. Byrant d. Dunlop

147. Occult fracture of neck femur is best diagnosed by
a. CT Scan
b. Bone scan *[PGMCET 2015]*
c. MRI
d. None of the above

148. "McMurray's Test" on knee is done to know integrity of
a. Anterior cruciate ligament *[PGMCET 2015]*
b. Posterior cruciate ligament
c. Meniscus
d. Medial collateral ligament

149. O'donoghue triad comprise of *[NIMSET 2015]*
a. Medial collateral ligament complete rupture with Anterior cruciate ligament and medial meniscus damage
b. Medial collateral ligament complete rupture with Posterior cruciate ligament and medial meniscus damage
c. Medial collateral ligament complete rupture with Posterior cruciate ligament and lateral meniscus damage
d. Medial collateral ligament complete rupture with Anterior cruciate ligament and Lateral meniscus damage

150. March fracture in Metatarsal following stress is seen in ____ of Second metatarsal *[AIIMS May 2017]*
a. Head
b. Neck
c. Shaft
d. Base

151. A patient came with Open wound with fractures of both bones of Right lower limb. He is classified as Class 3B of Gustilo Anderson Classification. So he must be having *[AIIMS November 2017]*
a. Open fracture with a wound < 1 cm long and clean
b. Open fracture with a laceration > 1 cm long without extensive soft tissue damage, flaps, or avulsions
c. Open fractures with extensive soft tissue injury loss with periosteal stripping and bone exposure, usually associated with massive contamination
d. Open fractures associated with arterial injury requiring repair

152. A 25-year-old male regular visitor to gymnasium develops pain in hip that aggravated while squatting. He provided a history of steroids and creatinine use since past 6 months. Flattening of Femoral head and subchondral cysts are seen on X-ray. Most likely diagnosis is
a. Tuberculosis hip *[AIIMS November 2017]*
b. Fracture neck of femur
c. AVN hip
d. Osteomalacia

NEET/NBE PATTERN MCQs ANSWERS WITH EXPLANATIONS

1. **Ans. (a) Bone Ingrowth/ongrowth over the surface of the stem**
   [Ref. Total Hip and Knee Arthroplasty by Berry, 1/e p472]

Cementless Arthroplasty Fixation

- Initial fixation of cementless femoral components relies on a press-fit design with contact pressure between the component and bone or a fit-and-fill design that attempts to fill the femoral canal
- Porous and textured surfaces allow for bony ingrowth or ongrowth, which provide the final fixation
- Cementless component geometry and the surface are aimed at obtaining optimal initial fixation and allowing for secondary fixation through bony ongrowth or ingrowth and must take into account the variable femur anatomy

2. **Ans. (d) Sub-capital fractures**
   [Ref. Rheumatology, Orthopaedics and Trauma at a Glance by Swales, 2/e]

- If the fracture is a sub-capital fractured neck of the femur, high under the head, then, in the elderly, the blood supply to the head is usually so badly compromised that even if the fracture is reduced, the head will die

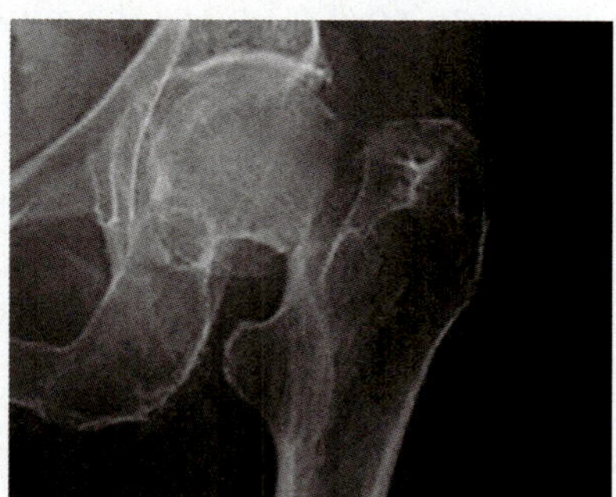

Fig. Fracture neck femur

3. **Ans. (b) TendoAchilles avulsion injury**
   [Ref. Rosen's Emergency Medicine, 8/e p733]

- **Achilles tendon rupture** results from direct trauma or indirectly transmitted forces, including sudden unexpected dorsiflexion, forced dorsiflexion of a plantar—flexed foot, and strong push—off of the foot with simultaneous knee extension and calf contraction

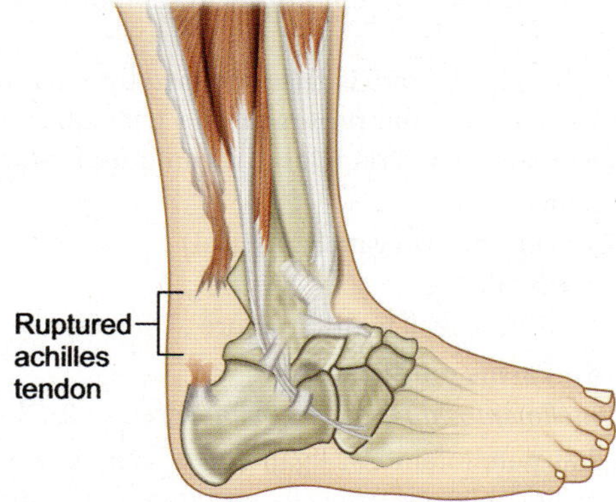

Fig. Achilles tendon rupture

4. **Ans. (b) Total knee Replacement**
   [Ref. Total Knee Arthroplasty by Bellemans, 1/e p63]

Patellar Clunk Syndrome

- A common complication relating to Patellofemoral articulation after Posterior stabilized total knee arthroplasty
- Patellar clunk syndrome occurs when a fibrous nodule develops just proximal to the patellar button
- At approximately 30–45 degrees from full extension, the nodule catches the anterior flange of the femoral prosthesis, resulting in the clunk and a painful range of motion

5. **Ans. (b) Fracture shaft femur in children**
   [Ref. Maheshwari, 4/e p132]

Gallows' traction

- Used for Fracture shaft of femur (Birth-2 years age group)
- Underlying principle: Hips are kept raised off the bed so that weight of body provides counter-traction, and fracture is reduced
- Maintenance till 3–6 weeks (Till Callus formation is sufficient)

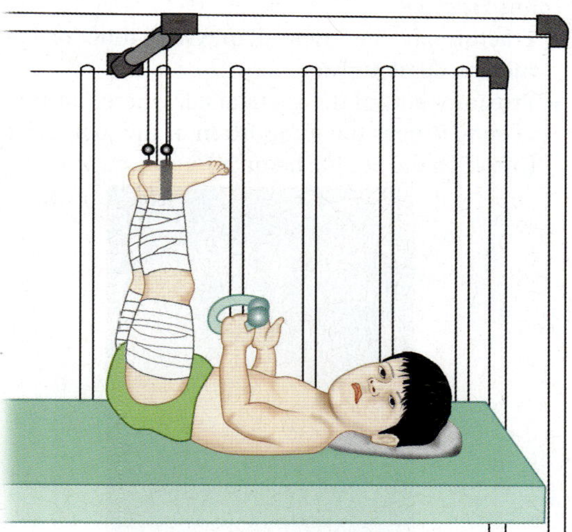

Fig. Gallow traction

6. **Ans. (b) Pelviacetabular fractures**
   [Ref. Orthopaedics and Orthopaedic Trauma by Pynsent, 2/e p237]

- Disruption of Pelvic ring is a serious injury that has high levels of associated morbidity and mortality
- In contrast, acetabular fractures have lower levels of mortality but high levels of morbidity due to associated pain, limited motion and degenerative changes

7. **Ans. (a) Fracture dislocation at the tarsometatarsal joint**
   [Ref. Mann's Surgery of Foot and Ankle by Saltzman, 9/e p1495]

Lisfranc Injuries/ Fracture-dislocations

- MC type of dislocation involving the foot
- Correspond to the dislocation of articulation of tarsus with metatarsal bases

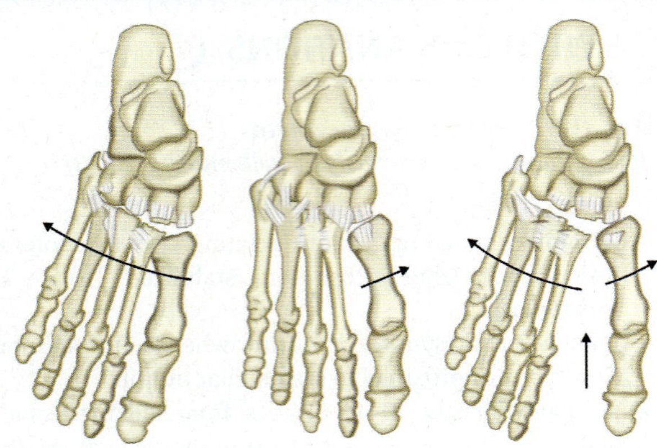

Fig. Lisfranc injury

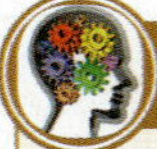

Also Remember

- Lisfranc joint: Articulation of the tarsus with the metatarsal bases, whereby the first three metatarsals articulate respectively with the three cuneiforms, and the 4th and 5th metatarsals with the cuboid

8. Ans. (b) Fracture base of 5th Metatarsal [Ref.

Jones Fracture

- Fracture in the meta-diaphyseal junction of the fifth metatarsal of the foot
- Proximal end of the metatarsal, where the Jones fracture occurs, is near the midportion of the foot, on the fifth ray (of which the 5th toe belongs)

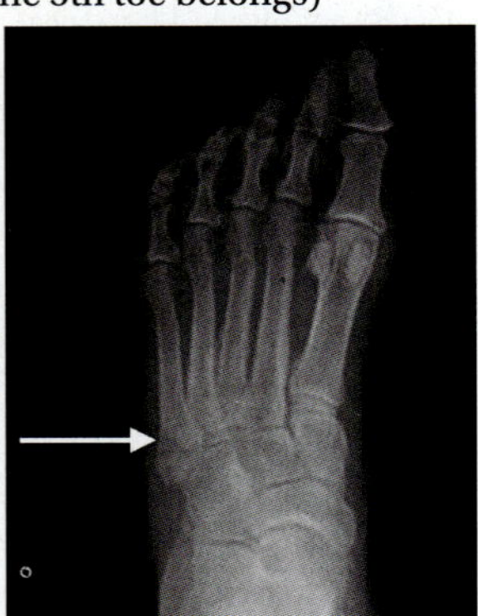

Fig. Jones fracture

9. Ans. (a) Posterior subluxation of tibia

[Ref. Practical Orthopedic Examination Made Easy by Kumar, 2/e p139]

- **Triple Deformity of Knee:** Flexion deformity of knee, Posterolateral subluxation of tibia, External rotation of tibia over femoral condyles
- **Quadruple deformity:** Triple deformity + Genu valgum

10. Ans. (b) Zygomaticomaxillary fracture

[Ref. Diagnostic Imaging by Broder, 1/e p59]

Tripod Fracture

- Zygomatic-complex fracture, Malar fracture, Zygomatico-maxillary fracture
- Fracture involves Zygomatic arch, Inferior orbital rim, Anterior & lateral walls of Maxillary sinus
- Typical feature: Free lambda-shaped fracture segment

11. Ans. (c) Femoral shaft fracture with proximal tibia metaphyseal fracture

[Ref. Skeletal Trauma by Browner, 5/e p1817]

- **Floating knee:** Flail knee joint segment resulting from a fracture of the shaft or adjacent metaphysis of the ipsilateral femur and tibia

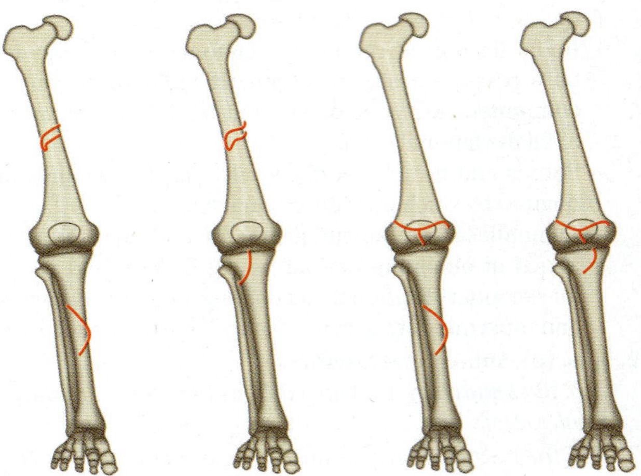

Fig. Floating knee injuries

12. Ans. (d) Osteoarthritis of subtalar joint

[Ref. Fundamentals of Orthopedics by Mohindra, 1/e p146]

Complications of Fracture Talus

- Avascular necrosis of body of Talus
- Malunion
- Non-union
- Osteoarthritis of Subtalar joint and Ankle joint: Due to damage to articular cartilage, malunion of fracture or osteonecrosis of talus

13. Ans. (a) Forward

[Ref. Sports Medicine and Science by Renström, 1/e p193]

Anterior Cruciate Ligament

- Main function is to prevent the leg bone (Tibia) from moving forward in relation to the thigh bone (Femur)
- In fact, the ACL absorbs 86% of the total strain in this direction
- ACL injuries are most serious ligament injuries in knee
- ACL is also the ligament most frequently surgically reconstructed

14. Ans. (c) Congenital coxa vara

[Ref. Fundamentals of Orthopedics by Mohindra, 1/e p411]

Fairbank's Triangle

- Congenital coxa vara is characterised by a decreased neck shaft angle and the presence of a triangular ossification defect (Fairbanks Triangle) of the inferior femoral neck
- Seen in:
  - Congenital coxa vara (Classical)
  - Perthes disease
  - Nonunion neck femur fracture

15. Ans. (a) Vastus medialis

[Ref. Patellofemoral Disorders by Biedert1/e p222]

- Medial patellofemoral ligament is dynamized by Vastus medialis obliquus muscle and the two function as a complex that acts to prevent Patellar dislocation

16. Ans. (c) Talus

[Ref. Maheshwari, 4/e p49]

Avascular Necrosis

- *Cause of Avascular necrosis*: Fracture of a part of bone compromising its vascularity
- *Common sites of Avascular necrosis*:

Site	Cause
Head of femur	Fracture neck of femur Posterior dislocation of hip
Proximal pole of scaphoid	Fracture through waist of scaphoid
Body of talus	Fracture through neck of talus

17. Ans. (c) Rupture of membranous urethra

18. Ans. (b) Longitudinal tear

19. Ans. (b) Calcaneum

20. Ans. (a) Fracture of 2nd metatarsal

21. Ans. (a) MCL

22. Ans. (d) Lateral tibial condyle

23. Ans. (a) Multiple screw fixation

24. Ans. (c) Avascular necrosis of body

[Ref. Maheshwari, 4/e p49, 160]

- *Anatomical relevance*: **Talus is the only bone of foot without any muscle attachment**, and blood supply is by anastomotic ring of blood vessels, osseous vessels entering its neck and runs within bone to supply its body. Thus, blood supply to body of talus is often cut-off following fractures occurring through neck.
- *Complication*: Avascular segment fails to unite, collapses and leads to deformity and ultimately osteoarthritis of ankle

25. Ans. (c) Anterior talofibular

[Ref. Maheshwari, 4/e p157-158 and Surgery by Bailey and Love, 25/e p462-463]

Ankle Sprains

- *Definition*: Ligament injuries of ankle
  - More commonly involved: Lateral collateral ligament (inversion injury)
  - Less commonly involved: Medial collateral ligament (eversion injury)
- *Most common ligament part involved*: Anterior talo-fibular ligament
- *Injury types and treatment*:
  - General functional treatment: **PRICE** routine (**P**rotect, **R**est, **I**ce, **C**ompression, **E**levation)
  - Specific treatment according to type:

Injury type	Treatment
Type I sprain	Below knee cast X 2 weeks + Immobilisation
Type II sprain	Below knee cast X 4 weeks + Immobilisation
Type III sprain	Below knee cast X 6 weeks + Immobilisation

26. Ans. (b) Bimalleolar ankle fracture

27. Ans. (c) 2nd metatarsal

[Ref. Maheshwari, 4/e p160]

Stress Fractures of Metatarsals

- *Type of fracture*: Fatigue/ stress fracture of metatarsals due to prolonged walking or running (army recruits)
- *Sites of stress fracture*:
  - 2nd metatarsal (*March fracture* - most common)
  - 5th metatarsal (*Jones fracture/ Dancer's fracture*)

28. Ans. (a) To prevent blood loss

29. Ans. (d) Posterior drawer test

[Ref. Maheshwari, 4/e p144, 356]

Tests of Anterior Cruciate Ligament

- Anterior drawer test
- Lachman test
- Pivot shift test

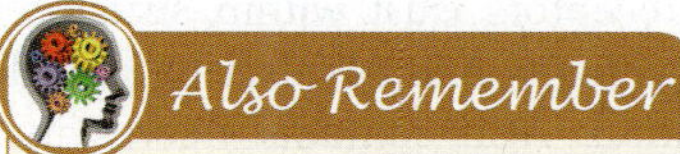

- *Test of Posterior cruciate ligament*: Posterior drawer test
- Test of Medial collateral ligament: Valgus stress test
- Test of Lateral collateral ligament: Varus stress test
- Tests of Meniscus injury: McMurray test, Apley's grinding test

30. Ans. (a) < 2 years

31. Ans. (b) Nonunion

32. Ans. (a) Common peroneal

33. Ans. (a) Anterior cruciate ligament injury

34. Ans. (a) Fracture of 2nd metatarsal

35. Ans. (b) 12 weeks

36. Ans. (d) Medial meniscus

37. Ans. (b) Complete fracture with undisplaced neck

38. Ans. (a) Anterior cruciate ligament injury

39. Ans. (d) Metatarsals

40. Ans. (d) Sub-talar and ankle arthrosis

[Ref. Orthopedic Trauma Surgery by Wiesel, 1/e p523]

- **Complications of Fracture Neck of Talus:**
  - Sub-talar and Ankle arthrosis (Most common)
  - Septic avascular necrosis
  - Malunion
  - Delayed union
  - Varus malalignment

41. Ans. (b) Posterior cruciate ligament

[Ref. Emergency Orthopedics by Sherman, 6/e p458]

- Injury to the MCL, ACL, and medial meniscus is referred to as **"unhappy triad"** because of the common association of these structures following a valgus stress to the knee

42. Ans. (b) Femur fracture

[Ref. Maheshwari, 4/e p24-25]

43. Ans. (c) Lateral collateral ligament

[Ref. Examination of Orthopedic and Athletic Injuries, 3/e]

- **Unhappy triad/ Terrible triad/ Horrible triangle/ O'Donoghue's triad/ Blown knee:** An injury to the anterior cruciate ligament, medial collateral ligament, and the meniscus

44. Ans. (a) It begins just behind the anterior horn of lateral meniscus on tibia

[Ref. CDTPMR by Maitin, 1/e p21]

Anterior Cruciate Ligament (ACL)

- ACL originates from medial aspect of Lateral femoral condyle in Intercondylar notch
  - *Two bundles of ACL: Anteromedial and Posterolateral*
  - *ACL attaches in front of the Intercondyloid eminence of Tibia, where it blends with the anterior horn of the Lateral meniscus*
- Anteromedial fibers are taut in flexion, whereas the larger Posterolateral fibers are tight in extension
- Intracapsular mechanoreceptors exist within structures such as the Cruciate ligaments and Menisci to provide proprioceptive information: ACL contains nerves that communicate proprioceptive input from the lower leg
- ACL is the only one of the four ligaments that is intrasynovial

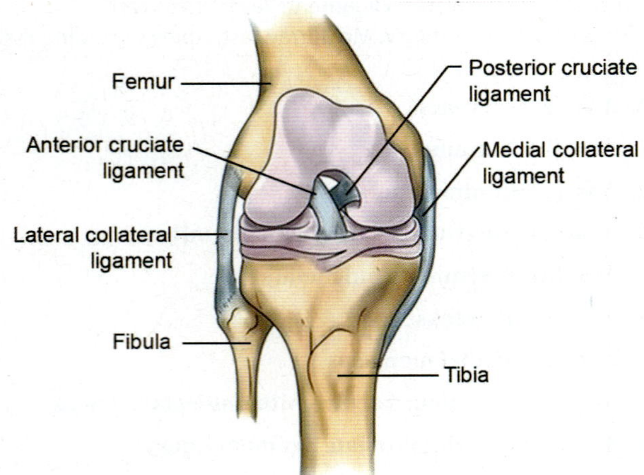

Fig. ACL

45. Ans. (a) Apophysitis of patellar tendon as it inserts in patella

[Ref. Bailey & Love's Surgery, 25/e p461]

Patellar tendinitis (Jumper's Knee)

- An apophysitis (inflammation) of the patellar tendon as it inserts into the patella
- A partial tear of the attachment of the patellar tendon to the lower pole of the patella
- A jumper or sprinter develops pain over the front of the knee
- This settles with rest and then recurs as activity is increased again
- Maximum performance is not possible
- Condition is one of an overload of the patellar tendon and its attachment to patella

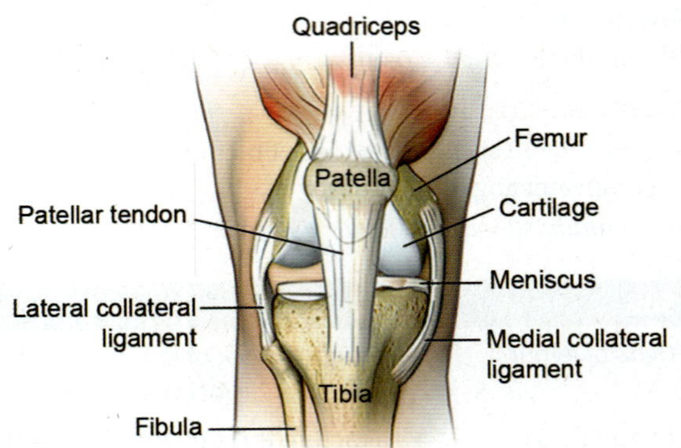

Fig. Patellar tendon

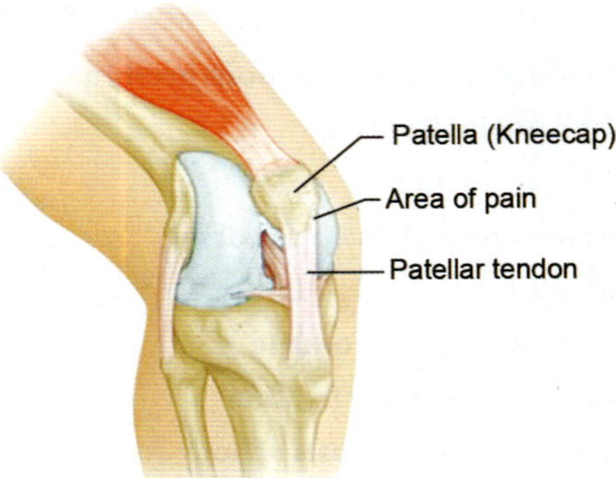

Fig. Patellar tendinitis

46. Ans. (b) It has straight medial border

[Ref. Orthopaedics Examination by Banerjee, 1/e p196]

CTEV SHOES

- Straight medial border
- No heel
- Slight (about 1/8") lateral sole raise
- Inner iron bar
- Outer T-strap
- Open toe

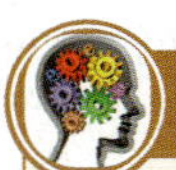

Also Remember

- When inner iron bar and T-strap is absent, it is a CTEV shoe
- When inner bar and T-strap is present, it is a Calliper

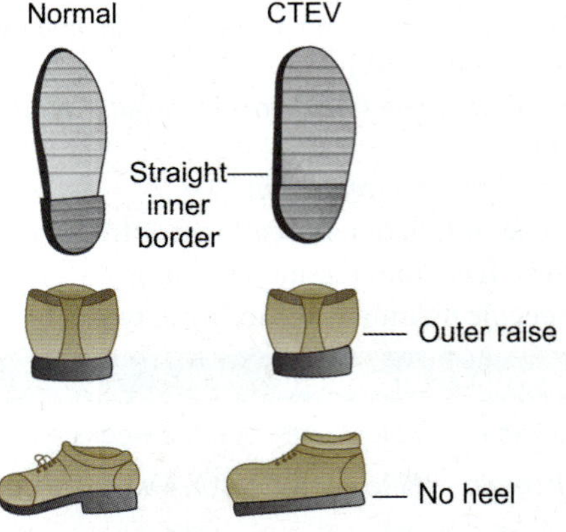

Fig. Normal vs CTEV shoes

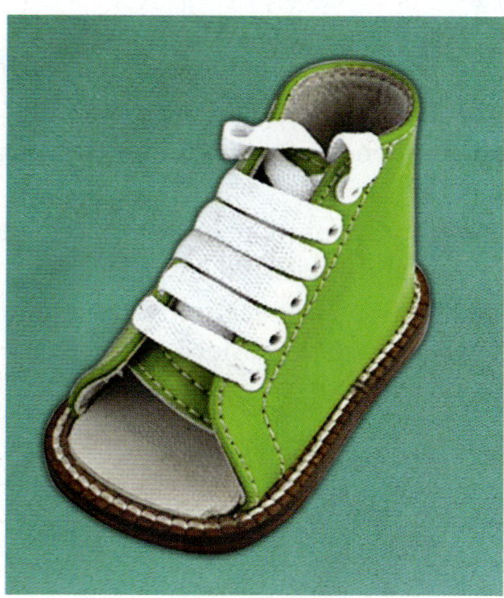

Fig. CTEV shoe

47. Ans. (a) Ortolani's test has two parts
[Ref. Maheshwari, 4/e p214]

Ortolani's Test

- Hips and knee are help in flexed position and gradually abducted
- Ortolani test positive in Congenital dislocation of hip: A 'click of entrance' will be felt as femoral head slips into acetabulum from position of dislocation

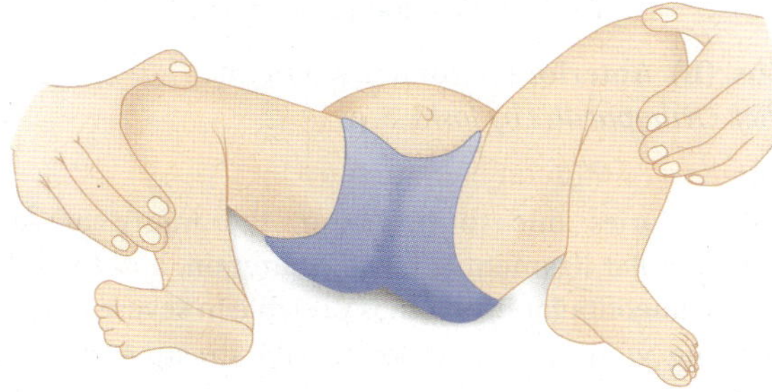

Fig. Ortolani test

48. Ans. (b) Lateral patellar subluxation
[Ref. Orthopedics by Mohindra, 2/e p179]

Quadriceps Angle (Q Angle)

- Q angle is angle subtended between a line drawn from Anterior superior Iliac spine to Centre of patella and a line from Centre of patella to Tibial tubercile
- **Normal Q angle: 14° males, 17° females**
- More is the Q angle (as when Tibial tuberosity is laterally shifted), more would be the lateral pull of the Quadriceps and more unstable would be the Patellofemoral joint
- A higher value predisposes the patient to lateral patellar instability

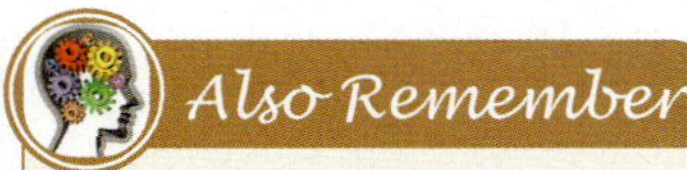

Also Remember

- Predisposing factors for Patellar Dislocation: Genu recurvatum, Patella alta, Increased Q-angle, Atrophy of the vastus medialis, Lateral insertion of the iliotibial tract, Increased internal femoral rotation, Increased femoral anteversion, and Genu valgum

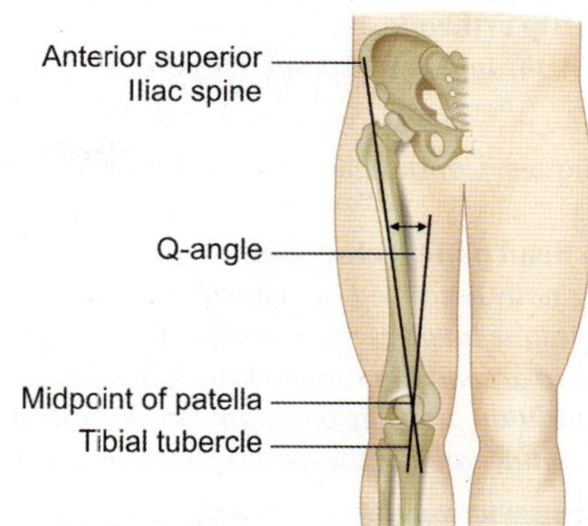

Fig. Q Angle

49. Ans. (b) Occurs more commonly in females
[Ref. Pediatric Radiology by Daldrup-Link, 1/e p134]

Legg-Calvé-Perthes disease

- Idiopathic **Avascular necrosis of the Femoral head**
- Boys are more commonly affected than girls and the peak age of occurrence is between 4 and 8 years age

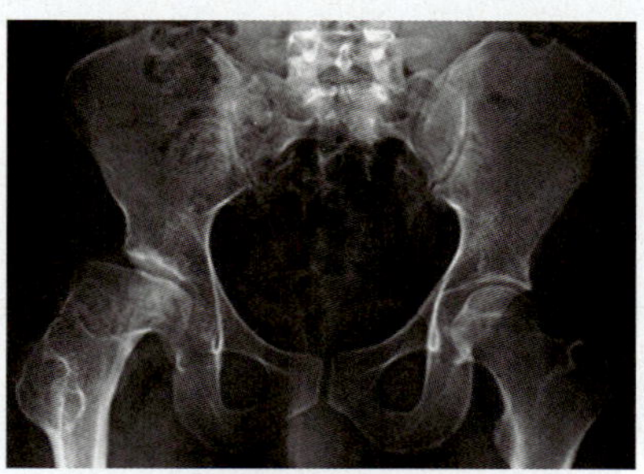

Fig. LCP Disease (Right hip)

50. Ans. (b) Extension is restricted
[Ref. Orthopaedic Examination Made Easy by Varshney, 2/e]

Slipped Capital Femoral Epiphysis (SCFE)

- Obese child, intermittent limp with or without pain
- History of minor trauma followed by typical course
- Shortening
- Attitude of flexion, abduction, external rotation with waddling gait
- Lower gluteal fold on same side
- Restriction of abduction, internal rotation and flexion
- Increased extension, adduction and external rotation
- Increased femoral retroversion
- Increased external rotation with straight leg raising

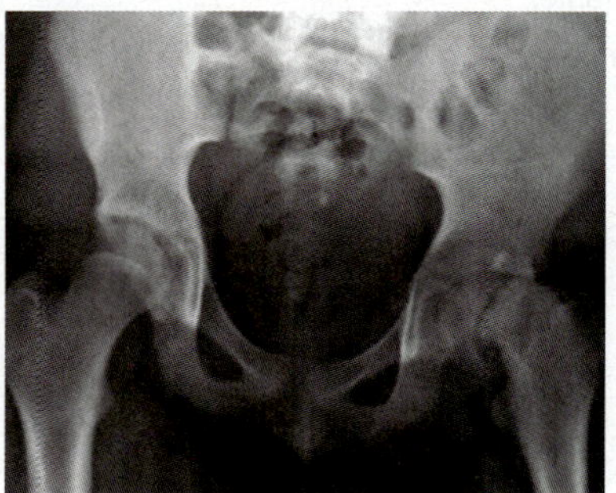

Fig. SCFE (Left hip)

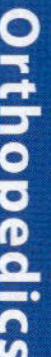

51. Ans. (a) Hip arthrodesis
[Ref. Hip Arthroplasty by Sporer, 1/e p39]

Surgical techniques for Hip Arthrodesis

- Techniques: Cobra head plate, anterior plating, and dual plating
- **Cobra head plate technique:**
  - *Originally described by Schneider*
  - *Technique involves release of the abductors from the iliac crest to accommodate a cobra-shaped plate*
  - *In addition, a pelvic osteotomy is performed to improve the contact area of the femoral head on the pelvis*

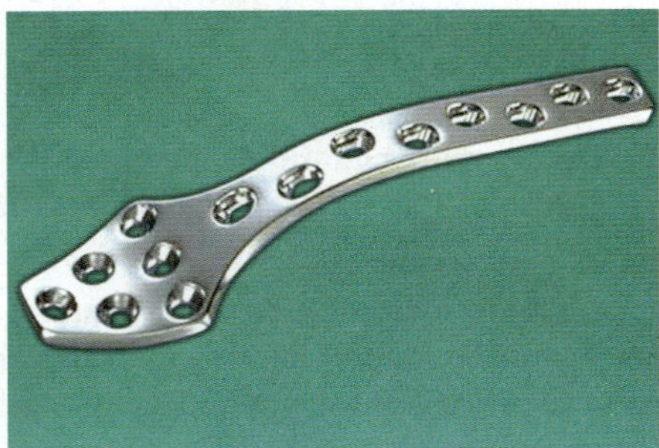

Fig. Cobra head plate

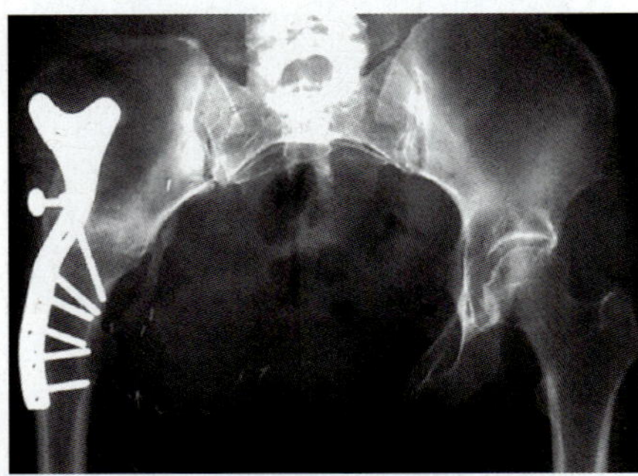

Fig. Hip Arthrodesis

52. Ans. (b) Malunion is common complication
[Ref. Musculoskeletal Imaging by McKinnis, 4/e p384]

- **Intracapsular fractures are especially vulnerable to post-traumatic vascular complications** because of the injury potential of blood vessels in close proximity
- Complications include Avascular necrosis, Non-union, Delayed union

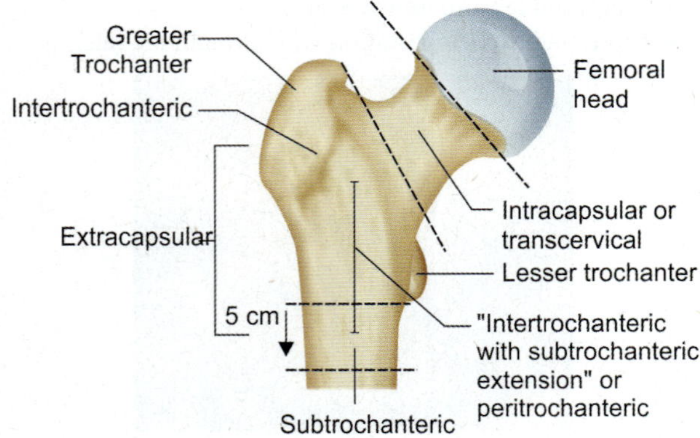

Fig. Hip fractures

53. Ans. (a) Anterior
[Ref. Insall & Scott Surgery of the Knee, 5/e p566]

- **Anterior dislocation is the most common and has the highest frequency of association with popliteal artery injury**
- Anterior dislocations more often result in traction injuries to the vessel and associated intimal tears
- A higher rate of arterial transection injury has been reported with Posterior dislocations

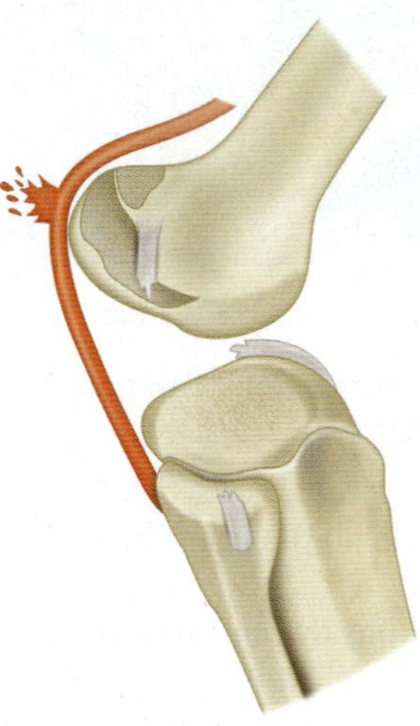

Fig. Anterior knee dislocation

54. Ans. (b) Anterior talofibular ligament
[Ref. Orthopaedics by Joshi, 3/e]

Anterior Talofibular Ligament (ATL)

- In injuries due to Inversion, the injury of Anterior talofibular ligament is mostly common, and the injury of Calcaneofibular ligament is possible in severe cases
- Being vertical and under tensile stress, ATL is usually damaged first
- If the stress continues, ATL tears completely

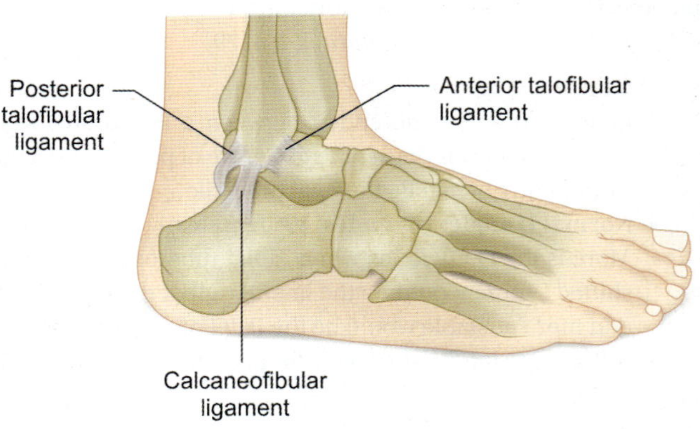

Fig. ATL

55. Ans. (c) Delayed union
[Ref. Orthopedics by Ebnezar, 5/e p256]

- Complications of Tibia Fractures include Delayed union
- This is a common complication and has an incidence of 1–17%

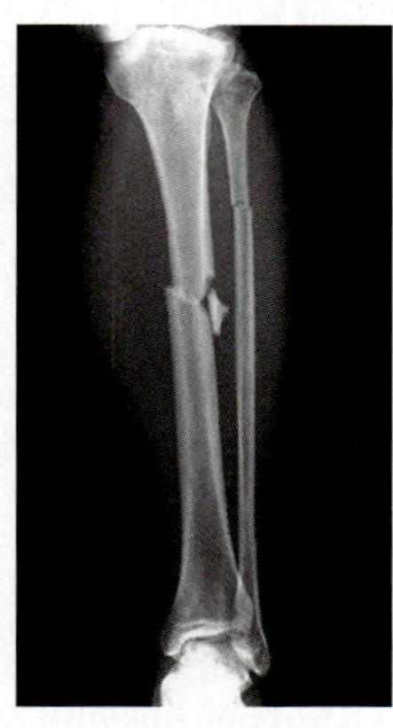

Fig. Tibial fracture

56. Ans. (b) **Sciatic nerve injury**

[Ref. Orthopedic Secrets by Brown, 3/e p296]

- Fractures of the neck of femur are more prone to serious complications than is any other fracture
- **Important complications are Avascular necrosis, Nonunion, and Late osteoarthritis**
- All these complications affect fractures with displacement rather than impacted abduction fractures

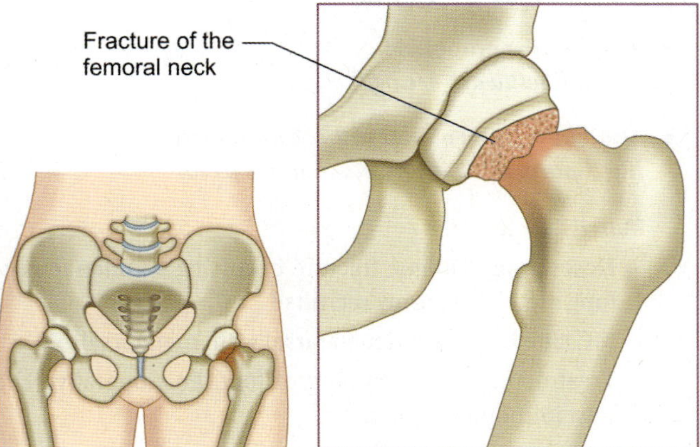

Fig. Fracture neck of femur

57. Ans. (d) **Anterior drawer test is the most sensitive test**

[Ref. Orthopedics by Mohindra, 2/e p503]

- Positive Lachman test is the **Most sensitive test** for ACL injury
- Pivot Shift test is the **Most specific test** for ACL injury

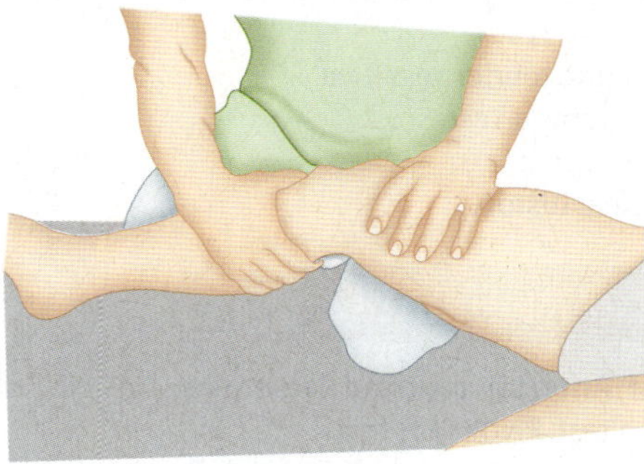

Fig. Lachman test

58. Ans. (b) **Varicose ulcers**

[Ref. Nursing Practice by Rice, 4/e p257]

Unna Boot

- Unna boot is often used to treat venous stasis ulcers
- Medicated dressing or layer compression dressing is used to control edema and to promote healing of poorly vascularized areas of the leg and foot

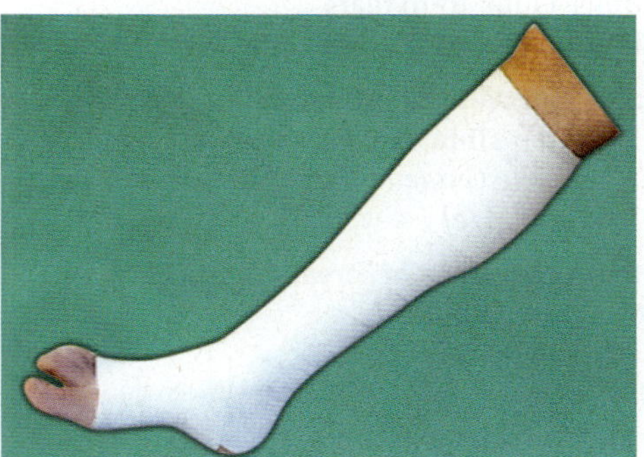

Fig. Unna boot

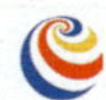

HIGH YIELD MCQs ANSWERS WITH EXPLANATIONS

1. **Ans. (a) Apley's test; (c) McMurray's test; (d) Thessaly test**
   [Ref. Evidence-based Orthopedics by Bhandari, 1/e p104]

Test for Injury of Meniscus Knee Joints
- Thessaly Test
- Joint line tenderness Test
- McMurray's Test
- Apley's Test
- Clinical history

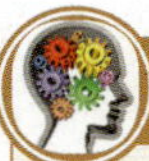

Also Remember

- **Tests of Anterior cruciate Ligament:** Anterior drawer test, Lachman test, Pivot shift test
- **Test of Posterior cruciate ligament:** Posterior drawer test
- **Test of Medial collateral ligament:** Valgus stress test
- **Test of Lateral collateral ligament:** Varus stress test
- **Test of Anterior shoulder dislocation:** Duga's test, Hamilton's ruler test

2. **Ans. (c) Outer area**
   [Ref. Rockwood and Wilkin's Fractures in Children by Kasser, 2/e p907]

Meniscal Repair Indications
- Adults: Outer third tears
- Children and adolescents: Middle third tears

3. **Ans. (a) Second metatarsal; (b) Fifth metatarsal; (d) Tibia; (e) Calcaneum**
   [Ref. Complete Guide to Soccer Fitness and Injury Prevention by Kirkendall, 1/e]

Common Locations of Stress Fractures
- Distal tibia/ fibula
- Calcaneus
- Navicular
- 2nd/ 5th metatarsals

4. **Ans. (b) Smith Petersen Nail**
   [Ref. Maheshwari, 4/e p132]
5. **Ans. (a) Upper third of shaft**
   [Ref. Medical Record, Volume 153, p86]
6. **Ans. (c) Flexion, abduction and external rotation**
   [Ref. Maheshwari, 4/e p136]
7. **Ans. (a) Ilizarov fixator**
   [Ref. Foot and Ankle Disorders by Saunders, 1/e p1141]
8. **Ans. (a) Fracture shaft femur**
   [Ref. Practical Fracture Treatment by Esser, 5/e]
9. **Ans. (c) Fracture will unite normally**
   [Ref. Injury 1977, British Journal of Residual Surgery p127]
   - A Fracture post-polio heals as rapidly as the normal bone
10. **Ans. (c) Tibial epiphyseal injury**
11. **Ans. (b) Laterally; (e) Anteriorly**
12. **Ans. (c) Gallow's traction**
   [Ref. Maheshwari, 4/e p138]
13. **Ans. (a) Hip Spica and if necessary internal fixation**
14. **Ans. (b) Gallow's splint**
   [Ref. Maheshwari, 4/e p138]
15. **Ans. (a) Intramedullary nail fixation**
   [Ref. Textbook of Orthopedic and Trauma by Kulkarni, 2/e p2091]
16. **Ans. (a) A transverse fracture**
   [Ref. Postgraduate Orthopedics by Kador, 2/e p401]
17. **Ans. (d) Compression plating with bone grafting**
   [Ref. Maheshwari, 4/e p139]
18. **Ans. (c) Bone grafting with internal fixation with K-Nail**
   [Ref. Maheshwari, 4/e p139]
19. **Ans. (a) Bone graft with internal fixation**
   [Ref. Maheshwari, 4/e p139]
20. **Ans. (d) Stress fracture**
21. **Ans. (d) Fat Embolism**
   [Ref. Maheshwari, 4/e p42]
22. **Ans. (a) Fat embolism**
   [Ref. Maheshwari, 4/e p42]
23. **Ans. (a) Involves shaft of 2 & 3 metatarsals**
   [Ref. Sports Medicine by Busconi, 1/e p110]

March Fracture
- Description: Fatigue fracture occurring spontaneously in long marches in army recruits
- MC site: Neck of 2nd metatarsal > 4th metatarsal
- Treatment: Rest, Strapping of foot, Post-operative shoe, Cast immobilization

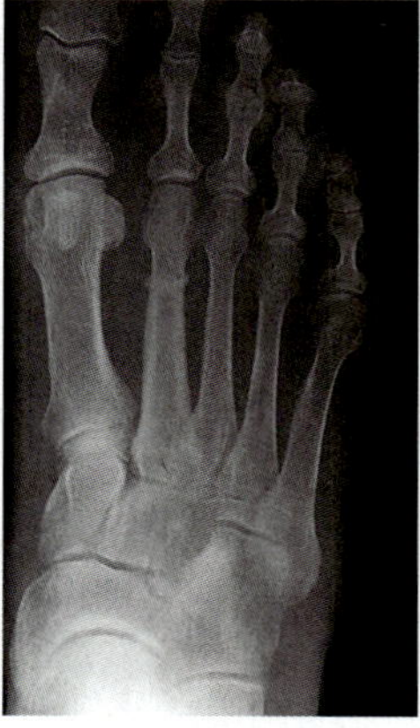

Fig. March fracture

24. **Ans. (b) Cast immobilization**
   [Ref. Manual of Sports Medicine by Stevens, 1/e p476]
25. **Ans. (a) Fracture of 2nd metatarsal**
   [Ref. Sports Medicine by Busconi, 1/e p110]

26. Ans. (d) 4-8 units
[Ref. Orthopedics Quick Review by Mehra, 1/e p22]

27. Ans. (c) Fat embolism
[Ref. Maheshwari, 4/e p42]

28. Ans. (d) Pulmonary Embolectomy
[Ref. Maheshwari, 4/e p42]

Treatment of Fat Embolism Syndrome
- Oxygen
- Steroids
- Heparin, Warfarin, Aspirin
- 5% dextrose with 5% alcohol
- LMW dextran

29. Ans. (d) He should be prepared for surgery and catheterization attempted in the O.T.
[Ref. Maheshwari, 4/e p122]

30. Ans. (c) Pelvis
[Ref. Fractures of Pelvis and Acetabulum by Kellam, 3/e p316]
- ***Suicidal Jumper's fracture*:** U-shaped or H-shaped fracture of upper sacrum with transverse fracture line normally at S1 or S2
  - Type 1: Flexion fracture with anterior bending
  - Type 2: Flexion fracture with posterior displacement
  - Type 3: Extension fracture

31. Ans. (d) Second metatarsal bone
[Ref. Foot and Ankle Injury by Parekh, 1/e p426]
- **Locations that are prone to stress fractures in the athlete:** Distal tibia, *Calcaneus*, Navicular, *Metatarsals*

32. Ans. (b) Metacarpals
[Ref. Foot and Ankle Injury by Parekh, 1/e p426]

33. Ans. (b) Pelvis
[Ref. Emergency radiology by Lucey, 1/e]

Pelvis Ring Injuries
- **Malgaigne injury:** Vertical shear injury resulting in disruption of Ipsilateral anterior and posterior arches
- **Bucket handle injury:** Disruption of Contralateral anterior and posterior arches
- **Open book injury:** Anteroposterior compression leading to Public diastasis along with lateral rotation of hemipelvis due to posterior arch disruption (Sacroiliac diastasis)

34. Ans. (d) Fracture of the iliac bone with sacroiliac disruption
[Ref. Fractures of Pelvis and Acetabulum by Morgan, 1/e p112]
- **Crescent fracture:** Posterior pelvic disruption passing through lower part of Sacroiliac joint, exiting through Ilium

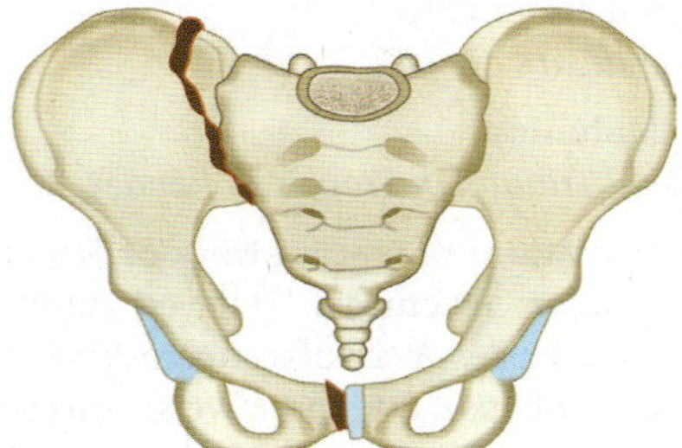

Fig. Crescent fracture

35. Ans. (d) Secondary osteoarthritis of hip joint
[Ref. Maheshwari, 4/e p121]
- **Secondary osteoarthritis** develop late in Acetabular fracture: Due to irregularity of the articular surface following injury

36. Ans. (d) Ischial tuberosities
[Ref. Maheshwari, 4/e p120]
- **Types of Type-A fractures of Pelvis:**
  - Ischio-pubic rami fractures
  - Iliac wing fractures
  - Avulsion fracture of Anterior inferior iliac spine
  - Acetabular fracture

37. Ans. (d) Morel-Lavallee lesion
[Ref. Bones and Joint Surgeries by Uranues, 1/e p218]

38. Ans. (d) Morel-Lavallee lesion
[Ref. Bones and Joint Surgeries by Uranues, 1/e p218]

Acetubular Fractures Management

Kocher-Langenbeck approach	Ilioinguinal approach
Posterior wall	Anterior wall
Posterior column	Anterior column
Transverse	Anterior column +
Posterior column + Posterior wall	Posterior hemitracts
Transverse + Posterior wall	Both columns
T-type	

39. Ans. (c) Superior exposure is very adequate
[Ref. Orthopedics Quick review by Mehra, 1/e p120]

40. Ans. (d) Retinacular branches of circumflex femoral arteries
[Ref. Instant Anatomy by Singh, 2/e p192]

Arterial Supply of Femoral Head
- Artery of head of femur (Ascending branch of Medial circumflex femoral artery)
- Nutrient artery (2nd perforating branch of Profunda femoris artery)
- Retinacular arteries: Most important source (Medial and lateral circumflex femoral arteries)

41. Ans. (c) Fracture neck of femur
[Ref. Maheshwari, 4/e p129]

Classification In Fracture Neck of Femur
- Anatomical classification: Based on Anatomical location of fracture (Subcapital, Transcervical, Basal)
- **Pauwel's classification:** Based on angle of inclination of fracture to horizontal plane (Type I 30 degrees, Type II 50 degrees, Type III 70 degrees)
  - More the angle, more the displacement, worse the prognosis

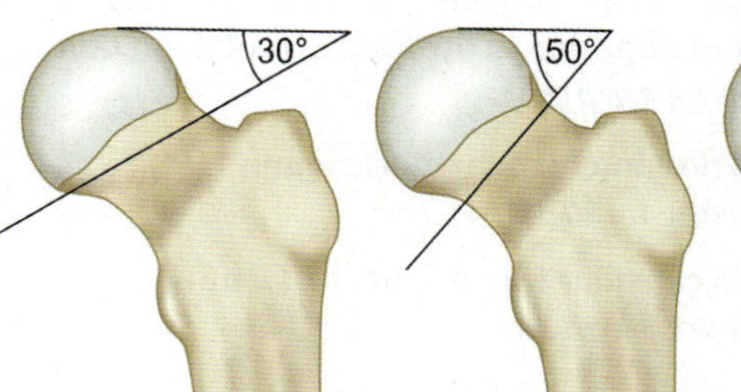

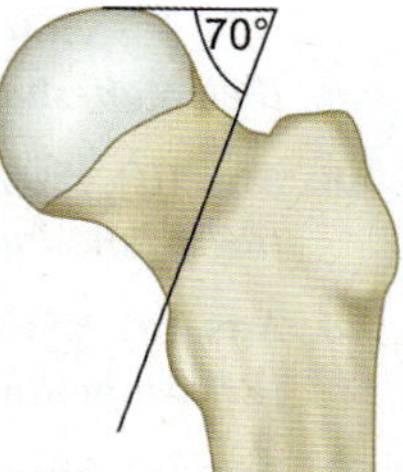

Fig. Pauwel's fracture

- **Garden's classification:** Based on degree of displacement of fracture and trabecular alignment (Acetabulum, Head, Neck trabeculae)

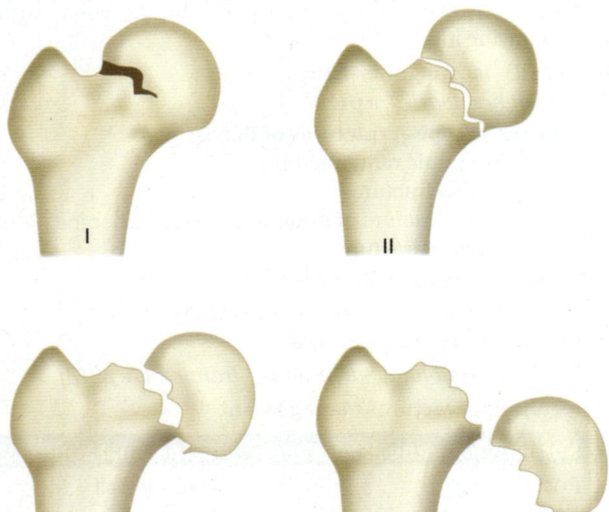

Fig. Garden's classification

Stage	Fracture	Trabeculae alignment
Stage 1	Incomplete (Valgus impacted fractures)	Bending only
Stage 2	Complete but undisplaced	Break in trabeculae with little angulation
Stage 3	Complete and partially displaced	All 3 sets of trabeculae out of alignment
Stage 4	Complete and fully displaced	Acetabular and head trabeculae in alignment

42. Ans. (b) Stage II
[Ref. Maheshwari, 4/e p129]

43. Ans. (c) More chances of displacement
[Ref. Maheshwari, 4/e p129]

44. Ans. (a) Intra capsular fracture neck of femur
[Ref. Maheshwari, 4/e p130]

45. Ans. (a) Neck of femur fracture
[Ref. Maheshwari, 4/e p130]

46. Ans. (b) Extracapsular fracture
[Ref. Maheshwari, 4/e p130]

47. Ans. (c) It can occur in young adults following severe violence applied in the long axis of the femur
[Ref. Maheshwari, 4/e p130]

48. Ans. (b) Fracture inter trochanteric femur
[Ref. Maheshwari, 4/e p134]

49. Ans. (a) Extra capsular fracture neck of femur
[Ref. Maheshwari, 4/e p130]

50. Ans. (c) Shortening and lateral rotation
[Ref. Maheshwari, 4/e p130]

Parameter	Fracture neck of femur	Inter-trochanteric fracture
Age/ Sex	>50 years	>60 years
Injury	Trivial	Significant
Ability to walk	May walk	Not possible
Pain	Mild	Severe
Swelling/ Ecchymosis	Absent	Severe
Tenderness	**In Scarpa's triangle**	**On Greater trochanter**
External rotation	<45 degrees	>45 degrees
Shortening	<1 inch	>1 inch
Treatment	Internal fixation	Traction
Complications	Non-union	Malunion

51. Ans. (b) MRI
[Ref. Skeletal Trauma by Jupiter, 5/e p1634]

Occult Femoral Neck Fractures

- MRI: 100% sensitivity for diagnosis of Hip fractures
- Technetium MDP scan: Good test but become positive after 2–3 days of fracture

52. Ans. (d) Stress at fracture site due to muscle spasm
[Ref. Maheshwari, 4/e p133]

53. Ans. (a) Malunion
[Ref. Maheshwari, 4/e p135]

54. Ans. (c) Malunion
[Ref. Maheshwari, 4/e p130]

55. Ans. (d) Fat embolism
[Ref. Maheshwari, 4/e p42]

56. Ans. (a) Avascular necrosis
[Ref. Hip Disorders in Children by Ratliff, 1/e p170]

57. Ans. (b) Transcervical
[Ref. Manual of Internal Fixation by Perren, 3/e p522]

- Transcervical neck fractures have a higher rate of Avascular necrosis than Subcapital "impacted" fractures

58. Ans. (c) Subcapital region
[Ref. Manual of Internal Fixation by Perren, 3/e p522]

59. Ans. (c) Non union
[Ref. Postmenopausal Osteoporosis by Meeta, 1/e p234]

60. All choices
[Ref. Smart Study Series Orthopedics by Rohilla, 1/e p124]

61. Ans. (a) Fat embolism
[Ref. Maheshwari, 4/e p42]

62. Ans. (b) Malunion
[Ref. Skeletal Trauma in Tropics by Pandey, 2/e p531]

Main Complications of Fractue Neck of Femur

- **Intracapsular fractures:** Delayed union, Nonunion, Fixation collapse, Avascular necrosis of femoral head, Segmental collapse, Degenerative arthrosis of hip
- **Extracapsular fractures:** Malunion, More systemic complications, More implant failure

63. Ans. (d) Hemireplacement arthroplasty
[Ref. Maheshwari, 4/e p131]

Treatment of Fracture Neck of Femur (<3 Weeks Old)

- Undisplaced fracture: Conservative, Multiple screws
- Displaced fracture physiologically less than 60 years age: Closed reduction under X-ray control
  - Reduction possible: Multiple screw fixation
  - Reduction not possible: Open reduction and Screw fixation
- Displaced fracture physiologically more than 60 years age: Prosthetic replacement
  - With otherwise normal hip: Hemi-arthroplasty
  - With pre-existing arthritis: Total hip replacement

Treatment of Fracture Neck of Femur (>3 Weeks Old)

- Patients aged more than 60 years: Replacement arthroplasty
- Patients aged less than 60 years:
  - If head is Vascular on MRI: Osteotomy (McMurray/ Pauwel's) or Reconstruction procedures (Meyer's operation)
  - If head is not Vascular on MRI: Bipolar prosthesis

64. Ans. (d) CR & IF
[Ref. Maheshwari, 4/e p131]

65. Ans. (a) Most common cause is child abuse; (b) Sclera must be examined; (d) Heals quite rapidly
[Ref. Maheshwari, 4/e p136]

66. Ans. (b) Closed reduction and Internal fixation by cancellous screws
[Ref. Maheshwari, 4/e p131]

67. Ans. (b) Closed reduction and internal fixation by cannulated cancellous screws
[Ref. Maheshwari, 4/e p133]

68. Ans. (c) Hemiarthroplasty
[Ref. Maheshwari, 4/e p131]

69. Ans. (d) Gallow's splint
[Ref. Maheshwari, 4/e p138]

70. Ans. (c) Internal fixation with bone graft
[Ref. Maheshwari, 4/e p139]

71. Ans. (d) Reduction of fracture and multiple pin or screw fixation
[Ref. Maheshwari, 4/e p131]

72. Ans. (d) Untreated femoral neck fracture in a patient over 65 years

73. Ans. (d) 65 years old male with non united fracture neck of femur

74. Ans. (b) Causes internal rotation of the leg
[Ref. Maheshwari, 4/e p130]

75. Ans. (a) Dynamic hip screw
[Ref. Maheshwari, 4/e p135]

Treatment of Intertrochanteric Fractures

- Conservative methods: Russell's traction, Skeletal traction in Thomas splint
- Operative methods: Dynamic hip screw, Ender's nails, Gamma nail, Proximal femoral nail, External fixation (if bed sores)

76. Ans. (b) Subcapital fracture neck femur

77. Ans. (d) Fracture neck of femur
[Ref. Maheshwari, 4/e p133]

Meyer's Procedure

- Indications:
  - Late presentations
  - Significant comminution
  - Non-union of femoral neck fractures
- Procedure:
  - Fracture reduced by exposing from behind
  - Fixed with multiple screws
  - Supplemented with Vascularized muscle-pedicle bone graft (Femoral attachment of Quadratus femoris muscle)

78. Ans. (b) Spica in abduction + internal rotation

79. Ans. (d) C.C. screw

80. Ans. (b) Distal fragment
[Ref. Gray's Anatomy Review by Abrahams, 2/e]

81. Ans. (d) Open reduction with Kirschner wire fixation of the fragment and tension band wiring
[Ref. Maheshwari, 4/e p142]

Treatment of Patellar Fractures

- **Undisplaced fracture:** Cylinder cast (knee in full extension for 3 weeks), Physiotherapy
- **Clean break with Separation of fragments:** Reduction of fragments, Tension band wiring, Repair of extensor retinaculae
  - If accurate reduction not possible, the Partial or Total patellectomy
- **Comminuted fracture:** Patellectomy (Excision of patella)

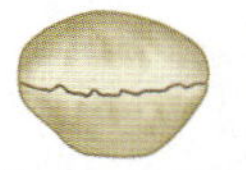

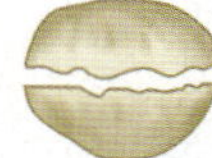

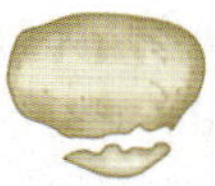

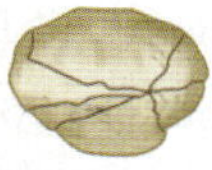

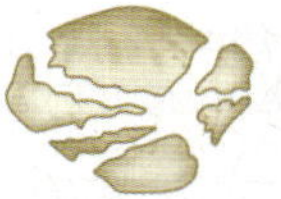

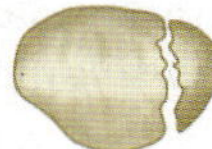

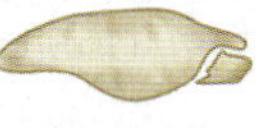

Fig. Patellar fractures

82. Ans. (b) Posterior dislocation is common
[Ref. Oxford's Handbook of Emergency Medicine by Graham, 4/e p468]

83. Ans. (c) Removal of all the patella
[Ref. Maheshwari, 4/e p142]

84. Ans. (b) Tension band wiring; (d) Patellectomy
[Ref. Maheshwari, 4/e p142]

85. Ans. (a) 5
[Ref. Handbook of Fractures by Egol, 4/e p471]

86. Ans. (a) Common peroneal nerve
[Ref. Clinical Neuropsychology by Misra, 2/e p80]

87. Ans. (a) Secure airway and treat the shock
[Ref. Trauma Manual by Rhodes, 4/e p254]

88. Ans. (b) Tibia
[Ref. Rockwood and Green's Fractures in Adults, Volume 1, 7/e p154]

- **Non-operative management of Tibial diaphysis:** Long leg cast, Patellar tendon bearing cast, Brace at 6-8 weeks

89. Ans. (a) Anterior talo-fibular ligament
[Ref. Functional Reconstruction of Foot and Ankle by Hansen, 1/e p43]

90. Ans. (b) Avascular necrosis
[Ref. Essentials of Skeletal Radiology by Rowe, 3/e p881]

91. Ans. (d) Fracture of vertebrae
[Ref. Emergency medicine by Adams, 2/e]

92. Ans. (c) Fibula

93. Ans. (d) Metatarsals
[Ref. Orthopedics for Physical Therapist Assistant by Dutton, 1/e p589]

94. Ans. (d) Do operative decompression of fascial compartment
[Ref. Maheshwari, 4/e p46]

Treatment of Compartment Syndrome

- Preventive measures: Limb elevation, Active finger movements
- Early surgical decompression:
  - Fasciotomy
  - Fibulectomy

95. Ans. (c) Normal sensation distally
[Ref. Maheshwari, 4/e p46]

96. Ans. (c) Toe dorsiflexion
[Ref. PGEE by Rohilla, 2008 p223]

97. Ans. (b) Right side

98. Ans. (b) Anterior component
[Ref. Adult Orthopedic Nursing by Schoen, 1/e p361]

99. Ans. (a) Rupture of anterior talo-fibular ligament
[Ref. Adult Orthopedic Nursing by Schoen, 1/e p361]

100. Ans. (a) Grade I
[Ref. Rockwood and Green's Fractures in Children by Kasser, 7/e p946]

Classification of Open Fractures

Grade I	Grade II
Low energy wound, <1 cm length Bone piercing skin from in/out Minimum muscle damage	Wound >1 cm length Moderate soft tissue injury

Contd...

Contd...

Grade III	Special cases
High energy wound >10 cms length Extensive muscle devitalization Bone widely displaced/ comminuted	Shotgun wound High speed gun shot Segmental fracture/ diaphyseal loss Associated vascular injury Farmyard environment

101. Ans. (b) Grade II
[Ref. Rockwood and Green's Fractures in Children by Kasser, 7/e p946]

102. Ans. (c) Sprain of Extensor digitorum brevis

103. Ans. (a) Abduction injury
[Ref. Radiology Review Manual by Dahnert, 7/e p96]

104. Ans. (b) Thorough debridement
[Ref. Textbook of Orthopedics by Kotwal, 1/e p321]

Treatment of Compound Tibial Fracture

- Thorough debridement of wound
- Stabilization of fracture by external fixation device
- Restoration of soft tissue cover by skin grafts/ flap

105. Ans. (b) Potts's fracture
[Ref. Maheshwari, 4/e p3]

106. Ans. (b) Lower end of tibia + fibula
[Ref. Maheshwari, 4/e p3]

107. Ans. (d) Fracture talus
[Ref. Essentials of Orthophysiotherapy for Upper and Lower Limb Fractures by Garg, 1/e p161]

Management of Fracture Talus

Type	Description	Management
Type I	Undisplaced	Short leg cast/ boot for 2–3 months
Type II	Subluxation-dislocation of Subtalar joint	Closed reduction, Plaster cast in Equinus position
Type III	Displaced with Subluxation-dislocation of Subtalar/ ankle joint	ORIF with leg screws
Type IV	Type III with Subluxation/ dislocation of Talonavicular joint	Debridement with Closed reduction, OR ORIF with K-wires, Leg screws

108. Ans. (a) Avascular necrosis
[Ref. Atlas Foot and Ankle Surgery by Wulker, 2/e p269]

109. Ans. (a) Osteoarthritis of ankle; (c) A vascular necrosis of body of talus; (e) Non union
[Ref. Maheshwari, 4/e p160]

110. Ans. (b) Increased
[Ref. Post Graduate Orthopedics by Ram, 1/e p138]

111. Ans. (a) Calcaneum
[Ref. Handbook of Foot and Ankle Surgery by Gould, 1/e p344]

112. Ans. (a) Type of fracture; (b) Subtalar joint dislocation; (c) Duration of presentation; (d) Degree of displacement

113. Ans. (a) Anterior cruciate ligament

[Ref. Articular Ligaments Acton, 2012 p9]

114. Ans. (c) Flexion and rotation movement

[Ref. Anatomy at a Glance by, 3/e p125]

115. Ans. (c) Menisci

[Ref. Adult Orthopedic Nursing by Schoen, 1/e p320]

- Bucket handle tear injury: Longitudinal tear of menisci when Femur and tibia trap it while knee is turning

116. Ans. (b) Lisfranc amputation

[Ref. Mann's Surgery of Foot and Ankle by Saltzman, 9/e p1495]

117. Ans. (c) Chronic osteomyelitis

[Ref. Undergraduate Surgery by Nan, 3/e p206]

Indications of Amputation

- Congenital: Supernumerary digits
- Traumatic: Grossly injured limb (Most common indication), Grossly lacerated gunshot wounds, Gas gangrene, Incarcerated limb, Charred limb, Uncontrollable secondary severe hemorrhage
- Vascular: Gangrene resulting from Buerger's disease, Arteriosclerotic disease, Diabetic gangrene, Embolism gangrene
- Infective: Acute osteomyelitis, Acute suppurative arthritis, Diabetic cellulitis, Madura foot, Chronic osteomyelitis (rare)
- Neoplastic tumours: Mesodermal origin (Osteosarcoma)
- Paralytic

118. Ans. (c) Arthroscopy

[Ref. Musculoskeletal Imaging by Pope, 1/e p405]

119. Ans. (a) Anterior talo-fibular

[Ref. Adult Orthopedic Nursing by Schoen, 1/e p361]

120. Ans. (a) Neutral

[Ref. First Aid and Emergency Management in Orthopedic Injuries by Dhillon, 1/e p21]

121. Ans. (d) Perianal stimulation

[Ref. PMR Board Review by Sara, 3/e p569]

122. Ans. (a) Lachman test; (c) Anterior drawer test

[Ref. Maheshwari, 4/e p356]

123. Ans. (a) Cruciate ligament injury

[Ref. Maheshwari, 4/e p356]

124. Ans. (a) Caisson's disease; (b) Sickle cell anaemia; (e) Intra-capsular fracture neck

[Ref. Diagnostic Imaging of Musculoskeletal Diseases by Khurana, 1/e p100]

125. Ans. (a) Walk downhill

[Ref. Smart Study Series Orthopedics by Rohilla, p101]

126. Ans. (c) Prevents posterior dislocation of tibia

127. Ans. (d) Fibular collateral ligament

[Ref. Smart Study Series Orthopedics by Rohilla, p102]

128. Ans. (d) Tibial collateral ligament

[Ref. Conservative Management of Sports Injuries by Hyde, 2/e p109]

129. Ans. (b) Rotation on a flexed knee

[Ref. Massage and Remedial Exercises by Tidy, 1/e p57]

130. Ans. (c) Flexion and rotation movement

[Ref. Techniques in Musculoskeletal Rehabilitation by Prentice, 1/e p545]

131. Ans. (b) Loose body in knee joint; (d) Medial meniscal partial tear

[Ref. SRB's Clinical Methods in Surgery by Bhat, 1/e p734]

132. Ans. (b) Meniscal tear

[Ref. Massage and Remedial Exercises by Tidy, 1/e p57]

133. Ans. (e) All of the above are correct

[Ref. Massage and Remedial Exercises by Tidy, 1/e p57]

134. Ans. (c) Lateral part of meniscus

[Ref. Netter's Collections of Medical illustrations by Parker, 2/e p140]

135. Ans. (a) Excessive forward glide

[Ref. Maheshwari, 4/e p146]

136. Ans. (a) Medial meniscus tear

[Ref. Maheshwari, 4/e p146]

137. Ans. (d) Arthroscopy

[Ref. Oxford's Handbook of Emergency Medicine by Graham, 4/e p434]

138. Ans. (a) Popliteal artery injury

[Ref. Surgery: A Case Based Clinical Review by Frank, 1/e p437]

139. Ans. All Choices

[Ref. Emergency Orthopedics by Sherman, 6/e p72]

140. Ans. (a) Inversion of foot

[Ref. Adult Orthopedic Nursing by Schoen, 1/e p361]

141. Ans. (a) Overuse

[Ref. Surgical Techniques in Sports Medicine by Neal, 1/e p647]

142. Ans. (d) Osteochondral defect of femur

[Ref. Cartilage Restoration by Gomoll, 1/e p44]

143. Ans. All Choices

[Ref. Surgical Techniques in Total Knee Arthroplasty and Alternative Procedures by Saverio, 1/e p6]

144. Ans. (a) Osteoarthritis of hip; (b) Ankylosis of elbow; (d) Ununited femoral neck fracture

[Ref. Best Orthopedics by Pramod, 1/e p100]

Indications and Contraindications of Arthroplasty

Indications	Contraindications
• Osteoarthritis of hip, knee • Ankylosis of elbow • Ununited femoral neck	• Sepsis of joint • Vascular insufficiency • Osteomyelitis • Neuropathic joint • Severe obesity • Previous surgery of joint • Well-functioning arthrodesis

145. Ans. (d) Thromboembolism

[Ref. Orthopedic Secrets by Brown, 3/e p34]

Thromboembolic Disease after Total Hip Arthroplasty

- Most common serious complication
- MCC of death within 3 months after surgery
- Cause >50% mortality

146. Ans. (d) Dunlop

[Ref. Pediatric Orthopedics by Staheli, 2/e p66]

- Dunlop traction is used for Supracondylar humeral fractures

147. Ans. (c) MRI

[Ref. Skeletal Trauma by Jupiter, 5/e p1634]

- Coronal MRI scan show a hip fracture with 100% sensitivity and is the best sequence to diagnose occult hip fracture

148. Ans. (c) Meniscus

[Ref. Knee Pain and Disability by Davis, 1/e p87]

- McMurray test, used to assess meniscal integrity, is performed with the patient supine and the examiner standing on the side of the affected knee
- To test the integrity of the medial meniscus, the physician "internally" rotates the lower leg on the femur and slowly extends the leg while internal rotation is maintained: A pop/ snap suggests Meniscal tear

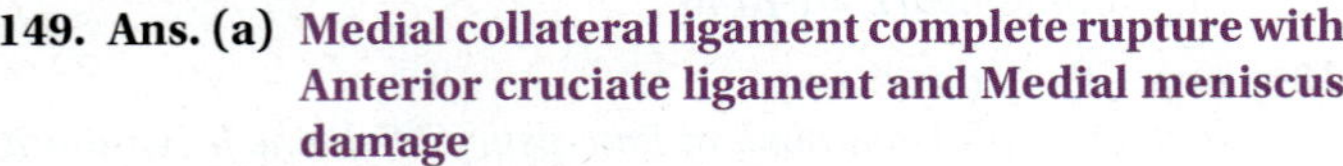

149. Ans. (a) Medial collateral ligament complete rupture with Anterior cruciate ligament and Medial meniscus damage

[Ref. Meniscus by Beaufils, 1/e p49]

- **Unhappy/Terrible/O'Donoghue's triad (Horrible triangle/Blown knee):** An injury to the anterior cruciate ligament, medial collateral ligament, and the medial meniscus

150. Ans. (b) Neck

[Ref. Churchill's Pocketbook of Surgery, 4/e]

March Fracture

- Stress fracture
- Usually affects the Second metatarsal neck
- Caused by stress of long hours of walking

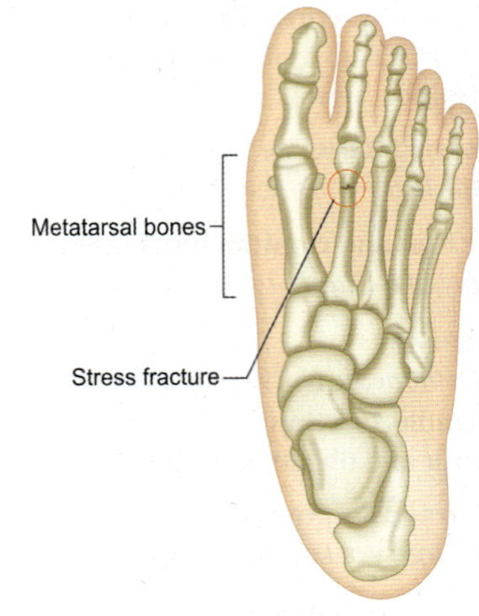

Fig. March fracture

151. Ans. (c) Open fractures with extensive soft tissue injury loss with periosteal stripping and bone exposure, usually associated with massive contamination

[Ref. Oxford Desk Reference - Major Trauma, 1/e p254]

Gustilo and Anderson Classification of Open Fractures

- Type I: Open fracture with a wound < 1 cm long and clean
- Type II: Open fracture with a laceration > 1 cm long without extensive soft tissue damage, flaps, or avulsions
- Type III: Either an open segmental fracture, an open fracture with extensive soft tissue damage (Laceration >10 cm), or a traumatic amputation
  - Type IIIA: Open fractures with adequate soft tissue coverage of a fractured bone despite extensive soft tissue laceration or flaps, or high-energy trauma regardless of the size of the wound
  - Type IIIB: Open fractures with extensive soft tissue injury loss with periosteal stripping and bone exposure, usually associated with massive contamination
  - Type IIIC: Open fractures associated with arterial injury requiring repair

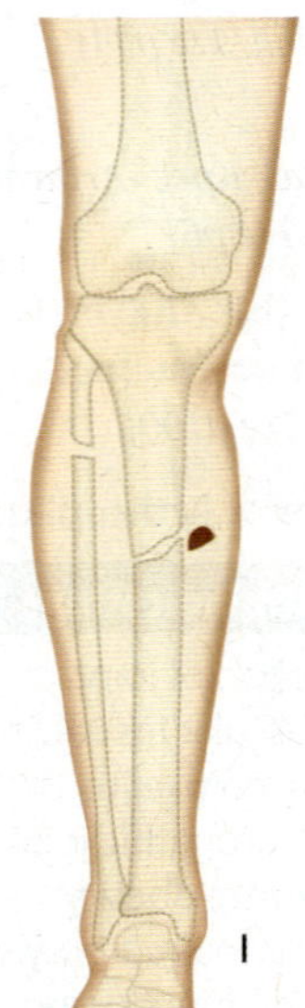

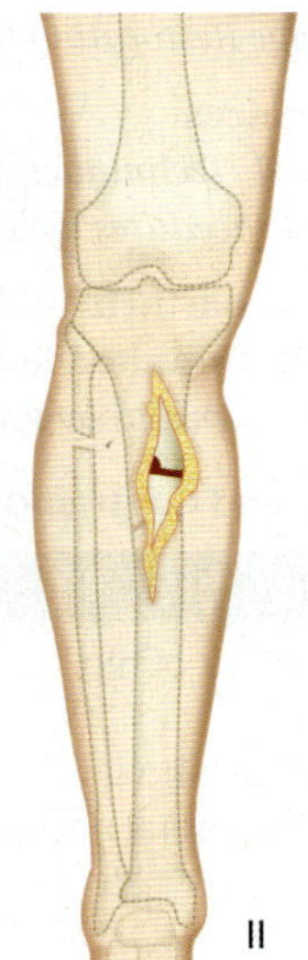

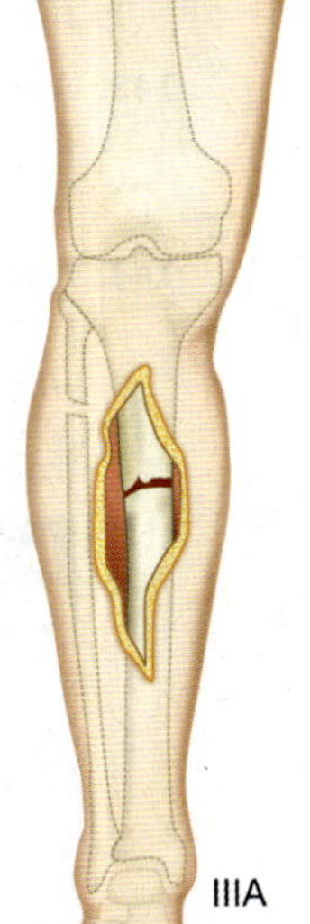

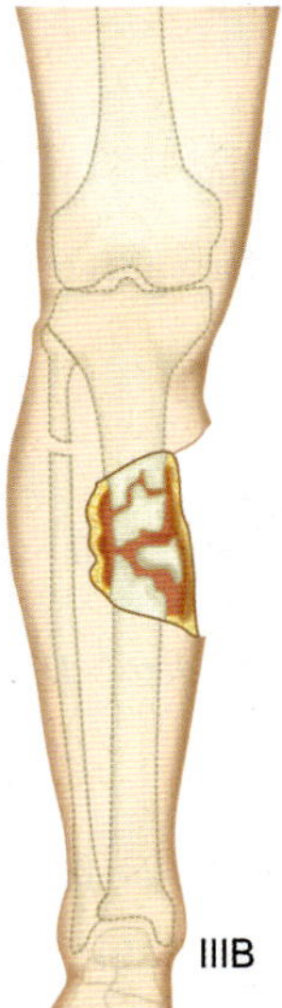

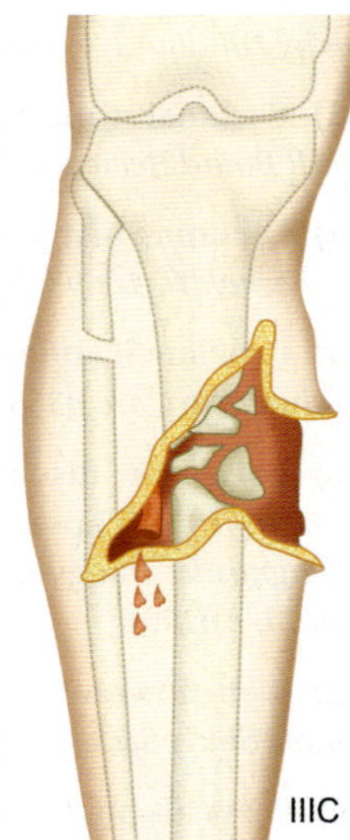

Fig. Gustilo and Anderson classification

152. Ans. (c) AVN hip

[Ref. Early Hip Disorders by McCarthy, 1/e p12]

- Primary cause of Avascular necrosis (AVN) of the femoral head after Direct hip trauma is an interruption of the arterial supply to the femoral head secondary to the injury
- One of the most recognized causes of AVN is long-term steroid use or alcohol use
- Other medical conditions that have been linked to avascular necrosis include connective tissue disease, vasculitis, long-term ethanol use, and trauma

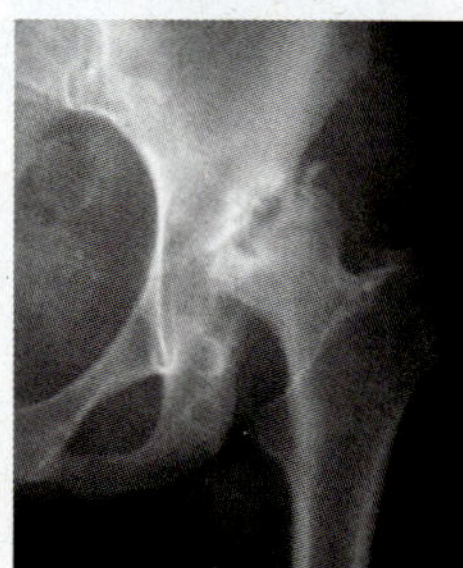

Fig. AVN hip

Chapter 5

Head, Neck, Trunk and Polytraumatology

THEORETICAL CONCEPTS

V A. SKULL FRACTURES

- ***Linear skull fracture*:** Traverse full thickness from outer to inner table
  - *Common mode of injury:* Blunt force trauma
  - *Depressed skull fracture*: Comminuted fractures with displaced bones[Q]
    - Compound type: Over a laceration
    - Complex type: Dura mater torn
    - May require surgery to lift bones if putting pressure on brain
- ***Diastatic skull fracture*:** Fracture line traverses one or more sutures[Q]
- ***Basilar skull fracture*:** Breaks in bones at base of skull **(MC involved: Temporal bone[Q])**
  - Battle's sign: Bruising over mastoid[Q]
  - Racoon's eyes: Bruising of orbits of eyes[Q]
  - CSF rhinorrhoea/Otorrhoea
  - Bleeding from nose and ears
  - Hemotympanum
  - Deafness, Nystagmus, Vomitus
  - Cranial nerve palsy (Facial/oculomotor/vestibule-cochlear): Bilateral facial nerve palsy is rare
- ***Growing skull fracture*:** Cystic mass filled with CSF
  - Usually involves parietal bones in children
- ***Compound skull fracture*:** Overlying laceration tears epidermis and meninges or runs through paranasal sinuses/middle ear structures
  - Most common complication: Infection[Q]
- ***Compound elevated skull fracture*:** Fractured bone is elevated above outer table of skull

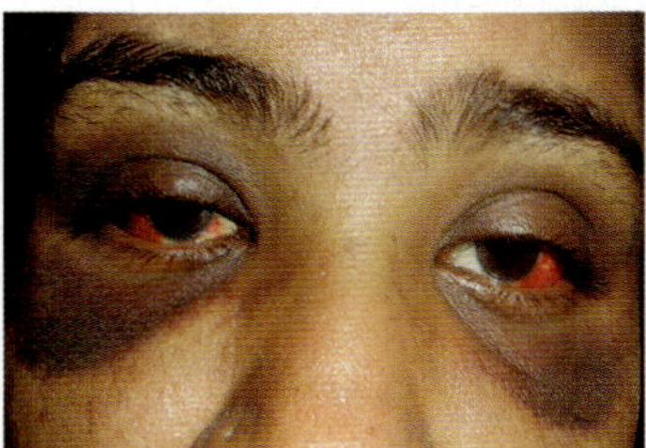

Fig. Racoon eyes

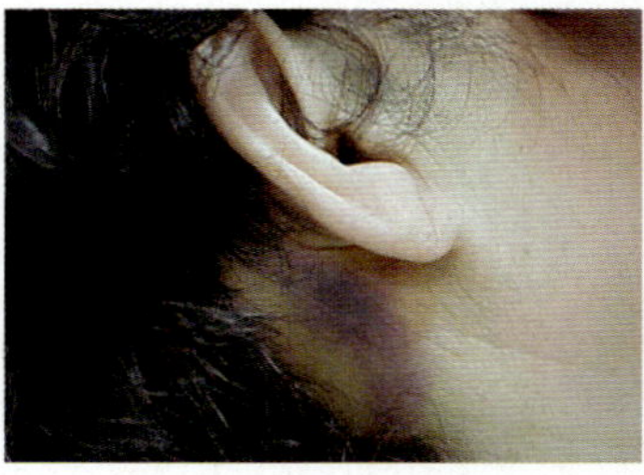

Fig. Battle sign

V B. LE FORT CLASSIFICATION OF MAXILLARY FRACTURES (TOP TO BOTTOM)

- **Le Fort I fracture:** Separates alveolus and palate from facial skeleton above
- **Le Fort II (pyramidal) fracture:** Involves orbital floor, bridge of nose, ethmoids, cribriform plate (leads to CSF rhinorrhea)
- **Le Fort III fracture:** Separates facial skeleton from base of skull (runs through nasal bridge, septum, ethmoids; may lead to CSF rhinorrhea)

I II III

V C. SPINAL INJURIES

Injury mechanism	Injury type	Common site
Flexion injury[Q]	**Compression fracture**	**L1, L2**
Flexion-rotation injury	Fracture dislocation	L1, D12
Vertical compression injury	Burst fracture	C5-C6
Extension injury[Q]	**Avulsion fracture**	**C5-C6**
Flexion distraction injury	Chance fracture	Dorsal spine
Direct injury	Fracture spinous/ transverse process	Any part

- ***MC spinal injury*:** Flexion injury
- ***Worst type of spinal injury*:** Flexion-rotation injury
- *Level of spinal injuries and effects*[Q]:

Level of injury	Muscles paralysed
Transection above C5	All respiratory muscles
C5 segment	Upper limbs, thorax, trunk, lower limbs
Below C5 segment	Thorax, trunk, lower limbs
D1-D10	Trunk, Lower limb
D10	Lower limb
D11-L1	Lower limb
Below L1	Flaccid paralysis, sensory loss, autonomic disturbances

Topper's Edge

Spinal Fractures

- **Jefferson fracture**[Q]**:** Burst fracture of C1 with fracture of anterior and posterior arches of C1 vertebra
- **Hangman's fracture**[Q]**:** Fracture pedicle-lamina of C2 vertebra
- **Clay-Shoveler's fracture**[Q]**:** Spinous process fracture of C6, C7 or T1
- **Anderson & D'Alonzo classification:** Odontoid process fracture
- McAfee's classification: Thoracolumbar fractures

IMAGE-BASED QUESTIONS

1. **Mechanism of Spine injury shown in Photograph is**

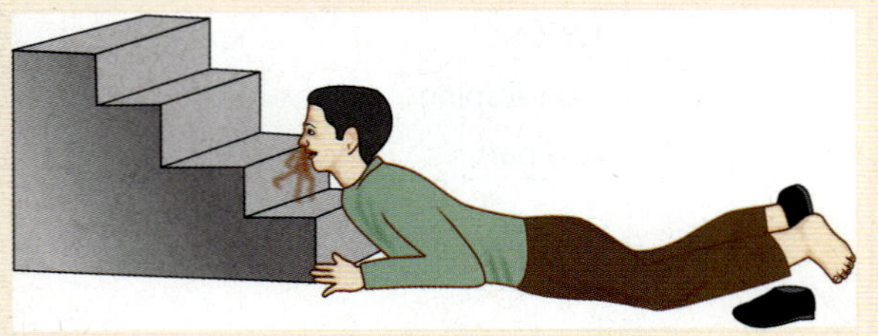

   a. Flexion extension injury
   b. Hyperextension injury
   c. Flexion rotation injury
   d. Flexion injury

2. **Identify the Fracture shown in Photograph** ***[Recent Question 2012]***

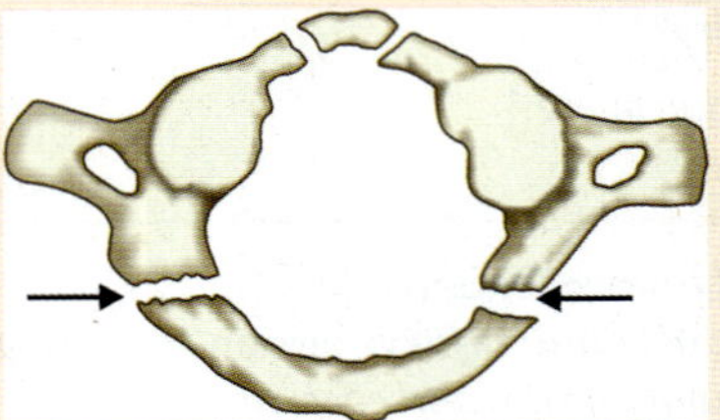

   a. Hangman's fracture
   b. Jefferson's fracture
   c. Clay-Shoveler's fracture
   d. Odontoid process fracture

3. **Clinical tests shown in Photograph are performed for**

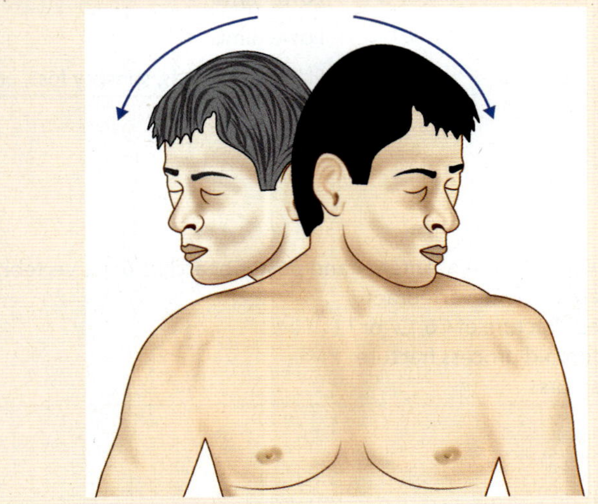

   a. Cervical rib
   b. Cervical disc syndromes
   c. Thoracic outlet syndrome
   d. Neck injuries

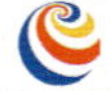 ANSWERS WITH EXPLANATIONS OF IBQs 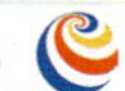

1. Ans. (b) Hyperextension injury *[Ref. Maheshwari, 4/e p260]*

- Extension injury of Spine:
  - MC seen in Cervical spine
  - Generally seen in Motor vehicle accidents, Shallow water diving

2. Ans. (b) Jefferson's fracture *[Ref. Maheshwari, 4/e p3]*

- Jefferson's fracture: Fracture of Anterior and Posterior arches of First cervical vertebra (Atlas)

3. Ans. (c) Thoracic outlet syndrome *[Ref. Plastic Surgery by Chang, Volume 6 p65]*

Tests For Thoracic Outlet Syndrome

- *Roo's test*: Patient stands and abducts shoulders to 90 degrees, externally rotates the shoulders, and flexes the elbows to 90 degrees, then opens and closes the hand slowly for three minutes; Test is positive if the patient is unable to complete the test or experiences heaviness, numbness, tingling or pain
- *Adson's test*: Examiner locates the radial pulse while arm is held in extension, external rotation and slight abduction. The patient is instructed to take a deep breath and turn head toward the test arm while extending the neck. If there is compression, the radial pulse will be diminished or absent
- *Costoclavicular test*: Examiner palpates the radial pulse and then draws the patient's shoulder down and back. If the pulse disappears, the test is positive
- *Halstead maneuver*: Examiner palpates the radial pulse and applies downward traction on the test extremity while the patient's neck is hyperextended and rotated to the opposite side; Absence of the pulse indicates a positive test
- *Wright test*: Examiner palpates the radial pulse and hyperabducts the arm so the hand is brought overhead with the elbow and arm in the coronal plane. The patient takes a deep breath and may rotate or extend the neck for additional effect
- *Allen maneuver*: Examiner palpates the radial pulse while positioning the shoulder in external rotation and horizontal abduction. The patient then rotates the head away from the test side.

NEET/NBE PATTERN MCQs

1. **Motorcyclist's Fracture is** *[Recent Question 2016]*
   a. Burst fracture of C2
   b. Burst fracture of Atlas
   c. Traumatic spondylolisthesis at Cl-C2 Level
   d. Hinge fracture at the base of skull
2. **Undertaker's fracture is** *[Recent Question 2016]*
   a. Traumatic spondylolisthesis of Cl over C2
   b. Spondylolisthesis of lower cervical spine with tearing of C6 C7 intervertebral disc
   c. Burst fracture of C3
   d. Spinous process fractures of lower cervical vertebrae
3. **Le Fort classification refers to** *[NBE DNB 2011]*
   a. Fractures of the mandible
   b. Soft issue injuries of the face
   c. Fractures of the maxilla
   d. Blow out fractures of the orbit
4. **Which of the following statements regarding Fracture of skull is correct?** *[NBE FMGE September 2008]*
   a. Most skull fractures require surgical treatment
   b. Depressed fractures are those in which patient's consciousness level is decreased or absent
   c. Compound fractures are those in which skull is fractured and underlying brain is lacerated
   d. Any bone fragment displaced >1 cm inward should be elevated surgically
5. **All of the following are frequently seen in a Basal skull fracture EXCEPT** *[NBE FMGE September 2008]*
   a. Facial nerve palsy b. Retro-auricular bruise
   c. CSF Otorrhoea d. Severe Epistaxis
6. **Hangman's fracture is** *[Recent Question 2012]*
   a. Subluxation of C5 over C6
   b. Fracture dislocation of C2
   c. Fracture dislocation of ankle joint
   d. Fracture of odontoid
7. **Jefferson's fracture is the fracture of** *[Recent Question 2012, 2013]*
   a. Odontoid b. C1
   c. C2 d. C3
8. **Le Fort classification is used for** *[NBE FMGE September 2007]*
   a. Fracture of mandible
   b. Fracture of maxilla
   c. Soft tissue injuries of the face
   d. Blow out fractures of the skull
9. **Compression fracture is most common in which part of spine?** *[NBE DNB 1992, 1994]*
   a. Upper thoracic b. Lower thoracic
   c. Cervical d. Lumbosacral
10. **Most common site for trauma of spine is** *[Recent Question 2012]*
    a. Cervical b. Thoracic
    c. Lumbar d. Sacrum
11. **In cervical spine injury, first to be done** *[Recent Question 2012, 2013]*
    a. Turn head
    b. Maintain airway
    c. Immobilization of spine
    d. None
12. **1Most common site for Vertebral Compression fractures is** *[Recent Question 2014]*
    a. C5-C6 b. C7-T1
    c. T12-L1 d. L5-S1
13. **Which of the following is not true about Jeffersons fracture?** *[Recent Question 2017]*
    a. It is a burst fracture of the ring of atlas vertebra
    b. It is the most common type of atlas fracture
    c. Fracture definition is particularly clear on CT scan image
    d. It is associated with injury elsewhere in spine in 25% of the cases
14. **Most dangerous type of Odontoid fracture as per Anderson and D'Alonzo classification and its respective management is** *[Recent Question 2017]*
    a. Type I Immobilization in rigid collar
    b. Type II Screw fixation
    c. Type III Halo vest immobilization
    d. Type IV Open reduction internal fixation
15. **Most common site for Osteoporotic vertebral wedge compression fracture is** *[Recent Question 2017]*
    a. Cervical spine
    b. Dorsolumbar spine
    c. Lumbosacral spine
    d. Lumbar spine
16. **Trendelenburg test is positive in** *[Recent Question 2017]*
    a. Dislocation of hip
    b. Fracture neck of femur
    c. Coxa vara
    d. All of the above

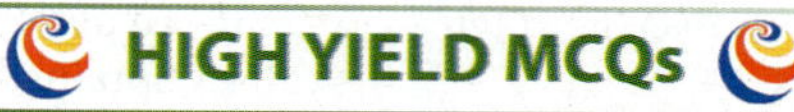

HIGH YIELD MCQs

1. **A 70 years old lady got compression fracture of L1 vertebra. There is no neurological deficit to this patient. What advise will you give for this patient?**
   a. Vitamin D supplementation *[PGI November 2016]*
   b. Do MRI scan
   c. Go for screw fixation of L1 vertebra
   d. To take Dexamethasone
   e. To take Alendronate
2. **All of the following lesions are seen in Battered baby syndrome except** *[AIIMS November 2016]*
   a. Corner fracture of metaphysis
   b. Microfractures at metaphysis
   c. Fractures of Epiphysiometaphyseal junction
   d. Bucket handle fracture of metaphysis
3. **'Signature fracture' refers to** *[All India PGMEE 2011]*
   a. Depressed skull fracture
   b. Contrecoup injury
   c. Fracture of foramen magnum
   d. Suture displacement fracture
4. **In multiple-fracture injury, most important is**
   a. Airway maintenance *[DPG 1988]*
   b. Blood transfusion
   c. I/v fluids
   d. Open reduction of fractures
5. **Severely injured patient with spinal fracture and unconsciousness, first to do is** *[AIIMS PG 1995, 1999]*
   a. Airway maintenance
   b. GCS scoring
   c. Mannitol drip
   d. Cervical collar to stabilise spine
6. **An 8 years old child is brought by parents to the casualty with a spiral fracture of Femur and varying degree of Ecchymosis all over body. The Etiology is** *[All India PGMEE 2000]*
   a. Hit & run accident
   b. Battered Baby Syndrome
   c. Hockey Stick injury
   d. Osteogenic imperfecta
7. **A one year old child presented with multiple fractures seen in various stages of healing. The most probable diagnosis in the case is** *[AIIMS PGMEE 2005]*
   a. Scurvy b. Rickets
   c. Battered baby syndrome d. Fall from height
8. **A 50 years old man presented with multiple pathological fractures. His serum calcium was 11.5 mg/dl and phosphate was 2.5 mg/dl. Alkaline phosphatase was 940 IU/dl. The most probable diagnosis is** *[AIIMS PGMEE 2005]*
   a. Osteoporosis b. Osteomalacia
   c. Multiple Myeloma d. Hyperparathyroidism
9. **A 4 years old female brought to casualty department with multiple fracture ribs, and inconspicuous history from parents. On examination show multiple bruise and healed fractures. The provable diagnosis is**
   a. Poly trauma for evaluation *[Kerala PGMEE 1999]*
   b. Flail chest
   c. Munchausen' syndrome
   d. Battered baby syndrome
10. **Fat embolism commonest occurs due to fracture of**
    a. Humerus b. Ulna *[AI 1999, 2005]*
    c. Femur d. Tibia
11. **A person with multiple injuries develops fever, restlessness, tachycardia, tachypnea and periumbilical rash. The likely diagnosis is** *[AIIMS PGMEE 2008]*
    a. Air embolism b. Fat embolism
    c. Pulmonary embolism d. Bacterial pneumonitis
12. **Correct order of priorities in the initial management of Head injury is** *[All India PGMEE 1992, 1999]*
    a. Airway, Breathing, Circulation treatment of extra cranial injuries
    b. Treatment of extra cranial injuries Airway, Breathing, Circulation
    c. Circulation airway, Breathing treatment of extra cranial injuries
    d. Airway, circulation, breathing treatment of extra cranial injuries
13. **Consider the following sign(s)** *[UPSC 1997]*
    1. Increasing pallor 2. Restlessness
    3. Air hunger 4. Water-hammer pulse

    Haemorrhagic shock due to Acute blood loss includes
    a. 1 & 4 b. 1 & 2
    c. 1, 2 & 3 d. 2, 3 & 4
14. **Polytrauma patient with open bleeding wound of right thigh should be managed first of all by** *[PGI 1994, JIPMER PGMEE 1999, AIIMS 1995]*
    a. Tourniquet application b. Tight bandage application
    c. Airway maintenance d. Blood transfusion
15. **Which of the following is not a component of the Crush syndrome?** *[AIIMS PGMEE 2002]*
    a. Myohemoglobinuria
    b. Massive crushing of muscles
    c. Acute tubular necrosis
    d. Bleeding diathesis
16. **Crush syndrome is managed by** *[AIIMS PGMEE 1993]*
    a. 20% Dextrose
    b. Hydrocortisone
    c. Maintaining high urine output
    d. Acidification of urine
17. **MC cause if spinal injuries in India is** *[AMU PGMEE 2002, PGI LUCKNOW 2003]*
    a. Road traffic accident b. Fall into well
    c. Fall from height d. House collapse
18. **Dislocation without fracture is seen in** *[DPG 1999]*
    a. Cervical spine b. Thoracic spine
    c. Lumbar spine d. Sacral spine

19. Whip-lash injury occurs due to *[AIIMS PGMEE 2003]*
a. A blow to top of head
b. Fall from height
c. Acute hyperextension of spine
d. Acute hyperflexion of spine

20. Jefferson's fracture is fracture of *[All India PGMEE 1999]*
a. C1 b. C2
c. C1-C2 d. C2-C3

21. Hangman's fracture is a fracture of *[All India PGMEE 1993, AIIMS PGMEE 1999]*
a. Spinous process b. Pars interarticularis
c. Lamina d. Dens

22. Hangman's fracture is *[Karnataka PGMEE 1998]*
a. Subluxation of C5 over C6
b. Fracture dislocation of C2 over C3
c. Fracture dislocation of ankle joint
d. Fracture of odontoid process

23. In shotgun injuries *[PGI 1996, AMU 1998, JIPMER PGMEE 2000]*
a. Each and every shot should be removed
b. All the shots within accessible limits may be removed and thorough debridement of the tissue done
c. Shots lodged in joints must be removed
d. All the above are true

24. Most common injury type to spinal cord is *[All India PGMEE 2007]*
a. Flexion b. Extension
c. Flexion rotation d. Compression

25. Seat belt injury is *[All India PGMEE 1990, PGI 1990, 1993]*
a. Tear drop fracture b. Wedge fracture
c. Whiplash injury d. Chance fracture

26. What type of fracture of petrous temporal bone has got the highest chance of facial nerve paralysis? *[AIIMS PGMEE 2008]*
a. Longitudinal b. Transverse
c. Oblique d. All have equal incidence

27. Motorcyclist's fracture *[All India PGMEE 2009]*
a. Ring fracture
b. Comminuted fracture
c. Separation of suture between anterior and posterior half of skull.
d. Fracture base of skull

28. In spinal cord injury, patient should be transferred with pad and bandage in the following position *[Orissa PGMEE 1998]*
a. Prone b. Supine
c. Lateral d. Semi-prone

29. Regarding Whiplash injury, a true statement includes *[JIPMER PGMEE 2000, All India PGMEE 1991]*
a. Contusion of the spinal cord and fracture of vertebra
b. Fracture of vertebral body
c. Spinal cord injury without vertebral fracture
d. Vertebral fracture without spinal cord injury

30. All are true regarding Whiplash injury except *[PGI 1996, PGI 1998]*
a. Lumbar spine is commonly involved
b. Fractures are not common
c. Paresthesia and chronic pain
d. Hyperextension injury
e. Sprains and strains without radiological findings

31. All of the following are true about Fracture of the Atlas vertebra, except *[All India PGMEE 2005]*
a. Jefferson fracture is the most common type
b. Quadriplegia is seen in 80% cases
c. Atlantooccipital fusion may sometimes be needed
d. CT scans should be done for diagnosis

32. True regarding Hangman's fracture is
a. Odontoid process fracture of C2
b. Spondylolisthesis of C2 over C3
c. Whiplash injury
d. Fracture of hyoid bone *[Manipal PGMEE 2000]*

33. Regarding Hangman's fracture true is *[JIPMER PGMEE 1999, AMU PGMEE 2002, SGPGI 2004]*
a. High post admission mortality
b. Most common axis fracture
c. Surgical treatment is necessary
d. Union almost always occurs

34. Burst fracture of cervical spine is due to
a. Whiplash injury *[Bihar PGMEE 1990, AIPGME 2007]*
b. Fall of weight on neck
c. Vertical compression injury
d. Car accident

35. Tear drop fracture of lower cervical spine implies *[AIIMS PGMEE 2005, 2006, Karnataka PGMEE 2002, MAHE PGMEE 2004]*
a. Wedge compression fracture
b. Axial compression fractures
c. Flexion-rotation injury with failure of anterior body
d. Flexion compression failure of body

36. In a patient with head injury, unexplained hypotension warrants evaluation of *[All India PGMEE 2002]*
a. Upper cervical spine b. Lower cervical spine
c. Thoracic spine d. Lumbar spine

37. Compression fracture is commonest in *[NBE DNB 1992]*
a. Cervical spine b. Upper thoracic spine
c. Lower thoracic spine d. Lumbosacral region

38. In case of unconscious patient, spinal injury is assessed by *[WB PGMEE 1998]*
a. Absence of response to painful stimulus
b. Absence of deep reflexes
c. Abdominal respiration
d. Spinal tenderness

39. Emergency treatment required in
a. Fracture humerus *[Rajasthan PGMEE 1992]*
b. Fracture pelvis
c. Vertical compression injury
d. Car accident

40. Careless handling of a suspected case of cervical spine injury may result in *[UPSC 1999]*
a. Injury to the spinal cord leading to quadriparesis or quadriplegia
b. Intracranial haemorrhage with cerebral imitation or unconsciousness.
c. Cervical haematoma with compression of brachial vessels
d. Complete paralysis of the affected upper extremity

41. A scooter is hit from behind. The rider is thrown off and he lands with his head hitting the kerb. He does not move, complains of severe pain in the neck and is unable to turn his head. Well-meaning on lookers rush up to him and try to make him sit up. What would be the best course of action in this situation? *[UPSC 1997]*

a. Be should be propped up and given some water to drink
b. He should not be propped up but turned on his face and rushed to the hospital
c. He should be turned on his back and a support should be placed behind his neck and transported to the nearest hospital
d. He should not be moved at all but carried to the nearest hospital in the same position in which he has been since his fall.

42. A young woman met with an accident and had mild quadriparesis. Her lateral X-ray cervical spine revealed C5-C6 fracture dislocation. Which of the following is the best line of management? *[All India PGMEE 2005]*

a. Immediate anterior decompression
b. Cervical traction followed by instrument fixation
c. Hard cervical collar and bed rest.
d. Cervical laminectomy.

43. Pathological changes in Caisson's disease is due to *[AIIMS PGMEE 1991]*

a. Oxygen gas b. Nitrogen gas
c. Carbon dioxide gas d. Carbon monoxide gas

44. MC site of Fracture mandible *[PGI November 2014]*

a. Ramus b. Coronoid process
c. Alveolar process d. Condyle, Body, Angle
e. Parasymphyseal region

45. All of the following methods are used for Removal of Vertebral disc, except *[AIIMS PG May 2015]*

a. Laminotomy b. Laminectomy
c. Laminoplasty d. Hemilaminectomy

46. A 42 years old man is diagnosed with irreparable tear of Rotator cuff. Treatment of choice *[AIIMS PG May 2015]*

a. Tendon transfer
b. Total shoulder replacement
c. Reverse shoulder replacement
d. Acromioplasty

47. Muscle affected in congenital torticollis is *[PGMCET 2015]*

a. Trapezius b. Rhomboideus Major
c. Rhomboideus Minor d. Sternocleidomastoid

NEET/NBE PATTERN MCQs ANSWERS WITH EXPLANATIONS

1. **Ans. (d)** Hinge fracture at the base of skull

   [Ref. Knight's Forensic Pathology, 4/e p178]

   Motorcyclist's Fracture
   - A **'hinge' fracture of the base of the skull** where the fracture line runs from side to side across the floor of the middle cranial fossa
   - Common in road accidents
   - At autopsy, base of skull may be appreciated to have divided into two halves, each moving independently of each other like a hinge

2. **Ans. (b)** Spondylolisthesis of lower cervical spine with tearing of C6 C7 intervertebral disc

   [Ref. Fundamentals of Orthopedics by Mohindra, 1/e p175]

   Undertaker's Fracture
   - A postmortem fracture which occurs due to careless handling of the dead body by undertakers
   - Cause: Falling of head backwards forcibly causing tearing of intervertebral disk and **subluxation of cervical spine most commonly at C6-C7 level**

3. **Ans. (c)** Fractures of the maxilla

4. **Ans. (c)** Compound fractures are those in which skull is fractured and underlying brain is lacerated
   - ***Compound skull fracture*:** Overlying laceration tears epidermis and meninges or runs through paranasal sinuses/ middle ear structures
     - Most common complication: Infection
   - ***Compound elevated skull fracture*:** Fractured bone is elevated above outer table of skull

5. **Ans. (a)** Facial nerve palsy

   [Ref. Short Practice of Surgery by Bailey and Love, 25th Ed., Pg 308]

6. **Ans. (b)** Fracture dislocation of C2

7. **Ans. (b)** C1

8. **Ans. (b)** Fracture of maxilla

   [Ref. Short Practice of Surgery by Bailey and Love, 25th Ed., Pg 329-30]

   Le Fort Classification of Maxillary Fractures (Top to Bottom)
   - **Le Fort I fracture:** Separates alveolus and palate from facial skeleton above
   - **Le Fort II (pyramidal) fracture:** Involves orbital floor, bridge of nose, ethmoids, cribriform plate (leads to CSF rhinorrhoea)
   - **Le Fort III fracture:** Separates facial skeleton from base of skull (runs through nasal bridge, septum, ethmoids; may lead to CSF rhinorrhoea)

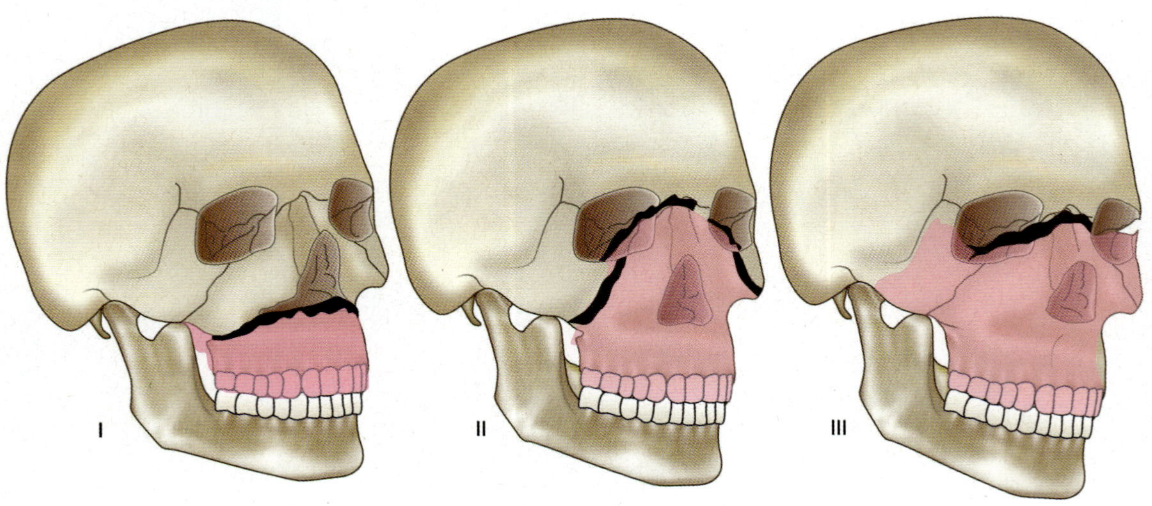

Fig. Le Fort fractures

9. **Ans. (b)** Lower thoracic

10. **Ans. (a)** Cervical

11. **Ans. (b)** Maintain airway

12. **Ans. (c)** T12-L1

    [Ref. Skeletal Radiology by Yochum, 3/e p683]
    - **MC site for vertebral compression fractures** is Thoracolumbar junction (T12-L1) as change in face provides poor resistance to anteroposterior displacement

13. **Ans. (d)** It is associated with injury elsewhere in spine in 25% of the cases

    [Ref. Maheshwari, 4/e p3]

Jefferson Fracture
- Burst fracture of C1 (Atlas vertebra) with fracture of anterior and posterior arches of C1 vertebra
- Result of an axial compression force, such as a fall onto the head vertex; fractures occur in the anterior or posterior arches of the atlas or both, typically in four places
- Patients complain with neck pain, cervical muscle spasms and neck tilt
- Atlas fractures are less common than Subluxation (MC are Jefferson's "burst" fracture, and anterior and posterior arch fractures)

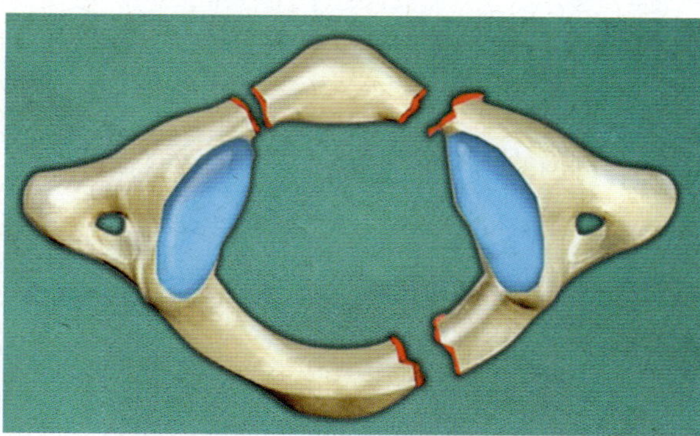

Fig. Jefferson fracture

14. Ans. (b) Type II Screw fixation

[Ref. Trauma and Orthopaedic Classifications by Lasanianos, 1/e p199]

Anderson and D'Alonzo classification of Odontoid Fractures

Types	Description	Outcome
Type 1	Oblique fracture through the odontoid tip	Stable
Type 2	Fracture through the base of the dens	Unstable. Higher risk of nonunion with comminuted fracture, age > 50 or more than 5 mm displacement
Type 3	Fracture through the body of C2	Will heal with immobilization, but may have residual spinal stenosis

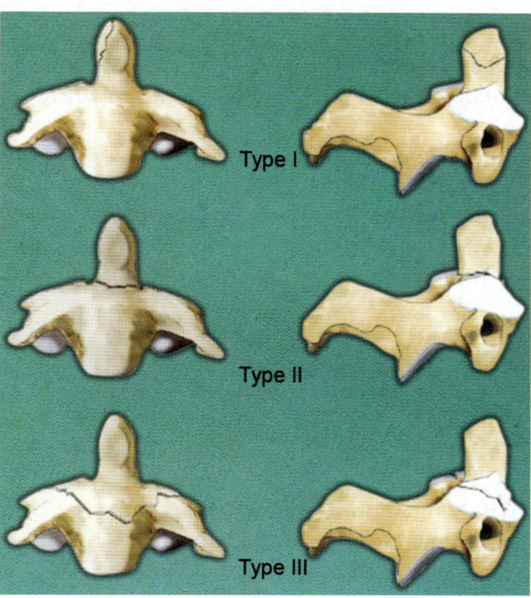

Fig. Odontoid fractures

Treatment of Odontoid Fractures

- Type I fractures Treatment: Hard-collar immobilization for 6-8 weeks
- Type II fractures Treatment: Halo immobilization, Internal fixation (Odontoid screw fixation) and posterior Atlanto-axial arthrodesis (C1-C2 Transarticular screw fixation)
- Type III fractures Treatment: Halo immobilization and Closed reduction (Deep, displaced, angulated fractures), Odontoid screw fixation (Uncomplicated shallow type fractures), C1-C2 arthrodesis

15. Ans. (b) Dorsolumbar spine

[Ref. Skeletal Imaging by Taylor, 2/e p327]

- Thoracolumbar region of the spine is the MC site of Osteoporotic compression fractures
- Wedge-shaped vertebral deformities occur due to compression fractures
- Uniform decrease in radiodensity, thinning of vertebral endplates, accentuation of vertical trabeculae

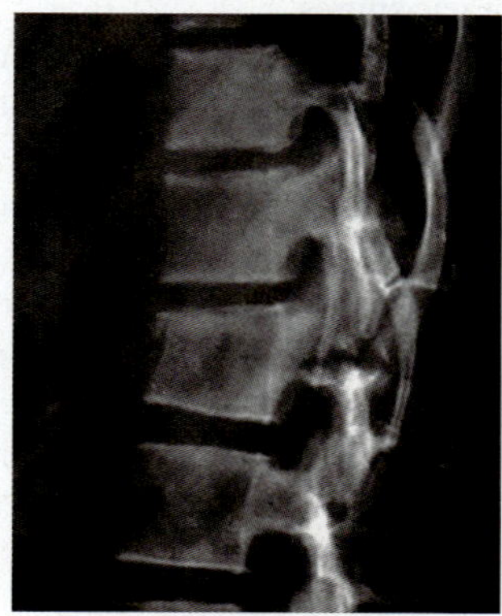

Fig. Vertebral fractures

16. Ans. (d) All of the above

[Ref. Hollinshead's Textbook of Anatomy, 5/e p334]

Trendelenburg Test

- An important maneuver for assessing the functional efficiency of the abductors
- A positive Trendelenburg test may result from other conditions besides abductor weakness
- Dislocation of the hip, for example, or coxa vara, or a femoral neck fracture that has not united, could all yield a positive result

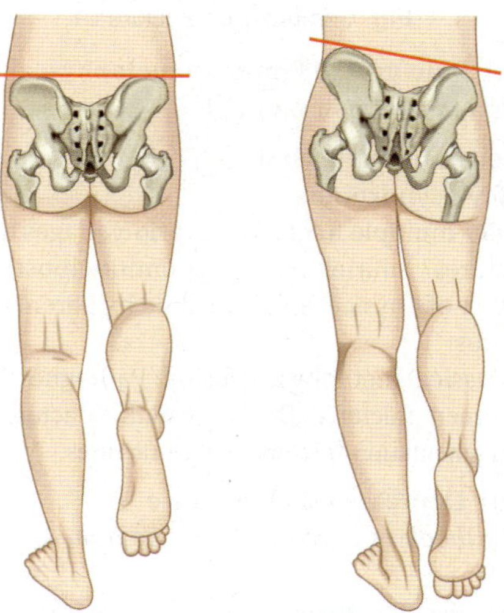

Fig. Trendelenburg test

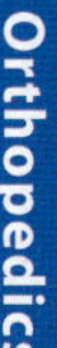

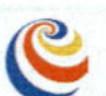

HIGH YIELD MCQs ANSWERS WITH EXPLANATIONS

1. Ans. (a) Vitamin D supplementation; (e) To take Alendronate
[Ref. Management of Fractures by Obrant, 1/e p221]

Compression Fracture L1 Vertebra

- **Diagnosis:**
  - Blood tests: CBC, PSA (middle-aged/ older men), ESR
  - Serum protein electrophoresis (Assessment of Multiple myeloma)
  - Urine: Markers of increased bone turnover, Bence-Jones proteins (Multiple myeloma)
  - X-ray: Anteroposterior and lateral views of the lumbar and thoracic spines
  - CT scanning: Evaluate complexity of fractures, Spot subtler fractures, Assess Spinal canal compromise & middle canal involvement
  - MRI scan: Only required in neurological deficits
- **Treatment:**
  - Parathyroid hormone, Anti-osteoporotic agents, Bisphosphonates (Alendronate), Selective estrogen modulators
  - L2 spinal nerve block (temporary relief of low back pain)

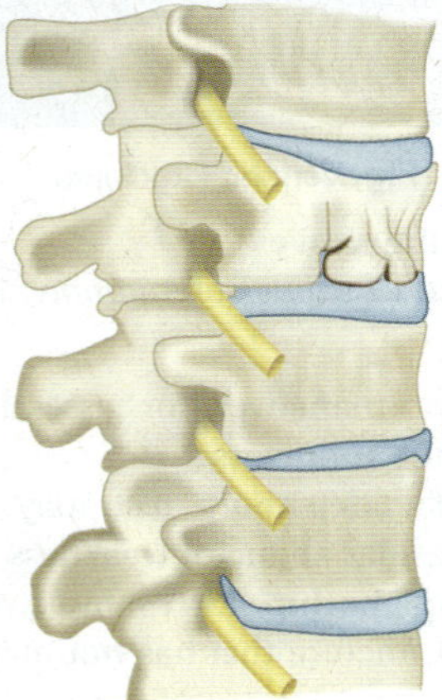

Fig. Compression fracture L1

2. Ans. (c) Fractures of Epiphysiometaphyseal junction
[Ref. Oski's Pediatrics, 4/e p154]

Battered Baby Syndrome

- **Caffey's syndrome**
- Single/ multiple fractures in various stages of healing
- Fractures/ injuries of ribs, extremities most diagnostic
- History of physical abuse of child by parents
- Injuires:
  - Classical metaphyseal lesion: Pathognomonic
  - Corner fracture, Bucket handle fracture, Metaphyseal fragmentation fracture, Microfractures

3. Ans. (a) Depressed skull fracture
[Ref. Textbook of Forensic Medicine and Toxicology by Rao, 1/e p194]

- **Signature fracture:** Depressed fracture of skull which provide clue about striking weapon

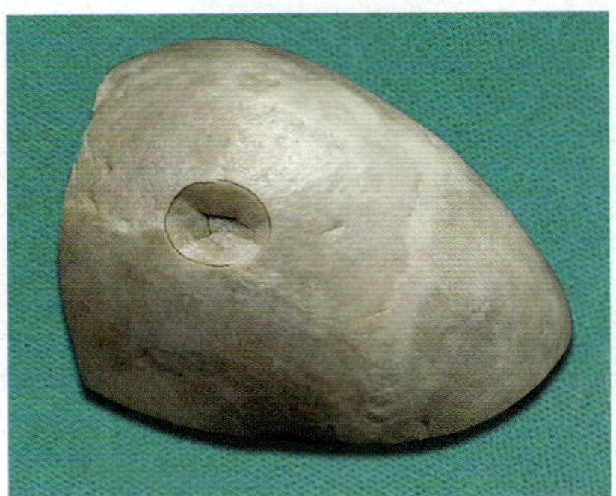

Fig. Signature fracture

4. Ans. (a) Airway maintenance
[Ref. Critical Decision in Trauma by Moore, 1/e p68]

5. Ans. (a) Airway maintenance
[Ref. Critical Decision in Trauma by Moore, 1/e p68]

6. Ans. (b) Battered Baby Syndrome
[Ref. Broken Bones by Galloway, 2/e p98]

Battered Baby Syndrome

- **Caffey's syndrome**
- Single/ multiple fractures in various stages of healing
- Fractures/ injuries of ribs, extremities most diagnostic
- History of physical abuse of child by parents

7. Ans. (c) Battered baby syndrome
[Ref. Broken Bones by Galloway, 2/e p98]

8. Ans. (d) Hyperparathyroidism

9. Ans. (d) Battered baby syndrome
[Ref. Broken Bones by Galloway, 2/e p98]

10. Ans. (c) Femur
[Ref. Rapid Review Pathology by Goljan, 4/e p121]

11. Ans. (b) Fat embolism
[Ref. Maheshwari, 4/e p42]

12. Ans. (a) Airway, Breathing, Circulation treatment of extra cranial injuries
[Ref. Trauma Manual by Rhodes, 4/e p254]

13. Ans. (c) 1, 2 & 3

14. Ans. (c) Airway maintenance
[Ref. Trauma Manual by Rhodes, 4/e p254]

15. Ans. (d) Bleeding diathesis
[Ref. Maheshwari, 4/e p43]

16. Ans. (c) Maintaining high urine output
[Ref. Disaster Medicine by Ciottone, 1/e p851]

Crush Syndrome

- **Etiology:** Massive crushing of muscles, Tourniquet application for excessive period
- **Causes:** Crushing of muscles lead to Myohemoglobin release in circulation; Its precipitation in renal tubules leading to Acute renal tubular necrosis

- **Consequences:** Deficient renal functions
- **Treatment:** Slow release of tourniquet, Treatment of ARF, Maintenance of high urine output (at around 200 ml per hour)

17. Ans. (c) Fall from height
[Ref. Neglected Musculoskeletal Injuries by Kumar, 1/e p161]

18. Ans. (a) Cervical spine
[Ref. Orthopedics Ready Recknor by Shenoy, 2/e p112]

19. Ans. (c) Acute hyperextension of spine
[Ref. Biomechanics of Musculoskeletal Injury by Zernicke, 2/e p268]

20. Ans. (a) C1
[Ref. Maheshwari, 4/e p3]

21. Ans. (b) Pars interarticularis
[Ref. Emergency radiology by Mirvis, 1/e p58]

22. Ans. (b) Fracture dislocation of C2 over C3
[Ref. Maheshwari, 4/e p3]

23. Ans. (b) All the shots within accessible limits may be removed and thorough debridement of the tissue done; (c) Shots lodged in joints must be removed

24. Ans. (a) Flexion
[Ref. Maheshwari, 4/e p259]

25. Ans. (d) Chance fracture
[Ref. Essentials of Orthopedics for Physiotherapist by Ebnezar, 1/e p183]

26. Ans. (a) Longitudinal
[Ref. Ballenger's Otorhinolaryngology, 1/e p397]

- **Most common type of Temporal bone fracture:** Longitudinal fracture
- **MC Temporal bone fracture** associated with Facial paralysis: Longitudinal fracture

27. Ans. (a) Ring fracture
[Ref. Textbook of Forensic Medicine and Toxicology by Vij, 5/e p300]

28. Ans. (b) Supine
[Ref. The Polytraumatized Patient with Fractures by Joseph, 1/e p82]

29. Ans. (c) Spinal cord injury without vertebral fracture
[Ref. APC Textbook of Forensic Medicine & Toxicology by Aggarwal, 1/e p344]

30. Ans. (a) Lumbar spine is commonly involved
[Ref. General Anatomy by Singh, 1/e p123]

- **Most common site of Whiplash injury:** Mid-cervical region

31. Ans. (b) Quadriplegia is seen in 80% cases
[Ref. Smart Study Series Orthopedics by Rohilla, 1/e p85]

32. Ans. (b) Spondylolisthesis of C2 over C3
[Ref. Maheshwari, 4/e p3]

33. Ans. (d) Union almost always occurs
[Ref. Apley's System of Orthopedics and Fractures by Solomon, 9/e p27]

34. Ans. (c) Vertical compression injury
[Ref. Radiology Illustrated: Spine by Kang, 1/e p216]

Mechanisms of Cervical Spine Injuries

Mechanisms	Injuries
Hyperflexion	Simple wedge compression fracture, Flexion teardrop fracture, Clay-Shoveler fracture, Anterior subluxation
Hyperflexion + Rotation	Unilateral facet dislocation (Locked vertebra)
Hyperextension	Hyperextension dislocation, Hangman's fracture, Laminar fracture, Extension teardrop fracture of Axis, Avulsion fracture of Anterior arch of Atlas
Hyperextension + Rotation	Pillar fracture
Vertical compression	Burst fracture, Jefferson's fracture
Lateral flexion	Uncinate process fracture

35. Ans. (d) Flexion compression failure of body
[Ref. Radiology Illustrated: Spine by Kang, 1/e p216]

36. Ans. (b) Lower cervical spine
[Ref. The Pediatric Emergency Medicine Resource, 4/e p296]

37. Ans. (c) Lower thoracic spine
[Ref. The Low Back and Pelvis by Howe, 1/e p76]

38. Ans. (a) Absence of response to painful stimulus; (b) Absence of deep reflexes; (c) Abdominal respiration

39. Ans. (c) Vertical compression injury

40. Ans. (a) Injury to the spinal cord leading to quadriparesis or quadriplegia
[Ref. Neurophysiological Basis of Movement by Latash, 2/e p310]

Consequences of Spinal Trauma

Level of Trauma	Likely consequence
Supraspinal	Hemiparesis, Hemiplegia (possibly spastic)
Cervical	Quadriparesis, Quadriplegia (possibly spastic)
Thoracic	Lower paraparesis, paraplegia (likely spastic)
Upper lumbar	Lower paraparesis, paraplegia (likely spastic)
Lower lumbar. Sacral	Lower paraparesis, paraplegia (flaccid)

41. Ans. (c) He should be turned on his back and a support should be placed behind his neck and transported to the nearest hospital

42. Ans. (b) Cervical traction followed by instrument fixation
[Ref AIPGMEE 2009 by Koli, 1/e]

43. Ans. (b) Nitrogen gas
[Ref. Pathology of Lungs by Corrin, 3/e]

44. Ans. (d) Condyle, Body, Angle
[Ref. Pediatric Emergency Medicine by Ludwig, 6/e p1309]

- Mandibular fractures are seen in:
  - Condyle
  - Body
  - Ramus
  - Angle

45. Ans. (c) Laminoplasty
[Ref. Postsurgical Neuroradiology by Ginat, 1/e p483]

Surgical Decompression Methods For Spine

- **Laminotomy:** Partial removal of lamina
- **Hemilaminectomy:** Removal of single lamina with exposure limited to one side of Interspinous ligament
- **Total Laminectomy:** Removal of bilateral lamina with spinous process
- **Laminoplasty:** Expansion of Spinal canal with preservation of dorsal laminar arch
- **Pediculectomy:** Removal of pedicle along with facet
- **Corpectomy:** Complete/ Partial removal of vertebral body
- **Vertebrectomy (Spondylectomy):** Complete/Partial removal of vertebra
- **Discectomy:** Removal of herniated disc

46. Ans. (a) Tendon transfer
[Ref. Shoulder Arthroscopy by Grasso, 1/e p505]

Treatment of Irreparable Rotator Cuff Tears

- Surgical decompression and debridement
- Tendon transfers: Latissimus dorsi (LD) tendon transfer represents often the best choice for treating massive and irreparable posterosuperior rotator cuff tears in young and active patients (Who are not suitable candidates for reverse shoulder arthroplasty)

47. Ans. (d) Sternocleidomastoid
[Ref. Orthopedic Secrets by Mehta, 4/e p186]

Congenital Torticollis

- **Torticollis:** Non-specific term used to describe tilting of the head and neck
- **Congenital muscular torticollis** is caused by contracture of the sternocleidomastoid muscle which cause head to tilt toward the affected side, with chin rotating towards opposite side
- **Congenital or infantile torticollis** primarily affects females aged 6 months to 3 years
- Underlying cause: Unilateral contraction of the SCM muscle caused by ischemic changes in the muscle

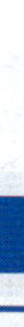
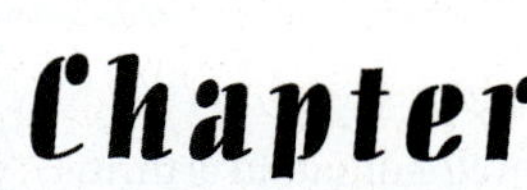

Chapter 6

Cold Orthopedics and Arthritic Disorders

THEORETICAL CONCEPTS

VI A. ARTHRITIC—DEGENERATIVE DISORDERS

Disorder	Sites involved
Rheumatoid arthritis	**MP joints of hand (Most common[Q])** PIP joints of fingers Wrists, knees, elbows, ankles
Ankylosing spondylitis *(Marie Stumpell disease)*	**Sacroiliac joints (Most common[Q])** Spine (above lumbar region) Hip, Knee, Manubrio-sternal joints
Gouty arthritis	**MP joint great toe (Most common[Q])** Olecranon bursa
Pseudogout	Menisci of knee[Q]
Psoriatric arthropathy	Distal IP joints[Q]
Alcaptonuric arthritis *(Ocronosis)*	Spine Shoulder joint
Hemophilic arthritis	Knee, elbow, ankle joint
Primary osteoarthritis	**Knee joint (Most common[Q])** Hip joint
Secondary osteoarthritis	Hip joint
Cervical spondylosis	C5-C6 intervertebral joint[Q]
Lumbar spondylosis	L5-S1 intervertebral joint[Q]

VI B. RHEUMATOID ARTHRITIS

- *Definition*: Chronic no-suppurative inflammation of synovial joints
- ***Diagnostic criteria***: (Four or more must be present[Q])
  - Morning stiffness
  - Swelling of ≥3 joints
  - Swelling of joints in hand/wrist
  - Rheumatoid nodule
  - Rheumatoid factor +ve
  - Erosion or osteopenia on X-ray
- *Underlying pathology*: Oedema of synovium

- *Clinical features*:
  - Polyarthritis in Rheumatoid arthritis
    - *Clinical presentation*: Pain and stiffness in multiple (>4) joints, usually in the morning
    - ***Most common joint involved*: Metacarpophalangeal joints (MC Index finger)**
    - *Joints affected in Rheumatoid arthritis*:

Involvement	Joints
Common[Q]	**MP joints of hand (Most common[Q])** PIP joints of fingers Wrists, knees, elbows, ankles
Less common	Hip joint Temporomandibular joint
Uncommon	Atlantoaxial joint Facet joints of cervical spine

    - *Deformities in Rheumatoid Arthritis*:

Site	Deformities
Hand	**Swan neck deformity[Q]** **Boutonniere deformity[Q]** **Z deformity[Q]**
Elbow	Flexion deformity
Knee	Triple subluxation
Ankle	Equinus
Foot	Wind-sweep deformity[Q] Hammer toe

  - *Extra-articular manifestations of Rheumatoid arthritis[Q]*:

Vasculitis	Digital arteritis Raynaud's phenomenon Peripheral neuritis Necrotising arteritis
Rheumatoid Nodules	**Olecranon (Most common site[Q])** Dorsal surface forearm
Serositis	Pleurisy, Caplan's syndrome Cardiomyopathy, Pericarditis Iridocyclitis Carpal tunnel syndrome
Others	Anaemia Felty's syndrome Sjogren's syndrome (Sicca syndrome) Amyloidosis

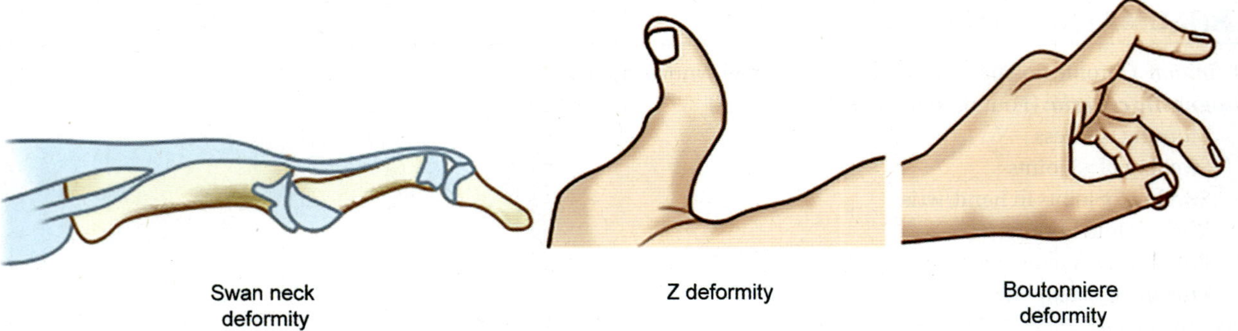

Topper's Edge

Rheumatoid Arthritis
- MC Inflammatory disease of joints[Q]
- 80% affected are women, Mean age 40 years
- Genetics role: HLA-DRW4 & HLA-DR1
- RA factor found in: 75% RA cases, 10% Healthy elderly people, 10% Malaria cases
- Most sensitive serological test[Q]: Inhibition test (Euglobulin)

VI C. RHEUMATOID FACTOR

- ***Rheumatoid factor is a type of autoantibody against*: Fc fragment of IgG**[Q]
  - *Most common sub*-type detected by most tests: IgM-RF
- *Tests for detection*:
  - Rose-Waaler test (sensitivity 60%)
  - Latex fixation test (sensitivity 80%)
- **Rheumatoid factor seen in** [**Mnemonic: R**heumatoid-factor **I**s **S**een **I**n **HEAT L**ike **S**ultry **S**ummers[Q]]
  - **R**hematoid arthritis (80% cases)
  - **I**nfectious mononucleosis
  - **S**LE
  - **In**fluenza
  - **H**epatitis
  - **E**ndocarditis
  - **A**IDS
  - **T**uberculosis
  - **L**iver disease
  - **S**arcoidosis
  - **S**yphilis

VI D. OTHER RHEUMATOID DISORDERS

- ***Ochronosis (Alcaptonuric Arthritis)***[Q]:
  - Underlying cause: Accumulation of homogentisic acid/ hydroquinione in connective tissues
  - Clinical features: **Urine darkens on standing**, pigmentation of sclera
  - Joints affected: Spine, Shoulder joint
  - X-ray findings: Disc space/ periarticular calcification in large joints[Q]
- ***Gout***:
  - Pathology: Accumulation of Uric acid in blood and **Sodium-monourate crystals in tissues**
  - MC site: Metacarpophalangeal joint **(Great toe)**, Bursitis **(Olecranon**[Q]**)**
- ***Pseudogout***:
  - Pathology: Accumulation of **Sodium-pyrophosphate crystals**[Q]
  - X-rays: Meniscal calcification[Q]

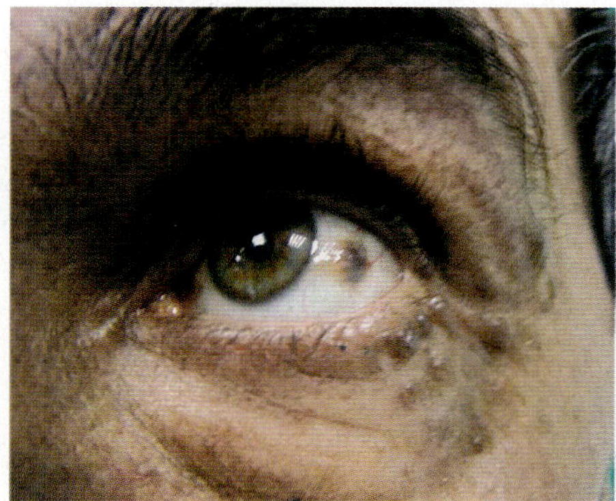

Fig. Ochronosis

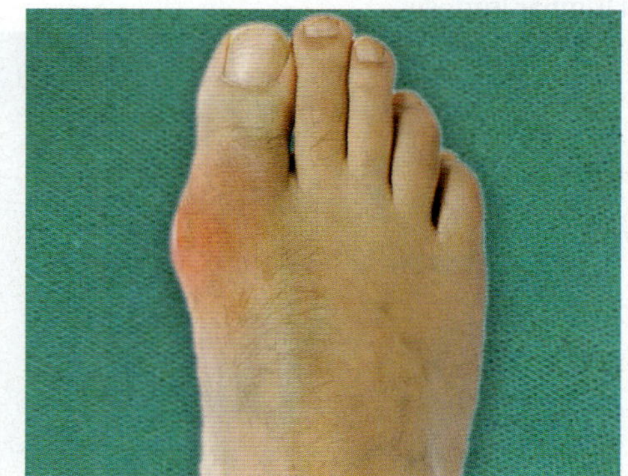

Fig. Gout

Orthopedics

VI E. ANKYLOSING SPONDLYLITIS

- *Definition*: Chronic progressive inflammatory stiffness of joints
- ***MC Site*: Sacroiliac joints[Q]**
- *Age group*: 15-30 years old males
- *Clinical presentation*:
  - Stiffness of lower back
  - SLRT +ve
  - Ganslen's test +ve
  - Pump-handle test +ve

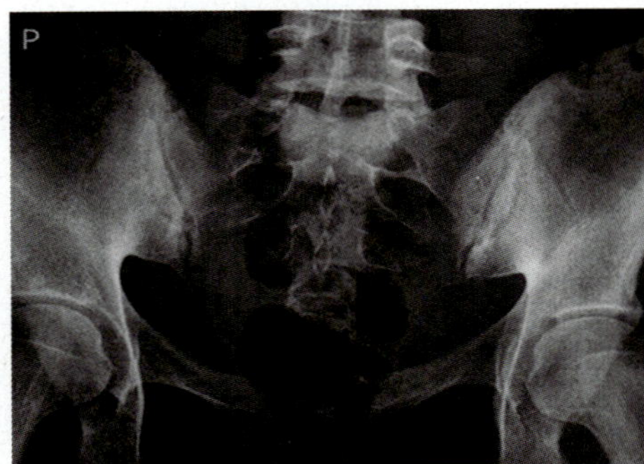

Fig. Sacroiliitis

- ***Extra-articular manifestations of Ankylosing spondylitis:***

Ocular	Acute iritis
Cardiovascular	Aortic incompetence[Q] Cardiomegaly Conduction defects Pericarditis
Neurological	Dislocation/ subluxation of atlanto-axial joint[Q]
Pulmonary	Costovertebral joints involvement Apical lobe fibrosis with cavitation
Systemic	Generalized osteoporosis Amyloidosis

- ***Radiology in Ankylosing spondylitis: X-ray pelvis***
  - Haziness of sacroiliac joints with subchondral erosions[Q]
  - Sclerosis of SI joints
  - Bony ankylosis of SI joints
  - Calcification of sacro-iliac and sacro-tuberous ligaments
  - Enthesopathy (calcification at attachments of muscles/ tendons/ ligaments)
- ***Radiology in Ankylosing spondylitis: X-ray lumbar spine***
  - **Squaring of vertebrae[Q]**
  - **Syndesmophytes (Bridging osteophytes[Q])**
  - **'Bamboo-spine appearance'[Q]**
  - Loss of lumbar lordosis

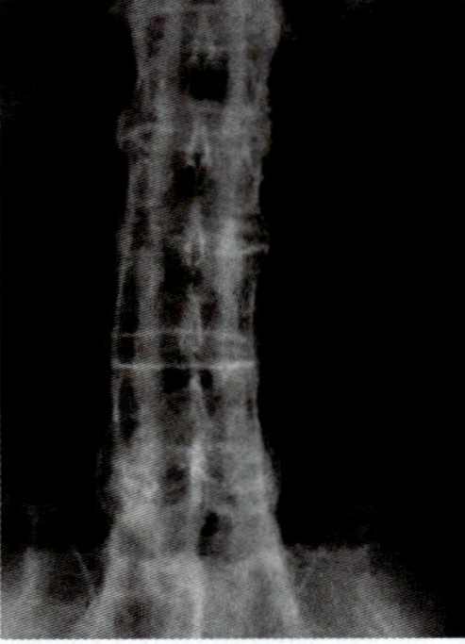

Fig. Bomboo-spine

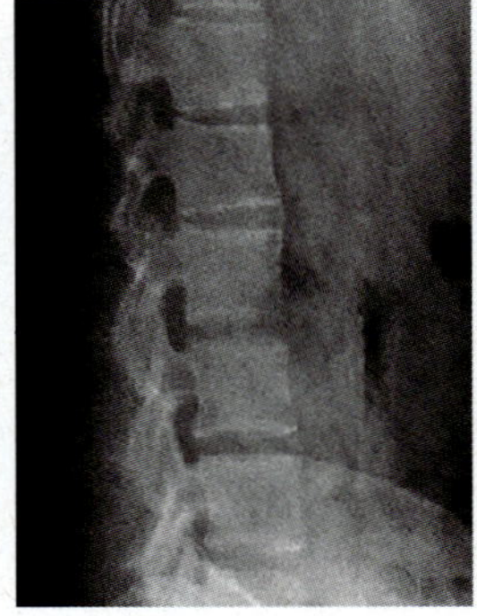

Fig. Squaring of vertebrae

Topper's Edge

Ankylosing Spondylitis
- **Marie-Strumpell disease**[Q]
- Chronic progressive inflammatory disease of Sacroiliac joints and Axial skeleton
- Male adults 15-30 years age group
- **HLA-B27 association in >85% cases**[Q]
- Intervertebral joints involved
- Uveitis, Conduction defects, Pulmonary complications

VI F. OSTEOARTHRITIS

- *Definition*: Degenerative disease of joints affecting articular cartilage (Fibrillation of cartilage)
- ***MC site*: Knee joint** (Hip joint in Western population[Q])
- *Underlying causes*:
  - Idiopathic
  - Post-traumatic
  - Steroids, Dialysis, Sickle cell anaemia
  - Coxa vara
  - CDH
  - Acetabular and malunited fractures
- *Clinical presentation*:
  - **Pain (First symptom[Q])**
  - Stiffness, swelling, tender joints
- *X-rays in Osteoarthritis*:
  - Narrowing of joint space (initially and mostly) in Medial compartment of tibiofemoral joint
  - Subchondral sclerosis
  - Subchondral cysts
  - Osteophytes formation
  - Loose bodies
  - Deformity of joint

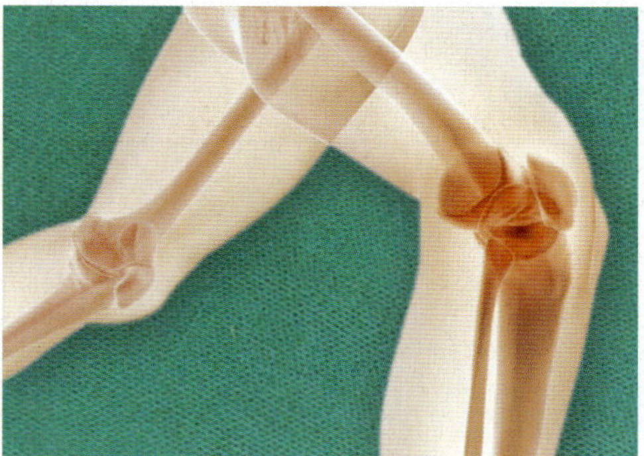

Fig. Osteoarthritis knee

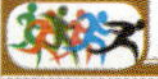
Topper's Edge

Osteoarthritis
- MC age group: Middle aged women
- **MC joint affected[Q]: Knee joint**
- Deformity in later stages: [Q] Varus deformity
- Most important diagnostic tool[Q]: Radiological investigation of knee joint (Loss of joint space, Subchondral cysts, Sclerosis, osteophytes, Loose bodies)
- **Causes of Secondary osteoarthritis:**
  - Obesity
  - Intraarticular fractures of knee

- Rheumatoid arthritis, Infection, Trauma, TB
- Hyperparathyroidism
- Hemophilia
- Syringomyelia
- Neurological disease (Diabetes)
- Overuse of intraarticular steroid therapy

OTHER ARTHRITIC DISORDERS OF JOINTS

Septic arthritis

- Infective arthritis/ Pyogenic infection of joint[Q]
- **MC organism responsible:**
  - **Overall: *Staphylococcus aureus*[Q]**
  - **Sickle cell anemia: *Salmonella*[Q]**
  - **Nail pricks: *Pseudomonas aeruginosa*[Q] (2nd Metatarsophalangeal joint)**
  - **Less than 2 years age: *H. influenzae*[Q]**
- **MC site affected[Q]:**
  - **Overall: Knee** (> Hip > Elbow > Shoulder)
  - Parenteral drug users: Sacroiliac joint, Sternal articulations, Pubic symphysis
- 90% cases are Monoarticular (10% polyarticular)
- Most accurate diagnostic tool[Q]: Joint aspirate and Synovial fluid analysis
- **Tom Smith arthritis[Q]: Septic arthritis of hip in infants**

Gonococcal arthritis

- *'Three-week infection'*
- 40% cases monoarticular
- Age group: 20-30 years age
- **MC site[Q]: Knee joint**

Charcot's joints

- **Neuropathic joints[Q]**
- Causes[Q]: Synringomyelia, Tabes dorsalis, Syphilis, rheumatoid arthritis, Intraarticular steroids, Traumatic division of Sciatic nerve, Chronic liver disease, Prolonged administration of drugs (Indomethacin)
- **MC joint[Q]: Knee joint** (> Ankle joint > Hip joint > Elbow joint > Shoulder joint)
- Treatment of choice: Charnley's compression

Hemophilic arthritis

- **Bleeder's joints[Q]**
- X-linked recessive disorder
- Normal bleeding time, prolonged clotting time

IMAGE-BASED QUESTIONS

1. Following X-ray is diagnostic of which of the following condition ***[AIIMS May 2016]***

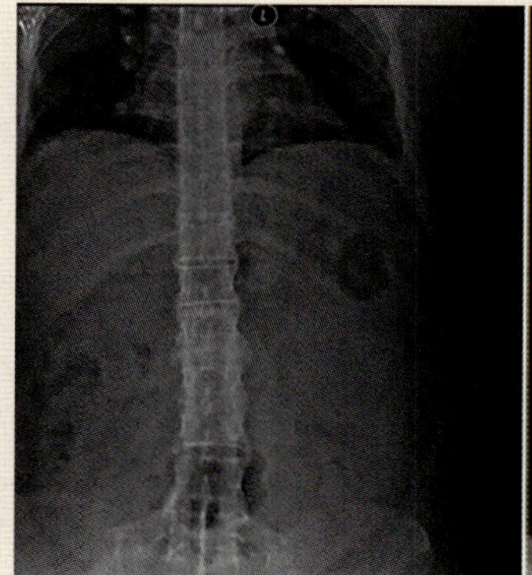

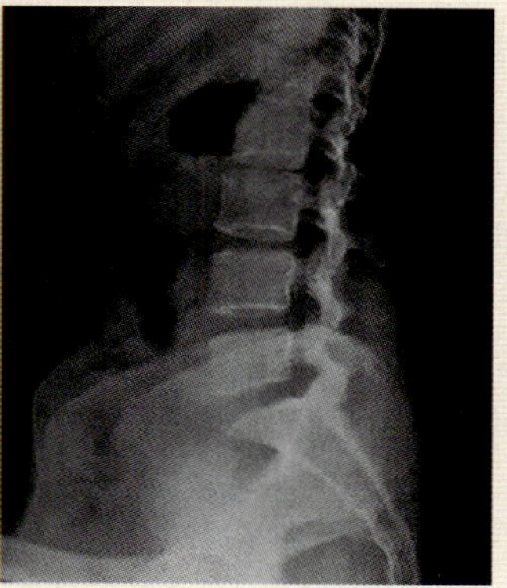

a. Rheumatoid arthiritis b. Ankylosing spondylitis
c. Hyperparathyroidism d. Pagets disease

2. Identify the Deformity shown in the Photograph ***[Recent Question 2013]***

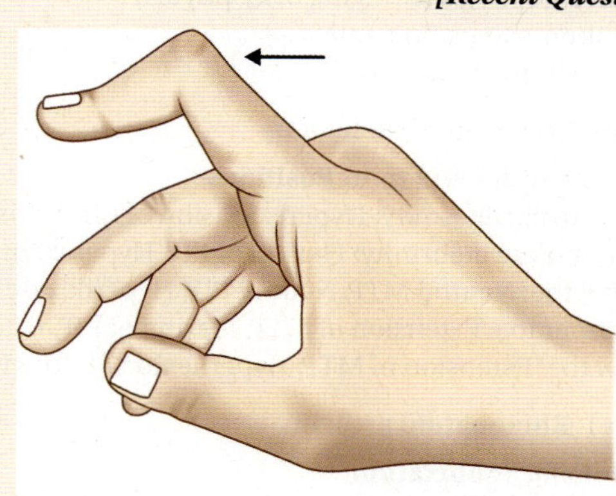

a. Trigger finger b. Mallet finger
c. Boutonniere deformity d. Swan-neck deformity

3. Deformity seen in Photograph is Most characteristic of

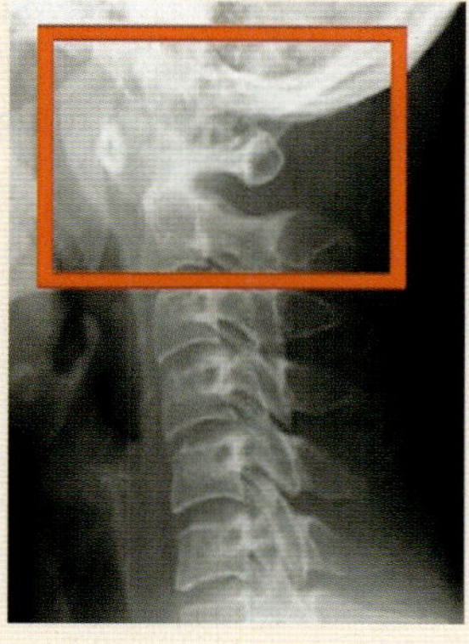

a. Rheumatoid arthritis b. Osteoarthritis
c. Fibrous dysplasia d. Ankylosing spondylitis

4. Bodies (Box) seen in Photograph is characteristic of

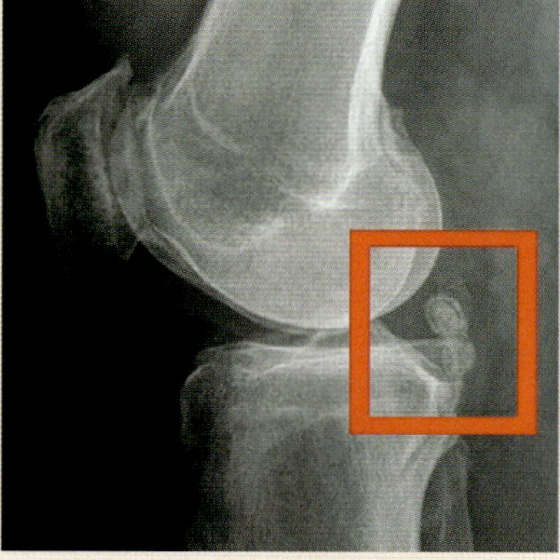

a. Osteoarthritis b. Rheumatoid arthritis
c. Ankylosing spondylitis d. Psoriatic arthritis

5. Deformity shown in Photograph is characteristic of ***[Recent Question 2014]***

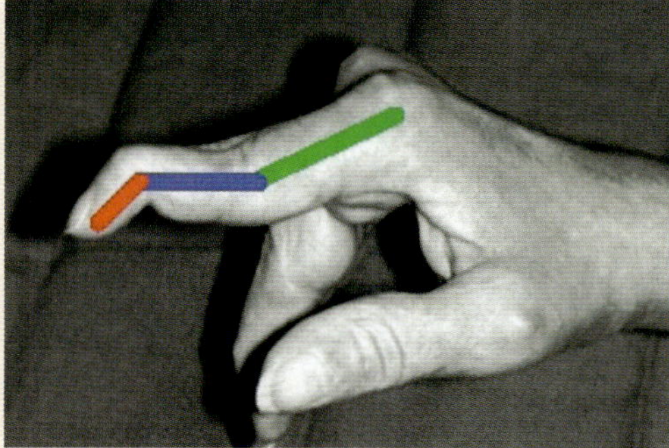

a. Osteoarthritis b Rheumatoid arthritis
c. Ankylosing spondylitis d. Psoriatic arthritis

ANSWERS WITH EXPLANATIONS OF IBQs 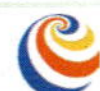

1. Ans. (b) Ankylosing spondylitis *[Ref. Maheshwari, 4/e p279]*

Radiology in Ankylosing spondylitis: X-ray lumbar spine (Photograph)

- Squaring of vertebrae
- Syndesmophytes (Bridging osteophytes)
- 'Bamboo-spine appearance'
- Loss of lumbar lordosis

2. Ans. (c) Boutonniere deformity *[Ref. Applied Therapeutics by Ernst, 10/e p1014]*

Key Deformities and Joint Positions

- Swan-neck deformity: Hyperextension of PIP, Hyperflexion of DIP
- Boutonniere deformity: Flexion of PIP, Hyperextension of DIP
- Mallet toe: Neutral MTP, Neutral PIP, Hyperflexion of DIP
- Hammer toe: Extension of MTP, Flexion of PIP, Extension of DIP
- Claw toe: Extension of MTP, Hyperflexion of PIP, Hyperflexion of DIP

3. Ans. (a) Rheumatoid arthritis *[Ref. Neurology of Older Adult by Joseph, 2/e p509]*

Atlantoaxial Subluxation

- MC Cervical spine abnormality in Rheumatoid arthritis
- Congenital causes: Down syndrome, Osteogenesis imperfecta, Neurofibromatosis, Morquio syndrome, Larsen syndrome, Spondyloepiphyseal dysplasia, Chondrodysplasia punctata, Metatropic dysplasia, Kniest syndrome

4. Ans. (a) Osteoarthritis *[Ref. Musculoskeletal Sonography by Martino, 1/e p127]*

- Loose bodies: *Osteoarthritis*, *Osteochondritis dessicans*, Osteochondral fractures, Osteonecrosis, S*ynovial* osteochondromatosis

5. Ans. (b) Rheumatoid arthritis *[Ref. Maheshwari, 4/e p280]*

Swan Neck Deformity of Rheumatoid Arthritis

- Finger postures with PIP hyperextension and DIP flexion; MP tends to be flexed, and the finger appears to zigzag when observed from the side
- IP positions are opposite to that of Boutonniere deformity

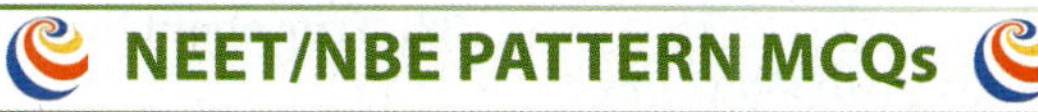

NEET/NBE PATTERN MCQs

1. In which of the following deformities is Distal interphalangeal joint extended? *[Recent Question 2016]*
a. Boutonniere deformity b. Swan neck deformity
c. Z deformity d. Claw Hand

2. Rheumatoid Arthritis affects which region of Spinal column? *[Recent Question 2016, 2017]*
a. Cervical Spine b. Thoracic Spine
c. Lumbosacral Spine d. Equally affects all regions

3. All of the following are radiological features of Rheumatoid arthritis except *[Recent Question 2016]*
a. Decreased Joint Space
b. Articular Erosions
c. Periarticular osteopenia
d. Fibrous Ankylosis

4. All of the following cause Erosive arthritis except
a. Rheumatoid Arthritis *[Recent Question 2016]*
b. Lupus Arthritis/Jaccoud arthritis
c. Tuberculous arthritis
d. Septic Arthritis

5. Hammer toe deformity is seen in *[Recent Question 2016]*
a. Rheumatoid arthritis
b. Fracture distal phalanx of great toe
c. Bunion
d. Osteochondritis

6. Tom smith's arthritis is due to *[Recent Question 2016]*
a. Pyogenic infection in infancy
b. TB
c. RA
d. OA

7. Pain and arthritis of Distal interphalangeal joint is seen in *[Recent Question 2016]*
a. Osteoarthritis b. Rheumatoid Arthritis
c. Ankylosing spondylitis d. Dequervain's disease

8. Which of the following is difference between Rheumatoid arthritis and Osteoarthritis? *[Recent Question 2016]*
a. Osteophytes are seen in osteoarthritis
b. Systemic symptoms are seen in osteoarthritis
c. Rheumatoid arthritis is uncommon in hands and feet
d. Osteoarthritis is an autoimmune disease

9. Swan-neck deformity is seen is *[NBE FMGE March 2008]*
a. Osteoarthritis b. Rheumatoid arthritis
c. Ankylosing spondylitis d. None of the above

10. Not seen in Osteoarthritis *[UPSC 2002]*
a. Osteophytes formation b. Cyst formation
c. Subchondral sclerosis d. Widening of joint spaces

11. Bony ankylosis usually occurs following *[NBE DNB June 2011]*
a. Tuberculosis b. Septic arthritis
c. Gouty arthritis d. Bechet's syndrome

12. Characteristic joint involvement in Rheumatoid arthritis is *[NBE FMGE September 2007]*
a. Knee joint b. Spine
c. Metacarpophalangeal joint
d. Hip joint

13. Earliest radiological change in RA *[Recent Question 2013]*
a. Decreased joint space b. Articular erosion
c. Periarticular osteopenia d. Subchondral cyst

14. Epiphyseal enlargement is seen in *[NBE DNB 1996]*
a. Stills' disease b. Rheumatoid arthritis
c. Down's syndrome d. Hypothyroidism

15. Osteoarthritis usually involves following compartment of the knee joint in the beginning *[NBE DNB June 2011]*
a. Lateral tibiofemoral b. Patellofemoral
c. Medial tibiofemoral d. All compartments

16. False regarding non-articular manifestations of Rheumatoid arthritis is *[NBE DNB 2009]*
a. Morning stiffness b. Tennis elbow
c. Fibrositis back/ neck d. Bursitis

17. Spondyloarthopathy which is seronegative are all except *[Recent Question 2012]*
a. AS b. Psoriasis
c. JRA d. Reiter syndrome

18. In Indian population which joint is most common affected in osteoarthritis *[NBE DNB 2011]*
a. Elbow b. Shoulder
c. Knee d. Hip

19. Sausage digits is seen in *[Recent Question 2012, 2013]*
a. Lyme arthritis b. Osteoarthritis
c. Psoriatic arthritis d. None

20. Heberdens nodules are seen in *[Recent Question 2016, NBE DNB 2009, AIPGME 2005]*
a. Proximal interphalangeal joints in Osteoarthritis
b. Distal interphalangeal joints in Osteoarthritis
c. Proximal interphalangeal joints in Rheumatoid arthritis
d. Distal interphalangeal joints in Rheumatoid arthritis

21. A young man presents with joint pain and backache. On X-ray of spine, sacroilitis is seen. Most probable diagnosis is *[NBE FMGE March 2007]*
a. Rheumatoid arthritis b. Ankylosing spondylitis
c. Psoriatic arthropathy d. Osteoarthritis

22. Tarsal tunnel syndrome is seen in *[NBE DNB 2010]*
a. Rheumatoid arthritis b. Osteoarthritis
c. Psoriatic arthritis d. Ankylosing spondylitis

23. Distal interphalangeal joints (DIP) hand, are typically involved in *[NBE DNB December 2011]*
a. Rheumatoid arthritis b. Osteoarthritis
c. Gout d. Ankylosing spondylitis

24. Resorption of distal phalanx is seen in
a. Scleroderma *[Recent Question 2012]*
b. Hyperparathyroidism
c. Reiter's syndrome d. All

25. All are true of Pseudogout EXCEPT *[NBE DNB 2010]*
a. Chondrocalcinosis
b. Calciumpyrophosphate deposition
c. Does not affect small joints
d. Does not affect large joints

26. Joint spared in RA *[Recent Question 2013, AIIMS PG 1998]*
a. PIP b. DIP
c. MCP d. Wrist

27. Which of the following constitute Felty's syndrome? *[UPSC 2011, AIIMS PG 1997]*
a. Rheumatoid arthritis, Neutropenia, Splenomegaly
b. Rheumatoid arthritis, Neutropenia, Hepatomegaly
c. Rheumatoid arthritis, Psoriasis, Anaemia
d. Reactive arthritis, Splenomegaly, Anaemia

28. In the beginning, which compartment of knee joint is involved in Osteoarthritis? *[NBE FMGE September 2006, NBE DNB June 2011]*
a. Lateral tibiofemoral b. Patellofemoral
c. Medial tibiofemoral d. All compartments

29. Which one of the following joints is typically spared in osteoarthritis? *[NBE DNB December 2011]*
a. Ankle
b. Cervical spine
c. Distal interphalangeal joint
d. Hip

30. In the Indian population, which joint is most commonly affected in Osteoarthritis? *[NBE FMGE September 2006, NBE DNB June 2011]*
a. Elbow b. Knee
c. Shoulder d. Hip

31. Which of the following is not a feature of Arthritis of Acute Rheumatic Fever? *[UPSC 2012]*
a. Elevated ASO titre
b. Involvement of large joints
c. Dramatic response to aspirin
d. Joint deformities are common sequel

32. Reiter's syndrome is characterized by all except *[UPSC 2012]*
a. Seronegative arthritis b. Non-specific urethritis
c. Conjunctivitis d. Lymphadenitis

33. The presence of 'Swan-neck' deformity, 'button-hole' deformity, 'Z' deformity of thumb and Baker's cyst suggest *[UPSC 2012]*
a. Reiter's syndrome b. Gouty urethritis
c. Psoriatric arthritis d. Rheumatoid arthritis

34. Joints of hand are not affected in *[Recent Question 2012]*
a. AS b. RA
c. OA d. Psoriatic arthritis

35. Ankylosing spondylitis is associated with *[NBE FMGE March 2006]*
a. Aortic stenosis b. Aortic insufficiency
c. Mitral insufficiency d. Mitral stenosis

36. Bamboo spine with sacroilitis *[Recent Question 2012, 2013]*
a. Ankylosing spondylitis b. RA
c. OA d. Psoriatic arthritis

37. Sicca syndrome is associated with *[NBE FMGE March 2006]*
a. Rheumatoid arthritis b. Laenec's cirrhosis
c. Scleroderma d. SLE

38. True about Psoriatic arthritis are all except *[Recent Question 2012]*
a. HLA-Cm6 association b. Involvement of DIP joint
c. More common in males d. DOC is methotrexate

39. Rheumatoid factor may be seen in all EXCEPT *[NBE FMGE March 2006]*
a. Syphilis
b. Tuberculosis
c. Infectious mononucleosis
d. Typhoid

40. Septic arthritis is diagnosed by *[Recent Question 2012, 2013]*
a. X-ray b. Joint aspiration
c. USG d. MRI

41. Most common site for Spondylolisthesis is *[NBE FMGE September 2005]*
a. C7 over T1 b. L3 over L4
c. L4 over L5 d. L5 over S1

42. Drug used in osteoarthritis *[Recent Question 2012, 2017]*
a. Methotrexate b. Glucosamine
c. Sulfasalazine d. All

43. Rheumatoid arthritis affects *[NBE FMGE March 2005]*
a. Cervical spine b. Thoracic spine
c. Lumbar spine d. Sacral spine

44. Rheumatoid arthritis is associated with all except *[Recent Question 2012]*
a. Cardiac involvement b. Bauchards nodes
c. Herberdens node d. Swan-neck deformity

45. Criteria for classification of rheumatoid arthritis include all of the following except *[NBE FMGE September 2011]*
a. Morning stiffness more than one hour
b. Symmetric arthritis
c. Symptoms for at least six months
d. Rheumatoid nodules

46. Pannus is seen in *[Recent Question 2012]*
a. OA b. RA
c. Gout d. None

47. All of the following are ocular features of juvenile rheumatoid arthritis EXCEPT *[NBE FMGE March 2012]*
a. Uveitis
b. Band shaped keratopathy
c. Cataract
d. Conjunctivitis

48. Effusion in knee is recognized by all of the following EXCEPT *[NBE FMGE March 2012]*
a. Patellar tap b. Filling of lateral fossae
c. Patellar shift d. Fluctuation

49. Characteristics of Osteoporosis include all except *[Recent Question 2014]*
a. Normal Serum calcium
b. Normal Serum phosphates
c. Normal Plasma Albumin
d. Normal Alkaline phosphatase

50. Joint erosions are seen in all except *[Recent Question 2015]*
a. SLE b. Gout
c. Rheumatoid arthritis d. Osteoarthritis

51. Psoriatic arthritis is associated with *[Recent Question 2015]*
a. HLA B13 b. HLA B16
c. HLA B27 d. HLA B17

52. Joint NOT involved in Osteoarthritis is *[Recent Question 2015]*
a. DIP b. Knee
c. PIP d. MCP

53. Consider the following statements about Polyarticular juvenile rheumatoid arthritis
1. It is more common in girls
2. Five or more joints are affected within the first six months of onset
3. Uveitis occurs in 95% patients
4. Rheumatoid factor may be negative

Which of the statements given above are true? *[UPSC CMS 2015]*
a. 1 and 4 only b. 1, 2 and 4
c. 2, 3 and 4 d. 2 and 3 only

54. Following features are suggestive of Behcet's syndrome except *[UPSC CMS 2015]*
a. Orogenital ulcers b. Polyarthritis
c. Uveitis d. Livedo reticularis

55. Most common type of Juvenile rheumatoid arthritis is *[UPSC CMS 2015]*
a. Rheumatoid factor positive polyarticular
b. Rheumatoid factor negative polyarticular
c. Pauciarticular type
d. Systemic onset type

56. Which of the following is not true regarding inflammatory arthritis? *[Recent Question 2017]*
a. Presence of morning stiffness
b. Sclerosis on X-ray
c. Anemia of chronic disease
d. Presence of fever, weight loss and elevated ESR

57. Which joint is rarely affected by Ankylosing spondylitis? *[Recent Question 2017]*
a. Ankle b. Hip
c. Shoulder d. Sacroiliac

58. Most commonly involved joint in Gout is *[Recent Question 2017]*
a. Knee
b. Metatarsophalangeal joint of big toe
c. Wrist
d. Metacarpophalangeal joint of thumb

59. Which of the following is not true about Osteoarthritis? *[Recent Question 2017]*
a. Inflammation of synovial joints
b. Most common joint disease
c. Affects shoulder joint
d. Narrowing of the joint space occurs

60. All are true about Marie-Strumpell disease except *[Recent Question 2017]*
a. Most commonly involves the Sacroiliac joints
b. Enthesitis is common
c. More common in males
d. Roentgenogram is the most sensitive investigation

61. Martels sign seen in which of the following condition? *[Recent Question 2017]*
a. Rheumatoid arthritis b. Osteoarthritis
c. Gouty arthritis d. Oochronosis

62. Most specific antibody seen in RA *[Recent Question 2017]*
a. Anti-CCP b. Rheumatoid factor
c. ANA d. Anti-dsDNA

63. In Rheumatoid arthritis, which type of cells are prominently present? *[Recent Question 2018]*
a. B cells
b. T cells
c. Macrophages
d. Dendritic cells

HIGH YIELD MCQs

1. Which of the statements are true about Polyarticular juvenile rheumatoid arthritis? *[UPSC CMS 2016]*
1. It is more common in girls
2. Five or more joints are affected within the first six months of onset
3. Uveitis occurs in 95% patients
4. Rheumatoid factor may be negative

a. 1 and 4 only
b. 1, 2 and 4
c. 2, 3 and 4
d. 2 and 3 only

2. Most common type of Juvenile Rheumatoid arthritis is *[UPSC CMS 2016]*
a. Rheumatoid factor positive polyarticular type
b. Rheumatoid factor negative polyarticular type
c. Pauciarticular type
d. Systemic onset type

3. True about Boutonniere deformity *[Recent Question 2017, PGI May 2016]*
a. Flexion of proximal interphalangeal joint & hyperextension of distal interphalangeal joint
b. Hyperextension of proximal interphalangeal joint & flexion of distal interphalangeal joint
c. Flexion at proximal interphalangeal & extension at metacarpophalangeal joint
d. Flexion deformity of the proximal interphalangeal joint occur due to tear in central slip of extensor tendon
e. May occur in rheumatoid arthritis

4. True about Ankylosing spondylitis *[PGI May 2016]*
a. Romanus lesion may be found
b. If left untreated, spine fusion may occur
c. Predilection of the joints of the axial skeleton
d. Bony erosions do not occur
e. None of the above

5. **A 65 years old lady presented with swollen, painful knee; on examination Grade III osteoarthritic changes are seen. Best course of action is** *[All India PGMEE 2011]*
   a. Conservative management
   b. Arthroscopic washing
   c. Partial knee replacement
   d. Total knee replacement

6. **Earliest radiological sign of the Osteoarthritis is** *[BIHAR PGMEE 1998]*
   a. Narrowing of joint space
   b. Osteophyte formation
   c. Sclerosis in subchondral bone
   d. Cystic lesion in cancellous bone

7. **Underlying cause of Rheumatoid arthritis is** *[PGI 2002]*
   a. Familial b. Infective
   c. Traumatic d. Immunological

8. **The following is involved in Rheumatoid arthritis** *[UP PGMEE 1999]*
   a. Subchondral bone b. Synovial fluid
   c. Synovial membrane d. Cartilage

9. **MC cause of tarsal tunnel syndrome is** *[AIIMS PGMEE 2009]*
   a. Osteoarthritis b. Rheumatoid arthritis
   c. Psoriatic arthritis d. Ankylosing spondylitis

10. **A young male presents with joint pains and backache. X-ray of spine shows evidence of sacroilitis. The most likely diagnosis is** *[UPSC 1998]*
    a. Rheumatoid arthritis
    b. Ankylosing spondylitis
    c. Polyarticular juvenile arthritis
    d. Psoriatic arthropathy

11. **One of the following is true regarding Ankylosing spondylitis** *[NBE DNB 1990]*
    a. Common in females b. Sacrolitis is common
    c. Anti-DNA and antinuclear antibodies are present
    d. Symmetrical peripheral arthritis

12. **Which is true about Ankylosing spondylitis?** *[UP PGMEE 1994]*
    a. Sacroliac joints unusually involved
    b. Peripheral joint is rarely involved
    c. Common manifestation in females
    d. Iritis is seen more frequently

13. **One of the following is not associated with Ankylosing spondylitis** *[NIMS PGMEE 1998]*
    a. Pain is more in the early morning period
    b. Pain is relieved in lying down position
    c. Morning stiffness more than 3 months
    d. PGMEE be associated with uveitis

14. **Which of the following agent has/have proven to be a value in treatment of Ankylosing spondylitis?** *[PGI 1990, JIPMER 1999]*
    a. Phenylbutazone b. Intramuscular gold
    c. Naproxen d. Penicillamine

15. **Proximal interphalangeal, distal interphalangeal and first carpometacarpal joints involvement and sparing of wrist is a feature of** *[AIIMS PGMEE 1995]*
    a. Rheumatoid arthritis b. Pseudogout
    c. Osteorthritis d. Psoriatic arthropathy

16. **Least common site involved in osteoarthritis is** *[All India PGMEE 1997, KERALA PGMEE 1996]*
    a. Shoulder joint
    b. Knee joint
    c. Hip joint
    d. Metacarpophalangeal joint
    e. Interphalangeal joint

17. **In patients with osteoarthritis of knee joint, atrophy occurs most commonly in** *[AIIMS PGMEE 2007, All India PGMEE 2007]*
    a. Quadriceps only
    b. Hamstrings only
    c. Both Quadriceps and Hamstrings
    d. Gastrocnemius

18. **True about osteoarthritis** *[PGI 2003]*
    a. Single joint involvement
    b. Commonly found in adult less than 50 years age
    c. Ankylosis is seen
    d. Lower limb deformity is seen
    e. Heberden's nodules are found

19. **Treatment of Osteoarthritis include all except** *[KERALA PGMEE 96]*
    a. Increase the weight bearing by the affected joint
    b. Graded muscle exercises
    c. Rest to the joint in acute phase
    d. Replacement of articular surface
    e. Correction of deformities

20. **Most common site of primary osteoarthrosis is** *[TN PGMEE 1997]*
    a. Ankle joint b. Shouder joint
    c. Hip joint d. Knee joint

21. **Most common arthritis that affects the wrists is** *[AP PGMEE 1993]*
    a. Osteoarthritis b. Rheumatoid arthritis
    c. Tuberculous arthritis d. Gouty arthritis

22. **Which joint is commonly affected in Ankylosing spondylitis?** *[TN PGMEE 1996]*
    a. Ankle b. Knee
    c. Shoulder d. All of the above

23. **Enthesopathy is commonly found in** *[PGI 1994]*
    a. Rheumatoid arthritis b. Rheumatic fever
    c. Ankylosing spondylitis d. Osteoarthritis

24. **All are true regarding Ankylosing spondylitis except**
    a. Sacroilitis b. HLA-B27 *[PGI 1997]*
    c. Iridocyclitis d. More common in females

25. **'Swan-neck deformity' is a feature of** *[All India PGMEE 1990]*
    a. Gouty arthritis b. Syphilitic arthritis
    c. Rheumatoid arthritis d. Osteoarthritis

26. **Wind-sweep deformity is seen in** *[Recent Question 2016, AIIMS PGMEE 1998]*
    a. Rheumatoid arthritis b. Rickets
    c. Ankylosing spondylitis d. Scurvy

27. **Boutonnière deformity occur due to** *[PGI 2008]*
    a. Flexion of Proximal Interphalangeal joint
    b. Flexion at Distal interphalangeal joint

c. Flexion at Metacarpophalangeal joint
d. Extension at Metacarpophalangeal joint
e. Extension at Distal interphalangeal joint

28. Joint commonly involved in syphilitic arthritis is *[All India PGMEE 1993]*
a. Hip b. Shoulder
c. Wrist d. Knee

29. What is pathognomonic feature of rheumatoid arthritis? *[AIIMS PGMEE 2005]*
a. Rheumatoid factor b. Ulnar drift of fingers
c. Rheumatoid nodule d. Morning stiffness

30. Type of anaemia in Rheumatoid arthritis *[AIIMS PGMEE 1997]*
a. Normocytic normochromic anaemia
b. Normocytic hypochromic anaemia
c. Microcytic hypochromic anaemia
d. Macrocytic hypochromic anaemia

31. Painless effusion in joints in Congenital Syphilis are called *[All India PGMEE 1995]*
a. Clutton's joint b. Charcot's joint
c. Barton'sjoint d. Chronic osteomyelitis

32. Erosion of bone is seen with all of the following except *[All India PGMEE 1994, AIIMS PG 1994]*
a. Gout b. SLE
c. Psoriasis d. Rheumatoid arthritis

33. Erosive arthritis is not noted in *[AP PGMEE 1993]*
a. Amyloidosis b. Hyperparathyroidism
c. Psoriasis d. Sickle-cell disorder

34. True about Rheumatoid arthritis is/are *[PGI 2006]*
a. Adrenal hyperplasia
b. Involves peripheral joints more commonly than axial joints
c. Does not decrease life expectancy
d. Associated with vasculitis
e. Involve only axial joints

35. Treatment of Rheumatoid arthritis include all except *[KERALA PGMEE 1996]*
a. Exercises
b. Give rest to the joints
c. Immunosuppressive drugs
d. Correction of deformities
e. Synovectomy

36. Multiple loose bodies are seen in *[PGI 2001]*
a. Osteogenesis imperfecta
b. Osteochondritis dessicans
c. Rheumatoid arthritis
d. Synovial chondrocalcinosis
e. Osteoarhritis

37. Deforming Polyarthritis is associated with all of the following except *[JIPMER PGMEE 1999]*
a. Rheumatoid arthritis b. Psoriatic arthritis
c. Behcet's syndrome d. Ankylosing spondylitis

38. Synovial fluid of low viscosity seen in *[PGI 2005]*
a. Gout
b. Septic arthritis
c. TB
d. Osteoarthritis
e. Rheumatoid arthritis

39. Tophi of gout is found in *[PGI 2003]*
a. Articular cartilage b. Synovium
c. Skin d. Muscle
e. Joint capsule

40. Clinical features of Gout are all except *[UP PGMEE 1993]*
a. Chronic patient with renal complication allopurinol is drug of choice
b. Positive birefringent crystal in the Synovial fluid
c. Hyperuricemia
d. Mostly affects smaller joint

41. The following is the commonest cause of loose body in a joint *[BIHAR PGMEE 1990]*
a. Osteoarthritis
b. Osteochondral fracture
c. Synovial chondromatosis
d. Osteochondritis dessicans

42. Disease where distal interphalangeal joint is characteristically involved *[Recent Question 2017, TN PGMEE 1990]*
a. Gout b. Rheumatoid arthritis
c. Psoriatic arthritis d. SLE

43. In Psoriatic arthropathy, treatment of choice is *[AIIMS PGMEE 1993]*
a. Indomethacin b. Methotrexate
c. Corticosteroids d. PUVA therapy

44. In Reiter's disease, untrue is *[AIIMS PGMEE 1993]*
a. Interstitial lung disease b. Conjunctivitis
c. After sexual contact d. Ulcer on palm & soles

45. Ankylosing spondylitis in associated with *[All India PGMEE 1999]*
a. HLA-DR3 b. HLA-B27
c. HLA-B8 d. HLA-DW4/DR4

46. A 35-year-old businessmen presents suddenly with severe pain, swelling and redness in left big toe in early morning. Most likely diagnosis is *[PGI 1994]* *[AIIMS PG 1992, 1995]*
a. Rheumatoid arthritis b. Gouty arthritis
c. Pseudogout d. Septic arthritis

47. All of the following drugs are used in an attack of Gout except *[AMU PGMEE 1992]*
a. Aspirin b. Indomethacin
c. Colchicine d. Phenylbutazone

48. All of the following diseases are associated with HLA-B27 and uveitis, except *[All India PGMEE 2000]*
a. Psoriasis b. Ankylosing Spondylitis
c. Reiter's syndrome d. Behcet's disease

49. Bamboo spine is seen in *[Recent Question 2017, AP PGMEE 1996]*
a. Tuberculosis spine b. Rheumatoid arthritis
c. Ankylosing spondylosis d. Ochronosis

50. The early X-Ray changes of Ankylosing spondylitis would be *[AMU PGMEE 1990]*
a. Disc space narrowing
b. Facetal joint ankylosis
c. Anterior osteophyte formation
d. Sacroiliac joint erosion

51. In a patient of gouty arthritis best investigation to detect it *[AIIMS PGMEE 1996, AIPGME 1998]*
a. Serum uric acid
b. Uric acid in urine
c. Urate crystal in synovial fluid
d. Serum calcium level

52. What is not true about gout? *[AIIMS PGMEE 1995]*
a. Abrupt increase in serum urate levels is more common a cause for acute gout than an abrupt fall in urate levels
b. Patient may be asymptomatic with high serum uric acid for years
c. Development of arthritis correlates with level of serum uric acid
d. Uric acid crystals are best seen by polarising light microscope

53. Specific test for gout is *[AIIMS PGMEE 1996]*
a. Raised serum uric acid level
b. Raised uric acid in synovial fluid of joint
c. Raised urea level
d. Raised urease enzyme level

54. Which is not involved in Ankylosing spondylitis? *[AIIMS PGMEE 1995]*
a. Knee & Ankle
b. Sacroiliac joint
c. Wrist & elbow
d. Spine

55. Most common charcot's joints involved in diabetes mellitus are those of *[All India PGMEE 1997]*
a. Shoulder
b. Foot
c. Ankle
d. Knee

56. A 35-year-old male patient develops involvement of proximal and distal interphalangeal joints and 1st carpometacarpal joints with sparing of wrist and metacarophalangeal joint. The diagnosis is *[All India PGMEE 2000]*
a. Osteoarthritis
b. Psoriatic arthropathy
c. Rheumatoid arthritis
d. Pseudogout

57. Osteoarthritis following is not a predisposing factor *[Kerala PGMEE 1996]*
a. Diabetes mellitus
b. Defective joint position
c. Weight bearing joints
d. Incongruity of articular surfaces
e. Old age

58. In Fracture acetabulum, late complication is *[Delhi PGMEE 1994]*
a. Osteoarthritis
b. Tardy sciatic nerve palsy
c. Recurrent Dislocation
d. None of the above

59. Clutton's joints are *[WB PGMEE 1997]*
a. Usually painful
b. Associated with trauma
c. Syphilitic joints
d. End stage Tuberculosis joints

60. The most common cause of Neuropathic joints is *[JIPMER PGMEE 1993, MANIPAL PGMEE 1994]*
a. Leprosy
b. Syphilis
c. Diabetes
d. Rheumatoid arthritis

61. Rheumatoid factor in rheumatoid arthritis is important because *[All India PGMEE 2002]*
a. RA factor is associated with bad prognosis
b. Absent RA factor rules out the diagnosis of rheumatoid arthritis
c. It is very common in childhood Rheumatoid arthritis
d. It correlates with disease activity

62. Joint not involved in Rheumatoid arthritis according to 1987 modified ARA criteria? *[AIIMS PGMEE 2008]*
a. Knee
b. Ankle
c. Tarsometatarsal
d. Metatarsophalangeal

63. All the following are true about Rheumatoid arthritis except *[All India PGMEE 1994]*
a. Positive for Anti-IgG antibody
b. Juxta-articular osteoporosis
c. Morning stiffness
d. C Reactive protein indicates better prognosis

64. Tertiary syphilitic arthritis most frequently involve *[TN PGMEE 1999]*
a. Hip
b. Ankle
c. Spine
d. Knee

65. All are true about gouty arthritis except *[AIIMS PGMEE 1993]*
a. Arthritis is manifested after long attack of hyperuricemia
b. There is good correlation between level of uric acid and severity of gouty arthritis
c. Synovial analysis is diagnostic
d. Allopurinol is treatment of choice in acute gout

66. Periosteal reaction is not common in *[AP PGMEE 1993]*
a. Syphilis
b. Gout
c. Osteomyelitis
d. Tuberculous dactylitis

67. How to differentiate gout with pseudogout? *[PGI 2000]*
a. Large joint involvement
b. Birefringent (Particles) crystals
c. Serum uric acid normal
d. Associated with hyperparathyroidism
e. Pain is very intense

68. Soft tissue calcification around the knee is seen in *[PGI 1990]*
a. Scurvy
b. Scleroderma
c. Hyperparathyroidism
d. Pseudogout

69. False about Charcot's joint in diabetes mellitus is *[All India PGMEE 2008]*
a. Limitation of movements with bracing
b. Arthrodesis
c. Arthrocentesis
d. Total ankle replacement

70. Which of the following is/are affected in gout? *[PGI 2000]*
a. Skin
b. Cartilage
c. Tendon
d. Muscle
e. Bursa

71. Para-articular erosion are most commonly seen in *[Delhi PGMEE 1996]*
a. Osteoarthirtis
b. Rheumatoid arthritis
c. Gout
d. Acute suppurative arthritis

72. Pain in small joints in an elderly lady is most likely due to *[UPSC 1993]*
a. Rheumatic arthritis
b. Rheumatoid arthritis
c. Psoriatic arthritis
d. Reiter's disease

73. All are features of Rheumatoid-arthritis, EXCEPT *[AIIMS PGMEE 1997]*
a. Osteosclerosis of joint
b. Soft tissue swelling
c. Narrowing of joint space
d. Periarticular osteoporosis

74. The most commonly involved joint in pseudo gout *[Rajasthan PGMEE 1993]*
a. Knee
b. Great toe
c. Hip
d. Elbow

75. A lady presents with right knee swelling. Aspiration was done in which CPPD crystals were obtained. Next best investigation is *[AIIMS PGMEE 2010]*
a. ANA
b. RF
c. CPK
d. TSH

76. In a patient with gouty arthritis, synovial fluid aspiration will show *[All India PGMEE 2009]*
a. Monosodium urate crystals
b. Calcium Pyrophosphate crystals
c. Mononuclear Leucocytosis
d. Polymorphonuclear Leukocytosis

77. All of the following are associated with CV junction anomalies except *[All India PGMEE 2007]*
a. Rheumatoid Arthritis
b. Ankylosing Spondylosis
c. Odontoid dysgenesis
d. Basal degeneration

78. In a gouty arthritis, the characteristic X-ray findings includes *[AP PGMEE 2000]*
a. Soft tissue calcification
b. Narrowing of joint space
c. Osteoporosis
d. Erosion of joint

79. Osteoarthritis all are true except *[PGI 2002]*
a. Occurs after 50 years of age
b. Single joint may be affected
c. Heberden's node present
d. Lower limb deformity seen
e. Ankylosis occurs

80. Severe disability in primary osteoarthritis of hip is best managed by *[PGI 1995]*
a. Arthrodesis
b. Arthroplasty
c. Mc Murray's osteotomy
d. Intra-articular hydrocortisone and physiotherapy

81. Involvement of PIP joint, DIP joint and the carpo-metacarpal joint of base of thumb with sparing the wrist is seen in *[All India PGMEE 2001, AIIMS 1999]*
a. Rheumatoid arthritis
b. Osteoarthritis
c. Psoriatic arthritis
d. Pseudogout

82. Which of the following is true regarding Rheumatoid arthritis? *[All India PGMEE 1994]*
a. Typically involves small and large joints symmetrically but spares the cervical spine
b. Causes pleural effusion with low sugar
c. Pulmonary nodules are absent
d. Enthesopathy prominent

83. All of the following are well known features of Rheumatoid arthritis except *[PGI 1992]*
a. Bilateral hip arthritis
b. Erosion of distal interphalangeal joints
c. Pleural effusion
d. Hypocomplementemia

84. Which is true regarding rheumatoid arthritis? *[PGI 2001]*
a. Small and large joints are affected mostly
b. Younger females are affected more commonly
c. Diagnosed only if Rheumatoid factor is positive
d. Life expectancy is unchanged
e. Hepatosplenomegaly is common

85. A person has severe pain & swelling in great toe. True statements is/ are *[PGI June 2009]*
a. Allopurinol used in acute control of gout
b. Colchicine cause gastrointestinal disturbances
c. High serum uric acid level may be not present
d. Joint Fluid aspiration is done for investigation
e. Colchicine acts slowly

86. Characteristic crystals in Pseudo-gout are *[All India PGMEE 1997]*
a. Sodium pyrophosphate
b. Calcium pyrophosphate
c. Sodium monourate
d. Potassium urate

87. Calcification of menisci is seen in *[All India PGMEE 1989]*
a. Hyperparathyroidism
b. Acromegaly
c. Pseudogout
d. Renal Osteodystrophy

88. Subluxation of atlanto-occipital joint is seen in all except *[DPG 1991]*
a. Gout
b. Parapharyngeal abscess
c. Rheumatoid arthritis
d. Ankylosing spondylitis

89. Extra articular clinical features of Rheumatoid Arthritis *[AIIMS PGMEE 1992]*
a. Splenomegaly
b. Fever
c. Subcutaneous nodules
d. Pleural effusion

90. In RA (Rheumatoid Arthritis) true is *[PGI 2006]*
a. MC in young
b. RF is diagnostic
c. Small & big joints involved
d. Felty syndrome associated

91. A woman presented with right shoulder pin and Rheumatoid factor test came as negative, but the pain responded to the Prednisolone therapy. The diagnosis include *[NBE DNB 1990, Delhi PGMEE 1999]*
a. Osteopetrosis
b. Seronegative Rheumatoid arthritis
c. Polymylagia
d. Polymyalgia rheumtica

92. A 65 years old man had history of back pain since last 3 months. ESR is raised. He also has marked stiffness on examination and mild restriction of chest movements. On X-ray, syndesmophytes are present in vertebrae. Diagnosis is *[AIIMS PGMEE 2010]*
a. Ankylosing spondylitis
b. Degenerative osteoarthritis of spine
c. Lumber canal stenosis
d. Tuberculosis

93. Most common site for pseudo-tumour like growth in haemophilic arthropathy is *[All India PGMEE 1998]*
a. Iliopsoas muscle
b. Quadriceps femoris muscle
c. Gastrocnemius muscle
d. Hamstring muscle

94. Still's disease is *[Bihar PGMEE 1991]*
a. Post traumatic bone formation in the lateral ligament of the knee
b. Spastic diplegia
c. Rheumatoid arthritis in child hood
d. Rheumatoid arthritis in the elderly

95. The following are rheumatoid disease modifying drugs except *[All India PGMEE 1995]*
a. Chloroquine b. Gold
c. Penicillamine d. BAL

96. Gold salts can be used in *[All India PGMEE 1994]*
a. Ankylosing spondylitis b. Rheumatoid arthritis
c. Osteoarthritis d. Behcet's syndrome

97. Indication of systemic steroids in rheumatoid arthritis is *[All India PGMEE 1997]*
a. Mononeuritis multiplex
b. Carpul tunnel syndrome
c. Presence of deformities
d. Articular cartilage involvement

98. Which is characteristic feature(s) of osteoarthritis on X-ray? *[JIPMER PGMEE 1997]*
a. Spurring
b. Subchondral sclerosis
c. Dimunition of cartilage space
d. All of these

99. Osteoarthritis is associated with all of the following except *[All India PGMEE 1999]*
a. Decrease joint space
b. Subchondral sclerosis
c. Osteophyte formation
d. Ca++ deposition in joint space

100. Which of the following is inflammatory arthritis? *[All India PGMEE 1994]*
a. Rheumatoid arthritis b. Osteoarthritis
c. Osteochondritis d. All of the above

101. One of the following is to be considered as differential diagnosis for foreign body in plain X-ray of knee joint *[NIMS PGMEE 2000]*
a. Fabella b. Calcified bursa
c. Patella d. Chondromatosis

102. True about osteochondromatosis *[PGI 2008]*
a. Malignant b. Manifest at adult
c. Seen at 4–6 years after disease
d. Common in women

103. Terminal interphalangeal joints of hands are commonly involved in *[All India PGMEE 1993]*
a. Psoriatic arthropathy b. Rheumatoid arthritis
c. Still diseases d. Ankylosing spondylitis

104. Tom smith's arthritis is due to *[PGI 1999, JIPMER PGMEE 2014, Recent Question 2018]*
a. Pyogenic infection in infancy
b. Tuberculosis
c. Rheumatoid arthritis
d. Osteoarthritis

105. Septic arthritis in a 2 year old child is often caused by *[AIIMS PGMEE 1994]*
a. Gonococci b. Pneumococci
c. *Haemophilous influenzae*
d. *Staphylococcus aureus*

106. Tom Smith arthritis manifests as *[All India PGMEE 1996]*
a. Increase hip mobility and unstability
b. Hip stiffness
c. A + D
d. Shortening of limb

107. Chondrolysis occurs commonly in *[PGI 1992]*
a. T.B. arthritis b. Syphilitic arthritis
c. Chondrosarcoma only d. Septic arthritis of infancy

108. Acute suppurative arthritis is associated with all except *[PGI 1994]*
a. Be caused by a penetrating wound
b. Be caused by a compound fracture involving a joint
c. Be due to blood-borne infection
d. Causes the joint to be held in the position of ease
e. Tends to end with the formation of a fibrous ankylosis

109. In rheumatoid arthritis, pathology starts in the *[All India PGMEE 1995]*
a. Articular cartilage b. Capsule
c. Synovium d. Muscles

110. A 35 year old male develops involvements of PIP, DIP and metacarpophalangeal joints with sparing of wrist and carpometacarpal joints. The probable diagnosis is *[AIIMS 1999]*
a. Psoriatic arthopathy b. Osteo arthritis
c. Rheumatoid arthritis d. Pseudo gout

111. All are true regarding psoriatic arthritis except *[PGI 2002, JIPMER PGMEE 2001]*
a. Arthritis mutilans b. DIP involvement
c. Ankylosis of small joints d. Sacroilitis
e. Lengthening of digit known as telescoping

112. Which one of the following is not associated with HLA B 27? *[UPSC 1999]*
a. Ankylosing spondylitis b. Reiter's syndrome
c. Sjogren's syndrome d. Psoriatic arthritis

113. All of the following are seen in inflammatory polyarthritis, except *[AIIMS PGMEE 1994]*
a. New bone formation b. Erythema
c. Increased ESR
d. Morning stiffness more than one hour

114. Distal interphalangeal joint is not involved in *[All India PGMEE 1998]*
a. Rheumatoid arthritis
b. Psoriatic arthritis
c. Multicentric histeocytosis
d. Neuropathic arthropathy

115. Most common cause of bony ankylosis is *[AIIMS PGMEE 1993, PGI 1995, 1997]*
a. Rheumatoid arthritis b. Pyogenic arthritis
c. Traumatic arthritis d. Osteoarthritis

116. Most common cause of nongonococcal septic arthritis is *[AIIMS PGMEE 1997]*
a. *Staphylococcus aureus* b. *H. influenzae*
c. Pseudomonas d. Streptococcus

117. Swan-neck deformity is *[AIIMS PGMEE 2000, PGI 1992 [Recent Question 2015]*
a. Flexion of Metacarpophalangeal joint and extension at interphalangeal joint
b. Extension at Proximal interphalangeal joint and flexion at Distal interphalangeal joint

c. Flexion at proximal interphalangeal joint and extension at distal interphalangeal joint
d. Extension at Metacarpophalangeal joint and flexion at interphalangeal joint

118. Hyperextension of PIP joints and hyperflexion of DIP joint is known as *[Kerala PGMEE 1990]*
a. Trigger finger
b. Boutonier's deformity
c. Swan-neck deformity
d. Mallet finger

119. A burn patient develop claw hand. Joint affected will be *[PGI 2008]*
a. Flexion at Proximal Interphalangeal Joint
b. Flexion at Distal Interphalangeal Joint
c. Thumb Abduction
d. Flexion at Metacarpophalangeal Joint
e. Extension at Metacarpophalangeal Joint

120. All are seronegative (spondyloepiphyseal) arthritis with ocular manifestations, except *[AIIMS PGMEE 2001]*
a. Ankylospondilitis
b. Ritter's disease
c. Rheumatoid arthritis
d. Psoriatic arthritis

121. HLA B27 is associated with *[All India PGMEE 1989]*
a. Rheumatoid arthritis
b. Ankylosing spondylitis
c. Rheumatic arthritis
d. Gouty arthritis

122. Positivity of HLA B 27 in Ankylosing spondylitis *[NIMS PGMEE 1996]*
a. 10%
b. 96%
c. 78%
d. 100%

123. In ankylosing spondylitis, the joint least commonly involved is *[AIIMS PGMEE 1993]*
a. Elbow
b. Sacroiliac
c. Ankle
d. Spinal

124. RA factor is used mainly *[PGI 1994]*
a. Screening patients for Rheumatoid arthritis
b. Predicting multisystem disease
c. Predicting severity of disease
d. Monitoring treatment

125. Flexion at distal interphalangeal joint in Rheumatoid arthritis is *[PGI November 2014]*
a. Equinus deformity
b. Boutonneire deformity
c. Swan neck deformity
d. Hammer toe
e. Mallet toe

126. HLA B27 is 90% positive in *[AIIMS November 2014]*
a. Ankylosing spondylitis
b. Reiter's syndrome
c. Rheumatoid arthritis
d. Psoriatic arthritis

127. 40 years old male presented with pain over great toe. X-ray shows erosions over phalanges extending into soft tissues. Most likely diagnosis is *[AIIMS November 2014]*
a. Gout
b. Psoriatic arthropathy
c. Rheumatoid arthritis
d. Charcot's joint

128. DMARD are useful in *[AIIMS November 2014]*
a. Rheumatoid arthritis
b. Resistant osteoarthritis
c. Gout
d. Hyperthyroidism

129. Bouchard's nodes are seen in *[ESI IMO 2014]*
a. Proximal IP joints
b. Distal IP joints
c. Sternoclavicular joints
d. Knee joint

130. All of the following conditions are observed in Gout except *[ESI IMO 2014]*
a. Uric acid nephrolithiasis
b. Deficiency of enzyme Xanthine oxidase
c. Increase is serum urate concentration
d. Renal disease involving interstitial tissues

131. Most common organism associated with Reactive arthritis is *[Recent Question 2016, ESI IMO 2014]*
a. Staphylococcus
b. Shigella
c. Chlamydia
d. Yersinia

132. A seven year old boy presents with acute onset of mild intermittent pain in the right groin and a limp. Abduction and internal rotation of the hip were restricted on the affected side. There was no fever. Radiographs of the pelvis were normal. The most likely diagnosis is *[UPSC CMS 2017]*
a. Transient monoarticular synovitis
b. Legg Calve Perthes disease
c. Slipped capital femoral epiphyses
d. Osteochondritis dissecans

ANSWERS WITH EXPLANATIONS OF MCQs

1. **Ans. (a) Boutonniere Deformity**
[Ref. Applied Therapeutics by Ernst, 10/e p1014]

Boutonnière (Buttonhole) Deformity (BD)

- Develop either in Acute setting (secondary to trauma) or Progressively (secondary to arthritis)
- Patient's finger exhibits pathologic flexion at Proximal interphalangeal (PIP) joint and hyperextension at Distal interphalangeal (DIP) joint

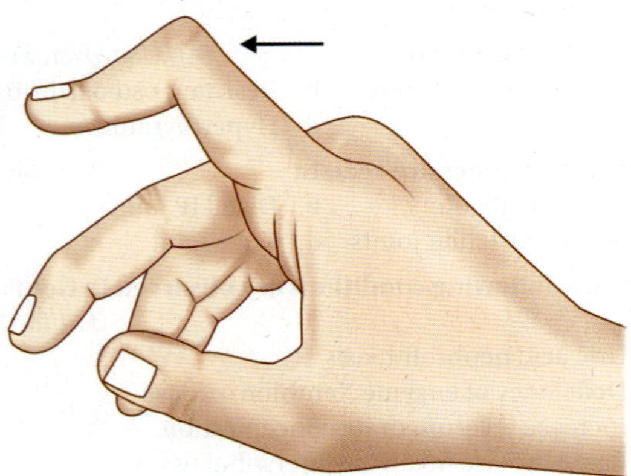

Fig. Boutonniere deformity

Also Remember

- Swan-neck deformity: DIP flexion with PIP hyperextension
- Z-thumb/deformity: Hyperextension of Interphalangeal joint, fixed flexion and subluxation of Metacarpophalangeal joint (MCP)
- Ulnar Claw hand: 4th and 5th fingers extended at MCP joints and flexed at Interphalangeal joints

2. **Ans. (a) Cervical Spine**
[Ref. Cervical Myelopathy by Passias, 1/e p93]

Rheumatoid Arthritis and Spine

- MC source of inflammatory disease of Cervical spine
- **Upper cervical spine is MC affected**
- Three hallmark disorders of RA Cervical spine:
  - Atlantoaxial subluxation
  - Vertical settling (Basilar invagination)
  - Sub-axial subluxation

3. **Ans. (d) Fibrous Ankylosis**
[Ref. Maheshwari, 4/e p280]

Rheumatoid Arthritis Radiology

- Joint space erosion **(Arrows in Photograph)**
- Erosion of articular margins
- Subchondral cysts
- Periarticular osteopenia, Juxta-articular rarefaction
- Soft tissue shadow at joint (Effusion or Synovial hypertrophy)
- Hand/ fingers deformities

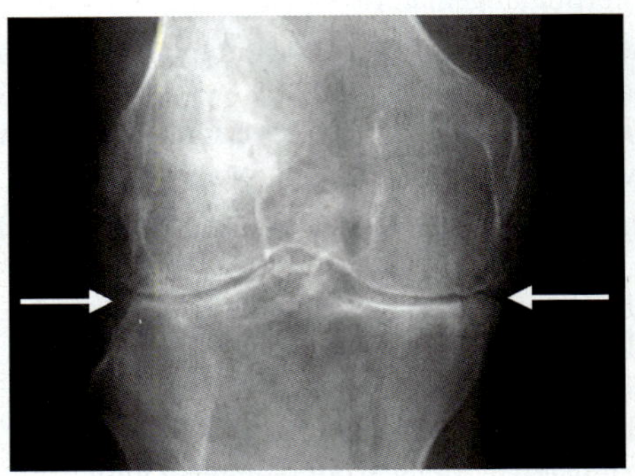

Fig. RA

Also Remember

Four Stages of Inflammation in RA

- **Stage 1 (Early stage RA):** Initial inflammation in the joint capsule and swelling of synovial tissue; Induces the clear symptoms of joint pain, swelling, and stiffness
- **Stage 2 (Moderate stage of RA):** Inflammation of synovial tissue becomes severe enough that it causes cartilage damage; Symptoms of loss of mobility and range of motion become more frequent
- **Stage 3 (Severe RA):** Inflammation in the synovium is destroying bone as well; Increased pain and swelling and a further decrease in mobility and even muscle strength with physical deformities on the joint may start to develop as well
- **Stage 4 (End RA):** Inflammatory process ceases and joints stop functioning altogether; Pain, swelling, stiffness and loss of mobility are still the primary symptoms

4. **Ans. (b) Lupus Arthritis/ Jaccoud arthritis**
[Ref. Cutaneous Medicine by Provost, 1/e p60]

Jaccoud's Type of Arthritis

- Nonerosive, deforming arthritis with Severe ulnar deviation
- Seen in Anti-Ro Lupus patients and SCFE patients

5. **Ans. (a) Rheumatoid arthritis**
[Ref. Clinical Primer of Rheumatology by Koopman, 1/e p52]

- **In hammer toe**, the proximal interphalangeal joint is flexed and the tip of the toe points downward

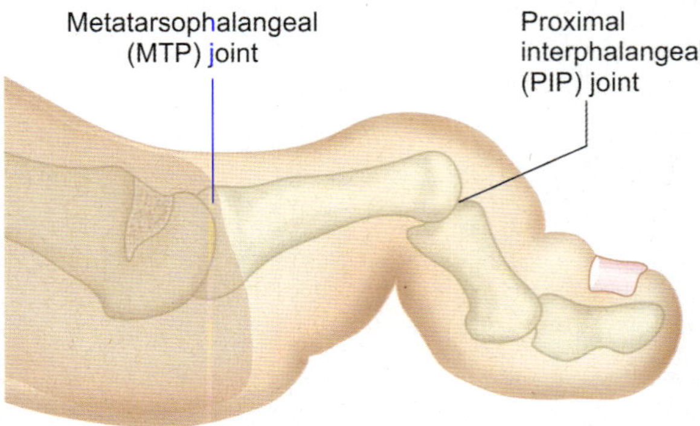

Fig. Hammer Toe

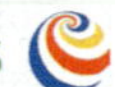

6. Ans. (a) **Pyogenic infection in infancy**
[Ref. IAP Textbook of Pediatrics by Parthasarathy, 6/e p1118]
- Acute septic arthritis of infancy (Tom Smith arthritis), seen in infancy, is generally secondary to a neighboring bone lesion

7. Ans. (a) **Osteoarthritis**
[Ref. Orthopedics for Primary Care by Anderson, 1/e p119]
- With age-related Osteoarthritis the distal interphalangeal joints (DIPs) are affected preferentially, with lesser involvement of the proximal interphalangeal joint

8. Ans. (a) **Osteophytes are seen in osteoarthritis**
[Ref. Orthopedic Secrets by Brown, 3/e p120]
- Large osteophytes seen in osteoarthritis are uncommon in rheumatoid arthritis

9. Ans. (b) **Rheumatoid arthritis**
[Ref. Maheshwari, 4/e p280]
- *Deformities in Rheumatoid Arthritis*:

Site	Deformities
Hand	Swan neck deformity, Boutonniere deformity, Z deformity
Elbow	Flexion deformity
Knee	Triple subluxation
Ankle	Equinus
Foot	Wind-sweep deformity, Hammer toe

10. Ans. (d) **Widening of joint spaces**
[Ref. Maheshwari, 4/e p288]
- **X-rays in Osteoarthritis**: Narrowing of joint spaces, Subchondral sclerosis, Subchondral cysts, Osteophytes, Loose bodies, Deformity of joint

11. Ans. (b) **Septic arthritis**
[Ref. Maheshwari, 4/e p171]
- Bony ankyloses is the usual outcome of a neglected Septic arthritis

12. Ans. (c) **Metacarpophalangeal joint**
[Ref. Maheshwari, 4/e p279]

Polyarthritis in Rheumatoid Arthritis
- *Clinical presentation*: Pain and stiffness in multiple (>4) joints, usually in the morning
- ***Most common joint involved*: Metacarpophalangeal joints (MC Index finger)**
- *Joints affected in Rheumatoid arthritis*:

Involvement	Joints
Common	**MP joints of hand (Most common)** PIP joints of fingers Wrists, knees, elbows, ankles
Less common	Hip joint Temporomandibular joint
Uncommon	Atlantoaxial joint Facet joints of cervical spine

13. Ans. (c) **Periarticular osteopenia**
[Ref. Core Radiology by Mandell, 1/e p351]
- **Earliest radiographic changes in Rheumatoid arthritis** are Soft-tissue swelling and Periarticular osteopenia (reflecting synovitis and hyperemia)

14. Ans. (a) **Stills' disease**
[Ref. Musculoskeletal Imaging by Chew, 2/e p23]

15. Ans. (c) **Medial tibiofemoral**
[Ref. Osteoarthritis by Moscowitz, 4/e p18]

16. Ans. (a) **Morning stiffness**
[Ref. Pathology of Rheumatic Diseases by Fassbender, 1/e p302]
- **ILAR International Classification for Rheumatic Disorders:**
  - Bursitis
  - Tendinitis, Tenosynovitis, Tenoperostitis
  - Fasciitis
  - Fibrositis
  - Myositis
  - Neuritis
  - Periarthritis
  - Panniculitis

17. Ans. (c) **JRA**
[Ref. Imaging of Arthritis and Metabolic Bone Disease by Weissman, 1/e p410]

Seronegative Spondyloarthropathies
- Ankylosing spondylitis (AS)
- Reactive arthritis/ Reiter's syndrome
- Psoriatic arthropathy
- Spondylopathy associated with Inflammatory bowel disease (Enteropathic)
- Undifferentiated spondylopathy
- Juvenile onset spondyloarthropathy

18. Ans. (c) **Knee**
[Ref. Maheshwari, 4/e p288]
- MC joint involved in Osteoarthritis in Western population: **Hip**
- MC joint involved in Osteoarthritis in Asian population: **Knee**

19. Ans. (c) **Psoriatic arthritis**
[Ref. The Cleveland Clinic Foundation: Intensive Review of Internal Medicine by Mendel, 5/e p353]
- **Sausage digits**: Combination of enthesopathy and dactylitis seen in Psoriatic arthritis and Reiter's syndrome

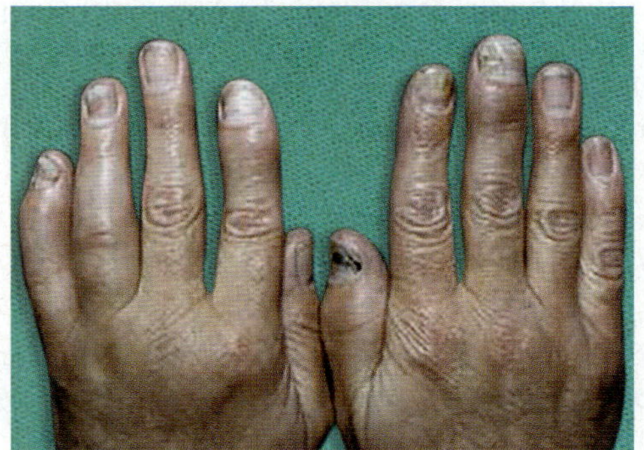

Fig. Psoriatic arthritis

Orthopedics

20. Ans. (b) **Distal interphalangeal joints in Osteoarthritis**
[Ref. Adult Orthopedic Nursing by Schoen, 1/e p60]

- **Heberden's Nodes**: Acute inflammation of Distal interphalangeal joints with prominent osteophytes as a consequence of Osteoarthritis

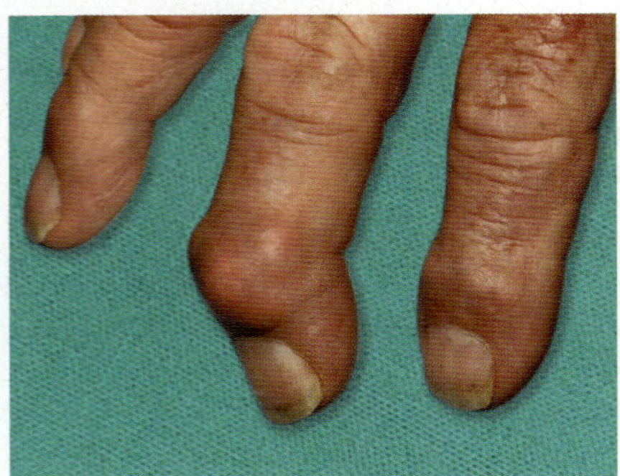

Fig. Heberdens nodes

21. Ans. (b) **Ankylosing spondylitis**
[Ref. Maheshwari, 4/e p279]

Sacroilitis

- Sacroilitis is an acute inflammation of sacro-iliac joint
- *Seen in spondyloarthropathies*:
  - **Ankylosing spondylitis (Most common)**
  - Psoriatic arthritis
  - Reactive arthritis
  - Inflammatory bowel disease (Ulcerative colitis, Crohn's disease)

Radiology in Ankylosing Spondylitis: X-Ray Pelvis

- Haziness of sacroiliac joints with subchondral erosions
- Sclerosis of SI joints
- Bony ankylosis of SI joints
- Calcification of sacroiliac and sacrotuberous ligaments
- Enthesopathy (calcification at attachments of muscles/ tendons/ ligaments)

Radiology in Ankylosing Spondylitis: X-Ray Lumbar Spine

- Squaring of vertebrae
- Syndesmophytes (Bridging osteophytes)
- 'Bamboo-spine appearance'
- Loss of lumbar lordosis

22. Ans. (a) **Rheumatoid arthritis**
[Ref. Rheumatoid Arthritis by Haynes, 1/e p18]

- **MC Compressive neuropathy in Rheumatoid arthritis: Carpal tunnel syndrome** (Median nerve compression - MC Neurologic manifestation of Rheumatoid arthritis)
- Other Compressive neuropathy in Rheumatoid arthritis: Tarsal tunnel syndrome (Posterior tibial nerve compression)

23. Ans. (b) **Osteoarthritis**
[Ref. Adult Orthopedic Nursing by Schoen, 1/e p60]

24. Ans. (d) **All**
[Ref. General Medicine Radiology by Prabhakar, 1/e p435]

- **Distal phalanx resorption (Acro-osteolysis)**: Scleroderma, Hyperparathyroidism, Reiter's syndrome, Psoriasis, Dermatomyositis, Thermal injury, PVC exposure, Epidermolysis bullosa, Rheumatoid conditions, Sarcoidosis, Leprosy, Pyknodysostosis, Progeria, Asymbolia, Syringomelia

25. Ans. (d) **Does not affect large joints**
[Ref. Rheumatology Secrets by West, 3/e p348]

26. Ans. (b) **DIP**
[Ref. Ferris Clinical Advisor 2016, p1084]

27. Ans. (a) **Rheumatoid arthritis, Neutropenia, Splenomegaly**
[Ref. Hematology/ Oncology Secrets by, 3/e p100]

28. Ans. (c) **Medial tibiofemoral**
[Ref. Maheshwari, 4/e p287-88]

Radiology in Osteoarthritis

- Narrowing of joint space (initially and mostly) in Medial compartment of tibiofemoral joint
- Subchondral sclerosis
- Subchondral cysts
- Osteophytes formation
- Loose bodies
- Deformity of joint

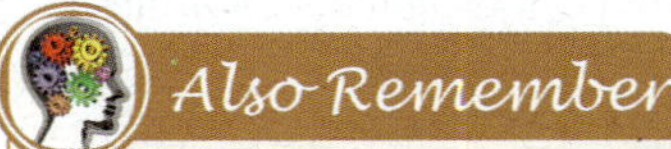

Also Remember

- In Osteoarthritis, due to more involvement of medial compartment of knee joint, *'genu varum deformity is more common'*

29. Ans. (a) **Ankle**
[Ref. Obesity: Science to Practice by Gareth, 1/e p323]

30. Ans. (b) **Knee**
[Ref. Maheshwari, 4/e p287]

Arthritic – Degenerative Disorders and Sites Involved

Disorder	Sites involved
Rheumatoid arthritis	MP joints of hand (Most common) PIP joints of fingers Wrists, knees, elbows, ankles
Ankylosing spondylitis (Marie Stumpell disease)	Sacroiliac joints (Most common) Spine (above lumbar region) Hip, Knee, Manubrio-sternal joints
Gouty arthritis	MP joint great toe (Most common) Olecranon bursa
Pseudogout	Menisci of knee
Psoriatic arthropathy	Distal IP joints
Alcaptonuric arthritis (Ocronosis)	Spine Shoulder joint
Hemophilic arthritis	Knee, elbow, ankle joint
Primary osteoarthritis	Knee joint (Most common) Hip joint
Secondary osteoarthritis	Hip joint
Cervical spondylosis	C5-C6 intervertebral joint
Lumbar spondylosis	L5-S1 intervertebral joint

31. Ans. (d) Joint deformities are common sequel
[Ref. Long Cases in Clinical Medicine by Abdullah, 1/e p457]

32. Ans. (d) Lymphadenitis
[Ref. Orthopedic Nursing Secrets by Michael, 1/e p55]

- **Reiter's syndrome**: Chronic form of arthritis, after infection, characterized by
  - Inflammation of joints (Seronegative arthritis)
  - Inflammation of conjunctiva (Conjunctivitis)
  - Inflammation of genital/ urinary system (Nonspecific urethritis/ cervicitis)

33. Ans. (d) Rheumatoid arthritis
[Ref. Maheshwari, 4/e p280]

34. Ans. (a) AS
[Ref. Hospital Medicine, Volume 65, p15]

35. Ans. (b) Aortic insufficiency
[Ref. Maheshwari, 4/e p284]

Extra-articular Manifestations of Ankylosing Spondylitis

Ocular	Acute iritis
Cardiovascular	Aortic incompetence Cardiomegaly Conduction defects Pericarditis
Neurological	Dislocation/ subluxation of atlanto-axial joint
Pulmonary	Costovertebral joints involvement Apical lobe fibrosis with cavitation
Systemic	Generalized osteoporosis Amyloidosis

36. Ans. (a) Ankylosing spondylitis
[Ref. Manual of Orthopedics by Stovitz, 7/e p76]

37. Ans. (a) Rheumatoid arthritis
[Ref. Maheshwari, 4/e p280]

Extra-articular Manifestations of Rheumatoid Arthritis

Vaculitis	• Digital arteritis • Raynaud's phenomenon • Peripheral neuritis • Necrotising arteritis
Rheumatoid Nodules	• Olecranon (Most common site) • Dorsal surface forearm
Serositis	• Pleurisy, Caplan's syndrome • Cardiomyopathy, Pericarditis • Iridocyclitis • Carpal tunnel syndrome
Others	• Anaemia • Felty's syndrome • Sjogren's syndrome (Sicca syndrome) • Amyloidosis

38. Ans. (c) More common in males
[Ref. Clinical Primer of Rheumatology by Koopman, 1/e p4]

39. Ans. (d) Typhoid
[Ref. Maheshwari, 4/e p280-281; Medicinenet.com]

Rheumatoid Factor

- *Rheumatoid factor is a type of autoantibody against*: Fc fragment of IgG
- *Most common sub*-type detected by most tests: IgM-RF
- *Tests for detection*:
  - Rose-Waaler test (sensitivity 60%)
  - Latex fixation test (sensitivity 80%)

Rheumatoid factor seen in

- [**Mnemonic: R**heumatoid-factor **Is S**een **In HEAT L**ike **S**ultry **S**ummers]
  - **R**hematoid arthtritis (80% cases)
  - **I**nfectious mononucleosis
  - **S**LE
  - **I**nfluenza
  - **H**epatitis
  - **E**ndocarditis
  - **A**IDS
  - **T**uberculosis
  - **L**iver disease
  - **S**arcoidosis
  - **S**yphilis

40. Ans. (b) Joint aspiration
[Ref. Current Therapy in Pain by Smith, 1/e p181]

41. Ans. (d) L5 over S1
[Ref. Maheshwari, 4/e p217, 277]

Spondylolisthesis

- *Definition*: Forward displacement of a vertebra over one below it (Most common: L5-S1)
- X-ray oblique view of spine: *Scottish dog 'head separated from neck' appearance*
- Vertebral slippage is PRESENT

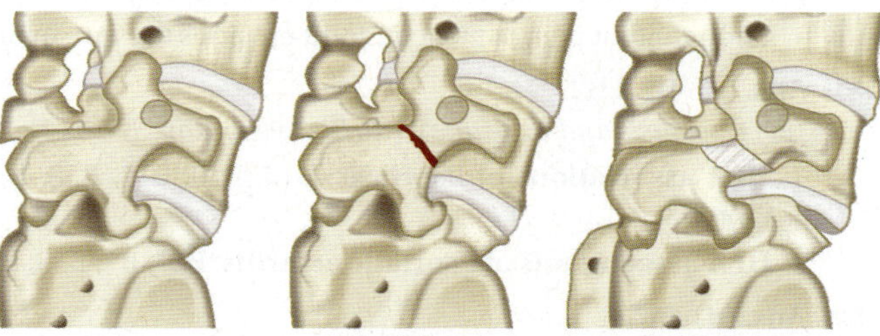

Normal Spondylolysis Spondylolisthesis

42. Ans. (b) Glucosamine
[Ref. Study Guide for Introduction to Clinical Pharmacology by Edmunds, 8/e p115]

43. Ans. (a) Cervical spine
[Ref. Maheshwari, 4/e p279]

44. Ans. (c) Herberdens node osteoarthritis
[Ref. Adult Orthopedic Nursing by Schoen, 1/e p60]

45. Ans. (c) Symptoms for at least six months
[Ref. Maheshwari, 4/e p278]

Diagnostic Criteria for Rheumatoid Arthritis: (Four or More Must be Present)

- Morning stiffness
- Swelling of >3 joints
- Swelling of joints in hand/ wrist
- Rheumatoid nodule
- Rheumatoid factor +ve
- Erosion or osteopenia on X-ray

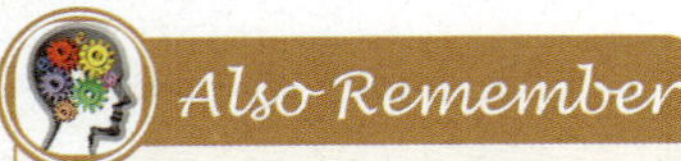

- *Sensitivity of these criteria*: 93%
- *Specificity of these criteria*: 90%

46. Ans. (b) RA
[Ref. Rheumatoid Arthritis by Haynes, 1/e p124]

47. Ans. (d) Conjunctivitis
[Ref. Handbook of Paediatric Renal Disease by Wright 1/e p357]

Ocular Manifestations of Juvenile Rheumatoid Arthritis

- Chronic iridocyclitis (predominant manifestation)
- Uveitis
- Glaucoma
- Band keratopathy
- Anterior, posterior synechiae
- Cataract
- Cystoid macular oedema

48. Ans. (b) Filling of lateral fossae
[Ref. Essential Orthopaedics by J. Maheshwari, 4th Ed., Pg 355]

Tests for Effusion in Knee Joint

- Patellar tap test ***('Dancing patella' sign)***
- Fluctuation test
- Stroke test (Brush test)
- Ballotment test
- Bulge sign (Filled up medial fossae)

49. Ans. (c) Normal Plasma Albumin
[Ref. Maheshwari, 4/e p298]

50. Ans. (a) SLE
[Ref. Basic Biomedical Science by Azer, 1/e p385]

- Though joint pain is present, Joint erosions are rare in SLE

51. Ans. (c) HLA B27
[Ref. Psoriasis and Psoriatic Arthritis by Gordon, 1/e p14]

- **HLA associations of Psoriasis**: B13, B16, B17, B38, B39, Cw6
- **HLA associations of Psoriatic arthritis**: B27, B7, B38, B39

52. Ans. (d) MCP
[Ref. MKSAP for Students 4, p306]

- Joints involved in Osteoarthritis: AC, PIP, DIP, 1st CMC, Hips, Knees, Midfoot, 1st MTP, Mid-to-low cervical spine, Lumbar spine
- Joints not involved in Osteoarthritis: MCP, Elbow

53. Ans. (b) 1, 2 and 4
[Ref. Rapid Review Pathology by Edward, 4/e p644]

- Uveitis is seen in only 40% cases of Juvenile Rheumatoid Arthritis

54. Ans. (b) Polyarthritis
[Ref. IBD by Bayless, 1/e p655]

Behcet's Syndrome

- **Criteria for diagnosis**: Recurrent oral ulceration, Recurrent genital ulceration, Skin lesions, Uveitis, Eye lesions, Positive pathergy
- **Additional features**: GIT disease, Peripheral arthritis (Oligoarticular, Large joint, Asymmetric), Sacroileitis, Thrombophlbitis, Epididymitis, Large vessel vasculitis, Stroke, Dementia

55. Ans. (c) Pauciarticular type
[Ref. RA by Batty, 1/e]

Pauciarticular JRA

- Affects four or fewer joints
- About 50 percent of children with JRA have the Pauciarticular type, making it the most common type
- Further subdivided into early onset and late onset

56. Ans. (b) Sclerosis on X-ray
[Ref. Sports Medicine by Waterbrook, 1/e p47]

Inflammatory Arthritis

- Systemic signs and symptoms of Inflammation: Elevates ESR/ CRP, fever, anemia of chronic disease, fatigue, and weight loss
- Warm, swollen joint and demonstrate painful crepitus in addition to tenderness
- Painful restriction of movements
- X-ray findings: Osteopenia, juxtaarticular erosions, symmetric joint space loss, cystic change and in severe cases central glenoid erosion, and humeral head elevation

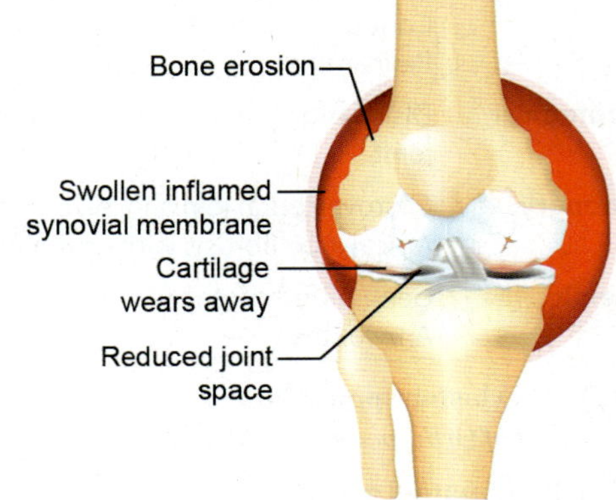

Fig. Inflammatory arthritis

57. Ans. (a) Ankle
[Ref. Joint Disease by Huskisson, 1/e p8]

- Shoulders and hips affected in 40%, peripheral joints in 25%, knees, commonest (15%), also ankles (10%), feet (5%), wrists (5%) and rarely fingers

58. Ans. (b) Metatarsophalangeal joint of big toe
[Ref. Ambulatory Medicine by Fiebach, 7/e p1243]

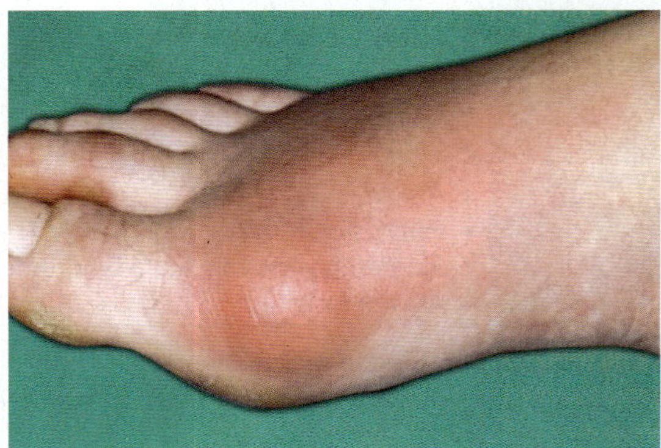

Fig. Gout

- Mostly monoarticular with swelling, tenderness, erythema, and intense inflammation
- Big-toe metatarsophalangeal joint commonly involved **(Podagra)**
- Forefeet, heels, ankles, knees, wrists, fingers, elbows, and other joints may be affected

59. Ans. (b) Most common joint disease
[Ref. Skeletal Radiology by Chew, 3/e p226]

Osteoarthritis

- OA is common, especially in the elderly, and women are affected more frequently than men
- Radiographically, the typical findings of OA: Joint space narrowing, Osteophytosis, Bony eburnation, Subchondral cyst formation, Intraarticular osteochondral bodies
- OA is classified into Primary or idiopathic and Secondary, and Inflammatory when there is significant synovial involvement with effusion

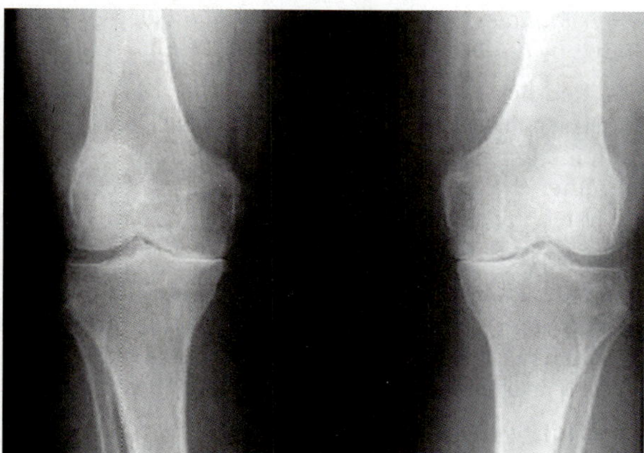

Fig. Joint space narrowing and osteophytes (OA)

60. Ans. (d) Roentgenogram is the most sensitive investigation
[Ref. Orthopaedics by Kotwal, 1/e p119]

Marie Strumpell Disease

- **Syn. Ankylosing Spondylitis**
- Common inflammatory enthesopathy and arthropathy preferentially affecting the axial skeleton, often beginning in Sacroiliac joints and ascending to involve the remaining spine
- MC Joint involved: Sacroiliac joint
- Aetiology is not known: Autoimmune disorder with a strong association with HLA-B 27
- More common in males (Male : Female ratio 9:1)
- Age of onset: 15-20 years

61. Ans. (c) Gouty arthritis
[Ref. Orthopedics by Mohindra, 2/e p435]

Martel's sign

- **Syn. Rat bite sign**
- X-ray finding seen in patients with Gout
- Well-defined, 'punched-out' type bony erosions with sclerotic margins, resulting from a long-standing, soft-tissue tophus in patients with Gout

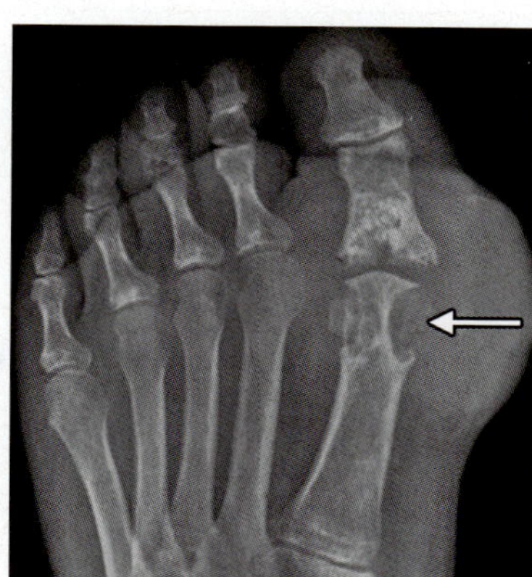

Fig. Martel's sign

62. Ans. (a) Anti-CCP
[Ref. Kelley and Firestein's Textbook of Rheumatology, 10/e p835]

Anti-CCP Antibodies

- High specificity for the diagnosis of RA
- In systematic reviews and meta-analyses, anti-CCP antibody positivity has been shown to be as sensitive as but more specific than RF in distinguishing RA from other forms of inflammatory arthritis
- Anti-CCP autoantibodies is an important predictor of development of RA: RA developed within 3 years in more than 90% of the patients with undifferentiated arthritis who tested positive for anti-CCP

63. Ans. (c) Macrophages
[Ref. Rheumatoid Arthritis by Henderson, 1/e p135]

- Rheumatoid Arthritis is characterized by hyperplasia of the synovial lining cells, prominent infiltration of monocyte/macrophages, neovascularization and fibroblast proliferation, and mast cells

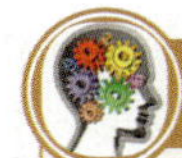

Also Remember

- All macrophages in rheumatoid tissue appear to be CD68 positive, but within the intima fibroblastic synoviocytes may carry modest amounts of CD68 as well

HIGH YIELD MCQs ANSWERS WITH EXPLANATIONS

1. Ans. (b) 1, 2 and 4
[Ref. Child's Foot and Ankle by McCarthy, 2/e p451]

Polyarticular Juvenile Rheumatoid Arthritis (PJRA)

- Five or more joints affected in first 6 months of illness
- 30% of JRA cases
- Symmetric involvement of wrists, knees, ankles
- Fatigue, low grade symptoms, joint symptoms
- Females: Males = 3 : 1
- Seronegative, Uveitis more common in children
- Only 7-15% PJRA show uveitis

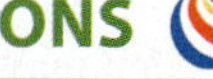

Also Remember

- Adolescents JRA present similar to Adult RA: RF Seropositivity, increased frequency of HLA antigens, Higher chance of Rheumatoid nodules/Joint erosions/Felty syndrome

2. Ans. (c) Pauciarticular type

[Ref. Pediatric Emergency Medicine by Fleisher, 6/e p1129]

- About 50 percent of children with JRA have Pauciarticular type, making it MC type of JRA

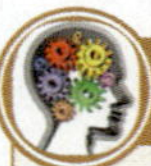

Also Remember

- **3 major types of Juvenile Rheumatoid arthritis:**
  - Polyarticular arthritis
  - Pauciarticular JRA
  - Systemic JRA

3. Ans. (a) Flexion of proximal interphalangeal joint & hyperextension of distal interphalangeal joint; (d) Flexion deformity of the proximal interphalangeal joint occur due to tear in central slip of extensor tendon; (e) May occur in rheumatoid arthritis

[Ref. Applied Therapeutics by Ernst, 10/e p1014]

Boutonniere Deformity

- Flexion of Proximal interphalangeal joint and hyperextension of Distal interphalangeal joint
- Flexion deformity of PIP occur due to tear in central slip of Extensor tendon
- May occur in rheumatoid arthritis

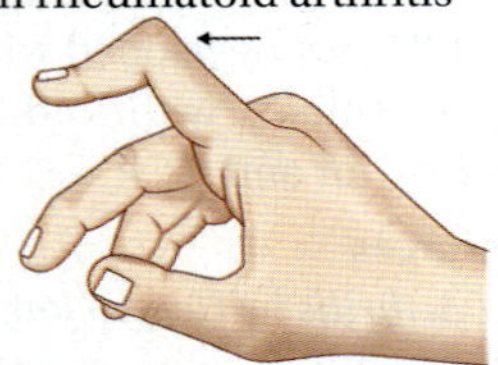

Fig. Boutonniere deformity

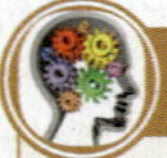

Also Remember

Key Deformities and Joint Positions

- Swan-neck deformity: Hyperextension of PIP, Hyperflexion of DIP
- Boutonniere deformity: Flexion of PIP, Hyperextension of DIP
- Mallet toe: Neutral MTP, Neutral PIP, Hyperflexion of DIP
- Hammer toe: Extension of MTP, Flexion of PIP, Extension of DIP
- Claw toe: Extension of MTP, Hyperflexion of PIP, Hyperflexion of DIP

4. Ans. (a) Romanus lesion may be found; (b) If left untreated, spine fusion may occur; (c) Predilection of the joints of the axial skeleton

[Ref. Spine Imaging by Saraf-Lavi, 3/e p192]

Ankylosing Spondylitis

- Bony erosions involve Posterior elements rather than Posterior aspect of vertebral bodies
- **Predilection for** the joints of Axial skeleton, especially **the Sacroiliac joints**
- If untreated, progression to fusion is typical, affecting facet joints as well as Anteior vertebral bodies

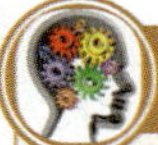

Also Remember

Romanus Lesion

- Represents an early finding in inflammatory spondyloarthropathies (Ankylosing spondylitis, Enteropathic arthritis), and appears as irregularity and erosion involving the anterior and posterior edges of the vertebral endplates
- Healing response to these inflammatory erosions appears radiographically as reactive sclerosis (Shiny corner sign)

5. Ans. (d) Total knee replacement

[Ref. Osteoarthritis by Roland, 4/e p404]

6. Ans. (a) Narrowing of joint space

[Ref. Radiology, Pathology and Immunology of Bones and Joints by Feldmann, 1/e p122]

Radiological Changes in Osteoarthritis

- **First change: Narrowing of joint space** (In weight-bearing joints)
- Other changes: Subchondral sclerosis, Subchondral cysts, Osteophytes formation, Loose bodies, Deformity of joints

7. Ans. (d) Immunological

[Ref. Medical Immunology by Variella, 6/e p347]

- Although *underlying cause* of *rheumatoid arthritis* is unknown, increasing evidence implicates both IL-1 and TNF in inflammatory/ destructive manifestations

8. Ans. (c) Synovial membrane

[Ref. Maheshwari, 4/e p279]

- **Synovial membrane in Rheumatoid arthritis:**
  - Synovial membrane edema, filled with fibrin exudates and cellular infiltrates
  - Hypertrophy of synovium, leading to Pannus formation
  - Pannus burrows into Subchondral bone
  - Cartilage wears off, Bone surface becomes raw

9. Ans. (b) Rheumatoid arthritis

[Ref. Neuromuscular Disorders in Clinical Practice by Bashar, 1/e p891]

- *Rheumatoid arthritis* is the ***most common*** systemic disorders associated with Tarsal tunnel syndrome

10. Ans. (b) Ankylosing spondylitis

[Ref. Maheshwari, 4/e p283]

11. Ans. (b) Sacrolitis is common

[Ref. Maheshwari, 4/e p283]

12. Ans. (b) Peripheral joint is rarely involved; (d) Iritis is seen more frequently

[Ref. Maheshwari, 4/e p283-284]

13. Ans. (b) Pain is relieved in lying down position

[Ref. Maheshwari, 4/e p283]

14. Ans. (a) Phenylbutazone

[Ref. Pharmacology in Clinical Practice by Lancaster, 1/e p263]

- **Phenylbutazone is the Drug of choice** for relieving the pain and reducing the stiffness associated with Ankylosing spondylitis

15. Ans. (c) Osteoarthritis
[Ref. Rheumatology Secrets by West, 3/e, p88]

Joint Involvement in Arthritis

Disease	Joints involved	Joints spared
Rheumatoid arthritis	Wrist, MCP, PIP, Elbow, Glenohumeral, Hip, Knee, Ankle, Tarsal, MTP, Cervical spine	DIP, Thoracolumbar spine
Osteoarthritis	1st CMC, DIP, PIP, Hip, Knee, 1st MTP, Toe IP, Cervical spine, Thoracolumbar spine	MCP, Wrist, Elbow, Ankle, Gleno-shoulder, Tarsal
Reactive arthritis	Knee, Ankle, Tarsal, MTP, 1st toe IP, Elbow, Axial	Hip
Psoriatic arthritis	Knee, Ankle, MTP, 1st toe IP, MCP, Hand IP, Axial	Wrist, CMC
Ankylosing spondylitis	Sacroiliac joint, Spine, Hip, Knee, Manubriosternal joint	Wrist, Elbow
Gout	1st MTP, Instep, Heel, Ankle, Knee	Axial
Lyme's arthritis	Knee, Shoulder, Wrist, Elbow	Axial
Hemochromatosis	MCP, Wrist, Shoulder, Ankle, Knee, Hip, Feet	

16. Ans. (d) Metacarpophalangeal joint
[Ref. Rheumatology Secrets by West, 3/e, p88]

17. Ans. (a) Quadriceps only
[Ref. Nursing and the Aged by Burnside, 1/e p284]

18. Ans. (a) Single joint involvement; (c) Ankylosis is seen; (d) Lower limb deformity is seen; (e) Heberden's nodules are found
[Ref. Maheshwari, 4/e p283]
- Osteoarthritis commonly occurs in Elderly people

19. Ans. (a) Increase the weight bearing by the affected joint
[Ref. Maheshwari, 4/e p288-289]

Treatment of Osteoarthritis
- Drugs: Analgesics
- Chondroprotective agents: Glucosamine, Chondroitin sulphate
- Viscosupplementation: Hylarunan
- Supportive therapy: Weight reduction, Avoidance of stress/strain to affected joint, Local heat, Exercises, Counter-irritants/ liniments
- Surgical treatment: Osteotomy, Joint replacement, Joint debridement, Arthroscopic procedures

20. Ans. (d) Knee joint
[Ref. Maheshwari, 4/e p287]

Sites of Osteoarthritis
- Primary Osteoarthritis: Weight-bearing joints (Knee – Most common, Hip), Hands
- Secondary Osteoarthritis: Hip – Most common, Elbow

21. Ans. (b) Rheumatoid arthritis
[Ref. Operative Techniques in Hand, Wrist, and Forearm Surgery by Weisel, 1/e p639]

22. Ans. (c) Shoulder
[Ref. The Complete Doctor's Healthy Back Bible by Reed, 1/e p100]

23. Ans. (d) Osteoarthritis
[Ref. Ankylosing Spondylitis by Khan, 1/e Table 4.1]

Causes of Enthesitis/ Enthesopathy
- Inflammatory causes **(Enthesitis)**: Ankylosing spondylitis, Reiter's syndrome, Psoriatic arthropathy, Enteric arthropathy (IBD), Juvenile spondyloarthropathy, Undifferentiated spondyloarthropathy
- Non-inflammatory causes **(Enthesopathy)**: Mechanical/ Degenerative, Trauma, Osteoarthritis
- Metabolic/endocrine/idiopathic enthesopathy: Acromegaly, Fluorosis, Hypoparathyroidism, Hyperparathyroidism, POEMS syndrome, X-linked hypophosphatemia
- Miscellaneous: Lyme's disease, Leprosy

24. Ans. (d) More common in females
[Ref. Maheshwari, 4/e p283]
- Ankylosing spondylitis: More common in Males
- Rheumatoid Arthritis: More common in Females

25. Ans. (c) Rheumatoid arthritis
[Ref. Maheshwari, 4/e p280]

Swan Neck Deformity of Rheumatoid Arthritis
- Finger postures with PIP hyperextension and DIP flexion; MP tends to be flexed, and the finger appears to zigzag when observed from the side
- IP positions are opposite to that of Boutonniere deformity

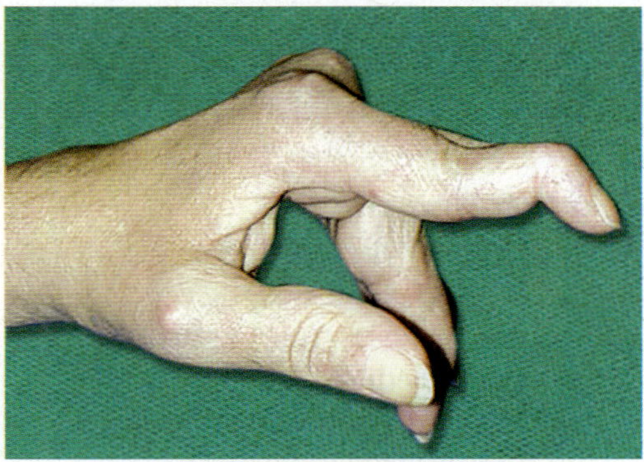

Fig. Swan neck deformity

26. Ans. (a) Rheumatoid arthritis; (b) Rickets
[Ref. Imaging of Arthritis and Metabolic Bone Disease by Weismann, 1/e p345]

Windswept Deformity
- Valgus deformity in one knee is associated with Varus deformity in another knee
- Seen in: Rheumatoid arthritis, nutritional rickets

27. Ans. (a) Flexion of Proximal Interphalangeal joint; (e) Extension at Distal interphalangeal joint
[Ref. Essential Orthopedics by Miller, 1/e p357]

28. Ans. (d) Knee
[Ref. Smart Study Series Orthopedics by Rohilla, 1/e p333]

29. Ans. (c) Rheumatoid nodule
[Ref. Textbook of Orthopedics and Trauma by Kulkarni, 2/e p853]

30. Ans. (a) Normocytic normochromic anemia
[Ref. DeGruchy's Clinical Hematology, 5/e p103]

Types of Anemia in Rheumatoid Arthritis

- Most common type: Normocytic normochromic
- Other types: Microcytic hypochromic, Hemolytic, Macrocytic

31. Ans. (a) Clutton's joint
[Ref. General Principles of Orthopedics and Trauma by Iyer, 1/e p36]

Syphilitic Arthritis

Inherited syphilis	Acquired early syphilis	Acquired late syphilis
• Osteochondritis • Clutton's joints • (Symmetrical hydrarthrosis)	• Arthralgia • Hydroarthrosis • Plastic arthritis	• Synovial form • Osseus form • Charcot's joints

32. Ans. (b) SLE
[Ref. New Trends in Image Analysis by Sansone, 1/e p145]

- **Bony erosions**: Rheumatoid arthritis, Psoriatic arthritis, Gout, Reiter's syndrome, Systemic sclerosis, Palindromic rheumatism, Osteoarthritis, Septic arthritis, SLE

33. Ans. (d) Sickle cell disorder
[Ref. Learning Radiology by Herring, 3/e p260]

- **Causes of Erosive arthritis**: Rheumatoid arthritis, Psoriatic arthritis, Gout, Ankylosing spondylitis (Spine), Reactive arthritis, Sarcoid, Hemophilia, Amyloidosis, Hyperparathyroidism

34. Ans. (b) Involves peripheral joints more commonly than axial joints; (d) Associated with vasculitis
[Ref. Maheshwari, 4/e p278-279]

35. Ans. (a) Exercises
[Ref. Maheshwari, 4/e p280-281]

Treatment of Rheumatoid Arthritis

- **Medical treatment**: NSAIDs, DMARDs, Steroids
- **Non-operative methods:**
  - Physiotherapy (Splintage, Heat, Joint mobilization exercises, Muscle building exercises)
  - Occupational therapy
  - Rehabilitation
- **Operative methods:**
  - Preventive surgery (Synovectomy of wrist, knee. MP joints)
  - Palliative surgery (Bone block operations, Tendon lengthening)
  - Reconstructive surgery (Tendon transfers, Interposition arthroplasties, Total joint replacement)
  - Salvage surgery

36. Ans. (b) Osteochondritis dessicans; (d) Synovial chondrocalcinosis; (e) Osteoarthritis
[Ref. Musculoskeletal Sonography by Martino, 1/e p127]

- **Loose bodies**: *Osteochondritis dessicans*, Osteochondral fractures, Osteonecrosis, *Osteoarthritis*, *Synovial* osteochondromatosis

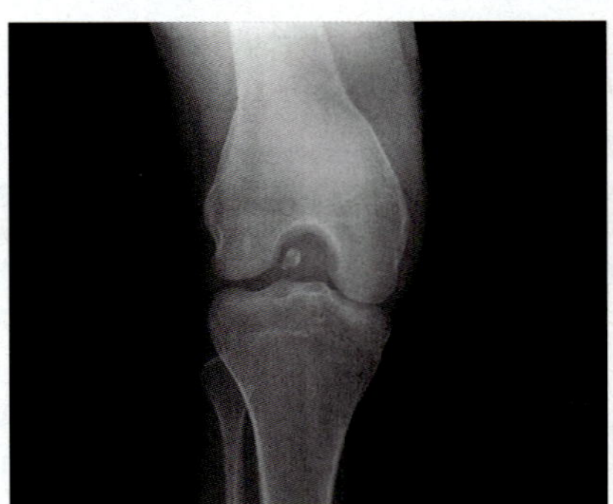

Fig. Loose bodies in joint

37. Ans. (d) Ankylosing spondylitis
[Ref. A Synopsis of Rheumatic Diseases by Golding, 5/e p204]

38. Ans. (a) Gout; (b) Septic arthritis; (c) TB; (e) Rheumatoid arthritis
[Ref. Oxford Handbook of Clinical and laboratory Investigation by Provan, 3/e p694]

- Synovial fluid with **low viscosity**: Gout, Septic arthritis, TB, Rheumatoid arthritis
- Synovial fluid with **high viscosity**: Osteoarthritis, Neuropathic arthropathy, Synovial chondropathy

39. Ans. (a) Articular cartilage; (b) Synovium; (c) Skin; (e) Joint capsule
[Ref. Cotran & Robbins Pathology, 9/e p1216]

40. Ans. (b) Positive birefringent crystal in the Synovial fluid
[Ref. Brigham Intensive Review of Internal Medicine by Singh, 2/e p297]

- ***Gout crystals*** are needle-shaped and display strongly negative birefringence (Yellow when parallel to axis of polarizer)

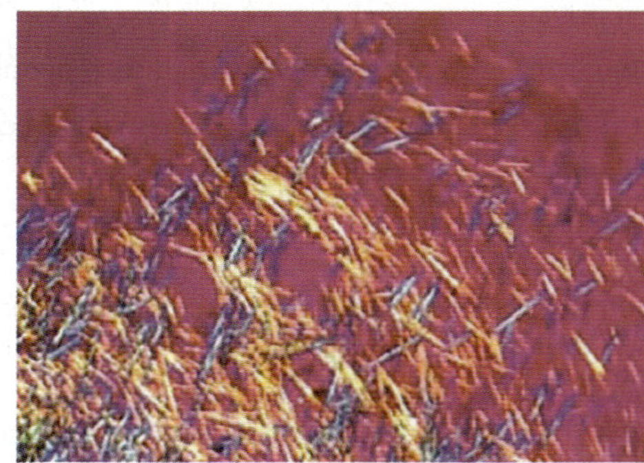

Fig. Gout crystals

41. Ans. (d) Osteochondritis dessicans
[Ref. Functional Soft Tissue Trauma and Treatment by Hammer, 2/e p311]

42. Ans. (c) Psoriatic arthritis
[Ref. Maheshwari, 4/e p286]

43. Ans. (b) Methotrexate
[Ref. Advances in Psoriasis by Lebwohi, 1/e p270]

44. Ans. (a) Interstitial lung disease
[Ref. Orthopedic Nursing Secrets by Michael, 1/e p55]

45. Ans. (b) HLA-B27
[Ref. Maheshwari, 4/e p283]

46. Ans. (b) Gouty arthritis
[Ref. Maheshwari, 4/e p283]
- **MC site of arthritis in Gouty arthritis**: MP joint of big toe

47. Ans. (a) Aspirin
[Ref. Pharmacology Recall by Ramachandran, 2/e p309]
- **Aspirin is Contraindicated in treatment of Gout**: Aspirin is salicylate, it inhibits uric acid secretion in renal tubules

48. Ans. (d) Behcet's disease
[Ref. Essentials of Rubin's Pathology by Reisner, 6/e p717]
- Behcet's disease associated is with **HLA B51**

49. Ans. (c) Ankylosing spondylosis
[Ref. Maheshwari, 4/e p283]
- **Radiology in Ankylosing spondylitis**: X-ray lumbar spine
  - Squaring of vertebrae
  - Syndesmophytes (Bridging osteophytes)
  - Bamboo-spine appearance
  - Loss of lumbar lordosis

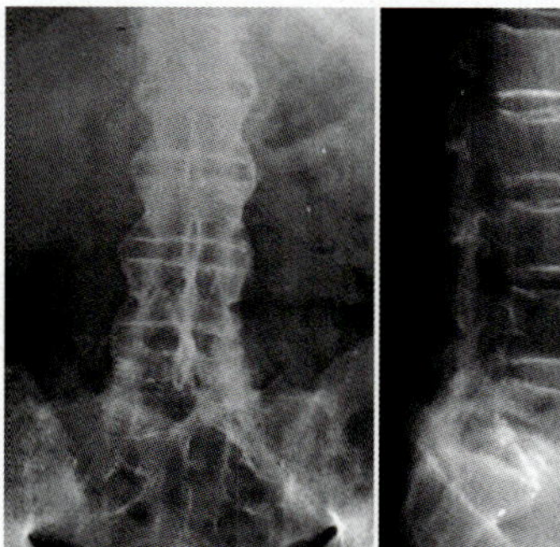

Fig. Bamboo spine

50. Ans. (d) Sacroiliac joint erosion
[Ref. Rheumatology Volume 2 by Hochberg, 1/e p105]

51. Ans. (c) Urate crystal in synovial fluid
[Ref. 100 Cases in Orthopedics and Rheumatology by Singh, 1/e p178]
- **Investigation of choice in Gouty arthritis**: Prompt aspiration of the joint with assessment of the *synovial fluid* for *crystals* or bacteria

52. Ans. (a) Abrupt increase in serum urate levels is more common a cause for acute gout than an abrupt fall in urate levels
[Ref. Maheshwari, 4/e p285]

53. Ans. None
[Ref. Nurse Practitioner for Long Term Care by Traux, 1/e p264]
- **Specific test for Gouty arthritis**: Urate crystal in synovial fluid

54. Ans. (c) Wrist & elbow
[Ref. Rheumatology Secrets by West, 3/e, p88]

55. Ans. (b) Foot
[Ref. Ferri's Clinical Advisor 2013, p234]

56. Ans. (a) Osteoarthritis
[Ref. Rheumatology Secrets by West, 3/e, p88]

57. Ans. (a) Diabetes mellitus

58. Ans. (a) Osteoarthritis
[Ref. Fractures of Acetabulum by Judet, 1/e p335]

59. Ans. (c) Syphilitic joints
[Ref. General Principles of Orthopedics and Trauma by Iyer, 1/e p36]

60. Ans. (c) Diabetes
[Ref. Primer on Rheumatic Disease by Klippel, 1/e p488]

61. Ans. (a) RA factor is associated with bad prognosis
[Ref. Maheshwari, 4/e p282]

62. Ans. (c) Tarsometatarsal
[Ref. Nutrition and Arthritis by Rayman, 1/e p12]

1987 ARA/ACR Criteria of Rheumatoid Arthritis (atleast 4 out of 7)

	Title	Description
1	Morning stiffness	Minimum 1 hour before improvement, Minimum 3 joints
2	Arthritis of 3 or more joints	Right or left PIP, MCP, Wrist, Elbow, Knee, Ankle, MTP
3	Arthritis of hand joints	Wrist, MCP or PIP
4	Symmetric arthritis	PIP, MCP, Wrist, Elbow, Knee, Ankle, MTP
5	Rheumatoid nodules	Over bony prominences or Extensor surfaces
6	Serum Rheumatoid factor	Abnormal amounts
7	Radiographic changes	Erosions, Decalcifications on Posterior hand & Wrists

63. Ans. (d) C Reactive protein indicates better prognosis
[Ref. Rheumatoid Arthritis by McNeil, 1/e p58]
- Higher level or Fluctuating level of CRP indicate higher chance of Erosive disease

64. Ans. (d) Knee
[Ref. Skeletal Impact of Disease by Martin, 1/e p38]
- **Joint involvement in Tertiary Syphilitic arthritis**: Knee > Hip > Ankle > Spine

65. Ans. (b) There is good correlation between level of uric acid and severity of gouty arthritis
[Ref. Bonica's Management of Pain by Fishman, 1/e p1122]

66. Ans. (b) Gout
[Ref. Skeletal Impact of Disease by Martin, 1/e p10]
- **Causes of Periosteal reaction**: Tuberculosis, Syphilis, Yaws, Rubella, Trauma, Scurvy, Rickets, Hypervitaminosis A, Vitamin D intoxication, Neuroblastoma, Leukemia,

67. Ans. (b) Birefringent (Particles) crystals; (e) Pain is very intense
[Ref. Current Therapy in Pain by Smith, 1/e p187]

Gout vs Pseudogout

	Gout	Pseudogout
Crystals composition	**Monosodium urate**	**Calcium pyrophosphate**
Refringence of crystals	Negative birefringent rods	Positive birefringent rhomboids
Pain	Intense	Moderate

Contd...

Orthopedics

Contd...

	Gout	Pseudogout
Joints	Inflamed	Swollen
Uric acid levels	Hyperuricemia	Normal

68. Ans. (d) Pseudogout
[Ref. Gout and Other Crystal Arthropathies by Robert, 1/e p313]

69. Ans. (d) Total ankle replacement
[Ref. Rheumatology and Immunology by Cohen, 1/e p343]

70. Ans. (a) Skin; (b) Cartilage; (c) Tendon; (e) Bursa
[Ref. Clinical Companion to Medical-Surgical Nursing by Bucher, 9/e p259]

- **Parts affected by Gout**: Joints, Synovium, Subchondral bone, Bursa (Olecranon bursa), Vertebra, Skin, Tendons, Cartilage

71. Ans. (b) Rheumatoid arthritis

72. Ans. (b) Rheumatoid arthritis
[Ref. Maheshwari, 4/e p279]

73. Ans. (a) Osteosclerosis of joint
[Ref. Maheshwari, 4/e p279]

74. Ans. (a) Knee
[Ref. Current Therapy in Pain by Smith, 1/e p187]

75. Ans. (d) TSH
[Ref. Current Therapy in Pain by Smith, 1/e p187]

76. Ans. (a) Monosodium Urate crystals
[Ref. Current Therapy in Pain by Smith, 1/e p187]

77. Ans. (b) Ankylosing Spondylosis
[Ref. Pediatric CV Disease by Akalan, 1/e p164]

- **Causes of Craniovertebral Junction Anomalies**: Rheumatoid arthritis, Achondroplasia, Paget's disease, Osteogenesis imperfecta, Osteomalacia, Hyperparathyroidism, Osteoblastoma, Neurofibromatosis, Basilar invasion, Odontoid dysgenesis, Fetal warfarin syndrome
- Ankylosing spondylitis is an extremely rare cause of CV junction anomaly

78. Ans. (d) Erosion of joint
[Ref. Surgery of Foot and Ankle by Mann, 9/e p924]

Radiography of Gouty Arthritis

- Soft tissue swelling
- **Bony erosions (First sign)**
- Lacy pattern of bony erosions in subcortical bone (Pathognomonic sign)
- **Overhanging edge sign (Characteristic sign)**
- Punched-out bony lysis
- Arthritic involvement of IP joint of Great toe

79. Ans. (a) Occurs after 50 years of age; (b) Single joint may be affected; (c) Heberden's node present; (d) Lower limb deformity seen
[Ref. Osteoarthritis by Moskowitz, 4/e p157]

- **Bony ankyloses is rare in Osteoarthritis** Except in Inflammatory OA or Non-inflammatory OA of Sacroiliac joint

80. Ans. (b) Arthroplasty
[Ref. Rheumatology by Weisman, 6/e]

81. Ans. (b) Osteoarthritis
[Ref. Rheumatology Secrets by West, 3/e, p88]

82. Ans. (b) Causes pleural effusion with low sugar
[Ref. The Netter Collection of Medical Illustrations by Parker, 2/e p175]

83. Ans. (b) Erosion of distal interphalangeal joints
[Ref. Rheumatology Secrets by West, 3/e, p88]

- **Rheumatoid arthritis generally involves** Wrist, MCP, PIP, Elbow, Glenohumeral, Hip, Knee, Ankle, Tarsal, MTP, Cervical spine
- **Rheumatoid arthritis typically spares** DIP joints & Thoracolumbar spine

84. Ans. (a) Small and large joints are affected mostly
[Ref. Rheumatology Secrets by West, 3/e, p88]

85. Ans. (b) Colchicine cause gastrointestinal disturbances; (c) High serum uric acid level may be not present; (d) Joint Fluid aspiration is done for investigation
[Ref. Portable Pathophysiology by Salamon, 1/e p506]

- **In Acute Gout**: Allopurinol is used for prevention and Colchicine is used fo treatment

86. Ans. (b) Calcium pyrophosphate
[Ref. Current Therapy in Pain by Smith, 1/e p187]

87. Ans. (c) Pseudogout
[Ref. Review of Orthopedics by Miller, 6/e p60]

88. Ans. (a) Gout
[Ref. Diagnostic Imaging of Musculoskeletal Diseases by Khurana, 1/e p447]

Causes of Atlanto-Axial Subluxation

- **Arthritis**: Rheumatoid arthritis, Ankylosing spondylitis, Psoriatic arthritis, SLE, Juvenile chronic arthritis
- **Congenital**: Down's syndrome, Morquio's syndrome, Congenital absence/ hypoplasia of dens, Atlanto-axial fusion
- **Infection**: Retropharyngeal abscess (Quinsy)
- **Trauma**: Fracture, Ligament rupture

89. Ans. All Choices
[Ref. Maheshwari, 4/e p280]

90. Ans. (c) Small & big joints involved; (d) Felty syndrome associated
[Ref. Mayo Clinic Internal Medicine Board Review by Ficalore, 10/e p380]

- **Classical triad of Felty's syndrome**: Rheumatoid arthritis, Splenomegaly, Leucopenia

91. Ans. (b) Seronegative Rheumatoid arthritis
[Ref. Mayo Clinic Internal Medicine Board Review by Ghosh, 9/e p875]

92. Ans. (a) Ankylosing spondylitis
[Ref. Maheshwari, 4/e p287-288]

93. Ans. (b) Quadriceps femoris muscle
[Ref. Pediatrics by Scheri, 1/e p295]

94. Ans. (c) Rheumatoid arthritis in childhood
[Ref. Differential Oral Diagnosis in Systemic Disease by Gardner, 1/e p267]

Still's Disease
- Rheumatoid arthritis in childhood
- Polyarthritis in children under 5-6 years age characterized by vascular and cardiac lesions, Leucopenia, Splenomegaly
- Severe complication: Blindness

95. Ans. (d) BAL
[Ref. Medical Therapeutics by Paulose, 2/e p107]
- **Nonsteroidal disease modifying drugs used in Rheumatoid arthritis**: Gold, Chloroquine, D-Penicillamine, Dapsone. Levamisole, Cyclophosphamide, Methotrexate, Salazopyrine, Azathioprine, Leflunomide, Cyclosporin

96. Ans. (b) Rheumatoid arthritis
[Ref. Medical Therapeutics by Paulose, 2/e p107]

97. Ans. (a) Mononeuritis multiplex
[Ref. Textbook of Systemic Vasculitis by Sharma, 1/e p380]

98. Ans. (d) All of these
[Ref. Apley's Orthopedics and Fractures by Solomon, 3/e p232]

99. Ans. (d) Ca++ deposition in joint space
[Ref. Maheshwari, 4/e p287-288]

100. Ans. (a) Rheumatoid arthritis
[Ref. Churchill's Pocketbook of Differential Diagnosis by, p]

Types of Degenerative Disorders of Bones & Joints
- Traumatic: Sprains, Fractures
- Infective: Pyogenic arthritis
- Inflammatory: Rheumatic arthritis, Reactive arthritis/ Reiter's syndrome, Ankylosing spondylitis
- Degenerative: Osteoarthritis
- Metabolic: Gout, Pseudogout
- Neuropathic: Charcot's joint
- Neoplastic: Osteogenic sarcoma
- Others: Bursitis, Cyst, Osteochondritis

101. Ans. (d) Chondromatosis
[Ref. Core Radiology by Mandell, 1/e p373]

102. Ans. (b) Manifest at adult; (c) Seen at 4-6 years after disease; (d) Common in women
[Ref. Core radiology by Mandell, 1/e p373]

103. Ans. (a) Psoriatic arthropathy
[Ref. Psoriasis and Psoriatic Arthritis by Ruderman, 1/e p76]

104. Ans. (a) Pyogenic infection in infancy
[Ref. Maheshwari, 4/e p172]

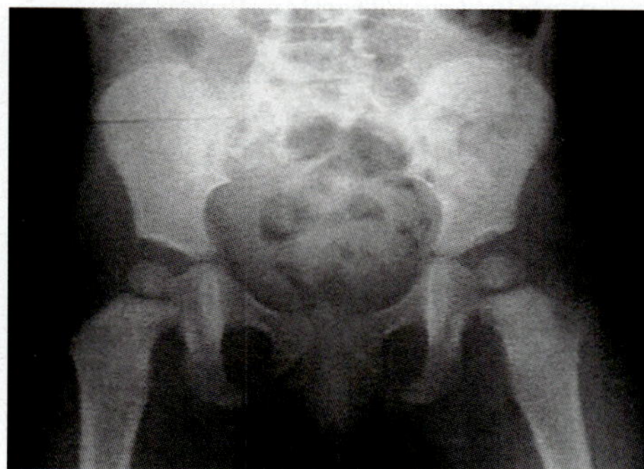

Fig. Tom Smith arthritis

Tom Smith Arthritis
- Description: Septic arthritis of hip in infancy
- Features: Cartilaginous femur head rapidly destroyed by pyogenic process
- Hip movements increased in all directions
- Affected limb shorter
- Telescopy test positive
- **X-ray: Complete absence of head and neck of femur**

105. Ans. (d) *Staphylococcus aureus*
[Ref. Textbook of Pediatric Rheumatology by Petty, 7/e]

Causes of Septic Arthritis in Children
- Less than 2 years age: Hemophilus influenzae B, *Streptococcus pneumoniae*
- After 2 years age: *Staphylococcus aureus*
- 6-10 years age: Group A Streptococci, Enterococci
- Septic arthritis with Sickle cell disease: Salmonella

106. Ans. (c) A + D
[Ref. Maheshwari, 4/e p172]

107. Ans. (d) Septic arthritis of infancy
[Ref. Maheshwari, 4/e p172]

108. Ans. (e) Tends to end with the formation of a fibrous ankyloses
[Ref. Apley's Concise System of Orthopedics and Fractures by Solomon, 3/e p23]

109. Ans. (c) Synovium
[Ref. Maheshwari, 4/e p279]

110. Ans. (a) Psoriatic arthopathy
[Ref. Rheumatology Secrets by West, 3/e, p88]

111. Ans. (e) Lengthening of digit k/ a telescoping

112. Ans. (c) Sjogren's syndrome
[Ref. Skeletal Radiology by Chew, 3/e p225]

HLA Associations
- **HLA B27** associations: Ankylosing spondylitis, Reiter's syndrome, Psoriatic arthritis, Enteropathic arthritis
- **HLA CW6** associations: Psoriasis, Psoriatic arthritis
- **HLA DR4** associations: Rheumatoid arthritis

113. Ans. (a) New bone formation
[Ref. Decision Making in Medicine by Mushlin, 3/e p516]

114. Ans. (a) Rheumatoid arthritis
[Ref. Rheumatology Secrets by West, 3/e, p88]

115. Ans. (b) Pyogenic arthritis
[Ref. Radiology of Joint Disease by Forrester, 1/e p180]

116. Ans. (a) *Staphylococcus aureus*
[Ref. Orthopedic Pathology by Vigorita, 2/e p257]

Common Causes of Non-Gonococcal Septic Arthritis
- **All ages: *Staphylococcus aureus***
- **Neonates: *Haemophilus influenzae***
- < 6 months: *Staphylococcus aureus*, Gram negative enteric bacteria
- 6 months – 2 years: *Staphylococcus aureus, Haemophilus influenzae*
- > 2 years: *Staphylococcus aureus*
- Adults: Gram positive cocci

117. Ans. (b) Extension at Proximal interphalangeal joint and flexion at Distal interphalangeal joint
[Ref. Maheshwari, 4/e p280]

118. Ans. (c) Swan-neck deformity
[Ref. Essential Orthopedics by Miller, 1/e p357]

119. Ans. (a) Flexion at Proximal Interphalangeal Joint; (b) Flexion at Distal Interphalangeal Joint; (e) Extension at Metacarpophalangeal Joint
[Ref. Clinical Anatomy for Students by Kulkarni, 1/e p105]

120. Ans. (c) Rheumatoid arthritis
[Ref. Multiple Sources]

- **Seronegative polyarthritis with Ocular manifestations:**
  - Ankylosing spondylitis
  - Reiter's disease
  - Psoriatic arthritis
  - Ulcerative colitis
  - Crohn's disease
  - Whipple's disease
  - Behcet's disease

121. Ans. (b) Ankylosing spondylitis
[Ref. Skeletal Radiology by Chew, 3/e p225]

122. Ans. (b) 96%
[Ref. Ankylosing Spondylitis and Klebsiella by Ebringer, p79]

- **Frequency of HLA B27 in Ankylosing spondylitis: 96%**
- Frequency of HLA B27 in General population: 8%

123. Ans. (a) Elbow
[Ref. Skeletal Imaging by Taylor, 2/e]

124. Ans. (b) Predicting multisystem disease; (c) Predicting severity of disease
[Ref. Pathology by Fuller, 4/e p448]

125. Ans. (c) Swan neck deformity; (e) Mallet toe
[Ref. Applied Therapeutics by Ernst, 10/e p1014]

Key Deformities and Joint Positions

- **Swan-neck deformity**: Hyperextension of PIP, Hyperflexion of DIP
- **Boutonniere deformity**: Flexion of PIP, Hyperextension of DIP
- **Mallet toe**: Neutral MTP, Neutral PIP, Hyperflexion of DIP
- **Hammer toe**: Extension of MTP, Flexion of PIP, Extension of DIP
- **Claw toe**: Extension of MTP, Hyperflexion of PIP, Hyperflexion of DIP

126. Ans. (a) Ankylosing spondylitis
[Ref. Rubin's Pathology by Reisner, 6/e p717]

- More than 90% of Ankylosing spondylitis patients have HLA-B27 (Normal 4-8%)
- Only 1% of HLA-B27 haplotype develop Ankylosing spondylitis

127. Ans. (a) Gout
[Ref. Maheshwari, 4/e p285]

128. Ans. (a) Rheumatoid arthritis
[Ref. Maheshwari, 4/e p281]

- **Disease-modifying Anti-Rheumatic drugs (*DMARDs*)**: Drugs that retard or halt the underlying progression, limiting the amount of joint damage that occurs *inrheumatoid arthritis*
  - *Synthetic DMARDS:* Oral intake
  - Biological DMARDS: IV infusion or Subcutaneous route

129. Ans. (a) Proximal IP joints
[Ref. USMLE Step 1 Secrets by Brown 1/e p551]

- **Heberden's nodes** are seen on the distal interphalangeal joints
- **Bouchard's nodes** are seen at the proximal interphalangeal joints

130. Ans. (b) Deficiency of enzyme Xanthine oxidase
[Ref. Gout by Newcombe, 1/e p336]

131. Ans. (c) Chlamydia
[Ref. Molecular Medical Microbiology by Tang, 2/e p1411]

- **Most common infectious agents associated with reactive arthritis**: Salmonella, Shigella, Yersinia, Campylobacter, and Chlamydia (Overall MC) organisms
- Chlamydia-induced reactive arthritis may account for up to 50% of all infection-related reactive arthritis and primarily affects males

132. Ans. (a) Transient monoarticular synovitis
[Ref. Pediatric Nursing by Rudd, 1/e p465]

Transient Monoarticular Synovitis

- MCC of Acute-onset short-duration limping in children
  - More common in males than females
  - Average age of onset is 6 years (can range from 2-12 years age)
- Etiology: Nonspecific synovitis or hip irritation
  - Classified as: Allergic, Viral-like (following URI or other minor ailment) or result of a minor trauma
- Clinical Presentation: Anterior thigh/ knee pain, Mild limp, Mild fever, Irritable hip (Positive roll test)
- Diagnosis: X-ray is unremarkable
- Treatment: Bed rest, Traction, Bone scan

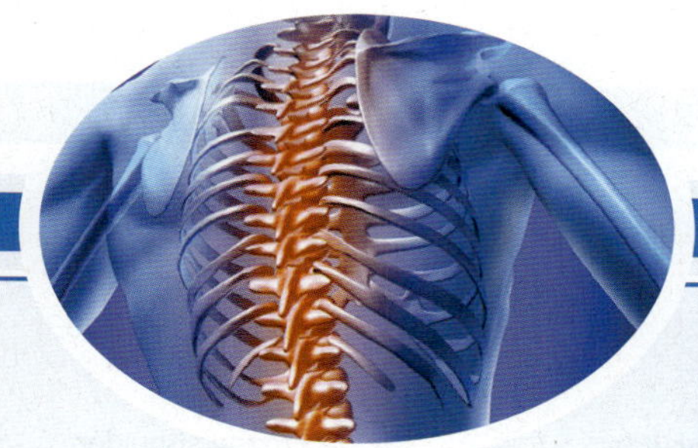

Chapter 7

Regional Conditions

THEORETICAL CONCEPTS

VII A. SHOULDER DISLOCATION

- *Types of shoulder dislocations*:
  - **Anterior dislocation: Most common** ; head of humerus in front of glenoid cavity
  - Posterior dislocation: Head behind glenoid cavity
  - Luxatio erecta: Head in sub-glenoid position
- *Lesions in shoulder dislocation*:
  - Hill-Sach's lesion[Q]
  - Bankart's lesion[Q]
- *Diagnosis*: Dugas test + X-ray
- ***Reduction of shoulder dislocation*: Kocher's manoeuvre**
- *Complications*:
  - ***MC early complication:* Injury to Axillary nerve**[Q]
  - MC late complication: Recurrence of dislocation
- *Treatment*: Putti-platt operation, Bankart's operation

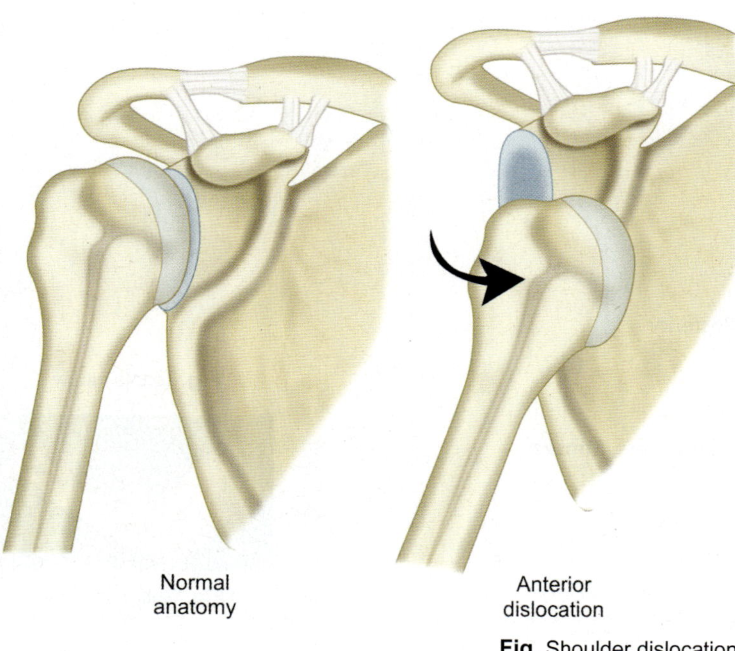

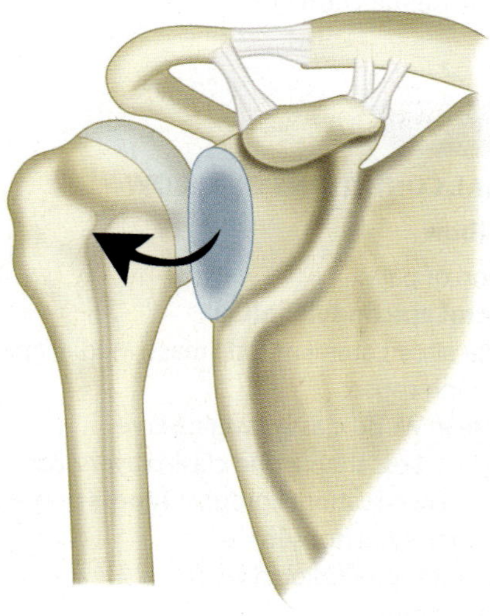

Fig. Shoulder dislocation

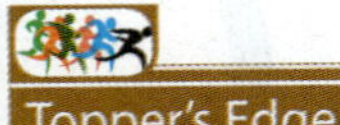

Topper's Edge

REGIONAL CONDITIONS OF SHOULDER

Frozen Shoulder

- **Humeroscapular periarthritis, Adhesive capsulitis**Q
- Underlying causes:
  - Shoulder causes: Tendinitis of rotator cuff, Bicipital tendinitis, Fractures, Dislocations
  - Non-shoulder causes: Diabetes, CVDs, Reflex sympathetic dystrophy
- Stages of Frozen shoulder:
  - Stage I: Stage of pain
  - Stage II: Stage of stiffness
  - Stage III: Stage of recovery
- **Pathognomonic radiologic sign**Q**: Golding's sign** (Dense sclerotic line on outer aspect of Head of humerus)
- Treatment:
  - Stage I: NSAIDs, Intra-articular steroids
  - Stage II: Active/passive exercises, Physiotherapy, Ultrasound/ Heat/ Shoulder wheel exercises
  - Stage III: Active/passive exercises, Physiotherapy, Short wave diathermy/ Ultrasound

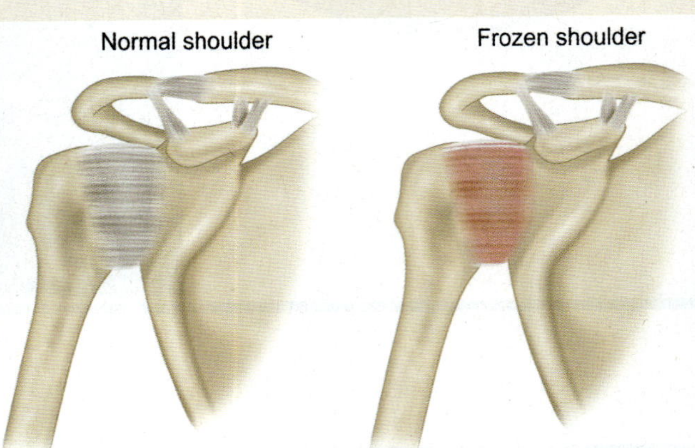

Fig. Frozen shoulder

Painful Arc Syndromes

- Pain in mid-range of abduction (60-120 degrees)
- **Underlying causes:**
  - **Rotator cuff lesions (MC**Q**)**
  - Supraspinatus tendinitis
  - Subacromial bursitis
  - Subdeltoid bursitis
  - Bicipital tenosynovitis
  - Fracture greater tuberosity
  - Calcific deposits

VII B. ELBOW DISLOCATION

- ***MC type*: Posterior dislocation**Q
- *Reversal of 3-point bony relationship*Q
- Bow-stringing of triceps

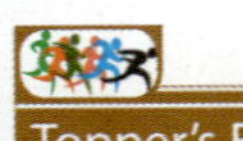

Topper's Edge

REGIONAL CONDITIONS OF ELBOW

Tennis Elbow

- Location of pain:
  - **Lateral epicondyle (MC**Q**)**
  - Other sites: Lateral muscle mass, Medial epicondyle, Posterior
- Underlying cause:
  - Cause in World class players: Serve
  - Cause in Less than world class players: Backhand stroke
  - Seen in occupational groups: **Tennis players (MC**Q**), Carpenters, Miners**
  - Seen in Indian housewives
  - Computer professional work
- Clinical features:
  - Local tenderness at Common extensor origin
  - Cozen's test positiveQ

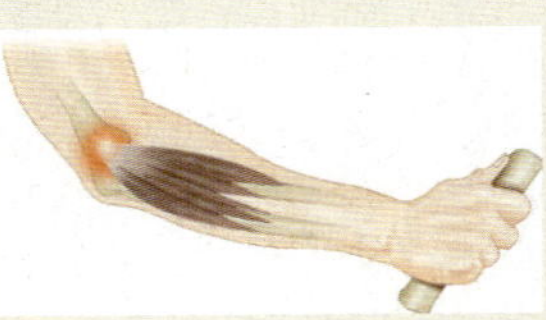

Fig. Tennis elbow

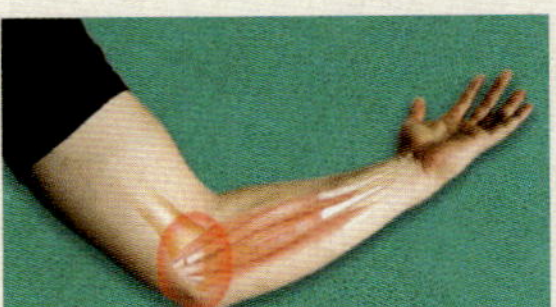

Fig. Golfer's elbow

Contd...

Orthopedics

Contd…

Golfer's Elbow

- Epitrochleitis, **Medial tennis elbow**[Q]

Students' Elbow

- **Olecranon bursitis**[Q]
- Cause: Infection due to chronic friction in students who tend to keep their elbow on table repeatedly during writing/ reading

REGIONAL CONDITIONS OF WRIST

deQuervain's Disease

- **Washerwoman's sprain**[Q]
- Tenovaginitis of common sheath of Abductor pollicis longus & Extensor pollicis brevis tendons[Q]
- Finkelstein's test positive[Q]: Tenderness elicited by sudden ulnar deviation of flexed hand

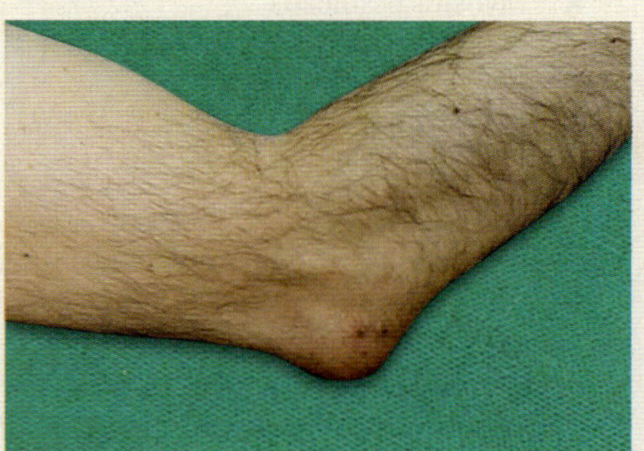

Fig. Student's elbow

Ganglion of Hand

- Localized, painless, tense, cystic swelling containing clear gelatinous fluid
- MC site: Dorsal wrist (Scapholunate ligament[Q]) > Volar ganglion > Sheath at a pulley

Carpal Tunnel Syndrome

- Causes: **[Mnemonic: PRAGMATIC]**
  - Pregnancy
  - **R**heumatoid arthritis
  - **A**rthritis degenerative
  - **G**rowth hormone anomalies (Acromegaly)
  - **M**etabolic causes (Gout, Diabetes, Myxedema)
  - **T**umors
  - **I**diopathic
  - **C**onnective tissue disorders (Amyloidosis)
- Tests done[Q]:
  - Wrist flexion (Phalen's) test[Q]
  - Tourniduet test
  - Two point discrimination test
  - Electrodiagnostic tests

REGIONAL CONDITIONS OF HAND

Dupuytren's Contracture

- Proliferative fibroplasia of subcutaneous palmar tissue forming nodules of cords along Ulnar border[Q]
- Causes: Hereditary, Chronic repetitive trauma, Drilling machine workers, Male sex, Epilepsy, Alcoholics

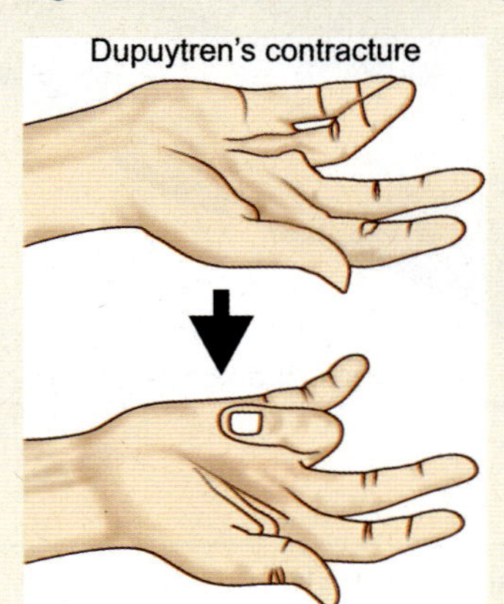

Compound Palmar Ganglion

- **Affects flexor fingers of Ulnar bursa**[Q]
- Cause: Tuberculosis, Rheumatoid arthritis
- **Hallmark**[Q]: Melon seed bodies (Resemble Grains of boiled sago)

Trigger Finger

- Constriction of fibrous digital sheath preventing free gliding of contained flexor tendon
- Locking of finger can be overcome by Passive stretching (Long sustained active effort)

VII C. POSTERIOR DISLOCATION OF HIP

- ***Underlying cause*: 'Dash-board injury'**[Q]
- *Clinical presentation*:
  - Flexion, Adduction, Internal rotation
  - Shortening of leg
- *Treatment*: Closed reduction
- *Complications*:
  - Avascular necrosis of femoral head
  - Sciatic nerve damage
  - Osteoarthritis
  - Myositis ossificans

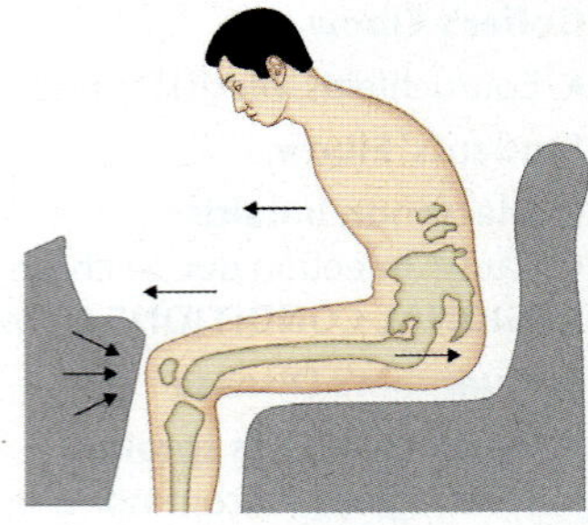

Fig. Dashboard injury

Topper's Edge

Posterior Dislocation of Hip

- More common (70%) than Anterior dislocation in Hip joint[Q]
- Mechanism of injury: Backward directed force a long line of femur in a flexed hip **(*Dashboard injury*)**[Q]
- Features:
  - **Flexion, adduction, medial rotation deformity**
  - **Marked shortening, Gross restriction of all hip movements**
- Reduction techniques:
  - Watson Jones technique (Classical method[Q])
  - Bigelow method of reduction
  - Allis method
  - Stimson's gravity method
- Early reduction prevent Post-traumatic osteonecrosis & Relieve Sciatic nerve compression

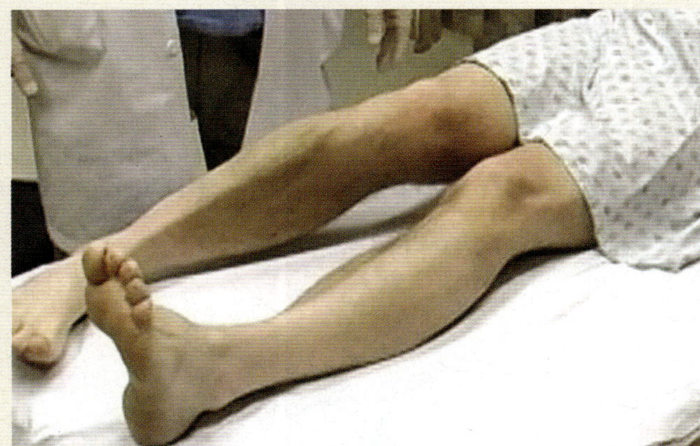

Fig. Posterior dislocation of hip

VII D. INFECTIONS OF HAND

- ***Acute paronychium*:** (Most common) Infection of nail-fold[Q]
- ***Whitlow/ Felon*:** Terminal pulp-space infection[Q]
- ***Frog hand*:** Deep palmar abscess[Q]
- ***Kanavel's sign*:** Ulnar bursa infection due to acute suppurative tenosynovitis of little finger[Q]

VII E. CONGENITAL TALIPES EQUINO VARUS (CTEV - CLUB FOOT)

- *Underlying cause*:
  - Idiopathic
  - Secondary (Poliomyelitis/ Spina bifida/ Arthrogryposis multiplex congenita[Q])

- *Joint deformities in CTEV*:

Deformity	Joint(s)
Equinus deformity	Ankle joint[Q]
Inversion deformity	Sub-talar joint[Q]
Forefoot adduction deformity	Talo-navicular joint[Q]
Forefoot cavus deformity	Mid-tarsal joint

- ***Tendons contracted in CTEV:***
  - Tibialis posterior
  - Flexor digitorum longus
  - Flexor hallucis longus
  - Tendochilles
- **X-ray: Kite's angle**[Q]
- *Treatment of CTEV*:

Situation	Treatment
At birth	
If corrected after manipulation	Dennis-Brown splint + CTEV shoes
If uncorrected after manipulation	Posteromedial soft tissue release, Dwyer's osteotomy
Old case[Q]	
1-3 years	Posteromedial soft tissue release
4-8 years	Dillwyn-Evan's operation
8-11 years	Wedge tarsectomy
>12 years	Triple arthrodesis
Recurrence post-surgery	Ilizarov technique

- **Triple Arthrodesis**[Q]
  - *Is one of the operative methods to correct*: Congenital Talipes Equino Varus (CTEV)
  - *Comprises of fusion of 3 joints*:
    - **Subtalar**
    - **Calcaneo-cuboid**
    - **Talo-navicular**
  - *Performed after the age of*: 12 years
  - *Most difficult joint fusion to achieve*: Talo-navicular

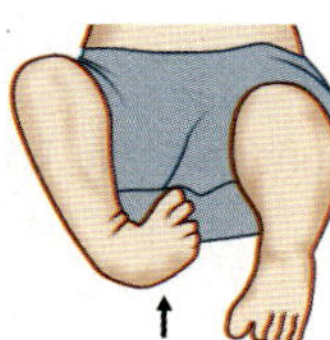

Fig. Club foot

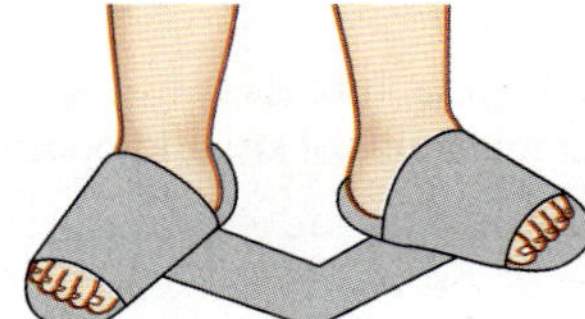

Fig. Dennis brown splint + CTEV shoes

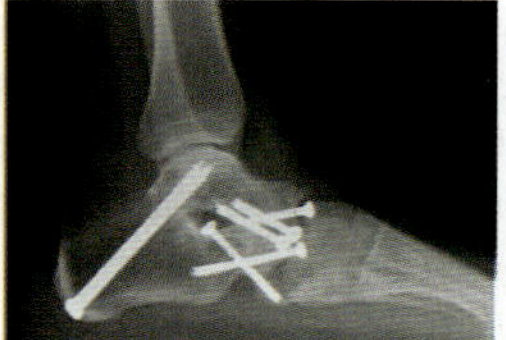

Fig. Triple arthrodesis

VII F. CONGENITAL DISLOCATION OF HIP

- *Underlying cause*:
  - **Maternal hormone (Relaxin) causes laxity of joint**[Q]
  - Breech presentation
- *Clinical presentation and Diagnosis*:
  - Peculiar gait on walking[Q]:
    - ***Trendelenburg's gait:*** Lurching on affected side in unilateral dislocation
    - ***Waddling gait:*** Alternate lurching on both sides in bilateral dislocation
  - Limited abduction of hip, asymmetrical thigh folds, lordosis of lumbar spine
  - ***Galeazzi's sign:*** Lowered knee while lying down with hips flexed to 70° and knees flexed[Q]
  - ***Ortolani's test, Trendelenburg' stest and Telescopy positive***[Q]
- *X-ray*:Von-Rosen's view, Andren's view[Q]

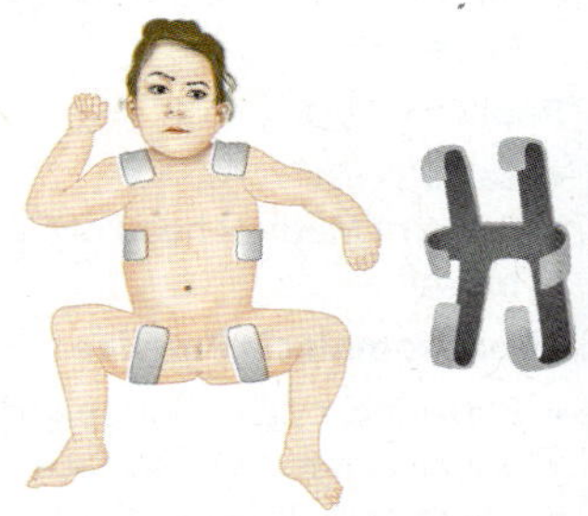

Fig. Von Rosen splint

- *Treatment*:
  - **Batchelor's cast**[Q]
  - **Lorenz (Frog leg) cast**[Q]
  - **Von-Rosen splint**[Q]
  - Salter's osteotomy

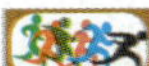

Topper's Edge

REGIONAL CONDITIONS OF HIP

Coxa Vara

- Defect of proximal shaft of femur characterized by decreased neck shaft angle[Q]
- Causes[Q]: Perthes' disease, Slipped femoral epiphysis, Rickets, Septic arthritis, Fibrous dysplasias
- Treatment: Lateral wedge osteotomy, Macewan and Shande's corrective osteotomy

Legg-Calve Perthes Disease

- Osteochondritis deformans juvenilis, **Coxa plana**[Q]
- MC form of Osteochondroses with AVN and enchondral ossification
- Two episodes of infarction: First episode cause unknown, Second episode due to sunchindral fracture
- Age group: 4-8 years old boys
- Classification: Catterall classification
- Tests: Thomas test, Internal rotation test, Trendelenburg test, Roll test
- Stages: Synovitis, AVN, Revascularisation, Healing

Slipped Capital Femoral Epiphysis

- Epiphyseal coxa vara, **Adolescent coxa vara**[Q]
- Slip mainly occur sin zone of hypertrophic cartilage
- Trethovan's sign positive[Q]

Varum Valgum Recurvatum

REGIONAL CONDITIONS OF KNEE

Genu Valgum

- **Knock knee**[Q]**:** Outward deviation of longitudinal axis of both tibia and femur
- Physiological genu valgum (75% cases): Appear by 4 years' age and disappears by 7 years' age
- Causes:
  - Causes of Unilateral Genu valgum[Q]: Trauma, Osteomyelitis, Tumours
  - Causes of Bilateral Genu valgum: Physiological, Congenital, Idiopathic (MC), Epiphyseal dysplasia, Thyroid disorders, Rickets, Paralytic/ Traumatic/ Infective/ Degenerative/ Inflammatory disorders

Genu Varum

- Lateral angulation of knee: Longitudinal axis of femur and tibia deviate medially[Q]
- Causes:
  - **Causes of Unilateral Genu varum**[Q]**:** Osteomyelitis, Trauma, Tumours
  - **Causes of Bilateral Genu varum:** Physiological, Osteoarthritis of knee, Idiopathic, Paget's disease, Blount's disease, Endocrine/ metabolic/ Degenerative/ Occupational disorders

Genu Recurvatum

- Backward bending of knee
- Causes: Congenital, Acquired (Polio, Post-injection quadriceps contracture)

Bursitis

- Suprapatellar bursitis
- Prepatellar bursitis **(Housemaid's knee**[Q]**)**
- Infrapatellar bursitis **(Clergyman's/ Parson's/ Carpet layer's knee**[Q]**)**

Popliteal Cyst

- Baker's cyst[Q]
- Bursa of Medical head of Gastrocnemius & Semimembranosus bursa[Q]

Chondromalacia Patellae

- Blistering, cystic change on Patella
- Usually affects Medial facet of patella
- Characteristic sign[Q]: Movie/ Theatre sign

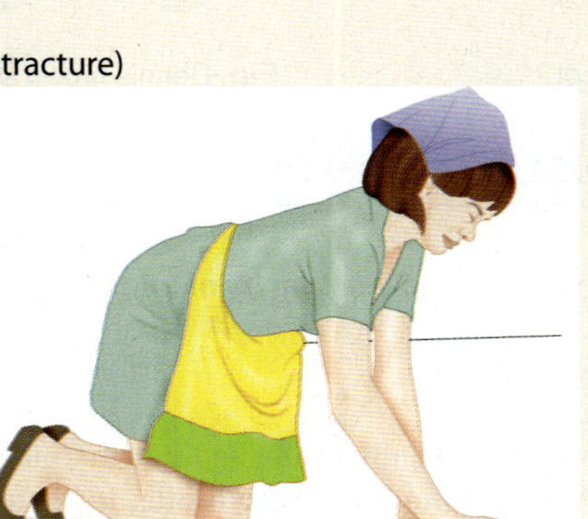

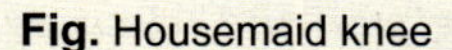

Fig. Housemaid knee

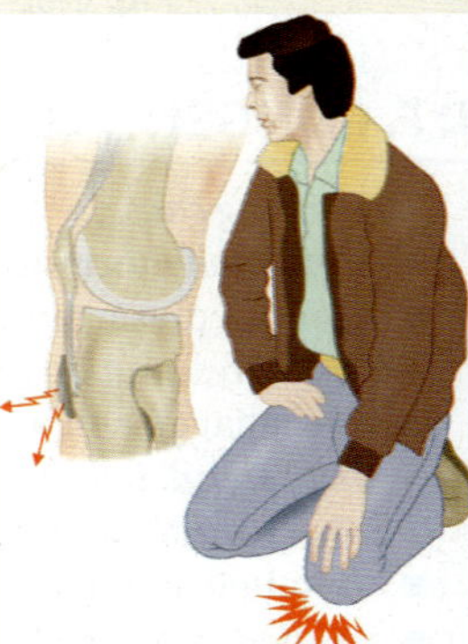

Fig. Clergyman knee

Orthopedics

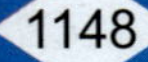

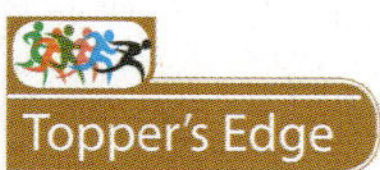

Topper's Edge

REGIONAL CONDITIONS OF FOOT

Pes Cavus

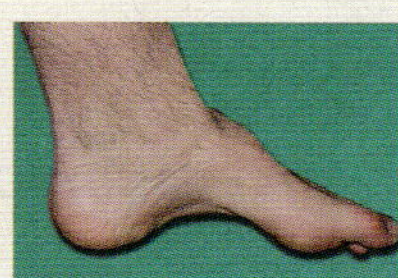

Fig. Pes cavus

- Deformity characterized by excessively high longitudinal arch due to Equinus position of forefoot in relation to hindfoot
- **Underlying cause:**
  - **Idiopathic** (80%): MC[Q]
  - Other causes: Secondary to neurological disorders (Cerebral palsy, Polio, Friedreich ataxia), CTEV, Trauma of foot
- Features: High medial longitudinal arch, 1st metatarsal drop & pronation, Tight plantar fascia, Cock-up deformities (MTP joints), Varus heel, Clawing of toes

Pes Planus

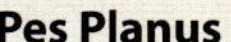

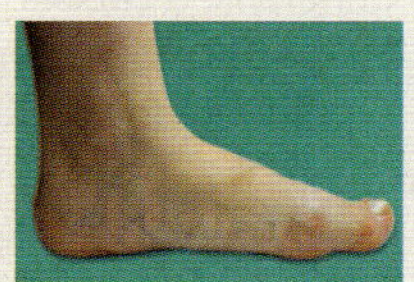

Fig. Pes planus

- Loss of Medial longitudinal arch of foot[Q]
- Predisposing factors: General muscle hypotonia, Excessive fatigue of foot muscles due to prolonged standing, Unsuitable footwear

Congenital Vertical Talus

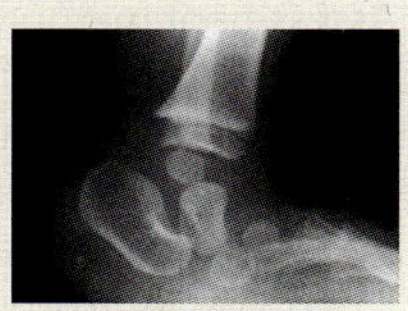

Fig. Congenital vertical talus

- **Rocker bottom foot**[Q]
- Recommended radiological views:
  - AP view: Increased talocalcaneal angle
  - Lateral view: Calcaneum & Talus vertically placed
  - Plantar flexion view: To assess Talar & Metatarsal calcaneal axes
  - Lateral dorsiflexion view: To assess heel equinus

Other Foot Disorders

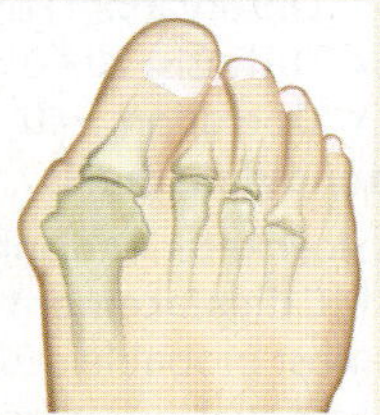

Fig. Hallux valgus

- Infantile Flatfoot: Congenital Ligament Laxity
- Metatarsalgia: Foot pain
- Morton's neuroma[Q]: Pinching of Lateral plantar nerve in 4th web space (Between 4th and 5th metatarsal heads)
- Calcaneal spurs: Spike of extra bone at Anterior edge of Calcaneal tuberosity (Medial)
- Hallus rigidus: Pain & stiffness in MTP joint of Great toe due to Osteoarthritis
- **Hallux valgus**[Q]**:**
  - Deviation of Great toe at Metatarsophalangeal joint, away from midline
  - Surgery: Keller's operation, Mayo's operation, Arthroplasty, Arthrodesis

VII G. OTHER CONGENITAL ANOMALIES

- *Spondylolysis*: Break in isthmus (pars interarticularis) of one of the lumbar vertebra (Most common: L5)
  - X-ray oblique view of spine: ***Scottish dog 'wearing a collar' appearance***[Q]
  - Vertebral slippage is ABSENT
- *Spondylolisthesis*: Forward displacement of a vertebra over one below it (Most common: L5-S1[Q])
  - X-ray oblique view of spine: ***Scottish dog 'head separated from neck' appearance***[Q]
  - Vertebral slippage is PRESENT
- *Phocomelia*: Lack of proximal part of limb (Thalidomide teratogenicity)
- ***Madelung's deformity***: Defect in epiphysial growth of distal radius
- ***Klippel-Feil syndrome***: Fused cervical vertebrae leading to short, stiff neck[Q]
- ***Rocker bottom foot***: Congenital vertical talus[Q]
- ***Sprengel's shoulder***: Congenitally high (descent-failure) scapula[Q]

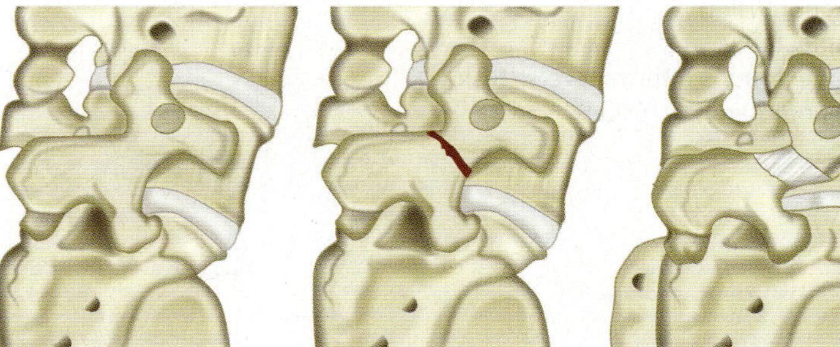

Fig. Spondylolysis & Spondylolisthesis

VII H. SPINAL DEFORMITIES

- ***Scoliosis***: Sideways curved spine
  - MC type: Idiopathic postural
  - X-ray: Reisser's sign + Cobb angle
  - Treatment: Milwaukee brace[Q]

- ***Kyphosis***: Backward convexity of spine
  - Postural (Most common)
  - Ankylosing spondylitis

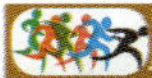

Topper's Edge

REGIONAL CONDITIONS OF SPINE

Kyphosis

- Increase in normal posterior convexity
- Localized causes: Fracture, Pott's disease, Secondaries
- Generalised causes: Ankylosing spondylitis, Osteomalacia, Paget's disease, Acromegaly
- **MC variety[Q]: Postural kyphosis**
- Types of kyphosis: Knuckle, Angular, Round

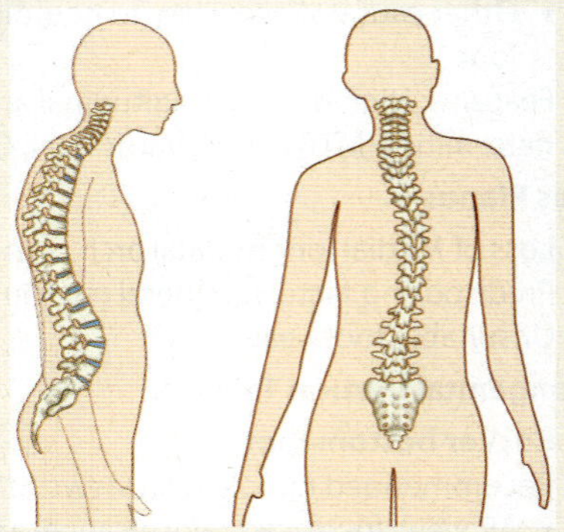

Fig. Kyphosis **Fig.** Scoliosis

Scoliosis

- Lateral curvature of spine in upright position
- **MC type of Structural scoliosis[Q]: Idiopathic (90% cases)**
- MC type of Nonstructural scoliosis: Postural scoliosis
- Assessment methods:
  - **Cobb's method[Q]:** Measure severity of curve
  - Nash & Moe's method: Measure vertebral rotation
  - Reisser's sign: Indirect measure of skeletal maturity; Earlier the Risser Grade, the greater the likelihood of a scoliosis progressing to the point it becomes clinically significant and requires intervention
  - Compensation: Formation of curves in opposite direction
- Treatment: **[Mnemonic: 3 O's]**
  - **O**bservation: For <20 degrees curve
  - **O**rthosis: 20-40 degrees curve
  - **O**peration: >40 degrees curve

Spondylolisthesis

- Slow anterior displacement of vertebra in lower lumbar spine[Q]
- **MC displacement[Q]: L5 vertebra slipping over S1 vertebra**
- Most probable cause[Q]: Defect in pars
- Essential lesion: Interruption of concavity of Pars interarticularis
- Wiltse, Macnab & Newman Classification:
  - Isthmic/ True (MC[Q])
  - Degenerative (Seen in adults)
  - Traumatic
  - Pathological
  - Dysplastic (Least common)
- Meyerding's Grading: G1 (25% forward displacement), G2 25-50%, G3 50-70%, G4 >75%
- Surgical management:
  - **Posterolateral fusion: Best method[Q]**
  - Posterior fusion
  - Laminectomy
  - Laminectomy & Intertransverse fusion
  - Anterior interbody fusion

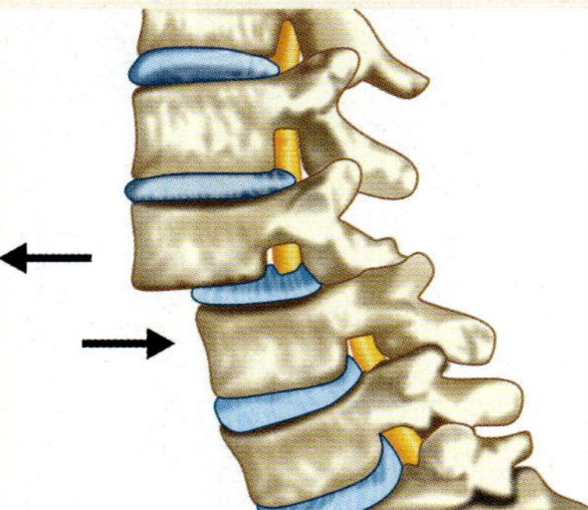

Fig. Spondylolisthesis

VII I. COMMON BURSITIS

Name	Bursitis
Housemaid's knee[Q]	Prepatellar bursitis
Clergyman's knee[Q]	Infrapatellar bursitis
Student's elbow[Q]	Olecranon bursitis (Most common)
Weaver's bottom	Ischial bursitis
Tailor's ankle	On lateral malleolus
Bunion[Q]	On great toe
Hip bursitis	Greater Trochanteric bursitis
Shoulder bursitis	Sub-acromial bursitis

VII J. CARPAL TUNNEL SYNDROME

- *Definition*: Syndrome characterised by *'compression of median nerve'* as it passes beneath flexor retinaculum[Q]
- *Causative agent*: [Mnemonic: In Carpal-tunnel Median-nerve is Rightly Affected at Wrist[Q]]
    1. **Idiopathic (Most common)**
    2. Post-traumatic causes (after Colles' fracture)
    3. Endocrine causes (Myxoedema, Acromegaly)
    4. Inflammatory causes (RA, Wrist osteoarthritis)
- *Clinical features*: Tingling, numbness of thumb and radial one-half of fingers
- *Examination*: Low median nerve compression found
- *Treatment*: Divide flexor retinaculum and decompress median nerve[Q]

IMAGE-BASED QUESTIONS

1. The below is X-ray pelvis of one year old baby. All of the following tests will be positive except

[AIIMS May 2016]

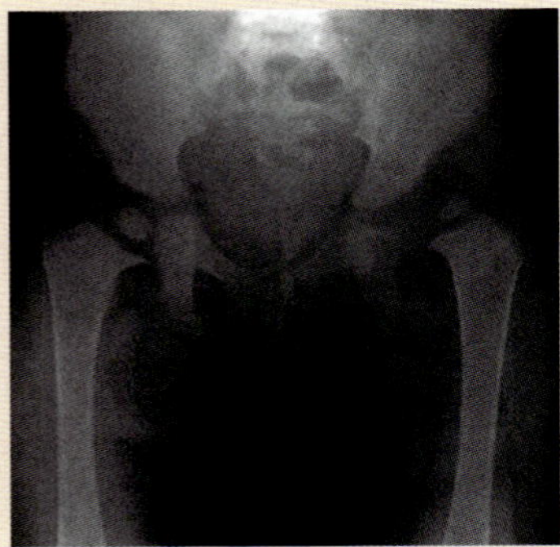

a. Narath test b. Ortolani test
c. Gaenslen test d. Barlow test

2. Orthopedic device shown in Photograph is

[Recent Question 2012]

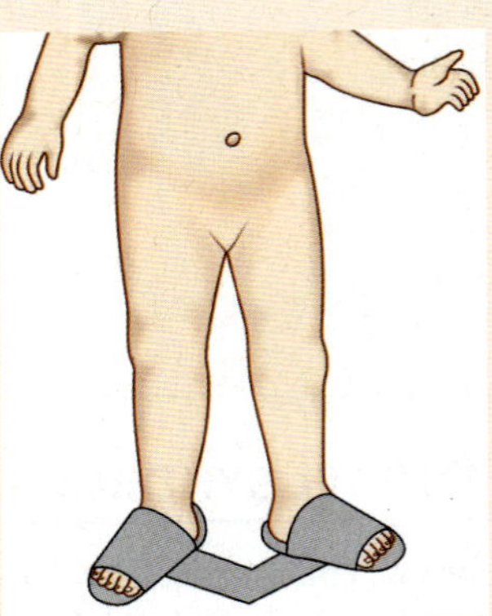

a. CTEV shoes b. Below knee calipers
c. Denis Browne splint d. Phelps brace

3. Sign shown in Photograph is characteristic of

[Recent Question 2013]

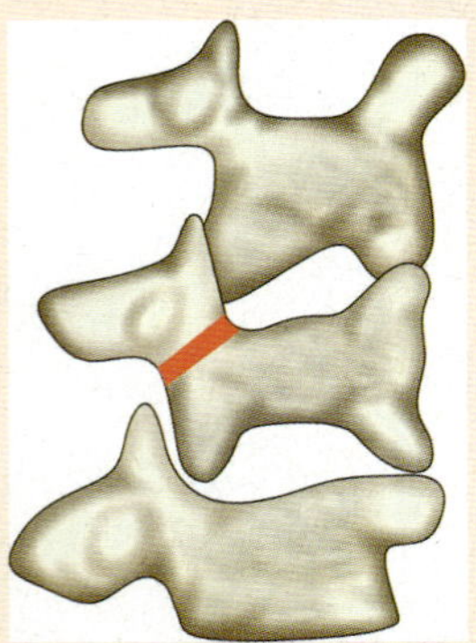

a. Scoliosis b. Kyphosis
c. Spondylolisthesis d. Spondylolysis

4. Identify the Orthopaedic device shown in Photograph

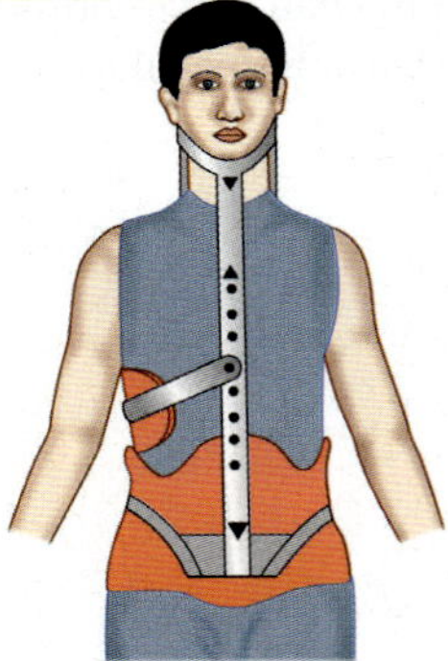

a. SOMI brace b. Halo-body orthosis
c. Lumbo-sacral belt d. Milwaukee brace

5. Bursa affected in the Mechanism shown in Photograph is

[Recent Question 2014]

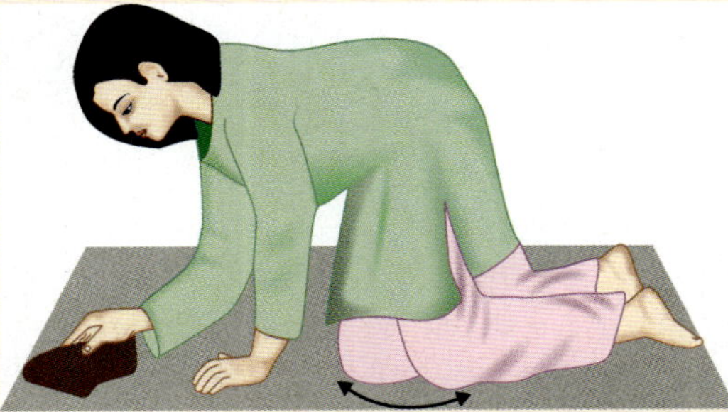

a. Suprapatellar bursa b. Prepatellar bursa
c. Infrapatellar bursa d. Olecranon bursa

ANSWERS WITH EXPLANATIONS OF IBQs

1. Ans. (c) Gaenslen test *[Ref. SRB's Clinical Methods in Surgery, 1/e p773]*

Also Remember

- Gaenslen test is positive in Ankylosing spondylitis

Tests Used in Congenital Dislocation of Hip (Photograph)

- Narath test
- Ortolani test
- Barlow test
- Telescopic test
- Useful lines: Perkin's line, Von Rosen femoral line, Acetabular angle

2. Ans. (c) Denis Browne splint *[Ref. Maheshwari, 4/e p209]*

Denis-Browne Splint (Foot Abduction Orthosis)

- Use: Maintenance of correction of CTEV (Club foot)
- Timing of use:
  - Throughout the day before child starts walking
  - During night time when child starts walking (CTEV shoes during day)

3. Ans. (d) Spondylolysis *[Ref. Maheshwari, 4/e p277]*

- Spondylolisthesis: *Scottish dog 'with collar' appearance*
- Spondylolisthesis: *Scottish dog 'head separated from neck' appearance*

4. Ans. (d) Milwaukee brace *[Ref. Maheshwari, 4/e p275]*

- Non-operative methods for Treatment of Scoliosis:
  - Milwaukee brace
  - Boston brace
  - Reisser's turn buckle cast
  - Localiser cast

5. Ans. (b) Prepatellar bursa *[Ref. Maheshwari, 4/e p292]*

Common Types of Bursitis

- Housemaid's knee: Prepatellar bursitis
- Clergyman's knee: Infrapatellar bursitis
- Student's elbow: Olecranon bursitis (Most common)
- Weaver's bottom: Ischial bursitis
- Tailor's ankle: On lateral malleolus
- Bunion: On great toe
- Hip bursitis: Greater Trochanteric bursitis
- Shoulder bursitis: Sub-acromial bursitis

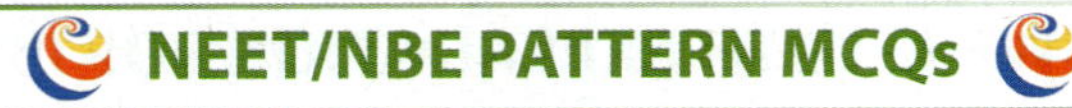

NEET/NBE PATTERN MCQs

1. Hamilton Ruler test sign is positive in which of the mentioned conditions? *[Recent Question 2016]*
a. Anterior dislocation of shoulder
b. Acromioclavicular joint dislocation
c. Posterior dislocation of shoulder
d. Luxatio erecta

2. Tennis elbow is *[Recent Question 2016]*
a. Medial epicondylitis
b. Lateral epicondylitis
c. Ulnar collateral ligament injury
d. Radial head subluxation

3. Snapping knee syndrome is due to involvement of *[Recent Question 2016]*
a. Pes Anserinus b. Quadriceps tendon
c. Gastrocnemius origin d. Lateral collateral ligament

4. Brace is used in Scoliosis is? *[Recent Question 2016]*
a. Milwaukee brace b. L S Belt
c. Taylors brace d. Four post collar

5. Investigation of choice to detect a Prolapsed intervertebral disc is ? *[Recent Question 2016]*
a. C T Scan b. MRI
c. Myelography d. Radiograph

6. Club foot clinically present as what deformity? *[Recent Question 2016]*
a. Calcaneovalgus b. Equinovarus
c. Equinocavovarus d. Calcaneovarus

7. Most common cause of Carpal tunnel syndrome is? *[Recent Question 2016]*
a. Pregnancy
b. Idiopathic
c. Alcoholism
d. Occupational-Excessive use of vibratory instruments

8. Milwaukee Brace is used in treatment of all except *[Recent Question 2016, 2017]*
a. Congenital kyphosis
b. Scheuermanns disease
c. Adolescent idiopathic scoliosis
d. Spondylolisthesis

9. Primary locus of Madelung deformity is located at *[Recent Question 2016]*
a. Distal end of radius
b. Distal end of humerus
c. Scaphotrapezial joint
d. 1st Carpometacarpal joint

10. All of the following are true regarding Congenital dislocation of Hip except *[Recent Question 2016]*
a. Asymmetric Thigh folds may be seen
b. Galeazzi sign and Ortolanis test may be positive
c. It may be bilateral
d. Polyhydramnios is a known risk factor

11. Cobb's angle is used to measure the degree of *[Recent Question 2016]*
a. Kyphoscoliosis
b. Angular deformity of the knee
c. Extent of depression in calcaneal fracture
d. Extent of spondylolisthesis

12. All of the following are described Surgical procedures for CTEV except *[Recent Question 2016]*
a. Dwyer's osteotomy
b. Posteromedial soft tissue release
c. Triple arthrodesis
d. Salter's osteotomy

13. Who devised correction of CTEV by Serial casting? *[Recent Question 2016]*
a. Ignasio Ponseti b. Gerhard Kuntscher
c. Gavril Ilizarov d. Hugh Owen Thomas

14. Ortolani's test is used to diagnose *[Recent Question 2016]*
a. Congenital coxa vara
b. Slipped Capital femoral epiphysis
c. Developmental dysplasia of the hip
d. Perthe's disease

15. Cozens test is used to detect *[Recent Question 2016, 2017]*
a. Golfer's elbow
b. Tennis elbow
c. Baseball pitcher's elbow
d. Posterior dislocation of elbow

16. Preferred treatment of Cubitus varus is *[Recent Question 2016]*
a. Medial closing wedge osteotomy
b. Lateral closing wedge osteotomy
c. Medial opening wedge osteotomy
d. Lateral opening wedge osteotomy

17. Pavlik harness is used to treat *[Recent Question 2016, 2017]*
a. Developmental dysplasia of hip
b. Perthe's disease
c. Slipped capital femoral epiphysis
d. Congenital coxa vara

18. All of the following are associated with Frozen shoulder except *[Recent Question 2016]*
a. Diabetes b. Hyperthyroidism
c. Psoriasis d. Hemiplegia

19. Irregular thigh folds are seen in *[Recent Question 2016]*
a. Developmental dysplasia of hip
b. Perthe's disease
c. Slipped capital femoral epiphysis
d. Congenital coxa vara

20. Last deformity to be corrected by Ponseti's method for CTEV is *[Recent Question 2016]*
a. Heel varus b. Equinus
c. Foot adduction d. Cavus

21. In Triple Arthrodesis, which of the following joints is not used? *[NBE FMGE September 2010]*
a. Talo-navicular b. Tibio-talar
c. Subtalar d. Calcaneo-cuboid

22. Spondylolysis involves which one of the following *[NBE DNB June 2011]*
a. Lamina b. Pars interarticularis
c. Spinous process d. Intervertebral disc

23. Housemaid's Knee is due to enlargement of
a. Supra-patellar bursa *[NBE FMGE September 2010]*
b. Sub-cutaneous pre-patellar bursa
c. Sub-cutaneous infra-patellar bursa
d. Deep infra-patellar bursa

24. Compound palmar ganglion is *[NBE DNB 1998]*
a. Ulnar bursitis (due to compound injury)
b. Ulnar bursitis (idiopathic)
c. Ulnar bursitis (pyogenic)
d. Ulnar bursitis (tubercular)

25. MC involvement in Volkmann's Ischemia seen is that of *[NBE DNB 1996, NBE DNB 2000]*
a. Flexor carpi radialis longus
b. Flexor digitorum superficialis
c. Flexor digitorum profundus
d. Pronator teres

26. Calcaneovalgus deformity develops usually because of *[NBE DNB June 2011]*
a. Paralysis of Gastrocnemius, soleus & tibialis posterior
b. Paralysis of ankle dorsi flexors
c. Paralysis of peroneal muscles
d. Contracture of gastrosoleus

27. Striated vertebra is seen in *[Recent Question 2013]*
a. TB spine b. Haemangioma
c. Chordoma d. Metastasis

28. Claw hand is a manifestation of *[NBE DNB 1995, 2005, 2006, Recent Question 2015]*
a. Median nerve injury b. Ulnar nerve injury
c. Radial nerve injury d. Carpal tunnel syndrome

29. Posterior dislocation of hip is characterized by
a. Marked shortening of limb *[Recent Question 2012]*
b. Lengthening of limb
c. No change in limb length
d. Extension deformity

30. Hill Sachs lesion is seen in *[NBE FMGE September 2007, NBE DNB June 2011]*
a. Recurrent dislocation of shoulder
b. Recurrent dislocation of patella
c. Perthes disease
d. Slipped capital femoral epiphysis

31. Most characteristic sign of Volkman's Ischemia is *[NBE DNB 2002, NBE DNB 2005]*
a. Absent arterial pulsation
b. Pain on passive movements
c. Disproportionate pain
d. Development of contracture

32. Most common involvement in Dupuytren's contracture is *[NBE DNB 1995, 1999, 2001, 2005, 2006, 2007]*
a. Ring finger b. Middle finger
c. Little finger d. Thumb

33. Position of the hip in posterior dislocation of the joint is *[NBE DNB 2002, 2011, NBE FMGE 2012, DPG 1988, 1993, JIPMER 1995, AIIMS 1997, 2000, AIPGME 2002]*
a. Flexion, abduction and external rotation
b. Flexion, abduction and internal rotation
c. Flexion, adduction and internal rotation
d. Flexion, adduction and external rotation

34. Most common cause of trigger finger *[Recent Question 2012]*
a. Trauma b. Alcohol
c. Smoking d. Drug abuse

35. MC reason for tendoachilles tendinitis is
a. Improper shoes b. Overuse *[NBE DNB 2010]*
c. Running and jumping d. Corticosteroids

36. Congenital Pseudoarthrosis Knee treatment is *[NBE DNB 2002, NBE DNB 2008]*
a. Immobilization of joint
b. Amputation
c. Vascularised fibular graft
d. Chaenye's implant

37. Investigation of choice for Congenital dislocation of hip is *[Recent Question 2015]*
a. X-ray b. USG
c. CT d. MRI

38. False about Pott's spine *[Recent Question 2012]*
a. Commonest at dorsolumbar junction
b. Always heals by chemotherapy
c. Back pain is an early symptom
d. There is disc space narrowing on X-ray

39. Nerve injured in anterior dislocation of shoulder is *[UPSC 2007, AIIMS 1995, AIPGME 1997, Recent Question 2012, 2017, NBE DNB 2011]*
a. Ulnar nerve b. Radial nerve
c. Median nerve d. Axillary nerve

40. Which nerve is involved in Carpal tunnel syndrome? *[Recent Question 2016, NBE FMGE September 2006, UPSC 2012]*
a. Radial nerve b. Ulnar nerve
c. Median nerve d. Posterior interosseus nerve

41. Part of glenoid labrum involved in Bankart's lesion is *[Recent Question 2017, NBE DNB 2009, AIIMS 2000, 2006, UPPG 2000]*
a. Anterior b. Antero-superior
c. Antero-inferior d. Posterior

42. In deQuervain's disease, there is tenosynovitis of *[NBE FMGE September 2011, Recent Question 2015]*
a. Extensor pollicis longus
b. Extensor pollicis brevis and abductor pollicis longus
c. Extensor carpi radialis longus and brevis
d. Brachiocardialis

43. Waddling gait is a feature of *[NBE DNB June 2011, Recent Question 2016, 2014]*
a. Bilateral DOH b. Bilateral genu varum
c. Bilateral CTEV d. Bilateral bowed tibia

44. Sprain of ankle joint results from injury to *[UPSC 2007 Recent Question 2012]*
a. Anterior talofibular ligament
b. Posterior talofibular ligament
c. Spring ligament
d. Deltoid ligament

45. Volkmanns contracture, which artery is involved *[Recent Question 2013]*
a. Radial b. Brachial
c. Ulnar d. Interosseus

46. Genu valgus deformity is seen when *[NBE DNB December 2011]*
   a. The long axis of tibia and fibula are deviated medially from that of the femur
   b. The long axis of tibia and fibula are deviated laterally from that of the femur
   c. The foot is deviated laterally from the long axis of tibia and fibula
   d. When the foot is plantar flexed

47. Trigger finger refers to *[NBE DNB 1998, 2000 2004, 2005, DPG 1991, Orissa 1990, WBPG 2000]*
   a. Stenosis and tenovaginits of flexor tendon of affected finger
   b. Injury to a finger while using a gun/ pistol
   c. Sensation loss in Carapl tunnel syndrome
   d. All of the above

48. In neglected cases of CTEV joint fused are *[Recent Question 2013]*
   a. Calcaneocuboid, talonavicular and talocalcaneal
   b. Tibiotalar, calcaneocuboid and talonavicular
   c. Ankle joint, calcaneocuboid and talonavicular
   d. None of the above

49. Spondylolysis involves which of the following? *[NBE FMGE September 2006]*
   a. Lamina b. Pars interarticularis
   c. Spinous process d. Intervertebral disc

50. In Hammer toe, flexion deformity is seen at
   a. Proximal interphalangeal joint *[NBE DNB 1998]*
   b. Distal interphalangeal joint
   c. Metatarsophalangeal joint
   d. Calcaneo-navicular joint

51. Provocative Test for detecting CDH? *[Recent Question 2013]*
   a. Peterson test b. Barlow test
   c. Perkin's test d. Von Rosen tests

52. After chronic use of steroids severe pain in right hip with immobility is due to *[Recent Question 2012, Recent Question 2013]*
   a. Avascular necrosis b. Perthes disease
   c. Hip dislocation d. Osteoarthritis

53. Deformity in posterior elbow dislocation *[Recent Question 2012]*
   a. Flexion b. Extension
   c. Both d. None

54. Erosion of hyaline cartilage is seen in all EXCEPT *[NBE FMGE March 2006]*
   a. Rheumatoid arthritis b. Gout
   c. SLE d. Psoriasis

55. Dysplastic hip in a child, investigation of choice *[Recent Question 2012, 2015]*
   a. X-ray b. MRI
   c. USG d. CT Scan

56. Complications of elbow dislocation are all except *[Recent Question 2012]*
   a. Myositis ossificans b. Median nerve injury
   c. Brachial artery injury d. Radial nerve injury

57. Investigation of choice for lumbar prolapsed disc *[Recent Question 2012]*
   a. X-ray b. CT Scan
   c. MRI d. Myelogram

58. Commonest dislocation of elbow *[Recent Question 2012, 2017]*
   a. Anterior b. Posterior
   c. Both same d. Medial

59. Commonest site for intervertebral disc prolapse in lumbar spine is *[FMGE September 2012]*
   a. L1-L2 b. L2-L3
   c. L3-L4 d. L4-L5

60. Caries sicca is seen in *[Recent Question 2012]*
   a. Hip b. Shoulder
   c. Knee d. None of the above

61. Winging of scapula is due to palsy of *[NBE FMGE September 2012, Recent Question 2015]*
   a. Long thoracic nerve b. Accessory nerve
   c. Axillary nerve d. Ulnar nerve

62. Damage to median nerve produces *[Recent Question 2013]*
   a. Claw hand b. Winging of scapule
   c. Ape thumb d. Wrist drop

63. False about Myositis ossificans
   a. Seen more in children *[NBE FMGE September 2005]*
   b. Stiffness of joints is present
   c. Mobilization of joints is advisable
   d. Surgery is treatment of choice

64. Most common nerve involved in Anterior dislocation of Humerus is *[Recent Question 2014]*
   a. Axillary b. Radial
   c. Scapular d. Musculocutaneous

65. Dupuytren's contracture involves *[Recent Question 2012, 2013, DPG 1994, AIPG 1994]*
   a. Dorsal fascia b. Palmar fascia
   c. Ulnar bursa d. Radial bursa

66. A 4-year-old child is brought with painful elbow and forearm held in pronation and extension. X-rays are normal. Most appropriate clinical diagnosis is *[NBE DNB December 2011]*
   a. Monteggia Fracture-dislocation
   b. Obstetric palsy
   c. Pulled elbow
   d. Cellulitis

67. Components of Posterior Dislocation of Hip include all except *[Recent Question 2014]*
   a. Flexion
   b. Adduction
   c. Internal rotation
   d. Limb lengthening

68. All are complications of Elbow dislocation EXCEPT
   a. Vascular injury *[NBE FMGE March 2004]*
   b. Median nerve injury
   c. VIC
   d. Myositis ossificans progressive

69. What is seen on X-ray with posterior elbow dislocation? *[Recent Question 2012]*
a. Coronoid process posterior to humerus
b. Coronoid process anterior to humerus
c. Coronoid process below humerus
d. None

70. Most common completely paralysed muscle in Poliomyelitis is *[FMGE September 2012]*
a. Opponens pollicis b. Quadriceps
c. Tibialis anterior d. Triceps

71. Injury to Supraspinatus muscle lead to *[Recent Question 2014]*
a. Frozen shoulder
b. Winging of scapula
c. Inability to adduct
d. Inability to bend to 90 degrees

72. Uncomplicated shoulder dislocation most commonly occurs in the following direction *[Recent Question 2013]*
a. Anterior b. Posterior
c. Superior d. Medially

73. Cubitus varus deformity is *[Recent Question 2014]*
a. Mallet finger b. Gun stock deformity
c. Dinner fork deformity d. Swan neck deformity

74. Pain and tenderness over the lateral condyle of humerus with a painful dorsiflexion of the wrist is indicative of *[NBE FMGE September 2011]*
a. Golfer's elbow b. Tennis elbow
c. Pitcher's elbow d. Cricket elbow

75. Posterior dislocation of Hip can damage which nerve *[Recent Question 2012]*
a. Superior gluteal b. Sciatic
c. Inferior gluteal d. Femoral

76. Felon most common complication is *[Recent Question 2012]*
a. Osteomyelitis b. Subungual hematoma
c. Infective arthritis d. None

77. Congenital vertical talus leads to *[FMGE September 2012]*
a. CTEV b. Spondylosis
c. Rocker bottom foot d. All of the above

78. Housemaid knee is bursitis of *[NBE FMGE September 2011, Recent Question 2012, Recent Question 2013]*
a. Prepatellar bursa b. Infrapatellar bursa
c. Olecranon d. Ischial bursa

79. Most common muscle damaged in rotator cuff *[Recent Question 2012, Recent Question 2013, 2017]*
a. Supraspinatus b. Infraspinatus
c. Subscapularis d. Teres minor

80. Felon is *[FMGE September 2012, Recent Question 2017]*
a. Infection of nail fold
b. Deep palmar abscess
c. Terminal pulp space infection
d. None of the above

81. Primary pathology in CDH *[Recent Question 2012, 2013]*
a. Large head of femur b. Shallow acetabulum
c. Excessive retroversion d. Everted limbus

82. Dupuytren's contracture of hand commonly start in *[NBE FMGE September 2011]*
a. Thumbs b. Index finger
c. Middle finger d. Ring finger

83. In posterior dislocation of elbow, most prominent part *[Recent Question 2012]*
a. Coronoid b. Radial head
c. Olecranon d. None

84. Avascular necrosis of hip, investigation of choice *[Recent Question 2012]*
a. MRI b. USG
c. CT d. X-ray

85. In elbow, osteochondritis usually involves *[Recent Question 2012, Recent Question 2013]*
a. Olecranon b. Trochlea
c. Radial head d. Capitulum

86. Thoracic outlet syndrome mainly occur due to compression of *[Recent Question 2015]*
a. Axillary vessels and Lower root
b. Subclavian vessels and Lower root
c. Axillary vessels and Upper root
d. Subclavian vessels and Upper root

87. Clergyman's knee affects *[Recent Question 2015]*
a. Prepatellar bursa b. Infrapatellar bursa
c. Olecranon d. Ischial bursa

88. Components of Clubfoot deformity include all except *[Recent Question 2016, 2015]*
a. Eversion b. Inversion
c. Equinus d. Adduction

89. Which of the following is not true about Impingement syndrome? *[Recent Question 2017]*
a. It is the tendinitis caused by inflammation of the rotator cuff tendons
b. Supraspinatus tendon is most often involved
c. Shoulder abduction in the arc of 60 - 120 degrees is particularly painful
d. Surgical decompression of the subacromial space is frequently indicated

90. Treatment of fresh case of CTEV in newborn is usually done by *[Recent Question 2017]*
a. Ponseti technique b. Kites technique
c. Kochers technique d. Wilsons technique

91. Dennis brown splint is used for *[Recent Question 2017]*
a. Manus varus b. Rocker bottom foot
c. Manus valgus d. CTEV

92. Genu recurvatum is seen in *[Recent Question 2017]*
a. Rheumatoid arthritis b. Poliomyelitis
c. Rickets d. All the above

93. Which of the following is not a cause for the development of Carpal tunnel syndrome? *[Recent Question 2017]*
a. Alcoholism b. Sarcoidosis
c. Gout d. Menorrhagia

94. Palpable femur head on per rectal exam is a feature of which of the following conditions? *[Recent Question 2017]*
   a. Posterior hip dislocation
   b. Anterior hip dislocation
   c. Central hip dislocation
   d. Inferior hip dislocation

95. Following is not a part of Ortolani test *[Recent Question 2017]*
   a. Examiners thumb rests on the medial thigh
   b. Examiners fingers lie on the greater trochanter
   c. Hips are flexed to 90 degrees and gently abducted
   d. Jerk is given to the knee to dislocate the femur head -jerk of exit

96. Which of the following is not true about the manipulation methods to correct CTEV? *[Recent Question 2017]*
   a. Involves serial casting and below knee plaster casting
   b. In Kites method deformities are corrected sequentially adduction → inversion → equinus
   c. Ponseti's technique has success rate of 90 – 98%
   d. Ponseti's method of correction involves cavus → adduction → heel varus → equinus

97. Which of the following is/are feature/s of Sprengel's deformity? *[Recent Question 2017]*
   a. Elevated shoulder on affected side
   b. Smaller than usual scapula
   c. Short neck
   d. All the above

98. Jumper's knee is due to *[Recent Question 2017]*
   a. Sacral fracture   b. Patellar tendonosis
   c. Tibial fracture   d. Fibular fracture

99. All are true regarding Carpal tunnel syndrome except *[Recent Question 2017]*
   a. Pregnancy is the most common cause
   b. More common in women
   c. Median nerve is compressed
   d. Symptoms often appear at night

100. Carpal tunnel syndrome is seen in all except *[Recent Question 2017]*
   a. Pregnancy   b. Alcoholism
   c. Colle's fracture   d. Smith's fracture

101. Which of the following is true about DDH? *[Recent Question 2017]*
   a. Male gender is a risk factor
   b. Limbs are in adduction, internal rotation and flexion in old children
   c. Femur neck is retroverted
   d. Ligamentum teres is atrophied

102. Which of the following is seen in Popliteal entrapment syndrome? *[Recent Question 2017]*
   a. Evidence of atherosclerosis
   b. Exercise induced calf claudication
   c. Abnormal relation between popliteal artery and lateral head of gastrocnemius
   d. Decreased ankle pulses with ankle extension

103. Ponseti technique failure in children should be managed with *[Recent Question 2017]*
   a. Posteromedial soft tissue release
   b. Anterolateral soft tissue release
   c. Triple arthrodesis
   d. Lateral closing wedge osteotomy of calcaneum

104. Bakers cyst is a type of *[Recent Question 2017]*
   a. Retention cyst
   b. Pulsion diverticulum of knee joint
   c. Bursitis
   d. Benign tumor

HIGH YIELD MCQs

1. Dupuytren's contracture occur in *[Kerala PGMEE 2007]*
   a. Diabetes mellitus
   b. Epilepsy
   c. Chronic pulmonary disease
   d. Alcohol   e. Rheumatoid arthritis

2. All are component of Complex regional pain syndrome except *[All India PGMEE 2008]*
   a. Pain   b. Swelling
   c. Anhydrosis   d. Osteoporosis

3. Commonest dislocation of the hip is *[Recent Question 2017, TN PGMEE 1989, TN PGMEE 1992]*
   a. Posterior   b. Anterior
   c. Central   d. None

4. Which is true about dislocation of hip joint? *[Karnataka PGMEE 1994]*
   a. Posterior dislocation is commoner
   b. In posterior dislocation whole lower limb is rotated medially
   c. In anterior dislocation whole lower limb is rotated laterally
   d. All of the above

5. A 50-year-old lady recovered after an ankle-sprain injury 2 months back. She now complains of severe pain in ankle joint with inability to flex the foot. On examination, there is local edema with shiny skin. Probable diagnosis *[All India PGMEE 2011]*
   a. Fibromyalgia
   b. Peripheral neuropathy
   c. Complex regional pain syndrome 1
   d. Complex regional pain syndrome 2

6. Luxatio erecta *[TN PGMEE 1998]*
   a. Tear of the glenoidal labium
   b. Inferior dislocation of shoulder
   c. Anterior dislocation of shoulder
   d. Defect in the humeral head

7. Recurrent dislocation is common in *[AIIMS PG 1997, AIPGME 1997]*
   a. Shoulder   b. Patella
   c. Hip joint   d. Elbow joint

8. Kienbock's disease is due to avascular necrosis of *[PGI 2004]*

a. Femoral neck b. Medial cuneiform bone
c. Lunate bone d. Scaphoid bone
e. Medial condyle of tibia

9. Which of the following is true about manifestation of Kienbock's disease? *[PGI 2005]*

a. Constant tenderness is present
b. Seen in old age
c. Restriction of joint movement is late sequelae
d. Tenderness in lunate bone
e. Ulna is shortened

10. Osgood-Schlatter disease is *[PGI 2013]*

a. A traction injury of femoral epiphysis
b. A traction injury of the posterior epiphysis of Os calcis
c. A traction injury of vertebral epiphysis
d. A traction injury of the tibial tubercle of the tibial epiphysis
e. None of the above is true

11. Osgood Schlatter disease affects *[PGI 2001]*

a. Upper tibia b. Lower tibia
c. Distal femur d. Proximal femur
e. Patella

12. Commonest type of shoulder dislocation *[PGI 1987]*

a. Subcoracoid b. Subglenoid
c. Posterior d. Subclavicular

13. A patient with hip in adduction and medial rotation and is unable to move probable diagnosis is

a. Posterior dislocation head of femur *[AP PGMEE 1994]*
b. Fracture shaft of femur
c. Fracture neck of femur
d. Sciatica

14. The pain around the hip with flexion, adduction & internal rotation and shortening of lower limb in a young adult after a road traffic accident is suggestive of *[AIIMS PGMEE 2005]*

a. Intracapsular fracture of the femoral neck
b. Extra capsular fracture of the femoral neck
c. Posterior dislocation of hip
d. Anterior dislocation of hip

15. Recurrent dislocation is least common in *[Delhi PGMEE 1994]*

a. Shoulder b. Knee
c. Patella d. None

16. Traumatic dislocation of hip is characterized by *[NBE DNB 1989, AMU PGMEE 1992, JIPMER PGMEE 1995]*

a. Adduction internal rotation deformity
b. Abduction external rotation deformity
c. Adduction external rotation deformity
d. Abduction internal rotation deformity

17. Dashboard injury results in *[AP PGMEE 1997]*

a. Anterior dislocation of hip
b. Posterior dislocation of hip
c. Central dislocation of hip
d. Fracture neck femur

18. MC type of shoulder dislocation seen is *[DPG 2004]*

a. Anterior (Sub-coracoid) b. Sub-glenoid
c. Posterior d. Sub-clavicular

19. Consider the following statements about Carpal tunnel syndrome *[UPSC 1999]*

1. It may occur in Acromegaly
2. It may occur in pregnancy
3. It causes delayed ulnar nerve conduction
4. It may be associated with wasting of abductor pollicis brevis of these statements,

a. 1, 2 and 3 are correct
b. 2, 3 and 4 are correct
c. 1, 2 and 4 are correct
d. 1, 3 and 4 are correct

20. Osteochondritis is not seen in .... disease *[Delhi PGMEE 1999]*

a. Pellegrini - Stieda b. Panner's
c. Calve's d. Kohler's

21. In carpal tunnel syndrome, features are of *[JIPMER PGMEE 1999]*

a. Compression of ulnar nerve
b. Compression of median nerve under the flexor retinaculum
c. Anaesthesia over thenar eminence
d. Atrophy of hypothenar muscles

22. Carpal tunnel syndrome can be caused by the following except? *[All India PGMEE 2009]*

a. Diabetes mellitus b. Amyloidosis
c. Addison's disease d. Hypothyroidism

23. Vascular sign of Narath is noticed in *[Recent Question 2016, 2017, NBE DNB 1991, WB PGMEE 1993]*

a. Fracture neck of femur
b. Perthes disease
c. Posterior dislocation of hip
d. All of the above

24. In a patient with a history of burning pain localized to the plantar aspect of the foot, the differential diagnosis must include *[AIIMS PGMEE 2003]*

a. Peripheral vascular disease
b. Tarsal coalation.
c. Tarsal tunnel syndrome
d. Planter fibromatosis

25. Classical flexion and rotation deformities at hip and knee joints, as a sequelae of poliomyelitis, are due to the contracture of *[AIIMS PGMEE 2002]*

a. Tensor fascia lata b. Gastrocnemius
c. Tendo Achilles d. Hamstrings

26. All are possible during contraction of Tensor fasciae latae except *[AIIMS PGMEE 1994]*

a. Adduction of Hip joint b. Flexion of Hip joint
c. Abduction of Hip joint d. Flexion of the knee

27. In a post-polio case, Ilio-tibial tract contracture is likely to result in *[All India PGMEE 2001, Recent Question 2017]*

a. Extension at the hip and knee
b. Extension at the hip
c. Flexion at the hip and the knee
d. Extension at the knee

28. In Pulled elbow, there is *[PGI 1994, AMU 1985, PGI 1979]*
a. Subluxation of proximal radio-ulnar joint
b. Subluxation of distal radio-ulnar joint
c. Disarticulation of elbow
d. Fracture Olecranon process

29. Recurrent dislocations are least commonly seen in *[All India PGMEE 2009]*
a. Ankle b. Hip
c. Shoulder d. Patella

30. Maximum shortening of limbs occur in *[AIIMS PGMEE 1997]*
a. Trochanteric fracture femur
b. Post dislocation of hip
c. Fracture neck femur d. Anterior dislocation of hip

31. Attitude in Subcoracoid dislocation of shoulder includes all EXCEPT *[AP PGMEE 1994]*
a. Adduction b. Limb on side of body
c. Abduction d. Elevation

32. A 7 years old boy with abrupt onset of pain in hip with hip held in abduction. Hemogram is normal. ESR is raised. What is the next line of management? *[AIIMS PGMEE 2009]*
a. Hospitalize and observe
b. Ambulatory observation
c. Intravenous antibiotics
d. USG guided aspiration of hip

33. Perthe's disease is *[AIIMS PGMEE 1994]*
a. Fracture of femoral shaft
b. Osteochondritis of femoral epiphysis
c. Infarction of femoral head
d. Fracture dislocation of femoral neck

34. A 10 years old male with pain in left hip & limping on examination restricted abduction & internal rotation, probable diagnosis is *[AIIMS PGMEE 1999]*
a. Septic arthritis of hip
b. Tuberculosis arthritis of hip
c. Cong dislocation of hip
d. Perthes disease

35. Perthe's disease is treated by *[AIIMS PGMEE 1993]*
a. High dose of calcium with steroids
b. Total hip replacement
c. Supervised containment of femora head in acetabulum
d. Relieving weight bearing

36. Position of arm in anterior dislocation of shoulder is *[AP PGMEE 1999]*
a. By the side b. In adduction
c. In abduction d. In external rotation

37. Sciatic nerve palsy may occur in the following injury *[All India PGMEE 2003]*
a. Posterior dislocation of hip joint
b. Fracture neck of femur
c. Trochanteric fracture
d. Anterior dislocation of hip

38. Attitude of limb in anterior dislocation of hip joint is *[DPG 1999, AIIMS PGMEE 1999]*
a. Flexion, adduction, internal rotation
b. Flexion, adduction, external rotation
c. Flexion, abduction, internal rotation
d. Flexion, abduction, external rotation

39. Following is true in treatment of posterior dislocation
a. Closed reduction under anaesthesia *[PGI 1990]*
b. Open reduction c. Skeletal traction
d. Soft tissue

40. Flexion, abduction and external rotation with limb length discrepancy is seen in *[Orissa PGMEE 1988, Orissa PGMEE 1990]*
a. Posterior dislocation of hip
b. Central dislocation of hip
c. Anterior dislocation of hip
d. Fracture neck of femur

41. Legg-Calves-Perthes' disease is *[Orissa PGMEE 1991]*
a. Mild pyogenic arthritis
b. Slipped femoral epiphysis
c. Avascular necrosis of head of femur
d. Low grade tuberculosis of hip

42. Commonest cause of limp in a child of seven years is *[UP PGMEE 2002]*
a. T.B. hip
b. C.D.H.
c. Perthe's disease
d. Slipped upper femoral epiphysis

43. Legg-Calve-Perthes' disease is *[UP PGMEE 1993]*
a. Femoral epiphyseal osteochondritis
b. Osteochondritis of tibial tubercle
c. Slipped upper femoral epiphysis
d. Spinal osteochondritis

44. Late radiographic changes seen in active Perthes' disease are all except *[NBE DNB 1990]*
a. Narrow joint space
b. A widened femoral neck
c. An irregular density of the epiphysis
d. An irregular epiphyseal line

45. Legg-Calve-Perthes disease is commonly seen in the age group of *[All India PGMEE 1989]*
a. 1-3 years b. 2-12 years
c. 12-22 years d. 20 year & above

46. In per rectal examination, femoral head is palpable in *[AP PGMEE 1998]*
a. Anterior dislocation of hip
b. Posterior dislocation of hip
c. Central dislocation of hip
d. Lateral dislocation of hip

47. Recurrent dislocation of shoulder occurs, because of *[AIIMS PGMEE 1993]*
a. Incomplete labrum
b. Superadded secondary infection
c. Crushed glenoidal labrum
d. Weak posterior capsule

48. Hill-sachs lesion is associated with *[JIPMER PGMEE 1992, JIPMER PGMEE 2014]*
a. Recurrent dislocation of shoulder
b. Recurrent dislocation of hip
c. Perthes' disease
d. Fracture neck of femur

49. Hill-Sachs lesion in recurrent shoulder dislocation is *[Recent Question 2017, AIIMS PGMEE 1992]*
a. Injury to humeral head
b. Rupture of tendon of supraspinatus muscle
c. Avulsion of glenoid labrum
d. None of the above

50. Foot drop occurs due to *[Recent Question 2016, 2017, PGI 1991]*
a. Anterior tibial nerve
b. Posterior tibial nerve
c. Superficial peroneal nerve
d. Deep peroneal nerve

51. Which one of the following is the investigation of choice for evaluation of suspected Perthes' disease? *[All India PGMEE 2005]*
a. Plain X-ray
b. Ultrasonography (US)
c. Computed Tomography (CT)
d. Magnetic Resonance Imaging (MRI)

52. Regarding Perthe's disease all of the following are correct except *[PGI 1995]*
a. Osteonecrotic osteochondritis
b. Decreased bone age
c. Male predominance
d. Restricted abduction
e. Age of onset has no affect on course

53. True about Perthe's disease is all except *[PGI PGMEE 2009]*
a. A vascular necrosis of femoral head
b. Onset before 10 years of age
c. Osteotomy is used for treatment
d. Limb shortening
e. Joint space obliterated

54. Bankart's lesion is seen in *[AIIMS PGMEE 2000]*
a. Anterior border of head of humerus
b. Posterior border of head of humerus
c. Anterior glenoid cavity
d. Posterior glenoid cavity

55. Avascular necrosis seen in *[PGI 2004]*
a. Fracture surgical neck of humerus
b. Fracture neck of scapula
c. Fracture neck of talus
d. Fracture neck of femur
e. Fracture neck of radius

56. Avascular necrosis can be a possible sequelae of fracture of all of the following bones, except *[All India PGMEE 2003]*
a. Femur neck
b. Scaphoid
c. Talus
d. Calcaneum

57. Most common site of fracture neck of femur that causes avascular necrosis is *[All India PGMEE 1996]*
a. Sub-capital
b. Intertrochanteric
c. Trans-cervical
d. Basal

58. All are related to recurrent shoulder dislocation except *[Karnataka PGMEE 1998, TN PGMEE 2000, Recent Question 2017, UP PGMEE 2002]*
a. Hill sachs defect
b. Bankart lesion
c. Lax capsule
d. Rotator cuff injury

59. Lesion associated with recurrent dislocation of shoulder include all, except *[AIIMS PGMEE 2006]*
a. Hill-Sach's lesion
b. Bankart's lesion
c. Capsular laxity
d. Supraspinatous tear

60. Recurrent dislocation is most common in the shoulder joint. Which one of the following is not an important cause for the same? *[Karnataka PGMEE 1989]*
a. Tear of the anterior capsule of the shoulder
b. Associated fracture neck of the humerus
c. Tear of the glenoid labrum
d. Freedom of mobility in the shoulder

61. Meralgia paraesthetica involves *[All India PGMEE 1994, AIIMS PG 2010, AIIMS PG November 2015]*
a. Median nerve
b. Axillary nerve
c. Sural nerve
d. Lateral cutaneous nerve of thigh

62. Which Joint is commonly involved in Osteochondritis dessicans? *[All India PGMEE 1995, NBE DNB 2003, 2009, JIPMER 2014]*
a. Elbow joint
b. Wrist joint
c. Knee joint
d. Ankle joint

63. Tennis elbow is *[Recent Question 2016, All India PGMEE 2007]*
a. Olecranon bursitis
b. Myositis ossificans
c. Pain over the medial epicondyle
d. Pain over the lateral epicondyle

64. De quervain's disease classically affects the *[AIIMS PGMEE 2005]*
a. Flexor pollicis longus and brevis
b. Abductor pollicis longus and brevis
c. Extensor carpi radialis and extensor pollicis longus
d. Extensor pollicis brevis and abductor pollicis longus

65. In Recurrent Anterior dislocation of shoulder, the movements that causes dislocation is *[All India PGMEE 1989]*
a. Flexion and internal rotation
b. Abduction and external rotation
c. Abduction and internal rotation
d. Extension

66. All of the following statements about dislocation of the shoulder are true, except *[Manipal PGMEE 1994]*
a. The injury is produced by a fall with the arm fully abducted
b. The commonest position for the head of the humerus to move into is the subspinous
c. The auxillary (circumflex humeral) nerve is likely to be injured
d. The easiest way to reduce it is by simple pressure with the patient under general anesthesia with muscle relaxation

67. About De Quervain's disease, which of the following is/ are correct *[PGI 2008]*
a. Tense mass may be visible
b. Steroid is used to relieve symptoms
c. Pain after straining at thumb base
d. Involve External pollicis longus
e. Involve Abductor pollicis longus

68. Dupuytren's contracture is *[All India PGMEE 1998]*
a. Thickening of palmar fascia
b. Base of little finger involved first
c. Seen in epileptics on hydantoin
d. All of the above

69. True about Dupuytren's contracture
a. Slight preponderance in males *[Delhi PGMEE 1994]*
b. Slight preponderance in females
c. Much more common in males
d. Much more common in females

70. Traumatic anterior dislocation of shoulder with sensory loss in lateral side of forearm and weakness of flexion of elbow joint, most likely injured nerve is *[AIIMS PGMEE 1999, AIPGME 2001]*
a. Radial nerve b. Ulnar nerve
c. Axillary nerve d. Musculocutaneous nerve

71. Traumatic glenohumeral instability on one direction with Bankarts lesion are treated by
a. Conservative methods *[NIMHANS PGMEE 2003]*
b. Surgery
c. Rehabilitation
d. Observation fib inferior capsule shift

72. Following statement regarding dislocation of shoulder are true except *[Karnataka PGMEE 1997]*
a. Head of humerus usually dislocates forward from shoulder joint
b. Injury is produced by forced extension & external rotation of abducted arm
c. In posterior dislocation, appearance of shoulder is not normal
d. None of the above

73. Dupuytren's Contracture of the hand commonly starts in *[Bihar PGMEE 1991]*
a. Thumbs b. Index finger
c. Middle finger d. Ring finger
e. Little finger only

74. Cause of Trigger finger is *[AIIMS PGMEE 1996]*
a. Thickening of the fibrous tendon sheath
b. Following local trauma
c. Unaccustomed activity
d. All of the above

75. In trigger finger the level of tendon sheath constriction is found at the level of *[Recent Question 2016, AIIMS PGMEE 2005, AIIMS PG 1996]*
a. Middle phalanx
b. Proximal interphalangeal joint
c. Proximal phalanx
d. Metacarpophalangeal joint

76. Osteonecrosis of femoral head seen in *[Recent Question 2016, PGI 2005, PGI 2005]*
a. Sickle cell disease b. Gaucher's disease
c. Polycythemia d. Hyperparathyroidism
e. Fracture neck of femur

77. Avascular necrosis of femur seen in *[PGI 2004]*
a. Steroid therapy b. Gaucher's disease
c. Fracture d. Pancreatitis

78. Avascular necrosis is seen in *[PGI 2002]*
a. Sickle cell disease b. Thalassemia
c. Polychthemia d. Hyperparathyroidism

79. Pulley involved in trigger finger *[AIIMS PGMEE 1993]*
a. A1 b. A2
c. A3 d. A4

80. Regarding Recurrent dislocation of the shoulder, which of the following is false? *[AP PGMEE 1992]*
a. All traumatic dislocations will be recurrent
b. Recurrent dislocation results when the capsule is stripped, not torn
c. The humeral head is always within the capsule
d. All of these

81. Which is true regarding shoulder dislocation? *[NIMHANS PGMEE 1999, SGPGI 2002]*
a. Posterior dislocation is often over-looked
b. Pain is severe in anterior dislocation
c. Radiography may be misleading in posterior dislocation
d. All of the above

82. Which is true about shoulder dislocation? *[MAHE PGMEE 2003, TN PGMEE 1998]*
a. Anterior dislocation is common than posterior
b. Fixed medial rotation in posterior dislocation
c. Kocher's manoeuvre is effective in anterior dislocation
d. All of the above

83. Which of the following is test of posterior glenohumeral instability *[AIIMS PGMEE 2009, AIIMS PGMEE 2010]*
a. Fulcrum test b. Sulcus test
c. Jerk's test d. Crank test

84. Trendelenberg's sign is negative in an Inter-Trochanteric fracture because of *[All India PGMEE 2000]*
a. Gluteus medius b. Gluteus maximus
c. Gluteus minmus d. Tensor fascia lata

85. A 6-year-old boy has a history of recurrent dislocation of the right shoulder. On examination, the orthopedician puts the patient in the supine position and abducts his arm to 9 degrees with the bed as the fulcrum and then externally rotates it but the boy does not allow the test to be performed. The test done by the orthopedician is *[AIIMS PGMEE 2001]*
a. Apprehension test b. Sulcus test
c. Dugas test d. McMurray's test

86. True regarding mallet finger is *[AIIMS PGMEE 2000]*
a. Avulsion of tendon at the base of the middle phalanx
b. Avulsion of extensor tendon at the base of the distal phalanx
c. Fracture of distal phalanx
d. Fracture of the proximal phalanx

87. A 30-year-old man involved in a fisticuff, injured his middle finger and noticed slight flexion of DIP joint. X-rays were normal. The most appropriate management at this stage is *[AIIMS PGMEE 2004]*
a. Ignore
b. Splint the finger in hyperextension
c. Surgical repair of the flexor tendon
d. Buddy strapping

88. A child is spinned around by holding his hand by his father. While doing this the child started crying and does not allow his father to touch his elbow. The diagnosis is *[AIIMS PGMEE 2001]*
a. Pulled elbow
b. Radial head dislocation
c. Annular ligament tear
d. Fracture olecranon process

89. True about ganglion *[PGI 2003]*
a. Common in volar aspect
b. Seen adjacent to tendon sheath
c. Communicates with joints cavity and sheath
d. It is Unilocular

90. Hallux valgus is associated with all except *[PGI 2000]*
a. An exostosis on the medial side of the head of the first metatarsal
b. A bunion
c. Osteoarthritis of the metatarsophalangeal joint
d. Over-riding or under-riding of the second toe by the third

91. In Hallux valgus surgery, the patients who are likely to be most satisfied are *[AIIMS PGMEE 1995]*
a. Those with pain
b. Those with hammertoe
c. Those with metatarsus primus varus
d. Young age

92. The primary pathology in Athletic Pubalgia is *[All India PGMEE 2009]*
a. Abdominal muscle strain
b. Rectus femoris strain
c. Gluteus medius strain
d. Hamstring strain

93. Bleeding into joint cavities is not common in *[JIPMER PGMEE 1990]*
a. Christmas disease b. Hemophilia
c. ITP d. None of above

94. All are features of haemophilic knee joint, EXCEPT *[AIIMS PGMEE 1997]*
a. Juxta articular osteosclerosis
b. Sub chondral cyst formation
c. Widening of intercondylar notch
d. Squarring of patella

95. True about treatment of haemarthosis *[PGI 2007]*
a. Aspiration b. POP
c. Traction d. Compression bandage
e. Joint aspiration

96. Thoracic Outlet Syndrome is best Diagnosed By *[All India PGMEE 2009]*
a. CT scan
b. MRI
c. Digital subtraction angiography
d. Clinical examination

97. Trendelenburg's test positive in all EXCEPT *[AIIMS PGMEE 1998]*
a. Posterior dislocation of hip
b. Poliomyelitis
c. Fracture neck of femur
d. Tuberculosis of hip joint

98. In actinomycosis of the spine, the abscess usually erodes *[All India PGMEE 2003]*
a. Intervertebral disc
b. Into the pleural cavity
c. Into the reteropritoneal space
d. Towards the skin

99. A 3-year-old girl has developed painful elbow after being jerked by the forearm. The next thing to be done is *[AIIMS PGMEE 1993, AMU PGMEE 1999, JIPMER PGMEE 2001]*
a. Cuff & collar sling immobilization
b. Reduction setting and AEPOP application
c. X-Ray and elevation of limb in posterior slab
d. Fully supinate the forearm

100. A patient with swelling foot, pus discharge, multiple sinuses. KOH smear shares filamentous structures. Diagnosis is *[UPSC 1990]*
a. Osteomyelitis b. Madura mycosis
c. Anthrax d. None

101. A 5-year-old man sustained posterior dislocation of left hip in an accident. Dislocation was reduced after 3 days. He started complaining of pain in left hip after 6 months. X-ray of the pelvis were normal. The most relevant investigation at this stage will be- *[AIIMS PGMEE 2004]*
a. CRP Levels in blood
b. Ultrasonography of hip
c. Arthrography of hip
d. MRI of hip

102. A building contractor suddenly complains of lower backache which increase on bending down. He has *[UPSC 1990]*
a. Renal colic b. Tuberculosis of spine
c. Disc prolapse d. Fibrositis'

103. Most important single special investigation in lumbar disc prolapse is *[NBE DNB 1992]*
a. Epidurography b. Myelography
c. MRI d. Discography
e. Spinal venography

104. Most common type of Disc herniation is *[TN PGMEE 1996, All India PGMEE 1993]*
a. Central b. Postero-lateral
c. Intra-foraminal d. Extra-foraminal

105. A patient is using oral steroids for a period of 5 years and patient complaints of pain in the both hip regions. Which one of the following is a diagnostic modality for confirmation of diagnosis? *[WB PGMEE PGMEE, NIMS PGMEE 2000]*
a. Plain X ray b. CT scan
c. MRI d. Isotope Bone scan

106. A woman of 45, a known cause of pemphigus vulgaris on a regular treatment with controlled primary disease presented with pain in the right hip and knee. Examination revealed no limb length discrepancy but the patient has tenderness in the Scarpa's triangle and limitation of adduction and internal rotation of the right hip joint as compared to the other side. The most probable diagnosis is *[AIIMS PGMEE 2004]*
a. Stress fracture of neck of femur
b. A vascular necrosis of femoral head
c. Perthe's disease
d. Transient synovitis of hip

107. Patient developed breathlessness and chest pain, on second postoperative after a total hip replacement. Echocardiography showed right ventricular dilatation and tricuspid regurgitation. What is the most likely diagnosis. *[All India PGMEE 2010]*

a. Acute MI b. Pulmonary embolism
c. Hypotensive shock d. Cardiac tamponade

108. What is the most common cause of death after total hip replacement? *[All India PGMEE 2009]*

a. Infection b. Deep vein thrombosis
c. Pulmonary embolism d. Pneumonia

109. A 68 years old man came with pain and swelling of right knee. Ahlbeck grade 2 osteoarthritic changes were found on investigation. What is the further management *[AIIMS PGMEE 2010]*

a. Conservative b. Arthroscopic washout
c. High tibial osteotomy d. Total knee replacement

110. Which of the following movements are restricted in Frozen shoulder? *[AP PGMEE 2000]*

a. Abduction & Internal rotation
b. Adduction & external rotation
c. All range of movements
d. Only abduction

111. Painful arc syndrome is seen in all except *[AIIMS PGMEE 2001]*

a. Complete tear of supraspinatus
b. Fracture greater tuberosity
c. Subacromial bursitis
d. Supraspinatus tendinitis

112. Which movement at shoulder gets restricted when Supraspinatous torn? *(JIPMER PGMEE 1997]*

a. Flexion b. Adduction
c. Abduction d. Rotation only

113. All of the following statements about High Tibial Osteotomy are true, Except *[All India PGMEE 2009]*

a. Magnitude of correction achieved is greater than 30°
b. Indicated in Unicompartmental osteoarthritis
c. Performed through cancellous bone
d. Recurrence is a long term complication

114. A man aged 4 yrs presents with swelling over foot with multiple sinuses. What is most probable diagnosis *[AIIMS PGMEE 1996]*

a. TB b. Maduromycosis
c. Actinomycetoma d. Osteomyelitis
e. Tetanus unilateral

115. A 45-year-old was given steroids after renal transplant. After 2 years he had difficulty in walking and pain in both hips. Which one of the following is most likely cause? *[All India PGMEE 2005]*

a. Primary Osteoarthritis b. Avascular necrosis
c. Tuberculosis d. Aluminum toxicity

116. A five year old child is suffering from painful restriction of all movements of hip joint, the most likely cause in our country is *[Orissa PGMEE 1990)*

a. Congenital coax vara
b. Tuberculosis arthritis
c. Perthes' disease
d. Sequelae of septic arthritis of infancy

117. 'Light bulb sign' is seen in *[JIPMER PGMEE 2014]*

a. Anterior dislocation humerus
b. Posterior dislocation humerus
c. Anterior dislocation hip
d. Posterior dislocation hip

118. True about Club-foot is/are *[PGI November 2014]*

a. Associated with breech delivery
b. Extension of Tendoachilles
c. Adduction of forefoot
d. Detectable at birth
e. Denis Brown splint used

119. Nerve involved in 'Pronator teres syndrome'? *[AIIMS PG November 2015]*

a. Ulnar nerve b. Radius nerve
c. Median nerve d. Anterior interosseous nerve

120. Jersey finger is caused by rupture of *[Recent Question 2016, AIIMS PG May 2015]*

a. Flexor digitorum superficialis
b. Flexor digitorum profundus
c. Extensor digiti minimi
d. Extensor indicis

121. Part of spine involved in Rheumatoid arthritis is *[PGMCET 2015]*

a. Sacral b. Lumbar
c. Thoracic d. Cervical

122. Least helpful for the diagnosis of Spondylolisthesis is *[PGMCET 2015]*

a. Lateral X-ray of spine b. AP X-ray of spine
c. MRI d. CT

123. Identify the Abnormality shown in the following picture? *[AIIMS PG November 2015]*

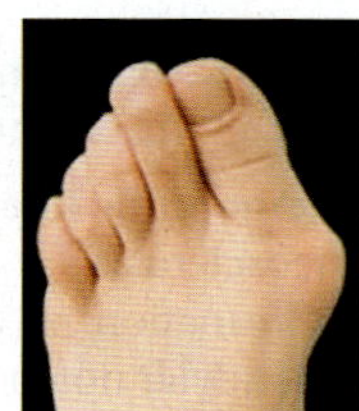

a. Hallux valgus b. Hallux varus
c. Rheumatoid nodule d. Subcutaneous nodule

124. Meralgia paresthetica is due to involvement of *[AIIMS PG November 2015]*

a. Lateral cutaneous nerve of thigh
b. Ilioinguinal nerve c. Genitofemoral nerve
d. Saphenous nerve

125. In Polio paralysis; hand, knee gait due to weakness of *[AIIMS May 2017]*

a. Gluteus maximus
b. Gluteus medius
c. Quadriceps
d. Gastrosoleus

126. Following is the MC sequel of Traumatic dislocation of shoulder *[AIIMS May 2017]*

a. Normal shoulder healing and normal movements
b. Recurrent dislocation of shoulder
c. Rotator cuff injury
d. Subcapsular tendinitis

Orthopedics

NEET/NBE PATTERN MCQs ANSWERS WITH EXPLANATIONS 

1. Ans. (a) Anterior dislocation of shoulder
[Ref. Maheshwari, 4/e p87]

Tests of Anterior Shoulder Dislocation

- Duga's test
- Hamilton's ruler test

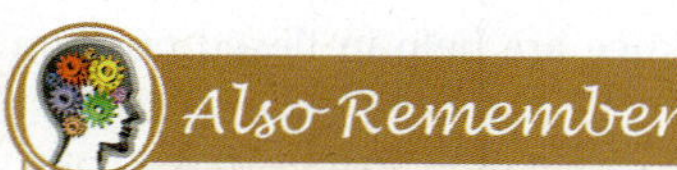

Hamilton ruler test

- Keep a straight ruler along lateral aspect of arm
- In Normal person, it does not touch acromion process
- In Dislocated shoulder, it touches acromion process

2. Ans. (b) Lateral epicondylitis
[Ref. Maheshwari, 4/e p293]

3. Ans. (a) Pes Anserinus
[Ref. Sports Medicine by Safran, 1/e p551]

- Medial knee pain is generally secondary to pes anserinus bursitis, or intraarticular medial bands (plica), which can snap over the femoral condyle after repetitive motion

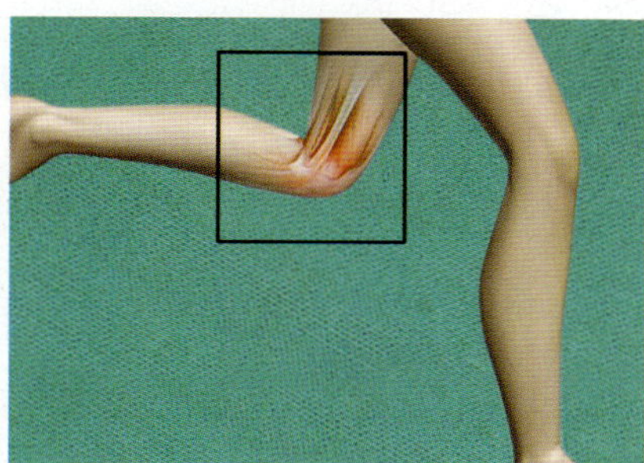

Fig. Pes Anserinus Tendinopathy

4. Ans. (a) Milwaukee Brace
[Ref. Maheshwari, 4/e p275]

Non-operative methods for Treatment of Scoliosis:

- Milwaukee brace (See Photograph)
- Boston brace
- Reisser's turn buckle cast
- Localiser cast

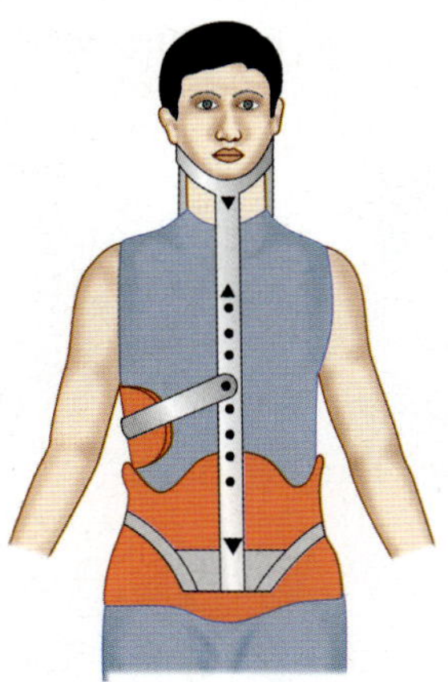

Fig. Milwaukee Brace

5. Ans. (b) MRI
[Ref. Oxford Textbook of Musculoskeletal Medicine, 2/e p232]

- **MRI is Investigation of choice** when it comes to imaging the spinal cord, spinal nerves, intervertebral discs (Prolapse) and ligaments of the spine
- Earlier Myelography was the IOC for Disc prolapse

6. Ans. (c) Equinocavovarus
[Ref. Essential Orthopedics Volume 1 by Varshney, 1/e p1300]

- Equino cavovarus: Typical deformity of uncorrected clubfoot

7. Ans. (b) Idiopathic
[Ref. Carpal Tunnel Syndrome by Acton, 1/e p9]

Idiopathic Carpal tunnel syndrome

- Common cause of carpal tunnel syndrome in Elderly
- Underlying reason: Chronic fibrosis and tenosynovial thickening

8. Ans. (d) Spondylolisthesis
[Ref. The Adolescent Spine by Keim, 2/e p155]

Milwaukee Brace

- **Cervico-Thoraco-Lumbo-Sacral-Orthosis brace**
- Contoured pelvic girdle attached by three uprights to an occipital pad and throat mould of chin piece
- Suspended from the uprights are the lumbar and thoracic pads as well as other accessories (shoulder flange, axillary sling, or subclavicular pads)
- Function: To redirect spinal growth by stimulating trunk muscle patterns, while three-point pressure systems play a lesser role
- **Uses:**
  - Congenital Kyphosis
  - Scheuermann's Disease
  - Adolescent Idiopathic Scoliosis

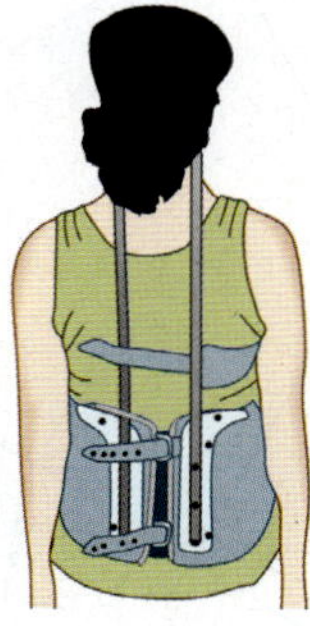

Fig. Milwaukee Brace

9. Ans. (a) Distal end of radius
[Ref. Nettler's Collections of Medical Illustrations by Parker, 2/e p146]

Madelung Deformity

- Growth disturbance in Volar-Ulnar distal Radial epiphysis at wrist
- Short and dorsolaterally curved radius, tilting of distal ulna, and dorsal subluxation/dislocation of ulna
- Limited wrist motion, prominence of the distal ulna and radial shortening

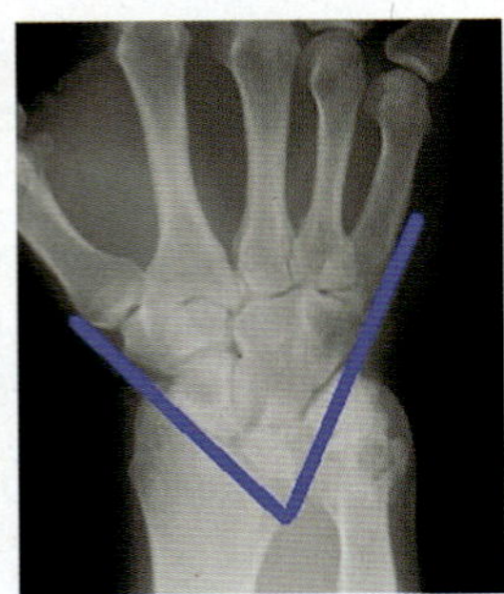

Fig. Madelung deformity

10. Ans. (d) Polyhydramnios is a known risk factor
[Ref. Practical Pediatrics by Roberto, 1/e p253]

Risk Factors of DDH

- Breech presentation
- Female baby
- Oligohydramnios
- Big baby (>4 kg)
- First born baby
- Family history

11. Ans. (a) Kyphoscoliosis
[Ref. Anesthesiology by Nag, 1/e p130]

Cobb's Method

- Utility: Identify the degree/ severity of Scoliosis
- **Interpretation of Cobb's angle:**
  - Angle >40 degrees: Indication for Surgery
  - Angle >65 degrees: Restrictive lung disease, Dyspnoea on exertion
  - Angle >100 degrees: Respiratory failure, Pulmonary hypertension, Right heart failure

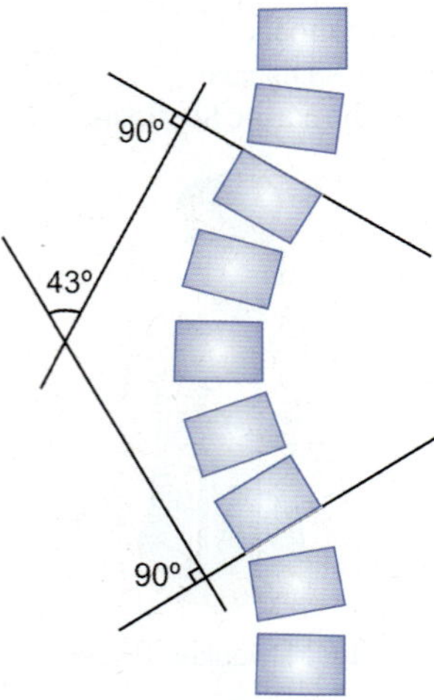

Fig. Cobb's Angle

12. Ans. (d) Salter's osteotomy
[Ref. Smart Study Series Orthopedics, 1/e p255]

Management of CTEV

- <1 year age: Manipulation and Above-knee casting
- 1-4 years age: Posteromedial soft tissue release
- 4-12 years age: Dillwyn-Even operation, Dwyer's osteotomy
- >12 years age: Triple arthrodesis, Talectomy (Severe uncorrected CTEV)

13. Ans. (a) Ignasio Ponseti
[Ref. Pediatric Orthopaedics by Wiesel, 1/e p636]

- In 1948 Dr. Ignacio Ponseti began manipulating clubfeet through Serial casting, completely correcting the Clubfoot deformity
- He abducted and dorsi-flexed the foot

14. Ans. (c) Developmental dysplasia of the hip
[Ref. Maheshwari, 4/e p214]

- **Ortolani test:** Hips and knee are help in flexed position and gradually abducted
- Ortolani test positive: In Congenital dislocation of hip, a 'click of entrance' will be felt as femoral head slips into acetabulum from position of dislocation

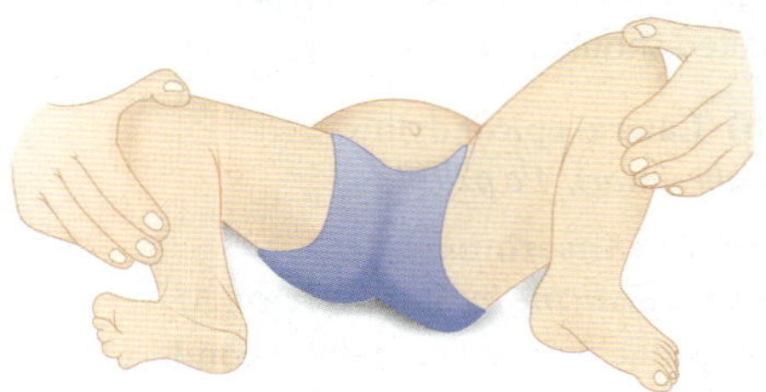

Fig. Ortolani Test

15. Ans. (b) Tennis elbow
[Ref. Orthopedic Physical Assessment by CTI Reviews, 5/e]

Cozen's Test

- A physical examination performed to evaluate for Tennis elbow
- It's said positive if a resisted wrist extension triggers pain
- Test is performed with extended elbow

16. Ans. (b) Lateral closing wedge osteotomy
[Ref. Rockwood and Wilkins' Fractures in Children Volume 3, 7/e p524]

- In general, a lateral closing wedge osteotomy with a medial hinge will correct Varus deformity, with minimal correction of Hyperextension

17. Ans. (a) Developmental dysplasia of hip
[Ref. Turek's Orthopaedics, 6/e p449]

- **Pavlik harness** prevents adduction and extension while allowing further flexion, abduction, and rotation
- This position allows for gentle spontaneous reduction of DDH

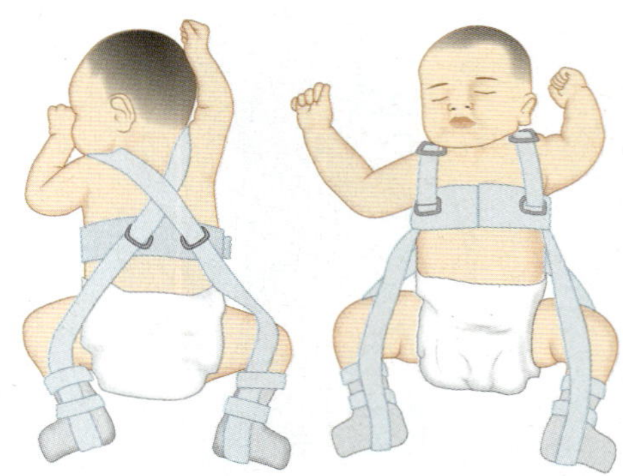

Fig. Pavlik Harness

18. Ans. (c) Psoriasis

[Ref. Orthopedic Imaging by Davies, 1/e p10.4.3]

Frozen shoulder (Periarthritis shoulder)

- **Adhesive capsulitis/ Periarthritis of shoulder**
  - Progressive pain and stiffness of the shoulder which usually resolves spontaneously after about 18 months
  - Disease occurs due to active fibroblastic proliferation in the anterior capsule, rotator interval and coraco-humeral ligament
  - This results in loss of resilience of the joint capsule with adhesion between the synovial folds
- **Etiology is unknown**
- The condition is particularly associated with:
  - Diabetes
  - Hyperlipidemia
  - Hyperthyroidism
  - Dupuytren's disease
  - Cardiac disease
  - Hemiplegia

19. Ans. (a) Developmental dysplasia of hip

[Ref. Paediatrics by Lissauer, 4/e p454]

- DDH presentation is usually with a limp or abnormal gait
- It may be identified from asymmetry of skinfolds around the hip, limited abduction of the hip or shortening of the affected leg

20. Ans. (b) Equinus

[Ref. Pediatrics by Tolo, 1/e p193]

- Unlike other forms of nonoperative treatment, the Ponseti method corrects all the components of the deformity simultaneously, with the exception of Equinus deformity which is corrected last
- **C**avus is corrected first, **A**dductus and **V**arus follow sequentially, and **E**quinus is the last to be corrected **[Mnemonic: CAVE]**

21. Ans. (b) Tibio-talar

[Ref. Maheshwari, 4/e p209]

Triple Arthrodesis

- Is one of the operative methods to correct: Congenital Talipes Equino Varus (CTEV)
- **Comprises of fusion of 3 joints:**
  - Subtalar
  - Calcaneo-cuboid
  - Talo-navicular
- **Performed after the age of: 12 years**
- *Most difficult joint fusion to achieve*: Talo-navicular

22. Ans. (b) Pars interarticularis

[Ref. Maheshwari, 4/e p217]

- ***Spondylolysis:*** *A* defect in the *pars interarticularis*, commonly involving the L5 and occasionally the L4 vertebrae

23. Ans. (b) Sub-cutaneous pre-patellar bursa

[Ref. Maheshwari, 4/e p292]

Common Bursites

Name	Bursitis
Housemaid's knee	Prepatellar bursitis
Clergyman's knee	Infrapatellar bursitis
Student's elbow	Olecranon bursitis (Most common)
Weaver's bottom	Ischial bursitis
Tailor's ankle	On lateral malleolus
Bunion	On great toe
Hip bursitis	Greater Trochanteric bursitis
Shoulder bursitis	Sub-acromial bursitis

24. Ans. (d) Ulnar bursitis (tubercular)

[Ref. Essentials of Orthopedics for Physiotherapist by Ebnezar, 1/e p239]

Compound Palmar Ganglion

- Condition affecting flexor tendons of the fingers (mainly *ulnar bursa)*
- Usually due to tuberculosis though rheumatoid arthritis may also be a cause
- Crepitus due to 'Melon seed bodies'

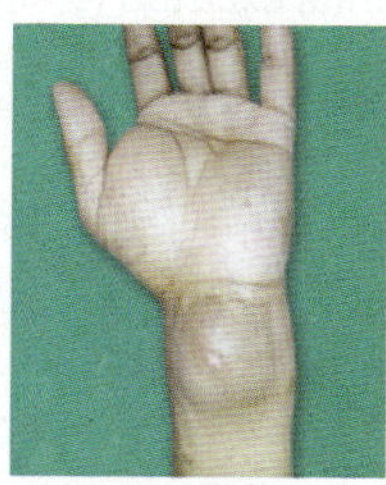

Fig. Compound Palmar Ganglion

25. Ans. (c) Flexor digitorum profundus

[Ref. Text and Atlas of Complications of Fractures by Ebnezar, 1/e p63]

- **Muscle involvement in Volkman's Ischemic Contracture:** Flexor digitorum profundus > Flexor pollicis longus > Flexor digitorum superficialis

26. Ans. (a) Paralysis of Gastrocnemius, soleus & tibialis posterior

[Ref. Orthopedic and Reconstructive Surgery by Albee, 1/e p622]

27. Ans. (b) Haemangioma

[Ref. Radiodiagnosis, Nuclear Medicine, Radiotherapy and Radiation Oncology by Daga, 1/e p388]

- **Striated vertebra** (Corduroy/ Accordion/ Honey comb vertebra): Vertebral hemangioma
- **Polka-dot sign on CT** (Punctate sclerosis in body of vertebra): Diagnostic of Vertebral hemangioma

28. Ans. (b) Ulnar nerve injury

[Ref. Maheshwari, 4/e p61]

29. Ans. (a) Marked shortening of limb

[Ref. Maheshwari, 4/e p126]

Posterior Dislocation of Hip

- Deformity: Flexion, Adduction, Internal rotation
- Shortening of leg

30. Ans. (a) Recurrent dislocation of shoulder
[Ref. Maheshwari, 4/e p87]

Pathological Changes in Anterior Dislocation of Shoulder

- *Bankart's lesion*: Stripping of glenoid labrum
- *Hill-Sachs lesion*: Depression on humerus head (postero-lateral quadrant)
- Rounding off of anterior glenoid rim
- Associated injuries: Fracture greater tuberosity, rotator cuff tear, chondral damage

31. Ans. (b) Pain on passive movements
[Ref. British Journal of Hospital Medicine, Volume 55, p326]

32. Ans. (a) Ring finger
[Ref. An Aid to MRCP by Freeman, 1/e p221]

Dupuytren's Contracture

- Description: Flexion deformity of finger(s) due to thickening or shortening of Palmar aponeurosis/ fascia
- Underlying conditions: Smoking, HIV/ AIDS, Alcoholism and Liver disease, Manual labor, Epilepsy, Phenytoin, Diabetes mellitus, COPD, Hypertension, Ischemic heart disease
- **Most common finger involved: Ring finger**
- Treatment: Subtotal excision (If significant deformity)

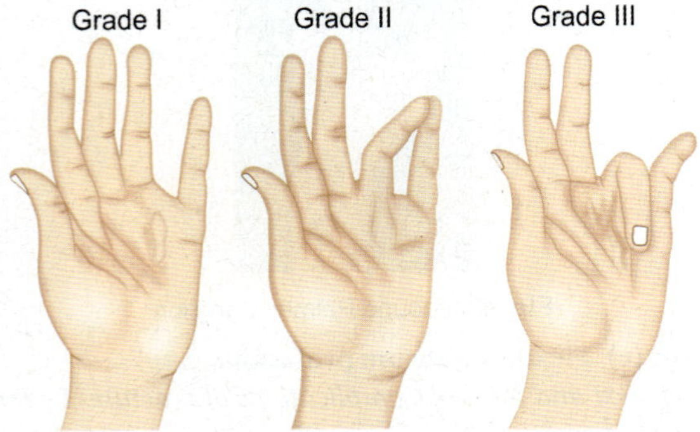

Fig. Dupuytren Contracture

33. Ans. (c) Flexion, adduction and internal rotation
[Ref. Maheshwari, 4/e p126]

34. Ans. (a) Trauma
[Ref. Physical Medicine and Rehabilitation Review by Kaplan, 2/e p222]

35. Ans. (b) Overuse
[Ref. Trauma and Sports Injuries by Lennox, 1/e p428]

36. Ans. (b) Amputation
[Ref. Rockwood and Wilkin' Fractures in Children by Kasser, 7/e p145]

37. Ans. (b) USG
[Ref. Imaging for Students by Lisle, 4/e p267]

- Investigation of choice for DDH: Dynamic USG

38. Ans. (b) Always heals by chemotherapy
[Ref. Maheshwari, 4/e p185]

39. Ans. (d) Axillary nerve
[Ref. Nerve and vascular Injuries in Sports Medicine by Herring, 1/e p92]

40. Ans. (c) Median nerve
[Ref. Maheshwari, 4/e p110, 294]

Carpal Tunnel Syndrome

- Definition: Syndrome characterised by 'compression of median nerve' as it passes beneath flexor retinaculum

Causation:

*[**Mnemonic:** In Carpal-tunnel Median-nerve is Rightly Affected at Wrist]*

- Idiopathic **(Most common)**
- Post-traumatic causes **(after Colles' fracture)**
- Endocrine causes (Myxoedema, Acromegaly)
- Inflammatory causes (RA, Wrist osteoarthritis)

- Clinical features: Tingling, numbness of thumb and radial one-half of fingers
- Examination: Low median nerve compression found
- Treatment: Divide flexor retinaculum and decompress median nerve

41. Ans. (c) Antero-Inferior
[Ref. Maheshwari, 4/e p87]

- **Bankart's lesion:** Dislocation cause stripping of Glenoid labrum and periosteum from Anterior surface of Glenoid and Scapular neck
- **Hill-Sach's lesion:** Depression on Humeral head in its Posterolateral quadrant caused by impingement of Anterior edge of Glenoid on head as it dislocates

42. Ans. (b) Extensor pollicis brevis and abductor pollicis longus
[Ref. Maheshwari, 4/e p294]

43. Ans. (a) Bilateral DOH
[Ref. Textbook of Orthopedics by Kotwal, 1/e p52]

Congenital Dislocation of Hip

In Older child	In Bilateral dislocation
Galeazzi's sign positive Trendelenburg's test positive Telescopy test positive Trendelenburg gait Waddling gait	Telescopy positive on both side Wider perineum Waddling gait

44. Ans. (a) Anterior talofibular ligament
[Ref. Adult Orthopedic Nursing by Schoen, 1/e p361]

45. Ans. (b) Brachial
[Ref. Mosby's Pathology for Massage Therapists, 2/e p149]

46. Ans. (b) The long axis of tibia and fibula are deviated laterally from that of the femur
[Ref. Maheshwari, 4/e p315]

47. Ans. (a) Stenosis and tenovaginits of flexor tendon of affected finger
[Ref. Maheshwari, 4/e p294]

48. Ans. (a) Calcaneocuboid, talonavicular and talocalcaneal
[Ref. Textbook of Orthopedics by Ebnezar, 4/e p509]

- **Triple arthrodesis:** Fusion of 3 joints, namely, Calcaneocuboid, Talonavicular and Talocalcaneal (Subtalar)in CTEV

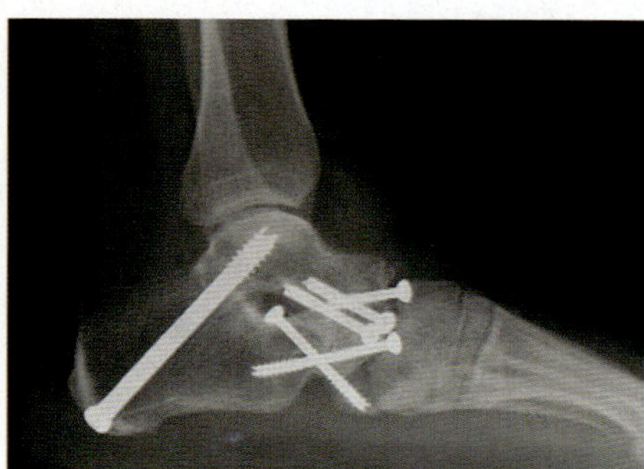

Fig. Triple Arthrodesis

49. Ans. (b) Pars interarticularis
[Ref. Maheshwari, 4/e p217, 277]

Spondylolysis

- Definition: Break in isthmus (pars interarticularis) of one of the lumbar vertebra (Most common: L5)
- X-ray oblique view of spine: *Scottish dog 'wearing a collar' appearance*
- Vertebral slippage is **ABSENT**

Spondylolisthesis

- Definition: Forward displacement of a vertebra over one below it (Most common: L5-S1)
- X-ray oblique view of spine: *Scottish dog 'head separated from neck' appearance*
- Vertebral slippage is **PRESENT**

50. Ans. (a) Proximal interphalangeal joint
[Ref. Maheshwari, 4/e p317]

- Hammer toe: Flexion deformity of an Interphalangeal joint of the toe, usually with callosity over prominent proximal joint

51. Ans. (b) Barlow test
[Ref. Essence of Pediatrics by Khan, 4/e p12]

52. Ans. (a) Avascular necrosis
[Ref. Understanding Medical Surgical Nursing by Hopper, 5/e p1085]

53. Ans. (a) Flexion
[Ref. Essentials of Orthopedics for Physiotherapist by Ebnezar, 1/e p95]

54. Ans. (c) SLE
[Ref. Maheshwari, 4/e p281]

Systemic Lupus Erythrematosus (SLE)

- Asymmetrical joint involvement
- Ankylosis not common
- Hyaline cartilage erosions not common

55. Ans. (c) USG
[Ref. Oxford Handbook of Clinical Surgery by Chikwe, 4/e p259]

56. Ans. (d) Radial nerve injury
[Ref. Clinical Procedures in Emergency Medicine by Roberts and Hedges, 6/e p973]

Complications of Elbow Dislocation

- Injury to Brachial artery (Most serious complication)
- Injury to Median nerve
- Injury to Ulnar nerve
- Myositis ossificans

57. Ans. (c) MRI
[Ref. Maheshwari, 4/e p248]

58. Ans. (b) Posterior
[Ref. Orthopedic Secrets by Brown, 3/e p139]

59. Ans. (d) L4-L5
[Ref. Manual of Practical Medicine by Alagappan, 5/e p724]

60. Ans. (b) Shoulder
[Ref. Textbook of Orthopedics and Trauma by Kulkarni, 2/e p376]

61. Ans. (a) Long thoracic nerve
[Ref. Maheshwari, 4/e p65]

Winging of Scapula

- Test: Pushing against wall with both hands make scapula on affected site more prominent
- Nerve involved: Long thoracic nerve
- Nerve root involved: C5, C6. C7

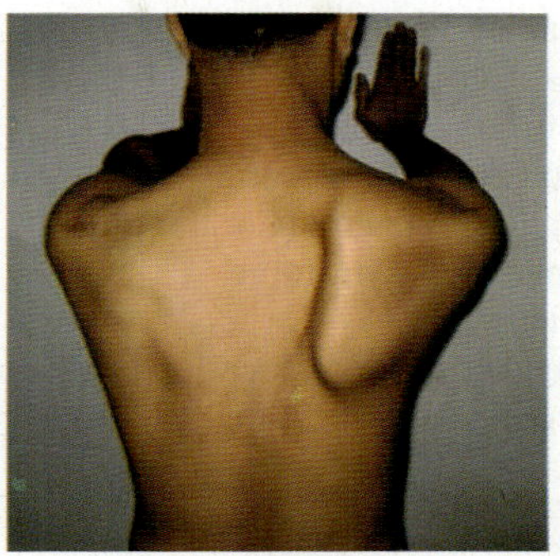

Fig. Winging of Scapula

62. Ans. (c) Ape thumb
[Ref. Clinical Anatomy for Students by Kulkarni, 1/e p108]

63. Ans. (c) Mobilization of joints is advisable
[Ref. Maheshwari, 4/e p51]

Myositis Ossificans

- *Description*: Is the *'post-traumatic ossification'* of a hematoma around a joint, resulting in formation of a bone-mass and restriction of joint movements
- *Causes*:
  - Severe injury to a joint (stripping of Periosteum)
  - Massage following trauma
- *Increased predisposition*:
  - Children (as Periosteum is loosely attached to bones)
  - Patients with prolonged neuronal damage due to head injury
  - Patients with paraplegia
- It can lead to stiff joints and extra-articular ankylosis
- *X-ray picture*:
  - Fluffy margins of bone mass (Active Myositis)
  - Trabeculated bone with well-defined margins (Mature Myositis)
- ***Treatment***:
  - **No massage after injury**
  - **Resting of limbs in early stages**
  - **Physiotherapy in late stages**
  - **Surgical excision of bone mass on maturity**

64. Ans. (a) Axillary
[Ref. The Shoulder by Rockwood, Volume 1, p677]

65. Ans. (b) Palmar fascia
[Ref. An Aid to MRCP by Freeman, 1/e p221]

66. Ans. (c) Pulled elbow
[Ref. Maheshwari, 4/e p101]

67. Ans. (d) Limb lengthening
[Ref. Maheshwari, 4/e p126]

68. Ans. (d) Myositis ossificans progressive
[Ref. Maheshwari, 4/e p101]

Dislocation of Elbow Joint

- ***Types of dislocations*:**
  - **Posterior (Most common)**
  - Postero-medial
  - Postero-lateral
  - Divergent
- *Associated complications*:
  - Median nerve palsy
  - Elbow stiffness
  - Myositis ossificans
  - Neurovascular compromise
  - Volkman's Ischaemic Contracture
  - Compartment syndrome
- *Occurrence*:
  - **Is Most common dislocation in children**
  - Is second MC dislocation in adults (after shoulder)

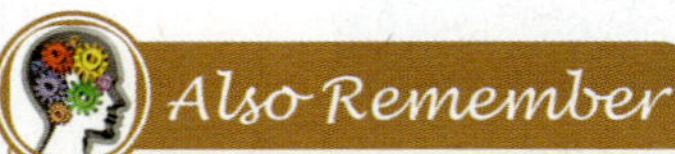

- Myositis ossificans progressive: Inherited autosomal dominant disorder

69. Ans. (a) Coronoid process posterior to humerus
[Ref. Rockwood and Wilkin's Fractures in Children by Kasser, 7/e p577]

70. Ans. (c) Tibialis anterior
[Ref. Maheshwari, 4/e p220]

Muscles in Poliomyelitis

- Type of paralysis: Descending asymmetric flaccid paralysis
- Sensory loss: Absebt
- MC muscle affected: Quadriceps (usually partially paralysed)
- MC muscle undergoing complete paralysis: Tibialis anterior
- MC muscle affcted in Hand: Opponens pollicis

71. Ans. (a) Frozen shoulder
[Ref. Clinical Mastery in Treatment of Myofascial Pain by Gerwin, 1/e p94]

72. Ans. (a) Anterior
[Ref. Maheshwari, 4/e p86]

73. Ans. (b) Gun stock deformity
[Ref. Maheshwari, 4/e p98]

- **Gun-stock deformity:** Cubitus varus deformity due to Malunion of Supracondylar fracture of humerus (MC complication)

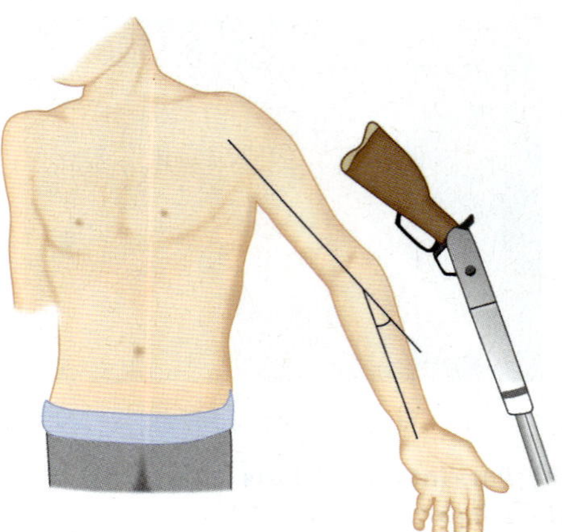

Fig. Gunstock Deformity

74. Ans. (b) Tennis elbow
[Ref. Maheshwari, 4/e p293]

Common Orthpedic Affections

Type of affection	Tissue involved	Remark
Bursitis	Bursa	MC Irritative type
Tenosynovitis	Synovial lining of tendon sheath	–
Dupuytren's contracture	Palmar aponeurosis contracture	MC Ring finger involved
Tennis elbow	Lateral epicondylitis	–
Golfer's elbow	Medial epicondylitis	–
de Quervain's tenovaginitis	Inflammed sheaths of APL, EPB*	Radial styloid process pain
Trigger finger/ thumb	Constricted fibrous digital sheath	Locking of finger
Carpal tunnel syndrome	Median nerve compression	Under flexor retinaculum
Frozen shoulder	Joint capsule (Gleno-humeral)	Periarthritis shoulder
Plantar fascitis	Inflammed plantar aponeurosis	Tender calcaneal tuberosity
Painful arc syndrome	Supraspinatous tendon	Tears, tendinitis
Meralgia paraesthetica	Entrapped Lateral cutaneous nerve	Thigh affected

*(*APL: Abductor pollicis longus; EPB: Extensor pollicis brevis)*

75. Ans. (b) Sciatic
[Ref. Surgery of the Hip by Berry, Volume 2 p615]

76. Ans. (a) Osteomyelitis
[Ref. Harwood-Nuss Clinical Practice of Emergency Medicine, 5/e p723]

77. Ans. (c) Rocker bottom foot
[Ref. Essentials of Skeletal Radiology by Rowe, 3/e p334]

78. Ans. (a) Prepatellar bursa
[Ref. Maheshwari, 4/e p292]

79. Ans. (a) Supraspinatus
[Ref. High Yield Gross Anatomy by Louis, 5/e p220]
- MC Injury in Rotator cuff injury: MC bursa affected: Acromian bursa

80. Ans. (c) Terminal pulp space infection
[Ref. Maheshwari, 4/e p98]

Felon/ Whitlow
- Description: Infection of terminal pulp space (Volar space of distal digit)
- **MC affected:** Index finger, Thumb
- **MC Cause:** Pin-prick
- Treatment: Conservative treatment, Abscess drainage
- Complications: Osteomyelitis, Pyogenic arthritis of distal IP joint, Suppurative tenosynovitis

81. Ans. (b) Shallow acetabulum
[Ref. Essentials of Orthopedics for Physiotherapist by Ebnezar, 1/e p339]

82. Ans. (d) Ring finger
[Ref. Maheshwari, 4/e p293]

Dupuytren's Contracture
- Condition: Contracture of palmar aponeurosis
- Cause: Hereditary predisposition
- Pathoanatomy:
  - Flexion of fingers at MP and PIP joints
  - MC affected finger: Ring finger
  - May be associated with: Thickened plantar fascia or penile fascia (Peyronie's disease)
- Clinical presentation: Flexion deformity of fingers
- Treatment: Sub-total excisio of palmar aponeurosis

83. Ans. (c) Olecranon
[Ref. The 5-Minute Sport Medicine Consult by Bracker, 2/e p136]

84. Ans. (a) MRI
[Ref. Imaging for Students by Lisle, 4/e p175]

85. Ans. (d) Capitulum
[Ref. Musculoskeletal MRI by Saif, 1/e p112]

86. Ans. (b) Subclavian vessels and Lower root
[Ref. Vascular and Endovascular Surgery by Loftus, 5/e p199]

Thoracic Outlet Syndrome
- Compression of the Brachial plexus or Subclavian vessels in their passage between Anterior scalene and Middle scalene muscles
- **MC involvement in Brachial plexus: C8, T1**
- **MC involvement in vessels: Subclavian artery** > Subclavian vein

87. Ans. (b) Infrapatellar bursa
[Ref. Maheshwari, 4/e p292]

88. Ans. (a) Eversion
[Ref. Rehabilitation by Nielsen, 3/e p190]

Clubfoot (Talipes Equinovarus)
- Varus deformity of both rear foot and fore foot
- Rear foot equinus
- Inverted forefoot
- Adducted forefoot

89. Ans. (d) Surgical decompression of the subacromial space is frequently indicated
[Ref. Anatomy and Kinesiology by Clippinger, 1/e p457]

Impingement Syndrome
- Three stages:
  - Stage I: Inflammation and/or tendinosis of the underlying tendons
  - Stage II: Partial rotator cuff tear along with underlying thickening or fibrosis of surrounding structures
  - Stage III: Full-thickness tear
- Supraspinatus tendon is most frequently involved, as the area of impingement is localized over the supraspinatus tendon insertion on the superior facet of the greater tubercle of the Humerus
- Tenderness near the insertion of the supraspinatus and aching pain that is magnified by shoulder abduction, especially between 60°-120°

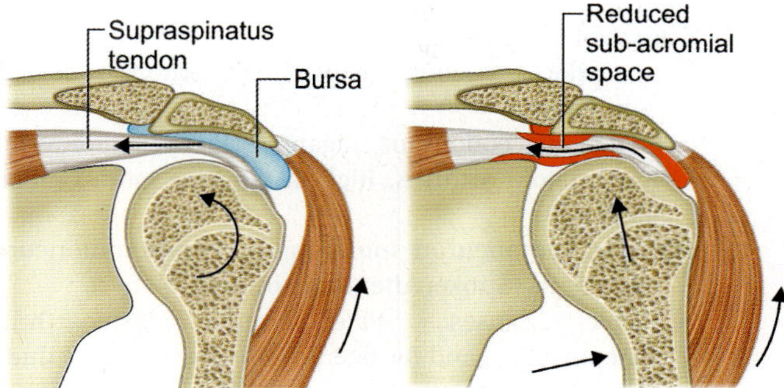

Fig. Impingement Syndrome

90. Ans. (a) Ponseti technique
[Ref. Pediatrics by Tolo, 1/e p193]
- Unlike other forms of nonoperative treatment, the Ponseti method corrects all the components of the deformity simultaneously, with the exception of Equinus deformity which is corrected last
- Cavus is corrected first, Adductus and Varus follow sequentially, and Equinus is the last to be corrected [Mnemonic: CAVE]

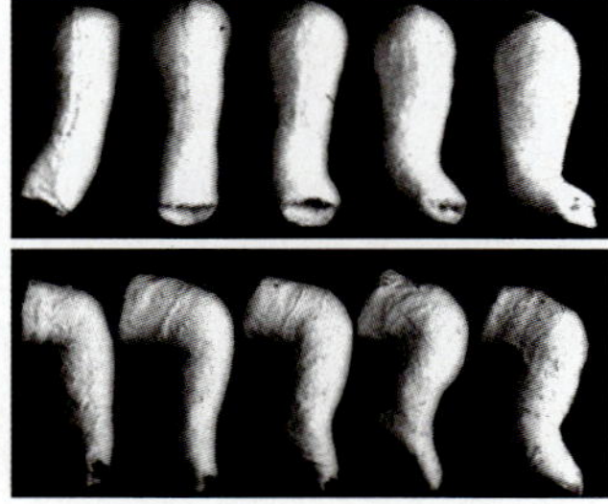

Fig. Ponseti Technique (Series of Plaster casts)

91. Ans. (d) CTEV
[Ref. Maheshwari, 4/e p209]

Denis-Browne Splint (Foot Abduction Orthosis)
- Use: Maintenance of correction of CTEV (Club foot)
- Timing of use:
  - Throughout the day before child starts walking
  - During night time when child starts walking (CTEV shoes during day)

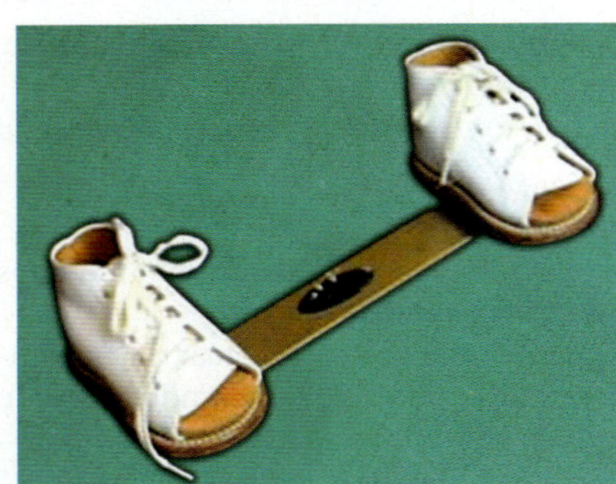

Fig. Denis-Browne Splint

92. Ans. (d) All the above

[Ref. Apley's System of Orthopaedics and Fractures, 9/e p558]

Genu Recurvatum

- Hyperextension of the knee joint: Knee extension greater than 5°
- Causes of Recurvatum:
  - Muscular, osseous, capsuloligamentous, or any combination
  - Congenital conditions, Ligament laxity, Poliomyelitis, Rheumatoid arthritis, Rickets, Charcot joint, Cerebral palsy (CP)
  - Lower motoneuron spinal injury, Upper motoneuron conditions (Stroke, After brain injury)
  - Other causes: Patellofemoral osteoarthritis, Osteomyelitis, and Iatrogenic after knee surgery due to injury to physeal plate

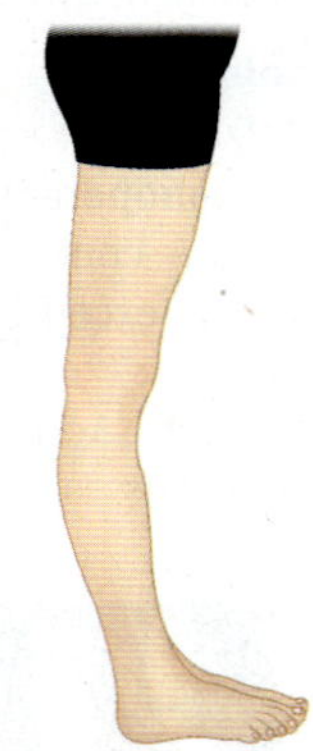

Fig. Genu Recurvatum

93. Ans. (d) Menorrhagia

[Ref. The 5-Minute Sports Medicine Consult by Bracker, 2/e p64]

Carpal Tunnel Syndrome Associated Conditions

- Idiopathic
- Local: Inflammation, Tumours, Trauma, Anatomic anomalies
- Regional: Osteoarthritis, Rheumatoid arthritis, Amyloidosis, and Gout
- Systemic: Diabetes, Obesity, Hypothyroidism, Pregnancy, Menopause, SLE, Scleroderma, Dermatomyositis, Renal failure, Long-term hemodialysis, Acromegaly, Multiple myeloma, Sarcoidosis, Leukemia, Alcoholism, and Hemophilia

94. Ans. (c) Central hip dislocation

[Ref. Orthopedics by Mohindra, 1/e p100]

- Femoral head may be palpable at Ipsilateral gluteal region in Posterior dislocation while it is palpable in groin in an Anterior dislocation
- In Central fracture dislocation (fracture of acetabular floor where head migrates into pelvis), the head can often be palpated on a per rectal examination

Also Remember

- Anterior dislocation: Femoral head losing contact with the acetabulum and is forced anteriorly, meaning to the front
- Posterior dislocation: Femoral head is displaced posteriorly, or forced backwards
- Central dislocation: Femoral head being forced downward, known as inferiorly

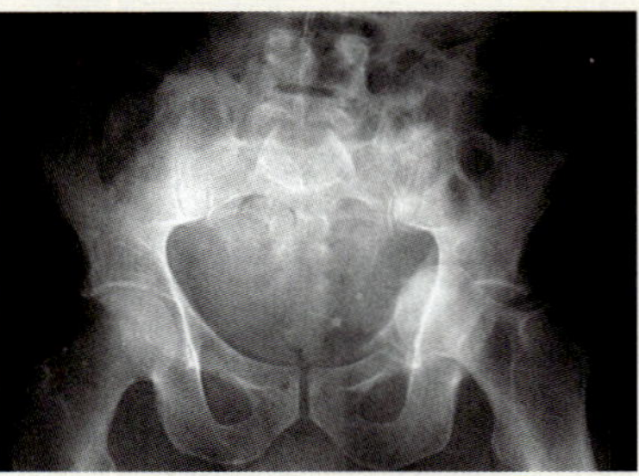

Fig. Central Dislocation of Hip

95. Ans. (d) Jerk is given to the knee to dislocate the femur head -jerk of exit

[Ref. Maheshwari, 4/e p214]

- Ortolani test: Hips and knee are help in flexed position and gradually abducted
- Ortolani test positive: In Congenital dislocation of hip, a 'click of entrance' will be felt as femoral head slips into acetabulum from position of dislocation

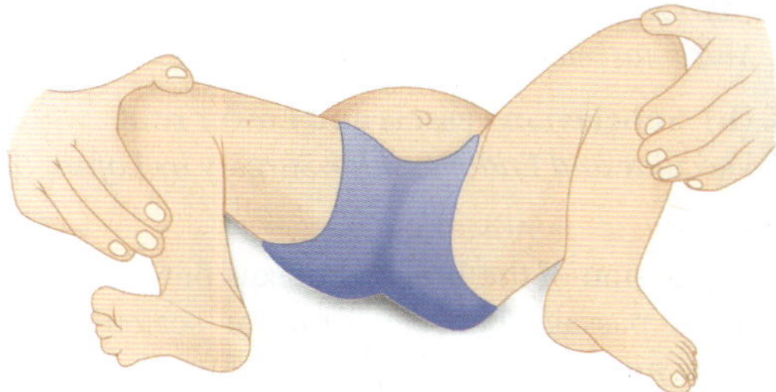

Fig. Ortolani Test

96. Ans. (a) Involves serial casting and below knee plaster casting

[Ref. Clubfoot by Miller, 1/e p13]

- In the Conventional Kite method, forefoot Adduction deformity is corrected first, followed by correction of heel Inversion, then Cavus and Equinus in the end [Mnemonic: A-ICE]
- Unlike other forms of nonoperative treatment, the Ponseti method corrects all the components of the deformity simultaneously, with the exception of Equinus deformity which is corrected last: Cavus is corrected first, Adductus

Orthopedics

and Varus follow sequentially, and Equinus is the last to be corrected [Mnemonic: CAVE]

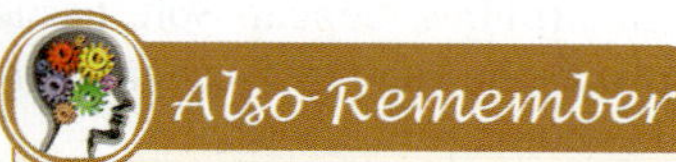

Ponseti Method

- Red Flag Casts used where each cast covers the entire leg from the toes up to the groin area
- During serial casting, short casts below the knee should not be used: They do not completely stabilize the tibius and talus bones

97. Ans. (d) All the above

[Ref. Medical Illustrations by Netter, 1/e p42]

Elevation of Scapula (Sprengel's Deformity)

- Scapula is elevated and hypoplastic
- Affected side of the neck is fuller and shorter than the uninvolved side
- Decrease in the cervicoscapular line and the appearance of torticollis
- Involved shoulder is typically smaller and the distance from the acromion to the spine is shorter than on the normal side.

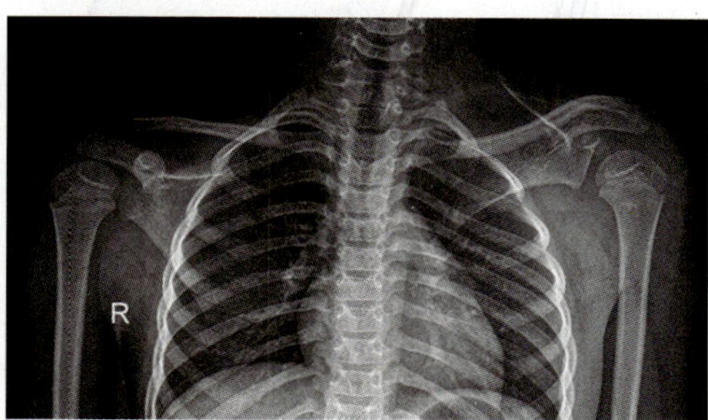

Fig. Sprengel's Deformity

98. Ans. (b) Patellar tendonosis

[Ref. Bailey & Love's Surgery, 25/e p461]

Patellar tendinitis (Jumper's Knee)

- An apophysitis (inflammation) of the patellar tendon as it inserts into the patella
- A partial tear of the attachment of the patellar tendon to the lower pole of the patella
- A jumper or sprinter develops pain over the front of the knee

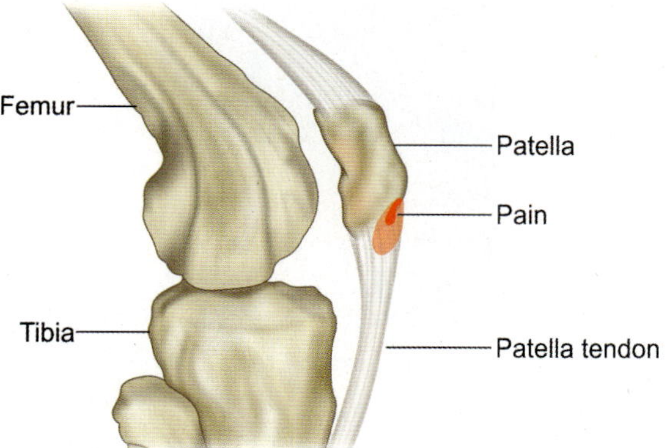

Fig. Jumper's Knee

99. Ans. (a) Pregnancy is the most common cause

[Ref. Orthopedics by Mohindra, 2/e p273]

Carpal Tunnel Syndrome (CTS)

- MC Compression neurology
- MCC of CTS: Repetitive strain of the flexor tendons, which control finger movements
- Usually caused by: Any activity that calls for repetitive hand movements (Repeatedly grasping, twisting, or turning objects with the hand)
- Causative associations:
  - MC association: Idiopathic
  - Other associations: Hypothyroidism (2nd MC), Pregnancy, Acromegaly, Diabetes, Amyloidosis, Rheumatoid arthritis, Hyperparathyroidism, Alcoholism, Colles fracture, Obesity, Malnutrition, Wrist injuries, Corticosteroids/ Estrogen use

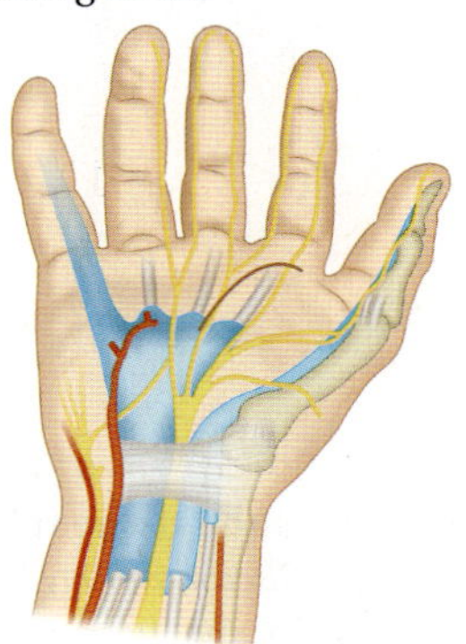

Fig. CTS

100. Ans. (d) Smith's fracture

[Ref. Orthopedics by Mohindra, 2/e p273]

Carpal Tunnel Syndrome (CTS) - Causative Associations

- MC association: Idiopathic
- Other associations: Hypothyroidism (2nd MC), Pregnancy, Acromegaly, Diabetes, Amyloidosis, Rheumatoid arthritis, Hyperparathyroidism, Alcoholism, Colles fracture, Obesity, Malnutrition, Wrist injuries, Corticosteroids/ Estrogen use

101. Ans. (b) Limbs are in adduction, internal rotation and flexion in old children

[Ref. Pathology by Goodman, 4/e p1181]

Developmental Dysplasia of Hip (DDH)

- History: Breech delivery, Female, Family history
- Gait: Waddling gait, Positive Trendelenburg sign, Pain
- Typical posture: Adduction, internal rotation and hip-flexion

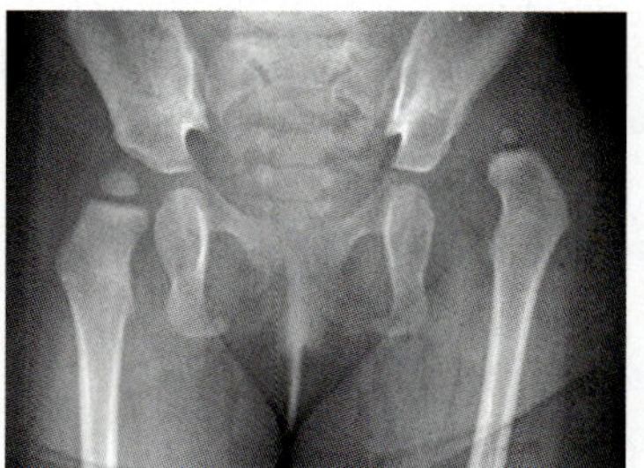

Fig. DDH

102. Ans. (b) Exercise induced calf claudication

[Ref. Interventional Radiology by Covey, 1/e p256]

Popliteal Artery Entrapment Syndrome (FAES)

- Presents with calf claudication exacerbated with exercise
- On physical examination distal pulses that decrease with plantar flexion
- Anatomical Popliteal entrapment occur due to deviation and compression of artery by Medial head of Gastrocnemius, which may result in adventitial thickening, fibrosis, aneurysm formation, thrombosis and distal embolization (Blue toe syndrome)

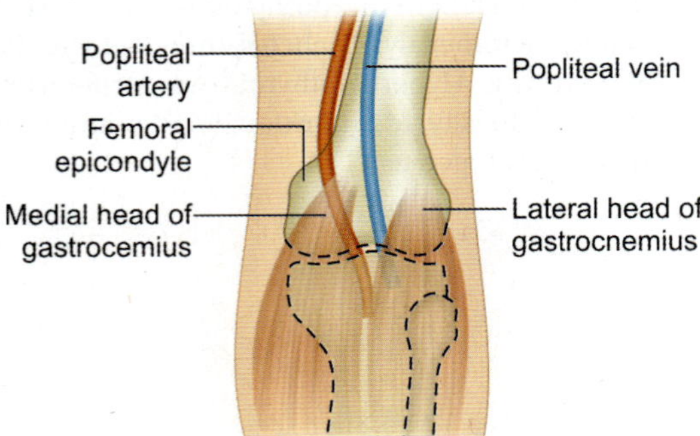

Fig. FAES

103. Ans. (a) Posteromedial soft tissue release

[Ref. Orthopaedics and Rheumatology by Singh, 1/e p98]

- In cases of failure of the Ponseti technique, a formal Posteromedial release is recommended even though the recurrence rate is high
- In cases where a Posteromedial release is not sufficient to obtain a plantigrade foot, then a Talectomy is advisable
- In cases of Recurrent deformities, repeat Soft tissue releases could be dangerous as the anatomy is completely distorted and neurovascular damage may ensue

104. Ans. (b) Pulsion diverticulum of knee joint

[Ref. Clinical Surgery by Sakr, 1/e p595]

Morrant Baker Cyst

- A pulsion diverticulum of the knee joint, caused by chronic disease in the joint
- It is a herniation of the synovial membrane of the knee
- Only occurs in connection with chronic inflammatory changes of the joint, often caused by Osteoarthritis or Rheumatoid arthritis

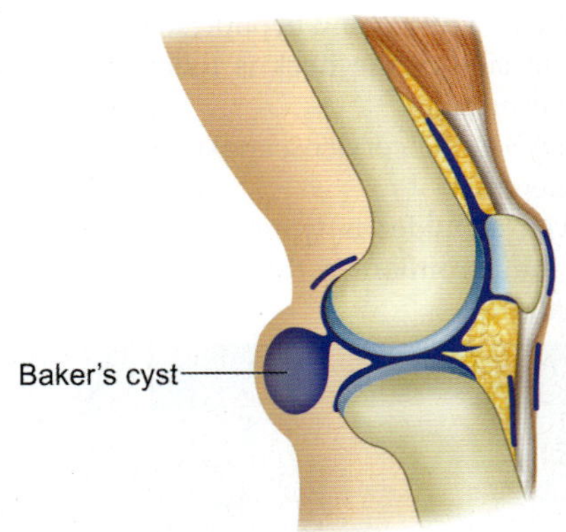

Fig. Baker's Cyst

HIGH YIELD MCQs ANSWERS WITH EXPLANATIONS 

1. Ans. (a) Diabetes mellitus; (b) Epilepsy; (c) Chronic Pulmonary disease; (d) Alcohol

[Ref. An Aid to MRCP by Freeman, 1/e p221]

2. Ans. (c) Anhydrosis

[Ref. Rockwood and Wilkin's Fractures in Children by Kasser, 7/e p602]

- **Complex Regional Pain Syndrome:** Post-traumatic pain syndrome with Osteoporosis, Edema and Trophic changes [Mnemonic: POET]
- Types of Complex Regional Pain Syndrome (CRPS):
  - CRPS-I (Reflex sympathetic dystrophy): No occurrence of nerve lesion
  - CRPS-II (Causalgia): Diagnostic and definable nerve lesion

3. Ans. (a) Posterior

[Ref. Maheshwari, 4/e p126]

4. Ans. (d) All of the above

[Ref. Maheshwari, 4/e p126-128]

5. Ans. (c) Complex regional pain syndrome 1

[Ref. Complex Regional Pain Syndrome by Scott, Thesis p37]

6. Ans. (b) Inferior dislocation of shoulder

[Ref. Orthopedic Emergencies by David, 1/e p305]

Luxatio Erecta

- Description: Inferior gleno-humeral dislocation, with Humeral head lying inferior to glenoid fossa
- Associated injuries: Avulsion of Supraspinatus/ Pectoralis major/ Teres minor, Brachial plexus injury

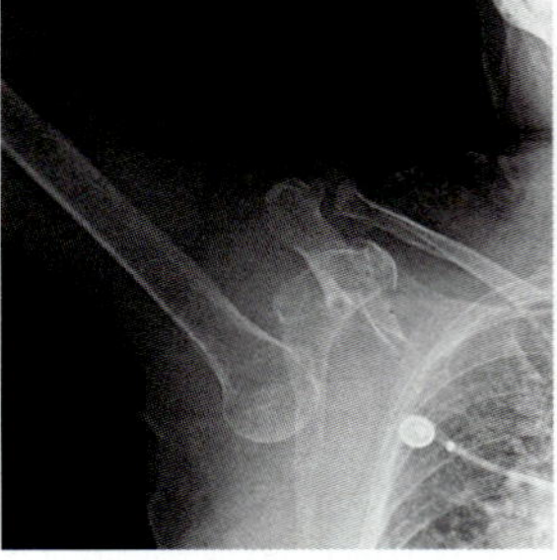

Fig. Luxatio Erecta

7. Ans. (a) Shoulder

[Ref. Quick Review Orthopedics by Mehra, 1/e p13]

- MC Site of Recurrent dislocations: Shoulder> Patella

8. Ans. (c) Lunate bone
[Ref. Maheshwari, 4/e p308]

Common Osteochondritis

Osteochondritis	Site
Perthes disease	Epiphysis of head of femur
Panner's disease	Capitulum
Kienbock's disease	Lunate
Osgood Schlatter disease	Tibial tuberosity
Kohler disease	Navicular
Frieberg's disease	Metatarsal head (2nd> 3rd)
Scheurmann's disease	Ring epiphysis of vertebrae
Calve's disease	Central body nucleus of Verterbral body

9. Ans. (c) Restriction of joint movement is late sequale; (d) Tenderness in lunate bone; (e) Ulna is shortened
[Ref. Maheshwari, 4/e p308]

10. Ans. (d) A traction injury of the tibial tubercle of the tibial epiphysis
[Ref. Maheshwari, 4/e p308]

11. Ans. (a) Upper tibia
[Ref. Maheshwari, 4/e p308]

12. Ans. (a) Subcoracoid
[Ref. Sports Injuries by Hyde, 2/e p516]
- **MC type of Shoulder dislocations: Subcoracoid** > Subglenoid > Subclavicular > Intrathoracic
- **MC Type of injury to Anterior shoulder:** Subcoracoid dislocation

13. Ans. (a) Posterior dislocation head of femur
[Ref. Maheshwari, 4/e p126]

14. Ans. (c) Posterior dislocation of hip
[Ref. Maheshwari, 4/e p126]

15. Ans. (b) Knee
[Ref. Orthopedic Surgery by Wiesel, 1/e]
- Less common dislocations: Ankle, Knee, Sternoclavicular joint

16. Ans. (a) Adduction internal rotation deformity
[Ref. Maheshwari, 4/e p126]

17. Ans. (b) Posterior dislocation of hip
[Ref. Maheshwari, 4/e p126]

18. Ans. (a) Anterior (Sub-coracoid)
[Ref. Sports Injuries by Hyde, 2/e p516]

19. Ans. (c) 1, 2 and 4 are correct
[Ref. Neurology by Sheth, 2/e p260]

Conditions Associated with Carpal Tunnel Syndrome

Endocrine conditions	Connective tissue disorders
Diabetes mellitus Hypothyroidism Acromegaly Pregnancy Obesity	Rheumatoid arthritis Amyloidosis Sarcoidosis Tuberculosis, Granulomatous diseases Trauma, Idiopathic Tenosynovitis

20. Ans. (a) Pellegrini - Stieda
[Ref. Maheshwari, 4/e p308]
- ***Pellegrini-Stieda disease:*** An ossification of the proximal MCL at the femoral condyle

21. Ans. (b) Compression of median nerve under the flexor retinaculum; (c) Anaesthesia over thenar eminence
[Ref. Maheshwari, 4/e p308]

22. Ans. (c) Addison's Disease
[Ref. Neurology by Sheth, 2/e p260]

23. Ans. (c) Posterior dislocation of hip
[Ref. Orthopedics by Biswas, 1/e p635]

24. Ans. (c) Tarsal tunnel syndrome
[Ref. Massage for Orthopedic Conditions by Hendrickson, 1/e p353]

25. Ans. (a) Tensor fascia lata
[Ref. Surgery of Hip Joint by Toronzo, 2/e p311]

26. Ans. (a) Adduction of Hip joint
[Ref. Myofascial Pain and Dysfunction by Simons, 1/e p217]

27. Ans. (c) Flexion at the hip and the knee
[Ref. Surgery of Hip Joint by Toronzo, 2/e p311]

28. Ans. (a) Subluxation of proximal radio-ulnar joint
[Ref. Conservative Management of Sports Injuries by Hyde, 2/e p565]
- **Pulled elbow/Nursemaid's elbow/Tantrum elbow:** Subluxation of proximal radio-ulnar joint

29. Ans. (a) Ankle
[Ref. Orthopedic Surgery by Wiesel, 1/e]

30. Ans. (b) Post dislocation of hip
[Ref. Maheshwari, 4/e p126]

31. Ans. (a) Adduction
[Ref. Medical Record by George, Volume 14, p426]

32. Ans. (d) USG guided aspiration of hip
[Ref. Joint Disease by Hart, 4/e p165]
- Condition described in the Question is Transient Synovitis of Hip

33. Ans. (b) Osteochondritis of femoral epiphysis
[Ref. Maheshwari, 4/e p308]

34. Ans. (d) Perthes disease
[Ref. Maheshwari, 4/e p308]

35. Ans. (c) Supervised containment of femoral head in acetabulum
[Ref. Maheshwari, 4/e p308]

36. Ans. (b) In adduction
[Ref. Medical Record by George, Volume 14, p426]

Attitude in Shoulder Dislocations
- Anterior dislocation: Arm in slight Abduction, External rotation
- Posterior dislocation: Arm in slight Adduction, Internal rotation
- Inferior dislocation: Arm fully Abducted, Elbow flexed

37. Ans. (a) Posterior dislocation of hip joint
[Ref. Skeletal Trauma by Browner, 4/e p1788]

38. Ans. (d) Flexion, abduction, external rotation
[Ref. Orthopedics Illustrated by Gupta, 2/e p76]

Deformities at Hip Joint

Condition	Deformity
Posterior dislocation of hip	Flexion, Adduction, Internal Rotation (FADIR)
Tuberculosis hip (Late stage)	Flexion, Adduction, Internal Rotation (FADIR)
Fracture neck of femur	Flexion, Abduction, External Rotation (FABER)
Intertrochanteric fracture	Flexion, Abduction, External Rotation (FABER)
Anterior dislocation of hip (Low)	Flexion, Abduction, External Rotation (FABER)
Tuberculosis hip (Early stage)	Flexion, Abduction, External Rotation (FABER)
Acute pyogenic arthritis of hip	Flexion, Abduction, External Rotation (FABER)
Transient synovitis	Flexion, Abduction, External Rotation (FABER)
Anterior dislocation of hip (High)	Extension, Abduction, External Rotation (EABER)
Slipped capital femoral epiphysis	Adduction, External rotation
Perthes' disease	Limited abduction, Internal rotation

39. Ans. (a) Closed reduction under anaesthesia
[Ref. Maheshwari, 4/e p126]

40. Ans. (c) Anterior dislocation of hip
[Ref. Orthopedics Illustrated by Gupta, 2/e p76]

41. Ans. (c) Avascular necrosis of head of femur
[Ref. Orthopedics for Physical Assistants by Hart, 1/e p331]

42. Ans. (c) Perthe's disease
[Ref. Colour Atlas of Pediatric Pathology by Stocker, 1/e p121]

- **Common Causes of Limp in Children:**
  - **Trauma: Fracture (Common cause)**, Soft tissue injury, Overuse injury
  - Infection: Septic arthritis, Syphilis
  - Rheumatic disease
  - Other disorders: Transient synovitis (Common cause), Legg-Calve-Perthes' disease (Common cause), Slipped capital femoral epiphysis

43. Ans. (a) Femoral epiphyseal osteochondritis
[Ref. 5-Minte Pediatric Consult by Schwartz, 6/e p645]

44. Ans. (a) Narrow joint space
[Ref. Gamuts in Radiology by Reeder, 3/e p293]

Joint Space Changes

Widened Joint Space	Narrow Joint Space
Congenital dislocation of hip Hemarthrosis Joint laxity (Neuromuscular disease) Legg-Calve-Perthes disease Pyogenic arthritis (early) Serous effusion (TB, RA, Collagen disease) Toxic transient synovitis Traumatic dislocation Acromegaly Early TB/ Hemophilic arthritis	Ankylosing synovitis Avascular necrosis Degenerative arthritis Advance chronic arthritis (TB, Lupus, Fungal) Psoriatic arthritis Septic arthritis Rheumatic arthritis Hemophilic arthritis Reiter's arthritis Pseudogout

45. Ans. (b) 2–12 years
[Ref. Pediatric Nurse Practitioner by Kreiger, 1/e p219]

Age-Wise Causes of Painful Limping

- 1–3 years age: Infection , Occult trauma, Neoplasm
- 4–10 years age: Infection, Transient synovitis, Legg-Calve-Perthes' disease, Rheumatologic disorder, Trauma, Infection
- 11+ years age: Slipped capital femoral epiphysis, Rheumatologic disorder, Trauma

46. Ans. (c) Central dislocation of hip
[Ref. Textbook of Orthopedics by Kotwal, 1/e p297]

47. Ans. (c) Crushed glenoidal labrum
[Ref. Sports Injury Guidebook by Gotlin, 1/e p82]

48. Ans. (a) Recurrent dislocation of shoulder
[Ref. Maheshwari, 4/e p87]

49. Ans. (a) Injury to humeral head
[Ref. Maheshwari, 4/e p87]

50. Ans. (d) Deep peroneal nerve
[Ref. Peripheral Neurology by Sackler, 3/e p108]

51. Ans. (d) Magnetic Resonance Imaging (MRI)
[Ref. SSS Radiology, p64]

52. Ans. (e) Age of onset has no effect on course
[Ref. Pediatric Orthopedics in Practice by Fritz, 2/e p240]

Prognostic Factors for Legg-Calve-Perthes Disease

- Major factors: Age, State of lateral pillar
  - If onset occur before 6 years age, prognosis is fairly good
- Minor factors: Lateral calcification, Subluxation, Overall extent of necrosis, Mobility
- Other factors: Sex, Metaphyseal involvement

53. Ans. (e) Joint space obliterated
[Ref. Gamuts in Radiology by Reeder, 3/e p293]

54. Ans. (c) Anterior glenoid cavity
[Ref. Maheshwari, 4/e p87]

55. Ans. (c) Fracture neck of talus; (d) Fracture neck of femur
[Ref. Essentials of Orthopaedics for Physiotherapists by Ebnezar, 1/e p42]

Common Sites of Avascular Necrosis

- Head of femur (Fracture neck of femur, Dislocation of hip)

Orthopedics

- Body of talus (Fracture neck of talus)
- Proximal pole of scaphoid (Fracture through waist of scaphoid)

56. Ans. (d) **Calcaneum**
[Ref. Essentials of Orthopaedics for Physiotherapists by Ebnezar, 1/e p42]

57. Ans. (a) **Sub-capital**
[Ref. ABC of Imaging in Trauma by King, 1/e]

58. Ans. (d) **Rotator cuff injury**
[Ref. Musculoskeletal MRI by Kaplan, 1/e p194]

59. Ans. (d) **Supraspinatus tear**
[Ref. Musculoskeletal MRI by Kaplan, 1/e p194]

60. Ans. (b) **Associated fracture neck of the humerus**
[Ref. Non-invasive Respiratory Support by Simonds, 3/e p307]

61. Ans. (d) **Lateral cutaneous nerve of thigh**
[Ref. Atlas of Nerve Conduction Studies and EMG by Leis, 1/e p246]

Meralgia Paraesthetica
- Cause: Compression of Lateral femoral cutaneous nerve of thigh (L2, L3) behind Inguinal ligament
- Predisposing factors: Obesity, Weight gain, Pregnancy, Prolonged hyperflexion of hip, Neoplasm, Penetrating injuries

62. Ans. (c) **Knee joint**
[Ref. Examination of Orthopedic and Athletic Injuries by Brown, 4/e p88]
- **Common sites of Osteochondritis dissecans:** Talus, Femur, Patella, Capitellum, Femoral head

63. Ans. (d) **Pain over the lateral epicondyle**
[Ref. Maheshwari, 4/e p293]

64. Ans. (d) **Extensor pollicis brevis and abductor pollicis longus**
[Ref. Maheshwari, 4/e p294]

65. Ans. (b) **Abduction and external rotation**
[Ref. Maheshwari, 4/e p86]

66. Ans. (b) **The commonest position for the head of the humerus to move into is the subspinous; (d) The easiest way to reduce it is by simple pressure with the patient under general anesthesia with muscle relaxation**
[Ref. Maheshwari, 4/e p87-88]
- **Treatment of Acute Shoulder Dislocation:** Reduction under Sedation or General anesthesia
  - Kocher's manoeuvre
  - Hippocrates manoeuvre

67. Ans. (b) **Steroid is used to relieve symptoms; (c) Pain after straining at thumb base; (d) Involve External pollicis longus; (e) Involve Abductor pollicis longus**
[Ref. Maheshwari, 4/e p294]

68. Ans. (d) **All of the above**
[Ref. Maheshwari, 4/e p293]

69. Ans. (c) **Much more common in males**
[Ref. Essential Orthopedics by Miller, 1/e p372]

70. Ans. (d) **Musculocutaneous nerve**
[Ref. The Netter Collections of Medical Illustrations by Parker, 2/e p27]

71. Ans. (b) **Surgery**
[Ref. Maheshwari, 4/e p88]

72. Ans. (c) **In posterior dislocation, appearance of shoulder is not normal**
[Ref. Essential Orthopedics and Trauma by Edwards, 5/e p196]

73. Ans. (d) **Ring finger**
[Ref. Practical Orthopedics by Mercier, 6/e p113]

74. Ans. (d) **All of the above**
[Ref. Maheshwari, 4/e p294]

75. Ans. (d) **Metacarpophalangeal joint**
[Ref. Essentials of PMR by Silver, 3/e p180]

76. Ans. (a) **Sickle cell disease; (b) Gaucher's disease; (c) Polycythemia; (e) Fracture neck of femur**
[Ref. Radiology Review Manual by Dahnert, 7/e p52]

Causes of Osteonecrosis
[Mnemonic: INFECTIVE GPS]
- Idiopathic (Perthes, Kohler)
- Neoplasia
- Fat Alcoholism
- Environmental (Frost bite, Thermal injury)
- Caisson's disease
- Trauma (Femoral neck fracture, Hip dislocation)
- Irradiation
- Vasculitis (SLE, PAN, Rheumatoid arthritis)
- End stage renal disease, Renal failure, Dialysis
- Gaucher disease
- Polycythemia, Pancreatitis
- Sickle cell disease, Steroids

77. Ans. **ALL CHOICES**
[Ref. Radiology Review Manual by Dahnert, 7/e p52]

78. Ans. (a) **Sickle cell disease; (b) Thalassemia; (c) Polycythemia**
[Ref. Radiology Review Manual by Dahnert, 7/e p52]

79. Ans. (a) **A1**
[Ref. Atlas of Ultrasound Guided Procedures by Samer, 1/e p311]
- Triggering occurs at First annular (*A1*) *pulley*, where there is an increase in friction or a mismatch in size between the flexor tendons and pulley
- *A1 pulley* consists of annular bands of connective tissue located at and proximal to and continuous to MCP flexor sheaths

80. Ans. (a) **All traumatic dislocations will be recurrent**
[Ref. Maheshwari, 4/e p86]

81. Ans. (d) **All of the above**
[Ref. Maheshwari, 4/e p86]

82. Ans. (d) **All of the above**
[Ref. Maheshwari, 4/e p86]

83. Ans. (c) **Jerk's test**
[Ref. Surgery of Shoulder Instability by Aroe, 1/e p25]

- **Tests for Posterior Glenohumeral instability:**
  - Posterior stress test
  - Jerk's test
  - Kim's test
- **Tests for Anterior Glenohumeral instability:**
  - Apprehension test
  - Relocation test
  - Surprise test

84. Ans. (d) Tensor fascia lata

85. Ans. (a) Apprehension test
[Ref. Orthopedic Shoulder Assessment by Magee, 6/e p301]

86. Ans. (b) Avulsion of extensor tendon at the base of the distal phalanx
[Ref. Maheshwari, 4/e p114]

87. Ans. (b) Splint the finger in hyperextension
[Ref. Maheshwari, 4/e p114]
- Treatment of Mallet finger: Immobilize the DIP joint in hyperextension with an Aluminum splint/ Plaster cast

88. Ans. (a) Pulled elbow
[Ref. Maheshwari, 4/e p101]

89. Ans. (b) Seen adjacent to tendon sheath;
(c) Communicates with joints cavity and sheath;
(d) It is Unilocular
[Ref. Maheshwari, 4/e p294]

90. Ans. (d) Over-riding or under-riding of Second toe by third
[Ref. Child's Foot and Ankle by Drennan, 1/e p270]

Hallux Valgus/Bunions
- Triad components:
  - Valgus deformity of Hallux
  - Exostosis on Medial side of 1st metatarsal head
  - Metatarsus primus varus
- Over-riding or under-riding of: Second toe by first toe

91. Ans. (a) Those with pain
[Ref. Foot Deformities by Acton, 2012 p3]

92. Ans. (a) Abdominal muscle strain
[Ref. Practical Orthopedics by Johnson, 1/e p533]

93. Ans. (c) ITP
[Ref. Textbook of Practical Physiology by Pravati, 2/e p112]

94. Ans. (a) Juxta articular osteosclerosis
[Ref. Pathology by Fuller, 4/e p479]
- Arnold-Hilgartner classification of Hemophilic Arthropathy:

Stage	Findings
0	Normal joint
I	No skeletal abnormalities, soft-tissue swelling is present
II	Osteoporosis and overgrowth of the epiphysis, no cysts, no narrowing of the cartilage space
III	Early subchondral bone cysts, squaring of the patella, widened notch of the distal femur or humerus, preservation of the cartilage space
IV	Findings of stage III, but more advanced; narrowed cartilage space
V	Fibrous joint contracture, loss of the joint cartilage space, extensive enlargement of the epiphysis, substantial disorganization of the joint

95. Ans. ALL CHOICES
[Ref. Advances in Pediatrics by Dutta, 1/e p437]

96. Ans. (d) Clinical examination
[Ref. Advanced Therapy in Thoracic Surgery by Putnam, 2/e p199]

97. NONE
[Ref. Maheshwari, 4/e p349]

98. Ans. (d) Towards the skin
[Ref. Microbiology Review Notes for PGMEE]

99. Ans. (d) Fully supinate the forearm
[Ref. Maheshwari, 4/e p101]

100. Ans. (b) Madura Mycosis
[Ref. Maheshwari, 4/e p172]

101. Ans. (d) MRI of hip
[Ref. Maheshwari, 4/e p172]
- Patient described has most likely developed Avascular necrosis of Femoral head, acomplication of Posterior dislocation of hip
  - X-ray changes appear after 1–2 years
  - Pain occurs after a painless period post-surgery

102. Ans. (c) Disc prolapse
[Ref. Maheshwari, 4/e p246]

103. Ans. (c) MRI
[Ref. Maheshwari, 4/e p248]

104. Ans. (b) Postero-lateral
[Ref. Textbook of Surgical Management of Lumbar Disc Herniation by Ramani, 1/e p110]
- **Most common site of Disc prolapse: Posterolateral (PL)**
  - Various combinations of disc compression, flexion and lateral bending lead to high pressures within Nucleus pulposus and localized points of high stress in Annulus; these are maximum in PL region
  - Least level of Chondroitin sulphate is in PL region

105. Ans. (c) MRI
[Ref. Drug Injury by Ahuja, 2/e p402]
- Patient described in question is a case of Avascular necrosis of hip
- *Investigation of choice for AVN hip:* MRI

106. Ans. (b) Avascular necrosis of femoral head
[Ref. Office Orthopedics for Primary Care by Anderson, 1/e p141]

107. Ans. (b) Pulmonary embolism
[Ref. Complications in Surgery by Doherty, 1/e p343]

Venous Complications after Orthopedic Surgery

Preceding Surgery	Incidence of DVT	Incidence of Pulmonary embolism
Total hip replacement	50%	20%
Total knee replacement	60%	5%
Hip fracture surgery	50%	15%

108. Ans. (c) Pulmonary embolism
[Ref. Venous Thromboembolism by Shirato, 1/e p159]

109. Ans. (d) Total knee replacement
[Ref. Clinical Trials in RA and OA by Miller, 1/e p85]

Grading in Osteoarthritis (Grade ≥ 2 define OA)

- Grade 0: No features of Osteoarthritis
- Grade 1: Minute osteophyte, Doubtful significance
- Grade 2: Definite osteophyte, Unimpaired joint space
- Grade 3: Moderate diminution of joint space
- Grade 4: Greatly impaired joint space; Sclerosis of subchondral bone

110. Ans. (c) All range of movements
[Ref. Maheshwari, 4/e p295]

- Initial movements restricted in Frozen shoulder: Abduction, Internal rotation of Shoudler
- Final movements restricted in Frozen shoulder: All movements

111. Ans. (a) Complete tear of supraspinatus
[Ref. Maheshwari, 4/e p295]

Painful Arc Syndrome

- Description: Pain in shoulder and upper arm during mid-range of Gleno-humeral abduction
- Causes:
  - Minor tears of Supraspinatus tendon
  - Supraspinatus tendinitis
  - Calcification Supraspinatus tendon
  - Subacromial bursitis
  - Fracture Greater tuberosity
- Treatment: Ultrasonics to point of tenderness, Anti-inflammatory drugs, Steroids injection

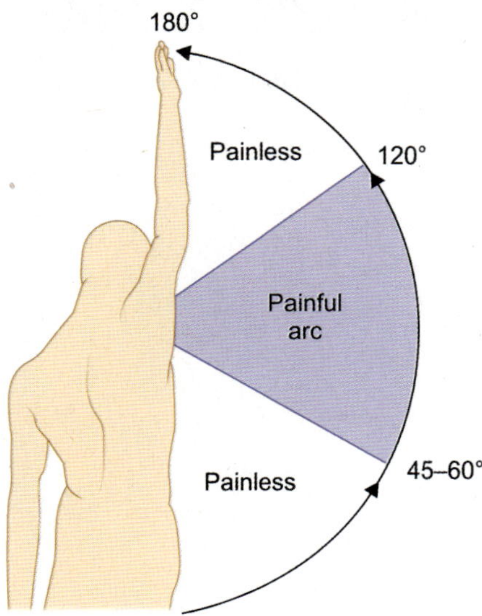

Fig. Painful arc syndrome

112. Ans. (c) Abduction
[Ref. Maheshwari, 4/e p295]

113. Ans. (a) Magnitude of correction achieved is greater than 30°

114. Ans. (b) Maduromycosis
[Ref. Maheshwari, 4/e p172]

115. Ans. (b) Avascular necrosis
[Ref. Drug Injury by Ahuja, 2/e p402]

116. Ans. (b) Tuberculosis arthritis
[Ref. Orthopedics Quick Review by Mehra, 1/e p75]

T.B. arthritis is the *most common cause* of reduced *joint movements* of *hip joints* in young patient in *India*

117. Ans. (b) Posterior dislocation humerus
[Ref. Radiology at Glance by Jones, 1/e p53]

- **Light-bulb sign** on plain X-ray: Humeral head exits glenid and rotates to give alight-bulb appearance on AP view

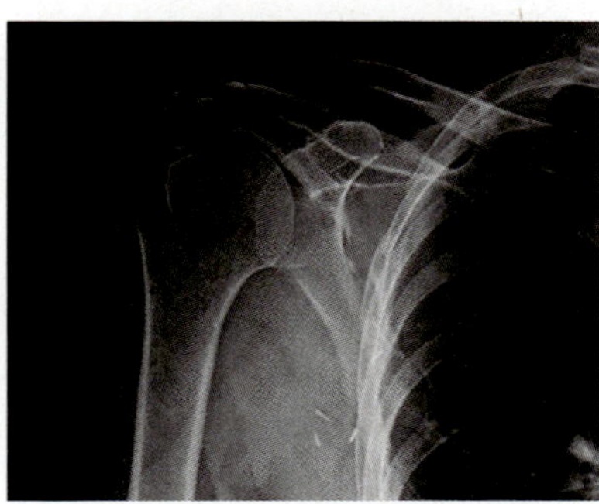

Fig. Light-bulb sign

118. Ans. (c) Adduction of forefoot; (d) Detectable at birth; (e) Denis Brown splint used
[Ref. Maheshwari, 4/e p204-208]

- In Clubfoot there is flexion of Tendoachilles, Tibialis posterior, Flexor hallucis longus, Flexor digitorum profundus
- Clubfoot has no association with Breech delivery, Oligohydramnios, Bicornuate uterus, Multiple gestations

119. Ans. (c) Median nerve
[Ref. Neurology in Clinical Practice by Bradley, 4/e p2314]

- **Pronator teres syndrome:** Median nerve is compressed in the proximal forearm between the two heads of Pronator teres muscle, Fibrous arcade of Flexor digitorum superficialis or Lacertus fibrosus

120. Ans. (b) Flexor digitorum profundus
[Ref. Family Medicine by Rudy, p149]

- **Jersey finger:** Avulsion of Flexor digitorum profundus tendon, caused by a violent hyperextension, such as the one that occurs when hurtling football strikes open hand's DIP or distal phalanx

121. Ans. (d) Cervical
[Ref. Rheumatoid Arthritis by Herman, p]

- Rheumatoid arthritis of the spine involves the cervical region more often than any other part (40% in adults)

122. Ans. (b) AP X-ray of spine
[Ref. The 5 Minute Sports Medicine Consult, 1/e p292]

Spondylolisthesis

- Oblique X-rays: Diagnostic
- Triple phase bone scan: Describes acuity of injury
- Single Photon Emission CT scan: Demonstrates Stress reactions at Pars
- CT scan: Delineate Bony pars defect or Neural compression
- MRI scan: Assess relationship of Cauda equina to Sacrum

123. Ans. (a) Hallux valgus

[Ref. Fundamentals of Pediatric Orthopedics by Lynn T. Staheli 4/e, p168]

- **Hallux valgus:** Medial deviation of the first metatarsal and lateral deviation and/or rotation of the hallux, with or without medial soft-tissue enlargement of the first metatarsal head

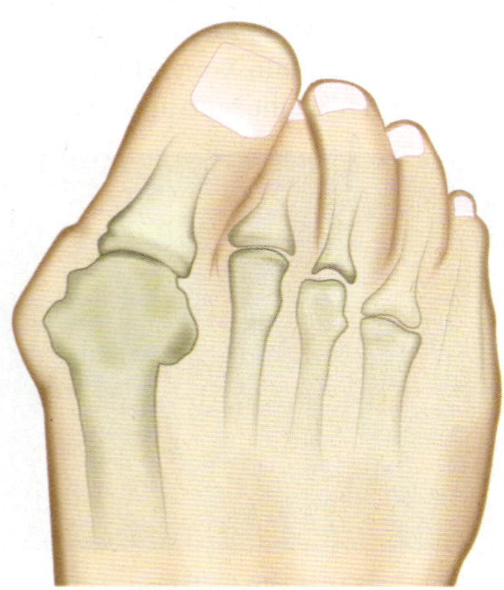

Fig. Hallux valgus

124. Ans. (a) Lateral cutaneous nerve of thigh

[Ref. Practical Orthopedics by Mercier, 6/e p205-206]

- **Meralgia paresthetica/Bernhardt-Roth syndrome:** One of large sensory nerves (Lateral femoral cutaneous nerve) to one of the legs is being compressed
- Compression results in a terrible burning sensation felt in outer thigh.

125. Ans. (c) Quadriceps

[Ref. Orthopedics by Mohindra, 2/e p121]

Hand-to-Knee Gait

- Seen in polio due to Quadriceps weakness with inability to lock the knee while walking
- Patient puts his hands on the knee to prevent it from buckling

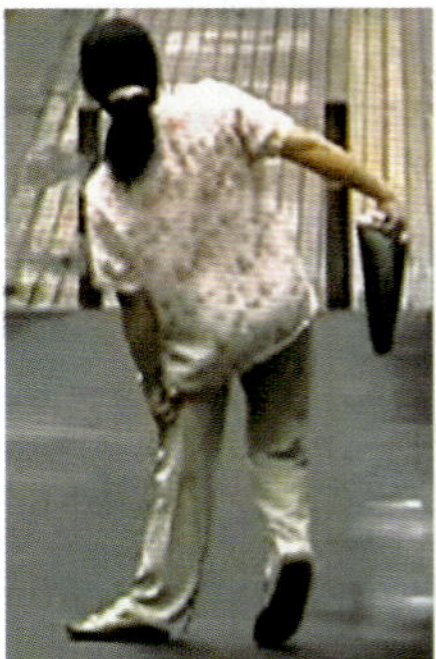

Fig. Hand-to-knee gait

126. Ans. (b) Recurrent dislocation of shoulder

[Ref. Pediatric Orthopaedics by Herring, 5/e p1261]

Recurrent Dislocation of Shoulder

- Recurrent subluxation or dislocation (shoulder instability) is the MC complication of Acute traumatic dislocation
- When the initial event occurs between the ages of 15–35 years, the dislocations usually become recurrent or habitual
- Once a second dislocation has occurred, the patient becomes a 'Recurrent dislocator'

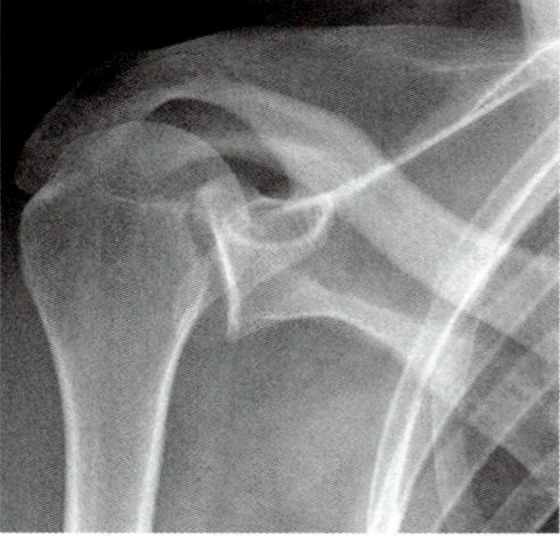

Fig. Posterior dislocation of shoulder

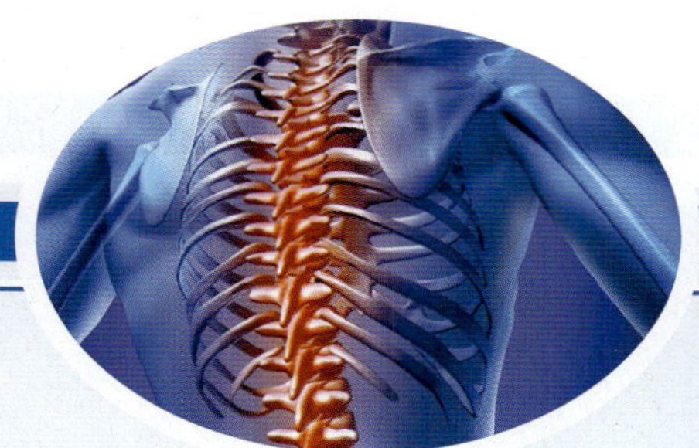

Chapter 8

Neuromuscular Disorders

THEORETICAL CONCEPTS

VIII A. SEDDON'S CLASSIFICATION OF NERVE INJURIES[Q]

- ***Neurapraxia***: Physiological disruption of conduction in nerve fibre; Spontaneous and complete recovery in few weeks[Q]
- ***Axonotmesis***: Axons damaged but nerve preserved; Partial spontaneous recovery in months
- ***Neurotmesis***: Cutting/ scarring of nerve with Wallerian degeneration; No spontaneous recovery requiring nerve repair

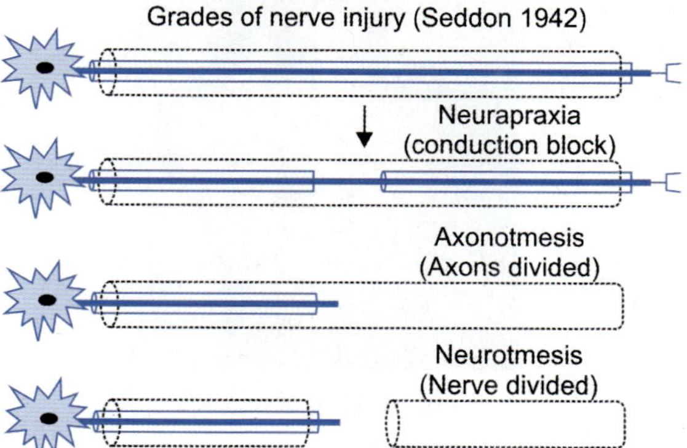

Fig. Seddon's Grading of Nerve Injuries

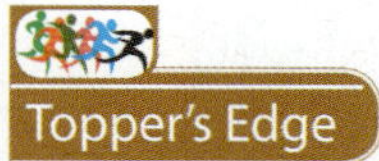

Topper's Edge

Peripheral Nerve Injuries

- Peripheral nerve is a mixed nerve
- Sunderland's classification is clinically accepted
- 40% bone and joint injuries are associated with Peripheral nerve lesions
- **MC peripheral nerve injured: Radial nerve**
- Treatment modalities:
  - Closed injuries: Conservative management is treatment of choice
  - Open injuries: Primary nerve repair (Clean wound), Delayed primary/ secondary nerve repair (Contaminated wound)
  - Methods of nerve suture: Epineural repair, Epiperineural repair, Perineural repair, Fascicular repair

VIII B. NERVE DEGENERATION AND REGENERATION

VIII B1. Nerve Degeneration

- Secondary/**Wallerian degeneration**: Degeneration of neuron distal to point of injury[Q]
- Primary/Retrograde degeneration: Degeneration of neuron proximal to point of injury, upto a single node

VIII B2. Signs of Nerve Regeneration

- ***Tinel's sign***: Distal progression of pins and needles sensation, on distal to proximal tapping of nerve
- ***Motor march***: Contraction of more distant muscles to the site of injury
- Electrodiagnostic test

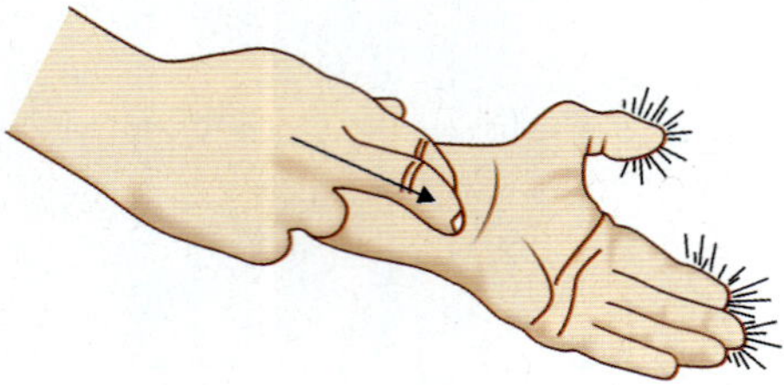

Fig. Tinel's sign

VIII C. CLASSICAL EXAMPLES OF PERIPHERAL NERVE INJURIES

- ***Wrist drop***: Radial nerve palsy[Q]
- ***Foot drop***: Common peroneal nerve palsy[Q]
- ***Winging of scapula***: Long thoracic nerve palsy[Q]
- ***Claw hand***: Ulnar + Median nerve palsy[Q]
- ***Ape-thumb deformity***: Median nerve palsy[Q]
- ***Pointing index***: Median nerve palsy[Q]

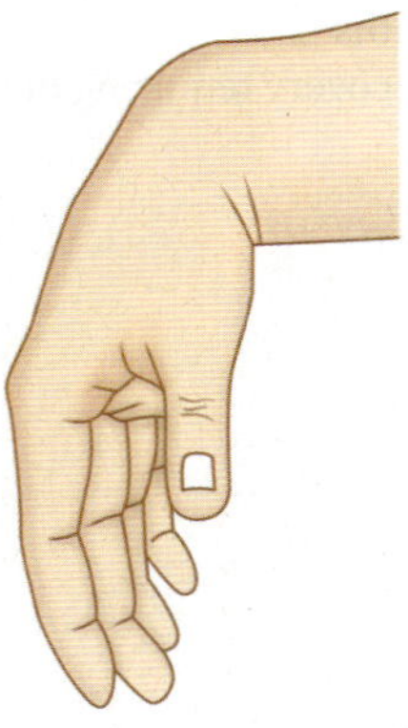

Fig. Wrist Drop

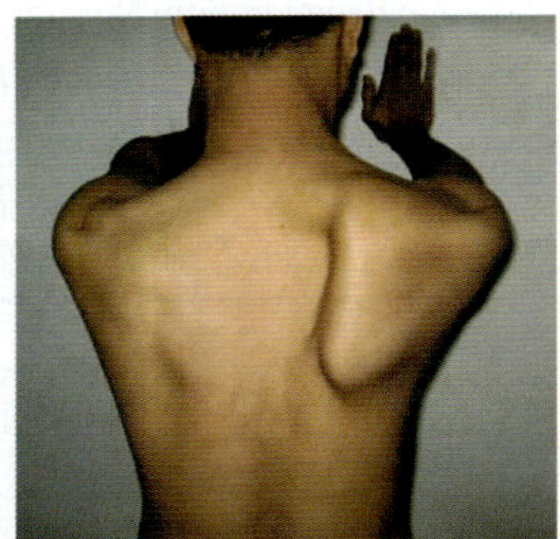

Fig. Winging of Scapula

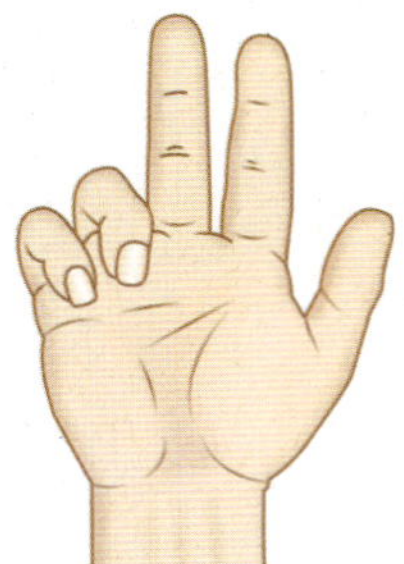

Fig. Claw Hand (Ulnar)

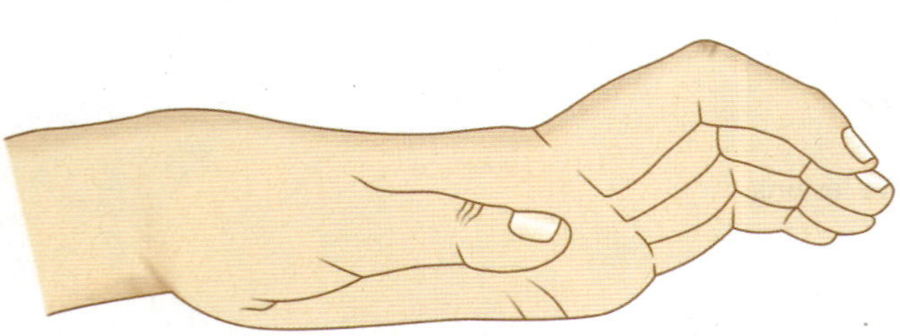

Fig. Ape Hand Deformity

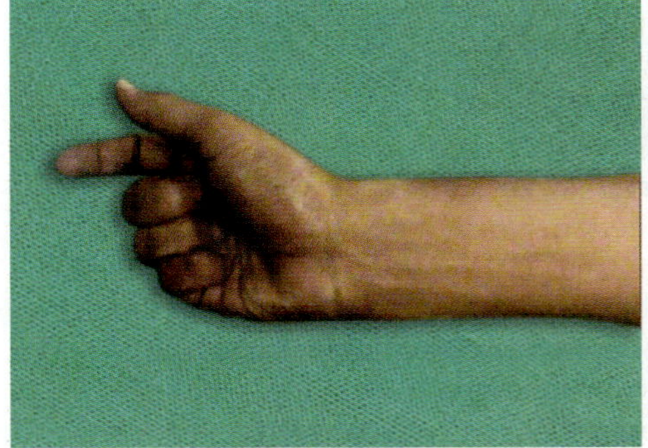

Fig. Pointing Index

VIII D. TESTS OF ULNAR NERVE (FOR MUSCLES PARALYSIS)

- *Palmar flexion of wrist against gravity*:Flexor carpi ulnaris
- *Abduction of little finger against resistance*: Abductor digiti minimi
- ***Egawa's test***: Dorsal interossei of middle finger (abductors)[Q]
- ***Card test***: Palmar interossei (adductors) of fingers[Q]
- ***Froment's sign/Book test***: Adductor pollicis[Q]

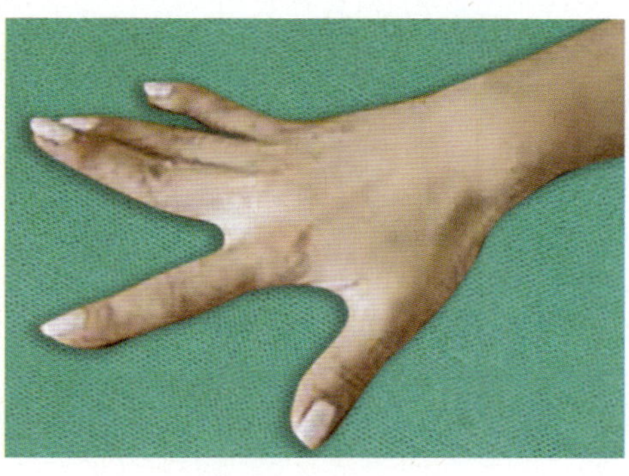

Fig. Egawa's Test

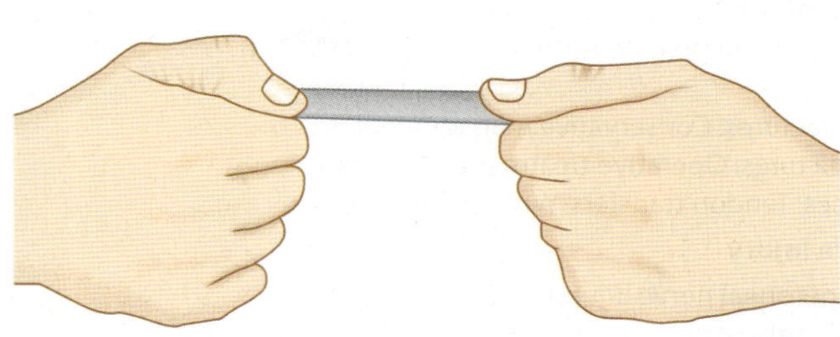

Fig. Froment's Sign

VIII E. TESTS OF MEDIAN NERVE (FOR MUSCLES PARALYSIS)

- *Flexion of terminal thumb phalanx against resistance*: Flexor pollicis longus
- *Pointing index*: Flexor digitorum superficialis and profundus
- ***Pen test***: Abductor pollicis brevis
- ***Apposition of thumb tip to other fingers***: Opponens pollicis

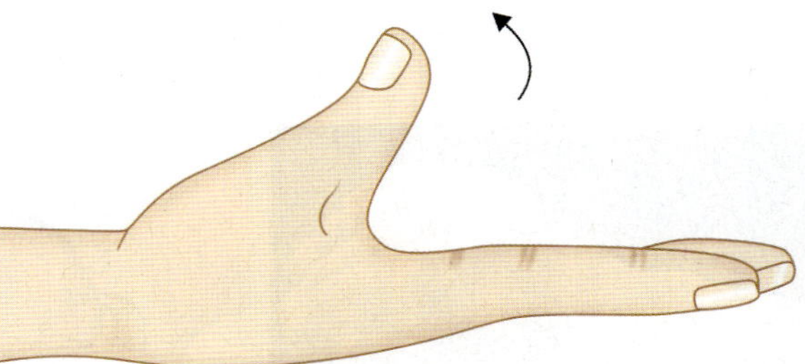

Fig. Pen Test

VIII F. TESTS OF OTHER NERVES

- ***Winging of scapula***: Long thoracic nerve (C5-6-7)[Q]
- ***Foot drop, High-step gait***: Common peroneal nerve (Sciatic nerve)[Q]

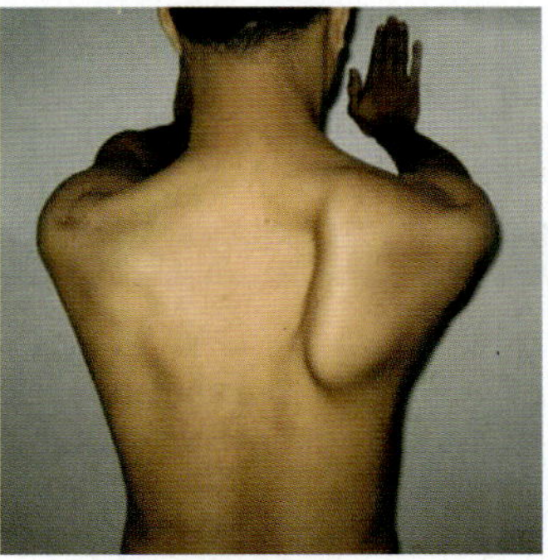

Fig. Winging of Scapula

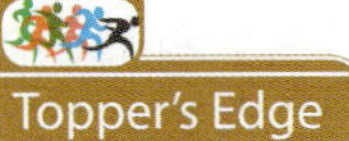

Topper's Edge

FEW CLASSICAL NERVE INJURIES

Ulnar Nerve Injury

- **Injury causes**[Q]: Ulnar clawing
- **Total clawing**[Q]: Ulnar nerve PLUS Median nerve affected
- **Reliable test**[Q]: Froment's test
- Quick clinical evaluation test: Test tip of little finger
- Ulnar paradox[Q]: Higher the lesion, lesser is the deformity an vice versa

Radial Nerve Injury

- MC peripheral nerve injured[Q]
- **MC site of injury[Q]**: Distal end of humerus
- Screening test: Thumb extension test (Hitchhiker's sign)
- Treatment:
  - Closed fractures: Conservative management
  - Open fractures: Operative treatment and repair
  - Late cases: Tendon transfers, Wrist arthrodesis

Sciatic Nerve Injury

- Common peroneal nerve injured at Fibular neck[Q]
- **MC cause[Q]: Leprosy**
- Foot drop: Complete or Incomplete
- **Characteristic gait[Q]: High-stepping gait**
- Treatment:
  - Main stay of Conservative treatment: Dynamic foot-drop splint
  - After 1 year: Tendon transfer for Mobile foot-drop

VIII G. SPLINTS FOR NERVE INJURIES

- *Cock-up splint*: Radial nerve palsy[Q]
- *Knuckle-Bender splint*: Ulnar nerve palsy

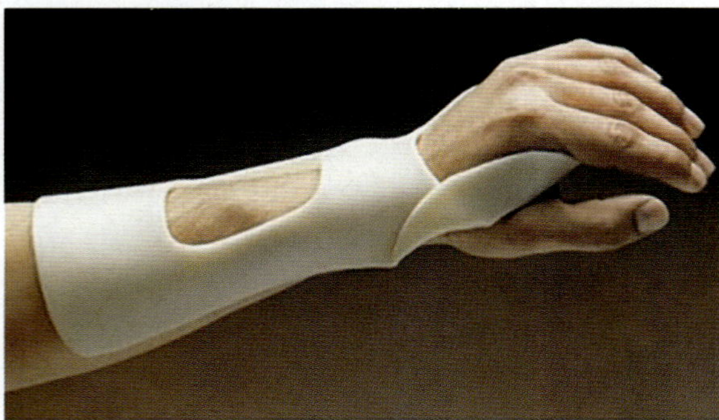

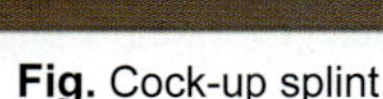

Fig. Cock-up splint

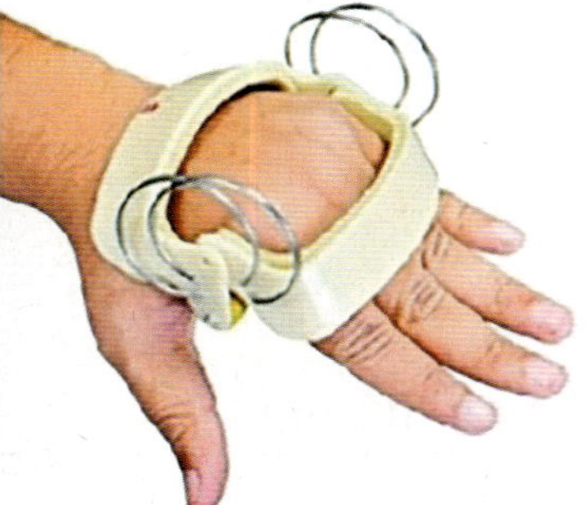

Fig. Knuckle-Bender splint

VIII H. SPINA BIFIDA

- *Underlying defect*: Failure of fusion of vertebral arches

Type	Features
Spina bifida occulta (Most common[Q])	
Lumbosacral (S1: Most common[Q])	Diastematomyelia +Myelodysplasia Investigation of choice: MRI[Q]
Spina bifida aperta	
Dorsolumbar	Myelocoele (Most common[Q]) Meningocoele Meningo-myelocoele Syringo-myelocoele

IMAGE-BASED QUESTIONS

1. **A 24 years old sustained the fracture shown in the X-ray below. The nerve most likely to be injured is** ***[AIIMS May 2016]***

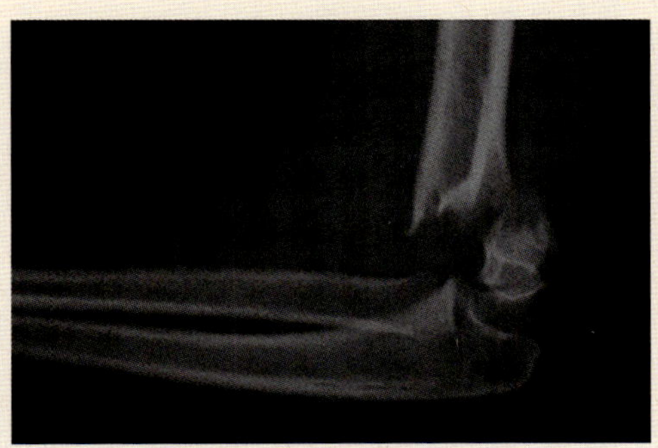

a. Ulnar nerve b. Median nerve
c. Radial nerve d. Musculocutaneous nerve

2. **Identify the Type of Splint shown in Photograph**

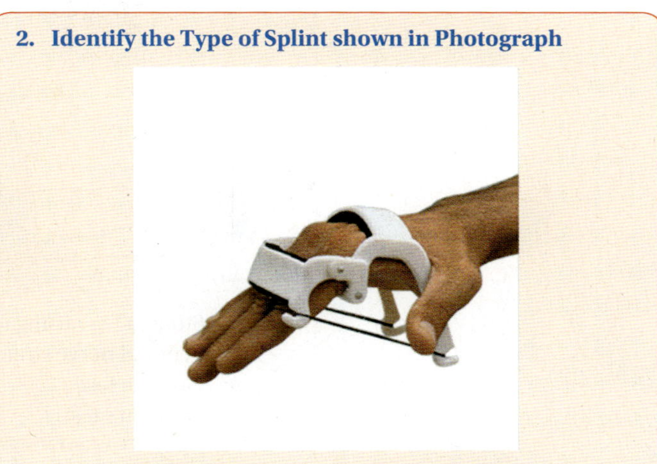

a. Aeroplane splint b. Thomas splint
c. Knuckle-bender splint d. Cock-up splint

3. **Nerve injured leading to Condition shown in Photograph** ***[Recent Question 2013, 2014, AIIMS May 2016]***

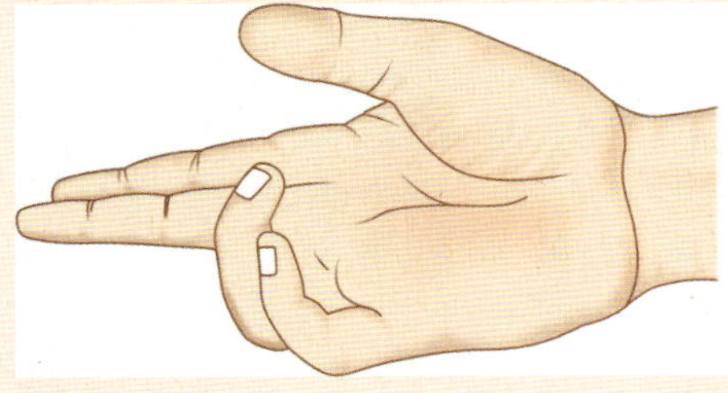

a. Radial nerve b. Median nerve
c. Ulnar nerve d. Axillary nerve

4. **Clinical test (Photograph) is used to test** ***[Recent Question 2013, 2014]***

a. Median nerve b. Radial nerve
c. Axillary nerve d. Ulnar nerve

5. **Nerve roots involved in Clinical condition shown in Photograph is**

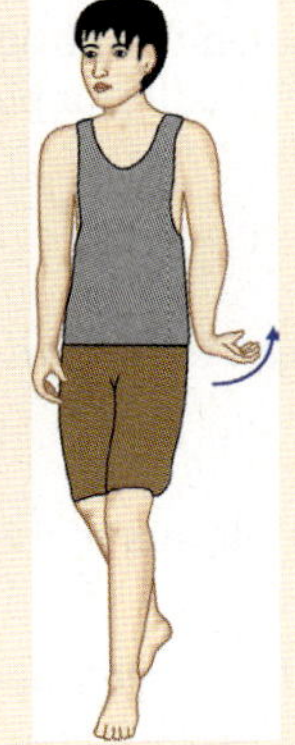

a. C5 C6 b. C7 C8
c. C8 T1 d. T5 T6

6. **Nerve injury caused by mechanism as shown in Photograph**

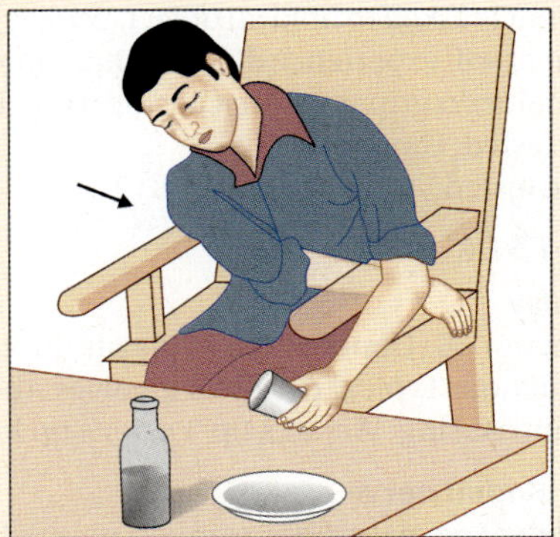

a. Median nerve b. Radial nerve
c. Axillary nerve d. Ulnar nerve

Orthopedics

7. Clinical Test doen in Orthopaedics clinic shown in Photograph is

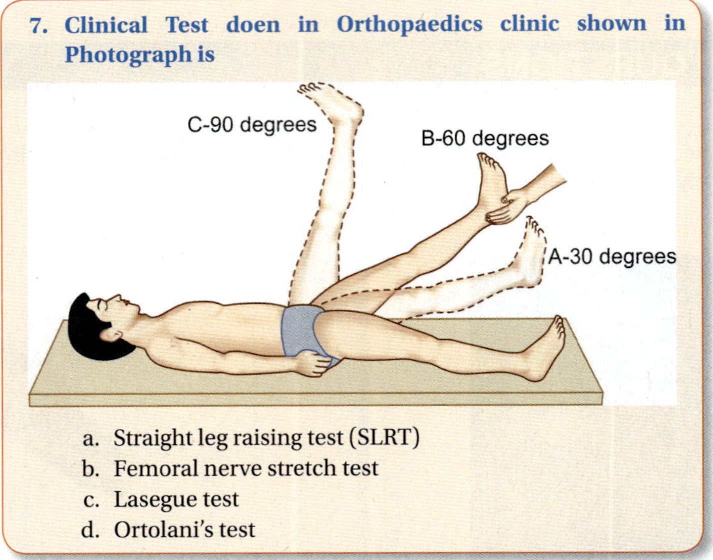

a. Straight leg raising test (SLRT)
b. Femoral nerve stretch test
c. Lasegue test
d. Ortolani's test

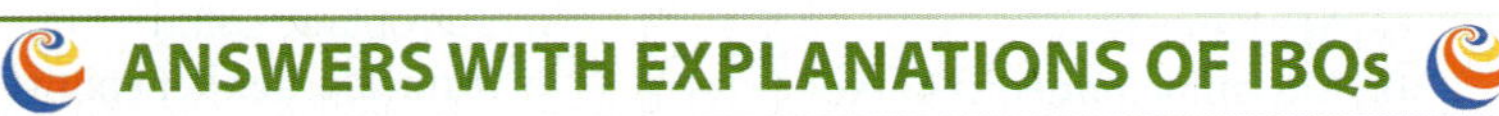

ANSWERS WITH EXPLANATIONS OF IBQs

1. Ans. (b) Median nerve *[Ref. Pediatric Emergency Medicine by Baren, 1/e p259]*

- Nerve injured in Supracondylar fracture humerus **(Photograph)**: Median nerve > Radial nerve > Ulnar nerve

2. Ans. (c) Knuckle-Bender splint *[Ref. Maheshwari, 4/e p294]*

Knuckle-Bender Splint

- Indications:
  - Ulnar claw hand (Ulnar nerve palsy)
  - Total claw hand (Median nerve + Ulnar nerve palsy)
- Function: Maintain MCP joint in 90 degree flexion and IP joints in extension
  - Immobilization of fingers
  - Stability of wrist in extension
  - Maintenance of transverse palmar arch

3. Ans. (c) Ulnar nerve *[Ref. Maheshwari, 4/e p61]*

Claw Hand (Main-En-Graffe)

- Hyperextension at MCP joint, Flexion at PIP & DIP joints
- Nerve palsy: Ulnar nerve
- Muscles paralyzed: Lumbricals

4. Ans. (d) Ulnar nerve *[Ref. Maheshwari, 4/e p65]*

Froment's Sign

- Method:
  - Patient is asked to hold an object, usually a flat object such as a piece of paper, between their thumb and index finger (pinch grip)
  - Patient will experience difficulty maintaining a hold and will compensate by flexing the FPL (flexor pollicis longus) of the thumb to maintain grip pressure causing a pinching effect
- Nerve tested: Ulnar nerve
- Muscle tested: Adductor pollicis

5. Ans. (a) C5 C6 *[Ref. Turek's Orthopedics by Buckwalter, 5/e p360]*

ERB's Palsy

- Lesion: C5, C6 (Upper brachial plexus injury)
- Presentation: Typical paralysis involves Abductors and external rotators of the shoulder, Flexors of the elbow, and Supinators of forearm, causing 'Waiter's tip/Porter's tip hand'

6. Ans. (b) Radial nerve *[Ref. Essentials of PMR by Silver, 3/e p129]*

- Saturday nerve palsy (Honeymoon palsy): Radial nerve prone to Injury in Spiral groove

7. Ans. (a) Straight leg raising test (SLRT)

- Positive STRAIGHT LEG RAISING TEST (SLRT) <40 degrees: Nerve root compression

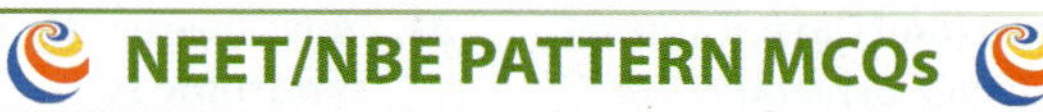

NEET/NBE PATTERN MCQs

1. Which of the following is used as a substitute for Wrist extensors in Radial nerve palsy? *[Recent Question 2016]*
a. Pronator Teres
b. Palmaris Longus
c. Flexor Digitorum Superficialis
d. Flexor Digitorum Profundus

2. A 45 years old carpenter with a blunt trauma to his arm sustained a fracture following which he developed wrist drop, loss of extension at fingers and loss of sensations on the lateral aspect of the wrist joint. Which of the following is true? *[Recent Question 2016]*
a. Patient has an injury to the Median nerve
b. He should have also lost Extension of the forearm
c. Patient has injured the Radial nerve in the spiral groove
d. There is combined involvement of Radial nerve and Median nerve

3. Wrist Drop is a feature of *[Recent Question 2016]*
a. Low radial nerve palsy
b. Posterior interosseous nerve palsy
c. High radial Nerve Palsy
d. Avulsion of triceps tendon

4. Which of the following nerve injury is most commonly associated with a Humerus shaft fracture? *[Recent Question 2016]*
a. Radial nerve
b. Median nerve
c. Axillary nerve
d. Ulnar nerve

5. Tinel's sign is seen in *[Recent Question 2016]*
a. Avascular necrosis of scaphoid
b. Kienbock's Disease
c. 1st carpometacarpal joint arthritis
d. Carpal tunnel syndrome

6. High stepping gait is due to *[Recent Question 2016]*
a. Quadriceps paralysis
b. Foot drop
c. Gluteus maximum paralysis
d. CDH

7. Seddon grading is used for *[Recent Question 2016]*
a. Classification of nerve injuries
b. Grading of open fractures
c. Classification Potts paraplegia
d. Grading of severity of malignant bone tumours

8. All of the following are Red flag signs of back pain except *[Recent Question 2016]*
a. Previous history of malignancy
b. Previous history of steroid use
c. Saddle anaesthesia
d. Age between 35 and 50

9. Disc prolapse is common in all sites except *[Recent Question 2016]*
a. L4-L5
b. L5-S1
c. C5-C6
d. T3-T4

10. In Neurapraxia, there is *[NBE FMGE September 2010]*
a. Loss of continuity of nerve
b. Loss of continuity of axon
c. Loss of conduction of nerve fibre
d. All of the above

11. Carpal tunnel syndrome is due to compression of ONE of the following nerves *[NBE DNB June 2011, AIPGME 2002, AIIMS 2008]*
a. Median nerve
b. Superficial branch of ulnar nerve
c. Deep branch of ulnar nerve
d. Superficial branch of radial nerve

12. Trendelenburg's sign is seen in *[NBE FMGE September 2012]*
a. Superior gluteal nerve injury
b. Inferior gluteal nerve injury
c. Sciatic nerve injury
d. Pudendal nerve injury

13. Wallerian degeneration is seen in *[NBE FMGE September 2009]*
a. Proximal cut-end of the nerve
b. Distal cut-end of the nerve
c. Both cut-ends of the nerve
d. Middle of the nerve

14. Klumpke's paralysis involves *[Recent Question 2012]*
a. C1-2　b. C4-5
c. C5-6　d. C8 T1

15. Cubital tunnel syndrome involves *[Recent Question 2012, 2013]*
a. Median nerve　b. Ulnar nerve
c. Tibial nerve　d. Common peroneal nerve

16. A young girl with ulnar nerve palsy will lead to all the following EXCEPT *[NBE DNB 2011]*
a. Presence of adduction of thumb
b. Loss of sensation of medial 1/3rd of hand
c. Claw hand
d. Hypothenar wasting

17. Injury to which of the nerves lead to 'Winging to scapula' *[UPSC 2007, NBE FMGE 2012]*
a. Axillary nerve　b. Radial nerve
c. Long thoracic nerve　d. Thoracodorsal nerve

18. Nerve showing best prognosis post-repair is *[NBE DNB 2010]*
a. Radial nerve　b. Ulnar nerve
c. Median nerve　d. Axillary nerve

19. Knuckle & Bender splint is for *[Recent Question 2012]*
a. Median nerve injury　b. Radial nerve injury
c. Ulnar nerve injury　d. None

20. Tinel's sign suggests *[NBE FMGE September 2007, FMGE September 2012, NBE DNB June 2011, December 2011, Recent Question 2017]*
a. Nerve degeneration　b. Nerve regeneration
c. Glomus tumour　d. Neurofibroma

Orthopedics

21. Nerve damage due to hamate dislocation (Carpal tunnel syndrome) is *[NBE FMGE September 2005]*
a. Median and ulnar b. Median
c. Ulnar d. Radial

22. MC cause of Tardy Ulnar nerve palsy *[NBE DNB 1996, AIIMS 1991, Recent Question 2014]*
a. Olecranon fracture
b. Supracondylar fracture humerus
c. Elbow dislocation (posterior)
d. Lateral Condylar fracture

23. MC nerve involved in Lunate dislocation in Carpal tunnel syndrome is *[Recent Question 2014]*
a. Anterior Interosseous b. Axillary
c. Radial d. Median

24. Cause of atonic bladder *[UPSC 1988]*
a. Injury to upper thoracic cord
b. Injury to sacral plexus
c. Urinary tract infection
d. Pregnancy

25. Inability to flex the index finger is a sign of *[UPSC 2011]*
a. Ulnar nerve injury b. Radial nerve injury
c. Median nerve injury d. Dupuytren's contracture

26. Match nerve injury and deformity *[NBE DNB 1993, NBE DNB 2003]*

A: Radial nerve; I: Claw hand
B: Ulnar nerve; II: Wrist drop
C: Axillary nerve; III: Porter tip hand
D: Upper trunk; IV: Flattened shoulder

a. A - I; B - II; C - IV; D - III
b. A - I; B - II; C - III; D - IV
c. A - II; B - I; C - III; D - IV
d. A - II; B - I; C - IV; D - III

27. Nerve injured in fracture of upper end of radius is *[UPSC 2006]*
a. Ulnar nerve b. Radial nerve
c. Median nerve d. Posterior interosseous nerve

28. Card test is used for paralysis of *[NBE FMGE March 2005]*
a. Radial nerve b. Median nerve
c. Ulnar nerve d. Musculocutaneous nerve

29. Wasting of intrinsic muscles of hand can be expected to follow the injury of *[UPSC 2009]*
a. Ulnar nerve b. Radial nerve
c. Brachial nerve d. Axillary nerve

30. Match the following sets *[NBE DNB 1998, NBE DNB 1999, NBE DNB 2001]*

A: Erb's palsy; I: Upper trunk injury
B: Klumpke's palsy; II: Lower trunk injury
C: Crutch paralysis; III: Ulnar nerve injury
D: Fracture surgical neck humerus; IV: Radial nerve injury

a. A - I; B - II; C - IV; D - III
b. A - I; B - II; C - III; D - IV
c. A - II; B - I; C - III; D - IV
d. A - II; B - I; C - IV; D - III

31. Most frequently involved cranial nerve in Guillain Barre syndrome is *[FMGE September 2012]*
a. Abducens nerve b. Trigeminal nerve
c. Oculomotor nerve d. Facial nerve

32. Froment's sign is characteristically seen in *[Recent Question 2013, 2014, NBE FMGE 2012, AIIMS 1997]*
a. Ulnar nerve injury
b. Median nerve injury
c. Radial nerve injury
d. Intercostobrachial nerve injury

33. Neuropathic joints are seen in all except *[FMGE September 2012, WB PG 1991]*
a. Diabetes mellitus b. Syphilis
c. Neurofibromatosis d. Myelomeningocoele

34. Tinel sign is used for *[Recent Question 2012, 2013]*
a. To assess the severity of damage of nerve
b. To classify the type of nerve injury
c. To locate the site of nerve injury
d. To assess the recovery

35. Neuropraxia is a condition characterized by *[NBE FMGE March 2012]*
a. Division of nerve sheath b. Division of axons
c. Division of nerve fibres d. Physiological paralysis

36. Tardy ulnar nerve palsy *[Recent Question 2013]*
a. Early onset
b. Late onset
c. Caused by shoulder dislocation
d. None

37. 'Ulnar paradox' is seen in *[Recent Question 2016, 2017, Recent Question 2012]*
a. High ulnar lesion b. Low ulnar lesion
c. Triple nerve disease d. None of the above

38. Carpal tunnel syndrome all are present except *[Recent Question 2013]*
a. Ulnar nerve dysfunction b. Tinel sign
c. Phalen's sign d. Pain & paraesthesia of wrist

39. Erb's paralysis involves *[Recent Question 2012, 2017]*
a. C5 C6 b. C8 T1
c. T1 T2 d. None

40. In axillary nerve paralysis, all the following are true except *[Recent Question 2012]*
a. Deltoid muscle is wasted
b. Extension of shoulder with arm abducted to 90 degrees is impossible
c. Small area of numbness is present over the shoulder region
d. Patient cannot initiate abduction

41. Ulnar nerve paralysis causes *[NBE FMGE March 2012]*
a. Ape thumb deformity b. Wrist drop
c. Claw finger deformity d. Madelung deformity

42. Sunderland Classification is used for *[Recent Question 2015]*
a. Maxillary fractures b. Pelvic ring injuries
c. Peripheral nerve injuries d. Epiphyseal injuries

43. Spina bifida is associated with *[Recent Question 2015]*
a. Cleft lip/palate b. Congenital hydrocephalus
c. Meningomyelocoele d. Leukemia

44. Keyboard operators and typists are especially susceptible to injury of the *[UPSC CMS 2015]*
a. Axillary nerve b. Median nerve
c. Ulnar nerve d. Radial nerve

45. An 18 years old boy had a closed lower limb injury while riding his motorbike. He was brought to hospital where on examination he had severe pain which increased on passive movement of effected limb with distal sensory disturbances. What is the probable diagnosis?
a. Degloving Injury *[UPSC CMS 2015]*
b. High Pressure Injection injury
c. Compartment syndrome
d. Deep Vein thrombosis

46. Tinel's sign is *[Recent Question 2017]*
a. Sensation on tapping the nerve
b. Numbness in the region of the nerve on inflating the pneumatic cuff
c. Tingling on flexion of the joint
d. Applying direct pressure

47. A patient presents with normal Babinski reflex with ankle areflexia with presence of saddle anesthesia and difficulty in micturition. What is the most probable diagnosis? *[Recent Question 2017]*
a. Cauda equina syndrome
b. Brown-Sequard syndrome
c. Leriche syndrome
d. Williams syndrome

48. What is the age of tendon transfer in Post-polio residual paralysis? *[Recent Question 2017]*
a. <6 months b. 1 year
c. 2 years d. >5 years

49. Crutch palsy is injury to which nerve? *[Recent Question 2017]*
a. Median nerve
b. Ulnar nerve
c. Radial nerve
d. Musculocutaneous nerve

HIGH YIELD MCQs

1. Not involved in entrapment neuropathy is
a. Ulnar nerve *[AIPGME 2007, 2009]*
b. Median nerve
c. Femoral nerve
d. Lateral cutaneous nerve of thigh

2. In Seddon's classification, complete division of nerve is *[ROHTAK PGMEE 1999]*
a. Neuropraxia b. Axonotmesis
c. Neurotmesis d. None of the above

3. Which one of the following statement is wrong about Erb's palsy? *[NIMS PGMEE 2000]*
a. Abductors of the shoulder are weak
b. Upper part of brachial plexus is involved
c. Supinators are normal
d. Internal rotation of arm

4. Erb's point is located at the junction of
a. Anterior primary rami of C5 and C6 *[WB PGMEE 2001]*
b. Anterior primary rami of C8 and T1
c. Superior and middle trunk of Brachial plexus
d. None of the above

5. Erb's palsy is due to involvement of *[UP PGMEE 1999]*
a. Upper trunk of brachial plexus
b. Middle trunk of brachial plexus
c. Lower trunk of brachial plexus
d. Long thoracic nerve

6. Commonest cause of wrist drop is *[Karnataka PGMEE 1997]*
a. Intramuscular injection b. Fracture humerus
c. Dislocation of elbow d. Dislocation of shoulder

7. Injury to which of the following nerves is most likely to result in Wrist drop? *[UP PGMEE 1994, Rajasthan PGMEE 1998, Recent Question 2014]*
a. Radial b. Ulnar
c. Median d. Musculocutaneous

8. Saturday night palsy involves nerve *[Recent Question 2016, AMU PGMEE 1989, Delhi PGMEE 1994]*
a. Radial b. Ulnar
c. Median d. Axillary
e. Any of the above

9. In fracture of distal half of humerus, the nerve injured is *[UP PGMEE 1999]*
a. Axillary b. Median
c. Radial d. Ulnar

10. After injury to radial nerve in radial groove, first sign of recovery is *[AIIMS PGMEE 1989]*
a. Tinel's sign
b. Power in extensor carpi radialis longus
c. Poorer in Brachioradialis
d. Power in Triceps

11. A young boy who was driving motorcycle at a high speed collided with a tree & was thrown on his right shoulder. Though there was no fracture, his right arm was medially rotated and forearm pronated. The following facts concerning this patient are correct, except
a. The injury was at Erb's point *[AIIMS PGMEE 2004]*
b. A lesion of C5 and C6 was present
c. The median and ulnar nerves were affected
d. Supraspinatus, Infraspinatus, Subclavius & Biceps brachii were paralyzed

12. **Best results of nerve suturing are seen in** *[UP PGMEE 1997]*
   a. Radial nerve b. Ulnar nerve
   c. Median nerve d. Sciatic nerve

13. **The nerve involved in anterior dislocation of the shoulder is** *[All India PGMEE 1996]*
   a. Radial nerve b. Axillary nerve
   c. Ulnar nerve d. Musculocutaneous nerve

14. **Complete transaction of the spinal cord at the C7 level produces all of the following effects except** *[All India PGMEE 2002]*
   a. Hypotension b. Limited respiratory effort
   c. Anaesthesia below the level of the lesion
   d. Areflexia below the level of the lesion

15. **A 40 years old male after RTA, attains spinal injury. His lower limb power is greater than that of upper limb and sacral sensations are present. Type of spinal cord lesion is** *[AIIMS PGMEE 1992, NIMHANS PGMEE 2003, JIPMER PGMEE 2005]*
   a. Central cord syndrome
   b. Anterior cord syndrome
   c. Posterior cord syndrome
   d. Complete spinal cord injury

16. **Feature of radial nerve injury at spiral groove** *[TN PGMEE 1999]*
   a. No wrist drop
   b. Sensory loss over deltoid
   c. Thumb, finger, wrist drop
   d. Wrist droop + Extensors of Forearm paralysis

17. **Radial nerve is most commonly injured in fracture of** *[UP PGMEE 1994]*
   a. Mid shaft of humerus
   b. Neck of humerus
   c. Lateral condyle of humerus
   d. Lower 1/3rd of humerus

18. **All of the following muscles undergo paralysis after injury to C5 and C6 spinal nerves except** *[AIIMS PGMEE 2004]*
   a. Biceps b. Coracobrachialis
   c. Brachialis d. Brachioradialis

19. **A 19 years old boy fell from the motor bike on his shoulder. The doctor diagnosed him a case of Erb's paralysis. The following signs and symptoms will be observed except** *[AIIMS PGMEE 2002]*
   a. Loss of abduction at shoulder joint
   b. Loss of lateral rotation
   c. Loss of pronation at radioulnar joint
   d. Loss of flexion at elbow joint.

20. **Lower branch of brachial plexus injury leads to** *[APPG 1988, 1997]*
   a. Erb's palsy b. Klumpke's palsy
   c. Bell's palsy d. Wrist drop

21. **Mode of injury of Klumpke's paralysis is** *[Bihar PGMEE 1988]*
   a. Forcible increase in the neck shoulder angle [As during child birth)
   b. Forcible rotation of upper arm
   c. Forcible hyperabduction of upper arm (falling person trying to catch an object)
   d. Fracture shaft humerus

22. **Injury to radial nerve - mid humerus level following occurs** *[PGI 1992]*
   a. Paralysis of extensors of hand & wrist
   b. Equally diagnosed by sensory and motor testing
   c. Can be approached by a lifting triceps
   d. Can be approached by splitting latissimus dorsi
   e. Paralysis of Triceps

23. **Damage to the radial nerve in the spinal groove spares which muscle** *[All India PGMEE 1994]*
   a. Lateral head of triceps
   b. Long head of triceps
   c. Medial head of triceps
   d. Anconeus

24. **Injury to radial nerve in lower part of spiral groove** *[All India PGMEE 2003]*
   a. Spares nerve supply to extensor carpi radialis longus
   b. Results in paralysis of anconeus muscle
   c. Leaves extensions at elbow joint intact
   d. Weakens pronation movement

25. **A patient presented with Saddle anaesthesia, bladder & bowel are normal and muscle power is normal. The diagnosis is** *[NIMS PGMEE 1998, AMU PGMEE 2000]*
   a. Cauda equina syndrome
   b. L3-L4 root involvement
   c. Conus medullaris lesion
   d. L4-L5 disc prolapse

26. **Most common nerve to be damaged in dislocation of shoulder is** *[All India PGMEE 1997, Orissa 1991]*
   a. Axillary nerve b. Radial nerve
   c. Median nerve d. Musculocutaneous nerve

27. **Anterior dislocation of shoulder is most commonly complicated by** *[AIIMS PGMEE 1992, PGI 1997]*
   a. Axillary artery injury
   b. Circumflex nerve injury
   c. Recurrent dislocation
   d. Radial nerve injury

28. **Cock up splint is used in management of** *[AIIMS PGMEE 1995, 1997, Recent Question 2014, 2017]*
   a. Ulnar nerve palsy
   b. Brachial plexus palsy
   c. Radial nerve palsy
   d. Combined ulnar & Median nerve palsy

29. **A 25 years old lady sustained a lacerated wound on the back of right thigh by a horn of a bull. The wound was sutured. Two months later she developed foot drop and an ulcer on the dorsum of the foot. The most likely diagnosis is** *[UPSC 1997]*
   a. Chronic ischaemia to limbs due to Popliteal artery injury
   b. Partial injury to sciatic nerve
   c. Complete division of sciatic nerve
   d. Injury to hamstring muscles

30. **Section of Lateral popliteal nerve at the neck of fibula causes** *[PGI 1990]*
   a. Foot drop b. Trophic ulcers on toes
   c. Atrophy of calf muscle d. Pain in the leg

31. Foot drop result because of injury to *[PGI 1991]*
a. Superficial peroneal nerve
b. Deep peroneal nerve
c. Posterior tibial nerve
d. Anterior tibial nerve

32. Sudden hyperflexion of thigh over abdomen (Mcroberts procedure), which of the following nerve is commonly involved *[AIIMS PGMEE 2008]*
a. Common peroneal nerve
b. Obturator nerve
c. Lumbosacral trunk
d. Lateral cutaneous nerve of thigh

33. Which of the following does not involve nerve damage? *[AIIMS PGMEE 1994]*
a. Guillain Barre syndrome b. Erb's paralysis
c. Volkmann's paralysis d. Neurotmesis

34. A 45 years male present with abrupt onset, pain weakness, loss of contour of shoulder and wasting of muscle of arm on 5th day of tetanus toxoid immunization in deltoid. Likely cause is. *[AIIMS PGMEE 2009]*
a. Radial nerve entrapment b. Thoracic outlet syndrome
c. Brachial neuritis d. Hysteria

35. All of the following are features of musculocutaneous nerve injury at axilla except *[All India PGMEE 1998]*
a. Loss of flexion of shoulder
b. Loss of flexion at elbow
c. Loss of supination of forearm
d. Loss of sensation on radial side of forearm

36. All of the following features can be observed after the injury to axillary nerve, except *[All India PGMEE 2003]*
a. Loss of rounded contour of shoulder
b. Loss of sensation along lateral side of upper arm
c. Loss of overhead abduction
d. Atrophy of deltoid muscle

37. Injury to the common peroneal nerve at the lateral aspect of head of fibula results in all of the following except: *[AIIMS PGMEE 2004]*
a. Weakness of ankle dorsi-flexion
b. Foot drop
c. Loss of ankle reflex
d. Sensory impairment on lateral aspect of leg extending to the dorsum of foot

38. Which of the following does NOT predispose to carpal tunnel syndrome *[AIIMS PGMEE 1994]*
a. Hypertension b. Hypothyroidism
c. Pregnancy d. Acromegaly

39. True about carpel tunnel syndrome *[PGI 2003]*
a. Paraesthesia of the lateral 2 fingers
b. Atrophy of the thenar eminence
c. Atrophy of the hypothenar eminence
d. Claw hand
e. Tinel sign is positive

40. Which of the following nerve injuries produce the deformities? *[NBE DNB 1993]*
I. Upper trunk I. Wrist drop
II. Ulnar nerve II. Porter's tip hand
III. Axillary nerve; III. Claw hand
IV. Radial nerve; IV. Flattening of the shoulder

Select the correct combination
a. I (i) II (ii) III(iii) IV (iv)
b. I (ii) II (iii) III (iv) IV (i)
c. I (iii) II (iv) III (ii) IV (i)
d. I (iv) II (iii) III (ii) IV (i)

41. Match the following *[NBE DNB 1999]*
i. Erb's paralysis; i. Lower trunk injury
ii. Klumpke's paralysis; ii. Axillary nerve injury
iii. Crutch paralysis; iii. Radial nerve injury
iv. Fractures surgical neck humerus; iv. Upper trunk injury

Select the correct combination
a. I (iv) II (iii) III (ii) IV (i)
b. I (iii) II (ii) III (iv) IV (i)
c. I (iv) II (i) III (iii) IV (ii)
d. I (i) II (iii) III (iv) IV (ii)

42. Symmetrical areflexic bladder bowel & lower limb occur in *[NIMHANS PGMEE 2002, MAHE PGMEE 2003]*
a. Cauda equina syndrome
b. Conus medullaris syndrome
c. Nerve root damage
d. Brown sequard syndrome

43. True about carpal tunnel syndrome is all except *[PGI 2009]*
a. More common in males
b. Acromegaly can cause
c. Positive tinel's sign
d. Nerve conduction study done
e. Transverse carpal ligament are cut to relieve symptom

44. Commonest cause for neuralgic pain in foot is *[All India PGMEE 2003]*
a. Compression of communication between medial and lateral planter nerves
b. Exaggeration of longitudinal arches
c. Injury to deltoid ligament
d. Shortening of planter aponeurosis

45. Cause of atonic bladder is *[UPSC 1988]*
a. Injury to sacral plexus
b. Injury to upper thoracic cord
c. Pregnancy
d. UTI

46. A paralysed bladder following spinal injury is best managed by *[AIIMS PGMEE 1993]*
a. Gibbon's catheter
b. Malecot catheter
c. Foley's catheter
d. Metallic catheter

47. Most common nerve involved in Volkmann's ischaemic contracture of forearm includes *[All India PGMEE 1999]*
a. Radial b. Ulnar
c. Median d. Posterior interosseous

48. Dislocation of which one of the following carpal bones can present as median nerve palsy? *[UPSC 1995]*
a. Scaphoid b. Hamate
c. Lunate d. Trapezium

49. Post Poliomyelitis, a patient has grade II power in Gastrocnemius, grade III is Peroneus, grade IV in Tibialis Anterior. The deformity is *[All India PGMEE 2000]*

a. Calcaneovalgus b. Equino varus
c. Calcaneovarus d. Genu valgus

50. In 3 years child with polio paralysis, tendon transfer operation is done at *[AIIMS PGMEE 1998]*

a. 2 months after the disease
b. 2 years after the disease
c. 6-12 months after the disease
d. After skeleton maturation

51. Injury of median nerve at wrist is best detected by *[All India PGMEE 1997]*

a. Action of abductor pollicis brevis
b. Action of flexor pollicis brevis
c. Loss of sensation of radial half of palm
d. Loss of sensation of tip of ring finger

52. Pointing index sign in seen in ...... nerve palsy *[UPSC 1986, Kerala PGMEE 1987, AIIMS PGMEE 1997, JIPMER PGMEE 2014]*

a. Ulnar b. Radial
c. Median d. Axillary

53. Spina bifida occulta is *[Karnataka PGMEE 1997]*

a. Infection of the spine
b. Traumatic fracture of the spine
c. Congenital fusion of the body of the Vertebra
d. Congenital non fusion of the spinal lamina

54. Hari Verdhman, 9 years old child, presents with scoliosis, hairy tuft in the skin of back and neurological deficit. Plain X-rays reveal multiple vertebral anomalies & a vertical bony spur overlying lumbar spine on AP view. The most probable diagnosis is *[All India PGMEE 2002]*

a. Dorsal dermal sinus
b. Diastematomyelia
c. Tight filum terminale
d. Caudal regression syndrome

55. Most common cause of neurological deficit in upper limb is *[AIIMS PGMEE 1993]*

a. Poliomyelitis b. Erb's palsy
c. C1-C2 dislocation
d. Fracture dislocation of cervical spine

56. Posterior interosseous nerve is injured in *[AP PGMEE 1999]*

a. Posterior dislocation of elbow
b. Monteggia fracture dislocation
c. Reverse monteggia fracture dislocation
d. Supracondylar fracture of humerus

57. A patient involved in a road traffic accident presents with quadriparesis, sphincter disturbance, sensory level up to the upper border of sternum and a respiratory rate of 35/ minute. The likely level of lesion is *[All India PGMEE 2010]*

a. C1-C2 b. C4-C5
c. Tl-T2 d. T3-T4

58. Median nerve is injured during *[JIPMER PGMEE 2000]*

a. Elbow dislocation
b. Fracture lateral epicondyle of humerus
c. Fracture medial epicondyle of humerus
d. Supracondylar fracture of humerus

59. Median nerve injury at the wrist causes *[PGI 1998]*

a. Claw hand
b. Loss of apposition of thumb
c. Policeman's tip deformity
d. Saturday night palsy

60. 'Ape thumb deformity' is observed in lesions of *[Bihar PGMEE 1991, All India PGMEE 2000]*

a. Radial nerve injury
b. Ulnar nerve injury
c. Median nerve injury
d. Circumflex humeral nerve injury
e. Posterior interosseous nerve injury

61. Compression of a nerve within the carpal tunnel products inability to *[AIIMS PGMEE 2005]*

a. Abduct the thumb
b. Adduct the thumb
c. Flex the distal phalanx of the thumb
d. Oppose the thumb

62. Median nerve lesion at the wrist causes all of the following, except *[All India PGMEE 2010]*

a. Thenar Atrophy
b. Weakness of adductor Pollicis
c. Weakness of 1st and 2nd Lumbricals
d. Weakness of Flexor Pollicis Brevis

63. Nerve roots involved in Erb's palsy *[TN PGMEE 1994]*

a. C3 C4 b. C4 C5
c. C5 C6 d. C7 C8

64. Most common nerve involvement is dislocation of Lunate is *[UP PGMEE 1998, PGI 2000]*

a. Median nerve b. Anterior interosseous
c. Posterior interosseous d. Median nerve

65. Which carpal bone fracture causes median nerve involvement? *[AIIMS PGMEE 2000]*

a. Scaphoid b. Lunate
c. Trapezium d. Trapezoid

66. Consider the following nerve injuries *[NBE DNB 1999]*

Axonotmesis
Neurotmesis
Neuropraxia

Correct sequence of these injuries in terms of 'increasing' severity of damage to the nerve fibres and sheath, is

a. 1, 2 and 3 b. 3, 2 and 1
c. 2, 1 and 3 d. 3, 1 and 2

67. Rate of regeneration of severed nerve is *[AP PGMEE 1991]*

a. 0.1 mm/day b. 1 mm/day
c. 1 cm/day d. None

68. Median nerve injury at wrist, is commonly tested by *[All India PGMEE 1997]*

a. Contraction of abductor pollicis brevis
b. Contraction of flexor pollicis brevis

Orthopedics

c. Loss of sensation on palm
d. Loss of sensation on ring finger

69. A cut injury on wrist causes inability of thumb to touch the tip of little finger, the nerve likely to be damaged is
a. Ulnar *[AIIMS PGMEE 1997]*
b. Radial
c. Median
d. Deep branch of ulnar nerve

70. A boy presents with complaints of hypoaesthesia and wasting of thenar eminence. The nerve most likely to damaged in this patient *[AIIMS PGMEE 2002]*
a. Musculocutaneous nerve b. Median nerve
c. Ulnar nerve d. Radial nerve

71. Tardy ulnar nerve palsy is due to *[Kerala PGMEE 1987, UPSC 1986, Bihar PGMEE 1990]*
a. Cubitus valgus
b. Fixation of nerve in the groove by
c. Excision of elbow joint
d. Fracture of internal condyle

72. "Tinel's sign" indicates *[Bihar PGMEE 1991]*
a. Neurofibroma
b. Injury to peripheral nerves
c. Atrophy of nerves
d. Regeneration of nerves

73. Disability of hand is maximum with lesion of *[PGI 1990]*
a. Median nerve at elbow b. Median nerve at wrist
c. Ulnar nerve at elbow d. Ulnar nerve at wrist
e. Radial nerve lesion

74. Cervical spondylosis *[Bihar PGMEE 1998]*
a. Most frequently results from an incidence of acute trauma
b. Causes compression of nerve roots to produce an upper motor neuron lesion in the lower limbs
c. Produces pain and Paresthesia over the lateral aspect of the forearm and thumb when affecting the 6th cervical nerve
d. Most frequently affects the upper cervical vertebrae

75. In cervical spondylosis which part of vertebral body involved *[Delhi PGMEE 1999]*
a. Inferior articular facet b. Pars interarticularis
c. Superior articular facet d. All of the above

76. Osteophytes developing at the joint at Luschka characteristically compress spinal nerves at *[NIMS PGMEE 1996]*
a. Intervertebral foramen
b. Anterior part of body
c. Posterior part of body
d. Paradural areas

77. Gradual painful limitation of shoulder movements in an elderly suggest that the most probable diagnosis is *[Orissa PGMEE 1990]*
a. Arthritis b. Osteoarthritis
c. Periarthritis d. Myositis Ossificans
e. Fracture - dislocation

78. Claw hand is caused by lesion of *[All India PGMEE 1991, 2007]*
a. Radial nerve b. Ulnar nerve
c. Median nerve d. Axillary nerve

79. Most common nerve involvement in fracture surgical neck humerus *[All India PGMEE 2002, AIIMS PGMEE 1997]*
a. Axillary nerve b. Radial nerve
c. Ulnar nerve d. Median nerve

80. A boy fell down from a tree and has fracture of neck of humerus. He cannot raise his arm because of the involvement of *[All India PGMEE 2000]*
a. Axillary nerve
b. Supraspinatus nerve
c. Musculocutaneous nerve
d. Radial nerve

81. Wrist drop occurs due to *[UP PGMEE 1994]*
a. Radial nerve b. Ulnar nerve
c. Median nerve d. Posterior interosseous nerve

82. Tardy ulnar nerve palsy seen in *[AIIMS PGMEE 1998]*
a. Medial condyle fracture humerus
b. Lateral condyle fracture humerus
c. Supracondylar condyle fracture humerus
d. Fracture shaft humerus

83. Tourniquet paralysis is an unfortunate complication leads to *[Karnataka PGMEE 1990]*
a. Neuropraxia b. Axonotmesis
c. Neurotmesis d. None of the above

84. Following are the recognized causes of Charcot's (Neuropathic) joint, EXCEPT for *[TN PGMEE 1994]*
a. Peripheral neuritis b. Syringomyelia
c. Tabes dorsalis d. Hysterical joint

85. Neuropathic joint of foot and ankle is most commonly due to *[TN PGMEE 1999]*
a. CTEV b. Hansen's disease
c. Polio d. Mycetoma

86. Charcot's joints have all of the following characteristics except *[UP PGMEE 1997]*
a. Copious effusion in the joint
b. Painful limitation of joint movements
c. Hypermobility of joint
d. Osteophyte formation

87. Nerve suturing in a clean cut injury is done best in *[NBE DNB 1999]*
a. 6 hours b. 12 hours
c. After one day d. After one day

88. In Seddon's Classification, complete division of nerve is *[Rohtak PGMEE 1989]*
a. Neuropraxia b. Axonotmesis
c. Neurotmesis d. None of the above

89. Following indicate better prognosis is in injury except *[JIPMER PGMEE 1993]*
a. Neuropraxia b. Younger age
c. Pure motor nerve injury d. Proximal injury

90. Most common cause of acute sciatica is due to *[AP PGMEE 1999]*
a. Syphilis of spine
b. Tuberculosis of spine
c. Secondaries of spine
d. Acute prolapsed Intervertebral disc

91. Ulnar nerve injury at wrist results in *[Manipal PGMEE 1997]*
a. Unable to grasp card between the fingers
b. Claw hand
c. Inability to abduct or adduct the fingers
d. All of the above

92. Ulnar nerve severed above elbow causes *[PGI 1991]*
a. Complete loss of sensation in 4th and 5th finger
b. Paralysis of all lumbricals
c. Paralysis of all interosseia
d. Paralysis of flexor carpi ulnaris
e. Paralysis of flexor profundus

93. A factory worker has laceration proximal to wrist with no opposition of thumb and fingers, loss of sensation over lateral aspect of thumb and fingers. Diagnosis is injury to *[UPSC 1991, 2000]*
a. Median nerve + Ulnar nerve
b. Median + Radial nerves
c. Radial + Ulnar nerves
d. Median nerve only

94. Prognosis after secondary nerve suturing is better in pure than in mixed ones. Based on this criterion, which one of the following nerves should be given the best result after suturing in identical conditions? *[Karnataka PGMEE 1990]*
a. Common peroneal nerve
b. Radial nerve
c. Ulnar nerve
d. Median nerve

95. Best results of nerve suturing are seen in *[AMU PGMEE 1992, UP PGMEE 1997]*
a. Median nerve
b. Ulnar nerve
c. Sciatic nerve
d. Radial nerve

96. All are true regarding brachial plexus injury, *except* *[Recent Question 2017, All India PGMEE 2006]*
a. Preganglionic lesions have a better prognosis than postganglionic lesions
b. Erb's palsy causes paralysis of the abductors and external rotators of the shoulder
c. In Klumpke's palsy, Horner's syndrome may be present on the ipsilateral side
d. Histamine test is useful to differentiate between the preganglionic and postganglionic lesions

97. Froment's sign is positive due to paralysis of *[AIIMS PGMEE 1993]*
a. Opponens pollicis
b. Abductor pollicis
c. Adductor pollicis
d. Adductor hallucis longus

98. A 60-year-old man with diabetes mellitus presents with painless, swollen right ankle joint. Radiographs of the ankle show destroyed joint with large number of loose bodies. The most probable diagnosis is *[All India PGMEE 2003]*
a. Charcot's joint
b. Clutton's joint
c. Osteoarthritis
d. Rheumatoid arthritis

99. In a patient suffering from Tabes dorsalis Charcot's joint occurs most commonly at *[Rajasthan PGMEE 1993]*
a. Elbow
b. Tarsometatarsal
c. Wrist
d. Knee

100. Dissociative sensory loss occurs in *[TN PGMEE 1993]*
a. Tuberculosis of spine
b. Disc prolapse
c. Tabes dorsalis
d. Syringomyelia

101. A boy presents with injury to medial epicondyle of the humerus. Which of the following would not be seen *[AIIMS PGMEE 2002]*
a. Weakness of the ulnar deviation and flexion
b. Complete paralysis of the IIIrd and IVth digits
c. Atrophy of the hypothenar eminence
d. Decreased sensation of the hypothenar eminence

102. All of the following muscles are paralyzed in trauma to median nerve at the wrist except *[AIIMS PGMEE 2008]*
a. Adductor pollicis
b. Abductor pollicis
c. First two lumbricals
d. Muscle of the Thenar eminence

103. Ulnar nerve injury at wrist involves following except *[PGI 1998]*
a. Palmar interossei
b. Opponens pollicis
c. Dorsal interossei
d. Adductor pollicis

104. Low ulnar nerve palsy is characterised by *[PGI 2003]*
a. Claw hand
b. Sensory loss of medial four digits
c. Weakness of grips
d. Inability to extend at MCP joint
e. Inability to abduct the thumb

105. A pole vaulter had a fall during pole vaulting and had paralysis of the arm. Which of the following investigations gives the best recovery prognosis? *[AIIMS PGMEE 2003]*
a. Electromyography
b. Muscle biopsy
c. Strength Duration Curve
d. Creatine phosphokinase levels

106. In a full term newly born male baby, on routine checkup soon after delivery has weak Moro's reflex on right hand but intact Grasp's reflex with weak abduction and supination movement of hand is found. This will suggest that most likely injury would be at *[AIIMS PGMEE 1999]*
a. C5, C6 nerve
b. C7, C8 nerve
c. C5, T1 nerve
d. T1, T2 nerve

107. Injury to the Ulnar nerve at the wrist causes paralysis of *[All India PGMEE 1995]*
a. Apposition of the thumb
b. Abduction of the carpometacarpal joint of the thumb
c. Adduction of the thumb
d. Flexion of the MCP joint of the middle finger

108. A patient with leprosy presents with clumsiness of hand. His ulnar nerve is affected. Clumsiness is due to palsy of which muscle *[AIIMS PGMEE 2000]*
a. Extensor carpi ulnaris
b. Abductor pollicis brevis
c. Opponens pollicis
d. Interosseous muscle

109. A person is not able to extend his metacarpophalangeal joint. This is due to injury to which nerve *[AIIMS PGMEE 2000]*
a. Ulnar nerve
b. Radial nerve injury
c. Median nerve injury
d. Posterior Interosseous nerve injury

110. A 44-year-old man presented with acute onset of low backache radiating to the right lower limb. Examination revealed SLRT <40° on the right side, weakness of extensor hallucis longus on the right side, sensory loss in the first web space of the right foot and brisk knee jerk. Which of the following is the most likely diagnosis? *[AIIMS PGMEE 2004]*

a. Prolapsed intervertebral disc L4-5
b. Spondylolysis L5-S1
c. Lumbar canal stenosis
d. Spondylolisthesis L4-5

111. A previously healthy 45 years old laborer suddenly develops acute lower back pain with right-leg pain & weakness of dorsiflexion of the right great toe. Which of the following is true *[All India PGMEE 2002]*

a. Immediate treatment should include analgesics muscle relaxants & back strengthening exercises
b. The appearance of the foot drop indicate early surgical intervention
c. If the neurological sign resolve within 2 to 3 weeks but low back pain persists, the proper treatment would include fusion of affected Lumbar vertebra
d. If the neurological signs fail to resolve within 1 week, Lumbar laminectomy and excision of any herniated nucleus pulposus should be done.

112. Which of the following is not recommended in the treatment of Chronic Low Back Pain? *[All India PGMEE 2009]*

a. NSAIDs
b. Bed Rest for 3 months
c. Exercises
d. Epidural steroid Injection

113. In spondylolisthesis, there is fracture of vertebra in

a. Spinous process *[Bihar PGMEE I998]*
b. Neural arch pars inter articularis
c. Transverse process
d. Body

114. True about spondylolisthesis is/are *[PGI 1991]*

a. Congenital defect of posterior arch
b. Slipping of L5 over S1
c. Progressive slipping
d. Abnormal congenital development

115. A 30-year-old male underwent excision of the right radial head. Following surgery, the patient developed inability to extend the fingers and thumb of the right hand. He did not have any sensory deficit. Which one of the following is the most likely cause? *[AIIMS PGMEE 2004]*

a. Injury to Posterior interosseous nerve
b. Iatrogenic injury to common extensor origin
c. Injury to anterior interosseous nerve
d. High radial nerve palsy

116. The most common nerve involvement in Volkmam's ischemic contracture is *[ESI IMO 2014]*

a. Ulnar nerve
b. Posterior interosseous nerve
c. Median nerve
d. Radial nerve

117. Which of the following nerve is involved in 'Pronator teres syndrome'? *[AIIMS PG November 2015]*

a. Ulnar nerve
b. Radius nerve
c. Median nerve
d. Anterior interosseous nerve

Orthopedics

NEET/NBE PATTERN MCQs ANSWERS WITH EXPLANATIONS 

1. Ans. (a) **Pronator Teres**
[Ref. Orthopaedics by Miller, 6/e p585]

Radial Nerve Palsy - Tendon transfers
- Wrist extension: Pronator teres to ECRB
- Finger extension: FCU or FCR to EDC II-IV
- Thumb extension: PL to EPL

2. Ans. (c) **Patient has injured the Radial nerve in the spiral groove**
[Ref. Clinical Anatomy for Students by Kulkarni, 1/e p58]

Radial Nerve Injuries Spiral groove Affects
- Brachioradialis
- Wrist extensors
- Supinator
- Wrist/Thumb extensors
- Sensory loss of Dorsum of hand (1st Interosseous space)

3. Ans. (c) **High radial Nerve Palsy**
[Ref. Orthopaedics & Applied Physiotherapy by Joshi, 3/e]

Radial Nerve Palsies
- **Above spiral groove**: Total wrist drop, Sensory loss over dorsum of thumb
- **Between spiral groove and lateral epicondyle**: Loss of wrist/ thumb/ finger extensors, Sensory loss over dorsum of first web space (Sparing of elbow extensors)
- **Below elbow**: Loss of thumb/ finger extensors, Sensory loss over first web space (Sparing of wrist/ elbow extensors)

4. Ans. (a) **Radial nerve**
[Ref. Musculoskeletal Trauma Simplified by Gupta, 1/e p42]
- Up to 20% of humerus shaft fractures are associated with radial nerve injury
- This is most commonly seen with injuries at the junction of the middle and distal thirds of the humeral shaft, because the radial nerve lies closely applied to the bone

5. Ans. (d) **Carpal tunnel syndrome**
[Ref. Viva Voce In Anatomy by Gangane, 3/e p31]

Tinel's Sign
- Seen in Carpal tunnel syndrome
- It is elicited by gentle percussion of the median nerve at wrist, leading to a tingling sensation radiating into hand

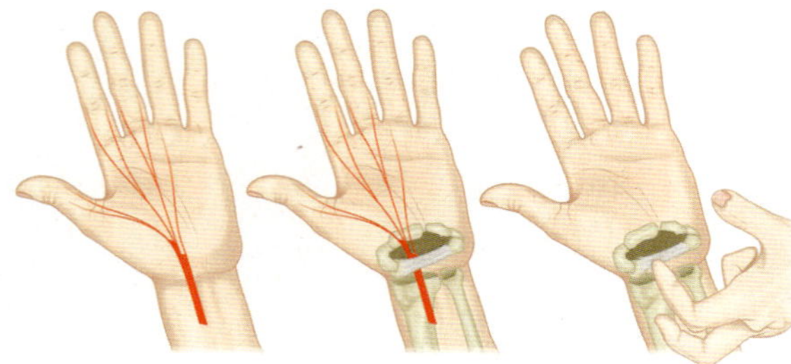

Fig. Tinel's Sign

6. Ans. (b) **Foot drop**
[Ref. A Dictionary of Neurological Signs by Larner, 4/e p303]
- Stepping gait occurs with a lower motor neuron type of Foot drop **("floppy" foot drop)**, e.g. due to Common peroneal nerve palsy or Peripheral neuropathy
- Because of the weakness of foot dorsiflexion (weak Tibialis anterior) there is compensatory overaction of hip and knee flexors during the swing phase of walking to ensure the foot clears the ground (hence **"High-stepping gait"**)

7. Ans. (a) **Classification of nerve injuries**
[Ref. Maheshwari, 4/e p60]
- **Seddon and Sunderland Classifications** are used for Peripheral Nerve Injuries and Clinical Correlations

8. Ans. (d) **Age between 35 and 50**
[Ref. Neuroimaging, Part 2 by Swaab, 1/e p1001]

Red Flags in Back Pain
- Features, signs and symptoms in a patient with back pain which indicate serious spinal pathology

Features	Signs	Symptoms
• History malignancy • Age <16 or >50 with NEW onset pain • Weight loss (unexplained) • Previous longstanding steroid use • Recent serious illness • Recent significant infection	• Saddle anaesthesia • Reduced anal tone • Hip or knee weakness • Generalised neurological deficit • Progressive spinal deformity • Urinary retention	• Non-mechanical pain (worse at rest) • Thoracic pain • Fevers/ rigors • General malaise • Urinary retention

9. Ans. (d) **T3-T4**
[Ref. Oxford Textbook of Rheumatology, 4/e p1348]

Common Sites of disc Prolapse
- L4/L5
- L5/S1
- C5/C6
- C6/C7

10. Ans. (c) **Loss of conduction of nerve fibre**
[Ref. Maheshwari, 4/e p60]

Seddon's Classification of Nerve Injuries
- ***Neurapraxia***: Physiological disruption of conduction in nerve fibre; Spontaneous and complete recovery in few weeks
- ***Axonotmesis***: Axons damaged but nerve preserved; Partial spontaneous recovery in months
- ***Neurotmesis***: Cutting/scarring of nerve with Wallerian degeneration; No spontaneous recovery requiring nerve repair

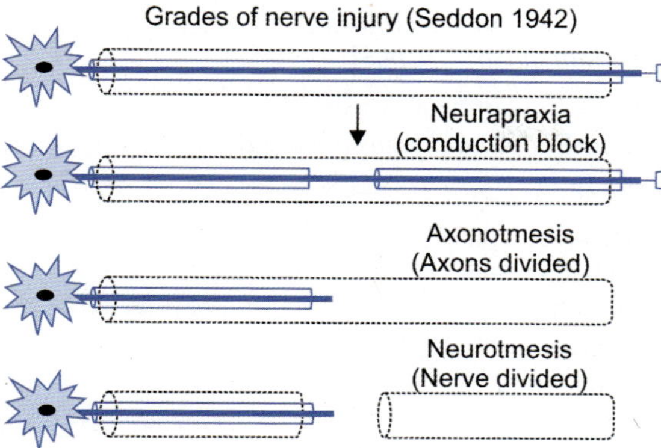

Fig. Seddon's Grading of Nerve Injuries

11. Ans. (a) Median nerve
[Ref. Maheshwari, 4/e p294]

Nerve Entrapments

- **Carpal tunnel syndrome**: Median nerve
- Anterior interosseous syndrome: Median nerve
- **Tarsal tunnel syndrome**: Posterior tunnel syndrome
- **Cubital tunnel syndrome**: Ulnar nerve
- **Guyon canal**: Ulnar nerve
- Foramen ovale: Trigeminal nerve
- Foramen rotundum: Trigeminal nerve
- Thoracic outlet: Brachial nerve
- Pelvic outlet: Sciatic nerve
- Fibular head: Common peroneal nerve
- **Meralgia paraesthetica** (Inguinal ligament): Lateral cutaneous nerve of thigh

12. Ans. (a) Superior gluteal nerve injury
[Ref. Total Hip Replacement by Ochsner, 1/e p169]

13. Ans. (b) Distal cut-end of the nerve
[Ref. Maheshwari, 4/e p59]

Nerve Degeneration

- *Secondary/Wallerian degeneration:* Degeneration of neuron distal to point of injury
- *Primary/Retrograde degeneration*: Degeneration of neuron proximal to point of injury, upto a single node

14. Ans. (d) C8 T1
[Ref. Anatomy by Bhatnagar, 3/e p155]

Brachial Plexus Injuries

Brachial plexus injury	Roots involved
Upper brachial plexus injury (Erb-Duchenne palsy)	C5, C6
Extended upper brachial plexus injury	C5, C6, C7
Lower brachial plexus injury (Dejerine-Klumpke paralysis)	C8, T1
Total brachial plexus lesion	C5, C6, C7, C8, T1
Peripheral brachial plexus lesion	Variable

15. Ans. (b) Ulnar nerve
[Ref. Foundations for Osteopathic Medicine by Ward, 2/e p445]

16. Ans. (a) Presence of adduction of thumb
[Ref. Splinting the Hand and Upper Extremity by Austin, 1/e p387]

Loss of Functions in Ulnar Nerve Palsy

High Ulnar Nerve Injury	Low Ulnar Nerve Injury
Ulnar wrist flexion Adduction, Abduction of all digits Adduction of thumb DIP, MP flexion of RF, SF MP flexion of thumb Grip, Pinch strength Sensory loss Dorsoulnar aspect of hand	Adduction, Abduction of all digits Adduction of thumb MP flexion of RF, SF MP flexion of thumb Grip, Pinch strength Sensory loss Ulnar aspect of hand
"Mild Claw deformity"	**"Significant claw deformity"**
PARALYSED MUSCLES Flexor carpi ulnaris Flexor profundus (Little/ Ring fingers) Lumbricals (Little/ Ring fingers) All Interossei Adductor of thumb Hypothenar muscles	PARALYSED MUSCLES Lumbricals (Little/ Ring fingers) All Interossei Adductor of thumb Hypothenar muscles

17. Ans. (c) Long thoracic nerve
[Ref. Maheshwari, 4/e p65]

18. Ans. (a) Radial nerve
[Ref. Trauma Surgery by Butterworths, Part 2, p639]

19. Ans. (c) Ulnar nerve injury
[Ref. Maheshwari, 4/e p68]

Splints used in Common Nerve Injuries

- Axillary nerve palsy (Deltoid paralysis): **Aeroplane splint**
- Radial nerve palsy (Wrist extensors, MP joints paralysis): **Cock-up splint**
- Ulnar nerve paralysis (Lumbricals paralysis): **Knuckle Bender splint**
- Sciatic N, Common peroneal N palsy: **Foot drop splint**

20. Ans. (b) Nerve regeneration
[Ref. Maheshwari, 4/e p66]

Signs of Nerve Regeneration

- ***Tinel's sign***: Distal progression of pins and needles sensation, on distal to proximal tapping of nerve
- *Motor march*: Contraction of more distant muscles to the site of injury
- Electrodiagnostic test

21. Ans. (c) Ulnar
[Ref. Short Practice of Surgery by Bailey and Love, 25th Ed., Pg 512]

- *Relevant anatomy*: The hook of the hamate (hamulus) is the distal border of Guyon's canal, which contains the ulnar artery and nerve. So any damage to hamate may lead to ulnar nerve injury.
- *Causes of hamate injury*:
  - Sports involving racquets, clubs and bats
  - Wrist compression between weights

- *Treatment of hamate injury*:
  - Surgical excision of humate hook
  - Internal fixation of bone

22. Ans. (d) Lateral Condylar fracture
[Ref. Postgraduate Orthopedics by Kader, 2/e p33]

23. Ans. (d) Median
[Ref. Carpal Tunnel Syndrome by Amadio, 1/e p4]

24. Ans. (b) Injury to sacral plexus
[Ref. Blueprints Neurology by Caplan, 3/e p65]
- **Atonic bladder**: Lower motor neuron lesion at the level of Conus medullaris, Cauda equina or Sacral plexus; or it may reflect Peripheral nerve dysfunction

25. Ans. (c) Median nerve injury
[Ref. Oxford Handbook of Clinical Specialties by Collier, 9/e p760]

26. Ans. (c) A - II; B - I; C - III; D - IV

27. Ans. (d) Posterior interosseous nerve
[Ref. Clinical Manual of Surgery by Rao, 1/e p906]

28. Ans. (c) Ulnar nerve
[Ref. Maheshwari, 4/e p64]

Tests of Ulnar Nerve (for Muscles Paralysis)

- *Palmar flexion of wrist against gravity*: Flexor carpi ulnaris
- *Abduction of little finger against resistance*: Abductor digiti minimi
- *Egawa's test*: Dorsal interossei of middle finger (abductors)
- *Card test*: Palmar interossei (adductors) of fingers
- *Froment's sign/ Book test*: Adductor pollicis

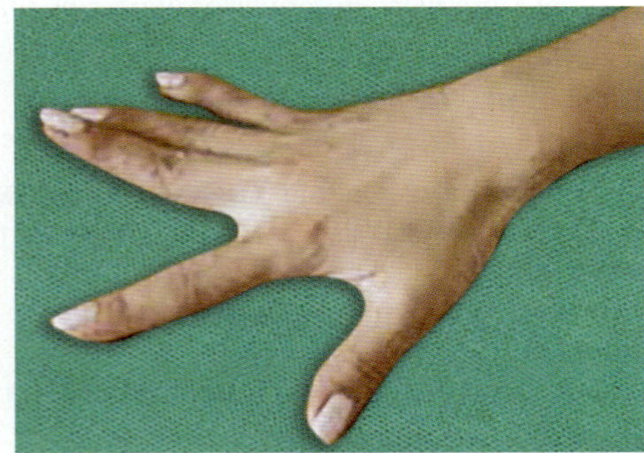

Fig. Egawa Test

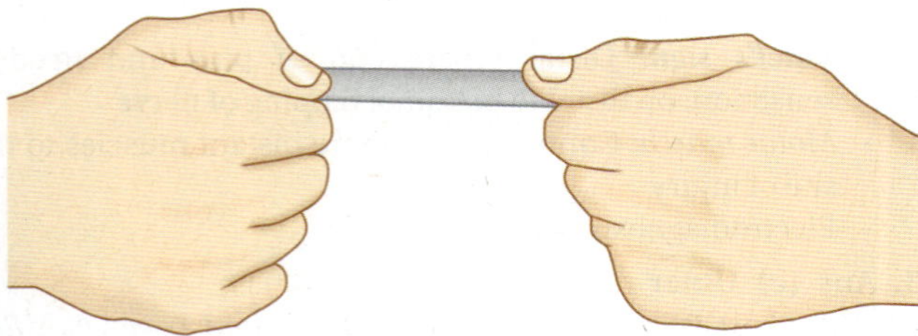

Fig. Froment's Sign

29. Ans. (a) Ulnar nerve
[Ref. Geriatric Rehabilitation Manual by Kauffman, 1/e p220]

30. Ans. (a) A - I; B - II; C - IV; D – III
[Ref. Essentials of PMR by Silver, 3/e p129]

31. Ans. (d) Facial nerve
[Ref. Localization in Clinical Neurology by Biller, 6/e p329]

32. Ans. (a) Ulnar nerve injury
[Ref. Maheshwari, 4/e p65]

33. Ans. (c) Neurofibromatosis
[Ref. Symptoms and Signs of Surgical Disease by Browse, 4/e p140]

Neuropathic Joints

- Diabetes mellitus
- Tabes dorsalis
- Syringomyelia
- Spina bifida
- Leprosy
- Yaws
- Cauda equina lesions (Meningomyelocele)
- Syphilis
- Multiple sclerosis
- Pernicious anemia
- Alcoholism, Amyloidosis
- Thalidomide
- Charcot-Marie-Tooth disease

34. Ans. (d) To assess the recovery
[Ref. Maheshwari, 4/e p66]

35. Ans. (d) Physiological paralysis
[Ref. Maheshwari, 4/e p60]

Seddon's Classification of Nerve Injuries

- ***Neuropraxia***: Physiological disruption of conduction in nerve fibres
  - No structural changes
  - Spontaneous complete recovery
- ***Axonotmesis***: Damage of axons
  - Internal architecture of nerve is preserved
  - Wallerian degeneration
  - Spontaneous recovery; may be incomplete
- ***Neurotmesis***: Structure of nerve is damaged by cutting/ scarring
  - Wallerian degeneration
  - Spontaneous recovery not possible
  - Nerve repair is required

36. Ans. (b) Late onset

Tardy Ulnar Nerve Palsy

- Description: Late onset Ulnar nerve palsy
- Causes:
  - Malunited Lateral condyle humerus
  - Displaced Medial condyle humerus
  - Elbow dislocations
  - Contusions of Ulnar nerve
  - Shallow ulnar groove
  - Hypoplasia of humeral tubercle

37. Ans. (a) High ulnar lesion
[Ref. ACES for PACES by Jayasekera, 1/e p510]
- **Ulnar Paradox**: Clawing of fingers less marked in High Ulnar nerve lesions
  - Weakness of Ulnar half of Flexor digitorum profundus
  - Weakened flexion of 4th, 5th fingers results in straighter fingers

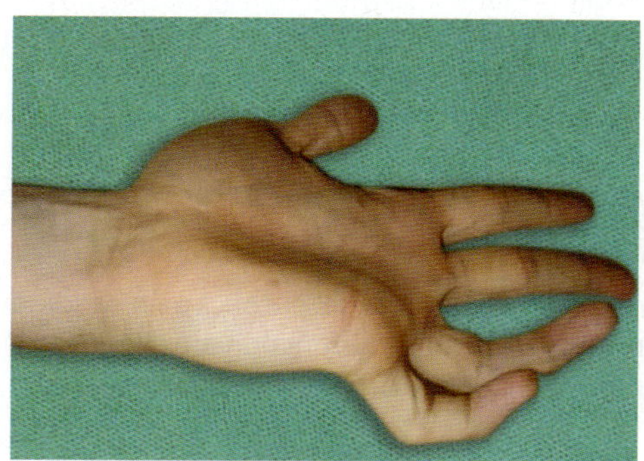

Fig. Ulnar Paradox

38. Ans. (a) Ulnar nerve dysfunction

[Ref. Double-Crush Syndrome by Vladimir, 1/e]

Five Most Used Tests/ Signs in Carpal Tunnel Syndrome

- **Tinel's sign**: Least sensitive, Most specific
- **Phalen sign**
- Reverse Phalen sign
- Carpal compression test
- Vibration test: Most sensitive, Least specific

39. Ans.(a) C5 C6

[Ref. Orthopedics by Biswas, 1/e p552]

40. Ans. (d) Patient cannot initiate abduction

[Ref. Human Anatomy by Halim, 1/e p82]

41. Ans. (c) Claw finger deformity

[Ref. Maheshwari, 4/e p61]

Attitudes in Nerve Injuries

Attitude	Nerve injury
Wrist drop	Radial nerve palsy
Foot drop	Common peroneal nerve palsy
Winging of scapula	Long thoracic nerve palsy
Claw hand	Ulnar nerve palsy
Ape thumb deformity	Median nerve palsy
Pointing index	Median nerve palsy
Policeman tip deformity	C5-C6 Upper trunk Brachial plexus injury
Claw hand	C8-T1 Lower trunk Brachial plexus injury

42. Ans. (c) Peripheral nerve injuries

[Ref. Peripheral Nerves by Barral, 1/e p30]

Sunderland Classification of Nerve Injuries

- First-degree (Seddon Class I): Seddon's neurapraxia
- Second-degree (Seddon Class II): Seddon's axonotmesis
- Third-degree (Seddon Class II): Nerve fiber interruption; Lesion of endoneurium, but epineurium and perineurium remain intact
- Fourth-degree (Seddon Class II): Only epineurium remain intact, Surgical repair is required
- Fifth-degree (Seddon Class III): Complete transection of the nerve; Recovery is not possible without an appropriate surgical treatment

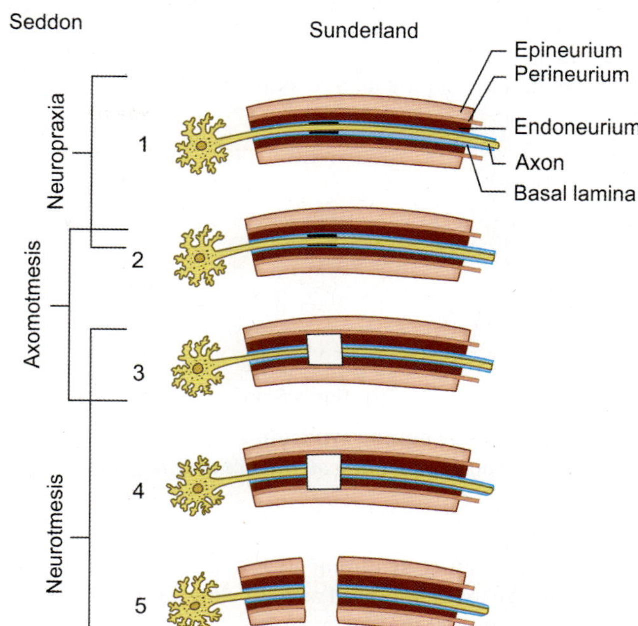

Fig. Sunderland Classification

43. Ans. (c) Meningomyelocoele

[Ref. Parameic Practice Today by Barbara, p43]

- Meningomyelocele (also called myelomeningocele) is the severest form of Spina bifida
- Meninges, CSF, and a portion of the spinal cord protrude from opening in spine

44. Ans. (b) Median nerve

[Ref. Health and Wellness by Edlin, 1/e p477]

Nerve Syndromes & Occupations

- Cervical radiculopathy: Computer work on screen
- Pronator syndrome: Mechanics, Barbers
- Carpal tunnel syndrome: Typists, Computer programmers, Potters
- Thoracic outlet syndrome: Violinists, Musicians
- Cubital tunnel syndrome: Truck drivers
- Distal ulnar neuropathy: Meat packers, Machine operators

45. Ans. (c) Compartment syndrome

[Ref. Essentials of PMR by Silver, 3/e p345]

Compartment Syndrome

- MCC: Trauma in young adult males
- Severe pain with passive movement of the muscles within the compartment
- Loss of voluntary movement of the muscles
- Sensory changes and paraesthesia in area supplied by nerve involved
- Pain out of proportion to swelling and injury (in early stages)

46. Ans. (a) Sensation on tapping the nerve

[Ref. Orthopedic Physical Assessment by Magee, 5/e p380]

- Tinel's sign: Reproducing tingling paresthesias by tapping on the nerve in the middle of the wrist and touching thumb to the fingertips to evaluate median nerve function
- Precipitation of a fleeting pain or sensory symptoms radiating into the palm and fingers when the Median nerve is tapped at the wrist

- In 1915, a French neurologist named Jules Tinel noticed that it was possible to generate a **"pins and needles" feeling by tapping on a recently injured nerve**

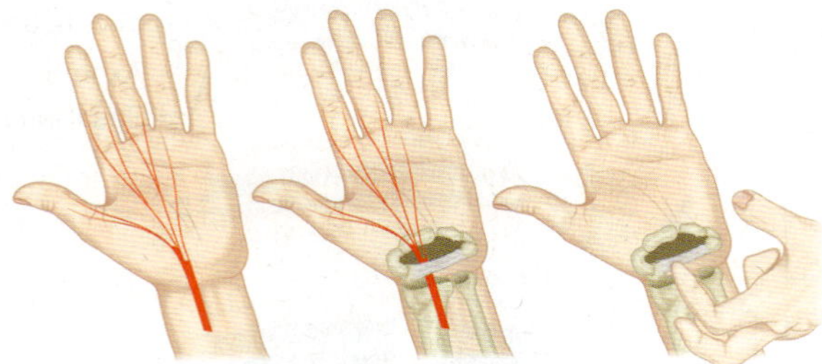

Fig. Tinel's Sign

47. Ans. (a) Cauda equina syndrome
[Ref. Harwood-Nuss' Clinical Practice of Emergency Medicine, 5/e p728]

Cauda Equina Syndrome

- Cauda equina syndrome (CES) is a condition due to damage to the bundle of nerves below the end of the spinal cord known as the cauda equina
- Features of CES:
  - Severe back pain
  - Saddle anesthesia: Anesthesia or paraesthesia involving S3-S5 dermatomes (Numbness or 'pins-and-needles' sensations of the groin and inner thighs which would contact a saddle when riding a horse)

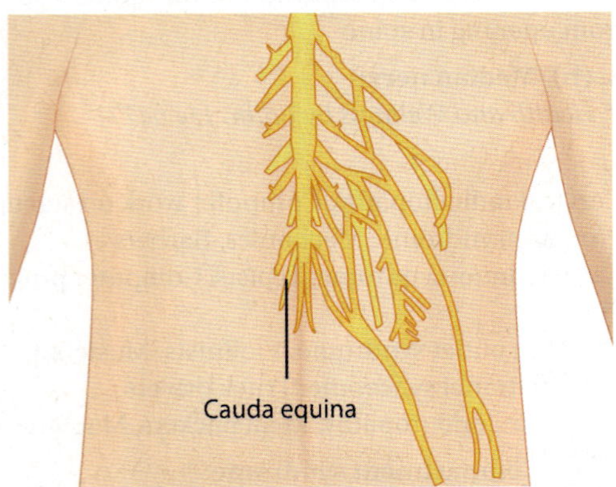

Fig. Cauda equina syndrome

  - Bladder and bowel dysfunction (Decreased tone of the urinary and anal sphincters)
  - Detrusor weaknesses (Urinary retention, Post-void residual incontinence)
  - Sciatica-type pain
  - Weakness of the muscles of the lower legs
  - Achilles (ankle) reflex absent (Both sides)
  - Sexual dysfunction
  - Absent anal reflex and bulbocavernosus reflex
  - Gait disturbance

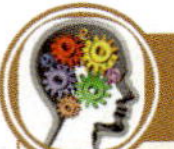

Also Remember

- In Cauda Equina Syndrome, severe back pain, saddle anesthesia, incontinence and sexual dysfunction are considered "red flags" (Features which require urgent investigation)

48. Ans. (d) >5 years
[Ref. Orthopedics by Mohindra, 2/e p387]

Treatment of Post-polio Residual Paralysis

- Once the paralysis is established and recovery has halted, the aim of treatment in this stage is to correct the deformities if they have developed and to provide maximum attainable function
- Tendon transfers are not to be done before 4 years of age as the rehabilitation exercises cannot be taught to a child of less than 4 years of age

49. Ans. (c) Radial nerve
[Ref. Hand Therapy by Cooper, 2/e p284]

Crutch Palsy

- Both the Radial nerve branches and the Main radial nerve suffer compression injury between a crutch and the underlying muscle tissue
- Axilla level, motor and sensory involvement
- Loss of triceps function at the elbow (that is, loss of elbow extension), weakness with supination, loss of digit MP/ thumb extension, radial abduction

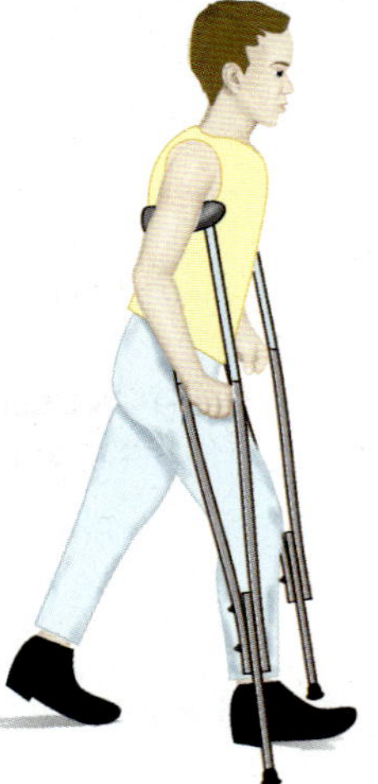

Fig. Crutch Palsy

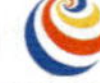 HIGH YIELD MCQs ANSWERS WITH EXPLANATIONS 

1. Ans. (c) Femoral nerve
[Ref. Multiple Sources]

- Ulnar nerve entrapment: Cubital tunnel syndrome
- Median nerve entrapment: Carpal tunnel syndrome
- Lateral cutaneous nerve entrapment: Meralgia paraesthetica

2. Ans. (c) Neurotmesis
[Ref. Maheshwari, 4/e p60]

3. **Ans. (c) Supinators are normal**
[Ref. Turek's Orthopedics by Buckwalter, 5/e p360]

Erb's Palsy
- Lesion: **C5, C6** (Upper brachial plexus injury)
- Presentation: Typical paralysis involves A*bductors* and external rotators of the shoulder, Flexors of the elbow, and *Supinators* of forearm, resulting in Waiter's tip/ Porter's tip hand

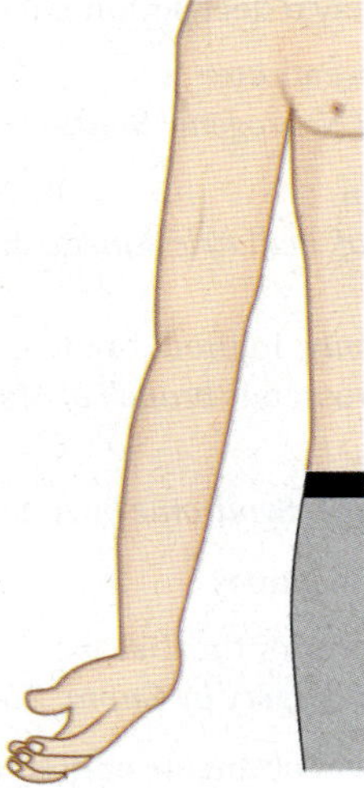

Fig. Erb's Palsy

4. **Ans. (a) Anterior primary rami of C5 and C6**
[Ref. Turek's Orthopedics by Buckwalter, 5/e p360]

5. **Ans. (a) Upper trunk of brachial plexus**
[Ref. Turek's Orthopedics by Buckwalter, 5/e p360]

6. **Ans. (b) Fracture humerus**
[Ref. Fundamentals of Hand Therapy by Cooper, 2/e p284]
- **Most common cause of radial nerve palsy**: Direct trauma to the nerve, often secondary to *fractures* of the *humerus*, elbow dislocations, and Monteggia-fracture dislocations
- **Most common cause of Radial nerve injury**: Fracture at Supracondylar humeral shaft

7. **Ans. (a) Radial**
[Ref. Fundamentals of Hand Therapy by Cooper, 2/e p284]

8. **Ans. (a) Radial**
[Ref. Essentials of PMR by Silver, 3/e p129]
- Saturday nerve palsy (Honeymoon palsy): Radial nerve prone to Injury in Spiral groove

9. **Ans. (c) Radial**
[Ref. Skeletal Trauma in Children by Marc, 5/e p264]
- Fracture at Junction of Middle and Distal third Humerus associated with injury to closely related Radial nerve

10. **Ans. (a) Tinel's sign**
[Ref. Rockwood and Wilkinsons' Fracture sin Children by Kasser, 7/e p666]

11. **Ans. (c) The median and ulnar nerves were affected**
[Ref. Turek's Orthopedics by Buckwalter, 5/e p360]

12. **Ans. (a) Radial nerve**
[Ref. Yearbook of Neurology, p591]
- Results of Nerve-suture repair results: Radial nerve > Median nerve > Ulnar nerve

13. **Ans. (b) Axillary nerve**
[Ref. Peripheral Nerve Injuries in the Athlete by Feinberg, 1/e p200]
- MC Nerve injured in Anterior shoulder dislocation: Axillary nerve
- MC Nerve injured in Shoulder dislocation: Axillary nerve

14. **Ans. (b) Limited Respiratory effort**
[Ref. Surgical Critical Care and Emergency Surgery by Forrest, 1/e p258]

15. **Ans. (a) Central cord syndrome**
[Ref. Neurological Disorders by Chipps, p116]

16. **Ans. (c) Thumb, finger, wrist drop**
[Ref. Clinical Anatomy for Students by Kulkarni, 1/e p58]

Radial Nerve Injuries
- **Injury in Axilla**: Weakness of Arm extension, Wrist extension (Wrist-drop), Finger/thumb extension
- **Injury in Spiral groove**: Affect Brachioradialis, Wrist extensors, Supinator, Wrist/Thumb extensors, Sensory loss of Dorsum of hand (1st Interosseous space)
- **Lesions of Posterior Interosseous nerve**: Finger drop, Thumb drop, Radial deviation of wrist

17. **Ans. (a) Mid shaft of humerus**
[Ref. Physical Medicine and Rehabilitation by Walsh, 4/e p906]
- **Mid-shaft fractures** are most commonly responsible for Radial nerve injuries (60% times associated)

18. **Ans. (b) Coracobrachialis**
[Ref. Concise Neurology by Biller, 1/e p284]

Impairments in Erb's Palsy (C5, C6 Injury)
- Shoulder abduction (Deltoid, Supraspinatus)
- External rotation of arm (Infraspinatus)
- Elbow flexion (Biceps, Brachioradialis, Brachialis)
- Forearm supination (Biceps)
- Biceps and Brachioradialis reflexes

19. **Ans. (c) Loss of pronation at radioulnar joint**
[Ref. Concise Neurology by Biller, 1/e p284]

20. **Ans. (b) Klumpke's palsy**
[Ref. Orthopedics by Biswas, 1/e p552]

21. **Ans. (c) Forcible hyperabduction of upper arm (falling person trying to catch an object)**
[Ref. Textbook of Surgery by Gupta, 2/e p429]

22. **Ans. (a) Paralysis of extensors of hand & wrist**
[Ref. Crush Step 1 by Blair, 1/e p414]

23. **Ans. (b) Long head of triceps**
[Ref. Anatomy and Exposure of Spinal Nerves by Hanna, 1/e p25]

24. **Ans. (c) Leaves extensions at elbow joint intact**
[Ref. Peripheral Nerve Injuries in the Athlete by Feinberg, 1/e p72]
- Radial Nerve injury in Spiral groove: Spares Anconeus muscle and Triceps muscle

25. Ans. (c) Conus medullaris lesion
[Ref. Neurology at the Bedside by Gunhild, 1/e p26]

26. Ans. (a) Axillary nerve
[Ref. Peripheral Nerve Injuries in the Athlete by Feinberg, 1/e p200]

27. Ans. (b) Circumflex nerve injury
[Ref. Essential Orthopedics and Trauma by Edwards, 5/e p193]

28. Ans. (c) Radial nerve palsy
[Ref. Maheshwari, 4/e p68]

29. Ans. (b) Partial injury to sciatic nerve

30. Ans. (a) Foot drop
[Ref. Skeletal Trauma in Tropics by Kumar, 2/e p668]

31. Ans. (b) Deep peroneal nerve
[Ref. Peripheral Neurology by Sackler, 3/e p108]

32. Ans. (d) Lateral cutaneous nerve of thigh
[Ref. Labor and Delivery Nursing by Murray, 1/e p105]

33. Ans. (c) Volkmann's paralysis
[Ref. Short Textbook of Surgery by Roy, 1/e p551]

34. Ans. (c) Brachial neuritis
[Ref. Bonica's Management of Pain by Fishman, 1/e p1038]

35. Ans. (a) Loss of flexion of shoulder
[Ref. Illustrated Clinical Anatomy by Abrahams, 2/e p181]

Musculocutanous Nerve Injury
- Usually seen after Dislocation of shoulder
- Cause paralysis of: Biceps, Brachialis, Coracobrachialis
- Lead to: Weakness in elbow flexion and Supination and Loss of sensation on Lateral side of forearm

36. Ans. (c) Loss of overhead abduction
[Ref. Neuroanatomical Basis of Clinical Neurology by Arslan, 2/e p244]

37. Ans. (c) Loss of ankle reflex
[Ref. Sammi's Essentials in Neurosurgery, 2/e p465]

38. Ans. (a) Hypertension
[Ref. Essentials of Skeletal radiology by Yochum and Rowe, 3/e p594]

Causes of Carpal Tunnel Syndrome
- Fractures (Colles, Hook of Hamate, Proximal metacarpal)
- Repetitive strain injury (Synovitis)
- Inflammatory arthritis (Gout, Pseudogout, Rheumatoid arthritis, Amyloidosis)
- Tumors of Median nerve (Fibromas, Neural sheath tumors)
- Space occupying lesions (Lipomas, Gangliomas)
- Other causes: Pregnancy, Hypothyroidism, Acromegaly, Diabetes mellitus

39. Ans. (a) Paraesthesia of the lateral 2 fingers; (b) Atrophy of the thenar eminence; (e) Tinel sign is positive
[Ref. Brigham Intensive Review of Internal Medicine by Singh, 2/e p982]

40. Ans. (b) I (ii) II (iii) III (iv) IV (i)

41. Ans. (c) I (iv) II (i) III (iii) IV (ii)

42. Ans. (b) Conus medullaris syndrome
[Ref. Textbook of Neurologic Bladder by Corcos, 3/e p276]

43. Ans. (a) More common in males
[Ref. Cumulative Trauma Disorders by Parker, 1/e p83]

44. Ans. (a) Compression of communication between medial and lateral planter nerves

45. Ans. (a) Injury to sacral plexus
[Ref. Blueprints Neurology by Caplan, 4/e p67]
- ***Atonic bladder*** implies a lower motor neuron lesion at the level of the conus medullaris, cauda equina, or *sacral plexus*; or it may reflect peripheral nerve dysfunction

46. Ans. (c) Foley's catheter
[Ref. Textbook of Neurogenic Bladder by David, 3/e p465]

47. Ans. (c) Median
[Ref. Textbook of Pediatric Emergency Procedures by King, 2/e p998]
- *Most commonly* injured branch of the *median nerve:* Anterior interosseous *branch of Median nerve*

48. Ans. (c) Lunate
[Ref. Carpal Tunnel Syndrome by Amadio, 1/e p4]

49. Ans. (c) Calcaneovarus

50. Ans. (b) 2 years after the disease
[Ref. Textbook of Surgery by Gupta, 2/e p123]

51. Ans. (a) Action of abductor pollicis brevis
[Ref. Short Textbook of Surgery by Roy, 1/e p551]

Median Nerve Injury at Wrist
- Paralysis of Abductor pollicis brevis (Pen test)
- Atrophy of Thenar eminence
- Paralysis of Opponens pollicis
- Sensory loss on palmar aspect lateral 3½ fingers
- Weakness 1st and 2nd lumbricals

52. Ans. (c) Median
[Ref. Maheshwari, 4/e p61]
- **Pointing index**: Index finger remains straight on trying to make a fist
  - Occurrence: Median nerve palsy (Level: Proximal to elbow)
  - Muscles paralyzed: Flexor digitorum superficialis, Flexor digitorum profundus (lateral half)

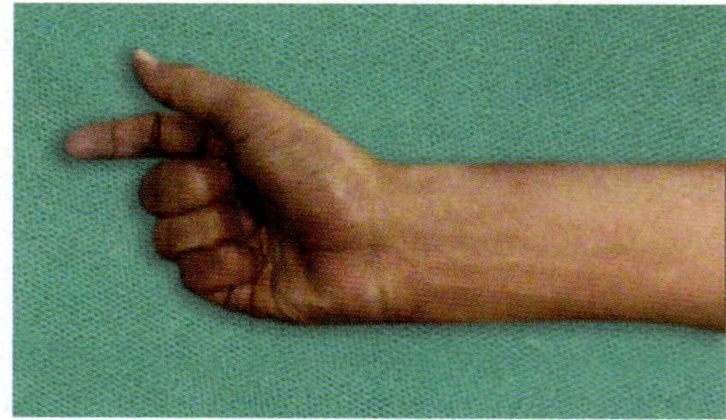

Fig. Pointing Index

53. Ans. (d) Congenital non fusion of the spinal lamina
[Ref. Pathophysiology by Clayton, 6/e p134]

Major CNS Malformations
- Neural tube defects: Arrest in development of brain and spinal cord

- Anencephaly: Absence of skull and parts of brain due to early closure of Anterior neural tube
- Encephalocoele: Herniation of Brain and meninges through a midline defect in skull
- Meningocoele: Protrusion of meninges through a vertebral defect
- Myelomeningocoele (Spina bifida): Herniation of meninges, spinal fluid, spinal cord and nerves through a vertebral defect (MC site: Lumbosacral region)
- Spina bifida occulta: Defect in Lumbar or sacral spine due to incomplete fusion of vertebral lamina
- Craniosynostosis: Premature closure of Cranial sutures during first 20 months of life
- Microcephaly: Defect in brain growth as a whole
- Congenital hydrocephalus: Increased volume of CSF due to overproduction, resorption defect or blockage of ventricular drainage system

54. Ans. (b) Diastematomyelia

[Ref. Spinal Imaging by Hauwe, 1/e p23]

- **Diastematomyelia (Split cord)**: MC abnormal midline notochordal integration with Variable elongated separation of Spinal cord into two
  - **Diastematomyelia Type I**: Two hemicords within two individual dural tubes separated by bony/ osteocartilaginous septum; presents with Hairy tuft on dorsum (Reliable clinical marker), Scoliosis, Tethered cord syndrome
  - **Diastematomyelia Type II**: Single dural tube housing both the hemicords; Less severe neurological impairment

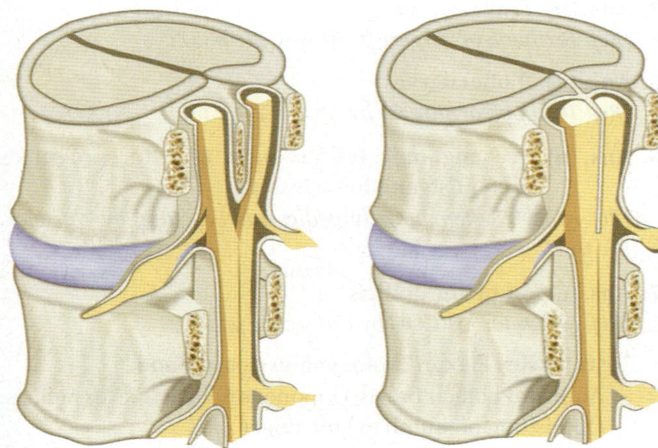

Fig. Diastematomyelia

55. Ans. (b) Erb's palsy

[Ref. Textbook of Surgery by Kaye, 3/e p481]

56. Ans. (b) Monteggia fracture dislocation

[Ref. Essentials of Orthopedics for Physiotherapist by Ebnezar, 1/e p105]

57. Ans. (b) C4-C5

58. Ans. (a) Elbow dislocation; (d) Supracondylar fracture of humerus

[Ref. Clinical Emergency Medicine by Garmel, 1/e p295]

Injuries and Nerve Deficits

Injury	Associated nerve deficit
Anterior shoulder dislocation/ fracture	Axillary N, Musculocutaneous N
Humeral shaft fracture	Radial N
Fracture distal 1/3 radius	Radial N
Supracondylar fracture radius	Median N, Radial N, Ulnar N
Posterior elbow dislocation	Median N, Ulnar N
Wrist fracture/ dislocation	Median N
Posterior hip dislocation	Sciatic N
Anterior hip dislocation	Femoral N
Knee fracture / dislocation	Peroneal N, Tibial N
Proximal fibular fracture	Peroneal N

59. Ans. (b) Loss of apposition of thumb

[Ref. Clinical Cases and Pearls in Medicine by Sainani, 1/e p394]

60. Ans. (c) Median nerve injury

[Ref. Clinical Cases and Pearls in Medicine by Sainani, 1/e p394]

61. Ans. (d) Oppose the thumb

[Ref. Clinical Anatomy by Kulkarni, 1/e p108]

62. Ans. (b) Weakness of adductor Pollicis

[Ref. Internal Medicine Practical Review by RCE Candidates, p162]

63. Ans. (c) C5 C6

[Ref. Textbook of Surgery by Kaye, 3/e p481]

64. Ans. (a) Median nerve

[Ref. Carpal Tunnel syndrome by Amadio, 1/e p4]

65. Ans. (b) Lunate

[Ref. Fractures of Distal Radius and Carpus by Osterman, 1/e p426]

66. Ans. (d) 3, 1 and 2

[Ref. Maheshwari, 4/e p60]

67. Ans. (b) 1 mm/day

[Ref. Neuroscience Year by Smith, 1/e p128]

68. Ans. (a) Contraction of abductor pollicis brevis

[Ref. Short Textbook of Surgery by Roy, 1/e p551]

69. Ans. (c) Median

[Ref. Short Textbook of Surgery by Roy, 1/e p551]

70. Ans. (b) Median nerve

[Ref. Short Textbook of Surgery by Roy, 1/e p551]

71. Ans. (a) Cubitus valgus

[Ref. Neglected Musculoskeletal Injuries by Kumar, 1/e p363]

72. Ans. (d) Regeneration of nerves

[Ref. Musculoskeletal Physical Examination by Malanga, 1/e p180]

73. Ans. (c) Ulnar nerve at elbow
[Ref. Fitness for Work by Brown, 4/e p277]

74. Ans. (c) Produces pain and Paraesthesia over the lateral aspect of the forearm and thumb when affecting the 6th cervical nerve
[Ref. Intensive Review of Internal Medicine by Stoller, 5/e p154]

75. Ans. (d) All of the above
[Ref. Cervical Spondylosis and Its' Complications by Smith, 1/e p35]

76. Ans. (a) Intervertebral foramen
[Ref. Textbook of Clinical Neuroanatomy by Singh, 1/e p92]
- In **Cervical spondylosis**, formation of Osteophytes from Neurocentral joints of Luschka project backwards into intervertebral foramina causing their narrowing
- Nerve roots are compressed leading to pain and muscle wasting along its' distribution

77. Ans. (c) Periarthritis
[Ref. Towards Earlier Diagnosis by Hodgkin, 1/e p390]

78. Ans. (b) Ulnar nerve
[Ref. Maheshwari, 4/e p61]

79. Ans. (a) Axillary nerve
[Ref. The Shoulder by Rockwood, 4/e p297]

80. Ans. (a) Axillary nerve
[Ref. The Shoulder by Rockwood, 4/e p297]

81. Ans. (a) Radial nerve
[Ref. Clinical Anatomy for Students by Kulkarni, 1/e p58]

82. Ans. (b) Lateral condyle fracture humerus
[Ref. Maheshwari, 4/e p100]
- In Lateral condyle of humerus, Diminished growth at lateral side of distal humerus epiphysis results in **Cubitus valgus deformity**: It may result in Late/ Tardy Ulnar nerve palsy due to friction neuritis of Ulnar nerve as it moves over medial epicondyle when elbow is flexed and extended

83. Ans. (a) Neuropraxia
[Ref. Complications of Regional Anesthesia by Brendan, 2/e p83]
- Post-tourniquet-application *neuropraxia* may occur, particularly in the setting of preexisting neuropathy

84. Ans. (d) Hysterical joint
[Ref. Symptoms and Signs of Surgical Disease by Browse, 4/e p140]

85. Ans. (b) Hansen's disease
[Ref. Orthopedics Manual by Thomas, 1/e p576]
- **MC Cause of Neuropathic joints in Upper extremity**: Syringomyelia > Leprosy
- MC Cause of Neuropathic joints in **Lower extremity Worldwide**: Leprosy >Diabetes mellitus
- MC Cause of Neuropathic joints in **Lower extremity Developed countries**: Diabetes mellitus

86. Ans. (b) Painful limitation of joint movements
[Ref. General Principles of Orthopedics and Trauma by Iyer, 1/e p156]

87. Ans. (a) 6 hours
[Ref. Textbook of Orthopedics by Ebnezar, 4/e, p334]

Types of Nerve Repair
- **Primary repair**: Within 6-8 hours if wound is clean cut
- **Delayed primary repair**: Between 7 and 18 days if wound is contaminated
- **Secondary repair**: After 18 days if injury is seen late, failure of conservative approach or incomplete injury

88. Ans. (c) Neurotmesis
[Ref. Maheshwari, 4/e p60]

89. Ans. (d) Proximal injury
[Ref. SRB's Surgical Operations by Bhat, 1/e p379]
- **Good prognostic factors in Nerve injury**: Distal injury, Younger age (Less than 10 years age), Lesser gap between cut ends, Nerves with pure motor/sensory function, Sharp mechanism of injury, Repair less than 6 months

90. Ans. (d) Acute prolapsed Intervertebral disc
[Ref. Case Presentations in Neurology by Bates, 1/e p76]

91. Ans. (d) All of the above
[Ref. Splinting the Hand and Upper Extremity by Austin, 1/e p387]

92. Ans. (b) Paralysis of all lumbricals; (c) Paralysis of all interossei; (d) Paralysis of flexor carpi ulnaris; (e) Paralysis of flexor profundus
[Ref. Splinting the Hand and Upper Extremity by Austin, 1/e p387]

93. Ans. (a) Median nerve + Ulnar nerve
[Ref. Human Anatomy and Physiology by Marieb, 6/e p364]

94. Ans. (b) Radial nerve
[Ref. Textbook of Surgery by Ahsan, 2/e p357]

95. Ans. (d) Radial nerve
[Ref. Textbook of Surgery by Ahsan, 2/e p357]

96. Ans. (a) Preganglionic lesions have a better prognosis than postganglionic lesions
[Ref. Apley's System of Orthopedics and Fractures by Warwick, 9/e p11]

97. Ans. (c) Adductor pollicis
[Ref. MCQs for MRCOG by Kanje, 2/e p447]

Tests for Key Flexor/Extensor Muscles in Hand
- Abductor pollicis brevis, Opponens pollicis, Flexor pollicis: Opposition of thumb to little finger
- Flexor pollicis longus: OK sign (Bring together tips of Thumb and Index finger together)
- Extensor pollicis longus: Lift thumb off table with palm flat on surface
- Adductor pollicis: Froment's sign

98. Ans. (a) Charcot's joint
[Ref. Maheshwari, 4/e p286]

99. Ans. (d) Knee
[Ref. Musculoskeletal Imaging by Disler, 4/e p271]

100. Ans. (d) Syringomyelia
[Ref. Neurologic Examination by Campbell, 7/e p545]

101. Ans. (b) Complete paralysis of the IIIrd and IVth digits
[Ref. Splinting the Hand and Upper Extremity by Austin, 1/e p387]

102. Ans. (a) Adductor pollicis
[Ref. Short Textbook of Surgery by Roy, 1/e p551]

103. Ans. (b) Opponens pollicis
[Ref. Splinting the Hand and Upper Extremity by Austin, 1/e p387]

104. Ans. (a) Claw hand; (c) Weakness of grips
[Ref. Splinting the Hand and Upper Extremity by Austin, 1/e p387]

105. Ans. (c) Strength Duration Curve
[Ref. Textbook of Orthopedics by Ebnezar, 4/e p332]

106. Ans. (a) C5,C6 nerve
[Ref. Manual of Neonatal Care by Cloherty, 7/e]

Duchenne-Erb's Palsy

- **Waiter's tip/ Porter's tip posture**: Arm adducted and internal rotated; Extension/ pronation of elbow and flexion of wrist/ fingers
- Moro's, biceps, radial reflexes absent on affected side
- Grasp reflex is intact

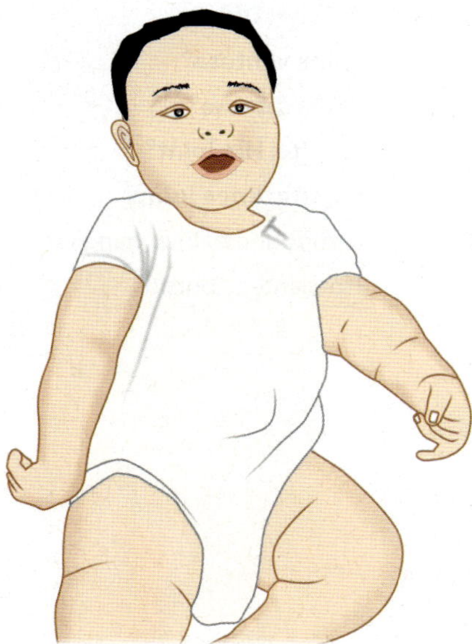

Fig. Porter's Tip Hand

107. Ans. (c) Adduction of the thumb
[Ref. Splinting the Hand and Upper Extremity by Austin, 1/e p387]

108. Ans. (d) Interosseous muscle
[Ref. Primer on Rheumatic Diseases by Klippel, 13/e p77]

109. Ans. (d) Post. Interosseous nerve injury
[Ref. Rehabilitation of Injured Combatant by Russ, 1/e p504]

110. Ans. (a) Prolapsed intervertebral disc L4-5
[Ref. Maheshwari, 4/e p246]

111. Ans. (b) The appearance of the foot drop indicate early surgical intervention
[Ref. Practice of Spinal Surgery by Crock, 1/e]

Indications for Surgery in Disc Prolapse

- Major neurological deficits: Acute Cauda equina compressions, Spinal canal stenosis
- Persistent or recurrent pain post-conservative treatment (MC indication)
- Progressive neurologic deficit: Foot drop
- Persistent spinal deformity: Lumbar scoliosis, Marked lumbar flexion deformity

112. Ans. (b) Bed Rest for 3 months
[Ref. Essentials of PMR by Silver, 3/e p247]

113. Ans. (b) Neural arch pars inter articularis
[Ref. Spondylolisthesis by Medifocus, 1/e p23]

114. Ans. (a) Congenital defect of posterior arch; (b) Slipping of L5 over S1; (c) Progressive slipping
[Ref. Spondylolisthesis by Medifocus, 1/e p23]

115. Ans. (a) Injury to Posterior interosseous nerve
[Ref. Rehabilitation of Injured Combatant by Russ, 1/e p504]

116. Ans. (c) Median nerve
[Ref. Fractures by Ebnezar, 1/e p63]

- **In VIC**, Median nerve is more commonly affected than the ulnar nerve: Median nerve is more susceptible to ischemia and subsequent fibrosis

117. Ans. (c) Median nerve
[Ref. Netters Concise Orthopaedic Anatomy, Chapter 5]

- **In Pronator teres syndrome**, Median nerve is compressed in the proximal forearm between the two heads of Pronator teres muscle, Flexor digitorum superficialis, Lacertus fibrosus

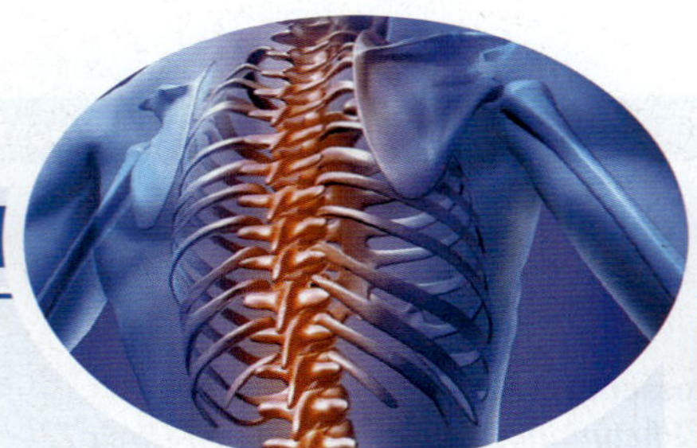

Chapter 9

Bone and Joint Tuberculosis

THEORETICAL CONCEPTS

IX A. MUSCULOSKELETAL TUBERCULOSIS

Disease	Tissue	Remarks
TB osteomyeltits	Long bone	**MC site: Tibia[Q]**
TB dactylitis	Short bone (phalanges)	**Spina ventosa[Q]**
TB spondylitis	Spine	**Pott's disease[Q]**
TB arthritis	Joint	**MC site: Hip joint[Q]**
Synovial TB	Joint	**MC site: Knee joint[Q]**
TB tenosynovitis	Flexor tendons of wrist	Compound palmar ganglion
TB bursitis	Trochanteric bursa	Trochanteric bursitis

- *Mode of spread*:
  - **Hematogenous (Most common[Q])**
  - Direct extension from a neighbouring focus
- *Outcomes*:
  - Spine: Bony ankylosis
  - Other joints: **Fibrous ankylosis (Most common[Q])**

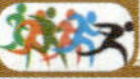

Topper's Edge

Skeletal TB

- Healing is by Fibrous ankylosis **(Except Spine where it is by Bony ankylosis[Q])**
- Usually monoarticular
- Always Secondary in nature
- **MC part affected[Q]: Spine**
- Cold abscess may be a feature
- Chemotherapy is mainstay of treatment

IX B. TUBERCULOSIS SPINE

- *Types*:
  - Anterior
  - Posterior
  - Central
  - **Para-discal (Most common[Q])**

- *Clinical features*:
  - Stiffness of back **(Earliest symptom[Q])**
  - Pain **(MC symptom[Q])**
  - Cold abscess
- *Investigations*:
  - X-rays: Reduction of disc space + abscesses
  - CT scan
  - MRI **(Investigation of choice[Q])**
- *Complications*:
  - Cold abscess (Most common)
  - Neurological compression

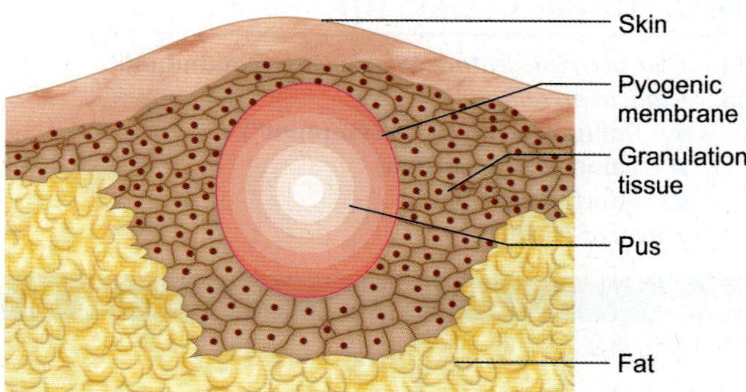

Fig. Cold abscess

Topper's Edge

Spinal Tuberculosis

- MC form of Skeletal TB[Q]
- **Regional distribution: Dorsal[Q]** (> Lumbar > Cervical/Dorsolumbar)
- **MC area in vertebrae involved[Q]: Metaphyseal or Intervertebral space**
- Cold abscess composition (No inflammation): Serum, WBCs, Caseous material, Granulation tissue, TB bacilli
- Typical attitudes:
  - Upper cervical: Wry neck
  - Lower cervical: Military position
  - Lower thoracic: Alderman's gait
  - Upper lumbar: Prominent abdomen
  - Lower lumbar: Increased lordosis
- **Spine irregularities: Kyphosis (MC[Q])**, Scoliosis, Lordosis, Boarding, Paravertebral thickening
- Only detectable radiological anomaly[Q]: Fine calcification in Paravertebral soft tissue shadow

IX C. POTT'S PARAPLEGIA

- *Definition*: TB spine with neurological involvement[Q]
- ***MC site*: Dorsal spine[Q]**
- *MC cause of early onset Pott's paraplegia*: Abscess
- *Most prominent early sign*: Ankle/Patellar clonus
- ***Investigation of choice*: MRI[Q]**
- *Surgical management*:
  - Hong Kong Operation
  - **Anterolateral decompression (Most common[Q])**
  - Costotransversectomy

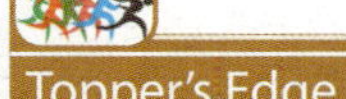

Topper's Edge

TB Spine with Paraplegia

- **MC site[Q]: Dorsal spine**
- Classification used: Seddon's classification (Early onset, Late onset paraplegia)
- Grading of Paraplegia used: Kumar's grading
- **Earliest prominent sign[Q]: Clonus**
- **Gold standard for diagnosis[Q]: MRI**
- Treatment:
  - Bosworth regime: Immobilization and Early arthrodesis
  - Hodgson radical regime: Anterior decompression and Arthrodesis
  - Tuli and Kumar's Middle path regime: Triple drug therapy (with Surgery only for Neurological complications, recrudescence, non-responsive patients)
- Surgical techniques:
  - **Anterolateral decompression (Surgery of choice)**
  - Costotransversectomy
  - Anterior decompression
  - Laminectomy

IX D. TUBERCULOSIS HIP

- *Characteristic feature*: **Wandering acetabulum**[Q]
- *Clinical presentation*:
  - Stiffness of hip **(First symptom**[Q]**)**
  - Lameness **(First sign)**
  - Shortening of limb
- *Stages of TB Hip*

Stage	Attitude
I—Synovitis	Flexion, Abduction, External rotation
II—Arthritis	Flexion, Adduction, Internal rotation
III—Erosion	Flexion, Adduction, Internal rotation

- *X-rays*:
  - Haziness of bones **(First sign**[Q]**)**
  - Wandering acetabulum with ***'Pestle and mortar appearance'***[Q]
  - Reduced joint space
- *Treatment*:
  - Girdlestone arthroplasty
  - Debridement of joint
  - Osteotomy

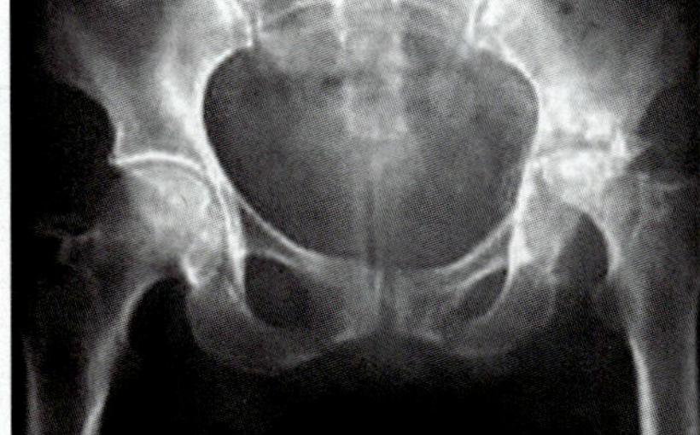

Fig. Wandering Acetabulum

Topper's Edge

TB OF HIP

TB of Hip Joint

- 2nd MC type of Skeletal TB (After Spinal TB[Q])
- **Earliest symptom of TB Hip**[Q]**: Limp**
- **3 Classical deformities**[Q]**:** Flexion deformity, Adduction deformity, Abduction deformity
- 7 types of TB Hip in Advanced arthritis: Normal appearance, Travelling/wandering acetabulum, Dislocated hip, Perthes type, Atrophic type, Protrusio acetabuli type, Mortar and pestle type
- Complication[Q]: Fibrous ankylosis

IX E. TUBERCULOSIS KNEE JOINT

- ***Characteristic feature*: Triple displacement**[Q]
  - Flexion
  - Posterior subluxation
  - External rotation

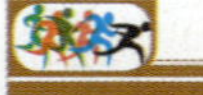

Topper's Edge

TB OF KNEE JOINT

TB of Knee Joint

- 3rd MC type of Skeletal TB (After Spinal TB, TB Hip joint)
- **MC site**[Q]**: Synovium**
- **5 Classical deformities**[Q]: Flexion, Posterior subluxation, Lateral subluxation, Lateral rotation, Abduction of tibia

IX F. TUBERCULOUS ADENITIS

- *Most commonly affected age*: Children or young adults
- ***Most common nodes affected***: Deep upper cervical lymph nodes
- *Causative agent*:
  - *Mycobacterium tuberculosis*
  - *Mycobacterium bovis*

- *Collar stud abscess*: Cold abscess in neck is not just confined to deep fascia; pus flows into space beneath superficial fascia
- *Treatment*:
  - Antibiotic therapy
  - Surgical excision with removal of lymph nodes

IMAGE-BASED QUESTION

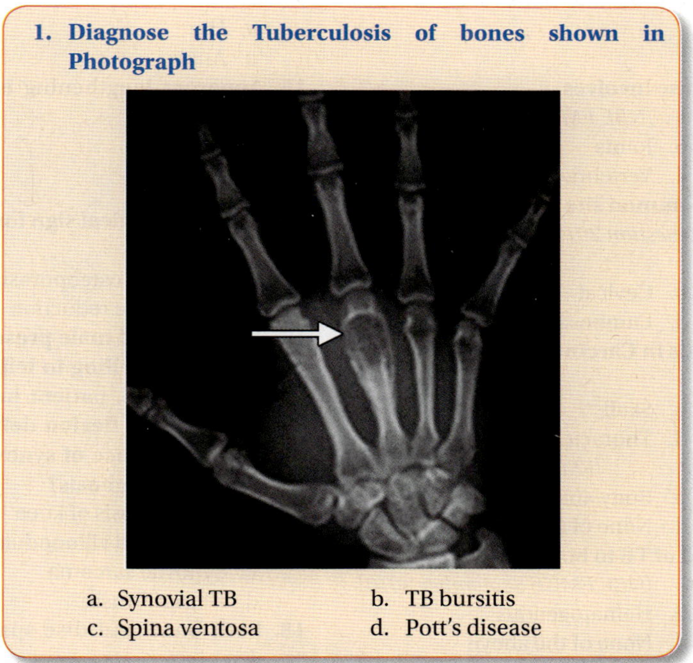

1. Diagnose the Tuberculosis of bones shown in Photograph

a. Synovial TB b. TB bursitis
c. Spina ventosa d. Pott's disease

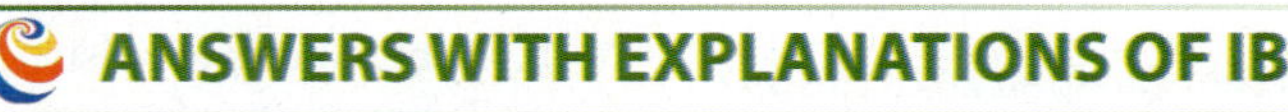

ANSWERS WITH EXPLANATIONS OF IBQ

1. Ans. (c) Spina ventosa *[Ref. Maheshwari, 4/e p176]*

- Spina ventosa/TB dactylitis: Tuberculosis of short bones (Phalanges)
  - Lytic expansile lesion in diaphysis
  - Gradual healing by sclerosis
  - Periosteal reaction is not common

NEET/NBE PATTERN MCQs

1. **Most common site for tuberculosis of skeletal system is** *[NBE FMGE September 2010]*
   a. Hip b. Spine
   c. Ankle d. Knee
2. **TB spine results in paraplegia of (most common)** *[NBE DNB 1997]*
   a. Cervical part b. Upper thoracic part
   c. Lower thoracic part d. Lumbar part
3. **Spina ventosa is** *[NBE DNB December 2011]*
   a. TB of the ventral aspect of the spinal cord
   b. Malunion of fracture of the spinous process of C7
   c. Spindle-shaped expansion of the bone seen in TB dactylitis
   d. TB of sacroiliac joint
4. **In Tuberculosis, Pott's disease involves** *[NBE FMGE September 2010]*
   a. Spleen b. Joints
   c. Femur d. Vertebrae
5. **Tuberculosis spine; most-common site is** *[Recent Question 2012, 2013, AIIMS 1995, AIPGME 1995]*
   a. Sacral b. Cevical
   c. Dorsolumbar d. Lumbosacral
6. **MC site of skeletal metastasis in Carcinoma breast is** *[UPSC 2011]*
   a. Pelvis b. Skull
   c. Lumbar vertebrae d. Thoracic vertebrae
7. **TB arthritis of joints causes** *[FMGE September 2012]*
   a. Fibrous ankylosis b. Bony ankylosis
   c. Loosening of joints d. None of the above
8. **Commonest route of spread of TB to bones is** *[NBE FMGE September 2010]*
   a. Direct b. Hematogenous
   c. Lymphatics d. None of the above
9. **Anterolateral decompression is done for** *[Recent Question 2012, 2013]*
   a. Spinal tuberculosis b. Chest TB
   c. Hand TB d. Foot TB
10. **Complication of joint TB** *[Recent Question 2012, 2013]*
    a. Fibrous ankylosis b. Bony ankylosis
    c. Normalhealing d. None
11. **Most common site seen in skeletal tuberculosis is** *[NBE FMGE September 2008, Recent Question 2012]*
    a. Hand b. Hip
    c. Knee d. Spine
12. **TB hand** *[Recent Question 2012]*
    a. Spina ventosa b. Caries sicca
    c. Pott's disease d. None
13. **Collarstud abscess is seen in** *[NBE FMGE March 2007]*
    a. Tuberculosis b. Syphilis
    c. AIDS d. Actinomycosis
14. **Besides spine, most common site of Tuberculosis of bones is** *[NBE FMGE March 2006]*
    a. Hip b. Knee
    c. Ankle d. Shoulder
15. **Apparent lengthening is seen in which stage of TB Hip** *[Recent Question 2012]*
    a. Stage I b. Stage II
    c. Stage III d. None
16. **First radiological sign for active tubercular arthritis is** *[Recent Question 2017]*
    a. Localized osteoporosis b. Sclerosis
    c. Joint space reduction d. Osteophytes
17. **A 20-year-old male presents with history of gradual onset pain and swelling in left knee since 6 months. Now since last 1 month, patient has started limping while walking and also has flexion deformity of knee. Ultrasonography shows presence of synovial thickening. What is the most probable diagnosis?** *[Recent Question 2017]*
    a. Tuberculosis of knee
    b. Pigmented villonodular synovitis
    c. Synovial sarcoma
    d. Hemarthrosis
18. **Both bone and disc spaces are involved in which spine disease** *[Recent Question 2017]*
    a. Tuberculosis b. Osteoporosis
    c. Osteoid osteoma d. Eosinophilic granuloma
19. **Caries sicca refer to** *[Recent Question 2017]*
    a. Tuberculosis of shoulder
    b. Tuberculosis of wrist
    c. Tuberculosis of ankle
    d. Tuberculosis of calcaneum

HIGH YIELD MCQs

1. **False about TB osteomylitis is** *[All India PGMEE 2008]*
   a. Abundant periosteal reaction
   b. Abundant sequestrum
   c. Minimal signs of inflammation
   d. Usually secondary from elsewhere
2. **Site of TB bursitis is/are** *[PGI 2007]*
   a. Trochanteric b. Prepatellar
   c. Subacromial d. Subdeltoid
   e. Subpatellar
3. **Which of the following is NOT TRUE regarding tubercular osteomyelitis?** *[All India PGMEE 2008]*
   a. It is a secondary TB
   b. Periosteal reaction is seen
   c. Sequestration is uncommon
   d. Inflammation is minimum
4. **The most common site of skeletal tuberculosis is** *[KERALA PGMEE 2004]*
   a. Tibia b. Humerus
   c. Vertebrae d. Radius

5. **Tuberculosis of the spine commonly affects all of the following parts of the vertebra except** *[All India PGMEE 2004]*
   a. Body b. Lamina
   c. Spinous process d. Pedicle
6. **Tuberculosis of the spine is thought to originate from** *[Bihar PGMEE 1998]*
   a. By extension from the paravertebral structures
   b. In the cancellous vertebral body
   c. In the ligamentous structures
   d. In the nucleus pulposus
7. **Early features of spinal tuberculosis in a child includes** *[UP PGMEE 1999]*
   a. Pain on sudden movement
   b. Gradual deformity
   c. Night cries
   d. Sudden deformity
8. **In TB spine, the first symptom is** *[ORISSA PGMEE 1992, AIIMS PGMEE 1995]*
   a. Decreased sensation
   b. Decreased motor power
   c. Pain
   d. Increased deep tendon reflexes
9. **First symptom in tuberculous cord compression is** *[All India PGMEE 1997]*
   a. Sensory change b. Decrease tendon reflex
   c. Spasticity d. Lower limb weakness
10. **Which of the following causes paravertebral abscess?** *[TN PGMEE 1999]*
   a. Brucella b. Tuberculosis
   c. Kala-azar d. Typhoid
11. **Paraplegia due to Tuberculosis of spine most commonly occurs at** *[NBE DNB 1997, Recent Question 2017]*
   a. Cervical spine b. Upper thoracic spine
   c. Lower thoracic spine d. Lumbar spine
12. **Paraplegia is common in Tuberculosis of dorsal spine, because** *[WB PGMEE 1995]*
   a. Incidence of Tuberculosis is commoner in dorsal spine
   b. Natural tendency for kyphosis
   c. Canal is narrow
   d. Spinal cord ends at L1
   e. All of the above
13. **In tuberculosis of spine, which one of the following is not a cause for paraplegia?** *[NIMS PGMEE 2000]*
   a. Stretching of spinal cord in gibbus deformity
   b. Spinal artery compression
   c. Compression by granulation tissue
   d. Oedema of spinal cord
14. **Most common cause of Paraplegia of early onset of Tuberculosis of spine is** *[Karnataka PGMEE 1992]*
   a. Spinal artery thrombosis
   b. Sudden collapse of vertebra
   c. Granulation tissue pressing on cord
   d. Cold abscess pressing on the cord
15. **Most common cause of Kyphosis in a male is** *[NBE DNB 1997]*
   a. Congenital b. Tuberculosis
   c. Trauma d. Secondaries
16. **Most common sequelae of tuberculous spondylitis in an adolescent is** *[All India PGMEE 2005)*
   a. Fibrous Ankylosis b. Bony-Ankylosis
   c. Pathological dislocation d. Chronic osteomyelitis
17. **Clinical features of TB spine is/are** *[PGI 2003, 2004, 2006]*
   a. Night sweat b. Reduced appetite
   c. Loss of lordosis d. Back pain
   e. Increased height
18. **True about TB spine is all except** *[PGI 2000]*
   a. Early paraplegia is good prognosis
   b. Insidious onset paraplegia is good prognosis
   c. Dorsolumbar spine is commonest site
   d. It is commonest site for TB of bone in the body
19. **Poor prognostic factors in pott's paraplegia** *[PGI 2003]*
   a. Acute onset of paraplegia
   b. Sudden progression of paraplegia
   c. Motor paralysis alone
   d. Long-standing paraplegia
   e. Paraplegia in children
20. **Indicator(s) of poor prognosis in the pott's spine is/are** *[PGI 2009]*
   a. Healed vertebral lesion
   b. Grade IV Pott's spine
   c. Kyphotic angle >60°
   d. Short duration
   e. Acute onset
21. **Commonest infective lesion of the spine in India as** *[AIIMS PGMEE 1996]*
   a. Pyogenic infection b. Typhoid
   c. Fungal d. Tuberculosis
22. **Tuberculosis of the spine in known as** *[JIPMER PGMEE 1997]*
   a. Perthes disease b. Pott's disease
   c. Scheuermann's disease d. Frieberg's disease
23. **The 1st sign of TB is** *[CUPGEE 1995, CUPGEE 1999]*
   a. Narrowing of intervertebral space
   b. Rarefaction of vertebral bodies
   c. Destruction of laminae
   d. Fusion of spinous processes
24. **Compression of single vertebra with narrow joint space is characteristic of** *[Orissa PGMEE 1988]*
   a. Caries spine
   b. Fracture spine
   c. Prolapsed intervertebral disc
   d. Secondaries spine
25. **A 46-year-old, known alcoholic, presented with pain in the dorsal spine. On examination, there is tenderness at the-dorso-lumbar junction. Radiograph shows destruction of the 12th dorsal vertebra with loss of disc space between D12–L1 vertebrae. The most probable diagnosis is** *[AIIMS PGMEE 2004]*
   a. Metastatic spine disease b. Pott's spine
   c. Missed trauma d. Multiple myeloma
26. **X-ray showing decreased Intervertebral space and presence of paravertebral shadow. What could be the diagnosis?** *[NIMS PGMEE 2000]*
   a. Tuberculosis of spine b. Ankylosing spondylitis
   c. Eosinophilic granuloma
   d. Multiple myeloma

27. Treatment of Pott's paraplegia is *[UPSC 1988]*
a. Lateral decompression b. Posterior decompression
c. Excision of vertebra d. Antituberculous drugs

28. Commonest site for tuberculous spondylitis is *[All India PGMEE 1998]*
a. T12–L1 b. C6–C7
c. L4–L5 d. S1–S2

29. Pott's spine is commonest in spine *[DPG 1994]*
a. Cervical b. Thoracic
c. Lumbar d. Sacral

30. Most common type of spinal Tuberculosis is *[BIHAR PGMEE 1994]*
a. Anterior b. Posterior
c. Central d. Paradiscal

31. Tuberculosis of the spine starts in *[BHU PGMEE 1998]*
a. Nucleous pulposus b. Annulus fibrosis
c. Paravertebral fascia d. Vertebral body

32. Cold abscess in chest wall most commonly occurs in *[AIIMS PGMEE 1998]*
a. TB spine b. TB ribs
c. Kala-azar d. Typhoid

33. Feature of Bony ankylosis *[UP PGMEE 1998]*
a. Painless with no movement
b. Painful complete movement
c. Painless complete movement
d. Painful incomplete movement

34. Earliest radiological sign of spinal tuberculosis is *[BIHAR PGMEE 1999]*
a. Decreased joint space
b. Wedging of vertebra
c. Syndesmophyte formation
d. Formation of paravertebral abscess

35. Spina ventosa results from *[BIHAR PGMEE 1997]*
a. Sarcoidosis b. Tuberculosis
c. Histiocytosis X syndrome d. Both A+B but not C

36. Tuberculosis of spine is best treated by *[TN PGMEE 1994]*
a. Anterior fusion b. Posterior fusion
c. Anterolateral decompression
d. Aspiration of Paraspinal abscess and instillation of streptomycin

37. Ideal surgical treatment for Pott's paraplegia is *[Recent Question 2017, UPSC 1997]*
a. Laminectomy and decompression
b. Anterior decompression and bone grafting
c. Anterolateral decompression
d. Costotransversectomy

38. Surgical treatment in Pott's spine is indicated, if there is *[PGI 1991]*
a. Progressive loss of function in spite of medical treatment
b. No improvement in motor power in spite of 3 months of treatment
c. There is no improvement in fever in 3 months of treatment
d. Patient who is an adult or middle aged

39. All of the following movements of the hip are painful in a patient with psoas abscess, except *[TN PGMEE1994]*
a. Extension
b. Adduction to abduction
c. Abduction to adduction
d. Fixed flexion to further full flexion

40. A psoas abscess present on the right side, the correct statement is *[NIMS PGMEE 1992]*
a. Opposite hip flexion relieves pain
b. Same side hip flexion relieves pain
c. Same side extension relieves pain
d. Kyphosis may occur

41. Short long bones of hand and foot are commonly infected by the following organism *[TN PGMEE 1994]*
a. Pyogenic b. Tuberculous
c. Fungal d. All of the above

42. Most common cause of monoarthritis in children is *[AP PGMEE 1989]*
a. Septic arthritis b. Tuberculous arthritis
c. Osteoarthritis d. Rheumatoid arthritis
e. Any of the above

43. Tuberculous arthritis in advanced cases lead to *[TN PGMEE 1989]*
a. Bony ankylosis b. Fibrous ankylosis
c. Loose joints d. Charcots joints

44. All are features of joint Tuberculosis except *[PGI 1991]*
a. Synovium is involved
b. Synovial fluid has < 20% blood sugar
c. Kissing arthritis—subchondral bone is involved
d. Pain is a common feature
e. Lymphocyte/Monocyte ratio is decreased

45. Most appropriate for a 20-year-old man suffering from old tuberculosis arthritis of knee with triple deformity is *[ORISSA PGMEE 1990)*
a. Plaster immobilization b. Joint clearance and traction
c. Total knee replacement d. Charnley's arthrodesis

46. Caries sicca is seen in *[ROHTAK PGMEE 1996]*
a. Shoulder b. Hip
c. Knee d. Ankle

47. Most common site of skeletal tuberculosis is *[AMU PGMEE 1992]*
a. Cervical spine b. Hip + Spine
c. Knee + Hip joints d. Knee joint

48. Triple deformity of knee is classically seen in *[AIIMS PGMEE 1994]*
a. Fracture patella b. Tuberculosis
c. Rheumatic arthritis d. Rheumatoid arthritis

49. Wandering acetabulum is seen in *[AIIMS PGMEE 1993, JIPMER PGMEE 2014]*
a. Dislocation of femur b. Fracture acetabulum
c. Tuberculosis of hip d. CDH

50. Usual site of Tubercular bursitis *[PGI 2003]*
a. Prepatelar b. Subdeltoid
c. Subpatellar d. Trochanteric
e. None

51. Composite deformity in Neglected cases of TB knee is due to *[NIMSET 2015]*
a. Posterior and Lateral dislocation/subluxation, External rotation, Fixed flexion
b. Anterior and Medial dislocation/subluxation, Internal rotation, Fixed flexion
c. Posterior and Medial dislocation/subluxation, Internal rotation, Fixed flexion
d. Anterior and Lateral dislocation/subluxation, External rotation, Fixed flexion

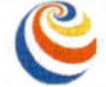 NEET/NBE PATTERN MCQs ANSWERS WITH EXPLANATIONS 

1. **Ans. (b)** Spine
[Ref. Maheshwari, 4/e p179]
   - ***Most common site of bone and joint tuberculosis***: Spine (Pott's disease)
   - ***Most common site of spinal TB***: Dorsolumbar region

2. **Ans. (c)** Lower thoracic part
[Ref. Textbook of Surgery by Gupta, 2/e p421]

3. **Ans. (c)** Spindle-shaped expansion of the bone seen in TB dactylitis
[Ref. Textbook of Orthopedics by Kulkarni, 2/e p384]

TB Dactylitis
- Description: TB infection of Metacarpal, Metatarsal and Phalangeal bones
- Seen less than 5 years age group
- **First incoculum**: Centre of marrow cavity leading to Granuloma formation
- **Spina ventosa**: TB granuloma leads to Spindle-shaped expansion of the bone

4. **Ans. (d)** Vertebrae
[Ref. Maheshwari, 4/e p176]

Musculoskeletal Tuberculosis

Disease	Tissue	Remarks
TB osteomyelitits	Long bone	**MC site: Tibia**
TB dactylitis	Short bone (phalanges)	Spina ventosa
TB spondylitis	Spine	Pott's disease
TB arthritis	Joint	**MC site: Hip joint**
Synovial TB	Joint	**MC site: Knee joint**
TB tenosynovitis	Flexor tendons of wrist	Compound palmar ganglion
TB bursitis	Trochanteric bursa	Trochanteric bursitis

5. **Ans. (c)** Dorsolumbar
[Ref. Essential Handbook of Practical Orthopedic Examination by Banerjee, 1/e p80]

Tuberculosis in India
- **MC sites of TB**: Lungs > Lymph nodes > Skeletal TB
- **MC Sites in Skeletal TB**: Spine > Hip > Knee
- **MC sites in Spinal TB**: Dorsolumbar spine

6. **Ans. (c)** Lumbar vertebrae
[Ref. Tumours by Louis, 1/e p106]
   - **MC cancers causing skeletal metastases**: Breast > Prostate > Kidney > Thyroid
   - **MC sites of Skeletal metastases**: Vertebrae > Paravertebral spaces > Epidural > Interdural/Intramedullary
   - **MC sites in Metastases to Vertebrae**: Lumbar > Thoracic > Cervical > Sacrum

7. **Ans. (a)** Fibrous ankylosis
[Ref. Joint Imaging in Childhood and Adolescence by Machada, 1/e p115]
   - **MCC Bony ankyloses**: Septic arthritis
   - MCC Peripheral joints Bony ankyloses: Septic arthritis
   - MCC Peripheral joints Fibrous ankyloses: TB arthritis
   - **MCC Spine Bony ankyloses**: TB arthritis

8. **Ans. (b)** Hematogenous
[Ref. Maheshwari, 4/e p176]
   - Bone and joint tuberculosis is ALWAYS secondary to primary focus in lungs, lymph nodes, etc.
   - *Mode of spread*:
     - **Hematogenous (Most common)**
     - Direct extension from a neighbouring focus

9. **Ans. (a)** Spinal tuberculosis
[Ref. Textbook of Orthopedics and Trauma by Kulkarni, 2/e p437]

Surgical Approaches to Tuberculous Spine
- Cervical spine: Anterior decompression
- Lumbar spine: Anterior decompression
- Dorsal spine:
  - Thoracotomy
  - Anterolateral/Extrapleural decompression

10. **Ans.(a)** Fibrous ankylosis
[Ref. SAMJ, Volume 22, p97]

11. **Ans.(d)** Spine
[Ref. Maheshwari, 4/e p179]

12. **Ans. (a)** Spina ventosa
[Ref. Textbook of Orthopedics by Kulkarni, 2/e p384]

13. **Ans. (a)** Tuberculosis
[Ref. Short Practice of Surgery by Bailey and Love, 25th Edn., Pg 731]

Tuberculous Adenitis
- *Most commonly affected age*: Children or young adults
- *Most common nodes affected*: Deep upper cervical lymph nodes
- *Causative agent*:
  - *Mycobacterium tuberculosis*
  - *Mycobacterium bovis*
- ***Collar stud abscess***: Cold abscess in neck is not just confined to deep fascia; pus flows into space beneath superficial fascia
- *Treatment*:
  - Antibiotic therapy
  - Surgical excision with removal of lymph nodes

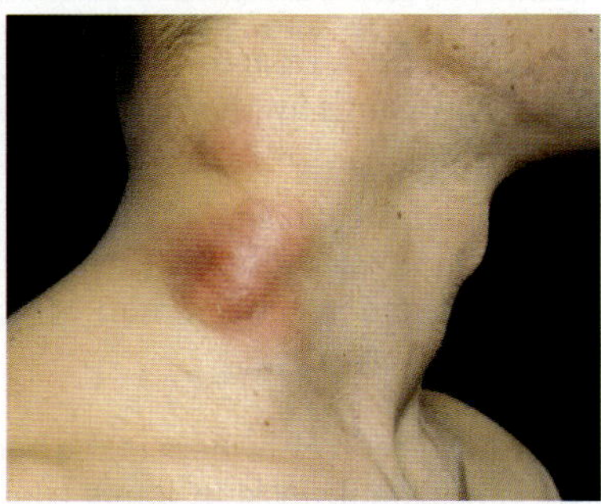

Fig. Collar stud abscess

14. Ans. (a) Hip

[Ref. Maheshwari, 4/e p188]

After spine, hip is most commonly after by Tuberculosis of bones

15. Ans. (a) Stage I

[Ref. Essential Handbook of Practical Orthopedic Examination by Banerjee, 1/e p70]

Stages of Tuberculosis Hip

- Stage I (TB Synovitis): Flexion + Abduction + External rotation, Apparent lengthening, Effusion
- Stage II (Early arthritis): Flexion + Adduction + Internal rotation, Apparent shortening or True shortening < 1 cm, Destruction of articular cartilage
- Stage III (Advanced arthritis): True shortening > 1 cm, Gross restriction of movements, Fixed deformities
- Stage IV (Complications): Destruction of Capsule/ligaments, Wandering acetabulum

16. Ans. (a) Localized osteoporosis

[Ref. Fundamentals of Orthopedics by Mohindra, 2/e p298]

Tuberculous Arthritis

- Localized osteoporosis is the **first radiological sign of active disease**
- Articular margins and bony cortices become irregular and hazy with no periosteal reaction or new bone formation
- Bony destruction in the absence of periosteal new bone formation is pathognomonic of TB
- Synovial fluid, thickened synovium and pericapsular tissues may cause a soft tissue swelling. With the destruction of articular cartilage, the joint space is reduced.

17. Ans. (a) Tuberculosis of knee

[Ref. Orthopedics by Mohindra, 1/e p248]

Tuberculosis Knee Joint

- **Characteristic feature:** Triple displacement (Flexion, Posterior subluxation, External rotation)
- **5 Classical deformities:** Flexion, Posterior subluxation, Lateral subluxation, Lateral rotation, Abduction of tibia
- **MC site:** Synovium

18. Ans. (a) Tuberculosis

[Ref. Orthopaedic Pathology by Vigorita, 2/e p236]

- TB in the spine is characterized by changes in the disc space and adjacent vertebral bodies
- When both neighbouring vertebral bodies are involved, the disc may lose its nutrition and be involved secondarily

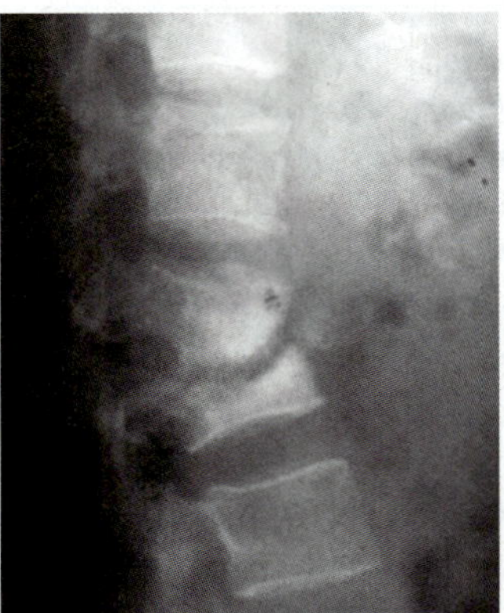

Fig. TB spine

19. Ans. (a) Tuberculosis of shoulder

[Ref. Orthopedic Pathology by Vincent, 2/e p236]

Caries Sicca

- An erosion (literally a "Dry hole") seen as a common finding in humeral heads involved by long-standing and probably burnt-out TB
- Tuberculosis of shoulder joint belongs to the Osseous type in most cases and develops frequently in the humeral head and around the bicipital groove; Periosteal type is found in only a small number of cases, and its characteristic is manifestation of caries sicca.

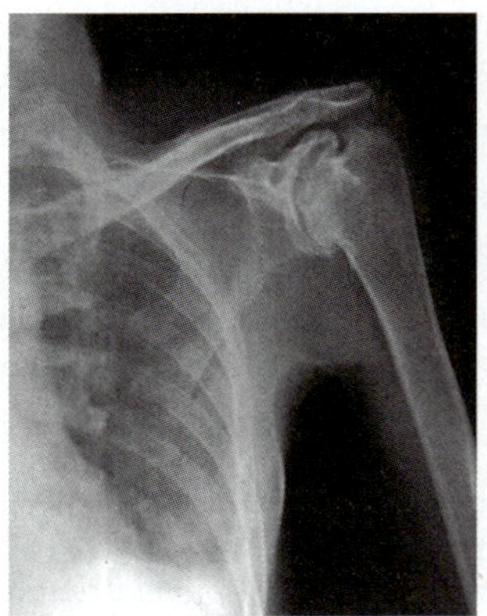

Fig. Caries sicca

HIGH YIELD MCQs ANSWERS WITH EXPLANATIONS 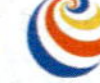

1. Ans. (a) Abundant Periosteal reaction

[Ref. Orthopedic Diagnosis by Murray, 1/e p112]

Tuberculous Osteomyelitis

- Little or none periosteal reaction
- Little or none bone sclerosis
- Sequestrum formation uncommon (Sequestrum type seen: Sandy/Feathery type)
- Minimal inflammation
- Secondary to TB lesion elsewhere in the body
- Outcome: Fibrous ankylosis in joints (Bony ankylosis in spine)

2. Ans. (a) Trochanteric; (d) Subdeltoid

[Ref. Tuberculosis by Madkour, 1/e p600]

3. Ans. (b) Periosteal reaction is seen

[Ref. Orthopedic Diagnosis by Murray, 1/e p112]

4. Ans. (c) Vertebrae

[Ref. Pediatric Orthopedics by Herring, 5/e p1062]

5. Ans. (c) Spinous process

[Ref. Essential Handbook of Practical Orthopedic Examination by Banerjee, 1/e p92]

Types of Vertebral Tuberculosis

- **Paradiscal (Most common type)**: Involves tow contiguous vertebrae with intervening disc
- Central: Inside of body
- Anterior: Anterior part of body
- Posterior: Pedicle, Transverse process, Lamina, Spinous process (Least common)

6. Ans. (b) In the cancellous vertebral body

[Ref. Adolescent Spine by Keim, 2/e p102]

Tuberculous **infection of** ***spine*** usually begins in *Cancellous* bone of *vertebral body*, and only rarely in Posterior neural arch/Transverse process

7. Ans. (d) Sudden deformity

[Ref. Pediatrics by Holt, 1/e p1373]

8. Ans. (c) Pain

[Ref. Maheshwari, 4/e p181]

9. Ans. (c) Spasticity

10. Ans.(b) Tuberculosis

[Ref. The Imaging of Tuberculosis by Palmer, 1/e]

11. Ans.(b) Upper thoracic spine

[Ref. Textbook of Orthopedics by Ebnezar, 4/e p562]

12. Ans. (e) All of the above

[Ref. Textbook of Orthopedics by Ebnezar, 4/e p562]

Paraplegia of TB Spine Most Common In Dorsal Spine

- TB more common in dorsal spine
- Spinal cord terminated below L1
- Spinal cord smallest in this region
- Normal curve encourages marked Kyphosis
- Anterior longitudinal ligament in dorsal region loosely confines the abscess

13. Ans. (b) Spinal artery compression

[Ref. Textbook of Neurosurgery by Tandon, 3/e p756]

Causes of Paraplegia of TB Spine

- Cord compression in Active disease:
  - Abscess - Fluid or Caseous (MCC of paraplegia: Cold abscess)
  - Granulation tissue
  - Sequestered bone and disc
  - Pathological subluxation or dislocation of vertebrae
- Cord compression in Healed disease:
  - Transverse ridge or bone anterior to spinal cord
  - Stretching/attrition of cord due to spinal deformity (Gibbus)
  - Dural fibrosis
- Other causes:
  - Infective thrombosis of cord
  - Spinal tumor syndrome

14. Ans. (d) Cold abscess pressing on the cord

[Ref. Textbook of Surgery by Gupta, 2/e p421]

15. Ans. (b) Tuberculosis

[Ref. Spondylitis by Acton, Scholarly paper 2012 p1]

- MCC of Kyphosis in Males: Tuberculosis
- MCC of Kyphosis in Females: Osteoporosis

16. Ans. (b) Bony-Ankylosis

[Ref. Joint Imaging in Childhood and Adolescence by Machada, 1/e p115]

17. Ans. (a) Night sweat; (b) Reduced appetite; (c) Loss of lordosis; (d) Back pain

[Ref. Foundations of Osteopathic Medicine by Chila, 3/e p979]

18. Ans. (b) Insidious onset paraplegia is good prognosis

[Ref. Orthopedics for Undergraduate by Crabbe, 1/e p102]

- Early sudden onset paraplegia in TB has good prognosis: Cord is compressed but not damaged
- Late insidious onset paraplegia in TB has poor prognosis: Irreversible with high chance of permanency

19. Ans. (b) Sudden progression of paraplegia; (d) Long-standing paraplegia

[Ref. Spinal Infections and Trauma by Jain, 1/e p173]

Poor Prognostic Factors in Pott's Paraplegia

- Late onset
- Sudden progression
- Age >50 years
- Complete paraplegia or Flaccid paraplegia at presentation
- Involvement of thoracic spine
- Duration >6 months
- Intrinsic cord changes
- Poor general health

20. Ans. (b) Grade IV Pott's spine; (c) Kyphotic angle >60 degrees

21. Ans.(d) Tuberculosis

[Ref. Diagnostic Radiology by Berry, 2/e p140]

22. Ans. (b) Pott's disease

[Ref. Maheshwari, 4/e p179]

23. Ans. (a) Narrowing of intervertebral space

[Ref. Maheshwari, 4/e p183]

24. Ans. (a) Caries spine

[Ref. Maheshwari, 4/e p183]

25. Ans. (b) Pott's spine

[Ref. Maheshwari, 4/e p183]

26. Ans. (a) Tuberculosis of spine

[Ref. Maheshwari, 4/e p183]

27. Ans. (a) Lateral decompression; (d) Antituberculous drugs

[Ref. Maheshwari, 4/e p178-179]

28. Ans. (a) T12–L1

[Ref. Essential Handbook of Practical Orthopedic Examination by Banerjee, 1/e p80]

29. Ans. (b) Thoracic

[Ref. Orthopedic Nursing Secrets by Michael, 1/e p81]

30. Ans.(d) Paradiscal

[Ref. Maheshwari, 4/e p180]

31. Ans.(d) Vertebral body

[Ref. Medicine in Africa by Parry, 3/e p329]

Tuberculosis starts as an inflammation of Intervertebral disc, which then spreads along anterior and longitudinal ligaments to involve adjacent vertebral bodies

32. Ans. (a) TB spine
[Ref. Short Textbook of Surgery by Roy, 1/e p143]

33. Ans. (a) Painless with no movement
[Ref. Undergraduate Surgery by Nan, 3/e p809]

34. Ans. (a) Decreased joint space
[Ref. Essentials of Skeletal Radiology, 3/e p1399]

35. Ans. (d) Both A+B but not C
[Ref. Musculoskeletal Radiology by Griffiths, 1/e p122]

36. Ans. (c) Anterolateral decompression
[Ref. Textbook of Orthopedics by Kotwal, 1/e p94]

Surgical Treatment of TB Spine

- Indications for surgery:
  - Lesion/abscess increasing in spite of chemotherapy
  - Paraplegia during chemotherapy
  - Worsening of paraplegia with adequate chemotherapy
  - Sudden onset paraplegia
- Surgical approaches:
  - Aspiration
  - Costotransversectomy
  - **Anterolateral decompression (Most common method used)**
  - Anterior decompression and stabilization with strut graft and implant (Ideal for Pott's paraplegia)
  - Laminectomy (only done if posterior elements of vertebra involved)

37. Ans. (b) Anterior decompression and bone grafting
[Ref. SAMJ, Volume 73 p562]

38. Ans. (a) Progressive loss of function in spite of medical treatment; (b) No improvement in motor power in spite of 3 months of treatment
[Ref. Textbook of Orthopedics by Kotwal, 1/e p94]

39. Ans. (d) Fixed flexion to further full flexion
[Ref. The 5-Minute Clinical Consult Premium 2015, 23/e p6]

40. Ans. (b) Same side hip flexion relieves pain
[Ref. The 5-Minute Clinical Consult Premium 2015, 23/e p6]

41. Ans. (b) Tuberculous
[Ref. Maheshwari, 4/e p176]

42. Ans. (b) Tuberculous arthritis
[Ref. Bone and Joint Infections by Zimmerli, 1/e p208]

- MC cause of monoarthritis in Children (Rheumatic): Juvenile idiopathic arthritis
- MC cause of monoarthritis in Children (Non-Rheumatic): Tuberculosis

43. Ans. (b) Fibrous ankylosis
[Ref. Surgical Diseases in Tropical Countries by Sood, 1/e p166]

44. Ans. (b) Synovial fluid has < 20% blood sugar
[Ref. Manual of Tropical Pediatrics by Seear, 1/e p225]

In Tuberculous arthritis, synovial blood sugar is <75% of Blood glucose

45. Ans. (d) Charnley's Arthrodesis
[Ref. Operative Orthopedics by Chapman, Volume 4 p3384]

46. Ans. (a) Shoulder
[Ref. Orthopedic Pathology by Vincent, 2/e p236]

Caries sicca: An erosion (literally a **"dry hole"**) seen as a common finding in humeral heads involved by long-standing and probably burnt-out TB

47. Ans. (b) Hip + Spine
[Ref. Essential Handbook of Practical Orthopedic Examination by Banerjee, 1/e p80]

MC Sites in Skeletal TB: Spine > Hip > Knee

48. Ans. (b) Tuberculosis
[Ref. Practical Orthopedic Examination Made Easy by Kumar, 2/e p139]

Triple Deformity of Knee

- Components: Flexion deformity of knee, Posterolateral subluxation of tibia, External rotation of tibia over femoral condyles
  - **Quadruple deformity**: Triple deformity + Genu valgum
- Conditions showing triple deformity:
  - Tuberculosis (Classic example)
  - Rheumatoid arthritis
  - ITB contracture

49. Ans. (c) Tuberculosis of hip
[Ref. Maheshwari, 4/e p189]

50. Ans.(d) Trochanteric
[Ref. Tuberculosis by Madkour, 1/e p600]

51. Ans. (a) Posterior and lateral dislocation/subluxation, External rotation, Fixed flexion
[Ref. Apley's, 9/e p20]

Classical Neglected Cases of TB (Composite Deformity)

- Posterior and lateral subluxation or dislocation
- External rotation
- Fixed flexion

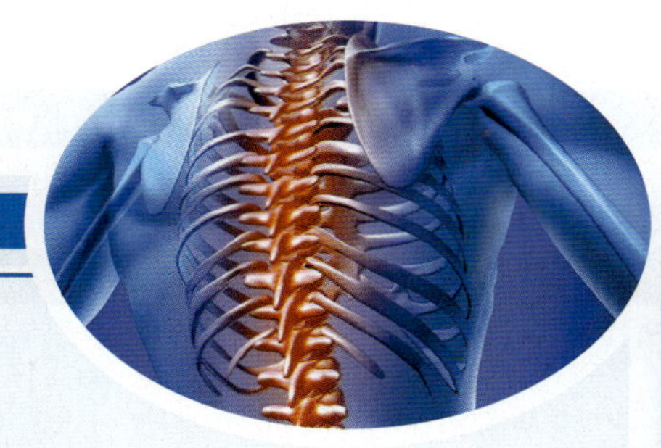

Chapter 10

Tumors

THEORETICAL CONCEPTS

X A. COMMON SITES OF BONE TUMORS IN BODY

Tumour	Common sites
BENIGN TUMORS	
Osteoma	Skull bones Facial bones
Osteoid osteoma	**Diaphysis of Tibia** (Most common[Q]) Posterior elements of vertebrae
Osteoblastoma	**Jaw bone**[Q] Spine
Hemangioma	**Vertebrae**[Q] Skull bones
Adamantinoma	**Jaw bone** (Most common[Q]) Lower half tibia
Chordoma	Sacrum Cervical spine
Giant cell tumour (Osteoclastoma)	**Epiphysis lower end femur**[Q] Epiphysis upper end tibia Epiphysis lower end radius
MALIGNANT TUMORS	
Osteogenic sarcoma (Osteosarcoma)	**Lower end femur** (Most common[Q]) Upper end tibia Upper end humerus
Ewing's sarcoma	**Diaphysis long bones** (Most common[Q]) Flat bones (pelvis[Q]) Calcaneum
Multiple myeloma	Flat bones (pelvis, vertebrae, skull, ribs[Q])
Chondrosarcoma	Flat bones (scapula, pelvis, ribs)
Synovial sarcoma	Knee bones
Reticulum cell sarcoma	Long bones (Most common[Q]) Flat bones

Contd…

Contd…

Tumour	Common sites
Secondaries in bone	**Spine** (Most common[Q]) Ribs Extremities
TUMOUR-LIKE CONDITIONS	
Chondroblastoma	Knee bones
Osteochondroma	Knee bones
Enchondroma	Small bones of hand and foot
Simple bone cyst	**Upper end humerus** (Most common[Q])
Aneurysmal bone cyst	Ends of long bones
Fibrous dysplasia	Upper end femur Upper end tibia Ribs

X B. COMMON BONE MALIGNANCIES

- ***Most common primary bone malignancy:*** Multiple myeloma[Q]
- *Second most common primary bone malignancy:* Osteosarcoma
- *Most common **benign tumour of bone:*** Osteochondroma[Q]
- *Most common **'TRUE' benign tumour of bone:*** Osteoid osteoma[Q]
- *Most common **malignant bone tumour**:* Secondaries to bone[Q]
- *Most common **bone tumour in Hand***: Enchondroma[Q]

	Site	Location[Q]	Most common age	Radiology	Management
Simple bone cyst	Metaphysis	Humerus upper	5–20 years	–	Curettage + Bone grafting
Aneurysmal bone cyst	Metaphysis	Humerus	10–40 years	Balloon-cortex	
Fibrous dysplasia	Metaphysis	Femur neck	20–30 years	**Ground-glass**[Q]	
Giant cell tumour	Epiphysis	Upper tibia	20–40 years	**Soap-bubble**[Q]	Excision
Osteoid osteoma	Diaphysis	Tibia	5–25 years	Sclerotic zone	
Osteosarcoma	Metaphysis	Femur lower	15–25 years	**Sun-ray**[Q]	Chemotherapy
Ewing's sarcoma	Diaphysis	Femur	5–15 years	**Onion-peel**[Q]	Radiotherapy

Topper's Edge

Osteogenic Sarcoma

- Highly malignant bone tumour
- 2nd most common primary bone tumor (After Multiple myeloma[Q])
- Arise from: Multipotent cells
- **MC site[Q]: Metaphysis (90%)**
- MC variety: Mixed type of both osteosclerotic and osteolytic varieties
- Characteristic features[Q]:
  - First symptom: Pain
  - Sunray appearance
  - Codman's triangle
  - Leg of mutton appearance

X C. METASTASIS/ SECONDARIES IN BONE

- *MC tumors to give rise to sclerotic secondaries in bone*: Carcinoma of prostate (males) and breast (females)
- *Common sites in body*:
  - **Vertebral bodies (Most common site[Q])**
  - Ribs

- Pelvis
- Humerus
- Femur

***Common origins of bony secondaries*:**	***Common sites of bony secondaries*:**
• **Breast (Most common in females[Q])** • **Prostate (Most common in males[Q])** • Lung • Renal • Thyroid	• **Spine (Most common[Q])** • Proximal femur • Proximal humerus
***Osteoblastic secondaries in men*:** • Carcinoma prostate[Q] • Seminoma	***Osteoblastic secondaries in women*:** • Carcinoma breast[Q] • Carcinoma uterus • Carcinoma ovary
***Osteoblastic secondaries in both men and women*:** Neurogenic tumors Carcinoid tumors Osteosarcoma	***Osteolytic secondaries*:** Carcinoma lung Carcinoma kidney Carcinoma thyroid Carcinoma breast Carcinoma stomach Carcinoma colon

X D. EOSINOPHILIC GRANULOMA

- *EG is a rare neoplastic proliferation of*: **Langerhans cells**[Q]
- *Types of Eosinophilic granulomas*[Q]:
  - Unifocal: *Eosinophilic granuloma*
  - Mutlifocal: *Hand-Schüller-Christian disease*
  - Disseminated: *Letterer-Siwe disease*
- *Bones affected*:
  - Skull
  - Diaphyses of long bones
  - Spine (shows vertebral collapse – ***Vertebra plana***[Q])
- *X-ray picture*:
  - Punched-out lesions
  - Periosteal reaction

Fig. Vertebra plana

X E. EWING'S SARCOMA

- *Type*: Highly malignant round cell sarcoma of diaphyses
- *Age group affected*: 10-20 years
- *Bones affected*: Femur, Tibia, Flat bones (pelvis, calcaneum)
- *Histopathology*: Pseudorosette formation
- *X-ray picture*: Moth-eaten with ***'Onion-peel appearance***[Q]***'***
- *Treatment*: Highly radiosensitive but recurs with poor prognosis

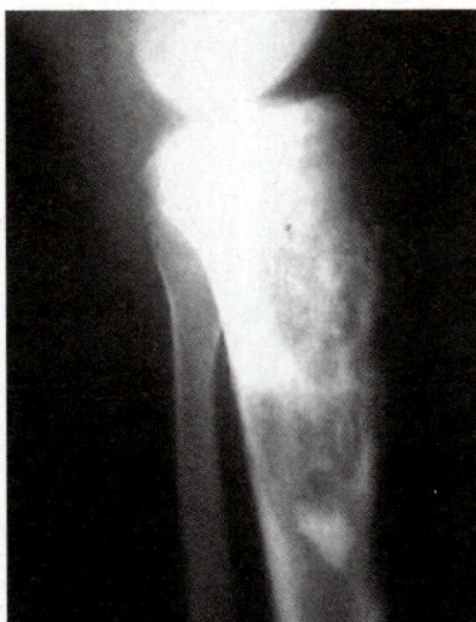

Fig. Onion-peel appearance

Orthopedics

X F. FIBROUS DYSPLASIA

- *Type of disorder*: Normal bone replaced by fibrous tissue
- *Associated with*: Hormone disorders
  - McCune-Albright's syndrome (most severe form)
  - Cushing's disease
- *Hormonal abnormalities*:
  - Parathyroid hormone
  - Growth hormone
  - Gonadotropins
- *Fibrous dysplasia can affect*:
  - **Tibia (Long bones)**
  - Ribs
  - Skull
  - Maxilla
  - Fibrous dysplasia is premalignant

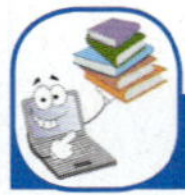

IMAGE-BASED QUESTIONS

1. A 20-year-old male with complaint of pain and swelling in right hip. X-ray pelvis of the patient is given below. Most probable diagnosis is *[AIIMS May 2016]*

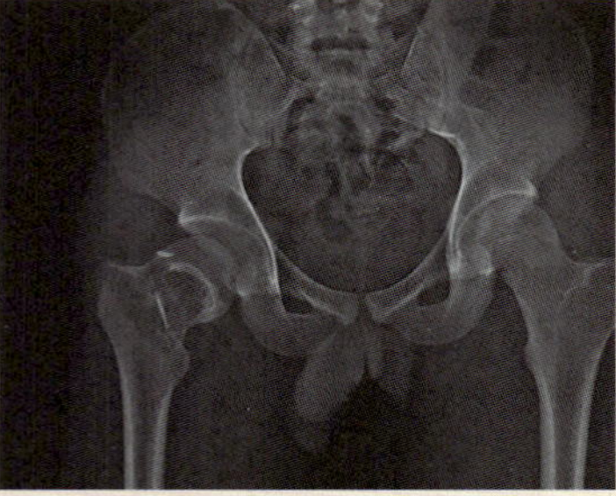

a. Simple bone cyst
b. Ewing's sarcoma
c. Giant cell tumour
d. Adamantinoma

2. Diagnose the Developmental disorder shown in Photograph

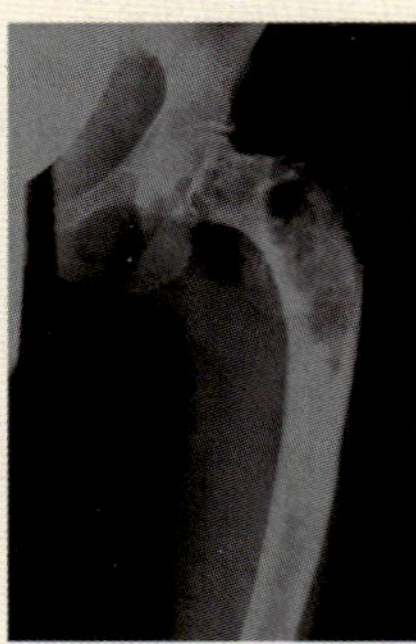

a. Marfan's syndrome
b. Fibrous dysplasia
c. Achondroplasia
d. CDH

3. Condition (Arrow) shown in Photograph is *[Recent Question 2012, Recent Question 2013]*

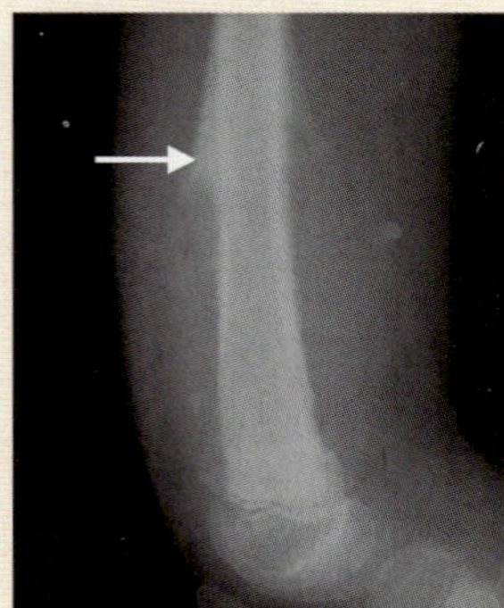

a. Chondroblastoma
b. Chondrosarcoma
c. Osteosarcoma
d. Giant cell tumour

4. Diagnose the Bone tumor shown in Photograph *[Recent Question 2013]*

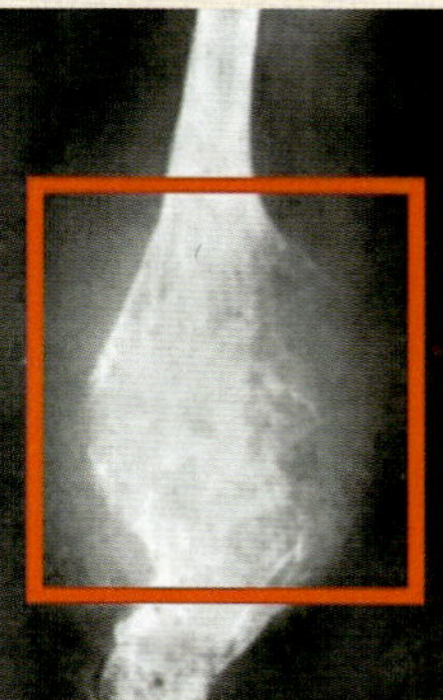

a. Osteosarcoma
b. Giant cell tumour
c. Ewing's sarcoma
d. Osteoid osteoma

5. Diagnose the bone tumor shown in Photograph

[Recent Question 2014, 2015]

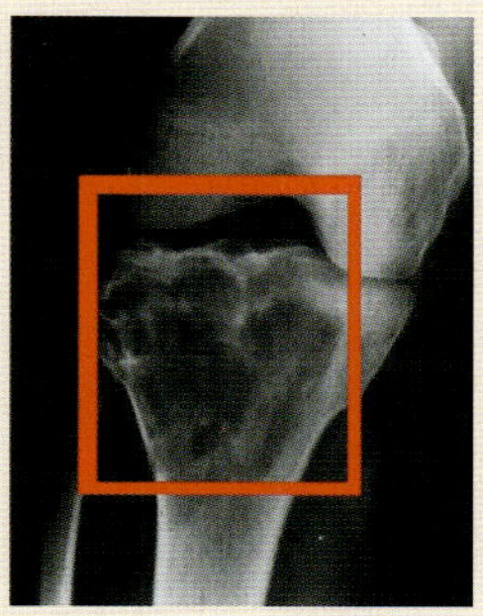

a. Osteosarcoma
b. Giant cell tumour
c. Ewing's sarcoma
d. Osteoid osteoma

6. Diagnose the Bone tumor shown in Photograph

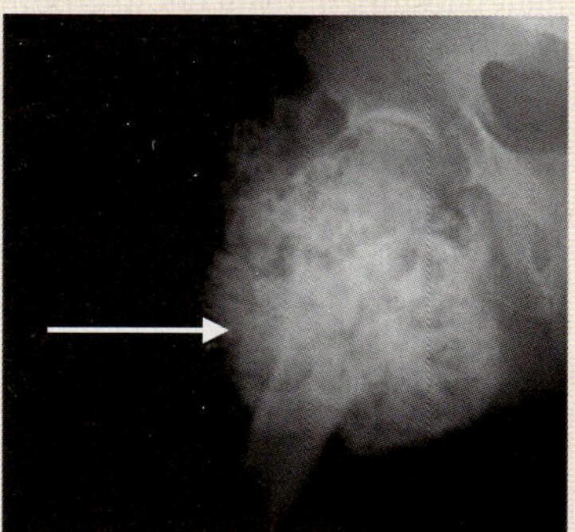

a. Osteoid osteoma
b. Osteochondroma
c. Chondrosarcoma
d. Unicameral bone cyst

7. Diagnose the underlying disorder as shown in Photograph ***[Recent Question 2012]***

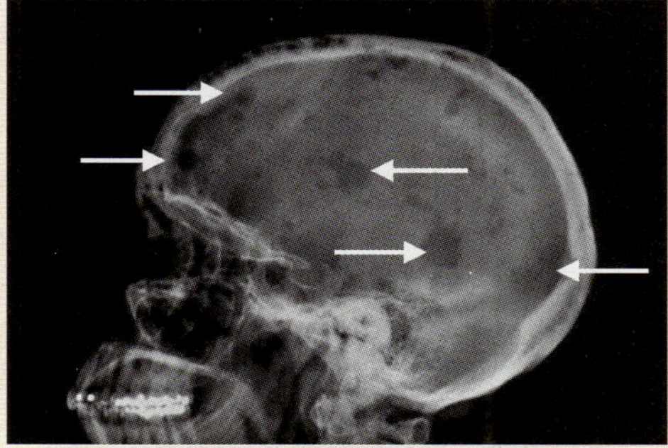

a. Osteogenic sarcoma
b. Enchondroma
c. Multiple myeloma
d. Giant cell tumour

ANSWERS WITH EXPLANATIONS OF IBQs 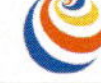

1. Ans. (a) Simple bone cyst *[Ref. Radiology Recall by Gay, 1/e p379]*

Simple Bone Cyst

- MC in adolescents (10–20 years age)
- Ends of the long bones are the favorite sites: MC being upper-end of Humerus
- X-ray: **(Photograph)**
  - At times, the cortex may be so thin that it is invisible on plain radiographs, and thus this benign lesion may be mistaken for a malignant bone tumor
  - Well-defined geographic lucent lesions with narrow zone of transition, which are centrally located and show sclerotic margin in majority of cases with no periosteal reaction or soft tissue component
  - They sometimes expand the bone with thinning of the endosteum without any breach of the cortex, unless there is a pathologic fracture
  - Prominent ridges of bone can appear as pseudotrabeculation on X-ray but its actually made of one contiguous cystic space
- Pathologic fractures may occur with a benign cause of weakened bone (Simple bone cyst, enchondroma, aneurysmal bone cyst, or fibrous dysplasia)
- 40% simple bone cysts may recur

2. Ans. (b) Fibrous dysplasia *[Ref. Maheshwari, 4/e p242]*

Fibrous Dysplasia

- Description: Normal bone is replaced by fibrous tissue which erodes cortices of bone from within, with subperiosteal bone around mass

- Radiology:
  - Multiloculated lesion, translucent to ground glass, expanding the cortex of bone
  - *Shepherd crook deformity*: Coxa varus angulation of the proximal femur, classically seen in femoral involvement by fibrous dysplasia (Also seen in Paget's disease of bone, Osteogenesis imperfecta)
- Treatment: Curettage and Grafting

3. Ans. (c) Osteosarcoma *[Ref. Radiology Review Manual by Dahnert, 7/e p11]*

Codman' Triangle
- Osteosarcoma
- Ewing's sarcoma
- Acute osteomyelitis
- Fracture
- Hemorrhage

4. Ans. (c) Ewing's sarcoma *[Ref. Maheshwari, 4/e p236]*
- 'Onion-peel appearance' on X-ray is characteristic of: Ewing's sarcoma
- Bony changes: Lytic lesion in medullary zone of mid-shaft of along bone, with cortical destruction; new bone formation occurs in new concentric layers

5. Ans. (b) Giant cell tumour *[Ref. Maheshwari, 4/e p230]*

Soap bubble appearance in Giant cell tumor: Homogeneously lytic tumor with trabeculae of bone traversing it, giving rise to loculated appearance

6. Ans. (c) Chondrosarcoma *[Ref. Orthopedics by Biswas, p138]*

Radiology of Chondrosarcoma
- Central lytic lesion with calcification gives fluffy *'Cotton-wool/ Popcorn/Bread-crumb' appearance*
- Invasion of soft tissue
- Little or none periosteal reaction

7. Ans. (c) Multiple myeloma *[Ref. Maheshwari, 4/e p238]*

Radiology in Multiple Myeloma
- Multiple punched out lesions in skull and other flat bones
- Wedge collapse of vertebrae (Most common: Thoracic spine)
- Erosion of border of ribs
- Rarefaction of bones

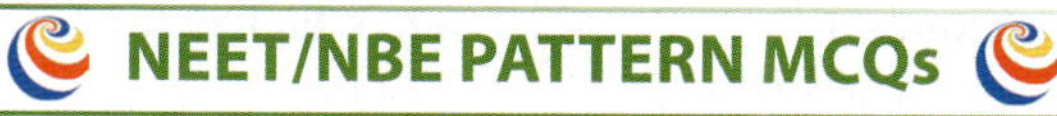

NEET/NBE PATTERN MCQs

1. **Commonest site of occurrence of Chondrosarcoma is** *[Recent Question 2016]*
   a. Pelvis b. Femur
   c. Ribs d. Proximal tibia
2. **All of the following are true regarding Paget's disease except** *[Recent Question 2016]*
   a. Pelvis is the most common site
   b. Cranial nerve involvement may be seen
   c. High output cardiac failure is one of the complications
   d. It may progress to a Secondary chondrosarcoma
3. **Sunray appearance and Codman's triangle are radiological features of which of the following tumors?** *[Recent Question 2016]*
   a. Osteosarcoma b. Ewing's Sarcoma
   c. Chondrosarcoma d. Multiple Myeloma
4. **All of the following are features of Pyle disease except** *[Recent Question 2016]*
   a. It is an autosomal recessive disease
   b. It is an epiphyseal dysplasia
   c. Mental retardation is uncommon
   d. Dental caries and mandibular prognathism
5. **Dripping Candle Wax lesion on spine is seen in** *[Recent Question 2016]*
   a. Metastasis b. TB spine
   c. Osteopterosis d. Melorheostosis
6. **Secondary osteosarcoma is associated with** *[Recent Question 2016]*
   a. Paget's disease b. Osteogenesis imperfecta
   c. Melorheostosis d. Ankylosing spondylitis
7. **Which of the following is bone forming malignant tumour?** *[Recent Question 2016]*
   a. Osteoid osteoma b. Osteosarcoma
   c. Chondrosarcoma d. Giant cell tumour
8. **Most common malignant lesion in vertebral bodies is** *[NBE FMGE September 2008]*
   a. Ewing's sarcoma b. Osteosarcoma
   c. Secondary deposits d. Multiple myeloma
9. **Surgical staging system for musculo-skeletal tumors is done through** *[NBE DNB 2010]*
   a. Edmonton staging b. Manchester staging
   c. TNM staging d. Enneking staging
10. **MC site of osteomas in paranasal sinuses is** *[NBE DNB 2011]*
    a. Frontal b. Maxillary
    c. Ethmoid d. Sphenoid
11. **Commonest primary malignant bone tumour is** *[NBE FMGE March 2008]*
    a. Multiple myeloma b. Giant cell tumour
    c. Osteosarcoma d. Ewing's sarcoma
12. **MC site seen for Osteogenic sarcoma in India is** *[NBE DNB 2010, AIIMS 2000, AIPGME 2001]*
    a. Lower end humerus b. Lower end tibia
    c. Upper end femur d. Lower end femur
13. **Epiphyseal tumour is** *[NBE DNB 2009]*
    a. Osteogenic sarcoma b. Giant cell tumour
    c. Ewing's sarcoma d. Osteoblastoma
14. **Commonest malignant bone tumour is** *[NBE DNB 2011]*
    a. Metastatic secondaries
    b. Multiple myeloma
    c. Osteosarcoma
    d. Chondrosarcoma
15. **Osteoblastic secondaries most commonly originate from** *[NBE DNB 2010]*
    a. Carcinoma prostate b. Carcinoma breast
    c. Carcinoma GIT d. Carcinoma lung
16. **Bone tumour most commonly arising from pelvis is** *[NBE FMGE March 2008]*
    a. Osteogenic sarcoma b. Chondrosarcoma
    c. Ewing's sarcoma d. Giant cell tumour
17. **A middle-aged man with lower jaw swelling. On clinical examination, there is expansion of left ramus of mandible. X-ray shows Soap-bubble appearance. Clinical diagnosis is** *[UPSC 2010]*
    a. Keratocyst b. Admantinoma
    c. Aneurysmal bone cyst d. Odontogenic myxoma
18. **Tumor with maximum bone matrix** *[Recent Question 2012]*
    a. Osteoid osteoma b. Chondrosarcoma
    c. Enchondroma d. None
19. **Tumour showing 'Sun-ray appearance' is** *[NBE DNB 1993, 2003, 2008, AIIMS 1995]*
    a. Ewing's tumour b. Osteosarcoma
    c. Osteoclastoma d. Osteochondroma
20. **Most likely primary site for carcinomatous metastasis to lumbar spine is** *[NBE FMGE September 2008]*
    a. Colon b. Breast
    c. Kidney d. Prostate
21. **Paget's disease after 10 years develops into** *[Recent Question 2012]*
    a. Osteosarcoma b. Fibrous cortical defect
    c. Osteoid osteoma d. Ankylosing spondylitis
22. **Onion-skin layering on X-ray is characteristic of** *[NBE FMGE March 2006]*
    a. Osteogenic sarcoma b. Ewing's sarcoma
    c. Paget's disease d. All of the above
23. **Which is a correct combination?** *[NBE DNB 1995]*
    a. Ewing sarcoma: Diaphysis and Osteosarcoma: Metaphysis
    b. Ewing sarcoma: Metaphysis and Osteosarcoma: Diaphysis
    c. Ewing sarcoma: Diaphysis and Osteosarcoma: Epiphysis
    d. Ewing sarcoma: Epiphysis and Osteosarcoma: Diaphysis
24. **Metastasis not found in** *[Recent Question 2012]*
    a. Femur b. Humerus
    c. Fibula d. Spine
25. **Onion-peel appearance is seen in** *[Recent Question 2016, 2017, NBE FMGE September 2005]*
    a. Ewing's sarcoma b. Osteosarcoma
    c. Osteoclastoma d. Chondrosarcoma

26. Bone tumour with 'Soap bubble appearance' is *[NBE DNB 1998]*
a. Chordoma b. Chondroma
c. Osteoma d. Osteoclastoma

27. Codman's triangle is seen in *[Recent Question 2012]*
a. Osteosarcoma b. Osteoblastoma
c. Osteoclastoma d. GCT

28. In multiple myeloma, punched-out lesions are most common in *[NBE FMGE September 2005]*
a. Cervical rib b. Skull
c. Femur d. Pelvis

29. Hyperparathyroidism causes *[Recent Question 2012]*
a. Multiple bone cysts
b. Subperiosteal bone resorption
c. Brown's tumor
d. All of the above

30. Vertebra plana occurs in *[NBE FMGE September 2005]*
a. TB spine b. Secondaries in spine
c. Pyogenic osteomyelitis d. Eosinophilic granuloma

31. X-ray appearance of osteosarcoma are all except *[Recent Question 2013]*
a. Periosteal reaction b. Codman's triangle
c. Soap-bubble d. Sunray appearance

32. MC benign type of bone tumour seen is *[NBE DNB 1998, 2004, 2007]*
a. Bone cyst b. Osteoma
c. Chordoma d. Chondroma

33. Most radiosensitive tumour is *[NBE FMGE September 2005]*
a. Hodgkin's lymphoma
b. Carcinoma cervix
c. Malignant fibrous histiocytoma
d. Ewing's sarcoma

34. A patient presents with pain in the thigh, relieved by aspirin. X-ray shows a radiolucent mass surrounded by sclerosis. Diagnosis is *[Recent Question 2012]*
a. Osteoma b. Osteoid osteoma
c. Osteoblastoma d. Osteoclastoma

35. Which of the following is true about Giant cell tumor? *[Recent Question 2012, 2013]*
a. Usually presents as a lytic lesion with sclerotic rim
b. Always benign
c. Epiphyseal origin
d. Seen in age less than 15 years

36. Hormone-dependent bone tumour is *[NBE FMGE March 2005]*
a. Osteogenic sarcoma b. Ewing's sarcoma
c. Osteoclastoma d. Fibrous dysplasia

37. Tumour originating in Medullary canal of diaphysis is *[NBE DNB 2001, 2005]*
a. Osteosarcoma b. Osteoclastoma
c. Ewing's sarcoma d. Synovial sarcoma

38. Radiotherapy is useful in treatment of which of the following bone tumors? *[NBE DNB 2001, 2004, 2007]*
a. Osteosarcoma b. Osteoclastoma
c. Ewing's sarcoma d. Synovial sarcoma

39. Chemotherapeutic drug of choice in Osteosarcoma is *[NBE DNB 2002, 2007]*
a. Methotrexate b. 5-Fluorouracil
c. Cyclophosphamide d. Doxorubicin

40. Which of the following is epiphyseal tumor? *[Recent Question 2012, 2014]*
a. Giant cell tumor
b. Osteogenic Sarcoma
c. Ewing's Sarcoma
d. Osteoid osteoma

41. Following are seen in Fibrous dysplasia EXCEPT *[NBE FMGE September 2004]*
a. Café-au-lait spots
b. No premalignant change
c. Expanding rib lesions
d. Expanding lesions of maxilla

42. All are true about multiple exostosis EXCEPT *[NBE DNB 2009]*
a. Autosomal dominant disorder
b. Osteopenia present
c. Failure in re-modelling of ends of bones
d. Multiple bone lumps (exostoses) occur

43. Most common malignant bone tumour is *[NBE FMGE September 2003]*
a. Osteosarcoma
b. Osteoclastoma
c. Secondaries
d. Multiple myeloma

44. Osteoblastic secondaries arise from *[NBE FMGE March 2003]*
a. Renal carcinoma
b. Thyroid carcinoma
c. GIT carcinoma
d. Prostate carcinoma

45. Codman's triangle is seen in *[Recent Question 2014]*
a. Ewing's sarcoma b. Osteosarcoma
c. Acute osteomyelitis d. All of the above

46. MC benign tumor of bone in less than 20 years age group is *[Recent Question 2014]*
a. Osteoma
b. Osteoid osteoma
c. Osteoblastoma
d. Chondorblastoma

47. Ollier's disease is *[Recent Question 2015]*
a. Osteochondromatosis
b. Metaphyseal dysplasia
c. Multiple enchondromatosis
d. Osteopetrosis

48. Pulmonary metastasis occur from *[Recent Question 2015]*
a. Osteosarcoma
b. Ewing's sarcoma
c. Colorectal carcinoma
d. All of the above

49. Oncogenic osteomalacia is mediated by *[Recent Question 2017]*
a. Phosphatonin b. Calcitonin
c. Interleukin 2 d. Interleukin 6

50. Dense calcification is found in all except *[Recent Question 2017]*
a. Osteosarcoma
b. Chondroblastoma
c. Synovial sarcoma
d. Osteoblastoma

51. Which is Intramedullary tumor among Carcinoma of bone? *[Recent Question 2017]*
a. Classical Osteosarcoma b. Parosteal osteosarcoma
c. Periosteal osteosarcoma d. None of the above

52. Commonest malignancy of bones is *[Recent Question 2017]*
a. Ewing's sarcoma b. Metastases
c. Multiple myeloma d. Osteogenic sarcoma

53. Age group affected by Osteosarcoma *[Recent Question 2017]*
a. Upto 10 years b. 10-20 years
c. 30-40 years d. Older than 45 years

54. A 22-year-old male presents with bony mass in the metaphyseal region of right knee with typical Sunray appearance and CT scan of the chest reveals osteoblastic metastases. What is the most probable diagnosis? *[Recent Question 2017]*
a. Osteosarcoma b. Chondrosarcoma
c. Ewing's sarcoma d. Osteochondroma

55. Most common site of metastases in case of osteosarcoma is *[Recent Question 2017]*
a. Brain b. Lungs
c. Liver d. Bladder

HIGH YIELD MCQs

1. Which of the following is/are true about Giant cell tumour? *[PGI May 2016]*
a. Commonly occurs in bones around knee joint
b. Radiotherapy is given for treatment
c. Cause cortical thinning by expansion
d. Most commonly occur during puberty
e. None of the above

2. Which of the following is/are true about Simple bone cyst? *[PGI November 2016]*
a. Most commonly occur in adult
b. Commonest site is the upper end of the humerus
c. Cortex may be thin
d. Cause pathological fracture
e. No risk of recurrence after removal

3. Pulsating bone tumour is *[All India PGMEE 2007, AIIMS 2010]*
a. Osteosarcoma b. Osteoclastoma
c. Ewing's sarcoma d. Chondroma

4. Characteristic radiological feature of fibrous dysplasia is *[AIIMS PGMEE 2010]*
a. Bone enlargement b. Cortical calcification
c. Cortical thickening d. Ground glass appearance

5. Not a benign bone tumour *[All India PGMEE 1996]*
a. Chordoma b. Chondroma
c. Enchondroma d. Osteoid osteoma

6. MC tumour in hand is *[AIIMS PGMEE 1997]*
a. Giant cell tumour b. Enchondroma
c. Exostosis d. Synovial sarcoma

7. MC benign tumour of bone is *[Recent Question 2017, AIIMS PGMEE 1995]*
a. Enchondroma b. Osteochondroma
c. Simple bone cyst d. Giant cell tumour

8. Vertebra plana is seen in *[Recent Question 2016, PGI 2006]*
a. Trauma b. Malignancy
c. Paget's disease d. Ewing's sarcoma
e. Eosinophilic granuloma

9. Radioresistant malignant tumour is *[AP PGMEE PGMEE 2002]*
a. Neuroblastoma b. Ewing's sarcoma
c. Osteosarcoma d. Retinoblastoma

10. Benign bone tumors are *[PGI 2003]*
a. Osteoid osteoma b. Osteochondroma
c. Chondroblastoma d. Chondromyxoid fibroma
e. Multiple myeloma

11. All of the following tumor are benign tumour except *[All India PGMEE 1998]*
a. Chondroma b. Chordoma
c. Osteochondroma d. Enchondroma

12. According to a newer hypothesis Ewing's sarcoma arises from *[All India PGMEE 1999]*
a. Epiphysis b. Diaphysis
c. Medullary cavity d. Cortex

13. Bone tumors arising from diaphysis *[PGI 2000]*
a. Chondrosarcoma b. Ewing's tumor
c. Osteoclastoma d. Chondroblastoma
e. Osteoid osteoma

14. Solitary bone cyst is most common in the *[All India PGMEE 2004]*
a. Upper end of humerus b. Lower end of humerus
c. Upper end of fibula d. Lower end of femur

15. Chordoma can occur over all the following sites, except *[All India PGMEE 2000]*
a. Rib b. Clivus
c. Sacrum d. Vertebral body

16. True about bone tumour is *[AIIMS PGMEE 1999]*
a. Multiple myeloma- more than 55 years age and above
b. Osteogenic sarcoma- fourth decade
c. Chondrosarcoma- first decade
d. Osteoclastoma- fifth decade

17. A12-year-old boy, LEAST common cause of proximal lytic lesion of head of femur is *[AIIMS PGMEE 1997]*
a. Plasmacytoma b. Metastasis
c. Histiocytosis d. Bone tumour

18. Ramu, an 8-year-old boy presented with pain in the arm. On X-ray his upper end of humerus demonstrates an expansile lesion in the metaphysis with breech of the overlying cortex. Most likely diagnosis is *[AIIMS PGMEE 2002]*
a. Aneurysmal bone cyst
b. Unicameral bone cyst
c. Chondroblastoma
d. Osteoclastoma

19. A 8-year-child present with fracture humerus after trivial injury, X-ray shows lytic lesion diagnosis is *[AIIMS PGMEE 1999, AIPGME 2001]*

a. Osteoclastoma b. Osteomyelitis
c. Unicameral bone cyst d. Aneurysmal bone cyst

20. MC site of origin for Adamantinoma is *[AIIMS PGMEE 2001]*

a. Mandible near symphysis menti
b. Mandible near molar tooth
c. Hard palate
d. Middle alveolar margins

21. MC site of origin for Adamantinoma in long bones is *[AIIMS PGMEE 2002]*

a. Femur b. Tibia
c. Ulna d. Fibula

22. Chondroblastoma most commonly occurs in *[AIIMS PGMEE 2002]*

a. Epiphysis b. Metaphysis
c. Diaphysis d. Medullary cavity

23. All are true for Multiple myeloma *[PGI 2009]*

a. Monclonal M-band
b. Bone marrow plasma cells <5%
c. Hypercalcemia, Hyperuricemia
d. Increased ALP
e. Hyperglycemia

24. Lytic bevelled lesions in skull X-ray is due to *[AIIMS PGMEE 2000]*

a. Osteosarcoma b. Metastasis
c. Multiple myeloma d. Eosinophilic granuloma

25. Three most common cancers metastasising to bone are *[PGI 2007]*

a. Prostate b. Lungs
c. Kidneys d. Breast
e. Thyroid

26. Metastasis is commonly seen in all except *[PGI 2009]*

a. Skull b. Pelvis
c. Vertebrae d. Small bones of hand
e. Proximal part of long bones of upper limb

27. Most common cause of bone malignancy is *[PGI 2008]*

a. Osteosarcoma b. Osteoclastoma
c. Ewing's sarcoma d. Secondaries
e. Enchondroma

28. A classical expansile lytic lesion in the transverse process of a vertebra is seen in *[PGI 2004, AIPGME 2003]*

a. Osteosarcoma b. Aneurysmal bone cyst
c. Osteoblastoma d. Osteoclastoma
e. Metastasis

29. Which of the following conditions is least likely to present as an eccentric osteolytic lesion? *[Delhi PGMEE 2004]*

a. Aneurysmal bone cyst b. Giant cell tumor
c. Fibrous cortical defect d. Simple bone cyst

30. Differential diagnosis of simple bone cyst include *[PGI 2003]*

a. Giant cell tumour b. Non ossifying fibroma
c. Enchondroma d. Fibrous dysplasia
e. Eosinophilic granuloma

31. Histology of unicameral bone cyst *[PGI 2004]*

a. Blood-filled cavities b. Endothelial lining
c. Giant cells d. Bone formation

32. Histological features of unicameral bone cysts are *[PGI 2002]*

a. Blood-filled cystic spaces
b. Endothelial cell lining
c. Fibrous tissue with cystic spaces
d. Pseudocyst
e. Single cavity with connective tissue lining

33. Secondary aneurysmal bone cyst arises in *[PGI 2007]*

a. Osteoclastoma b. Chondroblastoma
c. Fibrous dysplasia d. None

34. Benign bone tumour(s) is/are *[PGI 2006]*

a. Osteoid osteoma b. Osteoclastoma
c. Osteochondroma d. Chondroblastoma
e. Endothelial hemangioma

35. Bone forming tumors is/ are *[PGI 2003]*

a. Chondrosarcoma b. Osteosarcoma
c. Osteoid osteoma d. Giant cell tumour
e. Osteoblastoma

36. Classification system of bone tumors is *[AIIMS PGMEE 2007]*

a. Enneking b. TNM
c. Manchester d. Edmonton

37. An 8-year-old boy presents with a gradually progressing swelling and pain since 6 months over the upper tibia. On X-ray, there is a lytic lesion with selerotic margins in the upper tibial metaphysis. The diagnosis is *[AIIMS PGMEE 2001]*

a. Osteogenic sarcoma b. Osteoclastoma
c. Brodie's abscess d. Ewing's sarcoma

38. In a young boy, X-ray of upper end of tibia shows a lytic lesion. The least likely diagnosis is *[AIIMS PGMEE 1994]*

a. Giant cell tumour b. Osteosarcoma
c. Solitary bone cyst d. Tuberculosis

39. When size of osteoclastoma exceeds the size of metaphysis *[PGI 2008]*

a. Tumor will be covered by cortex
b. Tumor will be covered by fibrous capsules
c. Covered by thin-layered bone
d. It is limited to metaphysis
e. Covered by periosteum

40. The differential diagnosis of lesion, histologically resembling giant cell tumour in the small bones of the hands or feet, includes all of the following except *[AIIMS PGMEE 2006]*

a. Aneursymal bone cyst b. Fibrosarcoma
c. Osteosarcoma d. Hyperparathyroidism

41. Treatment of histologically confirmed giant cell tumour *[PGI 2003]*

a. Excision, bone grafting and Chemical Cautery
b. Excision
c. Radiotherapy
d. Chemical excision

42. Which of the following bone tumour present secondaries in lung with pneumothorax? *[AIIMS PGMEE 1996]*

a. Osteosarcoma b. Ewing's sarcoma
c. Osteoclastoma d. Chondroblastoma

43. True about aneurysmal bone cyst *[PGI 2007, PGI 2009]*

a. Seen in older age b. Blood-filled spaces
c. Found in upper tibia d. Pulsatile in older age
e. Endothelial lining

44. Most common site of Simple bone cyst is *[Recent Question 2017, AIIMS PGMEE 1995]*
a. Humerus b. Radius
c. Tibia d. Femur

45. True about simple bone cyst is/are *[PGI 2005]*
a. Seen in young adults
b. Commonest site is diaphysis
c. Pathological fractures seen
d. Shaggy fibrous layering
e. Well demarcated radiolucent lesions

46. A patient presents with pneumothorax. Examination shows a swelling over knee. Chest X-ray shows lung nodules, give your most probable diagnosis *[AIIMS PGMEE 1995]*
a. Osteosarcoma b. Ewing sarcoma
c. Multiple myeloma d. Osteoclastoma

47. True regarding osteosarcoma is *[AIIMS PGMEE 2000]*
a. Occurs because of proliferation of osteoclasts
b. Sunray appearance in X-ray indicates new bone formation
c. Affects mainly males in 5th or 6th decade
d. Lymphatic metastasis is most common

48. A 15-year-old boy presented with mass in lower femur, which on X-ray was found to have Codman's triangle and sunray appearance. The diagnosis is
a. Ewing's Tumour *[All India PGMEE 2007]*
b. Osteosarcoma
c. Osteoclastoma
d. Osteomyelitis

49. Management plan for osteogenic sarcoma of the lower end of femur must include *[All India PGMEE 2004]*
a. Radiotherapy, amputation, chemotherapy
b. Surgery alone
c. Chemotherapy + Limb Salvage Surgery + Chemotherapy
d. Chemotherapy + radiotherapy

50. True about osteosarcoma *[PGI 2009]*
a. Involves epiphysis of long bones
b. Most commonly involve knee and distal femur
c. Spread to lung through hematogenous route
d. Exclusively found in adolescent and early adult life
e. X-ray sunray appearance

51. All are the predisposing factors of osteogenic sarcoma except *[PGI 2003]*
a. Paget's disease of bone
b. Radiation
c. Viral infection
d. Bone infarction

52. Features of parosteal osteosarcoma include *[PGI 2001]*
a. It invades the medullary cavity
b. Easily diagnosed by X-ray
c. Prognosis is same as in other forms of osteosarcoma
d. En bloc resection/amputation is the treatment of choice
e. Seen most commonly in younger age groups

53. 'T-10 Protocol' for treatment of osteosarcoma includes all of the following, except *[All India PGMEE 2009]*
a. High Dose Methotrexate
b. Bleomycin, Cyclophosphamide, Doxorubicin (BCD)
c. Vincristine
d. Etoposide

54. mic-2 mutation is associated with *[AIIMS PGMEE 2009]*
a. Osteosarcoma
b. Ewing sarcoma
c. Alveolar soft tissue sarcoma
d. Dermatofibrosarcoma protruberance

55. True about Ewing's sarcoma is *[PGI 2000]*
a. 5% cases reveals t (11-22)
b. Arise from medullary cavity of tubular bone
c. Arise from diaphysis
d. N-myc chromosome

56. Treatment of Osteoclastoma is *[PGI 2001]*
a. Excision b. Curettage
c. Chemotherapy d. Arthrodesis
e. Total bone replacement

57. Treatment for Soap-bubble appearance at lower end of radius is *[AIIMS PGMEE 1998]*
a. Amputation
b. Local excision
c. Excision and bone grafting
d. Radiotherapy

58. Chondroblastoma is a tumour of *[All India PGMEE 2000]*
a. Epiphysis b. Metaphysis
c. Diaphysis d. Flat bone

59. Bone tumors arising from diaphysis *[PGI 2000]*
a. Chondrosarcoma b. Osteoid osteoma
c. Ewing's tumor d. Osteoclastoma
e. Chondroblastoma

60. Which of the following occurs in epiphysis? *[PGI 2001]*
a. Osteoclastoma b. Chondroblastoma
c. Ewing's sarcoma d. Chodrosarcoma
e. Osteoid osteoma

61. Following tumors are seen in metaphysis *[PGI 2002]*
a. Osteoclastoma b. Ewing's sarcoma
c. Osteomyelitis d. Osteosarcoma
e. Chondrosarcoma

62. Osteosarcoma arise from *[PGI 2002]*
a. Diaphysis b. Metaphysis
c. Epiphysis d. Growth plate
e. Epiphyseal cortex

63. A child 10 yrs of age presents with a mass on his left thigh. The mass seems to be arising from diaphysis of femur, and involving the soft tissue of thigh. The child is having fever also. Give your most probable diagnosis
a. Osteosarcoma *[AIIMS PGMEE 2000]*
b. Ewing's sarcoma
c. Chondrosarcoma
d. Malignant fibrous histiocytoma

64. A 12-year-old girl complains of pain persisting in his leg for several weeks with a low-grade fever. A radiograph reveals a mass in the diaphyseal region of the left femur with overlying cortical erosion and soft tissue extension. A biopsy of the lesion shows numerous small round cells, rich in PAS positive diastase sensitive granules. The most likely histological diagnosis is *[AIIMS PGMEE 2003]*
a. Osteogenic sarcoma
b. Osteoblastoma
c. Ewing's sarcoma
d. Chondroblastoma

65. A 15-year-old boy is injured while playing cricket. X-rays of the leg rule out of a possible fracture. The radiologist reports the boy has an evidence of aggressive bone tumor with both bone destruction and soft tissue mass. The bone biopsy reveals a bone cancer with neural differentiation. Which of the following is the most likely diagnosis? *[AIIMS PGMEE 2006]*

a. Chondrablastoma b. Ewing's sarcoma
c. Neuroblastoma d. Osteosarcoma

66. A 7-year-old boy with h/o trauma 2 months back now presents with fever & acute pain over thigh. On X-ray femoral shaft shows lesions with multiple laminated periosteal 'reaction next line of management is *[AIIMS PGMEE 2009]*

a. CRP measurement b. Core biopsy
c. Tc99 MDP scan d. MRI

67. Most common lesion of the mandible is *[AIIMS PGMEE 2001]*

a. Ameloblastoma b. Squamous cell ca
c. Osteosarcoma d. Osteoclstoma

68. True about Ameloblastoma *[PGI 2006]*

a. Cystic lesion b. Rapidly growing
c. Malignant disease d. MC site is Tibia
e. Presented in children

69. A 33-year-old man presented with a slowly progressive swelling in the middle 1/3rd of his right tibia. X-rays examination revealed multiple sharply demarcated radiolucent lesions separated by areas of dense and sclerotic bone. Microscopic examination of a biopsy specimen revealed island of epithelial cells in a fibrous stroma. Which of the following is the most probable diagnosis? *[AIIMS PGMEE 2004]*

a. Adamantinoma b. Osteofibrous dysplasia
c. Osteosarcoma d. Fibrous cortical defect

70. Babu a 19 years old male has a small circumscribed sclerotic swelling over diaphysis of femur; likely diagnosis is *[All India PGMEE 2001, AIIMS 2001]*

a. Osteoclastoma b. Osteosarcoma
c. Ewing's sarcoma d. Osteoid osteoma

71. True statement (s) regarding Osteoid osteoma is/are *[PGI 2009]*

a. Malignant
b. MC bone involvement-tibia
c. Local excision or curettage cure
d. Bone pain relieved by aspirin
e. X-ray shows density surrounding radiolucent lesion

72. Jaw tumour is seen in *[AIIMS PGMEE 1992]*

a. Osteoporosis b. Osteomalacia
c. Osteopetrosis d. Caffey's disease

73. True about non-ossifying fibroma of bone *[PGI 2003]*

a. Present until 3rd and 4th decade
b. Eccentric
c. Prominent sclerotic margin
d. Histologically giant cell with areolar tissue
d. Metaphyseal lesion

74. True about non-ossifying fibroma *[PGI 2002]*

a. Prominent at 2nd and 4th decade
b. Prominent sclerotic margins
c. Fibrous tissue with areolar tissue
d. Centrally located
e. Risk of malignancy

75. Chordoma commonly involves *[PGI 2002]*

a. Dorsal spine b. Clivus
c. Lumbar spine d. Sacrum
e. Cervical spine

76. All are true about enchondroma except *[PGI 2014]*

a. Usually asymptomatic
b. Ollier's disease may be associated
c. Occurs only in short bones
d. Radiolucent lesion with flecks of calcification
e. Treatment is not always necessary

77. All of the following are the causes of sudden increase in pain in osteochondroma, except *[AIIMS PGMEE 2006]*

a. Sarcomatous change b. Fracture
c. Bursitis d. Degenerative changes

78. All the statements are true about exostosis, except *[All India PGMEE 2006]*

a. It occurs at the growing end of bone
b. Growth continues after skeletal maturity
c. It is covered by cartilaginous cap
d. Malignant transformation may occur

79. Which of the following statements is true about osteochondromatosis *[PGI 2001]*

a. Usually affects long bones, but can also occur in skull and pelvis.
b. Usual site is metaphyseal region
c. Also known as multiple exostoses, diaphyseal clasis
d. It does not interfere with general body stature
e. Autosomal dominant in inheritance

80. Which one of the following bone tumors typically affects the epiphysis of a long bone? *[AIIMS PGMEE 2005]*

a. Osteosarcoma
b. Ewing's sarcoma
c. Chondroblastoma
d. Chondromyxoid fibroma

81. Dense calcification is found in *[AIIMS PGMEE 1996]*

a. Osteosarcoma b. Chondroblastoma
c. Synovial sarcoma d. Osteoblastoma

82. A 15-year-old boy presented with painful swelling over the left shoulder. Radiograph of the shoulder showed an osteolytic area with stippled calcification over the proximal humeral epiphysis. Biopsy of the lesion revealed an immature fibrous matrix with scattered giant cells. Which of the following is the most likely diagnosis? *[AIIMS PGMEE 2004]*

a. Gaint cell tumor b. Chondroblastoma
c. Osteosarcoma d. Chondromyxoid fibroma

83. Radiological feature(s) of osteosarcoma is/are *[PGI 2006]*

a. New bone formation b. Soap bubble appearance
c. Codman's triangle d. Onion-peel appearance
e. Sun-ray appearance

84. Sunburst appearance is seen in *[PGI 2007]*

a. Osteoid osteoma b. Osteosarcoma
c. Osteoclastoma d. Ewing's sarcoma
e. Chondrosarcoma

85. Not useful for diagnosis of Osteosarcoma is *[All India PGMEE 2007]*

a. Bone scan b. MRI
c. CT scan chest d. Bone marrow biopsy

Orthopedics

86. A 45-year-old male presented with an expansile lesion in the centre of femoral metaphysis. The lesion shows Endosteal scalloping and punctuate calcifications. Most likely diagnosis is *[All India PGMEE 2002]*
a. Osteosarcoma b. Chondrosarcoma
c. Simple bone cyst d. Fibrous dysplasia

87. Which of the following statements is true regarding hemangioma of the bone *[PGI 2001]*
a. Occurs commonly in skull bones
b. Requires observation as I is premalignant
c. Hamartomatous in origin
d. Forms 10-12% of the bone tumors
e. Local gigantism occurs when it occurs in an extremity

88. A patient with pain in back. Lab investigation shows elevated ESR. X-ray skull shows multiple punched out lytic lesions. Most important Investigation to be done is *[AIIMS PGMEE 2000]*
a. Serum acid phosphatase b. CT head with contrast
c. Whole body scan d. Serum electrophoresis

89. A 60-year-old male has bone pain, vertebral collapse, fracture pelvis, the probable diagnosis is *[AIIMS PGMEE 1996]*
a. Multiple myeloma b. Secondaries
c. TB d. Hemangioma of bone

90. Which of the following usually produces osteoblastic secondaries? *[AIIMS PGMEE 2004]*
a. Carcinoma lung b. Carcinoma breast
c. Carcinoma urinary bladder
d. Carcinoma prostate

91. A patient developed paraplegia. On routine examination and X-ray, it was found that there are osteoblastic lesion in his spine. Most probable diagnosis is *[AIIMS PGMEE 2000]*
a. Carcinoma thyroid b. Carcinoma prostate
c. Breast carcinoma d. Pancreatic carcinoma

92. Expansile lytic osseous metastases are characteristics of primary malignancy of *[AP PGMEE 2012]*
a. Kidney b. Bronchus
c. Breast d. Prostate

93. Metastatic tumor least common in *[PGI 2004]*
a. Pelvis
b. Ribs
c. Small bone of lower limb
d. Vertebra
e. Skull

94. Bone metastases is common in which of the following *[PGI 2005]*
a. Nephroblastoma b. Neuroblastoma
c. RCC d. Clear cell sarcoma

95. Osteosclerotic bone metastasis is found most commonly in which carcinoma *[AIIMS PGMEE 2009]*
a. Kidney b. Thyroid
c. Lung d. Prostate

96. True about bone metastasis *[PGI 2009]*
a. 5% bone metastasis are symptomatic
b. Higher serum levels of alkaline phosphatase
c. Most common secondary in female is breast
d. Prostate produce osteosclerotic lesion
e. Commonly involves hand and feet bones

97. Which soft tissue sarcoma commonly gives to bone secondary? *[PGI 2008]*
a. Fibrosarcoma b. Liposarcoma
c. Osteosarcoma d. Neurofibroma
e. Synovial sarcoma

98. Most common soft tissue tumour in a child *[PGI 2000]*
a. Rhabdomyosarcoma b. Histiocytoma
c. Fibrosarcoma d. Liposarcoma

99. Regional lymph nodes are involved in which of these *[AIIMS PGMEE 1995]*
a. Ewing sarcoma b. Osteosarcoma
c. Adamantinoma d. Synovial cell sarcoma

100. Maffucci syndrome is characterized by *[Recent Question 2017, JIPMER PGMEE 2014]*
a. Osteopetrosis
b. Multiple fractures
c. Osteoporosis
d. Enchondromas with hemangiomas

101. Pathological fractures is not seen in *[PGI November 2014]*
a. Ewing's tumour b. Giant cell tumour
c. Osteochondroma d. Enchondroma
e. Osteosarcoma

102. True regarding Osteosarcoma is *[PGI November 2014]*
a. Common in age >60 years
b. Most common site Lower end of femur
c. Painless
d. Diaphyseal
e. Sun ray appearance

103. Sun-ray appearance of Osteosarcoma is due to *[AIIMS November 2014]*
a. Calcification of muscle
b. Bone deposition along vessels
c. Mild periosteal reaction
d. Bony necrosis

104. Bone dysplasia occurs due to *[AIIMS November 2014]*
a. Faulty development b. Faulty nutrition
c. Osteoporosis d. Trauma

105. A boy presented with small lytic lesion surrounded by sclerosing lesion in mid-shaft tibia. Most probable diagnosis is *[AIIMS November 2014, 2015]*
a. Ewing's sarcoma b. Osteofibrous dysplasia
c. Osteoid osteoma d. Fibrous cortical defect

106. Fallen fragment within a bone lesion is most common in *[Recent Question 2017, NIMSET 2015]*
a. Aneurysmal bone cyst
b. Unicameral (Simple) bone cyst
c. Giant cell tumor
d. Eosinophilic granuloma

NEET/NBE PATTERN MCQs ANSWERS WITH EXPLANATIONS 

1. Ans. (a) Pelvis
[Ref. Mosby's Oncology, 2/e p143]

Chondrosarcomas

- Group of malignant bone tumors that arise from Cartilage matrix
- MC primary sites of occurrence: Pelvis and Proximal femur

2. Ans. (d) It may progress to a Secondary chondrosarcoma
[Ref. Clinical Imaging by Sutton, 1/e p370]

Paget's Disease

- Common sites: Pelvis, hip, spine, skull, tibia, and humerus
- Typical neurologic deficits may include Eighth cranial nerve involvement (MC) with hearing loss
- Complications: Sarcomatous degeneration, Fracture, Osteoarthritis, Bony deformity, Cranial nerve palsies, Hyperuricemia and crystal formation, High output cardiac failure

3. Ans. (a) Osteosarcoma
[Ref. Practicals And Viva In Surgery by Ghosal, 1/e p197]

Radiological Features of Osteosarcoma

- Growth at metaphysis
- Erosion of cortex and irregular destruction of metaphysis
- Big soft tissue shadow
- Absence of clear line of demarcation with healthy bone
- New bone formation: Sun-ray spicules, Codman's triangle

4. Ans. (b) It is an epiphyseal dysplasia
[Ref. Genetic Disorders That Affect the Skeleton by Mankin, 1/e p64]

Pyle Disease

- Bone metaphyseal dysplasia
- Genu valgum, metaphyseal anomalies with broadening of the long bones extending into the diaphyses and giving the femora and tibiae an **'Erlenmeyer flask"** appearance
- Widening of the ribs and clavicles
- Platyspondyly
- Cortical thinning
- Dental caries, Mandibular prognathism

5. Ans. (d) Melorheostosis
[Ref. MRI of Bone and Soft Tissue Tumors by Meyers, 1/e p53]
Melorheostosis CT image shows smooth zones of cortical hyperostosis with a **"dripping candle wax"** appearance at the sides of involved vertebrae

6. Ans. (a) Paget's disease
[Ref. Bone Tumors and Tumor-Like Lesions by Davies, 1/e p295]

- **Secondary osteosarcomas** are associated with Paget's disease and previous irradiation
- Secondary malignancies associated with Paget's disease include osteosarcoma, chondrosarcoma, and fibrosarcoma

7. Ans.(b) Osteosarcoma
[Ref. Pathology of Bone by Revell, 1/e]

- An osteosarcoma is a malignant tumour showing evidence of osteoid or bone formation by the malignant tumour cells
- **Osteosarcoma or osteogenic sarcoma is the most common primary malignant tumour of the bone**

8. Ans. (c) Secondary deposits
[Ref. Maheshwari, 4/e p240]

Metastasis in Bone

- *MC tumors to give rise to sclerotic secondaries in bone*: Carcinoma of prostate (males) and breast (females)
- *Common sites in body*:
  - **Vertebral bodies (Most common site)**
  - Ribs
  - Pelvis
  - Humerus
  - Femur

9. Ans. (d) Enneking staging
[Ref. Bone Pathology by Khurana, 2/e p249]

Enneking Surgical Staging System

Stage	Grade	Site	Metastases
IA	Low (G1)	Intracompartmental (T1)	No (M0)
IB	Low (G1)	Extracompartmental (T2)	No (M0)
IIA	High (G2)	Intracompartmental (T1)	No (M0)
IIB	High (G2)	Extracompartmental (T2)	No (M0)
III	Any	Any	Yes (M1)

10. Ans. (a) Frontal
[Ref. Diseases of ENT by Bansal, 1/e p363]

PN Sinus, Nose, Jaws

- MC benign tumour of PN sinus: Osteoma
- **MC site of Osteoma: Frontal sinus**
- **MC site of Fibrous dysplasia: Maxilla**
- MC site of Malignancy in PN sinus: Maxillary sinus
- MC site of Mucocoele formation: Frontal sinus
- MC site of Hypoplasia/Aplasia: Frontal sinus

11. Ans. (a) Multiple myeloma
[Ref. Maheshwari, 4/e p228]

- *Most common primary bone malignancy*: Multiple myeloma
- *Second most common primary bone malignancy*: Osteosarcoma

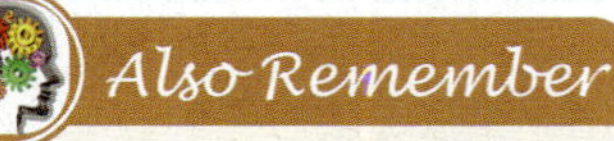

- **Most common benign tumour of bone:** Osteochondroma
- **Most common 'TRUE' benign tumour of bone:** Osteoid osteoma

12. Ans. (d) Lower end femur
[Ref. Maheshwari, 4/e p232]

- **MC site of Osteogenic sarcoma**: Lower end of femur > Upper end of tibia > Upper end of tibia

13. Ans. (b) Giant cell tumour
[Ref. Surgery by Bailey & Love, 26/e p534]

Orthopedics

Location of Common Bone Tumors

Diaphyseal	Metaphyseal	Epiphyseal
Eosinophil granuloma Osteoid osteoma Fibrous dysplasia Adamantinoma Ewing's sarcoma Osteoblastoma Lymphoma Primary Chondrosarcoma	Osteosarcoma Majority of tumors	Chondroblastoma Osteoclastoma Intra-articular Osteoid osteoma Giant cell tumour Clear cell chondrosarcoma
Flat bones Ewing's sarcoma Metastasis Myeloma Chondrosarcoma	**Vertebral bodies** Giant cell tumour Metastasis Ewing's sarcoma Eosinophilic granuloma	**Posterior elements of vertebra** Aneurysmal bone cyst Osteoid osteoma Osteoblastoma

14. Ans. (a) Metastatic secondaries
[Ref. French's Index of Differential Diagnosis by Ellis, 15/e p8]

15. Ans. (a) Carcinoma prostate
[Ref. Textbook of Bony Metastases by Jasmin, 1/e p41]

16. Ans. (b) Chondrosarcoma
[Ref. Maheshwari, 4/e p239]

Common Sites of Tumors in Body

Tumour	Common sites
BENIGN TUMORS	
Osteoma	Skull bones Facial bones
Osteoid osteoma	**Diaphysis of Tibia** (Most common) Posterior elements of vertebrae
Osteoblastoma	**Jaw bone** Spine
Hemangioma	**Vertebrae** Skull bones
Adamantinoma	**Jaw bone** (Most common) Lower half tibia
Chordoma	Sacrum Cervical spine
Giant cell tumour (Osteoclastoma)	Epiphysis lower end femur Epiphysis upper end tibia Epiphysis lower end radius
MALIGNANT TUMORS	
Osteogenic sarcoma (Osteosarcoma)	**Lower end femur** (Most common) Upper end tibia Upper end humerus
Ewing's sarcoma	**Diaphysis long bones** (Most common) Flat bones (pelvis) Calcaneum
Multiple myeloma	**Flat bones** (pelvis, vertebrae, skull, ribs)
Chondrosarcoma	Flat bones (scapula, pelvis, ribs)
Synovial sarcoma	Knee bones
Reticulum cell sarcoma	Long bones (Most common) Flat bones
Secondaries in bone	Spine (Most common) Ribs Extremities
TUMOUR LIKE CONDITIONS	
Chondroblastoma	Knee bones
Osteochondroma	Knee bones
Enchondroma	Small bones of hand and foot
Simple bone cyst	**Upper end humerus** (Most common)
Aneurysmal bone cyst	Ends of long bones
Fibrous dysplasia	Upper end femur Upper end tibia Ribs

Contd...

Contd...

17. Ans. (b) Adamantinoma
[Ref. Radiology by Hussain, 1/e p164]

- **Ameloblastoma/Adamantinoma**: Expansile multiloculated cyst with 'Honey-comb/Soap-bubble appearance' in 30–50 years age
- **Aneurysmal bone cyst**: Expansile multiloculated cyst with 'Soap-bubble appearance' in under 20 years age

18. Ans. (a) Osteoid osteoma
[Ref. Bone and Soft Tissue Tumors by Berndt, 1/e p410]

19. Ans. (b) Osteosarcoma
[Ref. Maheshwari 4/e p233]

Radiology in Osteosarcoma

- **Sunray/Sunburst appearance**: Periosteum unable to control the tumor, tumor grows into overlying soft tissues; New bone is laid down along blood vessels within tumour in centrifugal fashion
- **Codman's triangle**: Triangular area of subperiosteal bone formation seen at tumor-host cortex junction at end of tumor

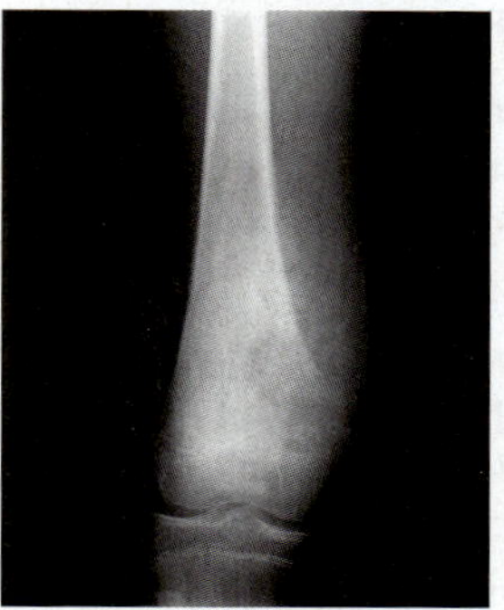

Fig. Sunburst Appearance

- Periosteal reaction
- Irregular destruction of metaphysis
- New bone formation

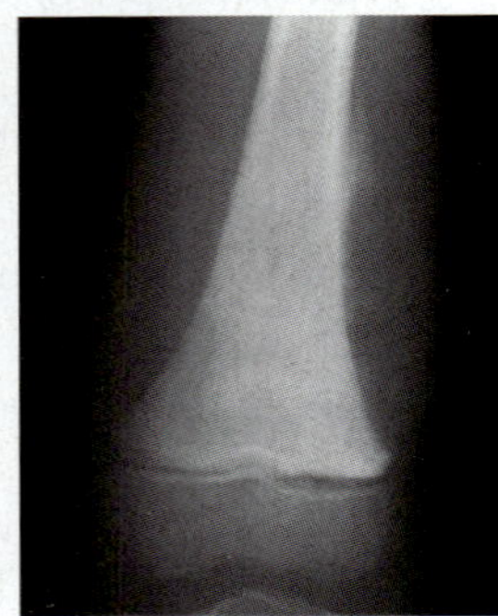

Fig. Codman triangle

20. Ans. (b) Breast

[Ref. Maheshwari 4/e p240]

Primary for Metastasis tumors in spine: Breast cancer > Lungs cancer MC subtype: Adenocarcinoma) > Prostate cancer > Renal cell carcinoma

21. Ans. (a) Osteosarcoma

[Ref. Maheshwari 4/e p232]

Premalignant conditions associated with osteosarcoma: Paget's disease, Multiple enchondromatosis, Fibrous dysplasia, Irradiation to bones, Multiple osteochondroma

22. Ans. (b) Ewing's sarcoma

[Ref. Maheshwari, 4/e p236]

- ***'Onion-peel appearance'*** *on X-ray is characteristic of*: Ewing's sarcoma
- *Bony changes*: Lytic lesion in medullary zone of midshaft of along bone, with cortical destruction; new bone formation occurs in new concentric layers

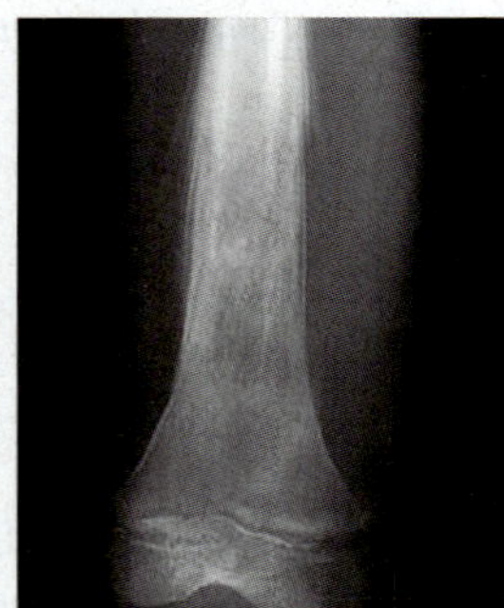

Fig. Onion peel appearance

23. Ans. (a) Ewing's sarcoma: Diaphysis and Osteosarcoma: Metaphysis

[Ref. Surgery by Bailey & Love, 26/e p534]

24. Ans. (c) Fibula

[Ref. Adult and Pediatric Urology by Young, 4/e p1479]

Seed and Soil Hypothesis of Paget: Radius/Ulna and Tibia/Fibula are deficient in Red marrow and therefore are relatively infertile sites of metastatic colonization

25. Ans. (a) Ewing's sarcoma

[Ref. Maheshwari, 4/e p236]

26. Ans. (d) Osteoclastoma

[Ref. Maheshwari, 4/e p230]

27. Ans. (a) Osteosarcoma

[Ref. Maheshwari 4/e p233]

28. Ans. (b) Skull

[Ref. Maheshwari, 4/e p238]

- ***Radiological picture in Multiple myeloma:***
  - **Multiple punched out lesions in skull** and other flat bones
  - Wedge collapse of vertebrae (Most common: Thoracic spine)
  - Erosion of border of ribs
  - Rarefaction of bones

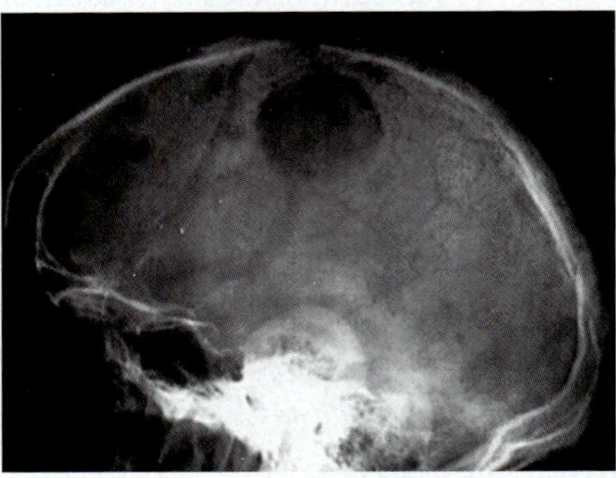

Fig. Punched-out lesions

29. Ans. (d) All of the above

[Ref. Maheshwari 4/e p303]

Radiology in Hyperparathyroidism

- **Salt-pepper appearance of skull**
- Subperiosteal resorption of phalanges
- Brown's tumour
- Clear cysts in pelvis
- Loss of lamina dura
- Central collapse of vertebral bodies

30. Ans. (d) Eosinophilic granuloma

[Ref. Short Practice of Surgery by Bailey and Love, 25th Edn., Pg 329-30]

Eosinophilic Granuloma

- *EG is a rare neoplastic proliferation of*: Langerhans cells
- ***Types of Eosinophilic granulomas:***
  - **Unifocal**: *Eosinophilic granuloma*
  - **Multifocal**: *Hand-Schuller-Christian disease*
  - **Disseminated**: *Letterer-Siwe disease*
- *Bones affected*:
  - Skull
  - Diaphyses of long bones
  - Spine (shows vertebral collapse – *Vertebra plana*)
- *X-ray picture*:
  - Punched-out lesions
  - Periosteal reaction

31. Ans. (c) Soap-bubble

[Ref. Maheshwari 4/e p233]

32. Ans. (b) Osteoma

[Ref. Maheshwari 4/e p228]

MC benign tumor of bone: Osteochondroma > Osteoma

- MC True benign tumor of bone: Osteoid osteoma
- MC tumor of bone: Metastasis
- MC Primary bone tumor: Multiple myeloma

33. Ans. (d) Ewing's sarcoma
[Ref. Maheshwari, 4/e p79, 236]

Ewing's Sarcoma

- *Type*: Highly malignant round cell sarcoma of diaphyses
- *Age group affected*: 10–20 years
- *Bones affected*: Femur, Tibia, Flat bones (pelvis, calcaneum)
- *Histopathology*: **Pseudorosette formation**
- *X-ray picture*: Moth-eaten with ***'Onion-peel appearance'***
- *Treatment*: Highly radiosensitive but recurs with poor prognosis

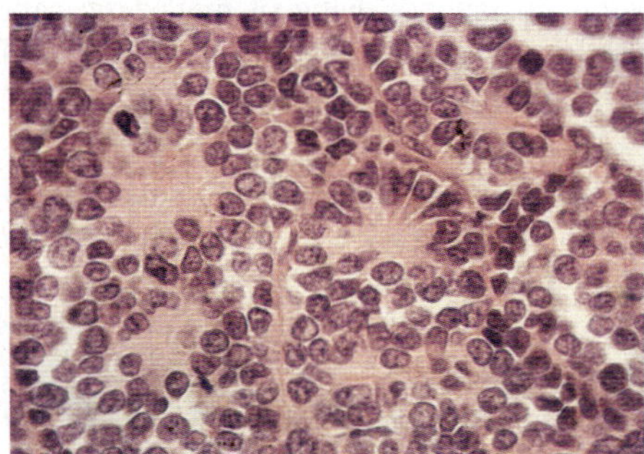

Fig. Pseudorosette formation

34. Ans. (b) Osteoid osteoma
[Ref. Maheshwari 4/e p228]

35. Ans. (c) Epiphyseal origin
[Ref. Surgery by Bailey & Love, 26/e p534]

36. Ans. (d) Fibrous dysplasia
[Ref. Maheshwari, 4/e p242-243]

Fibrous Dysplasia

- *Type of disorder*: Normal bone replaced by fibrous tissue
- *Associated with*: Hormone disorders
  - **McCune-Albright's syndrome (most severe form)**
  - Cushing's disease
- *Hormonal abnormalities*:
  - Parathyroid hormone
  - Growth hormone
  - Gonadotropins

37. Ans. (c) Ewing's sarcoma
[Ref. Surgery by Bailey & Love, 26/e p534]

38. Ans. (c) Ewing's sarcoma
[Ref. Maheshwari 4/e p236]

Radiosensitivity of tumors

Highly radiosensitive	Moderately radiosensitive
• Lymphoma • Seminoma • Myeloma • Ewing's sarcoma • Wilm's tumour	• Small cell cancer lungs • Breast cancer • Basal cell carcinoma • Medulloblastoma • Teratoma • Ovarian cancer (Most: Dysgerminoma)

Contd...

Contd...

Radiosensitivity of tumors

Relatively radioresistant	Extremely radioresistant
• Squamous cell carcinoma lung • Hypernephroma • Rectal carcinoma • Bladder carcinoma • Soft tissue sarcoma • Cervical cancer	• Melanoma • Osteosarcoma • Pancreatic carcinoma

39. Ans. (d) Doxorubicin
[Ref. Comparative Medicine, Volume 57 p263]

40. Ans. (a) Giant cell tumor
[Ref. Surgery by Bailey & Love, 26/e p534]

41. Ans. (b) No premalignant change
[Ref. Maheshwari, 4/e p242-243]

- *Fibrous dysplasia can affect*:
  - Tibia (Long bones)
  - Ribs
  - Skull
  - Maxilla
  - Fibrous dysplasia is premalignant
- *Fibrous dysplasia is associated with*: endocrine abnormalities

42. Ans. (b) Osteopenia present

43. Ans. (c) Secondaries
[Ref. Maheshwari, 4/e p239]

- *Most common malignant bone tumour*: Secondaries to bone
- *Most common primary bone malignancy*: Multiple myeloma
- *Second most common primary bone malignancy*: Osteosarcoma
- *Most common benign tumour of bone*: Osteochondroma
- *Most common 'TRUE' benign tumour of bone*: Osteoid osteoma
- *Most common bone tumour in Hand*: Enchondroma

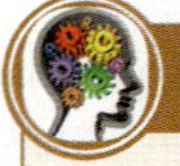

Also Remember

Bony Secondaries

Common origins of bony secondaries	Common sites of bony secondaries
• Breast (Most common in females) • Prostate (Most common in males) • Lung • Renal • Thyroid	• Spine (Most common) • Proximal femur • Proximal humerus

44. Ans. (d) Prostate carcinoma
[Ref. Several sources]

Bony Secondaries

Osteoblastic (Men)	Osteoblastic (Both Men and Women)
Carcinoma prostate	Neurogenic tumors
Seminoma	Carcinoid tumors
	Osteosarcoma

Contd...

Contd...

Osteoblastic (Women)	Osteolytic secondaries
Carcinoma breast	Carcinoma lung
Carcinoma uterus	Carcinoma kidney
Carcinoma ovary	Carcinoma thyroid
	Carcinoma breast
	Carcinoma stomach
	Carcinoma colon

45. Ans. (d) All of the above
[Ref. Radiology Review Manual by Dahnert, 7/e p11]

Codman's Triangle
- Osteosarcoma
- Ewing's sarcoma
- Acute osteomyelitis
- Fracture
- Hemorrhage

46. Ans. (b) Osteoid osteoma
[Ref. Pediatric Radiology by Parker, 3/e p189]

47. Ans. (c) Multiple enchondromatosis
[Ref. Bone Diseases by Adler, 1/e p60]
- **Enchondromas** are common intraosseous benign cartilaginous tumors, that develop in close proximity to growth plate cartilage
- When multiple enchondromas are present, the condition is called enchondromatosis, also known as Ollier's disease

48. Ans. (d) All of the above
[Ref. Thoracic Surgery by Feins, 7/e p1307]
Sources of pulmonary metastases: Colorectal carcinoma, Osteogenic sarcoma, Rhabdomyosarcoma, Ewing's sarcoma, Fibrosarcoma, Melanoma

49. Ans. (a) Phosphatonin
[Ref. Endocrinology by Bhansali1/e p303]

Tumor-induced Osteomalacia (Oncogenic Osteomalacia)
A paraneoplastic syndrome due to secretion of Phosphatonins (Fibroblast growth factor 23, FGF23) from mesenchymal tumors and results in severe hypophosphatemia and low 1,25$(OH)_2$D

50. Ans. (c) Synovial sarcoma
[Ref. Musculoskeletal Imaging by Chew, 3/e p325]
- Osteosarcoma may resemble a chondrosarcoma with dense calcifications, but the calcifications are usually more diffuse and ill-defined or linear with a 'Sun-ray appearance
- Chondroblastoma is composed of chondroid matrix with thread-like calcifications, lying in a dense cellular background that contains multinucleated giant cells
- Osteoblastomas CT scans show a round lesion, well circumscribed with regular calcified contours

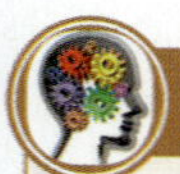

Also Remember

Osteoid matrix, which is produced by osteosarcoma, osteoid osteoma, and osteoblastoma, may calcify in an amorphous pattern, which is sometimes described as "cloud-like," "fluffy," or "cotton-wool"

51. Ans. (a) Classical Osteosarcoma
[Ref. Miller's Review of Orthopaedics, 7/e p744]

Types of Osteosarcomas (OS)
- MC type: High-grade Intramedullary OS (Classical OS)
- Other types: Paraosteal OS, Periosteal OS, Telangiectatic OS, OS with Paget's disease, Post-irradiation OS

52. Ans. (b) Metastases
[Ref. Orthopaedic Pathology by Vigorita, 2/e p527]
- Metastatic cancer to the skeleton is the MC malignant tumor affecting bone
- Bone is the third most common site of metastasis after the Lung and Liver, with up to 85% of cancer patients at autopsy revealing bone metastasis
- Most frequently seen tumor primaries affecting the skeleton in patients dying of metastatic cancer are the Breast, Prostate, Lung, Thyroid, and Kidneys (BPLTK)

53. Ans. (b) 10-20 years
[Ref. Orthopedics by Mohindra, 2/e p499]
- **Osteosarcoma has a bimodal age distribution**: The first peak occurs during adolescence, and the second occurs in older adults
- Primary in OS 10–20 years and secondary OS in 40–60 years

54. Ans. (a) Osteosarcoma
[Ref. Orthopedic Nursing Secrets by Zychowicz, 1/e p155]

Osteosarcoma (OS)
- OS generally affects Metaphysis
- Plain X-rays: Cortical destruction, bony expansion, calcification, 'Sunburst' appearance
- MC site for metastases of OS is the Lungs, and all patients with known OS should have chest imaging, preferably with CT

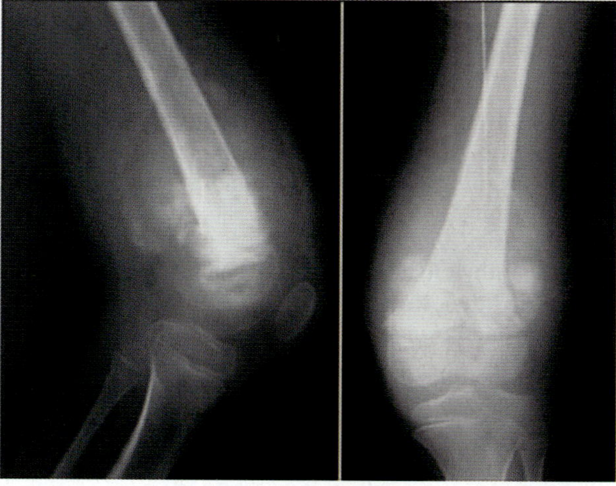

Fig. Osteosarcoma

55. Ans. (b) Lungs
[Ref. Duke Radiology, 2/e p249]
- MC site of Osteosarcoma: Intramedullary metaphyses of the long bones (Distal femur, Proximal tibia, and Proximal humerus)
- Osteosarcoma spreads hematogenously, with Lung followed by Bone being the MC sites of metastasis
- Other common sites of metastatic disease include regional and distal lymph nodes

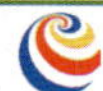

HIGH YIELD MCQs ANSWERS WITH EXPLANATIONS

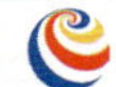

1. Ans. (a) Commonly occurs in bones around knee joint; (b) Radiotherapy is given for treatment; (c) Cause cortical thinning by expansion

[Ref. Pathophysiology by Porth, 1/e p1114]

Giant Cell Tumor

- Common around Knee joint (Distal femur, Proximal tibia)
- Common in 3rd decade
- 'Active' tumors have well-defined margins, but lack sclerosis; the cortex is thinned and expanded
- Treatment modalities:
  - Curettage
  - Curettage and bone grafting
  - Curettage and insertion of polymethylmethacrylate (PMMA)
  - Primary resection
  - Radiation therapy
  - Embolization of the feeding vessels

2. Ans. (b) Commonest site is the upper end of the humerus; (c) Cortex may be thin; (d) Cause pathological fracture

[Ref. Radiology Recall by Gay, 1/e p379]

Simple Bone Cyst

- MC in adolescents (10–20 years age)
- Ends of the long bones are the favorite sites: **MC being Upper-end of Humerus**
- At times, the cortex may be so thin that it is invisible on plain radiographs, and thus this benign lesion may be mistaken for a malignant bone tumor
- Pathologic fractures may occur with a benign cause of weakened bone (Simple bone cyst, enchondroma, aneurysmal bone cyst, or fibrous dysplasia)
- 40% simple bone cysts may recur

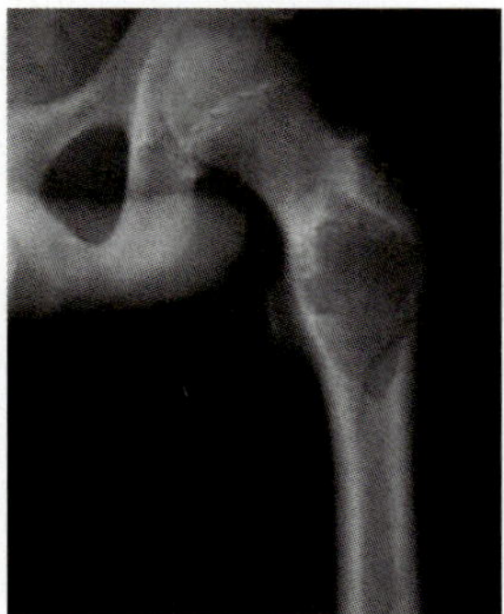

Fig. Simple bone cyst

3. Ans. (a) Osteosarcoma

[Ref. Clinical Surgery by Sakr, 1/e p557]

- **Pulsatile bone conditions**: Telangiectatic Osteosarcoma, Aneurysmal bone cyst, Highly vascular osteoclastoma, Hemangioma, Angioendothelioma

4. Ans. (d) Ground-glass appearance

[Ref. Rapid Review of Radiology by Hussain, 1/e p266]

5. Ans. (a) Chordoma

[Ref. Maheshwari 4/e p230]

- **Chordoma**: Locally malignant, sometimes actually malignant tumour arising from Notochord
  - Common sites: Sacrum, Cervical spine, Clivus
  - Hallmark feature: Bone destruction
  - Treatment: Complete excision, Radiotherapy

6. Ans. (b) Enchondroma

[Ref. MRI in Orthopedics Sports Medicine by Resnick, 1/e p257]

7. Ans. (b) Osteochondroma

[Ref. Maheshwari 4/e p228]

8. Ans. (a) Trauma; (b) Malignancy; (d) Ewing's sarcoma; (e) Eosinophilic granuloma

[Ref. Musculoskeletal Imaging by Joseph, 2/e Case 24]

Vertebra Plana

- Common conditions: Metastasis, Multiple myeloma, Traumatic fracture, Eosinophilic granuloma, Infection
- Less common conditions: Lymphoma, Hemangioma, Aneurysmal bone cyst
- Rare conditions: Ewing's sarcoma

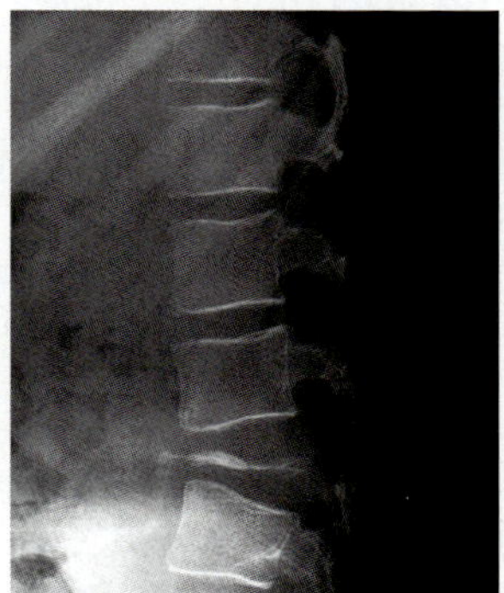

Fig. Vertebra plana

9. Ans. (c) Osteosarcoma

[Ref. Maheshwari 4/e p234]

10. Ans. (a) Osteoid osteoma; (b) Osteochondroma; (c) Chondroblastoma; (d) Chondromyxoid fibroma

[Ref. Maheshwari 4/e p229]

11. Ans. (b) Chordoma

[Ref. Maheshwari 4/e p230]

12. Ans. (c) Medullary cavity

[Ref. Pediatric Imaging by Newman, 1/e p370]

13. Ans. (b) Ewing's tumor; (e) Osteoid osteoma

[Ref. Surgery by Bailey & Love, 26/e p534]

14. Ans. (a) Upper end of humerus

[Ref. Disorders and Injuries of Musculoskeletal System by Salter, 3/e p398]

MC sites of Solitary bone cyst: Upper end humerus > Upper end femur > Upper end tibia > Lower end radius

15. Ans. (a) Rib

[Ref. Musculoskeletal Cytohistology by Crim, 1/e p129]

16. Ans. (a) Multiple myeloma—more than 55 years age and above
[Ref. Maheshwari 4/e p238]

Bone Tumors and Age Groups
- Ewing's sarcoma: 05–15 years
- Osteosarcoma: 15–25 years
- Osteoclastoma: 20–40 years
- Chondroma sarcoma: 30–60 years
- Multiple myeloma: 40–60 years

17. Ans. (a) Plasmacytoma
[Ref. Duke Radiology by Nelson, 2/e p283]
- Plasmacytoma is seen in 50–70 years age

18. Ans. (a) Aneurysmal bone cyst
[Ref. Pediatric Imaging by Coley, 1/e p438]

Benign Bone Lesions

	Unicameral bone cyst	Aneurysmal bone cyst
Initial manifestation	Pathological fracture, pain	Pain, Swelling
Bones affected	**Proximal Humerus >Proximal Femur**	**Distal femur >** Proximal tibia > Any bone
Lytic expansile lesion	Central, Well demarcated	Eccentric
Expansion	Lesser than growth plate	Wider than growth plate
Cortex	Cortical thinning	Cortical destruction, Periosteal elevation
Cavity	Multiple	Single
Histology	Yellow fluid, Endothelial lining, Fibrous tissue cystic spaces	Blood-filled spaces, No endothelial lining

19. Ans. (c) Unicameral bone cyst
[Ref. Pediatric Imaging by Coley, 1/e p438]

20. Ans. (b) Mandible near molar tooth
[Ref. Radiology Review Manual by Dahnert, 7/e p186]

21. Ans. (b) Tibia
[Ref. High Yield Orthopedics by Javad, 1/e p14]

22. Ans. (a) Epiphysis
[Ref. Surgery by Bailey & Love, 26/e p534]

23. Ans. (a) Monoclonal M-band; (b) Bone marrow plasma cells <5%; (c) Hypercalcemia, Hyperuricemia
[Ref. Maheshwari 4/e p238]

24. Ans. (c) Multiple myeloma
[Ref. Diagnostic Radiology by Berry, 2/e p10]
- **Eosinophilic granuloma**: Single lytic lesion, Sharp non-sclerotic border, beveled edge
- **Hand Schüller-Christian disease**: Multiple lytic, larger, punched-out lesions
- **Letterer-Siwe disease**: Multiple lytic, larger, punched-out lesions
- **Multiple myeloma**: Multiple lytic, punched-out lesions, beveled ledge

25. Ans. (a) Prostate; (b) Lungs; (d) Breast
[Ref. Maheshwari 4/e p239]

26. Ans. (d) Small bones of hand
[Ref. Maheshwari 4/e p239]

27. Ans. (d) Secondaries
[Ref. Maheshwari 4/e p239]

28. Ans. (b) Aneurysmal bone cyst
[Ref. Definitive Surgical Board Review by Moore, 1/e p202]

29. Ans. (d) Simple bone cyst
[Ref. Fundamentals of Diagnostic Radiology by Brant, 4/e p987]

30. Ans. (b) Non-ossifying fibroma; (c) Enchondroma; (d) Fibrous dysplasia; (e) Eosinophilic granuloma
[Ref. Bone and Soft Tissue Tumors by Mario, 2/e p831]

31. Ans. (b) Endothelial lining; (c) Giant cells
[Ref. Schwartz's Principles of Surgery, 9/e, p411]

32. Ans. (b) Endothelial cell lining; (c) Fibrous tissue with cystic spaces; (d) Pseudocyst
[Ref. Schwartz's Principles of Surgery, 9/e, p411]

33. Ans. (a) Osteoclastoma; (b) Chondroblastoma; (c) Fibrous dysplasia
[Ref. Ophthalmic and Plastic Reconstructive Surgery by Levine, 3/e p861]

Aneurysmal bone cyst associations: Fibrous dysplasia, Fibrous histiocytoma, Non-ossifying fibroma, Giant cell tumor, Osteoblastoma, Osteoclastoma, Osteosarcoma, Chondroblastoma

34. Ans. (a) Osteoid osteoma; (c) Osteochondroma; (d) Chondroblastoma
[Ref. Maheshwari 4/e p229]

35. Ans. (b) Osteosarcoma; (c) Osteoid osteoma; (e) Osteoblastoma
[Ref. Bone Cancer by Heymann, 1/e p163]

36. Ans. (a) Enneking
[Ref. Bone Pathology by Khurana, 2/e p249]

37. Ans. (c) Brodie's abscess
[Ref. Maheshwari 4/e p169]

38. Ans. (a) Giant cell tumour
[Ref. Maheshwari 4/e p230]
Giant cell tumor is seen in 20–40 years age

39. Ans. All Choices

40. Ans. (b) Fibrosarcoma
[Ref. Bone Tumors by Unni, 9/e p169]

41. Ans. All Choices
[Ref. Maheshwari 4/e p231-232]

42. Ans. (a) Osteosarcoma
[Ref. General Thoracic Surgery by Shields, 7/e p741]
Common sarcomas leading to Pneumothorax: Osteosarcoma, Synovial sarcoma

43. Ans. (b) Blood-filled spaces; (c) Found in upper tibia; (d) Pulsatile in older age
[Ref. Pediatric Imaging by Coley, 1/e p438]

44. Ans. (d) Femur
[Ref. Imaging of Bone Tumors and Tumor-like Conditions by Davies, 1/e p8]

45. Ans. (c) Pathological fractures seen; (d) Shaggy fibrous layering; (e) Well-demarcated radiolucent lesions
[Ref. Textbook of Oral Radiology by Ghom, 1/e p499]

46. Ans. (a) Osteosarcoma
[Ref. General Thoracic Surgery by Shields, 7/e p741]

47. Ans. (b) Sunray appearance in X-ray indicates new bone formation
[Ref. Maheshwari 4/e p233]

48. Ans. (b) Osteosarcoma
[Ref. Maheshwari 4/e p233]

49. Ans. (c) Chemotherapy + Limb Salvage Surgery + Chemotherapy
[Ref. Maheshwari 4/e p233]

50. Ans. (b) Most commonly involve knee and distal femur; (c) Spread to lung through hematogenous route; (e) X-ray sunray appearance
[Ref. Maheshwari 4/e p232-233]

51. Ans. (c) Viral infection
[Ref. Pediatric and Adolescent Osteosarcoma by Jaffe, 1/e p16]
Risk factors of Osteosarcoma: Ionizing radiation (most common), Alkylating agents, Paget's disease, Hereditary retinoblastoma, Li Fraumeni syndrome, Bone infarction, Multiple hereditary exostosis, Fibrous dysplasia, Multiple osteomyelitis.

52. Ans. (a) It invades the medullary cavity; (b) Easily diagnosed by X-ray; (d) En bloc resection/ amputation is the treatment of choice
[Ref. Tumors by Jain, 2/e p117]

53. Ans. (d) Etoposide
[Ref. Treatment of Cancer by Sikora, 6/e p721]

T-10 Protocol for Osteosarcoma
- Preoperative: Vincristine, High-dose Methotrexate, Doxorubicin
- Postoperative: Cyclophosphamide, Dactinomycin, Bleomycin, Vincristine, Methotrexate, Doxorubicin, Cisplatin (with/without)

54. Ans. (b) Ewing's sarcoma
[Ref. FNAC by Dey, 1/e p185]

55. Ans. ALL CHOICES
[Ref. Tumors by Jain, 2/e p138]

56. Ans. ALL CHOICES
[Ref. Maheshwari 4/e p231-232]

57. Ans. (c) Excision and bone grafting
[Ref. Maheshwari 4/e p231-232]
- Soap-bubble appearance of lesion at lower end of radius: Giant cell tumor

58. Ans. (a) Epiphysis
[Ref. Surgery by Bailey & Love, 26/e p534]

59. Ans. (b) Osteoid osteoma; (c) Ewing's tumor
[Ref. Surgery by Bailey & Love, 26/e p534]

60. Ans. (a) Osteoclastoma; (b) Chondroblastoma

61. Ans. (c) Osteomyelitis; (d) Osteosarcoma; (e) Chondrosarcoma
[Ref. Surgery by Bailey & Love, 26/e p534]
- Ewing's sarcoma is diaphyseal, osteoclastoma is Epiphyseal origin

62. Ans. (b) Metaphysis
[Ref. Surgery by Bailey & Love, 26/e p534]

63. Ans. (b) Ewing's sarcoma
[Ref. Surgery by Bailey & Love, 26/e p534]

64. Ans. (c) Ewing's sarcoma
[Ref. Maheshwari 4/e p236]

65. Ans. (b) Ewing's sarcoma
[Ref. Pediatric Neoplasia by Variend, Volume 22 p58]

66. Ans. (b) Core biopsy

67. Ans. (a) Ameloblastoma
[Ref. Oral Pathology by Sundaram, 7/e p277]

68. Ans. (a) Cystic lesion; (e) Presented in children
[Ref. Oral and Maxillofacial Surgery by Miloro, 3/e p823]

69. Ans. (a) Adamantinoma
[Ref. Diagnostic Histopathology of Tumors by Fletcher, 3/e p1626]

70. Ans. (d) Osteoid osteoma
[Ref. Maheshwari 4/e p228]

71. Ans. (b) MC bone involvement-tibia; (c) Local excision or curettage cure; (d) Bone pain relieved by aspirin; (e) X-ray shows density surrounding radiolucent lesion
[Ref. Maheshwari 4/e p231-232]

72. Ans. (d) Caffey's disease
[Ref. Maheshwari 4/e p310]

Caffey's Disease
- Synonym: Infantile Cortical Hyperostosis
- Feature: Subperiosteal bone formation on shaft of long bones and mandible
- Self-limiting course

73. Ans. (b) Eccentric; (c) Prominent sclerotic margin; (d) Histologically giant cell with areolar tissue; (d) Metaphyseal lesion
[Ref. Bone Tumors by Czernaik, 2/e]

74. Ans. (b) Prominent sclerotic margins; (c) Fibrous tissue with areolar tissue
[Ref. Bone Tumors by Czernaik, 2/e]

75. Ans. (b) Clivus; (d) Sacrum
[Ref. Maheshwari 4/e p230]

76. Ans. (c) Occurs only in short bones
[Ref. Maheshwari 4/e p240-241]

77. Ans. (d) Degenerative changes

78. Ans. (b) Growth continues after skeletal maturity
[Ref. Oncology and Basic Science by Damron, 1/e p133]
- Generally exostosis growth occurs till host bone reach skeletal maturity
- If growth continues after skeletal maturity, it should arouse suspicion of malignancy

79. Ans. (a) Usually affects long bones, but can also occur in skull and pelvis; (b) Usual site is metaphyseal region; (c) Also known as multiple exostoses, diaphyseal clasis; (e) Autosomal dominant in inheritance
[Ref. Oncology and Basic Science by Damron, 1/e p133]

80. Ans. (c) Chondroblastoma
[Ref. Surgery by Bailey & Love, 26/e p534]

81. Ans. (b) Chondroblastoma
[Ref. Diagnostic Radiology – Pediatric Imaging by Bhalla, 3/e p383]

82. Ans. (b) Chondroblastoma
[Ref. Diagnostic Radiology – Pediatric Imaging by Bhalla, 3/e p383]

83. Ans. (a) New bone formation; (c) Codman's triangle; (e) Sun-ray appearance
[Ref. Maheshwari 4/e p233]

84. Ans. (b) Osteosarcoma
[Ref. Maheshwari 4/e p233]

85. Ans. (d) Bone marrow biopsy
[Ref. The Shoulder by Rockwood, 4/e p1535]
Diagnosis of Osteosarcoma: Bone scan, MRI of extremity, CT scan of extremity, CT scan of Lung

86. Ans. (b) Chondrosarcoma
[Ref. Practical Orthopedic Pathology by Siegel, 1/e p142]
Typical features of Chondrosarcoma: Punctate/Popcorn calcification, Endosteal scalloping, Cortical thickening

87. Ans. (a) Occurs commonly in skull bones; (c) Hamartomatous in origin; (e) Local gigantism occurs when it occurs in an extremity
[Ref. Pathophysiology of Human Disease by Mitchell, 1/e p853]

Hemangioma of Bone
- Sites: Skull, Spine, Long bones
- MC age group: Middle age adults
- MC subtype: Cavernous
- Origin: Hamartomas (Vascular malformations)
- Radiology: Corduroy/Polka dot appearance (Vertical trabeculae among hypointense fat in spine)

88. Ans. (d) Serum electrophoresis
[Ref. Maheshwari 4/e p238]
Lower back pain with Multiple punched out lesions in skull, raised ESR indicate multiple myeloma

89. Ans. (a) Multiple myeloma
[Ref. Maheshwari 4/e p238]
- Old age male with bone pain, vertebral collapse and fracture pelvis indicate multiple myeloma

90. Ans. (d) Carcinoma prostate
[Ref. Cancer Chemotherapy by Longo, 5/e p741]

91. Ans. (b) Carcinoma Prostate
[Ref. Cancer Chemotherapy by Longo, 5/e p741]

92. Ans. (a) Kidney
[Ref. Textbook of Bone Metastases by Jasmin, 1/e p534]

93. Ans. (c) Small bone of lower limb
[Ref. Maheshwari 4/e p239]

94. Ans. (b) Neuroblastoma; (c) RCC
[Ref. head and Neck Surgery by Johnson, 4/e p1512]

95. Ans. (d) Prostate
[Ref. Textbook of Pathology by Dutta, 2/e p991]

96. Ans. (b) Higher serum levels of alkaline phosphatase; (c) Most common secondary in female is breast; (d) Prostate produce osteosclerotic lesion
[Ref. Essentials of Skeletal Radiology by Rowe, 3/e p1138]

Bony Metastases
- ESR is elevated
- Serum Calcium normal
- ALP elevated

97. Ans. (c) Osteosarcoma; (e) Synovial sarcoma

98. Ans. (a) Rhabdomyosarcoma
[Ref. Imaging of Soft Tissue Tumors by Schepper, p258]

99. Ans. (d) Synovial cell sarcoma
[Ref. Treatment of Bone and Soft Tissue Sarcoma by Tunn, 1/e p25]
Sarcomas associated with regional lymphatic spread: Clear cell sarcoma, Synovial sarcoma, Rhabdomyosarcoma, Epitheloid sarcoma

100. Ans. (d) Enchondromas with hemangiomas
[Ref. Limb Malformations by Horn, 1/e p126]

101. Ans. (c) Osteochondroma
[Ref. Maheshwari 4/e p4]

Pathological Fractures
- Localized diseases:
  - Inflammatory causes: TB osteomyelitis, Pyogenic osteomyelitis
  - Benign tumors: Giant cell tumor, Enchondroma
  - Malignant tumors: Osteosarcoma, Ewing's tumor
  - Secondary metastases: Lung, Prostate, Kidney, Breast
  - Miscellaneous: Simple bone cyst, Aneurysmal bone cyst, Monostotic fibrous dysplasia
- Generalized diseases:
  - Hereditary causes: Osteopetrosis, Osteogenesis imperfecta, Ollier's disease
  - Acquired causes: Rickets, Scurvy, Osteoporosis, Osteomalacia, Multiple myeloma, Diffuse metastatic carcinoma
  - Miscellaneous: Paget's disease, Polyostotic fibrous dysplasia, Eosinophilic granuloma

102. Ans. (b) Most common site Lower end of femur; (e) Sun-ray appearance
[Ref. Maheshwari 4/e p232]

103. Ans. (b) Bone deposition along vessels

[Ref. Essentials of Pediatrics by Khan, 4/e p315]

Sun-ray appearance in Osteosarcoma occur due to: Deposition of Osteoid along new blood vessels

104. Ans. (a) Faulty development

[Ref. Basic facts in Orthopedics by Brown, 2/e p47]

Dysplasias of *bone result* from the *faulty* maturation of the cells involved in *developing bone, namely* fibroblasts and other cells

105. Ans. (b) Osteofibrous dysplasia

[Ref. Musculoskeletal Cytohistology by Crim, 1/e p202]

Osteofibrous dysplasia: Lytic lesion in Anterior cortex of Tibia causing cortical expansion and reactive surrounding sclerosis

106. Ans. (b) Unicameral (Simple) bone cyst

[Ref. Tumors by Park, 1/e p26]

In Unicameral bone cyst, with fracture, there can be a characteristic **"fallen fragment sign,"** which is a piece of cortical bone seen dependently within the fluid-filled cyst.

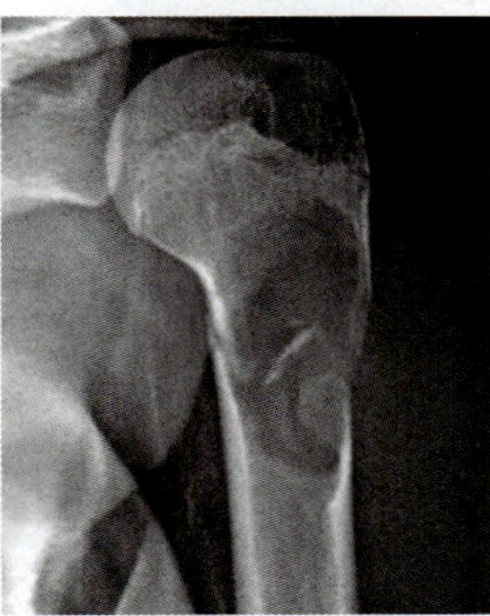

Fig. Fallen fragment sign

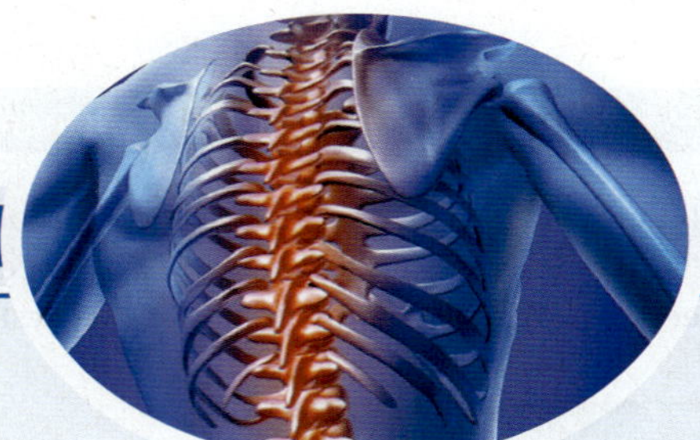

Chapter 11

Common Orthopedic Problems

THEORETICAL CONCEPTS

XI A. ACUTE OSTEOMYELITIS

- *Definition*: Infection of bone, mainly in metaphysis
  - Primary OM: **Hematogenous (Most common[Q])**
  - Secondary OM: Post fracture/ surgery
- *Organisms causing Acute Hematogenous Osteomyelitis*:
  - **Staphylococcus aureus (Most common[Q])**
  - Streptococcus
  - Pneumococcus
- *Sites of Acute Hematogenous Osteomyelitis* ***(Most common in Metaphyses)***:
  - **Lower femoral metaphysic (Most common)**
  - Upper tibial metaphysis
  - Upper femoral metaphysis
  - Upper humeral metaphysis
- *Diagnosis*:
  - X-ray: Periosteal reaction (new bone formation) **[First sign[Q]]**
  - Tc-99 bone scan
- *Treatment*:
  - < 48 hours: Rest + antibiotics
  - 48 hours: Surgical exploration + drainage
- *Complications*:
  - **Chronic osteomyelitis (Most common[Q])**
  - Pyogenic arthritis

XI B. OTHER OSTEOMYELITIS

- ***Salmonella osteomyelitis***: Sub-acute osteomyelitis in convalescence of typhoid
  - Diaphysial sclerosis
  - ***MC occurrence*: Sickle cell anaemia[Q]**
- ***Garre's osteomyelitis***: Chronic, sclerosing, non-suppurative osteomyelitis
  - Fusiform enlargement
  - Absence of discharging sinus
- ***Brodie's abscess***:
  - Chronic bone abscess surrounded by zone of sclerosis in metaphysis[Q]
  - *MC site*: Upper end Tibia[Q]
- ***Septic arthritis of infancy (Tom Smith arthritis)*:[Q]**
  - **Site: Hip[Q]**
  - X-ray: Complete absence of head and neck of femur

- ***Gonococcal arthritis*:**
  - **MC site: Knee joint[Q]**
- ***Syphilitic arthritis*:**
  - Periosteitis (Most common[Q])
  - Metaphysitis
  - *Sabre tibia*: Convexity of tibia (diaphysitis[Q])
  - *Clutton's joints*: Painless synovitis at puberty (late manifestation of Congenital Syphilis)
  - *Charcot's joints*: Neuropathic joints[Q]
  - *Hot cross bun skull*: Sclerotic frontal/ parietal bones

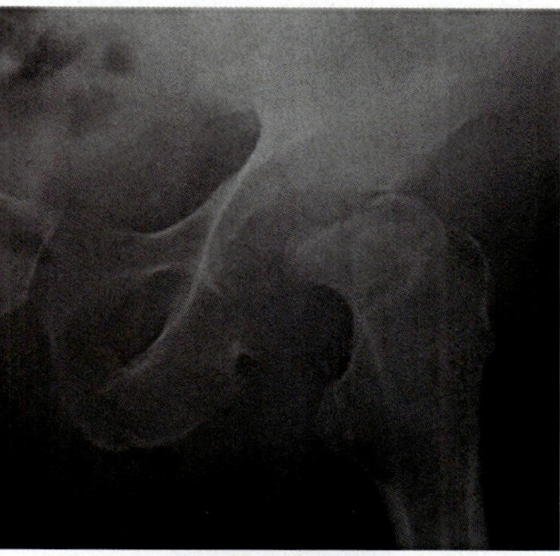

Fig. Tom-Smith arthritis

XI C. POLIOMYELITIS

- Underlying affection: Anterior horn cells of spinal cord
- Features in a Poliomyelitis case:

Early stage of poliomyelitis	
Paralysis[Q]	Asymmetric flaccid (lower limbs)
***Most common muscle affected*[Q]**	**Quadriceps femoris**
Most common muscle with complete paralysis	Tibialis anterior
***Most common muscle affected in hand*[Q]**	**Opponens pollicis**
Sensory loss	Absent
Bulbo-spinal polio	Motor neurons of medulla affected
Late stage of poliomyelitis	
Deformity at hip[Q]	Flexion, abduction, external rotation
***Deformity at knee*[Q]**	***'Triple deformity*'***
Deformity of foot (Most common)	Equinovarus

*(*Flexion, posterior subluxation, external rotation)*

- *Treatment of a Poliomyelitis case*:
  - Calipers
  - Modified Jones' operation (Tendon transfer[Q])

XI D. OSTEOPOROSIS

- *Definition*: Diffuse reduction in bone density
- *Underlying causes*:
  - Senility (Most common in **Males**[Q])
  - Menopause (Most common in **Females**[Q])
  - Drug induced (Phenobarbitone/ Steroids)

- Protein deficiency
- Endocrinal causes
- Post-immobilisation

- *Clinical presentation*:
  - **Fractures (Dorsolumbar spine: Most common[Q])**
  - Kyphosis
  - Serum calcium, phosphate and alkaline phosphatase: Normal[Q]
- *X-rays*: **COD FISH VERTEBRAE**
- *Treatment of Osteoporosis* **[Mnemonic: $A^2BC^2D^2E^2F^Q$]**
  - **A**ndrogens
  - **A**lendronate
  - **B**races
  - **C**alcitonin
  - **C**alcium supplementation
  - Vitamin **D** (along with Vitamin K – as a cofactor for carboxylase activity, vitamin K can facilitate the conversion of glutamyl to gamma-carboxyglutamyl residues and influence the synthesis and excretion of gamma-carboxylation of osteocalcin to increase the formation of bone)
  - High protein **D**iet
  - **E**strogens
  - **E**xercises
  - **F**luoride

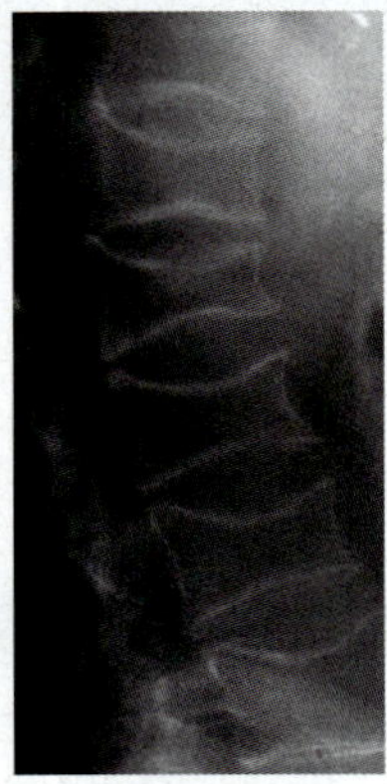

Fig. Cod-fish vertebrae

XI E. RICKETS

- *Definition*: Failure of proper mineralisation of bone matrix
  - Type I: Deficiency of Vitamin D or metabolism defect
  - Type II: Deficiency of phosphate
- *Underlying causes*: **Nutritional deficiency (Most common)**
- *Clinical presentation*:
  - **Bossing of frontal and parietal bones[Q]**
  - Broad ends of long bones
  - **Craniotabes[Q]**
  - Delayed teeth eruption
  - Deformities **(Knock-knees/ Bow legs[Q])**
  - **Harrison sulcus[Q]**
  - Pigeon chest[Q]
  - Pot belly
  - Rachitic rosary
- *X-rays*:
  - **Splaying[Q]**
  - **Cupping[Q]**
  - **Fraying[Q]**
  - **Rachitic rosary[Q]**
  - **Looser's zones[Q]**
  - **Wind-swept deformity[Q]**

- *Treatment*:
  - Vitamin D[Q]
  - Osteotomies

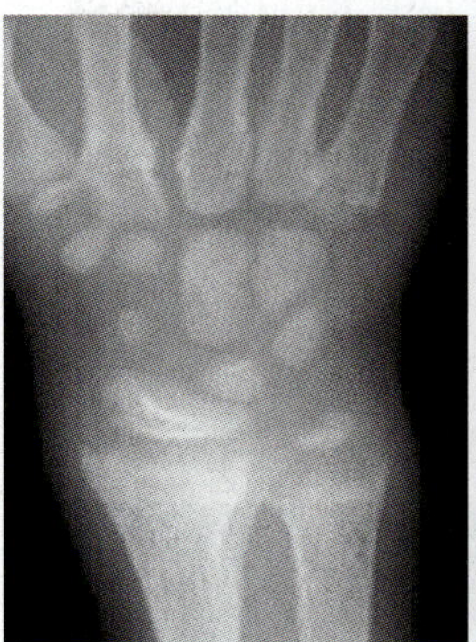
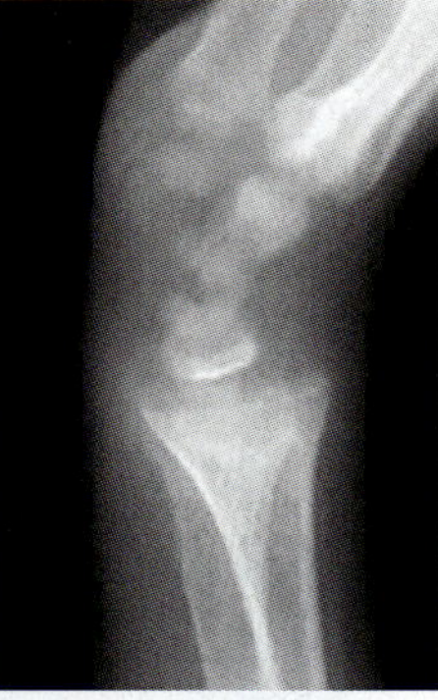

Fig. Rickets

XI F. OSTEOMALACIA

- *Definition*: Softening of bones in adults
- *Underlying causes*: Inadequate sunlight exposure
- *Clinical presentation*:
  - Spine fractures/ Kyphosis
  - Muscular weakness
  - Bone pains
- *X-rays*[Q]:
  - **Looser's zones**[Q]
  - **Triradiate pelvis**[Q]
  - Protrusion acetabuli
- *Treatment*:
  - Vitamin D
  - Osteotomies

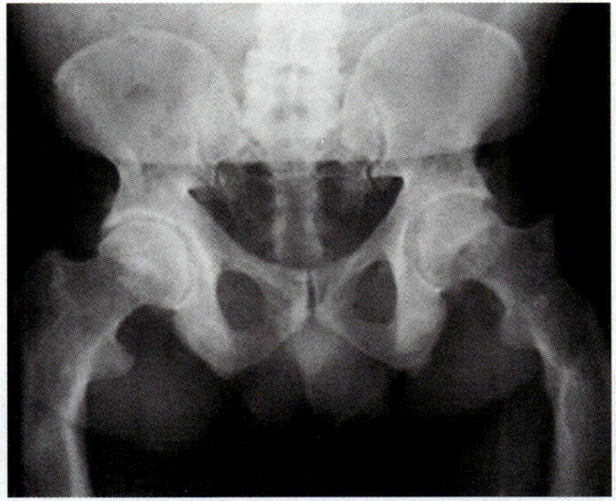

Fig. Triradiate pelvis

Topper's Edge

Looser's Zones

- **Pseudofractures**[Q], **Milkman's lines**[Q]
- Transverse, bilaterally symmetrical, incomplete
- Fracture heal with defective callus
- Common sites of stress[Q]:
  - Axillary border of scapula
  - Ramus of pubis/ ischium
  - Neck of femur
  - Ribs

XI G. HYPERPARATHYROIDISM

- *Clinical presentation*:
  - Bone pain (Most common)
  - Brown's tumor
  - Serum calcium, alkaline phosphatase normal + High ALP
- *X-rays*:
  - **Pepper-pot (Salt-pepper) skull**[Q]
  - Chondrocalcinosis
  - Rugger-Jersey spine
  - Brown's tumor in maxilla/ mandible
  - Subperiosteal resorption of phalanges (Pathognomonic feature)

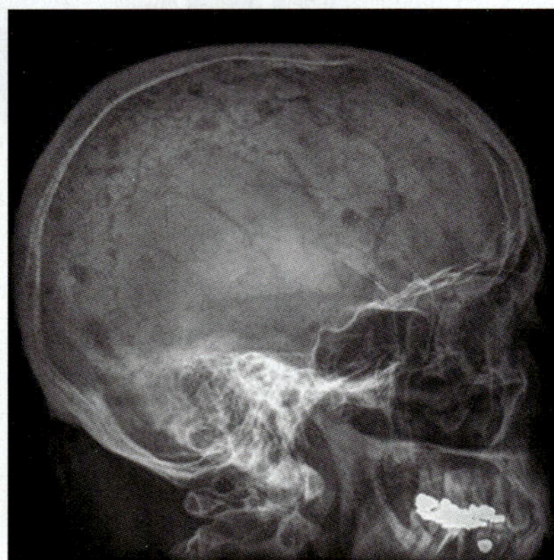

Fig. Pepper pot skull

XI H. SCURVY

- *Underlying cause*: Deficiency of Vitamin C
- *Clinical features*[Q]:
  - Perifollicular hemorrhages
  - Swollen gums
  - Bleeding tendencies
- *X-rays*:
  - **Pencil-thin cortex**[Q]
  - **White line of Frankel**[Q]
  - **Zone of Trummerfeld**[Q]
  - **Pelkan spurs**[Q]
  - **Halo sign of Wimberger**[Q]

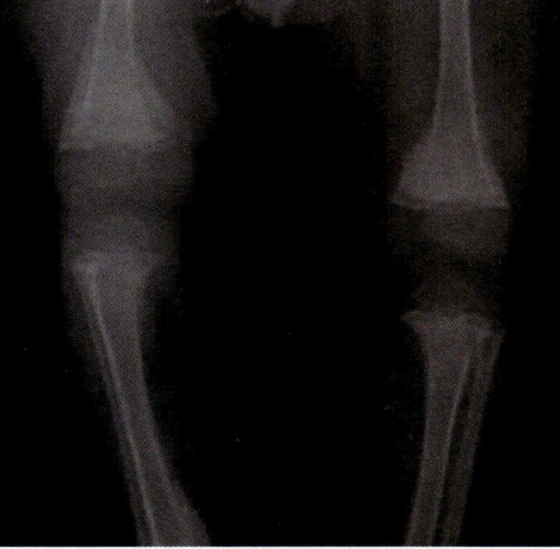

Fig. Scurvy

XI I. OSTEOGENESIS IMPERFECTA (FRAGILITAS OSSIUM)

- Tendency for frequent fractures due to ***'defective collagen synthesis'***
- Usually an Autosomal dominant disorder
- *Associated features*: Blue sclera[Q], Otosclerosis, Joint laxity[Q]

XI J. HISTIOCYTOSIS

- Definition: Proliferation of histiocytes
- Types:
  - Eosinophilic granuloma (Single bone involved)
  - Hand-Schuller-Christian disease
  - Litterer-Siwe disease (Most serious)

XI K. OSTEOCHONDRITIS

Osteochondritis	Site
Perthes disease	Epiphysis of head of femur
Panner's disease	Capitulum
Kienbock's disease[Q]	**Lunate**
Osgood Schlatter disease	**Tibial tuberosity**
Kohler disease	Navicular

XI L. POTT'S PUFFY TUMOUR

- *PPF is* ***osteomyelitis of*****: Frontal bone**[Q]
- *Characteristic feature*: Periosteal abscess
- *Cause of PPF*:
  - Complication of acute/ chronic frontal sinusitis
  - Trauma
  - Intranasal cocaine/ methamphetamine abuse
- *Diagnostic test*: CT scan
- *Surgical treatment*: Endoscopic frontal sinusotomy/Frontal sinus trephining

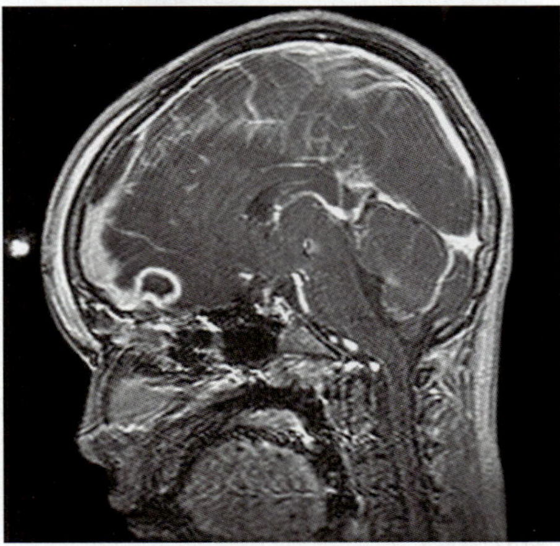

Fig. Pott's puffy tumor

XI M. ARACHNODACTYLY

- *Definition*: Elongated and slender tubular bones of hands and feet ***('Spider fingers')***[Q]
- *Measured by*: **Metacarpal Index**
  - Normal metacarpal index: 5.4–7.9
  - Arachnodactyly: 8.4–10.4

- *Arachnodactyly is seen in*[Q]:
  - **Marfan's syndrome**[Q]
  - Homocystinuria
  - Ehlers Danlos syndrome

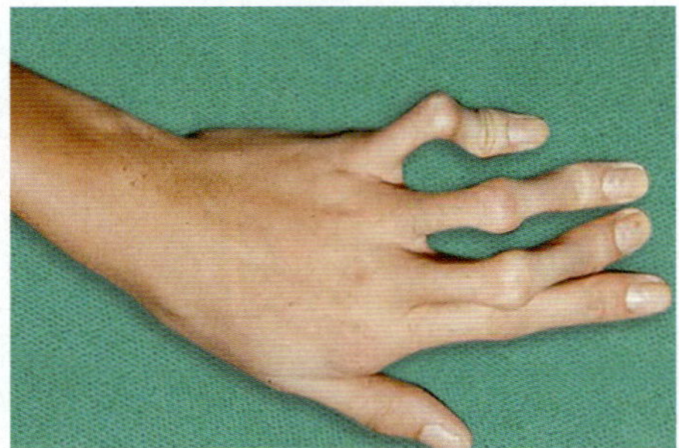

Fig. Spider fingers

XI N. ATLANTO-AXIAL SUBLUXATION [MNEMONIC: NOON DAY GRASS RUMINATES SALIVA][Q]

- **N**eck trauma (Most common)
- **O**dontoid process aplasia/hypoplasia
- **O**steogenesis imperfecta
- **N**eurofibromatosis
- **D**own's syndrome
- **G**out (Tophaceous)
- **R**heumatoid arthritis
- **A**nkylosing spondylitis
- **S**evere pneumonia
- **S**pinal surgery
- **R**etropharyngeal abscess
- **S**till's disease (Juvenile rheumatoid arthritis)

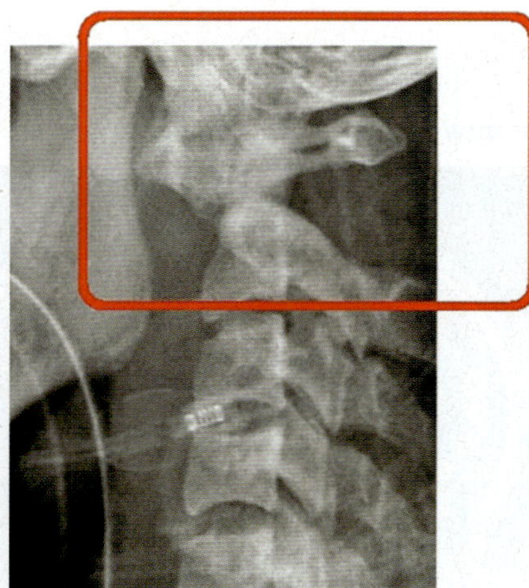

Fig. Atlantoaxial dislocation

XI O. INTERVERTEBRAL DISC PROLAPSE

- *Definition*: Protrusion of nucleus pulposus through annulus fibrosus
  - **MC site of exit: Posterolateral**
- ***MC site in body*: L4-L5**[Q]
  - Less common: C5-C6
- *Clinical presentation*:
  - Low back pain (Most common[Q])
  - Neurological symptoms
  - SLRT (Straight leg raising test) positive

- *Investigation of choice*: MRI[Q]
- *Treatment*:
  - Conservative: Rest + Physiotherapy[Q]
  - Surgical: Laminectomy[Q]

XI P. COMMON AFFECTIONS OF SOFT TISSUES

Type of affection	Tissue involved	Remark
Bursitis	Bursa	MC Irritative type
Tenosynovitis	Synovial lining of tendon sheath	-
Dupuytren's contracture[Q]	Palmar aponeurosis contracture	**MC Ring finger involved**[Q]
Tennis elbow[Q]	**Lateral epicondylitis**	-
Golfer's elbow[Q]	**Medial epicondylitis**	-
de Quervain's tenovaginitis[Q]	**Inflammed sheaths of APL, EPB***	Radial styloid process pain
Trigger finger/ thumb[Q]	**Constricted fibrous digital sheath**	Locking of finger
Carpal tunnel syndrome[Q]	**Median nerve compression**	Under flexor retinaculum
Frozen shoulder[Q]	**Joint capsule (Gleno-humeral)**	Periarthritis shoulder
Plantar fascitis	Inflammed plantar aponeurosis	Tender calcaneal tuberosity
Painful arc syndrome	Supraspinatous tendon	Tears, tendinitis
Meralgia paraesthetica[Q]	**Entrapped Lateral cutaneous nerve**	Thigh affected

*(*APL: Abductor pollicis longus; EPB: Extensor pollicis brevis)*

XI Q. USEFUL AIDS/ PROCEDURE IN ORTHOPEDICS

Orthopedic aid/ procedure	Used in
Austin-Moore prosthesis[Q]	Fracture neck of femur
Kirschner wire	Small bone fixation
Kuntscher nail	Fracture shaft of femur
Bankart's procedure[Q]	Recurrent dislocation of shoulder
Dwyer's osteotomy[Q]	CTEV
Meyer's operation[Q]	Fracture neck of femur
Thomas splint[Q]	Immobilisation of hip and thigh injuries
Cock-up splint[Q]	Radial nerve palsy
Von Rosen's splint[Q]	Congenital dislocation of hip
Dennis Brown splint[Q]	CTEV
Milwaukee brace[Q]	Scoliosis
Gallow's traction[Q]	Fracture shaft of femur (Age <2 years)
Hip spica	Fracture shaft of femur
Russel's traction[Q]	Trochanteric fractures
Frog's cast	Congenital dislocation of hip
Batchelor's cast[Q]	Congenital dislocation of hip
Hanging cast[Q]	Fracture shaft of humerus
Minerva jacket	Immobilization of injured cervical spine

XI R. ATTITUDES IN NERVE INJURIES

Attitude	Nerve injury
Wrist drop[Q]	Radial nerve palsy
Foot drop	Common peroneal nerve palsy
Winging of scapula[Q]	Long thoracic nerve palsy
Claw hand[Q]	Ulnar nerve palsy
Ape thumb deformity[Q]	Median nerve palsy
Pointing index[Q]	Median nerve palsy
Policeman tip deformity[Q]	C5-C6 Upper trunk brachial plexus injury
Claw hand	C8-T1 Lower trunk brachial plexus injury

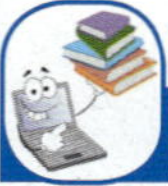

IMAGE-BASED QUESTIONS

1. Underlying Orthopedic disorder based on Characteristic (Arrow) shown in Photograph ***[AIIMS November 2016]***

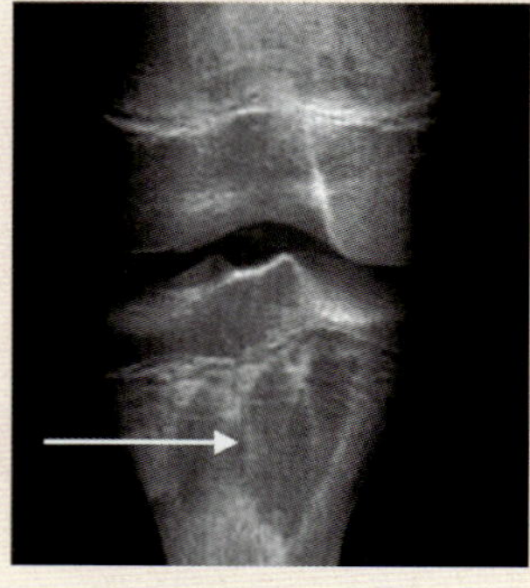

a. Acute Osteomyelitis
b. Chronic Osteomyelitis
c. Brodie's abscess
d. Tuberculous Osteomyelitis

2. Diagnose the disorder shown in the X-ray Photograph

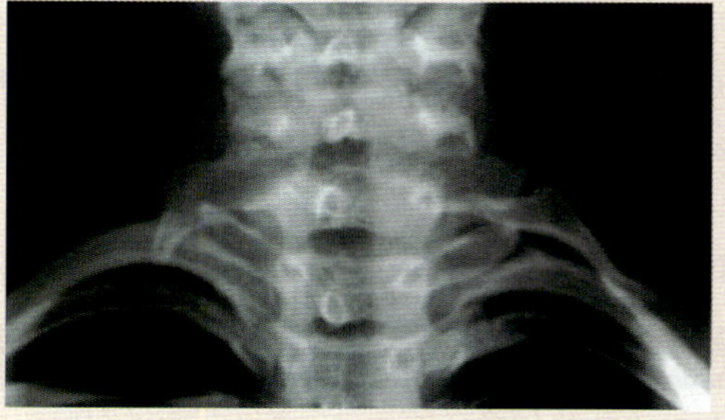

a. Cervical rib
b. Cervical disc syndromes
c. Thoracic outlet syndrome
d. Neck injury

3. Line used in Slipped capital femoral epiphysis as shown in Photograph is known as

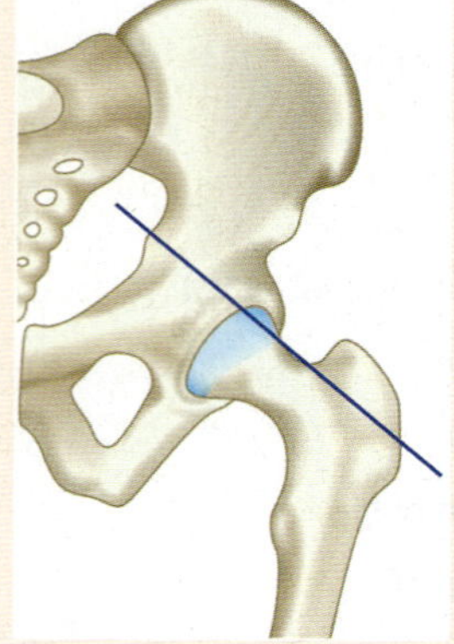

a. Shenton's line
b. Trethowan's line
c. Salter's line
d. Von Rosen's line

4. Clinical test shown in Photograph is ***[Recent Question 2013]***

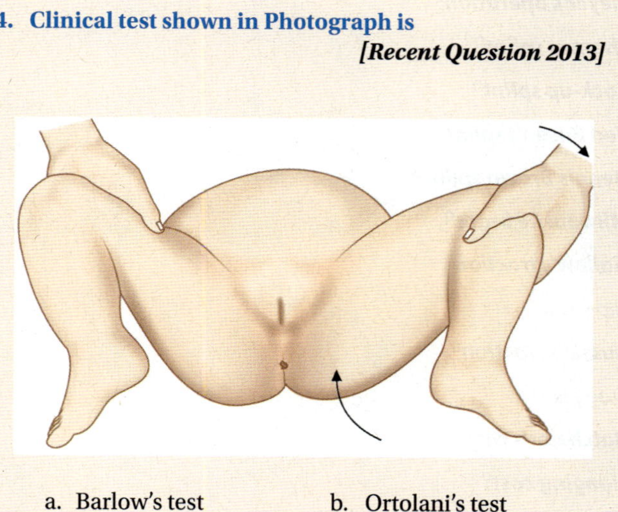

a. Barlow's test
b. Ortolani's test
c. Galeazzi test
d. Allen's test

5. Clinical test shown in Photograph is

[Recent Question 2013]

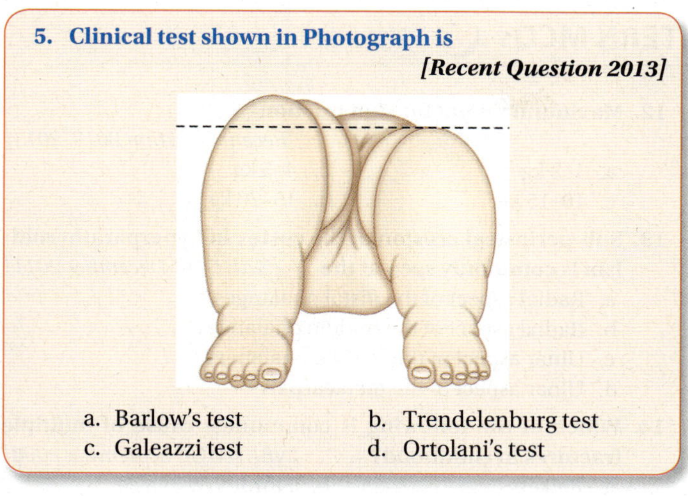

a. Barlow's test
b. Trendelenburg test
c. Galeazzi test
d. Ortolani's test

6. Identify the Test being performed in the image below

[AIIMS PG November 2015]

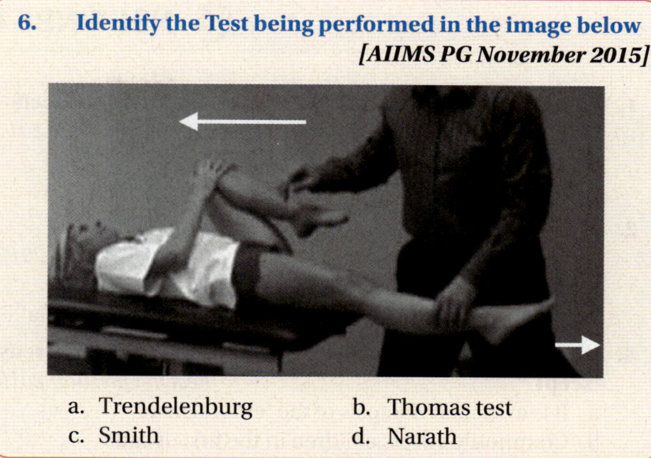

a. Trendelenburg
b. Thomas test
c. Smith
d. Narath

ANSWERS WITH EXPLANATIONS OF IBQs

1. Ans. (c) Brodie's abscess *[Ref. Maheshwari, 4/e p169]*

Brodie's Abscess

- Description: Osteomyelitis where body's defence mechanism is able to contain infection, thereby creating chronic bone abscess containing granulation tissue surrounded by a zone of sclerosis
- Radiology: Circular/ oval lucent area surrounded by a zone of sclerosis

2. Ans. (a) Cervical rib *[Ref. Myofascial Pain and Dysfunction by Travell and Simon, 2/e p520]*

Cervical Rib (Neck Rib)

- Description: A supernumerary (or extra) rib which arises from the 7thcervical vertebra
- Importance:
  - Congenital abnormality located above the normal first rib
  - May be associated with Thoracic outlet syndrome

3. Ans. (b) Trethowan's line *[Ref. Practical Orthopedics by Ebnezar, 1/e p290]*

- Trethowan line: Line drawn along upper neck of femur
- Importance: Epiphysis lie below Trethowan line in Slipped capital femoral epiphysis

4. Ans. (b) Ortolani's test *[Ref. Maheshwari, 4/e p214]*

- Ortolani test: Hips and knee are help in flexed position and gradually abducted
- Ortolani test positive: In Congenital dislocation of hip, a 'click of entrance' will be felt as femoral head slips into acetabulum from position of dislocation

5. Ans. (c) Galeazzi test *[Ref. Maheshwari, 4/e p214]*

- Galeazzi sign: Levels of knees are compared in a child lying with hips flexed to 70 degrees and knees flexed
- Galeazzi sign positive: In Congenital dislocation of hip, there is lowering of knee on affected side

6. Ans. (b) Thomas test *[Ref. Maheshwari, 4/e p349-350]*

Positive Thomas Test

- Tight Iliopsoas: Flexion of Contralateral hip
- Tight Tensor fascia lata: Abduction of hip during test
- Tight Rectus femoris: Knee extension occurs
- Tight Biceps femoris: Lateral rotation of tibia

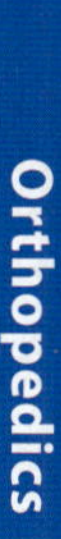

NEET/NBE PATTERN MCQs

1. Acute Osteomyelitis in children most commonly affects *[Recent Question 2016, 2017]*
a. Metaphysis b. Diaphysis
c. Epiphysis d. Physis

2. Osteosclerosis is a feature of which of the following? *[Recent Question 2016]*
a. Rickets b. Hyperparathyroidism
c. Paget's Disease d. Osteogenesis Imperfecta

3. All of the following are true regarding Perthes' disease except *[Recent Question 2016]*
a. It is avascular necrosis of the femoral head
b. Commonly affects children in the first decade
c. Limp and restricted rotations of the hip are common clinical features
d. MRI is not a good confirmatory investigation

4. Primary Hyperparathyroidism is associated with *[Recent Question 2016]*
a. Increased serum PTH and Hypercalcemia
b. Decreased serum PTH and Hypercalcemia
c. Increased serum PTH and Hypocalcemia
d. Decreased serum PTH and Hypocalcemia

5. Total duration of antibiotics in Acute osteomyelitis *[Recent Question 2016]*
a. 4 weeks b. 2 weeks
c. 6 weeks d. 8 weeks

6. Loosers zones/ Pseudofractures are commonly seen in the following areas except- *[Recent Question 2016]*
a. Scapula b. Ribs
c. Pelvis d. Radius

7. Vitamin beneficial in Osteoporosis in combination with Vitamin D is *[NBE FMGE March 2010]*
a. Vitamin A b. Vitamin B
c. Vitamin E d. Vitamin K

8. Pott's puffy tumor is *[NBE DNB June 2011]*
a. Osteomyelitis of skull bone
b. Basal cell carcinoma
c. Cylindroma
d. Squamous cell carcinoma

9. Not a feature of Rickets is *[NBE FMGE September 2009]*
a. Metaphyseal widening b. Bowing of legs
c. Cupping d. Frankel's line

10. Osteomalacia is characterized by *[NBE DNB June 2011]*
a. Defect in matrix mineralization
b. Increased bone resorption
c. Sub-periosteal bone resorption
d. Increased osteoclastic activity

11. Most common organism responsible for Acute Hematogenous Osteomyelitis is *[Recent Question 2016, NBE FMGE September 2008, PGI November 2014]*
a. Staphylococcus aureus
b. Streptococcus
c. Pneumococcus
d. Mycobacterium tuberculosis

12. Maximum weight for skin traction *[Recent Question 2012, 2013]*
a. 1–2 kg b. 4–5 kg
c. 10–15 kg d. 15–20 kg

13. Sub-periosteal erosion of the cortex in hyperparathyroidism is commonly seen at the *[NBE DNB December 2011]*
a. Radial aspect of the distal phalanges
b. Radial aspect of the middle phalanges
c. Ulnar aspect of the middle phalanges
d. Ulnar aspect of the metacarpals

14. Which of the following is commonest cause of multiple fractures in childhood? *[NBE FMGE September 2008]*
a. Rickets b. Fibrous dysplasia
c. Osteogenesis imperfecta d. Enchondromatosis

15. Anti-acetylcholine receptor antibodies are found in *[FMGE September 2012]*
a. SLE b. Myasthenia gravis
c. Diabetes mellitus type 1 d. Pemphigus vulgaris

16. Pott's puffy tumour is *[NBE FMGE September 2007]*
a. Squamous cell carcinoma
b. Basal cell carcinoma
c. Osteomyelitis of skull bone
d. Cylindroma

17. Allen test is used for assessment of *[FMGE September 2012]*
a. Integrity of Palmar arch b. Integrity of Foot arch
c. Radial nerve injury d. Median nerve injury

18. Waddling gait is a feature of *[NBE FMGE September 2006]*
a. Bilateral DOH
b. Bilateral genu varum
c. Bilateral CTEV d. Bilateral bowed tibia

19. 8 years old child with Genu valgum, Cranial bossing, widening of wrist joint. Most likely diagnosis is *[Recent Question 2014]*
a. Scurvy b. Fluorosis
c. Rickets d. Hyperthyroidism

20. CPPD crystals are seen in which disease? *[Recent Question 2013]*
a. Hypothyroidism
b. Primary hyperparathyroidism
c. Hemochromatosis
d. All of the above

21. Most commonly affected lower limb muscle in Poliomyelitis is *[NBE FMGE March 2006]*
a. Tibialis anterior b. Tibialis posterior
c. Quadriceps femoris d. Peroneus longus

22. Painful effusion of joints in Congenital syphilis is known as *[NBE FMGE March 2006]*
a. Hill Sach's lesion b. Charcot's joint
c. Cluttons' joint d. Morquio's disease

23. Fairbank triangle is seen in *[Recent Question 2012]*
a. CDH b. Congenital coxa vara
c. Perthe's disease d. SCFE

24. Abnormal metacarpal index is a feature of *[NBE FMGE March 2006]*
a. Down's syndrome b. Turner's syndrome
c. Marfan's syndrome d. All of the above

25. In EMG/NCV study, H. reflex correlates with *[Recent Question 2012, Recent Question 2013]*
a. L3 radiculopathy b. L4 radiculopathy
c. L5 radiculopathy d. S1 radiculopathy

26. MC cause of Anterior compartment syndrome is *[NBE DNB 1998, NBE DNB 2000]*
a. Fractures
b. Superficial muscular injury
c. Surgical operative trauma
d. Gas gangrene

27. Atlanto-axial subluxation is seen in all EXCEPT *[NBE FMGE March 2006]*
a. Still's disease b. Turner's syndrome
c. Retropharyngeal abscess d. Ankylosing spondylitis

28. Chronic persistent neutrophilic discharge is seen *[Recent Question 2012]*
a. Chronic osteomyelitis b. Acute osteomyelitis
c. Septic arthritis d. None

29. Earliest site of bony involvement in Acute hematogenous osteomyelitis is *[NBE DNB 2010, AIIMS 2009]*
a. Epiphysis b. Diaphysis
c. Metaphysis d. None

30. Brodie's abscess is *[Recent Question 2012]*
a. Acute osteomyelitis b. Subacute osteomyelitis
c. Chronic osteomyelitis d. Septic arthritis

31. Following hallmarks characterise Diaphyseal achalasia except *[UPSC 2011]*
a. Pseudoarthrosis common
b. Genu valgum can be found
c. Chondrosarcoma may occur in <1% cases
d. It is inherited as autosomal dominant dysplasia

32. 'Bag of bones' effect is seen in *[NBE FMGE March 2006]*
a. Osteopetrosis b. Paget's disease
c. Rheumatoid arthritis d. Charcot's joint

33. Marble bone disease is *[Recent Question 2012]*
a. Osteoporosis b. Paget's disease
c. Osteopetrosis d. Osteogenesis

34. Codfish vertebrae are seen in *[NBE FMGE March 2006]*
a. Osteopetrosis b. Hyperparathyroidism
c. Morquio's syndrome d. All of the above

35. Osteitis fibrosa cystica is a type of *[UPSC 2010, AIPGME 1996]*
a. Hyperthyroidism b. Hyperparathyroidism
c. Milk alkali syndrome d. Rickets

36. Which change will be seen in vertebral column in Ochronosis? *[Recent Question 2012]*
a. Calcification of disc b. Bamboo spine
c. Increased disc space d. None

37. Sudeck's dystrophy symptoms are all except *[Recent Question 2012]*
a. Pain b. Increased bone density
c. Sweating d. Stiffness

38. Calcification of menisci of knee joints is seen in *[NBE FMGE March 2006]*
a. Ochronosis b. Osteoarthritis
c. Hyperparathyroidism d. Gout

39. In Rickets all are seen except *[Recent Question 2012]*
a. Bowing of legs b. Rachitic rosary
c. Bleeding d. Craniotabes

40. Neuropathic joint is seen in all except *[Recent Question 2012]*
a. DM b. Tabes Dorsalis
c. Syringomyelia d. Hypertension

41. Osteomalacia can be caused by which of the following drugs? *[NBE FMGE September 2005]*
a. Phenytoin b. Quinidine
c. Lignocaine d. Chloramphenicol

42. In scoliosis degree of deformity is calculated by *[Recent Question 2012]*
a. Cobbs' method b. Hamburger method
c. Haldane method d. Milwaukee method

43. Alkaline phosphatase is increased in all EXCEPT *[NBE FMGE September 2005]*
a. Osteoporosis b. Osteomalacia
c. Rickets d. Vitamin D deficiency

44. Posterior scalloping of vertebrae is not seen *[Recent Question 2012]*
a. Neurofibromatosis b. Astrocytoma
c. Aortic aneurysm d. Ependymoma

45. 'Bone within bone appearance' is seen in *[NBE FMGE September 2004]*
a. Scurvy b. Congenital syphilis
c. Gaucher's disease d. All of the above

46. Windswept deformity is seen in *[Recent Question 2013]*
a. Achondroplasia
b. Ankylosing spondylitis
c. Rickets d. Scurvy

47. Cast syndrome is due to *[Recent Question 2012]*
a. Above elbow cast b. Below elbow cast
c. Hip Spica d. Above knee cast

48. Atlantoaxial subluxation is seen in all EXCEPT *[NBE FMGE September 2004]*
a. Gout b. Still's disease
c. Retropharyngeal abscess d. Ankylosing spondylitis

49. 60 degree angle of Z plasty causes how much increase in length? *[Recent Question 2012]*
a. 25% b. 50%
c. 75% d. 100%

50. A 30 years old female has low serum calcium and phosphate with elevated parathormone. Diagnosis is *[Recent Question 2012]*
a. Vitamin D deficiency
b. Primary hyperparathyroidism
c. Osteoporosis
d. Paget's diseases

51. 'Bag of bones' is seen in *[NBE FMGE September 2004]*
a. Osteopetrosis b. Charcot's joints
c. Rheumatoid arthritis d. Paget's disease

52. Drug used in acute gout *[Recent Question 2012, 2013]*
- a. Allopurinol
- b. Probenacid
- c. Colchicine
- d. Sulfapyrazone

53. Which of the radiological features are seen in scurvy? *[UPSC 2005]*
1. Diaphyseal fracture
2. Ground glass appearance
3. Rarefied zone at metaphysis
4. Sub-periosteal hemorrhages

- a. 1 only
- b. 2 and 3
- c. 2, 3 and 4
- d. 1, 2, 3 and 4

54. Not useful in treatment of osteoporosis *[NBE DNB 1992, Karnataka 1992]*
- a. Sodium chloride
- b. Potassium
- c. Phosphate
- d. Calcium

55. Codfish vertebrae are pathognomonic of *[NBE FMGE March 2004]*
- a. Osteopetrosis
- b. Hyperparathyroidism
- c. Morquio's syndrome
- d. All of the above

56. Albers Schonberg disease is also known as *[Recent Question 2012]*
- a. Osteoporosis
- b. Osteopetrosis
- c. Osteogenesis imperfecta
- d. Paget's disease

57. Painful arc syndrome is not caused by *[UPSC 2000]*
- a. Sub-acromial bursitis
- b. Supraspinatus tendinitis
- c. Acromio-clavicular arthritis
- d. Rupture supraspinatus tendon

58. Slipped capital femoral epiphysis is seen most commonly in which age group? *[Recent Question 2012, 2013]*
- a. Infants
- b. Adolescents
- c. Old age
- d. Childhood

59. Loosers-zone are seen in *[Recent Question 2016, NBE DNB 1992, NBE DNB 2003]*
- a. Osteomalacia
- b. Hyperparathyroidism
- c. Pagets disease
- d. Scurvy (Vit C deficiency)

60. Lengthening of calcaneus is done in which deformity? *[NBE DNB 1993]*
- a. Flat foot
- b. Foot drop
- c. Equinus deformity
- d. Cuboid deformity

61. Calcification of menisci of knee joints is seen in *[NBE FMGE March 2004]*
- a. Ochronosis
- b. Osteoarthritis
- c. Hyperparathyroidism
- d. Gout

62. Abnormal metacarpal index is seen in *[NBE FMGE March 2003]*
- a. Down's syndrome
- b. Turner's syndrome
- c. Marfan's syndrome
- d. All of the above

63. All of the following statements regarding Chikungunya arthritis is true, EXCEPT *[NBE FMGE September 2011]*
- a. Affects small joints most often
- b. Causes early morning pain and swelling
- c. Can persist for months
- d. Early institution of steroids is essential

64. Subperiosteal erosions are seen in *[NBE DNB 1994]*
- a. Scurvy
- b. Rickets
- c. Hypoparathyroidism
- d. Hyperparathyroidism

65. MC site for acute osteomyelitis seen in infants is *[NBE DNB 1994, 1999, 2003]*
- a. Shoulder joint
- b. Hip joint
- c. Tibia
- d. Olecranon process

66. All of the following are true of osteomalacia except *[NBE FMGE March 2012]*
- a. Proximal myopathy
- b. Raised serum calcium
- c. Bone biopsy shows increased demineralized bone matrix
- d. Vitamin D deficiency

67. Least common cause of osteomyelitis is *[NBE DNB 1995]*
- a. Staphylococccus
- b. Streptococcus
- c. Hemophilus influenzae
- d. Escherichia coli

68. Sub-periosteal bone absorption is best seen in *[NBE FMGE March 2012]*
- a. Radius
- b. Metacarpals
- c. Phalanges
- d. Ulna

69. "Bone within bone" appearance is classically seen in *[NBE FMGE March 2012]*
- a. Osteogenesis imperfecta
- b. Osteopetrosis
- c. Renal osteodystrophy
- d. Achondroplasia

70. Treatment of Club foot *[NBE DNB 1997, NBE DNB 2000]*
- a. Should be started immediately after birth
- b. Should be started 1 month after birth
- c. Should be started 1 year after birth
- d. Should be started in adulthood

71. Which of the following is not a feature of Turner's Syndrome? *[NBE FMGE March 2012]*
- a. Adult stature less than 145 cms
- b. Long 4th metacarpals and metatarsals
- c. Medial tibial exostosis
- d. Lymphedema of dorsum of hands

72. Defect in collagen synthesis is seen in *[NBE FMGE March 2012]*
- a. Marfan's syndrome
- b. Osteogenesis imperfecta
- c. Scurvy
- d. Hunter's syndrome

73. Neuropathic joints are most commonly seen in *[NBE DNB 1997, 1999, 2001, 2003, 2005, 2007]*
- a. Syphilis
- b. Diabetes mellitus
- c. Leprosy
- d. Rheumatoid arthritis

74. Osteoporosis has all of the following features EXCEPT *[NBE FMGE March 2012]*
- a. Reduction of bone tissue mass
- b. Increased serum alkaline phosphatase
- c. Involves multiple bones
- d. Causes backache

75. Poliomyelitis mainly affects *[Recent Question 2014]*
- a. Anterior horn cells
- b. Posterior horn cells
- c. Basal ganglia
- d. Peripheral nerves

76. Charlie Chaplin gait is seen in *[Recent Question 2014]*
- a. Phenylketonuria
- b. Alcaptonuria
- c. Tay Sachs disease
- d. Marfans syndrome

77. Jaipur foot was invented by *[Recent Question 2014]*
a. JH Gibbon b. J Maheshwari
c. PK Sethi, RK Sharma d. Nicolas Andry

78. A child presents with multiple fractures and Blue sclera. He is a case of *[Recent Question 2015]*
a. Battered baby syndrome b. Wilson's disease
c. Osteogenesis imperfecta d. Marfan's syndrome

79. Polymyositis is characterized by all except *[Recent Question 2016, 2015]*
a. Distal muscle weakness b. Increased CPK
c. Fiber regeneration d. Fiber degeneration

80. Reflex sympathetic dystrophy is seen in *[Recent Question 2015]*
a. Osteoarthritis b. Rheumatoid arthritis
c. Osteoporosis d. Sarcoidosis

81. Collagen deficiency in Osteogenesis imperfecta *[Recent Question 2015]*
a. Type I b. Type II
c. Type III d. Type IV

82. Age group of Perthes' disease *[Recent Question 2015]*
a. 0–1 years b. 4–12 years
c. 12–28 years d. 45–65 years

83. Osteoporosis is seen in all the following except *[Recent Question 2017]*
a. Hyperprolactinemia b. Thalassemia
c. Homocystinuria d. Systemic sclerosis

84. False about Osteogenesis imperfecta is *[Recent Question 2017]*
a. Defective collagen formation
b. Associated with cataract formation
c. Autosomal dominant
d. Known as Brittle bone disease

85. Which of the following is the most metabolically active part of long bone? *[Recent Question 2017]*
a. Epiphysis b. Metaphysis
c. Diaphysis d. All of the above

86. Osteomyelitis in Sickle cell anemia is due to *[Recent Question 2017]*
a. Salmonella b. Streptococcus
c. Hemophilus d. Neisseria

87. Bunion is *[Recent Question 2017]*
a. Delayed union of base of 1st metatarsal
b. Bursitis
c. Bone dysplasia
d. Union of base ball finger

88. Hooked vertebrae seen in *[Recent Question 2017]*
a. Achondroplasia
b. Osteogenesis imperfecta
c. Congenital hypothyroidism
d. All of the above

89. Ankle reflex is affected in Prolapsed intervertebral disc at what level? *[Recent Question 2017]*
a. L3-L4 b. L4-L5
c. L5-S1 d. S1-S2

90. Pseudofracture can be seen in the following conditions *[Recent Question 2017]*
a. Hereditary hyperphosphatasia
b. Pagets disease
c. Fibrous dysplasia
d. All the above

91. Paprika sign during debridement is crucial in management which of the following condition? *[Recent Question 2017]*
a. Chronic osteomyelitis b. Osteosarcoma
c. Osteoid osteoma d. Brodies abscess

92. A 40 years old female presents with urine darkening on standing, joint pain and stiffness, and pigment deposition in joints. What is the probable diagnosis? *[Recent Question 2017]*
a. Phenylketonuria b. Tyrosinemia
c. Alkaptonuria d. Tyrosinemia

93. Patient has history of RTA 2 years back. Now at the same site, he has developed pain and swelling. X-ray shows the following features as given in Photograph. What will be the diagnosis? *[Recent Question 2018]*

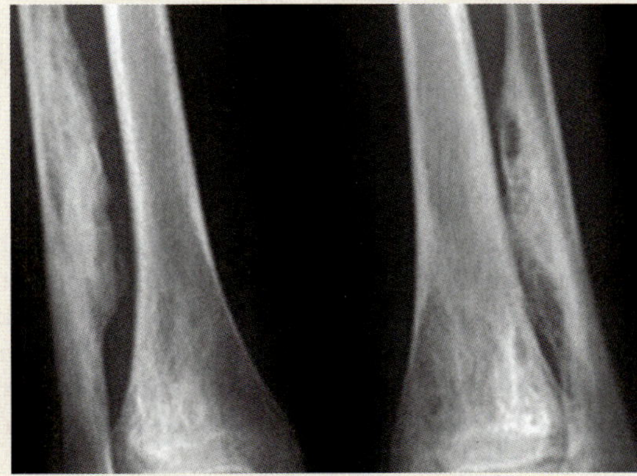

a. Multiple myeloma
b. Ewing's sarcoma
c. Chronic osteomyelitis
d. Osteogenic sarcoma

HIGH YIELD MCQs

1. Compound palmar ganglion is *[UP PGMEE 1997]*
a. Ulnar bursitis due to compound injury
b. Tuberculosis affection of ulnar bursa
c. Pyogenic affection of ulnar bursa
d. Nonspecific affection of ulnar bursa

2. A teenage girl complains of knee pain on climbing stairs and on getting-up after sitting for long duration. Most probable diagnosis is *[All India PGMEE 2011]*
a. Plica syndrome b. Bipartite patella
c. Chondromalacia patellae
d. Patello-femoral osteoarthritis

3. Commonest cause of hematogenous Osteomyelitis *[JIPMER PGMEE 1998]*

a. H. influenzae
b. Streptococcus
c. Staphylococcus aureus
d. Salmonella typhi

4. In a newborn child, abduction and internal rotation produces a click sound. It is *[AP PGMEE 1993, Delhi PGMEE 1993]*

a. Ortolani sign b. Telescoping sign
c. Lachman's sign d. Mc Murray's sign

5. Prenatal determination of osteogenesis imperfecta is done by *[PGI 2007]*

a. Acid phosphatase b. Alkaline phosphatase
c. Abnormal Pro - *a* chain d. None

6. In congenital dislocation of hip, not true is *[AMU PGMEE1989]*

a. Real shortening b. Telescoping
c. Trendelenburg test d. Head of femur downwards
e. Asymmetrical crease

7. Congenital dislocation of hip is more commonly seen in *[AP PGMEE 1989]*

a. Caucasians b. Negroes
c. Japanese d. Eskimos

8. Acute Osteomyelitis of long bones commonly affects the *[PGI 1998]*

a. Epiphysis b. Diaphysis
c. Metaphysis d. Any of the above

9. Calcitonin is used in the treatment of *[AIIMS PGMEE 1991, Manipal PGMEE 1997]*

a. Post menopausal osteoporosis
b. Malignant hyper calcemia
c. Paget's disease
d. All of the above

10. A 67-year-old man on biochemical analysis found to have three fold rise of level of serum alkaline phosphatase that of upper limit of norm value during a routine checkup but serum calcium and phosphorous concentration and liver function test results and normal. He is asymptomatic. The probable cause is *[AIIMS PGMEE 1999, APPG 1991]*

a. Multiple myeloma
b. Paget's disease of bone
c. Primary hyperparathyroidism
d. Osteomalacia

11. Acute Osteomyelitis is most commonly caused by *[All India PGMEE 2002, UP PGMEE 1998]*

a. Staphylococcus aureus b. Borrelia Vincentii
c. Actinomyces bovis d. Nocardia asteroids

12. A 3-old year male presented with progressive anemia, hepatosplenomegaly and osteomyelitis of jaw with pathological fracture, X-ray shows chalky white deposits on bone, probable diagnosis is *[AIIMS PGMEE 1993]*

a. Osteopetrosis
b. Osteopoikilocytosis
c. Alkaptonuria
d. Myositis- ossificans progressiva

13. Raju, a 10 years old child, presents with predisposition to fractures, anemia, hepatosplenomegaly and a diffusely increased radiographic density of bones. The most likely diagnosis is *[All India PGMEE 2002]*

a. Osteogenesis imperfecta b. Pycnodysostosis
c. Myelofibrosis d. Osteopetrosis

14. Most common organism causing osteomyelitis in drug abusers is *[PGI 1997]*

a. E. coli b. Pseudomonas
c. Klebsiella d. Staphylococcus aureus

15. Commonest deformity in congenital dislocation of hip *[PGI 1997]*

a. Small head of femur
b. Angle of torsion
c. Decreased neck shaft angle
d. Shallow acetabulum

16. All of the following statements regarding Paget's disease are correct except *[Manipal PGMEE 1997]*

a. Females are affected more than males
b. It frequently leads to Osteogenic sarcoma
c. Serum alkaline phosphates level is elevated
d. All called as Osteitis deformans

17. Which is not true about Paget's disease of bone? *[Delhi PGMEE 2000]*

a. Often there is no symptom
b. Alkaline phosphates is low
c. Thickening of bone due to widening of cortex
d. All of these

18. Which of the following is not true regarding Paget's disease of bone? *[Kerala PGMEE 1990, Karnataka PGMEE 1996]*

a. Serum alkaline phosphatase is low
b. It frequently leads to Osteogenic sarcoma
c. Males are affected more than females
d. Involved area shows rapid formation and resorption of bone.

19. All of the following features are characteristic of Osteopetrosis except *[AIIMS PGMEE 2008]*

a. Pancytopenia
b. Abnormally slow rates of fracture healing
c. Compression of cranial nerves
d. Mandibular osteomyelitis

20. Muscle most commonly affected by congenital absence is *[All India PGMEE 2009]*

a. Pectoralis major b. Semi membranosus
c. Teres minor d. Gluteus maximus

21. All of the following statements are true about development dysplasia (DOH) of the hip, except *[All India PGMEE 2006]*

a. It is more common in females
b. Oligohydramnios is associated with a higher risk of DDH
c. The hourglass appearance of the capsule may prevent a successful closed reduction
d. Twin pregnancy is a known risk factor

22. The treatment of Congenital dislocation of hip after childhood is *[AP PGMEE 1991]*

a. Leave alone
b. Surgery should be done if symptomatic
c. Conservative measures to be taken
d. None of the above

23. Increased bone density in X-ray seen in *[PGI 2008]*
a. Collapse cancellous bone
b. Periosteal reaction c. Paget's disease
d. AVN e. Osteomyelitis

24. Increased bone density occurs in *[UP PGMEE 1988, PGI 1990]*
a. Cushing syndrome
b. Hypoparathyroidism
c. Fluorosis
d. Hyperthyroidism
e. Renal osteodystrophy

25. Paget's disease *[Bihar PGMEE 1990]*
a. Is painless
b. Begins as an osteoblastic
c. Is frequently complicated by osteogenic sarcoma
d. Does not affect bones singly (e.g. Only the clavicle)

26. 60 years old male with bony abnormality at upper tibia associated with sensorineural hearing loss. On laboratory examination serum alkaline phosphatase levels are (44 mU/1] elevated and serum Ca^{++} and PO_4^- are normal. Skeletal survey shows ivory vertebrae and cotton wool spots in X- ray skull. Diagnosis is *[AIIMS PGMEE 2007]*
a. Fibrous dysplasia b. Paget disease
c. Osteosclerotic metastasis d. Osteoporosis

27. Which of the following is seen in osteoporosis? *[AIIMS PGMEE 2000]*
a. Low Ca, high PO_4, high alkaline phosphatase
b. Low Ca, low PO_4, low alkaline phosphatase
c. Normal Ca, normal PO_4, normal alkaline phosphatase
d. Low Ca, low PO_4, normal alkaline phosphatase

28. All are causes of Osteoporosis, except *[All India PGMEE 2000]*
a. Thyrotoxicosis b. Hypothyroidism
c. Chronic heparin therapy d. Old age

29. Coxa vara is found in *[PGI 1996]*
a. TB b. Rickets
c. Perthes disease d. Rheumatoid arthritis
e. Osteogenesis imperfecta

30. Movement restricted in Congenital dislocation of hip in infants *[JIPMER PGMEE 1993]*
a. Flexion b. Extension
c. Rotation d. Full abduction in 90°

31. Deafness in cases of Paget's disease is due to *[PGI 1981, NBE DNB 1989]*
a. Thickened cranium
b. Narrowing of foramina of skull
c. Brain compression d. Otosclerosis

32. Drug therapy of Paget's disease (Osteitis Deformans) include all except *[Karnataka PGMEE 2001]*
a. Alendronate b. Etidronate
c. Calcitonin d. Plicamycin

33. The histopathologic feature of Paget's disease includes *[Bihar PGMEE 1989]*
a. Simultaneous osteoblastic activity at places
b. Osteoclastic resorption
c. Replacement of bone marrow by fibro vascular tissue
d. All of the above

34. Congenital dislocation of hip occurs due to *[PGI 1997]*
a. Small neck of femur b. Small head of femur
c. Rotation of femur d. Large acetabulum

35. What is the diagnostic radiological finding skeletal fluorosis? *[JIPMER PGMEE 1998]*
a. Sclerosis of sacroiliac joint
b. Interosseous membrane ossification
c. Osteosclerosis of vertebral body
d. Ossification of ligaments of knee joint

36. Osteoporosis may be seen in all except *[All India PGMEE 1998]*
a. Hyperparathyroidism b. Hypoparathyroidism
c. Thyrotoxicosis d. Heparin administration

37. Osteoporosis is seen in *[All India PGMEE 1994]*
a. Thyrotoxicosis b. Cushing's disease
c. Menopause d. All of the above

38. Following is a radiological feature of Skeletal Fluorosis *[JIPMER PGMEE 2000]*
a. Intervertebral ligament calcification
b. Sacral sclerosis
c. Osteolytic lesion in pelvis
d. None

39. Manifestations of Fluorosis includes *[PGI 1990]*
a. Stiffness of back ligaments
b. Caries teeth (due to deficiency of fluorine)
c. Genu valgum
d. Dental changes
e. Stiffness of bones and tendons

40. Test useful for diagnosis of Congenital dislocation of hip *[PGI 1999]*
a. Thomas test b. Barlow's test
c. Hibb's test d. Laguerres test
e. Ortolani's test

41. Absolute indication of X-ray of pelvis in case of congenital dislocation of hip are all EXCEPT *[AIIMS PGMEE 1999]*
a. Positive family history b. Breech presentation
c. Unstable hip d. Shortening of limb

42. True about B/L CDH *[PGI 1990, 2000, 2004, 2006, 2007, 2009]*
a. Exaggerated lordosis b. B/L genu valgum
c. Wadding gait d. Shenton's line broken
e. Short stature

43. MC presentation of Congenital dislocation of knee is *[AIIMS PGMEE 1996]*
a. Flexion b. Hyperextension
c. Varus d. Valgus

44. Caffey's disease occurs in *[NIMS PGMEE 1996]*
a. Infants below 6 months b. Above years
c. Above 10-20 years d. 20–40 years

45. Osteomyelitis of Jaw is seen in *[AIIMS PGMEE 1992]*
a. Osteomalacia b. Osteopoikilosis
c. Osteoporosis d. Caffey's disease

46. All of following conditions may be responsible for osteoporosis except *[All India PGMEE 1996]*
- a. Steroid therapy
- b. Prolonged weightlessness in spaceship
- c. Hyperparathyroidism
- d. Hypoparathyroidism

47. Osteoporosis is seen in following except *[TN PGMEE 1995]*
- a. Old age
- b. Prolonged Heparin administration
- c. Hyperthyroidism
- d. Steroid intake

48. Rugger jersey spine in CRF is due to *[PGI 2004]*
- a. Osteomalacia
- b. Trauma
- c. Hyperparathyroidism
- d. Aluminium osteodystrophy
- e. Osteopetrosis

49. Pappu, 7 years old young boy, had fracture of lateral condyle of femur. He developed malunion as the fractUre was not reduced anatomically. Malunion will produce *[All India PGMEE 2002]*
- a. Genu vulgum
- b. Genu varum
- c. Genu recurvatum
- d. Dislocation of knee

50. Which statement is true regarding Genu varum (Bowleg)? *[PGI 2001]*
- a. In infants, it may be considered normal
- b. Occurs due to epiphyseal dysplasia
- c. Seldom associated with tibial angulation
- d. Affects only tibia but never femur
- e. Does not require any treatment

51. Most common cause of Genu valgum in children *[AIIMS PGMEE 1993]*
- a. Rickets
- b. Osteoarthritis
- c. Paget's disease
- d. Rheumatoid arthritis

52. Blount's disease is *[Recent Question 2016, PGI 2000]*
- a. Rickets
- b. Flat foot
- c. Tibia vera
- d. Genu valgus
- e. Genu recurvatum

53. A Bald child with swollen abdomen, hyperosteous bones with mental retardation has *[Karnataka PGMEE 1998]*
- a. Hypervitaminosis A
- b. Hypervitaminosis D
- c. Down's syndrome
- d. Tuberous sclerosis

54. Most common deformity seen in Club foot is *[Bihar PGMEE 1999]*
- a. Equines
- b. Equino valgus
- c. Calcaneo equino varus
- d. Talipes equino varus

55. Treatment of CTEV in newborn is *[AIIMS PGMEE 1993]*
- a. Observation till 6 months age
- b. Tendon release surgery
- c. Corrective splint
- d. Manipulation and corrective splint

56. All are false regarding genu varum except *[PGI 1994, JIPMER PGMEE 1995]*
- a. Orthosis is a must only during weight bearing
- b. Orthosis is recommended during day time
- c. Orthosis is recommended during night time
- d. Orthosis is recommended full time

57. Critical age of osteotomy for genu varum is *[AMU PGMEE 1997, JIPMER PGMEE 1998]*
- a. 4 years
- b. 6 years
- c. 8 years
- d. 10 years

58. Osteomalacia is associated with *[All India PGMEE 2003]*
- a. Decreases in osteoid volume
- b. Decrease in osteoid surface
- c. Increase in osteoid maturation time
- d. Increase in mineral apposition rate

59. The cause of osteomalacia is/ are *[PGI 1994]*
- a. Phenytoin
- b. Malabsorption
- c. Vincristine
- d. Cushing's syndrome

60. Most common manifestation of osteoporosis is *[All India PGMEE 1994]*
- a. Compression fracture of the spine
- b. Asymptomatic, detected incidentally by low serum Calcium
- c. Bowing of legs
- d. Loss of weight

61. MC site of fracture of the following bones occur in senile osteoporosis is *[TN PGMEE 1990]*
- a. Vertebra
- b. Neck of femur
- c. Radius
- d. Shaft off emur

62. Not a complication of menopause *[Kerala PGMEE 1995]*
- a. Fracture spine
- b. Colles fracture
- c. Fracture neck of femur
- d. Supra condylar fracture humerus

63. Nail patella syndrome is characterized by *[PGI 2002]*
- a. Iliac horn
- b. Sacral horn
- c. Absent patella
- d. Knee deformity
- e. Dislocation of patella

64. Rocker bottom foot is seen in *[PGI 2008]*
- a. Congenital vertical talus
- b. Excessive correction of Grice procedure
- c. Arthrogryposis
- d. Holding club foot in too long corrected position
- e. Force dorsiflexion against equinus varus

65. CTEV is caused by *[PGI 2001] [PGI 2001]*
- a. Neurological disorder
- b. Idiopathic
- c. Spina bifida
- d. Cubitus varus
- e. Arthrogryposis multiplex

66. Club foot is commoner among *[Rajasthan PGMEE 1992]*
- a. Males
- b. Binovular twins
- c. Females
- d. Uniovular twins

67. Chronic club foot is treated by *[JIPMER PGMEE 1995]*
- a. Amputation
- b. Triple arthrodesis
- c. Dorso-medial release
- d. None of the above

68. Osteomalacia causes include *[PGI 1991]*
- a. Phenytoin
- b. Malabsorption
- c. Indoor stay
- d. Vincristine
- e. Cushing's syndrome

69. Treatment of Osteoporosis include *[PGI 2009]*
a. Alendronate b. Teriparatide
c. Denosumab d. Strontium renalate
e. Calcitonin

70. Osteomalacia / Rickets my be seen in all except *[JIPMER PGMEE 1999]*
a. Neurofibroma b. Osteoblastoma
c. Hemangiopericytoma d. Ewings sarcoma

71. Rickets is seen in all except *[TN PGMEE 1996, UP PGMEE 1995]*
a. Dietary deficiency b. Hypocalcemia
c. Malabsorption d. Fanconi's syndrome

72. All are seen in Klippel-Feil syndrome EXCEPT *[All India PGMEE 2005, Recent Question 2014]*
a. Bilateral neck webbing
b. Low hair line
c. Bilaterally shortened sternocleidomastoid muscles
d. Grossly limited neck movement

73. Wormian bones are found in *[AP PGMEE 1999]*
a. Scurvy b. Osteogenesis imperfecta
c. Cretinism d. Rickets

74. Club foot characteristically involves
a. Foot and ankle *[Bihar PGMEE 1999]*
b. Foot, ankle and leg
c. Foot only
d. Foot, ankle, leg and knee joint

75. Treatment of postmenopausal osteoporosis *[PGI 2004]*
a. Calcitonin b. Alendronate
c. Progesterone d. Tamoxifence
e. Androgen

76. Bone density is decreased in which of the following? *[PGI 2002]*
a. Osteoporosis b. AVN of bone
c. Osteopetrosis
d. Fracture and collapse of cancellous bone
e. Fluorosis

77. Denosumab, a monoclonal antibody against RANKL receptor is used in treatment of *[AIIMS PGMEE 2006, Recent Question 2015]*
a. Rheumatoid arthritis b. Osteoporosis
c. Osteoarthritis d. SLE

78. Osteoporosis is characterized by *[PGI 2005]*
a. Increased serum alkaline phosphatase
b. Decreased bone density c. Wasting of muscles
d. Looser's zone seen e. Decreased serum Ca^{2+}

79. Various congenital deformity of the ankle joint occurs at *[Bihar PGMEE 1999]*
a. Calcanionavicular joint b. Talocalcaneal joint
c. Talonavicular joint d. Tarsonavicular joint

80. Not seen in Osteogenesis imperfecta *[All India PGMEE 1998]*
a. Blue sclera
b. Osteoporosis
c. Lax ligament
d. Bilateral hip dislocation

81. Defective mineralization of proximal zone of cartilage and epiphysis is a feature of *[All India PGMEE 1999, 2000]*
a. Rickets b. Scurvy
c. Osteomalacia d. Syphilis

82. Rickets of vitamin D deficiency is associated with *[UP PGMEE 1998]*
a. Subperiosteal haemorrhage
b. Ricketirosary at costochondral junction produced by subluxation of sternal plate
c. Apt to develop during growth in low birth weight infants
d. Inorganic serum phosphate concentration 4.5–6.5 mg/dL

83. Hypervitaminosis causing bony abnormalities
a. Vitamin A b. Vitamin C *[PGI 2006]*
c. Vitamin D d. Vitamin E
e. Vitamin K

84. Causes of Osteomalacia is/ are *[PGI 1991]*
a. Indoor stay b. Vincristine
c. Phenytoin d. Malabsorption
e. Cushing's syndrome

85. Most important pathology in club foot is *[TN PGMEE 1990]*
a. Congenital talonavicular dislocation
b. Tightening of Tendoachilles
c. Calcaneal fracture
d. Lateral derangement

86. Talipes equino varus is *[PGI 1997]*
a. Equinus, inversion, abduction
b. Equines, inversion, adduction
c. Equines, eversion, abduction
d. Equines, eversion, abduction

87. Which of the following is true of Talipes calcane ovalgus? *[JIPMER PGMEE 1991]*
a. Dorsiflexed and inverted b. Dorsiflexed and everted
c. More serious than CTEV d. Plantar flexed

88. In nutrional rickets changes occurs at the *[PGI 1995]*
a. Metaphysis b. Epiphysis
c. Diaphysis d. All of these

89. Rickets in infancy is characterised by the following except *[AIIMS PGMEE 2007]*
a. Craniotabes b. Rachitic rosary
c. Wide open fontanelles d. Bow legs

90. Not seen in Rickets *[Delhi PGMEE 2001]*
a. Cupping of ends of bones
b. Instability c. Craniotabes
d. Decreased alkaline phosphatase

91. True regarding Osteomalacia is/ are *[PGI 2009]*
a. Normal serum calcium b. Increased serum calcium
c. Increased serum phosphate
d. Pseudofractures e. Osteosclerotic lesions

92. A thirty one year old male with Nephrotic syndrome complains of pain in right hip joint of 2 months duration. The movements at the hip are free but painful terminally. The most likely diagnosis is
a. Tuberculosis of hip *[AIIMS PGMEE 2003]*
b. Avascular necrosis of femoral head
c. Chondrolysis of hip
d. Pathological fracture of femoral neck

93. A patient of nephrotic syndrome taking steroids for 6 years presented with a limp gait and of limitation of abduction and internal rotation. He most probably has *[AIIMS PGMEE 2001]*
a. Renal osteodystrophy b. Avascular necrosis of hip
c. Septic arthritis d. Osteomyelitis of hip joint

94. Which of the following is a Persistent biochemical marker of rickets? *[All India PGMEE 1998]*
a. S.Ca^{++} b. S. Alkaline phosphate
c. S. Acid phosphate d. S. phosphate

95. The crucial component of the club foot deformity is *[TN PGMEE 1990]*
a. Contracture of Tendoachilles
b. Under development of calf and personeal muscles
c. Subluxation of the talo-navicular joint
d. Lateral derangement of tarsal bones

96. Rocker-bottom foot is seen in all except *[Recent Question 2016, PGI 2008]*
a. Arthrogryposis
b. Congenital vertical talus
c. Improper correction of CTEV
d. Overcorrection of CTEV
e. Excessive correction of Grice procedure

97. Pseudo fracture is seen in *[Orissa PGMEE 1992]*
a. Pseudo parathyroidism b. Hypoparathyroidism
c. Osteomalacia d. Osteoprosis

98. Which is true about Osteomalacia? *[PGI 1995]*
a. Alkaline phosphatase is raised
b. Serum phosphate is low
c. Serum calcium is low or normal
d. All the above

99. Trident hand is seen in *[AIIMS PGMEE 1998]*
a. Mucopolysachharidosis b. Achondroplasia
c. Diaphyseal achalasia d. Cleidocranial dysostosis

100. Absent clavicle is seen in *[AIIMS PGMEE 1990]*
a. Oliver's disease b. Achondroplasia
c. Cleidocranial dysostosis d. Moriquo's disease

101. Ideal treatment of bilateral idiopathic clubfoot in a newborn is *[All India PGMEE 2006]*
a. Manipulation by mother
b. Manipulation and Dennis Brown splint
c. Manipulation and casts
d. Surgical release

102. Treatment of clubfoot in newborn is *[BHU PGMEE 1987, AIIMS PGMEE 1993, 1995, AP PGMEE 1993]*
a. Manipulation and corrective splint
b. Corrective splint
c. Nothing to be done for 6 months
d. Surgical

103. Increased alkaline phosphate in seen in *[All India PGMEE 1999]*
a. Multiple myeloma
b. Primary hyperparathyroidism
c. Chronic renal failure d. Osteoporosis

104. During a routine check up, a 67-year-old man is found to have a level of serum alkaline phosphatase three times the upper limit of normal. Serum calcium and phosphorus concentrations and liver function test results are normal. He is asymptomatic. The most likely diagnosis is *[AIIMS PGMEE 1999]*
a. Metastatic bone disease
b. Primary hyperparathyroidism
c. Paget's disease of bone d. Osteomalacia

105. Early CTEV is treated by *[UP PGMEE 1999]*
a. CTEV cast from 1st postnatal day
b. Manipulation
c. Manipulation & Strapping
d. Operative repair as early as possible

106. Osteogenesis imperfecta is due to *[MANIPAL PGMEE 1999]*
a. Defective mineralisation of bone
b. Defective collagen c. Excessive osteoid formation
d. Fracture mobilization of calcium from bone

107. Multiple fractures in newborns is found in *[DPG 1998, 1999]*
a. Syphilis b. Scurvy
c. Morquio's syndrome d. Osteogenesis imperfecta

108. A 65-year-old female presented with fracture of T12 vertebra with increased alkaline phosphatase and parathormone level along with low calcium and low phosphate level, diagnosis is *[AIIMS PGMEE 1999]*
a. Osteoporosis
b. Paget's disease
c. Primary hyperparathyroidism
d. Vitamin D deficiency

109. A young patient presents with enlargement of costochondral junction and with the white line of Fraenkel at the metaphysis. The diagnosis is *[Karnataka PGMEE 2000]*
a. Scurvy b. Rickets
c. Hyperparathyroidism d. Osteo malacia

110. CTEV is caused by *[PGI 2001]*
a. Idiopathic b. Cubitus varus
c. Arthrogryposis multiplexa
d. Spina bifida e. Neurological disorders

111. True about Paget's disease of bone is/ are *[PGI 2009]*
a. Increased alkaline phosphatase
b. More common among females
c. Mostly adolescent girls 10–16 years are affected
d. Associated with chondrosarcoma
e. Associated with hypercalcemia and hypophosphatemia

112. Seen in Osteoporosis *[AIIMS 2000]*
a. Low calcium, High phosphate, High alkaline phosphate
b. Low calcium, Low phosphate, Normal alkaline phosphate
c. Low calcium, Low phosphate, Low alkaline phosphate
d. Normal calcium, Normal phosphate, Normal alkaline phosphate

113. Ring sign is seen in *[NIMHANS PGMEE 1999]*
a. Rickets b. Barlow's disease
c. Scurvy d. Fibrous dysplasia

114. Which is/ are X-ray finding of infantile scurvy? *[JIPMER PGMEE 1997]*
a. A dense line between metaphysis and epiphysial cartilage
b. A clear band of rarefaction on the diaphysial side
c. Both of these
d. None of these

115. Metaphyseal fracture is commonly seen in *[Delhi PGMEE 1992]*
a. Osteogenesis imperfecta b. Scurvy
c. Rickets d. None

116. Soft tissue calcification occurs in all except *[Kerala PGMEE 1995]*
a. Hyper parathyroidism
b. Scleroderma
c. Hyperthyroidism
d. Hyper Vitaminosis D

117. Osteitis fibrosa cystica is due to *[JIPMER PGMEE 1995]*
a. Paget's disease of bone b. Polyostotic fibrous dysplasia
c. Parathyroid adenoma d. All of the above

118. True about osteoporosis *[PGI 2007]*
a. Codfish vertebra seen
b. It decreases with increase in age
c. Is always associated with hormonal anomalies
d. Due to dietary deficiency of calcium
e. Commonly presents with fracture

119. Treatment of club foot should begin *[PGI 1990, JIPMER PGMEE 1995, UPSC 1993, Karnataka PGMEE 1995]*
a. As soon as possible after birth
b. 1 month after birth
c. 1 year after birth d. None of the above

120. In correction of clubfoot by manipulation, which deformity should be corrected first? *[AMU PGMEE 1995]*
a. Forefoot adduction b. Varus
c. Upper end tibia d. Calcaneum

121. Child 3½ years is treated for CTEV by *[TN PGMEE 1997]*
a. Triple arthrodesis
b. Postero medial soft tissue release
c. Lateral wedge resection
d. Tendo Achilles lengthening and posterior capsulatomy

122. Treatment for chronic cases of club foot is *[JIPMER PGMEE 1995]*
a. Triple arthrodesis
b. Dorso medial release
c. Amputation
d. None

123. Osteoporosis is seen in all of the following except *[All India PGMEE 1994]*
a. Hypoparathyroidism b. Steroid therapy
c. Thyrotoxicosis d. Rheumatoid arthritis

124. Spinal shock is associated with *[AIIMS PGMEE 1990]*
a. Increased spinal reflexes b. Absent spinal reflexes
c. Loss of autonomic reflexes
d. Bizarre reflexes

125. Most common cause of primary hyperparathyroidism is *[All India PGMEE 1997]*
a. Solitary adenoma b. Chief cell hyperplasia
c. Multiple adenoma d. Werner's syndrome

126. Which is not a feature of Osteitis fibrosa cystica? *[AP PGMEE 1989]*
a. Fracture b. Tetany
c. Increased srum calcium
d. Increased alkaline phosphatase

127. Sub-Periosteal erosions of middle phalanges at the radial aspect in characteristic of *[AP PGMEE 1993]*
a. Hypothyroidism b. Hyperthyroidism
c. Hypoparathyroidism d. Hyperparathyroidism

128. In spinal shock *[NIMHANS PGMEE 1999]*
a. Knee jerk is the first reflex to return
b. High thoracic lesions are commonly associated with more severely associated with more severe neurological deficits
c. Failure of return offord activity within 48 hours in a very poor prognostic sign
d. Both B & C

129. True about CTEV is *[JIPMER PGMEE 1999]*
a. Bilateral b. Associated with Spina bifida
c. Bones normal in thickness
d. All of the above

130. Osteoporosis is characterized most commonly by *[All India PGMEE 1999]*
a. Fracture vertebra b. Abdominal pain
c. Bowing of legs d. Backache

131. All of the following fractures are associated with Osteoporosis except *[MANIPAL PGMEE 1999]*
a. Vertebral fracture b. Colles fracture
c. Fracture neck of femur d. Fracture of clavicle

132. Club foot seen in a 15 year old could be treated successfully by a *[Recent Question 2017, PGI 1978, 1983]*
a. Appropriate footwear b. Soft tissue operation
c. Triple arthrodesis d. Quadrple fusion

133. 'Pseudoarthrosis' in Triple fusion is seen at the joint of *[Delhi PGMEE1990]*
a. Calcaneocuboid b. Calcaneonavicular
c. Naviculocuboid d. Talonavicular

134. Subperiosteal erosion is seen in *[NBE DNB 1994]*
a. Scurvy b. Hyperparathyroidism
c. Hypoparathyroidism d. Rickets

135. In hyperparathyroidism bone resorption is seen in all except *[Orissa PGMEE 1991]*
a. Jaws b. Metacarpals
c. Ribs d. End of long bones

136. Soft tissue calcification with hypercalcemia is observed in *[Bihar PGMEE 1998]*
a. Hyperparathyroidism b. Alkaptonuria
c. Gout d. Cushing's disease

137. Tufting of the terminal phalanges is seen in *[All India PGMEE 1995]*
a. Hypoparathyroidism b. Hyperparathyroidism
c. Hyperthyroidism d. Hypothyroidism

138. Resorption of the terminal phalanx is not seen in *[Kerala PGMEE 1998]*
a. Hyperparathyroidism b. Reiter's syndrome
c. Scleroderma d. Psoriasis

139. Drug of choice for senile osteoporosis is *[JIPMER PGMEE 1990]*
a. Androgens b. Estrogens
c. Etidronate d. Calcitonin

140. Treatment of postmenopausal osteoporosis *[PGI 2006]*
a. Alendronate
b. Progesterone
c. Estrogen
d. Tamoxifen
e. Calcitonin

141. The characteristic triad of Klippel-Feil syndrome includes all of the following, Except *[All India PGMEE 2010]*
a. Short neck
b. Low hair line
c. Limited neck movements
d. Elevated scapula

142. Sprengel's deformity of scapula *[AIIMS PGMEE 1980, 1984, UP PGMEE 2000, TN PGMEE 2002]*
a. Undescended/ Elevated scapula
b. Undescended neck of scapula
c. Exostosis scapula
d. None of the above

143. Which is true of bones in scurvy? *[AIIMS PGMEE 2010]*
a. Decreased mineralisation of bone
b. Reduced formation of osteoid matrix
c. Loss of calcium from mineralised matrix
d. Normal X-rays

144. Which is not a deep heat therapy? *[AIIMS PGMEE 2007]*
a. Short wave diathermy b. Ultrasound therapy
c. Infrared therapy d. Microwave therapy

145. Erosion of ungula tufts in terminal phalanges of hand may be due to *[PGI 1988]*
a. Rheumatoid arthritis b. Gout
c. Hyperparathyroidism d. Psoriasis

146. Brown Tumor is seen in *[AIIMS PGMEE 2009]*
a. Hypothyroidism b. Hyperthyroidism
c. Hypoparathyroidism d. Hyperparathyroidism

147. Sclerotic lesion in the bone is seen in all except *[All India PGMEE 1991, 1993]*
a. Osteitis fibrosa b. Osteopetrosis
c. Melorheostosis d. Caffey's disease

148. Absence of lamina dura in the alveolus occurs in *[TN PGMEE 1991]*
a. Rickets b. Osteomalacia
c. Deficiency of vitamin C d. Hyperparathyroidism

149. Epiphyseal enlargement occurs in *[AIIMS PGMEE 1994]*
a. Paget's disease
b. Sheurmann's disease
c. Epiphyseal dysplasia d. Hemophilia

150. Epiphyseal dysgenesis is a feature of *[AIIMS PGMEE 1993]*
a. Hyperparathyroidism b. Hypoparathyroidism
c. Hypothyroidism d. Hyperthyroidism

151. Sclerosis of bone is seen in all except *[Kerala PGMEE 1994]*
a. Secondaries from prostate
b. Fluorosis
c. Hyperparathyroidism
d. Osteopetrosis

152. All the following are true in infantile torticollis, EXCEPT *[PGI 1997]*
a. It arises before birth
b. There is facial asymmetry
c. Commonest form of wryneck
d. Infarction of sterno-cleidomastoid muscle

153. Which of the following is not true in case of congenital torticollis? *[All India PGMEE 2007]*
a. Seen only in cases of breech vaginal delivery
b. It can disappear spontaneously
c. It is also known as sternomastoid tumour
d. Untreated, neglected cases can result in plagiocephaly

154. Causes of Congenital torticollis include *[PGI 2012]*
a. Prenatal injury
b. Malposition of head in utero
c. Fibroma
d. Ruptured blood supply
e. Fibrotic rupture of SCM

155. Most Common site of osteochondritis dessicans *[AIIMS PGMEE 1998]*
a. Medial part of the lateral femoral condyle
b. Medial part of the medial femoral condyle
c. Lateral part of the medial femoral condyle
d. Lateral part of the lateral femoral condyle

156. Treatment of choice for Paget's disease of the bone is *[All India PGMEE 1995]*
a. Vitamin D
b. Immobilization of the limb
c. Surgical treatment
d. Calcitonin

157. Paget's disease also known as *[PGI 2000]*
a. Osteitis deformans
b. Osteitis fibrosa cystica
c. Osteochondritis
d. Osteomalacia
e. Marble bone disease

158. Kienbock disease is due to avascular necrosis of *[All India PGMEE 2003, NIMSET 2015]*
a. Scaphoid bone b. Femoral neck
c. Lunate bone d. Trapezium bone

159. Osteocondritis is Osgood Schlatter disease affect which bone? *[UP PGMEE 1993]*
a. Tibial tuberosity b. Capitulum's
c. Metatarsal d. Navicular

160. Cause of congenital pseudoarthrosis is *[AP PGMEE 1994]*
a. Intrauterine fracture b. Neurofibromatosis
c. Fibrous dysplasia d. Unknown

161. Musculoskeletal abnormalities in neurofibromatosis is *[UP PGMEE 2001]*
a. Hypertrophy of limb b. Scoliosis
c. Pseudo arthrosis d. All

162. The common features of Neurofibromatosis include all, except *[TN PGMEE 1999]*
a. Optic glioma
b. Dumbbell neurofibroma
c. Scoliosis
d. Periventricular calcifications

163. Congenital pseudo arthrosis is seen in the following *[TN PGMEE1993]*
a. Hip joint b. Femur
c. Radius-ulna d. Tibia-fibula

164. Pseudoarthrosis can be due to all except *[PGI 1993]*
a. Congenital b. Post inflammatory
c. Trauma d. None of the above

165. Chondrocalcinosis is seen in *[AIIMS PGMEE 2002]*
a. Rickets b. Ochronosis
c. Hyperparathyroidism d. Hypervitaminosis D

166. The earliest manifestation of Alkaptonuria is
a. Ankylosis of lumbodorsal spine *[UP PGMEE 2002]*
b. Prostatic calculi
c. Pigmentation of tympanic membrane
d. Ochronotic arthritis

167. Pseudoarthrosis is seen in all of the following except *[All India PGMEE 1998]*
a. Idiopathic b. Fracture
c. Osteomyelitis d. Neurofibromatosis

168. Pseudoarthrosis of tibia is best treated by
a. Internal fixation *[Delhi PGMEE 1996]*
b. Internal fixation and bone grafting
c. Above knee POP cast
d. Below knee POP cast

169. Progression of congenital scoliosis is least likely in which of the following vertebra anomalies?
a. Fully segmented Hemivertebra *[All India PGMEE 2010]*
b. Wedge vertebra
c. Block vertebra
d. Unilateral unsegmented bar with Hemivertebra

170. Causes of a painless limb since infancy includes
a. Congenital dislocation of hip *[TN PGMEE 1992]*
b. Infantile coax vara
c. Poliomyelitis d. All of the above

171. All the following are causes of a painful limb except
a. Slipped femoral epiphysis *[All India PGMEE 1995]*
b. TB of the hip
c. Perthes disease
d. Infantile coxa vara

172. Antalgic hip gait is related to which of the following? *[TN PGMEE 1994]*
a. Waddling gait b. Trendelenberg gait
c. Painful hip gait d. Short leg gait

173. Paget's disease of bone commonly affects *[PGI 2000, 2001, 2006]*
a. Skull b. Vertebra
c. Pelvis d. Femur
e. Humerus

174. Pain in Pagets disease is relieved best by *[AIIMS PGMEE 1986]*
a. Simple analgesics b. Narcotic analgesics
c. Radiation d. Calcitonin

175. The complications of Paget's disease is *[AIIMS PGMEE 1987]*
a. Osteogenic sarcoma b. Deafness
c. Heart failure d. All of the above

176. Congenital Coxa vara is treated by *[PGI 2004]*
a. Fixation by SP Nail
b. Osteotomy c. Bone grafting
d. Traction e. Splint

177. Coxa vara is found in *[PGI 1986]*
a. Perthe's disease
b. Tuberculosis
c. Rickets
d. Rheumatoid arthritis

178. X-ray of a young man shows heterotopic calcification around bilateral knee joints. Next investigation would be
a. Serum phosphate *[AIIMS PGMEE 2007]*
b. Serum calcium
c. Serum PTH
d. Serum Alkaline phosphatase

179. The best treatment for Dupuytren's contracture is
a. Fasciotomy *[AP PGMEE 1994]*
b. Fasciectomy
c. Incision and release
d. Fasciectomy + Skin transplantation

180. Risser Localiser cast is used in the management of *[AIIMS PGMEE 2008]*
a. Kyphosis b. Spondylolysthesis
c. Idiopathic scoliosis d. Lordosis

181. Bone dysplasia is due to *[Bihar PGMEE 1998]*
a. Faulty nutrition b. Faulty development
c. Trauma d. Parathyroid tumour

182. Following is false of Achondroplasia *[JIPMER PGMEE 1991]*
a. Autosomal dominant b. Mental retardation
c. Due to gene mutation d. Shortening of limbs present

183. Mode of inheritance for Achondroplasia is *[PGI 1996]*
a. Autosomal dominant b. Autosomal recessive
c. X-linked dominant d. X-linked recessive

184. True about Osteomyelitis is/ are *[PGI 2009]*
a. Sequestrum is piece of deal bone
b. Involucrum is dense sclerotic bone overlying a sequestrum
c. Epiphysis most commonly involved region of bone
d. In sickle cell anemia, Salmonella is causative organism
e. Staphylococcus aureus is most common cause

185. Complications of acute osteomyelitis *[PGI 2005]*
a. Fracture of the affected bone
b. Malignancy
c. Chronic osteomyelitis
d. Sepsis
e. Chronicity

186. Acute Hematogenous Osteomyelitis is treated with
a. Antibiotics b. Splinting *[PGI 1998]*
c. Analgesics d. Surgery
e. Antihistaminics

187. True about HIV, Osteomyelitis is all EXCEPT
a. Necrosis absent *[AIIMS PGMEE 1997]*
b. Often bilateral
c. Periosteal new bone formation
d. Most common cause is staph aureus

188. When osteomyelitis disseminates by Hematogenous way the most affected part of bone is *[JIPMER PGMEE 1995, AP PGMEE 1997]*

a. Metaphyses b. Epiphyses
c. Diaphyses d. Any of the above

189. Chronic osteomyelitis is diagnosed mainly by *[Manipal PGMEE 1997]*

a. Sequestrum b. Bone fracture
c. Deformity d. Brodie's abscess

190. Pain & tenderness over the lateral condyle of humerus with a painful dorsi flexion of the wrist is indicative of *[AIIMS PGMEE 2005]*

a. Golfer's Elbow b. Tennis Elbow
c. Pitcher's Elbow d. Cricket Elbow

191. A 40 year-old man was repairing his wooden shed on Sunday morning. By afternoon, he felt that the hammer was becoming heavier and heavier. He felt pain in lateral side of elbow and also found that squeezing water out of sponge hurt his elbow. Which of the muscles are most likely involved? *[AIIMS PGMEE 2002]*

a. Biceps brachii and supinator
b. Flexor digitorum superficialis
c. Extensor carpi radialis longus and brevis
d. Triceps brachii and anconeous

192. About Sequestrum not true is *[PGI 1998]*

a. Infection nidus
b. Lighter than live bone
c. Dead piece of bone
d. Heavier than live bone & trabeculated

193. Involucrum means *[Manipal PGMEE 1998]*

a. Fragment of dead bone
b. Hole formed in the bone during the formation of a draining sinus
c. Osteomyelitis of spine
d. Periosteal new bone formation around necrotic sequestrum

194. A short statured patient brought to Orthopaedics OPD with a X ray showing flattened vertebra with beak. The probable diagnosis is *[NIMS PGMEE 2000]*

a. Achondroplasia b. Ochronosis
c. Eosinophilic granuloma d. Calve's disease

195. The features of Achondroplasia include all, except *[UP PGMEE 2002]*

a. Defective head b. Mental retardation
c. Autosomal recessive d. Familial

196. Absent lateral 1/3rd of clavicle is seen in *[PGI 2002]*

a. Hyperparathyroidism b. Turner's syndrome
c. Fibrous dysplasia d. Cleidocranial dysostosis

197. Cleidocranial dysostosis may show *[AMU PGMEE 1987, PGI 1981]*

a. Wide foramen magnum b. Absence of clavicles
c. Coax vara d. All of the above

198. Involucrum is found *[AP PGMEE 1997]*

a. Underneath the sequestrum
b. Around the sequestrum
c. At metaphysis
d. Beneath the periosteum

199. Non-healing sinus is a common clinical feature is chronic osteomyelitis. The most common frequent cause for this presentation is *[Karnataka PGMEE1988]*

a. Resistant organisms b. Retained foreign body
c. Presence of sequestrum d. Intraosseous cavities

200. All are associated with chronic osteomyelitis except *[All India PGMEE1999]*

a. Amyloidosis b. Sequestrum
c. Metastatic abnormality d. Myositis ossificans

201. Which of the following terms is inappropriate to the condition of Osteomyelitis? *[AMU PGMEE 1989]*

a. Cloacae b. Involucrum
c. Sequestrum d. Myelocoele

202. When does the lesion of Osteomyelitis appear on X-ray *[Delhi PGMEE 1990]*

a. 2 hours b. 24 hours
c. 1 week d. 2 week

203. True regarding acute osteomyelitis in a child *[PGI 2002]*

a. Diagnosis by X-ray is 8–10 days after onset
b. There is diffuse tenderness at the site
c. Antibiotic therapy should be at least for 4 weeks
d. Salmonella is the most common cause

204. A 9-year old child with high arched palate has shoulders meeting in front of his chest. He has *[NBE DNB 2009]*

a. Erb's palsy b. Cleidocranial dysostosis
c. Chondro-Osteodystrophy d. Cortical hyperostosis

205. Absent calvicles are seen in *[AIIMS PGMEE 1990]*

a. Cleidocranial dysostosis b. Achondroplasia
c. Moriquo's disease d. Oliver's disease

206. The characteristics of Morquio's disease include *[Kerala PGMEE1989]*

a. Spinal kyphosis
b. Subnormal/normal intelligence
c. Excessive excretion of keratosulphate in urine
d. Dwarfism e. All of the above

207. Osteogenesis imperfecta is due to *[Manipal PGMEE 1999, PGI 1998]*

a. Defective mineralization of bone
b. Fracture mobilization of calcium from bone
c. Abnormal collagen defect
d. Excessive osteoid formation

208. Osteogenesis imperfecta is due to the following *[Tamil Nadu PGMEE 1994]*

a. Excessive Osteoblastic activity
b. Defective Osteoid formation
c. Defective osteoclast function
d. Defective mineralisation of bone

209. Which is false regarding acute Osteomyelitis? *[Kerala PGMEE1989]*

a. Staphylococcus is the usual organism
b. Rest and elevation relieves pain
c. Parenteral antibiotics are given
d. Surgery is the only treatment

210. Ideal treatment for acute Osteomyelitis of long bones is *[UP PGMEE 1993]*

a. Antibiotics only
b. Drilling of bone
c. Decompression
d. Antibiotics and delayed decompression

211. Instillation treatment in Osteomyelitis is *[JIPMER PGMEE 1994]*
a. Continuous suction + continuous drainage
b. Intermittent suction + continuous drainage
c. Continuous suction + intermittent suction
d. Intermittent suction + intermittent drainage

212. Sclerosis of a long bone may suggest *[PGI 1988]*
a. Osteoid osteoma
b. Sclerosing Osteomyelitis
c. Both are correct
d. None of the above

213. Metaphyseal lesion in children include *[PGI 1991]*
a. Fracture
b. Osteomyelitis
c. Dislocation
d. Ewing's tumour
e. Osteosarcoma

214. Osteogenesis imperfecta *[PGI 1990]*
a. Autosomal dominant [AD)
b. Autosomal Recessive [AR)
c. Both AD and AR
d. Sex linked dominant
e. None of the above

215. Multiple bone fractures are seen in *[AMU PGMEE 1991, Delhi PGMEE 1998]*
a. Rickets
b. Osteomalacia
c. Scurvy
d. Osteogenesis imperfecta

216. What is Brodie's abscess? *[JIPMER PGMEE 1990]*
a. Long standing localized pyogenic abscess in the bone
b. Cold abscess
c. Subperiosteal abscess
d. Soft tissue abscess

217. Treatment of triple deformity is *[AMU PGMEE 1995]*
a. ATT
b. ATT + Immobilisation
c. ATT + Immobilisation + Debridement
d. None

218. An 11-year-old 70 kg child presents with limitation of abduction and internal rotation. There is tenderness in scarpas triangle. On flexing the hip the limb is abducted. The diagnosis is *[PGI 1995, AIIMS PGMEE 2001, JIPMER PGMEE 2002]*
a. Perthes disease
b. Slipped capital femoral epiphyses
c. Observation hip
d. Tuberculosis hip

219. Which the following movement is restricted in congenital dislocation of hip (CDH) in infant? *[JIPMER PGMEE 1993]*
a. Flexions
b. Extension
c. Rotation
d. Full abduction in 90° flexion

220. Wormian bones are not noted in *[AP PGMEE 1993]*
a. Fibrous dysplasia
b. Osteogenesis imperfecta
c. Cretinism
d. Rickets

221. Not true about Osteogenesis imperfecta *[UP PGMEE 2000]*
a. Impaired healing of fracture
b. Deafness
c. Laxity of joints
d. Fragile fracture

222. Following are true about Osteogenesis imperfecta except *[MP PGMEE 1998]*
a. Usually green stick fracture
b. Generally do not unite without treatment
c. Fracture frequency decreases during puberty
d. Fracture seen intrauterine life and during parturition

223. All are seen in osteogenesis imperfecta except *[All India PGMEE 1998]*
a. Blue sclera
b. Bilateral Hip dislocation
c. Lax ligament
d. Osteoporosis

224. Which of the following test is useful in diagnosis of cogenital dislocation of hip? *[PGI 1999]*
a. Barlow's test
b. Thomas test
c. Hibb's test
d. Laguerres test

225. Not true about Osteogenesis imperfecta is *[UP PGMEE 2000, AIIMS PGMEE 1997, TN PGMEE 1998]*
a. Deafness
b. Fractures
c. Cataract
d. Blue Sclera

226. Osteogenesis imperfecta is characterized by *[PGI 2003] [PGI 2004]*
a. Blue sclera
b. Also known as brittle bone disease
c. Collagen defect
d. Otosclerosis
e. Autosomal dominant

227. False about Marfan's syndrome *[PGI November 2014]*
a. Autosomal recessive
b. Scoliosis
c. Ectopia lentis
d. Short limbs
e. Archanodactyly

228. True about Osteogenesis imperfecta *[PGI November 2014]*
a. White sclera
b. Fractures rare
c. Defective collagen synthesis
d. Autosomal dominant
e. Laxity of joints

229. A 45-years-old female presents with lytic lesions in bone and clavicular fracture. She has resorption of phalanges. Most likely diagnosis is *[AIIMS November 2014]*
a. Osteomalacia
b. Hyperthyroidism
c. Hyperparathyroidism
d. Renal osteodystrophy

230. Brown tumor of bone is seen in *[ESI IMO 2014]*
a. Hyperparathyroidism
b. Hypoparathyroidism
c. Hypothyroidism
d. Hyperthyroidism

231. Following is seen in Osteoporosis *[AIIMS PG May 2015]*
a. Normal Calcium, Decreased ALP
b. Decreased Calcium, Increased ALP
c. Normal Calcium, Normal ALP
d. Decreased Calcium, Decreased ALP

232. Diaphyseal aclasis is aetiologically *[PGMCET 2015]*
a. Congenital
b. Developmental
c. Metabolic
d. Inflammatory

233. Brodie's abscess is a terminology for *[PGMCET 2015]*
a. Subungual infection
b. Chronic osteomyelitis
c. Web space infection
d. Infected hematoma

234. Not a feature of Osteopoikilosis *[NIMSET 2015]*
a. Sclerotic bone islands
b. Involves Epiphysis and Metaphysis
c. X-linked inheritance
d. Autosomal dominant inheritance

235. Haglund deformity is seen in _____ joints *[AIIMS May 2017]*
a. Knee
b. Wrist
c. Elbow
d. Ankle

236. Sprengel's deformity is associated with all except *[AIIMS November 2017]*
a. Klippel Feil syndrome
b. Diastematomyelia
c. Dextrocardia
d. Congenital scoliosis

237. A six-year-old boy presents with short neck, low hairline and restriction of neck movements. The child also has Sprengel anomaly, scoliosis, and fused cervical vertebrae. The most likely diagnosis is *[UPSC CMS 2017]*
a. Atlantoaxial instability
b. Klippel Feil syndrome
c. Noonan syndrome
d. Sandifer syndrome

 NEET/NBE PATTERN MCQs ANSWERS WITH EXPLANATIONS 

1. Ans (a) Metaphysis
[Ref. Maheshwari, 4/e p162]

Acute Hematogenous Osteomyelitis in Children

- Age distribution is Bimodal, generally affecting children younger than age 2 years and 8-12 years
- Metaphysis has relatively fewer phagocytic cells than Physis or Diaphysis, allowing infection to occur more easily in this area
- **Hip joint is MC affected in young patients** (Physes proximal humerus, radial neck, and distal fibula may also be affected)
- MC bones affected: Tibia, Femur
- MC organism: Staphylococcus aureus

2. Ans. (c) Pagets Disease
[Ref. Rheumatology by O'Neill, 1/e p254]

- **Blastic (Late inactive) phase of Paget's disease** manifests as Osteosclerosis and presents predominantly sclerotic changes and bony enlargement

3. Ans. (d) MRI is not a good confirmatory investigation
[Ref. Paediatric Emergency Medicine by Cameron, 1/e p618

- Magnetic resonance imaging (MRI) is excellent for detailed delineation of soft- tissue and bony pathology in Perthes' disease, especially when surgery is planned

4. Ans. (a) Increased serum PTH and Hypercalcemia
[Ref. Endocrinology and Metabolism by Becker, 3/ep957]

- Typically, Primary hyperparathyroidism is confirmed with an elevated serum calcium and PTH level

5. Ans. (c) 6 weeks
[Ref. Infectious Diseases by Mainous III, 2/e p321]

- Optimal duration of therapy in osteomyelitis is unknown
- Many experts advocate a total duration of 4–6 weeks

6. Ans. (c) Pelvis
[Ref. Diagnostic Imaging by Bennett, 2/e p171]

Loosers zones/Pseudofractures Sites

- Ribs
- Lateral scapula
- Clavicles
- Pubic rami
- Radius/ Ulna
- Medial femoral cortices

7. Ans. (d) Vitamin K
[Ref. Maheshwari, 4/e p299-300]

Treatment of Osteoporosis

[Mnemonic: $A^2BC^2D^2E^2F$]

- **A**ndrogens
- **A**lendronate
- **B**races
- **C**alcitonin
- **C**alcium supplementation
- Vitamin **D** (along with Vitamin K – as a cofactor for carboxylase activity, vitamin K can facilitate the conversion of glutamyl to gamma-carboxyglutamyl residues and influence the synthesis and excretion of gamma-carboxylation of osteocalcin to increase the formation of bone)
- High protein **D**iet
- **E**strogens
- **E**xercises
- **F**luoride

8. Ans. (a) Osteomyelitis of skull bone
[Ref. Outpatient Medicine by Francis, 1/e p80]

- *Pott's puffy tumor: A* circumscribed area of edema surrounding areas of *osteomyelitis* of the *skull*

9. Ans. (d) Frankel's line
[Ref. Maheshwari, 4/e p300-301]

Features of Rickets

- Bossing of skull
- Broadening of wrists and knees
- Craniotabes
- Delayed teeth eruption
- Deformities
- Harrison's sulcus
- Pigeon chest
- Rachitic rosary
- Muscular hypotonia
- Radiological features:
  - Delayed appearance of epiphysis
  - Widening of epiphyseal plates
  - Cupping of metaphysis

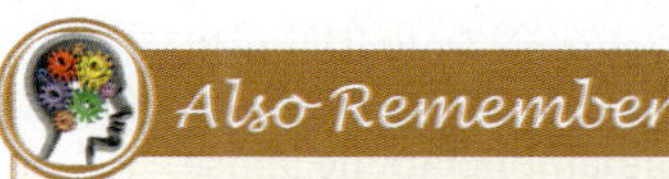

- *Frankel's line*: Increased opacity of distal epiphysis (between epiphysis and metaphysis) seen in Scurvy

10. Ans. (a) Defect in matrix mineralization
[Ref. Maheshwari, 4/e p303]

- **Rickets**: Defective bone matrix mineralization of newly formed bone and growth plate cartilage seen in children
- **Osteomalacia**: Defective bone matrix mineralization at the sites of bone remodeling seen in both children and adults

11. Ans. (a) Staphylococcus aureus
[Ref. Maheshwari, 4/e p300-301]

- *Organisms causing Acute Hematogenous Osteomyelitis*:
  - **Staphylococcus aureus (Most common)**
  - Streptococcus
  - Pneumococcus
- *Sites of Acute Hematogenous Osteomyelitis (Most common in Metaphyses)*:
  - **Lower femoral metaphysic (Most common)**
  - Upper tibial metaphysis
  - Upper femoral metaphysis
  - Upper humeral metaphysis

12. Ans. (b) 4–5 kg
[Ref. Orthopedics by Bentley, Part 1 p78]

13. Ans. (b) Radial aspect of the middle phalanges
[Ref. Imaging of Arthritis and Metabolic Bone Disease by Weismann, 1/e p643]
- Earliest occurrence of *subperiosteal resorption* occurs along the *radial aspect of middle phalanges* of index and middle fingers

Also Remember

- *Tendency for easy fractures*:
  - Osteogenesis imperfecta
  - Osteoporosis
  - Osteopetrosis
  - Osteomalacia
  - Poliomyelitis limb

14. Ans. (c) Osteogenesis imperfecta
[Ref. Maheshwari, 4/e p300-301]

Osteogenesis Imperfecta (Fragilitas Ossium)
- Tendency for frequent fractures due to *'defective collagen synthesis'*
- Usually an Autosomal dominant disorder
- Associated features: Blue sclera, Otosclerosis, Joint laxity

15. Ans. (b) Myasthenia gravis
[Ref. Clinical Anesthesia by Barash, 6/e]

16. Ans. (c) Osteomyelitis of skull bone
[Ref. Journal of Craniofacial Surgery, 2008; Pg 1694-1697]

Pott's Puffy Tumour
- PPF is osteomyelitis of: Frontal bone
- Characteristic feature: Periosteal abscess
- Cause of PPF:
  - Complication of acute/chronic frontal sinusitis
  - Trauma
  - Intranasal cocaine/ methamphetamine abuse
- Diagnostic test: CT scan
- Surgical treatment: Endoscopic frontal sinusotomy/ Frontal sinus trephining

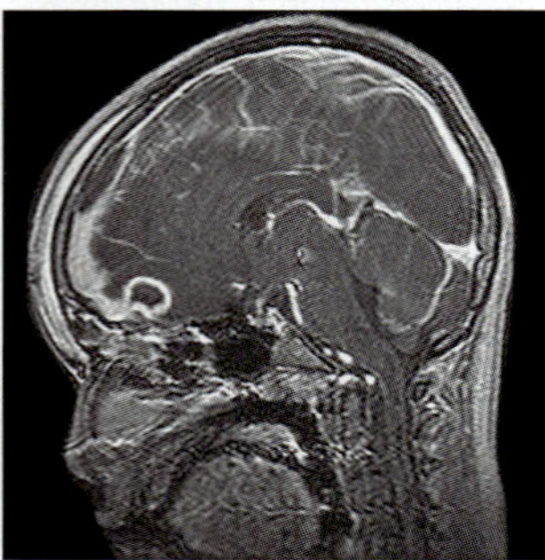

Fig. Pott's puffy tumor

17. Ans. (a) Integrity of Palmar arch
[Ref. Vascular Diseases by White, 1/e p310]

18. Ans. (a) Bilateral DOH
[Ref. Maheshwari, 4/e p214]

Clinical Presentation of Congenital Dislocation of Hip
- Peculiar gait on walking:
  - Trendenleburg's gait: Lurching on affected side in unilateral dislocation
  - Waddling gait: Alternate lurching on both sides in bilateral dislocation
- Limited abduction of hip, asymmetrical thigh folds, lordosis of lumbar spine
- Galeazzi's sign: Lowered knee while lying down with hips flexed to 70° and knees flexed
- Ortolani's test, Trendelenburg' stest and Telescopy positive

19. Ans. (c) Rickets
[Ref. Maheshwari, 4/e p300-301]

20. Ans. (d) All of the above
[Ref. Internal Medicine Board Review by Ghosh, 9/e p900]
- **Calcium Pyrophosphate deposition (CPPD)**: Hypothyroidism, Primary hyperparathyroidism, Hemochromatosis, Hemosiderosis, Gout, Hypomagnesia, Hypophosphatasia, Wilson's disease, Ochronosis

21. Ans. (c) Quadriceps femoris
[Ref. Maheshwari, 4/e p220]

Features in a Poliomyelitis Case

Early stage of poliomyelitis	
Paralysis	Asymmetric flaccid (lower limbs)
Most common muscle affected	**Quadriceps femoris**
Most common muscle with complete paralysis	Tibialis anterior
Most common muscle affected in hand	**Opponens pollicis**
Sensory loss	Absent
Bulbo-spinal polio	Motor neurons of medulla affected
Late stage of poliomyelitis	
Deformity at hip	Flexion, abduction, external rotation
Deformity at knee	*'Triple deformity*'*
Deformity of foot (Most common)	Equinovarus

*(*Flexion, posterior subluxation, external rotation)*

22. Ans. (c) Cluttons' joints
[Ref. Maheshwari, 4/e p172]

Cluttons' Joints
- Seen in: Late congenital syphilis
- Characteristic feature: Painless synovitis at puberty
- **Most commonly affects: Knee (bilateral)**

Also Remember

- ***Hill Sach's lesion***: Depression on humerus head (posterolateral quadrant) seen in anterior dislocation of shoulder
- ***Charcot's joint***: Neuropathic arthropathy seen in Daibetes mellitus (most common) and acquired syphilis
- ***Morquio's disease***: Autosomal recessive lysosomal storage disorder (X-ray: Tonguing of lumbar vertebrae)

23. Ans. (b) Congenital coxa vara
[Ref. Concise System of Orthopedics and Trauma by Solomon, 4/e p253]

- **Fairbank's triangle**: Physeal line is too vertical; typically, in the infant, there is a separate triangular fragment of bone in the inferior portion of the metaphysis in Congenital coxa vara

24. Ans. (c) Marfan's syndrome
[Ref. Maheshwari, 4/e p310]

Archnodactyly

- *Definition*: Elongated and slender tubular bones of hands and feet *('Spider fingers')*
- *Measured by*: **Metacarpal Index**
  - Normal metacarpal index: 5.4–7.9
  - **Arachnodactyly: 8.4–10.4**
- *Arachnodactyly is seen in*:
  - Marfan's syndrome
  - Homocystinuria
  - Ehlers Danlos syndrome

25. Ans. (d) S1 radiculopathy
[Ref. Pocket EMG by Pohlman, 1/e p36]

26. Ans. (a) Fractures
[Ref. Compartment Syndromes by Styf, 1/e p49]

27. Ans. (b) Turner's syndrome
[Ref. Wheeless Textbook of Orthopaedics, www.wheelessonline.com]

Causes of Atlanto-Axial Subluxation

[**Mnemonic: NOON D**ay **GRASS R**uminates **S**aliva]

- **N**eck trauma (Most common)
- **O**dontoid process aplasia/hypoplasia
- **O**steogeneis imperfecta
- **N**eurofibromatosis
- **D**own's syndrome
- **G**out (Tophaceous)
- **R**heumatoid arthritis
- **A**nkylosing spondylitis
- **S**evere pneumonia
- **S**pinal surgery
- **R**etropharyngeal abscess
- **S**till's disease (Juvenile rheumatoid arthritis)

28. Ans. (a) Chronic osteomyelitis
[Ref. Basic Surgical Training by Raftery, 1/e p2]

29. Ans. (c) Metaphysis
[Ref. Maheshwari, 4/e p162]

Osteomyelitis Begins in Metaphysis

- Venous system of bones begin in metaphysis and drain towards diaphysis
- Vessels in metaphysis are arranged in form of a Hair-pin loop arrangement: Blood stasis allow bacteria to settle and lead to Acute osteomyelitis

30. Ans. (b) Subacute osteomyelitis
[Ref. Imaging of Arthritis and Metabolic Bone Disease by Weisman, 1/e p316]

Brodie's Abscess

- *Description: A* focus of *subacute osteomyelitis* that is usually in metaphysis of a long bone usually tibia or femur
- Radiology: Sharply defined radiolucent lesion with sclerotic margin
- Treatment: Surgical evacuation and Curettage

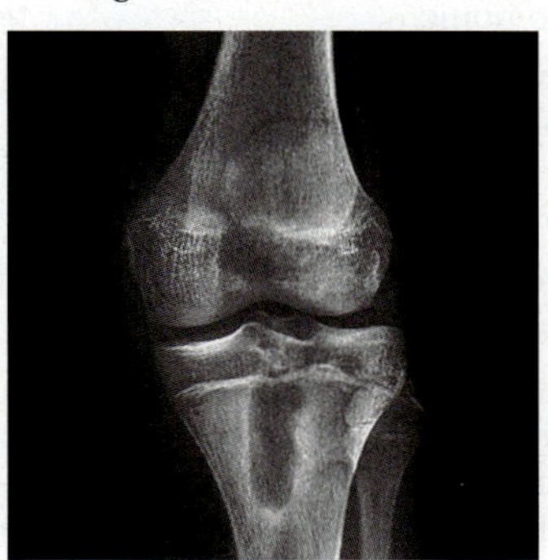

Fig. Brodie abscess

31. Ans. (a) Pseudoarthrosis common
[Ref. SBAs for Final FRCR 2A, 1/e p232]

- **Pseudoarthrosis**: Non-union or False joint is a bone fracture that has no chance of union without intervention

32. Ans. (d) Charcot's joint
[Ref. The Merck Manual]

- ***Bag of bones effect***: Movement of joint produce a grating sound due to bone fragments floating in the joint; seen in Charcot's joint (Neurogenic arthropathy)

33. Ans. (c) Osteopetrosis
[Ref. Maheshwari, 4/e p307]

- **Marble bone disease**: Osteopetrosis/ Albers Schonberg disease is characterized by dense, brittle bones

34. Ans. (b) Hyperparathyroidism
[Ref. Maheshwari, 4/e p303]

- ***Codfish vertebrae***: Exaggerated concavity of upper and lower endplates of vertebrae, as seen in several types of osteopenia
- *Cod-fish vertebrae are seen in*:
  - Osteogenesis imperfecta
  - Osteoporosis
  - Osteomalacia
  - Sickle cell disease
  - Homocystinuria
  - Hyperparathyroidism

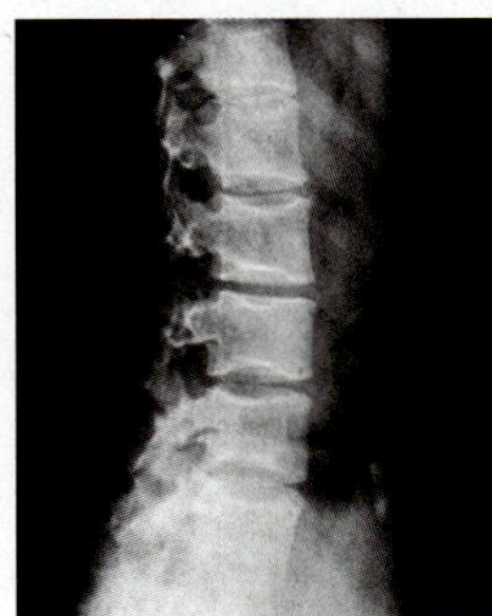

Fig. Codfish vertebrae

35. Ans. (b) Hyperparathyroidism
[Ref. Pathology by Rubin, 5/e p552]

36. Ans. (a) Calcification of disc
[Ref. Clinical Imaging by Eisenberg, 5/e p1208]

- **Ochronosis**: Dense laminated *calcification* of multiple intervertebral *discs* (beginning in the *lumbar spine* and extending to the dorsal and cervical regions) is virtually pathognomonic

37. Ans. (b) Increased bone density
[Ref. Maheshwari, 4/e p60-61]

- In Sudeck's dystrophy there are patchy areas of decreased bone density

38. Ans. (a) Ochronosis
[Ref. Maheshwari, 4/e p286]

Ochronosis (Alcaptonuric Arthritis)

- Underlying cause: Accumulation of homogentisic acid/ hydroquinione in connective tissues
- Clinical features: **Urine darkens on standing,** pigmentation of sclera
- Joints affected: Spine, Shoulder joint
- X-ray findings: Disc space/ periarticular calcification in large joints

39. Ans. (c) Bleeding
[Ref. Maheshwari, 4/e p300-301]

40. Ans. (d) Hypertension
[Ref. Symptoms and Signs of Surgical Disease by Browse, 4/e p140]

41. Ans. (a) Phenytoin
[Ref. Nutrition in prevention and treatment of disease by AM Coulston, 2nd Ed., Pg 821]

- Several anti-epileptic drugs can cause osteomalacia by reducing body's Vitamin-D level and bone density
  - Carbamazepine
  - Primidone
  - Phenobarbital
  - Phenytoin
  - Topiramate
  - Sodium valproate

42. Ans. (a) Cobbs method
[Ref. Anesthesiology by Nag, 1/e p130]

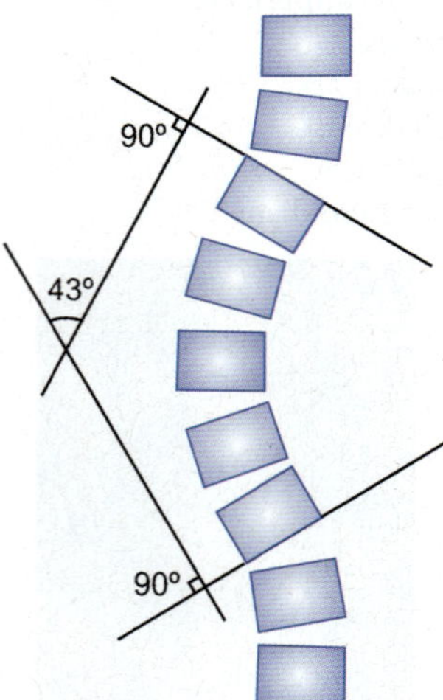

Fig. Cobbs angle

Cobb's Method

- Utility: Identify the degree/ severity of Scoliosis
- Methods used:
  - Lippmann-Cobb method
  - Risser-Ferguson method
- Interpretation of Cobb's angle:
  - Angle >40 degrees: Indication for Surgery
  - Angle >65 degrees: Restrictive lung disease, Dyspnoea on exertion
  - Angle >100 degrees: Respiratory failure, Pulmonary hypertension, Right heart failure

43. Ans. (a) Osteoporosis
[Ref. Maheshwari, 4/e p299]

- ***Biochemical picture of Osteoporosis*:**
  - Normal Serum Calcium, Phosphorus, ALP
  - Low Total plasma proteins, albumin

44. Ans. (c) Aortic aneurysm
[Ref. Imaging Modalities in Spinal Disorders by Kricun, 1/e p87]

Scalloping of Vertebra

Anterior scalloping	Posterior scalloping
• Down' syndrome • Abdominal aortic aneurysm • Chronic leukemia • Lymphoma • Tuberculosis	• Achondroplasia • Astrocytoma • Ependymoma • Spina schwannoma • Paraganglioma • Neurofibromatosis (MC Cause) • Acromegaly • Mucopolysacchridosis • Marfan;s syndrome • Ehler Danlos syndrome • Osteogenesis imperfecta tarda

45. Ans. (c) Gaucher's disease
[Ref. Medcyclopedia]

Bone within a Bone Appearance

[Mnemonic: STOP D GHOST]

- **S**ickle cell disease
- **T**horotrast
- **O**steopetrosis
- **P**aget's disease
- Hypervitaminosis **D**
- **G**aucher's disease
- **H**eavy metal poisoning
- **O**steonecrosis
- **S**arcoidosis
- **T**halassemia

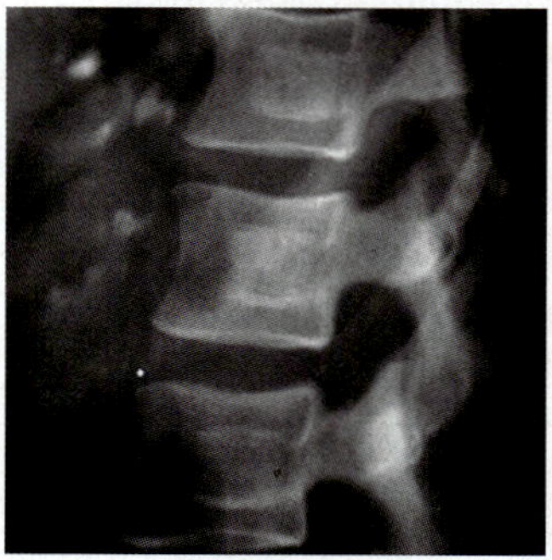

Fig. Bone within bone

46. Ans. (c) Rickets

[Ref. Diet, Nutrients and Bone Health by Anderson, 1/e p435]

- ***Windswept Deformity***: Condition in which a valgus deformity in one knee is associated with a varus deformity in the opposite knee seen in Rickets

47. Ans. (c) Hip Spica

[Ref. Skeletal Trauma in Children by Green, 4/e p113]

- **Cast syndrome/ Superior mesenteric artery syndrome**: Acute gastric dilation and vomiting due to Hip-spica or Body-cast

48. Ans. (a) Gout

[Ref. Wheeless Textbook of Orthopaedics, www.wheelessonline.com]

- Atlantoaxial subluxation is seen in Chronic (tophaceous) gout

49. Ans. (c) 75%

[Ref. Essentials of Plastic Surgery by Jones, 1/e p31]

Z-Plasty

- Description: Transposition flap with two adjacent triangular flaps that are reversed
- Gains in Central limb length:

Angle of Z-Plasty (Degrees)	Increase in Limb length (%)
30 degrees	25%
45 degrees	50%
60 degrees	75%

50. Ans. (a) Vitamin D deficiency

[Ref. Hypoparathyroidism by Brown, 1/e p158]

51. Ans. (b) Charcot's joints

[Ref. Clinical Radiology by Hartman, 4/e p417]

52. Ans. (c) Colchicine

[Ref. Practical Drug Therapy by Richards, 2/e p640]

- **Drugs used in Treatment of Acute Gout**: NSAIDs, Colchicine, Corticosteroids, Corticotropin (ACTH)

53. Ans. (d) 1, 2, 3 and 4

[Ref. Orthopedics by Biswas, 1/e p63]

Radiology in Scurvy

- Pencil-thin cortex
- White line of Frankel
- Zone of Trummerfeld (Zone of rarefaction)
- Pelkan spurs
- Halo sign of Wimberger
- Diaphyseal fracture
- Subperiosteal fractures
- Ground glass translucency of bones

54. Ans. (c) Phosphate

[Ref. Osteoporosis by Rosen, 3/e p1294]

Medical Treatment of Osteoporosis

- High protein diet
- Calcium, Vitamin D, Fluoride, Calcitonin
- Androgens, Estrogens, Sodium chloride
- Commonly used drugs: Alendronate, Risedronate
- Newer drugs: Denosumab, Strontium renalate, Zoledronic acid, Teriparatide

55. Ans. (b) Hyperparathyroidism

[Ref. Maheshwari, 4/e p303]

56. Ans. (b) Osteopetrosis

[Ref. Maheshwari, 4/e p307]

57. Ans. (c) Acromio-clavicular arthritis

[Ref. Ferri's Clinical Advisor 2016, 1/e p1091]

58. Ans. (b) Adolescents

[Ref. Pediatric Emergency Medicine Secrets by Selbst, 3/e p402]

- ***Slipped capital femoral epiphysis*** is the *most common* disorder of the hip in *adolescents, more common in Obese males*

59. Ans. (a) Osteomalacia

[Ref. The Adult Hip by Callaghan, 2/e p522]

- *Looser's zones* are radiolucent areas of bone that are the result of multiple microstress fractures that heal by the formation of *osteomalacic (unmineralized) bone*

60. Ans. (c) Equinus deformity

[Ref. Atlas, Foot and Ankle Surgery by Wulter, 2/e p272]

- If marked *equinus deformity* of the *calcaneus*is present, Achilles tendon lengthening should be performed prior to triple arthrodesis

61. Ans. (a) Ochronosis

[Ref. Maheshwari, 4/e p286]

62. Ans. (c) Marfan's syndrome

[Ref. Maheshwari, 4/e p310]

63. Ans. (d) Early institution of steroids is essential

[Ref. Zoonosis by Krebbs & Weber, 3rd Ed., Pg 18]

Chikungunya Arthritis

- *Differences of Rheumatoid and Chikungunya arthritis*:

	Rheumatoid arthritis	Chikungunya arthritis
Affects	Bones, lungs, heart, skin	Bones, muscles, joints
Steroids treatment	Usually prescribed	Not prescribed

- *Treatment of Chikungunya arthritis*:
  - Usually symptomatic
  - Aspirin and NSAIDs are not useful
  - Steroids are not used
  - Chloroquine phosphate has shown best results

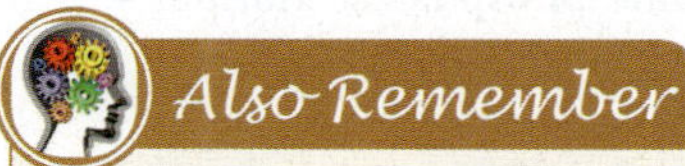

WHO Guidelines for Chikungunya Fever Treatment

- Treatment is entirely symptomatic
- There is no specific antiviral drug
- Paracetamol is the drug of choice
- In acute stage, Steroids are not usually indicated because of the adverse effects
- Aspirin is preferably avoided for fear of side effects like Reye's syndrome.
- Mild forms of exercise and physiotherapy allowed in recovery
- Treatment instituted in all suspect cases without waiting for confirmation
- During an epidemic, do not subject all cases to investigations.
- All suspected cases should be kept under mosquito nets during the febrile period
- Communities should be sensitized about mosquito control measures

64. Ans. (d) Hyperparathyroidism
[Ref. Maheshwari, 4/e p303]

65. Ans. (b) Hip joint
[Ref. Platinum Notes USMLE Step-2 by Hassan, p386]
- *Most common site* of *acute osteomyelitis* in *infants:Hip*
- *Most common site* of *acute osteomyelitis* in *children*: Femur

66. Ans. (b) Raised serum calcium
[Ref. Maheshwari, 4/e p302]

Osteomalacia
- Definition: Softening of bones in adults
- Underlying causes: Inadequate sunlight exposure
- Clinical presentation:
  - Spine fractures/ Kyphosis
  - Muscular weakness
  - Bone pains
- *Serum changes*:
  - Low serum calcium
  - Serum alkaline phosphatase high
- ***X-rays***:
  - **Looser's zones**
  - **Triradiate pelvis**
  - **Protrusion acetabuli**
- *Treatment*:
  - Vitamin D
  - Osteotomies

67. Ans. (d) Escherichia coli
[Ref. Musculoskeletal Imaging by Pope, 2/e p791]
- **Common causes of Osteomyelitis**: Staphylococcus aureus **(Most common cause)**, Group B Streptococcus, Group A Streptococcus, Hemophilus influenza, Pseudomonas, Proteus, Salmonella, Kingella, E. coli (Rare cause)

68. Ans. (c) Phalanges
[Ref. Maheshwari, 4/e p303]

Hyperparathyroidism
- *Clinical presentation*:
  - Bone pain (Most common)
  - Brown's tumor
  - Serum calcium, alkaline phosphatase normal + High ALP
- *X-rays*:
  - Pepper-pot (Salt-pepper) skull
  - Chondrocalcinosis
  - Rugger-Jersey spine
  - Brown's tumor in maxilla/ mandible
  - Subperiosteal resorption of phalanges (Pathognomic feature)

69. Ans. (b) Osteopetrosis
[Ref. Rapid Review of Radiology by Hussain, Abdel and Hall, 1/e p260]

70. Ans. (a) Should be started immediately after birth
[Ref. The Netter's Collection of Medical Illustrations by Parker, 2/e p229]

71. Ans. (b) Long 4th metacarpals and metatarsals
[Ref. Differential Diagnosis in Paediatric Radiology by Ebel & Blickman, 1/e p801]

Turner's Syndrome
- *Underlying abnormality*: Missing one entire X sex chromosome (XO)
- *Clinical presentation*:
  - Short stature (only up to 143–145 cms)
  - Lymphoedema
  - Shield-chest (widely spaced nipples)
  - Sterility, amenorrhoea
  - Obesity
  - Webbed neck
  - Shortened 4th metacarpal
  - Coarctation of aorta
  - Horse-shoe shaped kidney
  - Medial tibial exostosis

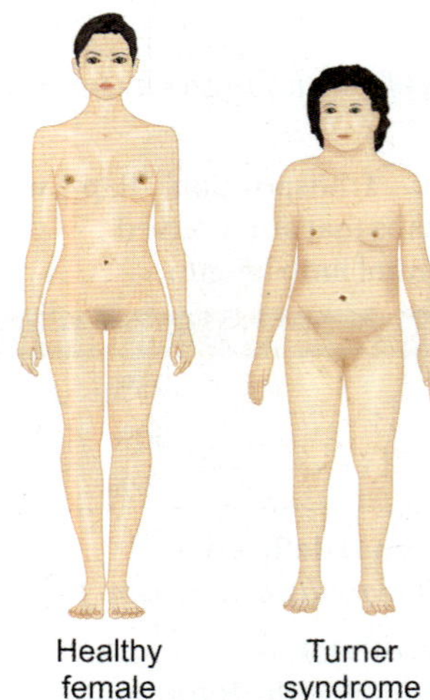

Fig. Turner syndrome

72. Ans. (b) Osteogenesis imperfecta
[Ref. Textbook of Medicine by Souhami & Moxham, 4th Ed., Pg 71]

Collagen Synthesis Disorders

Disorder	Defect
Ehler Danlos Syndrome	Type III collagen synthesis deficiency
Marfan's Syndrome	Defect in fibrillin
Osteogenesis imperfecta	Type I collagen synthesis defect
Cutis laxa	Defect in elastin
Pseudoxanthoma elasticum	Abnormal collagen and elastin

73. Ans. (b) Diabetes mellitus
[Ref. Ferri's Clinical Advisor 2016, 1/e p313]

74. Ans. (b) Increased serum alkaline phosphatase
[Ref. Maheshwari, 4/e p299]

Osteoporosis
- *Definition*: Diffuse reduction in bone density
- *Underlying causes*:
  - Senility (Most common in Males)
  - Menopause (Most common in Females)

- Drug induced (Phenobarbitone/ Steroids)
- Protein deficiency
- Endocrinal causes
- Post-immobilisation

- *Clinical presentation*:
  - Fractures (Dorsolumbar spine: Most common)
  - Kyphosis
  - Serum calcium, phosphate and alkaline phosphatase: Normal
  - Plasma proteins, albumin low
- *X-rays*:
  - Looser's zones (Pseudo-fractures- Hallmark)
  - Cod fish vertebrae
  - Triradiate pelvis

75. Ans. (a) Anterior horn cells
[Ref. Maheshwari, 4/e p219]

76. Ans. (b) Alcaptonuria
[Ref. Practical Orthopedic Examination by Kumar, 2/e p509]

Charlie Chaplin GAIT

- Alkaptonuria
- External rotation deformity of tibia
- Flat feet with Valgus deformity of knee

77. Ans. (c) PK Sethi, RK Sharma
[Ref. Engineering Applications by Striebig, SI/e p663]

78. Ans. (c) Osteogenesis imperfecta
[Ref. Maheshwari, 4/e p306]

Osteogenesis Imperfecta

- Major feature: Multiple fractures due to Osteoporosis, Excessive bone fragility
- Other features: Blue sclera, Lax ligaments, Skeletal deformities, Congenital deafness, Joint laxity, Otosclerosis

79. Ans. (a) Distal muscle weakness
[Ref. HIV infected Patient by Mills, 1/e p158]

Polymyositis

- Description: A condition marked by inflammation and degeneration of skeletal muscle throughout the body
- Characteristic feature: Proximal muscle weakness
- Lab features: Increased CPK, Abnormal EMG
- Pathology: Lymphocytic infiltration of muscles, Degeneration and regeneration of fibres

80. Ans. (c) Osteoporosis
[Ref. Musculoskeletal Imaging by Imhof, 1/e p30]

- **Reflex sympathetic dystrophy** is a painful Acute osteoporosis with Soft-tissue swelling or atrophy

81. Ans. (a) Type I
[Ref. Collagen Disease, 2012 Scholarly Edition p36]

Osteogenesis Imperfecta

- More prevalent autosomal dominant forms are caused by primary defects in Type I collagen
- Autosomal recessive forms are caused by deficiency of proteins which interact with type I procollagen for post-translational medication/ folding

82. Ans. (b) 4-12 years
[Ref. Practical Orthopedic Examination, 3/e p72]

83. Ans. (d) Systemic sclerosis
[Ref. Osteoporosis by Slon, 1/e p6]

Secondary Osteoporosis

- Osteoporosis resulting from a medical condition or the use of certain medications
- Associated conditions include Hemochromatosis, Marfan's syndrome, Systemic mastocytosis, Chronic metabolic acidosis, Hemophilia, Multiple myeloma, Thalassemia, Cushing's syndrome, Homocystinuria, Multiple sclerosis, Thyrotoxicosis, Cystic fibrosis, Hypercalciuria, Muscular dystrophy, Turner's and Klinefelter's, Diabetes

84. Ans. (b) Associated with cataract formation
[Ref. Maheshwari, 4/e p300-301]

Osteogenesis Imperfecta

- Fragilitas Ossium/ Brittle bone disease
- Tendency for frequent fractures due to 'defective collagen synthesis'
- Usually an Autosomal dominant disorder
- Associated features: Blue sclera, Otosclerosis, Joint laxity

85. Ans. (b) Metaphysis
[Ref. Skeletal Radiology by Yochum & Rowe, 3/e p827]

- Metaphysis is the most metabolically active region of a bone and, as a result, is the most common site for tumors and infections of bone
- Endosteum can be considered as the most metabolically active part of a bone
- Trabecular bone is the more metabolically active because it has about 8–10 times more total surface area than a similar mass of cortical bone

86. Ans. (a) Salmonella
[Ref. Rheumatology Secrets by West, 2/e p355]

- Salmonella infections account for 50% of osteomyelitis in Sickle cell disease (2nd MCC is Staphylococcus aureus)
- Probable site of entry for Salmonella: Intestinal wall (Microinfarctions allow the organism to enter the circulation)
- Children with Sickle cell anemia are more prone to Osteomyelitis and Septic arthritis because of multiple factors, namely, functional asplenia, frequent tissue infarctions and failed opsonization

87. Ans. (b) Bursitis
[Ref. Orthopedics by Anderson, 1/e p214]

Bursitis Bunion

- An inflammation of a bursa, a sac containing fluid about the consistency of the white of an egg; this bursa acts as a lubricant between the skin and bones

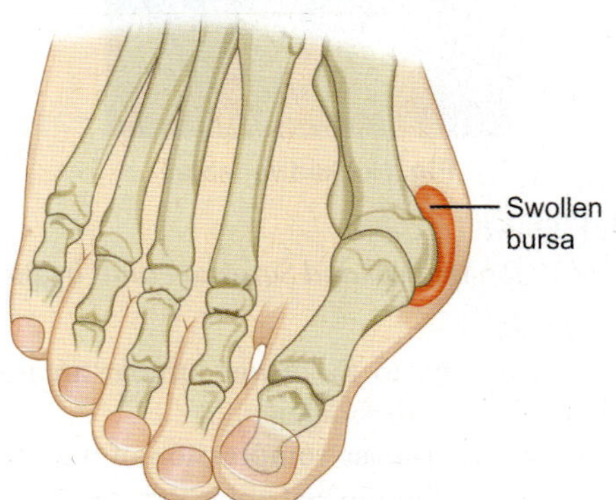

Fig. Bunion

- Continual irritation by external pressure such as an ill-fitting shoe causes the sac to become inflamed, and the condition gets acute and painful (Bursitis)

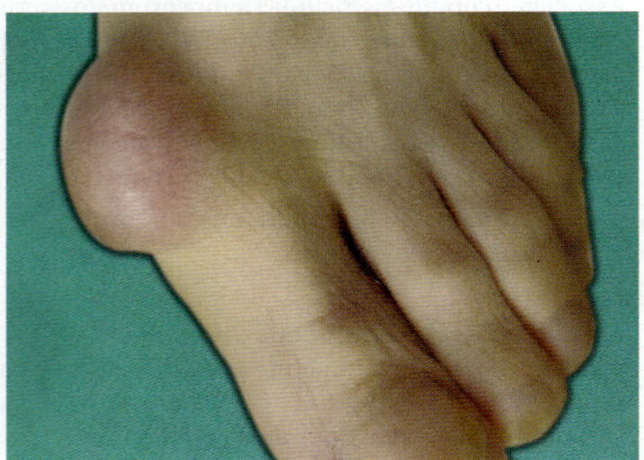

Fig. Bunion

88. Ans. (d) All of the above

[Ref. Skeletal Impact of Disease: Bulletin 33 by Rothschild, p13]

Hooked/ Notched/ Beaked Vertebrae

- Occur maximum in stress area in Thoraco-lumbar junction (T11-L3), suggesting response to Mechanical stimuli: Likely related to exaggeration of normal "physiologic" kyphosis
- **Represent deformity secondary to hyperflexion of the spine**, with or without anterior herniation of the nucleus pulposus
- Seen in Hurler's disease, Congenital hypothyroid, Morquio's disease, Spondyloepiphyseal dysplasia, Osteogenesis imperfecta, Achondroplasia
- Other associations: Mongolism, Phenylketonuria, Niemann Pick disease, Werdnig Hoffman disease, Hypotonia

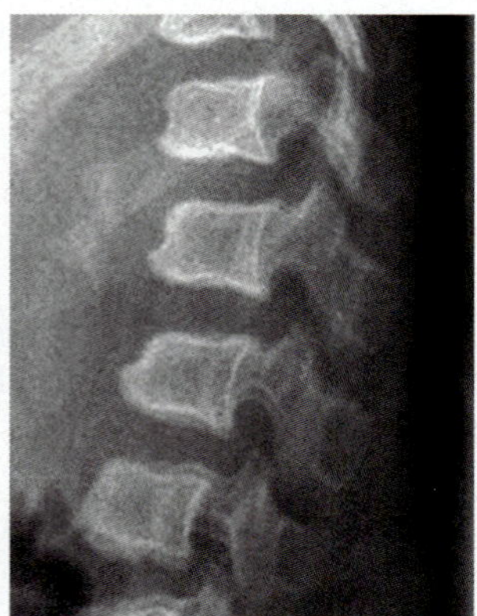

Fig. Hooked vertebrae

89. Ans. (c) L5-S1

[Ref. OSCEs for Medical and Surgical Finals by Bora, 1/e p39]

Disc Prolapse

- Pain is confined to the lower lumbar area and/or may radiate to the buttock or leg
- L5-S1 prolapse causes compression of the S1 root, which may result in a diminished ankle jerk, weakness of plantar flexion, sensory loss against lateral border of foot and sole

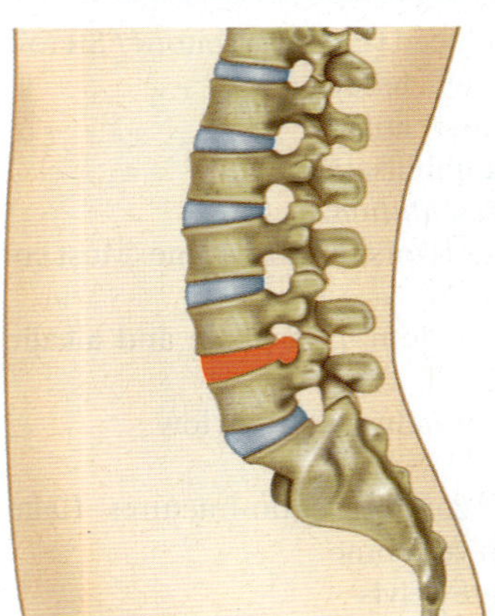

Fig. L5-S1 disc prolapse

90. Ans. (d) All the above

[Ref. Conventional Radiology by Burgener, 2/e p59]

Pseudofractures

- Vitamin D deficiency (Osteomalacia, Rickets), renal osteodystrophy, Paget's disease, Fibrous dysplasia, and Hereditary hyperphosphatasia (Juvenile Paget's disease) or are rarely idiopathic
- Located in the femur (neck and shaft), pubic and ischial ramus, scapula, clavicle, ribs, ulna (proximal shaft), radius (distal shaft), metacarpals, metatarsals, and phalanges

91. Ans. (a) Chronic osteomyelitis

[Ref. Skeletal Trauma by Browner, 4/e p599]

Paprika Sign

- Punctate haversian bleeding (Sign of viable bone)
- Used as a sign of healthy bone and helps establish the limits of debridement; debridement of bone carried down until uniform haversian or cancellous bleeding is visualized
- Sign is not useful during debridement of dense cortical bone or operations where tourniquet is used

92. Ans. (c) Alkaptonuria

[Ref. Rheumatology by Watts, 1/e p516]

Alkaptonuria

- Cause: Deficiency of Homogentisate 1,2-dioxygenase (an enzyme that converts homogentisic acid (HGA) to maleylacetoacetic acid in the tyrosine degradation pathway)
- 3 major features:
  - Oxidation of the HGA excreted in the urine produces a melanin-like product and causes the **urine to turn dark on standing**
  - Ochronosis (bluish-black pigmentation in connective tissue): Occurs only after age 30 years
  - Arthritis of the spine and larger joints: Often begins in the third decade
- Other manifestations: Pigment deposition, aortic or mitral valve calcification or regurgitation and occasionally aortic dilatation, renal stones, and prostate stones

93. Ans. (c) Chronic osteomyelitis

[Ref. Orthopaedic Pathology by Vigorita, 2/e p253]

Chronic Osteomyelitis

- Garré sclerosing osteomyelitis, or Chronic nonsuppurative sclerosing osteomyelitis, is a form of Chronic osteomyelitis
- Mild inflammation and infection lead to Subperiosteal bone deposition
- Disease is frequently asymptomatic.
- Onion skin appearance: Characteristic radiographic appearance is an area of periosteal proliferation surrounded by successive layers of condensed cortical bone

HIGH YIELD MCQs ANSWERS WITH EXPLANATIONS 

1. **Ans. (b) Tuberculosis affection of ulnar bursa**
   [Ref. Essentials of Orthopedics for Physiotherapist by Ebnezar, p239]

   Compound Palmar Ganglion
   - Description: A condition which affects flexor tendons of fingers mainly the ulnar bursa
   - Cause: Usually due to tuberculosis though rheumatoid arthritis may also be a cause
   - Hallmark; Melon seed bodies

2. **Ans. (c) Chondromalacia patellae**
   [Ref. Pediatrics by Paulson, 1/e p253]
   - **In chondromalacia patellae**, there is knee pain that is worse after sitting, climbing stairs, jumping, or squatting
     - There may be patellar instability on examination and there is tenderness of the undersurface of the patella

3. **Ans. (c) Staphylococcus aureus**
   [Ref. Pediatric Nursing by Nicki, 3/e p1313]

4. **Ans. (a) Ortolani sign**
   [Ref. Maheshwari, 4/e p214]

5. **Ans. (c) Abnormal Pro - α chain**
   [Ref. Perinatal Nutrition by Lindblad, 1/e p79]

6. **Ans. (d) Head of femur downwards**
   [Ref. Clinical Methods in Surgery by Bhat, 1/e p773]
   - In Dislocation of hip, head of femur is dislocated upwards and backwards

7. **Ans. (a) Caucasians**
   [Ref. Emergency Medicine Review by Harrigan, 1/e p241]
   - Dislocation of hip is more common in Native Americans and Caucasians, especially females

8. **Ans. (c) Metaphysis**
   [Ref. Maheshwari, 4/e p162]

9. **Ans. (d) All of the above**
   [Ref. Medicinal Chemistry by Williams, 7/e p979]

10. **Ans. (b) Paget's disease of bone**
    [Ref. Maheshwari, 4/e p307]

11. **Ans. (a) Staphylococcus aureus**
    [Ref. Maheshwari, 4/e p162]

12. **Ans. (a) Osteopetrosis**
    [Ref. Maheshwari, 4/e p307]

13. **Ans. (d) Osteopetrosis**
    [Ref. Maheshwari, 4/e p162]

14. **Ans. (b) Pseudomonas**
    [Ref. A Practical Approach to Infectious Diseases by Chapman, 5/e p129]

    Common Organisms in Osteomyelitis
    - **Hematogenous osteomyelitis: Staphylococcus aureus**
    - **Acute osteomyelitis: Staphylococcus aureus**
    - Osteomyelitis in Children: Group A Streptococci
    - Osteomyelitis in Neonates: Group B Streptococci
    - Osteomyelitis due to Gram negative organisms in Neonates: Enterobacteriaceae
    - Osteomyelitis due to Gram negative organisms in Sickle cell disease: Salmonella
    - Osteomyelitis due to Gram negative organisms in IV Drug users: Pseudomonas
    - **Vertebral osteomyelitis: Mycobacterium tuberculosis**

15. **Ans. (a) Small head of femur; (d) Shallow acetabulum**
    [Ref. Pediatric Orthopedic Deformities by Shapiro, 1/e p181]

16. **Ans. (a) Females are affected more than males**
    [Ref. Bone and Soft Tissue Tumors by Mario, 2/e p733]

17. **Ans. (b) Alkaline phosphates is low**
    [Ref. Maheshwari, 4/e p307]

18. **Ans. (a) Serum alkaline phosphatase is low**
    [Ref. Maheshwari, 4/e p307]

19. **Ans. (b) Abnormally slow rates of fracture healing**
    [Ref. Maheshwari, 4/e p307]
    - Osteopetrosis patients have a tendency for fracture

20. **Ans. (a) Pectoralis major**
    [Ref. USG of Musculoskeletal System by Bianchi, 1/e p285]

21. **Ans. (d) Twin pregnancy is a known risk factor**
    [Ref. Children's Orthopedic and Fractures by Benson, 3/e p437]
    - **Risk factors of Developmental dysplasia of Hip**: Female sex, First born girl child, Affected previous birth, Breech presentation, Oligohydramnios, Older primiparous mother

22. **Ans. (b) Surgery should be done if symptomatic**
    [Ref. Pediatric Secrets by Richard, 6/e]

23. **Ans. ALL CHOICES**
    [Ref. Learning Radiology by Herring, 3/e p231]

    Increased Bone Density
    - Carcinoma prostate
    - Avascular necrosis of bone
    - Paget's disease of bone
    - Compaction and collapse of dead cancellous bone
    - Chronic osteomyelitis
    - Osteopetrosis, Osteosclerosis
    - Fluorosis
    - Renal osteodystrophy
    - Hypoparathyroidism

24. Ans. (b) Hypoparathyroidism; (c) Fluorosis; (e) Renal osteodystrophy

[Ref. Learning Radiology by Herring, 3/e p231]

25. Ans. (c) Is frequently complicated by osteogenic sarcoma

[Ref. Practical Orthopedic Pathology by Siegel, 1/e p86]

26. Ans. (b) Paget disease

[Ref. Comprehensive Radiographic Pathology by Eisenberg, 6/e p113]

Radiology in Paget's Disease

- Ivory vertebra (Vertebrae with uniform dense sclerosis)
- Cotton wool spots (Irregular Sclerotic foci and Cortical thickening)
- Tam O' Shanter sign
- Squaring of vertebra
- Blade of glass/ Candle flame sign in Long bones

27. Ans. (c) Normal Ca, normal PO_4, normal alkaline phosphatase

[Ref. Maheshwari, 4/e p299]

28. Ans. (b) Hypothyroidism

[Ref. Maheshwari, 4/e p298]

Causes of Osteoporosis

- Senility (Old age)
- Postmenopausal
- Post immobilization
- Prolonged weightlessness in spaceship
- Protein deficiency (Inadequate intake, Malabsorption, Burns)
- Endocrinal (Cushing's syndrome, Hyperthyroidism, Hyperparathyroidism, Hyperprolactinemia, Hypercortisolism, Hypogonadism, Thyrotoxicosis)
- Drugs (Alcohol, Glucocorticoids, Heparin, Thyroxine, Anticonvulsants, Phenobarbitone)
- GIT system (Subtotal gastrectomy, Malabsorption, Primary biliary cirrhosis)
- Rheumatoid disorders: Rheumatoid arthritis, SLE

29. Ans. (c) Perthes disease; (e) Osteogenesis imperfecta

[Ref. Pediatric Orthopedics by Herring, 5/e p667]

Coxa Vara

- Congenital Coxa vara with Congenital femoral deficiency
- Congenital Coxa vara with Developmental dysplasias:
  - Cleidocranial dysplasia
  - Metaphyseal dysostosis
- Acquired Coxa vara:
  - Slipped capital femoral epiphysis
  - Avascular necrosis of femoral epiphysis: Legg-Calve Perthes disease, Femoral neck fracture, Traumatic hip dislocation, Septic necrosis
  - Pathologic bone disorders: Osteogenesis imperfecta, Fibrous dysplasia, Renal osteodystrophy, Osteopetrosis

30. Ans. (d) Full abduction in 90°

[Ref. Textbook of Surgery by Ahsan, 2/e p271]

- Normal hip abducts till 90 degrees whereas Congenitally dislocated hip abducts till 45 degrees only

31. Ans. (b) Narrowing of foramina of skull

[Ref. New Techniques in Metabolic Bone Disease by Stevenson, 1/e p269]

- Paget's disease of skull may affect individual cranial nerves by compression due to narrowing or distortion of their foramina, resulting in various neurological deficits
- Cause of deafness in Paget's disease:
  - Main mechanism: Compression of the auditory nerve
  - Other mechanisms: Narrowing/distortion of auditory meati, Invagination by cervical vertebrae (Paget's disease of ossicles, Paget's disease of base of skull)

32. Ans. (d) Plicamycin

[Ref. Endocrine Secrets by McDermott, 6/e p119]

Treatment of Paget's Disease

- Bisphosphonates: Etidronate, Aledronate, Risedronate, Pamidronate, Zoledronic acid
- Calcitonin
- Supplemental treatment: Calcium, Vitamin D

33. Ans. (d) All of the above

[Ref. Maheshwari, 4/e p307]

34. Ans. (b) Small head of femur

[Ref. Congenital Hip Disease in Adults by Babis, 1/e p16]

35. Ans. (b) Interosseous membrane ossification

[Ref. Diagnostic Radiology by Berry, 2/e p234]

Radiology in Fluorosis

- Osteosclerosis (Spine, Pelvis, Ribs)
- Thickening of cortex
- Ligamentous calcification and ossification (Intervertebral)
- Ossification of Interosseous membranes (Paired bones)
- Osteophytosis of vertebrae

36. Ans. (b) Hypoparathyroidism

[Ref. Maheshwari, 4/e p298]

37. Ans. (d) All of the above

[Ref. Maheshwari, 4/e p298]

38. Ans. (a) Intervertebral ligament calcification

[Ref. Diagnostic Radiology by Berry, 2/e p234]

39. Ans. (a) Stiffness of back ligaments; (d) Dental changes; (e) Stiffness of bones and tendons

[Ref. Diagnostic Radiology by Berry, 2/e p234]

40. Ans. (b) Barlow's test; (e) Ortolani's test

[Ref. PMR Board Review by, 3/e p749]

- Clinical exam maneuvers that assess hip dysplasia in children include: Galeazzi (Allis) test, Barlow test, Ortolani test

41. Ans. (b) Breech presentation

[Ref. Diagnostic Radiology - Pediatric Imaging by Bhalla, 3/e p356]

Radiology in Congenital Dislocation of Hip

Absolute indications	Relative indications (If more than two)
• Family history • Neonatal hip instability • Limb shortening • Limitation of hip abduction in flexion	• Breech presentation • First born child • Cesarean section • Congenital anomalies • Excessive foetal moulding

Orthopedics

42. Ans. (a) Exaggerated lordosis; (c) Wadding gait; (d) Shenton's line broken; (e) Short stature
[Ref. Pediatric Orthopedics by Flynn, 1/e p298]

43. Ans. (b) Hyperextension
[Ref. Knee Surgery by Aichroth, 1/e p513]

44. Ans. (a) Infants below 6 months
[Ref. Pediatric Orthopedic Diagnosis by Robb, 1/e p41]

45. Ans. (d) Caffey's disease
[Ref. Oral Medicine by Ghom, 1/e p437]

46. Ans. (d) Hypoparathyroidism
[Ref. Maheshwari, 4/e p298]

47. Ans. (c) Hyperthyroidism
[Ref. Maheshwari, 4/e p298]

48. Ans. (c) Hyperparathyroidism
[Ref. Spine by Kang, 1/e p492]

49. Ans. (a) Genu valgum
[Ref. Orthopedics by Perkins, 1/e p490]

50. Ans. (a) In infants, it may be considered normal; (b) Occurs due to epiphyseal dysplasia; (c) Seldom associated with tibial angulation; (e) Does not require any treatment
[Ref. Avery's Diseases of Newborn by Gleason, 8/e p1429]

51. Ans. (a) Rickets
[Ref. Orthopedics by Rohilla, 1/e p276]

52. Ans. (c) Tibia vera
[Ref. Maheshwari, 4/e p310]

- **Blount disease (Tibia vera)**: A bowing of the tibia and femur, affecting one or both knees mostly in obese persons

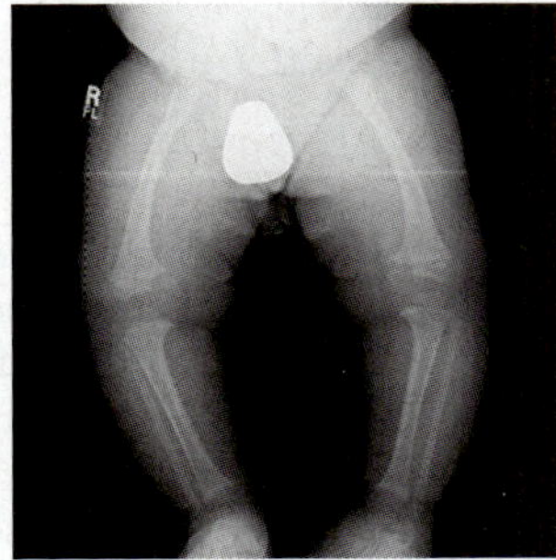

Fig. Blount disease

53. Ans. (b) Hypervitaminosis D
[Ref. Differential Radiological Diagnosis by Chapman, 6/e p336]

54. Ans. (d) Talipes equino varus
[Ref. Maheshwari, 4/e p203]

55. Ans. (d) Manipulation and corrective splint
[Ref. Maheshwari, 4/e p210]

56. Ans. (d) Orthosis is recommended full time
[Ref. Learning Radiology by Herring, 3/e p720]

57. Ans. (a) 4 years
[Ref. Fundamentals of Pediatric Orthopedics by Staheli, 4/e p143]

58. Ans. (c) Increase in osteoid maturation time
[Ref. Orthopedic Surgery, Excerpta Medica, Section 33 p230]

59. Ans. (a) Phenytoin; (b) Malabsorption
[Ref. Maheshwari, 4/e p298]

60. Ans. (a) Compression fracture of the spine
[Ref. Maheshwari, 4/e p298-299]

- Vertebral compression fractures are most common manifestation of osteoporosis of spine
  - MC Site: Lower thoracic and Upper lumbar vertebrae

61. Ans. (a) Vertebra
[Ref. Maheshwari, 4/e p298-299]

62. Ans. (d) Supra condylar fracture humerus
[Ref. Skeletal Trauma in Tropics by Kumar, 2/e p29]

63. Ans. (a) Iliac horn; (c) Absent patella; (d) Knee deformity; (e) Dislocation of patella
[Ref. Essentials of Skeletal Radiology by Rowe, 3/e p748]

Nail Patella Syndrome (Osteoonchodysostosis)

- Iliac horn, Iliac wings dysplasia
- Absent/ small patella, Dislocation of patella,
- Knee deformity, Genu valgum, Gait anomalies,
- Subluxation/dislocation of Radial head, Capiteller deformity
- Renal disease

64. Ans. (a) Congenital vertical talus; (c) Arthrogryposis; (d) Holding club foot in too long corrected position; (e) Force dorsiflexion against equinus varus
[Ref. Deformation by Lara, 4/e p32]

Rocker Bottom Foot

- Inheritance: Autosomal dominant
- Associated conditions: Congenital vertical talus, Arthrogryposis, Myelodysplasia, Trisomy 18, Sacral agenesis, 18q22q23 chromosome

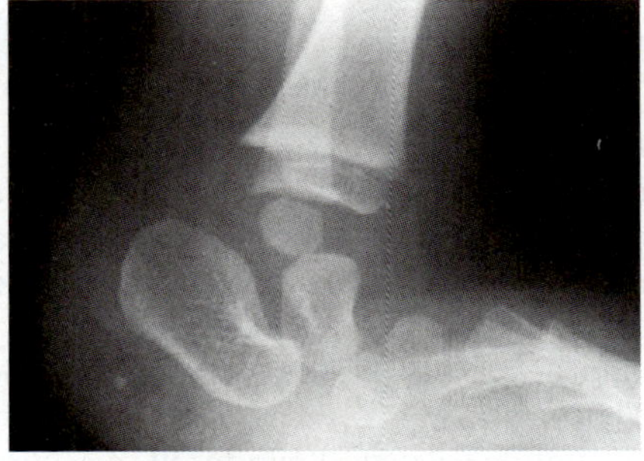

Fig. Rocker bottom foot

65. Ans. (a) Neurological disorder; (b) Idiopathic; (c) Spina bifida; (e) Arthrogryposis multiplex
[Ref. Maheshwari, 4/e p204]

Clubfoot Associations

- Idiopathic
- Congenital causes:
  - Spina bifida, Anencephaly, Hydrocephalus
  - Arthrogryposis multiplex congenita, Myelodyspalsia
  - Fredreich's ataxia

- Acquired causes:
  - Post-polio residual paralysis
  - Post-burn contractures
  - Volkman Ischemic contracture
  - Leprosy
  - Neurological disorders: Cerebral palsy
  - Post-traumatic

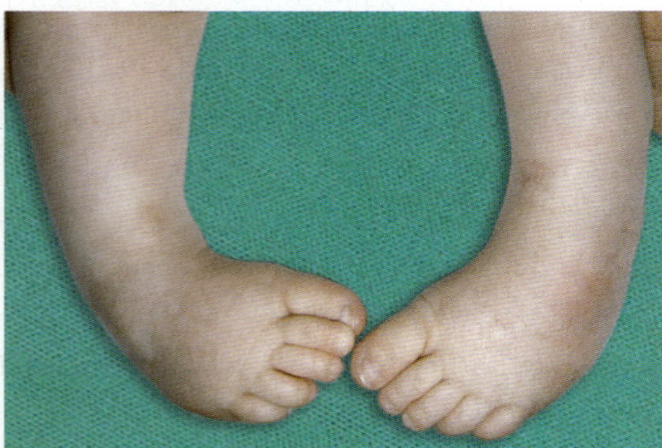

Fig. Club feet

66. Ans. (a) Males
[Ref. High Yield Orthopedics by Javad, 1/e p104]

67. Ans. (b) Triple arthrodesis
[Ref. Maheshwari, 4/e p209]

68. Ans. (a) Phenytoin; (b) Malabsorption; (c) Indoor stay
[Ref. Maheshwari, 4/e p298]

69. Ans. ALL CHOICES
[Ref. Nutrition in Prevention and Treatment of Disease by Coulston, 3/e p874]

70. Ans. (d) Ewings sarcoma
[Ref. Low Back and Neck Pain by Weisel, 3/e p590]

- **Tumors associated with Osteomalacia/Rickets**: Hemangiopericytoma, Giant cell tumor, Nonossifying fibroma, Osteoblastoma, Angiosarcoma, Neurofibroma, Osteosarcoma, Melorheostosis, Fibrous dysplasia

71. Ans. (b) Hypocalcemia
[Ref. Practical Pediatric Problems by Carachi, 1/e p442]

Causes of Rickets

- Vitamin D deficiency and failure: Dietary deficiency, Lack of sunlight exposure, Malabsorption (Celiac disease), 25-hydroxylase deficiency, 1alpha-hydroxylase deficiency, 1-25 dihydroxy D3 receptor defect
- Calcium deficiency: Preterm ill newborns, Sever dietary deficiency
- Phosphate deficiency: Preterm ill newborns, Fanconi syndrome, X-linked dominant hypophosphatemic rickets
- Distal renal tubular acidosis

72. Ans. (c) Bilaterally shortened sternocleidomastoid muscles
[Ref. Pediatric Ophthalmology and Strabismus by Speigel, 2/e p999]

Klippel-Feil Syndrome

- Synonyms: Congenital brevicollis, No neck-Head-on-shoulders appearance
- Underlying deformity: Fused or deformed cervical vertebrae
- Associated Features: (First three manifestations constitute classical triad)
  - Limited neck movement
  - Low posterior hairline
  - Short neck
  - Pterygium colli/ Webbed neck
  - Facial asymmetry
  - Hearing impairment

73. Ans. (b) Osteogenesis imperfecta
[Ref. Forensic Pathology of Fractures and Mechanism of Injury by Burke, 1/e p213]

Wormian Bones

- Description: Extra pieces of bones present within sutures
- **MC site: Lambdoid suture**
- Associated conditions: Osteogenesis imperfecta, Menkes' syndrome, Acro-osteolysis, Cleidocranial dysostosis, Prader Willi syndrome, Hydrocephalus, Hypothyroidism, Healing rickets, Trisomies

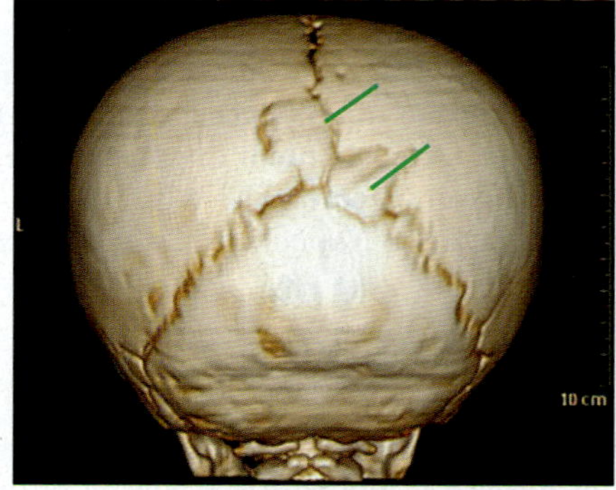

Fig. Wormian bones

74. Ans. (b) Foot, ankle and leg
[Ref. The Clubfoot by Simons, 1/e p292]

75. Ans. (a) Calcitonin; (b) Alendronate
[Ref. Osteoporosis by Gueldner, 1/e p78]

- **Treatment of Postmenopausal Osteoporosis**: Alendronate, Calcitonin (Nasal), Etidronate, Fluoride, Hormone replacement therapy, Parathyroid hormone, Raloxifene, Risedronate, Calcium, Vitamin D derivatives

76. Ans. (a) Osteoporosis
[Ref. Learning Radiology by Herring, 3/e p231]

77. Ans. (b) Osteoporosis
[Ref. Osteoporosis by Rosen, 3/e p1294]

78. Ans. (b) Decreased bone density
[Ref. Maheshwari, 4/e p299]

79. Ans. (c) Talonavicular joint
[Ref. McGlamry's Foot and Ankle Surgery, 4/e Chapter 60]

80. Ans. (d) Bilateral hip dislocation
[Ref. Maheshwari, 4/e p306]

Osteogenesis Imperfecta

- Major feature: Multiple fractures due to Osteoporosis, Excessive bone fragility
- Other features: Blue sclera, Lax ligaments, Skeletal deformities, Congenital deafness, Joint laxity, Otosclerosis

81. Ans. (a) Rickets
[Ref. Diagnostic Radiology by Berry, 2/e p202]

82. Ans. (b) Ricketrosary at costochondral junction produced by subluxation of sternal plate
[Ref. Pediatrics by Kabra, 1/e p53]

83. Ans. (a) Vitamin A; (c) Vitamin D
[Ref. The Vitamins by Combs, 4/e p133]

84. Ans. (a) Indoor stay; (c) Phenytoin; (d) Malabsorption
[Ref. Maheshwari, 4/e p298]

85. Ans. (a) Congenital talonavicular dislocation

86. Ans. (b) Equines, inversion, adduction
[Ref. Maheshwari, 4/e p204]

87. Ans. (b) Dorsiflexed and everted
[Ref. Pediatric Orthopedics by Herring, 5/e p774]

88. Ans. (a) Metaphysis
[Ref. Osteoporosis by Guglielmi, 1/e p27]
- **Classic radiographic changes in rickets** include Osteopenia and Changes in metaphysis (Cupping, Fraying, Splaying)

89. Ans. (d) Bow legs
[Ref. Nelson Textbook of Pediatrics, 20/e p340]

90. Ans. (d) Decreased alkaline phosphatase
[Ref. Maheshwari, 4/e p301]
- Laboratory parameters in Rickets: Low/normal Calcium, Low Phosphate, High Serum alkaline phosphatase

91. Ans. (a) Normal serum calcium; (d) Pseudofractures
[Ref. API Textbook of Medicine, 9/e p307]
- Laboratory parameters in Osteomalacia: Low/normal Calcium, Low Phosphate, High Serum alkaline phosphatase

92. Ans. (b) Avascular necrosis of femoral head
[Ref. Clinical Pediatric Nephrology by Kher, 2/e p183]
- Corticosteroid use in Nephrotic syndrome increase the risk of Avascular necrosis of femoral head

93. Ans. (b) Avascular necrosis of hip
[Ref. Clinical Pediatric Nephrology by Kher, 2/e p183]

94. Ans. (b) S. Alkaline phosphate
[Ref. Practical Pediatric Problems by Carachi, 1/e p352]

95. Ans. (c) Subluxation of the talo-navicular joint
[Ref. Children's Orthopedics and fractures by Benson, 3/e p543]

96. Ans. (e) Excessive correction of Grice procedure
[Ref. Pediatric Conditions in Practice by Heiti, 1/e p381]

97. Ans. (c) Osteomalacia
[Ref. Maheshwari, 4/e p302]
- **Loosers' zones (Pseudofractures)**: Radiolucent zones occurring at sites of stress
  - Commonly sites: Pubic rami, Axillary border of Scapula, Ribs, Medial cortex of neck of femur
  - Underlying cause: Rapid resorption and slow mineralization

98. Ans. (d) All the above
[Ref. Maheshwari, 4/e p302]

99. Ans. (b) Achondroplasia
[Ref. The Bedside Dysmorphologist by Reardon, 1/e p261]

Trident Hand
- Dwarfism with short extremities, particularly in the proximal (rhizomelic) segments
- Large head with frontal bossing
- Hypoplasia of the midface
- Trident hands (Splaying of fingers leading to index and ring finger pointing away from middle finger)

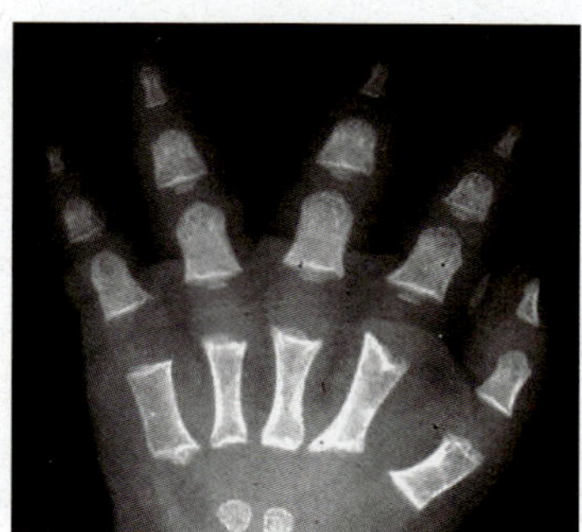

Fig. Trident hand

100. Ans. (c) Cleidocranial dysostosis
[Ref. The Netter's Collection of Medical Illustrations by Parker, 2/e p145]

101. Ans. (a) Manipulation by mother
[Ref. AIPGME 2006 by Koli]

102. Ans. (a) Manipulation and corrective splint
[Ref. Maheshwari, 4/e p207-209]

103. Ans. (b) Primary hyperparathyroidism; (c) Chronic renal failure
[Ref. MCQs in Pediatrics by Nayak, 1/e p511]

104. Ans. (c) Paget's disease of bone
[Ref. Principles and Practice of Endocrinology and Metabolism by Becker, 3/e p647]
- A markedly elevated serum alkaline phosphatase level in a healthy older patient with no evidence of liver disease and a normal serum Calcium level indicate Paget's disease of bone

105. Ans. (c) Manipulation & Strapping
[Ref. Orthopedics Illustrated by Gupta, 2/e p120]

106. Ans. (b) Defective collagen
[Ref. Maheshwari, 4/e p302]
- Osteogenesis imperfecta is due to defective collagen synthesis thus affecting collagen containing tissues like bones, skin, sclera, teeth, ligaments

107. Ans. (d) Osteogenesis imperfecta
[Ref. Maheshwari, 4/e p306]

108. Ans. (d) Vitamin D deficiency
[Ref. Mayo Clinic Internal Medicine Board review, 10/e p470]

109. Ans. (a) Scurvy
[Ref. Approach to Practical Pediatrics by Narang, 1/e p259]

Radiology in Scurvy
- Metaphyseal fractures
- Pencil-thin cortex
- White line of Frankel

- Zone of Trummerfeld
- Pelkan spurs
- Halo sign of Wimberger (Ring sign)

110. Ans. (a) Idiopathic; (c) Arthrogryposis multiplexa; (d) Spina bifida; (e) Neurological disorders
[Ref. Maheshwari, 4/e p204]

111. Ans. (a) Increased alkaline phosphatase; (d) Associated with chondrosarcoma
[Ref. Tumor Diagnosis by Nafussi, 2/e p68]

112. Ans. (d) Normal calcium, Normal phosphate, Normal alkaline phosphate
[Ref. Maheshwari, 4/e p299]

113. Ans. (c) Scurvy
[Ref. Approach to Practical Pediatrics by Narang, 1/e p259]

114. Ans. (c) Both of these
[Ref. Outline of Orthopedics by Adams, 1/e p112]

115. Ans. (b) Scurvy
[Ref. Approach to Practical Pediatrics by Narang, 1/e p259]

116. Ans. (c) Hyperthyroidism
[Ref. Imaging of Arthritis and Metabolic Bone Disease by Weismann, 1/e p681]

117. Ans. (c) Parathyroid adenoma
[Ref. Parathyroid Surgery by Terris, 1/e p23]

118. Ans. (a) Codfish vertebra seen; (e) Commonly presents with fracture
[Ref. Maheshwari, 4/e p298-299]

119. Ans. (a) As soon as possible after birth
[Ref. Maheshwari, 4/e p207]

- Ideally CTEV treatment should begin soon after birth but not later than 2 weeks

120. Ans. (a) Forefoot adduction
[Ref. Physical Therapist's Clinical Companion, 1/e p185]

- **Sequential corrections of CTEV**:
  - First: Forefoot adduction
  - Second: Varus (Inversion)
  - Third: Equinus (Plantar flexion)
- If Sequential corrections of CTEV are not followed it may result in Misshaped foot or Rocker bottom foot

121. Ans. (b) Postero medial soft tissue release
[Ref. Maheshwari, 4/e p207]

122. Ans. (a) Triple arthrodesis
[Ref. Maheshwari, 4/e p207]

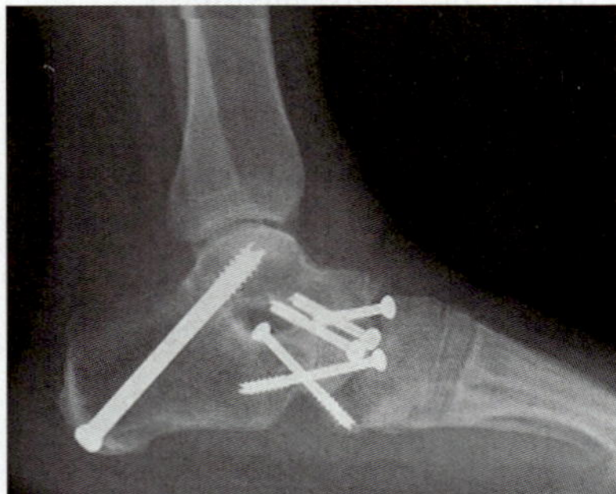

Fig. Triple arthrodesis

- **Triple arthrodesis** is performed after the age of 12 years as before this age bones are cartilaginous (so difficult to achieve fusion)
- Most difficult fusion to achieve: Talonavicular joint

123. Ans. (a) Hypoparathyroidism
[Ref. Maheshwari, 4/e p298]

124. Ans. (b) Absent spinal reflexes; (c) Loss of autonomic reflexes
[Ref. Neurology in Clinical Practice by Bradley, 4/e p360]

125. Ans. (a) Solitary adenoma
[Ref. Clinical Endocrine Oncology by Hay, 2/e p172]

126. Ans. (b) Tetany
[Ref. Orthopedics and Fractures by Blundell, 4/e p113]

- **Biochemical parameters in Osteitis fibrosa cystica**: High serum calcium, Low phosphate, Raised Alkaline phosphatase

127. Ans. (d) Hyperparathyroidism
[Ref. Imaging of Arthritis and Metabolic Bone Disease by Weismann, 1/e p643]

128. Ans. (d) Both B & C

129. Ans. (d) All of the above
[Ref. Maheshwari, 4/e p203-205]

130. Ans. (a) Fracture vertebra
[Ref. The Adult and Pediatric Spine by Weisel, 3/e p1180]

- Sagittal plane deformity due to Compression fracture of vertebrae is most characteristic feature of Osteoporosis Spine

131. Ans. (d) Fracture of clavicle
[Ref. Elder Care by Lewis, 2/e p71]

- Fractures associated with Osteoporosis: Vertebra, Distal forearm (Colles fracture), Neck of femur, Pelvis

132. Ans. (c) Triple arthrodesis
[Ref. Maheshwari, 4/e p209]

133. Ans. (d) Talonavicular
[Ref. Pediatric Orthopedics by Herring, 5/e p228]

134. Ans. (b) Hyperparathyroidism
[Ref. Maheshwari, 4/e p303]

135. Ans. (a) Jaws
[Ref. Radiology Illustrated by Kim, 1/e p1066]

- Subperiosteal resorption of bones in Hyperparathyroidism: Middle phalanges of hand, Metaphysis of tibia/ radius/ ulna, Femoral neck, Ribs, Clavicles, Metacarpals, Lamina dura

136. Ans. (a) Hyperparathyroidism
[Ref. Surgery by Bollinger, 1/e p869]

137. Ans. (b) Hyperparathyroidism
[Ref. Oral and Maxillofacial Diseases by Bagan, 4/e p10]

138. Ans. (b) Reiter's syndrome
[Ref. Oxford's Rheumatology by Watts, 1/e p25]

- Acro-osteolysis (Erosion of terminal tufts): Hyperparathyroidism, Scleroderma, Sjogren's syndrome, Psoriatic arthritis

139. Ans. (b) Estrogens
[Ref. Mayo Clinic Internal Medicine Board Review by Wilkins, 1/e p217]

140. Ans. (a) Alendronate; (c) Estrogen; (e) Calcitonin
[Ref. Osteoporosis by Rosen, 3/e p1294]

141. Ans. (d) Elevated scapula
[Ref. Pediatric Ophthalmology and Strabismus by Speigel, 2/e p999]

142. Ans. (a) Undescended/ Elevated scapula
[Ref. Maheshwari, 4/e p217]

- **Sprengel's shoulder**: Failure of descent of scapula, developmentally a cervical appendage i.e., Congenital high scapula

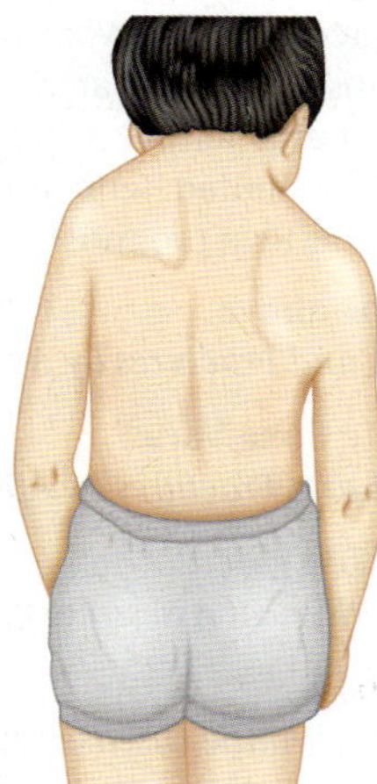

Fig. Sprengel deformity

143. Ans. (b) Reduced formation of osteoid matrix
[Ref. Applied Physiology of Mouth by Lavelle, 1/e p253]

Scurvy

- In the child suffering from scurvy bone growth is reduced because the formation of osteoid matrix is impaired
- Underlying reason: Insufficient amounts of dietary vitamin C (ascorbic acid) intake results in reduced hydroxylation of lysine and proline; it leads to impairment of collagen cross-linking further reducing secretion of collagen and formation of osteoid

144. Ans. (c) Infrared therapy
[Ref. Current Therapy in Pain by Smith, 1/e p533]

Heat Applications

Superficial Heat	Deep Heat
• Hydrocollator packs • Paraffin baths • Hydrotherapy • Heat wraps	• Diathermy ▪ Ultrasound ▪ Short wave diathermy ▪ Microwave diathermy) • Phonophoresis • Iontophoresis

145. Ans. (c) Hyperparathyroidism; (d) Psoriasis
[Ref. Oxford's Rheumatology by Watts, 1/e p25]

146. Ans. (d) Hyperparathyroidism
[Ref. Maheshwari, 4/e p217]

- **Brown's tumor**: Expansile lytic lesion, appearing like a bone tumor, generally affecting maxilla/ mandible is seen in Hyperparathyroidism

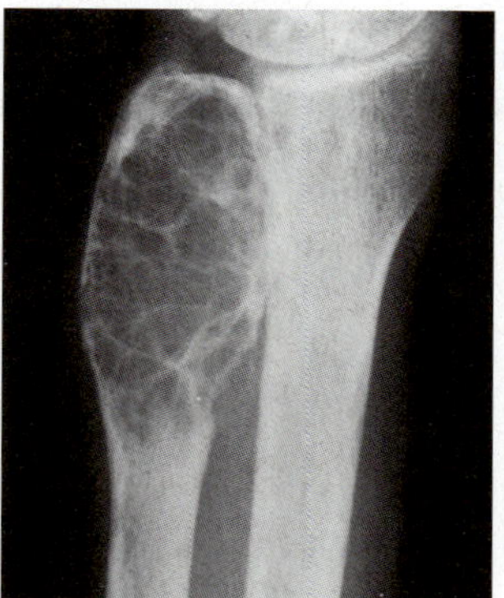

Fig. Brown tumor

147. Ans. (a) Osteitis fibrosa
[Ref. Radiology Review Manual by Dahnert, 7/e p2]

- **Sclerotic lesions in bones**: Osteopoikilosis, Enchondromatosis (Ollier's disease), Melorheotosis, Multiple osteomas (Gardener's syndrome), Osteopetrosis, Pyknodysostosis, Mastocytosis (Urticaria pigmentosa), Tuberous sclerosis, Infantile cortical hyperostosis (Caffey's disease), Traumatic, Osteosarcoma, Chronic osteomyelitis, Fluorosis, Paget's disease of bone, Renal osteodystrophy, Secondaries from Prostate, Engelman's disease

148. Ans. (d) Hyperparathyroidism
[Ref. Maheshwari, 4/e p303]

149. Ans. (d) Hemophilia
[Ref. MCQs in Clinical Radiology by Rajiah, 1/e p281]

Arnold Hilgatner Scale of Hemophilia in Knee

- Score 0: No change
- Score 1: Soft tissue swelling
- Score 2: Osteoporosis, Overgrowth of epiphysis
- Score 3: Subchondral cysts, Squaring of patella, Widened intercondylar notch
- Score 4: Narrowed cartilage space
- Score 5: Joint contracture, Loss of cartilage space, Disorganized joint, Gross epiphyseal enlargement

150. Ans. (c) Hypothyroidism
[Ref. Hutchison's Atlas of Pediatric Physical Diagnosis by Carachi, 1/e p333]

- **Epiphyseal dysgenesis is pathognomonic of hypothyroidism;** its' also seen in Panhypopituitarism

151. Ans. (c) Hyperparathyroidism
[Ref. Maheshwari, 4/e p304]

152. Ans. (a) It arises before birth
[Ref. Before We are Born by Moore, 9/e p241]

- Sternocleidomastoid muscle is sometimes injured at birth, resulting in Congenital torticollis

153. Ans. (a) Seen only in cases of breech vaginal delivery
[Ref. Children's Orthopedics and Fractures by Parsch, 3/e p583]

154. Ans. ALL CHOICES
[Ref. Professional Guide to Diseases by Wilkins, 9/e p368]

- **Causes of Congenital Torticollis:**
  - Prenatal injury
  - Malposition of head in utero
  - Fibroma
  - Interruption of blood supply
  - Fibrotic rupture of SCM with hematoma and scar formation

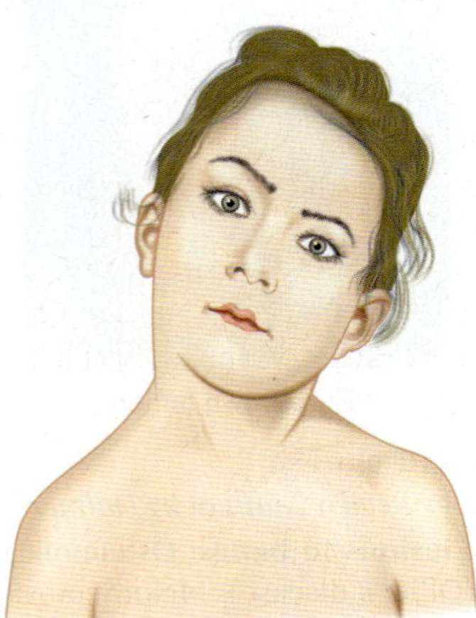

Fig. Congenital torticollis

155. Ans. (c) Lateral part of the medial femoral condyle
[Ref. Pediatric Orthopedic Deformities by Shapiro, 1/e p468]

156. Ans. (d) Calcitonin
[Ref. Pharmacology for Nursing Care by Rosenthal, 8/e p941]
- **Drug of choice for Paget's disease of bone**: Bisphosphonates > Calcitonin
- Drug of choice for Pain relief in Paget's disease of bone: Calcitonin

157. Ans. (a) Osteitis deformans
[Ref. Maheshwari, 4/e p307]

158. Ans. (c) Lunate bone
[Ref. Maheshwari, 4/e p308]

159. Ans. (a) Tibial tuberosity
[Ref. Maheshwari, 4/e p308]

160. Ans. (b) Neurofibromatosis
[Ref. Turek's Orthopedics by Buckwalter, 6/e p580]

161. Ans. (d) All
[Ref. 5-Minute Clinical Consult Premium 2015, 23/e p812]
- **Skeletal Abnormalities in Neurofibromatosis:**
  - Scoliosis and Vertebral angulation
  - Localised bone hypertrophy
  - Limb abnormalities (Pseudoarthrosis of tibia, Tibial dysplasia, Non-ossifying fibromas of long bones)

162. Ans. (d) Periventricular calcifications

163. Ans. (d) Tibia-fibula
[Ref. Musculoskeletal Imaging by Pope, 1/e p1071]
- **Congenital Pseudoarthrosis:**
  - Most common bone: Tibia
  - Other bones: Fibula, Radius, Ulna, Clavicle, Humerus

164. Ans. (b) Post inflammatory
[Ref. Abnormal Skeletal Phenotypes by Bruno, 1/e p321]

165. Ans. (c) Hyperparathyroidism
[Ref. Skeletal Radiology by Chew, 3/e p282]

166. Ans. (d) Ochronotic arthritis
[Ref. Nelson's Textbook of Pediatrics, 20/e p642]

167. Ans. (c) Osteomyelitis
[Ref. Turek's Orthopedics by Buckwalter, 6/e p580]

168. Ans. (b) Internal fixation and bone grafting
[Ref. Operative Orthopedics by Chapman, 1/e p3158]

169. Ans. (c) Block vertebra
[Ref. Pediatrics by Scheri, 1/e p65]
- **High rates of Progression of Congenital Scoliosis:**
  - Thoracic curve involvement
  - Unilateral thoracic unsegmented bars with contralateral fully segmented vertebra (Worst prognosis)
  - Unilateral unsegmented bar
  - Double ipsilateral hemivertebrae
  - Single fully segmented hemivertebra
  - Block vertebra (Best prognosis)

170. Ans. (d) All of the above
[Ref. Orthopedics and Fractures by Apley, 1/e p234]

171. Ans. (d) Infantile Coxa Vara
[Ref. Orthopedics and Fractures by Apley, 1/e p234]

172. Ans. (c) Painful hip gait
[Ref. Orthopedic Physical Assessment by Magee, 6/e p1007]

173. Ans. ALL CHOICES
[Ref. Primer on Rheumatic Diseases by Stone, 13/e p573]
- **Commonly affected bones in Paget's disease**: Pelvis, Femur, Skull, Tibia, Vertebra, Clavicle, Humerus

174. Ans. (d) Calcitonin
[Ref. Pharmacology for Nursing Care by Rosenthal, 8/e p941]

175. Ans. (d) All of the above
[Ref. Self-Assessment Questions in Rheumatology by Ali, p12]
- **Complications of Paget's disease**: Fracture, High-output heart failure, Deafness, Spinal nerve compression, Neuropathies, Deformities, Osteosarcoma (Rare)

176. Ans. (b) Osteotomy
[Ref. Surgery of Hip Joint by Tranza, 2/e p216]

177. Ans. (a) Perthe's disease
[Ref. Textbook of Orthopedics by Ebnezar, 4/e p410]

Types of Coxa Vara
- Congenital Coxa vara
- Acquired Coxa vara:
  - Capital coxa vara: Perthe's disease, Septic arthritis of Hip, Cretinism
  - Epiphyseal coxa vara: Slipped capital femoral epiphysis
  - Cervical coxa vara: Malunited trochanteric fracture, Rickets, Osteoporosis, Osteomyelitis, Paget's disease, Fibrous dysplasia

178. Ans. (d) Serum Alkaline Phosphatase
[Ref. Spinal Infections and Trauma by Jain, 1/e p559]
- **In Heterotopic ossification**, Serum alkaline phosphatase is used as a Marker of Osteoblastic activity and Early diagnosis (though its not specific)

179. Ans. (d) Fasciotomy + Skin transplantation
[Ref. Reoperative Hand Surgery by Duncan, 1/e p15]

180. Ans. (c) Idiopathic scoliosis
[Ref. Maheshwari, 4/e p275]
- Supports used in Scoliosis: Milwaukee brace, Boston brace, Reisser's turn-buckle cast, Localiser cast

181. Ans. (b) Faulty development
[Ref. Sclerosing Bone Dysplasias by Cremin, 1/e p15]

182. Ans. (b) Mental retardation
[Ref. Maheshwari, 4/e p306]
- Achondroplasia person has normal intelligence

183. Ans. (a) Autosomal dominant
[Ref. Maheshwari, 4/e p306]

184. Ans. (a) Sequestrum is piece of deal bone; (b) Involucrum is dense sclerotic bone overlying a sequestrum; (d) In sickle cell anemia, Salmonella is causative organism; (e) Staphylococcus aureus is most common cause
[Ref. Maheshwari, 4/e p162-165]
- MC region involved in Osteomyelitis: Metaphysis

185. Ans. (a) Fracture of the affected bone; (c) Chronic osteomyelitis; (d) Sepsis; (e) Chronicity
[Ref. Maheshwari, 4/e p165]

186. Ans. (a) Antibiotics; (b) Splinting; (c) Analgesics; (d) Surgery
[Ref. Maheshwari, 4/e p164-165]

187. Ans. (a) Necrosis absent
[Ref. Skeletal Trauma by Browner, 5/e p614]

188. Ans. (a) Metaphyses
[Ref. Maheshwari, 4/e p162]

189. Ans. (a) Sequestrum
[Ref. Maheshwari, 4/e p166]

190. Ans. (b) Tennis Elbow
[Ref. Maheshwari, 4/e p293]

191. Ans. (c) Extensor carpi radialis longus and brevis
[Ref. Maheshwari, 4/e p293]

192. Ans. (d) Heavier than live bone & trabeculated
[Ref. JAMA, Volume 64 p214]

193. Ans. (d) Periosteal new bone formation around necrotic sequestrum
[Ref. Maheshwari, 4/e p166]

194. Ans. (a) Achondroplasia
[Ref. Rapid Review of Radiology by Hall, 1/e p270]

Radiology in Achondroplasia
- Champagne glass pelvic inlet
- Squared iliac wings
- Vertebrae flattening
- Posterior vertebra scalloping
- Anterior inferior vertebral body beaks
- Macrocephaly with bulging forehead
- Shortened bowed long bones with 'Trumpet appearance'
- Brachydactyly
- Horizontal sacrum

195. Ans. (b) Mental retardation; (c) Autosomal recessive
[Ref. Maheshwari, 4/e p306]

196. Ans. (d) Cleidocranial dysostosis
[Ref. Musculoskeletal Imaging by Disler, 4/e p531]

197. Ans. (d) All of the above
[Ref. Musculoskeletal Imaging by Disler, 4/e p531]

198. Ans. (b) Around the sequestrum
[Ref. Maheshwari, 4/e p166]

199. Ans. (c) Presence of sequestrum
[Ref. Musculoskeletal MRI by Kaplan, 1/e p107]
- Most specific sign of active chronic osteomyelitis: Presence of a sequestrum

200. Ans. (d) Myositis ossificans
[Ref. Practical Surgery by Goel, 3/e p215]

201. Ans. (d) Myelocoele
[Ref. Maheshwari, 4/e p166]

202. Ans. (d) 2 week
[Ref. Maheshwari, 4/e p163-164]
- Earliest sign of Osteomyelitis to appear on X-ray is New bone deposition (Periosteal reaction) at metaphysis after 7–10 days

203. Ans. (a) Diagnosis by X-ray is 8–10 days after onset; (b) There is diffuse tenderness at the site; (c) Antibiotic therapy should be at least for 4 weeks
[Ref. Maheshwari, 4/e p162-164]

204. Ans. (b) Cleidocranial dysostosis
[Ref. Oral Pathology by Purkait, 2/e p459]

Cleidocranial Dysostosis
- Absent clavicles: Shoulders meet in front of chest
- High arched palate
- Slow skull ossification
- Coxa vara
- Absent sinuses
- Delayed eruption of teeth
- Maxillary hypoplasia
- 'Parrot beak' appearance of facial angle

205. Ans. (a) Cleidocranial dysostosis
[Ref. Oral Pathology by Purkait, 2/e p459]

206. Ans. (e) All of the above
[Ref. Maheshwari, 4/e p309]

Morquio's Disease
- Autosomal recessive disorder
- Dwarfism affecting limbs and trunk
- Spinal kyphosis
- Normal mental development
- Tonguing of vertebrae on X-ray
- Corneal opacity
- Keratan sulphate in urine

207. Ans. (c) Abnormal collagen defect
[Ref. Maheshwari, 4/e p306]

208. Ans. (b) Defective Osteoid formation
[Ref. Intercollegiate MRCS by Chan, 1/e p154]
- Osteogenesis imperfecta (brittle bone disease) is defective osteoid formation due to the congenital inability to

produce adequate intercellular substances, such as osteoid, collagen and dentine

209. Ans. (d) Surgery is the only treatment
[Ref. Maheshwari, 4/e p164-165]

210. Ans. (a) Antibiotics only
[Ref. Maheshwari, 4/e p164]

211. Ans. (a) Continuous suction + continuous drainage
[Ref. Pathophysiology by Rasta, 4/e p233]

Instillation-Suction Technique

- Infected bone is first exposed and all sequestra removed
- Two drainage tubes are perforated, inserted and brought out through the skin between 3 and 4 cm from the wound
- Perforated portions of the tubes are laid close to the infected area and the wound closed in layers
- One tube is connected to a drip bottle containing antibiotic solution and the second to a continuous suction pump
- Closed continuous steady flow instillation-suction is thus established

212. Ans. (c) Both are correct
[Ref. Radiology Review Manual by Dahnert, 7/e p2]

213. Ans. (b) Osteomyelitis; (e) Osteosarcoma
[Ref. Surgery by Bailey & Love, 26/e p534]

214. Ans. (c) Both AD and AR
[Ref. Oral Pathology by Sundaram, 7/e p699]

215. Ans. (d) Osteogenesis imperfecta
[Ref. Maheshwari, 4/e p306]

216. Ans. (a) Long standing localized pyogenic abscess in the bone

217. Ans. (b) ATT + Immobilisation
[Pediatrics by Pathasarathy, 3/e p1038]

218. Ans. (b) Slipped capital femoral epiphyses
[Ref. Maheshwari, 4/e p314]

219. Ans. (d) Full abduction in 90° flexion
[Ref. Orthopedics by Kotwal, 1/e p27]

220. Ans. (a) Fibrous dysplasia
[Ref. Musculoskeletal Imaging by Wilson, 1/e p891]

Wormian Bones

- Osteogeneis imperfecta
- Rickets
- Cretinism
- Pyknodysostosis
- Cleidocranial dysostosis
- Kinky hair syndrome
- Down's syndrome
- Hypophosphatasia

221. Ans. (a) Impaired healing of fracture
[Ref. Maheshwari, 4/e p306]

222. Ans. (b) Generally do not unite without T/t
[Ref. Maheshwari, 4/e p306]

223. Ans. (b) Bilateral Hip dislocation
[Ref. Maheshwari, 4/e p306]

224. Ans. (a) Barlow's test
[Ref. Maheshwari, 4/e p213]

225. Ans. (c) Cataract
[Ref. Maheshwari, 4/e p306]

226. Ans. ALL CHOICES
[Ref. Maheshwari, 4/e p306]

227. Ans. (a) Autosomal recessive; (d) Short limbs
[Ref. Orthopedics by Biswas, 1/e p34]

228. Ans. (c) Defective collagen synthesis; (d) Autosomal dominant; (e) Laxity of joints
[Ref. Maheshwari, 4/e p306]

229. Ans. (c) Hyperparathyroidism
[Ref. Maheshwari, 4/e p303]

Acro-osteolysis	Fingertip calcification
• Scleroderma • Hyperparathyroidism • Psoriatic arthropathy • Rheumatoid arthritis • Trauma • Thermal injury • Raynaud's disease • Syringomyelia • Diabetic neuropathy • Epidermolysis bullosa	• Scleroderma • Hyperparathyroidism • Raynaud's disease • Dermatomyositis

230. Ans. (a) Hyperparathyroidism
[Ref. Orthopedic Pathology by Vigorita, 2/e p187]

- Brown tumors are seen in the primary as well as secondary form of hyperparathyroidism (renal disease)

231. Ans. (c) Normal Calcium, Normal ALP
[Ref. Case Studies in OBG by Sanja, 1/e p52]

- Osteoporosis is characterized by Normal Calcium, Normal phosphate, Normal Alkaline phosphatase levels

232. Ans. (a) Congenital
[Ref. Orthopedics by Kotwal, p73]

Diaphyseal Aclasis

- A rare disorder of bone development in which multiple, cartilaginous exostoses develop and enlarge mainly on the ends of long bones
- Congenital multiple exostosis is an autosomal dominant disorder
- Underlying cause: Failure of remodeling of diaphysis

233. Ans. (b) Chronic osteomyelitis
[Ref. Mercer, 10/e p586]

Brodie's Abscess

- An insidiously developing chronic pyogenic osteomyelitis often occurring in the upper tibial metaphysis
- Underlying cause: Infection by organisms of low virulence in immunocompromised hosts

234. Ans. (c) X-linked inheritance
[Ref. Encyclopedia of Molecular Mechanisms of Disease by Lang, 1/e p1547]

- Osteopoikilosis is a rare and benign skeletal dysplasia with Autosomal dominant inheritance.

235. Ans. (d) Ankle

[Ref. McGlamry's Comprehensive Textbook of Foot and Ankle Surgery, 3/e p444]

Haglund's Deformity

- Also referred to as a **'Pump bump'**
- Bony prominence of the posterior superior portion of the calcaneal tuberosity anterior and adjacent to the Achilles tendon
- Bony prominence may be rubbed on by shoe leading to pain, callus, blisters

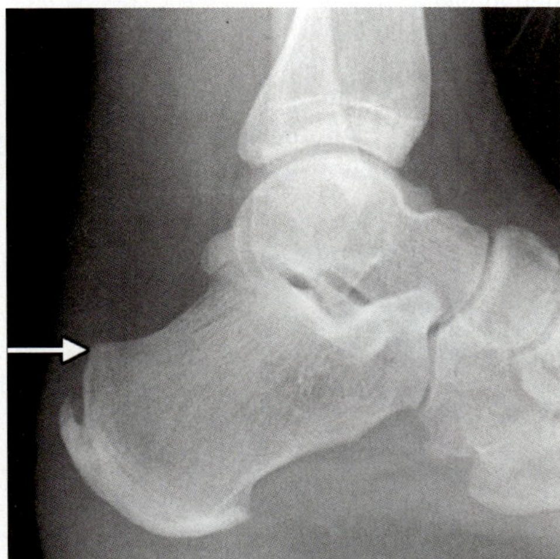

Fig. Haglund deformity

236. Ans. (c) Dextrocardia

[Ref. Pediatric Orthopaedics by Flynn, 1/e p362]

Sprengel's Deformity

- Congenital high elevation of the scapula and medial rotation of the inferior pole of the scapula
- Exact cause of the deformity is unknown
- Associated anomalies: Klippel-Feil syndrome, Rib deformities, Omovertebral bone formation, Muscle anomalies, Clavicle hypoplasia, Tracheoesophageal fistula, Anal stenosis, Kidney anomalies, Diastematomyelia, and Scoliosis

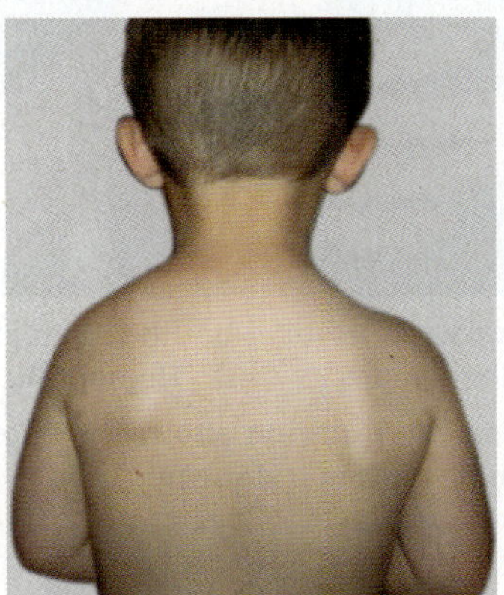

Fig. Sprengel's deformity

237. Ans. (b) Klippel Feil syndrome

[Ref. Campbell's Operative Orthopaedics, 12/e p1679]

Klippel-Feil Syndrome

- **Clinical Triad**: Low posterior hairline, Short neck, and Limited neck motion
- Several congenital problems have been associated with Congenital fusion of the Cervical vertebrae: **Scoliosis (MC)**, Renal abnormalities, Sprengel deformity, Deafness, Synkinesis, and Congenital heart defects

AIIMS PG 2018 MCQs

1. Diagnose the underlying disorder from the Image of the hands of a 55 years old lady shown below [AIIMS May 2018]

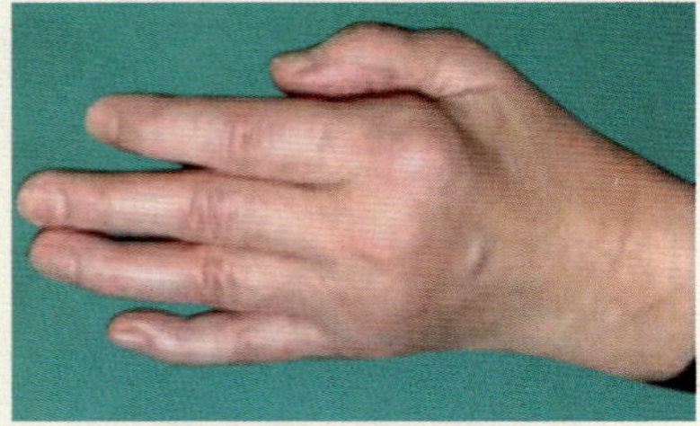

a. Primary osteoarthritis
b. Rheumatoid arthritis
c. Heberden's nodes
d. Hemophilic arthritis

2. Management of condition shown in Photograph in a 30 years old male patient is done by [AIIMS May 2018]

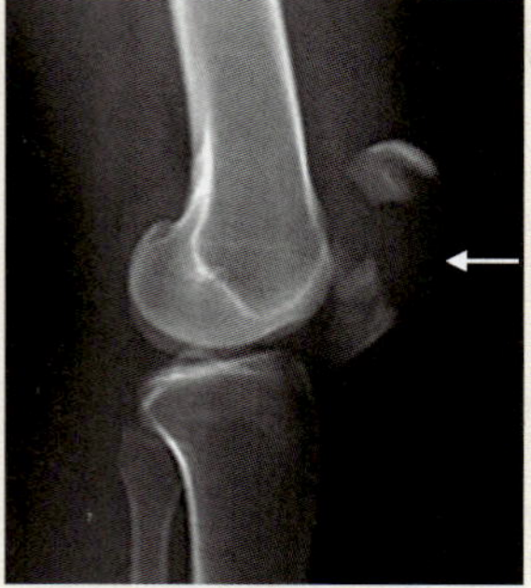

a. K-wire
b. Plating
c. Nails
d. Tension band wiring

3. Examine the Image of a deformity shown below. Diagnose the underlying preceding fracture type. [AIIMS May 2018]

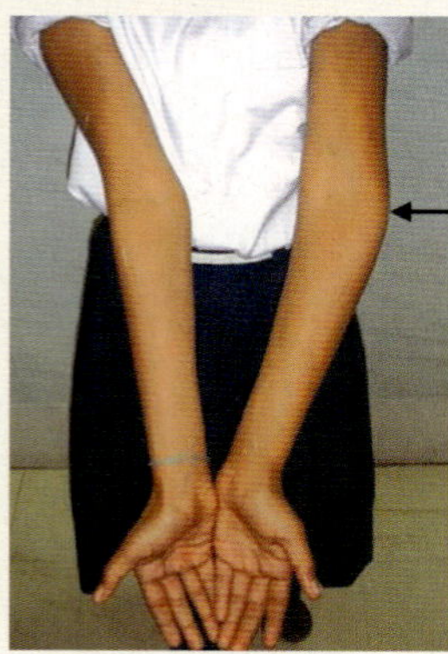

a. Fracture of 1st metacarpal bone
b. Fracture of lower end of radius
c. Supracondylar fracture of humerus
d. Lateral condylar fracture of humerus

4. A 25 years old male presents with absence of flexion on interphalangeal joint at thumb. Nerve injured is [AIIMS May 2018]

a. Radial nerve
b. Median nerve
c. Ulnar nerve
d. None of the above

5. Diagnose the X-ray Photograph of a 32 years old Patient presenting to Orthopedics OPD [AIIMS May 2018]

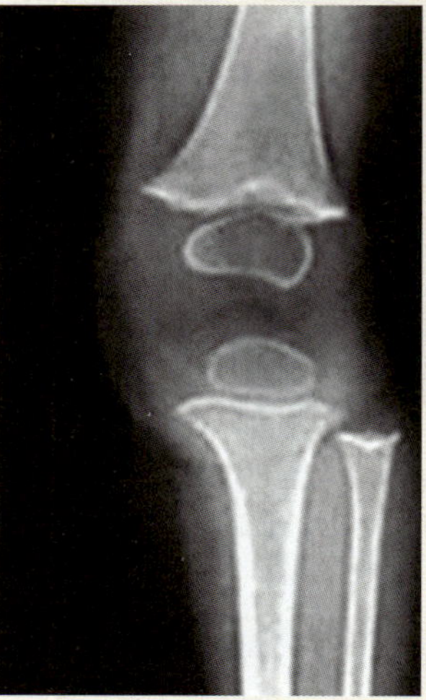

a. Rickets
b. Hyperparathyroidism
c. Scurvy
d. Osteosarcoma

6. Hip flexion contracture can be evaluated by [AIIMS May 2018]

a. Trendelenburg test
b. Thomas test
c. Ortolani test
d. Barlow test

EXPLANATORY ANSWERS

1. Ans. (b) Rheumatoid arthritis
[Ref. Maheshwari, 4/e p280]

Joints affected in Rheumatoid Arthritis

- Common: MP joints of hand (Most common), PIP joints of fingers, Wrists, knees, elbows, ankles
  - Deformities of hands: Swan neck deformity, Boutonniere deformity, Z deformity
- Less common: Hip joint, Temporomandibular joint
- Uncommon: Atlantoaxial joint, Facet joints of cervical spine

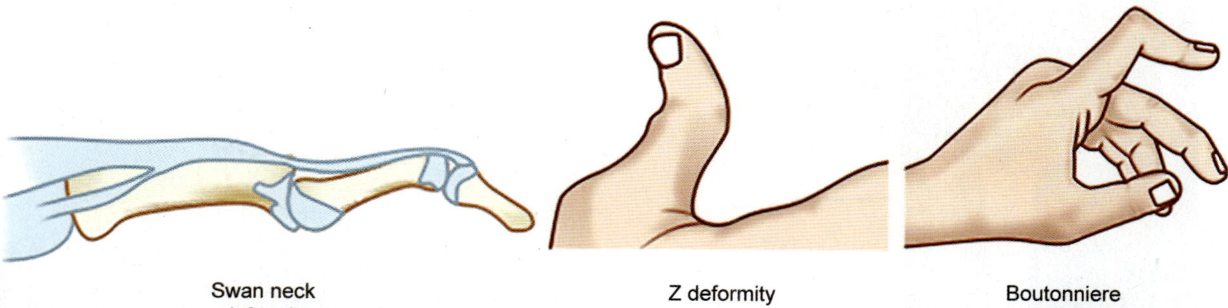

2. Ans. (d) Tension band wiring
[Ref. Maheshwari, 4/e p142]

Treatment of Patellar Fractures

- Undisplaced fracture: Cylinder cast (knee in full extension for 3 weeks), Physiotherapy
- Clean break with Separation of fragments (Photograph):
  - Reduction of fragments, Tension band wiring, Repair of extensor retinaculae
  - If accurate reduction not possible, the Partial or Total patellectomy
- Comminuted fracture: Patellectomy (Excision of patella)

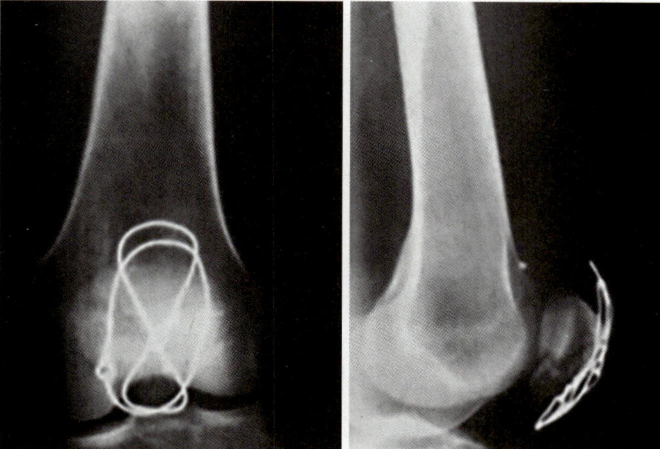

Fig. Tension Band Wiring (Patella)

3. Ans. (c) Supracondylar fracture of humerus
[Ref. Maheshwari, 4/e p98]

- Gunstock Seformity: Malunion of Supracondylar fracture of humerus leading to Cubitus varus deformity

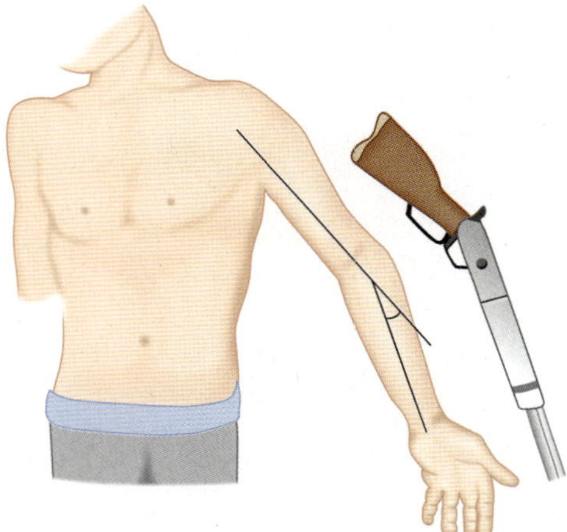

Fig. Gun-stock Deformity

4. Ans. (b) Median nerve
[Ref. Turek's Orthopaedics, 6/e p433]

Motor Strength Deficits of Median Nerve Injury

- Loss of Thumb opposition (Abductor pollicis brevis)
- Loss of Thumb interphalangeal (IP) joint flexion (Flexor pollicis longus muscle)
- Loss of Index distal interphalangeal joint flexion (Flexor digitorum profundus)

5. Ans. (c) Scurvy
[Ref. Orthopedics by Biswas, 1/e p63]

Radiology in Scurvy

- Subperiosteal hemorrhages (A)
- Zone of Trummerfeld (Zone of rarefaction) (B)
- White line of Frankel (C)
- Halo sign of Wimberger (D)

- Pelkan spurs (E)
- Pencil-thin cortex (F)
- Diaphyseal fracture
- Ground glass translucency of bones

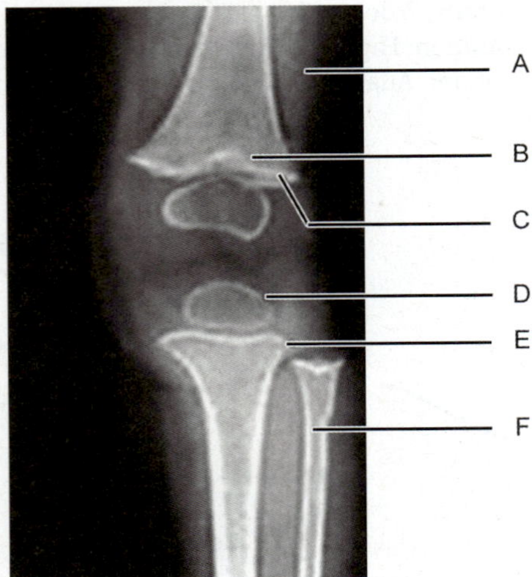

6. **Ans. (b) Thomas test**
[Ref. Practical Orthopedics by Ebnezar, 1/e p502]

Thomas Test

- Used to rule out Hip flexion contracture and Psoas syndrome
- Associated with runners, dancers, and gymnasts
- Steps:
  - *Step 1*: Patient lies supine on the examination table, Clinician passes the palm of his hand beneath the patients spine to identify lumbar lordosis
  - *Step 2*: Normal hip is flexed till the thigh just touches the abdomen to obliterate the lumbar lordosis
  - *Step 3*: Measure the angle between the affected thigh and the table to reveal the fixed flexion deformity of the hip

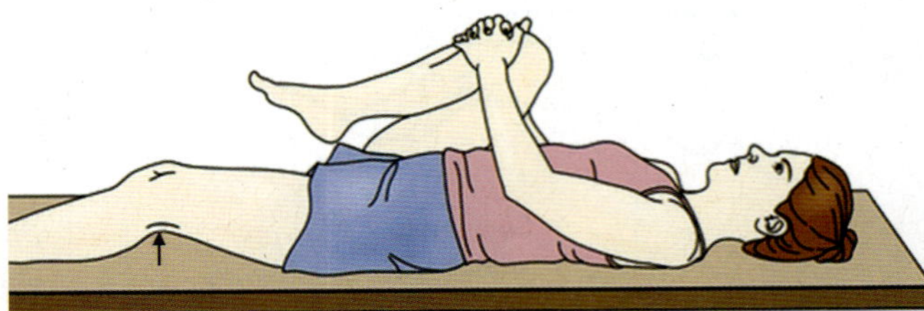

Fig. Thomas Test